617.56406 /BOR

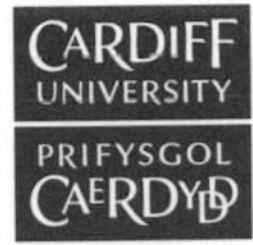

Sir Herbert Duthie Library
Llyfrgell Syr Herbert Duthie

University Hospital
of Wales
Heath Park
Cardiff
CF14 4XN

Ysbyty Athrofaol Cymru
Parc y Mynydd Bychan
Caerdydd
CF14 4XN

029 2074 2875
duthieliby@cardiff.ac.uk

Low Back and Neck Pain

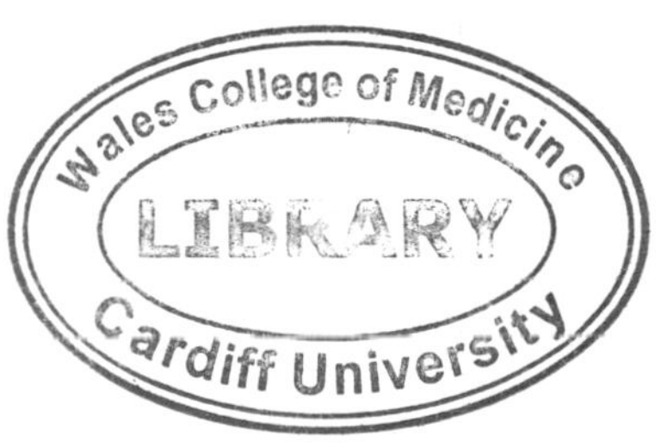

THIRD EDITION

Low Back and Neck Pain

Comprehensive Diagnosis and Management

David G. Borenstein, M.D.
Clinical Professor of Medicine
The George Washington University Medical Center
Washington, DC

Sam W. Wiesel, M.D.
Professor and Chairman
Department of Orthopaedic Surgery
Georgetown University Medical Center
Washington, DC

Scott D. Boden, M.D.
Professor of Orthopaedic Surgery
Director, The Emory Spine Center
Emory University School of Medicine
Atlanta, Georgia

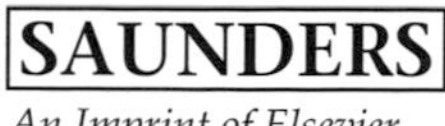

An Imprint of Elsevier

SAUNDERS
An Imprint of Elsevier

The Curtis Center
Independence Square West
Philadelphia, PA 19106

LOW BACK AND NECK PAIN: COMPREHENSIVE DIAGNOSIS AND MANAGEMENT

ISBN 0–7216–9277–X

Copyright 2004, 1995, 1989, Elsevier Inc. All rights reserved.

No part of this publication may be reproduced or transmitted in any form or by any means, electronic or mechanical, including photocopy, recording, or any information storage and retrieval system, without permission in writing from the publisher.

Permissions may be sought directly from Elsevier Inc. Rights Department in Philadelphia, USA: phone: (+1) 215 238 7869, fax: (+1) 215 238 2239, email: healthpermissions@elsevier.com. You may also complete your request on-line via the Elsevier homepage (http://www.elsevier.com), by selecting "Customer Support" and then "Obtaining Permissions."

Notice

Orthopaedics is an ever-changing field. Standard safety precautions must be followed, but as new research and clinical experience broaden our knowledge, changes in treatment and drug therapy may become necessary or appropriate. Readers are advised to check the most current product information provided by the manufacturer of each drug to be administered to verify the recommended dose, the method and duration of administration, and contraindications. It is the responsibility of the treating physician, relying on experience and knowledge of the patient, to determine dosages and the best treatment for each individual patient. Neither the Publisher nor the author assumes any liability for any injury and/or damage to persons or property arising from this publication.

The Publisher

First Edition 1989. Second Edition 1995.

Library of Congress Cataloging-in-Publication Data

Borenstein, David G.
Low back and neck pain: comprehensive diagnosis and management/David G. Borenstein, Sam W. Wiesel, Scott D. Boden—3rd ed.
p. ; cm.
Rev. ed. of 2nd ed.: Low back pain. c1995.
Includes bibliographical references and index.
ISBN 0–7216–9277–X (alk. paper)
1. Backache—Treatment. 2. Neck pain—Treatment. I. Borenstein, David G. Low back pain. II. Wiesel, Sam W. III. Boden, Scott D. IV. Title.
[DNLM: 1. Low Back Pain—diagnosis. 2. Low Back Pain—therapy. 3. Neck Pain—diagnosis. 4. Neck Pain—therapy. 5. Spinal Diseases. WE 755 B731L 2004]
RD771.B217B67 2004
617.5′6406—dc22 2003057378

Publishing Director: Richard Lampert
Acquisitions Editor: Daniel Pepper
Project Manager: Linda Van Pelt

KI/MVY

Printed in the United States of America.

Last digit is the print number: 9 8 7 6 5 4 3 2

For her support and understanding during the long process of writing this book as well as her companionship during my entire medical career, this book is dedicated to my wife, Dorothy Fait.

DAVID G. BORENSTEIN, M.D.

To Katie Holland Wiesel, who has brought so much joy into our family.

SAM W. WIESEL, M.D.

To Mary, Lauren, Stephanie, Allison, Susanne, and Michael for their continued and unwavering dedication and support of my professional endeavors.

SCOTT D. BODEN, M.D.

Foreword

In 1989, Drs. Borenstein and Wiesel broke new ground when they published the first major comprehensive textbook on the medical diagnosis and comprehensive management of low back pain. The textbook met a great need for specific and thorough information that could be used by physicians and other health professionals to evaluate patients with low back pain due to one or another of many different causes. The book was very well received, prompting a second edition, published in 1995. At that time, Dr. Borenstein was professor of medicine (rheumatology) and medical director of a newly formed Spine Center at the George Washington University Medical Center. Dr. Wiesel was professor and chairman of the department of orthopaedic surgery at the Georgetown University School of Medicine, and a preeminent surgeon for the treatment of back diseases. Dr. Boden, associate professor of orthopaedic surgery and director of The Spine Center at Emory University in Atlanta, was included as an additional author for his expertise. The authors then turned their attention to neck pain, employing a similar "medical" approach and format, leading to the publication of *Neck Pain: Medical Diagnosis and Comprehensive Management* in 1996.

The authors have now decided wisely some eight years later to combine these volumes into one new textbook on low back and neck pain, giving equal emphasis to both sets of conditions. There are many overlapping features in these two areas, such as anatomic structure and certain diseases (e.g., osteoarthritis), as well as distinctive aspects of each, such as variation in biomechanics, rheumatoid arthritis of the cervical spine, and lumbar spinal stenosis at the lower part of the spine.

Low back pain and neck pain are major health problems for the nation. The vast majority of Americans, at one point or another in their lives, are afflicted with pain (often severe) and/or disability caused by these disorders. National health surveys have revealed that back or neck pain is the leading cause of disability (limitation of activity) in the United States, especially in young adults (17 to 44 years of age) in the prime of their productive lives.

This new book includes a thorough discussion of the latest diagnostic techniques and therapeutic interventions for back and neck pain. It includes an excellent update on the neurophysiology of pain and pain receptors as well as the clinical interpretation of spinal pain. Particular attention has been paid to the newest imaging techniques, such as improved magnetic resonance imaging and other new technologies. A recommended approach to diagnosis and treatment of spinal pain is presented, along with helpful algorithms.

Perhaps most impressive is the multiplicity of conditions and diseases that underlie and lead to spinal pain and disability. They are comprehensively displayed in the chapters on mechanical disorders, rheumatologic diseases (there are 14 of them), infections, tumors (13 of these), and endocrine (7), hematologic, neurologic, and psychiatric disorders. Reading this book, one realizes the folly of the oft-heard remark, "she (he) just has back pain," as if it were due to only one cause.

Especially valuable is the discussion of the pitfalls in the evaluation of standard radiographic procedures (x-rays) in terms of both overreading films, such as diagnosing "arthritis" of the cervical spine, and noting deficiencies revealed by the newer imaging techniques. Another very helpful feature is an entire chapter devoted to referred pain, in which back pain is caused not by spine disease but rather to gastrointestinal, genitourinary, or cardiovascular disorders.

The third section of the book is devoted to therapy and is very comprehensive. Physical therapy and rehabilitation are thoroughly covered, including exercise, massage, traction, and supports such as neck collars, corsets, and braces. Chiropractic manipulation and other complementary techniques are reviewed. The efficacy of injections with anesthetic or anti-inflammatory agents is presented. The authors have paid a great deal of attention to alternative and complementary therapies such as acupuncture, herbal remedies, and nutritional supplements, with full appreciation that these newer treatments are just now beginning to be evaluated scientifically in proper clinical trials.

The medications sections are very much up-to-date. Drug therapy includes the administration of new COX-2 inhibitors for osteoarthritis of the spine; blockade of the pro-inflammatory cytokine, tumor necrosis factor alpha, for lumbar ankylosing spondylitis and cervical rheumatoid arthritis; and use of bisphosphonates and parathyroid hormone inhibitors to combat osteoporosis.

The last chapter of the text is concerned with surgical treatments. Here the emphasis is on the indications, now and in the future, for both neck and low back surgery, presented individually. For details of the surgical procedures, the reader is referred to the many surgical textbooks in this field. Helpful references are provided at the end of each chapter.

Drs. Borenstein, Wiesel, and Boden are to be very highly commended for providing health professionals with a most informative and well-organized book on the increasingly important subject of back and neck pain, vitally important for the health of the nation.

Lawrence E. Shulman, M.D., Ph.D.
Director Emeritus, National Institute of Arthritis
and Musculoskeletal and Skin Diseases
National Institutes of Health
Bethesda, Maryland

Preface

This third edition of *Low Back and Neck Pain: Comprehensive Diagnosis and Management* is an updated version of an amalgamation of the second edition of *Low Back Pain: Medical Diagnosis and Comprehensive Management* and the first edition of *Neck Pain: Medical Diagnosis and Comprehensive Management*. We have been pleased with the response of the medical and surgical communities to our efforts. Many health care providers have offered their unsolicited praise for the content of prior editions of this book. They remarked on how their copies were being worn out as they continually removed the volume from their shelves for frequent reference to problems affecting their patients. Professional organizations have also acknowledged the value of these volumes. The second edition of *Low Back Pain* was selected by the Medical Library Association for inclusion in its list of recommended books for medical libraries.

The authors brought the idea of combining both books into a single volume to our publisher, Elsevier. Their positive response resulted in a book that describes the similarities in the physiology and pathology that affect the cervical and lumbar spine. At the same time, in each chapter, specific differences between the separate areas of the spine are elucidated. Distinct diagnostic protocols are described for the lumbar and cervical spine areas. The appendix contains separate listings of disorders that involve the lumbar and/or cervical spine. Each chapter is updated with the latest pertinent references. This volume is not a compendium of all articles published on the axial skeleton. Instead, we have been selective in choosing papers included in this volume. We added insightful references that increase our understanding of the basic science involving the axial skeleton as well as those that offer practical and effective ways of treating spinal patients. In regard to therapy, we are willing to make our preferences known. In the therapy section, our recommendations regarding a specific therapy are listed at the conclusion of each section.

We realize that new medical information is published on an ongoing basis. On occasion, new data can have a significant effect on the choices we make for our patients. We did not want to wait until another edition of this book before making this information available. Therefore, in order to remain current with the latest important information, the authors developed Web sites that will update readers on clinical information that is a significant advance in the therapy of patients with axial disease. We invite the readers of this book to visit the following Web sites for the latest pertinent information on spinal disease:

www.drborenstein.com
www.georgetownortho.org
www.emoryhealthcare.org/departments/spine/index.html

As mentioned in the preface of the second edition, the publication of a book is like the birth and development of a child. This offspring has grown into its teens, having made great progress. We hope that our labor will continue to be recognized by the medical community as a worthy and valuable effort and will make the hard task of caring for patients with spinal disorders a bit easier.

David G. Borenstein, M.D.
Sam W. Wiesel, M.D.
Scott D. Boden, M.D.

Acknowledgments

The authors wish to recognize the individuals who supplied their support, encouragement, criticism, and knowledge to the three editions of this book.

The following physicians have shared their expertise, patient histories, and radiographs when requested. Their kindness and generosity is greatly appreciated. They have contributed to the wide array of disorders described in this volume. These individuals include Anne Brower, M.D., radiologist, author of *Arthritis in Black and White*, 2nd ed., Norfolk, Virginia; Alan Borenstein, M.D., private neurologist, Florida Medical Center, Plantation, Florida; Herbert Baraf, M.D., Norman Koval, M.D., and Werner Barth, M.D., rheumatologists, Arthritis and Rheumatism Associates, Wheaton, Maryland, and Washington, D.C.; William M. Steinberg, M.D., gastroenterologist, Chevy Chase, Maryland; Randall Lewis, M.D., orthopaedic surgeon, Washington, D.C.; Stanley C. Marinoff, M.D., obstetrician and gynecologist, Washington, D.C.; Ace Lipson, M.D., endocrinologist, Washington, D.C.; Laligam N. Sekhar, M.D., neurosurgeon, Long Island, New York; Arnold Schwartz, M.D., professor of pathology, Patience White, M.D., professor of medicine and pediatrics, Joseph M. Giordano, M.D., chairman, department of surgery, Michael Hill, M.D., professor of radiology, David O. Davis, M.D., professor of radiology, Edward M. Druy, M.D., professor of radiology, Thomas Dina, M.D., associate professor of radiology, and William O. Bank, M.D., professor of radiology, The George Washington University Medical Center, Washington, D.C; David Caldwell, M.D., professor of medicine, rheumatologist, Duke University Medical Center, Durham, North Carolina; Peter Levitin, M.D., rheumatologist, Greensboro, North Carolina; Eric Gall, M.D., professor and chairman, department of medicine, Chicago Medical School; Theodor Schifter, M.D., rheumatologist, Ramat-Gan, Israel; and Arnold Kwart, M.D., urologist, Washington, D.C.

Of equal importance and generosity was the expertise shared by allied health professionals and biomedical communicators. These individuals include Thomas Welsh, former chief physical therapist, The George Washington University Medical Center and Georgetown University Hospital, Chevy Chase, Maryland, who supplied the pictures of the exercises displayed in this book. He has taught all the authors the importance and benefit of physical therapy in the care of individuals with spinal disorders. Robert Irving, photographer; Judith Guenther, medical illustrator; Rhea Jett, word processing specialist; and Ann Bignell, artist, were patient and responsive to the exacting requests of the authors for the quality of pictures and drawings that has been associated with this effort. Michael Leong and other members of biomedical communications at the George Washington University Medical Center generated new drawings and photographs for this edition. Also acknowledged is Thelma Snider of Emory University School of Medicine for her invaluable help in organizing the many references used in this text.

UpToDate is a database of medical disorders that served as a resource for general information about a variety of illnesses discussed in this book.

We wish to acknowledge the encouragement and support of the editorial and production staff of Elsevier that comes from years of experience in medical publishing.

Contents

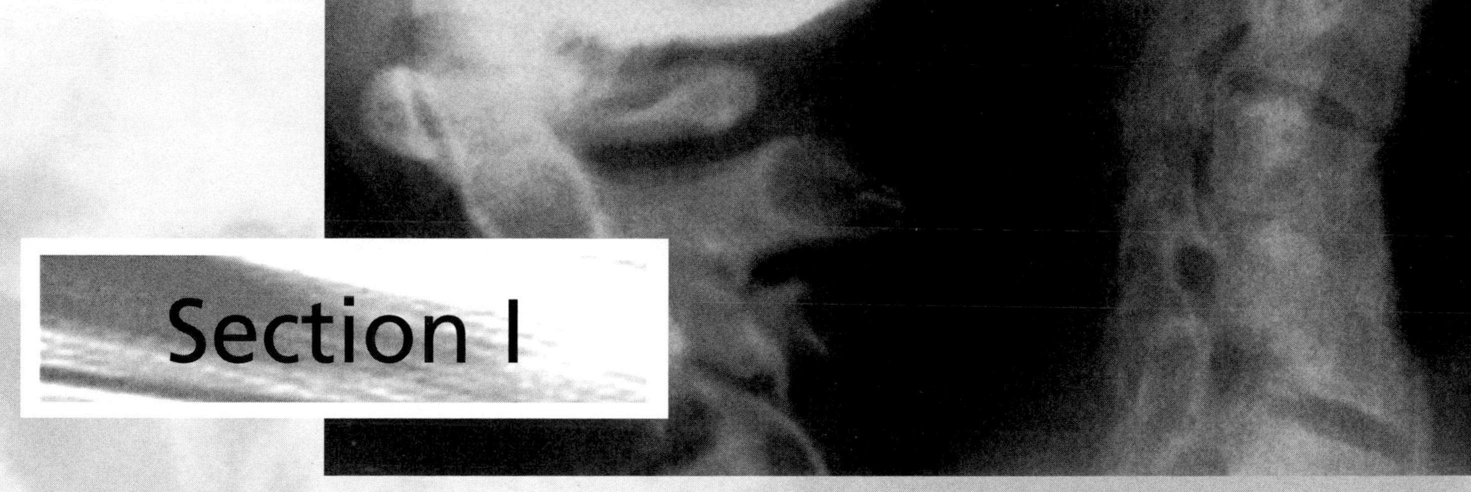

Section I

Anatomy, Biomechanics, Epidemiology, and Sources of Spinal Pain

Section I is a review of the fundamental information necessary to understand the anatomy and physiology of the axial skeleton. The epidemiology of spinal disorders quantifies the importance of this problem to both individuals and society. The complexity of low back and neck disorders is exemplified by the multiple pain generators in and around the spine and the various qualities of pain they produce. The information in this section forms a basic source of essential knowledge that allows for greater confidence in the evaluation and treatment of patients with spinal pain.

Knowledge of the basic anatomy of the cervical and lumbar spine is essential in organizing an approach to the care of the patient with spinal pain. The fine points of skeletal anatomy are frequently forgotten compared with that of single organs, however. The spine is composed of a number of structures, including bone, discs, ligaments, blood vessels, and nerves. Much of the fine detail of the axial skeleton has been described, but some of the important details relating structural components and the generation of symptoms remain unknown. For example, can the intervertebral disc be a source of pain if it contains no nociceptors? A study by Coppes and co-workers identified sensory fiber ingrowth into degenerative discs, but nociceptors were limited to the anterior longitudinal ligament and the outer portion of the annulus fibrosus.[2] The muscular system surrounding the spine is not divided into individual units. The muscles blend one into another (erector spinae, for example). Injury to one component frequently results in decreased function and pain in a much larger area supplied by the extent of the entire muscle. This anatomic characteristic of the spinous musculature makes it difficult to identify specific areas of damage as pain generators, as an example.

The axial skeleton is a beautifully engineered structure. The spine is built for protection of the neural elements while remaining flexible. In its normal functioning state, the human spinal column is capable of a wide variety of strenuous tasks. The spine is able to fly through the air, lift heavy objects, and bend into contorted shapes without suffering injury. The biomechanics of the spine allow a minimal amount of effort to be expended in maintaining an upright posture for extended periods of time. Any modification of this beautifully balanced system results in the expenditure of significant amounts of energy, which causes exhaustion and pain. In many circumstances, the cause of this imbalance in biomechanical efficiency cannot be discerned. Is it the leg length discrepancy that has been present for years? Is the curvature of the spine of such a marked degree to warrant scrutiny? Does palpable, increased muscle tension severe enough to cause an imbalance in muscle lengthening and shortening cause clinical symptoms? The answer is maybe. These are potential, but not absolute, causes of biomechanical dysfunction. Many individuals have these "abnormalities" but are totally asymptomatic. The bane of the physician who evaluates patients with spinal pain is "what you see is *not* what you get." Identifying an abnormality does not make it the cause of the patient's complaints. In most circumstances, maybe as many as 85%, the pain generator cannot be identified.[4]

Between 70% and 80% of the world's population experiences low back pain sometime during their lives. The incidence of low back pain in Western industrialized society has been reported to range from a high of 20% of adults in any given 2-week period to a "low" of 10% in a 2-year period.[6,7] Obviously, to determine the occurrence of back pain in any group, complete survey information must be obtained from the entire population at risk. The definition of spinal pain plays a great role in determining who will in fact have it; in addition, the definitions of the investigator and the patient may not coincide. In any case, we can agree that spinal back pain is a very common clinical problem that affects most of a physician's population, whether it consists of heavy laborers or sedentary office workers.[5,9,10] Back pain is second only to the common cold as the most common reason for visiting a physician.[3]

Cervical problems occur one half to one quarter as often as lumbar spine abnormalities.[8] The prevalence of neck pain in men and women is 8.2% among persons 25 to 74 years of age. In a study of 10,000 Norwegian adults, 34.4% reported neck pain over a 12-month period.[1] A total of 13.8% reported neck pain of 6 months' or longer duration.

Pain is a primary symptom that brings a patient for evaluation. Acute pain is one of the symptoms a physician will use to differentiate among various spinal disorders. The character of pain can be a reflection of damage to a spinal structure. Superficial somatic, deep somatic, radicular, neurogenic, viscerogenic referred, and psychogenic are the categories of spinal pain. Specific disorders (e.g., spondyloarthropathies, acute herniated disc with neural compression) are recognized by their pain patterns. Familiarity with these pain patterns helps the physician design an efficient evaluation. Chronic pain is not just acute pain that lasts longer; the physiology of chronic pain is associated with specific modification of the peripheral and central nervous systems. The complexity of chronic pain has only just started to be understood. The necessity for a variety of different therapies to control chronic pain can be explained by the wide-ranging change in the anatomy and function of the nociceptive system.

References

1. Bovim G, Schrader H, Sand T: Neck pain in the general population. Spine 19:1307-1309, 1994.
2. Coppes MH, Marani E, Thomeer RTWM, et al: Innervation of "painful" lumbar discs. Spine 22:2342-2350, 1997.
3. Cypress BK: Characteristics of physician visits for back symptoms: A national perspective. Am J Public Health 73:389-395, 1983.
4. Deyo RA, Weinstein JN: Low back pain. N Engl J Med 344:363-370, 2001.
5. Dillane JB, Fry J: Acute back syndrome: A study from general practice. Br Med J 3:82, 1966.
6. Frymoyer JW, Pope MH, Costanza MC, et al: Epidemiologic studies of low-back pain. Spine 5:419-423, 1980.
7. Nervell RLM, Turner JG: Orthopaedic Disorders in General Practice. Boston, Butterworths, 1985, pp 35-49.
8. Praemer A, Furner S, Rice DP, and American Academy of Orthopaedic Surgeons: Musculoskeletal Conditions in the United States. Rosemont, IL, American Academy of Orthopaedic Surgeons, 1999.
9. Troup JD, Martin JW, Lloyd DC: Back pain in industry. A prospective survey. Spine 6:61-69, 1981.
10. White AW: Low back pain in men receiving workmen's compensation. Can Med Assoc J 95:50-56, 1966.

CHAPTER 1

ANATOMY AND BIOMECHANICS OF THE CERVICAL AND LUMBAR SPINE

The structure of the spine is complex. To diagnose and treat this area effectively, one must have a clear knowledge of the normal anatomy. The purpose of this chapter is to present a working description of the anatomy and biomechanics of the cervical and lumbar spine. These two regions of the spine have quite unique anatomy and are discussed separately within this chapter. This information provides a keystone on which to build as the various pathologic entities affecting the spine are discussed.

CERVICAL SPINE

Cervical Vertebrae

The osseous anatomy of the cervical spine includes seven cervical vertebrae and the occiput (base of the skull). The first two cervical vertebrae, which compose the upper cervical segment, have a unique structure in comparison with other components of the spine. The lower cervical vertebrae (C3–C7) are similar and compose the lower cervical segment. Between each vertebral body below the second vertebra is an intervertebral disc. From cephalad to caudad, the size of each subsequent vertebra increases progressively.

The atlas, or first cervical vertebra, possesses no vertebral body (Fig. 1-1). The bone that comprises the body of the atlas is joined to that of the second cervical vertebra, the axis, to form the odontoid process, or dens. The atlas consists of an anterior and posterior arch, joining to form the heavy lateral masses that bear the superior and inferior articular surfaces. The superior facets articulate with the occiput, and the inferior facets with the axis.[25] The axial articular masses are broader and deeper than other masses because they bear the weight of the skull without any assistance from the odontoid process. Spanning the lateral masses anteriorly is the slender anterior arch, which lies in front of the dens. It has on its internal surface a facet for articulation with the dens, and in the front it has an anterior tubercle for muscular attachments. The posterior arch is longer and bears a small posterior tubercle in place of a spinous process. Each transverse process has a transverse foramen for the vertebral artery. The transverse processes of the atlas are wider than those of other vertebrae. This increased width provides greater leverage and mechanical advantage to the muscles inserted into the transverse process.[9] This transverse process is the only one in the cervical spine that is not grooved to allow exit of a nerve root.[37]

The second cervical vertebra, or axis, is identified by the projection of the odontoid process, or dens, that develops from the embryologic body of the first vertebra (Fig. 1-2). The dens is continuous with the body of the second vertebra. The dens acts as an eccentric point about which the atlas pivots. The posterior surface of the dens has a facet that accommodates the synovial bursa that separates it from the transverse band of the cruciate ligament. The spinous process of the dens is elongated and bifid. The superior articular surfaces are large and face upward, posteriorly, and laterally. They are placed on heavy masses arising from the body and pedicles. The axis does not form a neural foramen for spinal roots.

The third, fourth, fifth, and sixth vertebrae exhibit identical anatomic features (Fig. 1-3). The body of a typical cervical vertebra is elongated transversely so that its width is approximately 50% greater than its anteroposterior dimension. The upper surface is concave from side to side, and this concavity is deepened by an uncinate process, which is a bony protuberance projecting upward from the posterior lateral aspect of the rim of the body. These vertebral projections act as a barrier to the extrusion of disc material posterolaterally, preventing compression of the nerve roots. The upper surface is also concave in the anteroposterior direction. A prominent inferior overhanging lip is noted on the anteroinferior surface of the vertebral body. The inferior and slightly posterolateral aspects of the vertebral body are beveled and lie in apposition to the uncinate process of the body below, forming the bony components of the joints of Luschka, otherwise known as the *uncovertebral joints*. Bland has reported data from dissection of 191 cervical spines, stating that the joints of Luschka are not true synovial articulations.[9] This fact proves to be important in the consideration of areas of the cervical spine that may be at risk of being damaged by disorders that cause systemic synovitis, such as rheumatoid arthritis.

The seventh cervical vertebra is the vertebra prominens because its spinous process is usually larger than the process associated with the first thoracic vertebra. The C7 vertebra is the transitional vertebra of the cervicothoracic region. The C7 vertebra has anatomic characteristics that are similar to those of T1. The dimensions of the vertebrae increase with size, whereas the dimensions of the

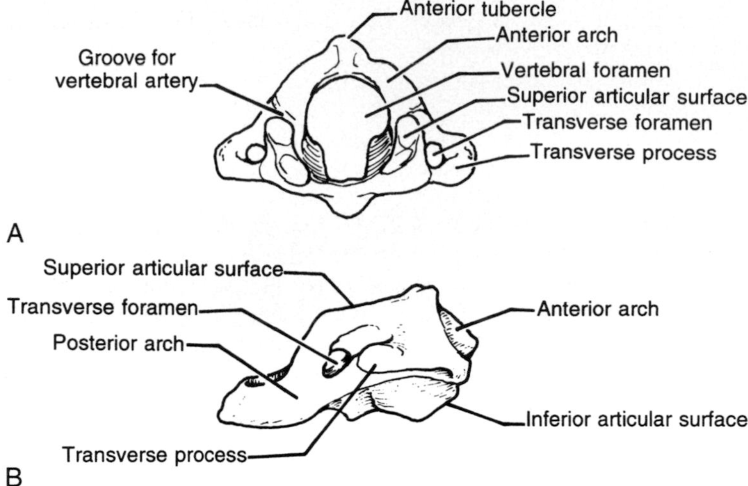

Figure 1-1 First cervical vertebra (atlas): *A*, cranial view; *B*, lateral view.

spinal canal decrease at C6 and C7, representing a transition from the cervical to the thoracic spine. The spinous process is large and single. The transverse process of the seventh vertebra does not contain a foramen for the vertebral artery and its accompanying veins and sympathetic nerves.

The pedicles of the lower cervical segment vertebrae are short and bear superior and inferior articular processes that form the zygapophyseal joints. The pedicles have a height of about 7 mm and a width of 6 mm.[50] In the cervical spine, the facet joints start at the C2–C3 level and range to the C7–T1 level. The articular processes of the superior facets face upward and posteriorly, whereas those of the inferior articular facets face downward and anteriorly at a 45-degree angle. Their surface area is about two thirds that of the intervertebral disc joints. The facet joints are enclosed in a fibrous capsule that is lax to allow movement in different planes. Synovial tissue lines the joint capsules. The joints contain a fibrofatty, fibrocartilaginous meniscus that separates the hyaline cartilage that covers the articular bone. The curvature of the facets allows for complex movements of these joints on lateral flexion and rotation of the neck, but the joints do not have the architectural stability of the joints of the thoracic or lumbar spine. A total of 37 separate joints allow movement of the head and neck, including 14 zygapophyseal joints and 12 joints of Luschka.[47]

On either side of the body are the transverse processes. The anterior portion of the transverse process is developmentally a rib, whereas the posterior portion is a true transverse process. These portions fuse, but between them persists the transverse foramen, which allows for passage of

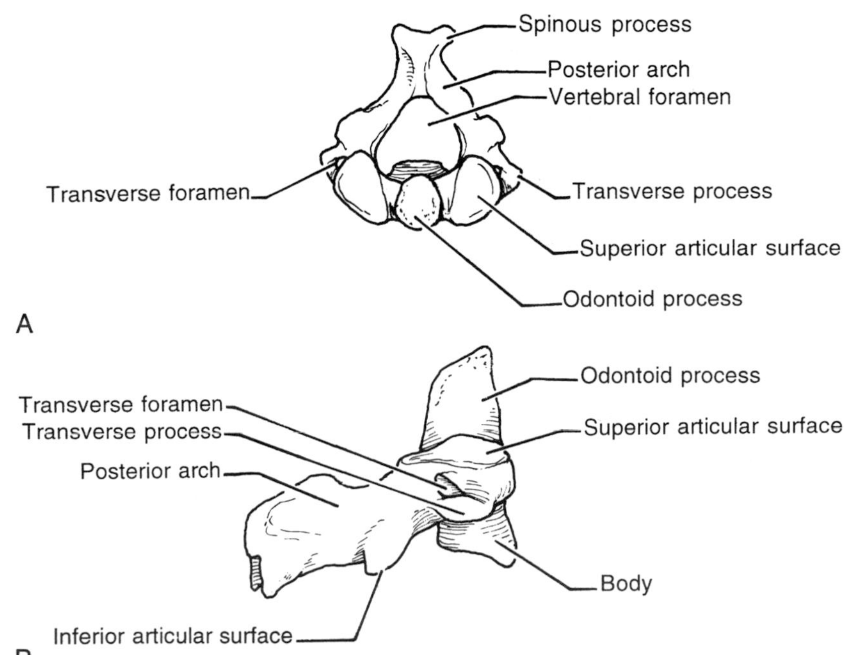

Figure 1-2 Second cervical vertebra (axis): *A*, cranial view; *B*, lateral view.

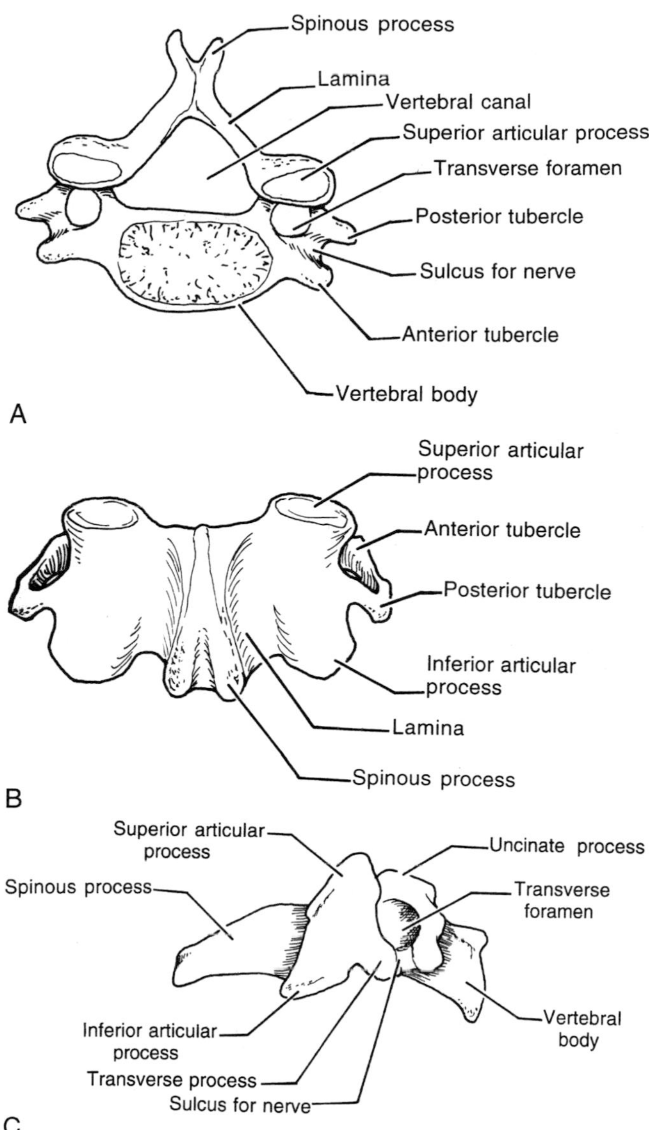

Figure 1-3 Fifth cervical vertebra: *A*, cranial view; *B*, dorsal view; *C*, lateral view.

the vertebral artery. One exception is the transverse foramen of the seventh vertebra, which does not generally contain the vertebral artery. The transverse processes contain a gutter that runs obliquely from back to front for the spinal nerves. Posteriorly the laminae terminate in a short, slender spinous process that is bifid; however, the large spinous process of the seventh vertebra is not bifid and is called the *vertebra prominens*.

At each cervical segment nerve roots exit from the spinal canal through the intervertebral foramina. Each foramen is bordered by the pedicles inferiorly and superiorly. The dorsal wall of the neural foramen consists of the facet joint and its capsule. Ventrally, it is defined by the posterolateral corner of the disc, the posterior portion of the uncovertebral joint, and the vertebral artery. The foramina are essentially small canals approximately 4 mm in length, and they exit obliquely in an anterior and inferior direction. They are ovoid in shape, and they have a vertical diameter of approximately 10 mm in height; the anteroposterior diameter is approximately half this. The foramina are largest at the C2–C3 level. They decrease in size progressively to the C6–C7 level. The roots and floors of the foramina fill the grooves in the bases of the adjacent vertebral arches (Fig. 1-4).

All of the cervical spinal nerves, except the first and second, are contained within the intervertebral foramina. The first cervical nerve exits the vertebral canal from an orifice in the posterior atlanto-occipital membrane just above the posterior arch of the atlas and posterior medially to the lateral mass of the atlas. The C1 ventral primary ramus unites with the C2 ventral primary ramus to contribute fibers to the hypoglossal nerve. The dorsal primary ramus of C1 enters the suboccipital triangle supplying the muscles of this region. C1 has no cutaneous branch.[32] The C2 nerve ganglion is found in the foramen formed by the arch of the atlas and the lamina of the axis. The C2 ganglion occupies 76% of the foramen height. This anatomy makes the C2 ganglion vulnerable to injury to the atlantoaxial joint. Injury in this location may be associated with cervicogenic headaches.[41]

In contrast with the nerves in the thoracic and lumbar spine, the nerves in the cervical spine take the name of the pedicle above which they exit. For example, the C5 nerve root exits between the fourth and fifth cervical vertebrae. The exception is the eighth cervical root, which exits between the seventh cervical and first thoracic vertebrae. The nerve roots and mixed spinal nerve completely fill the anteroposterior diameter of the intervertebral foramen. The nerve roots of the cervical spine pass almost directly laterally at each level to exit from the spinal canal at the same foraminal level as their origin from the spinal cord. The horizontal position contrasts with the more vertical orientation of the lumbar nerve roots. The upper quarter of the foramen is filled with areolar tissue and small veins. In addition to these structures, small arteries arising from the vertebral arteries and the sinuvertebral nerves traverse the canals. Any space-occupying lesion that encroaches on the anteroposterior diameter of the intervertebral foramen can be expected to cause compression of the nervous tissue elements traversing this limited space. The close proximity of the contents of the intervertebral foramen to the uncovertebral joints anteromedially and to the apophyseal (facet) joints posterolaterally should be noted because these are potential sites of hyperplastic processes that can constrict the canal. Flexion of the cervical spine increases the vertical diameter of the neural foramen, whereas extension decreases it.

The vertebral canal is triangular with rounded angles. The posterior aspect of the vertebral body is the base of the triangle. The pedicles and the transverse foramina compose part of the sides of the triangle, along with the zygapophyseal joints, the laminae, and the ligamenta flava. The canal has a funnel shape in the sagittal orientation. The canal is widest at the atlantoaxial level and narrowest at the lamina of C6. The lateral width of the canal is significantly greater than the anteroposterior depth at all levels. Normal sagittal diameters of the cervical spine are 17 to 18 mm at C3 through C6, and 15 mm at C7.[50] The cervical canal is capacious from the level of the atlas to C3. The cervical spinal cord enlargement extends from C3 to T2. The enlargement corresponds to the increase in nerves supplying the limbs. The transverse diameter and

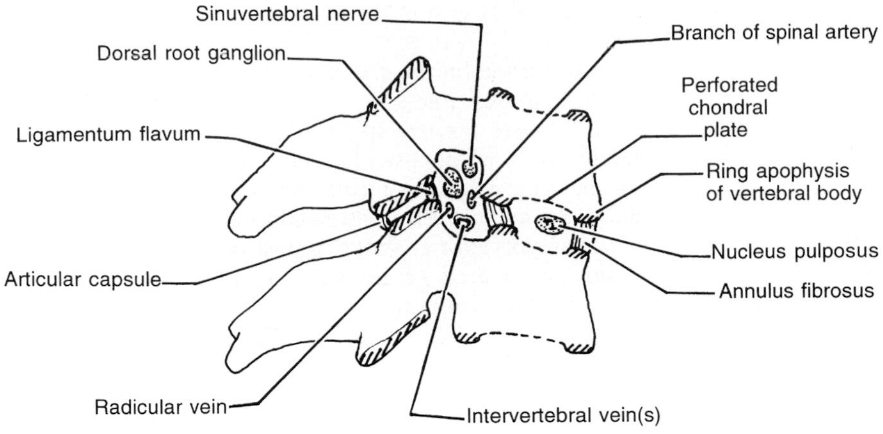

Figure 1-4 Schematic of a sagittal section of the cervical spine showing contents of an intervertebral foramen in relation to an intervertebral disc. The two vertebral bodies and disc along with the supporting structures constitute a motor unit, which includes all components of a somite in an embryo.

cross-sectional area of the spinal cord are maximal at C5. The cervical cord fills a greater portion of the canal in the area of the cervical enlargement. The relationship between the size of the canal and the size of the spinal cord differs significantly among individuals. However, the proportions of the spinal cord at specific levels remain constant individual to individual.[38] The vertebral canal is narrower in women than in men.[9] The size of the spinal cord is documented by postmyelographic computed tomographic (CT) measurements to be 15% to 20% smaller than dimensions measured in autopsy studies.[28]

Spinal Cord

The spinal cord is surrounded by the dura mater, which is firmly attached to the rim of the foramen magnum.[51] The dura merges with the periosteum of the skull inside the foramen magnum, but it is separated from the walls of the spinal canal by fat, forming the epidural space (Fig. 1-5). The dura is lined by the arachnoid. A capillary subdural space separates the dura from the arachnoid. The subarachnoid space is filled with cerebrospinal fluid. The pia mater covers the spinal cord and forms a linear fold that extends longitudinally the length of the spinal medulla. This fold is the source of 20 dentate ligaments that line both sides of the cord. The dentate ligaments extend between the ventral and dorsal nerve roots to attach to the dura and suspend the spinal medulla in the spinal fluid. This organization of ligaments limits the motion of the spinal cord while allowing movement of the dura.

The ventral motor roots exit the cervical spinal cord through the ventral lateral sulcus, and the dorsal sensory roots enter the cord through the lateral longitudinal sulcus. The dorsal root is three times thicker than the ventral root, except at C1 and C2, because of the greater amount of sensory input mirrored by the greater number of sensory fibers. The dorsal root ganglion may vary in its location more proximally or distally in the thecal sac. Distally situated ganglia may be more easily treated with

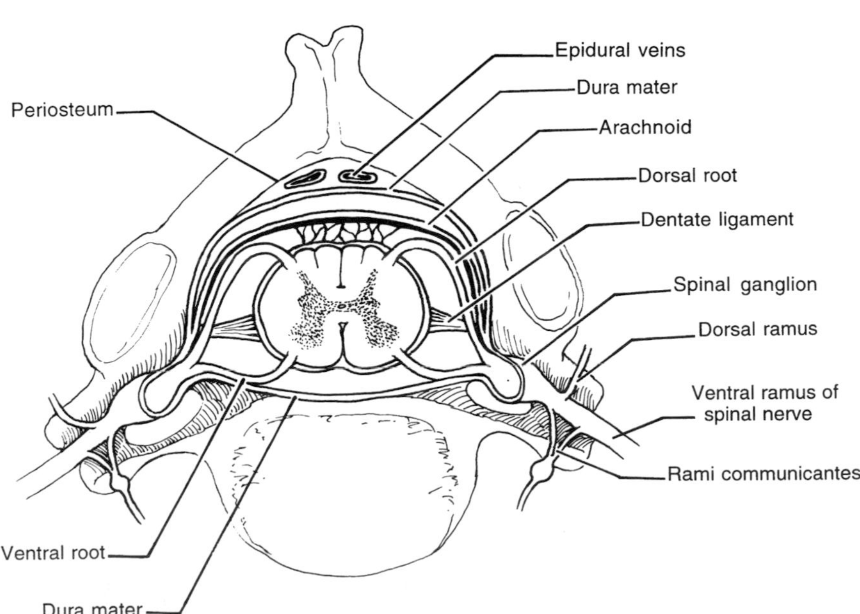

Figure 1-5 Cross-sectional view of the cervical spine demonstrating the position of the spinal cord, nerve roots, dorsal root ganglion, and spinal nerve. The dentate ligaments secure the spinal cord within the vertebral canal. The spinal cord is covered by the pia mater and suspended in the cerebrospinal fluid contained by the arachnoid membrane.

injection therapy.[66] The dorsal rami decrease in size from C3 to C7.[22] The six to eight rootlets at each level join together to be surrounded by the dura. Anastomoses may exist between contiguous levels of sensory nerve rootlets as they enter the spinal cord.[57] These anastomoses occur most frequently between the dorsal rootlets of C5, C6, and C7.[59] The presence of intrathecal anastomoses may explain some of the deviation from classic dermatome patterns found in patients with cervical spine disease. The two nerve roots independently enter an outpouching of the dura and exit the spinal canal. The dural sleeves are attached to the bony margin of the intervertebral foramen.[9] Within the confines of the intervertebral foramen, the dorsal spinal root is enlarged by the spinal ganglion cells. The ventral nerve root is in apposition to the uncinate process of the vertebral body; the dorsal root is in apposition to the zygapophyseal joint; and the vertebral artery is anterior to the nerve root. The dorsal roots exit near the anterolateral corner of the superior articular process 5 to 7 mm below the tip, a location used for the placement of surgical screws for fusion surgery. Damage to the dorsal rami may result in unilateral pain or paresthesias in the back of the neck.[22] The spinal root, containing motor and sensory fibers, loses its dural covering and splits into dorsal and ventral branches. The gray rami from the sympathetic cervical ganglia join the ventral primary divisions of the spinal roots lateral to the intervertebral foramen. No white rami communicantes are located in the cervical spine. The three sympathetic ganglia that supply nerve fibers to the gray rami in the cervical cord are in the connective tissue ventral to the transverse process of the cervical vertebra, are between the longus colli and the longus capitis, and are embedded in the dorsal aspect of the carotid sheath. The three ganglia are the superior cervical ganglion, the middle cervical ganglion, and the inferior ganglion. When the inferior and first thoracic ganglia are fused, the structure is referred to as the *stellate ganglion*. These ganglia are highly variable in their anatomic position. The cervical sympathetic system consists of preganglionic and postganglionic autonomic fibers. The preganglionic fibers originate in the interomediolateral gray column of the T1–T5 spinal cord segments. White rami communicantes leave the corresponding thoracic ventral roots and ascend in the sympathetic trunk. The largest ganglion is the superior ganglion, located at the C2–C3 level. The middle ganglion, the smallest, is located at C6. The inferior ganglion lies between the transverse process of C7 and the first rib.

Sympathetic nerves from the first four cervical nerve roots supply components of nerves innervating the pharynx. The fifth cervical spinal nerve root provides sympathetic innervation to the arteries of the head and neck. The sixth root has fibers to the subclavian artery and brachial plexus. The seventh root has components supplying the cardioaortic plexus, the subclavian and axillary arteries, and the phrenic nerves.[9] Sympathetic nerve fibers surrounding the internal carotid artery provide branches to the posterior orbit, orbital muscles, dilator muscles of the pupils, and smooth muscles of the upper eyelid. Those nerves surrounding the vertebral arteries reach the vestibular portion of the ear.[9]

Intervertebral Discs

The intervertebral discs form approximately 25% of the length of the vertebral column above the sacrum. In the cervical region the discs contribute 22% of the length of the column. The discs are the major structural link between adjacent vertebrae. They serve to allow greater motion between the vertebral bodies than would occur if the vertebrae were in direct apposition. More important, the discs distribute weight over a large surface of the vertebral body during bending motions—weight that would otherwise be concentrated eccentrically on the edge toward which the spine was bent.

Each intervertebral disc is composed of a gelatinous nucleus pulposus surrounded by a laminated, fibrous annulus fibrosus (Fig. 1-6). Each disc is situated between the cartilaginous endplates of two vertebrae. The discs are contained more closely in the cervical spine than at other levels owing to the deeply concave structure of the superior surface of the caudal vertebra and the more convex inferior surface of the rostral vertebra.

The annulus fibrosus forms the outer boundary of each disc. It is composed of fibrocartilaginous tissue and fibrous protein, which are arranged in concentric layers, or lamellae, and run obliquely from one vertebra to another. Successive layers of these fibers slant in alternate directions so that they cross each other at different angles depending on the intradiscal pressure of the nucleus pulposus. Thus, the annulus fibrosus can absorb stress by expanding and contracting like a Chinese finger trap. Its peripheral fibers pass over the edge of the cartilaginous endplate to unite with the bone of each vertebral body. The most superficial fibers blend with the anterior and posterior longitudinal ligaments. With age, these fibers deteriorate, become fissured, and lose their capacity to restrain the nucleus pulposus. If there is sufficient internal stress, the nucleus pulposus material can penetrate through the annulus, and the resulting injury is termed a *herniated disc*. Aging may also alter the integrity of the nucleus. After 50 years of age, the nucleus pulposus becomes a fibrocartilaginous mass that has characteristics

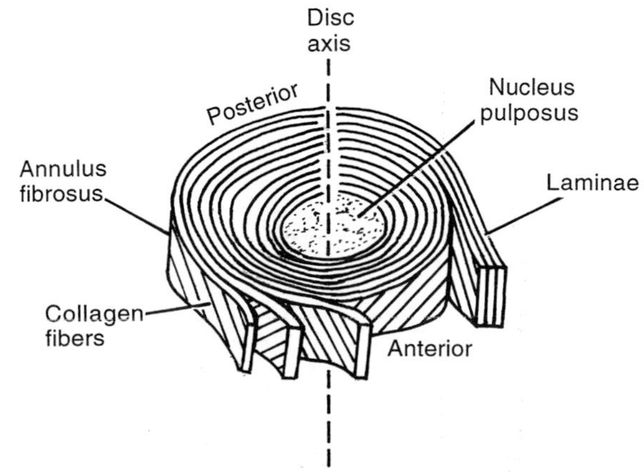

Figure 1-6 The intervertebral disc. The outer portion, the annulus fibrosus, is composed of 90 sheets of laminated collagen fibers that are oriented vertically in the peripheral layers and more obliquely in the central layers. Successive laminae run at angles to each other.

similar to those of the inner zone of the annulus fibrosus. The nucleus may no longer be distinguishable from the annulus in later life.[10]

The nucleus pulposus is situated posteriorly and centrally within the disc and consists of collagen fibrils enmeshed in a mucoprotein gel. The nucleus pulposus occupies about 40% of the disc's cross-sectional area. At birth, it has a high water content (88%), which mechanically allows it to absorb a significant amount of stress; however, with age, the percentage of water decreases, reflecting both an absolute decrease in available proteoglycans and a change in the ratio of the different proteoglycans present. This desiccation (loss of water) reduces the functional ability of the nucleus pulposus to withstand stress.

In the cervical spine, the discs are thicker anteriorly than posteriorly and are entirely responsible for the normal cervical lordosis. They do not conform completely to the surfaces of the vertebral bodies with which they are connected, being slightly smaller in width than the vertebral bodies. The discs bulge anteriorly beyond the adjacent vertebrae. The nucleus pulposus in the cervical spine is located more anteriorly than in other portions of the spine.

Ligaments of the Cervical Vertebral Column

The vertebral bodies are bordered front and back by two major ligaments. The anterior longitudinal ligament is a broad, strong ligament on the anterior and anterolateral aspects of the vertebral bodies from the atlas to the sacrum (Fig. 1-7). Superiorly, the ligament attaches to the anterior arch of the atlas and the anterior atlanto-occipital membrane. Its deepest fibers blend with the intervertebral disc and extend from the body of one vertebra, to the disc, and to the body of the adjacent vertebra. These deep fibers bind the disc and the margins of the vertebra. Most of the superficial fibers extend over several vertebrae, occasionally spanning as many as five. This ligament is most firmly attached to the vertebral bodies at their periphery. The edges of the ligament are thinner than the centermost portion.

The posterior longitudinal ligament lies on the posterior surface of the bodies of the vertebrae from the axis to the sacrum. The ligament is continuous with the tectorial membrane as it passes onto the occiput. The ligament is attached most firmly to the ends of the vertebrae and most deeply to the intervening discs. The midportion of the body is only loosely attached to this ligament. Unlike the anterior longitudinal ligament, which is ribbon-like, the posterior longitudinal ligament is waisted over the vertebral bodies and fans out over the intervertebral discs. The posterior longitudinal ligament is wider in the upper cervical spine than in the lower cervical spine.[51] The lateral expansions over the discs are rather weak and represent a more vulnerable area for disc herniation compared to the strong central band (Fig. 1-8).

The articulations between the vertebral arches are maintained by the supraspinous ligaments, which become the ligamentum nuchae in the cervical spine; the interspinous ligaments; the ligamentum flavum; and the synovial facet joints and capsules.

Supraspinous and interspinous ligaments are found between adjacent spinous processes. The supraspinous ligament is thin, is composed of a high percentage of elastic tissue, and runs over the tips of the spinous processes. In some quadruped animals, the ligamentum nuchae is an essential structure for maintaining the head in an extended position. In humans, this structure extends from the vertebra prominens to the external occipital protuberance, and although considered rudimentary compared with its configuration in quadrupeds, it is probably a major stabilizer of the head and neck. Its deeper fibers attach to the spinous process of each of the cervical vertebrae and reinforce the interspinous ligaments, which in the neck appear less developed than in other regions of the spine. The interspinous ligaments attach in an oblique orientation from the posterosuperior aspect of the anteroinferior aspect of the spinous process below.

The highly elastic ligamentum flavum, or yellow ligament, is found posteriorly between adjacent laminae. There are two of these ligaments at each level, a right and a left, and they are separated by a small cleft. The ligamenta flava merge with the interspinous ligaments posteriorly and with the fibrous capsule of the synovial facet joints anteriorly. They extend from the bases of the articular processes on one side to those on the opposite. They extend laterally into the intervertebral foramen, forming a

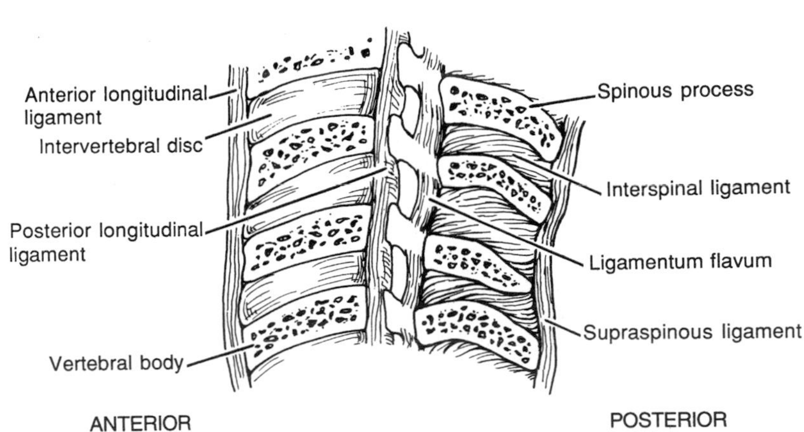

Figure 1-7 Lateral view of the cervical spine demonstrating the ligaments that support the anterior (anterior longitudinal, posterior longitudinal) and the posterior (supraspinous, interspinous) elements of the vertebral column. Note the position of the ligamentum flavum forming a smooth posterior wall of the neural foramen.

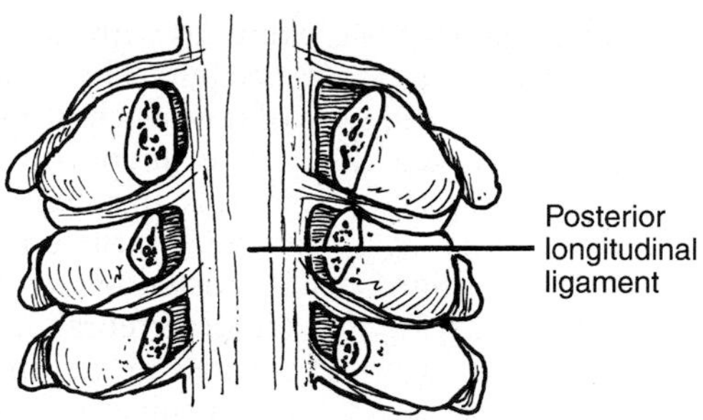

Figure 1-8 Posterior view of the cervical spine with the spinous processes removed. The posterior longitudinal ligament covers the posterior portion of the cervical vertebrae with lateral expansions to cover the intervertebral discs.

portion of the roof of the foramen. They are attached to the inferior aspect of the lamina above on the anterior surface and to the superior aspect of the lamina below on the dorsal surface. This unique attachment, combined with anterior tilting of the lamina, has the effect of creating an extremely smooth posteroinferior wall of the spinal canal, which remains smooth in the various postural positions and serves to protect the spinal cord.

The facet joints in the lower cervical spine are diarthrodial joints with typical synovial membranes and fibrous capsules. The joints are distinctive in that the facets are oriented more obliquely than in the thoracic or lumbar spine. In addition, the joint capsules are more lax than in other regions of the spine to permit a gliding motion. They contain menisci that protect articular surfaces from damage during cervical motion. These menisci may become entrapped in the joint and cause cervical dysfunction.[44,68]

The articulation of the occiput, atlas, and axis differs considerably from that of the lower cervical spine and must be considered separately. The occiput and the atlas articulate through two joints. Each of these joints is formed by the deeply concave, oval, superior articular surface of the lateral mass of the atlas and the corresponding convex condyle of the occiput. These joints are condyloid in configuration, and the articular surfaces are reciprocally curved. In spite of the massive size of the atlanto-occipital joint, strong accessory ligaments are necessary to provide stability.

The anterior atlanto-occipital membrane is a strong, dense band composed of thick fibers that stretch across the anterior margin of the foramen magnum above to the upper border of the anterior arch of the atlas below. In the midline there is a round, tough band of fibers connecting the anterior tubercle of the atlas with the occiput. This structure may be considered a continuation of the anterior longitudinal ligament. The posterior atlanto-occipital membrane is thinner than its anterior counterpart and connects the posterior margin of the foramen magnum with the upper border of the posterior arch of the atlas. Inferiorly and laterally, there is an arched defect that permits the passage of the vertebral artery and the first cervical nerve. The articular capsules of the atlanto-occipital joints are loose, thin structures connecting the condyles of the occiput with the superior articular processes of the axis (Fig. 1-9).

In addition to the stability provided by the ligaments between the occiput and the atlas, stability of the head on the vertebral column is further enhanced by a group of ligaments between the occiput and the axis. The alar ligaments are short, strong bundles of fibrous tissue directed obliquely upward and laterally from either side of the upper part of the odontoid process to the medial aspect of the condyles of the occiput. Because these ligaments restrict motion of the head on the atlas, they are often referred to as *check ligaments*. The apical odontoid ligament is a tough, fibrous cord arising from the apex of the odontoid process between the alar ligaments. It inserts into the anterior margin of the foramen magnum (Fig. 1-10).

The tectorial membrane, or occipitoaxial ligament, is a broad strong band in the vertebral column that lies immediately behind the body of the axis and its ligaments. Inferiorly, it is anchored to the posterior surface of the body of the axis and superiorly to the basilar groove of

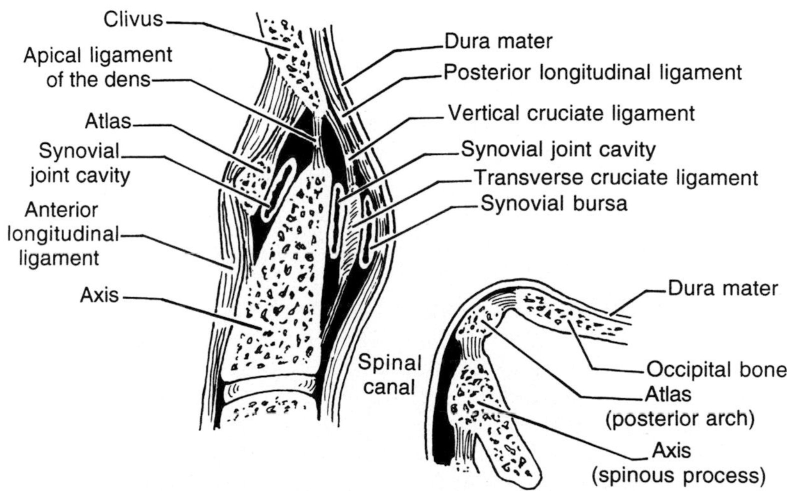

Figure 1-9 Sagittal view of the skull and upper cervical spine shows the atlantoaxial joint and surrounding synovial structures.

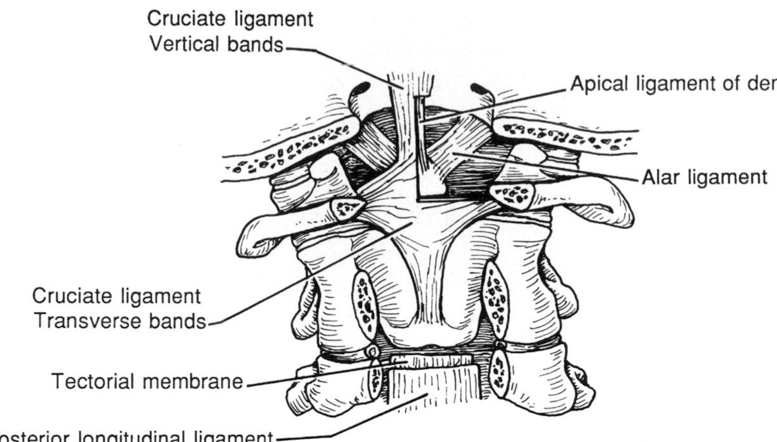

Figure 1-10 Coronal view of the skull and upper cervical spine shows the transverse-cruciate ligaments, the primary stabilizers of the odontoid process. Secondary stabilizers of the odontoid are the alar ligament, which arises from the sides of the dens to the condyles of the occipital bone, and the apical ligament, which arises from the apex of the dens to the foramen magnum as a remnant of the notochord.

the occiput. The structure is essentially a continuation upward of the posterior longitudinal ligament.

There are three true synovial articulations between the atlas and the axis—the two lateral atlantoaxial joints and the median atlantoaxial joint. The lateral joints are formed by the inferior articular surfaces of the atlas and the superior articular surfaces of the axis. They are a large mass of arthrodial, or gliding, joints. Their broad surfaces are directed slightly downward and laterally. The median atlantoaxial joint is essentially a pivot joint with two synovial cavities, one anteriorly between the odontoid and the posterior surface of the anterior arch of the atlas, and the other between the posterior aspect of the odontoid and the front of the transverse ligament of the atlas.

The transverse ligament of the atlas is undoubtedly the most important component of the ligamentous system in this region. It is a broad, strong, triangular ligament arching across the ring of the atlas and firmly anchored on each side to a tubercle in the medial surface of the lateral masses of the atlas. It divides the ring of the atlas into a small anterior and a large posterior compartment. In the anterior compartment lies the odontoid process, which is held firmly against the anterior arch of the atlas by the transverse ligament. There are two synovial cavities, one between the arch of the atlas and the odontoid anteriorly, and the other between the transverse ligament and the odontoid posteriorly (see Fig. 1-9). A bursa lined with synovium is interposed between the transverse ligament of the atlas and the posterior longitudinal ligament. The posterior compartment is occupied by the spinal cord and its membranes; this compartment is equally divided between free space and the spinal cord. The transverse ligament gives off two strong fasciculi. The superior fascicle is elongated upward to the basal part of the occiput. The inferior fascicle is attached to the posterior surface of the body of the axis. This gives the transverse ligament a cruciate configuration.

Blood Supply of the Cervical Spine

The vertebral artery is the major source of blood supply for the cervical spine and the cervical portion of the spinal cord. The vertebral arteries are usually the first and largest branch of the subclavian artery on each side. The vertebral arteries enter the foramen transversarium of C6 and ascend to the atlas, where they wind posteriorly around the lateral masses of the atlas and pass over the posterior arch of C1 just behind the lateral mass of that vertebra (Fig. 1-11). Good correlation is documented between the cadaveric location of the vertebral arteries and the CT images of the same specimens.[31] The left artery is larger in diameter than the right artery. The position of the vertebral artery in the transverse process is anterior to the exiting spinal nerve root just distal to the cervical ganglion. The vertebral arteries give off branches that supply the bone, joints, muscles, and neural elements. As a consequence of its relationship at the superior edge of the atlas, the vertebral artery is particularly vulnerable to injury during posterior surgery in the atlanto-occipital area (Fig. 1-12). Rotation of the cervical spine may compress the vertebral artery if it is atheromatous at this same location.[9]

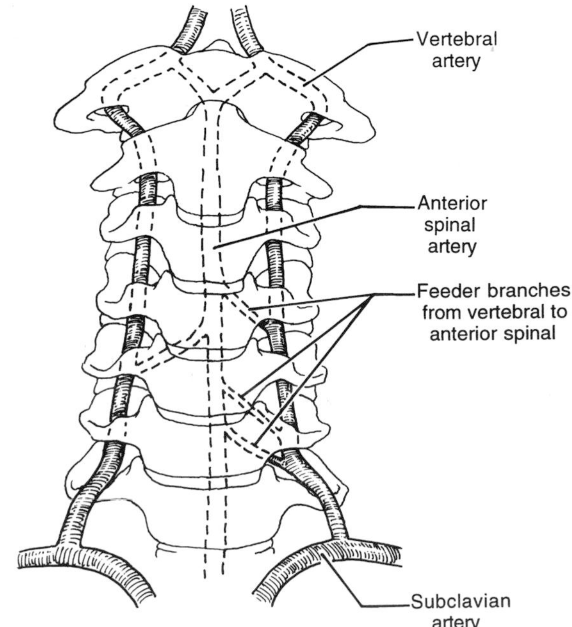

Figure 1-11 Anterior view of the cervical spine shows the course of the vertebral arteries from C6 to C1 through the transverse foramen. The course of the arteries is tortuous at the C1 and C2 levels, corresponding to a potential location for stenosis.

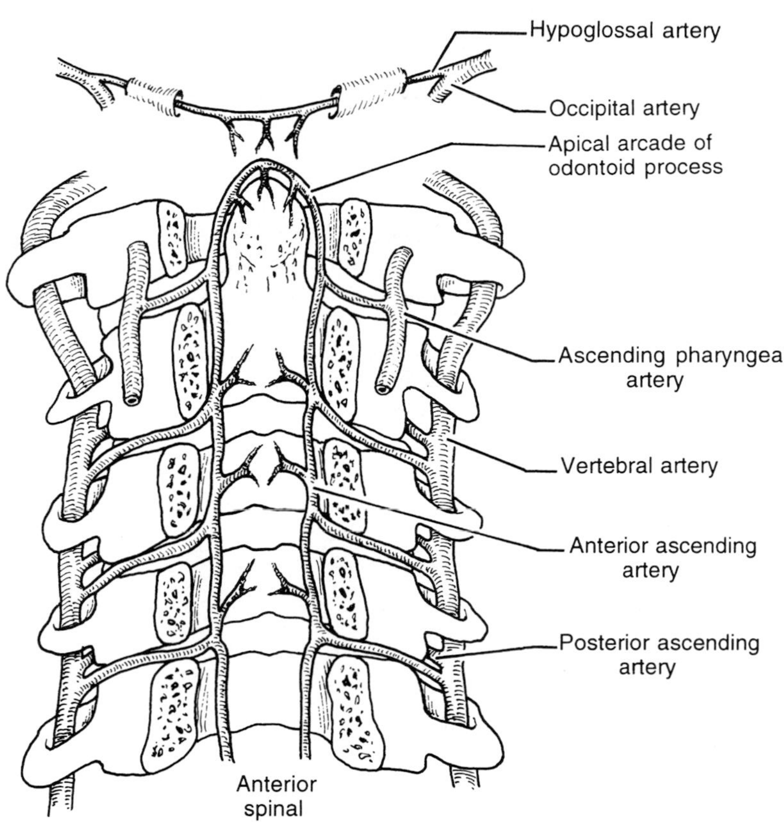

Figure 1-12 Posterior view of the upper cervical spine shows the vertebral arterial blood supply.

The vertebral arteries join together after passing through the foramen magnum to form the basilar artery. Just before joining, one or both of the vertebral arteries give off a branch that joins with the branch from the other side and descends in the ventral medial fissure on the anterior aspect of the spinal cord as the anterior spinal artery. The posterior cord is supplied by the two posterior spinal arteries that descend from the vertebral arteries and give rise to a plexus of vessels on the dorsal aspect of the cord. The vertebral arteries also give off medullary feeders to the anterior and posterior spinal arteries. The medullary feeders are inconsistent branches of the segmental arteries that are evident at each level of the spine. The segmental vessels enter the intervertebral foramen at each level and supply the vertebrae and surrounding soft tissues (Fig. 1-13). In neck flexion, an intervertebral disc herniation may cause compression of the spinal cord, with loss of pulsation and obliteration of venous channels. Neck extension allows for return of blood flow.

Venous blood returns from the spinal cord through a system analogous to the anterior and posterior arterial channels. The venous drainage of the vertebrae is divided

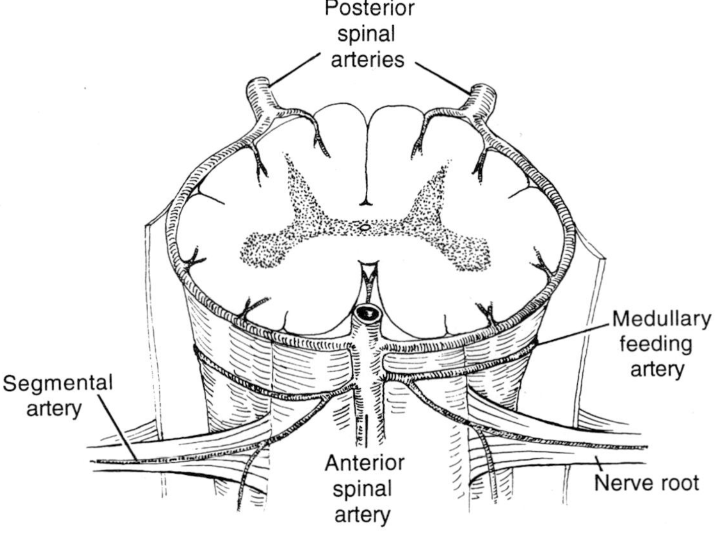

Figure 1-13 Anterior and posterior spinal artery blood supply to the spinal cord. A medullary feeding artery, originating from the segmental artery, also contributes to the vascularity of the spinal cord.

into an external and an internal system. The external system is arranged in the same distribution as the anterior, central, and posterior laminar arteries. The system inside the spinal canal consists of a series of valveless sinuses in the epidural space clustered anteriorly and just medial to the pedicles over the midportion of the vertebral bodies. The anterior portion of the external venous plexus drains into the venae comitantes of the vertebral arteries, and the posterior portion of the plexus drains into the deep cervical veins bilaterally. These venous systems drain into the brachiocephalic veins. The valveless complex of veins in the spine forms a continuous connection between the pelvis and the cerebral sinuses and connects with the caval and azygos systems. The absence of valves allows the reversal of blood from the pelvis to the cervical spine (Fig. 1-14).[6]

Muscles and Fascia of the Cervical Spine

The muscles of the neck can be defined by anatomic limits, innervation, or function. Because the cervical spine is the most mobile section of the spine, it contains the most elaborate and specialized muscle system of the spine. The complexity of the inner anatomy of the cervical spine muscles is elucidated in the work of Kamibayashi and Richmond.[39] For specific muscles, variations in attachments to different cervical bones were identified in cadaveric specimens. For example, considerable individual variations were found in the number and location of tendinous insertions of the scalenes and longissimus capitis muscles. A number of internal aponeurotic attachments shortened the effective length of individual muscles. The size of the neck muscles did not scale proportionately to body height and weight of individuals. These findings suggest that individual variation is the rule in identifying the role of neck muscle function in cranial stabilization and the muscles' ability to withstand injury.

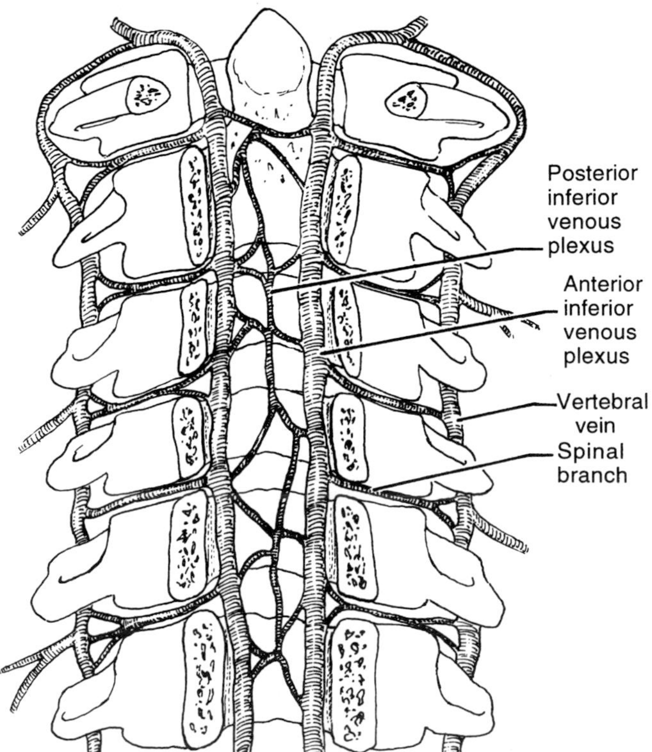

Figure 1-14 Posterior view of the cervical spine shows the internal and external system of venous channels that drain into the brachiocephalic veins.

The posterior muscles of the neck are divided into superficial, intermediate, and deep groups. The trapezius muscle is the most superficial muscle of the posterior group and is innervated by the spinal accessory nerve—the eleventh cranial nerve. This muscle originates from the spinous processes of C2 through T12 and occipital protuberance to insert on the scapula, acromion, and clavicle (Fig. 1-15). It functions to stabilize and elevate the scapula and extend the head. The trapezius muscle is a frequent source of pain in individuals with muscular strain of the cervical spine. Another muscle, the levator scapulae, elevates the medial scapula and rotates it medially. It is innervated by the nerve to the levator scapulae and runs from the transverse process of the upper cervical spine to the superior medial scapula.

The intermediate muscles surrounding the spine function primarily as spinal extensors. The muscles include the splenius capitis and the splenius cervicis. The muscles originate from the spinous processes of the lower cervical and upper thoracic spine and insert on the transverse processes of the upper cervical spine and the mastoid process (Fig. 1-16). Biomechanical studies have documented the importance of the splenius capitis and cervicis as prime muscles for extension of the head and neck.[48]

In the deep layer, the erector spinae muscles from the thoracolumbar spine continue to the cervical region, including the iliocostalis cervicis laterally; longissimus cervicis and longissimus capitis centrally; and spinalis cervicis, semispinalis capitis, and semispinalis cervicis medially (Fig. 1-17). The iliocostalis extends from the angles of the upper six ribs to the posterior tubercles of the transverse processes of the lower cervical vertebrae. The longissimus group extends from the transverse processes of the upper thoracic vertebrae to the posterior tubercles of the transverse processes of the lower cervical vertebrae and to the mastoid process as part of the longissimus capitis. The semispinalis group arises on the posterior tubercles of the transverse processes of the upper thoracic and lower cervical vertebrae and inserts into the area between the superior and inferior nuchal line of the occiput. Beneath the semispinalis muscle lie the multifidus from C4 to C7 and rotatores muscles that cross one segment of the spine and extend from the transverse process to the spinous process. In the upper cervical spine, suboccipital muscles (the rectus capitis posterior major and minor and the obliquus capitis inferior and superior) attach from the occiput to the C2 vertebra. Most posterior muscles are involved in producing extension of the neck and head; some muscles, particularly the deeper muscles, produce rotation and lateral flexion (Table 1-1). Posterior deep muscles are innervated segmentally by the branches of primary dorsal rami of one or more cervical nerves. This arrangement is related to the embryonic development and is termed *segmental innervation* (Fig. 1-18).

The anterolateral cervical muscles function to flex and rotate the head and neck. These muscles include the

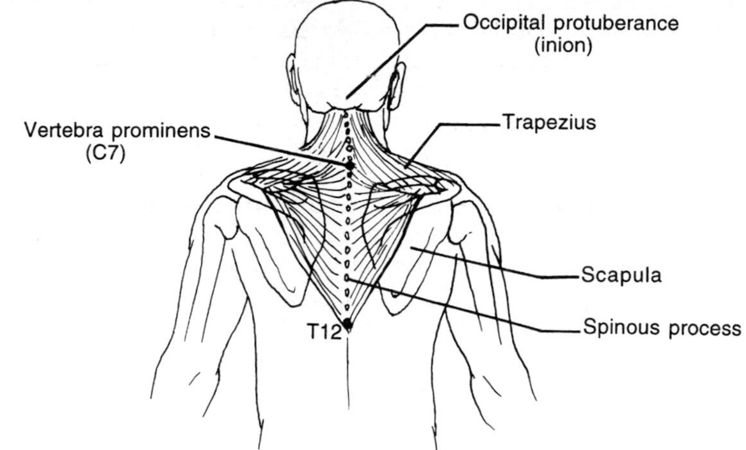

Figure 1-15 Posterior view of the cervical spine demonstrating the trapezius muscle, a primary extensor of the cervical spine.

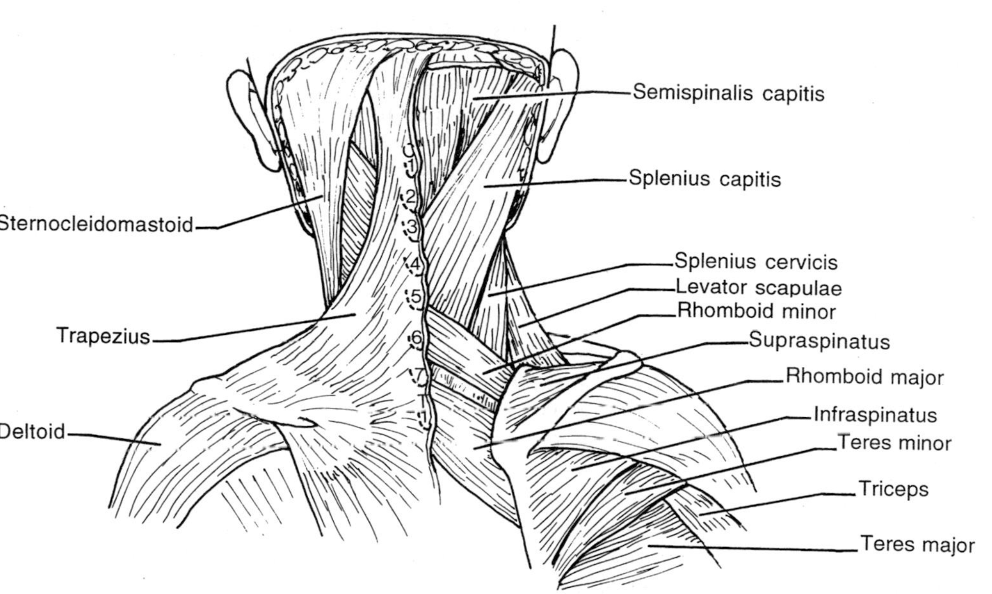

Figure 1-16 Posterior view of the superficial muscles of the cervical spine and shoulders.

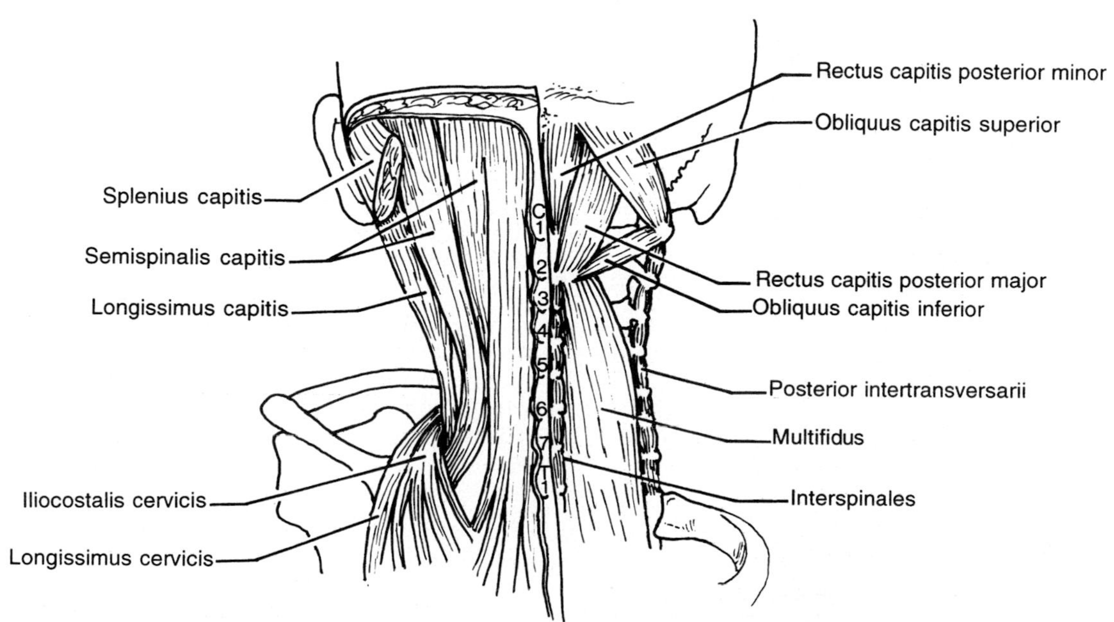

Figure 1-17 Posterior view of the deeper muscles of the cervical spine.

1-1 MUSCLES OF THE CERVICAL SPINE

FLEXION
Sternocleidomastoid
Longus colli
Longus capitis
Rectus capitis anterior

EXTENSION
Splenius capitis
Splenius cervicis
Semispinalis capitis
Semispinalis cervicis
Longissimus capitis
Longissimus cervicis
Trapezius
Interspinalis
Rectus capitis posterior major
Rectus capitis posterior minor
Obliquus capitis superior
Sternocleidomastoid

ROTATION AND LATERAL BENDING
Sternocleidomastoid
Scalene group
Splenius capitis
Splenius cervicis
Longissimus capitis
Levator scapulae
Longus colli
Iliocostalis cervicis
Multifidi
Intertransversarii
Obliquus capitis inferior
Obliquus capitis superior
Rectus capitis lateralis

platysma, sternocleidomastoid, and hyoid muscles; strap muscles of the larynx; and scalenes, longus colli, and longus capitis (Fig. 1-19). The platysma is a thin muscle below the subcutaneous tissue that spans the deltoid to the pectoral fascia and the clavicle, and it inserts on the mandible, muscles of the lip, and lower face skin. The platysma depresses the lower jaw and lip and tightens the skin of the anterior neck. The other anterolateral muscles are divided into two large triangles by the sternocleidomastoid muscle. The sternocleidomastoid is innervated by the spinal accessory nerve. The muscle arises from two heads: sternal and clavicular. When the sternocleidomastoid muscles contract simultaneously, the head is flexed or the thorax raised if the head is held in a fixed position. Medial and deep to the sternocleidomastoid muscle is the carotid sheath containing the internal carotid artery, vagus nerve, and internal jugular vein. The "strap muscles" attach to the hyoid, thyroid cartilage, and sternum and are medial to the sternocleidomastoid except for the posterior aspect of the omohyoid muscle (Fig. 1-20). These muscles are innervated by segmental branches of the cervical anterior primary rami. The muscles above the hyoid are innervated by the hypoglossal nerve and are rarely encountered in anterior cervical spine surgery. The hyoid muscles do not control motion of the cervical spine, but they are important in controlling movement of the hyoid bone and larynx. Deep and medial to the carotid sheath are the anterior cervical spine vertebral bodies, covered by a prevertebral fascia. The prevertebral muscles of the neck are the longus colli and longus capitis. These muscles are paired with one on each side of the spine. The longus colli muscles extend from C1 to T3, spanning the lateral portions of the vertebral bodies and having lateral attachment to the anterior tubercles of the lateral masses of C3–C6. The longus capitis muscles arise on the anterior tubercles of C3–C6 and extend cephalad to the basiocciput, where they are supplemented by the rectus capitis anterior and the rectus capitis lateralis. These muscles are flexors of the cervical spine.

The sternocleidomastoid is the dividing boundary for the anterior and posterior triangles of the neck (Fig. 1-21). The posterior triangle is formed by the sternocleidomastoid, trapezius, and clavicle, with a floor consisting of the semispinalis capitis, levator scapulae, splenius capitis, scalenus medius, and scalenus anterior. The omohyoid muscle runs obliquely across the inferior portion of the posterior triangle to form the omoclavicular triangle. The

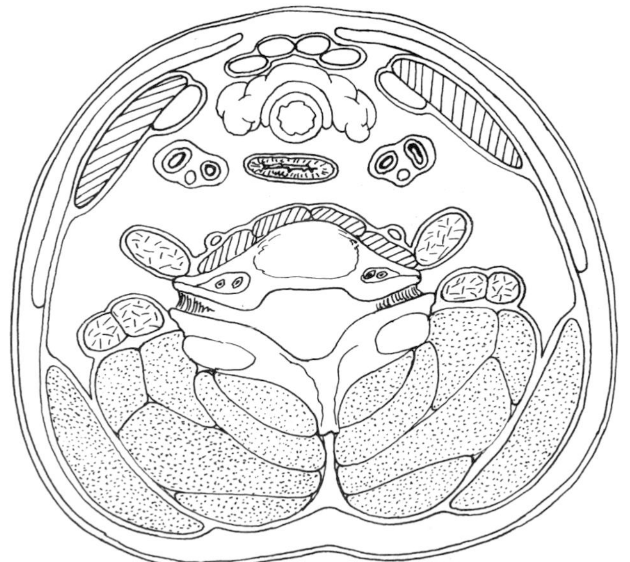

Figure 1-18 Cross section of body musculature through the sixth cervical vertebra. Flexors are anterior to the spine and extensors are posterior. The muscles that cause lateral bending and rotation are contiguous to the vertebral bodies in a lateral position.

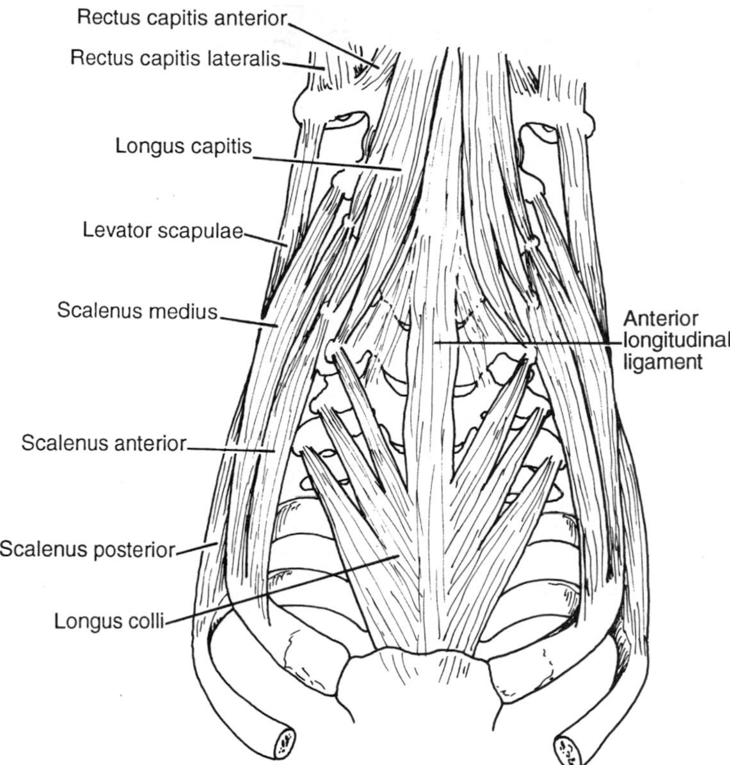

Figure 1-19 Anterior view of the superficial muscles of the cervical spine.

anterior triangle is bounded by the midline of the neck, the lower border of the mandible, and the sternocleidomastoid. The anterior triangle is further divided into the submental, submandibular, muscular, and carotid triangles. The carotid triangle is bounded by the anterior border of the sternocleidomastoid, the posterior belly of the digastric muscle, and the superior belly of the omohyoid muscle and contains the carotid sheath.

As in other parts of the body, muscles, blood vessels, nerves, and viscera of the neck are contained within fascial coverings of connective tissue. These fasciae form planes

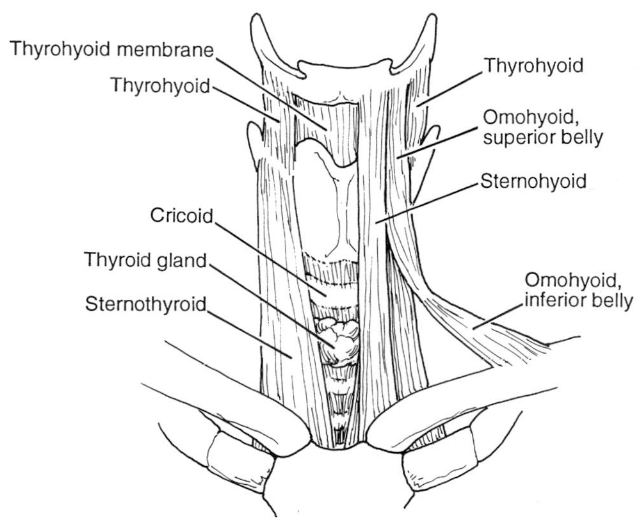

Figure 1-20 Anterior view of the deeper anterior muscles of the cervical spine.

and compartments in which deeper structures of the neck are organized (Fig. 1-22). The three fascial layers of the cervical spine are superficial, intermediate, and deep.[2] The superficial fascia surrounds subcutaneous fat, the platysma muscle, the external jugular vein, and cutaneous sensory nerves. The superficial layer surrounds all the deeper structures of the neck. The superficial fascia exists as a single sheet over the anterior and posterior cervical triangles. Immediately anterior to the cervical spine are the esophagus, trachea, and thyroid gland. These structures are covered by an intermediate fascial layer separate from the prevertebral fascia. The alar fascia spreads behind the esophagus and surrounds the carotid sheath. The carotid sheath encloses the carotid artery, the internal jugular vein, and the vagus nerve. The outer layer of the deep fascia extends from the trapezius muscle over the posterior triangle and then splits to enclose the sternocleidomastoid muscle. The middle layer of the deep cervical fascia encloses the strap muscles and extends laterally to the scapula. The deepest layer of the deep fascia is the prevertebral fascia, which covers the scalenus muscles, the longus colli muscles, and the anterior longitudinal ligament.

A number of important structures are located between these fascial layers. In the relatively avascular space between the anterior vertebral body and the carotid sheath pass several important nerves, arteries, and veins. The superior laryngeal nerve travels at the C3–C4 level with the superior thyroid artery. The inferior thyroid artery and vein pass caudally at about the C6–C7 level. The recurrent laryngeal nerve, a branch of the vagus nerve, provides an essential innervation to the vocal cord. The recurrent laryngeal nerve crosses this plane at different levels on the left and right sides. On the right side, the nerve loops

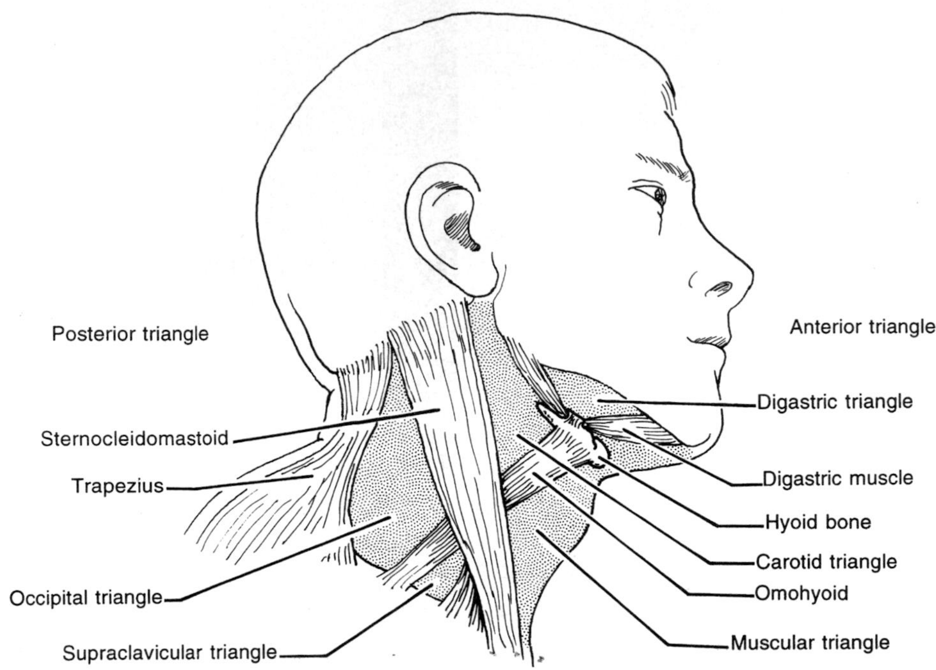

Figure 1-21 Triangle organization of the neck. The posterior triangle is formed by the trapezius, clavicle, and sternocleidomastoid, with the omohyoid muscle dividing this triangle into the occipital and supraclavicular areas. The anterior triangle is bounded by the midline of the neck, the lower border of the mandible, and the sternocleidomastoid. The anterior triangle is subdivided by the digastric and omohyoid muscles.

around the subclavian artery before it enters the visceral fascia between the esophagus and the trachea. Its course is somewhat variable. On the left side, the nerve loops around the arch of the aorta before entering the visceral fascia, as on the right. Its course is more predictable and lower in the interval between the vertebrae and the carotid sheath.

Nerve Supply of the Cervical Spine

The nerve supply to the spinal column is derived from the spinal nerve root once it passes out of the neural foramina. There are eight cervical nerve roots, and the first cervical nerve exits between the atlas and the occiput. Subsequently, the cervical nerve roots C2 to C8 exit from

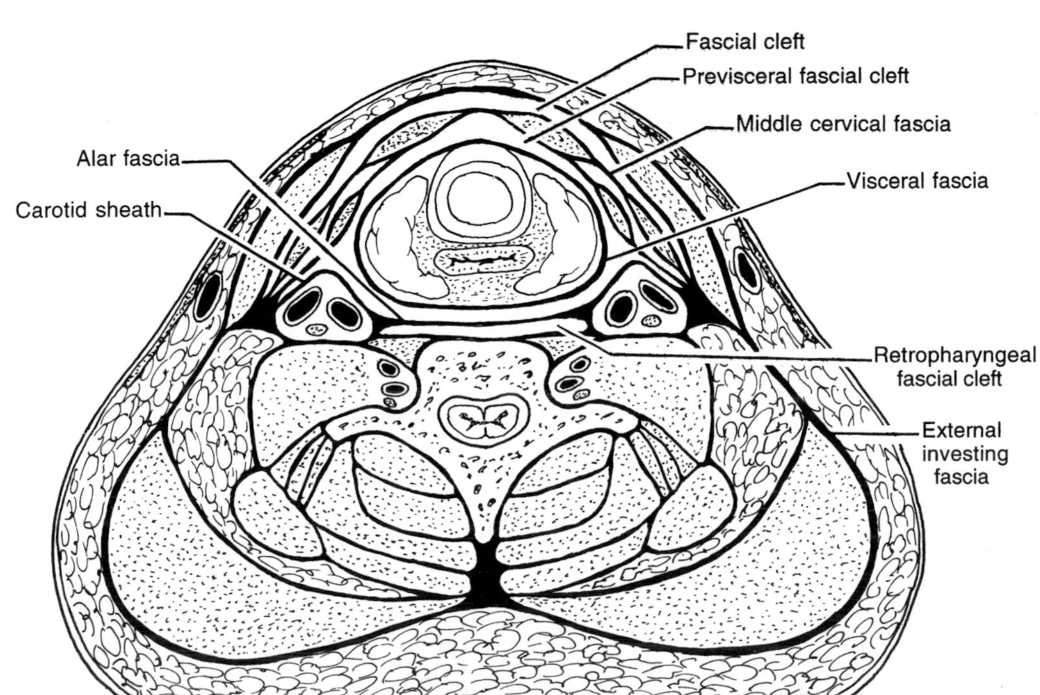

Figure 1-22 Sagittal view of the cervical spine demonstrating the division of neck structures into fascial planes.

the neural foramina so that the lower cervical nerve root exits after crossing the intervertebral disc numbered one higher (e.g., C5 crosses the C4–C5 disc).

The mixed spinal nerve contains motor fibers, sensory axons of the dorsal root ganglia, and preganglionic fibers from the autonomic nervous system. The main spinal nerve gives off three major branches before continuing into the brachial plexus: primary posterior rami, primary anterior rami, and sinuvertebral nerve of Luschka. The primary anterior and the posterior rami supply the muscles about the spine and chest wall. The sinuvertebral nerve contains only sensory and sympathetic fibers, and each nerve branches to two adjacent levels within the spinal canal. The cervical sinuvertebral nerves supply the level of entry and the disc above. Branches of the vertebral nerve supply the lateral aspects of the cervical discs. The nerve provides sensory endings for the posterior longitudinal ligament, annulus fibrosus, and ventral dura mater. Nerve fibers are present within the outer third of the annulus fibrosus.[12] The ventral nerve plexus, consisting of interconnections between the gray rami, the perivascular vertebral artery plexus, and the sympathetic trunk, innervates the anterior longitudinal ligament, the outer annulus fibrosus, and the anterior vertebral body (Fig. 1-23).[11] Structures that are not highly innervated include the nucleus pulposus and the ligamentum flavum. The sinuvertebral nerve is very sensitive to stretch and possibly ischemia. The facet joints are innervated by a branch of the primary dorsal rami and descend to at least one vertebral level below.

From the preceding discussion, it is obvious that there are several possible sources of pain in and around the spinal column. The phenomenon of referred pain, or pain distant from the source, follows the anatomic course of the given nerve. This helps demonstrate why cervical spine disease is often referred to the scapular area, the shoulder, or the chest wall. The concept of referred versus radicular pain is discussed in more detail in Chapter 3.

Neighboring Structures in the Cervical Spine

A working knowledge of the overall anatomy of the neck is helpful in understanding the possible sources of pain in this part of the human body. Structures other than the spine itself may cause neck or arm pain. Examples of the structures include the temporomandibular joints, the pharynx, the cervical lymph nodes, the esophagus, the thyroid, and the apex of the lungs. The clavicle and its articulations with the sternum and acromion process of the scapula may also be a source of cervical pain.

Correlating surface anatomy and structures in the neck and cervical spine is helpful in localizing important landmarks. The angle of the mandible is at the first cervical vertebra. The transverse process of the second cervical vertebra is between the angle of the mandible and the mastoid process. The hyoid bone is anterior to the third cervical vertebra. The thyroid cartilage is anterior to the fourth cervical vertebra. The sixth vertebra is at the level of the cricoid cartilage (Fig. 1-24).

Biomechanics of the Cervical Spine

Familiarity with the anatomy of the cervical spine helps identify those structures that are at risk of developing pain, but such familiarity is not adequate to explain all the mechanisms by which neck pain develops. The normal function of the cervical spine requires both flexibility to move the head and endurance of the musculature. The neck normally moves more than 600 times each hour, whether a person is awake or asleep.[47] Recognition of deviations from normal biomechanical function, such as a hypermobile segment and excessive cervical kyphosis, may help explain the source of pain in some individuals who do not have specific anatomic abnormalities. A basic understanding of the clinically relevant biomechanics of the cervical spine is necessary for making a complete assessment of the neck of patients who have cervical problems.

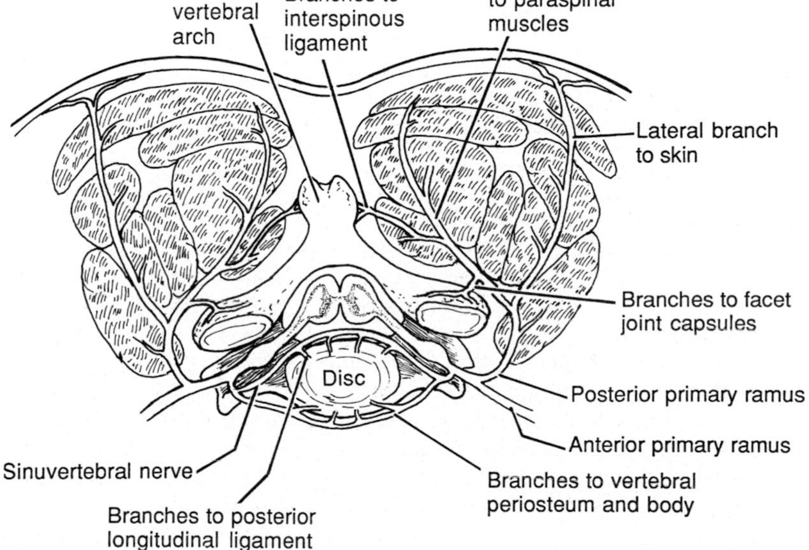

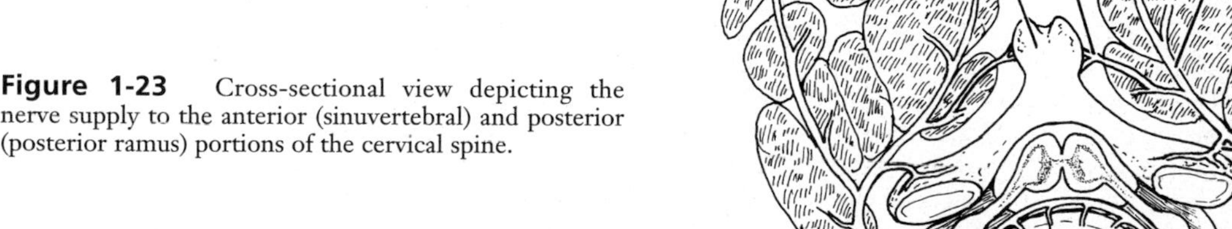

Figure 1-23 Cross-sectional view depicting the nerve supply to the anterior (sinuvertebral) and posterior (posterior ramus) portions of the cervical spine.

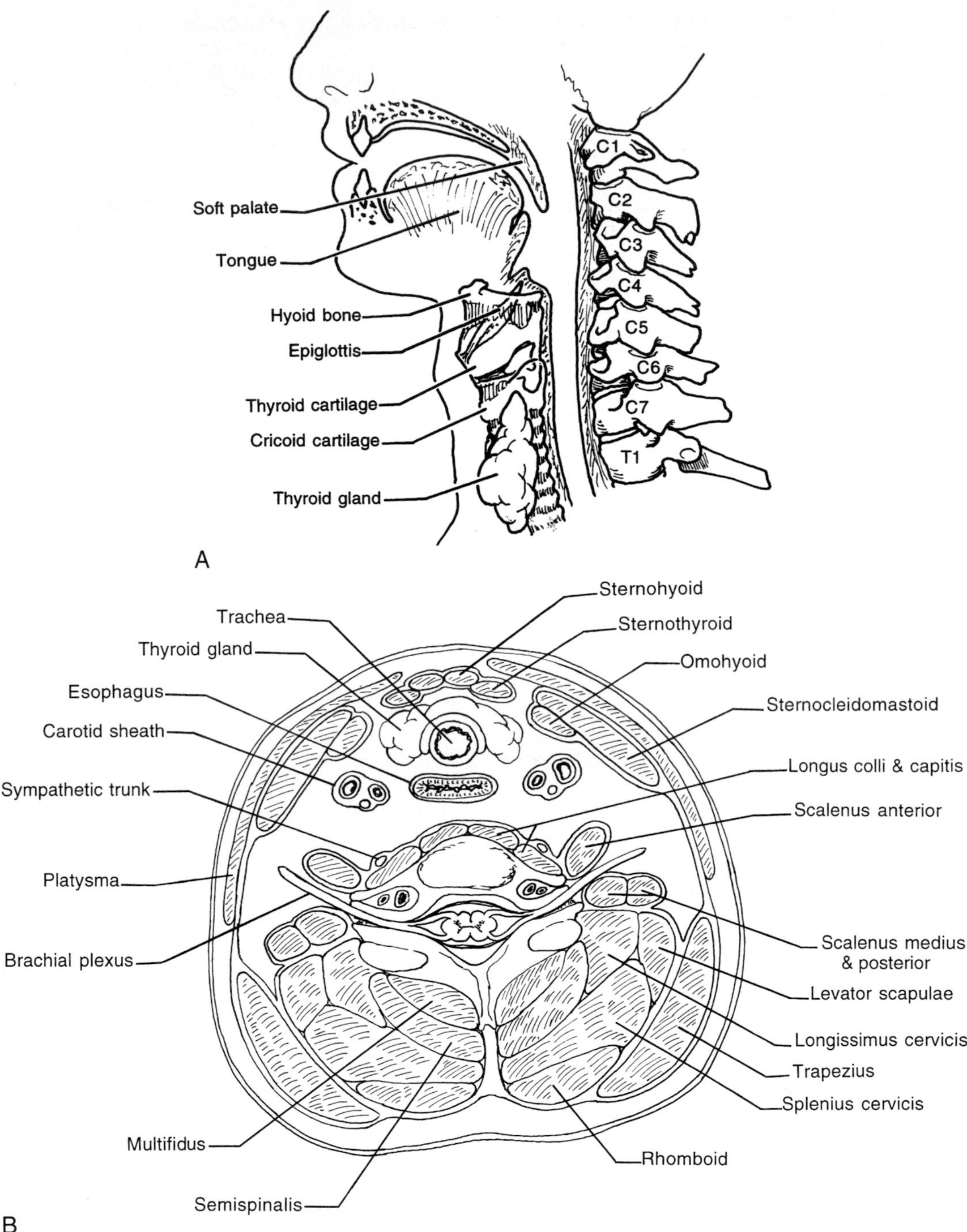

Figure 1-24 Diagrammatic views (*A* and *B*) of the anatomic relationships of the visceral organs in the anterior portion of the neck and the cervical spine.

Much of what is known about the normal biomechanics and pathomechanics of the cervical spine has been learned from static mechanical testing of cadaveric specimens in the laboratory. There is a wealth of information available about the dynamic mechanics of all aspects of the spine. It is well established that forces and stresses can be applied to the spine in any combination of flexion, extension, rotation, and shear. These stresses affect the entire motion segment, including the intervertebral disc, zygapophyseal joints and capsules, anterior and posterior longitudinal ligaments, uncovertebral joints, and other ligamentous structures. The muscles and the fascial attachments interact with the cervical spine to accommodate load, alter forces, and direct motion. Whereas the lumbar spine is well suited to accommodate heavy loads and provide stability, the cervical spine is better suited for mobility and is not required to transmit heavy loads. The head weighs only 5 to 7 pounds. However, all vital nerve centers are in the skull and allow coordination of vision, vestibular balance, and auditory direction. Precise control of head position and movement is essential for normal functioning of these senses.[15]

The architecture of the axial skeleton is designed to maintain the center of gravity in a functional position. The two lordotic curves, cervical and lumbar, and the two kyphotic curves, thoracic and sacral, balance each other. The center of gravity passes the external meatus of the ear and transects the odontoid process and the bodies of T1 and T12. The line then passes through the sacral promontory, courses slightly posterior to the center of the hip joint, passes anteriorly to the center of the knee joint through the calcaneocuboid joint of the foot, and ends slightly anterior to the lateral malleoli. In the coronal plane, the center of gravity descends from the foramen magnum and passes along the superior spinous processes of each vertebra and the tip of the sacrococcyx to a point midway between the two navicular bones of the feet.[15] Alterations in the degree of curvature in one area of the spine result in reciprocal alterations in curvature in other areas of the spinal column to preserve the orientation of the body over the center of gravity. For example, an increase in lumbar lordosis results in increased cervical lordosis.

The cervical spine is composed of functional units. Each functional unit consists of two contiguous vertebrae that may be divided into an anterior column, composed of the vertebral body, longitudinal ligaments, and intervertebral disc, and a posterior column, composed of the osseous canal, the zygapophyseal joints, and the erector spinae muscles. The anterior portion is a weight-bearing, shock-absorbing, flexible structure (Fig. 1-25). The posterior portion protects the neural elements, acts as a fulcrum, and guides movement for the functional unit (Fig. 1-26).

The biomechanical studies involving the cervical spine have concentrated on two major areas: clinical stability and kinematics. Stability as it applies to the spine may be defined as the ability of the spine under physiologic loads to limit patterns of displacement so as not to damage or irritate the spinal cord and nerve roots and, in addition, to prevent incapacitating deformity or pain due to structural changes.[63] Although the issue of clinical instability is particularly germane to traumatic injuries of the cervical spine, the subject also applies to inflammatory disorders such as rheumatoid arthritis and degenerative spondylolisthesis. Range of motion in the subaxial cervical spine can be helpful in making decisions about instability. The maximum anteroposterior translation on a lateral radiograph under physiologic loads has been measured. Direct measurements from cadavers suggest that the upper limit of normal is 2.7 mm. On a radiograph, with magnification due to tube distance, the guide for the upper limit of normal has been 3.5 mm.[62] An intervertebral disc space separation increase with traction of more than 1.7 mm is also abnormal.[64] A difference in angulation greater than 11 degrees between two cervical segments on a lateral radiograph also suggests abnormal motion.[62]

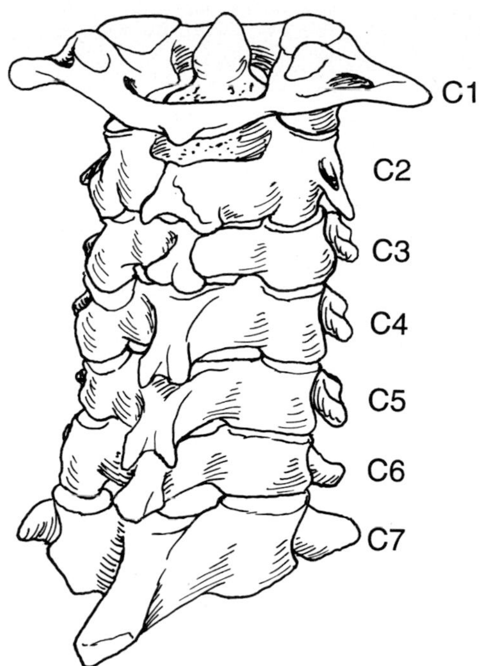

Figure 1-26 Posterior view of the entire cervical spine shows the posterior segments that offer maximum protection to the spinal cord and organized movement of the neck.

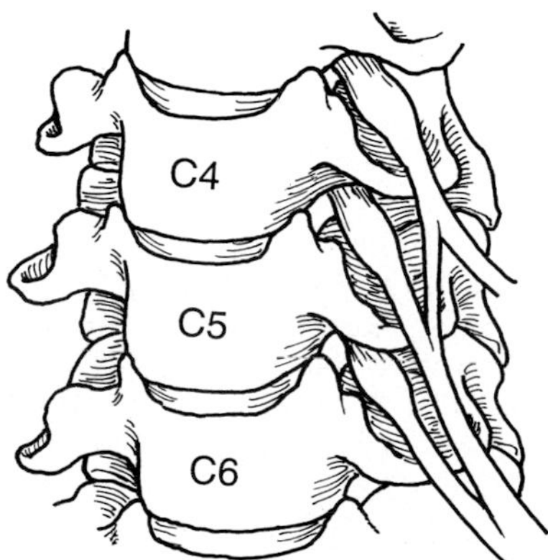

Figure 1-25 Anterior view of the cervical spine showing the anterior segments of C4 through C6 vertebral bodies. The structure of the anterior segment allows for the exit of spinal nerves and flexibility of the intervertebral discs for maximum motion.

Kinematics is the examination of the motion of bodies without consideration of the influencing forces. The two factors that determine the kinematics of vertebral motion are the geometry of the articulating surfaces and the mechanical properties of the connecting structures. At each level of the spine, the planes and extent of motion of each unit are dictated by the orientation of the articular surfaces as well as by the surrounding ligaments and integrity of the intervertebral disc. The motion in the cervical spine between the atlas and the axis, for example, is influenced by the specific geometry of the articular surfaces and the elastic properties of the ligaments.

The function of the cervical spine may be divided into two sections: that of the upper segment above C3 and that of the lower segment from C3 to C7. The upper cervical segment includes five articulations, consisting of two between the occiput and atlas, two between the atlas and axis, and one between the dens and atlas. The occipitoatlantoaxial complex is the most complicated series of articulations in the body. The occipitocervical angle is sharp so that the head is in a horizontal plane. The occipitoatlantal joint has about 13 degrees of flexion and extension and the atlantoaxial joint has about 10 degrees.[61] Thus, there are about 23 degrees of flexion/extension at the occipitoatlantoaxial complex. The

1-2 MEAN RANGE OF CERVICAL SPINE MOTION (DEGREES)

Level	Flexion/Extension	Lateral Bending	Rotation
0–C1	13	8	0
C1–C2	10	0	47
C2–C3	8	10	9
C3–C4	13	11	11
C4–C5	12	11	12
C5–C6	17	8	10
C6–C7	16	7	9
C7–T1	9	4	8

orientation of the condyles prevents any lateral flexion or rotation.

Most of the axial rotation in the upper cervical spine occurs at the atlantoaxial joint.[53] The articular surfaces are convex with a horizontal orientation, allowing for maximum mobility. Atlantoaxial rotation averages 47 degrees, which represents about 50% of the axial rotation in the neck, with the lower cervical spine contributing the other 50% of rotation. There are also about 4 degrees of axial rotation at the occipitocervical junction.[20] The rotation of C2 on C3 is physically limited by the anatomic locking of the anterior tip of the articular process of C3 on the lateral process of the axis. A summary of the normal range of motion of the various cervical segments is shown in Table 1-2.

The lower cervical segment includes C3 through C7 with foraminal openings for the spinal nerve roots that supply the upper extremities. Motion in the lower cervical spine includes flexion, extension, lateral flexion, and rotation. No motion occurs in a single plane. Cervical lateral flexion also requires rotation. Motion also requires deformation of the intervertebral disc. In forward flexion, the anterior disc space undergoes compression with widening posteriorly. Simultaneous separation and shear of the posterior elements occur. An anterior shearing force is placed on the disc with elongation of annular fibers. Forward gliding of the superior vertebra occurs on the inferior vertebra with widening of the facet joint. In extension of the cervical spine, the posterior aspect of the disc compresses and the anterior portion elongates. The facet joint glides posteriorly. Positions of the cervical spine affect intradiscal pressure: Pressure is least in the supine position, and extension of the cervical spine results in the greatest intradiscal pressure (Fig. 1-27).

The neural foramina are affected by the position of the cervical vertebrae. In cervical flexion, the vertebral bodies separate, thereby opening the neural foramina. In cervical extension, the foramina are narrowed. In lateral bending or rotation, the foramina close on the side toward which the neck moves, while opening on the contralateral side.

Flexion of the cervical spine is limited by the posterior longitudinal ligament, the posterior intervertebral ligaments that attach to the transverse processes, the posterior superior spine, and the limited elasticity of the fascia of the extensor musculature. Excessive extension of the cervical spine is limited by the direct contact of the vertebral laminae, the zygapophyseal joints, and the posterosuperior spinous process.[15]

Movement of the cervical spine affects the dura and the spinal cord. As the neck flexes, the spinal canal lengthens, with the posterior wall elongating to a greater degree than the anterior wall. Conversely, when the neck extends, the canal shortens, with the anterior wall lengthening in comparison with the posterior wall. The structures within the canal must follow a similar pattern. The spinal cord ascends and descends in the spinal canal as the neck is flexed and extended, respectively. In flexion, the plastic character of the cord allows elongation. Between a neutral posture and full flexion, the entire cord (C2–C7) elongates linearly with head flexion, increasing 10% and 6% of its initial length along the posterior and anterior surfaces, respectively. The upper shows caudad movement in the spinal canal, and the lower moves cephalad, again with larger movements on the posterior surface.[69] The dura unfolds its plications within flexion. In extension, the spinal cord shortens and descends in the canal. The dura shortens and becomes pleated. The nerves connected to

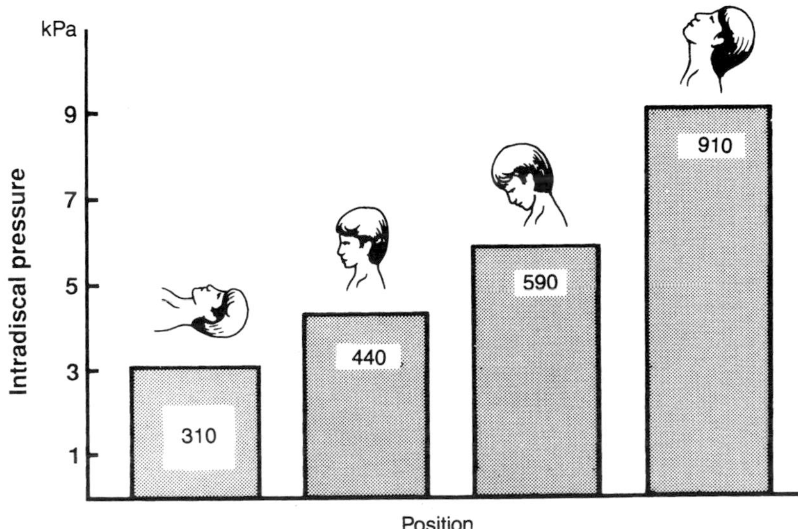

Figure 1-27 Normal intradiscal pressure in various positions of the cervical spine. *(Adapted from Hattori S, Oda H, Kawai S: Cervical intradiscal pressure in movements and traction of the cervical spine. J Orthop 119:568, 1981.)*

the spinal cord are affected in a manner similar to the cord. The nerve roots are elongated, assuming a more acute angle with the boundaries of the foramen. Compression of the nerve root is minimized because the flexion of the neck not only angulates the nerve but also widens the neural foramen, allowing greater room for the neural elements.

The combination of all these biomechanical factors results in a static and dynamic posture of the cervical spine. An individual has good posture if it can be maintained for extended periods in an effortless, nonfatiguing fashion. In the cervical spine, the antigravity action of the extensor muscles plays a predominant role as the source of support. Because the cervical curve is the uppermost curve in the axial skeleton, proprioceptive impulses from the lower extremities and the lower parts of the spine play a crucial role in determining the position of the neck and head by maintaining appropriate muscular tone. Posture is a neuromuscular reaction to proprioceptive impulses from the periphery, and the feeling that posture is appropriate is a learned process.[15] Mechanoreceptor endings are more common in cervical facet joints than the thoracic and lumbar joints, suggesting that the proprioceptive function of the cervical spine is of greater importance for the biomechanics of the spine.[43] Eventually, the position that is assumed during the years the musculoskeletal system develops results in the person's posture. This posture is considered "normal" by the nervous system even if it places the musculoskeletal system at a mechanical disadvantage. In later life, these positions may result in fatigue and neck pain. In addition, emotional states may have an effect on the physical position of the neck. Depression, anxiety, anger, or happiness are only a few of the psychological states that may result in the head being bent forward or upright. Consideration of these anatomic, biomechanical, and physiologic factors by the clinician may help in understanding the source of an individual's neck pain.

LUMBAR SPINE

Lumbar Vertebrae

The lumbar spine is composed of five vertebrae. Each vertebra consists of a body anteriorly and a neural arch posteriorly that encloses the vertebral canal (Fig. 1-28). The spinal cord and cauda equina pass through and are protected by the structures surrounding the vertebral canal.[40] The neural arch has two pedicles on its sides and a lamina posteriorly (see Fig. 1-28). The lumbar isthmus is the area between the superior and inferior apophyseal joints. The superior edge of the isthmus is longest at L5 and shortest at L2. The inferior edge is longest at L2 and shortest at L5. The diameter of the isthmus is smallest at L5. These anatomic characteristics may predispose the fifth lumbar vertebra to the pars defect associated with spondylolysis.[23] A spinous process projects posteriorly from the lamina in the midline and is usually palpable through the skin. A transverse process projects laterally from each side at the junction of the pedicle and lamina (Figs. 1-29 and 1-30).

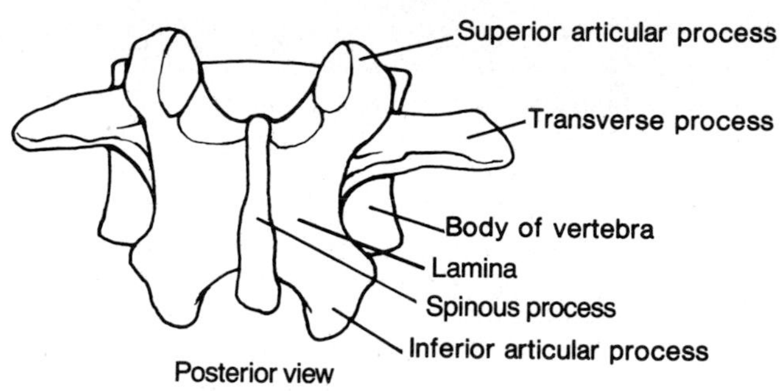

Figure 1-29 Posterior view of a typical lumbar vertebra.

The body of each vertebra has a dense bony cortex surrounding spongy medullary bone. The cortices of the inferior and superior aspects of the body are called the *vertebral endplates*. The endplate that is thicker in its center is covered by a cartilaginous plate. The periphery of the endplate is thickened to form a distinct rim that is derived from the epiphyseal plate and becomes fused to the body at 15 years of age. The endplates are smaller in women compared to men but are of identical shape.[30] The trabecular pattern of the spongy bone in the interior of the vertebral body follows the lines of force placed on the bone. In the frontal plane, vertical lines link the superior and inferior surfaces; horizontal lines, the lateral surfaces; and oblique lines, the inferior surface with the lateral surfaces. In the sagittal plane, the trabeculae follow a fanlike arrangement. The first arrangement transfers force from the superior surface to the two pedicles, superior articular surfaces, and spinous process. The second transfers force

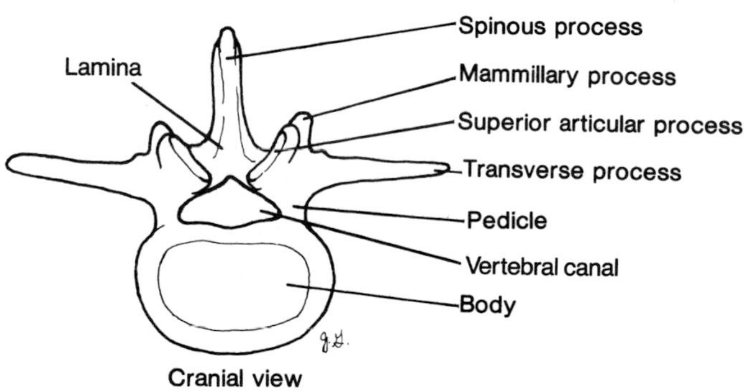

Figure 1-28 Cranial view of a typical lumbar vertebra.

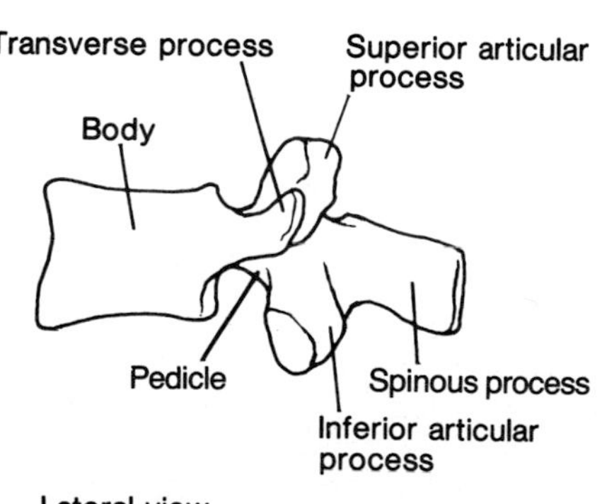

Figure 1-30 Lateral view of a typical lumbar vertebra.

from the inferior surface to the inferior articular surfaces and spinous process. The overlapping trabecular pattern leaves an area in the anterior portion of the vertebral body with a lesser number of trabeculae. This area of the vertebral body fractures at 75% of the force needed to fracture the posterior portion of the vertebral body (Fig. 1-31). The vertebral shell accounts for about 10% of body strength in vivo, with the trabecular centrum contributing the majority of stability.[58]

The facet joints are composed of articular processes arising from adjacent vertebrae. The articular processes project superiorly and inferiorly from the junction of the pedicles and the laminae. They form true synovial joints with synovial fluid (one superior process from below with one inferior process from above), and their purpose is to stabilize the motion between two vertebrae with respect to both translation and torsion while allowing sagittal plane flexion and extension. Each joint is enclosed in a fibrous capsule. The facet joint capsule consists of two layers: The outer layer is a dense connective tissue composed of parallel bundles of collagenous fibers, and the inner layer consists of elastic fibers similar to the ligamentum flavum. The fibers in the superior and middle portion of the joint align in the medial-to-lateral direction crossing the joint space. The inferior capsule consists of long, diagonal, thicker fibers covering the inferior articular recess.[67] The zygapophyseal or facet joints contain menisci that are rudimentary invaginations of the joint capsule that project into the joint space.[8] The menisci function as fillers that provide stability and distribute loads over greater articular areas. The menisci are rarely entrapped between the articular cartilage.

Nerve roots exit from the spinal canal through the intervertebral foramina. Each foramen is bordered by pedicles inferiorly and superiorly. The foramen is bordered anteriorly by the intervertebral disc and vertebral body and posteriorly by the lamina as well as the anterior aspect of the facet joint and its capsule. The intervertebral foramina are longer in their vertical dimension than in their horizontal, with the largest cross-sectional area at the L1–L2 foramen and the smallest at the L5–S1 foramen.

Because the spinal cord ends at the L1 level, the course of the exiting nerve roots becomes longer and more obliquely directed as they approach the lower segments (Fig. 1-32). Therefore, in the lumbar region, the nerve roots are located in the superior aspect of the foramen. The exiting nerve roots cross the disc immediately above the foramen from which they exit (Fig. 1-33). For example, the L4 nerve root crosses the L3–L4 foramen and then exits the foramen formed by the L4 and L5 vertebral bodies. The nerve leaves the foramen in a downward, anterolateral direction. At the lateral extent of the foramen, the dorsal root ganglion and anterior ramus have not yet joined to form the spinal nerve. The spinal nerve forms just lateral to the foramen. The dorsal (sensory) root is twice the thickness of the anterior (motor) root. The motor root is located anteriorly and inferiorly in the foramen. The nerve roots are covered by both arachnoid and dura. The arachnoid covers the nerve roots to the level of the dorsal root ganglion. The outer dura covers the roots through the foramen and continues along the spinal nerves as the perineurium. Within the foramen, the nerve and its sheath occupy 35% to 40% of the area. The largest of the lumbar spinal nerves is L5, which is housed in the smallest lumbar foramen. Consequently, the L5 spinal nerve is most vulnerable to compression by foraminal structures. Connective tissue, ligamentum flavum, arteries, veins, lymphatics, and the sinuvertebral nerve fill the remaining space (Fig. 1-34).[13]

The spinal canal in cross section is surrounded by the neural arch posteriorly and the posterior surface of the vertebral body anteriorly. The canal itself is triangular in shape with an anterior base. It progressively widens from L1 to the sacrum. However, the lateral angles of the triangle are smaller in the fourth and fifth lumbar vertebral bodies. These are locations of potential nerve impingement. The lumbosacral area of the spinal canal contains the cauda equina. The true spinal cord terminates with the conus medullaris approximately at the level of the inferior margin of the first lumbar vertebra. The canal also contains a posterior epidural fat pad that has special properties that allow sliding of neural structures.[7]

Sacrum and Coccyx

The sacrum is a large triangular bone (Figs. 1-35 and 1-36). It is composed of five fused vertebrae and is inserted like a wedge between the two pelvic bones. The cortical thickness is uniform throughout the bone. The alar area of the sacrum has the smallest amount of trabecular bone.[54] The strongest part of the sacrum is the anterior cortex.

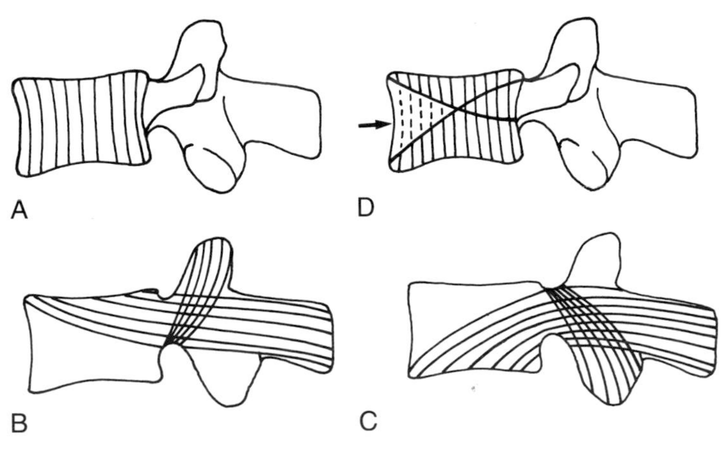

Figure 1-31 Lines of force in the interior of a vertebral body. *A*, Lines attaching vertebral endplates. *B*, Lines attaching the superior endplate with the pedicles, superior articular surface, and spinous process. *C*, Lines attaching the inferior endplate with inferior articular surface and spinous process. *D*, The arrow points to the weakest area of a vertebral body, a common location for vertebral fractures.

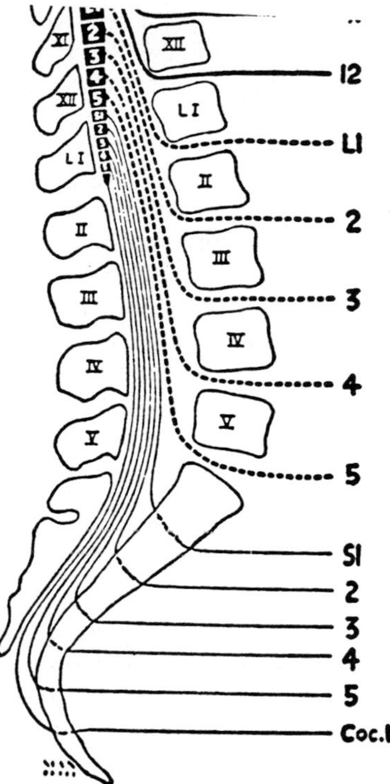

Figure 1-32 A lateral schematic of the spine showing the relationship of the conus medullaris to L1 and L2 and the relationship of the individual spinal nerves to each of the vertebral bodies at skeletal maturity. *(From Haymaker W, Woodhall B: Peripheral Nerve Injuries, 2nd ed. Philadelphia, WB Saunders, 1953.)*

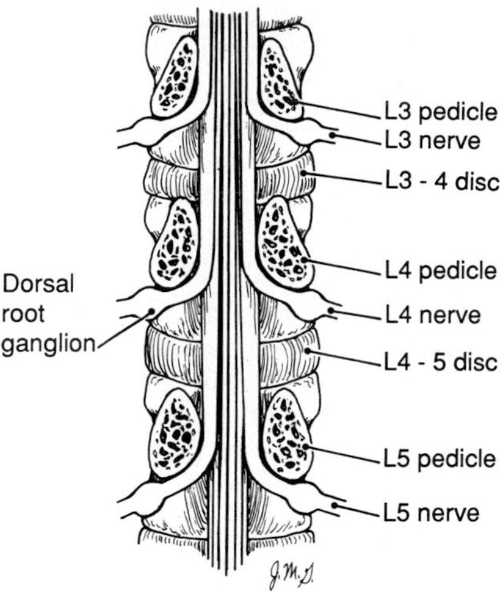

Figure 1-33 A coronal schematic view of the exiting lumbar spinal nerve roots. Note that the exiting root takes the name of the vertebral body pedicle under which it travels into the neural foramen. It is also evident why L4–L5 disc pathology generally affects the L5 root rather than the L4 root, which has already exited.

The weakest part of the sacrum is at the junction of S2 and S3. The alar area may be at greatest risk for fracture.[21]

The sacral and iliac sides of the sacroiliac amphiarthrodial joint are covered with thicker hyaline cartilage (1 to 3 mm) and thinner fibrocartilage (1 mm), respectively (Fig. 1-37).[8] The ventral, or anterior, portion of the joint is lined by synovial membrane, which produces a small amount of synovial fluid. The dorsal, or posterior, portion of the joint does not contain synovial tissue and is joined by fibrous attachments (Fig. 1-38). The most common segments articulating with the ilium include S1, S2, and S3. Occasionally, L5 may be an articulating segment, whereas S4 and L4 are rarely involved. Usually fewer sacral segments are involved in the female pelvis than in the male pelvis. There is a wedge-shaped intervertebral

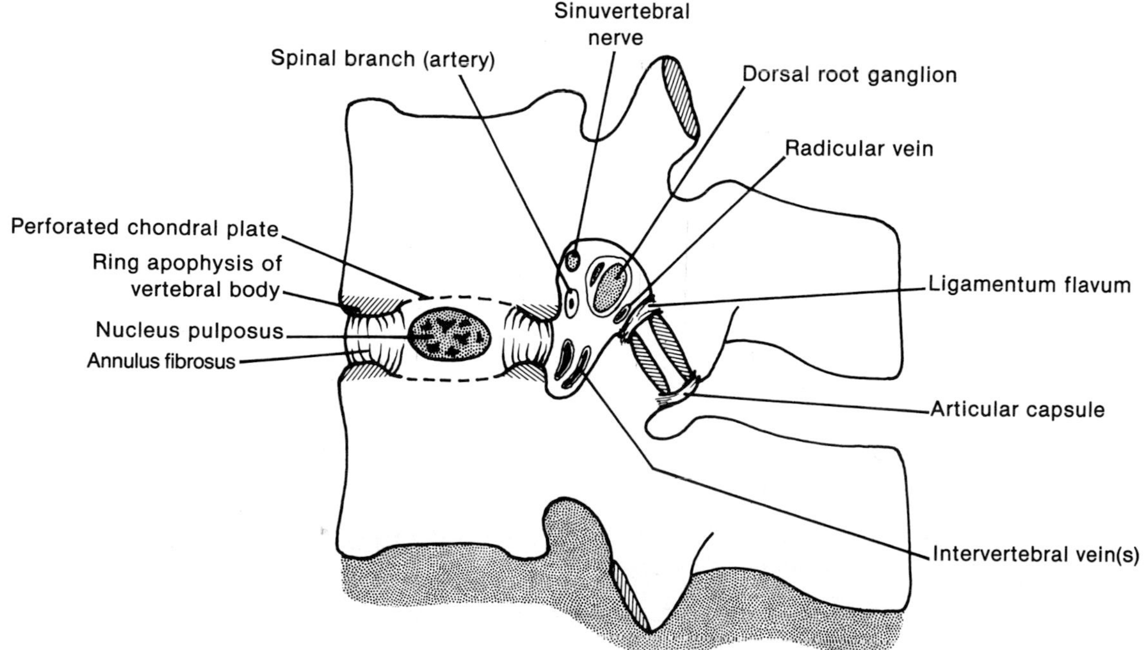

Figure 1-34 Schematic of a sagittal section of the spine showing contents of an intervertebral foramen in relation to a disc. The two vertebral bodies and intervertebral disc along with supporting structures constitute a motor unit, which includes all components of a somite present in an embryo.

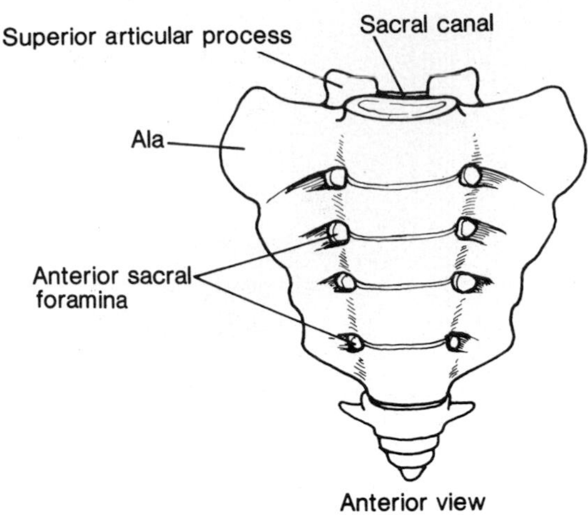

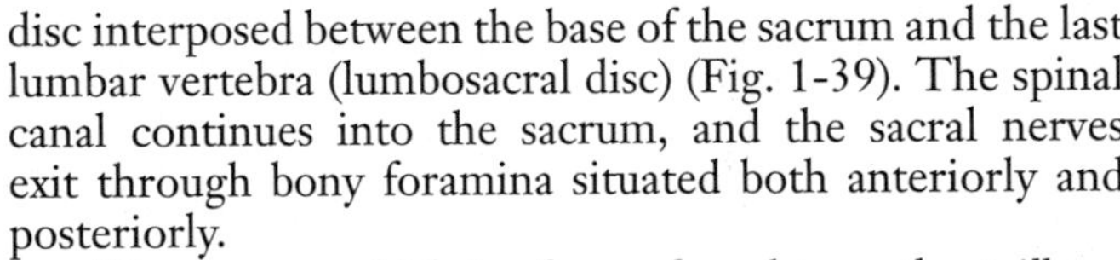

Figure 1-35 Anterior view of the sacrum and coccyx.

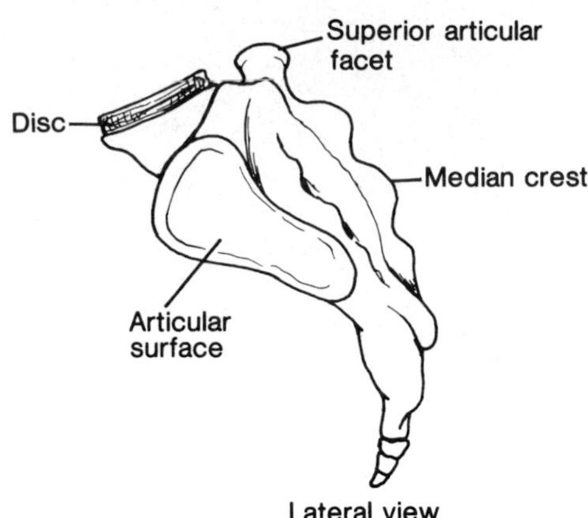

Figure 1-37 Lateral view showing the articular surface of the sacrum.

disc interposed between the base of the sacrum and the last lumbar vertebra (lumbosacral disc) (Fig. 1-39). The spinal canal continues into the sacrum, and the sacral nerves exit through bony foramina situated both anteriorly and posteriorly.

The coccyx, which is often referred to as the *tailbone*, is made up of four tiny fused vertebrae. It is connected to the inferior end of the sacrum and is solid. There is no spinal canal in the coccyx.

Intervertebral Discs

The intervertebral discs (see Fig. 1-6) are the major structural link between adjacent vertebrae. Together they make up 33% of the height of the lumbar spine.[13] They function as universal joints, permitting far greater motion between vertebral bodies than if the vertebral bones were in direct contact with each other.

Each intervertebral disc is made up of a gelatinous nucleus pulposus surrounded by a laminated, fibrous annulus fibrosus. Each disc is situated between the cartilaginous endplates of vertebrae above and below.

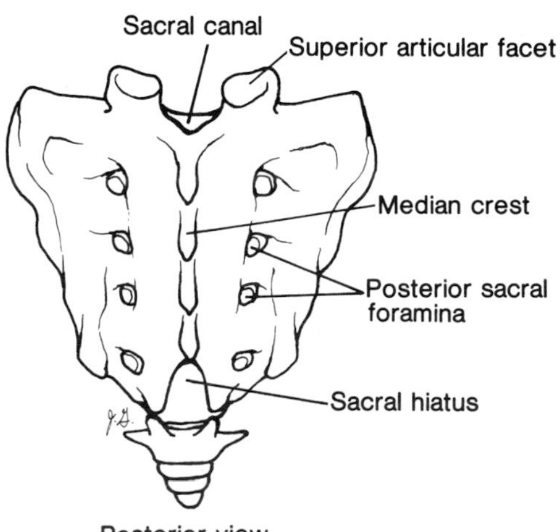

Figure 1-36 Posterior view of the sacrum and coccyx.

The nucleus pulposus is posterocentrally situated within the disc and consists of collagen fibrils enmeshed in a mucoprotein gel (see Fig. 1-6). The nucleus pulposus occupies about 40% of the disc's cross-sectional area. It has a high water content at birth (88%), which mechanically lets it absorb quite a bit of stress.[16,18] However, with age the percentage of water decreases, reflecting both an absolute decrease in available proteoglycans and a change in the ratio of the different proteoglycans present. This desiccation (loss of water) reduces the ability of the nucleus pulposus to function as a gel and withstand stress.

The annulus fibrosus forms the outer boundary of the disc.[29] It is composed of fibrocartilaginous tissue and fibrous protein arranged in concentric layers or lamellae that run obliquely from one vertebra to another. Successive layers of these fibers slant in alternate directions so that they cross each other at different angles that vary with the intradiscal pressure of the nucleus pulposus. Thus, the annulus fibrosus can absorb stress by expanding and contracting like a Chinese finger trap. Its peripheral fibers pass over the edge of the cartilaginous endplate to unite with the bone of each vertebral body. The most superficial fibers blend with the anterior and posterior longitudinal ligaments. With age, the annulus fibrosus fibers deteriorate, become fissured, and lose their capacity to contain the nucleus pulposus. If there is sufficient internal stress, the nucleus pulposus material can penetrate through the annulus; the resulting injury is termed a *herniated disc*.

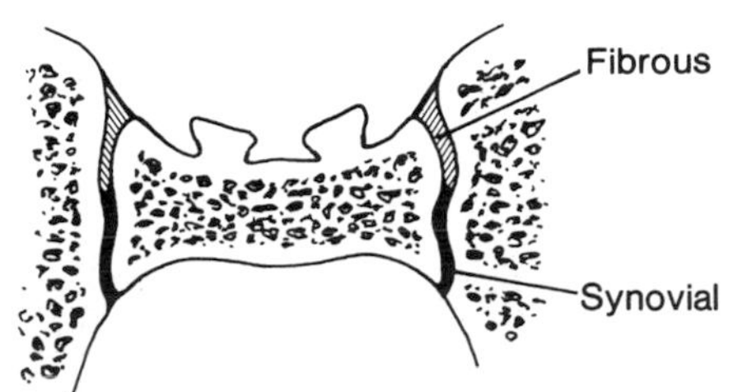

Figure 1-38 Transverse view of the sacroiliac joint. The anterior portion of the joint is lined by synovial tissue. The posterior portion is joined by fibrous tissue.

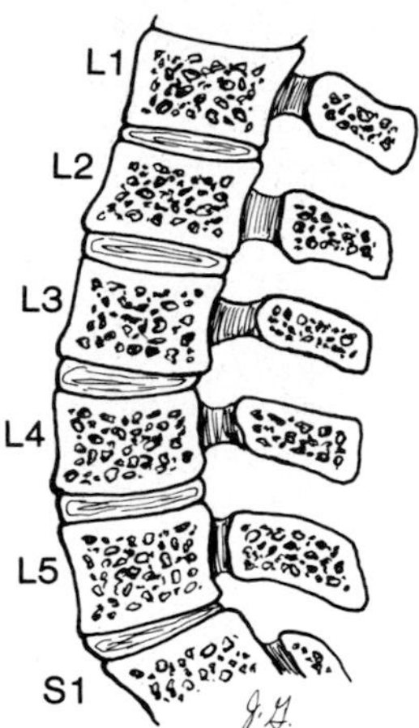

Figure 1-39 Lateral view of the lumbar spine including the lumbosacral articulation at the L5–S1 interspace.

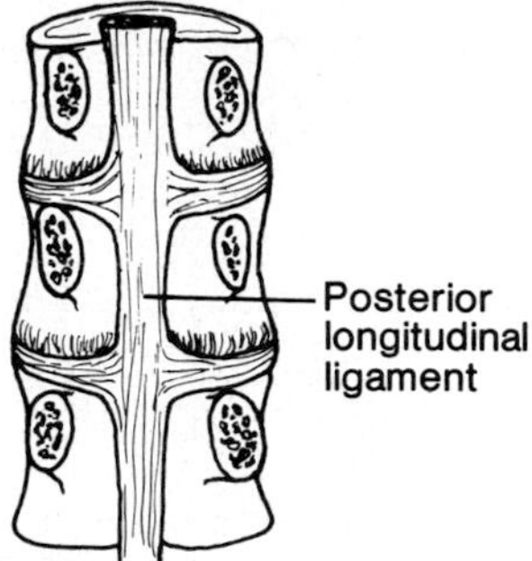

Figure 1-41 Posterior view of the lumbar vertebrae. The posterior longitudinal ligament expands laterally to cover the intervertebral discs. The posterior longitudinal ligament is weakest in this location.

Ligaments of the Lumbar Vertebral Column

The vertebral bodies are bordered front and back by two major ligaments.[34] The anterior longitudinal ligament is a broad, strong band of fibers extending along the front and sides of the vertebral bodies (Fig. 1-40). Its deepest fibers blend with the intervertebral discs and are firmly bound to each successive vertebral body. The ligament increases in thickness to fill the concavities formed by the configuration of the vertebral body.

The posterior longitudinal ligament extends along the posterior surface of the vertebral bodies (Fig. 1-41). It forms the anterior boundary of the spinal canal. In the lumbar canal, it becomes narrow as it passes over each vertebral body and then expands laterally as it passes over each disc. It thus takes on the configuration of a series of hourglasses, with the attenuated lateral expansions over the intervertebral discs being the weakest and most vulnerable to disc herniation. The posterior longitudinal ligament starts to narrow at the first lumbar level (L1) and becomes one half its original width at the L5–S1 interspace. A third ligament, the lateral vertebral ligament, lies between the anterior and posterior ligaments and passes from one vertebral body to the next, firmly adhering to the intervertebral disc.

The ligamenta flava run posteriorly between adjacent laminae (Fig. 1-42). These yellow, elastic ligaments extend from the base of the articular processes on one side to those on the opposite side, as well as laterally into the intervertebral foramina. They are attached inferiorly to the superior edges and posterosuperior surfaces of the laminae and superiorly to the inferior and anteroinferior surfaces of the laminae. This unique arrangement, combined with the anterior tilt of the laminae and elastic properties of the ligament that resist buckling, has the effect of creating an extremely smooth posteroinferior wall that remains smooth and protects the neural elements in spite of whatever position into which the spine is bent or twisted. Cadaveric studies have identified the ligamentum flavum to have a superficial and a deep layer. The superficial layer inserts on the superior edge and posterosuperior surface of the caudal lamina. The deep layer inserts for a variable distance onto the anterosuperior surface of the caudal lamina.[49]

In the posterior portion of the vertebrae, the intervertebral joints are strengthened by a series of ligaments that lie between adjacent transverse spinous processes (intertransverse ligaments) and spinous processes (interspinous and supraspinous ligaments) (Fig. 1-43). In the lumbar region, the supraspinous ligament is indistinct as it merges with the insertion of the lumbodorsal muscles. These ligaments help reduce the anterior force (shear) placed on the lumbar spine because of the lordotic curve and the lumbosacral angle. Iliolumbar ligaments that attach to the

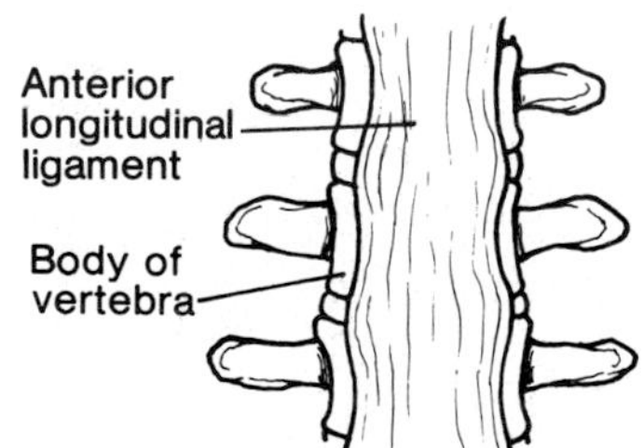

Figure 1-40 Anterior view of the lumbar spine. The anterior longitudinal ligament covers the anterior surface of the vertebral bodies and meshes with the anterior fibers of the annulus fibrosus.

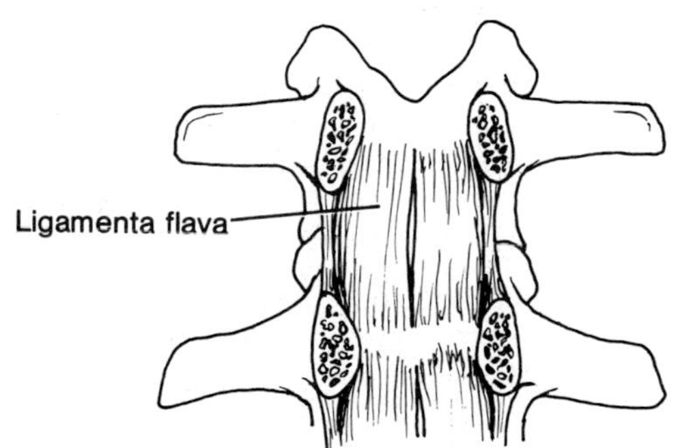

Figure 1-42 The ligamenta flava attach to the anterior surface of the lamina above and extend to the posterior surface of the upper margin of the lamina below.

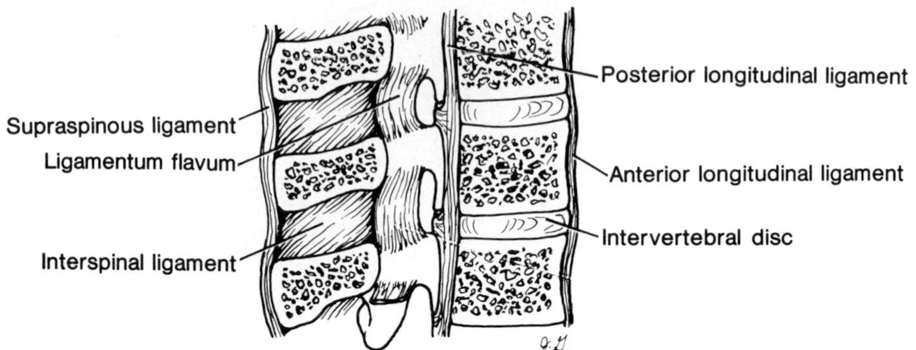

Figure 1-43 Lateral view of the lumbar spine demonstrating the ligaments that support the anterior (anterior longitudinal, posterior longitudinal) and the posterior (supraspinous, intraspinous) elements of the vertebrae. Note the position of the ligamentum flavum forming a smooth posterior wall of the neural foramen.

transverse processes connect the lower two lumbar vertebrae to the iliac crest, limiting the movement of the sacroiliac joint. During lateral flexion, the contralateral iliolumbar ligaments become taut, allowing on average only 8 degrees of movement of L4 relative to the sacrum. Flexion and extension of the lumbar spine is also limited but to a lesser degree than lateral flexion. More recent studies have identified this ligament as originating primarily from the L5 transverse process, and it is composed of a thicker anterior band and a thinner posterior band that may be more at risk of injury.[4]

The stability of the sacroiliac joint is dependent not only on the interdigitation of the articular surfaces of the ilium and sacrum but also on the several large accessory ligaments surrounding the joint. Ligaments attach the sacrum and ilium (anterior sacroiliac, posterior sacroiliac, and interosseous sacroiliac) and the sacrum and ischium (sacrotuberous and sacrospinous) (Fig. 1-44). The long dorsal sacroiliac ligament helps counterbalance stress on the sacrotuberous ligaments.[60] The relative strength of the ligaments is different between the sexes. After puberty, in contrast to the increasing strength of the ligaments in the male, the strength of the ligaments is sacrificed in the female for increased mobility, particularly during pregnancy and labor.

Blood Supply of the Lumbar Spine

The lumbar spine's blood supply arises directly from the aorta.[34] There are four paired lumbar arteries that arise directly from the posterior aspect of the aorta in front of the bodies of the first four lumbar vertebrae. In front of L5, a fifth pair may come off the middle sacral artery. These vessels (Fig. 1-45) curve posteriorly around the bodies of the vertebrae and give off posterior rami as they pass between the transverse processes. These posterior rami, in turn, furnish the vertebral or spinal branches, which supply the bodies of the vertebrae and their ligaments. The sacrum is supplied by medial branches of the

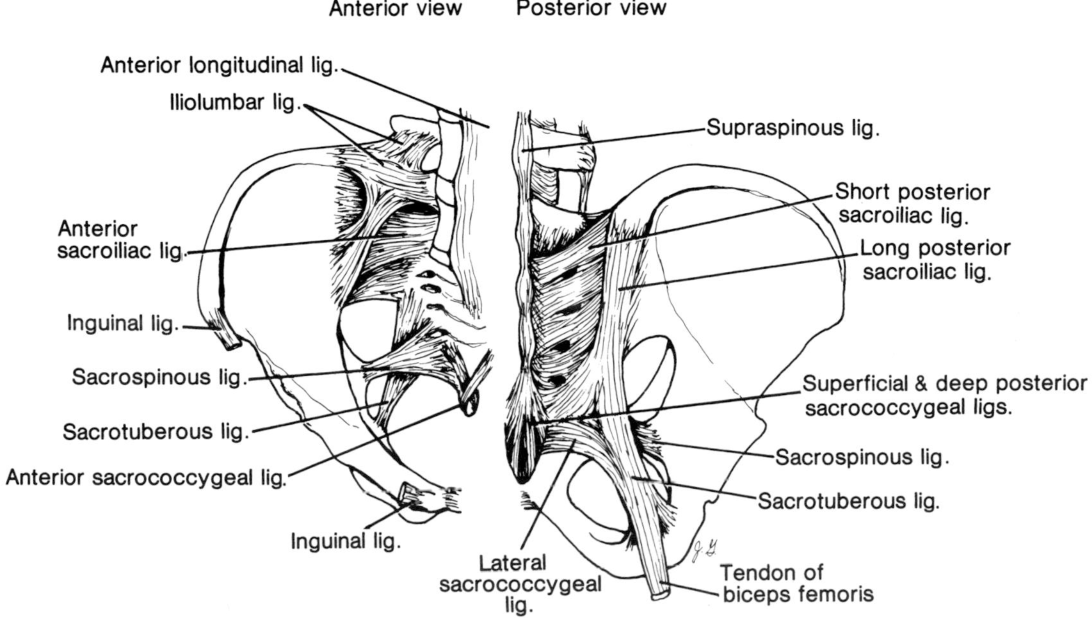

Figure 1-44 Anterior and posterior views of the sacroiliac joint ligaments. The anterior and posterior ligamentous attachments are very strong. Disruption of these attachments usually occurs only with severe trauma to the pelvis.

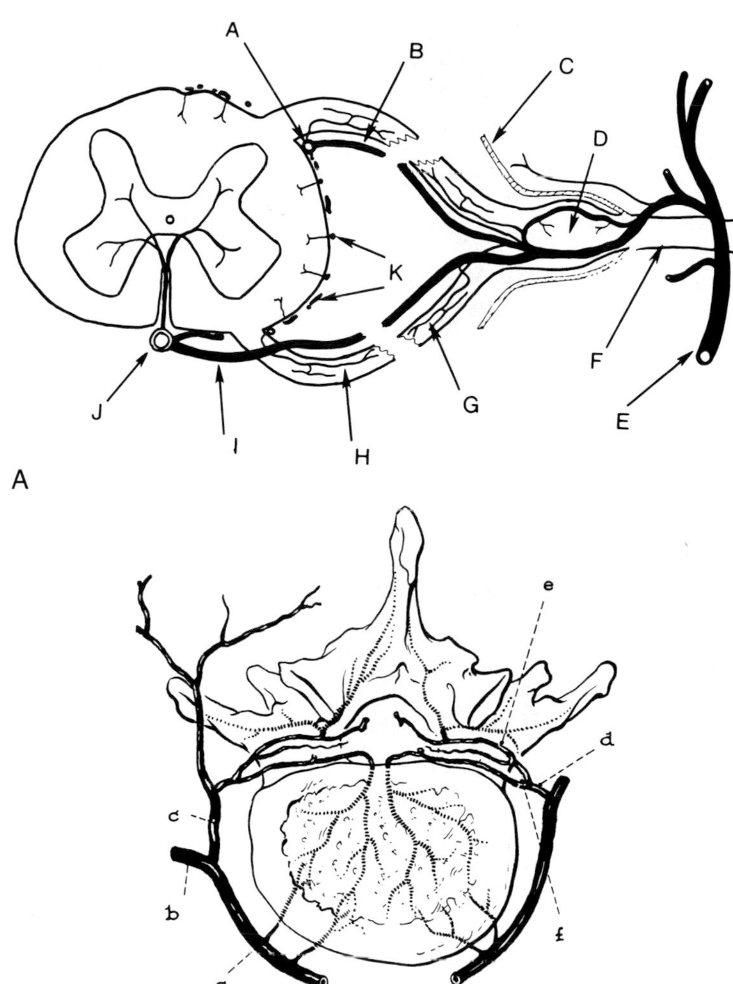

Figure 1-45 Arterial system of the lumbosacral spine. *A*, Schema illustrating all of the possible vascular relations of the spinal roots in which both medullary and radicular arteries are present. The break in the roots indicates that the schema applies to either the short cervical roots or the long lumbosacral elements of the cauda equina. The dorsolateral spinal artery (A) receives the dorsal medullary artery (B) and directly supplies the dorsal proximal radicular artery. The anterior spinal artery (J) receives the ventral medullary artery (I) and supplies the ventral proximal radicular artery (H) through the vasa corona (K). The segmental artery (E) gives a spinal branch that accompanies the spinal nerve (F) through the intervertebral foramen to supply the plexus of the dorsal root ganglion (D), which gives origin to the proximal radicular arteries (G) and (when present) the medullary vessels. The dura (C) receives fine meningeal branches. Note that medullary arteries usually do not supply roots in mid-course. *B*, Diagram of the blood supply to a vertebra as seen from below and from behind with the laminae removed: (a) is a segmental (in this case a lumbar) artery; (b) is its ventral continuation; (c) is its dorsal branch; (d) is the spinal branch; and (e) and (f) are the spinal branch's dorsal and ventral twigs to tissue of the epidural space and to the vertebral column; the unlabeled middle twig is to the nerve roots, and at some levels, to the spinal cord. *(A, From Parke W, Gammell K, Rothman R: Arterial vascularization of the cauda equina. J Bone Joint Surg Am 63:53, 1981; B, From Hollinshead WH: Anatomy for Surgeons, 3rd ed, Vol 3. Philadelphia, Lippincott, 1982.)*

superior gluteal or hypogastric arteries. The arteries follow the contour of the sacrum and send branches to each anterior sacral foramen. The arteries supply the sacral canal and exit the posterior sacral foramen to supply the lower back muscles.

The venous supply to the lumbar spine mirrors the arterial supply. The venous system is valveless, draining the internal and external venous systems into the inferior vena cava. The venous system is arranged in an anterior and posterior ladder-like configuration with multiple cross connections (Fig. 1-46). The functional result of this extensively anastomotic, valveless system is the constant shifting of blood from larger to smaller vessels and vice versa, depending on the degree of intra-abdominal pressure. Batson described retrograde venous flow from the lower pelvic organs to the lumbosacral spine.[5] He claimed that these venous connections provide the route for metastases to spread from pelvic neoplasms (prostate) to the spine. More recently, the anatomy of the internal and external venous plexuses has been identified on magnetic resonance imaging scans and correlated with anatomic sections, making noninvasive study of the venous anatomy possible.[19]

During the adult phase of life, there is no active blood supply to the intervertebral discs, although up to 8 years of age, there are small vessels supplying the discs that are gradually obliterated during the first three decades of life. By the time growth has stopped, the nucleus pulposus and annulus fibrosus no longer have an active blood supply and receive only marginal sustenance from the transfer of tissue fluid across the cartilaginous endplates.

Muscles and Fascia of the Lumbosacral Spine

The most superficial layer of tissue below the subcutaneous tissue contains the lumbodorsal fascia (Fig. 1-47). Medially it attaches to the dorsal spinous processes; inferiorly it attaches to the iliac crest and lateral crest of the sacrum; laterally it serves as the origin of the latissimus dorsi and transversus abdominis muscles; and superiorly it attaches to the angles of the ribs in the thoracic region. The fascia has extension cephalad to the rhomboids and the tendons of the splenius capitis.[3] It also surrounds the sacrospinalis muscles. Below the fascia lie superficial, multisegmental muscles, collectively named the *erector spinae muscle*. Its origin is a thick tendon attached to the posterior aspect of the sacrum, iliac crest, lumbar spinous processes, and supraspinous ligament. The muscle fibers split into three columns at the level of the lumbar spine: the lateral iliocostalis (insertion—angles of ribs), the intermediate longissimus (insertion—transverse processes of the lumbar and thoracic vertebrae), and the more medial spinalis (insertion—posterior spines) (Fig. 1-48). The muscle also

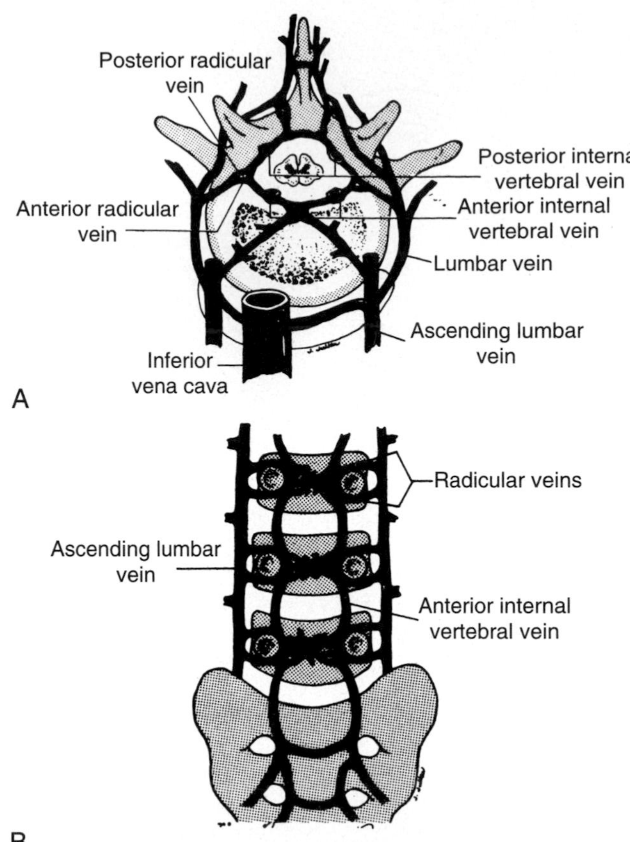

Figure 1-46 *A* and *B*, Venous system of the lumbosacral spine. *(A and B, From Wiesel SW, Bernini P, Rothman RH: The Aging Lumbar Spine. Philadelphia, WB Saunders, 1982.)*

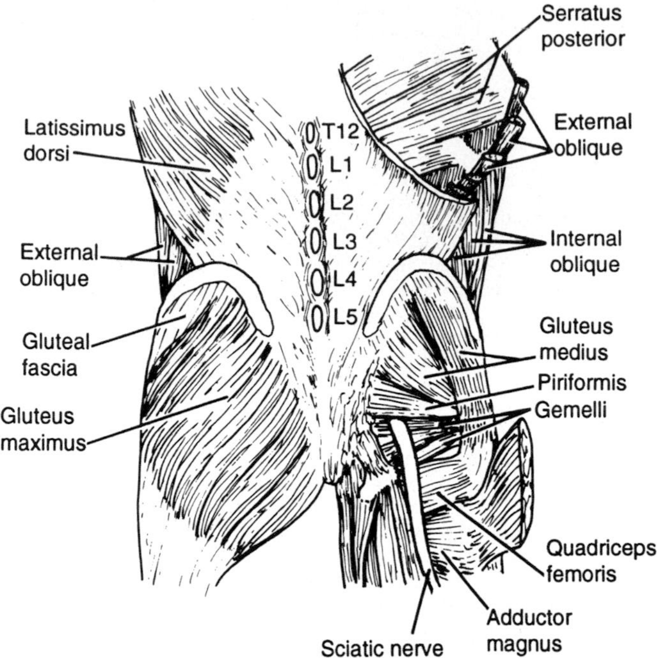

Figure 1-47 Posterior view of the superficial fascia and muscles of the lumbar spine and buttocks *(left)* and deeper posterior muscles of the lumbar spine and buttocks *(right)*.

is divided into distinct thoracic and lumbar portions.[52] The thoracic portions consist of tiny muscles with segmental origins from the thorax and the erector spinae aponeurosis. The lumbar portions insert into the ilium and arise from the accessory processes of the vertebrae. The action of this group of muscles is to extend the spine and, with unilateral action, bend the spinal column to one side.

Deep to the erector spinae lie the transversospinal muscles, including the multifidus and rotators. The multifidus originates from the posterior surface of the sacrum, aponeurosis of the sacrospinalis, posterior superior iliac spine, and posterior sacroiliac ligament and inserts two to four segments above their origin into spinous processes. The multifidus extends the spine and rotates it toward the opposite side. The rotators have similar attachments and action but ascend only one or two segments. Additional deep muscles include the interspinalis, connecting pairs of adjacent lumbar spinous processes, and the intertransversarii (medial, dorsal lateral, and ventral lateral groups), which connect pairs of adjacent transverse processes. They extend and bend the column to the same side.

The forward and lateral flexor muscles of the lumbar spine are located anterior and lateral to the vertebral bodies and transverse processes (Fig. 1-49). The iliopsoas consists of two separate muscular heads: the iliacus and psoas major. The origins of the psoas major arise from the intervertebral discs by five slips, each of which starts from adjacent upper and lower margins of two vertebrae, the transverse processes of the lumbar vertebrae, and membranous arches emanating from the bodies of the four upper lumbar vertebrae, permitting the lumbar arteries and veins and sympathetic rami communicantes to pass beneath them. The iliacus arises from the iliac fossa and joins the psoas under the inguinal ligament, crosses the hip joint capsule, and inserts into the lesser trochanter of the femur. These muscles flex the lumbar spine and bend it toward the same side. The quadratus lumborum lies lateral to the vertebral column arising from the posterior part of the iliac crest and iliolumbar ligament and inserts into the 12th rib and the tips of the transverse processes of the

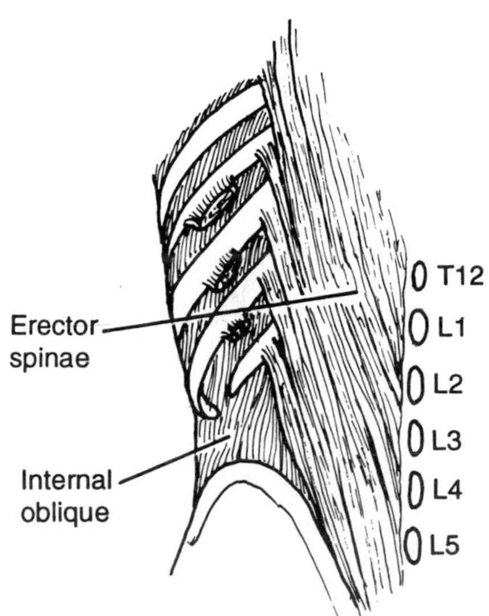

Figure 1-48 Posterior view of the erector spinae muscle, primary extensor muscle of the lumbar spine.

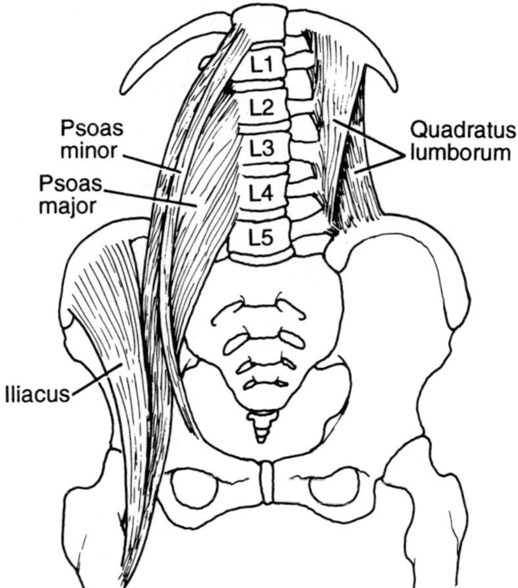

Figure 1-49 Anterior view of the intrinsic flexors of the lumbar spine. The quadratus lumborum contains two layers. The psoas major and iliacus muscles have a conjoined attachment on and around the lesser femoral trochanter.

upper four lumbar vertebrae. This muscle fixes the 12th rib down against traction exerted by the diaphragm during inspiration and bends the trunk toward the same side when acting alone.

Although not anatomically part of the low back, anterior abdominal muscles (such as the rectus abdominis, external abdominal oblique, and internal abdominal oblique), transversalis muscles (flexors of the lumbar spine), gluteal muscles (extensors of the hip and trunk), hamstrings (flexors of the knee), quadriceps (extensors of the knee), gastrocnemius muscle, and soleus muscle (plantar flexors of the foot) are important support structures of the lumbosacral spine. Abnormalities in these muscles (shortening, increased muscle tone) may result in abnormal kinetics of the lumbosacral spine and low back pain. The location and function of the lumbosacral and abdominal muscles that affect spinal motion are illustrated in Figure 1-50.

Nerve Supply of the Lumbosacral Spine

A familiarity with the neuroanatomy of the lumbosacral spine is essential in understanding the pain patterns that are associated with disease processes affecting individual anatomic components of the low back.[24,33,34,52] The sinuvertebral nerve is thought to be the major sensory nerve supplying the structures of the lumbar spine. It arises from its corresponding spinal nerve before it divides into posterior and anterior primary divisions. It is joined by a sympathetic branch from the ramus communicans and enters the spinal canal by way of the intervertebral foramen, curving upward around the base of the pedicle and proceeding toward the midline on the posterior longitudinal ligament (Fig. 1-51). The nerve divides into ascending, descending, and transverse branches, which anastomose with the contralateral side and sinuvertebral nerves at adjacent levels from above and below (Fig. 1-52). The sinuvertebral nerve innervates the posterior longitudinal ligament, the superficial layers of the annulus fibrosus, the blood vessels of the epidural space, the anterior but not the posterior dura mater (posterior dura is devoid of nerve endings), the dural sleeve surrounding the spinal nerve roots, and the posterior vertebral periosteum. The posterior longitudinal ligament is most heavily innervated, whereas the anterior, sacroiliac, and interspinous ligaments receive nociceptive (pain) nerve endings to a lesser degree.[36] The lumbar intervertebral discs are innervated posteriorly by the sinuvertebral nerves and laterally by branches of the ventral rami and gray rami communicantes.[1] Afferent sympathetic nerves may also supply the annulus fibrosus in the anterior portion of the intervertebral disc.[14] The anterior portion of the lower lumbar discs may be innervated by nerves from the L1 and L2 level. The innervation may explain groin pain experienced by individuals

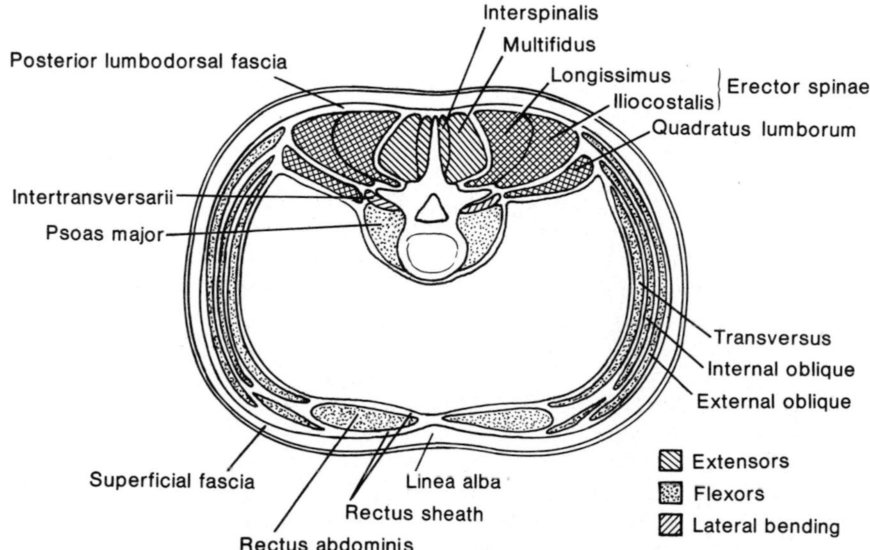

Figure 1-50 Cross section of body musculature and fascia through the third lumbar vertebra. The primary motions of the lumbar spine are flexion, extension, and lateral bending. (Only a small proportion of rotation occurs in the lumbar spine.) Flexors are anterior to the spine and extensors are posterior. The muscles that cause lateral bending are contiguous to the vertebral bodies in a lateral position.

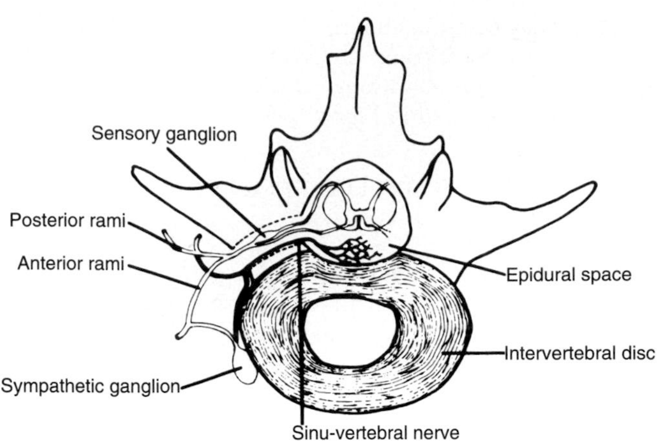

Figure 1-51 Axial view of the spine showing the sinuvertebral nerve. The nerve re-enters the neural foramen from the spinal nerve to innervate the posterior longitudinal ligament. *(From Wiesel SW, Bernini P, Rothman RH: The Aging Lumbar Spine. Philadelphia, WB Saunders, 1982.)*

with lower lumbar disc herniation.[45] Nociceptive fibers may grow into the annular portion of discs as they degenerate.[17]

The posterior primary rami arise from each corresponding spinal nerve and divide into medial and lateral branches. The medial (posterior) branch descends posteriorly at the back of the transverse and superior articular processes to supply sensory fibers to two facet joint levels. The sensory fibers supply the inferior portion of a posterior joint facet and the superior part of the joint capsule at the next lower level. Therefore, each facet joint is supplied by sensory nerves from spinal nerves from two different segments (Fig. 1-53). The medial branch continues caudally to supply innervation of dorsal muscles (including the multifidus, intertransversarii mediales, and interspinales), fascia, interspinous ligaments, blood vessels, and periosteum and anastomoses with sensory nerves from adjacent levels. The spinous processes and laminae are supplied by branches of the posterior primary rami (Fig. 1-54). The surface layer of the ligamentum flavum may receive sensory fibers from the posterior primary rami. The substance of the ligamentum flavum is not innervated. The interspinous and supraspinous ligaments are supplied by

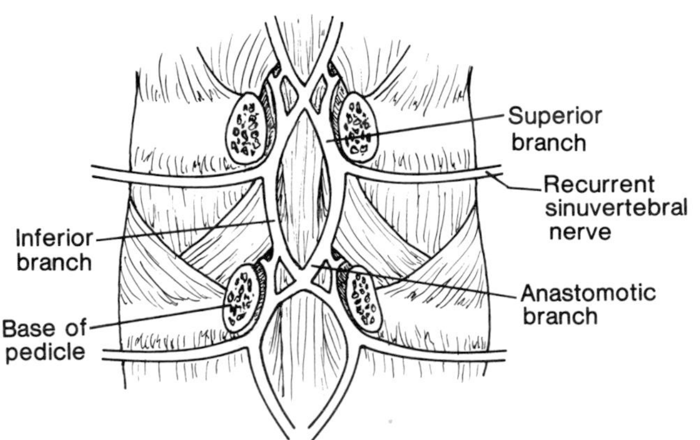

Figure 1-52 Branches of the recurrent sinuvertebral nerve anastomosing with nerve branches from above and below.

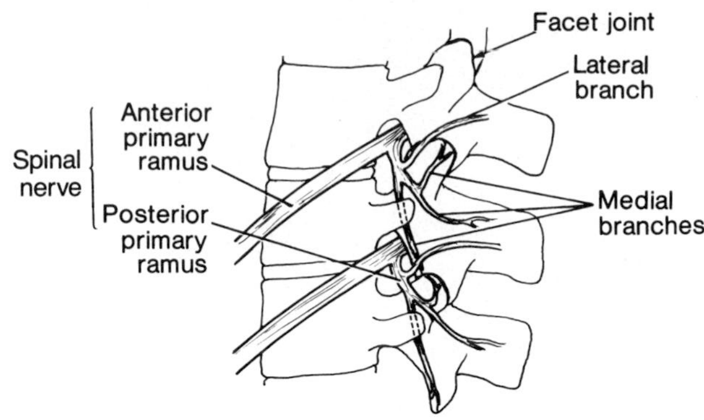

Figure 1-53 Lateral view of the posterior primary rami supplying facet joints at two vertebral levels.

branches arising from nerves that innervate surrounding muscles. The lumbodorsal fascia receives sensory innervation from cutaneous nerves of the posterior primary rami that originate at one level cephalad to the lumbar level.

The lateral (anterior) branches of the posterior primary rami supply small branches to the sacrospinalis muscle and continue to innervate cutaneous structures in the lumbar area (see Fig. 1-54). In the lumbar spine, only the posterior primary rami from the upper three lumbar levels supply cutaneous sensory nerves to the lumbar area. The cutaneous innervation may supply areas of skin as distal as the greater trochanter.

The nucleus pulposus of the intervertebral discs is devoid of any nerve endings. The posterior portion of the annulus fibrosus shares free nerve endings with the fibrous tissue that binds it to the posterior longitudinal ligament. Lesions of the nucleus pulposus cause no pain. Only when the nerve fibers near the annulus are stimulated are nociceptive impulses transmitted to the spinal cord.

RETROPERITONEAL ABDOMINAL STRUCTURES NEIGHBORING THE LUMBOSACRAL SPINE AND SURFACE ANATOMY

Anterior to the lumbosacral spine are a number of organs that are retroperitoneal in location. These structures may be enveloped in their own fascia or may be partially covered by peritoneum. During the embryonic development of the abdominal cavity, some organs come to lie relatively immobile against one another or against the retroperitoneal organs of the posterior body wall. The abdominal organs that are located posteriorly include the middle portion of the duodenum and the ascending and descending colon. Other retroperitoneal structures include the kidneys, ureters, aorta, inferior vena cava, bile duct, pancreas, and periaortic lymph nodes. Inferior to the abdominal cavity is the pelvic cavity. The rectum is directly anterior to the sacrum and coccyx. The anatomic relationships of the retroperitoneal structures and lumbosacral spine are depicted in Figure 1-55. The pancreas and duodenum lie anterior to the L1 vertebral body. The kidneys are at the same level in a paraspinous location. They extend to the L3 level. The ureters are also paraspinous in location, anterior to the aorta, running caudad to the bladder

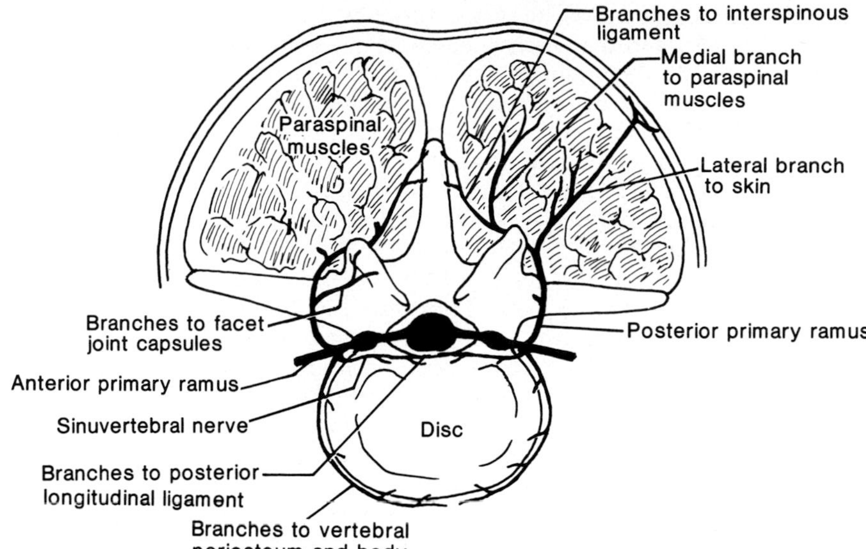

Figure 1-54 Cross-sectional view depicting nerve supply to the anterior (sinuvertebral) and posterior (posterior ramus) portions of the lumbar spine.

in the pelvis. The moveable portion of the sigmoid colon may reach the L1 vertebral level. The sigmoid colon enters the pelvis and is attached to the sacrum at the S2 level. The renal arteries take off from the aorta at the L1 level. The aorta branches into the common iliac arteries at the L4 vertebral body.

Superficial landmarks help localize portions of the lumbosacral spine. The L4 vertebral body is in the same plane as a line connecting the superior portions of the iliac crests. The junction of the lumbar spine with the sacrum is localized by the sacroiliac "dimples." On the anterior surface, in a patient without a panniculus, the umbilicus is situated anterior to the L5 vertebral body.

BIOMECHANICS OF THE LUMBOSACRAL SPINE

Familiarity with the anatomy of the lumbosacral spine helps identify those structures that are at risk of developing pain but is not adequate to explain all the mechanisms by which back pain develops. The normal function of the lumbosacral spine requires both great flexibility and strength. Recognition of deviations from normal function, such as hyperlordosis, helps explain the source of pain in those individuals who may not have specific anatomic abnormalities.

Better understanding of the biomechanics of back disorders has been garnered from laboratory studies of

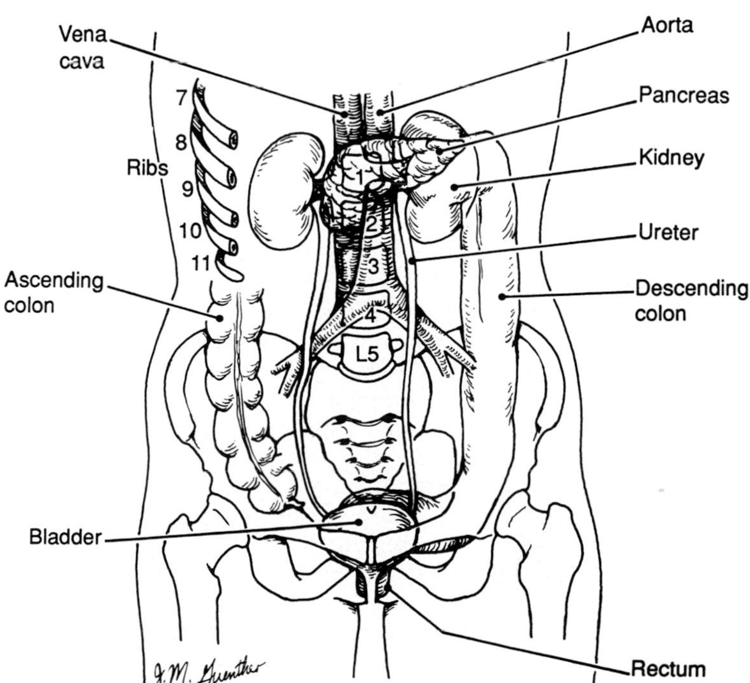

Figure 1-55 Diagrammatic view of the anatomic relationships of visceral organs in the retroperitoneum and the lumbosacral spine.

cadaveric spine segments. The whole vertebral column—cervical, thoracic, and lumbosacral components—supports humans in a balanced, upright position while allowing locomotion. The mobility of the spine is correlated with its organization, whereby multiple components (functional units) are superimposed on one another, interlocked by ligaments and muscles that allow flexion and extension. Flexor and extensor muscles also play a role in maintaining the rigidity of the spine.[56]

The function of the spine is divided between the anterior (static) and posterior (dynamic) portion of each functional unit. Each functional unit is composed of two vertebral bodies, an intervertebral disc anteriorly, and facet joints posteriorly. The anterior portion is a weight-bearing, shock-absorbing, flexible structure. The posterior portion protects the neural elements, acts as a fulcrum, and guides movement for the functional unit.

The intervertebral disc in the anterior portion of the functional unit gives the spine its flexibility. The disc is attached closely to the vertebral endplates. Between these endplates and the annulus fibrosus, the matrix (nucleus pulposus) of the disc is enclosed in a circle of unyielding tissues. Compressive pressure placed on the disc is dissipated circumferentially in a passive manner. In response to the greater axial forces exerted on the lumbar spine in comparison to the cervical and thoracic spines, the nucleus pulposus has its greatest surface area in the lumbar spine. The intervertebral disc is not the only structure that helps dissipate stresses placed on the spine. With flexion, extension, rotation, or shear stress, the load distribution on the functional unit is shared by the intervertebral disc, anterior and posterior longitudinal ligaments, the facet joints and capsules, and other ligamentous structures such as the ligamentum flavum and the interspinous and supraspinous ligaments that attach to the posterior elements of the functional unit. In addition, muscle attachments both intrinsic and extrinsic to the spine interact to accommodate the load-bearing requirements of the spine. The lower lumbar discs may need to bear a load of 1000 kg when stressed with pure compressive forces.[55] This degree of pressure generated by these compressive loads when progressively applied would fracture the vertebral endplates before herniating the nucleus pulposus. These fractures do not occur. The intrinsic muscles that help dissipate these compressive loads are the posterior segment muscles, which actively contract in response to load stresses. In addition, the excessive force is also borne by the abdominal muscles, which contract to increase intra-abdominal pressure.

The degree of pressure on the intervertebral disc varies depending on the position of the lumbar spine. Nachemson and Morris have recorded in vivo intradiscal pressures of volunteers in various positions, while exercising, and when wearing external supports (Fig. 1-56).[46] The load on a lumbar disc may vary from as little as 25 kg in the supine position to more than 250 kg in the seated, forward-flexed position. A more recent in vivo study of intradiscal pressure measurement documented higher intradiscal pressure in the standing position as opposed to the sitting position.[65]

The nucleus pulposus is spherical and acts like a ball between the two vertebral endplates. The nucleus acts like a "joint" from the standpoint of motion, allowing movement in many directions: flexion, extension, lateral flexion, rotation right and left, and gliding in the sagittal and frontal planes. In flexion, the nucleus pulposus migrates posteriorly in the disc. The opposite direction of the nucleus pulposus occurs with spine extension.[27] The nucleus pulposus may be thought of as a flattened tennis ball, constantly placing tension on the surrounding annular fibers. Examination of the disc under tension reveals that it is strongest in its anterior and posterior regions and weakest in its center.

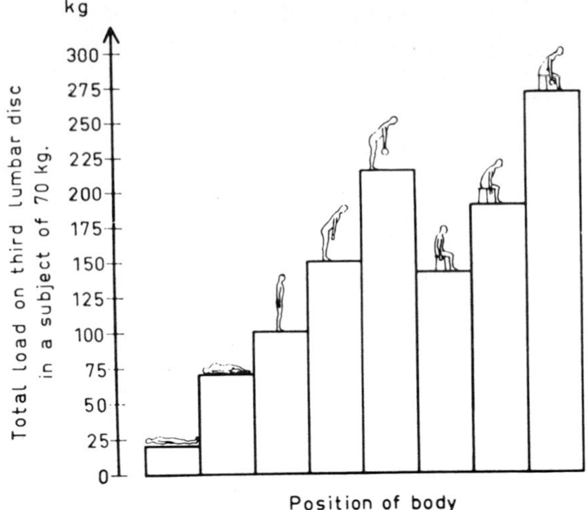

Figure 1-56 Total load on the third lumbar disc in a subject weighing 70 kg in a variety of positions. *(From Nachemson AL: In vivo discometry in lumbar discs with irregular nucleograms. Acta Orthop Scand 36:426, 1965.)*

While the nucleus pulposus affords shock absorbency to the disc, the annulus fibrosus allows for flexibility of the functional unit. With compressive forces, the nucleus pulposus stretches the annular fibers. Flexion or extension of the functional unit occurs in part because of the horizontal shift of fluid within the disc, resulting in the expansion of the annular fibers posteriorly or anteriorly, respectively. The annular fibers tend to oppose the movement of the nucleus pulposus, thereby tending to restore the functional unit to its resting state. As the disc ages, the annular fibers are replaced with fibrous elements with less elastic properties. The capability of the disc to recoil from compressive forces diminishes.

Resistance to stress by the vertebral column is further augmented by the vertebral ligaments. The ligaments run longitudinally along the anterior and posterior portion of the functional unit. The ligaments resist excessive movement in any direction and prevent any significant translational (shearing) action. Although the ligaments prevent excessive movement and support the annulus, they do not limit the normal motion and elasticity of the functional unit. Of pathologic importance is the narrowing of the posterior longitudinal ligament to half its original width at the lumbosacral interspace. The L5–S1 interspace undergoes the greatest static stress on the spine in general and the greatest movement of the lumbar spine yet is also the segment with the least posterior ligamentous support.

The posterior portion of the functional unit is composed of the two vertebral arches, two transverse processes, a spinous process, and paired superior and inferior facet joints. The posterior elements share some of the compressive loads and influence the pattern of spine motion. In cadaveric lumbar spines, Adams and Hutton determined the mechanical function of the facet, or apophyseal, joints to be resistance to intervertebral shear forces and compression.[1] Furthermore, the facet joints serve to prevent excessive motion from damaging the discs. In particular, the posterior annulus is protected in torsion by the lumbar facet surfaces and in flexion by the capsular ligaments of the facet joints.[1]

In the lumbar spine, the facet joint planes of motion are vertical, permitting flexion and extension of the spine. In the neutral lordotic position, lateral or rotational movements are prevented owing to the apposition of the joint surfaces. In a slightly forward flexed position (decreased lordosis), the facet surfaces separate, allowing some lateral and rotatory movement. With extension, the facet surfaces approximate, preventing any lateral or oblique movement. The extended posture decreases the volume of the lumbar spinal canal and neural foramina.[35]

The surface area of the posterior elements plays an important physiologic role as the site of muscular attachments. The pattern of muscular origins and insertions provides balance for the segments of the lumbar spine while allowing wide ranges of motion. The maintenance of erect posture is in part achieved by the support derived from the ligamentous structures of the lumbar spine as well as by the sustained, nonvoluntary tone generated by the surrounding lumbosacral muscles.

To understand the function of the lumbosacral spine, it must be viewed in its relationship to the other components of the vertebral column. In the sagittal plane, the vertebral column shows four curvatures: cervical (concave posterior), thoracic (convex posterior), lumbar (concave posterior), and sacral (fixed and nonmobile). These curves developed during phylogeny (evolution) with the transition from the quadruped to the biped state. Initially, the spine was concave anteriorly. The lumbar spine first became straight, then inverted. The same changes are observed during ontogeny (development of the individual). On the first day of life, the lumbar spine is concave anteriorly. At 5 months of age, the lumbar spine is slightly concave anteriorly, and at 13 months the concavity disappears. From the age of 3 years onward, the lumbar lordosis begins to appear, assuming its definitive adult state at age 10 (Fig. 1-57). The curvature of the vertebral column increases its resistance to axial compressive forces in comparison to the forces that could be sustained if the spine had remained with a completely straight orientation.

The entire spine with its three physiologic curves is balanced on the sacrum. The sacrum is part of the pelvis, which also includes the two iliac bones: the pubis and the ischium. The two sacroiliac joints and symphysis pubis and the attached bones form a closed ring that transmits forces from the vertical column to the lower extremities. The weight supported by L5 is distributed equally into the pelvic wing, ischium, and acetabulum on both sides. Back pressure from the weight of the body against the ground is transmitted to the acetabulum by the head and neck of the femur. Stress placed on both pubic bones is counterbalanced across the symphysis pubis.

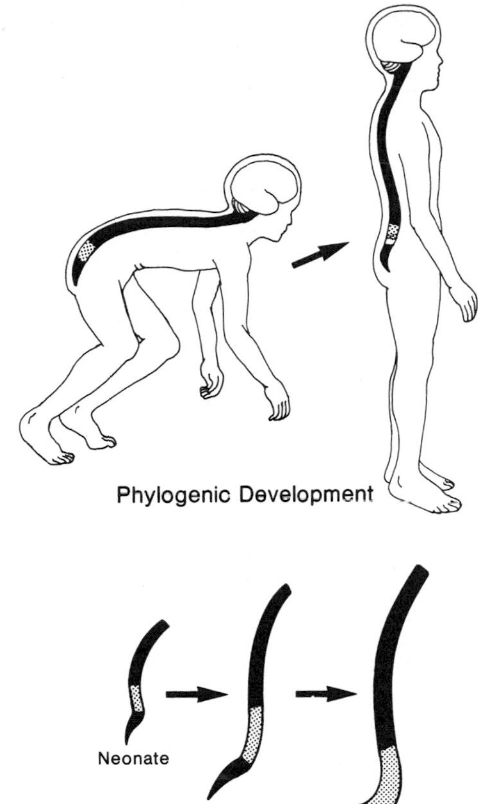

Figure 1-57 Phylogenic development of the lumbar lordosis (walking on all fours to upright position) is re-created in the development of the neonate to an adult (ontogenic development).

The sacrum and iliac bones move as one unit. The pelvis is balanced on a transverse axis between the hip joints, which allow rotatory motion in an anteroposterior plane. The anterior portion of the pelvis can rotate upward, lowering the sacrum with a decrease in the lumbosacral angle. A downward movement of the front portion of the pelvis elevates the rear portion of the pelvis and sacrum and increases the lumbosacral angle. The lumbosacral angle is determined as the line drawn parallel to the superior border of the sacrum measured in relation to a horizontal line (average 30 degrees).

The balance of the spine is related to the reciprocal physiologic curves in the three areas of the vertebral column. The balance in curvature results in an individual's posture. The lumbosacral angle plays a significant role in determining posture and the degree of spinal curvature. With a decrease in the lumbosacral angle, the angle between the lumbar spine and sacrum is decreased (decreased or flattened lordosis). An increase in the lumbosacral angle results in an increased lumbar lordosis (Fig. 1-58). The change in angle results in compensatory alterations in thoracic and cervical curves to maintain the head over the center of gravity. The shape of the lumbar lordosis is also influenced by the shape of the intervertebral discs, the supraspinous ligaments, the facet joints, the posterior erector muscles, and the traction of the hip flexors on the lumbar vertebral bodies.

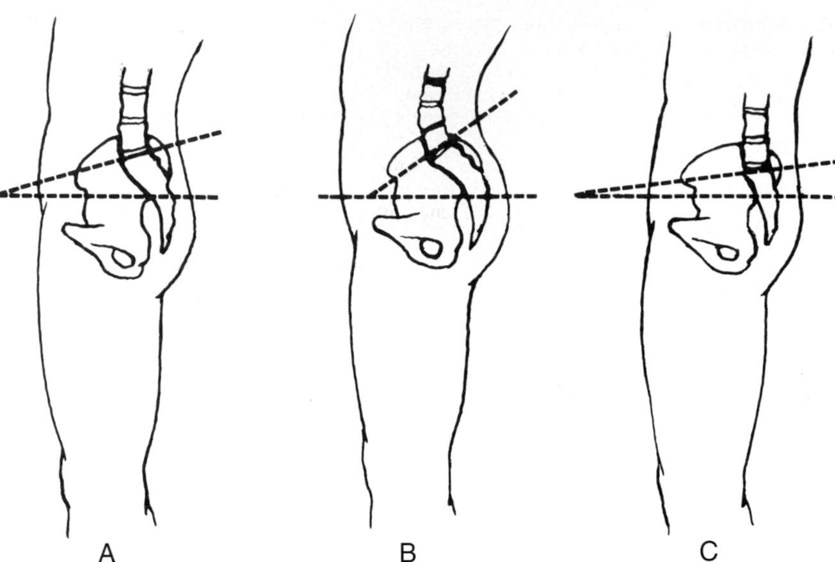

Figure 1-58 Lumbosacral angle: *A*, normal angle—normal lordosis; *B*, increased angle—increased lordosis; *C*, decreased angle—flattened lordosis.

An individual's posture is good if it can be maintained for extended periods in an effortless, nonfatiguing fashion. Maintenance of normal posture is essentially a ligamentous function relieved by intermittent small muscular contractions that are triggered by mechanoreceptors in the joints and ligaments.[14] Deviations from physiologic static spinal curves necessitate increased voluntary muscular action, which may result in fatigue, discomfort, and disability.

The proper alignment of posture requires the function of a number of structures in the lumbar spine, pelvis, and lower leg. Pelvic position is held in ligamentous balance by the anterior hip joint capsule and the iliopectineal ligament, which prevent hyperextension of the hip. The tensor fasciae latae also support the pelvis by limiting lateral shift. The tendency to increase the lumbosacral angle and increase the lumbar lordosis is also counterbalanced by the hamstrings and gluteus maximus, which decrease the lumbar lordosis.

The curvature of the lumbar spine tenses the anterior longitudinal ligament, which limits the degree of lordosis. Increased abdominal pressure generated by contracted abdominal muscles (rectus abdominis) also decreases the lumbar lordosis.

The knee joint is extended and locked during normal posture. The locking of the knee eliminates the need for muscular effort. The ankle cannot be locked in any position. Therefore, continued muscular effort from the gastrocnemius and soleus is needed to stabilize the foot.

In the resting static position, ligamentous, nonmuscular structures maintain posture. Rotation of the pelvis uncouples the balance of the ligaments and joints and necessitates the initiation of muscular effort.

The movements of the lumbar spine are flexion, extension, lateral bending, and rotation. The extent of motion in these planes is limited by the extensibility of the longitudinal ligaments, articular surface and capsule, fluidity of the disc, and pliability of the muscles. Extension of the lumbar spine has a range of 30 degrees and is limited by the anterior longitudinal ligaments. Forward flexion has a lumbar range of 40 degrees, which occurs to the greatest degree (75%) at the intervertebral space between L5 and S1. The remaining range of forward flexion is apportioned between the remainder of the lumbar vertebral interspaces. Lateral flexion is limited to 20 to 30 degrees. The segmental range is maximal between L3 and L4 and is minimal between L5 and S1. The degree of lumbar rotation exclusive of thoracic rotation is difficult to determine. For the lumbar column as a whole, the range of rotation is estimated to be only 10 degrees. Rotation is sharply limited by the orientation of the articular facet surfaces.

The movement of the lumbar spine is done in conjunction with other components of the spine and pelvis. The lumbar-pelvic rhythm is the simultaneous reversal of the lumbar lordosis and change in position of the pelvis. The lumbar component of the rhythm takes the lumbosacral spine from a concave, to flat, to convex configuration. During the progressional change, the pelvic component of the rhythm is rotating the pelvis around the transverse axis connecting the two hip joints, increasing the lumbar angle. In the normal individual, the rhythm is a smooth progression with equal alteration in lumbar reversal and pelvic rotation.

In forward flexion, the lumbar joints flex as the extensor muscles lower the torso. After 45 degrees of flexion, the tension in the ligaments has increased and contraction in the paraspinal muscles has decreased.[26] As flexion continues, the pelvis rotates further by the relaxation of the hamstring and gluteus muscles. As the trunk is returned to the upright position, the order of muscle recruitment is reversed with initial contraction of the hamstrings, then the glutei, which rotate the pelvis to 45 degrees of flexion, at which point the erector spinae muscles become active and return the torso to its fully upright position.

The flexion and extension of the lumbosacral spine are an unimpeded process when the various components of the spine and surrounding muscles are normal. The integrity of the discs must be intact to allow the migration of the nucleus pulposus in the annulus. Symmetrical facet joints permit smooth flexion and extension. The supporting ligaments must not be too long or too short. The paraspinous and hip girdle muscles must have matching elasticity, strength, and flexibility. Normal motion also requires good hip joint function. In addition, lower leg function must be normal. This normal function is ideal in the rested state. Fatigue with repeated lifting tasks may recruit other anatomic structures that are not used in the normal state.[42]

Abnormalities in any of these component parts result in static and/or kinetic dysfunction. Understanding of normal function pinpoints those factors that impede normal motion and identifies those structures that cause low back pain.

References

1. Adams MA, Hutton WC: The mechanical function of the lumbar apophyseal joints. Spine 8:327-330, 1983.
2. An HS: Anatomy of the cervical spine. In An HS, Simpson JM (eds): Surgery of the Cervical Spine. Baltimore, Williams & Wilkins, 1994, pp 1-39.
3. Barker PJ, Briggs CA: Attachments of the posterior layer of lumbar fascia. Spine 24:1757-1764, 1999.
4. Basadonna PT, Gasparini D, Rucco V: Iliolumbar ligament insertions: In vivo anatomic study. Spine 21:2313-2316, 1996.
5. Batson OV: The function of the vertebral veins and their role in the spread of metastasis. Ann Surg 112:138, 1940.
6. Batson OV: The vertebral vein system. AJR Am J Roentgenol 78:1957, 1957.
7. Beaujeux R, Wolfram-Gabel R, Kehrli P, et al: Posterior lumbar epidural fat as a functional structure? Histologic specificities. Spine 22:1264-1268, 1997.
8. Bellamy N, Park W, Rooney PJ: What do we know about the sacroiliac joint? Semin Arthritis Rheum 12:282-313, 1983.
9. Bland JH: Disorders of the Cervical Spine: Diagnosis and Medical Management, 2nd ed. Philadelphia, WB Saunders, 1994.
10. Bland JH, Boushey DR: Anatomy and physiology of the cervical spine. Semin Arthritis Rheum 20:1-20, 1990.
11. Bogduk N: The clinical anatomy of the cervical dorsal rami. Spine 7:319-330, 1982.
12. Bogduk N, Windsor M, Inglis A: The innervation of the cervical intervertebral discs. Spine 13:2-8, 1988.
13. Bradford FK, Spurling RG: The Intervertebral Disc: With Special Reference to Rupture of the Annulus Fibrosus with Herniation of the Nucleus Pulposus, 2nd ed. Springfield, IL, Charles C Thomas, 1945.
14. Cailliet R: Low Back Pain Syndrome, 4th ed. Philadelphia, FA Davis, 1988.
15. Cailliet R: Neck and Arm Pain, 3rd ed. Philadelphia, FA Davis, 1991.
16. Compere EL: Origin, anatomy, physiology, and pathology of the intervertebral disc. Am Acad Orthop Surg Instruction Lecture 18:15, 1961.
17. Coppes MH, Marani E, Thomeer RT, Groen GJ: Innervation of "painful" lumbar discs. Spine 22:2342-2349, 1997.
18. Coventry MB: The intervertebral disc: Its microscopic anatomy and pathology. I. Anatomy, development, and physiology. J Bone Joint Surg Am 27:105, 1945.
19. Demondion X, Delfaut EM, Drizendko A, et al: Radio-anatomic demonstration of the vertebral lumbar venous plexuses: An MRI experimental study. Surg Radiol Anat 22:151-156, 2000.
20. Dvorak J, Panjabi M, Gerber M, Wichmann W: CT–functional diagnostics of the rotatory instability of upper cervical spine. I. An experimental study on cadavers. Spine 12:197-205, 1987.
21. Ebraheim N, Sabry FF, Nadim Y, et al: Internal architecture of the sacrum in the elderly: An anatomic and radiographic study. Spine 25:292-297, 2000.
22. Ebraheim NA, Haman ST, Xu R, Yeasting RA: The anatomic location of the dorsal ramus of the cervical nerve and its relation to the superior articular process of the lateral mass. Spine 23:1968-1971, 1998.
23. Ebraheim NA, Lu J, Hao Y, et al: Anatomic considerations of the lumbar isthmus. Spine 22:941-945, 1997.
24. Edgar MA, Ghadially JA: Innervation of the lumbar spine. Clin Orthop 115:35-41, 1976.
25. Ellis JH, Martel W, Lillie JH, Aisen AM: Magnetic resonance imaging of the normal craniovertebral junction. Spine 16:105-111, 1991.
26. Farfan HF: Muscular mechanism of the lumbar spine and the position of power and efficiency. Orthop Clin North Am 6:135-144, 1975.
27. Fennell AJ, Jones AP, Hukins DW: Migration of the nucleus pulposus within the intervertebral disc during flexion and extension of the spine. Spine 21:2753-2757, 1996.
28. Fountas KN, Kapsalaki EZ, Jackson J, et al: Cervical spinal cord—smaller than considered? Spine 23:1513-1516, 1998.
29. Galante JO: Tensile properties of the human lumbar annulus fibrosus. Acta Orthop Scand Suppl 100:1-91, 1967.
30. Hall LT, Esses SI, Noble PC, et al: Morphology of the lumbar vertebral endplates. Spine 23:1517-1522, 1998.
31. Heary RF, Albert TJ, Ludwig SC, et al: Surgical anatomy of the vertebral arteries. Spine 21:2074-2080, 1996.
32. Heller JG, Pedlow FX Jr: Anatomy of the cervical spine. In Clark CR, Cervical Spine Research Society Editorial Committee (eds): The Cervical Spine, 3rd ed. Philadelphia, Lippincott-Raven, 1998, pp 15-16.
33. Hirsch C, Ingelmark B, Miller M: The anatomical basis for low back pain: Studies on the presence of sensory nerve endings in ligamentous, capsular, and intervertebral disc structures in the human lumbar spine. Acta Orthop Scand 33:1-17, 1963.
34. Hollinshead WH: Anatomy for Surgeons, 3rd ed. New York, Harper & Row, 1982.
35. Inufusa A, An HS, Lim TH, et al: Anatomic changes of the spinal canal and intervertebral foramen associated with flexion-extension movement. Spine 21:2412-2420, 1996.
36. Jackson HC, Winkelmann RK, Bickel WH: Nerve endings in the human lumbar spinal column and related structures. J Bone Joint Surg Am 48:1272-1281, 1966.
37. Jeffreys E: Disorders of the Cervical Spine, 2nd ed. Oxford, Butterworth-Heinemann, 1993.
38. Kameyama T, Hashizume Y, Sobue G: Morphologic features of the normal human cadaveric spinal cord. Spine 21:1285-1290, 1996.
39. Kamibayashi LK, Richmond FJ: Morphometry of human neck muscles. Spine 23:1314-1323, 1998.
40. Louis R: Surgery of the Spine: Surgical Anatomy and Operative Approaches. Berlin, Springer-Verlag, 1983, pp 32-42.
41. Lu J, Ebraheim NA: Anatomic considerations of C2 nerve root ganglion. Spine 23:649-652, 1998.
42. Marras WS, Granata KP: Changes in trunk dynamics and spine loading during repeated trunk exertions. Spine 22:2564-2570, 1997.
43. McLain RF, Pickar JG: Mechanoreceptor endings in human thoracic and lumbar facet joints. Spine 23:168-173, 1998.
44. Mercer S, Bogduk N: Intra-articular inclusions of the cervical synovial joints. Br J Rheumatol 32:705-710, 1993.
45. Morinaga T, Takahashi K, Yamagata M, et al: Sensory innervation to the anterior portion of lumbar intervertebral disc. Spine 21:1848-1851, 1996.
46. Nachemson A, Morris J: In vivo measurements of intradiscal pressure. J Bone Joint Surg Am 46:1077, 1964.
47. Nakano KK: Neck pain. In Kelley WN (ed): Textbook of Rheumatology, 4th ed. Philadelphia, WB Saunders, 1993, p 397.
48. Nolan JP Jr, Sherk HH: Biomechanical evaluation of the extensor musculature of the cervical spine. Spine 13:9-11, 1988.
49. Olszewski AD, Yaszemski MJ, White AA III: The anatomy of the human lumbar ligamentum flavum: New observations and their surgical importance. Spine 21:2307-2312, 1996.
50. Panjabi MM, Duranceau J, Goel V, et al: Cervical human vertebrae: Quantitative three-dimensional anatomy of the middle and lower regions. Spine 16:861-869, 1991.
51. Parke MM, Sherk HH: Normal adult anatomy. In Cervical Spine Research Society Editorial Committee (ed): The Cervical Spine, 2nd ed. Philadelphia, JB Lippincott, 1989, pp 11-32.
52. Pedersen HE, Blunck CFJ, Gardner E: The anatomy of lumbosacral posterior rami and meningeal branches of spinal nerves (sinu-vertebral nerves). J Bone Joint Surg Am 38:377-391, 1956.

53. Penning L: Normal movements of the cervical spine. AJR Am J Roentgenol 130:317-326, 1978.
54. Peretz AM, Hipp JA, Heggeness MH: The internal bony architecture of the sacrum. Spine 23:971-974, 1998.
55. Perey O: Fracture of vertebral endplates in the lumbar spine: An experimental biomechanical investigation. Acta Orthop Scand 25:10, 1957.
56. Quint U, Wilke HJ, Shirazi-Adl A, et al: Importance of the intersegmental trunk muscles for the stability of the lumbar spine: A biomechanical study in vitro. Spine 23:1937-1945, 1998.
57. Schwartz HG: Anastomoses between cervical nerve roots. J Neurosurg 13:190, 1956.
58. Silva MJ, Keaveny TM, Hayes WC: Load sharing between the shell and centrum in the lumbar vertebral body. Spine 22:140-150, 1997.
59. Tanaka N, Fujimoto Y, An HS, et al: The anatomic relation among the nerve roots, intervertebral foramina, and intervertebral discs of the cervical spine. Spine 25:286-291, 2000.
60. Vleeming A, Pool-Goudzwaard AL, Hammudoghlu D, et al: The function of the long dorsal sacroiliac ligament: Its implication for understanding low back pain. Spine 21:556-562, 1996.
61. Werne S: Studies in spontaneous atlas dislocation. Acta Orthop Scand Suppl 23:1, 1957.
62. White AA III, Johnson RM, Panjabi MM, Southwick WO: Biomechanical analysis of clinical stability in the cervical spine. Clin Orthop 109:85-96, 1975.
63. White AA III, Panjabi MM: The basic kinematics of the human spine: A review of past and current knowledge. Spine 3:12-20, 1978.
64. White AA, Panjabi MM: Clinical Biomechanics of the Spine. Philadelphia, JB Lippincott, 1978.
65. Wilke HJ, Neef P, Caimi M, et al: New in vivo measurements of pressures in the intervertebral disc in daily life. Spine 24:755-762, 1999.
66. Yabuki S, Kikuchi S: Positions of dorsal root ganglia in the cervical spine: An anatomic and clinical study. Spine 21:1513-1517, 1996.
67. Yamashita T, Minaki Y, Ozaktay AC, et al: A morphological study of the fibrous capsule of the human lumbar facet joint. Spine 21:538-543, 1996.
68. Yu SW, Sether L, Haughton VM: Facet joint menisci of the cervical spine: Correlative MR imaging and cryomicrotomy study. Radiology 164:79-82, 1987.
69. Yuan Q, Dougherty L, Margulies SS: In vivo human cervical spinal cord deformation and displacement in flexion. Spine 23:1677-1683, 1998.

CHAPTER 2

EPIDEMIOLOGY OF NECK AND LOW BACK PAIN

Epidemiology, the study of the incidence, prevalence, and control of disease in a population, can provide important insights to the physician caring for patients with back problems. Through epidemiology, the linkage between pain and individual or external factors can be determined, which allows risk factors to be identified and minimized. More important, epidemiology provides an understanding of the natural history of the condition, which is relevant to counseling patients about prognosis, and it provides a standard by which the efficacy of various treatments may be verified.

No discussion of epidemiology can begin without reviewing the two most basic concepts: incidence and prevalence. *Incidence* is the rate at which healthy people develop a new symptom or disease over a specified period. It is dependent solely on the rate at which the disease occurs. In contrast, *prevalence* is a measure of the number of people in a population who have a symptom or disease at a particular time. The 1-year prevalence of back pain, for example, is a measure of all those with back pain identified over a 1-year period, regardless of whether the problem began during or before the survey period. Lifetime prevalence is the percentage of those who can remember a symptom at some time during their lives. Therefore, prevalence depends on incidence and duration of disease.

Information on the prevalence and incidence of neck and back pain is available from multiple sources, including insurance and hospital data, interviews or questionnaires, and clinical studies. The quality of the databases is variable, especially if their primary purpose is financial rather than scientific. Individuals with more severe complaints are more likely to register a symptom than those with milder disease. Another problem that alters the measured prevalence is the lack of a uniform definition of the problem. For example, a study that defines low back pain as an episode lasting at least a week will report a much higher prevalence than one defining it as an episode lasting more than 2 weeks. Studies of neck pain frequently include individuals with shoulder symptoms.

Although information on the prevalence and incidence of neck pain is available, it is somewhat limited because often it is grouped with shoulder or back problems. Further, the information that is available is often confusing because of the variety of terms used to describe post-traumatic neck injuries. Terms such as *whiplash*, *acute neck sprain*, *acute cervical strain*, *cervical syndrome*, *hyperextension-hyperflexion neck injury*, *acceleration-deceleration neck injury*, *tension neck syndrome*, and others are frequently used to describe what appear to be similar conditions. These cervical injury syndromes have not been clearly defined, making meaningful analysis of the recorded neck injuries difficult.

PREVALENCE OF NECK PAIN

Neck pain is a far less frequent cause of work absenteeism than is low back pain, but in certain occupations it results in a substantial amount of lost productivity. The 1-year prevalence of neck pain is approximately 20% in most industrialized countries. Scandinavian studies have reported a 1-year prevalence rate of 16% in men and 18% to 20% in women.[117,127] In a study of 2684 male employees, Andersson reported cervical problems occurred one half to one quarter as often as lumbar spine abnormalities.[1]

If the definition of neck pain is an episode lasting 2 weeks, as it was in the National Health and Nutrition Examination Survey II, the prevalence of neck pain in men and women was 8.2% among persons 25 through 74 years of age (Table 2-1).[105] The highest prevalence (10.1%) was among persons 45 through 64 years of age. Rates were higher for white (8.6%) than either black (5.6%) or other racial groups (7.2%).

Bovim and colleagues reported on the results of a questionnaire inquiring about neck pain within the last year sent to 10,000 randomly selected Norwegian adults.[19] A total of 34.4% of the respondents had experienced back pain within that year. A total of 13.8% reported neck pain that continued for more than 6 months. In a study of a large population in Canada, the Saskatchewan Health and Back Pain survey was mailed to 2184 randomly selected adults aged 20 to 69 years measuring the prevalence and severity of neck and low back pain.[31] The lifetime prevalence of neck pain was 66.7% and the point prevalence was 22.2%. The frequency of severe disabling neck pain was 4.6%. The prevalence of low-intensity and low-disability neck pain decreased with age. This degree of neck pain was associated with individuals with headaches, low back pain, general better health, and a compensated motor vehicle accident. High-intensity, low-disability neck pain was associated with car accidents and current smoking. Most severe neck pain was strongly associated with co-morbidities including a history

2-1 PREVALENCE OF JOINT PAIN BY SITE OF JOINT AND SELECTED DEMOGRAPHIC CHARACTERISTICS*

	Back, Neck, or Other Joint Pain	Back Pain[1]	Neck Pain[2]	Other Joint Pain[3]
Total ages: 25–74 yr	21.0	16.0	8.2	19.0
Male	19.6	16.0	7.0	16.6
Female	22.4	16.0	9.4	21.3
Age (yr)				
25–44	15.8	12.3	6.6	12.3
45–64	38.4	20.3	10.1	25.1
65–74	40.1	18.2	9.3	28.1
Race				
White	21.9	16.5	8.6	19.4
Black	15.5	13.2	5.6	16.8
Other	13.7	11.3	7.2	12.5

[1]Have you ever had pain in your back on most days for at least 2 weeks?
[2]Have you ever had pain in your neck on most days for at least 2 weeks?
[3]Have you had pain or aching in any joint other than the back or neck on most days for at least 6 weeks?
*Rate per 100 persons.
From Praemer A, Furner S, Rice DP: Musculoskeletal conditions in the United States. Rosemont, IL, American Academy of Orthopaedic Surgeons, 1992, pp 23–33.
Source: National Center for Health Statistics, NHANES II, 1976–1980.

of neck injury during a car collision. The combination of chronic illnesses adds to the severity of neck pain.[32] More women develop high-disability neck pain than men. A study from Finland reported a similar lifetime prevalence of neck pain of 71%.[90]

PREVALENCE OF CERVICAL DISC HERNIATIONS AND ARM PAIN

The first step in establishing the prevalence of a disease is to define the clinical syndrome. Varied definitions of herniated disc are used in epidemiologic surveys. In general, brachialgia is considered to be pain radiating along the course of one of the cervical nerve roots to the shoulder or arm. A herniated nucleus pulposus is one but not the only cause of brachialgia. Arm symptoms are present in a minority of patients with neck problems.

The incidence of cervical disc herniations is difficult to estimate. A study in Rochester, Minnesota, showed an annual incidence of 5.5 per 100,000.[74] The most frequently affected disc level was C5–C6, followed by C4–C5 and C6–C7. Studies in New Haven and Hartford, Connecticut, surveyed people who had cervical disc herniation (confirmed by radiograph) and radicular pain.[66–68] These studies calculated odds ratios, showing an increased risk of herniation in men, frequent lifters, cigarette smokers, and springboard divers.

OCCUPATIONAL NECK PAIN

Prevalence

The relationship between occupational factors and neck pain is difficult to study because exposure to those factors is usually difficult or impossible to quantify. Workers may be exposed to multiple risk factors in the same job; workers in the same occupation may have substantially different exposure; and workers with neck pain may shift to less strenuous jobs, leaving healthy workers on the heavy tasks, thereby shifting the apparent prevalence of neck pain. In addition, workers' memory of occupational exposure is notoriously poor and is often influenced by financial manipulation of the insurance system.

Occupational neck pain represents less than 2% of all workplace injuries. The majority of work-related neck injuries are diagnosed as a sprain or strain. Certain occupations appear to have a predisposition to neck symptoms. For example, the lifetime prevalence of neck and shoulder symptoms is 81% for machine operators, 73% for carpenters, and 57% for office workers.[119] Manual workers have more symptoms than office workers, and the type of manual labor also seems to affect the risk. A history of twisting and bending during work and the age of the employee are strong risk indicators. Others have suggested that nonphysical factors, such as job satisfaction and general dissatisfaction, play an important role in neck pain syndrome.[72] Hult studied the experience of 1137 working men, aged from 25 through 54 years, who were evenly distributed between light- and heavy-duty jobs.[61] Neck pain occurred in 27% who were younger than 30 years of age and 50% who were older than 45 years of age. Arm pain occurred in only 8% of those younger than 30 years but in more than 38% of those older than 45 years. Heavy-duty laborers were not at a significantly increased risk of developing arm pain secondary to neck symptoms.

Risk Factors

Data from studies investigating the association of biomechanical and psychological factors in neck pain in the workplace reveal the importance of both. Other studies have shown an increased incidence of neck pain in dentists in comparison with office workers and farmers. Meat carriers, miners, and "heavy workers" have significantly higher rates of cervical degenerative changes in comparison with reference groups.[48] Keyboard operators have been shown to have an increase in tension neck syndrome.[47] Monotonous work is of particular risk for women early in their working career.[7] Women with increased levels of "perceived general tension" reported increased neck pain in customer relations employment with minimal biomechanical exposure. The question raised by the authors of this study is whether the general tension associated with neck pain should be considered work related versus an individual characteristic.[122]

Ariens and colleagues reported a 3-year prospective study of work-related neck pain in 1334 Dutch workers.[4] During the follow-up period, of the 997 workers who completed the study, 141 (14.4%) experienced neck pain. Neck pain was associated with psychological factors, such as high quantitative job demands (time pressure, deadlines), and low co-worker support with relative risks of 2.14 and 2.43, respectively. Physical factors of sitting and neck flexion also contributed to the development of neck pain with a similar magnitude of risk. Palmer and co-workers reported similar results from a study of 12,907 British respondents to a questionnaire regarding neck pain and the workplace.[102] In the past year 4438 had neck pain, with 2528 complaining of the symptoms in the last week. Symptoms were the most prevalent among male construction workers (past week, 24%, and past year, 38%), with 11% having pain interfering with activities. Work with arms above the shoulders longer than 1 hour per day was associated with a significant increase of symptoms, but no associations were found with typing, lifting, vibratory tool use, or professional driving. Stronger pain associations were noted with frequent headaches and frequent tiredness and stress.

Viikari-Juntura and associates studied the effect of work-related and individual risk factors affecting the development of radiating neck pain.[123] A total of 5180 Finnish forest industry workers responded to repeated questionnaires administered yearly from 1992 through 1995. The study outcome variable was the number of days with radiating neck pain during the preceding 12 months. The factors associated with increased radiating pain included increased body mass index (BMI), smoking, duration of work with a hand above shoulder level, mental stress, and other musculoskeletal pain.

The increased presence on radiographs of neck symptoms and cervical degenerative changes in various occupational groups is of great interest but limited practical value. Neck symptoms and cervical degenerative changes are quite prevalent in the general population, and it is often difficult to implicate a job-related accident as the root of the problem.

In summary, the risk factors for developing neck pain are multiple and are difficult to apply to an individual subject. The results of studies from one population may not apply to an individual from another population. Do time constraints and low co-worker support play a greater role in developing neck pain than lifting heavy, cumbersome objects overhead for longer than an hour per day? Improvements to the physical components of a job task may not be adequate to resolve all the episodes of neck pain in a workplace. On the other hand, improving co-worker support and diminishing time constraints will not prevent neck pain in individuals with a physically taxing job. Attempts at improving occupational neck pain must address physical and psychological factors.

PREVALENCE OF WHIPLASH INJURIES

Whiplash injuries have been known since the First World War, when airplane pilots were often injured during catapult-assisted takeoffs because of inadequate fixation of the cockpit seat. Following the early recognition and description of this condition, which then involved a limited number of people in a specialized occupational area, the prevalence of this type of injury has continued to increase. It is a frequently described injury almost universally associated with automobile accidents.

Whiplash is the most commonly used term to describe this type of post-traumatic, hyperextension-hyperflexion neck injury. *Whiplash* is a nonmedical term, first used by Crowe in 1928, to describe a hyperextension injury to the neck resulting from an indirect force, usually a rear-end automobile collision.[33] This syndrome was later redefined in 1953 by Gay and Abbott, and the term has been used extensively since then to describe this type of injury.[42] Therefore, the authors use the term, in spite of its lack of scientific specificity, because of its common public use and its frequent use in the medical literature. This term has also been accepted as a neck injury code for hospital discharges and for insurance reimbursement.

The National Safety Council has stated that 20% of all automobile accidents are rear-end impacts. It has been estimated that 85% of all neck injuries seen clinically result from automobile accidents. Of the automobile accidents that result in neck injuries, 85% are rear-end impacts. The remaining 15% of neck injuries result from some other type of impact.[62,63,113] MacNab estimated that one fifth of exposed occupants sustain neck injuries.[85]

The National Accident Sampling System (NASS) estimated that in 1979 there were 530,000 cases of minor whiplash injury.[103] These 530,000 people represented 2.8% of all victims in police-reported automobile accidents. The number of whiplash injuries to people in automobiles that did not require towing from the scene of the accident was significantly higher than the number of injuries to people in automobiles that did require towing. The NASS also found no correlation between the severity of damage to the automobile and the severity of an individual's complaints of neck pain.

When considering such statistics, one must also keep in mind the development of late whiplash syndrome.[5] This syndrome has been defined as a collection of symptoms and disabilities that occur more than 6 months after a neck injury resulting from an automobile accident. The physical and emotional implications of this syndrome are discussed at the end of the section on Neck Injuries and Litigation. Balla found a striking difference in the development of this syndrome when he compared individuals with acute neck injuries in Australia and Singapore.[5,6] When he compared groups of similar patients 2 years after the initial diagnosis, none of the Singapore patients had symptoms of late whiplash syndrome; however, it was a common finding among the Australian patients. The significance and possible causes of this finding are likely to be related to the rate of litigation in the local area. From this and similar studies, one certainly must conclude that the number of people suffering from late whiplash syndrome vary significantly in different cultural environments.

Factors Influencing Neck Injuries

Because the majority of acute neck injuries are the result of rear-end automobile accidents, it is appropriate to review certain factors concerning automobile accidents and automobile passengers that might influence the development of such injuries. These factors include the use of seat belts, shoulder straps, and head restraints; the sitting location of the injured individual; and the age, sex, and size of the occupants.

There is general agreement that acute neck injuries are more frequent among front seat passengers than among rear seat passengers.[73,113] The person most frequently injured is the front seat passenger. The number of injuries to drivers and rear seat passengers is essentially the same.

The influence of seat belts on acute neck injuries depends on other factors, the most important of which is the presence or absence of head restraints (head rests). If head restraints are present, the use of seat belts alone results in fewer injuries. Without head restraints, the use of seat belts alone appears to cause a slight increase in injuries.[113] Using seat belts with a shoulder strap reduces the incidence of injuries, even without head restraints. The combined use of seat belts, shoulder strap, and head restraint significantly reduces the number of injuries.

Various studies have evaluated the effectiveness of head restraints. Data from different sources show a reduction in neck injuries by 10% and more with the use of head restraints. In one study adjustable head restraints reduced injuries by approximately 10%, and head restraints that were an integral part of the seat reduced injuries by 17%.[64] This study noted that 72% of the cars sold during 1960 to 1981 had adjustable restraints, and 25% had head restraints that were an integral part of the seat. As a result of this mix of adjustable and integral head restraints, the study estimated that head restraints prevented more than 64,000 injuries per year. Other studies have estimated a significantly higher rate of protection with head restraints. Although an exact percentage cannot be given, the best estimate is that use of head restraints has reduced the incidence of acute neck injuries in rear-end automobile accidents by about 20%.

Studies have also shown that 75% of head restraints that are adjustable are kept in the lowest possible position, not an appropriate position for most automobile occupants.[64] A visual survey of drivers in 4983 moving domestic automobiles with adjustable head restraints in the Los Angeles and Washington, D.C. metropolitan areas indicated that in the former, 74% of the men drivers and 57% of the women drivers had their head restraints positioned improperly; in the latter, the respective figures were 93% of the men and 80% of the women.[101] Although this is a relatively small sample, it is evident that a significant majority of the head restraints now in use in automobiles in the United States are not in the appropriate position to protect the automobile occupants. Proper positioning would undoubtedly increase their protective value significantly.

The studies that have concentrated on the position of the head restraint have found that the restraint protects women more than men. This probably results from the restraints being in the lowest position and thereby providing more protection for women, whose height is less on average than that of men.

The possible use of head restraints in the rear seats of automobiles has also been considered. Many studies have shown, however, that their use in rear seats is not justified because they would not significantly reduce the number of acute neck injuries.

A relatively new safety feature in many cars is the driver- and/or passenger-side air bag. The air bag used together with a seat belt, shoulder strap, and head restraint will more than likely further reduce the incidence of cervical spine injuries from rear-impact accidents and may also play an important role in head-on collisions.

There are conflicting data concerning the incidence of neck injuries in men and women. A majority of studies show a higher incidence of whiplash injuries in women; some studies show the frequency of neck injury among women to be twice as high as among men.[73] Kahane found that significant injuries of the cervical spine were more common in men (in the ratio of 3:2) but that whiplash injuries occurred more often in women (70%).[64] This observation, which is apparently contradictory, has been confirmed by a number of other authors.[27,46,85] The reason for this may be that women travel more often as passengers and the injury occurs while they are in a state of muscular relaxation. The driver, more often a man, may anticipate the impact and be able to neutralize whiplash partially by keeping his head flexed and by gripping the steering wheel.

Age does not seem to be an important factor in acute neck injuries. The assumption that with increasing age and the development of osteoarthritic changes in the cervical spine there would be an increased incidence of acute neck injuries in older people has not been documented. The usual age distribution for whiplash injuries is between the ages of 30 and 50 years. Another explanation may lie in the decreased frequency of automobile accidents among older people, who spend less time driving.

Lightweight people appear to be more susceptible to acute neck injury than heavier people. There is also a positive correlation between increased height and neck injuries.[113]

Neck Injuries and Litigation

Effective litigation in acute neck injuries has received much attention.[27,45,58,63] Many articles have been written, with such titles as "The Whiplash: Tiny Impact, Tremendous Injury"[46] and "Whiplash Injury of the Neck—Fact or Fancy."[20] Television programs have shown characters in a minor automobile accident hiring a lawyer to sue for whiplash injury. Anecdotal incidents are prevalent, such as the city bus filled with passengers that is rear-ended by a small car with no damage to the car or bus and the only injury sustained being that of the bus driver, who suffers an acute whiplash injury. This has led to speculation that litigation and compensation are the most important factors in the incidence and severity of whiplash.

A unique factor is present in the type of accident that commonly leads to whiplash. The striking vehicle is almost invariably at fault and, therefore, this removes the burden of proof of liability for the accident. In addition, because the person with the injured neck rarely presents an objective, demonstrable abnormality, one is left with a blameless victim incapacitated by subjective symptoms, the existence of which are difficult to prove or disprove. This combination of accident events and subjective symptoms makes the accident victim a candidate for legal intervention and disability remuneration.

How frequently do people with whiplash injuries seek remuneration? This is difficult to determine because of the lack of follow-up in reporting of minor injuries and the current trend to settle out of court. However, in a few controlled studies, more than 50% of the accident victims eventually received some type of settlement.[101]

A number of studies have been undertaken to determine if the awarding of a monetary settlement has resulted in significant improvement of the symptoms of injured people. Among people with only subjective complaints, more than 50% improved significantly after litigation claims were settled. In patients with objective findings, such as reduced range of neck movement or evidence of neurologic loss, the percentage that improved is lower than 25% after settlement.[101]

Emotional factors that might contribute to a person's symptoms and disability cannot be overlooked. These might be classified as conscious malingering, conscious exaggeration of underlying complaints, or subconscious exaggeration or modification of an underlying acute neck injury. In studies of low back injuries, the conscious malingerer is relatively infrequent. The more frequent circumstance appears to be the conscious exaggeration of an underlying complaint.

Although it is sometimes difficult to separate the conscious from the subconscious exaggeration, under many circumstances this differentiation can be made fairly accurately by a careful examiner performing a detailed history and physical examination. The typical conscious manipulator is the person who arrives at the physician's office with extensive documentation of the accident or injury, demonstrates a persistently defensive attitude, is often overly hostile, withholds information, involves an attorney to the extent that simple questions are not answered without consulting the attorney, and shows variable and inconsistent hysterical symptoms.

The person with a subconscious emotional overlay often demonstrates a significantly different pattern. This person often shows a lack of concern for documentation and also starts with a defensive attitude. This attitude may alternate with transient episodes of anger, and the patient does not knowingly withhold information. If hysterical symptoms are present, they are usually constant. This person usually has an attorney but has a much more passive involvement.

Although these are general descriptions that do not apply in all cases, this type of differentiation has served the authors well in managing the course of treatment and particularly in the early use of independent medical examiners for employees suffering from acute neck injuries.

LONG-TERM OUTCOME OF NECK PAIN

Neck pain in the majority of patients resolves with time. Gore and colleagues reported on the evaluation of patients with neck pain 10 years after the initial episode.[44] Seventy-nine percent had decreased pain, 43% were free of pain, and 32% had moderate or severe pain. Patients who had an injury and severe pain in the initial episode were the individuals at greatest risk of developing persistent pain. Suissa and colleagues identified factors associated with delayed resolution of whiplash-associated neck pain from motor vehicle accidents in a study of 2627 individuals from Quebec, Canada.[114] Older women with neck pain with palpation, muscle pain, numbness radiating to the arms, or headaches had a median recovery time of 262 days versus 17 days for younger males (age 20) without these associated symptoms. A radiograph of the cervical spine did not predict the degree of pain an individual experienced. A prediction of final outcome based on initial symptoms or radiographic findings was not possible.

PREVALENCE OF LOW BACK PAIN

Back pain is the second leading cause of work absenteeism (after upper respiratory tract complaints) and results in more lost productivity than any other medical condition.[36,107,108] Spine or back impairments result in an annual average of 175.8 million restricted-activity days.[105] The lifetime prevalence of back pain exceeds 70% in most industrialized countries.[35] National statistics from the United States indicate a 1-year prevalence rate of 15% to 20% (Fig. 2-1).[34,37]

Using the definition of low back pain of the National Health and Nutrition Examination Survey II (NHANES II)—an episode lasting 2 weeks—the prevalence of back pain among both men and women is 16% for persons 25 to 74 years of age (see Table 2-1).[105] The highest prevalence was in the 45 to 64 age group. Rates were also higher for whites (16.5%) than for either blacks (13.2%) or other racial groups (11.3%). The primary site of pain was lower back (85.1%) with middle back pain reported in 7.9% and upper back pain in 7.0%.

Data from the National Center for Health Statistics show that 14.3% of new patient visits to physicians are for low back pain, and each year there are nearly 13 million physician visits for chronic low back pain.[2] The mean days of restricted activity due to back problems was 23.5. Eight days were completely lost from work. Chronic disability resulting from low back pain was reported to affect 2.4 million Americans permanently, with an additional 2.4 million temporarily disabled.

Data from NHANES II has been analyzed for the use of health professionals by subjects with back pain (Table 2-2). Overall, 84% of those with low back pain (> 2 weeks) had seen a health care professional, 30.9% had been admitted to a hospital, and 11.6% had undergone surgery.[37] It is worth noting that 75% to 85% of subjects reported success with the standard nonoperative treatments (excluding traction and cold application).

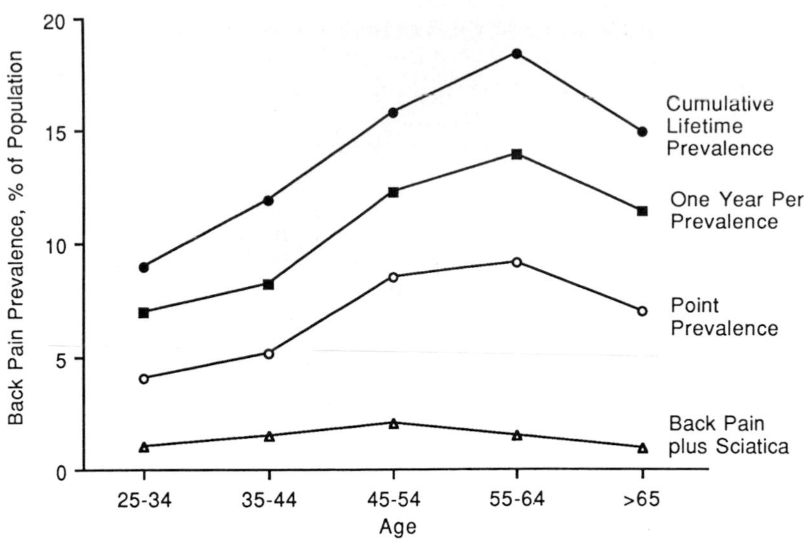

Figure 2-1 Prevalence of low back pain. Only episodes lasting for at least 2 weeks are included. Sciatica is defined as pain radiating to the legs, increasing with cough, sneeze, or deep breathing. *(From Deyo RA, Tsui-Wu YJ: Descriptive epidemiology of low back pain and its related medical care in the United States. Spine 12:264-268, 1987.)*

A prospective Swedish study analyzed all patients of Gothenburg with low back pain. Of 49,000 residents aged 20 to 65 years, a total of 7526 absence episodes were reported due to low back pain in an 18-month period.[29] This study also provided important natural history data for this condition: 57% of patients recovered in 1 week, 90% in 6 weeks, and 95% after 12 weeks. At the end of 1 year, 1.2% remained disabled and out from work. Recurrent pain and disability were common and occurred in 12% over the 18-month observation period. Data from a Danish population aged 30 to 50 years of age and a review of data from four surveys from Nordic populations revealed a lifetime prevalence of 66%, with 50% having an episode of back pain within the preceding year. Increased levels were not associated with a specific gender or greater age.[80]

Young Adult Population

The assumption of many individuals is that back pain is a problem for middle age or geriatric populations. Back pain is not a problem for younger individuals. A number of studies have reported data countermanding that assumption. In a Danish population of 34,076 twins born between 1953 and 1982, at least one episode of back pain occurred in more than 50% of girls by age 18 and by age 20 in boys. By age 25, the 65% of individuals who will have back pain at age 41 have had their episode.[81] In a study of Danish children ages 8 to 10 and adolescents from 14 to 16 years, the 1-month prevalence of back pain was 39%. Thoracic pain is most common in childhood, whereas thoracic and lumbar pain are equally common in adolescents. Neck pain was rare.[126] Feldman and co-workers studied the risk factors for the development of low back pain in 502 high school students in Montreal, Canada.[38] The frequency of back pain was 17% over an 18-month period. Those factors associated with the development of low back pain included rapid growth, smoking, tight leg muscles, and working during the school year.

Linton and associates studied the frequency of low back and neck pain in 3000 Swedish persons aged 35 to 45 years old over a 12-month period.[84] Questionnaires including items concerning location of pain, severity of pain, days lost from work, and visits to health care providers were returned by 2305 people (78.5%) from three rural communities. The prevalence of spinal pain was 66.3% in the respondents. The lower low back was the most common site (56%), followed by the neck (44%), and thoracic spine (15%). Approximately 25% of the study group reported substantial difficulties measured by more severe pain, sick days, and visits to health professionals. Men took more sick leave, whereas women visited health care providers.

Geriatric Population

Bressler and coauthors reviewed the medical literature to determine the prevalence of low back pain in individuals 65 years of age or older.[23] The frequency of back pain is estimated to be 13% to 49%, determined by a review of 12 available articles. The wide variability in reported frequencies related to the definitions of back pain and study design. The assumption is that all individuals who are older than 65 years have or develop low back pain. That is not the circumstance. Some individuals remain clear of back pain despite great longevity. Identifying those factors that predispose to a low back pain–free existence in later years would allow individuals to maximize their spine health while they are young.

2-2 USE OF HEALTH PROFESSIONALS BY NHANES II SUBJECTS WITH LOW BACK PAIN*

Type Of Health Professional	Percentage
General practitioner	58.6
Orthopedist	36.9
Chiropractor	30.8
Osteopath	13.8
Internist	7.6
Rheumatologist	2.5
Any	84.6

*$N = 1516$.
NHANES II, National Health and Nutrition Examination Survey II.
From Deyo RA, Tsui-Wu YJ: Descriptive epidemiology of low-back pain and its related medical care in the United States. Spine 12:264-268, 1987.

Economic Factors

Most epidemiologic studies for low back pain report frequencies in Western industrial countries. The frequency of spinal pain may not be similar in countries with middle or low income populations. Middle and low income countries are defined as those with gross national product per capita of $650 to $7829 and $350 to $650, respectively. Volinn completed a report of the frequency of back pain in middle and low income countries (Table 2-3) and found that the prevalence of back pain ranged from 7% to 28%.[124] The range of prevalence was explained by the lower prevalence in rural populations and higher prevalence in low income urban populations. The point prevalence of back pain was higher (12% to 68%) in specific classes of workers in urban settings in poor countries. This article would suggest that hard physical labor in low income populations is not associated with low back pain and is not a risk factor for this symptom. This study is a good attempt at describing the frequency of back pain in countries around the world but has methodologic flaws . The determination of the frequency of back pain in underdeveloped countries may depend on the definition of the disorder and the specific portions of the population (urban vs. rural) studied. This study does suggest that the societal organization of the industrialized countries may add to the problem rather than improve it.

The impact of back pain on society is staggering. Back pain is the most frequent cause of activity limitation in people younger than 45 years of age, the second most frequent reason for physician visits, the fifth most frequent for hospitalization, and the third ranking reason for surgical procedures.[95-99] About 1% of the United States population is chronically disabled because of back pain, and an additional 1% is temporarily disabled, representing a total of 400,000 compensable back injuries each year.

PREVALENCE OF SCIATICA AND DISC HERNIATIONS

The definitions of sciatica used in epidemiologic surveys vary. In general, *sciatica* is considered to be pain radiating along the course of the sciatic nerve to one or both legs to below the knee. A herniated nucleus pulposus is one cause, but not the only explanation, for sciatica. Sciatica is present in about 25% of those with back problems. The average work absence of patients with sciatica exceeds that of patients with back pain alone.

In the United Kingdom, the estimated prevalence of herniated disc is from 1% to 3%—3.1% of men and 1.3% of women.[78] In men 55 to 64 years of age, the prevalence was 9.6%; in women the maximum prevalence of 5% occurred after the age of 64. Similarly, in Sweden the lifetime prevalence of sciatica was found to be 3.6% in those younger than 25 and 22.4% among those aged 45 to 54.[56]

Sciatica usually resolves with nonoperative treatment, but a minority of patients may need hospitalization and surgery. Operation rates for herniated lumbar discs vary. It is estimated that the rate per 100,000 is 100 in Great Britain,[13,131] 350 in Finland,[54] 200 in Sweden,[92] and more than 450 in the United States.[39,71] More than 95% of operations are at the L4 and L5 levels.[112] The mean age at surgery is 40 to 45 years, with men being operated on twice as often as women.

2-3 PREVALENCE OF LOW BACK PAIN IN HIGH, MIDDLE, AND LOW INCOME POPULATIONS

Country	Income*	Prevalence (%)
Sweden	25,110	35
Germany	23,660	31
United States	22,240	20
Britain	16,550	14
Philippines	730	7
China	370	12
Nigeria	340	16
Nepal	180	18

*Gross national product per capita.
From Volinn E: The epidemiology of low back pain in the rest of the world: A review of surveys in low- and middle-income countries. Spine 22:1747-1754, 1997.

GENERAL RISK FACTORS

Back pain is a multifactorial disorder with many possible etiologies; consequently, determining risk factors for low back pain is difficult. In addition, many of the proposed risk factors have a high prevalence in the general (asymptomatic) population and require large database studies to make statistically valid statements about risk factors. Thus, the literature is filled with a myriad of studies with conflicting conclusions. The following discussion is intended to summarize the consensus of studies concerning risk factors.

The maximal frequency of low back pain symptoms appears to be in the age range of 35 to 55 years, whereas absences and duration of symptoms increase with increasing age.[3] Although gender seems to be of little importance with respect to low back symptoms,[9,60,115,116,121] surgery for disc herniations is performed about 1.5 to 3 times more often in men.[22,24,53,70,79,112,125] Postural deformities such as scoliosis, kyphosis, and leg-length discrepancy do not predispose to low back pain in general.[10,15-17,49,57,61,75,89,104,107,111] Studies of scoliosis have shown that there is no increased association with back pain unless the curve is severe (>80 degrees).[11,12,21,30,75,76,93,100] Anthropometric data are contradictory with no strong relationship between height, weight, body build, and low back pain.[8,67,106,129] Physical fitness is not a predictor of acute low back pain, but the physically fit have a lesser risk of chronic low back pain and a more rapid recovery after a pain episode.[25,26,94] In a prospective cohort study of 640 school children, Harreby and associates found that physical activity for at least 3 hours per week reduced the risk of low back pain measured as lifetime, 1-year, and point prevalence.[50] Several investigators have found an association between smoking, herniated discs, and low back pain.[40,41,65,66]

Obesity

Obesity has been implicated as a cause of low back pain, but epidemiologic studies have reported both positive and negative associations.[36,38,52] Leboeuf-Yde and coauthors correlated the association and dose-response connection between BMI and low back pain experienced over a 1-year period by 29,424 Danish identical twin subjects.[82] (Duration of back pain was divided into 7 days or less, 8 to 30 days, or more than 30 days. BMI was divided into < 20 [underweight], 20 to 24 [normal weight], 25 to 29 [overweight], and > 29 [severely overweight].) A modest positive association between BMI and low back pain occurred with increasing duration of pain. Underweight subjects consistently reported lower prevalence of low back pain. However, although the severely overweight group would have been expected to have the greatest frequency of back pain, the overweight group had the greatest frequency of pain. Individuals with more than 30 days of back pain were most likely to be women older than 20 years who worked sitting, standing, and walking, or men in jobs involving primarily sitting. When monozygotic twins who had different BMIs were compared, the odds ratio was 1, suggesting that genetic factors play a greater role than environmental factors in the perpetuation of low back pain. Obesity may be a minor factor in the causation of back pain but is associated with chronicity. Obesity may be associated with sedentary lifestyle, low occupational status, and psychological distress, as well as physical strain in spinal structures that facilitate the chronicity of back pain.

Smoking

Smoking is associated with a wide range of serious illnesses. A number of studies have attempted to correlate the degree of cigarette smoking with the severity of back pain.[41,65,66] For example, smoking was associated with exacerbations of back pain in adolescents who developed scoliosis. Smoking may have a greater impact on those individuals with co-morbid spine conditions.[109] However, the effect may be related to nonspecific back pain. Inadequate information is available to document the association with herniated intervertebral discs and sciatica. The mechanism of smoke-associated spinal damage remains to be elucidated.[43] Leboeuf-Yde and co-workers also studied the role of smoking in the development of back pain in 29,424 Danish identical twins. There is a definite link between smoking and low back pain that increases with the duration and frequency of the low back pain problem.

OCCUPATIONAL RISK FACTORS

The relationship between occupational factors and low back pain is difficult to study because exposure is usually difficult or impossible to quantify. The problem is further complicated by several factors: (1) workers may be exposed to multiple risk factors in the same job; (2) workers in the same industry or occupation may have substantially different exposure, and (3) workers with back pain may shift to less strenuous jobs leaving a preponderance of healthy workers on the heavy tasks and shifting the apparent prevalence of back pain. In addition, the recall of occupational exposures is notoriously poor and often influenced by financial manipulation of the insurance system.[65]

Physical factors found to be associated with increased risk of low back pain include heavy work, lifting, static work postures (prolonged sitting or standing), bending and twisting, and vibration.[3,28,41,69,86,87,110,120] Flexion and rotation of the trunk and lifting at work were found to be moderate risk factors in a study of 861 workers in 34 companies in the Netherlands.[59] A study of more than 6000 volunteers first interviewed at age 18 and followed up at age 40 was revealing; the prevalence of low back pain increased from 38% to 74% during the 20-year period.[55] This prospective study found that early back pain causing absence from work, reduced activity levels because of the pain, and heavy workloads showed a significantly increased risk for frequent pain problems at follow-up examination. Thorbjornsson and colleagues completed a 24-year retrospective study of physical and psychosocial factors associated with the development of low back pain.[118] A total of 46% of subjects became patients. Among women, heavy physical workload, sedentary work, smoking, whole-body vibrations, and low influence over work conditions was associated with back pain. Men were more at risk if they had a heavy physical workload, sedentary work, heavy workload outside of employment, poor social relations, and overtime. These data suggest that physical tasks do play a role in the development of low back pain.

Psychological and psychosocial work factors including monotony at work, job dissatisfaction, and poor relations with co-workers have been found to increase complaints about low back pain.[14,88,115,128] Prospective studies have concluded that these psychological risk factors were more predictive than any of the physical risk factors.[11,18] Linton reviewed the literature involving psychological risk factors and the development of low back pain.[83] These factors are usually associated with the development of chronic low back pain. Linton suggested that evidence exists associating psychological factors with acute pain and the transition from acute to chronic pain. The point in time in the course of back pain may be important in determining the significance of a specific physical or psychological risk factor.

Krause and co-workers reported on the importance of physical and psychological factors in the persistence of low back pain.[77] This prospective study determined the effect of physical workload and psychological factors in the development of back pain in urban transit workers from San Francisco. A total of 1871 workers had medical evaluations for a commercial driver's license between 1983 and 1985. A total of 1449 completed a voluntary job survey, whereas 405 did not. Psychological and job factors investigated included type of shift, overtime work, break time, frequency of job problems, psychological demand, job strain, job dissatisfaction, co-workers' support, and supervisory support. The worker categories included drivers of diesel buses, electric trolley buses, light rail trains, and cable cars. During the study period, 320 drivers reported an initial episode of back pain. A back pain episode was predicted by psychological job demands, job dissatisfaction, and frequency of job problems. Less significant were low supervisory support and female gender. Compared with full-time work, part-time work was associated with a 2.7-fold reduced risk for back pain. Cable car crews performing the heaviest physical labor had a threefold increased risk for injury compared to bus drivers.

The study demonstrates the independent importance of physical and psychological factors in the identification of individuals at risk for back pain.

Occupational low back pain may be decreasing in frequency. Murphy and Volinn reported data from Liberty Mutual Insurance Company (1987–1995), a workers' compensation carrier, the Washington State Department of Labor and Industry (1991–1995), and the Bureau of Labor Statistics (1992–1995) regarding industrial-related low back pain.[91] The U.S. estimate of annual low back pain claims decreased by 34% between 1987 and 1995. Annual costs decreased during this period by 58% (Fig. 2-2). However, the frequency of claims remained at 1.8 per 100 workers, with an estimated cost of \$8.8 billion in 1995.

The distribution of the costs of occupational back pain is skewed to a small number of workers with chronic back conditions. Williams and colleagues reported data derived from the National Council on Compensation Insurance on health care use and indemnity costs within the natural history of low back pain.[130] Health care costs were disproportionately distributed along the disability curve with 20% of claimants with low back pain for 4 months or more accounting for 60% of health care costs. The most costly services were diagnostic procedures (25%), surgery (21%), and physical therapy (20%). Physician evaluation was 15% of the total, whereas medication costs were 2%.

The frequency of physician visits for low back pain was reviewed by Hart and co-workers.[51] Data from the National Ambulatory Medical Care Survey were grouped into three periods (1980–1981, 1985, and 1989–1990) and reviewed for frequency of visits for low back pain from 3000 office-based physicians, including internists, osteopaths, neurologists, orthopedic surgeons, family physicians, and neurologic surgeons. Low back pain accounted for 2.8% of office visits for mechanical low back pain (herniated disk, spinal stenosis, spondylosis, spondylolisthesis, lumbar strain), ranked fifth behind hypertension, pregnancy, general medical examinations, and upper respiratory infection for 1990 physician visits. Back pain accounted for the largest portion of patients for neurosurgeons (35%). Orthopedic surgeons (11%), neurologists (10%), osteopaths (5%), family physicians (3%), and internists (2%) had back pain patients as a smaller component of their clinical practices.

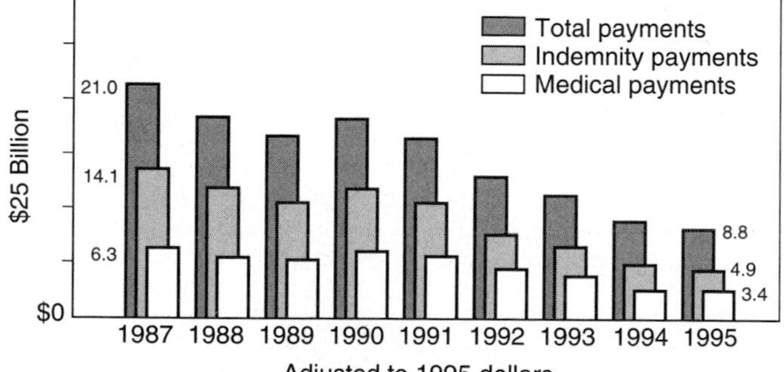

Figure 2-2 U.S. estimated payments for claims related to low back pain, 1987–1995. *(From Murphy PL, Volinn E: Is occupational low back pain on the rise? Spine 24:691-697, 1999.)*

Cervical and Lumbar Spine Impairment Ratings

The determination of impairments of the cervical and lumbar spine is a complicated procedure with specific requirements in regard to measurements of motion. This determination is beyond the scope of this book. The reader is referred to the most current edition of *Guides to the Evaluation of Permanent Impairment* (American Medical Association) for the standard accepted method for determining physical impairments.

SUMMARY

The epidemiology of neck pain, low back pain, brachialgia, and sciatica is both critical and confusing. All epidemiologic information on this topic must be carefully analyzed relative to the source from which it is taken as well as to the potential motivation for gain on the part of the patients or physicians who provide the information. Knowledge of the incidence, prevalence, and natural history of degenerative neck problems is much more extensive than knowledge of the frequency of true acute neck injuries. In addition, acute neck injuries have resulted in a great deal of discussion but little verifiable medical information. Although it is apparent that the most common initiating factor is a rear-end automobile impact, it also appears clear that the number of resulting injuries could be significantly reduced by the proper use of the safety equipment in the automobiles. Patients with neck strain or whiplash injury should be treated according to the same protocols that are presented in the following chapters. The physician should recognize that those with a whiplash injury may have a protracted recovery of 12 to 18 months compared with those with more acute exacerbations of degenerative problems, which tend to be more often an acute strain unrelated to litigation and generally resolve within several weeks. Understanding and knowledge of the physical and psychosocial risk factors that have been confirmed can help prevent and minimize the severity of recurrences.

Most episodes of low back pain or sciatica resolve spontaneously within the first 2 weeks, and a relative minority take 6 to 12 weeks. Only 1% to 2% of cases should require evaluation for operative management. Knowledge of the physical and psychosocial risk factors can help prevent and minimize the severity of recurrences.

References

1. Anderson JAD: Rheumatism in industry: A review. Br J Ind Med 28:103, 1971.
2. Andersson GB: The epidemiology of spinal disorders. In Frymoyer JW (ed): The Adult Spine: Principles and Practice. New York, Raven, 1991, pp 107-146.
3. Andersson GB: Epidemiologic aspects on low back pain in industry. Spine 6:53-60, 1981.
4. Ariens GA, Bongers PM, Hoogendoorn WE, et al: High quantitative job demands and low coworker support as risk factors for neck pain: Results of a prospective cohort study. Spine 26:1896-1901, 2001.
5. Balla JI: The late whiplash syndrome. Aust N Z J Surg 50:610-614, 1980.
6. Balla JI: The late whiplash syndrome: A study of an illness in Australia and Singapore. Cult Med Psychiatry 6:191-210, 1982.

7. Barnekow-Bergkvist M, Hedberg GE, Janlert U, et al: Determinants of self-reported neck-shoulder and low back symptoms in a general population. Spine 23:235-243, 1998.
8. Battié MC: The reliability of physical factors as predictors of the occurrence of back pain reports: A prospective study within industry [thesis]. Goteborg, Sweden, University of Goteborg, 1989.
9. Battié MC, Bigos SJ, Fisher LD, et al: Isometric lifting strength as a predictor of industrial back pain reports. Spine 14:851-856, 1989.
10. Battié MC, Bigos SJ, Fisher LD, et al: A prospective study of the role of cardiovascular risk factors and fitness in industrial back pain complaints. Spine 14:141-147, 1989.
11. Battié MC, Bigos SJ, Fisher LD, et al: Anthropometric and clinical measures as predictors of back pain complaints in industry: A prospective study. J Spinal Disord 3:195-204, 1990.
12. Battié MC, Bigos SJ, Fisher LD, et al. The role of spinal flexibility in back pain complaints within industry: A prospective study. Spine 15:768-773, 1990.
13. Benn RT, Wood PH: Pain in the back: An attempt to estimate the size of the problem. Rheumatol Rehabil 14:121-128, 1975.
14. Bergenudd H, Nilsson B: Back pain in middle age—occupational workload and psychologic factors: An epidemiologic survey. Spine 13:58-60, 1988.
15. Biering-Sorensen F: A prospective study of low back pain in a general population. I. Occurrence, recurrence, and aetiology. Scand J Rehabil Med 15:71-79, 1983.
16. Biering-Sorensen F: A prospective study of low back pain in a general population. III. Medical service—work consequence. Scand J Rehabil Med 15:89-96, 1983.
17. Biering-Sorensen F: The Prognostic Value of the Low Back History and Physical Measurements. Copenhagen, Denmark, University of Copenhagen, 1983.
18. Bigos SJ, Spengler DM, Martin NA, et al: Back injuries in industry: A retrospective study. III. Employee-related factors. Spine 11:252-256, 1986.
19. Bovim G, Schrader H, Sand T: Neck pain in the general population. Spine 19:1307-1309, 1994.
20. Braaf MM, Rosner S: Whiplash injury of neck—Fact or fancy. Int Surg 46:176-182, 1966.
21. Bradford DS, Moe JH, Winter RB: Scoliosis and kyphosis: Operative management of idiopathic scoliosis. In Rothman RH, Simeone FA (eds): The Spine, 2nd ed. Philadelphia, WB Saunders, 1982, pp 316-349.
22. Braun W: Ursachen des lumbalen Bandscheiberverfalls: Die Wirbelsaule in Forschung und Praxis 43, 1969.
23. Bressler HB, Keyes WJ, Rochon PA, Badley E: The prevalence of low back pain in the elderly: A systematic review of the literature. Spine 24:1813-1819, 1999.
24. Brown JR: Factors contributing to the development of low back pain in industrial workers. Am Ind Hyg Assoc J 36:26-31, 1975.
25. Cady LD, Bischoff DP, O'Connell ER, et al: Strength and fitness and subsequent back injuries in firefighters. J Occup Med 21:269-272, 1979.
26. Cady LD Jr, Thomas PC, Karwasky RJ: Program for increasing health and physical fitness of firefighters. J Occup Med 27:110-114, 1985.
27. Cammark KV: Whiplash injuries to the neck. Am J Surg 93:663, 1957.
28. Chaffin DB, Park KS: A longitudinal study of low back pain as associated with occupational weight-lifting factors. Am Ind Hyg Assoc J 34:513-525, 1973.
29. Choler U, Larsson R, Nachemson A, Peterson LE: Back Pain [in Swedish]. SPRI Report No. 188. Stockholm, Sweden, SPRI, 1985.
30. Collis DK, Ponseti IV: Long-term follow-up of patients with idiopathic scoliosis not treated surgically. J Bone Joint Surg Am 51:425-445, 1969.
31. Cote P, Cassidy JD, Carroll L: The Saskatchewan Health and Back Pain Survey: The prevalence of neck pain and related disability in Saskatchewan adults. Spine 23:1689-1698, 1998.
32. Cote P, Cassidy JD, Carroll L: The factors associated with neck pain and its related disability in the Saskatchewan population. Spine 25:1109-1117, 2000.
33. Crowe HE: Injuries to the cervical spine. Paper presented at the Meeting of the Western Orthopaedic Association, San Francisco, 1928.
34. Cunningham LS, Kelsey JL: Epidemiology of musculoskeletal impairments and associated disability. Am J Public Health 74:574-579, 1984.
35. Damkot DK, Pope MH, Lord J, Frymoyer JW: The relationship between work history, work environment, and low back pain in men. Spine 9:395-399, 1984.
36. Deyo RA, Bass JE: Lifestyle and low back pain: The influence of smoking and obesity. Spine 14:501-506, 1989.
37. Deyo RA, Tsui-Wu YJ: Descriptive epidemiology of low back pain and its related medical care in the United States. Spine 12:264-268, 1987.
38. Feldman DE, Shrier I, Rossignol M, et al: Risk factors for the development of low back pain in adolescence. Am J Epidemiol 154:30-36, 2001.
39. Frymoyer JW: Back pain and sciatica. N Engl J Med 318:291-300, 1988.
40. Frymoyer JW, Pope MH, Clements JH, et al: Risk factors in low back pain: An epidemiological survey. J Bone Joint Surg Am 65:213-218, 1983.
41. Frymoyer JW, Pope MH, Costanza MC, et al: Epidemiologic studies of low back pain. Spine 5:419-423, 1980.
42. Gay JR, Abbott KH: Common whiplash injuries of the neck. JAMA 152:1098, 1958.
43. Goldberg MS, Scott SC, Mayo NE: A review of the association between cigarette smoking and the development of nonspecific back pain and related outcomes. Spine 25:995-1014, 2000.
44. Gore DR, Sepic SB, Gardner GM, et al: Neck pain: A long-term follow-up of 205 patients. Spine 12:1-5, 1987.
45. Gotten N: Survey of one hundred cases of whiplash injury after settlement of litigation. JAMA 162:856, 1956.
46. Guy JE: The whiplash: Tiny impact, tremendous injury. IMS Ind Med Surg 37:668-691, 1968.
47. Hagberg M, Sundelin G: Discomfort and load on the upper trapezius muscle when operating a word processor. Ergonomics 29:1637-1645, 1986.
48. Hagberg M, Wegman DH: Prevalence rates and odds ratios of shoulder-neck diseases in different occupational groups. Br J Ind Med 44:602-610, 1987.
49. Hansson T, Bigos S, Beecher P, et al: The lumbar lordosis in acute and chronic low back pain. Spine 10:154-155, 1985.
50. Harreby M, Hesselsoe G, Kier J, et al: Low back pain and physical exercise in leisure time in 38-year-old men and women: A 25-year prospective cohort study of 640 school children. Eur Spine J 6:181-186, 1997.
51. Hart LG, Deyo RA, Cherkin DC: Physician office visits for low back pain: Frequency, clinical evaluation, and treatment patterns from a U.S. national survey. Spine 20:11-19, 1995.
52. Heliövaara M, Makela M, Knekt P, et al: Determinants of sciatica and low back pain. Spine 16:608-614, 1991.
53. Heliövarra M, Knekt P, Aromaa A: Incidence and risk factors of herniated lumbar intervertebral disc or sciatica leading to hospitalization. J Chronic Dis 40:251, 1987.
54. Heliövarra M: Epidemiology of Sciatica and Herniated Lumbar Intervertebral Disc. Helsinki, Research Institute for Social Security, 1988, 1-47.
55. Hellsing AL, Bryngelsson IL: Predictors of musculoskeletal pain in men: A twenty-year follow-up from examination at enlistment. Spine 25:3080-3086, 2000.
56. Hirsch C, Jonsson B, Lewin T: Low back symptoms in a Swedish female population. Clin Orthop 63:171-176, 1969.
57. Hodgson S, Shannon HS, Troup JDG: The Prevention of Spinal Disorders in Dock Workers: Report to National Dock Labour Board. London, National Dock Labour Board, 1974.
58. Hohl M: Soft tissue injuries of the neck in automobile accidents: Factors influencing prognosis. J Bone Joint Surg Am 56:1675-1682, 1974.
59. Hoogendoorn WE, Bongers PM, de Vet HC, et al: Flexion and rotation of the trunk and lifting at work are risk factors for low back pain: Results of a prospective cohort study. Spine 25:3087-3092, 2000.
60. Horal J: The clinical appearance of low back disorders in the city of Gothenburg, Sweden: Comparisons of incapacitated probands with matched controls. Acta Orthop Scand Suppl 118:1-109, 1969.
61. Hult L: Cervical, dorsal, and lumbar spinal syndromes. Acta Orthop Scand Suppl 17:1, 1954.

62. Jackson R: The positive findings in alleged neck injuries. Am J Orthop 6:178, 1964.
63. Jackson R: Crashes cause most neck pain [newspaper article]. Am Med News 1966.
64. Kahane CJ: An evaluation of head restraints. 2982, 308. 1982. Federal Motor Vehicle Safety Standard 22. Technical Report.
65. Kelsey JL: An epidemiological study of the relationship between occupations and acute herniated lumbar intervertebral discs. Int J Epidemiol 4:197-205, 1975.
66. Kelsey JL, Githens PB, O'Conner T, et al: Acute prolapsed lumbar intervertebral disc: An epidemiologic study with special reference to driving automobiles and cigarette smoking. Spine 9:608-613, 1984.
67. Kelsey JL, Githens PB, Walter SD, et al: An epidemiological study of acute prolapsed cervical intervertebral disc. J Bone Joint Surg Am 66:907-914, 1984.
68. Kelsey JL, Githens PB, White AA III, et al: An epidemiologic study of lifting and twisting on the job and risk for acute prolapsed lumbar intervertebral disc. J Orthop Res 2:61-66, 1984.
69. Kelsey JL, Hardy RJ: Driving of motor vehicles as a risk factor for acute herniated lumbar intervertebral disc. Am J Epidemiol 102:63-73, 1975.
70. Kelsey JL, Ostfeld AM: Demographic characteristics of persons with acute herniated lumbar intervertebral disc. J Chronic Dis 28:37-50, 1975.
71. Kelsey JL, White AA III: Epidemiology and impact of low back pain. Spine 5:133-142, 1980.
72. Kiesler S, Finholt T: The mystery of RSI. Am Psychol 43:1004-1015, 1988.
73. Kihlberg JK: Flexion-torsion neck injury in rear-end impacts. Proceedings of 13th Annual Conference of American Association for Automotive Medicine, Minneapolis, MN, 1969.
74. Kondo K, Molgaard CA, Kurland LT, Onofrio BM: Protruded intervertebral cervical disk: Incidence and affected cervical level in Rochester, Minnesota, 1950 through 1974. Minn Med 64:751-753, 1981.
75. Kostuik JP, Bentivoglio J: The incidence of low back pain in adult scoliosis. Spine 6:268-273, 1981.
76. Kostuik JP, Israel J, Hall JE: Scoliosis surgery in adults. Clin Orthop 93:225-234, 1973.
77. Krause N, Ragland DR, Fisher JM, Syme SL: Psychosocial job factors, physical workload, and incidence of work-related spinal injury: A 5-year prospective study of urban transit operators. Spine 23:2507-2516, 1998.
78. Lawrence JS: Rheumatism in Populations. London, Heinemann Medical, 1977.
79. Lawrence JS, Graft R, deLaine VAI: Degenerative joint diseases in random samples and occupational groups. In Kellgren JH, Council for International Organizations of Medical Sciences (eds): The Epidemiology of Chronic Rheumatism: A Symposium Organized by the Council for International Organizations of Medical Sciences, Vol 1. Oxford, Blackwell Scientific Publications, 1983.
80. Leboeuf-Yde C, Klougart N, Lauritzen T: How common is low back pain in the Nordic population? Data from a recent study on a middle-aged general Danish population and four surveys previously conducted in the Nordic countries. Spine 21:1518-1525, 1996.
81. Leboeuf-Yde C, Kyvik KO: At what age does low back pain become a common problem? A study of 29,424 individuals aged 12–41 years. Spine 23:228-234, 1998.
82. Leboeuf-Yde C, Kyvik KO, Bruun NH: Low back pain and lifestyle. II. Obesity: Information from a population-based sample of 29,424 twin subjects. Spine 24:779-783, 1999.
83. Linton SJ: A review of psychological risk factors in back and neck pain. Spine 25:1148-1156, 2000.
84. Linton SJ, Hellsing AL, Hallden K: A population-based study of spinal pain among 35- to 45-year-old individuals: Prevalence, sick leave, and health care use. Spine 23:1457-1463, 1998.
85. MacNab I: Acceleration injuries of the cervical spine. J Bone Joint Surg Am 46:1797, 1964.
86. Magora A: Investigation of the relation between low back pain and occupation. III. Physical requirements: Sitting, standing, and weight lifting. IMS Ind Med Surg 41:5-9, 1972.
87. Magora A: Investigation of the relation between low back pain and occupation. IV. Physical requirements: Bending, rotation, reaching, and sudden maximal effort. Scand J Rehabil Med 5:186-190, 1973.
88. Magora A: Investigation of the relation between low back pain and occupation. V. Psychological aspects. Scand J Rehabil Med 5:191-196, 1973.
89. Magora A: Investigation of the relation between low back pain and occupation. VII. Neurologic and orthopaedic condition. Scand J Rehabil Med 7:146-151, 1975.
90. Makela M, Heliovaara M, Sievers K, et al: Prevalence, determinants, and consequences of chronic neck pain in Finland. Am J Epidemiol 134:1356-1367, 1991.
91. Murphy PL, Volinn E: Is occupational low back pain on the rise? Spine 24:691-697, 1999.
92. Nachemson A, Eck C, Lindstrom H, et al: Chronic low back disability can largely be prevented: A prospective randomized trial in industry. AAOS 56th Annual Meeting, Las Vegas, 1989.
93. Nachemson AL: Back problems in childhood and adolescence [in Swedish]. Lakartidningen 65:2831, 1968.
94. Nachemson AL: Report to the Swedish Department of Economy [in Swedish]. 1989.
95. National Center for Health Statistics: Physician visits, volume, and interval since last visit, United States, 1971. Series 10, No. 97. Hyattsville, MD, U.S. Department of Health and Human Services, 1975.
96. National Center for Health Statistics: Inpatient utilization of short stay hospitals by diagnosis, United States, 1973. Series 13, No. 25. Hyattsville, MD, U.S. Department of Health and Human Services, 1976.
97. National Center for Health Statistics: Surgical operations in short stay hospitals, United States, 1973. Series 13, No. 24. Hyattsville, MD, U.S. Department of Health and Human Services, 1976.
98. National Center for Health Statistics: Limitation of activity due to chronic conditions, United States, 1974. Series 10, No. 111, 1977.
99. National Center for Health Statistics: Prevalence of selected impairments, United States, 1977. Series 10, No. 134. Hyattsville, MD, U.S. Department of Health and Human Services, 1981.
100. Nilsonne U, Lundgren KD: Long-term prognosis in idiopathic scoliosis. Acta Orthop Scand 39:456-465, 1968.
101. O'Neill B, Haddon W Jr, Kelley AB, et al: Automobile head restraints—frequency of neck injury claims in relation to the presence of head restraints. Am J Public Health 62:399-406, 1972.
102. Palmer KT, Walker-Bone K, Griffin MJ, et al: Prevalence and occupational associations of neck pain in the British population. Scand J Work Environ Health 27:49-56, 2001.
103. Partyka S: Whiplash and other inertial force neck injuries in traffic accidents. Paper presented at the Meeting of the Mathematical Analysis Division, National Center for Statistics and Analysis, 1981.
104. Pope MH, Bevins T, Wilder DG, et al: The relationship between anthropometric, postural, muscular, and mobility characteristics of males ages 18–55. Spine 10:644-648, 1985.
105. Praemer A, Furner S, Rice DP, American Academy of Orthopaedic Surgeons: Musculoskeletal Conditions in the United States, 2nd ed. Rosemont, IL, American Academy of Orthopaedic Surgeons, 1999.
106. Riihimaki H, Wickstrom G, Hanninen K, Luopajarvi T: Predictors of sciatic pain among concrete reinforcement workers and house painters—a five-year follow-up. Scand J Work Environ Health 15:415-423, 1989.
107. Rowe ML: Low back pain in industry—a position paper. J Occup Med 11:161-169, 1969.
108. Salkever DS: Morbidity costs: National estimates and economic determinants. NCHSR Research Summary Series, October 1985. Publication No. (PHS) 86-3393. Bethesda, MD, Department of Health and Human Services, 1986.
109. Scott SC, Goldberg MS, Mayo NE, et al: The association between cigarette smoking and back pain in adults. Spine 24:1090-1098, 1999.
110. Snook SH: Low back pain in industry. In White AA, Gordon SL, American Academy of Orthopaedic Surgeons (eds): Symposium on Idiopathic Low Back Pain, Miami, Florida, December 1980. St. Louis, Mosby, 1982, pp 23-28.
111. Sorensen KH: Scheuermann's juvenile kyphosis [doctoral dissertation]. Copenhagen, Munksgaard, 1964.
112. Spangfort EV: The lumbar disc herniation: A computer-aided analysis of 2,504 operations. Acta Orthop Scand Suppl 142:1-95, 1972.

113. States JD, Korn MW, Masengill JB: The enigma of whiplash injury. N Y State J Med 70:2971-2978, 1970.
114. Suissa S, Harder S, Veilleux M: The relation between initial symptoms and signs and the prognosis of whiplash. Eur Spine J 10:44-49, 2001.
115. Svensson HO, Andersson GB: Low back pain in 40- to 47-year-old men: Work history and work environment factors. Spine 8:272-276, 1983.
116. Svensson HO, Andersson GB, Johansson S, et al: A retrospective study of low back pain in 38- to 64-year-old women: Frequency of occurrence and impact on medical services. Spine 13:548-552, 1988.
117. Takala J, Sievers K, Klaukka T: Rheumatic symptoms in the middle-aged population in southwestern Finland. Scand J Rheumatol Suppl 47:15-29, 1982.
118. Thorbjornsson CB, Alfredsson L, Fredriksson K, et al: Physical and psychosocial factors related to low back pain during a 24-year period: A nested case-control analysis. Spine 25:369-374, 2000.
119. Tola S, Riihimaki H, Videman T, et al: Neck and shoulder symptoms among men in machine operating, dynamic physical work, and sedentary work. Scand J Work Environ Health 14:299-305, 1988.
120. Troup JDG, Roantree WB, Archibald RM: Survey of cases of lumbar spinal disability: A methodological study. Medical Officers' Boardsheet: National Goal Board, 1970.
121. Valkenburg HA, Haanen HCM: The epidemiology of low back pain. In White AA, Gordon SL, American Academy of Orthopaedic Surgeons (eds): Symposium on Idiopathic Low Back Pain, Miami, Florida, December 1980. St. Louis, Mosby, 1982, pp 9-22.
122. Vasseljen O, Holte KA, Westgaard RH: Shoulder and neck complaints in customer relations: Individual risk factors and perceived exposures at work. Ergonomics 44:355-372, 2001.
123. Viikari-Juntura E, Martikainen R, Luukkonen R, et al: Longitudinal study on work-related and individual risk factors affecting radiating neck pain. Occup Environ Med 58:345-352, 2001.
124. Volinn E: The epidemiology of low back pain in the rest of the world: A review of surveys in low- and middle-income countries. Spine 22:1747-1754, 1997.
125. Weber H: Lumbar disc herniation: A controlled, prospective study with ten years of observation. Spine 8:131-140, 1983.
126. Wedderkopp N, Leboeuf-Yde C, Andersen LB, et al: Back pain reporting pattern in a Danish population-based sample of children and adolescents. Spine 26:1879-1883, 2001.
127. Westerling D, Jonsson BG: Pain from the neck-shoulder region and sick leave. Scand J Soc Med 8:131-136, 1980.
128. Westrin CG: Low back sick-listing: A nosological and medical insurance investigation. Acta Sociomed Scand 2:127-134, 1970.
129. Westrin CG: Low back sick-listing: A nosological and medical insurance investigation. Scand J Soc Med Suppl 7:1-116, 1973.
130. Williams DA, Feuerstein M, Durbin D, et al: Health care and indemnity costs across the natural history of disability in occupational low back pain. Spine 23:2329-2336, 1998.
131. Wood PHN: Epidemiology of back pain. In Jayson MIV (ed): The Lumbar Spine and Back Pain, 3rd ed. Edinburgh, Churchill Livingstone, 1987, pp 1-15.

CHAPTER 3

SOURCES OF SPINAL PAIN

Advances in pain research since the first edition of this book have increased our understanding of the basic human complaint of spinal pain. The early concept of pain presented by Descartes as little strings (petits filets) connecting the periphery with the ventricles of the brain has been superseded by an ever-increasing number of networks of multiple synapses throughout the neuraxis mediated by a variety of amino acids, electrolytes, inflammatory mediators, and neurochemicals.[13]

PAIN—THE FIFTH VITAL SIGN

The importance of pain as a clinical entity has been recognized by a number of professional scientific organizations. For example, in the hospital setting, the Joint Commission on Accreditation of Healthcare Organizations has added the measurement of pain as a fifth vital sign in addition to temperature, pulse, respirations, and blood pressure.[43]

Acute pain is the warning sign of acute injury and has its associated mediators recognizing damage, with immediate recognition by the sensory nervous system. This results in reflex actions in the motor system to limit the damage. The psychological response of fear is usually contained as the damaging elements are removed or relieved. The neuraxis is otherwise unmodified.

Initially, chronic pain was thought to be acute pain that went on for an extended period, usually more than 6 months or beyond the time for normal healing. This concept is not correct.[41] Chronic pain is a separate entity associated with major alterations in the nervous system. The tonic stimulation of the nervous system results in its modification. The plasticity of the nervous system is manifested by changes in the physical anatomy and physiology of the sensory system stretching from the peripheral sensory fibers to the anterior cingulate cortex of the brain where pain is experienced.[69]

Pain to be diagnosed and treated must be placed in its appropriate context. Acute pain has its own implications for evaluation and treatment. Investigation of chronic pain may result in no further identification of a damaged tissue or injury. That should not mean to the health care provider that pain does not exist. The therapy of chronic pain requires a different range of interventions. Those interventions that may be very effective with acute pain may not be useful with chronic pain. Therapies not effective for acute pain may be essential to modification of the psychological response to chronic pain. Although these designations may not have had importance in the past, identification of the type, character, and duration of pain is essential for selection of the most appropriate therapy. The concern about acute pain as a marker of disease and the need for investigation have been paramount in the conscientiousness of the health care provider. The need for treatment of acute pain to preempt chronic pain was considered ill advised. For example, treating postsurgical pain before an operation would only cloud the clinical symptoms and make evaluation more difficult. These concepts are no longer absolutely true. The use of nonnarcotic analgesics that do not affect coagulation prior to surgery decreases the doses of postoperative narcotics to relieve acute pain.

The patient with spinal pain presents a challenge to the family practitioner, internist, rheumatologist, orthopedist, neurosurgeon, physiatrist, psychiatrist, osteopathic physician, occupational therapist, and physical therapist. The patient's complaint is a symptom, not a diagnosis. The number of anatomic parts of the lumbar and cervical spine that have the potential to cause pain is substantial. In addition, the spectrum of disease processes that may affect paraspinal structures is broad. Compounding the problem are the patients who have spinal pain that is associated with a work-related or motor vehicle injury. The extent and intensity of symptoms may be exaggerated by nonphysiologic factors. The physician's task in treating patients with spinal pain is to identify the likely source of pain and the pathologic process causing it. Only then may the physician feel reasonably confident in implementing appropriate therapy.

Unfortunately, in many circumstances, a physician may not fully examine a patient with spinal pain. There are many reasons for an incomplete history and physical examination, including the number of patients with the symptom of spinal pain, the natural history of gradual improvement of spinal pain, the effect of nonphysiologic factors on the severity and duration of symptoms, and the physician's degree of knowledge of the functional anatomy of that part of the body.

Physicians see many patients with low back and/or neck pain. Low back pain is second to the cold as the most common affliction of humankind. The natural history of spinal pain is one of rapid improvement. Eighty percent to

90% of patients with spinal pain are better within 2 months, with or without intervention of a physician. The need for making a specific diagnosis at the initial visit is not important from a practical standpoint. Most patients will improve, and most patients have a mechanical, noninflammatory cause for their spinal pain (muscle strain, annular tear of an intervertebral disc), not an underlying serious, systemic illness. Identifying the source of a patient's pain to be ligamentous, muscular, or articular in origin in this acute circumstance does not significantly alter therapy or hasten recovery. Furthermore, some physicians may have developed a skepticism about the severity of patients' symptoms of spinal pain. Physicians are taught to believe that patients will be honest about the severity of their symptoms because it is in their self-interest. When that honesty seems questionable, the physician believes there is a breach of trust. This skepticism occurs among physicians whose patients are involved in motor vehicle accidents or work-related injuries. Some physicians see so many of these patients that they have stopped "evaluating" them. A patient may have a motive for continuing to have pain to increase a monetary reward or to get a light-duty job at work. This distrust is destructive to the physician-patient relationship and results in patients who might be helped being denied appropriate care. The manipulation of workers' compensation or insurance systems by a few individuals should not influence the way a physician treats patients with spinal pain.

It is not uncommon for a physician to be more familiar with the functional anatomy of organs of the chest and abdomen than with those of the spine. It is left to the orthopedists and neurosurgeons to be concerned with anatomic relationships and sensory innervation of the structures of the spine. Unfortunately, this is a shortsighted view of a complicated problem. Only with familiarity with anatomic sources of pain in the lumbar and cervical spine and the mechanism of pain transmission and inhibition can any physician adequately evaluate patients with spinal pain. With greater knowledge of functional anatomy and pathophysiologic effects of disease processes on the structures of the spine, a physician is better able to differentiate those individuals with a potentially more ominous cause of spinal pain from those with mechanical abnormalities. The physician may also be better able to differentiate the various causes of mechanical spinal pain. The significant differences between acute and chronic pain take on greater importance in regard to goals for therapy. Not only does understanding of the sources of pain help in the differential diagnosis of diseases of the spine, but it also provides a rationale for a variety of therapeutic modalities used for patients with spinal pain. These therapies treat the mechanisms that cause continued pain in areas of healed, structural injury. The purpose of this chapter is to review pain neuroanatomy and physiology and to discuss the sources and character of pain associated with abnormalities involving the structures of the spine.

PAIN PRODUCTION AND TRANSMISSION

Pain is defined by pain specialists (algologists) as an unpleasant sensory and emotional experience associated with actual or potential tissue damage, or an experience described in terms of such damage.[39] Pain is a subjective, individual perception related to mechanical and chemical alterations of body tissues. This means that pain is perceived in the cortical portions of the central nervous system; it is not dependent on the precise nature or absolute amount of tissue destruction peripherally. This potential separation of tissue destruction from the perception of pain emphasizes the fact that pain messages can be modified at many levels of the nervous system.

Peripheral Nerve Fibers

The peripheral nervous system contains a wide range of nerve fibers. Myelinated somatic nerves are called *A fibers* and are subdivided into four groups according to decreasing size: alpha, beta, gamma, and delta. The largest are the alpha fibers, which conduct impulses that serve motor function, proprioception, and reflex activity. Beta fibers also innervate muscle and convey touch and pressure sensations. For example, in the skin, A-beta fibers respond to light touch and the bending of hairs. Gamma fibers control muscle spindle tone. Delta fibers subserve pain and temperature functions. The thinly myelinated B fibers are preganglionic autonomic axons that innervate smooth muscle. The unmyelinated C fibers transmit nociceptive impulses (Table 3-1).

Bare nerve endings and specialized corpuscular receptors are the two kinds of receptor organs serving body sensory function.[38] They differ in their capacity to transform mechanical, thermal, and chemical energy into electrical impulses. The corpuscular receptors (mechanoreceptors) are most sensitive to mechanical vibratory energy. They are larger myelinated fibers (A-alpha and A-beta) that rapidly transmit information about innocuous mechanical stimuli to the cerebral cortex.

Nociceptors

Another set of fibers responds only to stimuli associated with actual tissue damage. These fibers are called *nociceptors*. Mechanoreceptors and polymodal nociceptors are two primary forms of these nerve fibers. Mechanoreceptors transmit information about mechanical forces that cause tissue injury. Bare nerve endings, in contrast, are sensitive to all physical modalities (such as heat and chemical injury) but differ in their individual sensitivity and threshold to different stimuli.

Nociceptors have two mechanisms to differentiate innocuous from noxious stimuli. These mechanisms are the association of intensity of tissue damage with frequency of nerve impulses and a high threshold for stimulation. The highest neural firing rates occur when nociceptors respond to stimuli in the noxious range.

Nociceptive impulses are carried by two sizes of nerve endings. The larger of the two types of pain fiber is the A-delta fiber, 6 to 8 μm in diameter, which is thinly myelinated and conducts impulses relatively quickly (12 μm/sec). Some A-delta fibers respond mainly to mechanical energy and accurately locate a site of injury.

3-1 PERIPHERAL NERVE FIBER CHARACTERISTICS

	Myelination	Receptor Type	Transmission (m/sec)	Threshold	Distribution	Modality
A-alpha	+	Mechanoreceptor	Rapid (70–120)	Low	Local	Vibration (proprioception) Pain (prick)
A-beta	+	Mechanoreceptor	Rapid (40–70)	Low	Local	Vibration (proprioception) Reflex withdrawal
A-gamma	+	Mechanoreceptor	Rapid (20–40)	Low	Local	Muscle spindle
A-delta	+	Mechanonociceptor	Slow (5–15)	High	Local	Damaging pressure
A-delta	+	Thermal mechanonociceptor	Slow (5–15)	High	Local	Noxious Temperature (sharp)
B	+	Autonomic	Slow (10–15)	High	Diffuse	Preganglionic fibers
C	–	Mechanonociceptor	Slow (0.2–1.5)	High	Diffuse	Noxious
C	–	Polymodal nociceptor	Slow (0.2–1.5)	High	Diffuse	Pressure (sharp) Any noxious stimulus (dull)

Others respond to chemical or thermal stimulation in proportion to the degree of injury. More frequent nerve firings are associated with greater tissue damage.[15] Some A-delta fibers may be polymodal responders, which fire after a high threshold has been reached and tissue damage has occurred. These fibers lower their active thresholds once they have been exposed to other noxious stimuli.[27] In the sensitized state, innocuous mechanical stimuli that previously evoked no response produce nociceptive impulses that continue following cessation of the stimulus. Sensitization plays a role in the prolongation of acute pain and the development of chronic pain. Complete destruction of a receptor does not block the sensitized transmission of impulses from undamaged receptors of the same axon.[82] Focal areas of demyelination caused by chronic irritation may give rise to spontaneous action potentials that travel in an anterograde or retrograde direction. In these injured nerves, normal stimulation may evoke sustained afterdischarges.

The smaller, unmyelinated C fibers, 0.3 to 1.0 μm in diameter, conduct impulses slowly (0.4 to 1.0 m/sec), are polymodal responders (mechanical, chemical, heat), and are activated only by tissue destruction. These receptors show continued or delayed firing after the physical stimulus has been discontinued. After repeated or prolonged stimulation, their threshold for activation can diminish to levels of intensity that are usually innocuous.[7] *Allodynia* is pain generated by an innocuous stimulation in an area of sensitized nociception. Humoral mediators and chemical substances released during acute inflammation and tissue destruction may play a role temporally in C fiber transmission. Peptides, such as bradykinin, are released after a latency of 15 to 30 seconds and reach a peak 15 seconds after the latency period, which may contribute to the delayed and continued firing of high-threshold receptors. Other factors that may play similar roles in nociceptive potentiation are potassium, histamine, substance P, serotonin, and prostaglandins.[24,44] In combination, these nociceptive A-delta and C fibers detect noxious stimuli that damage body structures. For example, muscle pain is mediated by both A-delta and C fibers. The A-delta fibers are activated by release of histamine, serotonin, and bradykinin during intense exercise. The C fibers respond to rapid contractions of muscle but not to byproducts of muscle metabolism.

Inflammation and Pain

The interaction of the chemical mediators of inflammation, peripheral inflammatory cells, and neuropeptides that mediate nociceptive stimulation is complex.[1] Products of inflammation released during tissue destruction sensitize and stimulate peripheral nociceptors. The nociceptors produce neurotransmitters that stimulate the C fiber (Table 3-2).[11] The excitation of the primary afferent also produces an axon reflex that results in the peripheral release of neuropeptides such as substance P, neurokinin A, and calcitonin gene–related peptide. Other identified sensitizing factors include interleukin-1, neutrophil-chemotactic peptides, and nerve growth factor–derived octapeptide.[53] A combination of chemical mediators and peripheral white blood cells affects the transmission of nociceptive impulses (Fig. 3-1). Activated immune cells release soluble proinflammatory cytokines (interleukin-1, interleukin-6, and tumor necrosis factor [TNF]-alpha) that activate peripheral nerves.[84] Some of these neuropeptides are the same mediators that stimulate second-order neurons in the spinal cord. The tissue damage caused by the direct stimulation of peripheral nociceptive fibers by dorsal horn cells is called *neurogenic inflammation*.[54] Painful inflammatory conditions can also induce the appearance of peripheral opioid receptors on peripheral sensory nerve endings. Resident immune cells in inflamed tissues can upregulate the production of their endogenous ligands—opiate peptides. The result is local analgesia. The clinical importance of this finding is the potential of opiates to mediate analgesia topically in a location distant from the central nervous system.[78]

Peripheral immune cytokines have effects not only locally on nociceptors but also centrally in the cerebral cortex. However, cytokines are large lipophobic proteins that have difficulty crossing the blood-brain barrier. Direct penetration is unlikely. Immune activation to the central nervous system may be mediated through the subdiaphragmatic vagus nerve and primary afferent neurons in

3-2 MEDIATORS OF PERIPHERAL NOCICEPTIVE TRANSMISSION

Type	Ligands	Sources
Amino acids	Glutamate	PAF, macrophages
	GABA	PAF, plasma
Cholinergic	Acetylcholine	PAF, keratinocytes
Biogenic amines	Norepinephrine	Sympathetic nerves
	Serotonin	Mast cells, platelets
	Histamine	Mast cells
Nucleotides	Adenosine	PAF, cell damage
Purines	ATP	PAF, cell damage
Vanilloids	Capsaicin	Exogenous
Prostanoids	PGE_2	Macrophages
Ions	Hydrogen	Cell damage
Cytokines	Interleukin-1β	Macrophages
	Interleukin-6	Macrophages
Corticosteroids	Glucosteroids	Serum
Neuroactive peptides	Substance P	PAF
	Neurokinin A	PAF
	Bradykinin	Plasma
	Cholecystokinin	PAF
	Somatostatin	PAF
	Bombesin	PAF
	Angiotensin II	Serum
	Neuropeptide Y	PAF
	CRF	Hypothalamus
Opioid peptides	Endorphins	PAF, immunocytes
	Enkephalins	PAF, immunocytes
	Dynorphin	PAF, immunocytes
Growth factors	NGF	Fibroblasts
	BNF	PAF
	GNF	Schwann cell
	FGF	Fibroblasts, Schwann cells

GABA, gamma-aminobutyric acid; PAF, primary afferent fiber; ATP, adenosine triphosphate; PGE_2, prostaglandin E_2; CRF, corticotropin-releasing factor; NGF, nerve growth factor; BNF, brain-derived neurotrophic factor; GNF, glial-derived neurotrophic factor; FGF, fibroblast growth factor.
Modified from Byers MR, Bonica JJ: Peripheral pain mechanisms and nociceptor plasticity. In Loeser JD (ed): Bonica's Management of Pain. Philadelphia, Lippincott Williams & Wilkins, 2001, pp 26-72.

skin, joints, and muscles.[84] The vagus contains a large number of afferent nerves that respond to the binding of cytokines to glomus cells of the abdominal paraganglia. The projection of these neurons is to the nucleus tractus solitarius, which stimulates the raphe magnus nucleus. Descending signals are transmitted to the dorsal horn of the spinal cord. In addition, activation of these cells results in increases in brain cytokines produced by glial cells. The end result is pain facilitation through hyperalgesia, an increased response to a noxious stimulus.

Peripheral Nociceptive Transmission

The two groups of pain fibers are associated with two dissociable types of sensory input. The pinprick type of sensation, which is quick in onset and well localized, is carried in the larger, myelinated A fibers. These fibers belong to a phylogenetically newer sensory system that ascends to the sensory cortex with few interposed relays. This type of pain results in rapid movement, quick protection, and reflex withdrawal from a potentially damaging stimulus. The later, dull, aching, less localized sensation is carried by the unmyelinated C fibers. These smaller fibers belong to a phylogenetically older sensory system with multiple relays in the medulla and thalamus.[8] The pain associated with C fiber stimulation produces tonic contraction, which functions to guard and protect the injured part.

The Dorsal Horn

Dorsal horn neurons are classified according to their response to primary afferent input. Low-threshold neurons respond only to non-noxious stimuli such as hair movement or touch. High-threshold neurons are nociceptive specific, responding to excessive joint movement. Dorsal horn neurons stimulated by noxious and non-noxious stimuli are classified as wide-dynamic-range neurons. These neurons have graded responses that increase with increasing intensities of stimulation. Wide-dynamic-range neurons respond to hair movement, pressure, pinch, or pinprick.

The nociceptive A-delta and C fibers with nerve endings in the periphery and their cell bodies in the dorsal root ganglion have destination points in the dorsal horn of the spinal cord.[55] Of the six specialized layers (laminae) of

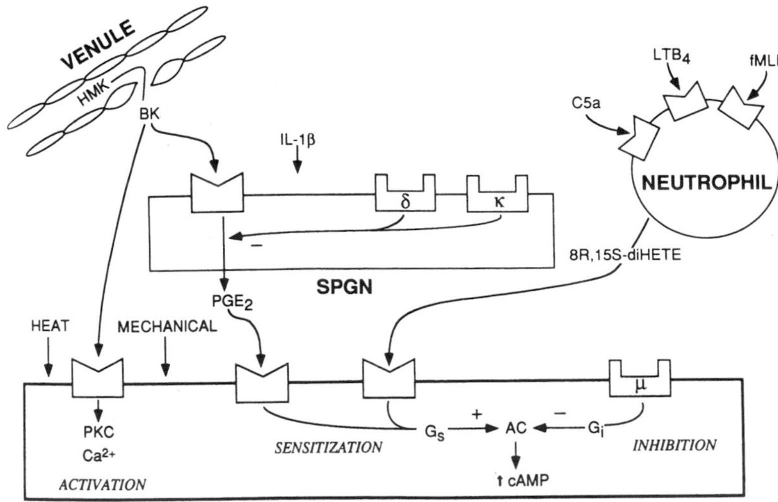

Figure 3-1 Sites of peptide action in peripheral pathways of pain and hyperalgesia. The inflammatory peptide bradykinin (BK), cleaved from high-molecular-weight kininogen (HMK) circulating in the venules, can activate the primary afferent nociceptor (PAN) in a protein kinase C (PKC)– and Ca^{2+}-dependent mechanism or sensitize the PAN through the production of prostaglandin E_2 (PGE_2) in sympathetic postganglionic neurons (SPGNs). Opioid ligands can do so at the level of the PAN via the inhibitory G protein. IL-1β, interleukin-1β; LTB_4, leukotriene B_4; fMLP-f-met-leu-phe. *(From Levine JD, Fields HL, Basbaum AI: Peptides and the primary afferent nociceptor. J Neurosci 13:2275, 1993.)*

nerve endings that are laminated in the dorsal horn, layers I, II, and V receive nociceptive fibers (Fig. 3-2). Laminae III and IV receive primary afferent input from large-fiber, low-threshold neurons involved with spinal cord processing of proprioception. Lamina VI has low-threshold and wide-dynamic-range neurons that may share some function with lamina V in transmission of nociceptive information to supraspinal sites. This organization of the dorsal horn has physiologic importance. Small-caliber myelinated fibers ascend or descend in Lissauer's tract for one or two segments before entering the dorsal gray matter. They terminate in lamina I and the bottom of lamina II. Lamina I receives A-delta mechanoreceptors and some polymodal C afferents. The sensory input is from the skin and muscle nociceptors that have a small peripheral receptive field. These neurons are important in signaling the presence of pain, but they are unlikely to transmit information concerning the intensity or nature of the painful stimulus.[14] In contrast, cells in lamina V receive more specific information because of the convergent input of rapidly conducting A-beta fibers and of the more slowly conducting A-delta and C nociceptive fibers (wide-dynamic-range neurons). These fibers respond to mechanical or thermal stimuli, steadily increasing their discharge frequency with the intensity of the noxious stimulus. Lamina V conveys the information concerning the location, intensity, and form of harmful stimuli.

Substance P

These lamina V axons contain substance P, a neurotransmitter that is most highly concentrated in the superficial layers of the dorsal horn.[50] Substance P plays an important role in dorsal horn transmission of nociception. Dorsal horn nociceptors are substantially stimulated by substance P. Capsaicin, the active ingredient in hot peppers, has a significant effect on the transmission of nociceptive impulses.[75] Initially, capsaicin activates nociceptors selectively. A later effect of capsaicin on nerve fibers is the depletion of substance P. Depletion of substance P in the spinal cord with capsaicin is associated with decreased transmission of nociceptive impulses.[83]

Substance P is an undecapeptide that is present in 20% of dorsal root ganglion neurons. Substance P is a member of a group of peptides, the tachykinins or neurokinins. Although substance P is present in nociceptors, this neurotransmitter is not solely associated with pain transmission because it is also found in non-nociceptive fibers.[68] Dorsal root ganglion nerves contain a variety of neurotransmitters. Afferents innervating different organs differ consistently in their peptide content. The peptide content of primary afferents is determined by specific factors in the tissues they innervate. In addition, peptide content changes dramatically in response to certain prolonged stimuli or nerve damage. However, control of substance P

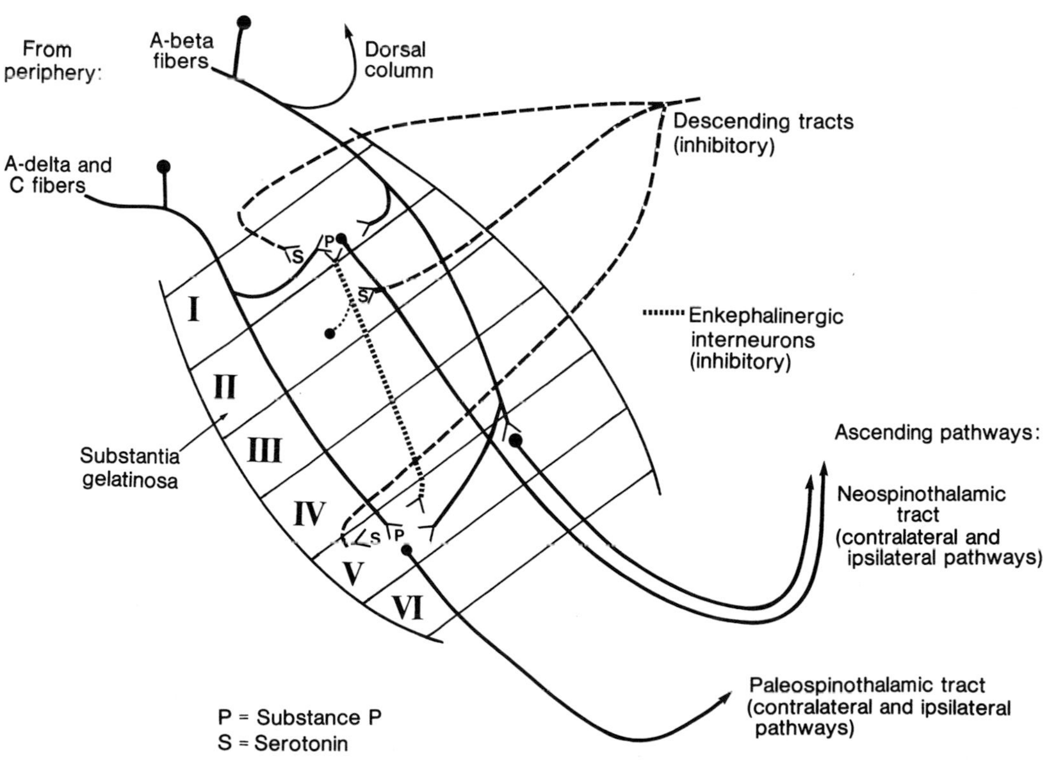

Figure 3-2 The dorsal horn. This graphic demonstrates the organization of the pain-related fibers in the dorsal horn. Nociceptive A-delta and C fibers carry pain messages from the periphery to laminae I and V. These nerves release substance P. These neurons synapse with second-order relay neurons, which ascend in the rapid pathway (neospinothalamic tract) and/or the slow pathway (paleospinothalamic tract). The nociceptive messages of these neurons are modified presynaptically by collateral branches of the large low-threshold cutaneous mechanoreceptors (A-beta fibers), whose main branches ascend in the ipsilateral dorsal columns. The nociceptive fibers are also inhibited by enkephalinergic interneurons whose cell bodies are situated in lamina II. The enkephalinergic cells are driven by the large peripheral A afferents or the serotoninergic fibers descending in the dorsolateral white funiculus of the spinal cord. Descending tracts also attach presynaptically to nociceptors in laminae I and V to inhibit pain transmission.

levels does not totally eliminate the production of pain transmission in the nociceptor.

Substance P, along with other chemical mediators, may contribute to the severity of injury associated with joint inflammation.[61] Depletion of substance P concentrations in animal models of arthritis is associated with less severe joint damage.[4] Substance P is only one of an ever-increasing number of neuropeptides associated with modulation of sensory input in the spinal cord (Table 3-3).[8] Many fibers produce more than one neuropeptide. For example, substance P and calcitonin gene–related peptide are released simultaneously by neurons in the spinal cord.[63] Excitatory amino acids, such as aspartate and glutamate, are also neurotransmitters in the spinal cord. One hypothesis has suggested that excitatory amino acids are the mediators of fast nociceptive transmission, and the neuropeptides are the mediators of slow transmission.[83] The repertoire of neuropeptides and excitatory amino acids associated with a specific noxious stimulus has not been determined. Not only do these neuropeptides have effects at the level of their nerve source, but they may also diffuse to act at a distance from their site of release (Fig. 3-3).

The unmyelinated fibers from lamina V supply not only the skin and muscles but also other somatic structures such as joints and ligaments. In addition, visceral afferents converge on the wide-dynamic-range neurons in lamina V that supply sensory innervation for somatic structures, including skin. On entering the spinal cord, the visceral fibers travel caudally or cranially for several segments in the posterior horn of gray matter before synapsing with neurons in the dorsal horn. The "referred pain" associated with visceral disease processes occurs secondarily to "cross talk" between visceral sensory afferents and the wide-dynamic-range neurons that supply sensation to cutaneous structures. This convergence of afferent nerves allows for the summation of nociceptive input on a spatial and temporal basis. Stimulation of the visceral afferents results in a wide field of cutaneous nerve stimulation, which activates secondary neurons ascending to the midbrain. This diffuse stimulation results in the perception that the skin has been stimulated when in fact the actual source of the sensory input is the visceral afferents.[70]

Lamina II (substantia gelatinosa) receives the majority of the slow, unmyelinated C afferents. Although a small number of cells in this lamina have projections that reach the cortex, most cells in the substantia gelatinosa have local connections with other neurons in other laminae at the same segmental level and with the substantia gelatinosa on the opposite side of the spinal cord. This connection is accomplished through commissural fibers that cross the spinal cord. These nerves have inhibitory effects on pain transmission. Most of the C fibers interconnect with descending inhibitory neurons.[12]

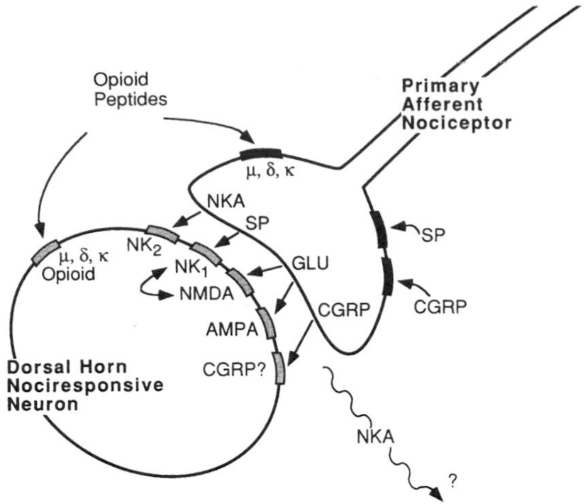

Figure 3-3 Primary afferents and peptide actions in the central nervous system. The primary afferent nociceptor releases a variety of co-occurring neuropeptides (NKA, SP, CGRP) and excitatory amino acids (e.g., glutamate [GLU]). These act at several postsynaptic receptors: the NK_1 and NK_2 tachykinin receptors, the CGRP receptor, and the NMDA and AMPA excitatory amino receptors. NKA may diffuse to act at a distance from its site of release. There is evidence that SP and CGRP also act at autoreceptors at neuropeptide-containing primary afferent terminals. In addition, opioid peptides act on both presynaptic and postsynaptic μ-, δ-, and κ-opioid receptors to modulate transmitter release and the firing of second-order nociresponsive neurons. *(From Levine JD, Fields HL, Basbaum AI: Peptides and the primary afferent nociceptor. J Neurosci 13:2279, 1993.)*

3-3 NEUROPEPTIDES MODULATING NOCICEPTIVE INPUT IN THE SPINAL CORD

Stimulatory	Inhibitory
Substance P	Serotonin
Neurokinin A	Somatostatin
Glutamate	Cholecystokinin
Aspartate	Norepinephrine
Vasoactive intestinal polypeptide	Gamma-aminobutyric acid
Glycine	Endogenous opioid peptides
Calcitonin gene–related peptide	β-endorphin
	Enkephalin
	Dynorphin

Spinothalamic Tract

The majority of the second-order neurons connect with incoming afferent neurons in laminae I and V of the dorsal horn and cross to the contralateral side at the same spinal cord level to ascend rostrally in the anterolateral spinothalamic tract (neospinothalamic tract) (Fig. 3-4). Phylogenetically, the neospinothalamic tract is the newer pain sensory tract in the human nervous system. The neospinothalamic tract courses upward in the spinal cord with new fibers, at each spinal level, joining medially, pushing axons from more caudal segments laterally. This organization preserves the somatotopic organization of the tract in the spinal cord. These fibers terminate in the posterior nuclear group of the thalamus, particularly the ventral posterolateral nucleus. Third-order neurons carry impulses from the thalamus to the posterior central gyrus of the parietal cortex. This rapid system, with its somatotopic organization, allows for analysis of the site, intensity, and nature of pain (pricking, pressing, throbbing, stabbing, or burning). However, this rapid transit system provides no means to mediate reflexes to activate the motor system for evasive action or to alter cortical function to

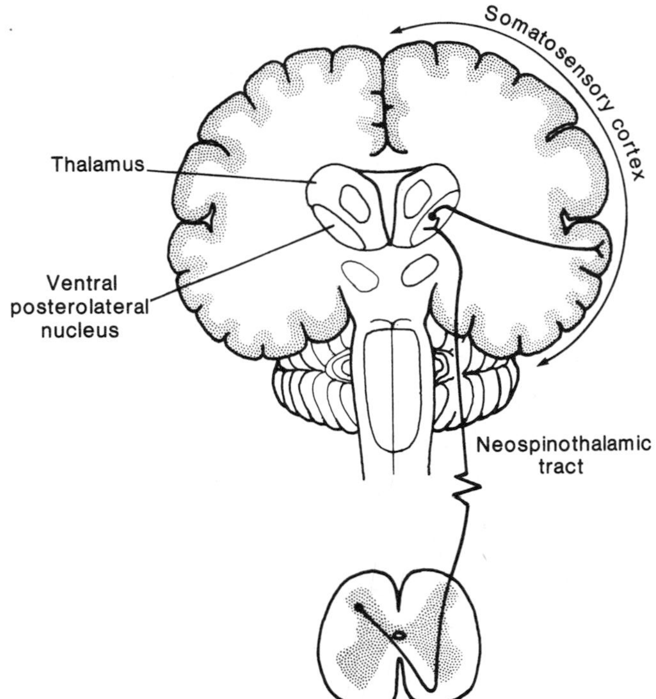

Figure 3-4 The neospinothalamic tract consists of a rapid three-neuron relay system from the dorsal horn to the ventral posterolateral nucleus of the thalamus to the somatosensory cortex. This rapid system, with its somatotopic organization, allows for analysis of the site, intensity, and nature of pain but provides no means to activate evasive motor action.

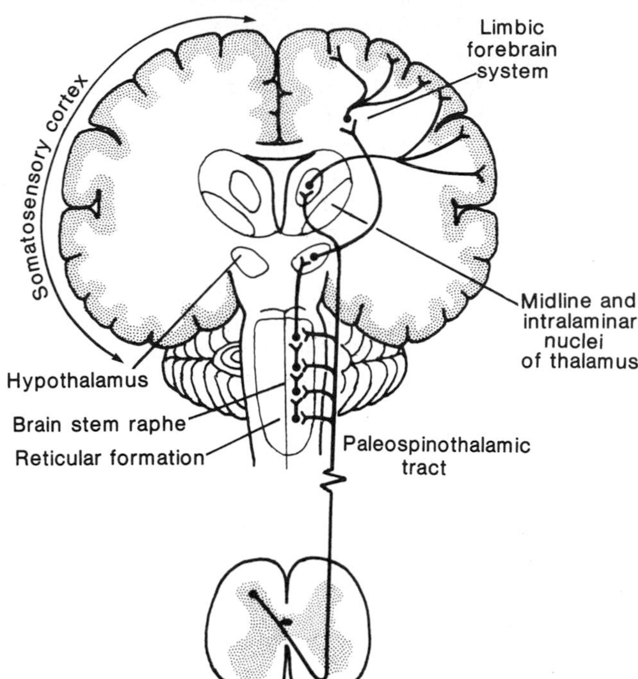

Figure 3-5 The paleospinothalamic tract consists of a slow multineuron relay system from the dorsal horn to the brain stem, hypothalamus, thalamus, and limbic forebrain system. This tract mediates reflexes and integrated responses (fear, memory, suffering) related to nociceptive impulses.

increase alertness. The neospinothalamic tract also has a polysynaptic portion with fibers branching with collaterals that enter the reticular system of the brain stem. Some of these collaterals synapse on cells that provide nociceptive information to the descending inhibitory system.[86]

The phylogenetically older anterior division, the paleospinothalamic tract, supplies the connections for the cortical response to pain (Fig. 3-5). These include suffering, which is a negative affective response to pain; fear; and depression. The second-order neurons of this tract send multiple connections to the reticular formation of the brain stem while traveling to the midline and intralaminar nuclei of the thalamus. The higher-order neurons that emerge from the reticular formation and thalamic nuclei connect with other thalamic nuclei, the hypothalamus, the basal ganglia, and the midbrain central gray area. From these structures, a multitude of higher-order neurons synapse with a number of cortical areas, including the frontal lobe (pain perception), temporal lobe (recent and long-term memory), and hypothalamus (autonomic sympathetic and parasympathetic reflexes).[88] These cortical functions work independently of each other; the intensity of nociceptive input does not necessarily result in a specific emotional response or autonomic reflexes such as increased heart rate and blood pressure or increased gastrointestinal secretion and motility.

Cerebral Cortex

The connections of the nociceptors with a number of different areas of the cerebral cortex underscore the definition of pain as a subjective response that is a summation of total sensory input. Pain has sensory-discriminative, motivational-affective, and cognitive-evaluative dimensions.[58] The neospinothalamic tract contributes to the sensory-discriminative dimension. The cortical projection of this system transmits information that characterizes the spatial, temporal, and magnitude properties of a noxious stimulus. The brain stem reticular formation and the limbic system play a significant role in the motivational-affective dimension. The paleospinothalamic tract supplies the nerves with multiple synapses in the reticular system. These nerves do not carry spatial or temporal information because target cells in the brain stem and cortex have wide receptive fields covering half or more of the body surface. Effects of sight and sound on pain perception occur through connections in the reticular system. Escape and protective behaviors are mediated through the reticular-limbic system. This system acts as an intensity monitor and contributes to the quality of unpleasantness, mobilizes internal defenses, and elicits behavior geared to avoiding or stopping the distress.

Cognitive functions—memory, cultural values, and anxiety—also play a significant role in the perception of pain. A new pain with little associated damage may be perceived as severe because of the fear of the unknown, whereas a pain associated with greater tissue damage may not elicit the same degree of discomfort because its cause is familiar. This central cognitive system evaluates and analyzes input in terms of past experience, probability of outcome, and symbolic importance. This system facilitates or inhibits activities in the sensory and motivational systems by modulating activity of inhibitory neurons in the substantia gelatinosa.

The activation of the somatosensory cortices of the brain relates to the appreciation of intensity and affective quality of pain. Multiple ascending pathways from the spinal cord project to several cortical regions that mediate these effects. Nociceptive projections lead to the thalamic nuclei as well as to the limbic cortical areas such as anterior cingular and insular cortex (Fig. 3-6). The anterior cingular cortex is an important cortical area more closely associated with pain unpleasantness compared with the parietal cortices.[69]

Psychosocial events during the time the neuraxis is developing in an individual have an effect on the subsequent formation of linkages between spinal tracts. Pain pathways will be matured to a greater degree if pain is severe during the first 22 years of life. Those individuals who have experienced severe physical or emotional traumas (sexual abuse) during these years will be at greater risk of experiencing chronic pain.

Spinal Cord Reflex

Another important connection between nerves at the level of the dorsal horn is the synapse between dorsal horn sensory fibers and anterior horn motor fibers. Through direct synapse with internuncial nerves, input from sensory nerves stimulates motor neurons at the same or neighboring segmental levels. This stimulation may result in reflex action that causes an instantaneous contraction of a muscle or a more tonic contraction (spasm) with repeated stimulation of nociceptive fibers.

Descending Analgesic Pathways

In addition to the two distinct sensory pathways that transmit nociceptive signals to brain stem and cortical structures, the cortex and midbrain have descending pathways that modulate pain input at the level of the dorsal horn (Fig. 3-7).[71] Neurons surrounding the cerebral aqueduct of the midbrain and the brain stem raphe in medullopontine reticular formation terminate on interneurons present in lamina II (substantia gelatinosa).[25] The entire descending network extends from the frontal cortex and hypothalamus, through the periaqueductal gray zone to the rostral ventromedial medulla, and then via the dorsolateral funiculus to the dorsal horn of the spinal cord. The dorsolateral pontomesencephalic tegmentum is a parallel system projecting to the rostral ventromedial medulla that also

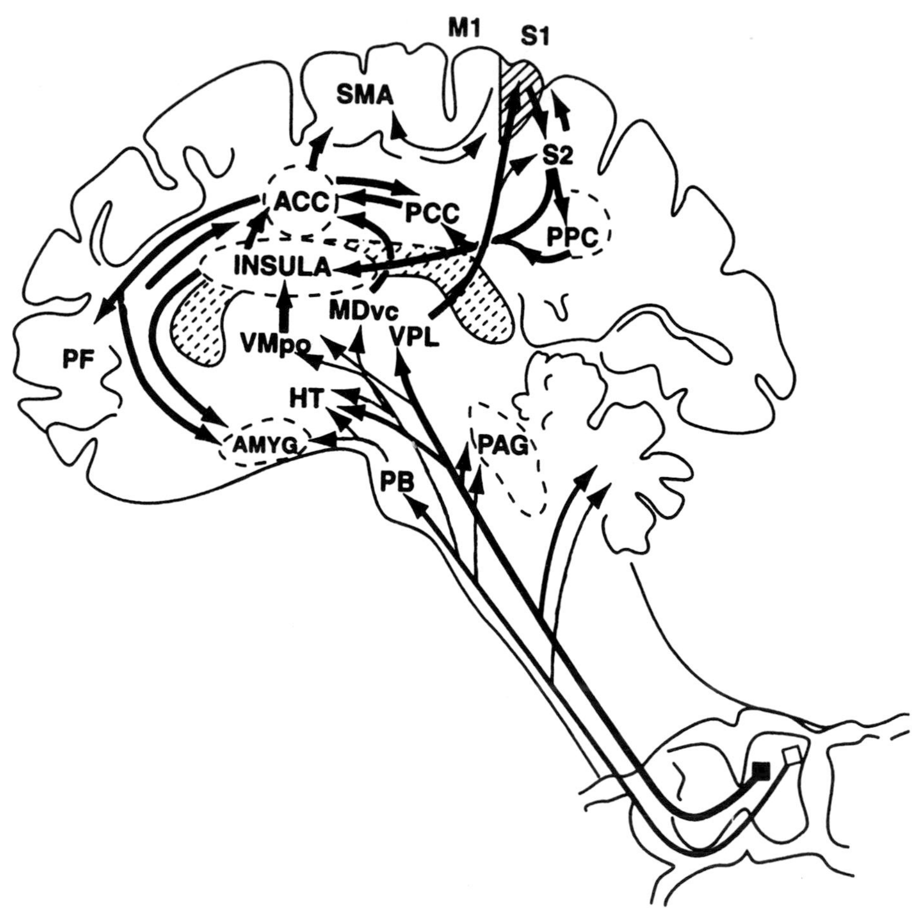

Figure 3-6 Schematic of ascending pathways, subcortical structures, and cerebral cortical structures involved in processing pain. ACC, anterior cingulated cortex; AMYG, amygdala; HT, hypothalamus; MDvc, ventrocaudal part of the medial dorsal nucleus; PAG, periaqueductal gray; PB, parabrachial nucleus of the dorsolateral pons; PCC, posterior cingulated cortex; PF, prefrontal cortex; PPC, posterior parietal complex; S1 and S2, first and second somatosensory cortical areas; SMA, supplementary motor area; VMpo, ventromedial nuclear complex; VPL, ventroposterior lateral nucleus. *(From Price DD: Psychological and neural mechanisms of the affective dimension of pain. Science 288:1769-1772, 2000.)*

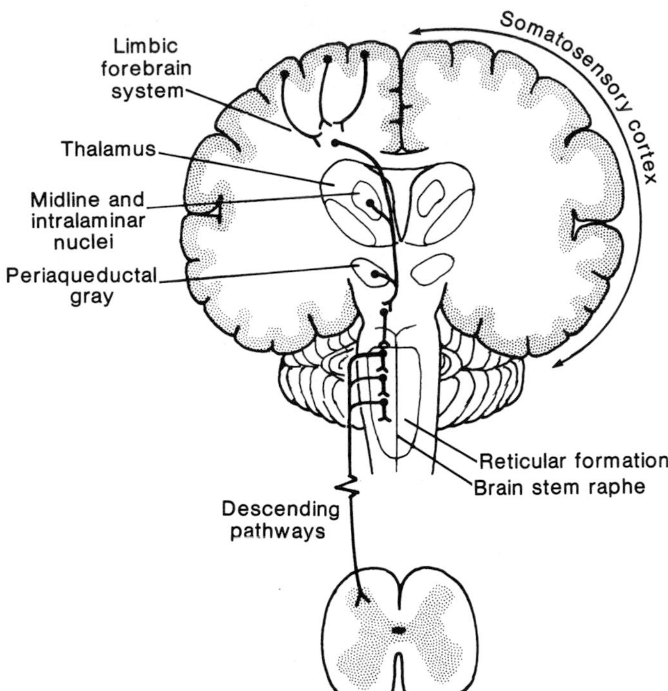

Figure 3-7 Descending pathways carry signals from higher brain centers through the periaqueductal gray and the brain stem raphe back to the dorsal horn, whereas its associated neurons release serotonin and inhibit pain transmission through nociceptive fibers.

modulates pain signals generated in the spinal cord.[26] The neurotransmitter for this descending pathway is serotonin (5-hydroxytryptamine). Serotoninergic cells activate enkephalinergic interneurons that exert presynaptic inhibition of the small unmyelinated nociceptors that produce substance P.

Endogenous Opioids (Endorphins)

The enkephalins, dynorphins, and beta-endorphins are the three major classes of endogenous opioids.[81] Leucine (leu) or methionine (met) enkephalins are pentapeptides (cleaved from proenkephalin A) that are secreted by neurons with opiate receptors.[3] The enkephalins are located in the dorsal horn and supraspinal regions, corresponding to the neurons with opiate receptors. Substance P is produced by unmyelinated nociceptive fibers.[36] The release of enkephalin inhibits substance P–sensitive nociceptors, decreasing the ascending signals. This inhibitory process relies on opiate receptors for its action. Naloxone, an opiate antagonist, temporarily reverses the analgesic effects of activation of the periaqueductal gray and raphe neurons. Two other descending analgesic fiber systems include neurons from the locus ceruleus (neurotransmitter—norepinephrine) and Edinger-Westphal nucleus (neurotransmitter—cholecystokinin). The exact location for the interaction of these systems and neurons in the dorsal horn is unknown.

Dynorphins are a group of molecules numbering between 8 and 17 peptides. Proenkephalin B is the precursor for these endogenous opioids. Dynorphin-containing cells are located in the periaqueductal gray zone, mesencephalic reticular formation, and medullary and spinal dorsal horns.[81] Intrathecal injection of dynorphins results in prolonged analgesia. However, the exact mechanism of dynorphins in the mediation of analgesia is not clear. The distribution of dynorphin-producing cells and cells with dynorphin receptors suggests both presynaptic and postsynaptic input on primary afferent neurons. Dynorphins affect nociceptive processing, but the range of dynorphin concentrations may result in a diminished or enhanced effect on analgesia.

Beta-endorphins range in size from 17 to 31 amino acids. Proopiomelanocortin is the precursor of beta-endorphin, along with adrenocorticotropic (ACTH) and melanocyte-stimulating hormones. Beta-endorphin neurons are concentrated in the basal hypothalamus, with axons extending to the limbic system rostrally, and the periaqueductal gray, midbrain, and locus ceruleus caudally. Effects of stress that result in the release of ACTH also cause the release of beta-endorphins. This is an adaptive response to potential injury. This same mechanism also causes sympathetic activation resulting in catecholamine release.

Opioid Receptors

Opioid peptides exert their effects on cell membrane opioid receptors.[81] These receptors have mu, kappa, and delta subclasses. Specific subtypes respond preferentially to different endorphins, which results in a variety of clinical effects. The delta opiate receptor binds leu and met enkephalin. Dynorphin binds to the kappa receptor. The mu receptors have high affinity for the endomorphins, two 4–amino acid peptides. An epsilon receptor is proposed for beta-endorphin.

The subclasses mediate different beneficial and detrimental effects. For example, the mu_1 receptor mediates pain relief, whereas the mu_2 receptor is responsible for respiratory depression. $Delta_1$ and $delta_2$ receptors mediate spinal and supraspinal antinociception, respectively. Delta receptor agonists have epileptogenic toxicities. Kappa receptors mediate dysphoric effects.

Spinal opiate receptors are 70% mu, 24% delta, and 6% kappa. Presynaptic receptors make up approximately 70% of all mu and delta receptors. Kappa receptors are localized to postsynaptic structures.

Opiate receptor activation results in inhibition of the associated cell's function. Activation of the opioid receptor results in activation of the G protein coupled to the receptor. Opiates open potassium channels or close calcium channels. These actions result in less transmitter release presynaptically, resulting in difficulty in reaching postsynaptic action potentials.

Gate Theory of Pain

In addition to the descending analgesic pathways, segmental input from myelinated mechanoreceptors that synapse with small-diameter nociceptive afferents inhibits pain transmission. The modulation of nociceptive input by massage, compression, or vibration of tissues is known as *diffuse noxious inhibitory control.* This effect is the cornerstone of the "gate theory of pain."[60] A limited amount of sensory information can activate ascending fibers terminating in the brain stem and cortical portions of the nervous system. A gate at the level of the spinal cord can swing open to allow nociceptive impulses or proprioceptive impulses to pass through. Stimulation of myelinated A-beta (mechanoreceptor) fibers inhibits (closes the gate to) transmission of A-delta and C nociceptive fibers. The substantia gelatinosa (lamina II), including wide-dynamic-field neurons, is the location for this interaction. This inhibition is not related to opioid receptors because this effect is independent of naloxone (narcotic antagonist).[76] The enkephalinergic interneurons and the descending inhibitory neurons also serve to close the gate to pain transmission.

The clinical correlation of pain moderation by proprioceptive stimulation is the practice of rubbing the area after it has been injured. This maneuver activates large low-threshold fibers, reducing the effects of small-fiber input to a level at which pain is less severe. The procedure of transcutaneous electrical nerve stimulation in diminishing pain is based on this principle. On the other hand, disease processes that diminish large-fiber input may magnify painful stimuli. Herpes zoster viral infection, which preferentially damages large-fiber vibratory dorsal ganglion cells, may result in hyperesthesia in the sensory field of the affected nerve secondary to the loss of large-fiber, proprioceptive input. Fibromyalgia patients may also have diffuse noxious inhibitory control that is deficient. Fibromyalgia patients are unable to tolerate a tonic stimulus of sufficient intensity to stimulate an inhibitory response.[51]

Visceral Sensory System

The sensory nerves for the thoracic, abdominal, and pelvic viscera have cell bodies in the dorsal root ganglia but do not use the spinal nerves to reach the target organ. Instead these nerves pass through the pathways of the sympathetic and parasympathetic nervous systems. The sympathetic trunks are longitudinal strands of nerve fibers and sympathetic ganglia that lie anterolateral to the vertebral column from the level of the first cervical vertebra to the front of the coccyx. The sympathetic trunk in the neck does not receive white rami communicantes, but it contains three cervical sympathetic ganglia (inferior, middle, and superior) that receive their preganglionic fibers from the upper thoracic spinal nerves via white rami communicantes, whose fibers leave the spinal cord on the ventral roots of thoracic spinal nerves. From the sympathetic trunk in the neck, fibers pass to the structures as postganglionic fibers in cervical spinal nerves or leave as direct visceral branches (e.g., to the thyroid gland). Branches to the head run with arteries, especially the internal and external carotid arteries (Fig. 3-8).

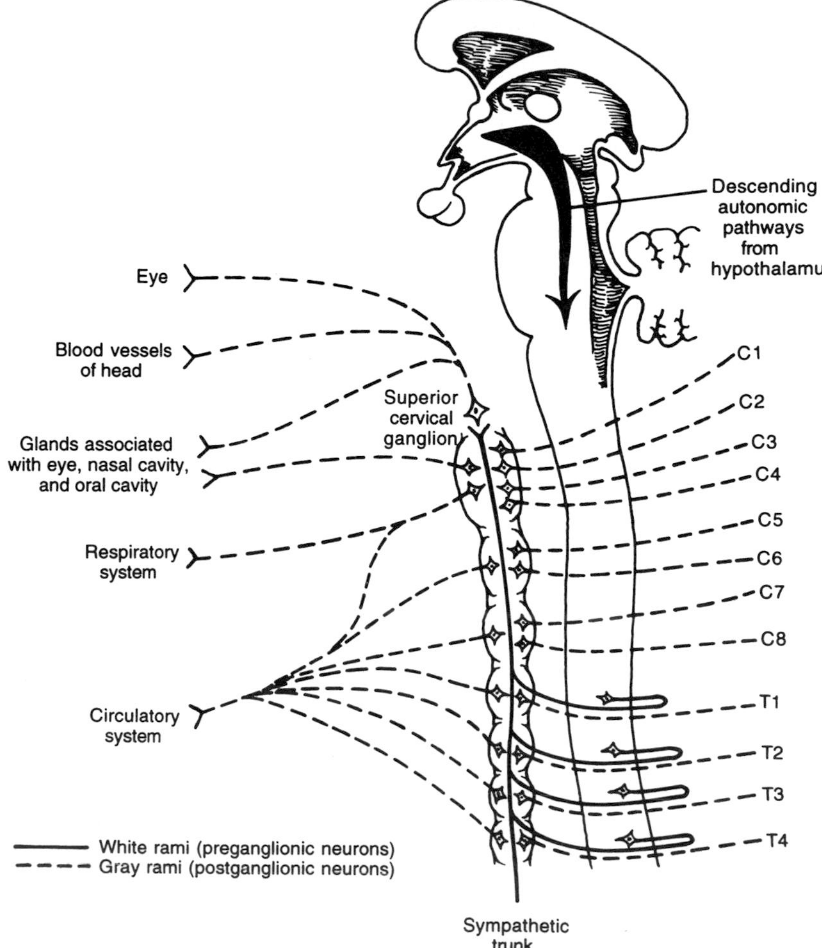

Figure 3-8 The sympathetic (thoracolumbar) division of the autonomic nervous system. Preganglionic fibers extend from the intermediolateral nucleus of the spinal cord to the peripheral autonomic ganglia, and postganglionic fibers extend from the peripheral ganglia to the effector organs as shown. Sympathetic outflow from the spinal cord is illustrated. The preganglionic fibers are shown in heavy lines, and the postganglionic fibers are in dashed lines.

The inferior cervical ganglion lies at the level of the neck of the first rib, where it is wrapped around the posterior aspect of the vertebral artery. It is usually fused with the first thoracic ganglion (and sometimes the second) to form a large ganglion known as the *cervicothoracic ganglion* (stellate ganglion). It lies anterior to the transverse process of C7, just above the neck of the first rib on each side, posterior to the origin of the vertebral artery. Some postganglionic fibers from this ganglion pass into the seventh and eighth cervical nerves and to the heart and the vertebral plexus around the vertebral artery.

The middle cervical ganglion is small and lies on the anterior aspect of the middle thyroid artery at about the level of the cricoid cartilage and the transverse process of C6, just anterior to the vertebral artery. Postganglionic branches pass from it to the fifth and sixth cervical nerves and to the heart and the thyroid gland.

The superior cervical ganglion is large. It is located at the level of the atlas and axis. Postganglionic branches from it pass along the internal carotid artery and enter the head. It also sends branches to the external carotid artery and into the upper four cervical nerves.

There are four paired lumbar ganglia, four paired sacral ganglia, and one single coccygeal ganglion. The sympathetic trunks are anterolateral to the spinal column, pass medially in the sacrum, and join centrally at the ganglion impar at the coccyx (Fig. 3-9). Arising from the thoracic and first two lumbar spinal nerves are white rami communicantes that pass to the trunk or ganglia. These rami allow the passage of peripheral processes of the visceral dorsal root ganglion cells to the sympathetic chain. These visceral sensory nerves do not synapse in the sympathetic ganglia but pass directly through them, each on its way to its visceral destination by way of the associated artery. The peripheral processes may ascend or descend through the sympathetic chain, eventually exiting through splanchnic nerves arising from the sympathetic trunk, which contain autonomic nerves with various functions. Thoracic segments on both sides form the greater, lesser, and least splanchnic nerves, which run from the thorax through the

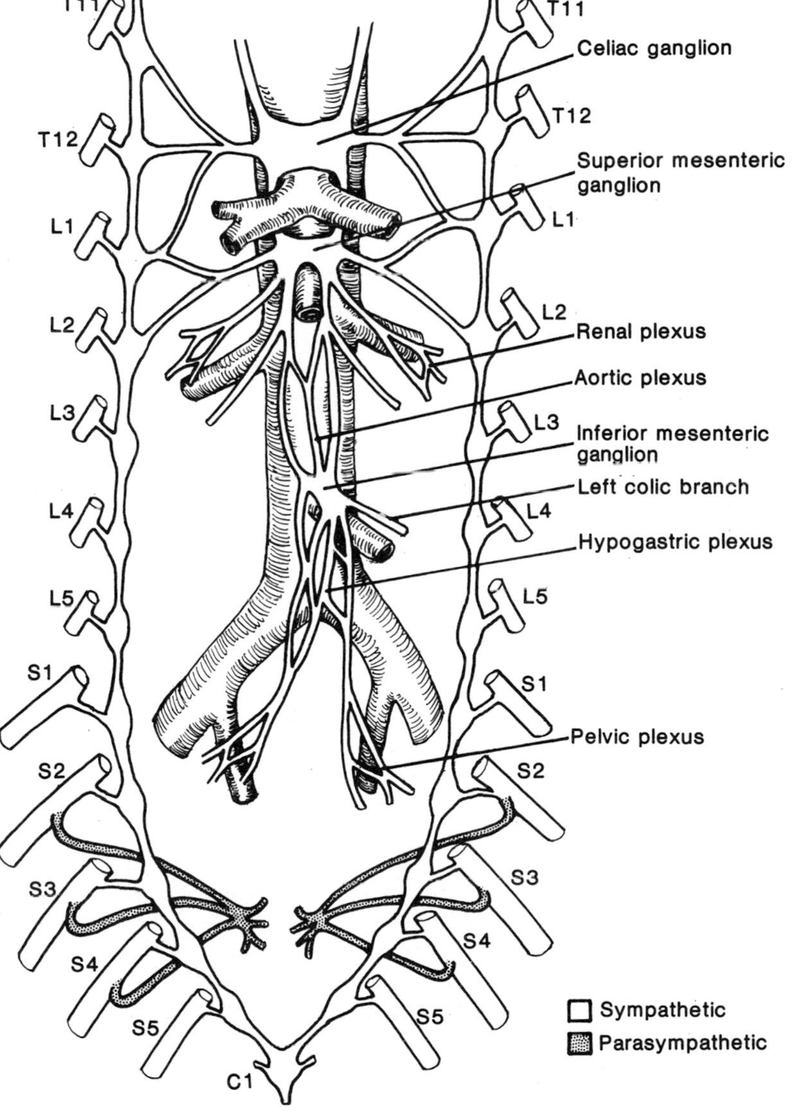

Figure 3-9 Sympathetic nerve trunks with bilateral ganglia at each spinal level are located lateral to the spinal column. The sympathetic nerves pass from the bilateral nerve chains to the aortic plexus, which consists of the celiac, superior mesenteric, and inferior mesenteric ganglia. The hypogastric and pelvic plexuses are located at the level of the aortic bifurcation and below. The parasympathetic nerves travel through the second, third, and fourth sacral nerves to supply organs in the pelvis.

diaphragm to the abdomen, reaching the aortic plexus. The preaortic plexus is a large, elongated, dense network of nerve fibers and ganglion cells located on the anterior aspect of the aorta and its branches. Increased densities of cells on the aorta as it travels to its bifurcation are arbitrarily designated *celiac*, *superior mesenteric*, and *inferior mesenteric ganglia*. Below the level of the bifurcation of the aorta at the fourth lumbar vertebra, the hypogastric plexus runs over the sacral promontory and passes into the pelvis, where it divides into bilateral pelvic plexuses that supply the rectum and genitourinary organs (see Fig. 3-9).

The parasympathetic autonomic nervous system also supplies sensory innervation to the pelvic organs. The cell bodies for the sensory parasympathetic nerves are, like the sympathetic system, found in the dorsal root ganglia of the corresponding segment. However, in contrast to passing through the sympathetic chain of splanchnic nerves, the parasympathetic nerves pass through the splanchnic branches of the third, fourth, and fifth sacral nerves (nervi erigentes). These nerves pass to the pelvic plexus and inferior mesenteric plexus (see Fig. 3-9).

The segmental innervation of a visceral organ is not dependent on its location in the fully mature human but rather on its embryologic segment of origin because sensory nerves grow into the viscera early in their development before they migrate to their final anatomic destination. An example is subdiaphragmatic irritation, which presents as referred pain to the shoulder. In addition, the organization of visceral afferents in the dorsal horn also plays an important role in the distribution of visceral pain. Visceral afferents synapse in lamina V with wide-dynamic-range neurons. These visceral neurons have a wide field of innervation. A single visceral fiber may synapse with a number of cutaneous afferents. Stimulation of the visceral afferent activates a wide field of cutaneous nociceptors whose activity is perceived as referred pain (see Fig. 3-8). The visceral afferents are also closely associated with activation of sympathetic and parasympathetic nerves. Stimulation of visceral afferents, in the appropriate circumstances, activates autonomic nerve fibers, resulting in, for example, vasoconstriction, vasodilation, flushing, or tachycardia. The field of activated nociceptors may be transmitted to several segmental levels, whereas somatic pain is transmitted to a single level.

Segmental Innervation

A brief review of the embryologic origin of the axial skeleton and the peripheral nervous system provides the anatomic background for understanding the clinical symptoms associated with disorders of the cervical and lumbar spine. By the end of the second week, the notochord forms on the dorsum of the embryonic disc between the endoderm and ectoderm. The notochord is the central framework of the spine and is eventually absorbed into the vertebral column where its remnants form the nucleus pulposus of the intervertebral disc. By the third week, mesodermal cells that parallel the notochord start to segment into individual somites. The somites subsequently differentiate into three primary parts: skin (dermatome); muscle, tendon, and ligaments (myotome); and bone (sclerotome). Simultaneously, the corresponding spinal nerve for each somite develops from the neural tube, supplying innervation for three components of the somite. As the skin, muscle, and bone develop and migrate to their final location in the body, each segment takes along its corresponding nerve supply in its cells. Structures from one somite, which includes parts of the neck, shoulder, arm, and cervical spine, and parts of the buttock, posterior thigh, leg, and lumbosacral spine, all may become painful if one component is damaged.

The embryologic organization of segmental structures is evident in the innervation of skin, muscle, and bones of the spine and limbs. The sensory nervous system is organized segmentally. Each dorsal root ganglion supplies a particular segment. Topographically, on the surface of the body, the segments are ordered into cutaneous dermatomes. The same dermatomes cover areas both in the cervical and lumbar spine as well as the upper and lower extremity, respectively. This organization may seem confusing when viewing the body in an upright position; the organization becomes clearer when the body is placed in a quadruped orientation (Fig. 3-10). Dermatomes stretch from areas in the cervical spine to contiguous areas in the upper extremity and lumbar spine to the lower extremity. The C6, C7, and C8 segments have no cutaneous branches in the cervical spine. They supply cutaneous structures in the arm situated between the C5 and T1 segments. The L4 and L5 segments have no cutaneous structures in the lower leg situated below L3 and S1 segments.

The distribution of these dermatomes is not absolute and may vary from individual to individual. The dermatomes overlap each other and extend slightly past the midline (Figs. 3-11 and 3-12). For deeper somatic structures (muscles, joint capsule, tendons), the sensory fibers correspond with the same spinal cord segment that supplies motor nerves to those muscles. On the other hand, as previously mentioned, the segmental innervation of the viscera that are supplied with visceral afferents corresponds with the level of embryologic origin rather than with the actual anatomic location. Table 3-4 lists the cutaneous, somatic, and visceral innervation for cervical, lumbosacral, thoracic, and abdominal structures. Figures 3-13 through 3-29 list the dermatome, myotome, and sclerotome for the cervical, thoracic, lumbar, and sacral nerves. Review of these figures reveals the extent of the innervation of structures from individual spinal cord levels and marked overlap among the levels. The complexity of innervation of the spine and surrounding organs occurs because of structural duplication and individual variation. It is important for physicians evaluating patients with neck or back, shoulder or buttock, or arm or leg pain to keep the overlap and variation of innervation from individual to individual in mind when evaluating referred pain.

CLINICAL INTERPRETATION OF SPINAL PAIN

The challenge for the clinician is to translate the patient's description of pain into anatomic and physiologic correlates that will identify the structure that has been "injured" and the pathologic process that has resulted in pain. Anatomically, structures of the cervical or lumbar spine receive specific types of sensory innervation that are asso-

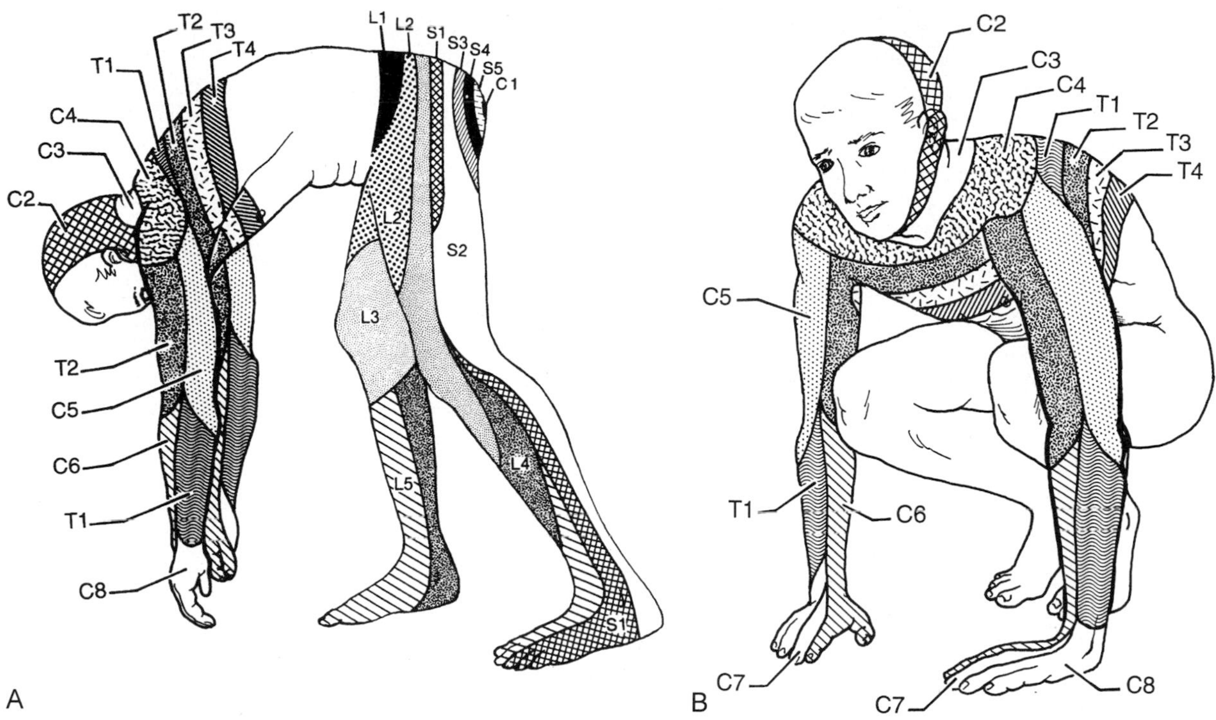

Figure 3-10 *A* and *B*, Organization of the cervical and lumbosacral dermatomes in the quadruped orientation.

ciated with distinct qualities of pain (i.e., sharp, dull, aching, throbbing, burning). An understanding of the quality of pain associated with pathologic processes in specific structures helps identify the source of the pain. In addition to quality, pain may be categorized by its intensity, location, onset and duration, aggravating and alleviating factors, and behavioral response (Table 3-5).[9,21,56] The sources of spinal pain are superficial somatic, deep somatic (spondylogenic), radicular, neurogenic, viscerogenic referred, and psychogenic.

Superficial Somatic Pain

The skin and subcutaneous fibers of the neck are innervated by nociceptive nerve fibers that cover small areas. Pathologic processes in the skin result in localized lesions whose intensity correlates with the extent of tissue distention and damage. The involvement of superficial tissues of the neck or back with trauma (laceration, burning, compression), ulceration, superficial neoplasms, or infections (cellulitis) is usually recognized rapidly because of location and is not of great diagnostic difficulty. The exception may be patients who present with the burning pain of herpes zoster infection prior to the appearance of vesicles. The acute onset and distribution in a dermatomal pattern should alert the clinician to this possibility.

Deep Somatic (Spondylogenic) Pain

The parts of the spine that are the sources of deep somatic pain are the structures of the vertebral column, the surrounding muscles, and the attaching tendons, ligaments, and fascia. Processes that mechanically disrupt these structures result in spinal pain. In addition, inflammatory processes that destroy tissue or increase tissue tension cause pain. Increased vascular pressure that results in distended vessels may also cause pain.

In general, with the exception of inflammatory and neoplastic processes, spondylogenic pain is characterized by a deep, dull ache that is maximum over the involved site. The pain is exacerbated by specific motions and is relieved by recumbency. The most common cause of spondylogenic pain is the production of high tensions in the muscles surrounding the cervical and lumbar spine, which leads to avulsion of tendinous attachments of muscles to bony structures or rupture of muscle fibers or tearing of muscles sheaths (sudden recruitment of muscle bundles when muscles are flexed and relaxed).[28] Pain associated with tendinous lesions is more severe than that associated with muscle injury proper. Either injury is associated with a sharp stab of pain at the moment of injury, followed by a dull ache that may persist for weeks along with tenderness on palpation and reflex muscle spasm. The initial pain originates in the unmyelinated nerve fibers that are stimulated by the mechanical disruption of the tendons, fascial sheaths of muscles, or the surrounding intramuscular blood vessels. The prolonged aching pain is a result of the same nerve endings being stimulated by chemical mediators associated with the healing inflammatory response.[88]

Muscle pain may occur in the absence of true muscle injury. Persistent use of muscle groups results in muscle pain and, potentially, tonic contraction (spasm). The chronic use of a muscle, which occurs more commonly in untrained than in trained muscles, results in increased metabolic activity and the production of chemical byproducts

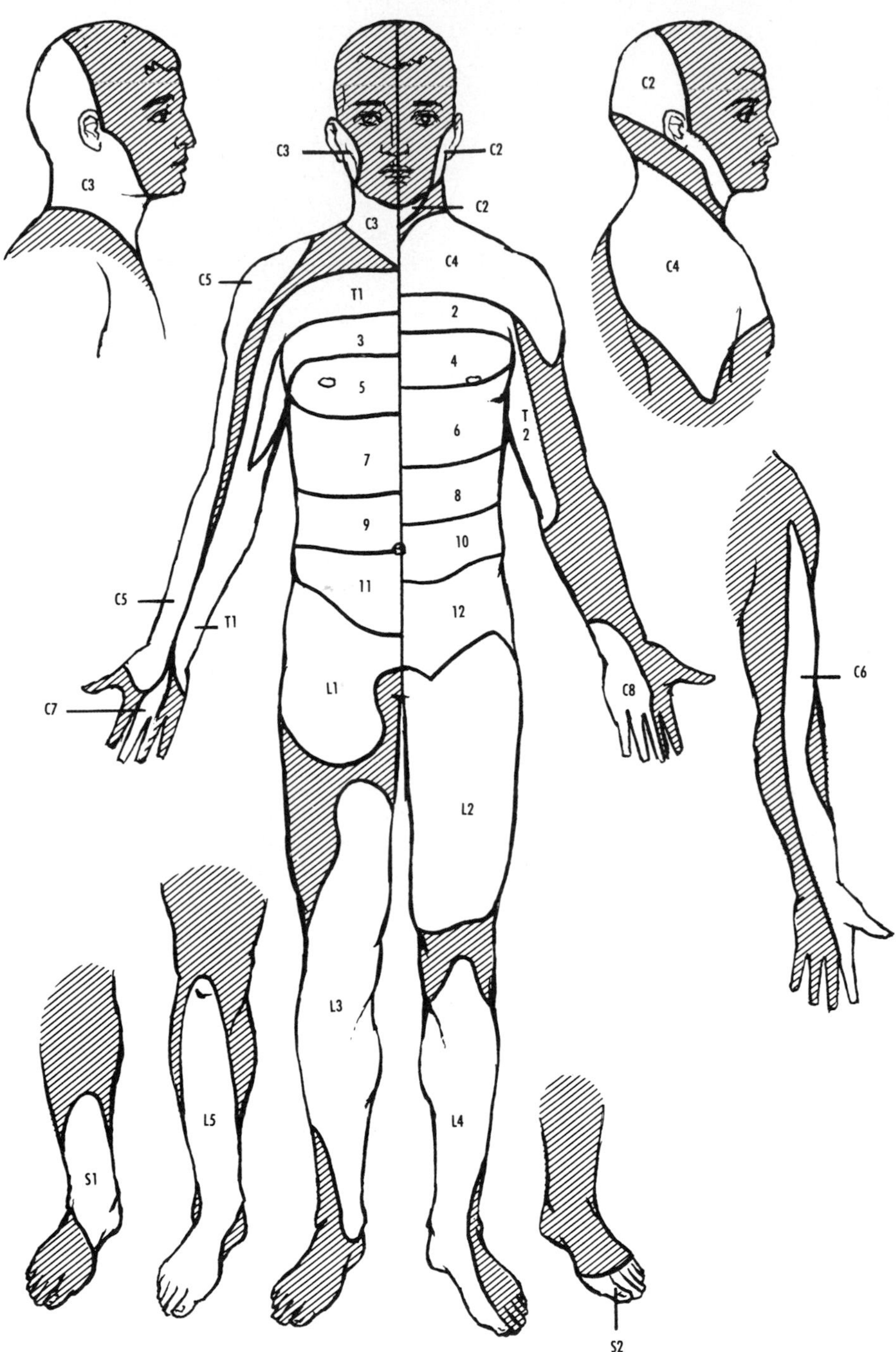

Figure 3-11 Dermatomal distribution (frontal view). The right and left halves show the total distribution of the alternating dermatomes, illustrating the overlap that may involve two or more dermatomes. The insets demonstrate the broad distribution of certain dermatomes. *(Adapted from Gardner E, Gray DJ, O'Rahilly R: Anatomy, 4th ed. Philadelphia, WB Saunders Co, 1975.)*

that may stimulate unmyelinated nerve fibers. These byproducts may include lactic acid and potassium. Physical factors (ambient temperature) and muscle training (sedentary vs. athletic) may explain the reason for spondylogenic pain in the person whose abnormal posture results in persistent contraction of posterior cervical muscles, as often occurs with poorly designed data entry environments for typists, or erector spinae muscles, as often occurs in pregnancy. With increasing fatigue, primary muscles are unable to complete physical tasks, necessitating the recruitment of secondary muscle groups, at a greater risk for injury. The endurance of muscles may be more important as a predictor of pain than absolute strength of muscles.

Muscle hyperactivity may also develop secondary to nociceptive input from nonmuscular sources. Pathologic processes resulting in inflammatory or degenerative processes in facet joints, periosteum, skeleton, or visceral organs may cause muscle pain. It is difficult to differentiate reflex spasm secondary to mechanical, structural abnormalities from inflammatory lesions of the cervical spine or viscera. Taking a careful history and physical examination may help in suggesting the primary source of tissue injury. Of great importance in separating traumatic muscle spasm from reflex spasm is a history of partial injury. However, an episode of trauma is not always remembered by patients. In other circumstances, patients

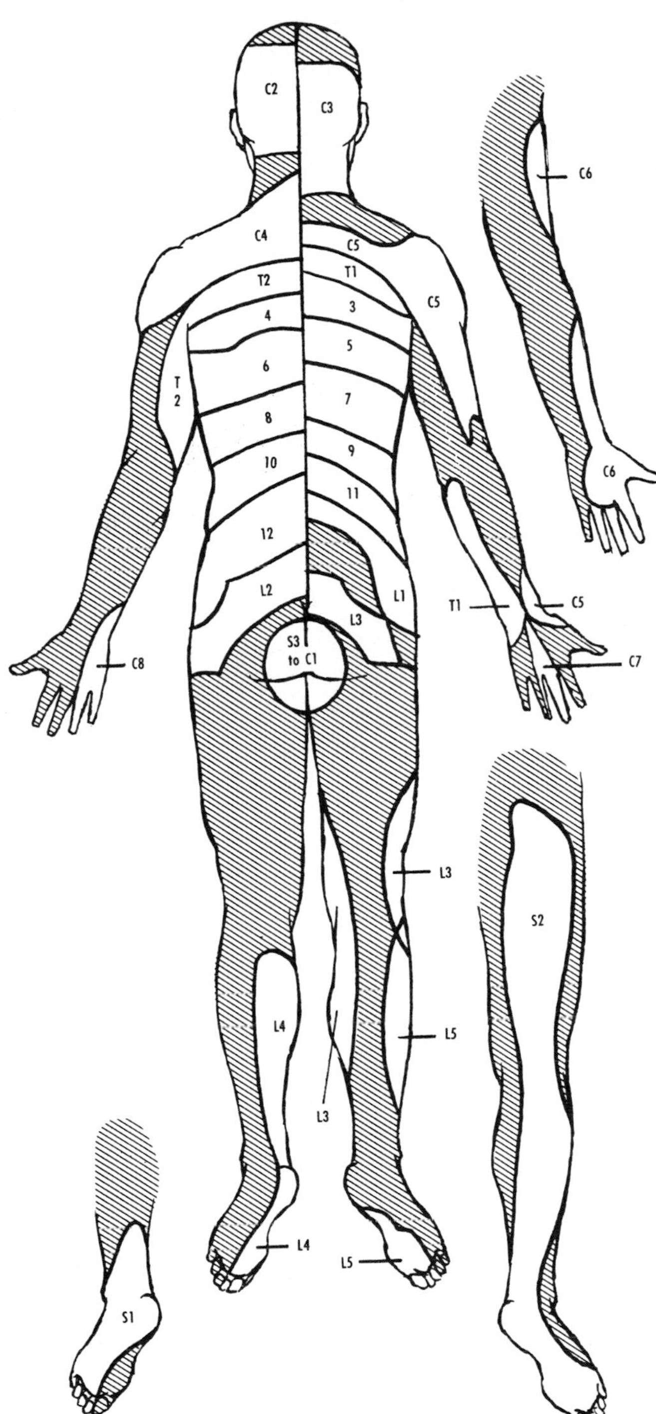

Figure 3-12 Dermatomal distribution (posterior view). *(Adapted from Gardner E, Gray DJ, O'Rahilly R: Anatomy, 4th ed. Philadelphia, WB Saunders Co, 1975.)*

ascribe their symptoms of muscle pain to an insignificant episode of trauma when in fact their symptoms are secondary to a more serious illness (metastasis).

Other sources of spondylogenic nociceptive input are the anatomic components of the vertebral column, including joints, ligaments, bone, vessels, and the dural and epidural structures. Mechanical injury and resultant inflammation of the apophyseal joint capsule and ligamentous structure of the spine may cause pain. Nerves that supply joints with sensory innervation frequently also supply surrounding muscle, bones and skin. There is usually an overlap of nerve innervation, with several nerves supplying a single joint (see Fig. 1-54 in Chapter 1). Terminal branches of unmyelinated and myelinated fibers are distributed through the synovium and periosteum. The joint capsule is richly supplied with sensory innervation. Sensory innervation to the joints includes mechanoreceptors in the joint capsule and nociceptors surrounding blood vessels and near the surface of synovial cells. The most painful stimuli to a joint are twisting, tearing, and stretching of the joint capsule or surrounding ligaments. The unmyelinated C nerve fibers of the posterior primary rami of multiple segments supply these structures. Therefore, patients have difficulty identifying the exact location for sources of their pain. Usually patients point to the midline or the occipitocervical joint area. Percussion tenderness does not cause as much discomfort in the joints as percussion over muscles in spasm. However, because of the distribution of the sensory and motor nerves, patients with articular and ligamentous disease may develop reflex spasm on both sides of the spine and cutaneous hyperesthesia over the same areas.

Mechanical or inflammatory processes may cause joint pain. Mechanical stresses that stimulate nociceptors in the joint capsule may occur secondary to prolonged sitting or standing in inappropriate postures (hyperlordosis with high-heeled shoes, soft chair, sagging mattress), atrophy of paraspinous muscles, excess joint motion secondary to decreased disc or vertebral body height, or malformations. Inflammatory diseases of the axial skeleton joints may cause the production of joint swelling along with release of inflammatory mediators that are irritating to nociceptors in the fibrous capsule. Structural changes affecting articular cartilage and synovium may not be associated with pain because these tissues contain no free nerve endings. The clinical correlate of this fact is the lack of relationship between the extent of structural joint changes on radiographic evaluation of the spinal column and the severity of pain.[52]

Another source of spondylogenic pain are ligaments surrounding the vertebral column and fascia that attach muscles to each other and bone. Although noncontractile tissue, the ligaments of the spine play an essential role in the static postural support of the neck and low back in the upright, sitting, and flexed positions. When the cervical and lumbar spine are in their normal configuration (normal lordosis), the ligaments stretch to a natural length that supports the neck and low back without muscular contraction other than what is generated by autonomic muscle tone. Pain is generated by nociceptors in the ligaments if they are placed under mechanical stress by poor posture, chronic contraction, excessive force, or a loss of elasticity due to aging. The same inflammatory disease that affects joints may also engulf ligamentous structures, resulting in pain that may spread beyond the margins of articular structures. The exact segmental distribution of pain arising from ligamentous structures is hard to define. Experiments injecting hypertonic saline into ligamentous structures have described locations of pain, but it is unclear whether the tension caused by the injection or the chemical irritation was the source of pain.[45] Whether pain

3-4 INNERVATION OF CUTANEOUS, SOMATIC, AND VISCERAL STRUCTURES OF THE CERVICAL SPINE, LUMBOSACRAL SPINE, ABDOMEN, THORAX, AND PELVIS

	Dermatome	Motor	Serosal Surface	Visceral
Cervical 1	Posterior scalp	Head flexors, extensors, rotators	—	—
Cervical 2	Lateral scalp	Head flexors, extensors, rotators Scapular rotators	—	—
Cervical 3	Anterolateral neck, clavicle	Head flexors, extensors, rotators Lateral flexors	Diaphragm	Heart, apex of lung, diaphragm, distal esophagus
Cervical 4	Shoulder, clavicle	Head and neck flexors and extensors Lateral flexors	Diaphragm	Heart, apex of lung, diaphragm, gallbladder, distal esophagus
Cervical 5	Arm	Shoulder flexors, abductors, adductors Scapular elevators	Diaphragm	Heart, apex of lung, diaphragm, gallbladder, aorta, distal esophagus
Cervical 6	Arm	Wrist extensors Arm adductors Forearm flexors and pronators	—	Heart, gallbladder, aorta
Cervical 7	Hand, forearm	Arm adductors Forearm extensors Wrist flexors Finger extensors	—	Aorta
Cervical 8	Hand, forearm	Finger flexors, abductors, adductors	—	—
Thoracic 1	Forearm	Finger abductors, adductors	—	—
Lumbar 1	Groin Level of L1 vertebral body descending to flanks	Iliopsoas	Anterior and lateral abdominal wall	Kidney, ureter, body of uterus, abdominal aorta, small intestine
Lumbar 2	Anterior thigh Level of L2–L3 vertebral body to lateral thigh (L5 dura—posterior longitudinal ligament)	Iliopsoas, sartorius, adductors	Posterior abdominal wall	Vault of bladder, abdominal aorta, ascending colon
Lumbar 3	Lower anterior thigh to anterior knee Level of L4–L5 vertebral body	Iliopsoas, quadriceps femoris, sartorius, adductors	Posterior abdominal wall	Abdominal aorta
Lumbar 4	Inner calf to medial portion of foot (first two toes)	Tibialis posterior, quadriceps femoris, gluteus medius, gluteus minimus, tensor fasciae latae	Posterior abdominal wall	Abdominal aorta
Lumbar 5	Dorsum of foot and big toe (lateral side of lower leg)	Tibialis anterior, extensor hallucis longus, gluteus maximus, hamstring, extensor digitorum longus	—	—
Sacral 1	Sole, heel, and lateral edge of foot	Gastrocnemius, gluteus maximus, hamstring, foot muscles, peroneus longus, peroneus brevis	Pelvic walls	—
Sacral 2	Posterior medial lower and upper leg	Flexor digitorum longus, hallucis longus Foot muscle	Pelvic walls	—
Sacral 3	Medial portions of buttocks	—	Pelvic walls	Rectum, upper anus, base of bladder, cervix, upper vagina, prostate
Sacral 4	Perirectal	—	Pelvic walls	Rectum, upper anus, base of bladder, cervix, upper vagina, prostate
Sacral 5	Perirectal	—	Pelvic walls	—
Coccyx 1	Tip of coccyx	—	Pelvic walls	—

C1

DERMATOME
- Posterior scalp
- Retro-orbital area
- Forehead

MYOTOME
Muscles
- Head flexors
- Head extensors
- Head rotators

SCLEROTOME
Bones
- Atlas
- Occiput

Ligaments
- Atlanto-occipital
- Medial atlanto-occipital
- Alar
- Apical dental
- Cruciform
- Accessory atlantoaxial
- Articular capsule
- Nuchal
- Atlanto-occipital (anterior, posterior)

(Pain perceived: forehead, retro-orbital area, and temple)

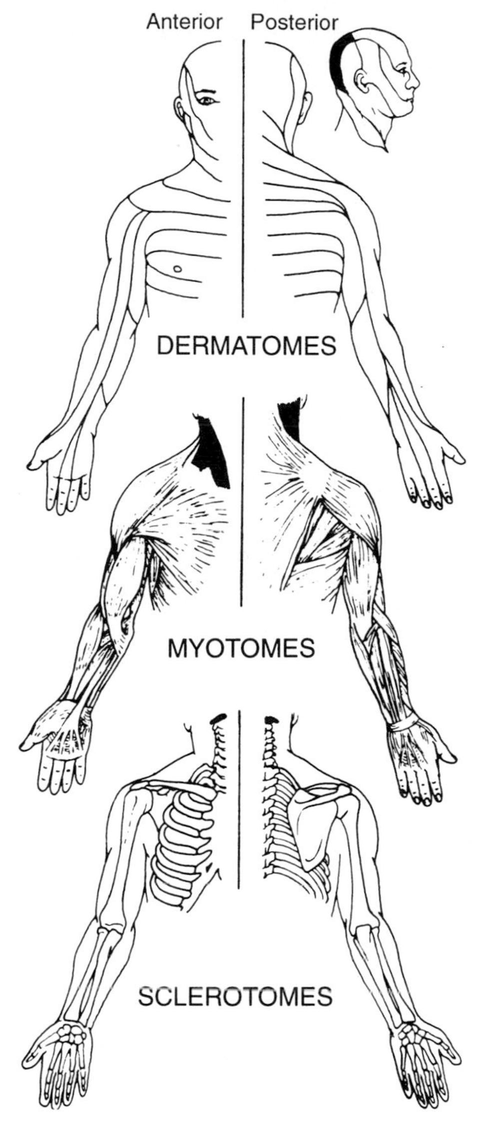

Figure 3-13 Dermatome, myotome, and sclerotome distribution for C1.

generated in this fashion is the same as pain generated by a mechanical injury is conjecture because pain is related not only to the location of injury but also to the form of the noxious stimulus.

Bone pain is particularly intense when the periosteum is disrupted. Mechanical trauma, crush fractures, neoplasms, or infections may be causes of pain. For example, spinal extension may cause pain by impaction of contiguous spinous processes or an inferior articular process on the lamina below. Pain from a vertebral body may be insignificant despite destruction and replacement of trabecular bone if the process is slowly progressive and does not cause fractures or irritation of the periosteum. Once bone has been replaced to a significant degree, minor trauma may result in a pathologic fracture and intense pain.

Another potential cause of somatic spine pain is the distention of veins of the vertebral plexus.[88] Nociceptive fibers supply the venous plexus. When sufficiently stretched by prolonged coughing, vomiting, parturition, or obstructed micturition, these fibers produce a dull, deep pain that may be associated with headache. In patients with herniated nucleus pulposus or intraspinal tumor, a moderate degree of increased pressure may provoke or exacerbate existing pain. These are patients who describe increased neck or back pain secondary to coughing or straining with a bowel movement.

The nociceptive innervation of the dura explains the association of pain with pathologic processes affecting the anterior dural membrane. The posterior dura has no nociceptive innervation. The anterior dura and the dural sleeves, which extend into the neural foramina, are densely innervated. Pain associated with dural lesions is of a deep, aching quality, located near the midline.

The annulus fibrosus receives nociceptive innervation, which is limited to the outer fibers of the annulus. Tears of the annulus fibrosus produce somatic pain that is predominantly located in the central neck or low back. Abnormalities of the nucleus pulposus unassociated with disruption of annular fibers are devoid of pain. The nucleus pulposus does not receive any sensory innervation.

Kuslich and colleagues reported their observations made during lumbar disc procedures performed under progressive local anesthesia on the pain sensitivity of various

C2

DERMATOME
- Scalp (lateral, posterior)
- Jaw area
- External ear
- Anterolateral area

MYOTOME
Muscles
- Head flexors
- Head extensors
- Head rotators
- Scapular rotators

SCLEROTOME
Bones
- Atlas
- Axis

Joints
- Intervertebral
- Atlantoaxial

Ligaments
- Anterior longitudinal
- Atlantoaxial
- Capsular
- Cruciform

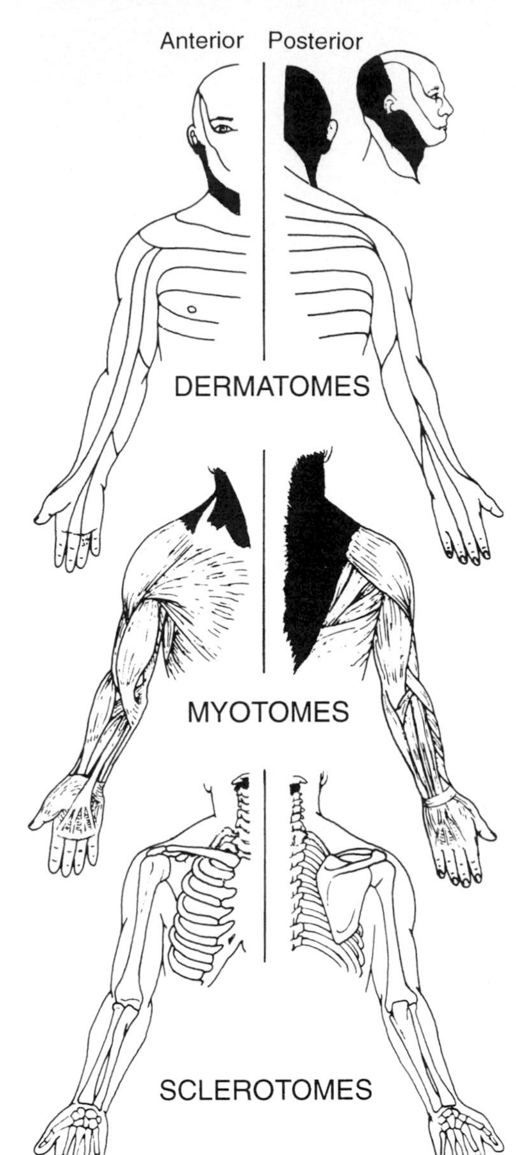

Figure 3-14 Dermatome, myotome, and sclerotome distribution for C2.

structures in the lumbar spine.[49] Compressed and inflamed nerve roots were painful. The ventral dura mater, posterior longitudinal ligament, and annulus fibrosus were frequently pain sensitive. Lesions on the left side of the annulus caused left-sided back pain, and right-sided lesions caused right-sided back pain. The facet capsule, articular cartilage, and bone were less often pain sensitive. These patterns of pain lend evidence in support of sclerotomal sensory innervation.

Radicular Pain

The source of radicular pain is not the peripheral sensory nerves but the proximal spinal nerves that form from the ventral and dorsal roots. Processes that decrease blood flow to the spinal nerve (ischemia) cause radicular pain. The large mechanoreceptor fibers, because of their large diameters, have greater metabolic activity and are more sensitive to disturbances of blood flow. This results in the loss of inhibitory pain impulses, allowing for preferential nociceptive input into the dorsal horn. Another mechanism of pain production is inflammatory chemical irritation. Traction on a normal, noninflamed nerve root does not produce pain. However, slight tension on an inflamed root is associated with production of radicular pain.

Radicular pain has a lancinating, shooting, burning, sharp, tender quality that may radiate from the neck to the arm and hand, or from the back to the leg and the foot, in the distribution of the compromised spinal nerve. This pain that radiates from the neck to the arm is commonly called *brachialgia*. In addition to arm pain, achiness and spasm may be experienced in neck and shoulder muscles. In the lumbar spine, pain radiating from the back, to the leg, to the foot, is called *sciatica*. Additional pain is experienced in the thigh and calf muscles. Radicular pain is exac-

Figure 3-15 Dermatome, myotome, and sclerotome distribution for C3.

C3

DERMATOME
- Posterior, anterolateral neck
- Posterior scalp
- Clavicle

MYOTOME
Muscles
- Head flexors
- Head extensors
- Head rotators
- Lateral flexors

SCLEROTOME
Bones
- Vertebrae axis-C3

Joints
- Discs
- Luschka
- Sternoclavicular
- Zygapophyseal

Ligaments
- Anterior, posterior longitudinal
- Capsular
- Nuchal
- Ligamenta flava
- Interspinous

(Pain perceived: upper neck, jaw area, and anterior upper neck)

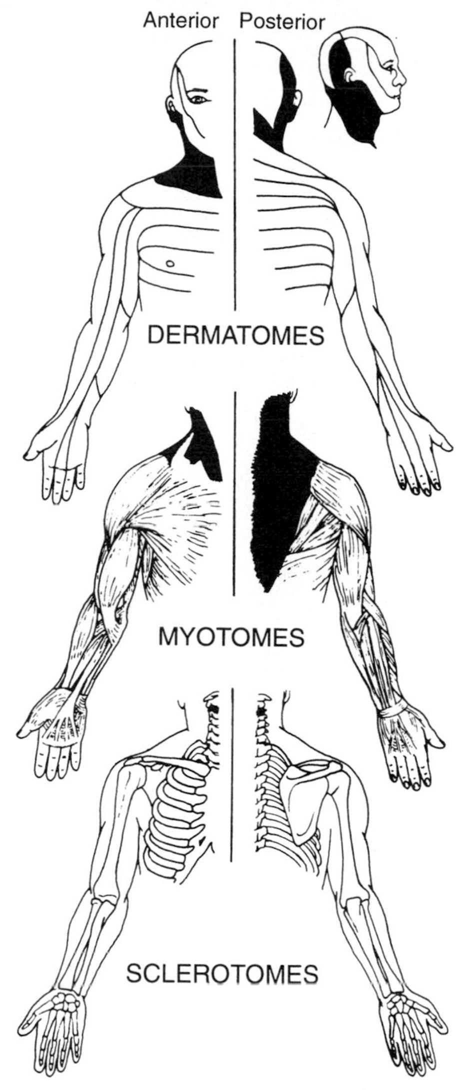

erbated by any motion that increases tension on the involved nerve root; immobilization and decreased axial loading relieve pain.

A frequent cause of compressive lesions, which result in radicular pain, are lesions of the intervertebral discs (most commonly the C5–C6, L4–L5, and L5–S1 discs). Factors that cause disruption of normal disc architecture facilitate degeneration of discs and increase the potential of rupture and the production of radicular pain. The majority of research in this area has involved the lumbar spine, and much of the work has been focused on the behavior of healthy and degenerated discs. The research effort has been multidisciplinary, focusing on biomechanical, biochemical, nutritional, immunologic, and nociceptive factors. A review of these factors helps in recognizing individuals who are at risk of developing this problem.

Disc Biomechanical Factors

Most of what is known about the pathomechanics of spinal disorders has been gleaned by studying the mechanical behavior of cadaveric spinal motor segments. A motor segment is composed of two adjacent vertebral bodies, the interposed disc, and surrounding structures. It seems clear that under flexion, extension, rotation, and shear stress, the load distribution in the motor segment is not confined to the intervertebral disc alone but is shared among the strong anterior and posterior longitudinal ligaments, the facet joints and their capsules, and the other ligamentous structures, such as the ligamentum flavum and the interspinous and supraspinous ligaments. In vivo, these same structures, as well as the muscle and fascial attachments intrinsic and extrinsic to the vertebral column, interact to accommodate the load-bearing requirements of the cervical and lumbar spine.

When pure compressive loads are progressively applied to an intervertebral disc, the vertebral endplate gives way before the nucleus pulposus herniates. The disc itself behaves like a viscoelastic structure and protrudes circumferentially. It should be appreciated that there is no difference in the failure pattern between normal and degenerated intervertebral discs.

It has been suggested that abnormal torsional stresses, applied particularly to the lordotic motion segments, may be the mechanism by which radial and circumferential fissures are produced within the annulus fibrosus.

C4

DERMATOME
- Summit of shoulder
- Region of clavicle
- Anterolateral neck

MYOTOME
Muscles
- Head and neck flexors
- Head and neck extensors
- Lateral flexors

SCLEROTOME
Bones
- Clavicle
- Vertebrae C3-C4

Joints
- Discs
- Luschka
- Zygapophyseal
- Sternoclavicular

Ligaments
- Anterior, posterior longitudinal
- Capsular
- Nuchal
- Ligamenta flava
- Interspinous

(Pain perceived: posterior neck, scapular area, high thoracic spine)

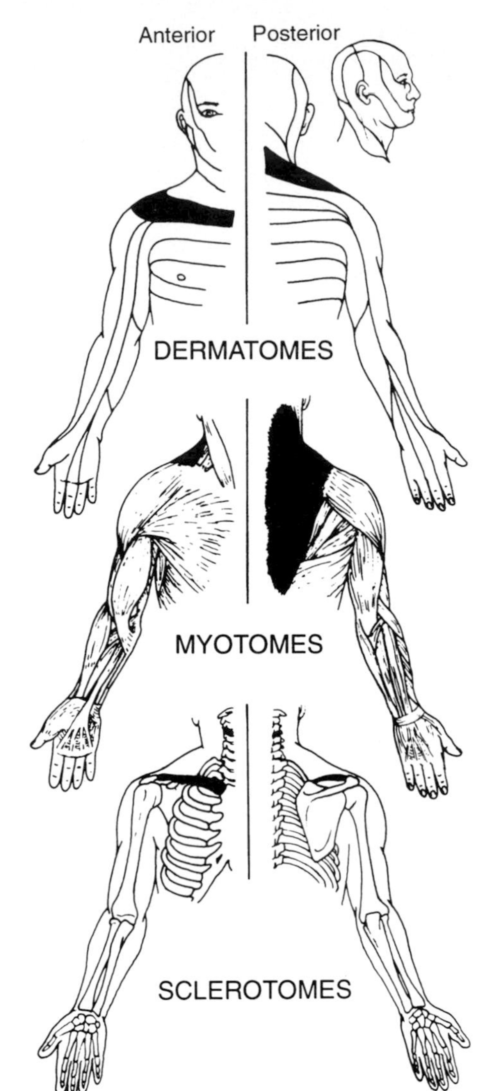

Figure 3-16 Dermatome, myotome, and sclerotome distribution for C4.

Furthermore, these fissures tend to occur in the posterolateral segments of the annulus because of the eccentric geometry of the intervertebral disc. The effects of this torsional stress concentration are also intensified in the presence of asymmetry of the facet joints as well as when there is advanced degeneration of the disc. In these situations the disc tends to fail after a few degrees of torsion.

Under tension, the disc is strongest in the anterior and posterior regions and weakest in the center. It is somewhat paradoxical to note that the tensile strength of the annulus has been found to be greatest in its posterolateral segment, which is usually the location where the nucleus pulposus herniates. This is the location where the posterior longitudinal ligament is weakest.

Most of the biomechanical knowledge of the cervical and lumbar spine deals with the normal and abnormal function of the intervertebral disc. The bony elements have only recently been evaluated. It appears that the anterior elements provide the major support for the spinal column and absorb various impacts. The posterior structures share some of the loads, but they mainly influence the potential patterns of motion.

The facet joints resist most of the intervertebral shear force and in lordotic postures share in resisting intervertebral compression. The facet joints also serve to prevent excessive motion from damaging the discs. In particular, the posterior annulus is protected in torsion by the facet surfaces and in flexion by the capsular ligaments of the facet joints.

Krismer and associates completed a study to determine the relative importance of anterior and posterior elements in disc herniation.[48] This cadaveric study measured the rotational movement of six spinal segments with an intact disc, a disc with dissected annular fibers angled in one direction, and after bilateral facetectomy. In another six segments, bilateral facetectomy was performed before annular dissection. The rotational motion was greater with dissection of the annular fibers than with bilateral facetectomy. In normal discs, the annular fibers restrict axial rotation more than the facet joints. The initiating event in the process of degeneration of the lumbar motion segment is loss of annular fibers. With greater rotational forces, the facet joints degenerate secondarily.

The configuration of vertebral endplates may also have biomechanical consequences for disc herniation.[33]

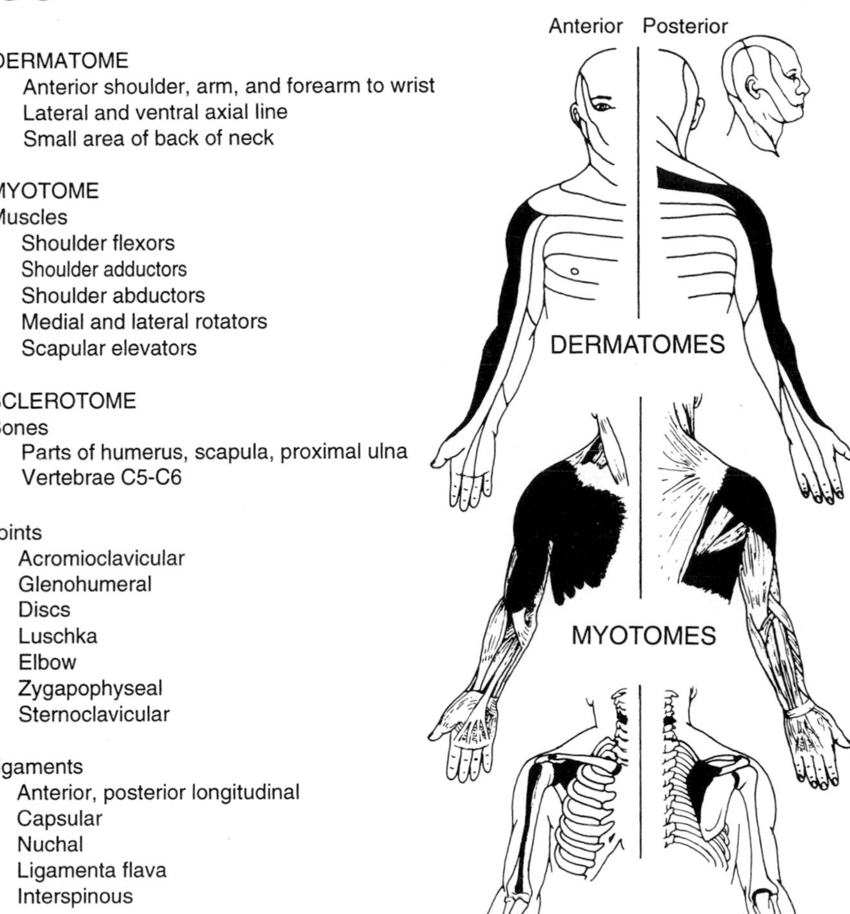

Figure 3-17 Dermatome, myotome, and sclerotome distribution for C5.

The law of Laplace states that tension in a fluid-filled tube is directly related to the radius, or in an ovoid tube, to the radius of curvature. Harrington and colleagues suggested that rounder endplates would be associated with a greater risk of disc herniation.[33] Evaluation of 97 computed tomographic scans revealed a strong association between a rounder endplate shape (L4–L5, L5–S1) ($P < 0.000001$) and disc area (L5–S1) ($P < 0.018$) with disc herniation.

Disc Biochemical Factors

On a microscopic level, the intervertebral disc consists of two adjacent hyaline cartilage endplates, an annulus fibrosus composed of collagen fibers obliquely aligned in layered sheets at angles varying between 40 degrees and 80 degrees, and a nucleus pulposus consisting of a loosely arranged network of collagen fibers and cells in an extracellular matrix. The annular fibers are attached to the endplates and, for a short distance, into the vertebral bodies. The annulus is thicker anteriorly than posteriorly and gradually thins out as it approaches the nucleus pulposus internally.

To function efficiently, the disc depends largely on the physical properties of the nucleus pulposus, which in turn are closely related to its water-binding capacity. The higher the hydration content, the more effectively the disc functions. Unfortunately, the hydration of the disc drops progressively from early life, when the water content is 88%, to a level of 69% in the eighth decade of life.[22] Ultrastructurally, 99% of the tissue mass of the disc is formed by its matrix, which contains glycoproteins, proteoglycans, collagen, and other proteins. It is presently believed that structural insufficiency of the disc is accompanied by an alteration in this biochemical composition.

The bulk of the connective tissue matrix in an intervertebral disc is collagen. There are seven major subtypes of collagen identified in the intervertebral discs. The annulus fibrosus contains types I, II, III, V, VI, IX, and XI and the nucleus pulposus types II, VI, IX, and XI.[5] Type I, found predominantly in tendons, skin, bones, and ligaments,

C6

DERMATOME
- Upper arm and forearm lateral to ventral axial line
- Thumb
- Small area of posterior neck and shoulder

MYOTOME

Muscles
- Wrist extensors
- Arm adductors
- Medial rotators
- Forearm flexors and pronators

SCLEROTOME

Bones
- Parts of radius, humerus, first metacarpal, scapula
- Vertebrae C6-C7

Joints
- Glenohumeral
- Discs
- Luschka
- Elbow
- Zygapophyseal

Ligaments
- Anterior, posterior longitudinal
- Capsular
- Nuchal
- Ligamenta flava
- Interspinous

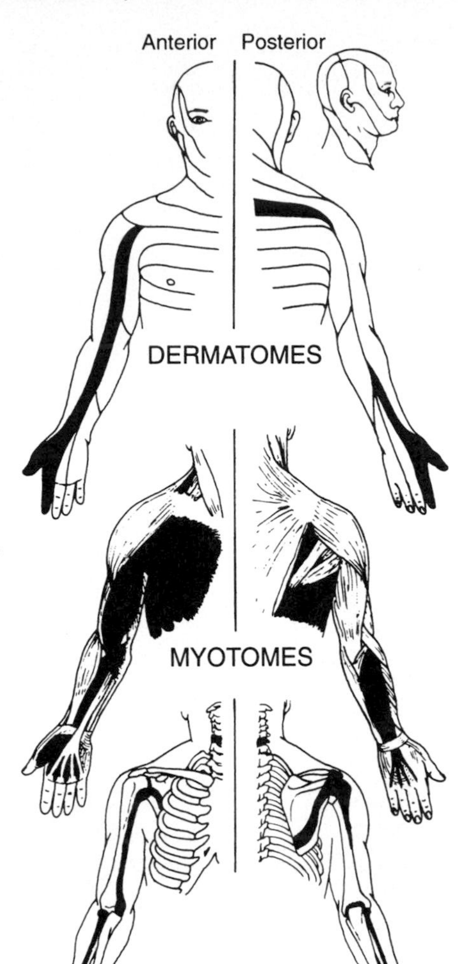

Figure 3-18 Dermatome, myotome, and sclerotome distribution for C6.

accounts for about 90% of the collagen in the body. Type II is absent from these tissues but is found in high concentrations in hyaline cartilage. In the human, the collagen in the annulus fibrosus is predominantly type I, with the remainder being type II. More than 80% of the collagen in the nucleus pulposus is type II. The significance is that type I collagen has a restricted water content and is thus better able to handle tensile stress; conversely, type II, with its hydrophilic physical properties, is ideally suited to absorb compressive forces. Types II, V, and XI are fibril-forming collagens. Type III is found in both the nucleus and the inner annulus fibrosus. Type V is distributed in noncartilaginous tissues in combination with type I collagen. Type V collagen forms a scaffold for type I, and these are copolymerized within the same fibril network in the annulus. Type XI copolymerizes with type II to control fibril diameter and may also serve as the site of binding of cartilage proteoglycans, heparin, and chondroitin sulfate. Type VI collagen is located in the nucleus pulposus and encircles interstitial collagen fibers, forming an independent network for organization of extracellular components, including proteoglycans. Type IX is found primarily in the nucleus pulposus and cross-links type II to bridge collagen fibrils covalently. In addition, collagens VI, IX, and XI form a porous capsule around chondrocytes that provides a compliant but inelastic barrier during compression. The interactions of the component collagens result in a three-dimensional meshwork of fibrils that influence the biologic properties of the disc.[5]

Nerlich and co-workers studied the age-related changes of collagen production in intervertebral disc.[64] The investigation determined the modification of distribution patterns of collagen types I, II, III, IV, V, VI, IX, and X, along with the production of *N*-(carboxymethyl)lysine (CML) as a biomarker of oxidative stress. A total of 229 lumbar motion segments from 47 individuals from fetal age to 86 years was the focus of the study. CML modification of extracellular collagen was first observed in the nucleus pulposus of a 13-year-old child. CML deposition increased with age and was accentuated in areas of macroscopic and histologic disc degeneration. CML deposition was followed with alterations in collagen-type pattern with initial increase in nuclear collagen types II, III, and VI and a subsequent loss of collagen type II, the manufacture of

C7

DERMATOME
- Dorsum of hand and forearm
- Dorsal and palmar 2nd and 3rd digits

MYOTOME
Muscles
- Arm adductors
- Forearm extensors
- Wrist flexors
- Finger extensors

SCLEROTOME
Bones
- Radius, ulna, humerus, scapula

Joints
- Discs
- Luschka
- Elbow
- Zygapophyseal

Ligaments
- Anterior, posterior longitudinal
- Nuchal
- Ligamenta flava
- Interspinous

(Pain perceived: below elbow in area overlapping and much larger than dermatome)

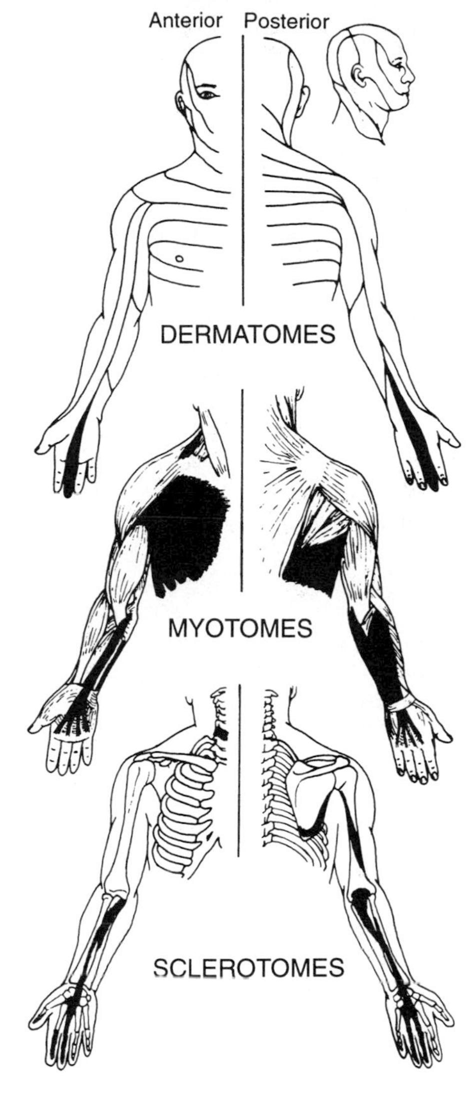

Figure 3-19 Dermatome, myotome, and sclerotome distribution for C7.

collagen type I, and the persistence of collagen types III and VI. The phenotypic expression of disc cells is modified in the pericellular matrix with early expression of basement membrane collagen IV in adolescents, changing to type X hypertrophic cartilage collagen in mature adults with increasing disc degeneration. Cumulative oxidative stress contributes to disc degeneration and alteration of repertoire of disc collagens. Therapies that lower oxidative stress may be helpful in slowing the progression of disc degeneration. Antoniou and associates have also described similar variations of collagen production in vertebral endplates at different ages.[2]

After collagen, the proteoglycans make up the major component of the extracellular matrix of the disc. These molecules consist of noncollagenous protein cores along with the attached sulfated glucose aminoglycans of chondroitin 4-sulfate, chondroitin 6-sulfate, and keratan sulfate. The proteoglycans are, in turn, attached to long chains of hyaluronic acid by small glycoprotein links. These molecules are found in great abundance within the nucleus pulposus but form only a small proportion of the dry weight of the annulus fibrosus. They are hydrophilic and therefore regulate the fluid content of the nucleus.

Proteoglycans are synthesized in chondrocytes. After the protein core is manufactured, up to 100 chondroitin sulfate and 50 keratan sulfate chains are added during post-translational processing in the chondrocyte.[5] The proteoglycan monomers aggregate as they encounter hyaluronate. The process of aggregation immobilizes the proteoglycans within the extracellular matrix. A link protein cements the proteoglycan to hyaluronate. Approximately 100 to 200 proteoglycan monomers are bound to a single hyaluronate chain.

Many age-related changes have been noted in disc proteoglycans. With time, these molecules lose their ability to associate with collagen, have a lower molecular weight, have a reduced aggregation potential, and develop an increased keratan sulfate content. These changes adversely affect the ability of the disc to imbibe water, which in turn decreases its capacity to dissipate energy when loaded. The changes in disc composition may also be related to topographic variations in the synthesis of disc proteoglycans.[6] Proteoglycan synthesis rates for annulus fibrosus in fetal discs are five times greater than for similar locations in adult discs. Synthesis rates are highest in the inner annulus for fetal discs and the midannulus for adult

C8

DERMATOME
- Ulnar aspect of arm and forearm
- Palmar and dorsal 4th and 5th digits

MYOTOME

Muscles
- Finger flexors
- Metacarpal abductors (thumb and little finger)
- Finger abductors and adductors

SCLEROTOME

Bones
- Parts of ulna, humerus
- 4th and 5th fingers (all bones)
- Vertebrae C7-T1

Joints
- Discs
- Luschka
- Zygapophyseal
- Elbow
- Wrist
- Hand

Ligaments
- Anterior, posterior longitudinal
- Ligamenta flava
- Interspinous
- Supraspinous
- Nuchal

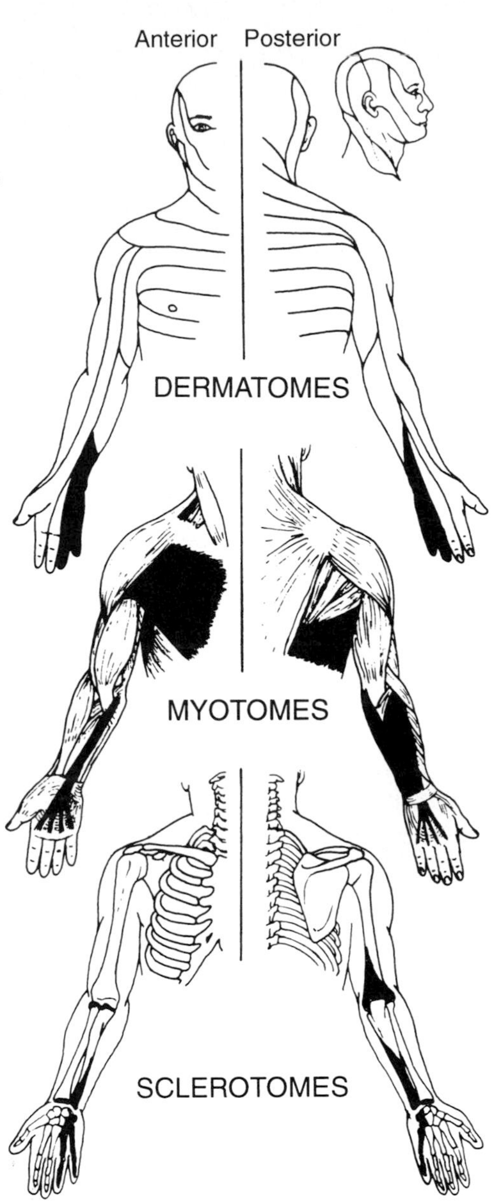

Figure 3-20 Dermatome, myotome, and sclerotome distribution for C8.

discs. Proteoglycans produced by fetal and newborn cells are larger than those of adults. Adult cells make smaller proteoglycan products that vary between regions of a disc. Adult proteoglycans also have poor aggregating properties compared with those from immature tissues.[42] The clinical correlate is that certain portions of an intervertebral disc are at risk of persistent injury secondary to inadequate production of proteoglycan. Injuries to the annulus fibrosus are unable to heal.[32] A greater understanding of the mechanisms by which chondrocytes synthesize and degrade extracellular matrix and collagen may help in differentiating between normal aging and pathologic degeneration of intervertebral discs.

Matrix metalloproteinases are other biochemical factors that play a role in the aging of intervertebral discs. Collagenase-1 (MMP-1) and stromelysin (MMP-3) are present in intervertebral discs. These enzymes play a key role in modifying disc collagens. A number of cytokines stimulate (interleukin-1) or inhibit (tissue inhibitors of metalloproteinases) metalloproteinase function. Control of these enzymes may offer a therapeutic means to delay disc degeneration.[29]

Disc Nutritional Factors

The intervertebral disc is a relatively avascular structure and, beyond 15 through 20 years of age, has no direct blood vessels. Diffusion is the main transport mechanism for disc nutrition in the adult. Small uncharged solutes, such as glucose and oxygen, mainly gain access to the metabolizing cells through the vertebral endplates. The diffusion of negatively charged solutes such as sulfates, which are important for proteoglycan production, occurs mainly through the annulus fibrosus. Because the area available for diffusion of these negatively charged solutes is smaller in the posterior region of the annulus, turnover of both collagen and proteoglycan is slower in this critical zone. It is believed that this nutritional inadequacy in

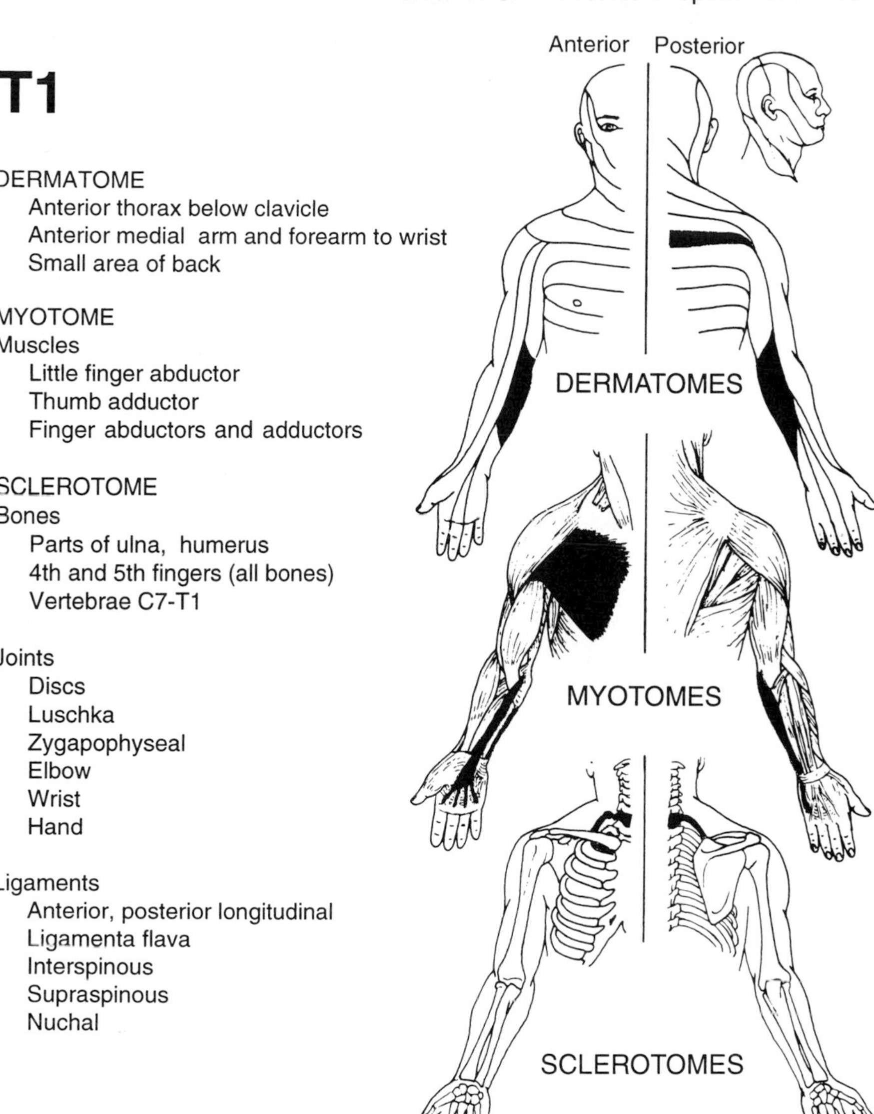

Figure 3-21 Dermatome, myotome, and sclerotome distribution for T1.

conjunction with the concentration of mechanical stress in the posterolateral annulus accounts for the high incidence of intervertebral disc ruptures in this area. Also, it is most likely that when fissures and cracks do occur in this area, even prior to the stage of rupture, the propensity for healing is liable to be low or inadequate at best.

Decreased oxygen concentrations throughout intervertebral discs result in increased lactate concentrations. The increased lactate levels result in decreased pH. The acid milieu causes decreased matrix synthesis and increased degradative enzyme activity. The eventual consequence of inadequate nutrients is degeneration and poor healing of disc constituents.[23]

In a tissue culture model, Horner and Urban demonstrated the effects of nutrient supply on the viability of disc chondrocytes.[37] With higher cell densities, the cells in the center of the culture died. The viable distance from the nutrient supply fell with an increase in cell density. Glucose was the critical nutrient. An acidic environment promoted cell death. Disc cells were able to live without oxygen for up to 13 days but were unable to produce proteoglycans. This model supported the idea that the number of disc cells is limited by nutritional constraints and that a diminution in nutrient supply reduces viable cells and promotes disc dissolution.

Disc Immunologic Factors

In its normal state, the intervertebral disc, owing to its avascular structure, seems to be an immunologically privileged site. However, as the disc degenerates, its chemical constituent parts are exposed to the host's normal immune defense mechanism, causing an autoimmune reaction to some extent. The phenomenon was first demonstrated in rabbits when it was found that their nucleus pulposus can induce the production of autoantibodies. This autoimmune reaction has been confirmed in the human, and there is particularly strong evidence that this sequestration within the spinal canal elicits a strong cell-mediated immune response to the autogenous disc material. Habtemariam and colleagues identified increased levels of IgM and IgG in the form of immune complexes in

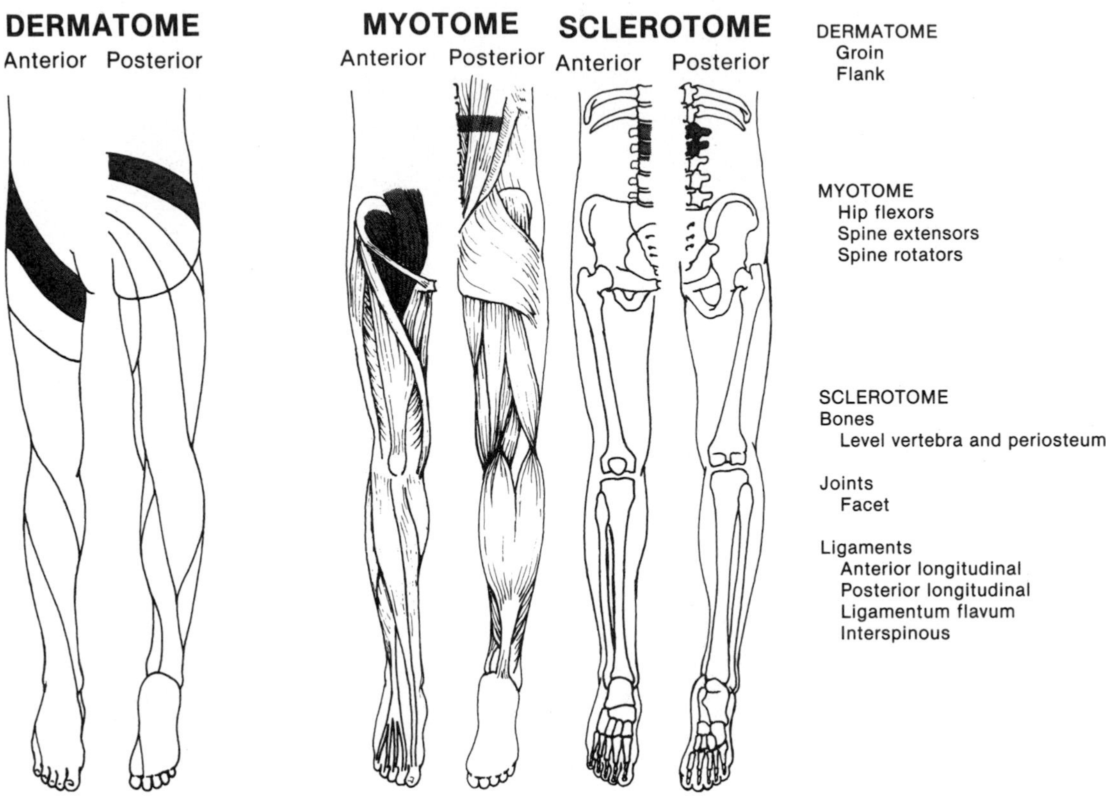

Figure 3-22 Dermatome, myotome, and sclerotome distribution for L1.

herniated discs compared to normal discs.[31] Satoh and coworkers studied the immunochemistry of eight patients with lumbar disc herniations.[72] Antigen-antibody complexes were observed in the pericellular capsule of herniated disc tissue compared with control disc tissue. However, proof has not been offered that the deposition of immunoglobulins or immune complexes causes disc herniation as opposed to an event that occurs in response to tissue damage.

Willburger and Wittenberg demonstrated the ability of tissues from intervertebral discs, apophyseal cartilage, and bone to generate mediators of inflammation, prostaglandins.[85] The capacity of these tissues to generate these metabolites does not equate with the presence of these factors in the pathologic states associated with spinal disorders.[30] Gronblad and associates measured phospholipase A_2 in normal discs, degenerated discs, and herniated discs. Neither degenerated nor herniated disc tissue samples had greater phospholipase A_2 activity than control disc tissues. In a parallel study, inflammatory lymphocytes immunoreactive for interleukin-2 receptors were identified in only 15% of disc herniations.

These findings can help explain, in part, the etiology of the acute radicular pain associated with disc ruptures. It seems clear that the mechanical compression on the nerve root that is being irritated by the herniated disc material is an important factor in the production of pain. As for the inflammation that occurs around the nerve root, no one is certain whether it is related to an autoimmune phenomenon, ischemic neuropathy from alteration in blood flow patterns, or defects in the neuronal transport mechanism of the nerve root itself. Regardless, it has been shown that inflammation is a necessary ingredient in the production of root pain from disc herniations. This was demonstrated by the use of thin silk threads that were passed around lumbar nerve root sheaths at times of surgery for the removal of herniated discs. The threads were brought out through the skin during wound closure. Postoperatively, when pressure was applied to the roots that had not been compressed by the disc herniation, the patient experienced only paresthesias in the dermatomal distribution of the nerve. There was no pain. When tension was applied to the inflamed root that had previously been compressed by the disc herniation, radicular pain was perceived. This perhaps explains the reason why many patients with radicular symptoms can be treated effectively with anti-inflammatory medications.[77]

Radicular pain may occur in the absence of nerve root compression secondary to nucleus pulposus extrusion. The nucleus pulposus may have properties that inflame nerve roots without direct compression. Olmarker and colleagues developed a porcine model of nucleus pulposus herniation without mechanical compression.[67] The epidural application of nuclear material to a nerve root

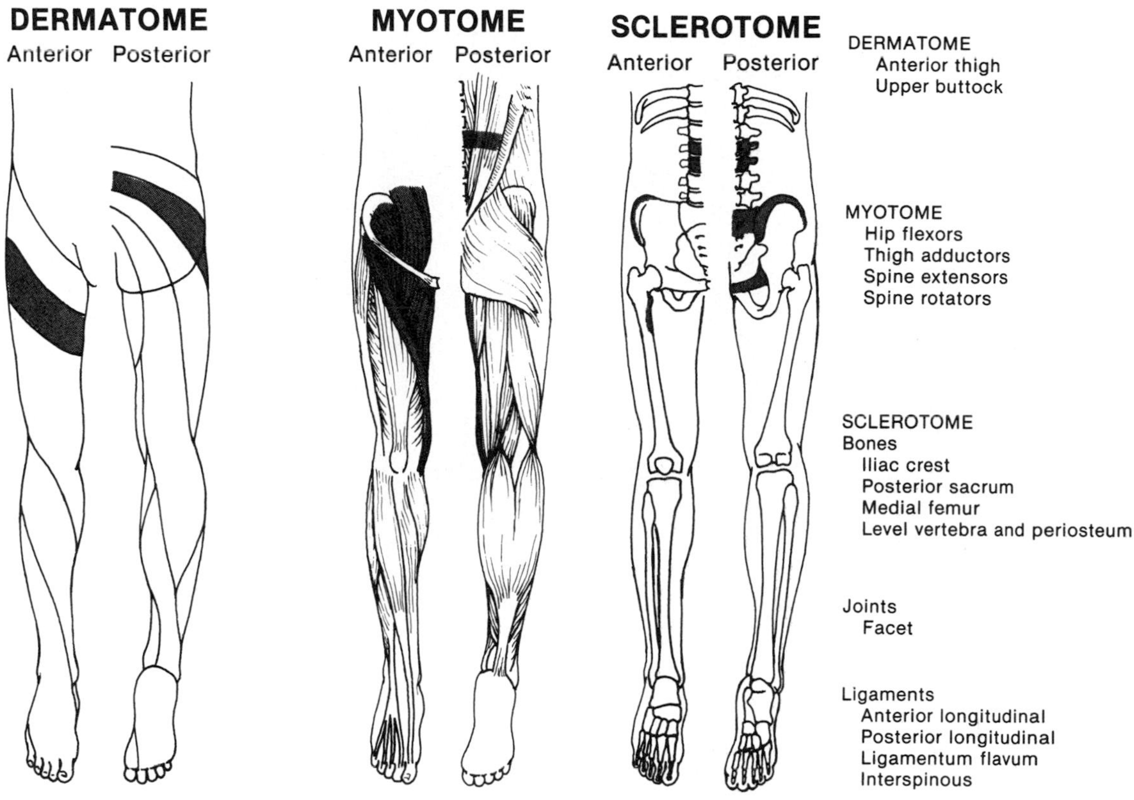

Figure 3-23 Dermatome, myotome, and sclerotome distribution for L2.

causes a pronounced reduction in nerve conduction velocity compared with application of retroperitoneal fat. Histologic evaluation of affected nerve roots could not explain the nerve conduction delay because of breakdown of axons and myelin sheaths in a minority of myelinated nerve fibers. This suggests that spinal nerve root dysfunction with disc herniation may be mediated by a number of factors, including autoimmune reactions, microvascular changes, and inflammatory phenomena independent of mechanical compression. The implication of this study is that nerve root dysfunction may occur without compression, suggesting that therapy of nerve root dysfunction may not always be improved by elimination of compression alone and should include anti-inflammatory drugs.

Additional work by Olmarker and Larsson has demonstrated the potential role of TNF-alpha as a mediator of nerve root dysfunction.[65] The porcine model revealed the nucleus pulposus as a source for TNF. Antibody directed to TNF limited the reduction of nerve conduction velocity generated by the application of nucleus pulposus to the cauda equina. In the same porcine model, TNF inhibitors (etanercept or infliximab) inhibited nerve fiber injury, intracapillary thrombus formation, and intraneural edema formation, compared to a heparin analogue (enoxaparin) or placebo. This study suggests that control of the effects of TNF on spinal roots has potential as a means of managing sciatica.[66]

Disc Nociceptive Factors

In the cervical and lumbar regions, free nerve endings supplied by the sinuvertebral nerve and posterior primary ramus provide sensory innervation to the anterior and posterior longitudinal ligaments, the facet joint capsules, the superficial lamellae of the annulus fibrosus, the dural envelope, the periosteum of the vertebrae, and the blood vessels. A review of the anatomy of the neural foramina elucidates the structures at risk from compression by a herniated disc.

As the nerve roots descend from the C4 level, they cross the disc immediately at the level of the foramen they exit. They enter the foramen below the pedicle and leave the foramen in a downward and forward fashion. In the lower cervical spine, the roots exit at a more horizontal angle and the T1 root exits in a slightly cephalad direction. By virtue of this configuration, the nerve is located in the superior portion of the foramen. The nerve carries the arachnoid along with it until the confluence of the ventral and dorsal roots, and the dura, which invaginates in the foramen. The dura continues along the distal nerve and forms the outer sheath, the perineurium. There is some question whether the dural sleeves are firmly or loosely attached to the walls of the foramen.[88] At the L1 level where the true spinal cord terminates, they cross the disc immediately above the foramen they exit.

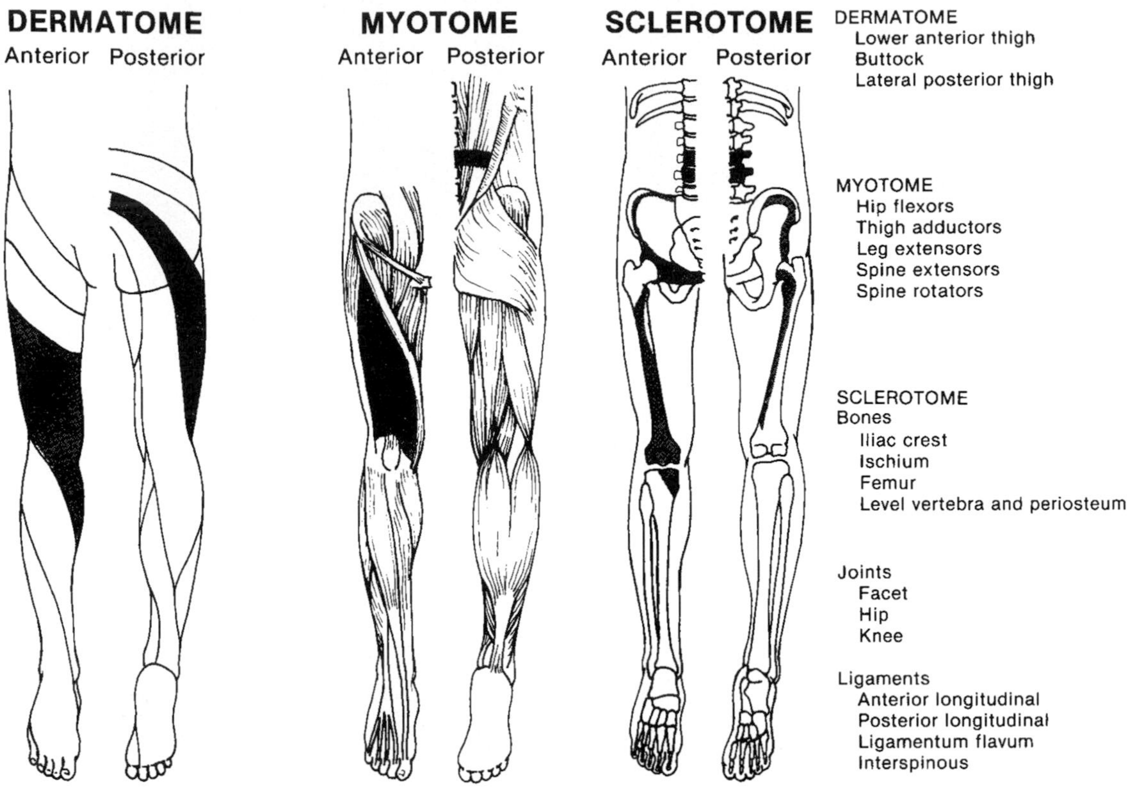

Figure 3-24 Dermatome, myotome, and sclerotome distribution for L3.

Flexion of the spine allows motion of these elements in the foramina. When tension is placed on the structures, the nerve will elongate, and the dura increases in tension. In the foramen, about 50% of the space is occupied by the nerve and its sheath. Connective tissue, adipose tissue, vessels, lymphatics, and the sinuvertebral nerve fill the remainder. The sinuvertebral nerve winds back into the foramen, supplying the posterior longitudinal ligament, fibrous tissue near the annulus, and the anterior but not the posterior dural sheath. The posterior dura has no nociceptive innervation.

In the initial stage of protrusion, the sinuvertebral nerve on the posterior longitudinal ligament is irritated, which gives rise to pain in the lower neck without brachialgia, or the lumbar spine without sciatica. As the impingement increases, the dural sleeves and nerve root are involved. As a result, neck or back pain becomes more severe and widely distributed. With greater pressure, pain in a radicular distribution is elicited along with paresthesias and numbness, and the motor fibers in the inferior portion of the spinal nerve are compressed, resulting in reflex muscle spasm. With greater duration and extent of nerve pressure, numbness replaces pain as a symptom and muscle weakness replaces spasm. Additional clinical features of herniated vertebral discs are discussed in Chapter 10.

It is known that not all radicular-like pain is related to disc herniation. Distention of degenerated lumbar intervertebral discs or facet joints with injections of saline or contrast material can produce pain in the low back that radiates down the leg.[35,62] This is not true radicular pain—it is referred pain that appears in mesenchymal structures of the same embryonic sclerotome in the injured tissue. When this type of pain is referred into the neck and arms, it has a dull, aching quality unlike the sharp, lancinating pain of true brachialgia.

Herniated vertebral discs are not the only cause of radicular pain. Overgrowth of bone from the facet joints intrudes into the spinal canal, decreasing the room for the neural elements. This is called *spinal stenosis*. A patient may experience neck and radicular pain in positions that decrease room in the spinal canal (positions of extension). In a severe case of central stenosis, spinal cord compression and clinical myelopathy may result. Alternatively, foraminal stenosis may be confined to an exiting nerve root.

Back pain and radicular pain may also occur secondary to obstruction of veins in the intervertebral foramen.[41] Direct compression of the nerve root may not be necessary to develop radicular pain. Intraforaminal venous dilation secondary to venous compression from a disc or osteophytes may result in adjacent neural fibrosis. Nerve root

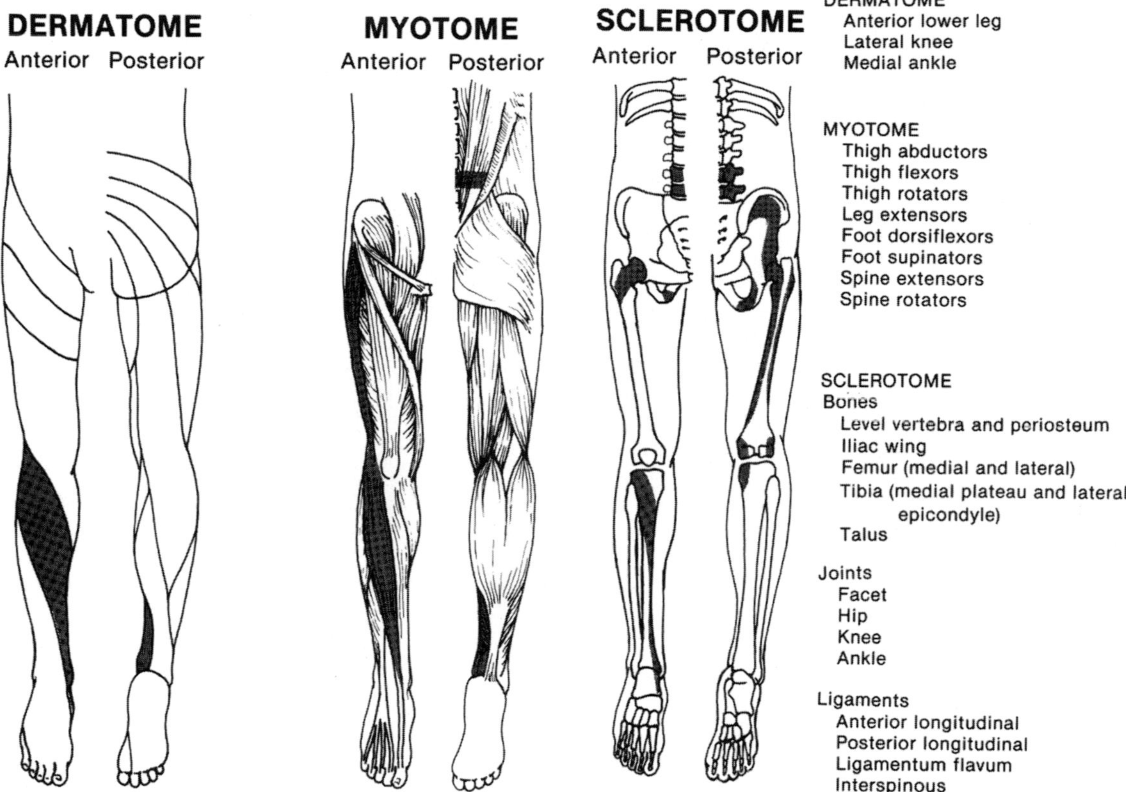

Figure 3-25 Dermatome, myotome, and sclerotome distribution for L4.

fibrosis may be a source of pain in patients with degenerative disc disease without herniation.

Nerve root compression is also seen with fracture-dislocation of the spine, infections, and neoplasms. Neoplasms that cause radicular pain are usually extradural (metastatic) or intradural (neurofibroma). Intramedullary tumors are associated with neurogenic symptoms.

Whether the intervertebral disc can be a generator of spinal pain has been a source of contention among spine specialists. The disagreement stems from the absence of pain fibers in the intervertebral disc. Sensory fibers are limited to the outer portions of the annulus fibrosus.[40] Coppes and colleagues suggested that histologic evaluation of nociceptive fibers in painful discs confirmed at discography was the appropriate material for study, not individuals who had died without back pain available for autopsy.[16] The intervertebral discs from 10 individuals undergoing anterior body fusion with an en bloc segment removal, including anterior longitudinal ligament, annulus fibrosus, and nucleus fibrosus after intense pain generated by discography, and 2 controls were studied for nociceptive fibers in the annulus fibrosus and nucleus pulposus. Substance P fibers were identified as single filaments in the anterior longitudinal ligament and the outer zone of the annulus fibrosus. Myelinated fibers and small free nerve fibers were noted in the inner portion of the annulus in two degenerated discs. The implication of this study is that ingrowth of sensory nerves, but not nociceptors, does occur in degenerated discs. The mechanism of pain production–associated intervertebral disc degeneration remains unknown.

Other questions concerning the generation of pain from disc herniation has surrounded the potential source of nociceptive messengers. A hypothesis proposed by Harrington and co-workers was that acidic amino acids from proteoglycans are the source for glutamate that diffuses to the dorsal horn to generate nociceptive signals. Glutamate was found in higher concentrations in herniated disc material compared to normal discs. Therapy that inhibits glutamate receptors may be beneficial in individuals with intervertebral disc herniations and radiculopathy.[34]

Neurogenic Pain

Neurogenic pain arises from abnormalities of the peripheral or central nervous system. The structures associated with neurogenic pain include the peripheral nerves, dorsal root ganglia, spinal cord, thalamus, and sensory area of the cerebral cortex. Damage to the sensory portion of the

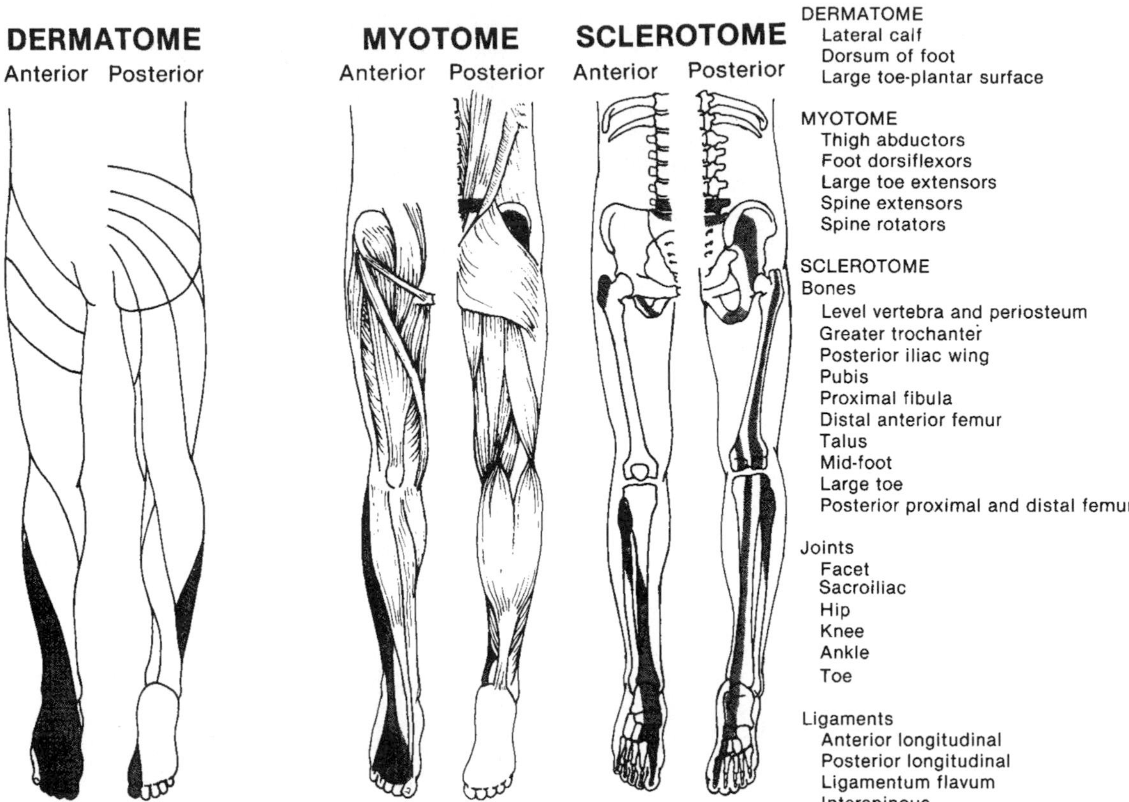

Figure 3-26 Dermatome, myotome, and sclerotome distribution for L5.

nervous system may result in pain produced spontaneously or by painless sensory stimulation (light touch—allodynia). The pain follows a distribution that corresponds to the damaged neural structure. The response to simple light touch can be excruciating pain similar to that experienced in a case of causalgia, reflex sympathetic dystrophy, or complex regional pain syndrome.[59] The pain may be delayed or occur in paroxysms. The pain may be sustained for some time after cessation of the stimulus (hyperpathia). Particularly in injuries of the central nervous system, pain may begin abruptly without evident peripheral stimulation. Hyperalgesia is a state associated with sustained painful stimuli with a short-duration stimulus. Neurogenic pain is described as burning, tingling, crushing, gnawing, or skin crawling (formication). In many circumstances, it is a unique pain that the patient has not experienced previously.[19] As opposed to what occurs in radicular pain, increases in intraspinal pressure produced by coughing or sneezing rarely exacerbate nerve pain. Instead, pain is intensified by sensory stimulation of the damaged nerve. Therefore, patients actively protect the limb from contact and develop behavior that protects the limb from the environment.

The abnormality causing neurogenic pain is the loss of the pain inhibitory system in the peripheral nerves and/or central nervous system. Those processes that diminish the large myelinated fiber input to the dorsal horn allow for increased transmission of nociceptive information. Loss of inhibitory interneurons may also result in persistent painful stimuli.[87] Also, nociceptive transmission is increased by diminished input from the nerves originating in the periaqueductal gray area of the midbrain.

An example of neurogenic pain is diabetic mononeuropathy of the femoral or sciatic nerve. The neuropathy presents with sudden onset of burning pain in the peripheral distribution of the nerve associated with loss of sensory and motor function. Herpes zoster preferentially affects dorsal root ganglion cells of mechanoreceptors and causes neurogenic pain distributed in a dermatomal pattern.

Viscerogenic Referred Pain

Viscerogenic referred neck or shoulder pain arises from abnormalities in organs that share segmental innervation with structures in the cervical spine. These organs include the thyroid, heart, esophagus, gallbladder, stomach, lungs, pancreas, and diaphragm. In the lumbosacral spine, the organs with shared segmental innervation include the pancreas, part of the duodenum, the ascending and descending colon, rectum, kidney, ureter, bladder, and pelvic

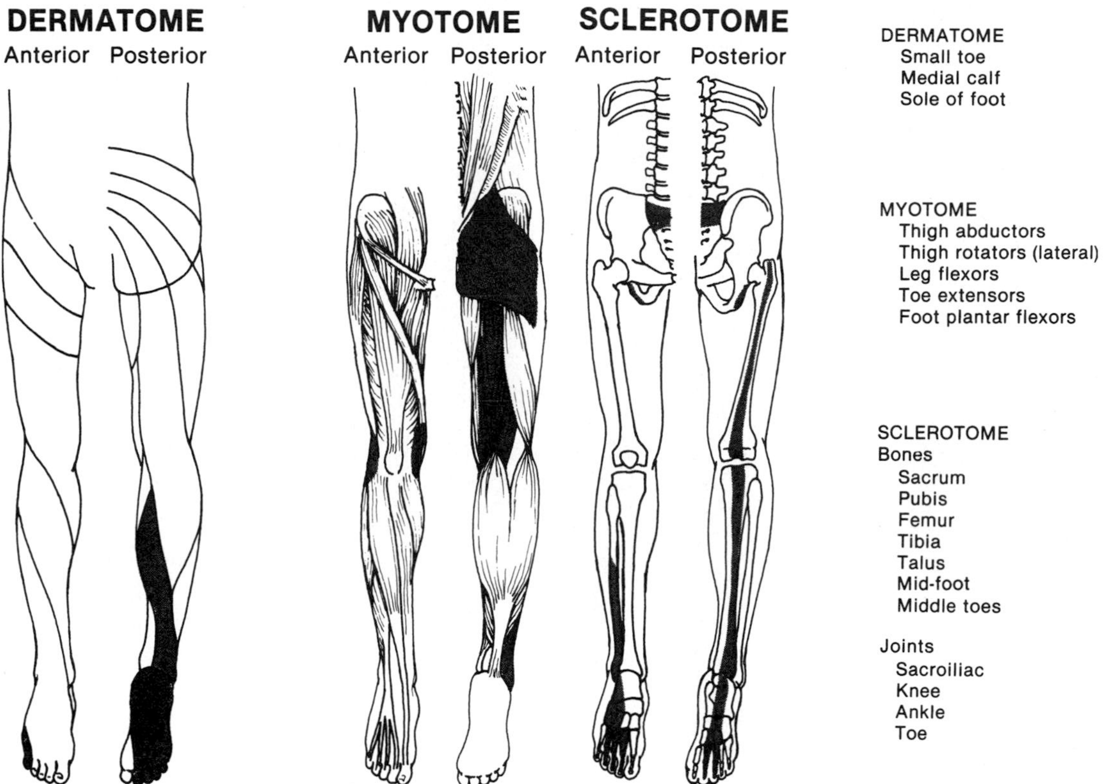

Figure 3-27 Dermatome, myotome, and sclerotome distribution for S1.

organs including uterus, cervix, and prostate. Visceral afferents that supply these organs transmit impulses to the dorsal horn, where somatic and visceral pain fibers share second-order neurons.[73] Impulses from visceral nerve endings arrive at the same reception point among the posterior horn cells as do impulses of somatic origin. Visceral pain is noted in the same somatic segment with which it shares neurons in lamina V of the dorsal horn.

The precise localization of somatic pain differs from the wider distribution of visceral pain because the latter is transmitted to multiple segments (Fig. 3-30). In addition to superficial cutaneous pain, reflex muscle spasm and vasomotor changes may also occur. The neck pain may have a gripping, cramping, aching, squeezing, crushing, tearing, stabbing, or burning quality, depending on the affected organ. The degree of tissue injury correlates with the intensity of the pain and is associated with recruitment of additional segmental levels above and below as well as those neighboring segments that have transmitted past or concurrent nociceptive impulses. A clinical correlate of this recruitment of segments is the radiating quality of visceral pain.

The duration and sequence of viscerogenic referred neck or low back pain are helpful in identifying its organ of origin. For example, neck pain caused by referred impulses follows the periodicity associated with the diseased organ. Rhythmic peristaltic waves of a hollow viscus attempting to expel its contents against resistance produce pain that rises quickly to its greatest intensity in 20 to 30 seconds, lasts 1 to 2 minutes, and quickly subsides, only to recur again in minutes. Lesions in the esophagus, ureter, uterus, or colon are associated with this pattern of pain. Vascular lesions are associated with throbbing pain. Lesions that result in inflammation and the release of chemical mediators that facilitate pain are associated with pain that increases in intensity and lasts extended periods.[44]

Neck or low back pain is rarely the sole symptom of visceral disease. Changes in gastrointestinal function may be clues to the potential source of pain. Viscerogenic pain may be differentiated from deep somatic pain by the response to activity and rest. Somatic pain is frequently exacerbated by activity and improved by rest. Patients with viscerogenic pain get no relief from bed rest. In fact, they may feel more comfortable by moving about, trying to achieve a comfortable position.

Psychogenic Pain

Psychogenic pain arises not from structures located in the cervical or lumbosacral spine but at levels of the cerebral

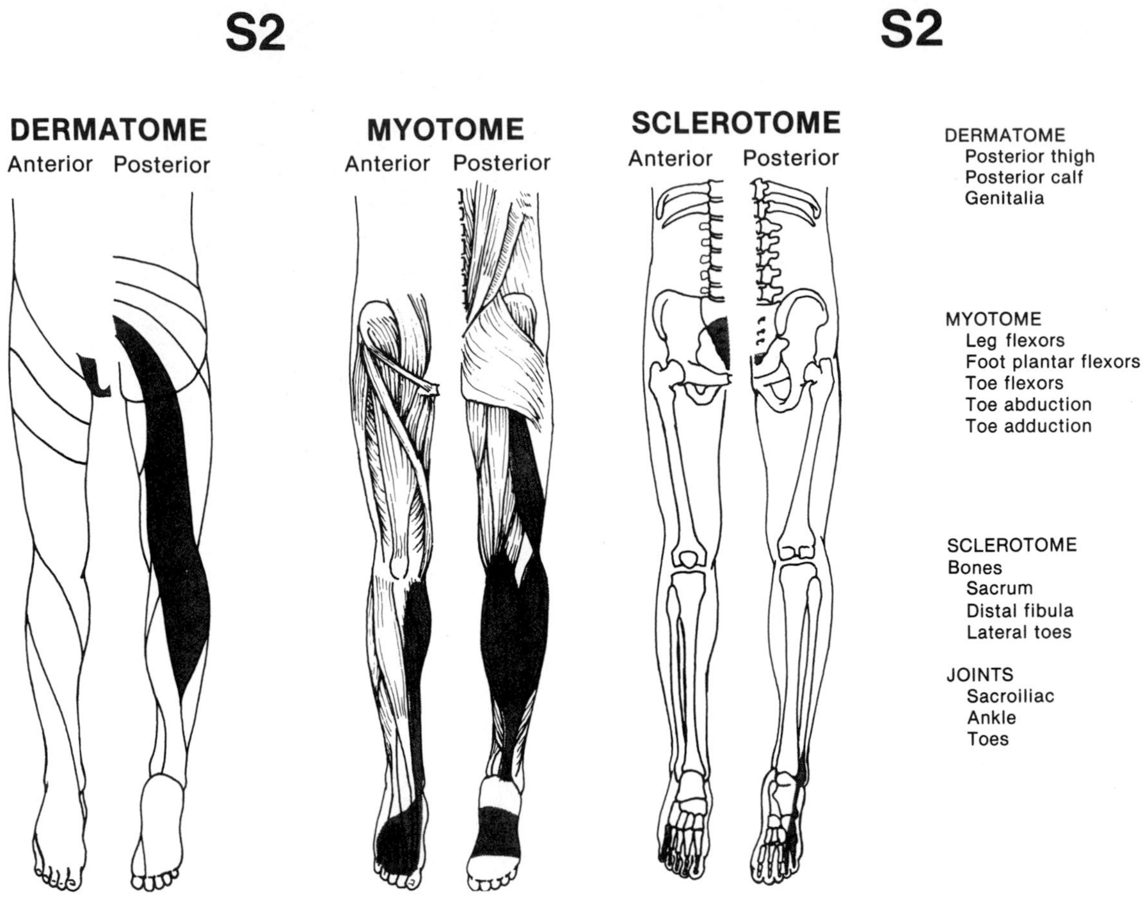

Figure 3-28 Dermatome, myotome, and sclerotome distribution for S2.

cortex. Patients with psychogenic pain experience discomfort, but the pain is not due to tissue damage. Patients with psychogenic pain may suffer from depression, hysteria, or conversion reaction. They respond to their environment with symptoms that help control their situation.[20] These individuals may have experienced physical or psychic damage earlier in life that increases their tendency to develop chronic pain

The pain is poorly defined and does not follow dermatomal patterns. It is superficial or deep, sharp or dull, radiating or nonradiating, constant or intermittent, excruciating or mild. Pain may be associated with specific social activities, such as work and sexual intercourse, whereas activities that require similar kinds of physical effort elicit little pain.

The duration of pain defies physiologic time sequences. Pain may last for seconds or for years. Pain may be unrelenting and unmoved by therapy during an extended time. The language used to describe the pain may reflect a patient's thoughts of suffering or punishment. The patient may speak of pain as a "knife sticking you," "being hit," "burned with a red hot poker," or "having your skin peeled off."[46]

Psychogenic pain resists most conventional therapies that are effective in somatic causes of spinal pain. Therapy must be directed not at the pain but at the reasons causing an agitated depression, conversion reaction, or reluctance to return to work. Patients with psychogenic pain experience pain that is just as incapacitating as that caused by muscle strain. These patients do not improve unless the source of their pain is recognized.

Duration of Pain

The function of pain as it affects the whole body is closely related to its duration. Acute pain frequently has an understandable cause (trauma), normally has a characteristic time course, and resolves once healing has occurred. The purpose of acute pain is to inform the host that tissue damage has occurred and to prevent further injury. The rapidly conducting systems (such as the neospinothalamic tract and dorsal column tract) are suited to the speedy relay of both nociceptive and light touch sensations necessary to determine the initial phase of tissue injury. The overlap between systems allows one to be responsive to proprioceptive stimuli and another to be primed to receive nociceptive stimulation. The organization of multiple ascending systems allows the individual to be constantly primed for nociceptive impulses, which are important to prevent injury while the central nervous system is flooded with non-nociceptive inputs.[18] This rapid system activates

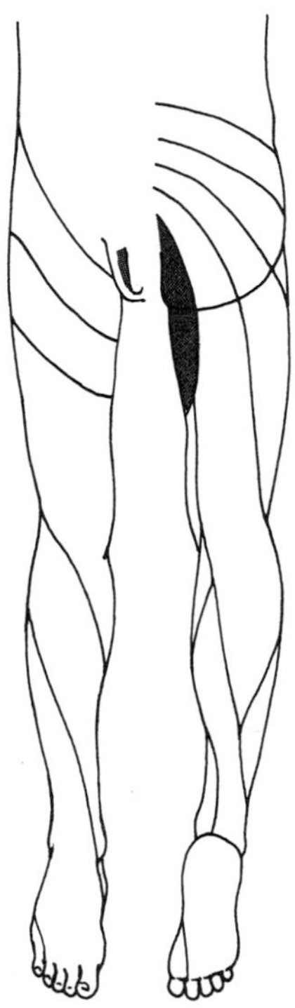

Figure 3-29 Dermatome, myotome, and sclerotome distribution for S3–C1.

appropriate motor responses that attempt to minimize damage to the affected part.

The slowly conducting system, including the paleospinothalamic tract, carries information about the state of the injury and its susceptibility to further damage. This tonic stimulation determines the general behavioral state of the individual to prevent further damage and foster rest and care of the damaged area to promote healing. Tonic pain also resolves with healing of the injury. The functions of the rapidly and slowly conducting systems may be controlled by different neurochemical mechanisms. This may have therapeutic implications because the phasic and tonic components of pain may respond to different drugs.[18]

Acute Pain Transmission

Acute pain is generated when a stimulus activates a high-threshold nociceptor.[57] The A-beta fibers contain only the excitatory amino acid, glutamate, contained in small, clear vesicles. C fibers include both glutamate and large dense-core vesicles containing substance P, calcitonin gene–related peptide, galanin, cholecystokinin, and brain- and glial-derived neurotrophic factor. With low-intensity noxious stimulation, only glutamate receptors are activated, with a rapid sensory response as an excitatory postsynaptic current. This fast response is mediated by glutamate acting on alpha-amino-3-hydroxy-5-methylisoxazole-4-propionic acid (AMPA) receptor. The AMPA receptor opens Na^{+},K^{+} channels. Kainate ligand-gated ion channels also mediate the fast excitatory synaptic transmission. Glutamate also stimulates the inhibitory pain system through activation of inhibitory neurons that co-release glycine and gamma-aminobutyric acid. This simultaneous stimulation focuses the excitation on the local area of damage.

Chronic Pain Transmission

As the noxious stimulus increases and persists, more glutamate and dense vesicle substances (substance P) are liberated. These vesicles have receptors on their surfaces. As a vesicle fuses with a membrane, a receptor becomes exposed, becoming susceptible to ligands excitatory to that receptor. This results in a slow excitatory postsynaptic current. The slow current, lasting seconds to minutes, is mediated by activation of a number of receptors, including *N*-methyl-D-aspartate (NMDA) receptor, as well as neurokinin-1 (NK-1), the substance P receptor. Continued stimulation by glutamate results in the release of the magnesium plug on the NMDA receptor. Activating the NMDA receptor allows for the influx of calcium into the nociceptor. The calcium activates intracellular kinases by G protein–coupled and tyrosine kinase–bound receptors activating protein kinase A or C. Activating protein C results in stimulation of nitric oxide synthase.[10] Nitric oxide diffuses through the dorsal horn membrane and synaptic cleft into the nociceptor that stimulates the closure of K^{+} channels by stimulating guanyl-synthase. Opioids inhibit pain by opening these channels. The production of nitric oxide also stimulates the release of substance P, which binds to the NK-1 receptor. Activation of the NK-1 receptor results in increased c-*fos* gene expression resulting in the sprouting of nociceptive fibers. The result of these changes is the development of chronic pain. The threshold for activation of dorsal horn neurons is lowered along with stimulation of wide-dynamic-field neurons that are non-nociceptive. The degree of response is exaggerated to light touch. The process results in physiologic and anatomic alterations to the central nervous system.

The changes associated with chronic pain that occur in the central nervous system are related to alterations in molecular control of neuropeptide synthesis and neuroreceptor production.[89] Immediate early genes (IEGs) are oncogenes that are activated by a variety of stimuli to nerve cells. IEGs, such as c-*fos* and c-*jun*, act as transcription messengers that control the transcription mechanisms of a cell. Repetitive noxious stimulation is a potent promoter of IEG activation.[74] Noxious stimulation of C fibers results in alterations in postsynaptic receptors for excitatory amino acids, such as NMDA. The ensuing increase in sensory nerve cell excitability is related to the emergence of NMDA receptors at the afferent synapses of dorsal horn neurons.[17] Increased excitability may persist for weeks following a transient peripheral injury. The development of chronic pain modifies transmission of stimuli in the nervous system. The persistence of chronic pain may become independent of ongoing nociceptive stimulation if neural

3-5 CLASSIFICATION OF SPINAL PAIN

Category	Sensory Nerves	Pathologic Entity	Quality
Superficial somatic (skin with subcutaneous tissue)	Cutaneous A fibers, small field	Cellulitis	Sharp
		Herpes zoster	Burning
Deep somatic (spondylogenic) (muscles, fascia, periosteum, ligaments, joints, vessels, dura)	Sinuvertebral	Muscular strain	Sharp (acute)
	Posterior primary ramus unmyelinated	Arthritis	Dull ache (chronic)
		Fracture Increased venous pressure	Boring
Radicular (spinal nerves)	—	Herniated vertebral disc	Segmental
		Foraminal stenosis Spinal stenosis	Radiating
			Shooting
Neurogenic	Mixed motor sensory nerves	Herpes zoster Brachial plexopathy Femoral nerve neuropathy	Burning
Viscerogenic referred (cardiac, carotid structures, abdominal and pelvic viscera, aorta)	Autonomic sensory, unmyelinated C fibers, large field	Myocardial infarction Pancreatitis	Deep, heaviness
		Carotidynia/Intestinal diseases Abdominal aneurysm Esophageal spasm	Boring Tearing Colicky
Psychogenic	—	Depression Conversion reaction Malingering	Variable

Modified from Engel GI: Pain. In Blacklow R (ed): Signs and Symptoms: Applied Pathologic Physiology and Clinical Interpretation. Philadelphia, JB Lippincott, 1983, pp 41–60; and Macnab I: Backache. Baltimore, Williams & Wilkins, 1983, pp 16–18.

cells have been modified to have a lower threshold for stimulation. The nervous system is malleable. It changes according to environmental stimuli. In the future, therapy for chronic pain may be directed at control of cellular gene products that normalize receptor distribution on cell membranes or neurotransmitter production.

Chronic pain may persist long after the injury has healed. Chronic pain, which is continuous over several months, results from habituation of the sensory system to nociceptive stimuli. Constant stimulation activates the cerebral cortex function of memory. The central nervous system becomes habituated to sensory input to such an extent that pain is perceived in the absence of a detectable lesion. As the duration of pain continues, the area affected may spread to adjacent or distal body areas. Chronic pain also results in autonomic responses that are depressive (vegetative) in quality: poor sleep, decreased appetite, irritability, withdrawal of interests, strained interpersonal relationships, and increased somatic preoccupation.[79] Therefore, chronic pain is associated with significant depression.[47] In addition, resolution or reduction of pain reverses the reactive depression caused by the pain.[80] The marked psychological effects, including depression and anxiety associated with chronic pain, do not serve a useful purpose.

SUMMARY

Pain is a complex, subjective experience that is mediated through multiple components of the peripheral and central nervous systems. Factors at all levels of the neuraxis modulate pain perception. The sum of these inputs results in a perception that can be described in terms of its intensity, location, onset and duration, aggravating and alleviating factors, and elicited emotional responses. In acute circumstances, pain marks the onset and location of damage. It serves the purpose of protection. With chronic pain, the pain itself becomes the disease because the injury that initiated the nociceptive response has healed. The goals for therapy for patients who experience spinal pain must take into account these anatomic, physiologic, and psychological factors. The choice of specific forms of therapy for patients with spinal pain should be made in light of these factors. The potential is great for individual patients

Location	Intensity	Onset and Duration	Aggravating and Alleviating Factors	Behavior
Well localized	Correlates with intensity of nerve stimulation (mild to moderate)	Acute	Intensified by direct contact	Mild concern
		Correlates with status of lesions	Diminished by light touch in adjacent areas	Able to see lesion
Diffuse	Correlates with intensity of nerve stimulation (mild to severe)	Acute or chronic	Intensified with movement	Avoidance of movement
Multiple segments affected			Diminished with rest	Abnormal posture secondary to protective spasm
Neck, low back pain	Mild to severe	Acute	Intensified with standing, sitting	Avoidance of movement
Afferent distribution of affected nerve root (superficial and deep)	Correlates with intensity of nerve impingement		Diminished with bed rest	Abnormal gait
Peripheral nerve	Severe	Chronic Persistent	Intensified with palpation	Apprehension
Segmental with radiation inside body	Mild to severe	Acute or chronic	Related to factors affecting each organ system	Movement to find comfortable position
	Correlates with intensity of nerve stimulation			
Nondermatomal	Variable	Persistent	No consistent correlation	Emphasis on suffering

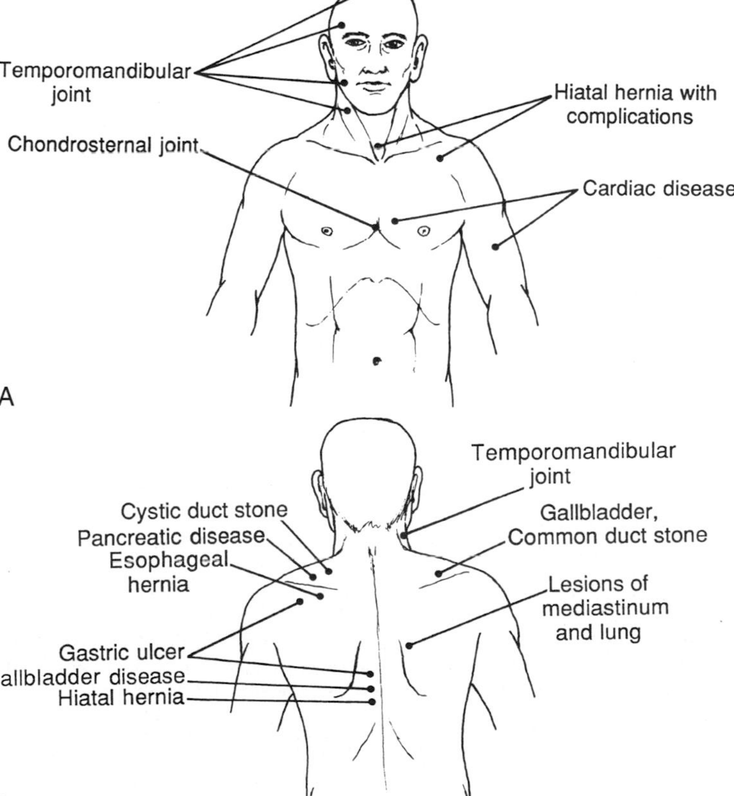

Figure 3-30 *A*, Anterior referral sites in the cervical spine arising from distant visceral or somatic structures. *B*, Posterior referral sites. *(A and B, Modified from Nakano KK: Neck pain. In Kelley WN, Harris ED Jr, Ruddy S, et al [eds]: Textbook of Rheumatology, 4th ed. Philadelphia, WB Saunders, 1993.)*

to respond to a wide variety of therapeutic interventions, given the multitude of factors that result in pain.

References

1. Aimone LD: Neurochemistry and modulation of pain. In Sinatra RS, Hord AH, Ginsberg B, Preble LM (eds): Acute Pain: Mechanisms and Management. St Louis, Mosby–Year Book, 1992, pp 29-43.
2. Antoniou J, Goudsouzian NM, Heathfield TF, et al: The human lumbar endplate: Evidence of changes in biosynthesis and denaturation of the extracellular matrix with growth, maturation, aging, and degeneration. Spine 21:1153-1161, 1996.
3. Aronin N, DiFiglia M, Liotta AS, Martin JB: Ultrastructural localization and biochemical features of immunoreactive leu-enkephalin in monkey dorsal horn. J Neurosci 1:561, 1981.
4. Basbaum AI, Levine JD: The contribution of the nervous system to inflammation and inflammatory disease. Can J Physiol Pharmacol 69:647-651, 1991.
5. Bayliss MT, Johnstone B: Biochemistry of the intervertebral disc. In Jayson MIV (ed): The Lumbar Spine and Back Pain. Edinburgh, Churchill Livingstone, 1992, pp 111-131.
6. Bayliss MT, Johnstone B, O'Brien JP: Proteoglycan synthesis in the human intervertebral disc: Variation with age, region, and pathology. Spine 13:972, 1988.
7. Bessou P, Perl ER: Response of cutaneous sensory units with unmyelinated fibers to noxious stimuli. J Neurophysiol 32:1025, 1969.
8. Bishop GH: The relation between nerve fiber size and sensory modality: Phylogenetic implications of the afferent innervation of the cortex. J Nerv Ment Dis 128:89, 1959.
9. Bogduk N: The sources of low back pain. In Jayson MIV (ed): The Lumbar Spine and Back Pain. Edinburgh, Churchill Livingstone, 1992, pp 61-88.
10. Brookoff D: Chronic pain. I. A new disease? Hosp Pract 35:45-59, 2000.
11. Byers MR, Bonica JJ: Peripheral pain mechanisms and nociceptor plasticity. In Loeser JD (ed): Bonica's Management of Pain. Philadelphia, Lippincott Williams & Wilkins, 2001, pp 26-72.
12. Cervero F, Iggo A: The substantia gelatinosa of the spinal cord: A critical review. Brain 103:717, 1980.
13. Chapman CR, Turner JA: Psychological aspects of pain. In Loeser JD (ed): Bonica's Management of Pain. Philadelphia, Lippincott Williams & Wilkins, 2001, pp 180-190.
14. Christensen BN, Perl ER: Spinal neurons specifically excited by noxious or thermal stimuli: Marginal zones of the dorsal horn. J Neurophysiol 33:293, 1970.
15. Collins WF, Nulsen FE, Randt CT: Relation of peripheral fiber size and sensation in man. Arch Neurol 3:381, 1960.
16. Coppes MH, Marani E, Thomeer RTWM, Groen GJ: Innervation of "painful" lumbar discs. Spine 22:2342-2350, 1997.
17. Davies SN, Lodge D: Evidence for involvement of *N*-methylaspartate receptors in "wind-up" of class 2 neurones in the dorsal horn of the rat. Brain Res 424:402, 1987.
18. Dennis SG, Melzack R: Pain-signaling systems in the dorsal and ventral spinal cord. Pain 4:97, 1977.
19. Denny-Brown D: The release of deep pain by nerve injury. Brain 88:725, 1965.
20. Devine R, Merskey H: The description of pain in psychiatric and general medical patients. J Psychosom Res 9:311, 1965.
21. Engel GL: Pain. In Blacklow R (ed): Signs and Symptoms: Applied Pathologic Physiology and Clinical Interpretation. Philadelphia, JB Lippincott, 1983, pp 41-60.
22. Eyre DE: Biochemistry of the intervertebral disc. Connect Tissue Res 8:227, 1979.
23. Eyre D, Benya P, Buckwalter J, et al: The intervertebral disc: Basic science perspectives. In Frymoyer JW, Gordon SL (eds): New Perspectives on Low Back Pain. Park Ridge, IL, American Academy of Orthopaedic Surgeons, 1988, pp 147-207.
24. Ferreira SH: Prostaglandins, aspirin-like drugs, and analgesia. Nature 240:200, 1972.
25. Fields HL, Basbaum AI: Brain stem control of spinal pain—transmission neurons. Annu Rev Physiol 40:217, 1978.
26. Fields HL, Basbaum AI: Central nervous system mechanisms of pain modulation. In Wall PD, Melzack R (eds): Textbook of Pain, 3rd ed. Edinburgh, Churchill Livingstone, 1994, pp 243-257.
27. Fitzgerald M, Lynn B: The sensitization of high threshold mechanoreceptors with myelinated axons by repeated heating. J Physiol (Lond) 65:549, 1977
28. Floyd WF, Silver PHS: Function of erectores spinae and flexion of the trunk. Lancet 1:133, 1951.
29. Goupille P, Jayson MIV, Valat J, Freemont AJ: Matrix metalloproteinases: The clue to intervertebral disc degeneration? Spine 23:1612-1626, 1998.
30. Gronblad M, Virri J, Ronko S, et al: A controlled biochemical study of human synovial-type (Group II) phospholipase A_2 and inflammatory cells in macroscopically normal, degenerated, and herniated human lumbar disc tissues. Spine 21:2531-2538, 1996.
31. Habtemariam A, Gronblad M, Virri J, et al: Immunocytochemical localization of immunoglobulins in disc herniations. Spine 21:1864-1869, 1996.
32. Hampton D, Laros G, McCarron R, Franks D: Healing potential of the annulus fibrosus. Spine 14:398, 1989.
33. Harrington JF, Sungarian A, Rogg J, et al: The relation between vertebral endplate shape and lumbar disc herniation. Spine 26:2133-2138, 2001.
34. Harrington JF, Meissier AA, Bereiter D, et al: Herniated lumbar disc material as a source of free glutamate available to affect pain signals through the dorsal root ganglion. Spine 25:929-936, 2000.
35. Hirsch C, Inglemark BE, Miller M: The anatomical basis for low back pain: Studies on the presence of sensory nerve endings in ligamentous, capsular, and intervertebral disc structures in the human lumbar spine. Acta Orthop Scand 33:1, 1963.
36. Hökfelt T, Kellerth JO, Nilsson G, Pernow B: Substance P: Localization in the central nervous system and in some primary sensory neurons. Science 190:889, 1975.
37. Horner HA, Urban JPG: 2001 Volvo award winner in basic science studies: Effect of nutrient supply on the viability of cells from the nucleus pulposus of the intervertebral disc. Spine 26:2543-2549, 2001.
38. Iggo A: Activation of cutaneous nociceptors and their actions on dorsal horn neurons. Adv Neurol 4:1, 1974.
39. International Association for the Study of Pain: Pain terms: A list of definitions and notes on usage. Recommended by the IASP Subcommittee on Taxonomy. Pain 16:249, 1979.
40. Jackson HC, Winkelmann RK, Bickel WM: Nerve endings in the human lumbar spinal column and related structures. J Bone Joint Surg Am 48:1271-1281, 1966.
41. Jayson MIV: Presidential address: Why does acute back pain become chronic? Spine 22:1053-1056, 1997.
42. Johnstone B, Bayliss MT: The large proteoglycans of the human intervertebral disc changes in their biosynthesis and structure with age, topography, and pathology. Spine 20:674-684, 1995.
43. Joint Commission on Accreditation of Healthcare Organization's Pain Standards for 2001. http://www.jcaho.org/
44. Keele CA: Chemical causes of pain and itch. Annu Rev Med 21:67, 1970.
45. Kellgren JH: On the distribution of pain arising from deep somatic structures, with charts of segmental pain areas. Clin Sci 41:46, 1939.
46. Klein RF, Brown W: Pain descriptions in medical settings. J Psychosom Res 10:367, 1967.
47. Krishnan KR, France RD, Pelton S, et al: Chronic pain and depression. I. Classification of depression in chronic low back pain patients. Pain 22:279, 1985.
48. Krismer M, Haid C, Rabi W: The contribution of annulus fibrosus fibers to torque resistance. Spine 21:2551-2557, 1996.
49. Kuslich SD, Ulstrom CL, Michael CJ: The tissue origin of low back pain and sciatica: A report of pain response to tissue stimulation during operations on the lumbar spine using local anesthesia. Orthop Clin North Am 22:181, 1991.
50. LaMotte CC, de Lanerolle N: Substance P, enkephalin, and serotonin: Ultrastructural basis of pain transmission in primate spinal cord. In Bonica JJ, Lindblom V, Iggo A (eds): Advances in Pain Research and Therapy, Vol 5. New York, Raven, 1983, pp 247-256.
51. Lautenbacher S, Rollman GB: Possible deficiencies of pain modulation in fibromyalgia. Clin J Pain 13:189-196, 1997.
52. Lawrence JS, Bremner JM, Bier F: Osteoarthrosis: Prevalence in the population and relationship between symptoms and x-ray changes. Ann Rheum Dis 25:1, 1966.

53. Levine JD, Fields HL, Basbaum AI: Peptides and the primary afferent nociceptor. J Neurosci 13:2273, 1993.
54. Lynn B: Neurogenic inflammation. Skin Pharmacol 1:217, 1988.
55. Maciewicz R, Landrew BB: Physiology of pain. In Aronoff GM (ed): Evaluation and Treatment of Chronic Pain. Baltimore, Urban & Schwarzenberg, 1985, pp 17-38.
56. Macnab I: Backache. Baltimore, Williams & Wilkins, 1983, pp 16-18.
57. Mannion RJ, Woolf CJ: Pain mechanisms and management: A central perspective. Clin J Pain 16:S144-S156, 2000.
58. Melzack R: Neurophysiological foundation of pain. In Sternbach RA (ed): The Psychology of Pain. New York, Raven, 1986, pp 1-24.
59. Melzack R, Loeser JD: Phantom body pain in paraplegics: Evidence for a central "pattern-generating mechanism" for pain. Pain 4:195, 1978.
60. Melzack R, Wall PD: Pain mechanisms: A new theory. Science 150:971, 1965.
61. Meyer RA, Campbell JN, Raja SN: Peripheral neural mechanisms of nociception. In Wall PD, Melzack R (eds): Textbook of Pain, 3rd ed. Edinburgh, Churchill Livingstone, 1994, pp 13-44.
62. Mooney V, Robertson J: The facet syndrome. Clin Orthop 115:149, 1976.
63. Morton CR, Hutchison WD: Release of sensory neuropeptides in the spinal cord: Studies with calcitonin gene–related peptide and galanin. Neuroscience 31:807, 1989.
64. Nerlich AG, Schleicher ED, Boos N: 1997 Volvo award winner in basic sciences studies: Immunologic markers for age-related changes of human lumbar intervertebral discs. Spine 22:2781-2795, 1997.
65. Olmarker K, Larsson K: Tumor necrosis factor-alpha and nucleus pulposus–induced nerve root injury. Spine 23:2538-2544, 1998.
66. Olmarker K, Rydevik B: Selective inhibition of tumor necrosis factor prevents nucleus pulposus–induced thrombus formation, intraneural edema, and reduction of nerve conduction velocity: Possible implications for future pharmacologic treatment strategies of sciatica. Spine 26:863-869, 2001.
67. Olmarker K, Rydevik B, Nordborg C: Autologous nucleus pulposus induces neurophysiologic and histologic changes in porcine cauda equina nerve roots. Spine 18:1425, 1993.
68. Plenderleith MB, Haller CJ, Snow PJ: Peptide coexistence in axon terminals within the superficial dorsal horn of the rat spinal cord. Synapse 6:344-350, 1990.
69. Price DD: Psychological and neural mechanisms of the affective dimension of pain. Science 288:1769-1772, 2000.
70. Procacci P, Zopp M: Pathophysiology and clinical aspects of visceral and referred pain. In Bonica JJ, Lindblom V, Iggo A (eds): Advances in Pain Research and Therapy, Vol 5. New York, Raven, 1983, pp 643-660.
71. Reynolds DV: Surgery in the rat during electrical analgesia induced by focal brain stimulation. Science 164:444, 1969.
72. Satoh K, Konno S, Nishiyama K, et al: Presence and distribution of antigen-antibody complexes in the herniated nucleus pulposus. Spine 24:1980-1984, 1999.
73. Selzer M, Spencer WA: Convergence of visceral and cutaneous afferent pathways in the lumbar spinal cord. Brain Res 14:331, 1969.
74. Sheng M, Greenberg E: The regulation and function of c-*fos* and other immediate early genes in the nervous system. Neuron 4:477, 1990.
75. Simone DA, Baumann TK, La Motte RH: Dose-dependent pain and mechanical hyperalgesia in humans after intradermal injection of capsaicin. Pain 380:99-107, 1989.
76. Sjolund BH, Eriksson MBE: The influence of naloxone on analgesia produced by peripheral conditioning stimulation. Brain Res 173:295, 1979.
77. Smyth MJ, Wright V: Sciatica and the intervertebral disc: An experimental study. J Bone Joint Surg 40:1401, 1958.
78. Stein C: The control of pain in peripheral tissue by opioids. N Engl J Med 332:1685-1690, 1995.
79. Sternbach RA: Clinical aspects of pain. In Sternbach RA (ed): The Psychology of Pain. New York, Raven, 1986, pp 223-239.
80. Sternbach RA, Timmermans G: Personality changes associated with reduction of pain. Pain 1:177, 1975.
81. Terman GW, Bonica JJ: Spinal mechanisms and their modulation. In Loeser JD (ed): Bonica's Management of Pain. Philadelphia, Lippincott Williams & Wilkins, 2001, pp 72-152.
82. Thalhammer JG, LaMotte RH: Spatial properties of nociceptor sensitization. Brain Res 231:257, 1982.
83. Yaksh TL, Farb D, Leeman S, Jessell T: Intrathecal capsaicin depletes substance P in the rat spinal cord and produces prolonged thermal analgesia. Science 206:481, 1979.
84. Watkins LR, Maier SF, Goehler LE: Immune activation: The role of pro-inflammatory cytokines in inflammation, illness responses, and pathological pain states. Pain 63:289-302, 1995.
85. Willburger RE, Wittenberg RH: Prostaglandin release from lumbar disc and facet joint disease. Spine 19:2068-2070, 1994.
86. Willis WD, Maunz RA, Foreman RD, Coulter JD: Static and dynamic responses of spinothalamic tract neurons to mechanical stimuli. J Neurophysiol 38:587, 1975.
87. Woolf CJ, Salter MW: Neural plasticity: Increasing the gain in pain. Science 288:1965, 2000.
88. Wyke B: Neurological aspects of low back pain. In Jayson MIV (ed): The Lumbar Spine and Back Pain. New York, Grune & Stratton, 1976, pp 189-256.
89. Zimmermann M: Basic neurophysiological mechanisms of pain and pain therapy. In Jayson MIV (ed): The Lumbar Spine and Back Pain. Edinburgh, Churchill Livingstone, 1992, pp 43-59.

Section II

Clinical Evaluation of Neck and Low Back Pain

Spinal pain in the cervical and lumbar regions is a ubiquitous problem.[4] Most individuals reading this book have personally experienced this disorder. It is also fair to say that a physician with a busy general practice will evaluate patients with spinal back pain on a daily basis. Low back pain occurs more commonly than neck pain in the general population, and it causes a greater number of physician visits.

Even though most of the population is affected by this clinical problem, many individuals will not seek the advice of a physician in the diagnosis and treatment of this malady. Most spinal pain is self-limited. Of those individuals who are evaluated by their physician, 40% to 50% are better in 1 week, 51% to 86% in 1 month, and 92% within 2 months.[3] A similar pattern is also seen in work-related low back pain, with 70% to 90% of affected individuals being better within 2 months. Another study suggests that only about 14% of adults who do develop back pain have an episode that has a duration greater than 2 weeks.[2] Most individuals believe that their spinal pain is related to bad posture or a strain that will be transient in duration and is not of such a significant degree of discomfort as to warrant a visit to a physician's office. Those with more severe degrees of pain may choose to do nothing or to treat themselves with limited activity, over-the-counter medications, or temperature modalities (ice, hot packs). Others bypass the family physician and go to the chiropractor, "the practitioner with an interest in spine problems." All of these interventions seem to work, since the natural history of the symptom is resolution over a short period. Some patients place too much confidence in their own understanding of the source of their pain and their initial response to therapy. The 50- or 60-year-old patient who develops persistent back pain after a minor trauma may ascribe all subsequent symptoms to the injury. Such patients may overlook the symptoms of fatigue, anorexia, and weakness, which have more ominous significance. They optimistically believe that the increasing doses of analgesics will eventually be effective and that their pain will subside.

In contradistinction to patients who belittle their symptoms, other patients may amplify their symptoms and express great anxiety in regard to the presence of spinal pain. These patients have unreasonably high expectations. They believe that 100% pain relief should be the end result of therapy even though their pain has been present for months. They want to undergo simultaneous therapies without forethought to a progression of modalities that offer a range of benefits and risks. These are the patients who undergo many of the more than

400,000 back operations done each year in the United States.[1] The vast majority of these operations are done for appropriate indications and result in good outcomes. However, many patients with persistent spinal pain of unknown etiology undergo exploratory spine surgery, usually with poor results.

The clinician is faced with a constant dilemma. Back pain is common and affects any group of patients. Most episodes of back pain are related to mechanical regional abnormalities. Up to 95% of patients who have mechanical, self-limited back pain will improve. In 85% of patients, no specific diagnosis can be determined despite a thorough history, physical examination, and radiographic evaluation.[7] Some researchers have suggested that the absence of pathoanatomic abnormalities implicates psychosomatic mechanisms for the source of back pain.[5,6] Although psychosomatic disorders may play a role in the perpetuation of pain, the initiating factor is usually physical in origin. Spinal pathology must be excluded before psychological disorders are considered the source of a patient's pain. Therefore, an appropriate medical evaluation, including history and physical examination, is essential in the initial investigation of every patient with spinal pain. The therapy chosen for this common problem should relieve symptoms, with toxicities limited to a minimum, while natural healing occurs. Intermixed in this large population of patients are individuals (2% to 10%) with potentially more serious causes of their pain.[2] Overlooking the correct diagnosis in these patients can have dire consequences.

Through careful review of the history, physical examination, and appropriate laboratory and radiographic tests, it should be possible for the clinician evaluating the patient's symptoms of spinal pain to formulate a logical diagnosis and implement an appropriate treatment plan.

References

1. Cypress BK: Characteristics of physician visits for back symptoms: A national perspective. Am J Public Health 73:389-395, 1983.
2. Deyo RA, Rainville J, Kent DL: What can the history and physical examination tell us about low back pain? JAMA 268:760-765, 1992.
3. Dillane JB, Fry J: Acute back syndrome: A study from general practice. BMJ 3:82, 1966.
4. Horal J: The clinical appearance of low back disorders in the city of Gothenburg, Sweden: Comparisons of incapacitated probands with matched controls. Acta Orthop Scand Suppl 118:1-109, 1969.
5. Sarno JE: Etiology of neck and back pain: An automatic myoneuralgia? J Nerv Ment Dis 169:55-59, 1981.
6. Waddell G: Understanding the patient with backache. *In* Jayson MIV (ed): The Lumbar Spine and Back Pain, 4th ed. Edinburgh, Churchill Livingstone, 1992, p 485.
7. White AA III, Gordon SL: Synopsis: Workshop on idiopathic low back pain. Spine 7:141-149, 1982.

CHAPTER 4

HISTORY

TAKING THE HISTORY

Taking the history is the essential initial step in evaluating the patient with the symptom of neck or back pain. The history should include the patient's chief complaint, family history, past history, social history, review of systems, and present illness. Some physicians may concentrate only on the present illness, leaving out parts of the review of systems or social history. Others use reproduced forms that list a succession of questions that are complete for evaluating the patient's pain but do not integrate the neck symptoms with other medical, social, or psychological problems. In circumstances involving patients with acute spinal cord compression (from tumor, infection, or trauma), or cauda equina symptoms (saddle anesthesia, progressive muscular weakness, incontinence), the necessity to do a complete history is reduced in the face of the need to evaluate the patient for emergency surgical decompression. In other patients with chronic pain, a thorough review of all the components of the patient's history is essential to understanding the patient's difficulties. Historical evaluation and physical examination are the major means of gathering data in diagnosing spinal disorders, and they are done superficially in many circumstances.[5] In fact, the history taking has proven to be a highly variable art with a kappa coefficient of only 0.40 in one study.[24] The reproducibility between clinicians increased to a kappa coefficient of 0.66 after addition of the physical examination to the history.

Common sense is an essential component of this process. The astute clinician allows patients to tell their story in their own words and also steers them in directions that elicit the essential information needed for the diagnostic process. The clinician knows when the history must be abbreviated to administer essential therapy or prolonged to gather all the facts that may pertain to the patient's problem.

The expenditure of time in obtaining a complete history reaps the clinician great dividends in understanding the patient's disease. If not all the information is obtained during the initial evaluation, it is worthwhile to review the history on subsequent visits. The patient may have forgotten an essential piece of history. Repeated questions about the spinal pain may jar the patient's memory. It also allows the patient to monitor response to therapy.

Chief Complaint

The recording of the chief complaint describes the patient's age, sex, and location and duration of pain. It is at this point that the possibility of a life-threatening cause of neck or low back pain needs to be considered.

Emergency Evaluation

A tumor, infection, or traumatic disruption of the cervical spine is one of the few catastrophic causes of neck pain that may require emergency intervention. In addition to neck pain, progressive motor weakness, incontinence, progressive gait abnormalities, and lower extremity pain should be recognizable by the emergency department physician or general practitioner as findings indicative of cauda equina syndrome. A leaking or ruptured abdominal aneurysm is one of the few catastrophic causes of acute low back pain that requires emergency intervention. Patients with an expanding aneurysm develop abdominal pain, distention, and circulatory collapse. This might include history of prior vascular surgery, anticoagulant therapy, or severe hypertension. In such instances only essential history needs to be obtained. Another potentially life-threatening emergency associated with low back pain is abrupt paraplegia. Acute paraplegia occurs secondary to a major insult to the spinal cord. In addition to muscle weakness, bladder, bowel, and sexual function need to be assessed. Disorders associated with acute paraplegia include spinal cord tumors, epidural hemorrhage, epidural abscess, embolus, spinal artery thrombosis, and central herniation of a nucleus pulposus (cauda equina syndrome).[15] These disorders are associated with a history of progressive muscle weakness, anticoagulant therapy, fever, or cardiac disease (atrial fibrillation or atherosclerosis). Physical examination helps establish the potential causes of the paraplegia and spinal cord compression. Neurologic dysfunction, although not life threatening, results from a spinal cord insult and requires immediate evaluation. If the level of insult to the spinal cord is high up in the cervical spine, it may present respiratory difficulties and thus become a life-threatening emergency. After the life-threatening causes of neck or low back pain have been eliminated as potential diagnoses, a complete history should be obtained.

Age

Figure 4-1 lists the various causes of spinal pain arranged by the age range at which they most frequently occur. Spondyloarthropathies, including ankylosing spondylitis, reactive arthritis, spondylitis associated with inflammatory bowel disease, and benign tumors of the spine (aneurysmal bone cyst, osteoid osteoma, osteoblastoma, and giant cell tumor) occur between the third and fourth decades. Trauma and spasmodic torticollis occur more commonly in younger individuals. Diseases of middle age include diffuse idiopathic skeletal hyperostosis, gout, Paget's disease, and osteomyelitis. A different set of diseases occurs more commonly during and following the sixth decade. These diseases include malignant disease (metastases), metabolic disease (chondrocalcinosis), and degenerative diseases (expanding aortic aneurysm). Approximately 80% of patients with malignant disease affecting the lumbar spine are older than 50 years of age.[10] Cervical angina is one of the few disorders exclusively limited to the neck and arm in older populations.

Gender

Spinal pain is common in men and women. Some studies indicate that the frequency of neck injuries may actually be higher in women. Occupational exposure for women who work at a desk and frequently type at computers may explain some of the increased prevalence of this symptom. Back pain occurs predominantly in men. Occupational exposure to heavy-duty labor explains some of the increased prevalence of this symptom. Many medical illnesses, including the spondyloarthropathies, infections, and malignant and benign tumors, occur more commonly in men. Endocrinologic disorders, including parathyroid disorders and muscle disease (polymyalgia rheumatica and fibromyalgia), are more likely to occur in women. Psoriatic spondylitis, spondylitis associated with inflammatory bowel disease, hemangioma, herpes zoster, and skeletal metastases occur with equal frequency in men and women. A listing of illnesses associated with neck and back pain according to sexual predominance is presented in Table 4-1.

FAMILY HISTORY

Familial predisposition does occur in certain medical illnesses that are associated with spinal pain. A prime example of a group of illnesses with such a predisposition is the spondyloarthropathies. In the presence of a particular histocompatibility locus antigen (HLA-27), members of a family are at risk of developing ankylosing spondylitis, reactive arthritis, psoriatic spondylitis, and spondylitis associated with inflammatory bowel disease. Other spondyloarthropathies, such as those occurring in familial Mediterranean fever and Whipple's disease, occur more commonly in family members without any specifically associated genetic factor. The ethnic background of the family may predispose members to specific illnesses. White women of northern European extraction are at greater risk of developing osteoporosis. Ashkenazic Jews may develop Gaucher's disease. Many of the other illnesses that cause spinal pain have no specific familial predilection. However, it is always prudent for the examining physician to inquire about other family members with similar symptoms and the diagnoses that have been associated with their complaints. This information can help direct the clinician in formulating the diagnostic evaluation of the patient.

OCCUPATIONAL/SOCIAL HISTORY

The occupational history is essential for evaluating the risk of the patient for developing mechanical neck or back pain. Workers who have been required to do repetitive tasks with their upper extremity as well as prolonged sitting with their head in a flexed position, such as during typing, are at risk of developing mechanical neck pain. In addition, occupations that involve vibration or exposure to an environment filled with smoke may also predispose workers to this problem. However, neck pain is common and does not require occupational exposure to occur. Workers doing heavy lifting at their job are at risk of developing mechanical low back pain, but this symptom also occurs in sedentary workers. Lifting a light object from a rotated position or stretching far overhead to reach an object on a shelf may be associated with the onset of low back pain. The association of work and the onset of pain is important in evaluating the patient in regard to compensation. Whether or not the symptom of spinal pain is related to the patient's work, it is important to discuss the association of the two from the patient's viewpoint.

Ankylosing spondylitis is not caused by any work-related actions. Patients may have difficulty accepting that the work they have been doing has no correlation with the onset of their illness. A positive therapeutic outcome has a better chance of occurring when patients realize the source of their difficulties and do not have false expectations about compensation for their symptoms. It is also appropriate to inquire about any pending litigation in regard to the patient's spinal pain. It is incumbent on the physician not to assume that, because workers' compensation is involved or litigation is pending, the patient's symptoms are fictitious or exaggerated. Physicians should give the patient the benefit of the doubt. Patients who are hurt on the job or have an accident develop spinal pain secondary to mechanical or medical causes. An incidental trauma may be assumed to be the source of pain while the actual cause of pain, such as a pathologic fracture secondary to a tumor, goes unrecognized. Only a thorough examination by the patient's physician can discover the true cause of the patient's spinal pain.

Pressures to return to work may be different for the salaried employee versus the self-employed person. A self-employed individual may push the physician into cutting corners of evaluation and therapy to obtain the "quick fix" needed to allow a return to normal activities. On the other hand, the salaried employee may delay return because of the fear of reinjury. The treating physician must keep these concerns of patients in mind when developing an appropriate diagnostic and therapeutic program.

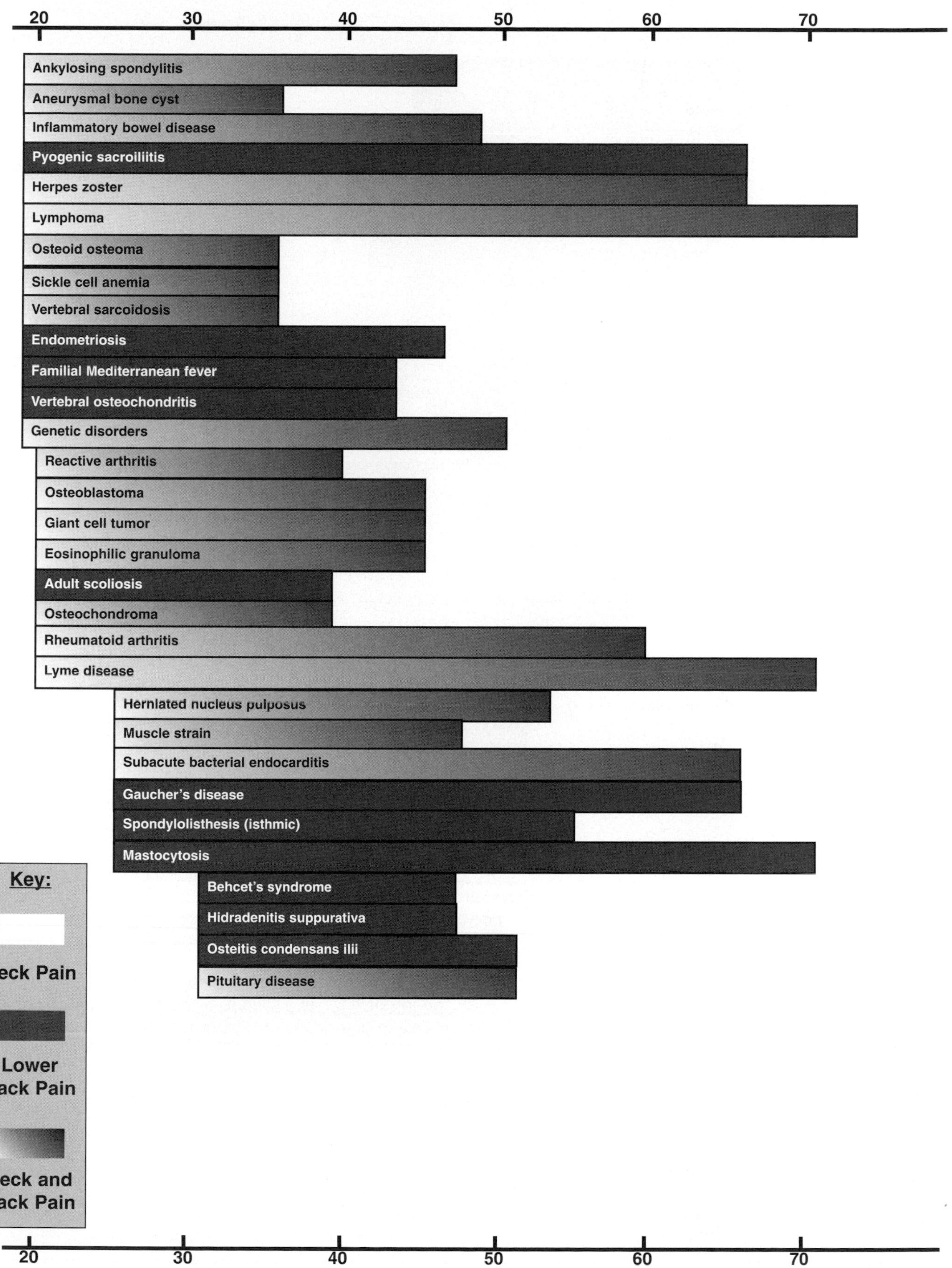

Figure 4-1 Age at peak incidence of neck and low back pain associated with mechanical and nonmechanical disorders.

Continued

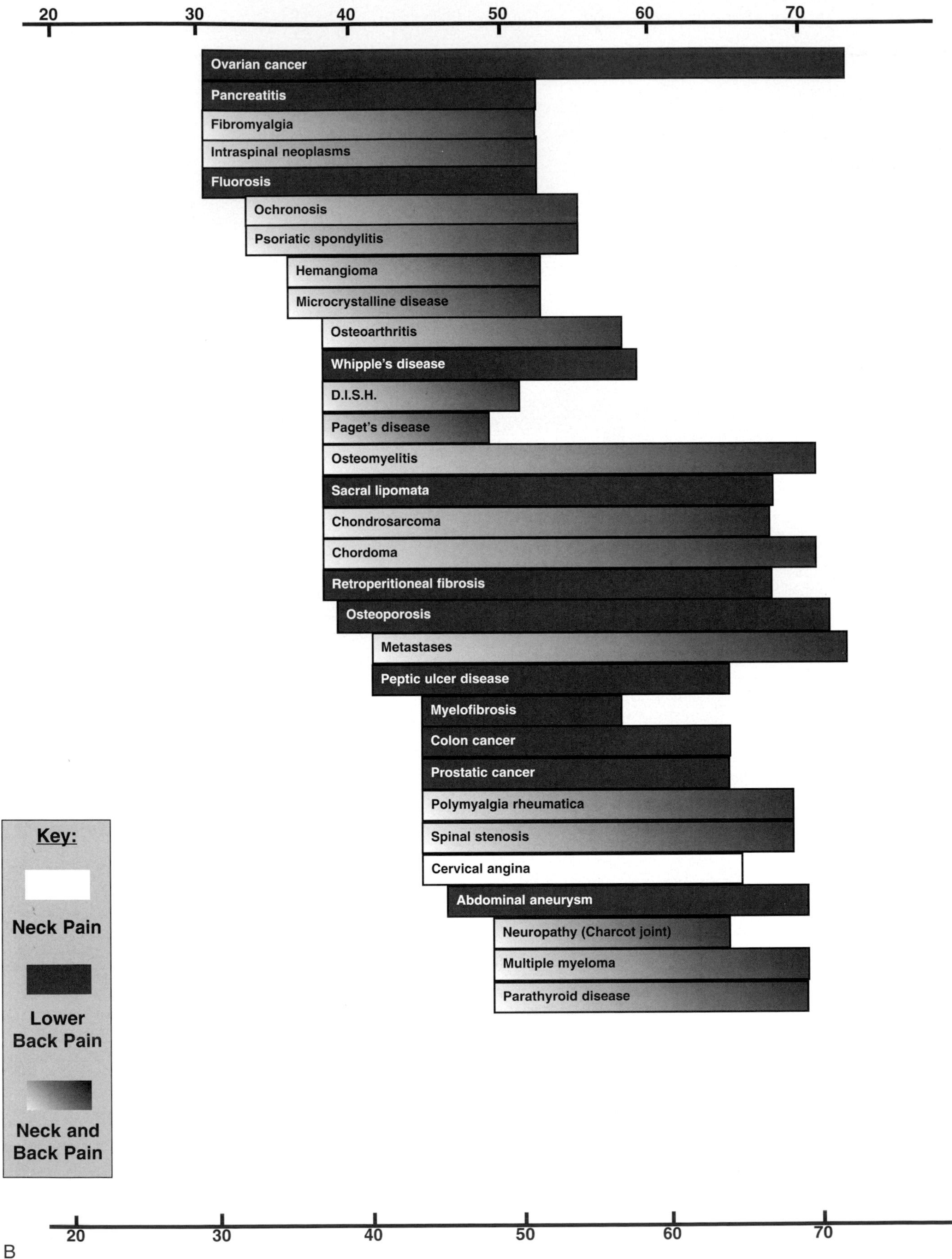

B

Figure 4-1, cont'd

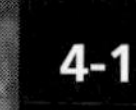

4-1 SEX PREVALENCE FOR ILLNESSES ASSOCIATED WITH SPINAL PAIN

MALE PREDOMINANT
Ankylosing spondylitis
Reactive arthritis
Familial Mediterranean fever
Behçet's syndrome
Whipple's disease
Diffuse idiopathic skeletal hyperostosis
Osteomyelitis
Discitis
Pyogenic sacroiliitis
Paget's disease
Osteoblastoma
Eosinophilic granuloma
Osteoid osteoma
Multiple myeloma
Chondrosarcoma
Chordoma
Lymphoma
Ochronosis
Gout
Abdominal aneurysm
Prostatic cancer
Vertebral sarcoidosis
Retroperitoneal fibrosis
Peptic ulcer disease
Osteochondroma
Vertebral osteochondritis

FEMALE PREDOMINANT
Rheumatoid arthritis
Osteitis condensans ilii
Polymyalgia rheumatica
Fibromyalgia
Giant cell tumor
Aneurysmal bone cyst
Sacroiliac lipomata
Osteoporosis
Parathyroid disease
Calcium pyrophosphate deposition disease
Endometriosis
Pregnancy
Ovarian cancer
Adult scoliosis

EQUAL FREQUENCY
Psoriatic spondylitis
Enteropathic arthritis
Hemangioma
Gaucher's disease
Pituitary disease
Subacute bacterial endocarditis
Herpes zoster
Mastocytosis
Skeletal metastases
Mechanical disorders
Muscle strain
Herniated disc
Osteoarthritis/spinal stenosis
Spondylolysis

Social history also includes quantification of consumption of alcohol, coffee, cigarettes, and recreational drugs. Increased consumption of alcohol, coffee, or cigarettes is associated with osteoporosis, and illicit drug use results in immunosuppression and predisposition to infection. Smoking may also be associated with increased risk for herniated intervertebral disc and low back pain.[7]

Review of leisure time activities is another important way to measure level of function before the onset of spinal pain. Are recreational activities limited to the same degree as work-related tasks? Response to therapy can often be measured by the patient's resumption of recreational activities. Inquiries about the new use of bifocals may also be significant. Repeated flexion and extension of the cervical spine may result in neck pain, occipital pain, or retro-orbital discomfort.[3]

PAST MEDICAL HISTORY

Past medical history should list in chronologic order all operations, hospitalizations, and previous severe injuries that affected the spine. Neck injuries remembered from childhood are usually significant in the amount of damage sustained by anatomic structures. A history of slipping on ice and hitting the head or "cracking" the back, resulting in bed rest for a few days, may be the initial episode that results in the development of disc disease in adulthood. Individuals may remember a swimming accident in which the neck was severely bent during bodysurfing or diving. Similarly, a car accident or any high-speed trauma with a whiplash injury may, in some instances, predispose to later degeneration, although this association has not been linked. All general medical problems should be reviewed. Certain diseases, including diabetes, other endocrinopathies, malignancies, and metabolic bone disease, may have a direct effect on structures in the spine. A past history of cancer has high specificity as the cause of back pain but has low sensitivity, with only one third of patients with an underlying malignancy having this history.[9] Other disorders may not have a direct effect on the neck or back pain per se, but they may be associated with physical disorders (congestive heart failure and angina) or require specific medications (anticoagulants) that limit the therapeutic options for the treating physician. In addition, allergies to medications are listed on the history.

REVIEW OF SYSTEMS

Although frequently thought to be redundant or superfluous, review of systems is an essential part of neck or back pain history. A complete negative review is added evidence for the regional or mechanical nature of the pain. Positive responses help organize symptoms into patterns associated with systemic illness that cause spinal pain. The presence of constitutional symptoms is a worrisome finding and requires a more thorough evaluation. Fever in the setting of new-onset neck or back pain may be associated with influenza, pyogenic discitis, or osteomyelitis. The sensitivity of fever as a marker of spinal infection runs the gamut from 27% for tuberculous osteomyelitis to 83% for spinal epidural abscess.[10]

Review of the integumentary system may reveal a history of scaling patches over the elbows that respond to topical agents (psoriasis) or nail opacification that never responded to antifungal therapy (reactive arthritis). History of conjunctivitis, iritis, or oral ulcers should raise the possibility of a spondyloarthropathy as the cause of neck or back pain. Temporomandibular joint dysfunction may be associated with a painful bite or limited jaw opening resulting in neck pain. Decreased cardiopulmonary function may be a manifestation of the spondyloarthropathy or endocrinopathy. Lesions of segments C3, C4, and C5 may affect the diaphragm and thus breathing. Patients may complain of dyspnea when the nerve supply to respiratory muscles is affected. Visceral causes of neck or back pain should be considered in the patient with a positive history for gastroesophageal reflux, diffuse esophageal spasm, lower gastrointestinal disorders, or malignancy. Dysphagia may be caused by disorders affecting the cervical spine. Pain with swallowing may be related to anterior disc protrusion, vertebral osteophyte, or vertebral subluxation into the esophagus. Difficulty forming a bolus of food may be related to muscular weakness secondary to a primary muscle disorder (polymyositis) or a neurologic disorder (myasthenia gravis). A history of anemia may be related to a systemic illness, gastrointestinal blood loss of an iatrogenic nature (drugs), or a primary hematologic disorder (sickle cell disease). A history of peptic ulcer disease may alter the ability to tolerate anti-inflammatory medications. Nausea and vomiting may accompany spinal cord compression.

A cardiovascular system history is relevant. Cervical angina consists of cardiac ischemic symptoms referred to regions innervated by the C5–T1 nerve roots, thereby mimicking an acute cervical radiculopathy.[19] Pain may radiate to the left shoulder or arm and be accompanied by upper extremity numbness. These symptoms are usually exacerbated by exertion, relieved by nitrates, and unaffected by neck movement. In older individuals, the coexistence of true angina and pseudoangina must be considered. Irritation of the C4 nerve root, which supplies the diaphragm and pericardium, may result in palpitations or tachycardia. Episodes of syncope may be indicative of insufficiency of vertebral circulation secondary to cervical spine disease.

Neuropsychiatric history should not be skipped. Headache is common in cervical syndromes. The occipital region is affected and is dull and aching in character. The headache pain may spread to the eye region on one or both sides. This pain may be related to occipital neuralgia. The pain is aggravated by straining, sneezing, and coughing, as well as by movements of the head and neck. Headache may result from nerve root or sympathetic nerve compression, vertebral artery pressure, autonomic dysfunction, muscle spasm, or osteoarthritis of the apophyseal joints affecting the upper three cervical vertebrae.[11] In its most severe form, headache may awaken individuals from sleep. A number of factors should alert the clinician to potential, dangerous forms of headache that are unassociated with abnormalities in the cervical spine (Table 4-2).[23] Eye symptoms, such as blurred vision, increased tearing, eye pain, or retro-orbital pain, may be associated with cervical disorders. Irritation of the cervical sympathetic nerves that supply eye structures that are innervated by plexuses surrounding the vertebral and internal carotid arteries may cause neck symptoms. Abnormalities in equilibrium may also result from disorders of the sympathetic plexus surrounding the vertebral arteries. These abnormalities of gait may also be associated with decreased auditory acuity or tinnitus. These symptoms of autonomic disorders may persist during pain-free intervals.[2]

Descriptions of local versus generalized sensory and motor abnormalities help categorize neck or back symptoms as a component of a systemic neurologic disease or as a regional disturbance associated with local nerve dysfunction. Review of any psychiatric disturbance is also essential. During this part of the examination it is helpful to have the patient describe his or her personality. Is the patient obsessive, compulsive, or driven? Is the patient passive? Is the patient depressed about the physical condition? Is the patient overly anxious or unconcerned about the potential cause of the neck or back pain (anxiety neurosis or hysteria)? Answers to these questions alert the physician to the individual who may have psychogenic spinal pain.

PRESENT ILLNESS

The majority of the history taken about the present illness is directed toward the elaboration of the chronologic development of the neck or back pain and its character, review of the results of previously obtained diagnostic tests, and response to therapy.

Onset

Mechanical causes of spinal pain (muscle strain and herniated nucleus pulposus) usually have an acute, sudden onset. The onset of pain is frequently associated with a specific task done in a mechanically disadvantaged position. Muscle bundles may be torn, fasciae stretched, and facet joints or uncovertebral joints irritated. Pain starts instantaneously or may come on gradually within a few hours.

Medical causes of spinal pain tend to have a more gradual onset of pain. Tumor pain, for example, starts insidiously, except for episodes of acute pain associated with pathologic fractures of skeletal structures. Pain from inflammatory spondyloarthropathy may develop over months or years.

4-2 DANGEROUS SIGNS INVOLVING HEADACHES

1. Headache is a new symptom or has markedly changed in character over the past 3 months.
2. Presence of sensory or motor deficits accompanying headache other than the typical visual prodromata of migraine with aura.
3. Headache solely on one side of the head.
4. Headache associated with unconsciousness after a trauma.
5. Headache is constant and unremitting.
6. Patient with tension-like headache has pain intensity steadily increasing over a period of weeks to months with little relief; worse in the morning and less severe during the day and accompanied by vomiting.
7. Headache occurs in a patient with a history of cancer.
8. Headache is associated with change in personality, behavior, or intellectual function.
9. Headache is a new complaint in an individual who is older than 60 years of age.
10. Headache pain is sudden in onset and occurs during conditions of exertion.
11. Headache occurs in an individual with a family history of cerebral aneurysm, other vascular anomalies, or polycystic kidneys.

Modified from Andrasik F: Assessment of patients with headaches. In Turk DC, Melzack R (eds): Handbook of Pain Assessment. New York, Guilford, 1992, p 345.

Duration and Frequency

Mechanical spinal pain generally has a duration of a few days to a few months. Most muscle strains are relieved within 1 or 2 weeks. Disc herniations may require 8 weeks for resolution. Disc degeneration may cause a low-grade chronic discomfort that is exacerbated during acute attacks that last for 2 to 4 weeks. Most mechanical spinal pain is intermittent. The frequency of episodes depends to a certain extent on exposure of the individual to mechanical stresses that worsen the condition.

Medical conditions, in contrast, cause chronic pain that is persistent rather than episodic. Patients with spondyloarthropathies develop chronic aching pain that has a long duration measured in months. Pain may extend to other portions of the spine. Tumors of the spine cause pain that is persistent, building in intensity over months. In addition, a history of night pain is also frequent.

Psychogenic pains are constant and unrelenting. Histories of years of constant, excruciating pain are not uncommon.

Location and Radiation

Most mechanical and medical causes of spinal pain are localized to the spine. Damage to the musculoskeletal structures (discs and posterior apophyseal joints) may cause referred pain in surrounding areas of the neck and shoulders or lumbosacral spine. These structures include adjacent paraspinous, anterior, and posterior cervical muscles in the neck as well as buttock and thigh muscles in the low back. Abnormalities in facet joints, annular disc fibers, and supporting ligaments may also result in neck or low back pain. Pain can be localized to a specific midline structure, such as a spinous process, or may be more lateral in the paraspinal tissues. The identification of the point of maximum tenderness in the midline often helps differentiate bone lesions from soft tissue lesions with paraspinal pain.

Cervical Intervertebral Disc Herniation

Pain that radiates into the arm from the cervical spine or that is exclusively in the arm is more suggestive of a cervical nerve root irritation. Lesions from C5 and below may cause arm symptoms. Discs that disrupt annular fibers cause pain in the neck. As the disc impinges the nerve root, pain is referred down the arm. Once the disc is extruded and the pressure on the annulus from disc protrusion is relieved, arm pain continues while neck pain may resolve. Spinal canal narrowing also causes radiation of pain into the arm. Disc herniation causes radiating pain that is present at rest, whereas radiating pain with canal narrowing occurs in positions that extend the spine or decrease room in the spinal canal for the neural elements.

Radiation of pain to the upper extremity is not limited to mechanical abnormalities exclusively. Compression of the brachial plexus may occur from thoracic outlet syndrome, a cervical rib, or hypertrophy of the scalene muscles. Pathologic conditions in and around the shoulder may also result in nerve compression as well as compression of any point distally in the extremity itself. Common causes are compression of the ulnar nerve in the cubital tunnel and the median nerve in the carpal tunnel syndrome. In general it is easy to distinguish these problems from a herniated cervical disc, if their diagnosis is thought of and checked for. It is important to elicit a history of shoulder and arm pain that is related to position or movement of the arm. It is also important to remember that a subdiaphragmatic process such as an abscess can cause referred pain in the shoulder.

Lumbar Intervertebral Disc Herniation

Pain radiating to the lower leg from the lumbar spine or exclusively in the lower limb is more suggestive of a lumbar nerve root irritation. Lumbar discs that disrupt annular fibers cause pain in the low back. As the disc impinges the nerve root, pain is referred down the leg. Once the disc is extruded and the pressure on the annulus from disc protrusion is relieved, leg pain continues while back pain resolves. Lumbar spinal stenosis also causes radiation of pain into the lower extremity. Disc herniation causes radiating pain at rest, while with spinal stenosis radiating pain occurs in positions that extend the spine and decrease room in the spinal canal for the neural elements.

Radiating pain to the lower extremity is not limited to mechanical abnormalities. The piriformis syndrome includes leg pain associated with back pain but without persistent abnormal neurologic signs. The sciatic nerve is compressed by the piriformis muscle. The muscle undergoes sustained contraction because of its attachment to an inflamed sacroiliac joint. Therapy that decreases joint inflammation reduces muscle contraction, resulting in diminished radicular symptoms. This syndrome is easily confused with a herniated disc. If the existence of pseudosciatica is not recognized, unnecessary diagnostic tests are done.

In contrast to pain from nerve root irritation, psychogenic pain is not well localized. Large nondermatomal areas are affected. Radiation of pain follows no consistent pattern.

Aggravating and Alleviating Factors

Characteristically, mechanical lesions of the cervical spine improve with recumbency and worsen with increased activity. Increased activity includes long sitting or standing with the neck unsupported, particularly when looking down at a keyboard or reading. Patients with muscle strain improve with bed rest or controlled immobilization of the neck with a soft cervical collar. Characteristically, mechanical lesions of the lumbosacral spine improve with rest and worsen with increased activity. Increased activity includes prolonged sitting with forward flexion if the patient has a herniated disc or prolonged standing in an extended position if the patient has spinal stenosis. Patients with muscle strain improve with modified activity. Not all spine movements necessarily exacerbate muscle strain pain. Careful history defines those motions that are painless and put no stress on damaged muscles and those that irritate the injured muscle and result in reflex spasm.

Increases in cerebrospinal fluid pressure increase nerve root irritation caused by disc herniation. Coughing, sneezing, and Valsalva's maneuver increase pressure and may exacerbate radicular pain. Sudden, reflex motions associated with coughing or sneezing may increase muscle strain as well. However, pain caused by muscle strain remains localized and does not radiate into the extremities.

Some patients with mechanical neck or back pain feel worse with bed rest. Patients with spondyloarthropathy have exacerbated pain after they have been in bed for a few hours. Not infrequently they wake up during the night because of pain associated with rolling over in bed. Early morning is the worst time of day for the patient with spondyloarthropathy.

Pain from tumors involving bone, muscle, or the spinal cord is often increased with recumbency. Patients with such tumors seek relief by sleeping in a chair or pacing the floor.

Other patients do find relief of pain with recumbency. These individuals find relief only with absolute immobility. This is a sign of acute infection, compression fracture related to metabolic bone disease, or pathologic fracture secondary to a tumor or infiltrative disease.

Patients with viscerogenic referred pain rarely describe any association of the discomfort with position. Patients with colic are constantly moving, trying to find a comfortable position. Interventions that are effective at reducing genitourinary symptoms (antibiotics) or gastrointestinal symptoms (antacids) control back pain in these individuals. Patients with psychogenic pain have difficulty describing factors that relieve or worsen their pain. The pain is present all the time. There is no position that is comfortable. Activities that involve little physical effort have an exaggerated effect on their pain.

Do weather changes have an effect on the severity of spinal symptoms? An attempt at the answer was repeated by McGorry and associates.[17] Over a 6-month period, 121 back pain sufferers from Boston, Massachusetts, completed a diary of their discomfort that was matched with weather conditions on the same days. Individuals who believed that pain is affected by weather described greater pain with colder temperatures and low vapor pressure. This study did not study weather effects during winter with lower temperatures and barometric pressure. A study to really determine the effect of weather will have to be 12 months in duration as a minimum. The effects of weather were small. In general, patients with chronic spinal conditions experience some variability of symptoms that can be correlated with changes in barometric pressure and temperature.

Time of Day

Mechanical disorders (muscle strain, degenerative disc disease, spinal stenosis, and osteoarthritis) cause pain that increases with activity. The end of the day, after the patient has been up and around, is associated with the most pain. Diurnal changes in spinal mechanics may also explain maximal stresses on structures in the lumbar spine that correlate with patient symptoms.[1] The risk of disc herniation is greatest in the morning when the disc is extended to its greatest degree. At the end of the day, when the disc is less tense, symptoms related to joint compression are more likely. Medical disorders are problematic in the morning or after the patient has gone to sleep. Classically, inflammatory arthropathies cause morning stiffness. Patients have great difficulty getting out of bed in the morning because of stiffness and pain. As the patient ambulates, the stiffness and pain lessen.

Tumors of the spine and spinal cord cause pain that increases with recumbency. Therefore, most individuals with cervical or lumbar spine tumors complain of pain that is maximal during the night. This characteristic of tumors is not solely reserved to malignant processes. Benign tumors, a prime example being an osteoid osteoma, cause severe nocturnal pain. Patients with spinal tumors may get up and ambulate at night to diminish their discomfort.

Sleeping position of the patient may have a significant effect on the extent of neck pain. Individuals with large pillows may be in a flexed posture for extended periods. An arm hyperabducted under the pillow may be associated with shoulder pain.

Quality and Intensity

Description of the quality of the pain can be helpful in identifying its source. The adjectives used to describe neck and back pain are numerous. Initially patients should describe the quality of pain themselves without suggestions from the examining physician. A list of words from the physician may alter the patient's responses to a category of terms that cannot really describe the discomfort. However, some patients are unable to describe their pain in their own words. At this point it would be helpful to supply them with a list of choices. One example of such a list of pain descriptions is the McGill Pain Questionnaire (Fig. 4-2).[18] The questionnaire divides words into three major groups: (1) those that describe the sensory quality of pain in terms of temporal, spatial, pressure, thermal, and other properties; (2) those that describe the affective qualities of pain in terms of tension, fear, and autonomic properties; and (3) those that describe the subjective, overall intensity of pain. In each category the words are listed according to increasing intensity. In addition a line drawing of the body is included, demarcating the location of pain. A pain rating index is determined by adding together the rank values of origin in each subclass. The number of words chosen is quantified. The scale can be administered on successive visits to help quantify response to therapy. If the McGill Pain Questionnaire is not used, the examining physician should include a line drawing of the body in the patient's history. The pictorial representation of the patient's pain helps delineate its extent. The patient's response to therapy may also be monitored by review of the extent of painful areas on serial line drawings. Pain mapping can be especially helpful in patients with low back pain of uncertain etiology that has been refractory to nonoperative therapies.[20]

The intensity of pain may also be measured by visual means. The visual analogue scale (Fig. 4-3) is a visual way to quantify pain.[14] A visual analogue scale is a line, 10 cm

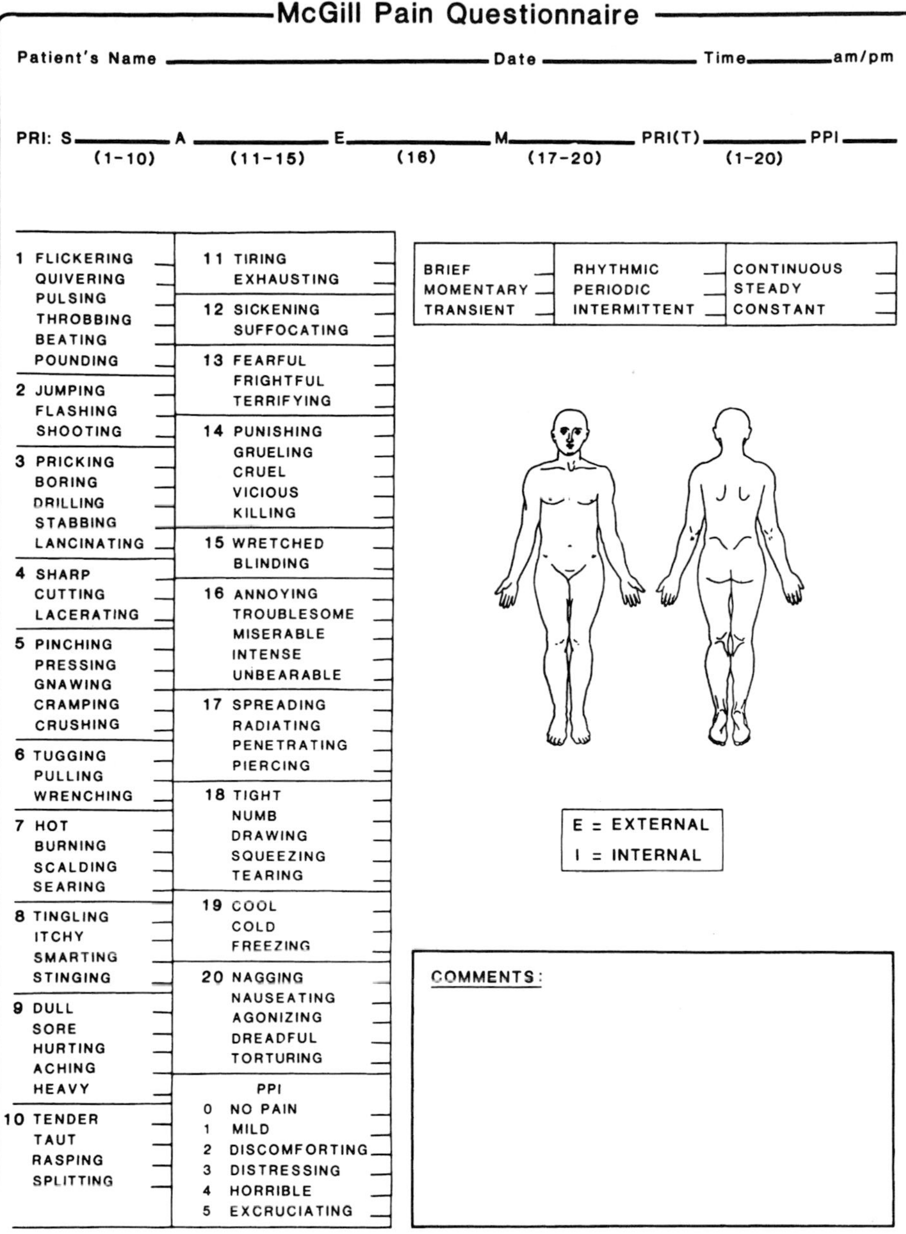

McGill Pain Questionnaire

Patient's Name ______ Date ______ Time ______ am/pm

PRI: S ______ (1-10) A ______ (11-15) E ______ (16) M ______ (17-20) PRI(T) ______ (1-20) PPI ______

1 FLICKERING, QUIVERING, PULSING, THROBBING, BEATING, POUNDING
2 JUMPING, FLASHING, SHOOTING
3 PRICKING, BORING, DRILLING, STABBING, LANCINATING
4 SHARP, CUTTING, LACERATING
5 PINCHING, PRESSING, GNAWING, CRAMPING, CRUSHING
6 TUGGING, PULLING, WRENCHING
7 HOT, BURNING, SCALDING, SEARING
8 TINGLING, ITCHY, SMARTING, STINGING
9 DULL, SORE, HURTING, ACHING, HEAVY
10 TENDER, TAUT, RASPING, SPLITTING
11 TIRING, EXHAUSTING
12 SICKENING, SUFFOCATING
13 FEARFUL, FRIGHTFUL, TERRIFYING
14 PUNISHING, GRUELING, CRUEL, VICIOUS, KILLING
15 WRETCHED, BLINDING
16 ANNOYING, TROUBLESOME, MISERABLE, INTENSE, UNBEARABLE
17 SPREADING, RADIATING, PENETRATING, PIERCING
18 TIGHT, NUMB, DRAWING, SQUEEZING, TEARING
19 COOL, COLD, FREEZING
20 NAGGING, NAUSEATING, AGONIZING, DREADFUL, TORTURING

PPI
0 NO PAIN
1 MILD
2 DISCOMFORTING
3 DISTRESSING
4 HORRIBLE
5 EXCRUCIATING

BRIEF	RHYTHMIC	CONTINUOUS
MOMENTARY	PERIODIC	STEADY
TRANSIENT	INTERMITTENT	CONSTANT

E = EXTERNAL
I = INTERNAL

COMMENTS:

Figure 4-2 The McGill Pain Questionnaire. *(From Melzack R [ed]: Pain Measurement and Assessment. New York, Raven, 1983.)*

in length, in which one end represents no pain and the other severe, incapacitating pain. Patients mark a point on the line corresponding to the severity of their pain. The distance from this point to the end of the line represents pain severity. The visual analogue scale has greater sensitivity quantifying pain than verbal descriptors. It is a continuum, whereas verbal descriptors correspond to points along a line. There are not enough words to describe all the possible points along a line.

Leak and colleagues at Northwick Park Hospital in London, England, developed a validated questionnaire to measure neck pain and disability (Fig. 4-4).[16] Questions on duration and intensity of pain were good indicators

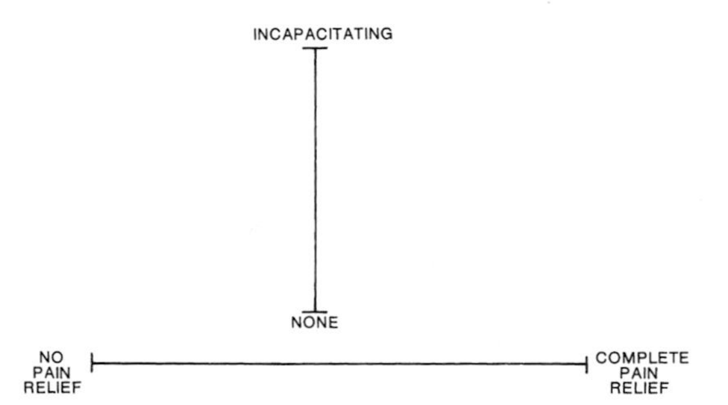

Figure 4-3 Visual analogue scales for pain (*top*) and pain relief (*bottom*). The physical orientation of the scales may be vertical or horizontal.

of patients' global assessment of their condition. Improvement of symptoms over time was associated with a decrease in the severity of pain as measured by the questionnaire. This questionnaire is a useful tool to objectify the degree of neck pain experienced by patients with cervical spine disease.

Another differentiation is between organic and psychogenic pain. A standardized way to differentiate psychogenic from organic pain is to use the Minnesota Multiphasic Personality Inventory (MMPI). The MMPI is a 566-question, self-administered true-false test formulated to identify psychological traits, for example, hypochondriasis, depression, hysteria, or psychopathic deviance, associated with elevated scale scores in patients with chronic pain.[22] Although the MMPI may help differentiate organic from functional pain, the test does not correlate well with patient physical findings. A test that validates the presence of pain is the Mensana Clinic Back

NECK PAIN QUESTIONNAIRE

Label

Surname: OTHER NAMES:
HOSPITAL NO:

DATE OF BIRTH:
CONSULTANT:
DATE COMPLETED:

Please read:
This questionnaire has been designed to give us information as to how your NECK PAIN has affected your ability to manage in everyday life.

Please answer every section and mark in each section ONLY THE ONE BOX which applies to you. We realize you may consider that two of the statements in any one section relate to you, but PLEASE JUST MARK THE BOX WHICH MOST CLOSELY DESCRIBES YOUR PROBLEM.

Remember, just mark ONE box in each section.

1. NECK PAIN INTENSITY

- ☐ I have no pain at the moment
- ☐ The pain is mild at the moment
- ☐ The pain is moderate at the moment
- ☐ The pain is severe at the moment
- ☐ The pain is the worst imaginable at the moment

2. NECK PAIN AND SLEEPING

- ☐ My sleep is never disturbed by pain
- ☐ My sleep is occasionally disturbed by pain
- ☐ My sleep is regularly disturbed by pain
- ☐ Because of pain I have less than 5 hours sleep in total
- ☐ Because of pain I have less than 2 hours sleep in total

3. PINS & NEEDLES OR NUMBNESS IN THE ARMS AT NIGHT

- ☐ I have no pins & needles or numbness at night
- ☐ I have occasional pins & needles or numbness at night
- ☐ My sleep is regularly disturbed by pins & needles or numbness
- ☐ Because of pins & needles I have less than 5 hours sleep in total
- ☐ Because of pins & needles or numbness I have less than 2 hours sleep in total

4. DURATION OF SYMPTOMS

- ☐ My neck and arms feel normal all day
- ☐ I have symptoms in my neck or arms on waking, which last less than 1 hour
- ☐ Symptoms are present on and off for a total period of 1–4 hours
- ☐ Symptoms are present on and off for a total of more than 4 hours
- ☐ Symptoms are present continuously all day

5. CARRYING

- ☐ I can carry heavy objects without extra pain
- ☐ I can carry heavy objects, but they give me extra pain
- ☐ Pain prevents me from carrying heavy objects, but I can manage medium weight objects
- ☐ I can only lift light weight objects
- ☐ I cannot lift anything at all

6. READING & WATCHING T.V.

- ☐ I can do this as long as I wish with no problems
- ☐ I can do this as long as I wish, if I'm in a suitable position
- ☐ I can do this as long as I wish, but it causes extra pain
- ☐ Pain causes me to stop doing this sooner than I would like
- ☐ Pain prevents me from doing this at all

7. WORKING/HOUSEWORK ETC

- ☐ I can do my usual work without extra pain
- ☐ I can do my usual work, but it gives me extra pain
- ☐ Pain prevents me from doing my usual work for more than half the usual time
- ☐ Pain prevents me from doing my usual work for more than a quarter the usual time
- ☐ Pain prevents me from working at all

8. SOCIAL ACTIVITIES

- ☐ My social life is normal and causes me no extra pain
- ☐ My social life is normal, but increases the degree of pain
- ☐ Pain has restricted my social life, but I am still able to go out
- ☐ Pain has restricted my social life to the home
- ☐ I have no social life because of pain

9. DRIVING (Omit 9 if you never drive a car when in good health)

- ☐ I can drive whenever necessary without discomfort
- ☐ I can drive whenever necessary, but with discomfort
- ☐ Neck pain or stiffness limits my driving occasionally
- ☐ Neck pain or stiffness limits my driving frequently
- ☐ I cannot drive at all due to neck symptoms

10. Compared with the last time you answered this Questionnaire, is your neck pain:

- ☐ Much better
- ☐ Slightly better
- ☐ The same
- ☐ Slightly worse
- ☐ Much worse

Thank you very much for your help.

DATE: . . . .

TIME: . . . .

SIGNED . . . .

Figure 4-4 Neck pain questionnaire. *(From Leak AM, Cooper J, Dyer S, et al: The Northwick Park Neck Pain Questionnaire, devised to measure neck pain and disability. Br J Rheumatol 33:474, 1994. By permission of Oxford University Press.)*

4-3 MENSANA CLINIC BACK PAIN TEST*

		Points
1	**How did the pain that you now experience occur?**	
	(a) Sudden onset with accident or definable event	0
	(b) Slow, progressive onset without acute exacerbation	1
	(c) Slow, progressive onset with acute exacerbation without accident or event	2
	(d) Sudden onset without an accident or definable event	3
2	**Where do you experience the pain?**	
	(a) One site, specific, well-defined consistent with anatomic distribution	0
	(b) More than one site, each well-defined and consistent with anatomic distribution	1
	(c) One site, inconsistent with anatomic considerations, or not well-defined	2
	(d) Vague description, more than one site, of which one is inconsistent with anatomic considerations, or not well-defined or anatomically explainable	3
3	**Do you ever have trouble falling asleep at night, or are you ever awakened from sleep?** If the answer is "no," score 3 points and go to question 4. If the answer is "yes," proceed.	
3a	**What keeps you from falling asleep?**	
	(a) Trouble falling asleep every night due to pain	0
	(b) Trouble falling asleep due to pain more than three times a week	1
	(c) Trouble falling asleep due to pain less than three times a week	2
	(d) No trouble falling asleep due to pain	3
	(e) Trouble falling asleep that is not related to pain	4
3b	**What awakens you from sleep?**	
	(a) Awakened by pain every night	0
	(b) Awakened from sleep by pain more than three times a week	1
	(c) Not awakened from sleep by pain more than twice a week	2
	(d) Not awakened from sleep by pain	3
	(e) Restless sleep, or early morning awakening with or without being able to return to sleep, both unrelated to pain	4
4	**Does weather have any effect on your pain?**	
	(a) The pain is always worse in both cold and damp weather	0
	(b) The pain is always worse with damp weather or with cold weather	1
	(c) The pain is occasionally worse with cold or damp weather	2
	(d) The weather has no effect on the pain	3
5	**How would you describe the type of pain that you have?**	
	(a) Burning; or sharp, shooting pain; or pins and needles; or coldness; or numbness	0
	(b) Dull, aching pain, with occasional sharp, shooting pains not helped by heat; or the patient is experiencing hyperesthesia	1
	(c) Spasm-type pain, tension-type pain, or numbness over the area, relieved by massage or heat	2
	(d) Nagging or bothersome pain	3
	(e) Excruciating, overwhelming, or unbearable pain, relieved by massage or heat	4
6	**How frequently do you have your pain?**	
	(a) The pain is constant	0
	(b) The pain is nearly constant, occurring 50–80% of the time	1
	(c) The pain is intermittent, occurring 25–50% of the time	2
	(d) The pain is only occasionally present, occurring less than 25% of the time	3
7	**Does movement or position have any effect on the pain?**	
	(a) The pain is unrelieved by position change or rest, and there have been previous operations for the pain	0
	(b) The pain is worsened by use, standing, or walking and is relieved by lying down or resting the part	1
	(c) Position change and use have variable effects on the pain	2
	(d) The pain is not altered by use or position change, and there have been no previous operations for the pain	3
8	**What medications have you used in the past month?**	
	(a) No medications at all	0
	(b) Use of non-narcotic pain relievers, nonbenzodiazepine tranquilizers, or antidepressants	1
	(c) Use of a narcotic, hypnotic, or benzodiazepine less than three times a week	2
	(d) Use of a narcotic, hypnotic, or benzodiazepine more than four times a week	3
9	**What hobbies do you have, and can you still participate in them?**	
	(a) Unable to participate in any hobbies that were formerly enjoyed	0
	(b) Reduced number of hobbies or activities relating to a hobby	1
	(c) Still able to participate in hobbies but with some discomfort	2
	(d) Participates in hobbies as before	3
10	**How frequently did you have sex and orgasms before the pain, and how frequently do you have sex and orgasms now?**	
	(a^1) Sexual contact, prior to pain, three to four times a week, with no difficulty with orgasm; now sexual contact is 50% or less than previously, and coitus is interrupted by pain	0
	(a^2) (For people > 45 years of age) Sexual contact twice a week, with a 50% reduction in frequency since the onset of pain	0
	(a^3) (For people > 60 years of age) Sexual contact once a week, with a 50% reduction in frequency since the onset of pain	0
	(b) Prepain adjustment as defined above (a^1–a^3), with no difficulty with orgasm; now loss of interest in sex and/or difficulty with orgasm or erection	1
	(c) No change in sexual activity now as opposed to before the onset of pain	2
	(d) Unable to have sexual contact since the onset of pain, and difficulty with orgasm or erection prior to the pain	3
	(e) No sexual contact prior to the pain, or absence of orgasm prior to the pain	4

Continued

4-3 MENSANA CLINIC BACK PAIN TEST*—cont'd

	Score
11 Are you still working or doing your household chores?	
(a) Works every day at the same prepain job or same level of household duties	0
(b) Works every day but the job is not the same as prepain job, with reduced responsibility or physical activity	1
(c) Works sporadically or does a reduced amount of household chores	2
(d) Not at work, or all household chores are now performed by others	3
12 What is your income now compared with before your injury or the onset of pain, and what are your sources of income?	
(a) Any one of the following answers scores	
1. Experiencing financial difficulty with family income 50% or less than previously	0
2. Was retired and is still retired	
3. Patient is still working and is not having financial difficulties	
(b) Experiencing financial difficulty with family income only 50–75% of the prepain income	1
(c) Patient unable to work, and receives some compensation so that the family income is at least 75% of the prepain income	2
(d) Patient unable to work and receives no compensation, but the spouse works and family income is still 75% of the prepain income	3
(e) Patient does not work, yet the income from disability or other compensation sources is 80% or more of gross pay before the pain; the spouse does not work	4
13 Are you suing anyone, or is anyone suing you, or do you have an attorney helping you with compensation or disability payments?	
(a) No suit pending and does not have an attorney	0
(b) Litigation is pending but not related to the pain	1
(c) The patient is being sued as the result of an accident	2
(d) Litigation is pending or workmen's compensation case with a lawyer involved	3
14 If you had three wishes for anything in the world, what would you wish for?	
(a) "Get rid of the pain" is the only wish	0
(b) "Get rid of the pain" is one of the three wishes	1
(c) Does not mention getting rid of the pain, but has specific wishes usually of a personal nature such as for more money, a better relationship with spouse or children, etc.	2
(d) Does not mention pain, but offers general, nonpersonal wishes such as for world peace	3
15 Have you ever been depressed or thought of suicide?	
(a) Admits to depression, or has a history of depression secondary to pain and associated with crying spells and thoughts of suicide	0
(b) Admits to depression, guilt, and anger secondary to the pain	1
(c) Prior history of depression before the pain or a financial or personal loss prior to the pain; now admits to some depression	2
(d) Denies depression, crying spells, or feeling blue	3
(e) History of a suicide attempt prior to the onset of pain	4

*Each test question is asked by an examiner, who assigns the appropriate points for each response.

Score 17 or less: Patient is in the objective-pain category and reporting a normal response to chronic pain and is willing to participate in all modalities of therapy, including exercise and psychotherapy. This individual is a good surgical candidate. The patient with conversion reaction or post-traumatic neurosis may score less than 18 points. The person scoring 14 or less usually is considered more of an objective-pain patient than one scoring between 14 to 18.

Score 18 to 20: This group has features of the objective-pain and the exaggerating-pain patient and personality difficulties. Organic lesions result in a more extreme response because of a premorbid condition.

Score 21 to 31: Patient is in the exaggerating-pain category. This type of patient has a prepain personality that may increase the likelihood of obtaining secondary gain from the complaint of pain. This patient responds to therapy that alters his or her attitude toward chronic pain. Surgery should be undertaken with caution.

Score above 32: Patient is the affective-pain category and has considerable difficulty in coping with chronic pain. This individual may need psychiatric consultation.

Modified from Hendler N, Viernstein M, Gucer P, Long D: A preoperative screening test for chronic back pain patients. Psychosomatics 20:801, 1979.

Pain Test (MPT).[13] MPT is a 15-item questionnaire that takes about 10 minutes to complete (Table 4-3). Patients are classified as objective-pain patients, exaggerating-pain patients, and affective-pain patients corresponding to increasing test scores.[12] The MPT is more successful than MMPI in differentiating organic from functional low back pain and is useful for patients with chronic low back pain.[12] It also predicts the presence or absence of physical abnormalities better than MMPI. Other tests developed to measure the validity of the presence of pain rather than the patient's personality profile include the Oswestry Disability Questionnaire, the Sickness Impact Profile, and the Waddell Disability Index.[6]

Another means of testing the severity of pain is to measure the degree of disability an individual experiences with the discomfort. Roland and Morris developed a questionnaire consisting of 24 items (Table 4-4).[21] The test not only measures disability resulting from back pain but also measures response to therapy.

Outcome Measures

The literature evaluating the efficacy of therapeutic interventions uses a variety of measurement tools to quantify improvement. The determination of the best-outcome measure is a source of constant refinement dependent on the component of spinal disease to be evaluated. No single instrument fits all circumstances since spinal disease is associated with a variety of disorders and has no specific

4-4 ROLAND DISABILITY QUESTIONNAIRE*

1. I stay at home more of the time because of my back.
2. I change position frequently to try and get my back comfortable.
3. I walk more slowly than usual because of my back.
4. Because of my back I am not doing any of the jobs that I usually do around the house.
5. Because of my back, I use a handrail to get upstairs.
6. Because of my back, I lie down to rest more often.
7. Because of my back, I have to hold on to something to get out of an easy chair.
8. Because of my back, I try to get other people to do things for me.
9. I get dressed more slowly than usual because of my back.
10. I only stand up for short periods of time because of my back.
11. Because of my back, I try not to bend or kneel down.
12. I find it difficult to get out of a chair because of my back.
13. My back is painful almost all the time.
14. I find it difficult to turn over in bed because of my back.
15. My appetite is not very good because of my back pain.
16. I have trouble putting on my socks (or stockings) because of the pain in my back.
17. I only walk short distances because of my back pain.
18. I sleep less well because of my back.
19. Because of my back pain, I get dressed with help from someone else.
20. I sit down for most of the day because of my back.
21. I avoid heavy jobs around the house because of my back.
22. Because of my back pain, I am more irritable and bad tempered with people than usual.
23. Because of my back, I go upstairs more slowly than usual.
24. I stay in bed most of the time because of my back.

*The questions should be answered as your back feels today.
From Roland M, Morris R: A study of the natural history of back pain. I. Development of a reliable and sensitive measure of disability in low back pain. Spine 8:141, 1983.

laboratory quantitative measurement of success.[4] Deyo and colleagues presented a listing of six basic questions to be asked to determine the outcomes of a back pain study.[8] These questions (Table 4-5) are a simple tool to use in the clinical setting to monitor the clinical course of a patient.

Superficial somatic, deep somatic, neurogenic, viscerogenic referred, and psychogenic pain have qualities that differentiate them. Those qualities have been described in Chapter 3. Refer to that chapter for the characteristics of the various pain categories. Cramping, dull, aching pain is associated with muscle damage. Sharp, shooting pain is linked to nerve root disorders. Burning, stinging, pressure sensations are caused by disorders affecting sympathetic nerves. Deep, nagging, dull pain symptoms are associated with bone disorders, and severe, sharp pain is caused by fractures. Diffuse, throbbing pain is associated with vascular lesions.

Patients should list the physicians who have been consulted about their spinal pain. Sometimes the length of this list is instructive in making the diagnosis of a malingerer. In addition, information about the diagnostic tests used for evaluation of the patient's spinal pain and efficacy of previous therapies should be obtained from the patient. Finally, the history is not complete unless the physician has a clear understanding of why the patient "really" came to see the physician and what are the patient's true expectations from the encounter.

SUMMARY

The history is the foundation on which the rest of the diagnostic process is built. By listening carefully to the patient's description of the chief complaint, the clinician should be able to generate a list of potential diagnoses that could be causing the difficulties. The time spent in understanding the patient's pain is worth the investment. The next step in the process is a complete and appropriate physical examination. With the myriad of tests that can be done during the physical and laboratory evaluations, the history allows the clinician to select those parts of the examination that will help the clinician most efficiently make the correct diagnosis from the possibilities included in the differential diagnosis list.

4-5 CORE QUESTIONS FOR OUTCOME MEASUREMENT

1. During the past week how bothersome have each of the following symptoms been?					
	Not at all bothersome	Slightly bothersome	Moderately bothersome	Very bothersome	Extremely bothersome
a. Low back pain	1	2	3	4	5
b. Leg pain (sciatica)	1	2	3	4	5
2. During the past week, how much did pain interfere with your normal work (including both work outside the home and housework)?					
	Not at all	A little bit	Moderately	Quite a bit	Extremely
3. If you had to spend the rest of your life with the symptoms you have right now, how would you feel about it?					
	Very dissatisfied	Somewhat dissatisfied	Neither satisfied or dissatisfied	Somewhat satisfied	Very satisfied
4. During the past 4 weeks, about how many days did you cut down on the things you usually do for more than half the day because of back pain or leg pain (sciatica)? ___ Number of days					
5. During the past 4 weeks, how many days did low back pain or leg pain (sciatica) keep you from going to work or school? _____ Number of days					
6. Over the course of treatment for your low back pain or leg pain (sciatica), how satisfied were you with your overall medical care?					
	Very dissatisfied	Somewhat dissatisfied	Neither satisfied or dissatisfied	Somewhat satisfied	Very satisfied

References

1. Adams MA, Dolan P, Hutton WC, Porter RW: Diurnal changes in spinal mechanics and their clinical significance. J Bone Joint Surg Br 72:266-270, 1990.
2. Appenzeller O: The autonomic nervous system in cervical spine disorders. *In* Bland JH (ed): Disorders of the Cervical Spine: Diagnosis and Medical Management, 2nd ed. Philadelphia, WB Saunders, 1994, pp 313-327.
3. Bland JH: Clinical methods. *In* Bland JH (ed): Disorders of the Cervical Spine: Diagnosis and Medical Management, 2nd ed. Philadelphia, WB Saunders, 1994, pp 113-146.
4. Bombardier C: Outcome assessments in the evaluation of treatment of spinal disorders: Summary and general recommendations. Spine 25:3100-3103, 2000.
5. Brain WR: Some unsolved problems in cervical spondylosis. BMJ 1:771-777, 1963.
6. Deyo RA: Measuring the functional status of patients with low back pain. Arch Phys Med Rehabil 69:1044-1053, 1988.
7. Deyo RA, Bass JE: Lifestyle and low back pain: The influence of smoking and obesity. Spine 14:501-506, 1989.
8. Deyo RA, Battie M, Beurskens AJ, et al: Outcome measures for low back pain research: A proposal for standardized use. Spine 23:2003-2013, 1998.
9. Deyo RA, Diehl AK: Cancer as a cause of back pain: Frequency, clinical presentation, and diagnostic strategies. J Gen Intern Med 3:230-238, 1988.
10. Deyo RA, Rainville J, Kent DL: What can the history and physical examination tell us about low back pain? JAMA 268:760-765, 1992.
11. Edmeads J: The cervical spine and headache. Neurology 38:1874-1878, 1988.
12. Hendler N, Mollett A, Talo S, Levin S: A comparison between the Minnesota Multiphasic Personality Inventory and the "Mensana Clinic Back Pain Test" for validating the complaint of chronic back pain. J Occup Med 30:98-102, 1988.
13. Hendler N, Viernstein M, Gucer P, Long D: A preoperative screening test for chronic back pain patients. Psychosomatics 20:801-808, 1979.
14. Huskisson EC: Visual analog scales. *In* Melzack R (ed): Pain Measurement and Assessment. New York, Raven, 1983, pp 33-40.
15. Kostuik JP, Harrington I, Alexander D, et al: Cauda equina syndrome and lumbar disc herniation. J Bone Joint Surg Am 68:386-391, 1986.
16. Leak AM, Cooper J, Dyer S, et al: The Northwick Park Neck Pain Questionnaire, devised to measure neck pain and disability. Br J Rheumatol 33:469-474, 1994.
17. McGorry RW, Hsiang SM, Snook SH, et al: Meteorological conditions and self-report of low back pain. Spine 23:2096-2102, 1998.
18. Melzack R: The McGill Pain Questionnaire. *In* Melzack R (ed): Pain Measurement and Assessment. New York, Raven, 1983, pp 41-47.
19. Mitchell LC, Schafermeyer RW: Herniated cervical disk presenting as ischemic chest pain. Am J Emerg Med 9:343-346, 1991.
20. Pang WW, Mok MS, Lin ML, et al: Application of spinal pain mapping in the diagnosis of low back pain—analysis of 104 cases. Acta Anaesthesiol Sinica 36:71-74, 1998.
21. Roland M, Morris R: A study of the natural history of back pain. I. Development of a reliable and sensitive measure of disability in low back pain. Spine 8:141-144, 1983.
22. Sternbach RA, Wolf SR, Murphy RW, Akeson WH: Traits of pain patients: The low-back "loser." Psychosomatics 14:226-229, 1973.
23. Turk DC, Melzack R (eds): Handbook of Pain Assessment, 2nd ed. New York, Guilford, 2001.
24. Vroomen PC, de Krom MC, Knottnerus JA: Consistency of history taking and physical examination in patients with suspected lumbar nerve root involvement. Spine 25:91-96, 2000.

CHAPTER 5

PHYSICAL EXAMINATION

After completion of the medical history, the physical examination is the next step in the diagnostic process. The history has alerted the physician to those individuals who have medical emergencies and require therapy to begin after only an abbreviated examination.

MEDICAL EMERGENCIES

Cases of medical emergency include patients with a lesion causing acute, progressive cord compression (herniated intervertebral disc), ruptured abdominal aneurysm, acute cauda equina syndrome, or infection (meningitis). Patients with cervical spine cord compression may present with acute paraplegia, lower extremity weakness or awkwardness of gait, and urinary incontinence. These patients are evaluated expeditiously so that therapy may be instituted to minimize permanent damage to the spinal cord. The history of severe, tearing pain and dizziness associated with an abdominal pulsatile mass alerts the physician to the problem of an expanding aneurysm. Patients with the cauda equina syndrome present with acute paraplegia, saddle anesthesia, and rectal or urinary incontinence. These patients are evaluated expeditiously for abnormalities of the aorta and spinal cord so that therapy may be instituted before a life-threatening bleed or permanent neurologic damage occurs. Fortunately, the number of patients who present in this manner is extremely small.

GENERAL MEDICAL EXAMINATION

Examination of the cervical and lumbar spine is done after completion of the general physical examination. This is a useful sequence of events for a number of reasons. Examining the part of the body that is painful is best left for the last portion of the evaluation. Putting the patient through various maneuvers needed to evaluate spine function may leave the patient in a condition that limits cooperation in completing portions of a general medical examination. It also allows the physician an opportunity to observe the patient's motions and posture at a time when the spine is not being examined. The patient may be unaware of the fact that observation is the initial portion of the physical examination. In fact, unbeknownst to the patient, the chief complaint is being evaluated starting with the physician's introduction to the patient.

Vital Signs

Clues to the systemic character of neck or back pain are discovered during the general physical examination. Vital signs can document the presence of fever associated with an infection or neoplasm. Tachycardia may be the sympathetic nervous system's response to the patient's pain. Normotension in a patient with hypertension suggests acute blood loss. Discrepancies in blood pressure between the arms occurs in neck pain patients who have compression of vascular structures in the cervical spine. A reduction of blood pressure in one arm and bruit heard in one or both subclavian arteries suggests the diagnosis of subclavian steal syndrome.[1]

Dermatologic Examination

The skin examination is particularly helpful in alerting the physician to the presence of systemic illness. A number of the spondyloarthropathies cause dermatologic abnormalities: keratoderma blennorrhagicum, a rash over the palms and soles, is characterized by hyperkeratotic, yellowish, confluent plaques. Psoriasis causes erythematous raised plaques with overlying scales that occur on extensor surfaces (elbows and knees) and on the scalp, umbilicus, and perianal area. Erythema nodosum (erythematous raised nodules, particularly noted on the lower extremities) is associated with inflammatory bowel disease and sarcoidosis. Dermal plaques are also associated with sarcoidosis. Painful vesicles distributed in a dermatomal pattern are a telling sign of herpes zoster. Petechiae raise the possibility of thrombocytopenia, associated with a primary hematologic disorder (multiple myeloma), secondary metastatic tumor, or subacute bacterial endocarditis. The presence of small skin ulcers or needle marks raises the possibility of intravenous drug use, although the patient may deny substance abuse. Erythema migrans, a large, raised, erythematous skin lesion, is the cutaneous hallmark of Lyme disease.

HEENT Examination

The eye examination may reveal the presence of conjunctivitis (reactive arthritis) or iritis (ankylosing spondylitis).

Asymmetrical pupillary signs may indicate irritability of sympathetic nerves in the neck supplying the ciliary muscles. Complete paralysis of the sympathetic fibers (Horner's syndrome) is associated with miosis, vasomotor instability, increased perspiration, and ptosis. Examination of the oropharynx may reveal painless (reactive arthritis) or painful (Behçet's syndrome) oral ulcers. Examination of the neck may reveal thyromegaly, indicative of thyroid gland dysfunction. Lymphadenopathy may be associated with neoplastic processes (lymphoma), infectious processes (tuberculosis and subacute bacterial endocarditis), or idiopathic processes (sarcoidosis). Cervical ribs may be palpated in the supraclavicular area.

Cardiopulmonary Examination

Excursion of the chest wall is important to measure. Arthritis of the costovertebral joints associated with a spondyloarthropathy limits motion, decreasing chest excursion and lung capacity. Chest excursion should be measured with the patient's arms held straight up over the head, with a tape measure pulled tight and placed at the fourth intercostal space in men and just below the breasts in women. The patient is then requested to take in a deep breath (normal excursion is < 2.5 cm). Auscultation of the lung fields may result in discovery of abnormal breath sounds indicative of fibrosis. Pulmonary fibrosis is found in patients with spondyloarthropathies, sickle cell anemia, and sarcoidosis. Cardiac examination may demonstrate cardiomegaly, gallops, and murmurs. These abnormal findings may be associated with cardiac disease related to ankylosing spondylitis (aortic insufficiency), sickle cell disease (cardiomyopathy), and subacute bacterial endocarditis (valve insufficiency).

Gastrointestinal Examination

Abdominal examination is necessary to identify pathologic processes associated with back pain. These processes include gallbladder, pancreatic, and ulcer disease. A pulsatile mass, particularly in the horizontal plane, should make the examiner suspicious of an expanding abdominal aneurysm. Abnormalities of bowel sounds should be noted. Organomegaly or masses are of diagnostic importance and need to be evaluated in greater detail. The inguinal area is examined for the presence of a direct or indirect hernia. Palpation of the costovertebral angles will elicit pain in patients with kidney abnormalities. Rectal and/or gynecologic examination is done after the completion of the lumbosacral spine evaluation.

Musculoskeletal Examination

The musculoskeletal examination is helpful in identifying peripheral joint arthritis, which is often associated with cervical spine disease. For example, distal interphalangeal (DIP) joint arthritis is characteristic of psoriatic arthritis. Proximal interphalangeal joint disease in conjunction with DIP joint arthritis is commonly found in patients with osteoarthritis. Reactive arthritis causes lower extremity arthritis in addition to sacroiliitis and spondylitis. Ankle arthritis associated with erythema nodosum is associated with sarcoidosis. During the musculoskeletal examination, it is appropriate to check for peripheral pulses.

The lumbosacral spine examination is essential for evaluating cervical spine disorders and vice versa. The axial skeleton works as a unit to support the head and maintain balance. Abnormalities in the lumbar spine in the form of a list, or loss of lordosis, result in mechanical alterations in the cervical spine that may cause pain. Abnormalities in cervical spine position can also place additional strain on the lumbar spine. At a minimum, the lumbar spine should be moved through its full range of motion and palpated for any areas of tenderness and increased muscle tension.

EXAMINATION OF THE CERVICAL SPINE

Once the general examination is completed, the examination of the cervical spine should proceed. Common sense needs to be used in conducting the physical examination. Some patients who are in extreme pain do not tolerate an extensive general medical examination before evaluation of the cervical spine. In these patients an examination that concentrates solely on the cervical spine is appropriate. The remainder of the examination may be completed after evaluation of the cervical spine or on a subsequent visit.

The objective of the physical examination of the cervical spine is a demonstration of those physical abnormalities that help sort out the possible disease entities causing pain that were suggested from the medical history. Abnormalities of the cervical spine may be discovered while the spine is static or in motion. Unless the tests are done in orderly fashion, important observations may be missed. Therefore, it is helpful to evaluate the patient in a series of positions that test the function of musculoskeletal and neurologic structures of the cervical spine. In circumstances where involvement is unilateral, the uninvolved side should be compared to the affected side.

It is helpful to observe the patient disrobing. The head should move naturally with body movements. If the head is held stiffly to one side to protect or splint an area of pain, there may be a pathologic reason for such a posture. The neck region should then be inspected for normal characteristics as well as abnormalities, such as blisters, scars, and discoloration. Surgical scars on the anterior portion of the neck most often indicate previous thyroid surgery, and irregular pitted scars in the anterior triangle are likely events of previous tuberculous adenitis. Facial expression of the patient often gives the examiner an indication of the amount of pain the patient is experiencing.

The patient is initially examined standing. The patient should be undressed. Initially, gait is observed to detect any asymmetry or any list or limp. The patient can be asked to walk approximately 5 to 10 feet on the toes and then to return walking on the heels. This is a quick and cursory test of distal motor strength. Some of the earliest findings of cervical cord compression may be simply an abnormality in a patient's gait.

The spine is then viewed from behind, laterally, and anteriorly to see if the alignment is normal. From behind, the levels of the shoulders and any lateral spinal curves (scoliosis) should be noted. The patient stands with the head centered over the feet and the eyes level. Therefore, any deviation of the spine from the vertical is compensated by an opposite deviation elsewhere in the spine. The spine is compensated if the first thoracic vertebra is centered over the sacrum. A list occurs if that vertebra is not centered. The degree of list may be measured by dropping a perpendicular line from the first thoracic vertebra and measuring how far to the right or left of the gluteal cleft it falls. Pain in the neck may cause deviation that can be toward or away from the painful side.

The position of the scapulae should be noted. Asymmetry of the scapular height may be related to trapezius muscle weakness (spinal accessory nerve dysfunction), leg-length discrepancy, or long thoracic nerve neuritis.

Laterally, any exaggeration or decrease of the normal cervical curvature is noted. Does the patient have a hyperlordosis (increased concavity) at the back of the neck or flattened cervical lordosis (lack of the normal curve in the posterior portion of the neck)? Is frank cervical kyphosis present as is seen with ankylosing spondylitis, whose severest form produces a chin-on-chest deformity? Torticollis causes the head to be tilted toward the side with the contracted sternocleidomastoid muscle.

During this portion of the examination, the examiner should engage the patient in some conversation. Typically, patients turn their head to speak to the physician. Discrepancies between ranges of motion should be noted.

The neck should be palpated while the patient is supine. Because muscles overlying in the deeper prominences of the neck are relaxed in that position, the bony structures become more sharply defined. To palpate the anterior bony structures of the neck, it is best to support the patient's neck from behind at the base with one hand and to examine with the opposite hand. The hyoid bone, a horseshoe-shaped structure, is situated above the thyroid cartilage. On a horizontal plane, it is opposite the C3 vertebral body. This can easily be palpated just above the thyroid cartilage—if the patient is asked to swallow, the movement of the hyoid bone becomes palpable.

Moving inferiorly in the midline allows the fingers to come in contact with the thyroid cartilage and its small, identifiable superior notch. The upper portion of the cartilage, commonly known as the *Adam's apple*, corresponds with the level of the C4 vertebral body, and the lower portion designates the C5 level.

The first cricoid ring is situated immediately inferior to a lower border of the thyroid cartilage and lies opposite C6. It is the only complete ring of the cricoid series that is an integral part of the trachea, and is immediately above the site for an emergency tracheostomy. This structure should be palpated gently because vigorous pressure may cause the patient to gag.

Moving laterally about 1 inch from the first cricoid ring, the examiner will come across the carotid tubercle, also known as *Chassaignac's tubercle*. The carotid tubercle is small and lies away from the midline, deep under the overlying muscles, but is palpable. The carotid tubercle of C6 should be palpated separately because simultaneous palpation can restrict the flow of blood in both carotid arteries, which run adjacent to the tubercles. The carotid tubercle is frequently used as an anatomic landmark for an anterior surgical approach to the C5–C6 level, and it is a site for the injection of the stellate cervical ganglion.

While exploring the anterior portion of the neck, it is possible to locate a small, hard bump of the C1 transverse process that lies between the angle of the jaw and the skull styloid process just behind the ear. As the broadest transverse process in the cervical spine, it is readily palpable and, although it has little clinical significance, it serves as an easily identifiable point of orientation.

The posterior landmarks of the neck are more accessible to palpation if the examiner stands behind the patient's head and cups the hands under the neck so that the fingertips meet at the midline. Because tense muscles can limit the palpation of the neck, the patient's head should be held in such a way that the neck muscles need not be used for support, and the patient should be encouraged to relax. Palpation of the posterior aspect of the cervical spine should begin at the occiput, the posterior portion of the skull. The inion, a dome-shaped bump, lies in the occipital region in the midline and marks the center of the superior nuchal line. As the examiner palpates laterally toward the end of the superior nuchal line, the rounded mastoid processes of the skull are felt. Next, the spinous processes of the cervical vertebrae lie along the posterior midline and should be palpated. Because no muscle tissue crosses the midline, these bony prominences are generally easily palpated. Beginning at the base of the skull, the C2 spinous process is the first one that is palpable, since the C1 spinous process is only a small tubercle and lies deep within the soft tissue. As the spinous processes are palpated from C2 through T1, the normal lordosis of the cervical spine should be noted. In some patients the spinous processes of C3 through C5 may be bifid (with two posterolateral projections rather than one midline projection of bone). The C7 and T1 spinous processes are larger than those above them, and the C7 spinous process is also known as the *vertebra prominens*. The processes are normally in line with each other. A shift in the normal alignment may be due to a unilateral facet dislocation or to a fracture of the spinous process following trauma.

When the examiner moves laterally from the spinous processes approximately 1 inch, the joints of the vertebral facets that lie between the cervical vertebrae may be palpated. These joints often can cause symptoms of pain in the neck region. The joints feel like small domes and lie deep beneath the trapezius muscle. The facet joints are not always clearly palpable, and the patient must be completely relaxed to enable them to be palpated.

In general, when examining the cervical spine for posterior tenderness, it is important to determine whether the tenderness is midline, which is most often related to an intrinsic spinal problem, or whether it is paraspinal or off the midline and related to soft tissue pathology.

The remainder of the physical examination can be performed with the patient sitting. The sternocleidomastoid muscle extends from the sternoclavicular joint to the mastoid process and may be frequently stretched in hyperextension injuries of the neck that occur during automobile accidents. This muscle becomes more prominent when the patient turns the head to the side opposite the muscle to be examined. Palpable local swellings within the muscle may be due to hematoma and may cause the head to turn abnormally to one side (torticollis).

A chain of lymph nodes is situated along the medial border of the sternocleidomastoid muscle. In normal circumstances lymph nodes are either nonpalpable or only slightly so, and they are usually not tender. Lymph nodes may be palpable as small lumps that become tender to the touch when they are enlarged or inflamed.

The thyroid cartilage lies in a central position along the anterior midline of the neck anterior to the C4–C5 vertebrae. The thyroid gland lies superficial to the cartilage in a bilobed pattern, with a thin isthmus between them crossing the midline. A normal thyroid gland feels smooth and indistinct, whereas a gland with some pathologic changes may contain unusual local enlargements due to cysts or nodules that may also be tender to palpation. The thyroid gland is most easily felt by standing behind the patient.

The carotid artery is situated next to the carotid tubercle (C6). The carotid pulse is palpable if the examiner presses at this point with the tips of the index and middle fingers. As mentioned earlier, it is important to palpate only one side at a time to avoid an excessive decrease in flow to the brain. The pulses in each side of the neck should be approximately equal and both should be checked to determine the relative strengths.

The parotid gland overlies the sharp angle of the mandible. The gland is generally not palpable. If, however, the parotid gland is swollen (as in the case of mumps or Sjögren's syndrome), the angle of the mandible no longer feels sharp as it is covered by a larger soft tissue structure.

The supraclavicular fossa lies superior to the clavicle and lateral to the suprasternal notch. It is important to palpate this region for any unusual swellings or lumps. Although the platysma muscle crosses the fossa, it is not stretched tautly across it and therefore does change its concave shape. Swelling within the fossa may be caused by edema, secondary to trauma in the soft tissues about the shoulder as seen with a clavicular fracture. Small lumps in the fossa may be due to an enlargement of the lymph glands or may be an indicator of an apical disorder in the lung. If a cervical rib is present, it may be palpable in this fossa and can cause vascular or neurologic symptoms in the upper extremity.

In palpating the posterior aspect of the neck, it is important to note the broad origin of the trapezius muscle from the ending of the skull to T12. The muscle's insertions must be palpated laterally under the clavicle, acromion, and spine of the scapula. It is most important to note any asymmetry from one side to the other when examining musculature. Any discrepancy in the size or shape on either side and any tenderness, unilateral or bilateral, should be noted. Tenderness most often is found in the superolateral portion of the muscle.

It is also important to feel for the exit point of the greater occipital nerves. This can be found by moving from the trapezius muscle to the base of the skull, probing both sides of the inion. If these nerves are inflamed, as may be the case following a whiplash injury, the nerves may be distinctly palpable. Inflammation of the greater occipital nerves may result in headache, with pain that radiates from the occipital ridge toward the apex of the skull.

The final structure to be palpated is the superior nuchal ligament, which arises from the inion at the base of the skull and extends to the C7 spinous process. Although this is not a distinctly palpable structure, the area in which it lies can be palpated to elicit tenderness. This structure runs between the tips of the spinous processes and the posterior aspect of the cervical spine. Tenderness at any one level may indicate either a stretched ligament as a result of a neck flexion injury or perhaps a defect within the ligament itself.

Range of Motion

The normal range of motion of the neck provides an extremely flexible mechanism for positioning the head in space to direct a wide scope of vision as well as an acute sense of balance. It is important to assess the range of motion in the cervical spine in all the basic planes (Fig. 5-1).

First, test active flexion-extension of the neck. Instruct the patient to nod forward and place the chin on the chest. The normal range of flexion should allow the chest to be touched with the chin. The patient is then asked to look directly at the ceiling; with a normal range of motion, this should be possible with extension of the cervical spine. As the patient's head moves, it is important to watch to see if the arc of motion is smooth rather than halting or jerking. An auto accident may cause soft tissue trauma around the cervical spine, which may result in limitation of the range of motion and a disruption of the normal smooth arc. For an exact measurement of neck flexion and extension, a cervical range of motion goniometer is an effective tool. Tousignant and associates matched goniometer and radiographic measurements in healthy individuals. The ranges of motion were highly correlated (flexion, $r = 0.97$, $P < 0.001$; extension, $r = 0.98$, $P < 0.001$).[48]

Next, rotation should be assessed. The patient should be able to move the head far enough to both sides so that the chin is almost in line with the shoulder. Again, the smoothness of the motion should be observed.

Active lateral bending can be tested by asking the patient to touch ear to shoulder, making sure the patient does not compensate for limited motion by lifting shoulder to ear. In normal circumstances the patient should be able to tilt the head approximately 45 degrees toward each shoulder.

The physician should observe the patient carefully during active bending to identify any specific arcs of limited motion. The patient may repeat the range of motion while the physician palpates the neck muscles for increased muscle tension that may limit motion.

Testing for passive range of motion in the cervical spine is seldom necessary. In fact, if the patient has an unstable cervical spine as a result of trauma, passive range of motion examination may cause neurologic damage.

Scapular and shoulder movements should also be tested. The following scapular movements are tested: a full shrug (trapezius and levator scapulae muscles); forward movement (pectoralis major and minor and serratus anterior muscles); backward movement (rhomboids and lower trapezius muscles); upward and lateral movements of arms over the head, palms together; and forward movement pressing against a wall (serratus anterior). Approximation of the scapulae stretches the dura mater through traction in the upper thoracic nerve roots, sometimes causing pain

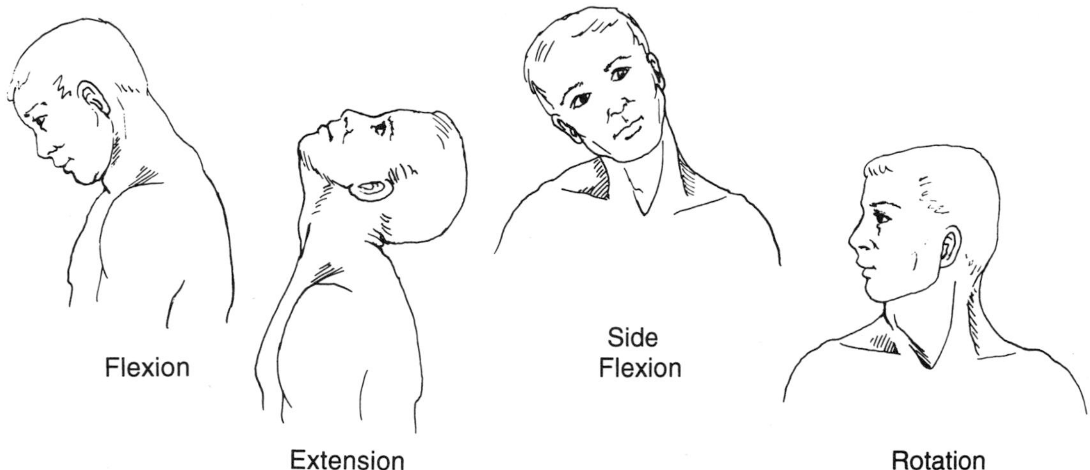

Figure 5-1 Range of motion tests for examination of movement of the cervical spine.

in the chest, suggesting a thoracic disc lesion.[4] These motions may also identify areas of joint disease in the shoulder or acromioclavicular joints. Paresthesias in the hands with arm elevation to 90 degrees suggest thoracic outlet syndrome.

The age, sex, body weight, and athletic activity influence the range of motion of the cervical spine. Castro and colleagues used an ultrasound system to establish reference ranges of motion for subjects grouped by age and sex.[11] The range of motion decreased with increasing age, increasing body weight, and decreasing athletic activity. The rotation in the upper cervical spine increases with age to compensate for the reduced range in the lower cervical segments. After age 70, women demonstrated better mobility than men of the same age.

Neurologic Examination

There are three phases to a neurologic examination of the cervical spine (Table 5-1): motor strength testing, sensory examination, and reflex examination.

Motor Strength Testing

The first part of the motor portion of the neurologic examination concerns testing the intrinsic muscles of the neck, cervical spine, and functional groups. In this respect, muscle testing indicates the presence of any motor weakness affecting the motion of the neck and, in addition, may demonstrate the integrity of the nervous supply. Muscles of the cervical spine are innervated by multiple

5-1 CERVICAL RADICULOPATHY SYMPTOMS AND FINDINGS

Disc Level	Nerve Root	Symptoms and Findings
C2–C3	C3	Pain: Back of neck, mastoid process, pinna of ear Sensory change: Back of neck, mastoid process, pinna of ear Motor deficit: None readily detectable except by EMG Reflex change: None
C3–C4	C4	Pain: Back of neck, levator scapulae, anterior chest Sensory change: Back of neck, levator scapulae, anterior chest Motor deficit: None readily detectable except by EMG Reflex change: None
C4–C5	C5	Pain: Neck, tip of shoulder, anterior arm Sensory change: Deltoid area Motor deficit: Deltoid, biceps Reflex change: Biceps
C5–C6	C6	Pain: Neck, shoulder, medial border of scapula, lateral arm, dorsal forearm Sensory change: Thumb and index finger Motor deficit: Biceps Reflex change: Biceps
C6–C7	C7	Pain: Neck, shoulder, medial border at scapula, lateral arm, dorsal forearm Sensory change: Index and middle fingers Motor deficit: Triceps Reflex change: Triceps
C7–T1	C8	Pain: Neck, medial border of scapula, medial aspect of arm and forearm Sensory change: Ring and little fingers Motor deficit: Intrinsic muscles of hand Reflex change: None

EMG, electromyography.
From Boden SD, Wiesel SW, Laws ER Jr, et al: The Aging Spine: Essentials of Pathophysiology, Diagnosis, and Treatment. Philadelphia, WB Saunders, 1991, p 46.

levels (Fig. 5-2). Muscle strength may not be perceived to be diminished if only a portion of the segmental innervation to an individual muscle is disrupted. The primary flexors of the neck are the sternocleidomastoid muscles, innervated by the spinal accessory nerve, and the secondary flexors are the splenius muscles and the prevertebral muscles. Resistive muscle testing in the cervical spine is no different from that in any other area. Essentially, the patient is asked to perform a motion against a resistive force. In the case of cervical flexion, the examiner's palm is placed on the patient's forehead and the patient is asked to flex the neck slowly.

Primary extensors in the cervical spine consist of the paravertebral extensor muscles and the trapezius muscle, and the secondary extensors consist of the small intrinsic neck muscles. Resistive testing of extension is performed by placing the examiner's hand over the midline of the patient's upper posterior thorax and scapula; the other hand is placed in the back of the skull. The patient is then asked to extend the neck actively.

The primary lateral rotators of the neck are the sternocleidomastoid muscles. The secondary rotators are the small intrinsic neck muscles. To test the strength of rotation, the examiner places one hand on the shoulder and the other hand on the opposite jaw, asking the patient to actively turn toward the side with the hand on the jaw. The strength of a resistive lateral motion should be compared from side to side.

The primary lateral benders in the neck are the three splenius muscles, which are innervated by the anterior primary divisions of the lower cervical nerves. The secondary lateral benders include some of the small intrinsic muscles in the neck. To test the strength of lateral bending, the examiner places one hand on the patient's shoulder and

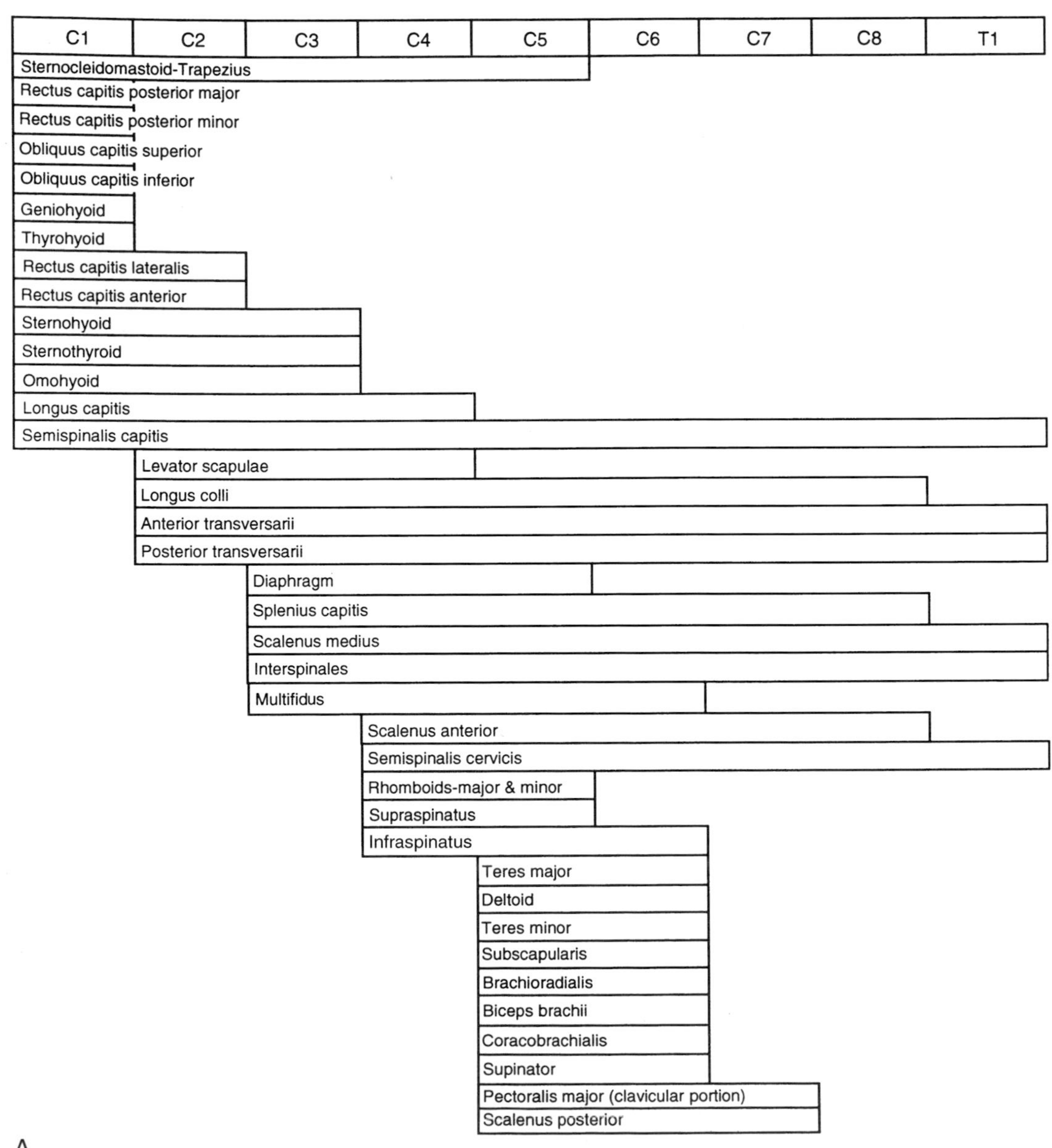

Figure 5-2 Segmental motor innervation of muscles supplied by C1 through T1 spinal nerves. The innervation of muscles from multiple (minimally two, and more commonly three) spinal cord levels is evident.

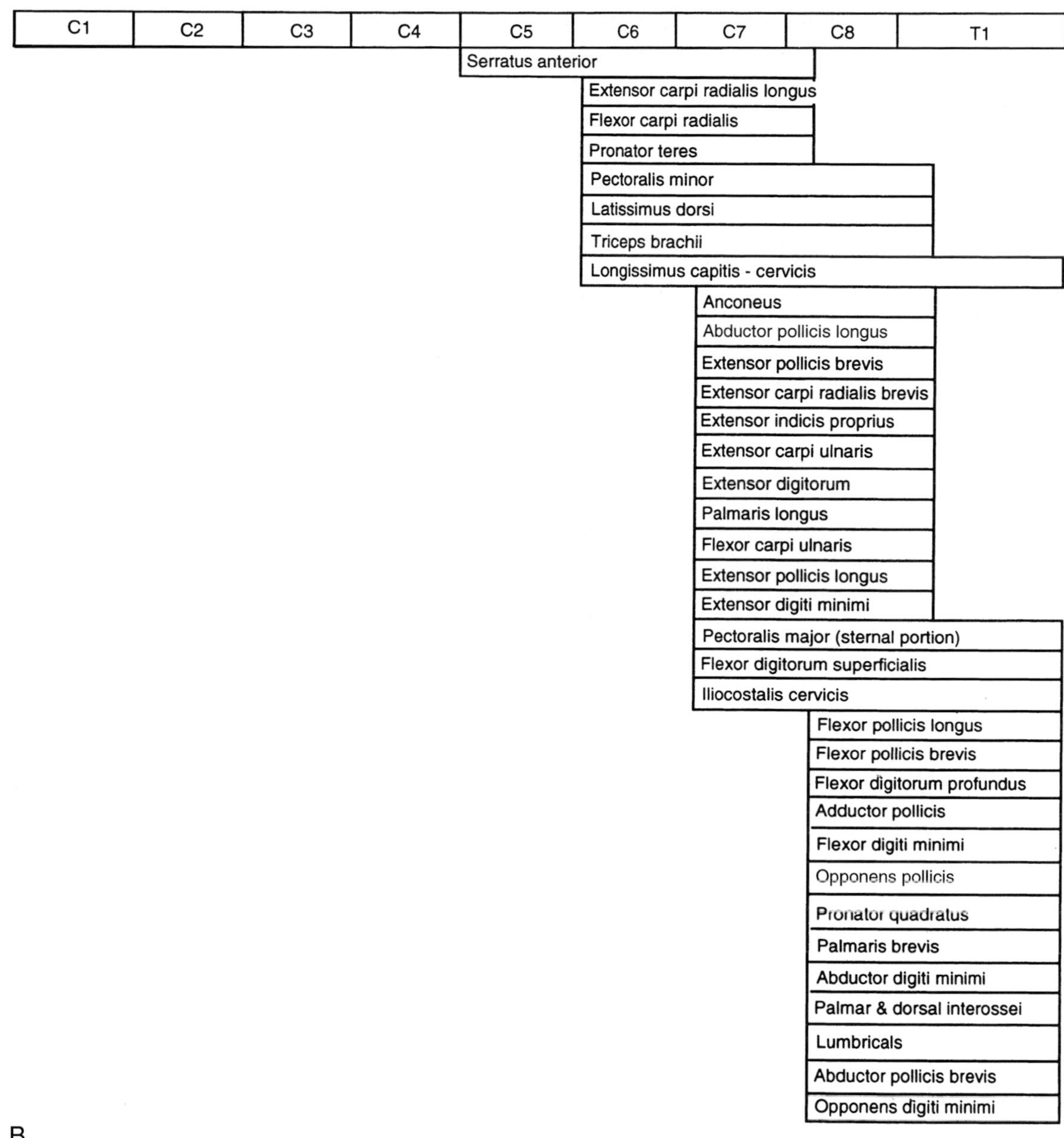

Figure 5-2, cont'd

places the other hand on the superior lateral aspect of the patient's skull on the same side. The patient is then asked to bend laterally toward that side and is resisted by the examiner's hand on the skull. In all these resistive muscle tests it is important to assess symmetry on both sides and get a sense of the maximal force that is attainable by the patient.

The second phase of the motor examination is designed to test motor strength of the muscles innervated by the nerve roots of the mid to lower cervical spine, which comprise the brachial plexus. Each nerve root, as it leaves the spinal canal through the neural foramen, is enclosed within a sleeve that contains spinal fluid and very small blood vessels about and within the nerve. This sac, referred to as the *dural sleeve*, provides nourishment to the nerve root. Any compression or traction on the dura will compress its contents and encroach on the nerve and its blood supply. Secondary to compression, pain is perceived along the course of the peripheral nerve and is accompanied by dysesthesias, motor weakness, and decreased reflex function associated with the affected nerve root. The goal of many of the maneuvers done during this phase of the examination is to increase nerve compression to uncover neurologic dysfunction. One of the possible neurologic abnormalities, true muscle weakness, is one of the most reliable indicators of persistent nerve compression with loss of nerve conduction.[45] In contrast, sensory changes are subjective and are easily affected by the emotional and energy state of the patient. As a patient fatigues, consistent sensory findings are difficult to reproduce. In addition, reflex changes may be lost from a previous episode of nerve root compression, and they may not return even with the recovery of sensory and motor function.[5] With age, reflexes are more difficult to elicit even without any prior history of nerve compression. However, the loss of reflexes is generally symmetrical with increasing age. Patients who lose reflexes in both lower extremities because of compression may have a central herniation of a disc.

In addition to nerve root lesions, upper motor neuron and peripheral nerve disease can cause abnormalities that may be discovered during the neurologic examination. Thus, it is also important to evaluate the cranial nerves and the brachial plexus. With upper motor neuron lesions, fine control of muscles is lost while the trophic effects of the peripheral nerves remain intact. Muscle strength is maintained initially, but patients develop spasticity of muscles (tonic contractions) and hyperreflexia. Patients also develop a positive Babinski's reflex (extension of the large toe and spreading of the other toes with stroking of the sole of the foot) or a positive Hoffmann's reflex (involuntary flexion of the thumb and fifth digit on quick flexion of the DIP joint of the long finger). Cervical spine abnormalities, including herniated disc or spinal cord compression, are closely associated with a positive Hoffmann's reflex. A proportion of these individuals are asymptomatic.[46]

Peripheral nerve injuries may cause sensory or motor abnormalities, depending on the damaged nerve. Peripheral nerves receive neurofibrils from a number of nerve root levels. The locations of nerve roots and peripheral nerve lesions affecting cutaneous structures in the upper extremity are depicted in Figures 5-3 and 5-4. A lesion at one nerve root may cause a minor change in function if a structure is supplied by multiple spinal cord levels. However, if a peripheral nerve is injured, innervation in specific muscles and cutaneous areas is interrupted (Table 5-2). In this circumstance specific muscles may become paralyzed and areflexic or specific cutaneous areas may be anesthetized. The differentiation of upper motor neuron, nerve root, and peripheral nerve lesions is an important one. The locations of the abnormalities causing these neurologic manifestations are different. Also, the category of pathologic process causing upper motor neuron, nerve root, and peripheral nerve abnormalities may be different (multiple sclerosis, disc herniation, and diabetes, respectively).

Although conceptually it is easiest to think about performing the neurologic examination of the upper extremities on a nerve root level innervation basis, it is much more practical to perform an overall examination of the entire motor system, then the entire sensory distribution, and finally all the reflexes together (Fig. 5-5).

Motor strength quantification by physical examination is not precise, and some studies have suggested that as much as 30% to 40% of motor strength must be absent before any consistent detection of weakness is made on the basis of a physical examination. In any case, one of the more common grading systems is a six-tier system, with 5 being normal strength; 4 being decreased strength against active resistance but ability to move against gravity; 3 being the ability to move only in the plane of gravity, not being able to move against gravity; 2 being the ability to contract the muscle but without purposeful motion; and 1 being the presence of muscle fibrillations. Grade 0 is the absence of any activity in the muscle group. When testing muscle power, it is important to test the muscles with the intervening joints in a neutral position. Pressure is applied to a nonarticular structure for a minimum of 5 seconds.

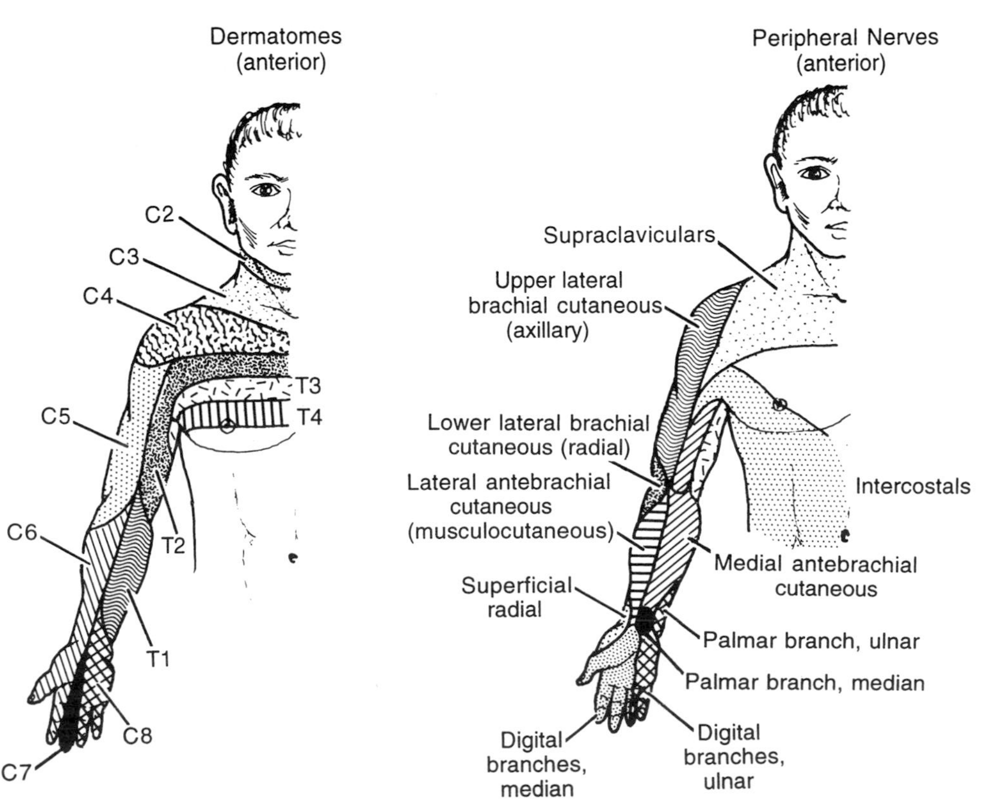

Figure 5-3 Anterior view of the upper extremities depicting skin areas innervated by nerve roots *(left)* and peripheral nerves *(right)*.

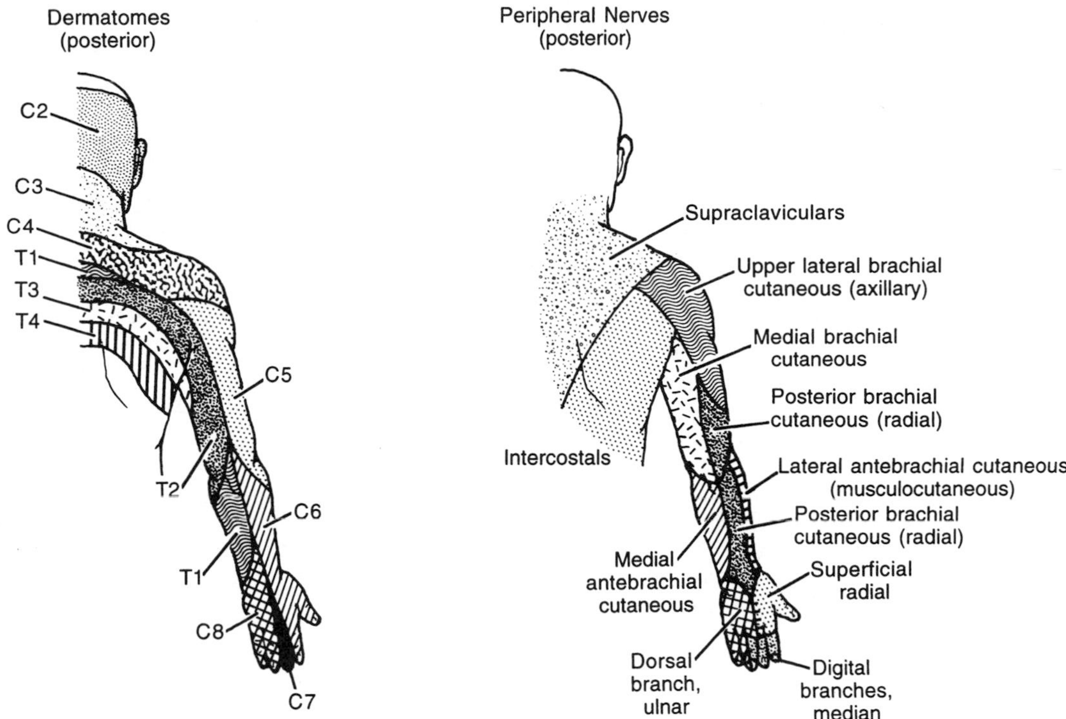

Figure 5-4 Posterior view of the nerve root *(left)* and peripheral nerve *(right)* areas of the upper extremities.

When feasible, it is preferable to test both sides simultaneously.

An overlap of nerve innervation to muscles exists through the upper extremity. A general location of a lesion may be suspected with muscle weakness, but further evaluation is required to identify a specific location of nerve dysfunction. Testing the muscles innervated by the brachial plexus begins with the deltoid and biceps muscles, which are the two muscles with C5 innervation that are easily evaluated. Whereas the deltoid is innervated almost entirely by C5, the biceps has a dual innervation from both C5 and C6. The deltoid muscle has three parts: anterior, middle, and posterior. To test deltoid strength, resisted motion of the shoulder should be performed in flexion, adduction, and extension. The biceps acts as a flexor for the shoulder and elbow and as a supinator of the forearm.

5-2 THE MAJOR PERIPHERAL NERVES

Nerve	Motor Test	Sensation Test
Radial nerve finger	Wrist extension Thumb extension	Dorsal web space between thumb and index finger
Ulnar nerve	Abduction—little finger	Distal ulnar aspect—little finger
Median nerve	Thumb pinch Opposition of thumb Abduction of thumb	Distal radial aspect—index finger
Axillary nerve	Deltoid	Lateral arm—deltoid patch on upper arm
Musculocutaneous nerve	Biceps	Lateral forearm

Biceps strength can be tested relative to elbow flexion to determine the integrity of the C5 root. Because the brachialis muscle, the other main flexor of the elbow, is also innervated by the musculocutaneous nerve, a flexion test of the elbow should provide an adequate indication of C5 integrity. To test elbow flexion, the patient should flex the elbow slowly with the forearm supernated, as the examiner resists motion.

The next muscle group that should be tested is the wrist extensors. This muscle group does not have pure C6 innervation; it has partial innervation by C7. The wrist extensor group is composed of three muscles: the extensor carpi radialis longus (C6), the extensor carpi radialis brevis (C6), and the extensor carpi ulnaris (C7).

Next, the C7 nerve root can be evaluated by testing elbow extension, a function of the triceps, as innervated by the radial nerve, as well as the wrist flexor group innervated by C7 root, median, and ulnar nerves. The wrist flexor group is composed of two muscles: the flexor carpi radialis (median nerve) and the flexor carpi ulnaris (ulnar nerve). The flexor carpi radialis is the more significant of these two muscles because it powers most of the wrist flexion. Flexor carpi ulnaris (C8) is less powerful. Wrist flexion strength can be tested by asking the patient to make a fist and then flexing the wrist as the examiner resists against the palmar aspect of the fist. Finger extension is also a test of the C7 root and radial nerve innervation.

The next motor group to be tested is the finger flexors. The two muscles that flex the fingers are the flexor digitorum superficialis and the flexor digitorum profundus. The superficialis muscle receives innervation from the median nerve, and the profundus muscle receives half its innervation from the ulnar nerve and half from the median nerve. To test the strength of finger flexion, ask the patient

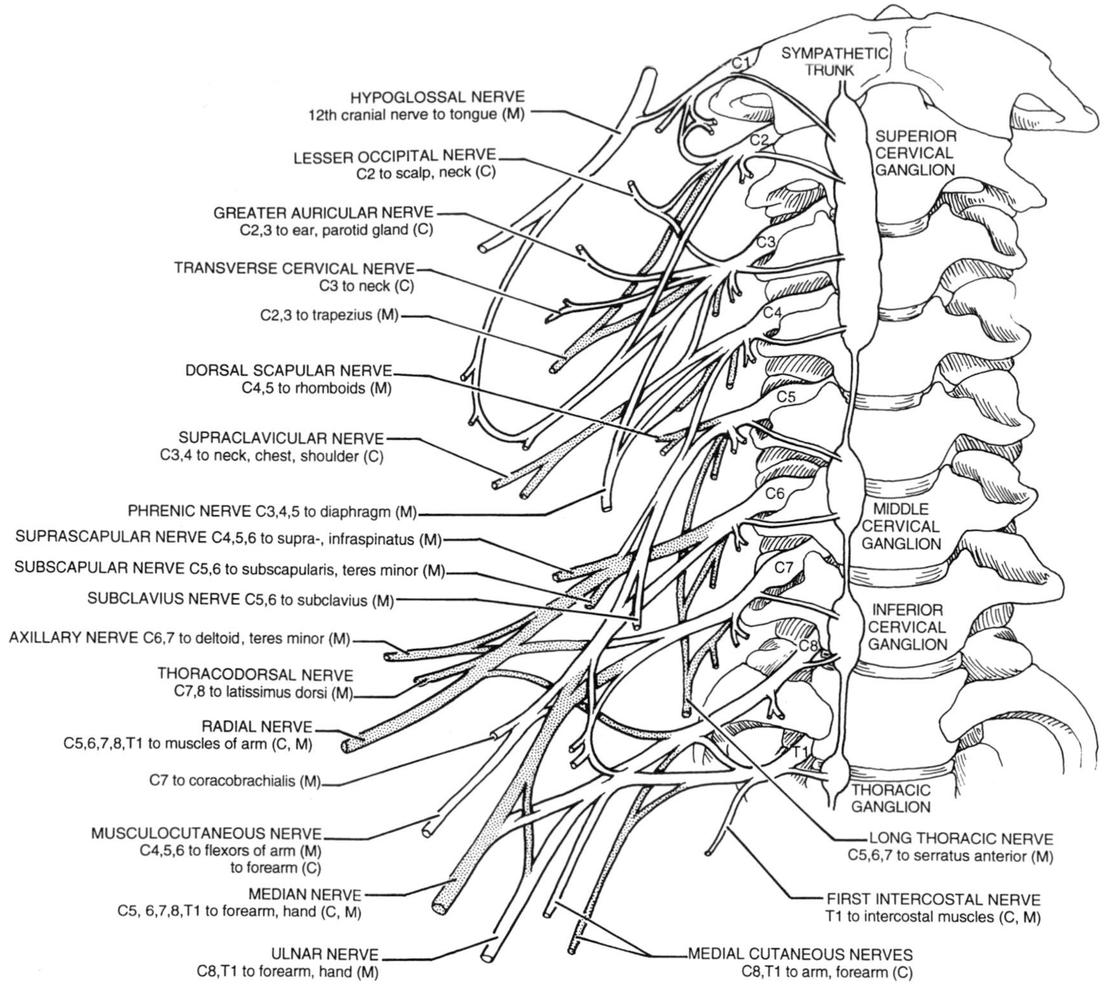

Figure 5-5 Nerves originating in the cervical spine. The plexus, roots, branches, divisions (anterior and posterior), terminal branches, and autonomic nervous system components of the brachial plexus are included. The cutaneous (C) and motor (M) components of the peripheral nerves are noted. The functions of muscles are listed under the associated nerves.

to curl the fingers around the examiner's index and long finger, while the examiner tries to pull out of the grip.

The T1 neurologic level is tested by examining the intrinsic muscles of the hand. The finger abductors, innervated by the ulnar nerve and largely the T1 root, consist of the dorsal interossei and abductor digiti quinti. Finger abduction strength can be tested by asking the patient to abduct the fingers and then have the examiner attempt to squeeze them together at the level of the proximal phalanx of the index and little finger of the patient (Fig. 5-6).

Reflex Testing

The scapulohumeral reflex tests the integrity of the cord segments from C4 to C6. The reflex is elicited by striking the lower end of the medial border of the scapula. The response is adduction and lateral rotation of the arm. This reflex tests the supply of the suprascapular (axillary) nerve to the infraspinatus and teres minor.

The biceps reflex primarily indicates the neurologic integrity of the C5 nerve root. However, the reflex also has a C6 component. Because the muscle has two major levels of innervation, even a slightly diminished reflex in comparison with the opposite side indicates potential pathologic changes. The biceps reflex may be tested by the examiner placing a thumb over the biceps tendon and then tapping the reflex hammer on the examiner's thumb.

The brachioradialis reflex is tested proximal to the wrist where the muscle becomes tendonless just before it inserts into the radius. This tendon can be tapped directly with the blunt end of the reflex hammer and may result in wrist extension and elbow flexion. The primary innervation of this reflex is C6.

The triceps reflex is predominantly a C7 root reflex. To test the triceps reflex, it is necessary to tap the tendon of the triceps muscle where it crosses the olecranon fossa, just proximal to the elbow joint on the posterior aspect of the arm.

Because C8 has no reflex, muscle strength and sensory tests are used primarily to determine the integrity of the C8 nerve root. Similarly, T1, like C8, has no identifiable reflex, so it is evaluated for its motor and sensory components only.

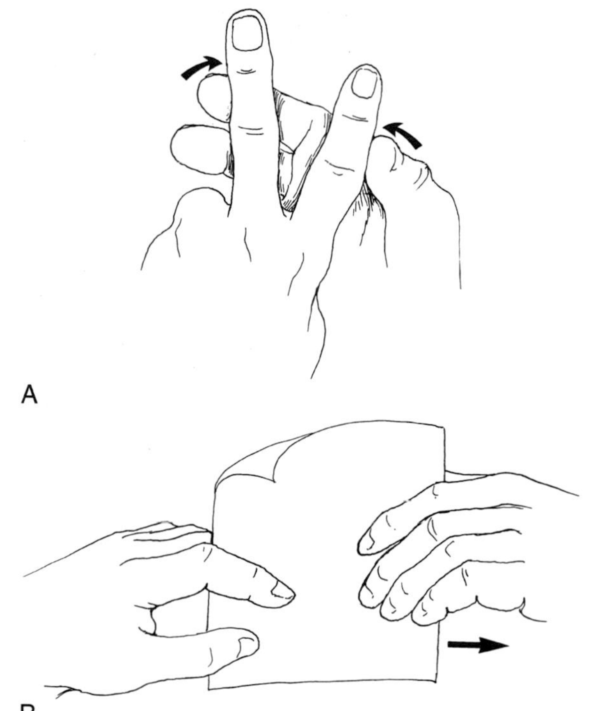

Figure 5-6 *A* and *B*, Motor examination of T1 nerve root, testing the strength of intrinsic hand muscles.

It is also important to test for evidence of upper motor neuron lesions, and these can be detected through several additional reflexes. The Hoffmann's sign is the equivalent of the Babinski's sign in the lower extremity. This test can be performed by placing the patient's middle phalanx of the long finger across the DIP joint of the examiner's long finger on the dominant hand, with the palm facing down. Next, by placing the patient's long finger in slight extension, the DIP joint is flicked downward by the examiner's thumb. An involuntary flexion of the DIP joints of the patient's thumb and little finger at the same time represents a positive Hoffmann's reflex. Another reflex that can be tested for upper motor neuron lesions is the jaw reflex, which can be tested by having the patient relax the open jaw. The examiner places a finger over the mental area of the chin and taps with the reflex hammer. The normal reflex should result in the jaw closing. A brisk reflex may be due to an upper motor neuron lesion somewhere along the course or above the level of the fifth cranial nerve (Fig. 5-7). If pathologic reflexes are present, motor examination should be expanded to determine signs of paralysis or weakness of voluntary motion, and increased muscle tone is indicative of an upper motor neuron lesion. Sensory examination may determine sensory loss on one side of the body with contralateral analgesia and thermesthesia a few segments below. These findings are compatible with Brown-Séquard syndrome.

One final reflex is the Chvostek's sign. This can result from tapping over the facial nerve as it passes through the parotid gland, anterior to the ear. A hyperactive reflex in this area may result from hypocalcemia or other systemic metabolic abnormality.

Sensation Testing

The C5 neurologic level supplies sensation to the lateral aspect of the arm. The purest patch of axillary sensation is located on the lateral arm and the skin covering the lateral portion of the deltoid muscle. This localized area is useful in diagnosing injuries to the axillary nerve or general C5 nerve root injury.

Testing the sensation of the C6 nerve root can be performed by examining the sensory function to the lateral forearm, thumb, index, and half of the middle finger. An easy way to remember the sensation to the fingers of the hand, from the purist's standpoint, is that C6 innervates thumb and index finger, C7 the middle finger, and C8 the ring and little finger. The ulnar side of the little finger is the purest area for ulnar nerve sensation (predominately C8).

Sensation is supplied to the medial side of the upper half of the forearm and the arm by T1. T2 supplies the axillary area, T3 supplies the anterior chest, and T4 supplies the area approximately at the level of the nipple on the anterior chest wall.

In general, sensory innervation can be tested in a cursory fashion by examining light touch in all the areas mentioned in this section. In addition, a pin can be used to test sensation to pinprick. Although posterior column function, position, and vibratory sense are not routinely tested, these sensory modalities become more relevant in patients who have any suggestion of cord compression or any posterior canal impingement.

If abnormalities are found in any component of the neurologic examination, additional tests should be completed, including tests of cranial nerves and thoracic nerve

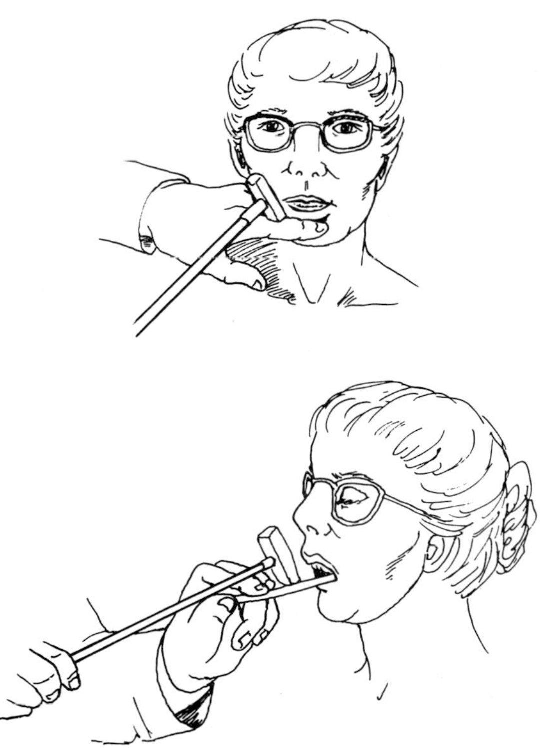

Figure 5-7 Jaw jerk obtained by alternative methods.

roots. These additional tests may be able to better define the location of a lesion in the upper spinal cord or thoracic spine that may be associated with neck pain.

Special Tests

Distraction Test. This test demonstrates the effect that neck traction might have in relieving a patient's neck pain. Distraction relieves pain, which is caused by a narrowing of the neural foramen and resulting nerve root compression, by widening the foramen. Distraction also relieves pain in the cervical spine by decreasing pressure on the joint capsules around the facet joints. In addition, it may help alleviate muscle spasm by relaxing the contractive muscles, although this is less reliable.

To perform the cervical spine distraction test, the examiner places the open palm of one hand under the patient's chin and the other hand on the patient's occiput. The head is then gently lifted to remove its weight from the neck (Fig. 5-8*A*). Distraction is continued for 30 to 60 seconds.

Compression Test. A narrowing of the neural foramen, pressure on the facets, or muscle spasm can cause increased pain on compression. In addition, a compression test may reproduce pain referred to the upper extremity from the cervical spine and, in so doing, may locate the neurologic level of any existing pathologic problem that may not be evident on routine examination without such a provocative test.

To perform the compression test, press down on the top of the patient's head while the patient is either sitting or lying down. If there is an increase in pain in either the cervical spine or the extremity, it is important to note its exact distribution and whether it follows any of the previously described dermatomal patterns (Fig. 5-8*B*).

Valsalva's Test. This test increases the intrathecal pressure. If a space-occupying lesion, such as a herniated disc or tumor, is present in the cervical canal, the patient may develop pain in the cervical spine secondary to increased pressure. Pain may also radiate into the dermatome distribution that corresponds to the neurologic level of the intracanal pathology. Abnormalities in the supraclavicular fossa, such as enlarged lymph glands, may also become prominent with the Valsalva's test.[33]

To perform the Valsalva's test, the patients are instructed to hold their breath and to bear down as if moving their bowels. The examiner asks if the patient feels any increase in pain and, if so, asks the patient to describe its character and location.

Spurling's Maneuver. This is a test of nerve root compression or irritation. This maneuver may be carried out by performing an extension and rotation movement of the head or extension and bending of the cervical spine to the right or left. A positive result is noted by reproduction of the patient's radicular pain.[8] Tong and co-workers completed Spurling's test on 235 consecutive individuals referred for electrodiagnosis of upper extremity nerve disorders.[47] The Spurling's test had a sensitivity of 30% and a specificity of 93%. The Spurling's test is not sensitive but is specific for cervical radiculopathy. The test is useful in confirming the presence of a cervical radiculopathy.

Lhermitte's Sign. This is the sensation of lightning-like paresthesias or dysesthesias in the hands or legs on cervical flexion. This sensation is most often caused by a large disc herniation impinging the anterior spinal cord or by bony compression of the anterior cord in patients with a narrow canal diameter. This sign may also be associated with instability associated with rheumatoid arthritis. Similar sensations are reported in patients with multiple

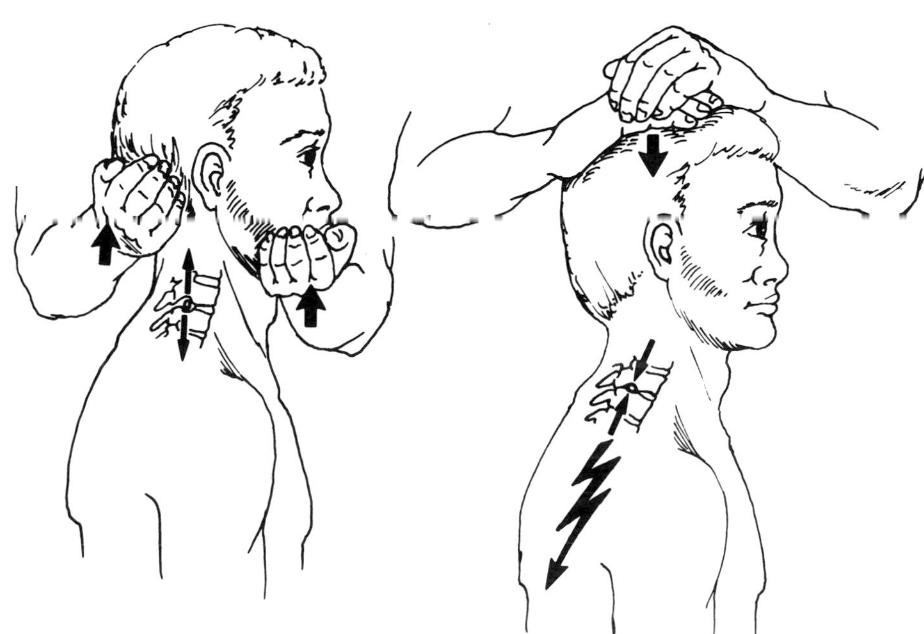

Figure 5-8 Distraction test *(A)* is positive when radicular pain is relieved with upward traction on the neck. Compression test *(B)* is positive when radicular pain is increased with downward pressure on the cervical spine.

sclerosis affecting the spinal cord. Lhermitte's sign has also been associated with a variety of spinal cord lesions, including neoplasm, arachnoiditis, syringomyelia, and subacute combined degeneration.[9]

Shoulder Depression Test. This is a test of nerve root irritation. The neck is laterally flexed while downward pressure is placed on the shoulder. The test stretches nerve roots that cause radicular pain or paresthesias with lesions of the spinal nerve roots.

Shoulder Abduction Test. This test relieves pressure on nerve roots. The arm on the painful side is placed on top of the head. This shortens the distance between the cervical spine and coracoid process, releasing tension on the nerve roots. Some authors have suggested that the relief of pain is an indicator of cervical extradural compressive disease that may be related to disc herniation or osteophytes.[32] Others have suggested that relief of pain is related to cervical disc herniation. Pain associated with foraminal stenosis secondary to spondylosis is not improved with shoulder abduction.[3]

Adson's Test. This test is used to determine any potential compression of the subclavian artery, which may be caused by an extra cervical rib or by tightened scalene muscles. Compression may occur at the thoracic outlet where the artery passes between the chest and the upper extremity.

To perform the Adson's test, the patient's radial pulse is examined at the wrist. While the pulse is continuously palpated, the arm is then abducted, extended, and externally rotated. The patient is then instructed to take a deep breath and turn the head toward the arm being tested. If there is compression in the subclavian artery, there is a marked diminution or disappearance of the radial pulse. Auscultation, above and below the clavicle, may discover bruits that are only audible with critical narrowing of the subclavian artery by arm abduction.

Sharp-Purser Test. This test is accomplished by placing a hand on the patient's forehead and the thumb of the other hand on the tip of the spinous process of the axis. As the patient flexes the neck against the hand on the forehead, a sound may be appreciated as the atlantoaxial subluxation is reduced.[44] This test may exacerbate neurologic symptoms. The determination of subluxation may be better quantified by flexion and extension radiographs of the cervical spine.

PERIPHERAL NERVE ENTRAPMENT SYNDROMES

Peripheral nerves in the upper extremity may be compressed in predictable areas of disease, giving rise to upper extremity numbness, paresthesias, and sensory and motor loss. Although these radicular-type signs and symptoms may mimic cervical radiculopathy owing to pathologic problems of the cervical spine, concomitant neck pain may be noncontributory, simply occurring simultaneously. It is important to be able to differentiate peripheral nerve entrapment from more central root compression. The most reliable method of making this differentiation is through careful history and physical examination (Table 5-3).

Median Nerve

The median nerve may be compressed anywhere along its course. However, there are three common points. The

5-3 PERIPHERAL NERVE ENTRAPMENT SYNDROMES

Nerve	Pain	Sensory	Weakness
MEDIAN NERVE			
Pronator syndrome (C6 + C7 mimic)	Proximal volar forearm	Radial 3½ digits	Pronator teres Flexor carpi radialis
Anterior interosseous syndrome (C8 mimic)	Proximal forearm	None	Flexor pollicis longus Pronator quadratus Flexor digitorum profundus (index)
Carpal tunnel syndrome (C6 + C7 sensory mimic) (T1 motor mimic)	Hand	Radial 3½ digits	Thenar muscles
ULNAR NERVE			
Cubital tunnel syndrome (C8 or T1 mimic)	Medial elbow	Ulnar 1½ digits	Flexor carpi ulnaris Flexor digitorum profundus (long + ring) Interossei Hypothenar muscles
Guyon's canal (C8 or T1 mimic)	Ulnar wrist	Volar, ulnar 1½ digits	Hypothenar muscles Interossei Abductor pollicis
RADIAL NERVE			
Posterior interosseous syndrome (C7 mimic)	Proximal forearm	None	Extensor digitorum communis Extensor carpi ulnaris Abductor pollicis longus Extensor pollicis longus

most proximal level of compression may produce the pronator syndrome, which is associated with pain in the proximal volar forearm and sensory signs and symptoms in the radial 3½ digits of the hand. Weakness of all median nerve–innervated muscles occurs because the compression is proximal to the branching of the anterior interosseous nerve. Symptoms are generally aggravated by flexion of the elbow against resistance from 90 degrees to 135 degrees of flexion and may be caused by compression from the ligament of Struthers or the lacertus fibrosus. Symptoms that are worsened by resistance to forced voluntary pronation of the forearm combined with simultaneous wrist flexion may indicate compression by the pronator teres muscle. This muscle may cause compression of the median nerve by hypertrophy or by the sharp aponeurotic edge of the deep head or reflected head muscle fascia forming fibrous bands. Symptoms elicited by resistive flexion of the long finger flexor digitorum superficialis muscle may be referable to compression from a deep tendinous aponeurotic arch of the muscle, underneath which the median nerve passes. Sensory symptoms and signs of the pronator syndrome typically mimic C6 and C7 radiculopathy. Although the pronator syndrome may affect the function of the median nerve–innervated muscles in the C6 and C7 distribution, it spares the radial nerve–innervated muscles in the C6–C7 distribution (elbow, wrist, and finger extensors). In addition, it may induce abnormalities in muscles innervated by the median nerve but not in the C6–C7 distribution (finger flexors and thenar muscles).

Since the anterior interosseous nerve is essentially a motor branch of the median nerve, anterior interosseous syndrome is not characterized by sensory abnormalities. Pain in the proximal forearm is typically aggravated by exercise and abates with rest. Motor abnormalities are manifested as weakness and are referable to those muscles innervated by this nerve (flexor pollicis longus, pronator quadratus, and flexor digitorum profundus of the index finger). This syndrome may mimic a C8 radiculopathy because this is the root through which they are all innervated. Other C8-innervated muscles unaffected by the anterior interosseous nerve syndrome include the flexor digitorum superficialis (median nerve proximal to anterior interosseous nerve), the flexor carpi ulnaris, and the flexor digitorum profundus to the ring and little fingers (ulnar nerve). Electrodiagnostic evaluation may also be helpful in differentiating a C8 radiculopathy from this syndrome.

Compression of the median nerve in the carpal tunnel typically causes sensory symptoms. Night pain, paresthesias, and numbness in the hand in the radial 3½ digits are common and are caused by a thickened transverse carpal ligament. Carpal tunnel disease occurs most commonly in middle age and more frequently in women and those with occupations that require significant use and overuse of the hands and wrists. Symptoms may be referred proximally from the hand toward the forearm and even the elbow and may be reproduced or elicited by Phalen's maneuver or Tinel's sign. Thenar muscle weakness and atrophy represent advanced disease. Sensory symptoms may mimic C6 and C7 radiculopathy, but no C6 or C7 muscles demonstrate abnormalities because they are all innervated proximal to the carpal canal. Thenar motor weakness may mimic T1 radiculopathy because of abnormalities of the opponens pollicis and the abductor pollicis brevis; however, other T1-innervated muscles are normal, including the hypothenar muscles and the first dorsal interosseous (ulnar nerve).

Ulnar Nerve

The ulnar nerve has two common areas of entrapment. The most common location of ulnar nerve entrapment is the elbow in the cubital tunnel. The most typical symptom of cubital tunnel syndrome is aching pain on the medial aspect of the elbow, although radiation of the pain and paresthesias may migrate distally on the ulnar forearm and into the ulnar 1½ digits of the hand. Symptoms may be elicited by percussion of the nerve behind the medial epicondyle or by acute, prolonged flexion of the elbow. The weakness is manifested in muscles innervated by the ulnar nerve distal to the elbow (flexor carpi ulnaris, flexor digitorum profundus to the long and ring fingers, and the interossei and hypothenar muscles). All these muscles are innervated by the C8 and T1 nerve roots. However, because the sensory changes also occur in the distribution of the C8 and T1 roots, cubital tunnel syndrome may be difficult to differentiate from C8 or T1 radiculopathy. Clinical tenderness and pain referable to the medial aspect of the elbow and electrodiagnostic studies demonstrating a significant conduction delay across the elbow may be useful in this regard. Furthermore, abnormalities in C8-innervated muscles or T1-innervated muscles that are not innervated by the ulnar nerve, such as the flexor pollicis longus, the thenar muscles, and the index and long finger flexors (median nerve), may signal C8 or T1 radiculopathy rather than ulnar nerve entrapment.

The ulnar nerve may also be compressed at the wrist in Guyon's canal. Compression at this level usually affects both the superficial and deep branches of the ulnar nerve. Therefore, sensory symptoms are referred to the volar aspect of the ulnar 1½ fingers. The dorsal aspect of these digits remains unaffected because that area of skin is supplied by the dorsal sensory branch of the ulnar nerve, which originates proximal to the wrist and does not traverse Guyon's canal. The deep branch is essentially all motor, and the superficial branch is essentially all sensory. Therefore, motor symptoms, weakness, and atrophy are referable only to those muscles innervated by the deep branch of the ulnar nerve. These include the hypothenar muscles, the interossei, and the abductor pollicis. Because the sensory symptoms are in the C8 distribution and the abnormal muscles are innervated by T1 and C8, the syndrome may mimic T1 and C8 radiculopathy. In this syndrome, however, sensation over the dorsum of the ulnar 1½ fingers is normal. In addition, median nerve–innervated muscles in the T1 distribution (thenar) are normal.

Radial Nerve

The radial nerve is most commonly compressed at the elbow. Radial tunnel syndrome is a compression neuropathy of the radial nerve between the supinator muscle and the radial head just proximal to its entrance into the supinator muscle. The radial nerve gives motor branches to the brachioradialis, extensor carpi radialis longus and brevis, and supinator muscles, and then splits into a superficial sensory branch that does not enter the radial tunnel and the all-motor deep branch, the posterior interosseous nerve. Because only the motor branch is compressed, sensory symptoms are rare, although aching over the site of compression is felt and may be elicited by full extension of the elbow with the forearm in supination and the wrist in neutral. These symptoms may be aggravated by full flexion of the wrist with the forearm held in full pronation. Motor weakness may be seen in those muscles supplied by the posterior interosseous nerve (extensor digitorum communis, extensor carpi ulnaris, abductor pollicis longus, and extensor pollicis longus), all of which are supplied by the C7 root. C7 radiculopathy may be ruled out by noting no abnormalities in median nerve–innervated C7 muscles (flexor carpi radialis and pronator teres). In addition, the triceps (C7) muscle should be spared because it receives its radial nerve innervation in the upper arm, a significant distance proximal to the typical site of compression.

EXAMINATION OF RELATED AREAS

In most cases it is the cervical spine that refers pain to other areas of the upper extremity; however, it is possible for pathologic problems of the temporomandibular joint; infections of the lower jaw, teeth, or scalp; and pathologic problems of the intrinsic shoulder to refer pain to the neck.

The temporomandibular joint is the most frequently used joint in the body. This joint may be palpated by placing an index finger into the patient's external auditory canal, pressing anteriorly, and instructing the patient to open and close the mouth slowly. As the patient does so, the motion of the mandibular condyle becomes palpable to the tip of the examiner's finger. Both sides should be palpated simultaneously, and the motion should feel smooth and symmetrical. A palpable crepitation or clicking may be due to a damaged meniscus in the temporomandibular joint or to synovial swelling secondary to trauma. Asymmetrical dentition or poor occlusion can overload the joint and cause palpable clicking in the external auditory canal. Constant grinding or clenching of the teeth may also overload the joint and eventually cause clinical problems. Normal range of motion of this joint should allow the patient to open and close the mouth to admit a minimum of three fingers inserted between the incisor teeth (approximately 35 to 40 mm).

A tooth abscess of the lower jaw may refer pain to the temporomandibular joint and the neck but, more commonly, pathologic changes and dysfunction of the temporomandibular joint refer pain to the head and neck and cause headache or mandibular pain. In addition to pathologic problems about the jaw, intrinsic shoulder pathology and strain may cause pain that refers to the neck. The shoulder joint should be examined completely in any patients with lower cervical problems. This can be performed in a cursory fashion by principles similar for any physical examination. First, inspection of the shoulder joint from anterior to posterior is helpful. It is important to note any muscle atrophy. Second, the examiner should palpate all the joint complexes of the shoulder, including the sternoclavicular joint, the acromioclavicular joint, and the glenohumeral joint. Pain from biceps or rotator cuff tendinitis can also be detected by palpation of the biceps tendon in its groove. Shoulder tendinitis may be detected by a provocative movement, such as the palm-down shoulder abduction test, in which the shoulder is abducted to 90 degrees and internally rotated maximally; or the forward-flexed abduction test, in which the shoulder is externally rotated, flexed, and abducted anteriorly in an attempt to impinge the greater tuberosity on the acromial process. Production of pain in the shoulder on either of these provocative maneuvers may be an indication of rotator cuff tendinitis. It is particularly important to note whether motions of the shoulder reproduce, in total or in part, any of the pain that is associated with the person's cervical problems. It is a common error to mistake intrinsic shoulder pathology for radicular symptoms of the cervical spine. In such cases, management of the cervical spine may not result in resolution of the patient's shoulder problems.

In cases in which it is difficult to differentiate intrinsic shoulder pathologic changes from referred cervical pain, it is possible to do an intra-articular injection of lidocaine (with or without steroid). Within 10 to 15 minutes of injection, it is generally possible to eliminate the component of pain that is due to intrinsic shoulder pathologic changes. The patient can then be re-examined and a determination can be made whether or not the majority of the pain is from within the shoulder joint or being referred from the cervical spine.

EXAMINATION OF THE LUMBOSACRAL SPINE

The patient is examined initially *standing*.[23] The patient should be undressed. The spine is viewed from behind, as well as laterally and anteriorly, to see if the alignment is normal. From behind, the levels of the shoulders and any lateral spinal curves (scoliosis) should be noted. The patient stands with the head centered over the feet and the eyes level. Therefore, any deviation of the spine from the vertical is compensated by an opposite deviation elsewhere in the spine. The spine is compensated if the first thoracic vertebra is centered over the sacrum. A list occurs if the first thoracic vertebra is not over the center of the sacrum. The degree of list may be measured by dropping a perpendicular line from the first thoracic vertebra and measuring how far to the right or left of the gluteal cleft it falls. In one study, 52% of patients had a detectable lumbar scoliosis.[38] The posterior superior iliac spines should be of equal height. Any prominence of bones in the thorax or pelvis should be listed. Infection, fracture, or congenital abnormalities cause bony prominences. The gluteal folds and knee joints should be at an equal height. The feet should be in normal alignment without any limitation of movement from the Achilles tendons. The patient with lumbar muscle spasm may demonstrate a list to one side, with loss of normal spinal contours. Movement of the sacroiliac joint may be examined with the patient standing. The examiner places one thumb on the posterior superior iliac spine and the other on the sacral spine. The patient flexes the ipsilateral hip. Normally, the iliac spine moves downward. Upward motion is indicative of a fixed sacroiliac joint (Fig. 5-9).

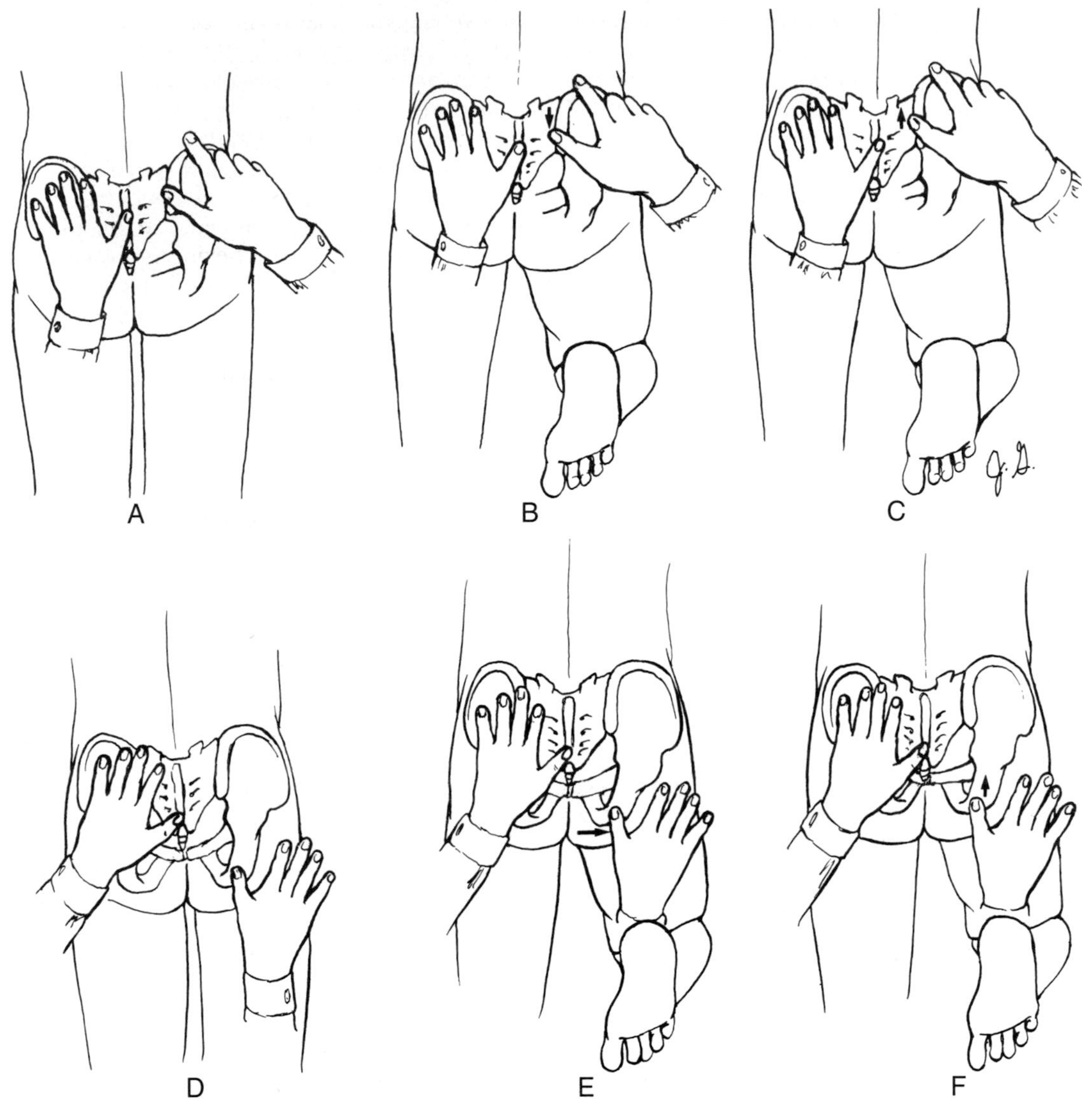

Figure 5-9 Sacroiliac joint movement. The upper row of figures depicts movement of the upper part of the joint. The lower row depicts movement of the lower part of the joint. *A*, The examiner places one thumb on the posterior superior iliac spine and the other thumb over one of the sacral spinous processes. *B*, Normal movement is associated with downward movement of the iliac spine with flexion of the ipsilateral hip. *C*, Abnormal movement associated with a fixed joint results in an upward motion of the iliac spine with flexion of the ipsilateral hip. *D*, The examiner places one thumb over the ischial tuberosity and the other thumb over the apex of the sacrum. *E*, Normal movement is associated with lateral movement of the ischial tuberosity with hip flexion. *F*, Abnormal movement associated with a fixed joint results in an upward movement of the ischial tuberosity with flexion of the hip.

Laterally, any exaggeration or decrease of normal spinal curvatures is noted. Does the patient have hyperlordosis (increased lumbosacral angle) or a flattened lumbosacral curve (decreased lumbosacral angle)? Is kyphosis present with drooped shoulders, as seen in Scheuermann's disease? In the lower extremity, are the legs straight or bent with flexion or extension deformities of the knees? Abnormalities in the lower extremity will be mirrored with similar abnormalities in the lumbosacral spine (flexion or extension deformity, respectively).

Anteriorly, the head should be straight, with level shoulders. The highest points on the flanks or the iliac wings should be of equal height. There should be no tilt to the pelvis. Anatomic structures in the lower extremities (patellae, malleoli) should be of equal height and aligned appropriately.

Abnormalities of any superficial structures are noted. These abnormalities include a tuft of hair over the spine, which may indicate a congenital abnormality, such as diastematomyelia or spina bifida occulta. Vesicles in a dermatomal pattern are suggestive of herpes zoster. Café au lait spots are associated with neurofibromatosis.

The patient should squat in place. This maneuver tests not only general muscle strength but also the integrity of function of the joints from the hips to the feet in the lower extremity. Specific areas of decreased function must be identified if the patient is unable to complete this maneuver.

With the patient in the standing position, the range of motion of the lumbosacral spine in forward flexion, extension, lateral bending (side flexion), and rotation is observed. The normal range of motion for forward flexion is 40 to 60 degrees, for extension 20 to 35 degrees, for lateral bending 15 to 20 degrees, and for rotation 3 to 18 degrees.

Spinal motion is important in terms of symmetry and rhythm. The absolute range of motion is not of major diagnostic significance because of wide individual variance. The statement is frequently made that the patients bend forward and reach to within 6 inches of the floor or 12 inches of the floor or place their palms to the floor. The important part of the observation of the patients as they bend toward the floor is the quality of spinal flexion in terms of the smooth reversal of the normal lumbar lordosis as the spine flexes forward. This is termed *lumbosacral rhythm*, and when abnormal (patients keep their lumbar lordosis and bend from the hips) signifies local back disease. Although limitation of spine flexion is of limited diagnostic value, the improvement of spine flexion is a means to monitor response to therapy of an individual patient.[36]

Also important in assessment is the time of day and degree of activity prior to the examination. Malko and associates used magnetic resonance imaging to measure the volume of discs during load cycles of five healthy volunteers, aged 27 to 52 years, without back pain.[35] The load cycle consisted of bed rest, followed by wearing a 20-kg backpack for 3 hours, followed by 3 hours of bed rest. The average changes in volumes of the L2 through L5 disc were 5.4%. The discs regained volume over 3 hours after removal of the compressive force. The changes in disc volume may affect the degree of spinal mobility. In a similar investigation, Ensink and colleagues measured lumbar spine motion in 29 chronic back pain patients in the morning and afternoon.[18] Total lumbar range of motion increased significantly during the course of the day. Flexion was increased to the greatest degree during the day, whereas extension was independent of time of measurement. These measurements were not affected by the gender, age, height, or weight of the patients.

Forward flexion of the spine is a segmental motion, with bending occurring at each functional unit (a functional unit comprising two adjacent vertebrae along with their interposed disc). These units also contain the ligaments, nerves, and facet joints of the two adjacent vertebrae. The most movement occurs at the lumbosacral L5–S1 and L4–L5 levels. As a result, most of the damage and most symptoms relate to these two functional units. In forward bending, each unit flexes about 8 to 10 degrees. This means that the entire lumbar spine has only 45 degrees of excursion, and as a person reaches to touch the ground, the rest of the motion comes from the pelvis rotating through the hip joints.

When a person with an injury to one of the functional units attempts to bend forward, the flexion will frequently be inhibited by protective muscle spasm. The lumbar spine will not have the normal curve in the erect position, nor is there any reversal of the sway of the back on attempting to bend forward. As the patient attempts to touch the floor, all of the motion occurs at the hip joints.

Although this inability to flex the lumbar spine can be due to injury, it also may be voluntary in that the patient either is afraid or does not wish to bend forward. Consequently, this restriction is not necessarily indicative of an injury. A good examiner can generally differentiate between actual spasm and just a reflex, protective response. Flexion from an upright position should be compared with similar movement while kneeling. In the kneeling position, the sciatic nerve is not under tension and the hamstring muscles are relaxed; thus, the back can move untethered.

It also should be appreciated that flexion is relative and its limitation may be only an indication of poor conditioning. The patient's perceived stiffness may actually represent very little loss of flexibility in respect to a preinjury state.

If the protective spasm is unilateral owing to injury of the tissues on one side of the spine, scoliosis develops. The spine is tilted to one side because of one-sided muscle spasm. Scoliosis is difficult to mimic and may go unnoticed by the patient with back pain. It frequently increases with forward flexion. Disc herniation can also cause scoliosis by irritating nerves on one side of the spine (Fig. 5-10). This usually occurs at the L4–L5 level. This diagnostic finding must be supplemented by other signs and symptoms to justify a diagnosis of a disc herniation. Scoliosis may be classified as structural or nonstructural. With structural scoliosis, anatomic changes in the vertebral column and thoracic ribs cause an asymmetry of structures, which

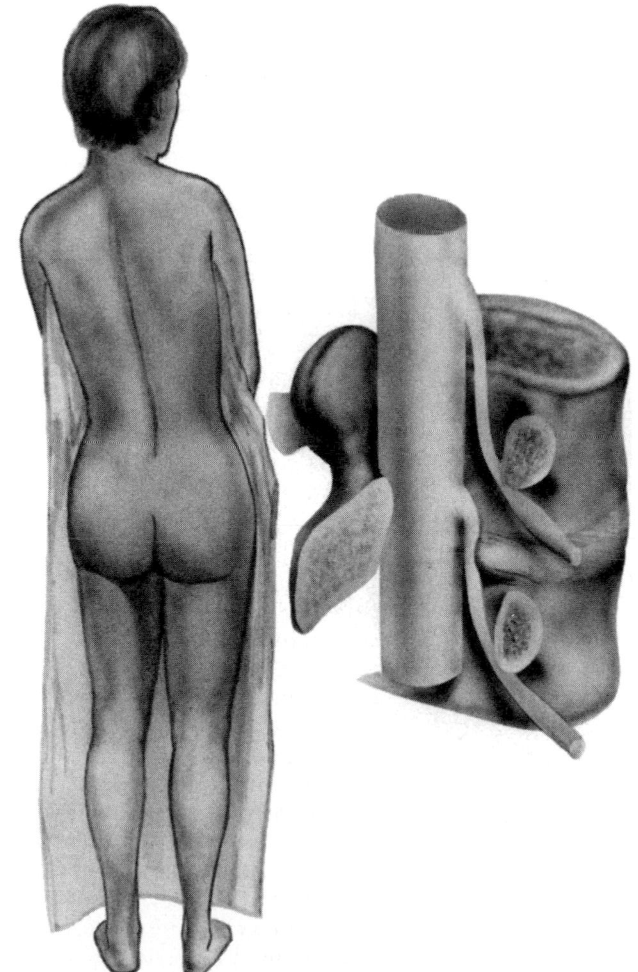

Figure 5-10 Herniation of a nucleus pulposus *lateral* to the corresponding nerve root. The sciatic list is away from the side of the irritated nerve root. *(From Rothman RH, Simeone FA: The Spine, 2nd ed. Philadelphia, WB Saunders, 1982.)*

appears with forward flexion. The high side (shoulder elevated) is on the convex side of the scoliotic curve. Nonstructural scoliosis is related to pain, has no associated anatomic change, and has no asymmetry with forward flexion. The scoliosis is of a lumbar variety if the apex of the curve is situated at the lumbar level.

Measurement of the distance from the floor to the patient's fingertips is an inexact measurement of lumbar flexion. However, the measurement is a useful way to follow the response of patients to therapy. Improvement in forward flexion will be manifested as a decrease in finger-to-floor distance whether the improvement is from decreased muscle spasm, increased hip motion, or decreased hamstring tightness.

After patients have fully flexed, it is helpful to observe how they regain the erect posture. How this maneuver is performed reflects past habits as well as the constraints of any tissue injury. Normally a return to erect position is accomplished by a derotation of the pelvis without alteration of the kyphosis of the spine until the person has raised up to 45 degrees. During the remaining 45 degrees of re-extension, the low back resumes its lordosis. Patients with legitimate back pain tend to resume the erect position with a fixed lordosis and without any spine movement. It is all done by the pelvis with the help of knee and hip flexion.

The ability to bend sideways in lateral flexion has no major diagnostic significance as long as the patient is not simultaneously flexing or extending. The patient is asked to run a hand down the side of the leg and not to bend forward or backward while performing the movement. Lateral bending simply causes ligamentous or muscular stretching and can be free or restricted without diagnostic significance. However, pain that increases with flexion to the ipsilateral side may be related to an articular disease or a disc protrusion lateral to the nerve root. If pain is increased with flexion to the contralateral side, the lesion may be articular, muscular (muscles are stretched), or a disc protrusion medial to the nerve root (Fig. 5-11). Quantification of right and left lateral flexion can be measured by noting the distraction of two points, 20 cm apart in the midaxillary line on contralateral flexion.[39]

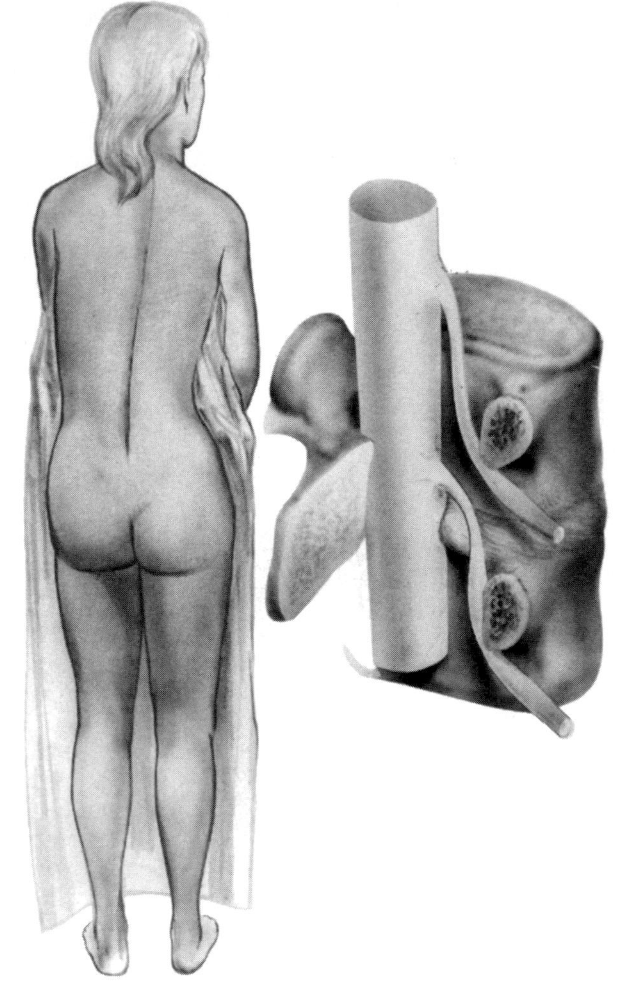

Figure 5-11 Herniation of a nucleus pulposus *medial* to the corresponding nerve root. The sciatic list is toward the side of the irritated nerve root. *(From Rothman RH, Simeone FA: The Spine, 2nd ed. Philadelphia, WB Saunders, 1982.)*

Hyperextension can cause pain by changing several anatomic relationships. Arching the back and increasing the lordosis forces the facet joints together, narrows the foramen through which the nerves exit the spine, and compresses the disc posteriorly. A combination of these three factors can create pressure on the nerves as they leave the spine and cause back pain, leg pain, or both.

Rotation may be examined in the standing position but care must be taken to stabilize the pelvis to eliminate accessory motion of the hips. Rotation may be examined more accurately in the seated position. The hips and pelvis are stabilized with seating, limiting rotating motion of the spine.

The strength and stamina of the back and leg muscles can be tested by repeated active movement, especially flexion and extension of the lumbosacral spine. The patient should perform 10 toe raises on both feet and 10 more on each foot separately. Repeated testing causes fatigue, which accentuates differences in strength in the lower extremities. The strength of the examiner's arms may be less than that of the patient's legs. By using the patient's own weight, instead of the examiner's strength, differences of strength between the legs are discovered.

Patients may also be asked to walk on their heels to test for strength of the dorsiflexors of the foot. These muscles are more appropriately tested with patients in the seated position. The Trendelenburg's sign may be elicited at this point. The patient is asked to stand on one leg. With a positive test, the buttock away from the affected muscle will fall when the patient is asked to stand on one leg. This may be related to an S1 nerve root lesion or hip disease (Fig. 5-12).

The physician should palpate the lumbosacral spine when the patient is standing, sitting, and during testing of motions. It is helpful to palpate both groups of paraspinous muscles simultaneously to discern differences of firmness or tenderness in the muscle bodies. Muscles become more prominent as they contract with spasm. Observation may demonstrate this muscle prominence on one side of the midline of the spine. Very localized areas of muscle tenderness, which may be trigger points for referred pain to other areas of the lumbosacral spine, should be identified. In the lumbosacral region, trigger points are located on both sides of the lumbosacral junction and in the superior

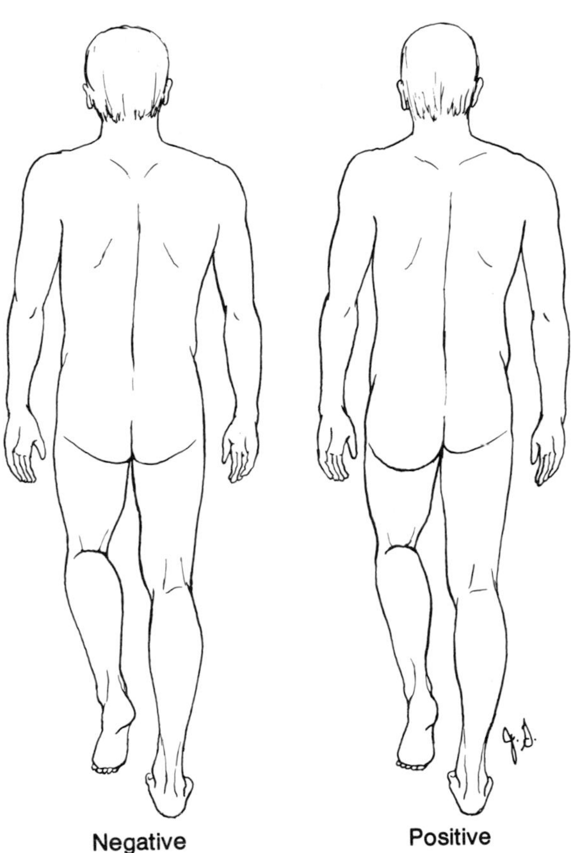

Figure 5-12 Trendelenburg's test measuring integrity of the S1 nerve root and ipsilateral hip joint. A positive test is associated with a fall of the buttock contralateral to the affected nerve root or hip joint. In this figure, the right side is affected.

portion of the buttocks near the iliac wings. Posterior thighs should also be palpated.

In addition to the soft tissue, bony structures should be palpated. The spinous processes are covered by ligamentous structures, not muscle, and are easily palpated. Localized tenderness suggests the presence of an isolated process, such as an infection, tumor, or fracture affecting that vertebral body. Pressure on the lateral surface of the vertebral body elicits pain if an abnormality has involved the transverse process of the vertebra.

Palpation of the lumbar spine in the midline usually elicits pain at the level of a symptomatic degenerative disc. Moving laterally from the midline 1 to 3 cm, palpation of the facet joints may generate pain in the patient with degenerative joint disease. Palpation should also be performed in the sciatic notch along the course of the sciatic nerve. Hyperesthesia along the irritated nerve is often found, and in addition, local tumors of the nerve may be discovered in this manner.

Vertebral tenderness may be a sensitive sign of spine pathology but is not discriminating in differentiating mechanical from medical disorders. Spinal pain with palpation may be from degenerative joint disease, spondyloarthropathy, or a vertebral infection.[6] Additional physical signs, such as fever and decreased chest expansion, help differentiate mechanical from medical causes of vertebral tenderness.

The patient should next be examined *kneeling*. The patient should kneel on a chair facing the back rest. The ankle reflex corresponding to the S1 level is more easily tested in this position. Reinforcement of the reflex is obtained by having the patient grab the back of the chair or having the examiner dorsiflex the foot.

Persistence of limited motion and muscle spasm may be evaluated in this position. Some patients voluntarily guard their back muscles and are unwilling to flex forward in the standing position. In the kneeling position, their muscles may relax and soften remarkably. The spine may become more mobile, allowing the patient to bend forward.

The patient is examined in the *seated* position with feet on the floor. The strength of the dorsiflexors of the foot is measured by the examiner maintaining steady downward pressure on the dorsum of the foot. The maneuver should be continued for a minute to allow for detection of weakness in the muscles supplied by the L5 nerve roots. The patient generates uniform resistance to pressure that is overcome in a smooth fashion. Patients who feign weakness may either resist pressure for a few seconds and then suddenly release the muscle or demonstrate a stepwise release of the muscle resulting in a cogwheel effect.[23]

Patients are asked to *bend forward* over the examining table, allowing their weight to rest on their abdomen. This position flattens the lumbar lordosis and tilts the sacrum, allowing examination of the inferior portion of the sacroiliac joint, ischial tuberosities, and sciatic notch. Palpation over these anatomic structures may elicit pain. Patients with inflammatory processes of the sacroiliac joints (ankylosing spondylitis) are among those who experience increased pain with percussion over the sacroiliac joints. The gait of the patients should be examined as they walk from the chair to the examining table. Back pain usually decreases the mobility of the lumbar spine and produces restriction of normal spinal movement. The back is stiff, as if frozen in one position. The patient walks in a stiff, guarded fashion, depending mainly on hip movement and lateral spine flexion rather than using a normal gait involving a more complete range of active spinal movements.

The positions of *sitting* with legs dangling, *lying supine*, *lying on one side*, and *lying prone* are used for the neurologic examination. Assessment of the neurologic status of the patient is important in the overall back evaluation. A positive neurologic finding gives objectivity to the patient's subjective complaints. Each nerve root must be examined. Abnormalities of motor, sensory, and reflex function are tested. Of the possible neurologic abnormalities, true muscle weakness is the most reliable indicator of persistent nerve compression with loss of nerve conduction.[45] Sensory changes are subjective and are easily affected by the emotional and energy state of the patient. As the patient fatigues, consistent sensory findings are difficult to reproduce. In addition, reflex changes may be lost in a previous episode of nerve root compression. Reflexes may not return even with recovery of sensory and motor function.[5] With age, reflexes are more difficult to elicit even without any prior history of nerve compression. However, the loss of reflexes is symmetrical. Patients who lose reflexes in both lower extremities on the basis of compression have a central herniation of a disc.

Peripheral nerve injuries may cause sensory and/or motor abnormalities, depending on the damaged nerve. Peripheral nerves receive nerve fibers from a number of nerve root levels. The locations of nerve root and peripheral nerve lesions affecting cutaneous structures in the lower extremity are depicted in Figures 5-13 and 5-14. A lesion at one nerve root level may cause a minor change in function if a structure is supplied by multiple spinal cord levels (hip flexion—psoas) (Fig. 5-15). However, if a peripheral nerve is injured, innervation to specific muscles and cutaneous areas is interrupted. In this circumstance, specific muscles may become paralyzed or areflexic (obturator nerve—thigh adduction) or specific cutaneous areas anesthetized (lateral femoral cutaneous nerve—lateral thigh) (Fig. 5-16). The differentiation of upper motor neuron, nerve root, and peripheral nerve lesions is an important one. The locations of the abnormalities causing these neurologic manifestations are different. Also, the category of pathologic process causing upper motor neuron, nerve root, and peripheral nerve abnormalities may be different (multiple sclerosis, disc herniation, and diabetes, respectively).

Sitting with legs dangling is the preferred position for testing knee reflexes (L4 nerve root). Minor differences in reflexes are usually caused by incomplete relaxation of the quadriceps or hamstrings by the patient. Reinforcing the reflex by having patients attempt to pull apart their locked hands will distract them, allowing for relaxation of muscles. True asymmetry of reflex action should be present on repeated testing. The Babinski's reflex may be tested in this position. This is done by lifting the leg to stroke the sole of the foot. By raising the foot, the examiner has performed a modified straight leg–raising test. Since the thigh is already flexed to 90 degrees in this position, straightening the knees to the horizontal places stretching forces on the nerve roots. The results of this sitting tension sign should correspond to those of the test done in the lying position.[40] This is a useful test in those situations where there is a suspicion of malingering. The patient with hamstring tightness may also experience leg pain. With extension of the knee, the patient will extend the trunk to relieve pressure (positive tripod sign). The patient with nerve root irritation has a similar response. The localization of pain to the thigh or lower leg helps differentiate these patients.

Straight Leg–Raising (SLR) Test

Lying supine on the examining table is an excellent position for testing the status of the nerve roots and peripheral nerves. The classic test of sciatic nerve (L4, L5, S1) irritation is the straight leg–raising test. Its purpose is to stretch the dura. The more useful straight leg–raising test is done by raising the leg with the knee extended, first described by J. J. Forst, a contemporary of Lasegue, in the late

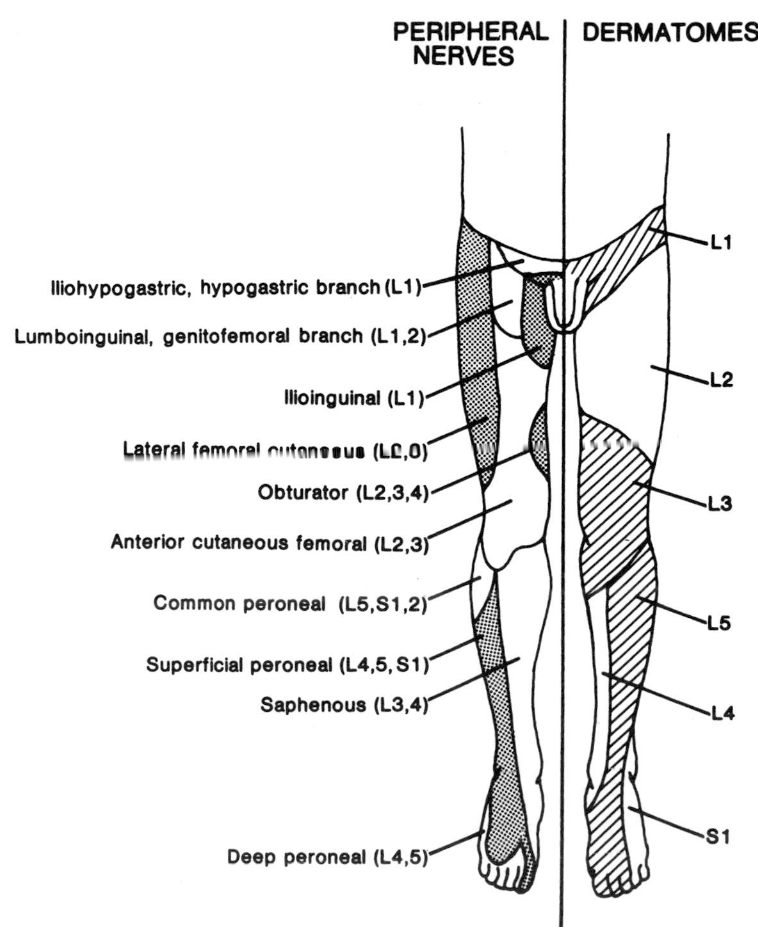

Figure 5-13 Anterior view of the lower extremities depicting skin areas innervated by nerve roots *(right)* and peripheral nerves *(left)*.

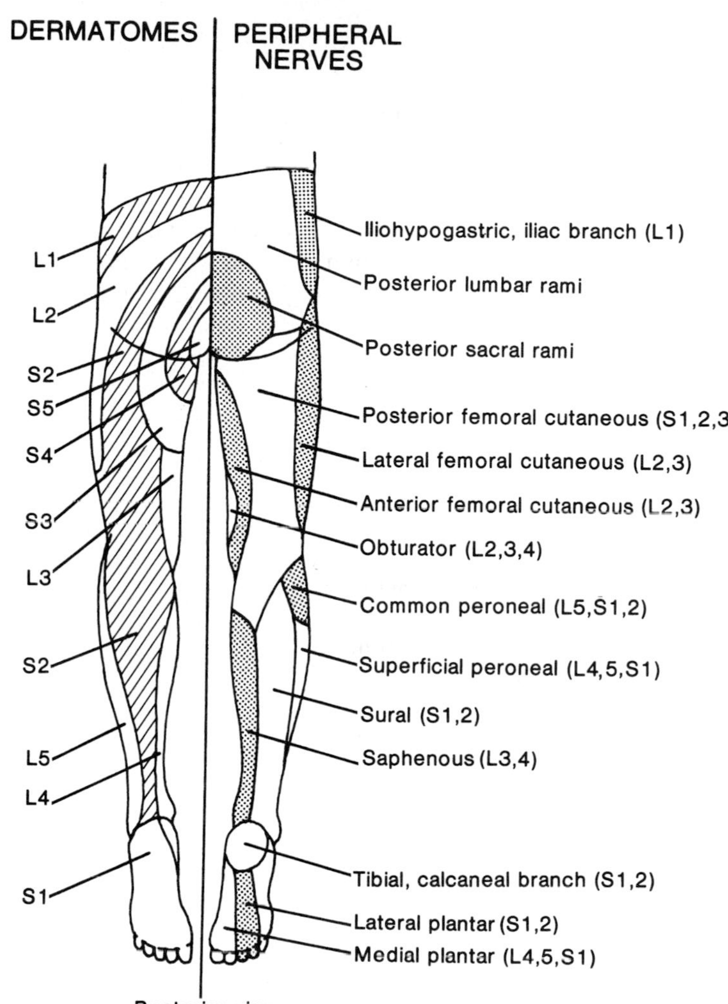

Figure 5-14 Posterior view of the nerve root *(left)* and peripheral nerve *(right)* areas of the lower extremities.

1800s.[20] When the sciatic nerve is stretched and its nerve roots and corresponding dural attachments are inflamed, the patient experiences pain along its anatomic course to the lower leg, ankle, and foot. Symptoms should not be produced in the lower leg until the leg is raised to 30 to 35 degrees. Until that elevation, these is no dural movement. Between 30 and 60 to 70 degrees, tension is applied to the dura and nerve roots (Fig. 5-17). The rate of deformation of the roots diminishes as the angle increases. Symptoms produced at elevations above 70 degrees may represent nerve root irritation but may also be related to mechanical low back pain secondary to muscle strain or to joint disease.[19] The test is considered positive when the patient's radicular symptomatology is reproduced; the production of back pain does not indicate a positive test. Some patients experience limitation of motion and posterior thigh pain secondary to hamstring muscle tightness. The degree of tightness is determined by raising the nonpainful side first, quantifying the degrees of painless motion.

Lasegue's Test

In Lasegue's test, which is frequently mistaken as a straight leg test, the patient is supine with the hip flexed to 90 degrees and the knee is slowly extended until sciatic pain is elicited (Fig. 5-18). This test is less valuable than the straight leg–raising test since both hip and knee joints are moved, resulting in greater difficulty in interpreting the test.

Bragard's Test

The patient with a positive straight leg–raising test will have pain that radiates to the lower leg. To confirm the presence of nerve irritability, the raised leg should be lowered until the pain is relieved. At that position, the foot is dorsiflexed, which causes a recurrence of pain as a result of stretching of the posterior tibial branch of the sciatic nerve (Fig. 5-19). Although this is not the test described by Lasegue, pain with dorsiflexion of the foot is commonly referred to as a *positive Lasegue's sign*. This test is also known as Bragard's test.

Bilateral SLR Test

A bilateral straight leg–raising test may also detect sciatic nerve irritation (Fig. 5-20). The test is performed in the supine position by raising both legs by the ankles with

SEGMENTAL MOTOR INNERVATION

L1	L2	L3	L4	L5	S1	S2	S3	S4	S5
Erector spinae									
Multifidus									
Interspinales									
Intertransversarii									
Quadratus lumborum									
Iliacus									
Psoas major									
Psoas minor									
	Pectineus								
	Sartorius								
	Quadriceps femoris								
	Gracilis								
	Adductor brevis								
	Adductor longus								
		Quadratus femoris							
		Adductor magnus							
		Obturator externus							
			Gluteus medius						
			Gluteus minimus						
			Tensor fasciae latae						
			Gemellus inferior						
			Extensor digitorum brevis						
			Plantaris						
			Popliteus						
			Tibialis anterior						
				Tibialis posterior					
				Gluteus maximus					
				Piriformis					
				Gemellus superior					
				Obturator internus					
				Biceps femoris					

A

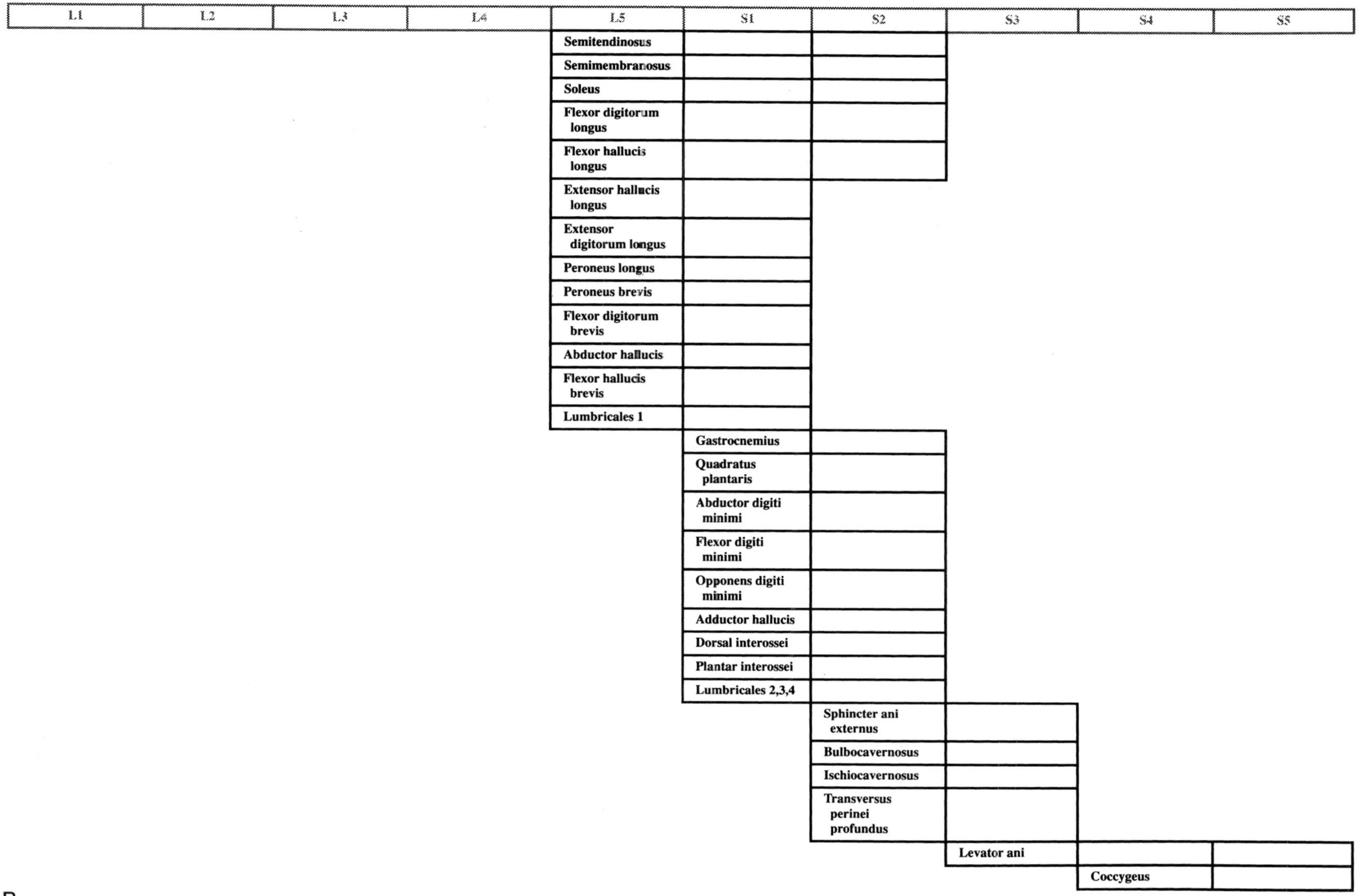

L1	L2	L3	L4	L5	S1	S2	S3	S4	S5
				Semitendinosus					
				Semimembranosus					
				Soleus					
				Flexor digitorum longus					
				Flexor hallucis longus					
				Extensor hallucis longus					
				Extensor digitorum longus					
				Peroneus longus					
				Peroneus brevis					
				Flexor digitorum brevis					
				Abductor hallucis					
				Flexor hallucis brevis					
				Lumbricales 1					
					Gastrocnemius				
					Quadratus plantaris				
					Abductor digiti minimi				
					Flexor digiti minimi				
					Opponens digiti minimi				
					Adductor hallucis				
					Dorsal interossei				
					Plantar interossei				
					Lumbricales 2,3,4				
						Sphincter ani externus			
						Bulbocavernosus			
						Ischiocavernosus			
						Transversus perinei profundus			
							Levator ani		
								Coccygeus	

B

Figure 5-15 Segmental motor innervation of muscles supplied by L1 through S5 spinal nerves. The innervation of muscles from multiple (minimally two, and more commonly three) spinal cord levels is evident.

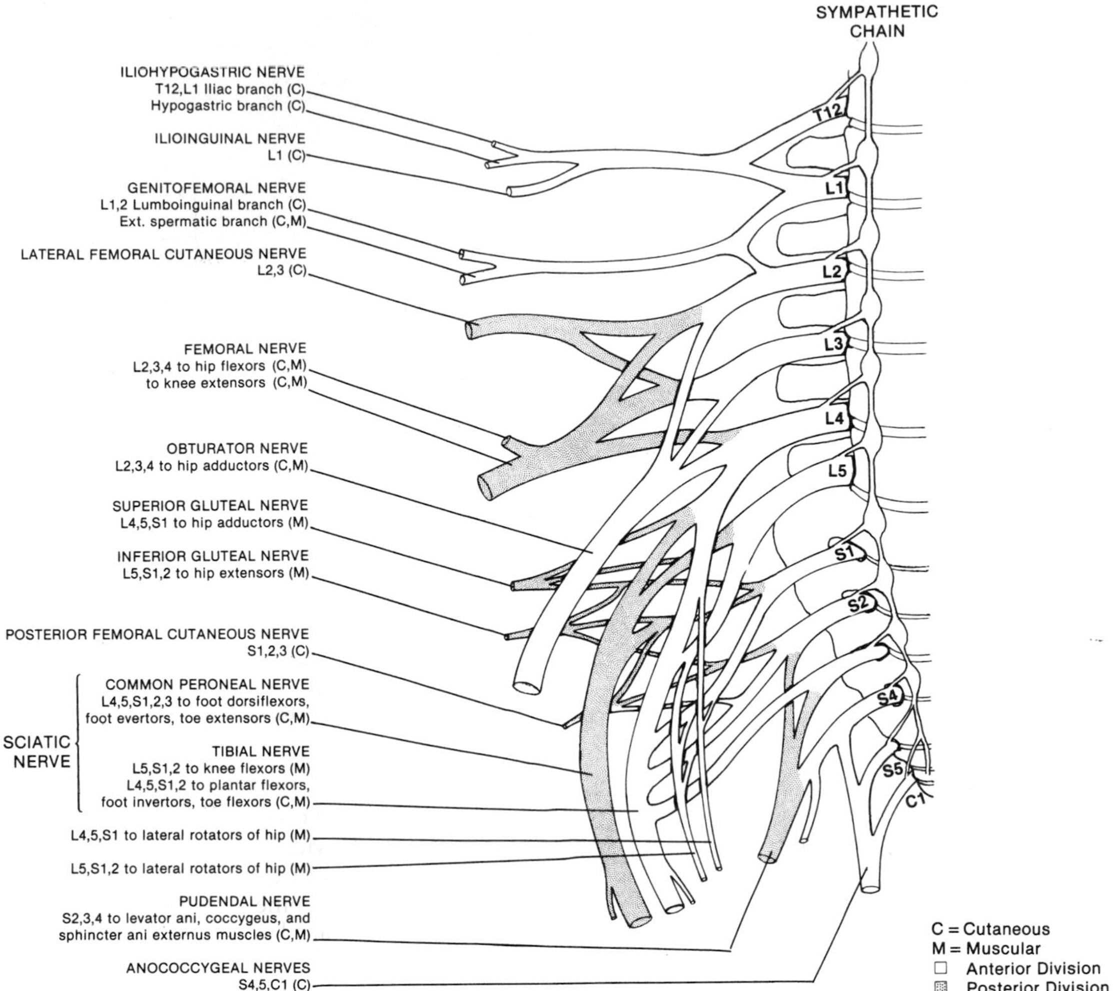

Figure 5-16 Nerves originating in the lumbosacral spine. The plexus, roots, branches, divisions (anterior and posterior), terminal branches, and autonomic nervous system components of the lumbosacral plexus are included. The cutaneous and motor components of the peripheral nerves are noted. The functions of muscles are listed under the associated nerves.

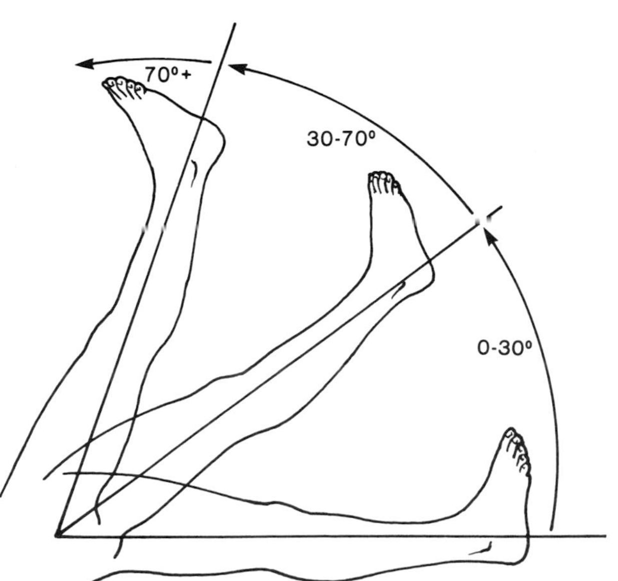

Figure 5-17 Dynamics of the single straight leg–raising test. Tension is applied to the sciatic roots at 30 degrees of elevation. Sciatic roots are maximally tightened over a herniated disc between 30 and 70 degrees. No additional tension is generated with angles greater than 70 degrees. Pain elicited at this height of elevation may be articular or muscular in origin.

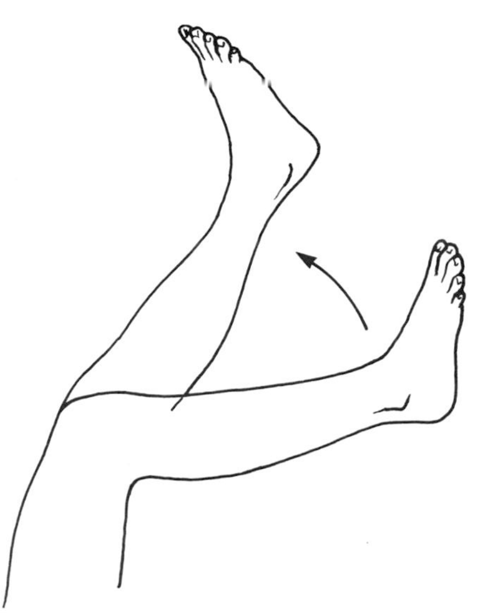

Figure 5-18 Lasegue's test.

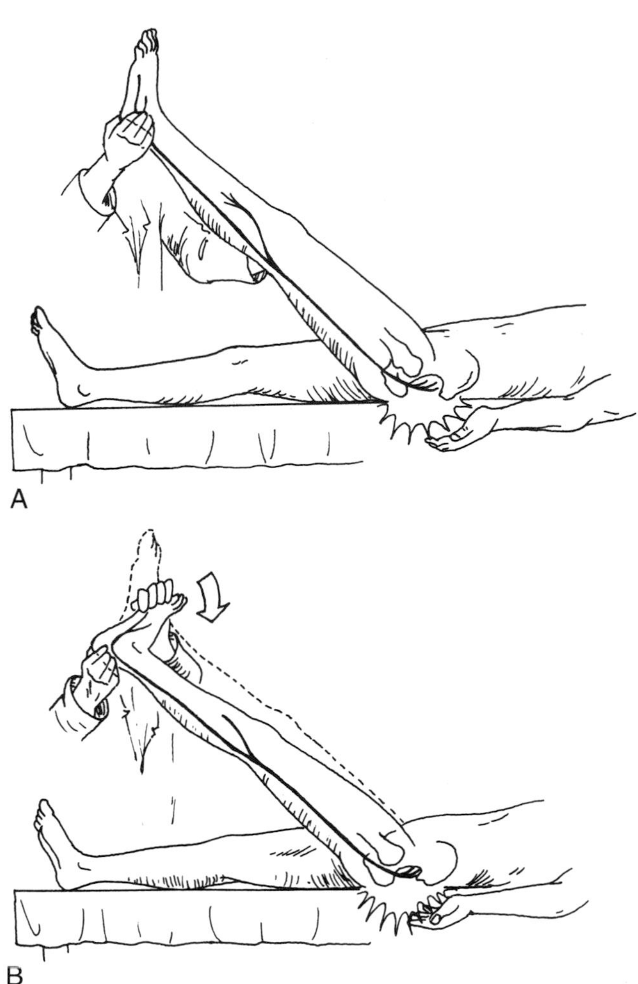

Figure 5-19 Confirmatory straight leg–raising test. *A*, The leg is raised until radicular symptoms are elicited. *B*, The leg is lowered until pain is relieved. The foot is then dorsiflexed; if this re-creates radicular pain, the test result is considered positive. *(From Reilly BM: Practical Strategies in Outpatient Medicine. Philadelphia, WB Saunders, 1984.)*

knees extended. Raising both legs simultaneously tilts the pelvis upward, diminishing some of the tethering of the sciatic nerve. Therefore, the legs may be raised to a greater angle before radicular pain appears. Pain that occurs before 70 degrees of motion is caused by stress on the sacroiliac joints. Above 70 degrees, pain is related to a lesion in the lumbar spine. When the examination reveals a psychogenic cause of pain, a bilateral straight leg–raising test is routinely painful at a lower elevation than a unilateral test.

The presence of a positive straight leg–raising test at 60 degrees is a sensitive sign but a nonspecific one for disc herniation.[31] Radicular pain at a lower angle of elevation is associated with a larger disc protrusion documented at the time of surgery.[19] A positive crossed straight leg–raising test is less sensitive but more specific for disc herniation.[52] Deville and colleagues reviewed 17 diagnostic studies of the sensitivity and specificity of the straight leg–raising test.[13] Individuals with more severe disease had positive tests, increasing the sensitivity of the test. The diagnostic accuracy of the straight leg–raising test is limited by its low specificity. The diagnosis of a radiculopathy

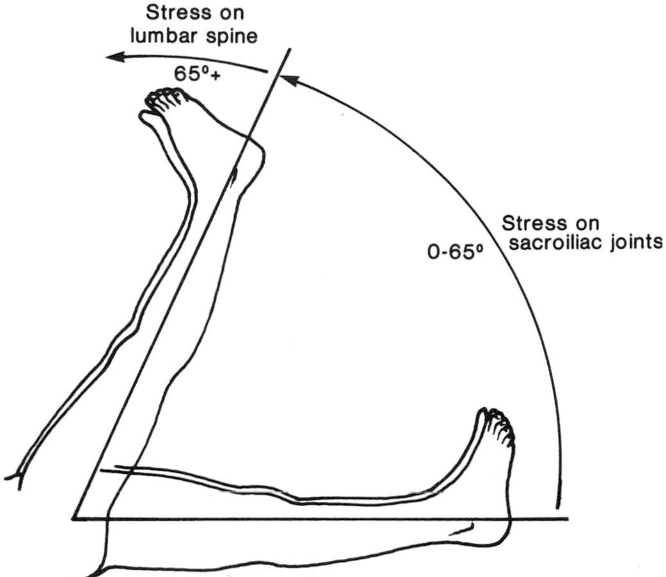

Figure 5-20 Bilateral straight leg–raising test. The movement from 0 to 65 or 70 degrees places stress on the sacroiliac joints. Above 70 degrees, stress is placed on structures in the lumbar spine. Patients with psychogenic pain and a positive single straight leg–raising test frequently develop pain at a smaller degree of elevation during the bilateral test.

should not be based on a straight leg–raising test alone but on the totality of evidence from all the physical findings.

Measurements of the lower extremity are made with the patient in the supine position. Leg lengths are measured using the bony landmarks of the anterior superior iliac spine and medial or lateral malleolus (Fig. 5-21). In addition, measurements of the thigh and calf at equivalent points above and below the patellae should be recorded.

Examination of the hip and sacroiliac joints is an essential part of the evaluation of the lumbosacral spine. Although hip pain may rarely be referred to the low back, it is more characteristically felt in the groin and down the anteromedial thigh to the top of the knee. Flexion of the hip is measured first. Normal flexion has a range to 120 degrees. As the examiner flexes the hip, a Thomas's test detects the presence of hip flexion contracture. As the hip is flexed, the lumbar lordosis is flattened. With flattening of the lordosis, a flexion contracture of the contralateral hip will appear with raising of that leg. The number of degrees the contralateral hip is above the horizontal is the extent of the flexion contracture. To evaluate abduction of the hip, the examiner places one hand on the iliac crest, grasps the ankle with the other, and moves the leg away from the midline, noting the angle at which the pelvis moves. Hip abduction is maximum at 45 degrees. Abduction may also be measured by quantifying the distance between the medial malleoli when both legs are maximally abducted. Adduction is measured with the examiner's hands in the same position, with note taken of when the pelvis moves after the leg is brought across the neutral position. Normal adduction ranges to 30 degrees.

Examination of the hip for internal and external rotation is particularly sensitive for detecting early abnormalities of the hip. Flexion and extension of the hip may be normal while first internal rotation and then external rotation

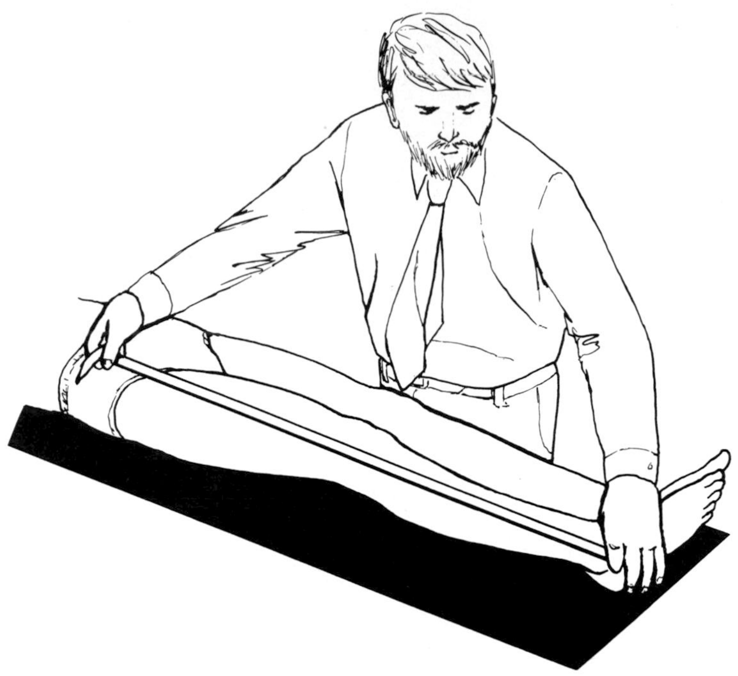

Figure 5-21 Measuring leg length.

become painful. The range of motion is 45 degrees for external rotation and 35 degrees for internal rotation. Rotation is measured with the hip and knee in 90 degrees of flexion. Internal rotation is measured by rotation of the lower leg away from the midline of the trunk, and external rotation is determined by rotation of the lower leg toward the midline of the trunk.

Patrick's Test

Another test that stresses both the hip and sacroiliac joint is the Patrick's or FABER (flexion, abduction, external rotation) test (Fig. 5-22). The test is done by positioning the lateral malleolus of the tested leg on the patella of the opposite leg. Downward pressure is then placed on the medial aspect of the knee. Pain associated with a quick pulse of downward pressure is usually localized to the lateral aspect of the lumbar spine and originates in the sacroiliac joint. Slow pressure may elicit groin pain indicative of hip joint dysfunction. Patients with iliopsoas spasm are unable to lower the leg and may also experience groin pain with pressure. A negative test is indicated by the test leg's falling to the table or being parallel with the opposite leg.

Sacroiliac Joint Tests

The integrity of the sacroiliac joints is tested by applying pressure down and out on the anterior superior iliac spines. This pressure stresses the anterior sacroiliac ligaments, and the test is positive if the patient complains of buttock or posterior leg pain. Compression of the iliac wings toward the midline stresses the posterior iliac ligaments, and the test is positive when the patient complains of low back pain. Strain on the sacroiliac joint may also be elicited by asking the patient to flex the hip and knee maximally and adduct the leg, bringing the knee toward the opposite shoulder. Pain in the stressed sacroiliac joint indicates a positive test. Gaenslen's test is another examination

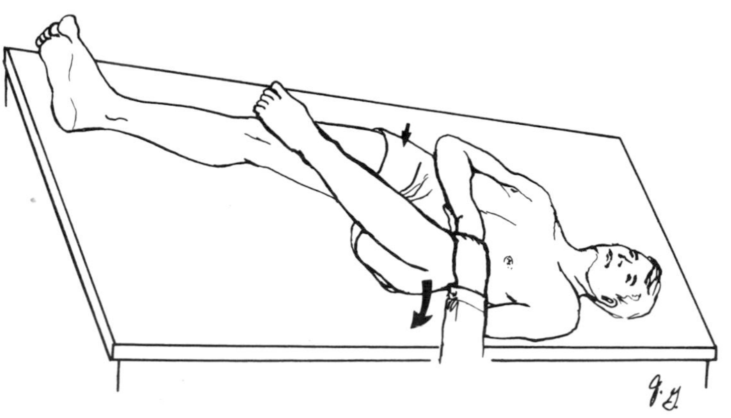

Figure 5-22 Patrick's test ("FABER maneuver"). The test is done by stabilizing the pelvis with downward pressure on the contralateral iliac wing (*small arrow*—arm not drawn) while lowering the ipsilateral flexed, abducted, and rotated leg. Rapid lowering tests the status of the sacroiliac joint, while slow lowering tests the hip.

for abnormalities of the sacroiliac joint. The hip farthest from the edge of the examination table is flexed to the chest, while the test hip is extended by lowering it off the table. Pain that is localized to the low back is due to sacroiliac joint disease. Lesions of the hip joint and L4 nerve root must be differentiated from sacroiliac disease. However, diseases specific to the sacroiliac joint remain difficult to determine by physical examination. Dreyfuss and co-workers tested 12 physical examination signs to exacerbate sacroiliac pain.[15] No specific combination of tests were specific for sacroiliac joint pain.

S1 Nerve Root Testing

Neurologic function associated with abnormalities of the lumbosacral spine should be tested when the patient is in the supine position. The examination may be conducted according to systems (motor, sensory, reflexes) or to nerve root lesions (Table 5-4). When the first sacral root is compressed, the patient can have gastrocnemius weakness. The Achilles reflex (ankle jerk) often is diminished or absent, and atrophy of the calf may be apparent. Another muscle innervated by the first sacral root is the gluteus maximus. It can be tested with the patient lying supine with the knee on the involved side flexed at 90 degrees. The strength of the gluteus maximus as well as the integrity of the S1 nerve can be evaluated unilaterally by having the patients raise their buttocks off the examining table five or six times—the affected side will be weaker as compared with the normal side. Sensory loss for the S1 root is confined to the posterior aspect of the calf and/or lateral side of the foot.

Bowditch and associates evaluated ankle reflexes in 1074 adult orthopedic patients with an age range of 16 to 99 years and without a history of sciatica or medical disorders (peripheral neuropathy) associated with absent ankle jerks.[7] The 543 men and 533 women were stratified by decade into nine groups. The earliest significant bilateral loss of ankle reflex occurred between the ages of 51 and 60 years, with 8% loss compared with 61 to 70 years with a 30% loss. Unilateral loss of reflex increased with age but never exceeded 10% of patients. The bilateral loss of ankle reflex obscures asymmetrical pathology as the patient ages. Unilateral loss of an ankle reflex is a significant neurologic sign, irrespective of age.

L5 Nerve Root Testing

Compression of the fifth lumbar nerve root may lead to weakness in extension of the great toe and, less often, to weakness of the everters and dorsiflexors of the foot. The sensory deficit may occur over the anterior tibia and the dorsomedial aspect of the foot down to the great toe. Primary reflex changes are uncommon, but sometimes a change in the posterior tibial reflex can be elicited. The absence of this reflex, however, must be asymmetrical for it to have any clinical significance. A superficial reflex associated with L5 lesions is the gluteal reflex; stroking the skin over the buttock will result in contraction of the gluteal muscles.

5-4 LUMBOSACRAL ROOT SYNDROMES

Root	Dermatome	Muscle Innervation	Muscle Action	Associated Reflex
L1	Back to trochanter Groin	Iliopsoas	Hip flexion	Cremasteric
L2	Back Anterior thigh to level of knee	Iliopsoas Sartorius Hip adductors (longus, brevis, pectineus, magnus, gracilis)	Hip flexion Hip adduction	Cremasteric Adductor
L3	Back Upper buttock to anterior thigh Medial lower leg	Iliopsoas Quadriceps femoris Sartorius Hip adductors	Hip flexion Hip adduction Knee extension	Patellar
L4	Inner calf to medial portion of foot (first 2 toes)	Tibialis anterior Gluteus medius Gluteus minimus Tensor fasciae latae Quadratus femoris	Knee extension	Patellar Gluteal
L5	Lateral lower leg Dorsum of foot First two toes	Extensor hallucis Tibialis posterior Hamstrings	Toe extension Ankle dorsiflexion	Tibialis posterior Gluteal
S1	Sole Heel Lateral edge of foot	Gastrocnemius Gluteus maximus Hamstrings Peroneus	Ankle plantarflexion Knee flexion	Ankle Hamstring
S2	Posterior and medial upper leg	Flexor digitorum longus Flexor hallucis longus	Ankle plantarflexion Toe flexion	None
S3	Medial portion of buttocks	—	—	Bulbocavernosus
S4	Perirectal	—	—	Bulbocavernosus
S5	Perirectal	—	—	Anal
C1	Tip of coccyx	—	—	Anal

L4 Nerve Root Testing

Involvement of the fourth lumbar nerve root may lead to quadriceps muscle weakness. This can present as weakness of knee extension and/or the complaint of an unstable knee. Atrophy of the thigh musculature can be marked, and the sensory loss is over the anteromedial aspect of the thigh. The patellar tendon reflex is affected.

Motor Strength Testing

When testing muscle power, it is important to test the muscles with the intervening joints in a neutral position. Pressure is applied by the examiner to a nonarticular structure for a minimum of 5 seconds. Where feasible, it is preferable to test both sides simultaneously. The innervation of muscles follows a sequential pattern, starting with the hip and ending with the ankle (Fig. 5-23). Hip flexion is supplied by L2 and L3 and hip extension by L4 and L5. Knee extension (forward movement) is a function of L3 and L4 and knee flexion (backward movement) of L5 and S1. Ankle dorsiflexion is associated with L4 and L5 and ankle plantarflexion with S1 and S2. Ankle inversion is a function of L4. Ankle eversion is associated with L5 and S1.

The presence of tender motor points in the lower extremity in patients with sciatic pain has diagnostic and prognostic importance (Fig. 5-24). The points represent the main neuromuscular junctions for the involved muscle groups and remain reliably constant in location from patient to patient. Patients with radiculopathy and tender motor points have a segmental nerve root lesion at the corresponding level within the affected myotome. In addition, patients with tender motor points remain symptomatic longer than those without them.[22]

Reflex Testing

Other superficial and deep reflexes may be tested in the supine position in addition to the patellar and Achilles reflexes. The bulbocavernous reflex is an indication of S3 and S4 nerve root function and is tested by pinching the skin over the dorsum of the glans penis. A normal response is contraction of the bulbous urethra. The superficial abdominal reflex is elicited by rubbing a sharp object in a rhomboid shape on the abdomen. A positive reflex results in the retraction of the umbilicus in the direction of the quadrant stroked. Unilateral absence of the reflex suggests a lesion of an ipsilateral nerve root between T7 and L2, depending on the quadrant affected. Total absence of the reflex is seen in normal or obese patients as well as in those with upper motor neuron lesions. If a positive Babinski's reflex is present, the absence of abdominal reflexes takes on greater significance. The adductor reflex indicates L2 function. The examiner's hand is placed over the medial femoral condyle and is struck with a reflex hammer. A normal response is adduction of the leg. The cremasteric reflex is elicited in males by stroking the inner aspect of the thigh with a sharp object. Upward retraction of the scrotal sac is the normal response. Lesions of L1 or L2 result in unilateral absence of the reflex.

Sensory Testing

Gross sensory function may be surveyed by running the examiner's hands lightly over all the exposed areas on the anterior and lateral aspects of the thighs, lower legs, and feet. If the patient describes differences in sensation, a careful examination differentiating dermatomal abnormalities from peripheral nerve dysfunction must be completed, testing pinprick, light touch, and vibratory function.

In the *lateral* position, the sacroiliac joints and hip abductors are tested. Pressure is applied to the iliac wing compressing the sacroiliac joint. This test causes forward pressure on the sacroiliac joint. Pain is felt in the sacroiliac joint suggestive of an intra-articular process or a strain of the posterior sacroiliac ligaments. Hip abduction, predominantly an L5 function, is tested as the patient elevates the upper leg against downward pressure applied below the knee by the examiner. The hip should be in a neutral position, not flexed or extended. The neutral position allows for sole testing of the hip abductors. These tests are repeated on the other side in a similar fashion.

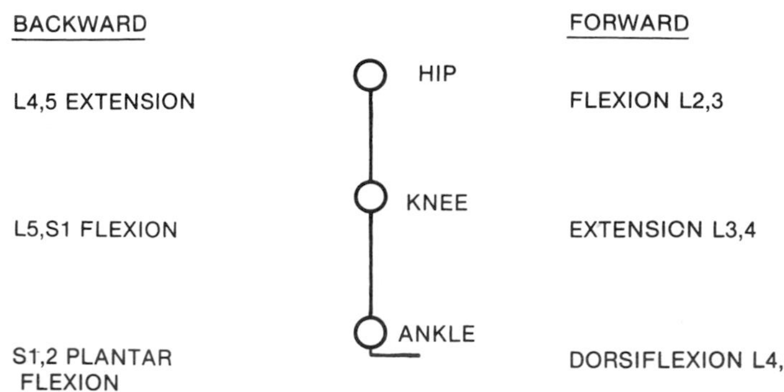

Figure 5-23 Sequential pattern of muscle innervation of the lower extremity.

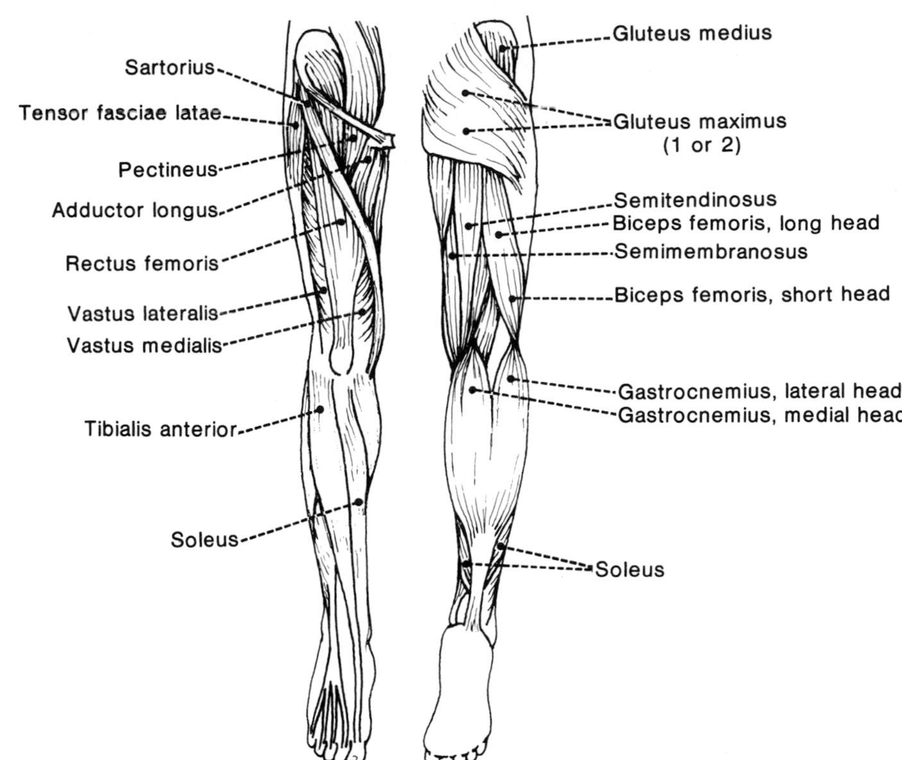

Figure 5-24 Anterior *(left)* and posterior *(right)* views of the lower extremity identifying location of motor points that become tender in association with corresponding nerve root lesions.

Femoral Stretch Test

In the *prone* position, the neurologic examination may be completed. For "high" discs (L2–L3 and L3–L4), dural irritability is checked by the femoral stretch test, which assesses irritation of the roots of the femoral nerve—L2, L3, and L4.[16] With the patient prone, the femoral nerve is stretched by bending the knee and passively elevating the thigh up from the examining table. The maneuver tethers the femoral nerve over the anterior portion of the pelvis. The test is positive if pain is reproduced in the front of the thigh (L2 and L3) or the medial aspect of the leg (L4). Pain that is localized to the back occurs secondary to the extension of the lumbosacral spine associated with extending the hip. The significance of the location of pain in the leg should not be overlooked.[25] Pain produced by leg extension, limited to an area just lateral to the midline, is frequently localized to vertebral apophyseal joints. This sign may occur in patients with early degenerative joint disease before spinal stenosis occurs.

The muscle power of the gluteus maximus (S1 root) should be tested in the prone position. The patient is asked to squeeze the buttocks tightly together while the examiner palpates the muscles to assess muscle tone. Inability to tense one side is objective evidence of a neurologic deficit. This test is another check on the patient's cooperation, since it is difficult to tighten only one buttock voluntarily. The gluteus maximus may be affected to the degree that it atrophies. The examiner observing the buttocks at the level of the feet may discover flattening that is secondary to atrophy. This is secondary to an L5, S1, or S2 inferior gluteal nerve lesion. This observation is a gluteal skyline test.[29]

The medial and lateral hamstring reflexes should be obtained. The knee is flexed and the lower leg is held by the examiner's arm. The hamstrings are supplied by L5 and S1. A loss of reflex may occur with lesions at either level. The findings from other tests (ankle reflex) may help localize the lesion.

Sensory examination of the skin over the lower legs, buttocks, and perianal area is important in determining the integrity of the upper (S1, S2) and lower (S3, S4) sacral nerve roots. The area tested is the perineum (saddle area). If saddle anesthesia is present, additional tests, including the well leg–raising test and a test of anal sphincter tone, must be completed. If results of these tests are abnormal, the patient must be evaluated for a massive central disc protrusion. These patients require immediate evaluation because expeditious operative decompression of the disc is necessary to preserve bladder and bowel continence. (Parasympathetic nerves have cell bodies in the lower part of the spinal cord and send peripheral fibers to supply the bladder and rectum through the S2, S3, and S4 roots.)

Nitta and colleagues identified the areas of sensory deficit associated with nerve blocks at three lumbar levels: L4 to S1.[41] A total of 71 patients received 86 lumbar spinal nerve blocks. Characteristic areas of numbness were noted on the medial side of the lower leg in 88% of L4 injections, on the dorsum of the first digit in 82% of L5 injections, and on the lateral aspect of the fifth digit in 83% of S1 injections. A continuous band of numbness was noted in the upper thigh and buttock in 42% of L4, 44% of L5, and 92% of S1 injections. This study demonstrates that L4 and L5 lesions may be associated with buttock and thigh dysesthesias.

The final part of the evaluation is the genital and rectal examination. In men, the testicles should be palpated for any nodules or masses. Men and women patients are placed on their side. The gloved finger is well lubricated and inserted into the rectum with gentle but persistent pressure. Rectal tone is determined by the pressure exerted on the inserted finger. The circumference of the rectum should be palpated. In men, the prostate is felt on the anterior wall of the rectum. A hard prostate suggests the presence of a malignancy. In women, the vagina is contiguous to the anterior wall of the rectum. The presence of firm nonfixed nodules suggests the presence of endometriosis. The examining finger should then move around the rectum, palpating the pelvic musculature. Increased tension, manifested by firmness in the palpated muscles (piriformis, coccygeus), may be determined. Finally, the coccyx and sacrum are palpated (Fig. 5-25). External pressure from the thumb on the sacrum tests for any abnormal motion in this portion of the spine. Sacral masses are palpated anterior to the sacrum through the posterior wall of the rectum. These masses will not be palpated unless the rectal examination is done. If the clinical history suggests a gynecologic source for back pain in a female patient, a complete pelvic examination is indicated. The examiner should palpate the uterus, cervix, and ovaries for any masses or adhesions associated with neoplastic or inflammatory lesions.

Commonly Used Low Back Tests

There are a number of other tests that may be added to the physical examination just described. For the most part these are just variations of tests previously described, but they need to be presented since they are commonly used to confirm positive test findings.

Schober's Test. The Schober's test (Fig. 5-26) measures the amount of flexion in the lumbar spine. Patients with spondyloarthropathies have decreased lumbar flexion and abnormal Schober's tests. A point between the sacroiliac dimples is marked along with another mark 10 cm above the lower one. The patient is asked to bend forward and the increased distance is measured. Patients with normal lumbar flexion increase the distance 4 to 5 cm. Patients with limited flexion have distances less than 4 cm. The validity of this test has recently been questioned.[24] The test may not accurately measure lumbar flexion. The test is also nonspecific, being positive in chronic back pain, spondyloarthropathies, and spinal tumors.[43] However, in another study, the modified Schober's test was the most repeatable test of four tests assessing lumbar spinal motion.[21]

Contralateral or Well Leg, Straight Leg–Raising Test (Fajersztajn's Test). This test (Fig. 5-27) is positive when pain is reproduced in the involved leg below the knee as the straight leg–raising test is performed on the opposite or uninvolved side.[26,27,51] This test is quite specific and sensitive to pressure on the nerve root; when positive, surgery is usually indicated to relieve the pain.

Voluntary Release. This test is used to differentiate the patient with true organic nerve damage from the one with an extensive emotional overlay. On attempting a sustained muscle contraction, such as dorsiflexion of the ankle, the patient with a functional problem holds up the ankle with intermittent quivering, breaking, contraction, and release in a jerky manner as opposed to the smooth release seen in a patient with an organic disorder. When this occurs, it is strongly suggestive of nonorganic pathology.

Bow String Sign (Cram's Test). The patient is seated with the knee flexed 70 degrees and the body bent forward so as to lengthen the course of the sciatic nerve. The examiner's finger is then pressed into the popliteal space to increase tension on the nerve. A positive test occurs when pain is increased down the leg and suggests the presence of a radiculopathy.[12]

Naffziger's Test. This test is done by compressing the jugular veins in the neck for approximately 10 seconds until the patient's face begins to flush. The patient is then asked to cough to increase the intrathecal pressure; sciatic pain will be aggravated if there is dural sensitivity.

Valsalva's Test. This test increases intrathecal pressure when patients are asked to bear down like they are trying to move the bowels. Sciatic pain occurs in the presence

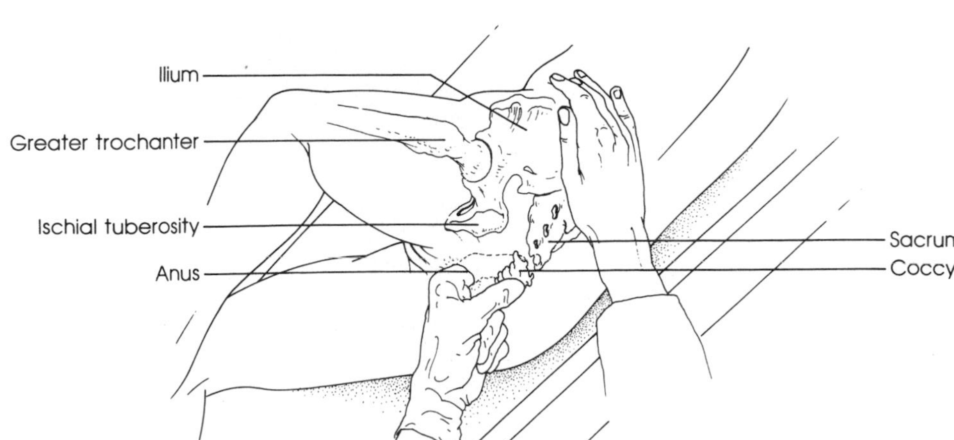

Figure 5-25 Palpation of the coccyx. *(From Magee DJ: Orthopedic Physical Assessment. Philadelphia, WB Saunders, 1987, p 199.)*

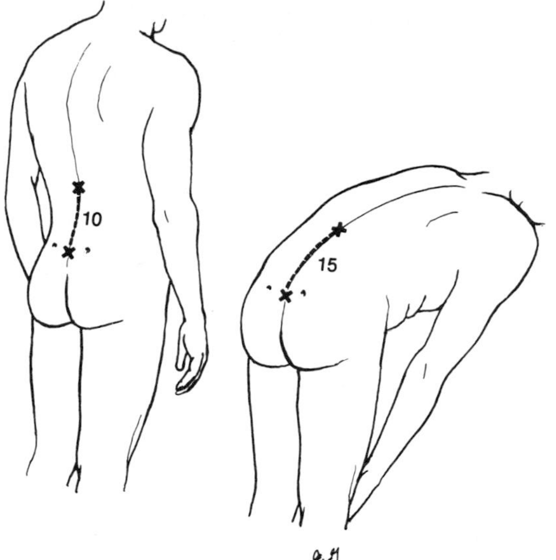

Figure 5-26 Schober's test measuring forward flexion of the lumbar spine. Normal expansion is 5 cm. This test is used in patients with spondyloarthropathies to monitor response to therapy.

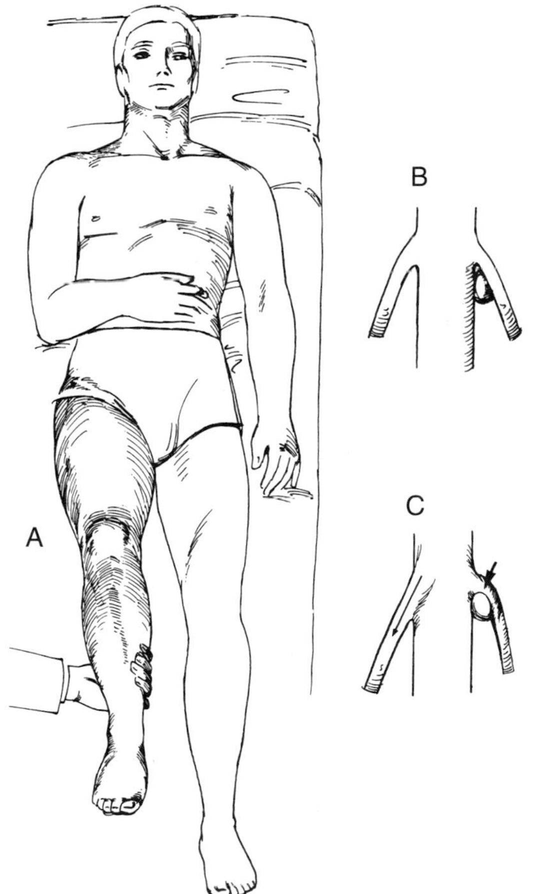

Figure 5-27 Contralateral or well-leg test of Fajersztajn. Movement of nerve roots when the leg on the contralateral side is raised: When the leg is raised on the unaffected side *(A)*, the roots on the opposite side slide downward and toward the midline *(B)*. In the presence of a medial disc herniation, this movement increases nerve root tension *(C)*. *(Modified from DePalma AF, Rothman RH: The Intervertebral Disc. Philadelphia, WB Saunders, 1970.)*

of dural irritation. Coughing and sneezing also raise intra-abdominal pressure and can be used as a modification of this test since leg pain will be produced in the same way.

Brudzinski/Kernig Test. With the patient lying supine, the head is passively flexed down on the chest. A positive test is reproduction of the patient's leg pain. The occurrence of neck pain is not significant. A positive Kernig's test occurs when supine patients extend their knee on a hip that is flexed at 90 degrees and develop back pain. Pain is secondary to meningeal nerve root or dural irritation.[10,30]

Milgram's Test. This is a further modification of the tension test. While in the supine position, the patient is asked to raise both extended legs about 1 to 3 inches from the examining table. This is another way to increase intra-abdominal pressure and thus intrathecal pressure. The patient is asked to hold the position for 30 seconds. The test is considered positive if the maneuver creates leg pain. Just as in the straight leg–raising test, however, a complaint of back pain does not make it significant.

Hoover's Test. This test checks the validity of a patient's attempt to raise one leg off the examining table. Normally as patients attempt to raise one outstretched leg, they must simultaneously press down with the opposite leg. Thus the downward pressure of the normal leg is a good indication of how hard they are trying. The examiner can check the sincerity of the effort by keeping a hand under the foot.[2]

Kneeling Bench Test. The patient, kneeling on a 12-inch-high bench, is asked to bend forward and touch the floor. Flexion at the hips is the only requisite to accomplish this. If the hips are normal and the fingers do not reach the floor, nonorganic back pain must be suspected.

Stoop Test. This test evaluates the association of intermittent claudication of neurogenic origin with exercise and position.[17] The patient is asked to walk briskly for 1 to 2 minutes. When back, posterior thigh, and lower limb pain appear, the patient sits and flexes forward. A positive test occurs if the pain is relieved with flexion. Reflexes may be absent during a period of neurogenic claudication. The reflexes must be examined expeditiously, since recovery of reflex function corresponds with the relief of pain, which may occur within 3 to 4 minutes.[28]

Oppenheim's Test. This test is used to detect upper motor neuron lesions. A dull object is run down the anterior portion of the tibia. A positive response is similar to that of Babinski's test, with extension of the big toe and splaying of the other toes. A positive test is secondary to an upper motor neuron lesion.

FUNCTIONAL DISORDERS

In some cases, objective findings associated with the neck problem do not match the subjective complaints. This is especially true in cases associated with psychogenic rheumatism, compensation, and litigation. These cases are termed *functional*, which is used medically in contradistinction to organic. For these functional cases, there is usually a psychological component as well as secondary gain involved.

Accentuation of symptoms for greater effect may be a sign of a patient with psychogenic difficulties. Lurching from one piece of office furniture to another, behavior associated with sudden paroxysms of twitching and pain in the cervical spine, is unusual for a patient with organic neck disease. Abrupt onset of total inability to move the head in any direction is suggestive of a psychogenic origin for neck dysfunction.[4]

To evaluate patients with these functional disorders, a list of physical signs was developed by Waddell and colleagues.[50] This provides a simple, rapid screen to help identify the few patients who require more detailed investigation. These signs were originally developed for patients with low back problems, and many of them are applicable to the cervical spine. Any of the individual signs count as one if positive. A finding of three or more of the five types is clinically significant. Isolated positive signs are ignored (Fig. 5-28).

1. Tenderness—when related to physical disease, tenderness is usually localized to a particular skeletal or neuromuscular structure. Nonorganic tenderness is nonspecific and diffuse.
   a. Superficial—the skin is tender to light pinch over a wide area of cervical skin.
   b. Nonanatomic—deep tenderness is felt over a wide area and is not localized to one structure; it often extends to the arms, thoracic spine, and lumbar spine.
2. Simulation tests—these tests should not be uncomfortable; if pain is reported, a nonorganic influence is suggested.
   a. There is a complaint of thoracic or low back pain with vertical pressure on the skull of a patient who is standing. This is least applicable to the cervical spine because intrinsic neck pathologic changes may in fact be exacerbated by axial loading. However, this should not cause pain in the low back in a patient with a cervical complaint.
   b. Rotation—neck or back pain should not be reported when the shoulders and pelvis are passively rotated in the same plane.
3. Distraction tests—first, a positive finding is demonstrated in the usual manner; next, this finding is rechecked while the patient's attention is distracted. Findings that are present only on formal examination

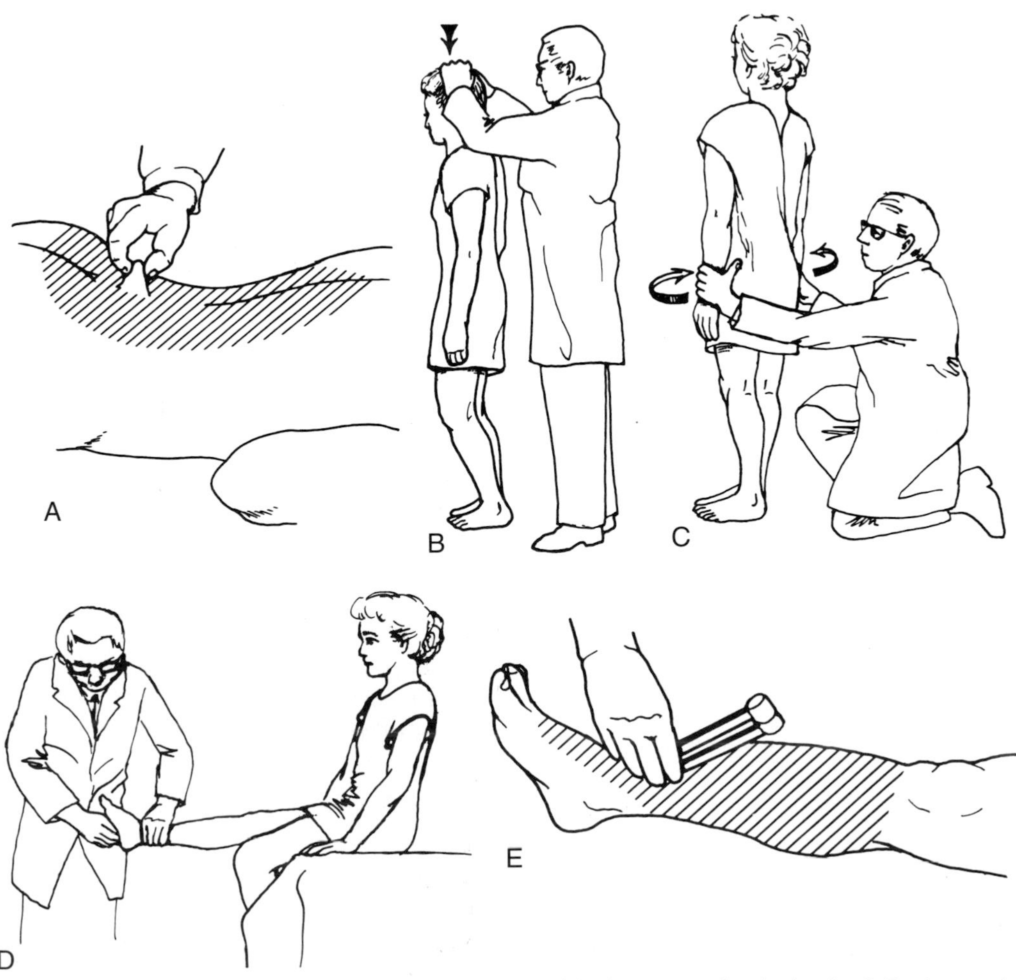

Figure 5-28 Waddell's tests. *A*, Superficial sensitivity to light pinch. *B*, Axial loading causing low back pain. *C*, Passive rotation of the shoulders and pelvis in the same plane causing back pain. *D*, Straight leg–raising test in the seated position. Stroking the skin on the bottom of the foot distracts the patient. *E*, Stocking distribution of sensory deficit.

and disappear at other times are considered positive. For example, the patient may describe an inability to use the hands because of muscular weakness but is able to lift off the examination table with the use of the wrists. Another example of a distraction test is the consistency of numbness in the forearm in the supinated and pronated positions.

4. Regional disturbances—findings that involve divergence from accepted neural anatomy.
   a. Weakness—nonanatomic (voluntary release) or unexplained (giving way) of muscle groups in the arms. Simultaneous strength testing of the hands may demonstrate equal strength (weak or strong) after finding weakness in one hand when tested one at a time. In true weakness, an antagonist muscle (triceps) should be relaxed when testing a weak agonist muscle (biceps). The tense antagonist muscle can be palpated while testing the weak agonist muscle.
   b. Sensory—sensory abnormalities fit a stocking rather than a dermatomal pattern.
5. Overreaction—this may take the form of disproportionate verbalization, jumping, cringing, excessive facial expression, and so on. Judgment should, however, be made with caution, because it is easy to introduce observer bias.

The preceding standardized group of nonorganic physical signs is easily learned and can be incorporated unobtrusively to add less than 1 minute to the routine physical examination. These tests are important, and when three are positive, the findings should be followed up.

Positive Waddell's signs do not always predict individuals who will be resistant to treatment. In the appropriate rehabilitation setting, individuals with functional signs can improve. Waddell's signs are useful in identifying those individuals with a component of psychosomatic disease.[42]

A distraction test may also be used for patients with a rigid neck.[34] The patient's range of motion is observed during the initial part of the examination. During the portion of the examination with the patient prone, a pillow is removed from under the patient's head. The head should have limited motion. Later in the examination with the patient supine, the pillow is replaced under the head. The range of motion should be noted.

Reproducibility of Physical Signs

Compared with physical signs in other fields of medicine, the physical findings associated with the examination of the lumbosacral spine are poorly defined in regard to performance and measurement.[14] The lack of definition makes it difficult for physicians to reproduce an abnormal physical finding in patients over time. Another concern is the reliability of physical signs to identify normal function and the presence of pathology.[49]

McCombe and associates evaluated the reproducibility between observers of 54 physical signs used in the evaluation of low back pain.[37] Three health professionals examined 83 back pain patients for specifically defined abnormalities of pain pattern, posture, movement, tenderness, sacroiliac and piriformis dysfunction, root tension signs, root compression signs, and inappropriate signs. Reliable signs consisted of measurements of lordosis, flexion range, determination of pain location on flexion and lateral bend, measurements associated with straight leg–raising test, determination of pain location in the thighs and legs, and sensory changes in the legs. Describing the location of pain increased the reliability of nerve root tension signs. Reproducibility of bone tenderness over the sacroiliac joint, spinous processes, and iliac crest was greater than that associated with soft tissue structures. Measurement of movement with a tape is a worthwhile way of reproducing results. Constant re-examination is needed to correlate the validity and reproducibility of physical findings with other components of patient evaluation for low back pain.

SUMMARY

With conclusion of the history and physical examination, the examining physician should have the answers to important questions concerning prior surgery, pre-existing injuries, the presence of malignancy or systemic illness, the presence of a nerve root irritation, and the possibility of a patient's being a malingerer. The physician should gather these facts and construct a list of diseases for the differential diagnosis. The diagnosis of neck or back pain of undetermined etiology is inadequate. Patients may have muscle strain, facet joint disease, discogenic disease with or without nerve root irritation, or systemic illness. In patients with mechanical abnormalities, no additional evaluation is necessary with the initial visit. Other patients with systemic symptoms and signs may require additional evaluation. Appropriate laboratory evaluation is useful in differentiating part of the myriad of systemic illnesses associated with neck or back pain. Laboratory evaluation is the subject of Chapter 6.

References

1. Anonymous: A neurovascular syndrome—the subclavian steal [Editorial]. N Engl J Med 264:912, 1961.
2. Archibald KC, Wiechec F: A reappraisal of Hoover's test. Arch Phys Med Rehabil 51:234-238, 1970.
3. Beatty RM, Fowler FD, Hanson EJ Jr: The abducted arm as a sign of ruptured cervical disc. Neurosurgery 21:731-732, 1987.
4. Bland JH: Clinical methods. In Bland JH (ed): Disorders of the Cervical Spine: Diagnosis and Medical Management, 2nd ed. Philadelphia, WB Saunders, 1994, pp 113-146.
5. Blower PW: Neurologic patterns in unilateral sciatica: A prospective study of 100 new cases. Spine 6:175-179, 1981.
6. Blower PW, Griffin AJ: Clinical sacroiliac tests in ankylosing spondylitis and other causes of low back pain: Two studies. Ann Rheum Dis 43:192-195, 1984.
7. Bowditch MG, Sanderson P, Livesey JP: The significance of an absent ankle reflex. J Bone Joint Surg Br 78:276-279, 1996.
8. Bradford FK, Spurling RG: The Intervertebral Disc: With Special Reference to Rupture of the Annulus Fibrosus with Herniation of the Nucleus Pulposus, 2nd ed. Springfield, IL, Charles C Thomas, 1945.
9. Brody IA, Wilkins RH: Lhermitte's sign. Arch Neurol 21:338-340, 1969.
10. Brudzinski J: A new sign of the lower extremities in meningitis of children (neck sign). Arch Neurol 21:217, 1969.
11. Castro WH, Sautmann A, Schilgen M, Sautmann M: Noninvasive three-dimensional analysis of cervical spine motion in normal subjects in relation to age and sex: An experimental examination. Spine 25:443-449, 2000.

12. Cram RH: A sign of sciatic nerve root pressure. J Bone Joint Surg Br 35:192, 1953.
13. Deville WL, van der Windt DA, Dzaferagic A, et al: The test of Lasegue: Systematic review of the accuracy in diagnosing herniated discs. Spine 25:1140-1147, 2000.
14. Deyo RA: Measuring the functional status of patients with low back pain. Arch Phys Med Rehabil 69:1044-1053, 1988.
15. Dreyfuss P, Michaelsen M, Pauza K, et al: The value of medical history and physical examination in diagnosing sacroiliac joint pain. Spine 21:2594-2602, 1996.
16. Dyck P: The femoral nerve traction test with lumbar disc protrusions. Surg Neurol 6:163-166, 1976.
17. Dyck P: The stoop-test in lumbar entrapment radiculopathy. Spine 4:89-92, 1979.
18. Ensink FB, Saur PM, Frese K, et al: Lumbar range of motion: Influence of time of day and individual factors on measurements. Spine 21:1339-1343, 1996.
19. Fahrni WH: Observations on straight-leg raising with special reference to nerve root adhesions. Can J Surg 9:44, 1966.
20. Finneson BE: Examination of the patient. In Finneson BE (ed): Low Back Pain, 2nd ed. Philadelphia, JB Lippincott, 1980, p 54.
21. Gill K, Krag MH, Johnson GB, et al: Repeatability of four clinical methods for assessment of lumbar spinal motion. Spine 13:50-53, 1988.
22. Gunn CC, Milbrandt WE: Tenderness at motor points: A diagnostic and prognostic aid for low back injury. J Bone Joint Surg Am 58:815-825, 1976.
23. Hall H: Examination of the patient with low back pain. Bull Rheum Dis 33:1-8, 1983.
24. Hendler N, Viernstein M, Gucer P, Long D: A preoperative screening test for chronic back pain patients. Psychosomatics 20:801-808, 1979.
25. Herron LD, Pheasant HC: Prone knee-flexion provocative testing for lumbar disc protrusion. Spine 5:65-67, 1980.
26. Hudgins WR: The cross-straight-leg–raising test. N Engl J Med 297:1127, 1977.
27. Hudgins WR: The crossed straight leg–raising test: A diagnostic sign of herniated disc. J Occup Med 21:407-408, 1979.
28. Joffe R, Appleby A, Arjona V: "Intermittent ischaemia" of the cauda equina due to stenosis of the lumbar canal. J Neurol Neurosurg Psychiatry 29:315-318, 1966.
29. Katznelson A, Nerubay J, Lev-El A: Gluteal skyline (GSL): A search for an objective sign in the diagnosis of disc lesions of the lower lumbar spine. Spine 7:74-75, 1982.
30. Kernig W: Concerning a little noted sign of meningitis. Arch Neurol 21:207, 1969.
31. Kosteljanetz M, Espersen JO, Halaburt H, Miletic T: Predictive value of clinical and surgical findings in patients with lumbago-sciatica: A prospective study. I. Acta Neurochir (Wien) 73:67-76, 1984.
32. Krishnan KR, France RD, Pelton S, et al: Chronic pain and depression. I. Classification of depression in chronic low back pain patients. Pain 22:279-287, 1985.
33. Kuiper DH, Papp JP: Supraclavicular adenopathy demonstrated by the Valsalva maneuver. N Engl J Med 280:1007-1008, 1969.
34. Macnab I, McCulloch JA: Back Ache and Shoulder Pain. Baltimore, Williams & Wilkins, 1994, pp 121-139.
35. Malko JA, Hutton WC, Fajman WA: An in vivo magnetic resonance imaging study of changes in the volume (and fluid content) of the lumbar intervertebral discs during a simulated diurnal load cycle. Spine 24:1015-1022, 1999.
36. Mayer TG, Tencer AF, Kristoferson S, Mooney V: Use of noninvasive techniques for quantification of spinal range of motion in normal subjects and chronic low back dysfunction patients. Spine 9:588-595, 1984.
37. McCombe PF, Fairbank JC, Cockersole BC, Pynsent PB: 1989 Volvo Award in clinical sciences: Reproducibility of physical signs in low back pain. Spine 14:908-918, 1989.
38. McKenzie RA: Prophylaxis in recurrent low back pain. N Z Med J 89:22-23, 1979.
39. Moll JM, Wright V: Normal range of spinal mobility: An objective clinical study. Ann Rheum Dis 30:381-386, 1971.
40. Nehemkis AM, Carver DW, Evanski PM: The predictive utility of the orthopedic examination in identifying the low back pain patient with hysterical personality features. Clin Orthop 145:158-162, 1979.
41. Nitta H, Tajima T, Sugiyama H, Moriyama A: Study on dermatomes by means of selective lumbar spinal nerve block. Spine 18:1782-1786, 1993.
42. Polatin PB, Cox B, Gatchel RJ, Mayer TG: A prospective study of Waddell signs in patients with chronic low back pain: When they may not be predictive. Spine 22:1618-1621, 1997.
43. Rae PS, Waddell G, Venner RM: A simple technique for measuring lumbar spinal flexion: Its use in orthopaedic practice. J R Coll Surg Edinb 29:281-284, 1984.
44. Sharp J: Spontaneous atlantoaxial dislocation in ankylosing spondylitis and rheumatoid arthritis. Ann Rheum Dis 20:47, 1961.
45. Spengler DM, Freeman CW: Patient selection for lumbar discectomy: An objective approach. Spine 4:129-134, 1979.
46. Sung RD, Wang JC: Correlation between a positive Hoffmann's reflex and cervical pathology in asymptomatic individuals. Spine 26:67-70, 2001.
47. Tong HC, Haig AJ, Yamakawa K: The Spurling test and cervical radiculopathy. Spine 27:156-159, 2002.
48. Tousignant M, de Bellefeuille L, O'Donoughue S, Grahovac S: Criterion validity of the cervical range of motion (CROM) goniometer for cervical flexion and extension. Spine 25:324-330, 2000.
49. Waddell G, Main CJ, Morris EW, et al: Normality and reliability in the clinical assessment of backache. BMJ 284:1519-1523, 1982.
50. Waddell G, McCulloch JA, Kummel E, Venner RM: Nonorganic physical signs in low back pain. Spine 5:117-125, 1980.
51. Woodhall R, Hayes GJ: The well leg–raising test of Fajersztajn in the diagnosis of ruptured lumbar intervertebral disc. J Bone Joint Surg Am 32:786, 1950.
52. Xin SQ, Zhang QZ, Fan DH: Significance of the straight leg–raising test in the diagnosis and clinical evaluation of lower lumbar intervertebral disc protrusion. J Bone Joint Surg Am 69:517-522, 1987.

CHAPTER 6

LABORATORY TESTS

The availability and expense of an ever-expanding variety of laboratory tests have complicated the professional life of the practicing physician. In the period when the laboratory evaluation was limited to blood counts, urinalysis, sedimentation rates, and serum chemistries, the physician obtained basic information about a patient for an inexpensive price. The present state of affairs is quite different. The number of available tests has grown at a great rate without a corresponding increase in diagnostic accuracy but with an appreciable increment in cost. In fact, the results of tests done at an inappropriate time or interpreted incorrectly may only confuse the physician and may hide the true diagnosis. For example, a patient with cryoglobulinemia secondary to multiple myeloma has an inappropriately "normal" erythrocyte sedimentation rate. Therefore, laboratory tests should be used in the situation in which a physician has developed a differential diagnosis by means of a history and physical examination for which laboratory data are needed to confirm or reject specific diagnoses.

In general, laboratory tests play a minor role in the diagnosis of spinal pain. They do have a role in separating mechanical from systemic diseases. They are also useful in distinguishing metabolic-endocrinologic disorders from those with more inflammatory characteristics. In rare circumstances, laboratory tests are required on an emergent basis to diagnose rapidly progressive disorders with life-threatening consequences. For example, in the evaluation of neck pain, laboratory tests are required for the expeditious diagnosis of meningitis.

The vast majority of individuals with spinal pain do not require laboratory studies with their initial evaluation. This is particularly true of a patient with a history of acute onset of back or neck pain related to physical activity. These patients may be given therapy for their pain without additional tests. They are candidates for laboratory evaluation if they fail to respond to medical therapy or develop a significant change in the character of their pain. The threshold for obtaining a laboratory evaluation at an initial visit is lowered for new-onset spinal pain in an elderly individual. Since medical etiologies (infections and tumors) for spinal pain occur commonly in older individuals, evaluation for systemic pathologic problems should be pursued earlier in the diagnostic process in this group. Occasionally, younger individuals present with severe systemic symptoms (fever, chills, and eye inflammation) that strongly suggest a local (infection) or systemic (spondyloarthropathy) inflammatory process as the source of their spinal pain. Laboratory evaluation during the initial evaluation may help confirm the inflammatory nature of their disease. Laboratory tests that are important in the study of disorders associated with spinal pain include acute-phase reactants, complete blood counts, blood chemistries, urinalysis, immunologic studies (cellular and humoral), body fluid analysis, cultures, and tissue biopsy. (For laboratory abnormalities associated with specific illnesses, refer to the relevant chapter and the appropriate listing in the Appendix.)

No specific consensus exists concerning the appropriate sequences or array of tests to obtain in the evaluation of a patient with spinal pain. Physicians from different specialties order tests with which they are familiar. However, these tests may not necessarily be appropriate for the evaluation. Cherkin and associates conducted a physician questionnaire regarding hypothetical patients with back pain.[4] The use of laboratory and radiographic tests were compared with guidelines suggested in the scientific literature. Rheumatologists ordered laboratory test twice as often as surgeons, neurologists, or physiatrists. These tests included "arthritis profiles," histocompatibility tests, and serum electrophoresis. The other physician groups ordered radiographic or electrophysiologic tests too early in the diagnostic evaluation. Physicians need to temper their enthusiasm for diagnostic tests too early in the course of pain that add no additional information to the evaluation of a spinal pain patient.

ACUTE-PHASE REACTANTS

Acute-phase reactants are a group of plasma proteins that increase or decrease by at least 25% during an inflammatory disorder (Table 6-1).[9] The magnitude of the elevation varies from 50% with ceruloplasmin to 1000-fold with C-reactive protein and serum amyloid A. The degree of increase is greatest with cancer, severe infections, vasculitis, and burns. Moderate changes occur with pregnancy, whereas small increases are associated with psychiatric illnesses.

The pattern of increases varies with different pathophysiologic states, corresponding to the cytokines induced with a specific disorder. Cytokines are intercellular signaling proteins produced by stimulated cells.[1] Cytokines stimulate the production of the wide array of acute-phase reactants. Many of these cytokines have a spectrum of biologic activities that overlap. An immune

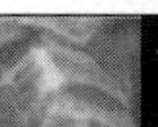

6-1 ACUTE-PHASE REACTANTS

INCREASED LEVELS

Complement System

C3, C4, C9
C1 inhibitor

Antiproteases

Alpha$_1$-protease inhibitor
Alpha$_1$-antichymotrypsin

Inflammatory Proteins

Phospholipase A_2
Lipopolysaccharide-binding protein
Interleukin-1 receptor antagonist
Granulocyte colony–stimulating factor

Coagulation and Fibrinolytic System

Fibrinogen
Plasminogen
Tissue plasminogen activator

Transport Proteins

Ceruloplasmin
Haptoglobin

Miscellaneous

C-reactive protein
Serum amyloid A
Alpha$_1$-acid glycoprotein
Fibronectin
Ferritin
Angiotensinogen

DECREASED LEVELS

Albumin
Transferrin
Alpha-fetoprotein
Thyroxine-binding globulin
Insulin-like growth factor-1

Modified from Gabay C, Kushner I: Acute-phase proteins and other systemic responses to inflammation. N Engl J Med 340:448-454, 1999.

cell interacts with a number of cytokines with a similar effect. The cytokines associated with the stimulation and inhibition of acute-phase reactants are listed in Table 6-2. Inflammatory process involves many different cell types and molecules; some initiate, amplify, or sustain inflammation, whereas others downregulate and resolve the process.[9] Current therapies for immune-mediated disorders (rheumatoid arthritis, spondyloarthropathies) are directed at the inhibition of these factors. However, from a diagnostic or therapeutic orientation, the measurement of inflammatory cytokines does not help identify specific disorders. The short plasma half-lives and the presence of blocking factors make quantification difficult. The lack of standardization, limited availability, and high cost deprive these tests of any advantage over more accessible and less expensive tests.

Erythrocyte Sedimentation Rate

The most useful test in helping to differentiate medical from mechanical spinal pain is the erythrocyte sedimentation rate (ESR). The ESR mirrors the state of activity of the acute-phase response. The acute-phase response is a reaction by the body to tissue injury. With tissue necrosis, a systemic response is initiated that results in the increase in concentration of glycoproteins of hepatic origin that affect complement and coagulation cascades. The acute-phase response has a beneficial effect of limiting the spread of tissue damage and facilitating wound healing. The increased concentration of plasma proteins causes an increased aggregation of erythrocytes, which forms stacks of discs (rouleaux). With rouleaux formation, erythrocyte mass is increased in relationship to cell surface area, resulting in an increased rate of fall of the cells.

6-2 ACUTE-PHASE CYTOKINES

Cytokine	Action
Interleukin-1-alpha/beta	Prostaglandin production Enhanced adhesion molecule expression Collagenase stimulation Stimulates B-cell proliferation Synergistic activation of natural killer cells with other cytokines
Interleukin-6	Major stimulator of hepatocyte-generated acute-phase reactants Induces growth and differentiation of T and B lymphocytes Enhanced immune globulin production
Interleukin-8	Chemotactic for neutrophils and T cells Enhanced adhesion molecule expression Oxygen radical production Release of lysosomal enzymes
Tumor necrosis factor-alpha/beta	Enhances gene expression of cytokines, transcription factors, receptors, and hepatocyte-generated acute-phase reactants Prostaglandin production Collagenase stimulation
Interferon-gamma	Activates macrophages and neutrophils Increases histocompatibility molecule expression
Transforming growth factor-beta	Chemotactic for monocytes Inhibits B cells, T cells, natural killer cells

The test is done by collecting blood from a patient and placing it in a specialized tube. The decrease in height of the column of erythrocytes is measured for 1 hour. The Wintrobe's method uses a tube 100 mm long and cannot measure ESR values greater than the patient's hematocrit.[47] The Wintrobe's method is most useful for mild elevations of ESR and may be more sensitive than the Westergren's method for minimal elevations.[26] The Westergren's method is the standard method for measuring ESR and involves diluting blood and using a tube that has a measuring length of 200 mm.[14] This method allows for the fall of erythrocytes to a distance greater than the packed height of the red blood cells (RBCs). Greater ESRs are more accurately determined by the Westergren's method.

In general, an elevated ESR suggests the presence of inflammation in the body. The ESR is elevated with tissue injury, whatever the source (Table 6-3). The ESR is used to screen for inflammatory diseases and to follow the response to therapy. For example, the spondyloarthropathies (ankylosing spondylitis and reactive arthritis) produce an elevation of the ESR. The ESR is normal in mechanical spinal pain (paraspinous muscle strain and osteoarthritis).

The ESR value must be interpreted according to the sex and age of the patient. The Westergren upper limits of normal are 15 mm/hr for men younger than 50 years of age and 20 mm/hr for men older than 50 years of age. The normal range is greater for women. The upper limit is 25 mm/hr to 50 years of age and up to 30 mm/hr after 50 years. The upper limit continues to rise as patients grow older. In patients older than 70 years of age, an ESR of 50 mm/hr or higher may be normal.[12] The change in ESR may be more important than the absolute value when a patient is evaluated by a clinician. A 70-year-old patient who had a Westergren ESR of 10 mm/hr who now has an ESR of 48 mm/hr is worthy of additional evaluation despite the ESR value being in the normal range.

ESR may be "falsely" normal with any process that alters RBC morphology, inhibiting rouleaux formation and slowing the rate of fall of erythrocytes despite the presence of increased concentrations of acute-phase reactants. Sickle cell anemia is associated with a normal ESR despite extensive tissue injury.

Markedly elevated ESR (≥100 mm/hr) is most commonly associated with malignancies, particularly those that are metastatic.[48] Other diseases associated with markedly increased ESR include connective tissue disease (polymyalgia rheumatica–temporal arteritis), acute bacterial infection (meningitis), and vertebral osteomyelitis with epidural abscess.

The ESR is the most valuable screening test for the detection of medical spinal pathologic conditions. In one series, an ESR of greater than 25 mm/hr had a false-positive rate of only 6%.[42]

The ESR also has utility as a means of following the progression or resolution of an inflammatory disorder. For example, in the setting of polymyalgia rheumatica, a decrease in ESR corresponds to an improvement in this inflammatory disorder. An increase in the ESR after a decrease toward normal suggests a change in the inflammatory state of the patient. For example, an increase in ESR during the healing phase of a surgical procedure suggests the presence of a postsurgical infection.[36]

The test has a number of flaws.[2] ESR is seldom the sole clue to systemic disease and is not a useful tool in asymptomatic individuals.[34] The ESR may be normal in patients with systemic diseases, including cancer. RBC morphology, a factor independent of the concentration of acute-phase reactants, influences the rate of cell sedimentation. ESR is an indirect measure of the concentration of acute-phase reactants. The activity of an illness is not always mirrored in the rise or fall of the ESR.[20] ESR may remain elevated for up to 3 to 5 weeks after spinal surgery, in the absence of infection.

Despite its shortcomings, ESR remains the most cost-efficient test for screening for systemic illness in patients with spinal pain. The continued use of the test is based on its availability in a wide variety of office and hospital laboratories, its simplicity, and the broad experience with test results in a multitude of medical conditions.

6-3 CONDITIONS ASSOCIATED WITH ELEVATED ERYTHROCYTE SEDIMENTATION RATE

RHEUMATIC DISEASES
Spondyloarthropathies
Rheumatoid arthritis
Rheumatic fever
Polymyalgia rheumatica
Systemic lupus erythematosus

MALIGNANT DISEASES
Multiple myeloma
Solid tumors (colon, breast)
Metastases

GASTROINTESTINAL DISEASES
Cholecystitis
Peptic ulcer disease
Inflammatory bowel disease

ACUTE INFECTIONS
Bacterial, including endocarditis and pyelonephritis
Lyme disease
Tuberculosis
Meningitis
Discitis
Vertebral osteomyelitis

TISSUE NECROSIS
Surgery
Myocardial infarction

MISCELLANEOUS
Endocrinopathies
Pregnancy
Vaccinations
Sarcoidosis

C-Reactive Protein

C-reactive protein (CRP) is an acute-phase protein synthesized by hepatocytes first described in 1930.[38] CRP is one of a variety of factors that are increased and decreased during an inflammatory response (see Table 6-1). CRP was named for its property of precipitating the somatic C-polysaccharide of the *Pneumococcus*. The protein is an aggregate of five identical subunits that are arranged in a planar, cyclic pentagon.[2] CRP may recognize inflammatory tissue damage by binding to phosphocholine, a cell membrane–based compound. Phosphocholine is part of endogenous damaged tissues and exogenous tissues, such as bacteria. The exact function of CRP in acute-phase response is not known. CRP does activate complement and interacts with phagocytic cells. CRP modulates neutrophils, suppressing superoxide production and degranulation and reducing phosphorylation of intracellular proteins. CRP also interacts with monocytes, platelets, and lymphocytes.

Levels of CRP in normal adult humans is less than 0.2 mg/dL, or 2 mg/L. Slight variations occur with minor injuries. Concentrations of less than 1 mg/dL are regarded as normal or insignificant elevations. Concentrations between 1 and 10 mg/dL are moderate increases and those higher than 10 mg/dL are marked increases. CRP increases within hours of an inflammatory stimulus. CRP usually reaches a peak in 2 to 3 days and then recedes in 3 to 4 days. CRP may remain elevated in chronic inflammatory states such as rheumatoid arthritis and tuberculosis. CRP may also be reported as high sensitivity in cardiac assays. The results are reported in milligrams per liter. Increases in risk for stroke and myocardial infarction start at levels of 0.56 to 1.14 mg/L. These are levels thought to be normal for other inflammatory conditions.

A study by Wener and co-workers reported the effects of age, sex, and race on the upper reference limits for CRP.[44] CRP are thought to be unaffected by age, sex, or race. This study reports higher levels of CRP as individuals age, independent of their inflammatory state. They suggest the upper limit of normal to be 0.95 mg/dL for men and 1.39 mg/dL for women. For ages 25 to 70 years, the age-adjusted upper reference limit (milligrams per deciliter) was CRP = age/50 for men and CRP = age/50 + 0.6 for women. Non-Hispanic black adults have an upper limit of normal of CRP = age/30 for men and CRP = age/50 + 1.0 for women. This study was based on results from 22,000 individuals. Higher reference levels should be considered in individuals as they age. Visser and associates demonstrated elevated CRP levels in obese individuals, even those aged 17 to 39 years.[41] Those individuals who are obese had an odds ratio of 2.13 for men and 6.21 for women for an elevated CRP. Elevated levels were those greater than 0.22 mg/dL. The source for this elevated CRP may be interleukin-6 that is expressed by human adipose tissue.

CRP levels have been slightly elevated within the normal range in individuals who subsequently developed angina and coronary artery events.[30] The CRP levels in these individuals was 1.51 mg/L. Some laboratories are reporting CRP results with a high sensitivity when used for cardiac patients. Levels of CRP reported in patients with rheumatoid arthritis are 10 times higher. Confusion can exist with the degree of CRP elevation if the absolute concentration is not designated. What remains to be determined is whether elevated CRP is merely a marker for arteriosclerosis or is directly involved with the development of plaques.[18]

CRP may be measured to levels as low as 0.2 mg/dL by a number of methods, including laser nephelometry, enzyme immunoassay, radial immunodiffusion, and radioimmunoassay. Latex agglutination, a test that was the measurement standard in the past, is not adequately sensitive to be currently useful in the clinical setting. CRP is more accurate than ESR in detection of infections after spinal surgery because it returns to baseline more quickly than ESR.[24,37] Serial determinations of CRP may also be helpful in following the course of acute and chronic inflammatory illnesses.[25] Elevated CRP after disc surgery has been associated with retrodiscal infection that has been detected with magnetic resonance evaluation.[31] With greater availability and accuracy of measurement techniques, CRP can be used more frequently in detecting inflammatory states in patients with spinal pain.

HEMATOLOGIC TESTS

Hematocrit

The hematocrit (Hct) level is normal in mechanical spinal pain, including herniated nucleus pulposus, spinal stenosis, and muscle strain. The presence of anemia suggests an inflammatory process of a systemic variety that has diminished erythrocyte production or hastened blood cell destruction. Rheumatologic disorders cause chronic inflammation and frequently cause so-called anemia of chronic disease, which is associated with inadequate production of RBCs. Malignancies, particularly those of hematologic origin (multiple myeloma), characteristically cause anemia. Hematologic disorders and hemoglobinopathies are also associated with decreased Hct levels.

Most laboratories determine Hct levels indirectly. Coulter machines measure mean erythrocyte volume (MCV) and hemoglobin (Hgb) concentration and derive the Hct level from these measurements. Changes in the MCV may have a significant effect on the Hct value. In serial determinations, the Hct level may vary widely, and the variation may be disconcerting to the physician. In these circumstances, following the measured Hgb concentration is helpful. A drop in Hgb level signifies a true change in the number of erythrocytes and requires further investigation.

Not all decreases in the Hct level are related to primary disorders of the axial skeleton. Many patients ingest nonsteroidal anti-inflammatory drugs (NSAIDs) for spinal pain. Many of these preparations are sold over the counter and contain aspirin. Patients may not mention these drugs to the physician, thinking that the medications are unimportant because they are nonprescription. However, these medications, as well as other NSAIDs, irritate the gastric mucosa, causing bleeding. In some patients, the amount of NSAID-associated bleeding is appreciable, causing a drop in the Hct level. Therefore, a falling Hct level may be more closely associated with therapy than with the lesion causing the pain. A decreased Hct level should be evaluated with RBC indices, reticulocyte count, serum iron level, total iron-binding capacity, haptoglobin level, and examination of the stool for occult blood.

In addition to the determination of the Hct level, levels of iron and transferrin saturation may be helpful in determining the cause of anemia. Low serum ferritin and low transferrin saturation suggest iron deficiency anemia. Elevated levels of ferritin above 400 μg/L and transferrin saturation of more than 55% are suggestive of hemochromatosis.[7] This determination may be useful in the patient with spinal pain and chondrocalcinosis.

Anemia of Chronic Disease

A decrease in Hct is a common finding associated with disorders mediated through chronic inflammation. The same cytokines that mediated the inflammatory response also cause changes in erythropoiesis. Anemia of chronic disease is a result of a number of factors affecting RBCs. Many patients have a mild anemia with an Hgb concentration of 10 to 11 g/dL. In about 20% of individuals anemia can be severe with an Hgb concentration of below 8 g/dL. RBC survival is shortened. Iron trapping in macrophages limits its mobilization for Hgb synthesis. Hypoferremia results from the sequestration of iron in macrophages by apoferritin mediated by cytokines interleukin-4 and interleukin-13. Erythropoietin levels are diminished. The response of erythroblasts to erythropoietin is impaired. Serum iron concentrations are low. The levels of iron-binding globulins are also diminished. The saturation levels are normal.[22] The preferred treatment for anemia of chronic disease is an improvement of the underlying condition. If levels of erythropoietin are below 500 IU, injections of recombinant human erythropoietin are helpful in ameliorating the anemia.[27]

White Blood Cell Count and Differential

The white blood cell (WBC) count is normal in mechanical spinal pain. The WBC count is also normal in many forms of medical spinal pain. An elevated WBC (leukocytosis) count suggests the presence of an infection, particularly if early forms of polymorphonuclear leukocytes (bands) are present. Increased numbers of WBCs are also seen in malignancies, particularly those of bone marrow or lymphatic origin. Elevations of WBC count occur less commonly in the spondyloarthropathies.

Drugs may alter the number and distribution of WBCs in the differential. Corticosteroids loosen the WBCs that line blood vessels (marginated pool). The pool is predominantly polymorphonuclear leukocytes. Corticosteroids are also lympholytic. Patients on corticosteroids have an increased WBC count in the 12,000 to 20,000 cells/mm^3 range (depending on the dose of medication). Polymorphonuclear leukocytes, as compared with lymphocytes, are present in greater number in the WBC differential. A rare toxicity of some of the drugs used in the treatment of spinal pain (i.e., immunosuppressives) is agranulocytosis or aplastic anemia. A WBC count obtained before the institution of therapy helps determine the patient's normal WBC level. A drop in WBC count after the institution of therapy requires close monitoring.

Platelets

Platelets are normal in mechanical spinal pain and most medical causes as well. In malignancies, platelets are commonly abnormal and may be elevated (thrombocytosis).[17] Platelet levels are frequently decreased (thrombocytopenia) in bone marrow and lymphatic tumors. Platelet counts may also be modified by drug therapy. A complete blood count obtained at the initiation of drug therapy establishes the patient's usual platelet count.

Blood Chemistry Tests

Blood chemistry tests are usually obtained as a battery of 12 or more tests. There is nothing mysterious about the selection of tests included in the chemistry profile other than the fact that they are frequently ordered and the process for their measurement is automated. Although the groupings of tests seem haphazard, combinations of tests help identify abnormalities associated with dysfunction in specific organ systems.[43] Disorders may be associated with specific tests as follows: renal—blood urea nitrogen, uric acid, creatinine, and glucose; hepatic—total bilirubin, alkaline phosphatase, lactic dehydrogenase, alanine aminotransferase (ALT), and aspartate aminotransferase (AST); parathyroid—calcium and phosphorus; bone—calcium; tumor—total protein, albumin, and lactic dehydrogenase; and hematologic—lactic dehydrogenase and total protein.

Serum Calcium and Phosphorus

An increase in serum calcium and decrease in serum phosphorus reflect activity of parathormone on bone and kidney. Patients with primary hyperparathyroidism have this relationship of calcium to phosphorus. Malignancies are associated with hypercalcemia. Malignancies with elevated serum calcium levels include those with parathormone activity (parathyroid adenoma and oat cell carcinoma of the lung), bone metastases, and multiple myeloma.

Metabolic bone disease may be associated with altered serum calcium and phosphorus concentrations. Osteomalacia (diminished vitamin D effect on bone) results in decreased serum calcium level and a range of changes in phosphorus levels. Phosphorus levels may be elevated in renal disease and acromegaly or diminished as in hereditary disorders, including hypophosphatemia. Osteoporosis is not associated with any serum alterations of serum calcium or phosphorus concentrations. Calcium and phosphorus levels are also unaltered in osteoarthritis and mechanical causes of spinal pain.

Serum Alkaline Phosphatase

Alkaline phosphatase (ALP) is produced to the greatest extent by osteoblasts. Any condition that increases osteoblastic activity increases ALP.[32,39] Disorders associated with ALP elevations include Paget's disease, metastatic carcinoma, hyperparathyroidism, osteomalacia, fractures during healing phase, and hypophosphatasia. Of the illnesses that cause spinal pain, metastatic tumors and Paget's disease cause the greatest increases (2 to 30 times normal). Up to 86% of patients with metastatic prostate carcinoma and 77% with metastatic breast cancer to bone have ALP elevations.[11] Not all bone tumors cause ALP elevations. Multiple myeloma, which causes little osteoblastic activity, is associated with increased ALP activity in less than 20% of patients. The ALP abnormalities in these myeloma patients may reflect healing bone fractures and may persist for several weeks.

The increase in ALP associated with Paget's disease is proportional to the activity of osteoblasts that are activated by increased osteoclastic resorption of bone. The extent of enzyme elevation is proportional to the extent of skeletal involvement. ALP increases with time in patients who are untreated. A rapid and marked elevation of enzyme activity is indicative of sarcomatous degeneration of a Paget's lesion.

Metabolic bone disease, particularly osteomalacia, is associated with abnormal levels of ALP. Osteomalacia is associated with increased enzyme levels with accompanying low-normal or decreased serum calcium concentration. Hyperparathyroidism is associated with increased ALP levels if the disease has caused bone disease. Radiographic changes of hyperparathyroidism may be present in the hands before serum elevations of ALP occur.[11]

Decreased levels of ALP are associated with an inherited deficiency of the enzyme (hypophosphatasia). The disease clinically resembles osteomalacia.

Not all elevations of ALP are associated with bone disease. Disease of the hepatobiliary system may be associated with marked increases of ALP activity. This is particularly evident in patients with obstructive lesions in the biliary system who may have concomitant abnormalities in other serum parameters of liver damage (ALT and AST, bilirubin, and cholesterol). An increased AST/ALT ratio is particularly suggestive of alcoholic liver disease.[23] Gamma-glutamyl transpeptidase (GGT) is another enzyme produced by biliary tubular cells. GGT is a highly sensitive but nonspecific test. Other tissues, including kidney, pancreas, heart, and brain, are sources. An isolated GGT may be indicative of iron overload or fatty liver. Women who are pregnant may develop increased ALP levels of placental origin during the second and third trimesters. Diseases of the intestinal mucosa, peptic ulcer, or ulcerative colitis may also cause enzyme elevations.

Serum Uric Acid

Uric acid determination is normal in the vast majority of patients with spinal pain. Serum uric acid level may be elevated in patients with tophaceous gout affecting the spine.[33] These patients usually have extensive gouty disease in peripheral joints. The diagnosis of gout is documented by the demonstration of sodium urate crystals in synovial fluid or from a tophus. Hyperuricemia alone is insufficient to make a diagnosis of gout. Increased uric acid concentrations are also associated with any process that causes rapid cell turnover. Lactate dehydrogenase may also be increased in these circumstances. These disease states include myeloproliferative and lymphoproliferative disorders, psoriasis, hypothyroidism, hyperparathyroidism, and Paget's disease. Chronic renal failure as well as a variety of drugs, including thiazide diuretics, furosemide, low-dose salicylate, phenothiazine, phenylbutazone, and corticosteroids, cause hyperuricemia.

Serum Glucose

The serum glucose determination obtained on a chemical profile has significance only if obtained when the patient is in a fasting state. Elevations of glucose in the fasting state require formal testing of glucose metabolism, including a 2-hour glucose tolerance test. A number of drugs may increase or decrease serum glucose concentrations. The drug history of the patient may help clarify abnormalities of glucose concentration observed with screening chemical evaluations.

Total Protein and Serum Albumin

Total protein and serum albumin concentrations are determined in most screening chemistry profile tests. In most patients with spinal pain, these tests are normal. However, in patients with chronic, systemic inflammatory diseases, the total protein concentrations may be altered. The same cytokines that cause the release of acute-phase reactants decrease the production of albumin.[9] With chronic inflammation or infection (tuberculosis), the total globulins of the total protein may be increased. Marked increase in total protein associated with elevated globulin levels should raise the possibility of multiple myeloma.

Patients with increased total protein should be evaluated with a serum protein electrophoresis. An increase in gamma globulins requires a serum immunoelectrophoresis test. An increase in globulins requires serum immunoelectrophoresis to characterize the increased component. Increased monoclonal immunoglobulins may occur with benign (monoclonal gammopathies) or malignant (multiple myeloma) disorders; a diffuse elevation of gamma globulins (polyclonal increase) suggests the presence of a chronic inflammatory process.

Blood Urea Nitrogen and Serum Creatinine

Elevations in blood urea nitrogen (BUN) and serum creatinine are associated with decreased renal function. Patients with visceral back pain of genitourinary origin may have elevations of these parameters. Additional evaluations, in the form of 24-hour urine collection for creatinine clearance and radiographic or sonographic examination, are helpful in defining the parenchymal or obstructive origin of the renal impairment. The drug history is important in a patient with abnormalities of BUN and creatinine. A number of drugs, including corticosteroids and NSAIDs, may cause elevations of these tests.[10,5] The cyclooxygenase-2 (COX-2) inhibitors were developed with the anticipation of having no effect on renal function. However, the COX-2 enzyme plays a role in the maintenance of renal function when kidney function is diminished. COX-2 inhibitors may increase BUN and creatinine levels in individuals at risk with limited function.[45]

IMMUNOLOGIC TESTS

Histocompatibility Typing

The human leukocyte antigens (HLAs) are present on all human nucleated cells.[3] HLA typing determines A, B, C, and D antigens. Specific haplotypes are associated with a wide variety of disorders. In regard to disorders of the lumbosacral spine, class IB antigens are most closely associated with the spondyloarthropathies. The histocompatibility antigen, HLA-B27, is present in more than 90% of patients with ankylosing spondylitis and 80% of patients with reactive arthritis, compared with 8% of the normal white and 4% of the normal black population. The HLA-B27 test is performed in vitro, using the patient's lymphocytes and antisera directed against specific HLA antigens. The presence of HLA-B27 is not diagnostic for any specific spondyloarthropathy. In general, the majority of patients with ankylosing spondylitis are more readily diagnosed on the basis of history, physical examination, and roentgenographic findings of sacroiliitis. HLA-B27 is a superfluous test. The test is most helpful for the young woman who presents with neck pain and equivocal changes of vertebral body squaring on plain radiographs. HLA-B27 positivity in a patient with neck pain and equivocal radiographs is additional evidence for the diagnosis of ankylosing spondylitis.

Four percent to 8% of normal people in the United States are HLA-B27 positive. The presence of HLA-B27 in a patient with noninflammatory back pain of bone or muscle origin is of no consequence.[15]

The HLA class II molecules are encoded in the HLA-D region. DR, DQ, and DP are the three major subregions of the D region. HLA class II molecules are expressed on a limited number of cells in the immune system, such as B lymphocytes and macrophages. Class II molecules play a central role in antigen recognition and effective collaboration between immunocompetent cells for an efficient immune response.[35] Histocompatibility testing for class II molecules is primarily used for research purposes. Like class I antigens, class II antigens are not found exclusively in patients with specific illnesses. A proportion of normal individuals have certain class II antigens.

6-4 DISEASES ASSOCIATED WITH RHEUMATOID FACTOR

RHEUMATIC DISEASES
Rheumatoid arthritis
Systemic lupus erythematosus
Sjögren's syndrome
Systemic sclerosis
Mixed connective tissue disease
CHRONIC BACTERIAL INFECTIONS
Tuberculosis
Subacute bacterial endocarditis
Salmonellosis
Brucellosis
Syphilis
Leprosy
HYPERGLOBULINEMIC STATES
Hypergammaglobulinemic purpura
Cryoglobulinemia
Chronic liver disease
Sarcoidosis
VIRAL INFECTIONS
Mononucleosis
Hepatitis
Influenza
AIDS
PARASITIC INFECTIONS
Trypanosomiasis
Kala-azar
Malaria
Schistosomiasis
Filariasis
NEOPLASMS
Post-therapy radiation or chemotherapy

Rheumatoid Factors

Rheumatoid factors (RFs) are a group of autoantibodies to human immunoglobulin G (IgG). RF may be of IgM, IgG, IgA, IgD, and IgE varieties. The classic RF is IgM antibody. RFs occur in a wide range of autoimmune and chronic infectious diseases (Table 6-4). The disease most closely associated with RF is rheumatoid arthritis. Approximately 80% of patients with rheumatoid arthritis are seropositive for RF. The cervical spine is commonly involved in patients with rheumatoid arthritis. Patients with cervical spine disease usually have joint inflammation in other locations, such as the wrists, fingers, and toes, that precedes neck involvement. The RF status of the patient is frequently known when the patient becomes symptomatic with neck pain.

The presence of RF activity may be important in the evaluation of patients with musculoskeletal pain secondary to subacute bacterial endocarditis. Patients with chronic endocarditis develop RF after 6 weeks of infection in the setting of hypocomplementemia and immune complex deposition manifested by glomerulonephritis.[46] RF titers play a greater role in following the response therapy than in diagnosing endocarditis. RF diminishes in titer as the patient's infection responds to antibiotic therapy.

RF in low titer may also be identified in an increasing proportion of normal individuals as they grow older. More than 40% of healthy individuals who are 75 years of age have detectable RF.[13] Therefore, RF determinations add little information to the evaluation of the patients with mechanical pain and should not be included in the laboratory examination of these individuals.

RF may also appear as part of a panel of tests combined to facilitate more accurate diagnosis when screening patients with musculoskeletal complaints. The three tests most commonly offered are the RF, antinuclear antibody, and uric acid level. The predictive value of these tests is only 35% in a population of individuals with joint disease and an estimated combined prevalence of the three resulting illnesses of 10%.[19] Therefore, 65% of individuals with a positive test would not have one of these illnesses. The use of panels of tests in the evaluation of spinal pain patients is not useful.

URINALYSIS

Abnormalities detected during a routine urinalysis are most helpful in identifying those individuals with viscerogenic-referred lumbar spine pain of genitourinary origin. The presence of protein in the urine may be indicative of a dysproteinemic state: multiple myeloma. The presence of proteinuria on a dipstick determination requires further evaluation. If the concentration of urinary protein is small, repeat urinalysis may detect no additional protein. If proteinuria persists, quantification of a 24-hour collection of urine is necessary. If multiple myeloma is suspected, a negative dipstick protein does not rule out the diagnosis because myeloma proteins are not detected by dipstick methods. The presence of myeloma proteins in urine is detected by adding sulfosalicylic acid to urine (nonspecific test for protein that turns urine turbid) or immunoelectrophoresis of urine, which identifies the specific protein present in increased concentration.

Twenty-four-hour urine collections may be helpful in patients with metabolic bone disease. Urine collection for calcium helps determine calcium excretion, degree of calcium absorption, and patient compliance with ingestion of calcium supplements. The value of the test result is only as good as the completeness of the collection. Partial collections are of no clinical value.

MISCELLANEOUS TESTS

The most crucial diagnostic procedure for bacterial meningitis is lumbar puncture for examination of cerebrospinal fluid (CSF). If the neurologic examination reveals meningismus and signs of increased intracranial pressure (papilledema), imaging of the central nervous system may be required to document the status of intracranial structures. Timely evaluation is essential to establish the diagnosis of meningitis so that antibiotic therapy can be initiated quickly.[21]

CSF is clear, colorless fluid that fills the subarachnoid space. The volume of CSF is 125 to 150 mL. Approximately 500 to 600 mL is produced by the choroid plexus each day.[40] The normal characteristics of CSF are listed in Table 6-5.

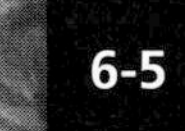

6-5 NORMAL CEREBROSPINAL FLUID (CSF) VALUES

PRESSURE

65–195 mm H_2O

CELL COUNT

Mononuclear cells 0–5/mm^3
 Borderline 5–10/mm^3
 Abnormal >10/mm^3

PROTEIN

0–45 mg/dL

GLUCOSE

Ratio of CSF to blood glucose ≥0.6
If blood glucose concentration is high, then ratio decreases (0.4)
If blood is present in CSF, correction for cells and protein:
 True CSF WBC = measured CSF WBC – blood WBC × CSF RBC/blood RBC
 True CSF protein = serum protein × CSF RBC/blood RBC

RBC, red blood cell; WBC, white blood cell.
Modified from Van Scoy RE: Evaluation of cerebrovascular fluid. In Schlossberg D (ed): Infections of the Nervous System. New York, Springer-Verlag, 1990, pp 381–388.

Abnormalities in CSF cells, glucose, protein, or pressure are noted in patients with infection, tumors, or other inflammatory lesions of the spinal cord or nerve roots. Subarachnoid bleeding may cause a centrifuged fluid to be xanthochromic for 2 to 4 weeks. CSF pressure may be increased by congestive heart failure, superior vena caval obstruction, thrombosis of the intracranial venous sinus, impaired resorption of CSF, or intracranial mass lesion. Low CSF pressure may occur in patients with dehydration, hypotension, subdural hematomas, spinal subarachnoid block, and barbiturate intoxication. The Queckenstedt's test is used to evaluate CSF pressure but is rarely used in the emergency setting of meningitis. The test is performed by occluding the jugular veins bilaterally for 10 seconds. Normal findings include an increase of pressure to 150 mm H_2O that returns to baseline in 15 to 20 seconds. No increase in pressure is associated with a positive test. Herniated discs, vertebral fractures, extradural abscesses, and neoplastic adhesions are associated with a positive test.[6] Decreased CSF glucose levels are most frequently associated with infections of the central nervous system, including meningitis, neurosyphilis, neoplasms, subarachnoid hemorrhage, sarcoidosis, and hypoglycemia. CSF protein levels are increased in a wide variety of disorders, including infections, multiple sclerosis, vasculitis, cerebrovascular accidents, encephalitis, and Guillain-Barré syndrome. Increased leukocyte count is most frequently associated with bacterial meningitis when the predominant cell is neutrophil. Lymphocytosis is most frequently associated with tuberculosis, fungal and viral meningitis, Guillain-Barré syndrome, vasculitis, and multiple sclerosis. Cultures for bacteria, tuberculosis, fungi, virus, and anaerobes should be obtained when adequate fluid is available. CSF should be examined with a Gram's stain, India ink stain, or acid-fast stain. The detection of bacterial antigens is increased with the use of counterimmunoelectrophoresis. The organisms most frequently detected by this technique include *Haemophilus influenzae*, *Neisseria meningitidis*, and *Streptococcus pneumoniae*.[8]

Polymerase chain reaction (PCR) techniques are becoming increasingly important in the detection of small amounts of DNA or RNA in a specimen.[28] PCR is a means to detect bacterial or viral genetic material. Enterovirus is an important cause of aseptic meningitis, and PCR CSF evaluation for enterovirus is now available.[29] The early detection of enterovirus decreases the need for prolonged antibiotic therapy and shortens hospital stays.

BIOPSY SPECIMENS

In certain patients with spinal pain, the diagnosis cannot be determined without histologic examination of tissue from the axial skeleton. Evaluation of biopsy specimens is most helpful in identifying benign and malignant tumors as well as obtaining bone, disc, or other tissues for culture to confirm the presence of infection. Tissue biopsy is indicated after noninvasive tests have been completed, the cause of the patient's pain remains in doubt, and examination of tissue becomes necessary to establish the diagnosis. Close cooperation is needed among the clinicians, radiologists, and surgeons to choose the appropriate site and method of biopsy.

Some lesions are accessible to needle biopsy and do not require an operation. Computed tomography–guided biopsy is an effective means of obtaining tissue for diagnosis.[16] Other lesions, particularly those in the anterior portion of vertebrae, are inaccessible to the biopsy needle and require an open biopsy. Careful handling of the biopsy material is necessary so the greatest amount of information is obtained from the invasive procedure.

SUMMARY

Laboratory test results should never replace a careful history and physical examination in the evaluation of the patient with spinal pain. In the majority of circumstances, the laboratory results help separate patients into categories (inflammatory vs. noninflammatory, bone vs. liver) but rarely establish specific diagnoses, except in the setting of infection. The clinician may place too much significance on laboratory findings, which results in inaccurate diagnoses. Laboratory tests are helpful when used appropriately. If their relative importance is kept in mind, the clinician will not be misled.

References

1. Alococer-Varela J, Valencia X: Cytokines in autoimmunity. In Lahita RG (ed): Textbook of the Autoimmune Diseases. Philadelphia, Lippincott Williams & Wilkins, 2000, pp 101-116.
2. Ballou SP, Kushner I: Laboratory evaluation of inflammation. In Kelley WN, Harris ED Jr, Ruddy S, Sledge CB (eds): Textbook of Rheumatology, 4th ed. Philadelphia, WB Saunders, 1993, pp 671-679.
3. Brenner MB, Glass DN: HLA polymorphisms and rheumatic disease. In Cohen AS (ed): Laboratory Diagnostic Procedures in the Rheumatic Diseases, 3rd ed. Orlando, Grune & Stratton, 1985, pp 249-271.
4. Cherkin DC, Deyo R, Wheeler K, Ciol MA: Physician variation in diagnostic testing for low back pain: Who you see is what you get. Arthritis Rheum 37:15-22, 1994.
5. Clive DM, Stoff JS: Renal syndromes associated with nonsteroidal anti-inflammatory drugs. N Engl J Med 310:563, 1984.
6. Dougherty JM, Roth RM: Cerebral spinal fluid. Emerg Med Clin North Am 4:516, 1986.
7. Edwards CQ, Kushner JP: Screening for hemochromatosis. N Engl J Med 328:1616, 1993.
8. Feldman WE: Relation of concentrations of bacteria and bacterial antigen in cerebrospinal fluid to prognosis in patients with bacterial meningitis. N Engl J Med 296:433, 1977.
9. Gabay C, Kushner I: Acute-phase proteins and other systemic responses to inflammation. N Engl J Med 340:448-454, 1999.
10. Galen RS: The effects of drugs on laboratory tests. Orthop Clin North Am 10:465, 1979.
11. Goldsmith RS: Laboratory aids in the diagnosis of metabolic bone disease. Orthop Clin North Am 3:545, 1972.
12. Hayes GS, Stinson IN: Erythrocyte sedimentation rate and age. Arch Ophthalmol 94:939, 1976.
13. Heimer R, Levin FM, Rudd E: Globulins resembling rheumatoid factor in serum of the aged. Am J Med 35:175, 1963.
14. International Committee for Standardization in Hematology: Recommendation for measurement of erythrocyte sedimentation rate of human blood. Am J Clin Pathol 68:505, 1977.
15. Kahn MA, Khan MI: Diagnostic value of HLA-B27 testing in ankylosing spondylitis and Reiter's syndrome. Ann Intern Med 90:70, 1982.
16. Kornblum MB, Weslowski DP, Fischgrund JS, Herkowitz HN: Computed tomography–guided biopsy of the spine: A review of 103 patients. Spine 23:81-85, 1998.
17. Levin H, Conley CL: Thrombocytosis associated with malignant disease. Arch Intern Med 114:497, 1964.
18. Levinson SS: What is C-reactive protein telling us about coronary artery disease? Arch Intern Med 162:389-392, 2002.
19. Lichtenstein MJ, Pincus T: How useful are combinations of blood tests in "rheumatic panels" in diagnosis of rheumatic diseases? J Gen Intern Med 3:436, 1988.
20. Malkiewitz A, Kushner I: Biochemical markers of inflammation in spondylitis. Spine State Art Rev 3:553, 1991.
21. Martin JB, Tyler KL, Scheld WM: Bacterial meningitis. In Tyler KL, Martin JB (eds): Infectious Diseases of the Central Nervous System. Philadelphia, FA Davis, 1993, pp 176-187.
22. Means RT Jr: Pathogenesis of the anemia of chronic disease: A cytokine-mediated anemia. Stem Cells 13:32-37, 1995.
23. Moseley RH: Evaluation of abnormal liver function tests. Med Clin North Am 80:887-905, 1996.
24. Mustard RA Jr, Bohnen JMA, Haseeb S, Kasina R: C-reactive protein levels predict postoperative septic complications. Arch Surg 122:69, 1987.
25. Okamura JM, Miyagi JM, Terada K, Hokama Y: Potential clinical applications of C-reactive protein. J Clin Lab Anal 4:231, 1990.
26. Pepys MB: Acute-phase phenomena. In Cohen AS (ed): Rheumatology and Immunology. Orlando, Grune & Stratton, 1979, p 85.
27. Pincus T, Olsen NJ, Russell IJ, et al: Multicenter study of recombinant human erythropoietin in correction of anemia in rheumatoid arthritis. Am J Med 89:16, 1990.
28. Post JC, Ehrlich, GD: The impact of the polymerase chain reaction in clinical medicine. JAMA 283:1544-1546, 2000.
29. Ramers C, Billman G, Hartin M, et al: Impact of a diagnostic cerebrospinal fluid enterovirus polymerase chain reaction test on patient management. JAMA 283:2680-2685, 2000.
30. Ridker PM, Cushman M, Stampfer MJ, et al: Inflammation, aspirin, and the risk of cardiovascular disease in apparently healthy men. N Engl J Med 336:973-979, 1997.
31. Schulitz KP, Assheuer J: Discitis after procedures on the intervertebral disc. Spine 19:1172, 1994.
32. Schwartz MK: Enzymes in cancer. Clin Chem 19:10, 1973.
33. Sequeira W, Bouffard A, Salgia K, Skosey J: Quadriparesis in tophaceous gout. Arthritis Rheum 24:1428, 1981.
34. Sox HC Jr, Liang MH: The erythrocyte sedimentation rate: Guidelines for rational use. Ann Intern Med 104:515, 1986.
35. Strominger JL: Biology of the human histocompatibility leukocyte antigen (HLA) system and a hypothesis regarding the generation of autoimmune disease. J Clin Invest 77:1411, 1986.
36. Takahashi J, Ebara S, Kamimura M, et al: Early-phase enhanced inflammatory reaction after spinal instrumentation surgery. Spine 26:1698-1704, 2001.
37. Thelander U, Larsson S: Quantitation of C-reactive protein levels and erythrocyte sedimentation rate after spinal surgery. Spine 17:400, 1992.
38. Tillet WS, Francis T Jr: Serological reactions in pneumonia with a non-protein somatic fraction of *Pneumococcus*. J Exp Med 52:561, 1930.
39. Van Lente F: Alkaline and acid phosphatase determinations in bone disease. Orthop Clin North Am 10:437, 1979.
40. Van Scoy RE: Evaluation of cerebrovascular fluid. In Schlossberg D (ed): Infections of the Nervous System. New York, Springer-Verlag, 1990, pp 381-388.
41. Visser M, Bouter LM, McQuillan GM, et al: Elevated C-reactive protein levels in overweight and obese adults. JAMA 282:2131-2135, 1999.
42. Waddell G: An approach to backache. Br J Hosp Med 28:187, 1982.
43. Ward PCJ: Chemical profiles of disease. Orthop Clin North Am 10:405, 1979.
44. Wener MH, Daum PR, McQuillan GM: The influence of age, sex, and race on the upper reference limit of serum C-reactive protein concentration. J Rheumatol 27:2351-2359, 2000.
45. Whelton A, Schulman G, Wallemark C, et al: Effects of celecoxib and naproxen on renal function in the elderly. Ann Intern Med 160:1465-1470, 2000.
46. Williams RC Jr, Kunkel HG: Rheumatoid factor, complement, and conglutinin aberrations in patients with subacute bacterial endocarditis. J Clin Invest 41:666, 1962.
47. Wintrobe MM, Landsberg JW: A standardized technique for the blood sedimentation test. Am J Med Sci 189:102, 1935.
48. Zacharski LR, Kyle RA: Significance of extreme elevation of erythrocyte sedimentation rate. JAMA 202:264, 1967.

CHAPTER 7

RADIOGRAPHIC EVALUATION

Evaluation of patients with spine-related pain frequently includes the use of radiographic techniques to visualize the structures of the spine. When obtained at the appropriate time in the diagnostic evaluation, and when interpreted correctly in the setting of the patient's clinical history and physical examination, radiographic images are extremely helpful in suggesting the possible location and source of a patient's pain (vertebral fracture, tumor, or osteoarthritis). On the other hand, radiographic images that are obtained too soon in the diagnostic process or are interpreted incorrectly may delay the determination of the true diagnosis. For example, the presence of degenerative disc disease on a radiograph may dissuade the clinician from fully evaluating a patient with new-onset spinal pain. The physician may ascribe the patient's pain to radiographic changes found in the spine associated with degenerative disc disease. The patient may not respond to therapy, and pain may persist. Does the physician continue therapy or take another radiograph? The patient may not like being exposed to additional radiation and may be resistant to reevaluation. Only the persistence of pain persuades the patient to undergo radiographic evaluation again later. At this time the process (infection, tumor, or joint inflammation) has destroyed enough bone for its presence to be detected with a plain radiograph. In this scenario, a roentgenogram taken between the initial and subsequent examinations may have detected the lesion at an earlier stage of development. Unless certain risk factors are present, which would suggest an infection or tumor, radiographs should be reserved until patients have documented that they are refractory to conservative management. Not only does this avoid unnecessary x-rays for those who respond to the usual maneuvers, but it also increases the chances that the source of the pathologic changes may be visible on a roentgenogram in patients who do not respond.

The underlying fact that complicates the relationship of spinal pain, particularly of a mechanical nature, and radiographic findings is the progressive anatomic changes that occur naturally in the axial skeleton over time and are not associated with pain. Although radiographic evidence of chronic disc degeneration is common in middle age, it is almost universal in the elderly. Degenerative disc disease of the spine is not seen as an isolated finding. Rather, it is part of a process that affects the structure of the entire spine. De Palma and Rothman reported gross microscopic and radiographic studies of aging spine specimens.[30] Severe disc degeneration was seen in 72% of the specimens older than 70 years of age. The most commonly affected level was C5–C6, with 86% of specimens having observable abnormalities. The C6–C7 level was the next most frequently affected, and the C2–C3 level was least often involved in chronic disc degeneration.[30,41]

The radiographic and morphologic findings of cervical spondylosis are as readily observed in asymptomatic patients. Gore and colleagues reported that by age 65, 95% of men and 70% of women had at least one degenerative change on their roentgenograms.[49] Anterior osteophyte formation and disc space narrowing were common findings. Anterior osteophyte formation was the only component of cervical spondylosis that occurred as an isolated finding. A similar study comparing groups of symptomatic and asymptomatic individuals found no difference between the two groups in the incidence of degenerative changes at the joints of Luschka, the intervertebral foramen, or the posterior articular processes.[40] In a study of asymptomatic patients ranging in age from 30 to 70 years, Friedenberg and Miller found that 35% had radiographic evidence of spondylosis.[40] Thus, it is important to remember that just because anatomic change is present and identifiable on radiographs, it is not necessarily the cause of any particular component of a patient's pain.

Similar findings of radiographic progression occur in the lumbosacral spine that are unassociated with pain. By age 50, up to 95% of adults who come to autopsy show evidence of aging changes in the lumbosacral spine with disc space narrowing, calcification, or marginal sclerosis (lumbar spondylosis).[59] Roentgenograms taken of living patients of a similar age demonstrate degenerative changes in 87%. The prevalence of lumbar spondylosis increases with age. Only 5% or less of people younger than 20 years of age have spondylosis. In a comparison of 238 patients with back pain with 66 patients without pain, there was no difference between the two groups in regard to the prevalence of spondylosis and disc degeneration.[142] Another study has demonstrated increased prevalence of roentgenographic findings of disc degeneration in individuals who are involved in heavy labor.[70] Although an anatomic change is present and is identifiable, it is not necessarily the cause of the patient's pain.

On the other hand, radiographic evaluation of the spine can be helpful in detecting specific abnormalities (lytic or blastic bone lesions, arthritis, expansive spinal cord tumors, disc space infections, and metabolic bone disease) that may be directly related to a patient's clinical symptoms and signs. Radiographic techniques are available to identify anatomic abnormalities associated with local destructive processes or systemic inflammatory illnesses that affect the skeletal system in general. The closest correlation between anatomic changes discovered with radiographic techniques and clinical symptoms occurs with medical diseases of the axial skeleton. The physician must not make the mistake of assuming the same close correlation between anatomy and symptoms when evaluating mechanical lesions in the spine.

Most neurodiagnostic imaging studies have a high sensitivity (the ability to detect anatomic abnormalities) but a low specificity (the ability to remain negative in the absence of clinical disease). The poor correlation between anatomic changes and clinical symptoms has been associated with computed tomography (CT) scan of the lumbosacral spine.[139] A study designed with neuroradiologists reading CT scans blinded to patients' symptoms reported a prevalence of 19% of patients younger than 40 years of age with a herniated nucleus pulposus. Diagnoses of canal stenosis and facet degeneration were reported in 50% of patients older than 40 years of age. Despite the scan "abnormalities," both groups of patients were asymptomatic without neurologic signs except for 6 of the 52 studied patients with surgically proven spine disease. In essence, the CT scan of the lumbosacral spine detects anatomic changes that are unassociated with symptoms in a significant proportion of patients.

Magnetic resonance (MR) is another technique that visualizes soft tissues in and around the spinal column. MR scan has been reported to detect herniated discs, epidural scar tissue, and spinal cord tumors.[84] The sensitivity of MR is equal to or greater than that of myelography. As with the CT scan, MR may identify structural abnormalities of the lumbosacral spine that are unassociated with clinical symptoms.

This introduction is presented with the hope that physicians who evaluate patients with spinal pain will temper their enthusiasm for radiographic evaluation as an easy way to diagnose the cause of pain. Radiographic studies of the spine play an important role in evaluation of pain associated with trauma and systemic disease, but the limitations of the technique must be considered. Strict adherence to the 1994 Acute Low Back Pain Guidelines to obtain plain roentgenograms for individuals with fever, unexplained weight loss, cancer history, neurologic deficits, drug abuse history, an age older than 50 years, or trauma results in overutilization of roentgenograms compared to usual ordering patterns.[123] Presence of degenerative disease in the spine may or may not be the cause of the patient's symptoms. Radiographic changes associated with systemic illnesses have greater diagnostic importance, particularly in those individuals with persistent spinal pain.

PLAIN ROENTGENOGRAMS OF THE CERVICAL SPINE

Plain roentgenograms remain the initial step in diagnostic imaging of the cervical spine because of their availability, speed, relatively low exposure of tissue to radiation, and reasonable costs. Conventional roentgenograms offer good spatial and contrast resolution of bony structures, but they are unable to image soft tissue structures clearly. The initial evaluation should consist of an anteroposterior (AP), lateral, oblique, and open-mouth odontoid view of the cervical spine. Other views, such as flexion-extension views, may be obtained later to confirm specific clinical suspicions of subluxation.

The lateral view of the cervical spine is the single most important in evaluating degenerative conditions, and it provides a wealth of information (Fig. 7-1). It is important that in a good-quality roentgenogram the bone and soft tissue, all seven cervical vertebrae, and the top of the first thoracic vertebra are visible. In a true lateral roentgenogram, the lateral masses should be superimposed so that these paired structures appear as a single posterior cortical line. Similarly, the facet joints should also be superimposed so that a single facet joint is seen on the lateral roentgenogram. The same is true for the posterior cortical margin of the body and the apophyseal joints. Even the slightest change in rotation of the patient disrupts this relationship and makes findings on the roentgenogram difficult to interpret.

When interpreting roentgenograms, an organized and orderly process should be used by the physician to avoid missing subtle findings. It is generally recommended to look at the area of highest interest last. Thus, the soft tissues should be examined first, to be sure there are no abnormal soft tissue calcifications, masses, or swellings anterior or posterior to the cervical spine. The upper limits of normal radiologic width for the prevertebral space are 7 mm for C2–C4 and 20 mm for C5–C7.[100] Next, the outline of all the bony structures should be examined to be

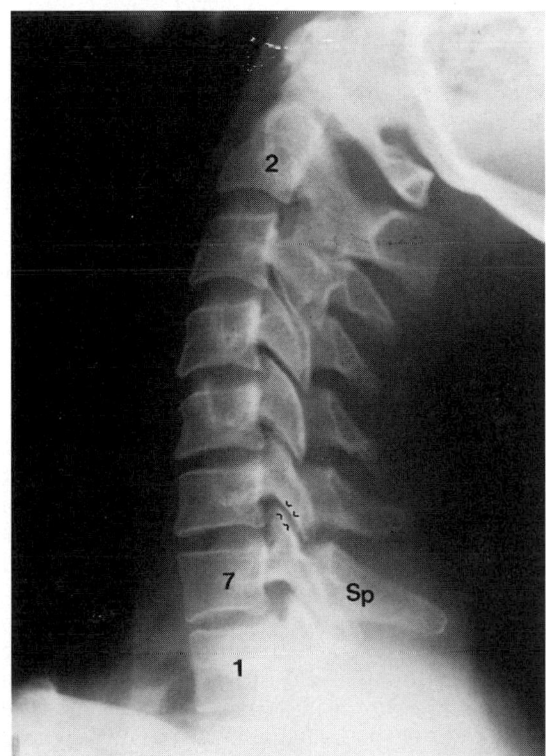

Figure 7-1 Lateral radiograph of a normal cervical spine shows all seven cervical vertebrae as well as the C7–T1 interspace. Also seen are the facet joints *(arrowheads)* and the spinous process (Sp), which is most prominent at C7 and is also known as the *vertebra prominens.*

sure there are no lytic or blastic lesions or fractures. In addition, the overall alignment of the cervical spine should be noted, including the normal lordosis and that there are no anterior or posterior translations of the cervical vertebrae relative to each other. This can be judged by looking at the anterior and posterior cortical margins of the cervical vertebra as well as at the smooth curve formed by the posterior spinolaminar line. The presence of osteophytes or syndesmophytes should be noted, and the heights of the disc spaces relative to each other should be observed.

The finding of disc space narrowing is facilitated by a comparison of the disc in question with the adjacent disc spaces. Disc space narrowing is the most constant feature of cervical spondylosis and is best seen on the lateral view in the lower portion of the cervical spine. Disc space narrowing can lead to relative loss of lordosis as the disc spaces decrease in height. Disc space narrowing is not pathognomonic of degenerative disc changes in the cervical spine and may be seen in other conditions, including rheumatoid disease, neuropathic joints, disc space infection, and traumatic disc herniation. The disc space is often spared with neoplastic involvement in contrast with an infectious process that generally involves the disc. The disc space should also be examined for the vacuum disc phenomenon, which is thought to be an accumulation of nitrogen in the center of a severely degenerative disc, because this is one of the findings that is strongly suggestive of spondylosis. In contrast, erosive changes of the discs and endplates are more suggestive of inflammatory lesions.

In examining the lateral roentgenograms for osteophytes, several types may be seen. Anterior osteophytes are the largest and may alter the overall shape of the vertebral body. Such large anterior osteophytes may be seen in diffuse idiopathic skeletal hyperostosis. On occasion, these anterior osteophytes may cause dysphagia. In contrast, posterior osteophytes or chondro-osseous spurs are smaller but more important clinically because these hypertrophic changes can project posteriorly into the ventral aspect of the spinal cord and nerve roots. As a general rule, on a standard lateral cervical spine film, the spinal canal as measured from the posterior aspect of the vertebral body to the narrowest point on the spinolaminar line should be about 17 mm. If this distance is narrowed by a posterior osteophyte to a diameter of 13 mm or less, it is likely that there is spinal cord compression. Such a narrowing would prompt further evaluation of this area with neurodiagnostic (CT or MR) imaging study.

Spondylosis is the term used to designate bone production in the spine associated with disc space narrowing and more advanced degenerative changes. This is most commonly manifested as the production of osteophytes occurring as a result of a breakdown in the outer annulus fibrosis of the intervertebral disc. This process must be distinguished from the formation of syndesmophytes in ankylosing spondylitis, reactive arthritis, and psoriatic arthritis. It is commonly thought that the formation of osteophytes is due to the pressure of disc material stretching and displacing the posterior annular fibers, causing stress at the ligament attachments and leading to ossification extending first horizontally, then vertically from the edges of the vertebra. In essence, this is an attempt by the disc to eliminate abnormal motion or to autostabilize.

Another component of degenerative disease of the cervical spine that can be evaluated on roentgenograms is the development of osteoarthritis in the synovial apophyseal joints. This predominates in the middle and lower cervical spine and is thought to be induced by excessive stress across these joints. In most instances, it is thought that changes in the disc space predate any facet joint changes. These facet changes result in joint space narrowing, marginal osteophytosis, bone fragmentation and, less commonly, capsular laxity with subluxation.

Uncovertebral joint arthrosis involves what are also known as the *joints of Luschka*, extending from C3 through C7. As loss in disc space height occurs, the bony ridges known as the *uncinate processes* can make contact at the back of the vertebral body, resulting in central clefts and a rounding off of the articular surface. Osteophytes that form in this area may project into the disc space or posteriorly into the intervertebral foramen, compressing nerve roots and producing radicular symptoms. Less commonly, osteophytes can encroach on the vertebral artery and cause vertebrobasilar insufficiency.

Although these entities—spondylosis, disc space degeneration, facet arthritis, and uncovertebral joint arthrosis—have been described as separate processes, they generally progress together at variable rates to produce a continuing range of changes in the cervical spine. Thus, the term *cervical spondylosis* is generally used to include all of these degenerative aspects. Each entity produces radiographically identifiable changes that are easily detected on plain films and can help confirm the diagnosis of cervical degenerative disease.

The AP view of the cervical spine shows the cervical vertebrae from C3 through T1 (Fig. 7-2). The first two cervical vertebrae are generally hidden from view by the superimposed mandible/occiput and must be evaluated separately on an open-mouth odontoid view. In the AP projection the disc spaces, the uncinate processes, and the uncovertebral joints are easily seen. In a correctly positioned AP view, the apophyseal or facet joints are generally not seen secondary to superimposed articular masses. The lateral margins of the articular masses should form what appears to be a continuous undulating pseudocortex at the lateral margin of the cervical spine. In addition, the spinous processes should be linear in the midline and without rotation.

The open-mouth odontoid view is useful for evaluating the relationship of the occiput, atlas, and axis; in addition, any erosive changes can be detected in the inflammatory arthropathies. In addition, this view is most useful for detecting arthritis between the articulations of the occiput and atlas or the atlantoaxial joint complex (Fig. 7-3). An abnormal relationship between the upper cervical spine and the base of the skull, resulting in basilar invagination, may be detected by this view.

Oblique views are used to evaluate the intervertebral foramina, the pedicles, the lateral masses, and apophyseal joints (Fig. 7-4). In addition, the relative relationship of the laminae can be evaluated. The oblique view is taken with the patient rotated approximately 45 degrees from the AP position. A recent study suggests that better visualization occurs with a 55-degree oblique view of the lower cervical spine neural foramina.[76] The foramina viewed on

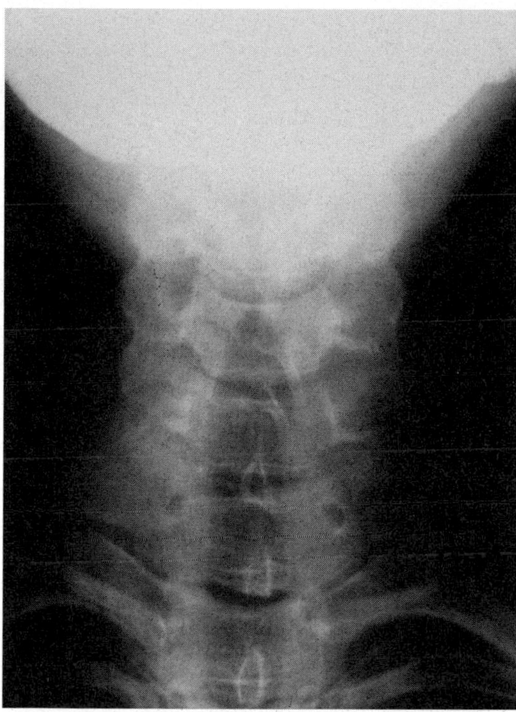

Figure 7-2 Anteroposterior view of a normal cervical spine shows C3 through T1 vertebral bodies. The lateral masses appear as a continuous pillar with a smooth, undulating outline on either side. The spinous processes can be seen in the midline and are bifid on C5 and C6.

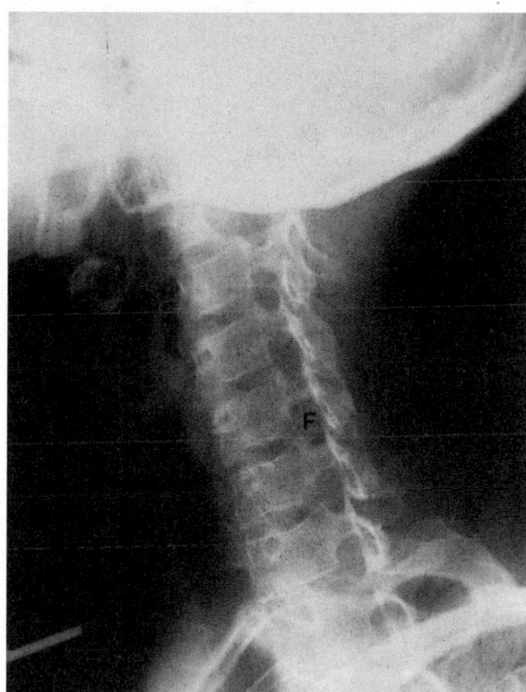

Figure 7-4 Oblique radiograph of a normal cervical spine shows the intervertebral foramina (F) and the facet joints just posterior to them, which have a normal shingling appearance. Spurs from the uncovertebral joints are frequently seen in this view, encroaching on the foramina where the nerve roots exit.

the roentgenogram are on the side opposite to the side of rotation of the chin. It is preferable that the entire body be rotated rather than just the head and neck. With a properly positioned oblique view, the intervertebral foramina become readily apparent, and any osteophytes that may be encroaching on their margins can be seen. The oblique views also allow the laminae to be viewed as an oval-shaped structure, which should be normally aligned like shingles on a roof.

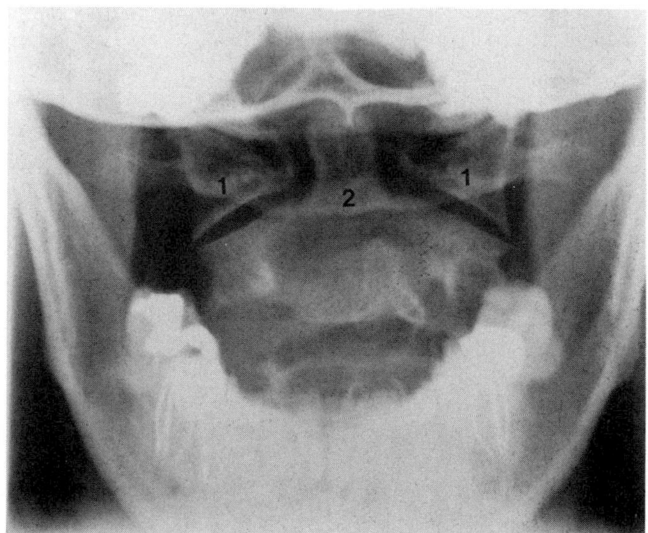

Figure 7-3 Open-mouth odontoid view shows the lateral masses of C1 (1) and the odontoid process (2) of the dens. The C1–C2 articulations are also clear.

Other views of the cervical spine, including flexion-extension views and the swimmer's views, can be obtained if specific areas need to be evaluated (Fig. 7-5). In general, flexion-extension views add little to the routine evaluation of the patient for cervical spondylosis, except in situations in which subluxation or instability is suspected on the basis of history or on the basis of static displacements on a standard roentgenogram. The swimmer's view is obtained with one arm elevated above the head.[110] The swimmer's view is preferred for investigating the cervicothoracic junction.

Normal variations in the configuration of the cervical spine may be identified on plain roentgenograms of the cervical spine.[62] Pointed configuration of the superior aspect of the tip of the odontoid process should not be confused with an erosive change. Fusion of posterior cervical elements may be produced with superimposed projections of the vertebral laminae. Rotation of the spine may also simulate posterior spinal ligament calcification. The superior articular surfaces of the fifth to seventh cervical vertebrae may show a groove or depression, which should not be confused with inflammatory changes.[63]

In summary, plain roentgenographic examination of the symptomatic degenerative cervical spine remains a beneficial, relatively inexpensive, and readily available diagnostic tool (Table 7-1). Plain roentgenograms can clearly exclude deformities, congenital anomalies, infection, and tumor. The standard views recommended for routine evaluation for degenerative problems in the neck include the AP, lateral, open-mouth odontoid, and 45-degree oblique roentgenograms. Flexion-extension views are not routinely recommended. Although the clinical symptoms of patients with neck pain, referred pain, or

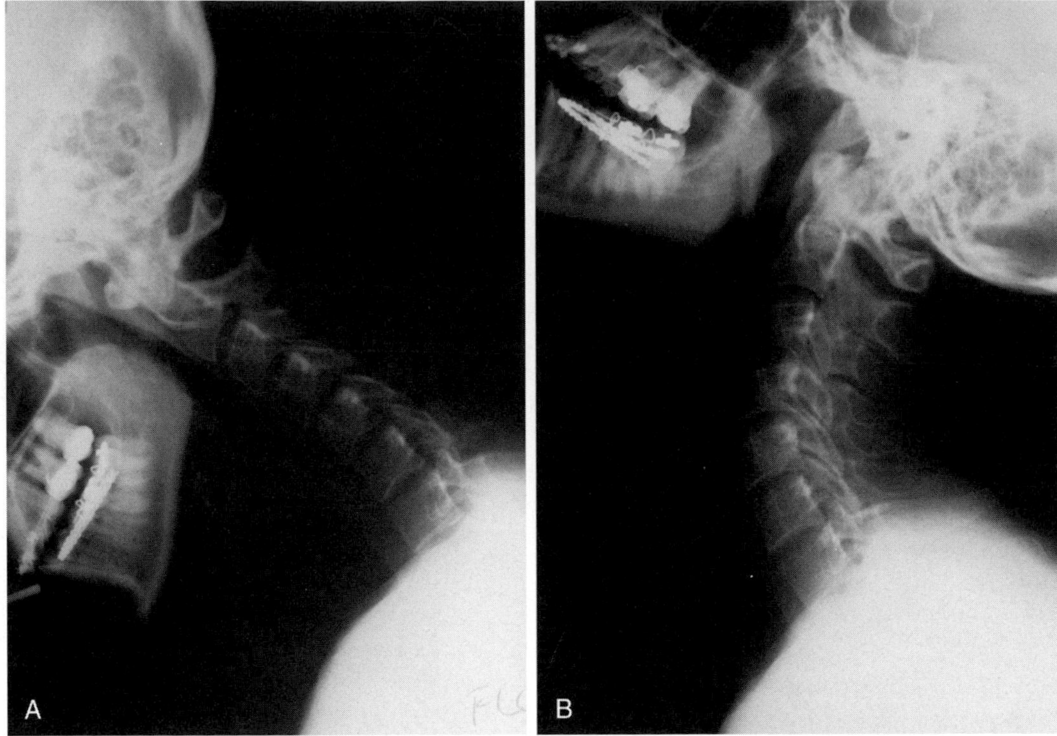

Figure 7-5 *A*, Lateral flexion view of a normal cervical spine. *B*, Lateral extension view of a normal cervical spine. These views show the normal range of motion with flexion and extension and can be useful in detecting instability at one or multiple levels when it is present. Instability can be noted either as a translation of one vertebra on another or as an increase in the posterior angular interspace distance between the spinous processes.

7-1 RADIOGRAPHIC STUDIES AND DISEASE CATEGORIES OF THE AXIAL SKELETON

Radiographs	Herniated Nucleus Pulposus	Spinal Stenosis (Osteoarthritis)	Spondylolisthesis	Spondyloarthropathy	Infection
PLAIN					
Radiation: 2.6 rads Cost: $150		1 (Motion)	1 (Sacroiliitis)	1	1
BONE SCAN					
Radiation: 0.15 rads Cost: $500				2	2*
COMPUTED TOMOGRAPHY					
Radiation: 3–5 rads Cost: $700	2	3	2	3	
MAGNETIC RESONANCE					
Radiation: None Cost: $1000	1†	2			3
MYELOGRAM					
Radiation: 6–7 rads Cost: $1200	3†	4			
DISCOGRAPHY					
Radiation: 2 rads (variable) Cost: $700	± (Disc degeneration)				
(NORMAL BACKGROUND)					
Radiation: 0.6 rads/year					

*Best method.
†Costs include mean technical and professional fee.

arm pain frequently correlate poorly with degenerative changes on plain roentgenograms of the cervical spine, the use of plain films still represents the best initial confirmatory test to direct further and more expensive radiographic evaluation in conjunction with history and physical findings.

PLAIN ROENTGENOGRAMS OF THE LUMBOSACRAL SPINE

In general, three roentgenographic views are all that are required to assess the lumbosacral spine. An AP view, a large port lateral view, and a small port lateral view to better visualize the lower two interspaces are needed. Two oblique views are also frequently taken because they occasionally help identify subtle spondylolysis. However, oblique views provide limited information and should not be routinely included.

The normal roentgenographic anatomy of the lumbar spine in the AP projection is shown in Figure 7-6. In this projection, the spinous and transverse processes, the pedicles, the facet joints, and the laminae are seen. The spinous processes are aligned in the middle of the vertebral bodies. The five lumbar processes should be counted. Rotation or lateral movement of the lumbar spine appears as a deviation in the alignment of the spinous processes.[4] The transverse processes project laterally from the middle of each vertebral body in a symmetrical fashion. Lytic or sclerotic lesions of the transverse processes are identified preferentially in the AP projection. The pedicles are perpendicular to the vertebral body and are projected end-on in the AP view.

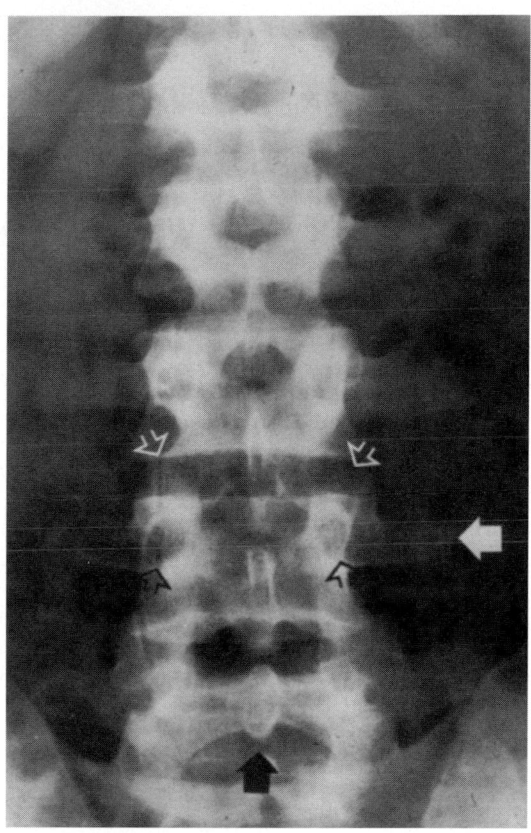

Figure 7-6 Anteroposterior view of a normal lumbar spine showing spinous process *(black arrow)*, transverse process *(white arrow)*, facet joints *(white open arrows)*, and pedicles *(black open arrows)*. *(Courtesy of Anne Brower, MD.)*

7-1 RADIOGRAPHIC STUDIES AND DISEASE CATEGORIES OF THE AXIAL SKELETON—cont'd

Radiographs	Tumor	Endocrinologic Disorder	Hematologic Disorder	Trauma	Other
PLAIN					
Radiation: 2.6 rads Cost: $150	1	1 (Osteoporosis, gout)	1	1	1
BONE SCAN					
Radiation: 0.15 rads Cost: $500	2* (Metastatic)	2 (Osteomalacia, CPPD)	2 (Hemoglobinopathy)	3	4
COMPUTED TOMOGRAPHY					
Radiation: 3–5 rads Cost: $700	4 (Myeloma)	3 (Mineral quantification)		2* (Intraspinal)	3* (Retroperitoneum)
MAGNETIC RESONANCE					
Radiation: None Cost: $1000	3* (Intraspinal)			3	
MYELOGRAM					
Radiation: 6–7 rads Cost: $1200	5* (Cord compression)				
DISCOGRAPHY					
Radiation: 2 rads (variable) Cost: $700					
(NORMAL BACKGROUND)					
Radiation: 0.6 rads/year					

*Numbers include sequence of radiographic studies used for diagnosis.
CPPD, calcium pyrophosphate dihydrate.

They appear as a dense cortical rim of bone in the superior and lateral portions of the vertebral bodies. The loss of a pedicle ("winking-owl" sign) is frequently seen in patients with metastatic disease to the spine. A short interpediculate distance may be associated with constriction of neural elements, while widening of the distance at a single level may indicate an expanding intraspinal lesion. The facet joints run in a vertical orientation and are located close to the pedicles. Sclerosis may be seen surrounding facet joints but may be difficult to see in the AP projection. The primary soft tissue structure seen in the AP projection is the psoas muscle. The psoas forms a triangular shape with the top at the transverse process of L1 and the base on the iliac crests. Asymmetrical visualization of the psoas muscle indicates clinical pathology in a minority of patients since positioning, muscle contraction, and spine rotation may affect the definition of the muscle border.

The lateral roentgenographic views visualize the lumbar and sacral spine and the L4–S1 area in a separate view. The normal roentgenographic anatomy of the lumbosacral spine is seen in Figure 7-7. In this projection, the bodies of the vertebrae, the pedicles, the spinous processes, and the intervertebral disc spaces are seen. The normal lumbar lordosis is observed with the posterior borders of the vertebral bodies lining up to form a smooth curve. Movement of a vertebral body in a horizontal plane in a forward or backward direction will be noted as a disruption of the curve and may be indicative of spinal instability. The slight concavity of the posterior surface of the vertebral bodies is noted. The disc spaces increase in size from L1 to L4. The L5–S1 disc space and intervertebral foramina are narrower than the spaces between the other lumbar vertebrae. The lumbar intervertebral foramina are best visualized in the lateral projection. Overlying shadows obscure posterior elements of the vertebral bodies. Soft tissues anterior to the spine may not be visualized well. However, examination of the area may discover calcification of structures, particularly of the aorta, which may have clinical significance.

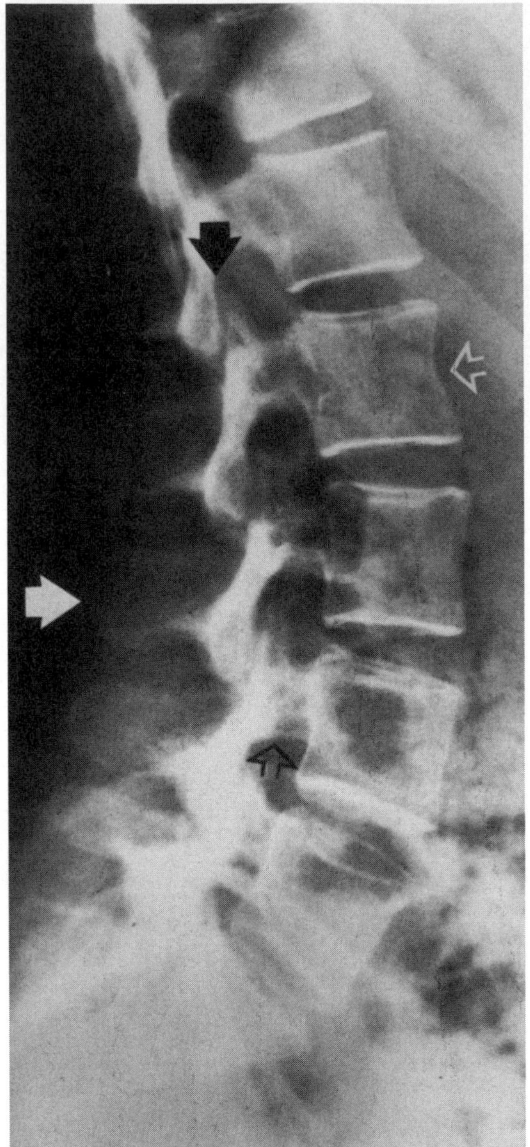

Figure 7-7 Lateral view of normal lumbar spine, showing spinous process *(white arrow)*, facet joint *(black arrow)*, laminae *(black open arrow)*, and vertebral body *(white open arrow)*. *(Courtesy of Anne Brower, MD.)*

The close-up view of the L5–S1 area provides information about the status of the intervertebral disc spaces and bone in the upper portion of the sacrum. An example is found in Figure 7-8.

The oblique projection is obtained to demonstrate the facet joints and pars interarticularis. In this view (Fig. 7-9), the posterior elements outline a shape that is reminiscent of a "Scotty dog." The nose is the transverse process, the eye the pedicle, the ear the superior articular process, the neck the pars interarticularis, the front legs the inferior articular process, and the body the laminae. A collar on the "dog" suggests the presence of spondylolysis. Other specialized views of the lumbosacral spine may be obtained. These include flexion (Fig. 7-10), extension (Fig. 7-11), and Ferguson (Fig. 7-12) views of the pelvis. These views are not obtained on a routine basis but are reserved for patients with specific symptoms and signs. The chapters describing certain disease entities include information about those special roentgenographic evaluations that are helpful in making specific diagnoses.

Usually plain roentgenograms of the lumbosacral spine do not add any information to the evaluation of many patients with mechanical low back pain but must be obtained if there is a suspicion of other pathology such as infection, tumor, hip arthritis, or urologic disease. Therefore, not everyone with acute low back pain requires a set of plain roentgenograms. If one is comfortable with diagnosis of an acute low back strain in a young patient (≤50 years of age), treatment may proceed without radiographic evaluation for the first 4 to 6 weeks after the onset of pain.[72] Roentgenograms are indicated if there is no response to the treatment. On the other hand, roentgenograms are indicated on the first visit if the patient is older (>50 years of age) or there is additional medical information that requires investigation. Roentgenograms are too often misread, or more specifically, "over-read." Normal asymptomatic people approaching 50 years of age frequently have disc narrowing. As previously described, the intervertebral disc has an 88% water content. It contains a gelatinous nucleus pulposus confined under great pressure between two cartilaginous endplates and by an elastic annulus fibrosus. The disc inevitably dehydrates with age. Numerous microscopic injuries occur with everyday wear and tear, which permits a certain amount of leakage of nuclear material from the central portion of the disc. As this occurs insidiously and gradually, the process evolves without symptomatology or impairment. Consequently, as the years pass, the disc spaces will narrow from repeated microtrauma and usually will remain symptom free. Thus,

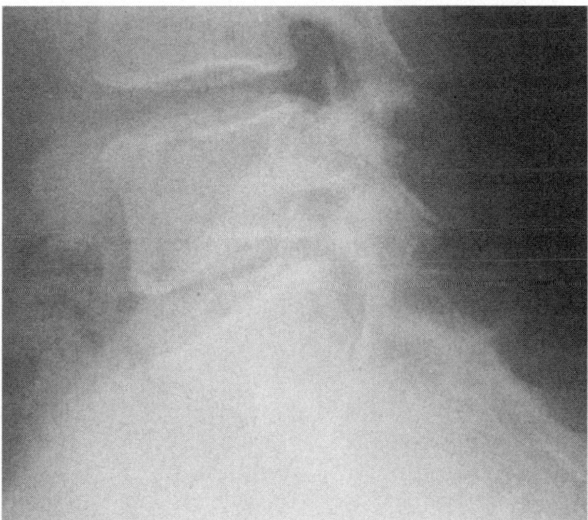

Figure 7-8 Coned-down view of a normal lumbosacral junction. The intervertebral disc between L5 and S1 may appear narrow compared with the other lumbar intervertebral discs.

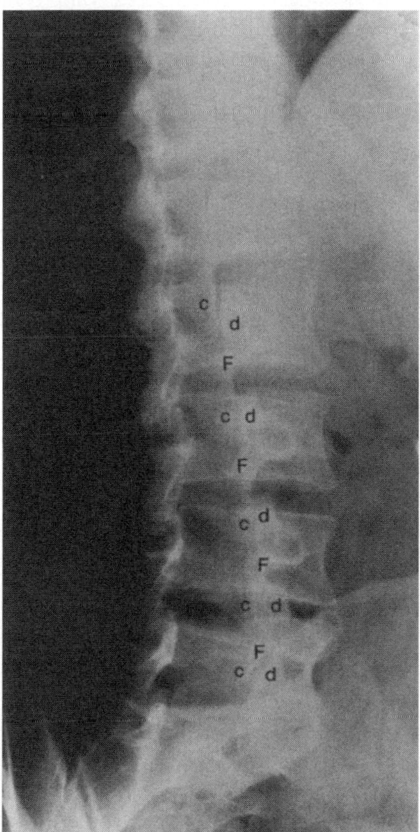

Figure 7-9 Oblique view of a normal lumbar spine. The inferior facet (c), the superior facets (d), and the pars interarticularis (F) are visualized on this view. *(From Wiesel SW, Bernini P, Rothman RH: The Aging Lumbar Spine. Philadelphia, WB Saunders, 1982.)*

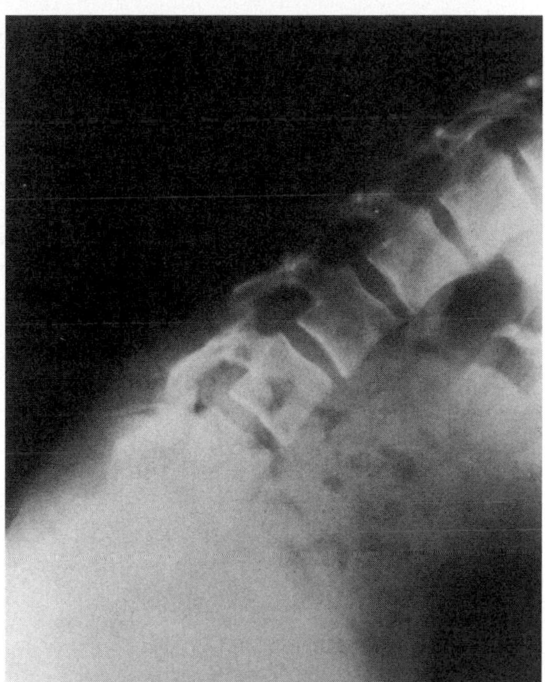

Figure 7-10 Flexion view of a normal lumbar spine in a 14-year-old girl.

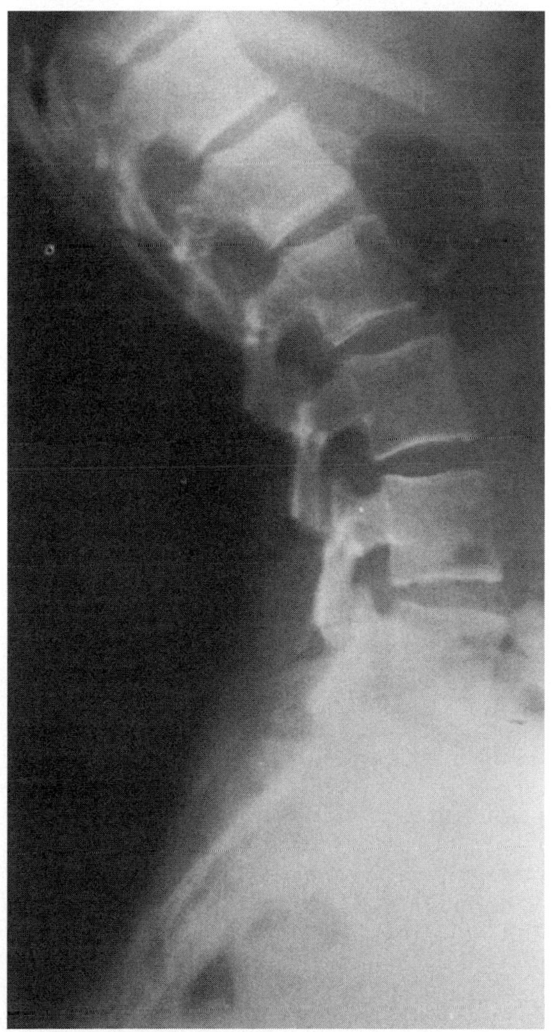

Figure 7-11 Extension view of a normal lumbar spine in a 14-year-old girl.

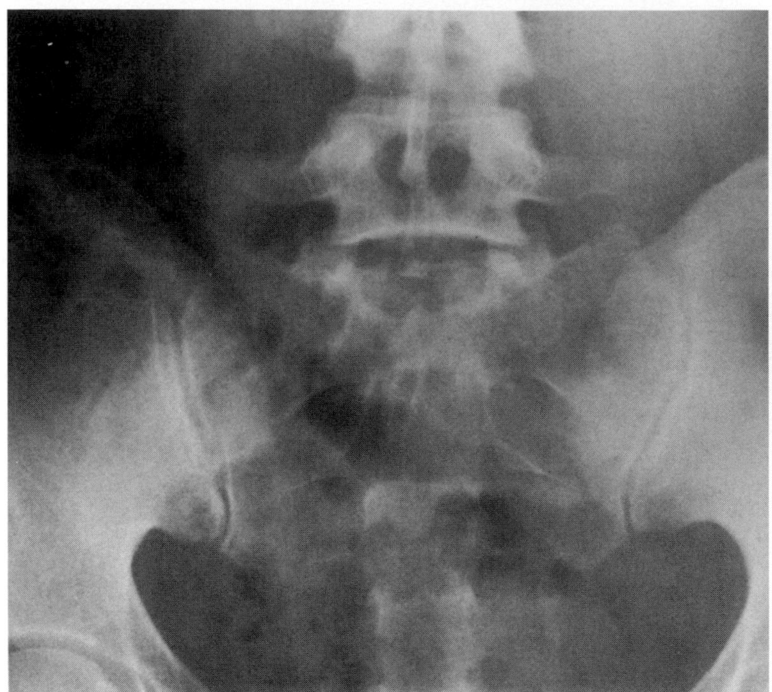

Figure 7-12 Ferguson view of normal sacroiliac joints in a 32-year-old woman.

the narrowing of a disc space on roentgenogram per se is not necessarily the etiology of the patient's complaint.

A recent study has reiterated the fact that general practitioners continue to use plain film radiographic examinations, despite their limited value in the diagnosis of low back pain.[102,108] Furthermore, a separate study concluded that an abnormal degenerative finding on lumbar radiography made no difference in clinical outcome as measured by the Roland score.[65] However, patients receiving radiographs were more satisfied with the care they received. The challenge for the treating physician is to increase patient satisfaction without ordering plain radiographs.

RADIONUCLIDE IMAGING (BONE SCAN)

Radionuclide imaging addresses function and tissue metabolism of organs by delivering to target structures a small dose of radioisotope material. This tracer emits radiation in proportion to its attachment to the target structure. This imaging is not invasive or associated with high risk, but it is relatively expensive. Radionuclide imaging is a good technique for the detection of bone abnormalities. Bone is a living tissue containing osteoblasts and osteoclasts. Normally the activities of these cells are balanced. Any process that disturbs the normal balance of bone production and resorption can produce an abnormality on bone scan. Increased osteoblastic activity is associated with greater concentration of radionuclide tracer on the bone scan. Interruption of blood flow to the bone results in the absence of tracer on the scan (cold spot). Interruption of metabolic activity also results in decreased activity on the bone scan. In addition to blood flow to the bone, a number of other factors affect the distribution of radionuclide in the normal adult skeleton. Bone turnover is an important factor. In children, the epiphyseal and metaphyseal growth plates are sites of active bone turnover in areas of increased radionuclide concentration. In adults, the metaphyses of long bones may show more activity than the diaphysis. Other factors, including the surface adsorption to bone, diffusion of tracer within bone tissue, and ion exchange between ionic tracers and the ions within the bone, also play a role.

The most commonly used radiopharmaceutical for bone scanning is technetium 99m (^{99m}Tc). This radiopharmaceutical is ideal for bone scans. It has a half-life of 6 hours, emits gamma rays, but has low radiation exposure, approximately 150 mrads.[29] The ^{99m}Tc compounds used for bone imaging are phosphates (inorganic compounds) or phosphonates (organic compounds). The phosphates have a greater propensity for protein binding, whereas diphosphonates are chemically more stable.[99] Examples of these compounds are methylene diphosphate or ethylene hydroxydiphosphonate. Pertechnetate may also be attached to technetium and may be used for radionuclide angiographic studies of bone. ^{99m}Tc pertechnetate binds primarily to serum albumin and is taken up rapidly by organs with increased blood flow.[136] Bone scan images must be taken within 5 to 15 minutes after injection of pertechnetate to allow this effect to be seen.

Bone scan images should be taken at variable times following injection of radionuclide. The most useful study is a form of three-phase scan that involves an immediate blood pool image that is obtained by sequential images 3 to 5 seconds apart. Images are then obtained after several minutes, at 2 to 4 hours after injection, and occasionally at 24 hours to detect residual increase of bone activity. In elderly osteoporotic patients, scintigraphy may be delayed until 72 hours to allow time for a measurable osteoblastic response that can be detected by the scan.

The normal bone scan image depends on the response of normal bone to mechanical pressure, the thickness of bone, and the excretion of 50% of the radionuclide in the kidney and bladder (Fig. 7-13). On the anterior view, nor-

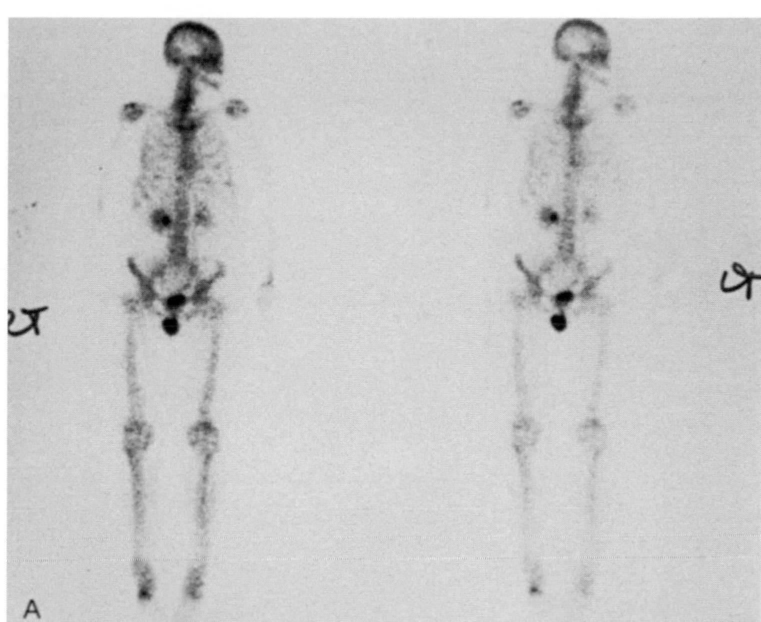

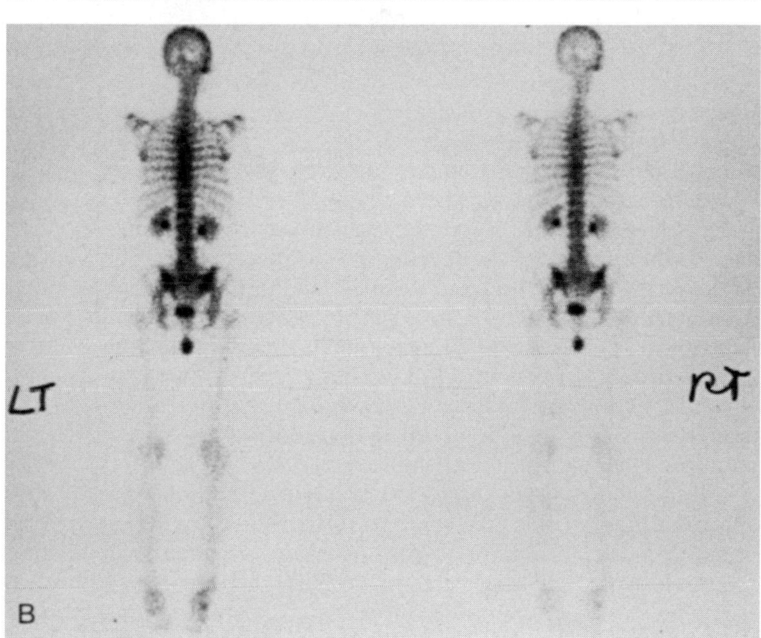

Figure 7-13 Normal bone scan using ^{99m}Tc methylene diphosphate. *A*, Anterior view—early image *(right)*, late image *(left)*. *B*, Posterior view—early image *(right)*, late image *(left)*.

mal concentrations of radionuclide are visible over the calvarium, facial bones, sternum, humeral heads, acromioclavicular joints, pelvis (particularly iliac wings), bladder and, to a lesser degree, the knees and ankles. On the posterior view the calvarium, axial spine, kidneys, and sacroiliac joints are prominent. Bone scans of reduced quality may occur secondary to dehydration, marked obesity, therapeutic agents (e.g., corticosteroids), increased age (patients > 30 years of age have progressively diminished uptake), and defective radionuclide preparations.[141]

In the clinical situation, radionuclide imaging is a useful technique for screening the entire skeletal system for abnormal activity. A bone scan is particularly useful in circumstances of radiographic changes lagging behind increased bone activity. The bone scan has been used most commonly for detecting metastatic disease (Fig 7-14). Approximately 80% of metastatic lesions are found in the axial skeleton.[79] From 10% to 40% of patients with metastatic disease with normal radiographs have abnormalities on bone scan, including areas that are painless.[32] One notable exception to early detection of metastatic bone lesions by bone scan is multiple myeloma. The neoplastic plasma cells do not induce an osteoblastic response by bone. Therefore, the lytic lesions of myeloma do not cause increased activity on bone scan until a fracture occurs.[143]

A lack of correlation between radiographic findings and bone scan activity also occurs in osteomyelitis. Radiographs may not be positive for 10 to 14 days after the onset of the disease, whereas the bone scan may be abnormal within the first day.[51] Radionuclide bone imaging is also useful for detecting the early stages of septic arthritis.

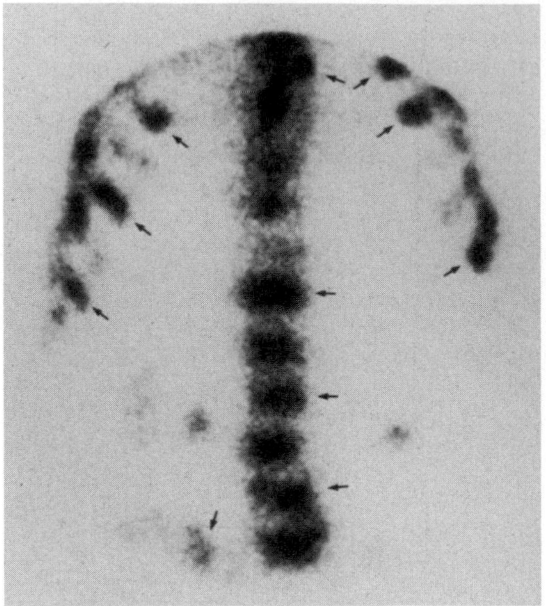

Figure 7-14 ^{99m}Tc methylene diphosphate bone scan of a 70-year-old man with metastatic prostate carcinoma. Increased uptake is noted in the ribs, vertebral column, and pelvis *(black arrows)*.

The bone scan images demonstrate increased activity in blood flow, and delayed static scans before radiographs show changes in infection other than capsular distention.

Trauma to bone, particularly stress fractures, may be difficult to detect by conventional radiography. Bone scintigraphy can detect lesions within 3 days of fracture. Activity at the fracture site may remain increased for an extended period but with a diminishing level of intensity on scan. The older the fracture, the milder the increase in uptake. This fact may be useful in determining the age of compression fractures of the spine.[77]

Generalized bone disease associated with metabolic abnormalities is often associated with diffuse increased uptake on bone scan. Bone scan is more sensitive than radiography in the detection of primary hyperparathyroidism, renal osteodystrophy, and osteomalacia. Osteoporosis is associated with a normal bone scan, unless a compression fracture has occurred.[37]

Arthritis may be detected by bone scan. Noninflammatory joint disease (osteoarthritis) is associated with osteoblastic activity in the form of sclerosis and osteophyte formation. Inflammatory arthropathies are associated with increased blood flow and increased activity on bone scan. The bone scan can quantitate increased activity in portions of the sacroiliac joints in patients with spondyloarthropathies.[48]

Other diseases associated with abnormal bone scans include Paget's disease, hemoglobinopathies, and aseptic necrosis of bone. Paget's disease is a generalized disease of bone associated with increased blood flow to the bone. The correlation between plain radiographs and bone scan abnormality is close. The activity of disease is reflected in the extent of bone scan intensity of the bone lesions.

Patients with sickle cell anemia have positive bone scans. In patients with acute infarcts of bone, the bone scan may demonstrate a cold spot. Within a few days, blood flow is restored and increased uptake appears.

Osteonecrosis of bone is associated with bone death, which may occur by a number of different mechanisms. Interruption of blood flow occurs secondary to disruption of vessels, increased pressure, or intraluminal occlusion. Early in the course of this lesion, blood flow is halted and an absence of radionuclide is noted on the scan. With revascularization, reparative processes are initiated, and increased blood flow is noted.

SPECT Scan

Single-photon emission computed tomography (SPECT) bone scanning is an useful adjunct in the diagnosis of spinal disorders. When compared with two-dimensional planar imaging, SPECT offers improved image contrast and more accurate localization of lesions. SPECT scanning sections the area under study, removing activity that originated in front of and behind the area of interest. Activity can be localized to specific positions, such as the vertebral body, pedicle, spinous process, or lamina.[43] SPECT scan can identify stress fractures of the pars interarticularis that result in spondylolysis. Facet joint arthritis can be highlighted by SPECT scans. These "hot" joints are more responsive to local anesthetic injections.[33] SPECT scan can also identify the location of bony lesions in vertebrae. Lesions that affect the pedicles are a strong indicator of malignancy, whereas lesions in the apophyseal joints are more likely to be benign.[105] SPECT scan is useful in the evaluation of vertebral lesions, spondylolysis, stress fractures, facet arthritis, sacroiliitis, pseudoarthrosis, and spinal fusion status.

PET Scan

Positron emission tomography (PET) is a nuclear medicine technique that demonstrates an increased rate of aerobic glycolysis by malignant cells. With the use of a glucose analogue (^{18}F fluorodeoxyglucose), tumor uptake is associated with increased metabolic activity. The increase in metabolic activity occurs prior to anatomic structural changes.[7] PET scans are utilized to the greatest degree to differentiate individuals with non-small cell lung cancer from those with benign solitary lung nodules. PET is also used to evaluate lymphoma, melanoma, and colorectal cancer. This technique will become more important in the diagnosis of spinal disorders as the scanners become available and increasingly discriminating.[52]

In general, radionuclide imaging is a useful technique for the evaluation of bone abnormalities in patients with neck or back pain. Although the bone scan is a highly sensitive test, the resolution of the image is relatively low. It also has less specificity than other radiographic techniques for diagnosing pathologic processes affecting the axial skeleton. With the advent of SPECT and PET scans, the localization of increased metabolic activity on bone scans may be more readily possible.

MYELOGRAPHY

The myelogram is the benchmark for evaluating neural compression within the spinal canal. The technique of spinal myelography consists of injecting radiopaque contrast media into the subarachnoid space and maneuvering this material into the appropriate spinal region under fluoroscopic guidance. Radiographs are then taken with the dye in the cervical or lumbar spine in the AP lateral and oblique planes. The flow characteristics and defects in the dye column of contrast material are observed fluoroscopically and then permanently recorded on images, using spot film techniques. Lumbar myelography may be performed with the patient hospitalized or on an outpatient basis. In most circumstances, a water-soluble, nonionic contrast medium is injected via a small, 22-gauge lumbar puncture needle. Approximately 10 to 15 mL of dye is injected.

Procedure

There are several contrast media available for myelography. When the technique was first developed, Pantopaque, an oil-based dye, was used. The oil-based dyes, however, were associated with a significant rate of long-term complications, including foreign body granulomas and chronic adhesive arachnoiditis.[116] Water-soluble contrast media, such as metrizamide, essentially eliminated the long-term complications but are associated with a few short-term side effects, including seizure activity.[104] Nonionic water-based contrast agents, such as iohexol, are associated with the fewest numbers of side effects and are being used routinely, often on an outpatient basis.[130]

The contrast material may be instilled into the subarachnoid space by either lumbar or lateral C1–C2 puncture. The lateral cervical route allows direct injection of contrast media into the cervical spinal canal; as a result, lower concentrations and a lower total dose of iodine may be used. The lateral C1–C2 puncture is somewhat more painful and hazardous than lumbar puncture.[53,91,92] For these reasons fluoroscopic-guided lumbar puncture is frequently recommended, using a 22-gauge needle and 10 mL of contrast media in 200 to 300 mg of iodine/mL concentration. The radiographs generally need to be completed within 20 to 30 minutes after the injection of dye to avoid dilution.

Certain precautions are necessary before and after myelography. Any drugs that lower seizure thresholds (e.g., phenothiazine derivatives) should be discontinued for 48 hours before the procedure. Patients with epilepsy should be maintained on their anticonvulsants. Patients should not eat for 4 hours before the procedure.

After the procedure patients should be in a semi-sitting position in bed for several hours. After that initial period the patient may lie down in bed, with the head raised 10 degrees. This helps prevent contrast material reaching the upper subarachnoid space. The most common complication is headache in 68% of patients. Nausea and vomiting occur in 38%, back pain in 26%, and seizures in 0.4%.[6] The complications with iohexol are less frequent, but if they occur they may be treated with analgesics along with caffeine, antiemetics, intravenous fluids, and intravenous diazepam for acute seizures.

Myelographic Findings

Neural compression shows up as a defect in the dye column. The possible locations for lesions are extradural, intradural-extramedullary, or intramedullary. A prime example of an extradural lesion is a herniated nucleus pulposus (Fig. 7-15). Other extradural lesions include osteophytes, abscesses, tumors, and hematomas. Neurofibromatosis causes intradural-extramedullary lesions, as do arachnoiditis and infection. Intramedullary lesions include spinal cord tumors, vascular malformations, and syringomyelia. Extradural lesions push the cord and subarachnoid space away from their normal course and interrupt the column of contrast material. Intradural-extramedullary lesions push the cord away from the dura. Intramedullary tumors cause expansion of the cord with symmetrical obliteration of the subarachnoid space.

The normal myelogram of the lumbar spine consists of one frontal, one lateral, and two oblique projections. The frontal view demonstrates the cauda equina and the nerve roots exiting along the inferior surface of the pedicles. The oblique view highlights the nerve roots surrounded by the nerve root sheath (Fig. 7-16). The lateral radiograph in the prone position shows the relationship of the subarachnoid space and dura to the posterior portions of the vertebral bodies and intervertebral discs. It should be remembered that the caudal limit of the subarachnoid spaces varies in position. It may end at the L5–S1 disc interspace or at the S3 level. At the L5–S1 interspace the interposition of epidural fat between the subarachnoid and vertebral bodies may limit the utility of myelography in detecting an L5–S1 disc herniation.

Like all diagnostic studies in the spine, the myelogram should be employed as a confirmatory study. An abnormal myelogram without substantiating historical and physical findings is not meaningful. It has been shown that 21% of asymptomatic people have an abnormal cervical myelogram (with Pantopaque contrast material) and 24% have an abnormal lumbar myelogram.[55] The experienced spine surgeon usually reserves the myelogram for preoperative assurance to confirm the location of the damaged disc or to check for congenitally anomalous nerve root tumor or double disc. If the myelogram is used as a screening test in the absence of objective clinical findings, exploratory surgery and disaster are the frequent results. Furthermore, patients who undergo a myelogram without positive physical findings (nerve root tension sign, motor weakness, or sensory deficit) are reported to have a significantly higher chance of developing side effects from the procedure itself (nausea, vomiting, or increased pain).

A particular advantage of the myelogram is that in addition to evaluating the cervical or lumbar spine, it can also evaluate the adjacent thoracic spine. Whereas the major advantage of myelography is that it provides visualization of the entire length of the cervical canal up to the level of the foramen magnum, as well as the remainder of the spine if necessary, the major disadvantage is its invasive

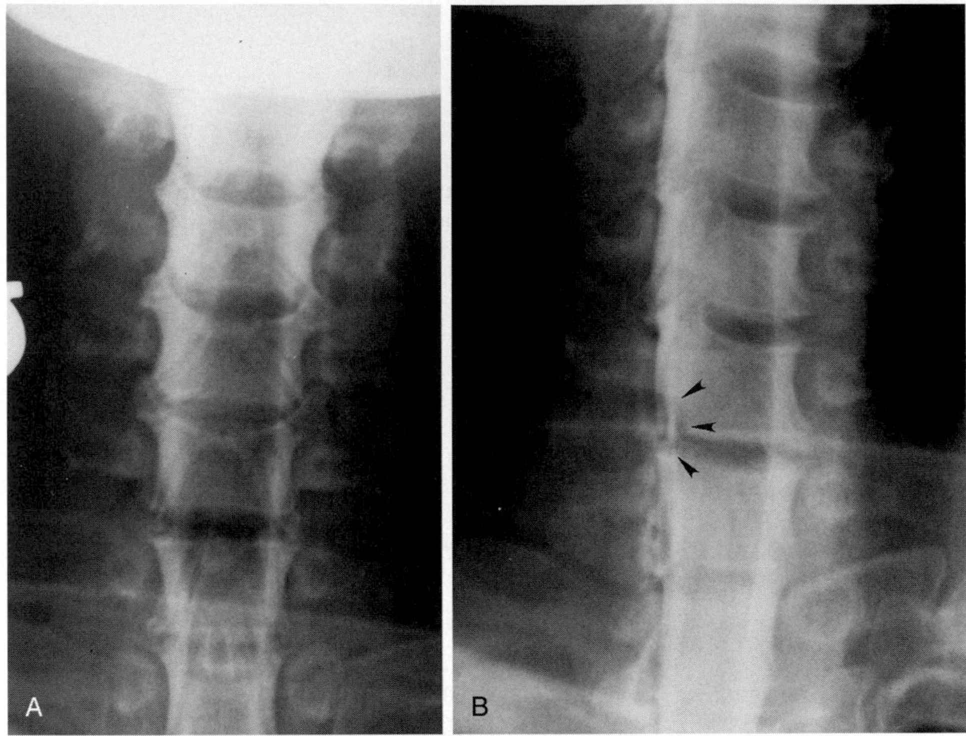

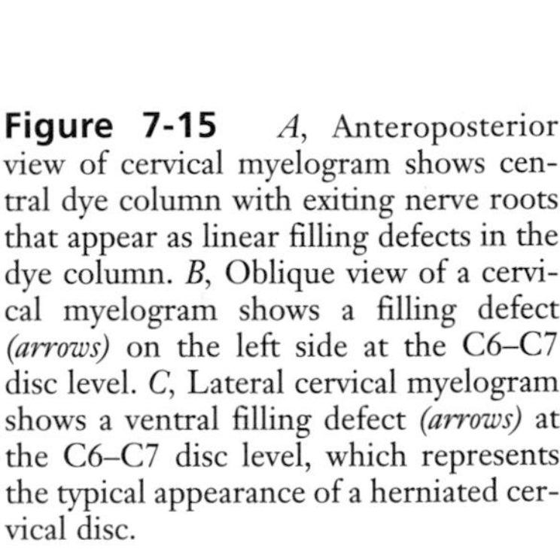

Figure 7-15 *A*, Anteroposterior view of cervical myelogram shows central dye column with exiting nerve roots that appear as linear filling defects in the dye column. *B*, Oblique view of a cervical myelogram shows a filling defect *(arrows)* on the left side at the C6–C7 disc level. *C*, Lateral cervical myelogram shows a ventral filling defect *(arrows)* at the C6–C7 disc level, which represents the typical appearance of a herniated cervical disc.

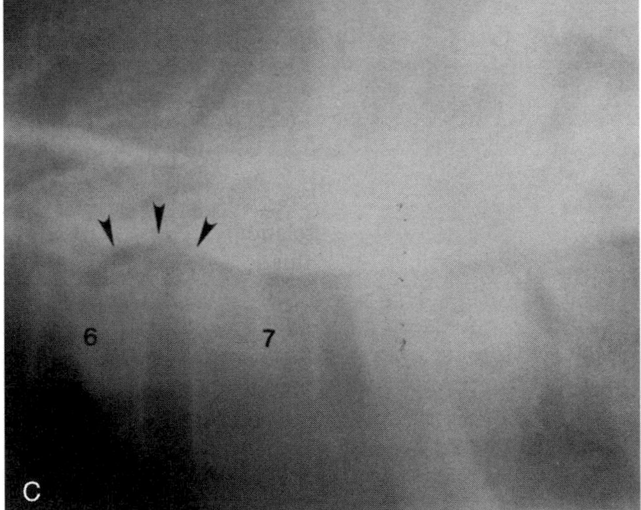

nature and, to some extent, its lack of diagnostic specificity. Accuracy rates for water-soluble nonionic cervical myelography in the diagnosis of nerve root compression range between 67% and 92%.[23,55,86,120] Difficulties in diagnostic accuracy can occur with small central disc protrusions. In addition, making the distinction between hard discs (bony spurs) and soft discs (herniations) can be difficult with the use of myelography alone. The metrizamide myelogram compares favorably with the CT scan in specificity and sensitivity as regards the diagnosis of herniated lumbar discs. A group of patients with surgically confirmed pathology of herniated lumbar discs underwent both preoperative metrizamide myelograms and CT scans. Each test was then evaluated by a neuroradiologist blinded to the patient's symptoms. Results indicated that myelography was more accurate than CT by 83% versus 72%.[10]

The use of myelography in combination with CT provides increased visualization of neural compression and its relation to the bony elements of the spine.

COMPUTED TOMOGRAPHY

CT has become extremely useful for evaluating abnormalities of the axial skeleton where the spatial anatomy is complex. CT creates cross-sectional images of the internal structure of the spine at various levels, and, with reformatting, one can also obtain coronal and sagittal sections. The CT scan assesses not only the bony configuration and structure-space relationship but also the soft tissue in graded shadings so that ligaments, nerve roots, free fat, and intervertebral disc protrusions can be evaluated as they

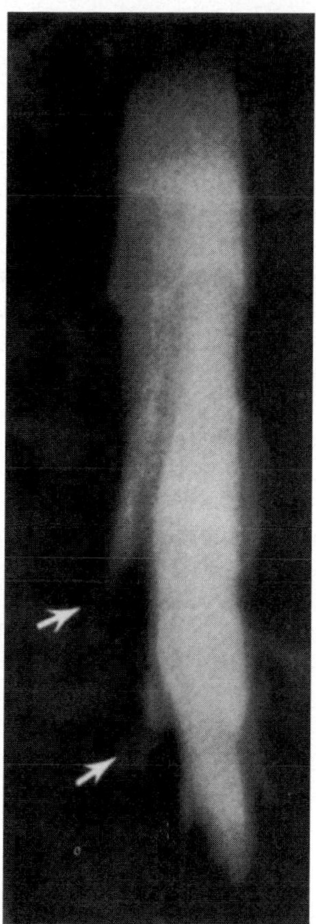

Figure 7-16 Example of a myelogram. An oblique view demonstrating nerve root sleeves (sheaths) *(arrows)* containing the exiting nerve roots (the linear filling defects) during a metrizamide myelogram. *(From Resnick D, Niwayama G: Diagnosis of Bone and Joint Disorders. Philadelphia, WB Saunders, 1981.)*

relate to their bony environment in a single scan. CT also permits excellent visualization of paraspinal soft tissues.

A CT image is produced by passing a tightly collimated beam of x-rays produced in an x-ray tube through the patient's body, which absorbs or attenuates portions of the beam to varying degrees, depending on the initial intensity of the beam and the density of the structures encountered. The attenuated beam is then picked up by a detector, amplified, and quantitated as electric signals that are then manipulated by a computer to produce the resulting image.

A CT/myelogram is a CT examination of the axial skeleton performed after intrathecal instillation of contrast media. The presence of radiopaque contrast media in the subarachnoid space significantly improves the diagnostic value of the CT examination, which can be performed either as an adjunct to standard myelography or as the primary procedure using lower dosages (3 to 5 mL) and lower concentrations (170 to 180 mg of iodine/mL) of contrast material. Using lower dosages of contrast media provides a safer method of studying patients on an outpatient basis. Although it has been shown that the anatomy of the neural foramina and contents may be demonstrated by conventional high-resolution CT, the addition of intrathecal contrast material allows the demonstration of swollen nerve roots and quantitative analysis of cord compression, which increases the specificity of this diagnostic modality.[5,97]

As opposed to bone scintigraphy, which generates a survey of the entire skeleton on one view, the CT scan is able to assess only one cross-sectional cut of the skeleton per view. Lesions that are not contained in the plane will not be viewed by the CT scanner. The scanner can be programmed to make axial cuts at varying distances. The usual amount required for the cervical spine is 2 to 3 mm in thickness because of the small size of the anatomic structures. In the lumbar spine, axial cuts are typically 5 mm in thickness.

CT of the Cervical Spine

A CT section of the cervical spine contains different anatomic structures, depending on the level of the cross section (Fig. 7-17). A scan through the superior portion of the vertebral body shows the transverse and spinous processes, laminae, inferior articular process of the cephalad vertebra, superior articular process of the caudad vertebra, pedicles, and vertebral body. A view in the middle of the vertebral body demonstrates cancellous bone in the center of the vertebral body along with pedicles and laminae—a complete bony ring of the spinal canal. The intervertebral foramina are shown in a view of the lower third of the vertebra. A section through the intervertebral disc demonstrates the inferior articular process of the cephalad vertebra and superior articular process of the caudad vertebra, the spinous process, and the intervertebral disc.

The significant advantage of the CT scan over the myelogram as a radiographic technique in evaluation of the cervical spine is not its resolution of structures but its ability to define the spatial relationships of the anatomic structures. CT is helpful in evaluation of spinal stenosis, infections with paraspinal abscesses, postsurgical epidural scarring, facet and uncovertebral joint arthritis, primary metastatic tumors of the cervical spine, and trauma to the spinal column. The facet joints and the size of the spinal canal are readily examined. CT can also visualize the medullary portion of the vertebral body and detect bone destruction before changes are visible on plain roentgenograms.

CT is particularly useful in the diagnosis and assessment of trauma because the patient is stationary during the procedure, limiting the hazards of moving the patient. Small fragments of bone that may not be detectable by plain roentgenogram are easy to localize on CT scan. Furthermore, evaluation of the craniocervical and cervicothoracic junctions is difficult on a plain roentgenogram but becomes quite clear on the CT examination.

The clinical significance of CT/myelographic findings in cervical spondylosis was studied by Penning and colleagues.[101] A 100% correlation was found between the site of disc herniation with an occlusion of the intervertebral foramen and the site of nerve root symptoms. Long-tract signs were noted after the cross-sectional area of the spinal cord had been reduced by 30% to a value of about 60 mm^2 or less. Penning and colleagues also noted that in the presence of a normal conventional plain film myelogram, post-CT/myelographic studies were superfluous. CT investigations in these cases may lead to false-positive interpretation of clinically irrelevant findings.

Reported accuracy rates for CT range from 72% to 91%.[23,34,69,86,88,120] Agreement rates between contrast-enhanced CT and myelography have been reported to range from 75% to 96%.[69,86,88] When a discrepancy exists between myelographic and CT findings, post-contrast CT is invariably the more accurate study.

CT of the Lumbosacral Spine

Careful study has revealed the potential pitfalls of making clinical decisions based on lumbar spine CT scan findings isolated from the patient's complete clinical picture.[139] CT scans of the lumbar area of 53 normal subjects with no history of back trouble and of 6 with back pain were submitted to three neuroradiologists who were unaware of the subjects' symptoms. Of the scans reviewed, 34.5% were read as abnormal and there was agreement among the interpreters in only 11% of the cases. The implication is that a patient with no history and physical findings indicative of spinal pathology has a 1 in 3 chance of having an abnormal CT scan. If a major therapeutic decision (to perform surgery) is made based only on the scan results, there is a 30% chance that the patient will be considered for unnecessary surgery. However, if the patient's history and physical findings correlate with the imaging findings of spine pathology, the CT scan frequently can be a helpful confirming diagnostic tool. The CT scan has the great advantage of being noninvasive and safely administered as an outpatient procedure. The radiation associated with a CT scan is 3 to 5 rads (see Table 7-1). Radiation exposure is increased with high-resolution, slow-speed scanning.

The CT scan is able to assess only one slice of the skeleton per view. Lesions that are not contained in the plane will not be viewed by the CT scanner. The machine takes slices every 0.5 cm. It is important to tell the radiologist which area of the skeleton needs to be examined so that the duration of the test and exposure of the patient to radiation are limited.

A CT image of the lumbar spine contains different anatomic structures depending on the level of the cross section (Fig. 7-18). A scan through the superior portion of the L4 vertebral body shows the transverse and spinous processes, laminae, inferior facet of L3, superior facet of L4, pedicles, and vertebral body (Fig. 7-19). A view in the middle of the vertebra demonstrates cancellous bone in the vertebral body along with the normal bone defect in the center of the posterior surface of the vertebral body caused by the basivertebral veins, pedicles, and laminae—a complete bony ring of the spinal canal (Fig. 7-20). The intervertebral foramina are shown in a view of the lower third of L4 (Fig. 7-21). A section through the interverte-

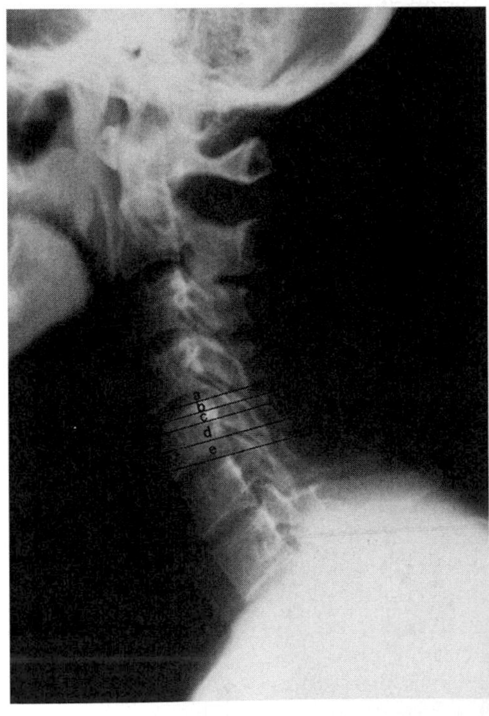

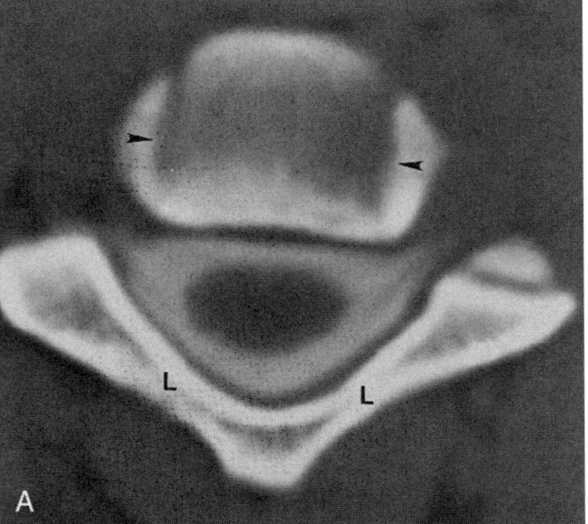

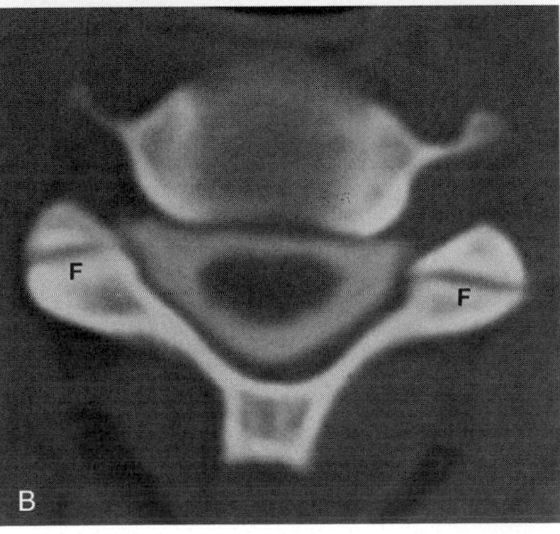

Figure 7-17 Myelogram and CT scan of a normal cervical spine. The lateral radiograph shows the linear cuts at the level of the vertebral body corresponding to the five cuts shown (a–e), which demonstrate the normal anatomy at each of the various levels. *A*, This axial cut through the level of the intervertebral disc space shows the spinal cord surrounded by the dye in the subarachnoid space anteriorly. The uncovertebral joints can be seen *(arrows)* posterior to the spinal canal. The lamina (L) can be seen. *B*, This axial cut just distal to the intervertebral joint space shows the top of the vertebral body and the beginning of the transverse processes. In addition, the facet joints (F) can be seen on each side as well as the foramen and exiting nerve roots.

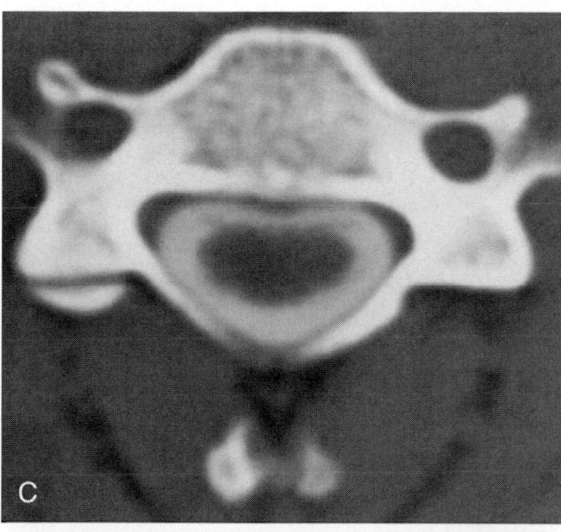

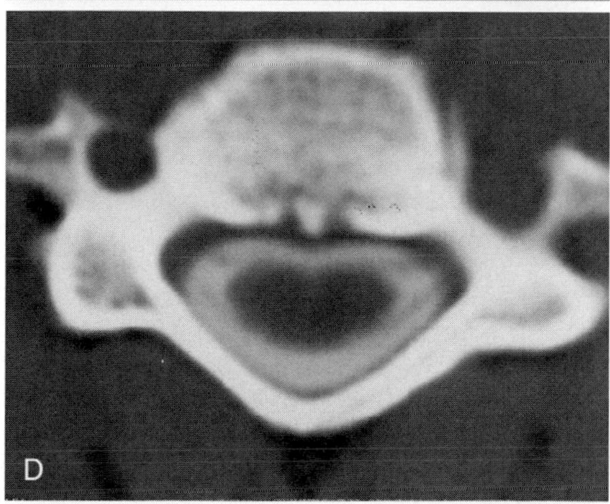

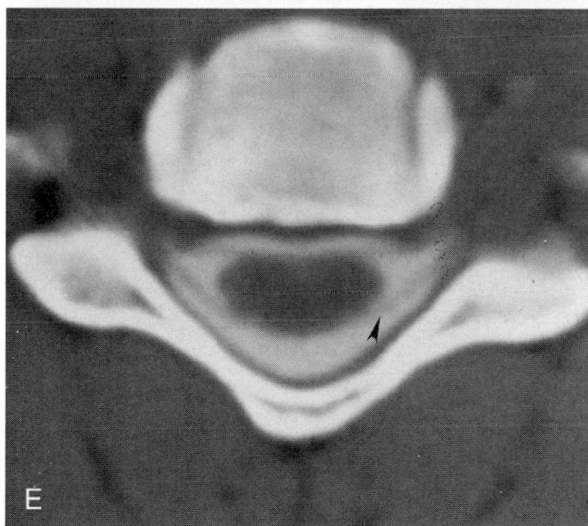

Figure 7-17, cont'd *C,* This axial cut through the midportion of the vertebral body shows the transverse process and the foramen transversarium, which contain the vertebral arteries on either side. *D,* This cut is at the lower third of the vertebral body and shows the inferior portion of the transverse process. *E,* This cut is at the inferiormost portion of the vertebral body bordering on the intervertebral disc space, again showing the uncovertebral joints. On this image the exiting spinal rootlets, both anterior and posterior, can be seen as a linear filling defect in the subarachnoid dye column *(arrow).*

bral disc demonstrates the inferior facet of L4, the superior facet of L5, the spinous process, and the intervertebral disc (Fig. 7-22).

Degenerative enlargement of facet joints may produce symptoms of spinal stenosis and is readily examined by

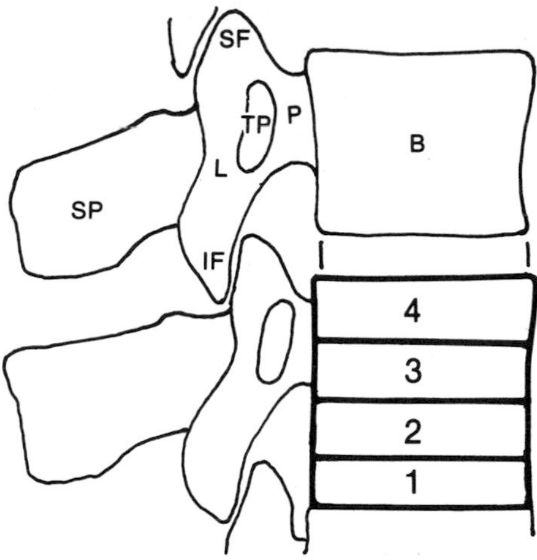

Figure 7-18 The four basic CT sections of the lumbar spine. The structures imaged by the scan include the spinous process (SP), inferior articular facet (IF), laminae (L), transverse process (TP), superior articular facet (SF), pedicle (P), and body (B).

CT.[21,129] CT scan can visualize the medullary portion of the vertebral body and can detect bone destruction before changes are visible on plain roentgenograms.[61] CT with or without contrast agent can detect the presence of epidural fibrosis, which can be differentiated from a recurrent herniated nucleus pulposus.[126] CT scan is able to visualize the sacroiliac joint in patients with sacroiliitis. This technique can be used with patients whose conventional

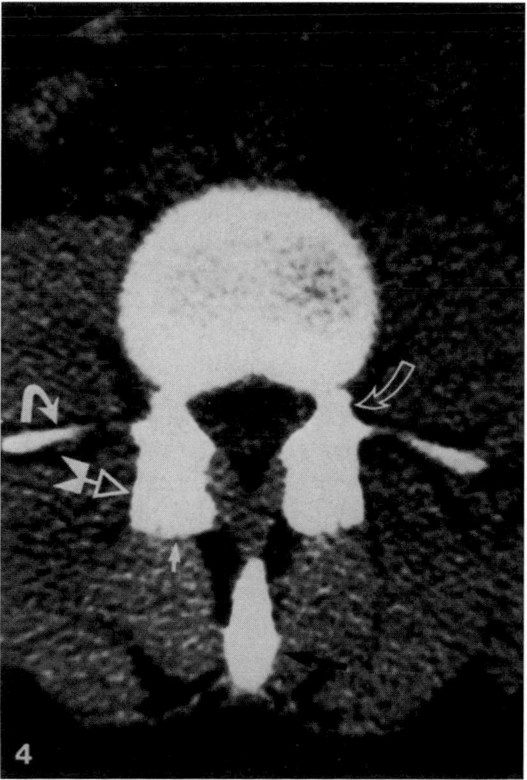

Figure 7-19 Section 4 contains the superior third of the vertebral body, the pedicles *(open curved arrow),* the transverse processes *(curved arrow),* the superior facets *(arrow with tail),* the spinous process *(black arrow),* and the inferior facet of the next higher vertebra *(short arrow).*

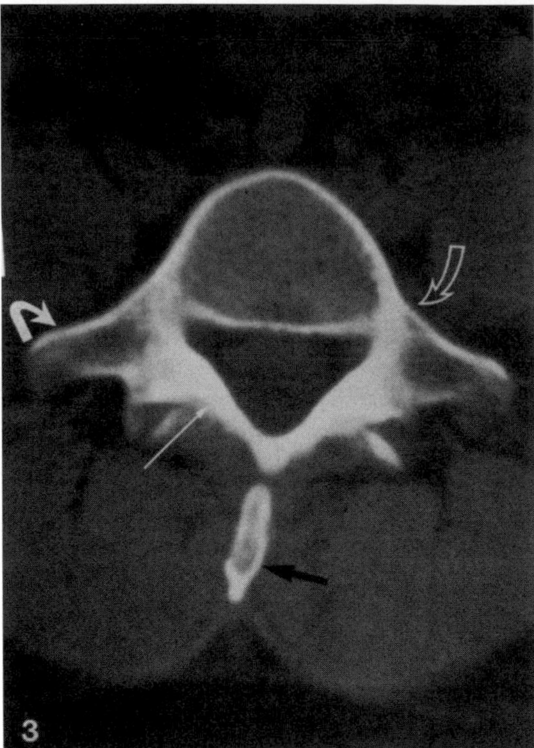

Figure 7-20 Section 3 contains the middle third of the vertebral body, the pedicles *(open curved arrow)*, the laminae *(long arrow)*, and the spinous process *(black arrow)*.

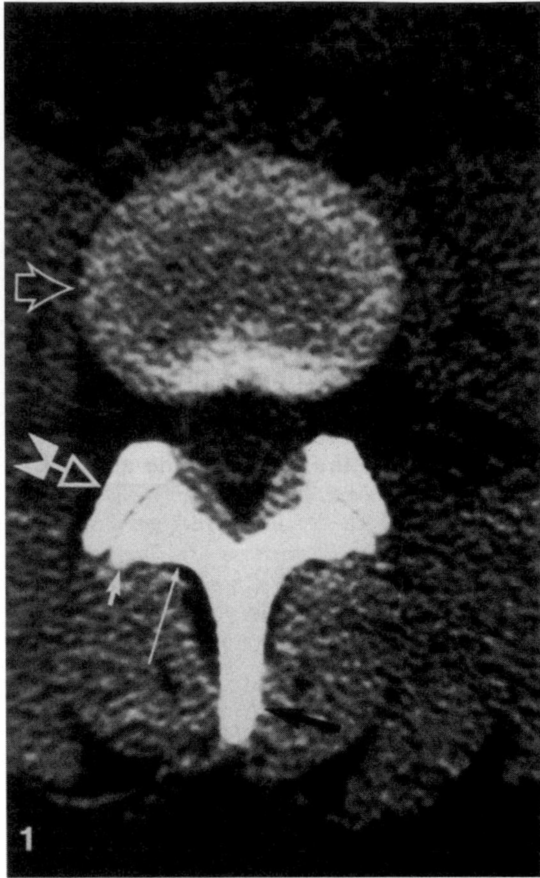

Figure 7-22 Section 1 contains the intervertebral disc *(open white arrow)* and the facet joints. The imaged osseous structures include the superior facet of the vertebra below the disc *(arrow with tail)* and the inferior facet *(short arrow)*, the laminae *(long arrow)*, and the spinous process *(black arrow)* of the vertebra above the disc.

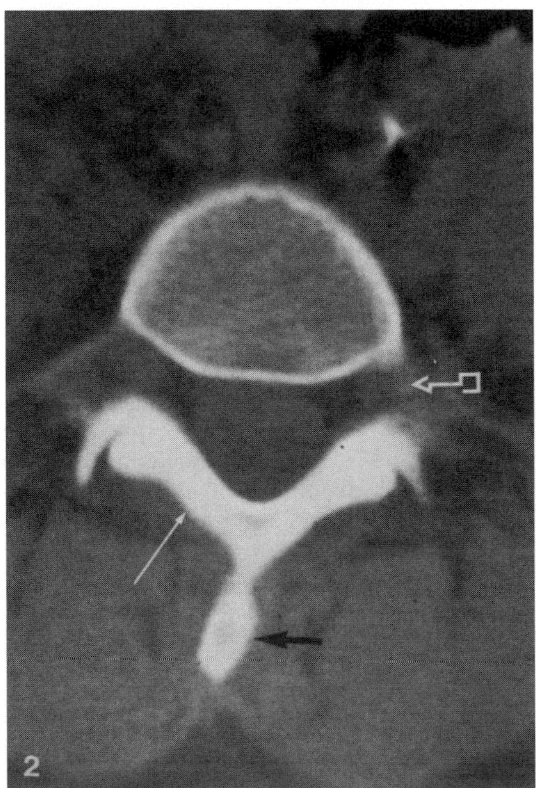

Figure 7-21 Section 2 contains the lower third of the vertebral body, the neural foramina and nerve roots *(arrow with square)*, the laminae *(long arrow)*, and the spinous process *(black arrow)*.

roentgenograms of the sacroiliac joints reveal equivocal findings of arthritis.[20]

CT is useful in the diagnosis of tumors of the lumbosacral spine for localizing the lesion, determining the intramedullary and extraosseous extent of the tumor, and defining its relationship with surrounding vital structures.[74] Plain roentgenographs may be better for spatial resolution but are unable to detect soft tissue extension. CT scan also may be able to detect intramedullary bone loss from multiple myeloma, for example, which may not be detectable by plain roentgenograms or bone scintiscan.

CT is useful in the diagnosis and assessment of trauma since the patient is stationary during the procedure, limiting the hazards of moving the patient. Fragments of bone that may not be detectable by plain roentgenograms are localized to the spinal canal by CT techniques.[24]

The use of myelography as an adjunct to the CT scan can significantly improve the assessment of neural compression. CT scan immediately following myelography allows an axial view with intrathecal contrast highlighting the precise edge of the dural sac. Bone or soft tissue can be evaluated in light of the degree of neural impingement on the dye column.[131]

The question of the ability of CT to identify a clinically significant herniated nucleus pulposus without the aid of a myelogram has not been answered. CT scans detect intervertebral discs that have expanded into the spinal canal. The CT can also identify compression of the dural sac, spinal nerves, root ganglia, and spinal veins. CT may be particularly helpful for lateral disc herniation beyond the dural sleeve, which may not cause an impression on the contrast column of the myelogram. Whether CT can totally replace the myelogram as the diagnostic test for herniated disc remains to be determined, but their use together exceeds the value of either alone.[140]

Axial CT scan data can be reconstructed into a three-dimensional image. Software technology produces an image of surface anatomy. The three-dimensional CT image adds no additional data, but it may allow greater appreciation of pathologic alterations to vertebrae, including neural foraminal narrowing.

Helical CT is the technique that allows for the continuous spiral motion of the x-ray gantry tube. This technique has been utilized for the diagnosis of abdominal and pulmonary disorders, including small bowel obstruction, appendicitis, ureteral colic, and pulmonary emboli and deep venous thrombosis, respectively. Helical CT is not used for the evaluation of spinal disorders. However, for detection of viscerogenic causes of low back pain, helical CT is an effective diagnostic tool. For example, helical CT imaging surpasses conventional roentgenograms for detection of ureteral stones. The techniques may also identify nonurinary causes of abdominal pain, including intestinal obstruction.[114]

MAGNETIC RESONANCE IMAGING

MR imaging is a diagnostic technique that displays small differences in tissue density with sharp contrast without exposing the patient to radiation or contrast material. MR has been clinically available since the middle 1980s. Since then, MR has been used increasingly for evaluation of the musculoskeletal system, including low back and neck pain.[98,112] MR has become the diagnostic imaging procedure of choice for certain disorders, including infection, disc herniations, and intramedullary tumors of the spinal cord. MR technology, owing to both hardware and software algorithmic manipulations, continues to be refined to decrease acquisition time of the scans and increase the spatial resolution.

The basic principle behind MR imaging involves the generation of a magnetic field by the nuclei of atoms with an odd number of protons. When placed between the poles of a strong magnet (up to 20,000 times the earth's magnetic field), the protons line up between the magnetic poles and vibrate at a frequency specific to each type of atom. Transmitting radio waves equal to the specific frequency of the target atoms and directed at a right angle to the static magnetic field causes the atoms to vibrate at an angle away from the vertical orientation. When the transmission of the radio waves is discontinued, the protons return to a state of relaxation (vertical position) by releasing radio waves. The radio waves generated by the atoms are detected by radio antennas, and the information is analyzed by computer to generate cross-sectional images of the body. Variations in proton density, radio frequency, and the time to return to a state of relaxation (relaxation time) modify the image produced by the MR scanner.

Proton density refers to the number of nuclei per unit volume of the structure to be examined. The most commonly measured atom is hydrogen. The hydrogen in water generates a different amplitude of MR image if it is loosely bound to tissue molecules than if tightly bound to specific molecules. Therefore, the amount and binding of water in the target tissue have a direct effect on the image generated by the MR scanner.

The proton relaxation times also play a major role in the generation of the MR image. When the aligned protons are deflected by the radio wave, they achieve a level of increased excitation by their axes spinning in the shape of a cone. The time it takes for the proton to regain its magnetization in its vertical position is the T1 relaxation time. The time it takes for the proton to lose its magnetization in the horizontal plane is the T2 relaxation time. It is possible to change the pulse sequences of radio waves to accentuate differences in T1 and T2 relaxation times. The weighting of the images to T1 or T2 relaxation time has a marked effect on the appearance of the MR image. With T1-weighted images, nerve tissue is white and cerebrospinal fluid (CSF) is gray. CSF is white and nerve tissue is gray in T2-weighted images.

The MR scan includes a sagittal and axial view of the cervical spine, frequently with T1 and T2 or some equivalent weighted image. Patients who are on life-support systems (metal machines) or who have cardiac pacemakers or metal clips on intracranial aneurysms are not suitable candidates for MR imaging: Pacemakers may revert from the demand mode to a fixed-rate mode of operation, and metal clips may twist or loosen. Although nonferromagnetic implants, such as stainless-steel appliances, are not attracted to the magnets, these objects cause artifacts that degrade the MR image. Claustrophobic individuals may have great difficulty in the closed space on the scanner and may need to be sedated with medications such as oral diazepam to complete the study. Open MR scanners are available for those individuals made uneasy with closed-tube machines. Images from open MR scanners lack some of the detail offered by closed scanners.

MR Imaging of the Cervical Spine

The normal MR image of the cervical spine visualizes the vertebral column, intervertebral discs, spinal canal, spinal cord, and CSF in the sagittal view (Fig. 7-23). The axial views generally show the paravertebral soft tissue structures, the disc or vertebral body, the spinal canal, and the spinal cord (Fig. 7-24). The choice of relaxation times (T1 or T2) and pulse sequences as well as other parameters may be modified to highlight specific structures or produce contrast that accentuates abnormalities associated with certain pathologic states.

MR imaging is an excellent technique for viewing the spinal cord within the spinal canal. It is the preferred imaging modality for syringomyelia, cord atrophy, cord infarction, traumatic injury to the cord, and intramedullary tumors or multiple sclerosis affecting the spinal cord. MR imaging is likely to be more accurate than CT at

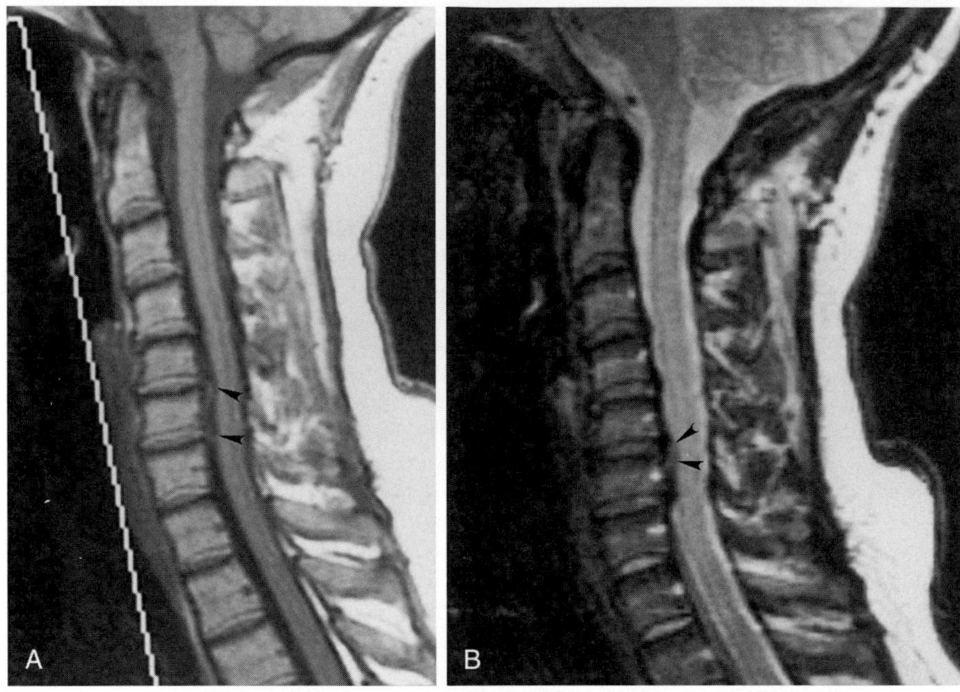

Figure 7-23 MR image of the cervical spine. *A*, T1-weighted sagittal image shows the vertebral bodies, intervertebral discs, spinal cord, and subarachnoid space. Small disc herniations are seen at C3–C4 and C4–C5. A larger disc herniation is seen at C5–C6 and C6–C7 *(arrows)*. *B*, T2-weighted sagittal image shows similar findings of a moderate herniated disc at C5–C6 *(arrows)*. Cerebrospinal fluid appears white instead of gray.

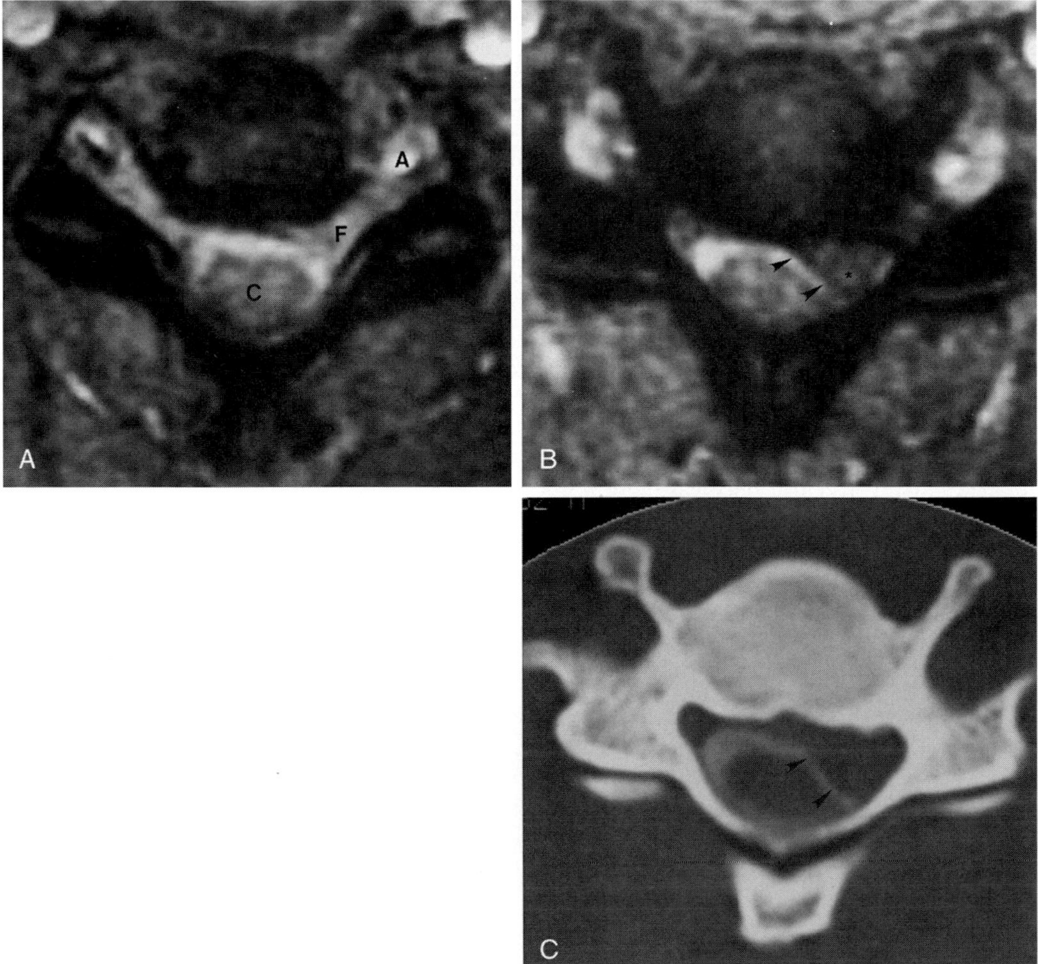

Figure 7-24 *A*, MR axial view of normal cervical level shows spinal cord (C) surrounded by cerebrospinal fluid. The bony facet joint is seen as a black area, with the disc seen at intermediate intensity, and between is the neural foramen (F) containing the exiting nerve root. Also seen are the vertebral arteries (A) in the foramen transversarium lateral to the intervertebral disc. *B*, MR axial view shows a large herniated disc (*), lateralized to the patient's left, which is causing posterolateral impression on the thecal sac *(arrows)*. *C*, CT scan of the same patient shows herniated disc and thecal sac impingement *(arrows)*.

characterizing extramedullary tumors. MR imaging delineates the extent of extradural tumor invasion of the spinal canal as well as compression or displacement of the spinal cord. It can identify the vertebral bodies in which bone marrow has been replaced with tumor.[103] It also shows early changes in discs and vertebral endplates with infectious discitis.[85] Most clinicians believe that CT scanning continues to offer better definition of the bony architecture of the spinal canal than does MR imaging (Fig. 7-25).

MR images may be obtained through traditional two-dimensional imaging or with more advanced three-dimensional acquisition techniques. Two-dimensional imaging may include the traditional spin-echo images or gradient-echo imaging techniques with partial flip angle. The difficulty, in general, with two-dimensional techniques in identifying foraminal disease is due to long echo times, thick image cuts, and the inability to view the course of the exiting nerve roots and planes other than axial. Although overall examination time tends to decrease with gradient-echo imaging, the length of examination continues to be problematic. One potential solution may be found in gradient-echo volume imaging (three-dimensional), which would allow short echo times with thin contiguous cuts and the ability to reformat the data in a desired viewing plane. Three-dimensional imaging techniques include fast low-angle shot (FLASH) and spoiled gradient recall acquisition in the steady state. Turbo-FLASH or magnetization-prepared rapid-acquisition gradient echo is a technique that uses short relaxation times and low flip angles for very rapid volume imaging. Another technique is fast imaging with steady-state precession, which can produce a hyperintense CSF signal (and a myelogram effect). In addition to providing new acquisition modalities, improved surface coils continue to increase the signal-to-noise ratio and improve the overall image quality.

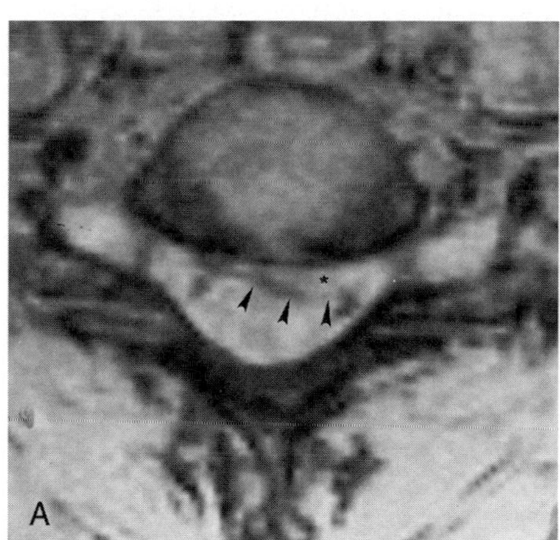

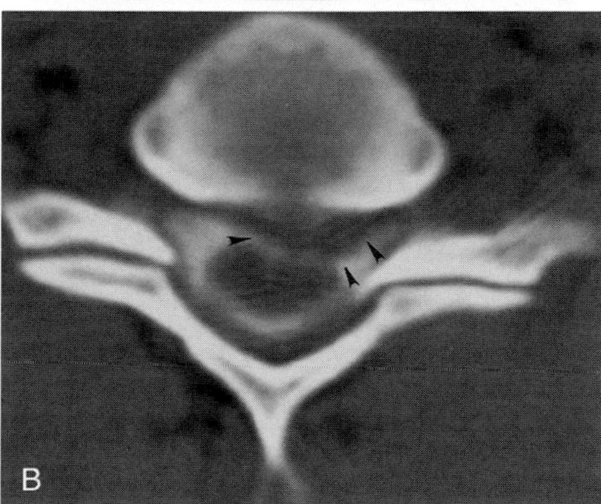

Figure 7-25 *A*, MR view shows axial posterolateral herniated disc (*) causing compression of the thecal sac and exiting nerve rootlet on the left *(arrows)*. *B*, CT/myelogram shows the same herniated disc and compression *(arrows)* of the exiting nerve rootlet on the left.

Many of the early-generation MR scanners that are still used produce what are considered to be inferior MR images. Such suboptimal images can be misleading in terms of false-positive diagnoses and can fail to detect more subtle problems. In general, a poor MR scan is worse than no MR scan, and the patient is better served with a standard myelogram followed by a high-resolution CT scan.

Two studies have documented the prevalence of degenerative changes in the cervical spine in asymptomatic subjects studied with MR imaging.[14,127] A wide variety of abnormalities were displayed in more than 20% of the asymptomatic subjects. Disc protrusion was seen in about 10% to 15% of subjects and may have increased frequency in older individuals. The prevalence of disc narrowing, disc degeneration, and spurs increased from 25% in subjects younger than 40 years of age to 60% in those older than 40 years of age.[14] Foraminal stenosis was present in 7% of subjects younger than 40 years of age and in 23% of those older than 40 years of age. Spinal cord impingement was seen in 10% to 15% of younger subjects and in 20% to 25% of older subjects. Spinal cord compression was seen in fewer than 5% and was due solely to disc protrusion. Cord area reduction averaged 7% and never exceeded 16%.[127] Thus, the cord appears to tolerate a certain amount of volume loss without demonstrating symptoms. In another study, degenerative disc disease of the cervical spine was noted to be more common in older individuals who were examined by MR imaging.[71] Degenerative disc disease begins at a later age in the cervical spine than in the lumbar region. Although asymptomatic anatomic abnormalities may be detected with MR evaluation, this technique remains the most sensitive for detecting bony and soft tissue changes in the cervical spine.[9]

MR Imaging of the Lumbosacral Spine

The normal MR of the lumbosacral spine visualizes the vertebral column, intervertebral discs, and the spinal canal along with the spinal cord in the sagittal view (Fig. 7-26). The axial view shows the paravertebral soft tissue structures, the disc or vertebral body, the spinal canal, and the spinal cord (Fig. 7-27). The choice of relaxation times (T1 or T2) and pulse sequences, among other factors, may be modified to highlight specific structures or produce contrast that accentuates abnormalities associated with certain pathologic states.

MR is an excellent technique to view the spinal cord within the spinal canal.[96] MR is the preferred imaging modality for syringomyelia, atrophy, cord infarction, traumatic injury, intramedullary tumors, or multiple sclerosis affecting the spinal cord. MR may be more accurate than CT scan at characterizing extramedullary tumors. MR

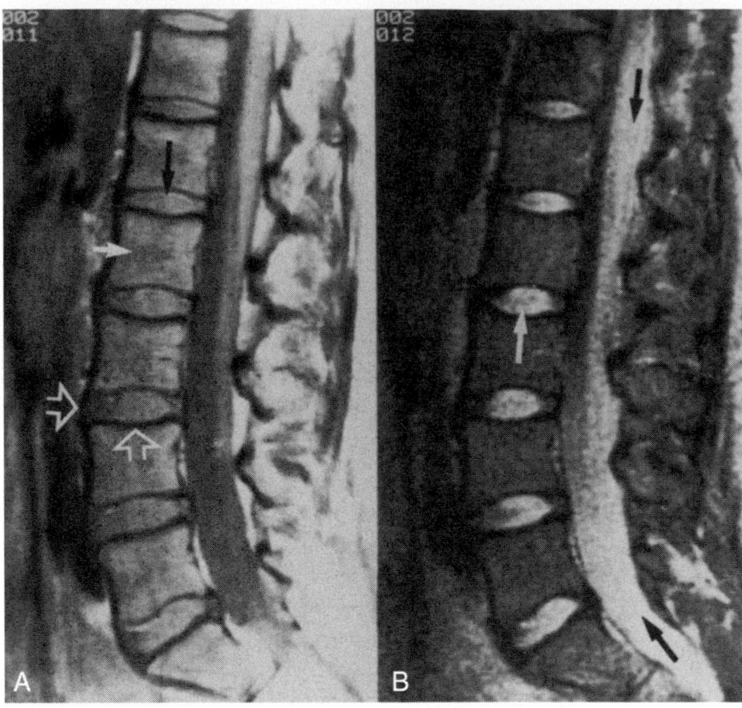

Figure 7-26 Normal MR scan of the lumbar spine, sagittal view. *A*, The T1-weighted image demonstrates bone marrow and fat as whiter structures *(white arrow)* with vertebral endplates (cortical bone) and ligaments as blacker images *(open white arrows)*. The intervertebral discs *(black arrow)* are intermediate in intensity. *B*, T2-weighted image demonstrates cerebrospinal fluid *(black arrows)* and nucleus pulposus *(white arrow)* as whiter structures. The nucleus pulposus can be separated from surrounding annular fibers and longitudinal ligaments.

delineates the extent of extradural tumor invasion of the spinal canal and compression or displacement of the spinal cord. MR can identify the vertebral bodies in which bone marrow has been replaced with tumor.[103] MR also shows early changes in discs and vertebral endplates with infectious discitis.[28] The importance of MR as a diagnostic tool for mechanical and systemic disorders has been further advanced by the availability of gadolinium-diethylenetriamine pentaacetic acid (Gd-DTPA) as an intravenous paramagnetic contrast agent. Epidural scar and recurrent herniated discs have similar appearances on unenhanced MRs. Gd-DTPA does not cross an intact blood-brain barrier. Pathologic processes (epidural scar, intramedullary tumors) that disrupt the blood-brain barrier result in leakage of Gd-DTPA and enhancement on MR.[45,73,124] CT scan continues to offer better definition of the bony architecture of the spinal canal than does MR. CT scan has been the radiographic method of choice for neural foraminal stenosis, posterior facet joint disease, and spinal stenosis.[75]

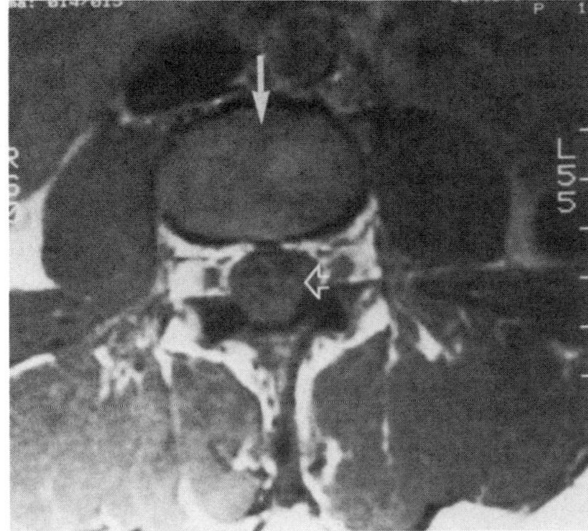

Figure 7-27 Normal MR scan of the lumbar spine, transaxial view. T1-weighted image demonstrates surrounding soft tissue structures, intervertebral disc *(white arrow)*, and the cauda equina *(open arrow)* surrounded by the spinal canal.

Numerous studies are under way to determine the sensitivity and specificity of MR in the diagnosis of lumbar spine disorders. Early studies that used MR scanners with poor resolution due to smaller magnets and body coils that did not allow thin imaging slices failed to demonstrate superiority of MR.[82] With the advent of surface coils, stronger magnets, and newer pulse sequences, MR scan resolution continues to improve and acquisition time continues to decrease. Most studies suggest that MR is more accurate in the detection of degenerative disc disease than discography or myelography.[46,137] Disc degeneration may also be associated with bone marrow changes associated with motion segment instability. Toyone and associates described the endplate and vertebral bone marrow changes associated with degenerative lumbar disc disease.[128] On T1-weighted images, decreased signal intensity was associated with thickened bony trabeculae and loss of fatty bone marrow. These individuals had hypermobility at the corresponding intervertebral space, with 27 (73%) of 37 having low back pain. Increased signal intensity was associated with fatty replacement of bone marrow. These patients had stable lumbar spine segments, with 4 (11%) of 37 having low back pain. These alterations of bone marrow content imaged by MR may permit detection of unstable segments that are sources of back pain. Albeck and colleagues compared myelography, CT, and MR imaging for the detection of lumbar disc herniations confirmed at surgery.[2] In a study of 80 patients, MR and CT supplied greater diagnostic information than myelography. MR is better at imaging soft tissue structures, whereas CT is superior for imaging bony structures.

MR has many advantages that may supersede both CT and myelography for the diagnosis of damaged discs. MR is more sensitive than CT for the diagnosis of herniated discs.[39] In 25 patients who underwent surgery at 31 levels for a herniated nucleus pulposus and who were evaluated by MR and simultaneous contrast CT scan, surgical findings supported the MR diagnosis at 28 of 31 levels (90.3% accuracy), whereas the CT diagnosis correctly reflected only 24 of 31 levels (77.4% accuracy). At 10 levels where MR and CT scanning had a discrepancy, MR was incorrect at three levels and CT scan at seven levels. This study demonstrated the superiority of MR over CT scan for evaluation of acute lumbar disc herniation.

Compared to CT, MR is at least as accurate in making the diagnosis of spinal stenosis, sequestered lumbar intervertebral discs, and far lateral disc herniation.[83,93,111] MR and contrast CT were similar in accuracy in detecting spinal stenosis in central canal, lateral recess, and foraminal locations.[111] In a retrospective study of 41 patients visualized by MR and contrast CT, a 96.6% agreement was demonstrated for level of stenosis. However, MR detected disc degeneration in 74 of 123 segments, whereas only 27 of 123 segments were designated on CT scan.

MR, especially when used with gadolinium, has clear advantages for demonstrating intraspinal tumors, detecting disc space infection, and distinguishing recurrent disc herniation from postoperative scar.[11,13,16,89] In a prospective investigation of operative low back pain patients, the greatest correlation of imaging studies (myelography, CT, MR) with surgical findings was 93%, achieved by the combination of CT and MR.[83]

As with the other diagnostic imaging modalities, MR also has been shown to have a high frequency of abnormalities in asymptomatic individuals. In a prospective, blinded study, 22% of the asymptomatic subjects younger than 60 years of age and 57% of those older than 60 years had significantly abnormal lumbar scans.[12] In addition, the prevalence of disc degeneration on the T2-weighted images was found to approach 98% in subjects older than age 60. Jensen and co-workers found only 36% of 98 asymptomatic individuals (mean age, 42.3 years) with normal lumbar MR scans.[60] Fifty-two percent had a disc bulge at one level, 27% had a protrusion, and 1% had an extrusion. Similar results were reported by Weishaupt and associates.[135] It is essential to understand the frequency and spectrum of imaging abnormalities that may exist without causing clinical symptoms to better interpret these studies in symptomatic patients. MR scans also have no value in predicting low back pain. Borenstein and colleagues reported on a 7-year follow-up of the 67 asymptomatic individuals reported by Boden in 1989.[15] A total of 50 individuals completed a questionnaire regarding the development of back pain. MR findings were not predictive of the development or duration of low back pain. Individuals with the longest duration of low-back pain did not have the greatest degree of anatomic abnormality on the 1989 scans.

MR is still a technique with continuing development. The potential for this procedure as a diagnostic tool in the evaluation of patients with neck and back problems is well established. Like CT scan, the sophistication of the radiologists using these machines will increase and the improvement in MR hardware and software will advance. For example, seated MR may more accurately simulate the pressures placed on the spine in stressed postures. Weishaupt and co-workers reported on positional MR in seated flexed and extended position in 30 individuals with disc abnormalities without neural compression.[134] Nerve root contact occurred in 34 of 152 instances in the supine position, in 62 instances in the seated flexed position, and in 45 instances in the seated extended position. Positional MR demonstrated minor neural compromise more consistently that conventional MR. However, our enthusiasm for the technique must be tempered by its high sensitivity for detecting asymptomatic as well as symptomatic spine pathology.[66] Despite the relatively high financial cost of an MR, the temptation to overuse this noninvasive imaging modality as a screening test must also be tempered.

DISCOGRAPHY

A discogram is performed by placing a fine-gauge spinal needle into the disc space, followed by injection of radiopaque dye (Fig. 7-28). The amount of dye accepted into the disc, the injection pressure, the radiographic appearance of the dye, and the reproduction of the patient's pain are important data generated during the test. Although a variety of complications are possible, disc space infection is the most common.

Since its introduction by Smith and Nichols in 1957, cervical discography has remained controversial.[118] Many authors believe the procedure has diagnostic value,[22,78,107,115,138] and others maintain that it is useless and misleading and should be discontinued altogether.[25,54,57,58,67,81,113,119,125] Advocates of the procedure state that a normal cervical disc accepts no contrast material or, at most, 0.1 to 0.2 mL. A normal lumbar disc accepts 1 to 2 mL of dye. Injection of a normal disc infrequently produces pain at the base of the neck. Injection of an abnormal disc, however, generally reproduces the type of pain and discomfort from which the patient is suffering. Injection of a local anesthetic promptly relieves this pain, which is confirmatory for the level of involvement. More than one disc is generally studied, and at least one level considered to be normal should not elicit pain and serve as a negative control level. Cervical discography may be useful in patients who present with chronic neck or radicular pain and shoulder and upper extremity pain, after noninvasive imaging has been inconclusive.[57] Unfortunately, the reliability and incidence of positive discograms in asymptomatic individuals remain a concern.[18,19]

Although some reports have suggested a close correlation among abnormal discograms, degenerative disc disease, and chronic neck or low back pain, other studies have reported little correlation between abnormal discograms and the local source of a patient's back pain.[56,115] Although a discographic study may reproduce a patient's spinal pain, results of spinal surgery for relief of back pain alone, without radicular symptoms of disc herniations caused by degenerative disease, have been unreliable.[121] A more recent study of discograms in normal, asymptomatic subjects demonstrated anatomic abnormalities in 17% of discs

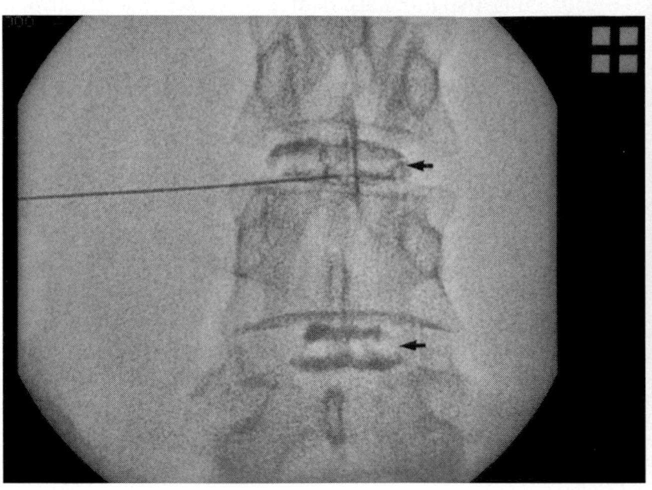

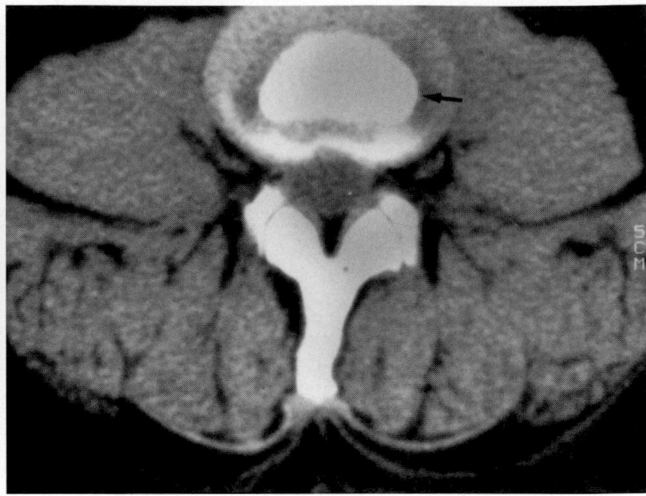

Figure 7-28 Normal discogram of a 45-year-old woman with low back pain after a fall at work. *A*, Fluoroscopic image of intradiscal dye in two intervertebral disc levels *(black arrows)*. *B*, CT scan with radiographic dye contained in an intact intervertebral disc *(black arrow)*.

examined. If pain with injection was the criterion for a positive test, only symptomatic patients had positive results. Discography revealed abnormal findings in 13 of the 20 discs studied in symptomatic individuals.[133] Discography may cause prolonged back pain as a result of the procedure. Individuals with significant emotional problems were at greater risk of having back pain 1 year after the procedure as compared to individuals with normal psychometric testing.[17] Discograms are less sensitive in identifying abnormal discs than are MR or CT. Therefore, reliance on data generated regarding the status of cervical and lumbar discs by noninvasive radiographic techniques (MR and CT) is usually adequate to define the integrity of the intervertebral space.[112] Discograms are less commonly indicated.

SPINAL ANGIOGRAPHY

Selective angiography of the blood supply to the vertebral column and spinal cord is now technically possible. Most spinal angiography is performed using mild sedation and local anesthesia. A femoral approach is used for most lumbar studies. Selective arterial catheterization is performed for vessels at least one level above and below the abnormality. Intra-arterial digital subtraction angiography reduces procedure time, contrast dosages, and patient discomfort.[144] Common uses for spinal angiography include mapping of the blood supply to the spinal cord and localization of feeder vessels for arteriovenous malformation.[80] Angiography is also used for preoperative planning of anterior approaches to the spine or preoperative embolization of vessels supplying a spinal tumor (Fig. 2-29).[35] Complications are rare but can include arterial spasm with subsequent spinal cord injury. The complications are sufficiently frequent, neurologic (8.2%), and nonneurologic (3.7%) that the procedure is performed only when absolutely necessary.[38]

MR angiography (MRA) is now used for the noninvasive assessment of vascular abnormalities. The thoracic and abdominal aorta, renal arteries, and lower extremity arteries are visualized with MRA techniques. Some techniques require gadolinium contrast, whereas others can be visualized without contrast. Gadolinium may be used with individuals with renal failure, which is an advantage over

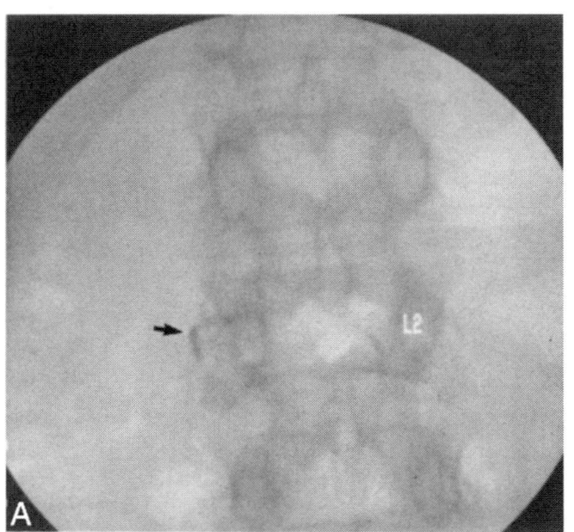

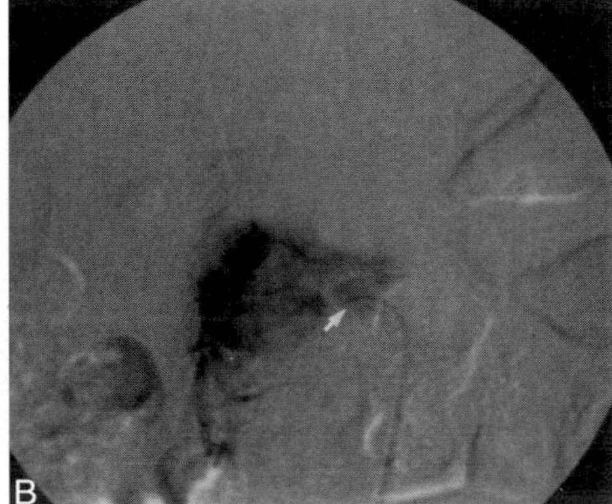

Figure 7-29 Spinal angiogram. A 31-year-old woman developed low back pain localized to L2. *A*, Anteroposterior view of L2 prior to injection. A gel foam has been placed in the right muscular radicular artery *(arrow)*. *B*, Digital subtraction angiogram. A microcatheter has been placed in vessels feeding a vertebral tumor prior to preoperative embolization to decrease bleeding *(arrow)*. The tumor was removed after embolization. The tissue diagnosis of the tumor was hemangioendothelioma.

iodinated contrast agents used in conventional angiography. This is a primary advantage over CT techniques. Evaluation of an abdominal aortic aneurysm is a common indication for MRA.[50] MRA provides the size of the aneurysm and the relationship of the aneurysm to the renal arteries, the inferior mesenteric artery, and the iliac arteries.

CLOSED BIOPSY OF THE SPINE

With the advent of more sophisticated technology, closed-needle biopsy of the spine has become a readily available procedure.[94] A successful closed biopsy obviates the need for open surgical biopsy, which is associated with the attendant risks, time, and expense. Closed-needle biopsy may use a thin needle for aspiration for cytologic or culture material or a cutting needle to obtain an intact section of tissue for histologic review.[1,87]

Advantages and disadvantages exist with closed biopsy in comparison to open biopsy. The closed procedure uses local anesthesia. The potential for infectious complications is limited. The time to complete the procedure is short and diminishes the period of hospitalization. The location of the lesion can be permanently recorded by radiographs taken at the time of biopsy. A major disadvantage of trocar biopsy is the size of the tissue specimen obtained for histologic evaluation. The amount of tissue recovered with a trocar is relatively small and may be insufficient for the pathologist to provide a specific diagnosis. Experience with the procedure on the part of the radiologist and pathologist helps in the decision regarding adequacy of the specimen for making specific diagnoses. Closed biopsy may also be a potential problem for sampling of malignant tumors. Theoretically, tumor cells may be implanted along the withdrawal path of the needle. In the clinical situation, tumor implantation rarely occurs. Open biopsy requires general anesthesia and creates a larger wound. These are clear disadvantages, but this approach is much more certain to provide sufficient biopsy material for diagnosis. Open biopsy also provides the surgeon the opportunity to visualize the extent of the lesion, which may not be apparent on radiographs.

Biopsy of a vertebra in the spine is indicated for lesions that are exclusively in the axial skeleton. Disease entities that may be diagnosed by closed-needle biopsy include metastatic lesions, infectious diseases, and articular or osseous abnormalities, including aseptic necrosis of bone. Metabolic bone disease usually causes generalized bone abnormalities. Bone in the iliac crest is easily accessible to percutaneous biopsy, obviating the need for vertebral body biopsy in bone diseases of a generalized nature. Other diseases that may cause localized lesions that may be diagnosed by histologic examination of a closed biopsy specimen include sarcoidosis, fibrous dysplasia, eosinophilic granuloma, and Paget's disease.

Contraindications to closed biopsy are vertebral lesions with extensive destruction where biopsy may be associated with hemorrhage and spinal instability. Lesions that may be associated with increased vascularity may bleed excessively when a closed biopsy sample is taken. Very vascular tumors, both benign (e.g., hemangioma) and malignant (e.g., renal cell carcinoma and thyroid carcinoma), may bleed with biopsy. Closed biopsy of the lumbar spine is also contraindicated if a lesion more accessible to percutaneous biopsy is present. Radionuclide studies are helpful in identifying lesions more accessible to closed-needle biopsy than those located in the spine.[26]

The procedure for closed biopsy of the spine may require hospitalization. Patients should not eat on the morning of the examination, and they require a sedative and pain medication. The radionuclide and radiographic studies of the biopsy site are reviewed to determine the location for the biopsy. Biplanar fluoroscopy or CT scan is used to localize the lesion. Local anesthesia to the area all the way down to the periosteum of the bone to be sampled is needed to allow for adequate pain control. The choice of biopsy needle is determined by the condition and type of lesion (soft vs. hard, vascular vs. nonvascular) to be biopsied. The Craig needle is used most frequently.[27] A right lateral approach is preferred at the appropriate level of the axial skeleton. The right lateral approach helps lessen the possibility of contacting the aorta. The patient is placed in a prone position, and a point 6.5 cm from the spinous process of the vertebra to be sampled is identified. At an angle of 145 degrees, a spinal needle is inserted until bone is contacted (Fig. 7-30). A fluoroscopic or CT image is taken to determine appropriate needle position. For biopsy of the posterior elements, a greater angle is needed.[106] After the biopsy sample is taken, the patient should be observed at bed rest for 24 hours.

Open surgical biopsy of the spine is a more complicated procedure. Cervical or thoracic vertebrae are approached anteriorly or posteriorly, depending on which side the pathology is present. Posterior elements of the lumbar vertebral bodies may be visualized through a midline or paramedian incision. Biopsy samples from anterior portions of L1–L4 may be taken using a posterior approach through a longitudinal incision just lateral to the paraspinous musculature. Dissection through the muscles leads to the transverse process, which may be followed onto the vertebral body. The lower lumbar segments and anterior lesions of the sacrum require an anterior approach through the retroperitoneum. Posterior lesions of the lower lumbar segments and sacrum may be reached through a posterior approach.[42]

Needle biopsy is an effective method to diagnose lesions of the skeletal system. Debnam and Staple reported an 81% rate of correct diagnoses in patients with bone lesions.[31] The high rate of success was related to a number of factors. These authors carefully selected patients for biopsy. Patients had careful roentgenographic and radionuclide investigation of their lesions, careful selection of the biopsy site, and careful histologic examination of the biopsy specimen. Kornblum and associates reported on 103 CT-guided spinal biopsies and found that adequate specimens were obtained in 90 individuals, a diagnosis was achieved in 71%, and greater success was obtained in the cervical and lumbar spine than the thoracic spine.[68] The need for biopsy of lesions of the lumbosacral spine is relatively uncommon. When necessary, closed-needle biopsy is a helpful diagnostic technique for physicians who are familiar with its advantages and disadvantages. Open biopsy should be undertaken if closed biopsy is contraindicated or if equivocal results are obtained with percutaneous methods.

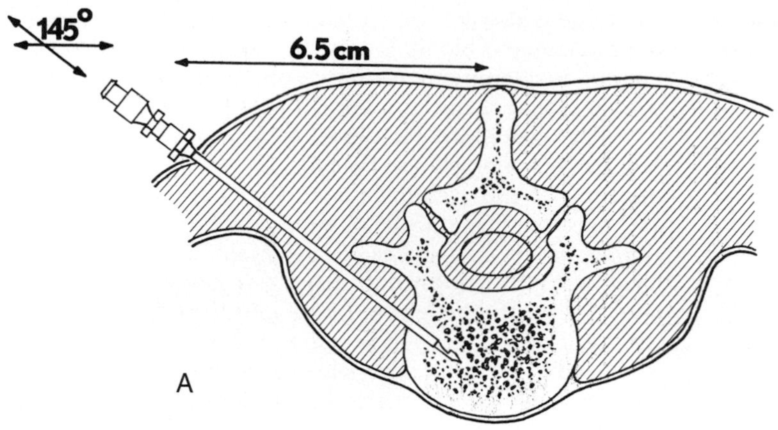

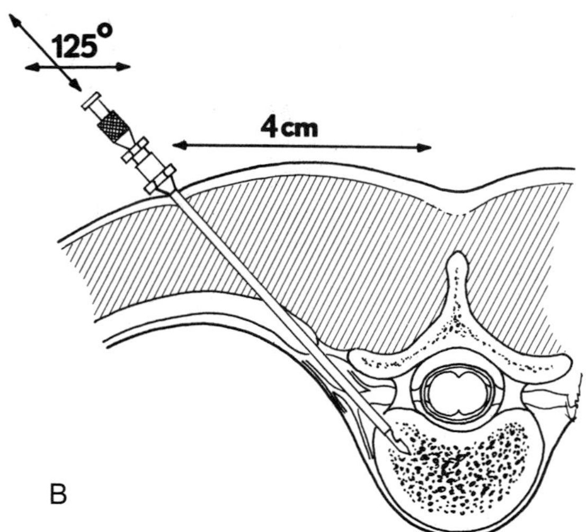

Figure 7-30 Technique of spinal biopsy. *A*, In the lumbar spine, the needle is inserted 6.5 cm from the spinous process at an angle of 145 degrees from the horizontal. Biopsy of the posterior elements requires an angle greater than 145 degrees. *B*, In the thoracic spine, needle placement is less lateral and directed more perpendicular to the skin. *(From Resnick D, Niwayama G: Diagnosis of Bone and Joint Disorders, 2nd ed. Philadelphia, WB Saunders, 1988.)*

BONE DENSITOMETRY

Four general methods are available for measuring bone mineral density in various anatomic sites, including the axial skeleton.[44] Single-photon absorptiometry is a technique limited to measurements of the peripheral skeleton and is not used for the spine. Dual-photon absorptiometry (DPA) uses two sources of photon energy to separate soft and bone tissue components of bone and surrounding tissues. DPA is used to measure the bone mineral density of the lumbar spine and long bones. The precision (reproducibility) of DPA spinal measurements is between 2% to 4%, with accuracy variability of 5% to 10%.[90,117] Quantitative computed tomography (QCT) measures bone calcium in trabecular bone in cross-sectional images of three to four vertebral bodies. The quantification of bone mineral is determined by comparison to a number of calibration phantoms containing mineral equivalents of known density. The precision error of QCT is 2% to 4%, with accuracy variability of 10% to 15%.[47,122] Dual-energy x-ray absorptiometry (DEXA) is based on the same principle as DPA but makes use of a dual-energy source of x-ray rather than a dual-photon source. The precision of DEXA for bone mineral density of the vertebral spine is 1%, with accuracy variability of 4% to 8%.[109,132]

Each technique is limited by technical factors. DPA long-term precision is affected by the decay of the radioactive source. DPA is also affected by anatomic abnormalities of the spine and vascular calcifications. QCT has increased levels of radiation exposure compared to other methods, and the accuracy is significantly affected by intravertebral marrow fat. The determination of bone mineral has progressed with more accurate assessment with less exposure to x-ray. The important determination that remains to be ascertained is the risk for fracture that is associated with specific amounts of vertebral body bone mineral. A combination of techniques (QCT for the diagnosis of osteoporosis and DEXA for sequential determinations and response to therapy) may be found to be the best way for quantifying bone mineral calcium and risk for fracture.[95] At one time DEXA was less sensitive than QCT in predicting vertebral fractures; however, the technique continues to improve and has really become the most popular modality for measuring bone density.[109] DEXA has become the method of choice to measure bone mineral density because it is accurate, precise, and fast and has low radiation exposure. Many osteoporosis guidelines including those of the World Health Organization and the American College of Rheumatology include recommendations based on DEXA measurements.[3]

Other measurement tools are available to measure bone mineral density, including heel ultrasonography. Although this technique is easily administered, has no radiation exposure, and describes the architecture of the measured bone, ultrasonography has not replaced DEXA measurements for spinal osteoporosis. When in doubt, a DEXA determination is preferred.

NORMAL ROENTGENOGRAPHIC VARIANTS

Normal roentgenographic variation is a common finding when investigation of large groups of asymptomatic individuals is undertaken. Roentgenographic variations may be a consequence of skeletal changes that occur during growth and development or may be positional artifacts. This is particularly true in the sacroiliac joints (Fig. 7-31). The margins of the sacroiliac joints are normally indistinct during adolescence and may be confused with changes consistent with those of the spondyloarthropathies. Obliquity of the joints may obscure them on an AP view. An oblique view of the sacroiliac joints demonstrates the normal state of the joint. In women exclusively, the bilateral indentation of the inferior portion of the iliac side of the sacroiliac joint (paraglenoid sulci) is a normal variant.

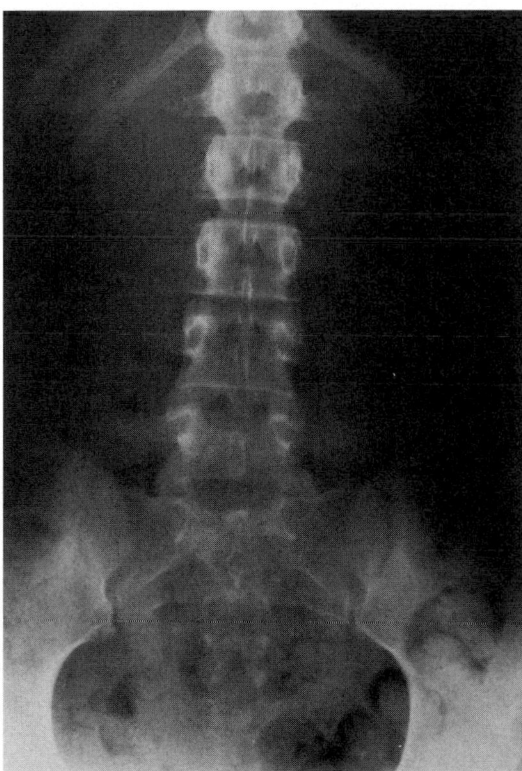

Figure 7-31 Normal anteroposterior view of the lumbosacral spine in a 14-year-old girl. The joint margins are less well defined than joint margins found in adults (see Fig. 7-12).

Normal variation may also be noted in the lumbar spine. Roentgenographic changes of the vertebral bodies may mimic findings associated with significant abnormalities, including infection and tumor. However, careful clinical and repeated radiographic evaluation of the patient demonstrates the benign nature of these x-ray changes. A few examples of these findings might include limbus vertebra, nondiscogenic sclerosis, and bone islands.[36,64]

PITFALLS OF RADIOGRAPHIC EVALUATION

The following case study is presented to temper the enthusiasm of clinicians for radiographic techniques as the method of choice in the diagnosis of low back pain.

CASE STUDY

A 54-year-old white man was evaluated for a chief complaint of a recurrence of severe low back pain. The patient first noted symptoms of left-sided sacroiliac pain when he was 20 years old. At age 26, he developed right-sided sacroiliac pain. Back pain was most severe in the morning and improved with activity. He developed abdominal pain with cramps and a diagnosis of Crohn's disease was made. An intravenous pyelogram at that time demonstrated bilateral sacroiliitis with fusion (Fig. 7-32). A lateral view of the lumbosacral spine revealed no syndesmophytes and a normal L5–S1 disc space (Fig. 7-33). The patient was started on indomethacin 25 mg three times a day with good relief of his symptoms.

The patient did well until 2 years later, when he developed sudden onset of severe midline low back pain radiating from the right buttock to the knee. Coughing or sneezing increased pain in the same distribution. Physical examination revealed normal vital signs. Moderate paraspinous muscle spasm along with a loss of lumbar lordosis was noted on examination of the axial skeleton. The sacroiliac joints were not tender to percussion. The straight leg–raising test was negative bilaterally. Motor strength and reflexes were normal. The patient had great difficulty arising from a supine position.

Plain roentgenograms demonstrated L5–S1 disc space narrowing and vertebral body sclerosis along with the possibility of vertebral endplate erosions (Fig. 7-34). A radionuclide scan was obtained when symptoms persisted and demonstrated markedly increased uptake over the L5–S1 region consistent with infection. Tomograms were obtained to better investigate the area for the presence of an infection. The tomograms demonstrated marked narrowing of the L5–S1 disc space with subchondral endplate sclerosis without destructive changes (Fig. 7-35). The radiologist suggested a gallium scan for detection of possible early osteomyelitis. The scan was normal. At this time the patient's radicular symptoms became more prominent. An electromyogram suggested the presence of very mild radiculopathy. A CT scan of the lumbosacral spine was obtained for detection of a herniated disc. The CT scan demonstrated a degenerative L5–S1 disc with a vacuum phenomenon (Fig. 7-36). The patient underwent lumbar myelography since surgical intervention for a correctable lesion was contemplated. The myelogram demonstrated a mild protrusion at the L4–L5 level (Fig. 7-37). The L5–S1 disc level showed no impingement of the neural elements. The patient refused any additional diagnostic tests. The possibilities of degenerative disc disease, spondylitis, and infection were reviewed with the patient. He decided on a therapeutic trial for radiculopathy including corticosteroids (prednisone, 25 mg/day) for 2 weeks, followed by indomethacin and a

CASE STUDY—CONT'D

lumbosacral corset. Over the next month, the patient's symptoms resolved.

In 1992, 6 years after the episode of radicular pain, the patient was admitted to the hospital for severe, diffuse back pain with radiating pain from the left buttock to the midthigh. In 1991, the patient developed biopsy-proven gastric cancer. An MR image was obtained to determine the presence and extent of metastatic disease. The MR image demonstrated findings that had been discovered on the plain roentgenograms, tomogram, CT scan, and myelogram. The L4–L5 disc was protruded as demonstrated on the myelogram, whereas the L5–S1 disc was severely degenerated. The new MR finding in all of the vertebral bodies was abnormal, a signal indicative of diffuse metastatic disease (Fig. 7-38).

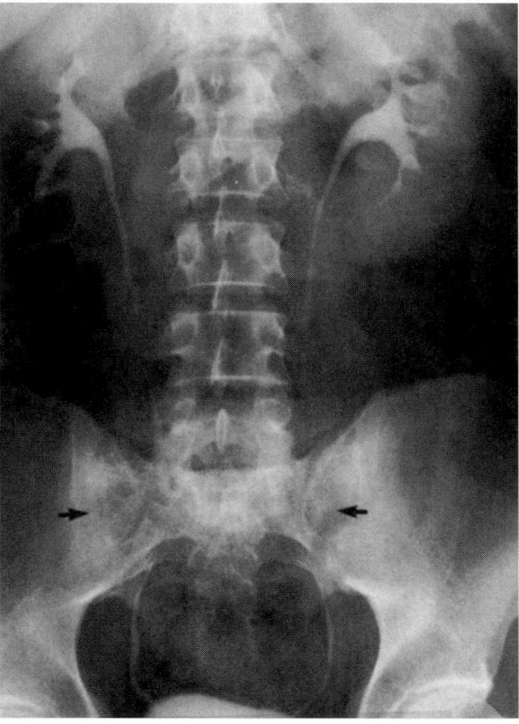

Figure 7-32 Intravenous pyelogram demonstrating fusion of both sacroiliac joints *(black arrows)*.

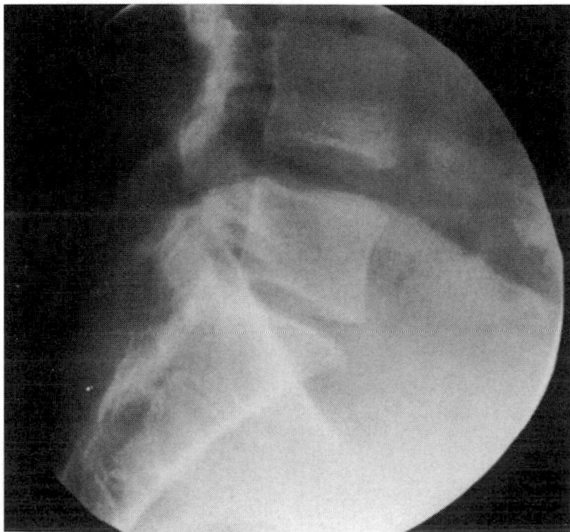

Figure 7-33 Coned-down view of the lumbosacral junction revealing an unremarkable L5–S1 intervertebral disc space.

We believe this case highlights the difficulties a physician may be faced with when obtaining too many diagnostic tests with conflicting results and the impact of MR on the radiographic evaluation of the lumbar spine. Radiologists may read films accurately describing the abnormalities they see. MR is a sensitive radiographic

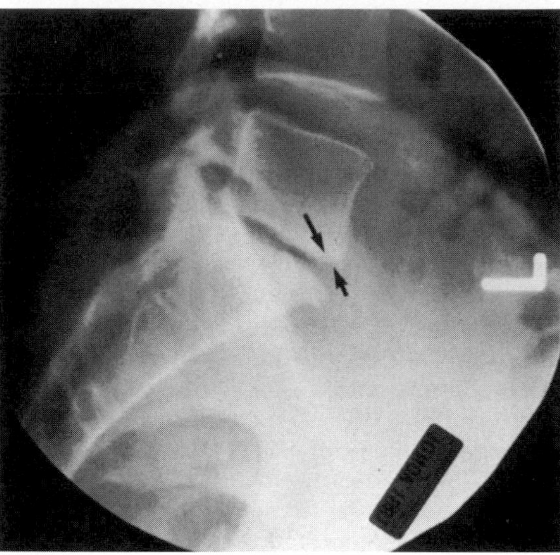

Figure 7-34 Coned-down view of the lumbosacral junction demonstrating disc space narrowing, bony sclerosis, and possible endplate erosion *(arrows)*.

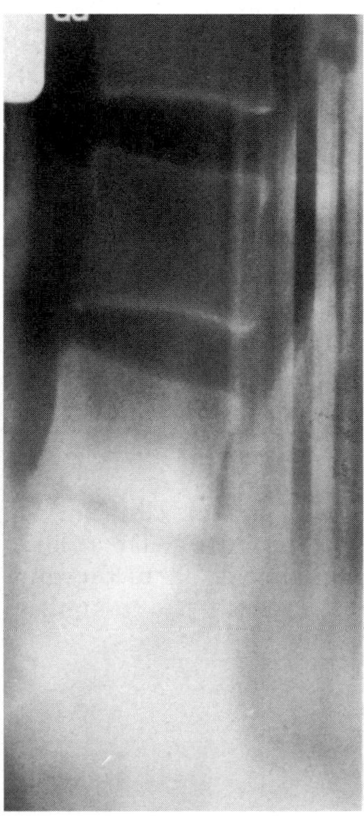

Figure 7-35 Tomographic view of the lumbosacral junction revealing marked disc space narrowing and surrounding bony sclerosis. No definite area of bony erosion was detected.

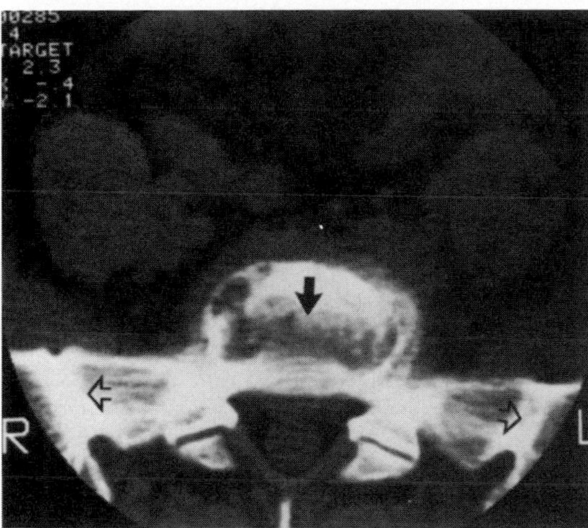

Figure 7-36 Transaxial view of the L5–S1 intervertebral disc space demonstrating a vacuum phenomenon in the disc proper *(arrow)*. Fused sacroiliac joints are also present *(open arrows)*.

technique that is able to identify abnormalities that, in the past, required a number of different examinations to detect. This patient would not have undergone the number of evaluations he did if MR imaging had been available in 1986. However, MR, like other radiographic techniques, may identify anatomic abnormalities that have little clinical importance. Radiographic findings become significant only when corroborating what is suspected by the history and physical examination of the patient.

The technology that is the basis of MR continues to improve.[8] In the future, improved imaging will be

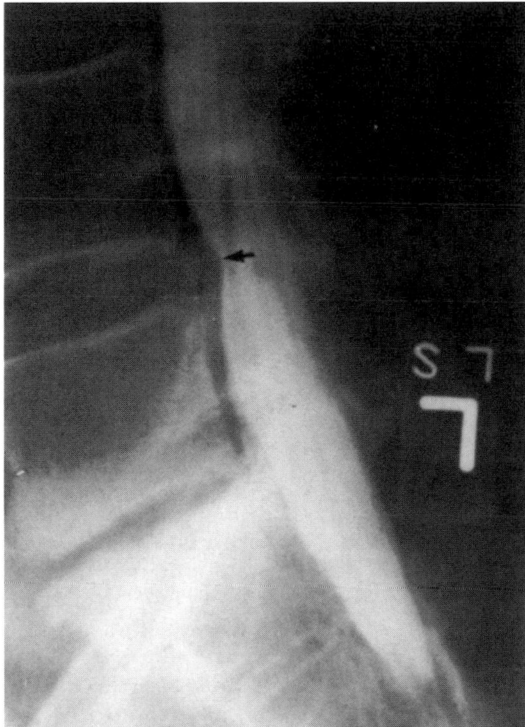

Figure 7-37 Lumbar myelogram, lateral view. The L4–L5 intervertebral disc is mildly protruded *(arrow)*. The L5–S1 disc is unassociated with any impingement of neural elements.

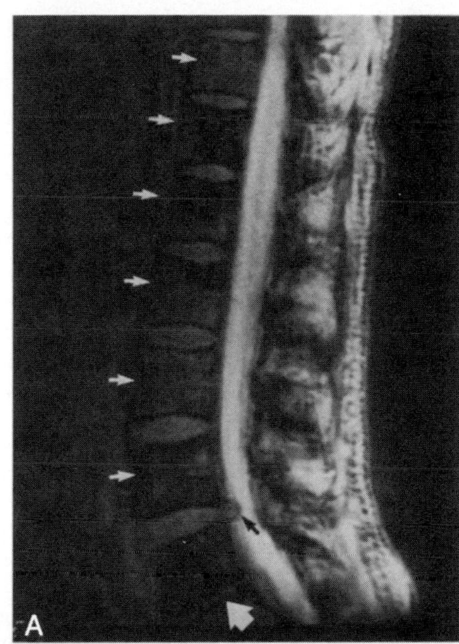

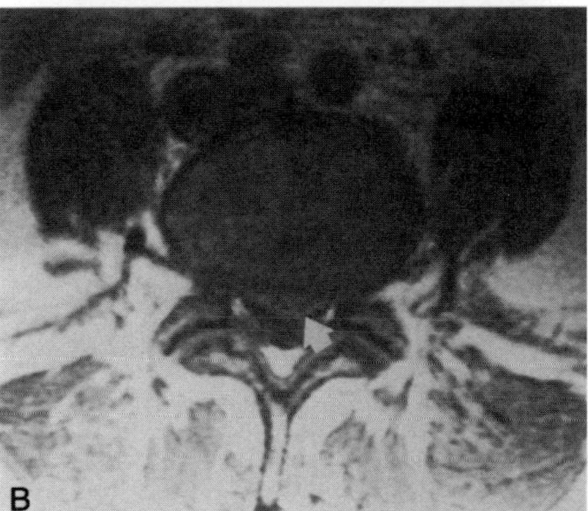

Figure 7-38 Lumbar MR. *A*, Sagittal view of T1-weighted image demonstrating disc herniation *(black arrow)* and severe disc space loss at the L5–S1 interspace *(large white arrow)*. Signal abnormalities are noted in most vertebral bodies indicative of metastatic disease *(small white arrows)*. *B*, Axial view of L4–L5 interspace demonstrating diffuse central disc protrusion *(arrow)*.

obtained through the use of perfusion imaging with new intravascular contrast agents, dynamic studies of CSF motion, and MR spectroscopy. These technologies will have to be evaluated as they become available to determine their appropriate place in the evaluation of spinal pain patients.

SUMMARY

The problem in patients with spinal pain is the identification of the level or levels that are productive of the symptomatology. The accuracy of the diagnostic tools that are employed is commonly compared to surgical findings. Although the surgeon can confirm or disprove the radiologic assessment of the anatomic status within the spinal canal, the surgeon is no more able than the radiologist to unequivocally ascertain that the patient's symptoms are etiologically related to the morphologic status of the canal.

In other words, both the radiologist and the surgeon are capable of describing the morphologic features of cervical or lumbar spondylosis, but neither can tell with certainty whether these features are responsible for the patient's symptoms. Accordingly, the results of an operation can provide an indication of the accuracy of these imaging modalities, but they are by no means conclusive. The importance of strict correlation of positive diagnostic studies with the patient's signs and symptoms cannot be overstressed. This is particularly important in light of the fact that a significant percentage of asymptomatic subjects have radiographic abnormalities on any of the imaging modalities that have been tested. In conclusion, imaging studies are useful for confirming a clinical diagnosis suggested by the history and physical examination, but they should never be interpreted in isolation from the overall clinical picture, and they should never be used as general screening tests.

References

1. Adler O, Rosenberger A: Fine-needle aspiration biopsy of osteolytic metastatic lesions. AJR Am J Roentgenol 133:15-18, 1979.
2. Albeck MJ, Hilden J, Kjaer L, et al: A controlled comparison of myelography, computed tomography, and magnetic resonance imaging in clinically suspected lumbar disc herniation. Spine 20:443-448, 1995.
3. Anonymous: Recommendations for the prevention and treatment of glucocorticoid-induced osteoporosis: American College of Rheumatology Task Force on Osteoporosis Guidelines. Arthritis Rheum 39:1791-1801, 1996.
4. Ardan GM: Bone destruction not demonstrable by radiography. Br J Radiol 24:107, 1951.
5. Badami JP, Norman D, Barbaro NM, et al: Metrizamide CT myelography in cervical myelopathy and radiculopathy: Correlation with conventional myelography and surgical findings. AJR Am J Roentgenol 144:675-680, 1985.
6. Baker RA, Hillman BJ, McLennan JE, et al: Sequelae of metrizamide myelography in 200 examinations. AJR Am J Roentgenol 130:499-502, 1978.
7. Bar-Shalom R, Valdivia AY, Blaufox MD: PET imaging in oncology. Semin Nucl Med 30:150-185, 2000.
8. Bates D, Ruggieri P: Imaging modalities for evaluation of the spine. Radiol Clin North Am 29:675-690, 1991.
9. Bell GR, Ross JS: The accuracy of imaging studies of the degenerative cervical spine: Myelography, myelo-computed tomography, and magnetic resonance imaging. Semin Spine Surg 7:9, 1995.
10. Bell GR, Rothman RH, Booth RE, et al: A study of computer-assisted tomography. II. Comparison of metrizamide myelography and computed tomography in the diagnosis of herniated lumbar disc and spinal stenosis. Spine 9:552-556, 1984.
11. Boden SD, Davis DO, Dina TS, et al: Contrast-enhanced MR imaging performed after successful lumbar disk surgery: Prospective study. Radiology 182:59-64, 1992.
12. Boden SD, Davis DO, Dina TS, et al: Abnormal magnetic resonance scans of the lumbar spine in asymptomatic subjects: A prospective investigation. J Bone Joint Surg Am 72:403-408, 1990.
13. Boden SD, Davis DO, Dina TS, et al: Postoperative diskitis: Distinguishing early MR imaging findings from normal postoperative disk space changes. Radiology 184:765-771, 1992.
14. Boden SD, McCowin PR, Davis DO, et al: Abnormal magnetic resonance scans of the cervical spine in asymptomatic subjects: A prospective investigation. J Bone Joint Surg Am 72:1178-1184, 1990.
15. Borenstein DG, O'Mara JW Jr, Boden SD, et al: The value of magnetic resonance imaging of the lumbar spine to predict low back pain in asymptomatic subjects: A seven-year follow-up study. J Bone Joint Surg Am 83:1306-1311, 2001.
16. Breger RK, Williams AL, Daniels DL, et al: Contrast enhancement in spinal MR imaging. AJNR Am J Neuroradiol 10:633-637, 1989.
17. Carragee EJ, Chen Y, Tanner CM, et al: Can discography cause long-term back symptoms in previously asymptomatic subjects? Spine 25:1803-1808, 2000.
18. Carragee EJ, Paragioudakis SJ, Khurana S: 2000 Volvo Award winner in clinical studies: Lumbar high-intensity zone and discography in subjects without low back problems. Spine 25:2987-2992, 2000.
19. Carragee EJ, Tanner CM, Yang B, et al: False-positive findings on lumbar discography: Reliability of subjective concordance assessment during provocative disc injection. Spine 24:2542-2547, 1999.
20. Carrera GF, Foley WD, Kozin F, et al: CT of sacroiliitis. AJR Am J Roentgenol 136:41-46, 1981.
21. Carrera GF, Haughton VM, Syvertsen A, Williams AL: Computed tomography of the lumbar facet joints. Radiology 134:145-148, 1980.
22. Cloward RB: Cervical discography: A contribution to the etiology and mechanism of neck, shoulder, and arm pain. Ann Surg 150:1052, 1959.
23. Coin CG: Cervical disk degeneration and herniation: Diagnosis by computerized tomography. South Med J 77:979-982, 1984.
24. Colley DP, Dunsker SB: Traumatic narrowing of the dorsolumbar spinal canal demonstrated by computed tomography. Radiology 129:95-98, 1978.
25. Collins HR: An evaluation of cervical and lumbar discography. Clin Orthop 107:133-138, 1975.
26. Collins JD, Bassett L, Main GD, Kagan C: Percutaneous biopsy following positive bone scans. Radiology 132:439-442, 1979.
27. Craig FS: Vertebral body biopsy. J Bone Joint Surg Am 38:93, 1956.
28. Davies SN, Lodge D: Evidence for involvement of *N*-methylaspartate receptors in "wind-up" of class 2 neurones in the dorsal horn of the rat. Brain Res 424:402-406, 1987.
29. Davis MA, Jones AL: Comparison of ^{99m}Tc-labeled phosphate and phosphonate agents for skeletal imaging. Semin Nucl Med 6:19-31, 1976.
30. De Palma AF, Rothman RH: The Intervertebral Disc. Philadelphia, WB Saunders, 1970.
31. Debnam JW, Staple TW: Trephine bone biopsy by radiologists: Results of 73 procedures. Radiology 116:607-609, 1975.
32. DeNardo GL, Jacobson SJ, Raventos A: ^{85}Sr bone scan in neoplastic disease. Semin Nucl Med 2:18-30, 1972.
33. Dolan AL, Ryan PJ, Arden NK, et al: The value of SPECT scans in identifying back pain likely to benefit from facet joint injection. Br J Rheumatol 35:1269-1273, 1996.
34. Dorwart RH, LaMasters DL: Applications of computed tomographic scanning of the cervical spine. Orthop Clin North Am 16:381-393, 1985.
35. Eskridge JM: Interventional neuroradiology. Radiology 172:991-1006, 1989.
36. Feldman F: The symptomatic spine: Relevant and irrelevant roentgen variants and variations. Orthop Clin North Am 14:119-145, 1983.
37. Fogelman I, Bessent RG, Turner JG, et al: The use of whole-body retention of Tc-99m diphosphonate in the diagnosis of metabolic bone disease. J Nucl Med 19:270-275, 1978.
38. Forbes G, Nichols DA, Jack CR, et al: Complications of spinal cord arteriography: Prospective assessment of risk for diagnostic procedures. Radiology 169:479-484, 1988.
39. Forristall RM, Marsh HO, Pay NT: Magnetic resonance imaging and contrast CT of the lumbar spine: Comparison of diagnostic methods and correlation with surgical findings. Spine 13:1049-1054, 1988.
40. Friedenberg Z, Miller W: Degenerative disc disease of the cervical spine. J Bone Joint Surg 45:1171, 1963.
41. Friedenberg ZB, Ediken J, Spenser N, et al: Degenerative changes in the cervical spine. J Bone Joint Surg Am 41:61, 1959.
42. Friedlaender GE, Southwick WO: Tumors of the spine. In Rothman RH, Simeone FA (eds): The Spine, 2nd ed. Philadelphia, WB Saunders, 1982, pp 1024-1025.
43. Gates GF: SPECT bone scanning of the spine. Semin Nucl Med 28:78-94, 1998.
44. Genant HK, Faulkner KG, Gluer CC: Measurement of bone mineral density: Current status. Am J Med 91:49S-53S, 1991.
45. Gero B, Sze G, Sharif H: MR imaging of intradural inflammatory diseases of the spine. AJNR Am J Neuroradiol 12:1009-1019, 1991.
46. Gibson MJ, Buckley J, Mawhinney R, et al: Magnetic resonance imaging and discography in the diagnosis of disc degeneration: A comparative study of 50 discs. J Bone Joint Surg Br 68:369-373, 1986.

47. Gluer CC, Genant HK: Impact of marrow fat on accuracy of quantitative CT. J Comput Assist Tomogr 13:1023-1035, 1989.
48. Goldberg RP, Genant HK, Shimshak R, Shames D: Applications and limitations of quantitative sacroiliac joint scintigraphy. Radiology 128:683-686, 1978.
49. Gore DR, Sepic SB, Gardner GM: Roentgenographic findings of the cervical spine in asymptomatic people. Spine 11:521-524, 1986.
50. Grist TM: MRA of the abdominal aorta and lower extremities. J Magn Reson Imaging 11:32-43, 2000.
51. Handmaker H, Leonards R: The bone scan in inflammatory osseous disease. Semin Nucl Med 6:95-105, 1976.
52. Hawkins RA, Hoh CK: PET FDG studies in oncology. Nucl Med Biol 21:739-747, 1994.
53. Hinck VC, Sachdev NS: Developmental stenosis of the cervical spinal canal. Brain 89:27-36, 1966.
54. Hirsch C, Schajowicz R, Galante J: Structural changes in the cervical spine: A study on autopsy specimens in different age groups. Acta Orthop Scand Suppl 109:7-77, 1967.
55. Hitselberger WE, Witten RM: Abnormal myelograms in asymptomatic patients. J Neurosurg 28:204-206, 1968.
56. Holt E: The question of lumbar discography. J Bone Joint Surg 50:720, 1968.
57. Holt EP Jr: Further reflections on cervical discography. JAMA 231:613-614, 1975.
58. Holt EP Jr: Fallacy of cervical discography. JAMA 188:799, 2001.
59. Hult L: The Munkfors investigation: A study of the frequency and causes of the stiff-neck-brachialgia and lumbago-sciatica syndromes, as well as observations on certain signs and symptoms from the dorsal spine and the joints of the extremities in industrial and forest workers. Acta Orthop Scand Suppl 16:1, 1954.
60. Jensen MC, Brant-Zawadzki MN, Obuchowski N, et al: Magnetic resonance imaging of the lumbar spine in people without back pain. N Engl J Med 331:69-73, 1994.
61. Kattapuram SV, Phillips WC, Boyd R: CT in pyogenic osteomyelitis of the spine. AJR Am J Roentgenol 140:1199-1201, 1983.
62. Keats TE: Plain film radiography: Sources of diagnostic errors. In Resnick D (ed): Diagnosis of Bone and Joint Disorders, 3rd ed. Philadelphia, WB Saunders, 1995, pp 41-43.
63. Keats TE, Johnstone WH: Notching of the lamina of C7: A proposed mechanism. Skeletal Radiol 7:233, 1982.
64. Keats TE: An Atlas of Normal Roentgen Variants that May Simulate Disease. Chicago, Year Book, 1984, pp 236-264.
65. Kendrick D, Fielding K, Bentley E, et al: Radiography of the lumbar spine in primary care patients with low back pain: Randomised, controlled trial. BMJ 322:400-405, 2001.
66. Kent DL, Larson EB: Magnetic resonance imaging of the brain and spine: Is clinical efficacy established after the first decade? Ann Intern Med 108:402-424, 1988.
67. Klafta LA Jr, Collis JS Jr: The diagnostic inaccuracy of the pain response in cervical discography. Cleve Clin Q 36:35-39, 1969.
68. Kornblum MB, Wesolowski DP, Fischgrund JS, Herkowitz HN: Computed tomography–guided biopsy of the spine: A review of 103 patients. Spine 23:81-85, 1998.
69. Landman JA, Hoffman JC Jr, Braun IF, Barrow DL: Value of computed tomographic myelography in the recognition of cervical herniated disk. AJNR Am J Neuroradiol 5:391-394, 1984.
70. Lawrence JS: Disc degeneration: Its frequency and relationship to symptoms. Ann Rheum Dis 28:121-138, 1969.
71. Lehto IJ, Tertti MO, Komu ME, et al: Age-related MRI changes at 0.1 T in cervical discs in asymptomatic subjects. Neuroradiology 36:49-53, 1994.
72. Liang M, Komaroff AL: Roentgenograms in primary care patients with acute low back pain: A cost-effectiveness analysis. Arch Intern Med 142:1108-1112, 1982.
73. Lim V, Sobel DF, Zyroff J: Spinal cord pial metastases: MR imaging with gadopentetate dimeglumine. AJNR Am J Neuroradiol 11:975-982, 1990.
74. Lukens JA, McLeod RA, Sim FH: Computed tomographic evaluation of primary osseous malignant neoplasms. AJR Am J Roentgenol 139:45-48, 1982.
75. Maravilla KR, Lesh P, Weinreb JC, et al: Magnetic resonance imaging of the lumbar spine with CT correlation. AJNR Am J Neuroradiol 6:237-245, 1985.
76. Marcelis S, Seragini FC, Taylor JA, et al: Cervical spine: Comparison of 45-degree and 55-degree anteroposterior oblique radiographic projections. Radiology 188:253-256, 1993.
77. Marty R, Denney JD, McKamey MR, Rowley MJ: Bone trauma and related benign disease: Assessment by bone scanning. Semin Nucl Med 6:107-120, 1976.
78. Massare C, Bard M, Tristant H: Cervical discography: Speculation on technique and indications from our experience. J Radiol 55:395, 1974.
79. McNeil BJ: Rationale for the use of bone scans in selected metastatic and primary bone tumors. Semin Nucl Med 8:336-345, 1978.
80. Merland JJ, Reizine D: Treatment of arteriovenous spinal cord malformations. Semin Intervent Radiol 4:281-290, 1987.
81. Meyer RR: Cervical diskography: A help or hindrance in evaluating neck, shoulder, arm pain? AJR Am J Roentgenol 90:1208, 1963.
82. Modic MT, Masaryk T, Boumphrey F, et al: Lumbar herniated disk disease and canal stenosis: Prospective evaluation by surface coil MR, CT, and myelography. AJR Am J Roentgenol 147:757-765, 1986.
83. Modic MT, Masaryk T, Boumphrey F, et al: Lumbar herniated disk disease and canal stenosis: Prospective evaluation by surface coil MR, CT, and myelography. AJNR Am J Neuroradiol 7:709-717, 1986.
84. Modic MT, Masaryk T, Paushter D: Magnetic resonance imaging of the spine. Radiol Clin North Am 24:229-245, 1986.
85. Modic MT, Pflanze W, Feiglin DH, Belhobek G: Magnetic resonance imaging of musculoskeletal infections. Radiol Clin North Am 24:247-258, 1986.
86. Modic MT, Ross JS, Masaryk TJ: Imaging of degenerative disease of the cervical spine. Clin Orthop 239:109-120, 1989.
87. Moore TM, Meyers MH, Patzakis MJ, et al: Closed biopsy of musculoskeletal lesions. J Bone Joint Surg Am 61:375-380, 1979.
88. Nakagawa H, Okumura T, Sugiyama T, Iwata K: Discrepancy between metrizamide CT and myelography in diagnosis of cervical disk protrusions. AJNR Am J Neuroradiol 4:604-606, 1983.
89. Nguyen CM, Ho KC, Yu SW, et al: An experimental model to study contrast enhancement in MR imaging of the intervertebral disk. AJNR Am J Neuroradiol 10:811-814, 1989.
90. Nilas L, Borg J, Gotfredsen A, Christiansen C: Comparison of single- and dual-photo absorptiometry in postmenopausal bone mineral loss. J Nucl Med 26:1257-1262, 1985.
91. Orrison WW, Eldevik OP, Sackett JF: Lateral C1–2 puncture for cervical myelography. III. Historical, anatomic, and technical considerations. Radiology 146:401-408, 1983.
92. Orrison WW, Sackett JF, Amundsen P: Lateral C1–2 puncture for cervical myelography. II. Recognition of improper injection of contrast material. Radiology 146:395-400, 1983.
93. Osborn AG, Hood RS, Sherry RG, et al: CT/MR spectrum of far lateral and anterior lumbosacral disk herniations. AJNR Am J Neuroradiol 9:775-778, 1988.
94. Ottolenghi CE: Aspiration biopsy of the spine: Technique for the thoracic spine and results of twenty-eight biopsies in this region and over-all results of 1050 biopsies of other spinal segments. J Bone Joint Surg Am 51:1531-1544, 1969.
95. Pacifici R, Rupich R, Griffin M, et al: Dual-energy radiography versus quantitative computed tomography for the diagnosis of osteoporosis. J Clin Endocrinol Metab 70:705-710, 1990.
96. Paushter DM, Modic MT, Masaryk TJ: Magnetic resonance imaging of the spine: Applications and limitations. Radiol Clin North Am 23:551-562, 1985.
97. Pech P, Daniels DL, Williams AL, Haughton VM: The cervical neural foramina: Correlation of microtomy and CT anatomy. Radiology 155:143-146, 1985.
98. Pech P, Haughton VM: Lumbar intervertebral disk: Correlative MR and anatomic study. Radiology 156:699-701, 1985.
99. Pendergrass HP, Potsaid MS, Castronovo FP: The clinical use of ^{99m}Tc-diphosphonate (HEDSPA): A new agent for skeletal imaging. Radiology 107:557-562, 1973.
100. Penning L: Prevertebral hematoma in cervical spine injury: Incidence and etiologic significance. AJR Am J Roentgenol 136:553-561, 1981.
101. Penning L, Wilmink JT, van Woerden HH, Knol E: CT myelographic findings in degenerative disorders of the cervical spine: Clinical significance. AJR Am J Roentgenol 146:793-801, 1986.
102. Peterson CK, Bolton JE, Wood AR: A cross-sectional study correlating lumbar spine degeneration with disability and pain. Spine 25:218-223, 2000.

103. Porter BA, Shields AF, Olson DO: Magnetic resonance imaging of bone marrow disorders. Radiol Clin North Am 24:269-289, 1986.
104. Ratcliff G, Sandler S, Latchaw R: Cognitive and affective changes after myelography: A comparison of metrizamide and iohexol. AJR Am J Roentgenol 147:777-781, 1986.
105. Reinartz P, Schaffeldt J, Sabri O, et al: Benign versus malignant osseous lesions in the lumbar vertebrae: Differentiation by means of bone SPET. Eur J Nucl Med 27:721-726, 2000.
106. Resnick D: Needle biopsy of bone. In Resnick D, Niwayama G (eds): Diagnosis of Bone and Joint Disorders: With Emphasis on Articular Abnormalities. Philadelphia, WB Saunders, 1981, pp 692-701.
107. Roth DA: Cervical analgesic discography: A new test for the definitive diagnosis of the painful-disk syndrome. JAMA 235:1713-1714, 1976.
108. Ryynannen OP, Lehtovirta J, Soimakallio S, Takala J: General practitioners' willingness to request plain lumbar spine radiographic examinations. Eur J Radiol 37:47-53, 2001.
109. Sartoris DJ, Resnick D: Dual-energy radiographic absorptiometry for bone densitometry: Current status and perspective. AJR Am J Roentgenol 152:241-246, 1989.
110. Scher A, Vambeck V: An approach to the radiological examination of the cervico-dorsal junction following injury. Clin Radiol 28:243-246, 1977.
111. Schnebel B, Kingston S, Watkins R, Dillin W: Comparison of MRI to contrast CT in the diagnosis of spinal stenosis. Spine 14:332-337, 1989.
112. Schneiderman G, Flannigan B, Kingston S, et al: Magnetic resonance imaging in the diagnosis of disc degeneration: Correlation with discography. Spine 12:276-281, 1987.
113. Shapiro R: Myelography, 4th ed. Chicago, Year Book, 1984.
114. Siegel MJ, Evens RG: Advances in the use of computed tomography. JAMA 281:1252-1254, 1999.
115. Simmons EH, Segil CM: An evaluation of discography in the localization of symptomatic levels in discogenic disease of the spine. Clin Orthop 108:57-69, 1975.
116. Skalpe IO: Adhesive arachnoiditis following lumbar myelography. Spine 3:61-64, 1978.
117. Slemenda CW, Johnston CC: Bone mass measurement: Which site to measure? Am J Med 84:643-645, 1988.
118. Smith GW, Nichols P Jr: The technique of cervical discography. Radiology 68:163, 1963.
119. Sneider SE, Winslow OP, Rogers WH: Cervical discography: Is it relevant? JAMA 185:163, 1963.
120. Sobel DF, Barkovich AJ, Munderloh SH: Metrizamide myelography and postmyelographic computed tomography: Comparative adequacy in the cervical spine. AJNR Am J Neuroradiol 5:385-390, 1984.
121. Spangfort EV: The lumbar disc herniation: A computer-aided analysis of 2,504 operations. Acta Orthop Scand Suppl 142:1-95, 1972.
122. Steiger P, Block JE, Steiger S, et al: Spinal bone mineral density measured with quantitative CT: Effect of region of interest, vertebral level, and technique. Radiology 175:537-543, 1990.
123. Suarez-Almazor ME, Belseck E, Russell AS, Mackel JV: Use of lumbar radiographs for the early diagnosis of low back pain: Proposed guidelines would increase utilization. JAMA 277:1782-1786, 1997.
124. Sze G, Stimac GK, Bartlett C, et al: Multicenter study of gadopentetate dimeglumine as an MR contrast agent: Evaluation in patients with spinal tumors. AJNR Am J Neuroradiol 11:967-974, 1990.
125. Taveras J: Is discography a useful diagnostic procedure? J Can Assoc Radiol 18:294-295, 1967.
126. Teplick JG, Haskin ME: CT of the postoperative lumbar spine. Radiol Clin North Am 21:395-420, 1983.
127. Teresi LM, Lufkin RB, Reicher MA, et al: Asymptomatic degenerative disk disease and spondylosis of the cervical spine: MR imaging. Radiology 164:83-88, 1987.
128. Toyone T, Takahashi K, Kitahara H, et al: Vertebral bone marrow changes in degenerative lumbar disc disease: An MRI study of 74 patients with low back pain. J Bone Joint Surg Br 76:757-764, 1994.
129. Ullrich CG, Binet EF, Sanecki MG, Kieffer SA: Quantitative assessment of the lumbar spinal canal by computed tomography. Radiology 134:137-143, 1980.
130. Vezina JL, Fontaine S, Laperriere J: Outpatient myelography with fine-needle technique: An appraisal. AJNR Am J Neuroradiol 10:615-617, 1989.
131. Voelker JL, Mealey J, Eskridge JM, Gilmor RL: Metrizamide-enhanced computed tomography as an adjunct to metrizamide myelography in the evaluation of lumbar disc herniation and spondylosis. Neurosurgery 20:379-384, 1987.
132. Wahner HW, Dunn WL, Brown ML, et al: Comparison of dual-energy x-ray absorptiometry and dual-photon absorptiometry for bone mineral measurements of the lumbar spine. Mayo Clin Proc 63:1075-1084, 1988.
133. Walsh TR, Weinstein JN, Spratt KF, et al: Lumbar discography in normal subjects: A controlled, prospective study. J Bone Joint Surg Am 72:1081-1088, 1990.
134. Weishaupt D, Schmid MR, Zanetti M, et al: Positional MR imaging of the lumbar spine: Does it demonstrate nerve root compromise not visible at conventional MR imaging? Radiology 215:247-253, 2000.
135. Weishaupt D, Zanetti M, Hodler J, Boos N: MR imaging of the lumbar spine: Prevalence of intervertebral disk extrusion and sequestration, nerve root compression, endplate abnormalities, and osteoarthritis of the facet joints in asymptomatic volunteers. Radiology 209:661-666, 1998.
136. Weiss TE, Shuler SE: New techniques for identification of synovitis and evaluation of joint disease. II. Joint imaging as a clinical aid in diagnosis and therapy. Bull Rheum Dis 25:786, 1974.
137. Weisz GM, Lamond TS, Kitchener PN: Spinal imaging: Will MRI replace myelography? Spine 13:65-68, 1988.
138. Whitecloud TS III, Seago RA: Cervical discogenic syndrome: Results of operative intervention in patients with positive discography. Spine 12:313-316, 1987.
139. Wiesel SW, Tsourmas N, Feffer HL, et al: A study of computer-assisted tomography. I. The incidence of positive CAT scans in an asymptomatic group of patients. Spine 9:549-551, 1984.
140. Williams AL, Haughton VM, Syvertsen A: Computed tomography in the diagnosis of herniated nucleus pulposus. Radiology 135:95-99, 1980.
141. Wilson MA: The effect of age on the quality of bone scans using technetium-99m pyrophosphate. Radiology 139:703-705, 1981.
142. Witt I, Vestergaard A, Rosenklint A: A comparative analysis of x-ray findings of the lumbar spine in patients with and without lumbar pain. Spine 9:298-300, 1984.
143. Woolfenden JM, Pitt MJ, Durie BG, Moon TE: Comparison of bone scintigraphy and radiography in multiple myeloma. Radiology 134:723-728, 1980.
144. Yeates A, Drayer B, Heinz ER, Osborne D: Intra-arterial digital subtraction angiography of the spinal cord. Radiology 155:387-390, 1985.

CHAPTER 8

MISCELLANEOUS EVALUATIONS

Many patients with spinal pain have clinical signs and symptoms that do not correlate with one another. In addition, neuroradiologic tests (plain roentgenograms, computed tomography [CT], myelograms, or magnetic resonance [MR] imaging) do not always provide data that pinpoint the specific nervous system structure that is the source of the patient's pain. Laboratory tests are also inadequate in this regard. In these circumstances, additional tests may be helpful in differentiating among the various sources of spinal pain. Some of these techniques have published data in the medical literature documenting their utility (electrodiagnostic tests), whereas the scientific basis of others (e.g., thermography) remains unproven.

ELECTRODIAGNOSTIC STUDIES

The spectrum of neurophysiologic assessments includes electromyography (EMG), conduction studies (electroneurography [ENG]), and somatosensory (SEP) and motor-evoked (MEP) potentials. EMG and ENG are useful for the evaluation of the peripheral nervous system. SEP and MEP are more helpful with the study of central nervous system pathways.[17] Intraoperative evoked-potential monitoring also plays a crucial role in limiting postsurgical neurologic deficits.[35]

Peripheral Nervous System

Electrodiagnostic studies are commonly used in the evaluation of disease affecting the peripheral nervous system. These studies are extensions of the neurologic examination and provide an objective measure of nerve damage. They can confirm the clinical impression of nerve root compression, define the severity and distribution of involvement, and document or exclude other illnesses of nerves or muscles that could contribute to the patient's symptoms and signs. Electrodiagnostic tests measure the integrity of the nerve-muscle relationship and do not, by themselves, offer a specific etiologic diagnosis or quantify the degree of nerve damage. For patients with neck and arm pain or back and leg pain, electrodiagnostic studies are helpful in documenting radiculopathy (disease located at the level of the spinal roots). These studies are also useful in differentiating abnormalities associated with entrapment neuropathies, distal peripheral neuropathies, myopathies, and myelopathies.[2]

Electrodiagnostic studies include evaluation of electrical activity generated by muscle fibers at rest and during contraction (electromyogram [EMG]) and speed of conduction of impulses electrically generated in peripheral nerves (nerve conduction studies—ENG). Studies of the integrity of the neuromuscular junction are not done in the evaluation of patients with spinal disease but are reserved for patients with neuromuscular abnormalities, such as myasthenia gravis.

EMG is the study of the action potentials of muscle fibers. The EMG machine consists of an amplifier, oscilloscope, audio system, and recording electrodes. The recording electrodes are needles, ranging from 18-gauge to 26-gauge, that are inserted into muscles. The procedure consists of inserting needle electrodes through the skin to varying depths of each muscle to be studied. Each muscle is examined at two or more locations and in three or more directions. The multiple locations and directions are needed because abnormalities are focal in distribution. The test is painful but usually does not require sedation or analgesics. The test takes more than an hour to complete and may cost up to $600 to $800.

Nerve conduction studies of motor and sensory nerves, ENG, may also be done as part of an electrodiagnostic study of a patient with peripheral neurologic symptoms. Surface electrodes are attached to the skin over a hand muscle, and electric shocks of increasing voltage are generated until the largest electrical potential response of the muscle is recorded. A point distal in the nerve is tested and is termed the *distal latency.* Latency is determined by stimulation of the same nerve at a proximal site. The distance between the points of stimulation is divided by the difference between the proximal and distal latencies to compute the conduction velocity of the tested peripheral nerve. Conduction is measured in the fastest-conducting fibers only. Conduction in slower fibers is masked by the faster velocity in the fast fibers. Sensory conduction velocities have low amplitude and are difficult to detect.

Central Nervous System

EMG and ENG studies are unable to detect the location of spinal cord lesions or sensory radiculopathy. Evoked potentials are electrical responses of the nervous system to external sensory stimuli.[12] Testing of evoked potentials demonstrates abnormalities of the sensory system when clinical signs and symptoms are ambiguous. Evoked potentials may identify the location of unsuspected lesions in the central nervous system and may monitor the response of the lesion to therapy.

Evoked potentials generate low amplitude electrical activity from 0.1 to 20 μV. These low-amplitude potentials are obscured by the background noise produced by muscle artifact, electroencephalographic activity, and environmental interference. The evoked potential occurs at the same time interval after a stimulus. Averaging of the signal response after repeated stimulation identifies the evoked potential that can be separated from background noise. The evoked response is characterized by peaks and waves that are identified by their polarity, latency, amplitude, and configuration. Normal values are influenced by patient factors, including gender, age, body size, and temperature.[64]

Somatosensory evoked potentials (SEPs) are a means to determine the conduction of potentials generated by stimulation of peripheral structures to the spinal cord or cerebral cortex. A stimulus is generated peripherally, travels through the dorsal root ganglion, and ascends in the ipsilateral dorsal column. The stimulus then ascends to the contralateral ventroposterolateral nucleus of the thalamus and then to the primary sensory cortex. The stimulus can be measured over the spinal cord or scalp overlying the cortex. A computer is able to average the small potentials generated by peripheral stimulation and determine the latency associated with the peripheral site. SEPs may test large mixed nerves, such as the median and ulnar nerves; small sensory nerves; or a single dermatome.[22]

Motor evoked potentials (MEPs) are a means to determine the conduction potentials generated by electrical or magnetic stimulation of the motor cortex.[4] For electrical stimulation of the motor cortex, surface or subdermal needle electrodes are located on the scalp or over the motor cortex. Stimulating coils are also placed to stimulate the cervical and lumbar nerve roots. Subdermal needles are placed in the peripheral muscles to be tested.[24] Alternatively, surface-recording electrodes may be placed over motor endplates.[13] Motor-evoked potentials are recorded in the abductor pollicis, adductor minimi, quadriceps, tibialis anterior, gastrocnemius, extensor hallicis, and abductor hallicis.[17]

To understand the significance of abnormal electrodiagnostic findings, a review of basic EMG and nerve conduction concepts is worthwhile.

EMG Studies

Motor Unit. The motor unit includes an anterior horn cell, axon terminal arborization, myoneural junction, and all the muscle fibers supplied by that single nerve cell.

Motor Unit Potential. The motor unit potential is a summation of electrical activity associated with the fibers in one motor unit. Motor unit fiber size varies from a few to thousands of fibers. Therefore, motor unit potentials vary in amplitude and duration. Normal motor unit potentials have two to four spikes, an amplitude up to 4.0 mV, and a duration up to 15 ms.

In a partially denervated muscle (commonly the circumstance with disc herniations) the remaining normal axons grow to innervate more of the muscle fibers than composed the original motor unit (Fig. 8-1). The increase in the number of muscle fibers per motor unit results in a longer duration and asynchronous depolarization of muscle fibers. The result is a motor unit potential of increased amplitude and longer duration. The slightly different time intervals of stimulation result in a polyphasic response with multiple spikes. The amplitude may vary up to 20 mV or greater.

Fibrillations are action potentials of small clusters of denervated, healthy muscle fibers awaiting reinnervation. Fibrillations have an amplitude of 20 to 300 μV and a short duration of less than 5.0 ms. They may fire up to 30 times per second. Fibrillations are abnormal but are a nonspecific finding (myopathies are also associated with fibrillations). Positive sharp waves are thought to come from denervated, healthy muscle fibers injured by the entry of the electrode needle. The amplitude of these waves is 4.0 mV or greater with a duration of 10 ms. Like fibrillations, positive waves are abnormal but a nonspecific finding (Fig. 8-2). Giant motor unit potentials are extremely high-voltage and long-duration motor unit potentials. In patients with denervated muscles, these potentials appear after reinnervation.

Interference. As muscle contraction increases, greater numbers of individual motor units come into play, resulting in generation of greater numbers of unit potentials. The potentials observe individual patterns on the screen, resulting in a blur of activity near the baseline level. This is normal and is referred to as interference.

Insertional Activity. The insertion of the needle electrode damages nerve fibers, which results in electrical activity. The activity is present only with movement of the needle. In normal fibers, action potential generation ceases once the needle electrode comes to rest.

In radiculopathies, the insertional activity persists with decreased intensity for a number of seconds. This phenomenon is termed *prolonged insertional activity* and may be the only indication of an abnormality. However, increased insertional activity is a subjective evaluation dependent on

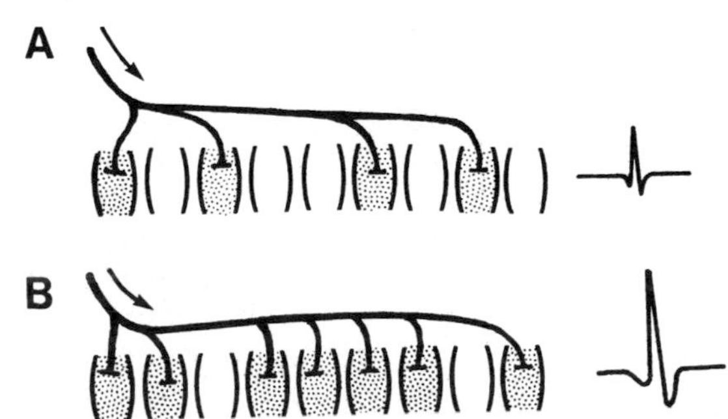

Figure 8-1 Schematic of a motor unit. The shaded muscle fibers are functional members of one motor unit with an axon that branches terminally to innervate the appropriate muscle fibers. The action potential produced by each motor unit is seen on the right. The unshaded muscle fibers belong to other motor units. *A*, A normal motor unit with four innervated muscle fibers, with corresponding action potential. *B*, Fibers that belonged to other motor units and had been denervated have been reinnervated by terminal sprouting from a normal, undamaged axon. The corresponding action potential has greater amplitude and duration.

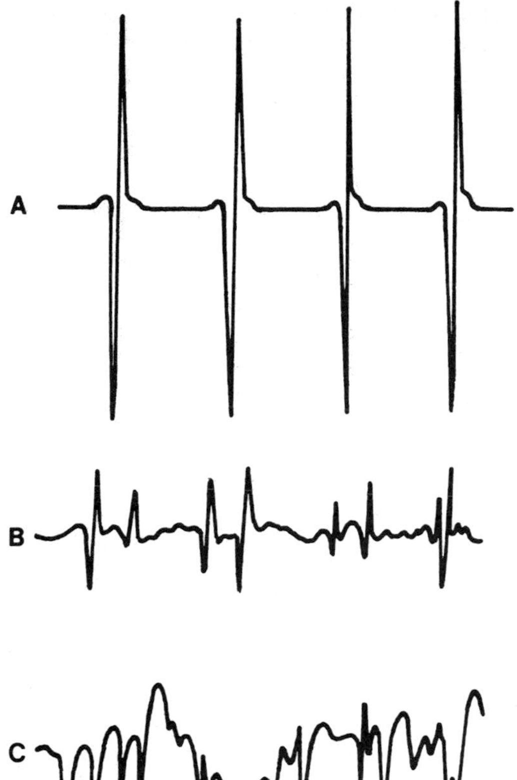

Figure 8-2 Electromyographic signals. *A*, Normal motor unit potential with four spikes, amplitude of 4.0 mV, and duration of 15 ms. *B*, Fibrillations consisting of small clusters of spikes with diminished amplitude and duration (200 μV). *C*, Positive sharp waves (250 μV).

observer criteria. This abnormality becomes significant only with other supporting EMG evidence.

A normal EMG, with the muscle relaxed, generates normal insertional activity only with electrode movement. Background fasciculations may be present. Motor unit potentials are normal in size, shape, and number. Maximum intensity of muscle contraction results in an interference pattern that observes individual action potentials.

Nerve Conduction Studies (Electroneurography)

H-Reflex. An H-reflex is an electrically elicited analogue of the tendon reflex (Fig. 8-3). By electrically stimulating large afferent fibers in a mixed nerve that synapses with alpha motor neurons, a monosynaptic reflex is evoked. The H-reflex is commonly used in the evaluation of S1 root lesions. The H-reflex is also used in the evaluation of C7 root lesions affecting the flexor carpi radialis.[48] The time latency (the period from time of stimulation until the impulse has traveled through the spinal cord to produce the reflex in the associated muscle) is standardized for the age and length of the limb or height of the patient. The difference between latencies of the upper extremities

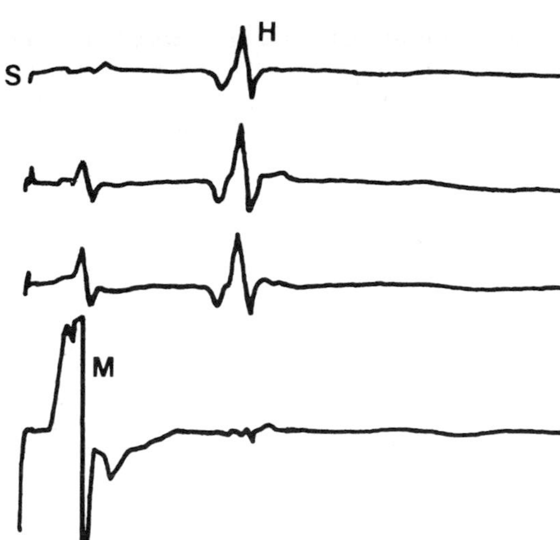

Figure 8-3 The H-reflex. The H wave (H) appears and becomes maximum as the stimulus (S) intensity increases, and it disappears at supraphysiologic levels of stimulation when the M wave is maximum.

is 1 ms or less. The differences between latencies of the lower extremities is 2 ms or less.

F Response. Antidromic activation of motor neurons after supramaximal stimulation of a peripheral nerve gives rise to an F response (Fig. 8-4). The F response travels along the motor nerve that supplies the innervation of the muscle. It is not a reflex because it does not involve sensory fiber. It is dependent on integrity of the motor unit only. Unlike the H-reflex, the F response is variable in the latency, and a number of repeated responses must be recorded. The most commonly reported result of the F response is the minimum response time or latency. The difference in the minimal latency between two extremities is usually less than 2 ms.

Sensory nerve action potential (SNAP) abnormalities do not occur with usual radiculopathy without dorsal root ganglion damage. However, discrepancies between

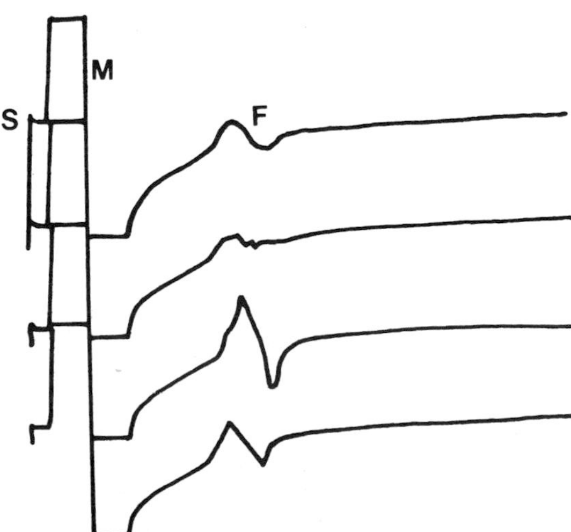

Figure 8-4 The F response. The F wave (F) is recorded after supraphysiologic stimulation (S). The amplitude, shape, and latency change with each stimulation.

latencies of SNAP of the two arms help differentiate plexopathy from radiculopathy. Plexus lesions cause damage at a location distal to the dorsal root ganglion. Therefore, SNAP is abnormal. Bilateral abnormalities suggest a diffuse process affecting nerves, such as peripheral polyneuropathy.

Electrodiagnostic Abnormalities Associated with Nerve Root Compression

In the first 3 days after compression, a decreased number of motor unit action potentials are noted during muscle contraction (Table 8-1). Also within the first week, H-reflex latency differences may appear in S1 radiculopathy before EMG changes are noted.[51] At day 7 to 10, the paraspinous muscles show the presence of positive waves along with polyphasic waves. Changes in the paraspinous muscles occur before changes in the extremities supplied by the same nerve root.[29] In about one third of patients, EMG abnormalities were found solely in the paraspinous muscles. Soon after the appearance of positive waves and fibrillations an increasing proportion of polyphasic waves is noted in muscles supplied by the corresponding nerve root.

Evaluation of the paraspinous muscles is helpful in localizing the area of nerve impingement. The paraspinous muscles are supplied by the posterior primary rami, which branch off the mixed peripheral nerve soon after its formation by the coalescence of the dorsal and ventral nerve root. There is marked anatomic segmental overlap in the superficial erector spinae muscles. The deepest layer, the multifidus layer, has the least degree of overlap. EMG studies done with electrodes placed 3 to 5 cm within the paraspinal muscle mass test the multifidus. Lesions of a single nerve root have abnormalities at one level only. Lesions that affect the anterior primary ramus, plexus, or peripheral nerve, distal to the division of the spinal root, have no effect on the paraspinous muscles.

Lesions that occur proximal to the branching of the primary rami result in abnormalities in both anterior and posterior divisions. Abnormalities may be limited to the paraspinous muscles in nerve root disease without anterior division abnormalities.

The most frequent abnormality found on an EMG for radiculopathy is the presence of positive waves. This is followed by an increased proportion of polyphasics and fibrillation potentials and a decreased number of motor units per contraction.[30]

8-1 ELECTROPHYSIOLOGIC ABNORMALITIES IN NERVE ROOT LESIONS

Day of Lesion	Abnormality
Day 3	Reduced muscle action potentials
	H-reflex delayed (C7)
	F response delayed (C7)
Day 7	Paraspinal fibrillations
Day 14	Paraspinal positive waves
	Associated proximal limb muscle positive waves
Day 21	Positive waves in entire myotome
Day 28	Fasciculations
Day 42	Prolonged polyphasic motor unit potentials

By the third week, paraspinous muscle fibrillation potentials are noted along with the emergence of positive waves in nerve root–associated limb muscles. With continued injury of 2 months or longer, motor unit amplitude and duration increase. In many patients, electrical signs of nerve damage do not appear until 21 days after the initial insult. EMG examination done too quickly in the course of events misses the lesion. An experienced electromyographer should be aware of this occurrence and should counsel the attending clinician on the appropriate time for electrodiagnostic studies.

EMG may not be helpful in chronic radiculopathies. Muscles may become reinnervated and not show spontaneous fibrillation potentials noted in acute radiculopathies. The severity of nerve dysfunction cannot be accurately determined by EMG. The cause of abnormal EMG findings cannot be specified by electrodiagnostic testing. Nerve root compression caused by a tumor, osteophyte, or herniated disc has similar findings. The level of a radicular injury can be localized to within one or two segments by EMG. The exact disc level can only be estimated.[25] EMG may also be of limited benefit after posterior spine surgery.

Relative contraindications for EMG examination are a patient with a bleeding tendency (hemophilia and thrombocytopenia) and a patient on anticoagulant therapy. The placement of needles through the skin may increase the possibility of cellulitis in those individuals particularly susceptible to infection. An EMG should be limited to one side of the body if a muscle biopsy is considered, because inflammation is associated with needle placement. The pathologic changes associated with needle examination may be confused with an acute inflammatory myositis.

Clinical Utility of Electrodiagnostic Results

Electrodiagnostic examination has a degree of accuracy in identifying patients with nerve root compression similar to that of myelography and clinical examination.[67] In studies comparing EMG and Pantopaque myelographic findings in patients undergoing surgery, EMG identified a root lesion and its level in 78% to 92% of patients, whereas the accuracy of myelography was 76% to 88%.[7,31,53] EMG was equally accurate in identifying root lesions at all lumbosacral levels, whereas myelography had greater accuracy at L4-L5 (85%) than at the L5-S1 level (60%).[32]

Partanen and colleagues studied 77 patients with suspected nerve root compression with EMG, myelography, and subsequent surgery.[43] Of these cervical spine patients, 26 had sensory impairment and only 34 had motor weakness. EMG identified abnormalities in 57%.

Motor nerve conduction and sensory nerve conduction velocities are normal in nerve root disease because peripheral nerves contain fibers from several roots and because root lesions from disc disease rarely produce complete loss of conduction through the involved roots. Damage to sensory nerves proximal to the dorsal root ganglia, as would occur in intervertebral disc herniation, produces no change in the peripheral sensory fibers. Conduction studies are of value in patients with suspected root disease because they exclude peripheral nerve disease as a potential cause of denervation changes.

H-Reflexes

H-reflexes are most sensitive to lesions of the sensory fibers in the S1 roots. Unilateral reduction of H-reflexes may be the sole electrophysiologic abnormality in some patients with S1 radiculopathy. The absence of an H-reflex correlates with an S1 radiculopathy with associated loss of ankle reflex.[22] H-reflex has an advantage over EMG in that H-reflex is abnormal almost immediately and is abnormal with sensory lesions. Milder S1 radiculopathies may be associated with subtle alterations in latency and amplitude that may be easily overlooked. An abnormal H-reflex is sensitive but not specific in determining the site of the lesion. Any abnormality of sensory roots, motor roots, spinal cord, sacral plexus, or sciatic nerve will demonstrate similar abnormalities. H-reflex has also been determined for L4 radiculopathies.[48]

H-reflexes are also useful in evaluation of cervical radiculopathies, particularly those affecting the C7 segment.[48] Unilateral reduction of H-reflexes may be the sole electrophysiologic abnormality in some patients with C7 radiculopathy. Because both motor and sensory pathways are tested, lesions limited to sensory fibers may be detected. Both extremities must be tested to detect abnormalities.[16] These abnormalities may be missed by the experienced electromyographer. An abnormal H-reflex is sensitive but not specific in determining the site of the lesion. Like a lesion in the lumbar spine, any abnormality of spinal cord, sensory roots, motor roots, brachial plexus, or peripheral nerves demonstrates similar abnormalities. The H-reflex is not positive in all radiculopathies. If large fibers are spared, the H-reflex may be normal. Once affected, the H-reflex tends to remain abnormal indefinitely, making it a less sensitive test for suspected radiculopathy.

F Response

One benefit of the F response is that it may become abnormal almost immediately after injury. However, the F response is relatively insensitive in detecting radiculopathy.[18] The F response tests a peripheral nerve served by several nerve roots. An abnormality in one nerve root may be overshadowed by normal function in the surrounding spinal nerves. The reliance on motor fibers alone may play a role in the relative insensitivity of F responses. Sensory tracts may play a significant role in radiculopathy. F waves evaluate the block or slow conduction through a few motor fibers at a time. The long distance tested may dilute the differences that may be detected side to side. Like the H-reflex, an abnormal F response is not synonymous with radiculopathy. Any lesion along the length of the affected nerve results in an abnormal F response. Acute and chronic radiculopathies cannot be distinguished by F responses.

A normal electrophysiologic examination does not exclude the possibility of a radiculopathy causing neurologic symptoms, but a definite abnormality points toward an organic origin of a patient's symptoms. This may be of particular importance in patients claiming disability or workers' compensation.

Electrodiagnostic studies may be helpful in detecting cervical spinal stenosis.[58] These tests may be particularly helpful in differentiating anterior motor horn cell disease from myelopathy. A number of findings, including upper and motor neuron signs, decreased reflexes in the arms and increased reflexes in the legs, fasciculations, and muscle atrophy, may be found in both groups. However, patients with cervical spinal stenosis should not have electrodiagnostic abnormalities above the foramen magnum, whereas anterior horn cell disease affects muscles in the head, including the tongue. Table 8-2 lists the electrophysiologic tests to differentiate between myelopathy, radiculopathy, and peripheral neuropathy.

Electrodiagnostic studies may also be used to differentiate individuals with shoulder and neck pain associated with upper extremity entrapment syndromes (carpal tunnel syndrome) from those with neck pain associated with cervical radiculopathy.[10,66] In some individuals, a double crush syndrome (median nerve compression and cervical nerve root compression) may explain the occurrence of neck, arm, and hand pain.[15] Electrodiagnostic testing is able to help detect the presence of two separate lesions.

Some non-neurologic disorders may be associated with EMG abnormalities. Metabolic disorders, particularly diabetes, may cause diffuse paraspinal abnormalities with no evidence of radiculopathy. Patients may improve with control of their diabetes. Paraspinal fibrillation and positive waves have been reported with metastatic disease.[38] EMG examination demonstrating marked segmental compromise of the posterior primary ramus distal to the spinal root with relative sparing of the anterior ramus may be the earliest evidence of paraspinal muscle metastases. Although CT scan may be unable to identify the presence of metastases, MR imaging is able to detect paraspinal lesions. Although a pattern of posterior primary ramus segmental compromise is not diagnostic of metastases, the abnormal EMG pattern may suggest MR examination.[33] Patients with arachnoiditis have also had abnormal paraspinal electrophysiologic studies.[23] Mechanical abnormalities such as muscle strains, ligamentous injury, and degenerative disc disease without nerve root compression should be associated with a normal EMG.

The role of serial EMG determinations in the management of patients is not well established compared with therapy decisions based on patients' symptoms and clinical findings. Once EMG changes of reinnervation occur, they may persist indefinitely. Denervation changes may also persist for many years after injury to the motor nerve, even when there is no evidence of continuing injury. It is difficult to determine the age or activity of a lesion once reinnervation changes appear. In addition, the extent of EMG abnormalities does not necessarily correlate with the extent of nerve damage.

8-2 ELECTROPHYSIOLOGIC TESTS FOR THE DIAGNOSIS OF MYELOPATHY, RADICULOPATHY, AND NEUROPATHY

	EMG	ENG	F Wave	EP
Myelopathy	(+)	–	+	+
Radiculopathy	+	–	+	(+)
Peripheral neuropathy	+	+	(+)	–

EMG, electromyography; ENG, electroneurography; EP, evoked potentials; ( ), less diagnostic benefit. Modified from Dvorak J: Epidemiology, physical examination, and neurodiagnostics. Spine 23:2663-2674, 1998.

Postsurgical Testing

Electrophysiologic studies obtained after laminectomy present particular difficulty in interpretation because of the injury associated with ischemia from retractors during surgery. In addition, patients may develop a recurrent cervical herniated disc after surgery. In 25% of all patients with lumbar root lesions from disc disease, denervation changes persist after surgery even in the absence of persistent impingement.[5] EMG abnormalities, particularly in the paraspinous muscles, are significant for a new lesion in a patient after laminectomy if the patient has acute recurrence of symptomatology and EMG abnormalities at a level different from the level affected during the previous episode of radiculopathy.

Somatosensory Evoked Potentials

Somatosensory evoked potentials (SEPs) of large mixed nerves measure the function of motor nerves and the sensory function of peripheral nerves. The most common nerves stimulated in the upper extremity are the median and ulnar nerves (Fig. 8-5). The most common nerves stimulated in the lower extremity are the posterior tibial and peroneal nerves. Theoretically, SEPs have advantages over peripheral nerve conduction studies for the diagnosis of cervical radiculopathies.[54] However, mixed nerve SEPs are not helpful for detecting single-level sensory radiculopathies because large mixed nerves carry nerves from multiple nerve roots. The findings from studies of SEPs in patients with cervical radiculopathies have been too inconsistent to be helpful in replacing any other test as a means of detecting spinal root dysfunction.[49] A more reliable method of detecting radiculopathies may be obtained with those of spinal rather than cortical somatosensory potentials.[52] However, mixed nerve SEPs are sensitive in detecting spinal cord abnormalities that affect cord pathways. Spinal cord tumors and multiple sclerosis are two types of pathologic pathways that result in abnormal mixed nerve SEPs. Cervical spondylodegenerative myelopathies may be detected by abnormal mixed nerve SEPs. A normal test does not exclude the possibility of a cord lesion, particularly one affecting motor function.[21]

Small Sensory Nerve Evoked Potentials

Small sensory nerve evoked potentials (SSEPs) are measured in the lower extremity. L4, L5, and S1 radicu-

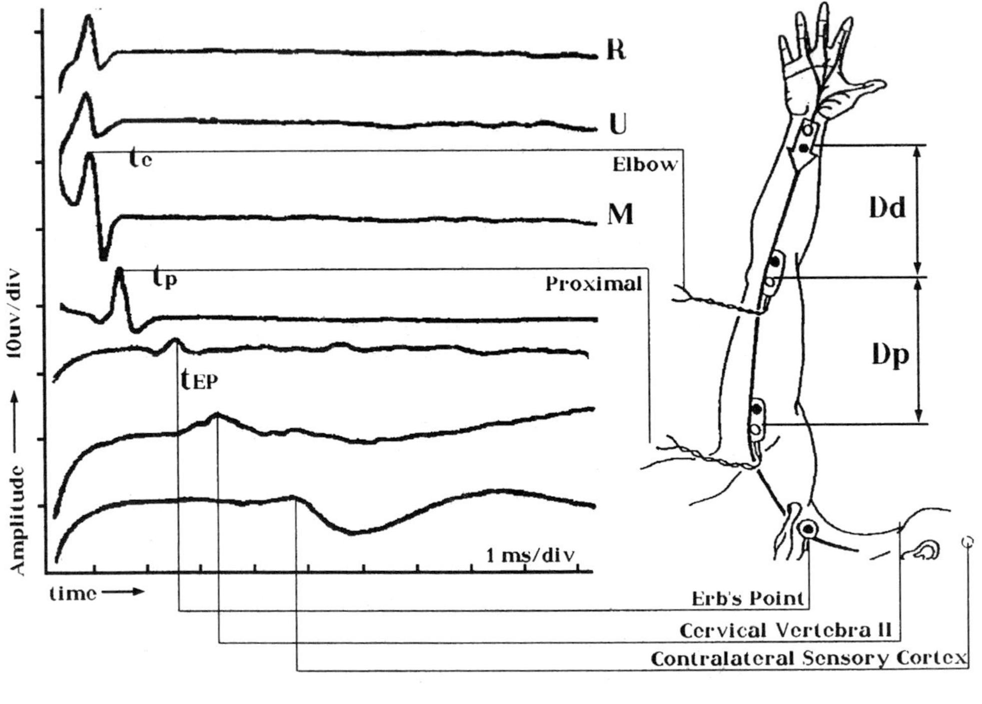

$$\frac{t_p - t_c}{D_d} = \text{Distal Conduction Velocity} \qquad \frac{t_{EP} - t_p}{D_p} = \text{Proximal Conduction Velocity}$$

Figure 8-5 Sensory evoked potentials, median nerve stimulation. The top three traces (t), labeled R, U, and M, reflect activity at electrodes placed at the elbow over the expected course for the radial, ulnar, and median nerves, respectively. Each of these traces contains a negative (that is, upward) potential at the latency t_c. The potential measured at R and U reflects volume conduction. The larger potential at M reflects the proximity of the median nerve action potential. The fourth trace shows a peak at t_p. This electrode is positioned in the biceps groove. Median and ulnar nerve stimulations result in a potential recorded in this electrode pair, but radial nerve stimulation does not because of its course on the far side of the humerus. The fifth tracing shows the latency as the potential passes the electrode at Erb's point (tEP) over the brachial plexus. The sixth tracing is derived from the electrode over C2 in the neck. The seventh tracing shows negative potential (that is, upward) at the time that the cortex is activated. The methods for calculating the distal and proximal conduction velocities are shown. The position of radial and ulnar pickup electrodes is not shown to avoid confusion. They are located lateral to the biceps tendon and just below the olecranon groove. *(Courtesy of Elizabeth Tidman.)*

lopathies are detected by abnormalities in the distribution of the saphenous, superficial peroneal, and sural nerves. Lower extremity SEPs are more sensitive than EMGs in some patients with lumbosacral radiculopathy. In a study of 59 patients with radiculopathy, 38 had an abnormal CT/myelogram, 32 had abnormal SEPs, whereas 11 had abnormal EMGs.[65] All 21 patients with normal CT/myelograms had normal SEPs. The SEP was less sensitive in patients in whom spinal stenosis was the only radiographic finding. The intermittent nature of nerve compression with spinal stenosis may explain the lessened sensitivity of SEPs in patients with spinal stenosis. SEP may be most helpful in patients with nondiagnostic EMG.

Dermatomal Somatosensory Evoked Potentials

A dermatomal somatosensory evoked potential (DSEP) is generated by direct stimulation of skin and recording of cortical responses. The accuracy of the test depends on the placement of stimulating electrodes. In the upper extremity, C6 is tested by stimulating the thumb, C7 by testing the middle finger, and C8 by testing the little finger. The recording of DSEPs is technically demanding, requiring an experienced technician. A DSEP is complementary to other electrodiagnostic tests. It does not evaluate motor nerve function and is not as sensitive as EMG for the diagnosis of nerve root lesions.[21] In the lower extremity DSEP test, S1 is tested by stimulating the lateral foot, L5 by testing the dorsum of the big and second toe, and L4 by testing the medial aspect of the calf above the ankle.

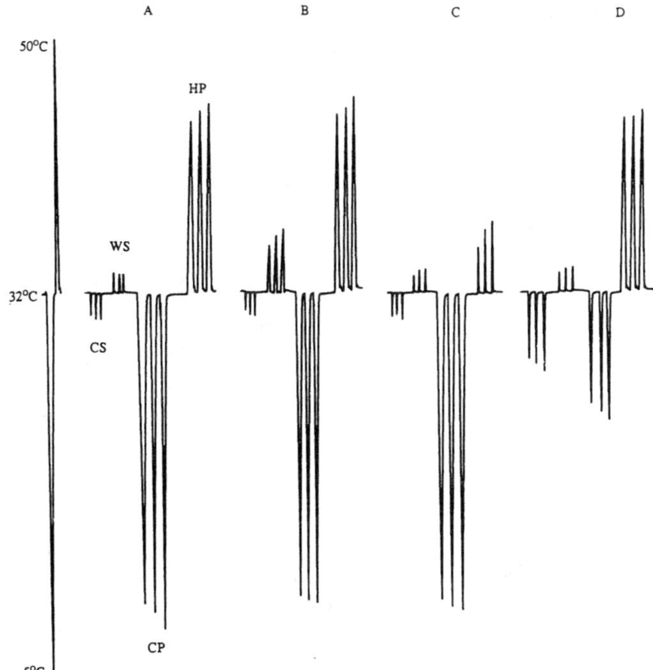

Figure 8-6 Quantitative somatosensory thermotest. Each peak represents one thermal stimulus ramp. A, Normal pattern; B, pure warm hypoesthesia; C, heat hyperalgesia; D, cold hypoesthesia associated with cold hyperalgesia. WS, warm sensation; CS, cold sensation; CP, cold pain; HP, heat pain. *(From Verdugo RJ, Ochoa JL: Use and misuse of conventional electrodiagnosis, quantitative sensory testing, thermography, and nerve blocks in the evaluation of painful neuropathic syndromes. Muscle Nerve 16:1058, 1993. By permission of Oxford University Press.)*

Pudendal Evoked Potentials

Sacral roots below S1 are tested by pudendal evoked potentials (PEPs). PEPs are generated by stimulating the dorsal nerve of the penis or clitoris using surface electrodes or by stimulating the urethra and anal sphincter using catheter electrodes. The major limitation of PEPs is that only sensory nerve fibers of the pudendal nerve are tested.[25] A bulbocavernosus reflex is needed to measure muscle function.

Quantitative Somatosensory Thermotest

Quantitative somatosensory thermotest is another form of somatosensory testing that measures the function of small afferent fibers in the peripheral nervous system.[62] The test is accomplished through the use of a Peltier device that supplies a controlled, progressively increasing or decreasing range of temperatures to the skin. The patient is asked to respond to the signal the instant of first sensation of cold, warmth, cold pain, or heat pain by pressing a switch that immediately returns the stimulator to baseline temperature. A recorder allows visual analysis of the temperatures associated with these sensations. Normal control values are available for rates of temperature change and standard stimulus area.[63] The function of different caliber sensory fibers is associated with different temperature sensations. Cold sensation is associated with small A-delta myelinated afferents, warm sensation with unmyelinated fibers, and cold and heat pain with unmyelinated C-fiber polymodal nociceptors and A-delta nociceptors. Abnormalities with each temperature modality are associated with a specific pattern (Fig. 8-6). For example, heat hyperalgesia (reduced threshold for heat pain) is associated with sensitization of C-unmyelinated nociceptors. The site of the test, distal or proximal in a limb, may be associated with a variety of findings. A distal site with more severe denervation may demonstrate warm, cold, and thermal hypoesthesia, whereas a more proximal lesion reveals sensitization of the remaining functioning afferent fibers with hyperalgesia to temperatures. The test measures function from the peripheral nerve endings to sensorium in the cerebral cortex. The test is reproducible in patients with organic neuropathic lesions. The test may be used to detect psychogenic disorders associated with thermal complaints of pain. Psychogenic pain patterns tend to be less consistent.

Intraoperative Monitoring

SEPs have been used during surgical procedures to determine the integrity of the function of components of the nervous system. SEPs analyze the sensory tracts. The MEPs monitor the spinal cord motor tracts. MEPs may elicit myogenic (MG) or neurogenic (NMEP) responses. A myogenic response is a muscle contraction that appears on EMG. A neurogenic response is the nerve action potential that elicits the contraction in the muscle innervated by that nerve. The myogenic response has a large amplitude and consistent latency but is modified by anesthesia and is not compatible with the surgical situation because muscles may contract while the patient is on the operating table. Significant changes on NMEPs are 10% increase in latency and 80% decrease in amplitude. The patient does not experience muscle contractions with this procedure.[34] The monitoring is used for procedures that correct spinal deformities, particularly scoliosis; decompress spinal stenosis lesions; repair spinal fractures; resect spinal tumors; and assess spinal cord injuries.[8]

Intraoperative monitoring includes a protocol for testing of a number of neurologic functions. The type of anesthesia has effects on the results of electrophysiologic tests.[55] The avoidance of muscle relaxants may be necessary depending on the measurement device. The electrophysiologic tests may be associated with false-positive and false-negative results. Both have great implications in regard to the outcome of spinal surgery that puts the spinal cord and spinal roots at risk. False-positive results will occur in patients being awakened to determine if nerve damage has occurred. False-negative results are noted in individuals developing nerve damage without the warning to correct the damage during surgery. Of the various tests, the NMEP is the one associated with no false-negative findings.[69]

Cooperation between the surgeon, anesthesiologist, and neurophysiologist is key to a successful outcome. The experience of the individuals working together is essential to good operative results. Recommending spine centers that do these procedures frequently is prudent for individuals who require surgery that puts their nervous system at risk.

Summary

Although they are not tests that pinpoint specific diagnoses, electrodiagnostic studies are helpful in the evaluation of patients with neurologic dysfunction. The procedure is performed in the outpatient department. These studies may identify a specific nerve root lesion when clinical symptoms suggest abnormalities at two levels. MR imaging tends to be more closely associated with electrodiagnostic abnormalities than myelograms. However, EMG tests may be abnormal when corresponding radiographic results are normal. An abnormal EMG is corroborative evidence of organic disease and helps the surgeon select patients who are candidates for surgery. EMG changes may recede after resolution of nerve impingement. Non-neurologic disorders have normal EMG findings. Electrodiagnostic tests help differentiate peripheral nerve lesions from radiculopathy. When used in the appropriate setting and with the limitations of the tests in mind, the clinician may rely on these procedures to supply information that is useful in the diagnosis and management of patients with neck and arm pain as well as those with back and leg pain.

THERMOGRAPHY

Thermography is a noninvasive procedure that images the infrared radiation (heat) emitted from the body surface. Thermography is based on the principle that alterations in a variety of body functions alter the cutaneous vascular supply that heats the skin. Postganglionic sympathetic cell bodies involved in the control of the cutaneous vessel are located in the sympathetic chain ganglia, which are connected to the spinal nerves distal to the dorsal root ganglia by the rami communicantes. The postganglionic nerve fibers from these cells travel to the cutaneous blood vessels by way of the peripheral nerves. Because the postganglionic nerves travel with peripheral nerves composed of multiple root fibers, sympathetic abnormalities spread beyond a single dermatome. Irritation of peripheral sensory nerves may affect sympathetic nerve fibers at the same segment level, resulting in alterations of blood flow to the skin. Factors that are associated with sensory activation of nociceptive fiber stimulation (substance P) may also have an effect on cutaneous blood flow. However, pain is a complex phenomenon that cannot be simplified to a direct correlation with cutaneous heat production. Thermography does not take a picture of pain itself; it does reveal pathophysiologic conditions associated with neurovascular, soft tissue, circulatory, and musculoskeletal disorders.

The two types of thermography are liquid crystal (contact) and electronic (noncontact) thermography. Contact thermography uses cholesterol crystals that change color with variations of surface temperature. The crystals are placed inside inflatable transparent boxes with one flexible, thermosensitive side that is applied to the body. Each box has a limited temperature range. An examination with liquid crystals requires selection of a box with the appropriate temperature range. A picture is taken of the box to record the patterns of surface temperature. The box is chosen by trial and error. The advantages of contact thermography include the absence of radiation exposure, ease of use, and lower cost than electronic thermography.

Electronic thermography uses an infrared radiation sensor that converts heat reading to electrical signals that are displayed on a black-and-white or color monitor. A picture can be taken of the video screen or can be stored on computer discs. This system has the advantage of viewing large areas of the body during a single examination.

The examination must be performed in an air-conditioned, draft-free room. The ambient temperature must be between 68° and 72° F. The patient should have refrained from smoking for the day of the test. In addition, the patient should refrain from pain medications, physical therapy, and exposure to strong sunlight for at least 24 hours. The patient must disrobe and be in equilibrium with room temperature for 30 to 60 minutes before the examination is started. The patient's temperature must be normal. If the patient is febrile, the examination must be postponed.

Examination of the lumbosacral spine and lower legs with liquid crystals consists of separate images of buttocks; anterior, lateral, and posterior thighs; lower legs; dorsa of the feet; and toes.[42] The examination requires 1 to 2 hours to complete.

Examination of the cervical spine and arms with liquid crystals consists of separate images of the posterior neck and superior shoulders; lateral oblique shoulders; lateral upper arms; posterior, lateral, anterior, and medial forearms; and dorsal and ventral aspects of the hands.[44] The examination requires 1 to 2 hours to complete.

The assessment of a thermogram is based on the distribution and temperature range of the skin. Both sides of the body have a temperature within 0.17° to 0.45° C in the healthy state.[60] The extent of thermal asymmetry between opposite sides of the body varies in different locations but remains less than 0.5° C. Values are reproducible for as long as 5 years. A thermogram is abnormal if a side-to-side difference of 1° C involving 25% of its evaluated area is present. Alterations in the physiologic temperature distribution patterns also indicate abnormalities.[45]

Acute pain is associated with increased heat, whereas chronic pain is linked with decreased temperatures. Increased temperature is found over areas involved with an inflammatory process. Increased muscle metabolism associated with spasm or tonic contraction can be detected as increased heat conveyed to the surface by circulation.

Artifacts are common. Skin folds conserve heat and appear "hot" on a thermogram. Sunburn alters the skin pattern. Alterations of the skin associated with injections, tattoos, or vaccinations change the normal thermographic patterns as well.[36]

Thermographic Abnormalities Associated with Spinal Pain

Thermographic diagnosis of spinal pain syndromes includes evaluation of the cervical spine and upper extremities or lumbar spine and lower extremities. Thermal asymmetry in patients with spinal pain is associated with a decrease in the affected limb's temperature. In one study of the lumbar spine, when the asymmetry of temperature exceeded one standard deviation from the mean temperature of homologous regions measured in 90 normal subjects, the positive predictive value of detecting root impingement was 94.7% and the specificity was 87.5%.[61]

The usefulness of thermography has been studied in patients with lumbar disc disease. Studies have reported a close correlation between abnormal thermograms and surgically proven herniated discs.[1a,17a] Investigators have also found that in patients with herniated discs, thermography and myelography have accuracy rates of 95% and 84%, respectively.[45] Infrared thermographic imaging has been compared to MR, CT, and myelography in patients with chronic back pain. Thermographic findings correlated with MR, CT, and myelographic abnormalities in 94%, 87%, and 80% of the time, respectively. Of 22 MR scans of patients with disc prolapse associated with nerve root lesions, 95% had leg abnormalities on thermography.[59] CT and thermographic findings were correlated in 15 asymptomatic volunteers and 19 patients with nerve root displacement.[9] The thermogram had 60% specificity and 100% sensitivity in detecting nerve root lesions. Thermographic accuracy in detecting nerve root irritation also has been reported to be greater than that of electromyography. This difference in sensitivity is thought to be related to thermographic capability to detect sensory nerve abnormalities.[61b]

Although some studies have reported a positive correlation between thermography and radiculopathy, a number of studies have appeared in the literature questioning the accuracy of thermography in the diagnosis of lumbosacral radiculopathy. For example, Mahoney and associates have reported the findings of an investigation of thermography in patients with sciatica.[36a, 36b] The thermograms of normal controls and patients with herniated discs were compared. The sensitivity of thermograms in identifying the side with the herniated disc was 35%. The "normal" controls showed "abnormal" or "asymmetrical" patterns in 75% of individuals studied. The thermogram was considered to be of no diagnostic value in evaluation of sciatica.[36a] In a comparison study, thermography was unable to document a correlation between pain and alteration in body temperature.[36b] A critique of this study by Uematsu and associates suggested that the poor results were related to failure to adhere to appropriate procedure in obtaining thermograms in the study patients. They stated that poor equipment, poor focusing, inadequate contrast, improper patient positioning, and improper preparation all played a role in the poor results of the study.[61a] Harper and So, in independent studies, were unable to demonstrate the reliability of thermography in the diagnosis of radiculopathy.[26,56] In the Harper study of 55 patients with radiculopathy and 37 normal controls, five readers reviewed thermograms in a blinded fashion. The specificity of thermography ranged from 20% to 44%. Thermography predicted the level of the radiculopathy correctly in less than 50% of the cases. In the So study, thermography abnormalities did not follow a dermatomal distribution and did not identify the clinical or electrophysiologic level of radiculopathy.

In a meta-analysis of the diagnostic accuracy and clinical usefulness of thermography for lumbar radiculopathy, significant methodologic flaws were identified in 27 of 28 studies reviewed.[27a] The one study of high quality found no discriminant value for liquid crystal thermography. The authors concluded that thermography could not be recommended for routine clinical investigation of low back pain.[27a]

Whereas a number of studies of thermography in the evaluation of lumbar spine pain and radiculopathy have been reported, cervical spine studies are fewer.[1,42,47,68] The thermogram had 60% specificity and 100% sensitivity in detecting lumbar nerve root lesions. Thermographic accuracy in detecting nerve root irritation has also been reported to be greater than electromyographic accuracy. This difference in sensitivity was thought to be related to thermographic ability to detect sensory nerve abnormalities.[61] Comparison of thermography and EMG in the diagnosis of cervical radiculopathy was not favorable.[57] In a study of 20 normal controls and 14 patients with cervical radiculopathy, thermography was abnormal in 43% and EMG was abnormal in 71%. Thermographic abnormalities were seen only in the hands and fingers, and the pattern did not follow the dermatome of the affected cervical root. In contrast, others have reported a higher frequency of positive thermographic tests in patients with cervical radiculopathy.[28] Hubbard and colleagues have suggested that a normal thermogram would negate the necessity for a CT scan for a patient with neck pain.[28] In the majority of circumstances, the thermogram has no diagnostic or predictive value in the evaluation of cervical radiculopathy. In another study, liquid crystal thermography was compared with nerve conduction studies for the evaluation of carpal tunnel syndrome. Thermography identified none of 9 patients with mild entrapment and 7 of 14 patients with marked entrapment. The sensitivity of thermography was significantly less than that of nerve conduction tests for the evaluation of carpal tunnel syndrome.[40] In a study of whiplash injury, Mahoney and colleagues found no significant difference in 28 symptomatic individuals when compared with 50 control subjects. In the two groups, only 1 of 28 whiplash subjects and 4 control subjects had abnormal thermograms.[37]

Psychogenic or functional spinal pain is difficult to differentiate from structural disease. Hendler and associates tried to differentiate psychogenic pain and malingering from true organic pain syndromes.[27] Forty-three (19%) of 224 patients referred with a diagnosis of psychogenic pain had abnormal thermograms corresponding to the symptomatic area. The thermogram was positive when other diagnostic tests, including an EMG, were normal.

Although a number of studies have reported on the usefulness and accuracy of thermography in musculoskeletal conditions, the procedure has not won acceptance by many physicians. The reasons for this lack of acceptance may be the need for special rooms in which to do the test, the array of equipment needed to do the examination, and the necessity of extensive experience with the technique to evaluate test results. However, the most important factor is that the exact role of the thermogram in diagnosis of spinal pain problems remains to be determined. Large prospective studies including control patients must be completed before the scientific merit of this diagnostic technique can be determined.

At present thermograms are not recommended for use in making routine decisions for diagnosis of patients with spinal pain. Thermograms detect autonomic dysfunction in different parts of the body. In the majority of individuals, determination of autonomic function is not necessary to adequately treat patients for their spinal pain. Interpretation of thermograms needs to be standardized. Additional prospective studies must be conducted to correlate the findings of thermography with the most sensitive radiographic techniques. The specificity and sensitivity of the thermogram need further definition. The value and role of thermography will be clarified as well-designed studies are completed that demonstrate diagnostic significance and effects on therapy. The technique will become more significant as it becomes more widely available and well-trained physicians can interpret thermographic results. Recent articles in Australia and a position paper by the American Medical Association's Council on Scientific Affairs question the use of thermography in the clinical setting at this time.[3,14]

DIFFERENTIAL NERVE BLOCKS

In patients who have intractable and chronic spinal pain, identification of the source of pain, whether somatic, sympathetic, or psychogenic, is essential in planning an appropriate treatment regimen. Differential nerve blocks are an invasive means for examining the central and peripheral components of a patient's pain. They are particularly helpful in localizing the source of pain in patients who have undergone multiple operations on their spine and continue to experience spinal pain.

The different susceptibilities of sensory fibers to anesthesia is the physiology on which differential blocks are based.[19] The different peripheral sensory fibers are classified into A (alpha and delta), B (preganglionic autonomic), and C (unmyelinated) groups. Different concentrations of local anesthetics have selective sensitivity for these fibers.[41] Fiber sensitivity in decreasing order is B, C, and A.[39] The sensitivity is related in part to the amount of myelination of the fibers. Unmyelinated fibers have exposure of the entire surface of the axon membrane to local anesthetics. In myelinated nerves, the membrane is exposed only at Ranvier's nodes because the myelin layer insulates the rest of the axon. Higher concentrations of local anesthetics are needed to penetrate the nerve to block transmission. Alternative explanations have suggested that large, fast-conducting fibers are more susceptible to conduction blockade than smaller, slower-conducting fibers.[20] The study concluded that conduction velocity is directly proportional to distance between Ranvier's nodes. The fastest fibers with the longest internodal distances should be affected before fibers with small diameters. The discrepancy between these conflicting findings may be explained by the location of nerve fibers in neural bundles. Small-diameter fibers are more superficial and surround large-diameter fibers in dorsal spinal roots. Anesthetics injected as part of a spinal block reach the small fibers first and affect their function before the large fibers.

Anesthetics may also be given that block sensory fibers but leave motor function intact. The local anesthetics with rapid onset, short duration of action, and ability to selectively block sympathetic, sensory, and then motor fibers with increasing concentrations are lidocaine and mepivacaine. Fiber size, degree of myelination, nerve fiber location, length of nerve fiber exposed to anesthetic, neuropathologic state of the nerve, and concentration and lipid solubility of the anesthetic all play a role in the effects of anesthetic blockade on nerve function.[42]

Differential Block Procedure

Lumbar Spine Procedure

Antegrade spinal block requires three concentrations (0.25%, 0.5%, and 1.0%) of local anesthetic (procaine) that are prepared before starting the procedure. The patient must have pain at the time of the procedure. If pain is absent, the procedure is postponed. Other contraindications include anticoagulation and local skin infection at the injection site. The patient is told that he or she will receive a series of medications that may or may not relieve the pain. A lumbar needle is placed into the subarachnoid space. A placebo is injected as the patient is told that he or she is receiving one of the drugs. After 20 minutes of no pain relief, a 5-mL injection of 0.25% procaine is administered. At this concentration of anesthetic, the sympathetic fibers are blocked. If there is pain relief without loss of sensory function other than sympathetic nerve function, a sympathetic mechanism of pain production is confirmed. If there is no pain relief despite sympathetic blockade, 5 mL of 0.5% procaine is injected. If there is no pain relief despite loss of pinprick sensation, 1% solution is injected for motor blockade. If pain continues despite sensory and motor paralysis, the site of the lesion is proximal to the site of the blocks. The pain may be related to malingering, psychogenic pain, or a central nervous system lesion.[47] Patients who continue to experience pain despite nerve blocks will not benefit from surgery or nerve blocks directed at peripheral structures.

The procedure for retrograde spinal block is slightly different. The patient receives the full dose of anesthetic after the placebo is injected. The benefit of doing the procedure in this fashion is that a catheter does not need to be left in the subarachnoid space for repeated injection. The patient will develop total motor and sensory loss. If pain persists, it is proximal to the site of the blockade. If pain is relieved, it is caused by somatic or sympathetic mechanisms. If pain relief continues after sensation returns, the mechanism of pain is sympathetic in origin.

The results of the test are most dramatic when the patient is completely relieved of pain with only saline or when no relief is obtained with 1% anesthetic that produces motor paralysis or affects a sensory level several dermatomes above the pain site. In these circumstances, a central nervous system defect, structural or psychiatric, is present.[68]

In one study, nerve blocks were helpful in making an appropriate diagnosis of organic versus functional disease in 35 (87.5%) of 40 patients. The results of the block helped the physicians plan appropriate therapy (medical or surgical, or both, versus psychiatric) for the appropriate patients.[1]

Cervical Spine Procedure

Differential nerve blocks may be able to differentiate pain of somatic and sympathetic nerve origin. Pain in the neck, upper extremity, and upper chest may be relieved with an injection of the stellate ganglion. Normal saline would be injected as the placebo. Relief of pain would be associated with a placebo effect. If there is no effect, a block with 10 to 15 mL of a local anesthetic is given. A successful sympathetic block would be manifested by the development of Horner's syndrome, including ptosis, miosis, and anhidrosis. If no pain relief is noted, a somatic block to the painful areas is completed. A successful somatic block is associated with peripheral motor and sensory loss. In the upper neck a block of the cervical plexus would be appropriate, whereas upper extremity pain would be helped by a brachial plexus injection.

Subarachnoid and Epidural Injections

Subarachnoid and epidural injections are used more commonly for differential spinal blockade in the evaluation of lumbar spine pain. Subarachnoid blockade is usually confined to the thoracic or lumbar spine. Blockade in the cervical spine would have the potential of affecting the function of the phrenic nerve, resulting in decreased breathing capacity. The effects of epidural blockade in the cervical spine are not useful in diagnosing the source of neck pain. Bilateral effects of epidural injection usually occur, and controlled manipulation of the area of action of the anesthetic is difficult. The epidural fluids do not flow freely or predictably. For these reasons, these techniques are not used for diagnosing the source of cervical spine pain.

Patients who do not experience any pain relief from differential nerve blockade may have pain of central or psychogenic origin. Techniques that affect central neurologic function are used to differentiate origins of pain central to the level of spinal blockade and those of psychogenic origin.[11] The tests are based on the assumption that patients in a light plane of sleep respond to pain in a pattern similar to when fully awake. Conversely, if the spinal pain resolves and the individual responds to other painful stimuli over other body locations, such as the anterior tibia, the implication is that the pain is of psychogenic origin. Sodium pentothal is slowly infused until the patient falls into a light plane of sleep. The infusion is stopped and the patient is allowed to wake up while being periodically tested for typical pain responses in areas other than the spine. When the patient responds to the pain stimulus, a stimulus that causes the typical spinal pain is given. If the stimulus does not cause typical spinal pain, the origin of the pain is psychogenic. Intravenous lidocaine at a dose of 1.2 to 2.0 mg/kg is given until tingling is reported by the patient. Two minutes later the patient's pain is assessed. A relief of pain that has been resistant to peripheral injections suggests a central origin. No relief suggests a psychogenic origin of pain. Few studies have been completed proving the validity of these intravenous tests for determining the source of spinal pain.[6,50]

Nerve blocks are invasive procedures with the potential for significant morbidity. The spread of injected materials is unpredictable. The exact site of the injection may not be known unless radiographic techniques document the site of the needle.[46] The complexity of the central nervous system makes discovering the source of spinal pain difficult. A positive response to a placebo injection does not absolutely demonstrate a central or psychogenic source of pain. Nerve blocks should be undertaken by experienced anesthesiologists in the evaluation of pain in patients with complicated symptomatology. In those difficult patients, the risks of surgery outweigh the risks associated with differential nerve block. The blocks should be undertaken if an unnecessary surgical procedure can be prevented based on the results of the procedure. Otherwise, the potential complications of the injections outweigh their benefits.

References

1. Ahlgren EW, Stephen R, Lloyd AC, McCollen DE: Diagnosis of pain with a graduated spinal block technique. JAMA 195:83, 1966.

1a. Albert SM, Glickman M, Kallish M: Thermography in orthopaedics. Ann N Y Acad Sci 121:157, 1964.

2. American Association of Electrodiagnostic Medicine: Guidelines in electrodiagnostic medicine. Muscle Nerve 15:229, 1992.

3. Awerbuch MS: Thermography—its current diagnostic status in musculoskeletal medicine. Med J Aust 154:441, 1991.

4. Barker AT, Jalinous R, Freestaon IL: Non-invasive magnetic stimulation of the human motor cortex. Lancet 1:1106-1107, 1985.

5. Blom S, Lemperg R: Electromyographic analysis of the lumbar musculature in patients operated on for lumbar rhizopathy. J Neurosurg 26:25, 1967.

6. Boas RA, Covino BG, Shahnarian A: Analgesic responses to I.V. lignocaine. Br J Anaesth 54:501, 1982.

7. Brady LP, Parker LB, Vaughn J: An evaluation of the electromyogram in the diagnosis of the lumbar disc lesion. J Bone Joint Surg Am 51:539, 1969.

8. Brown RH, Nash CL Jr: Intra-operative spinal cord monitoring. In Frymoyer JW (ed): The Adult Spine: Principles and Practice. New York, Raven Press, 1991, pp 549-562.

9. Chafetz N, Wexler CE, Kaiser JA: Neuromuscular thermography of the lumbar spine with CT correlation. Spine 13:922, 1988.
10. Cherington M: Proximal pain in carpal tunnel syndrome. Arch Surg 108:69, 1974.
11. Cherry DA, Gourlay GK, McLachlan M, Cousins MJ: Diagnostic epidural opioid blockade and chronic pain: Preliminary report. Pain 21:143, 1985.
12. Chiappa KH (ed): Evoked Potentials in Clinical Medicine, 2nd ed. New York, Raven Press, 1990.
13. Chomiak J, Dvorak J, Antinnes J, Sandler A: Motor evoked potentials: Appropriate positioning of recording electrodes for diagnosis of spinal disorders. Eur Spine J 4:180-185, 1995.
14. Cotton P: AMA's council on scientific affairs takes a fresh look at thermography. JAMA 267:1885, 1992.
15. Dawson DM: Entrapment neuropathies of the upper extremities. N Engl J Med 329:2013, 1993.
16. Deschuytere J, Rosselle N, DeKeyser C: Monosynaptic reflexes in the superficial forearm flexors in man and their clinical significance. J Neurol Neurosurg Psychiatry 39:555, 1976.
17. Dvorak J: Epidemiology, physical examination, and neurodiagnostics. Spine 23:2663-2674, 1998.
17a. Edeiken J, Wallace JD, Curley RF, Lee S: Thermography and herniated lumbar disks. AJR Am J Roentgenol 102:790, 1968.
18. Eisen A, Schomer D, Melmed C, et al: The application of F-wave measurements in the differentiation of proximal and distal upper limb entrapments. Neurology 27:662, 1977.
19. Gasser HS, Erlanger J: Role of fiber size in establishment of nerve block by pressure or cocaine. Am J Physiol 88:581, 1929.
20. Gissen AJ, Covino BG, Gregus J: Differential sensitivities of mammalian nerve fibers to local anesthetic agents. Anesthesiology 53:467, 1980.
21. Glantz RH, Haldeman S: Other diagnostic studies: Electrodiagnosis. In Frymoyer JW (ed): The Adult Spine: Principles and Practice. New York, Raven Press, 1991, pp 541-548.
22. Glantz RH, Haldeman S: Other diagnostic studies: Electrodiagnosis. In Frymoyer JW, Tucker TB, Hadler NM, et al (eds): The Adult Spine: Principles and Practice. New York, Raven Press, 1991, pp 541-548.
23. Grue BL, Pudenz RH, Sheldon CH: Observations on the value of clinical electromyography. J Bone Joint Surg Am 39A:492, 1957.
24. Gugino LD, Aglio LS, Segal ME, et al: Use of transcranial magnetic stimulation for monitoring cord motor paths. Semin Spine Surg 9:315-336, 1997.
25. Haldeman S: The electrodiagnostic evaluation of nerve root function. Spine 9:42, 1984.
26. Harper CM Jr, Low PA, Fealev RD, et al: Utility of thermography in the diagnosis of lumbosacral radiculopathy. Neurology 41:1010, 1991.
27. Hendler W, Uematsu S, Long D: Thermographic validation of physical complaints in "psychogenic pain" patients. Psychosomatics 23:283, 1982.
27a. Hoffman RM, Kent DL, Deyo RA: Diagnostic accuracy and clinical utility of thermography for lumbar radiculopathy: A meta-analysis. Spine 16:623, 1991.
28. Hubbard J, Maultsby J, Wexler C: Lumbar and cervical thermography for nerve fiber impingement: A critical review. Clin J Pain 2:131, 1986.
29. Johnsson B: Morphology, innervation and electromyographic study of the erector spinae. Arch Phys Med Rehabil 50:638, 1969.
30. Johnson EW, Melvin JL: Value of electromyography in lumbar radiculopathy. Arch Phys Med Rehabil 52:239, 1971.
31. Knuttson B: Comparative studies of electromyographic, myelographic and clinical-neurological examinations in the diagnosis of lumbar root compression syndrome. Acta Orthop Scand Suppl 49:1, 1961.
32. Knuttson B: Electromyographic studies in the diagnosis of lumbar disc herniations. Acta Orthop Scand 28:290, 1959.
33. LaBan MM, Tamler MS, Wang AM, Meerschaert JR: Electromyographic detection of paraspinal muscle metastasis: Correlation with magnetic resonance imaging. Spine 17:1144, 1992.
34. Lagattuta FP, Hudoba P: Electrodiagnostics. In Fardon DF (ed): Orthopaedic Knowledge Update: Spine 2. Rosemont, IL, American Academy of Orthopaedic Surgeons, 2002, pp 85-86.
35. Lenke LG: The clinical utility of intraoperative evoked-potential monitoring from a spinal surgeon's perspective. Semin Spine Surg 9:288-294, 1997.
36. LeRoy PL, Bruner WM, Christian CR, et al: Thermography as a diagnostic aid in the management of chronic pain. In Aronoff GM (ed): Evaluation and Treatment of Chronic Pain. Baltimore, Urban & Schwarzenberg, 1985, pp 232-250.
36a. Mahoney L, McCulloch J, Csima A: Thermography in back pain: 1. Thermography as a diagnostic aid in sciatica. Thermology 1:43, 1985.
36b. Mahoney L, Patt N, McCulloch J, Csima A: Thermography in back pain: 2. Relation of thermography to back pain. Thermology 1:51, 1985.
37. Mahoney L, Wiley M, McMiken D: Thermography in whiplash injuries of the neck. Advocates Q 10:1, 1988.
38. Massey EW: Coexistent carpal tunnel syndrome and cervical radiculopathy (double crush syndrome). South Med J 74:957, 1981.
39. McCollum DE, Stephen CR: Use of graduated spinal anesthesia in the differential diagnosis of pain of the back and lower extremities. South Med J 57:410, 1964.
40. Meyers S, Cros D, Sherry B, Vermeire P: Liquid crystal thermography: Quantitative studies of abnormalities in carpal tunnel syndrome. Neurology 39:1465, 1989.
41. Nathan PW, Sears TA: Some factors concerned in differential nerve block by local anesthetics. J Physiol (Lond) 157:565, 1961.
42. Nehme AE, Warfield CA: Diagnostic measures. In Warfield CA (ed): Principles and Practice of Pain Management. New York, McGraw-Hill, 1993, pp 53-61.
43. Partanen J, Partanen K, Oikarinen H, et al: Preoperative electromyography and myelography in cervical root compression. Electromyogr Clin Neurophysiol 311:21-26, 1991.
44. Pochaczevsky R: The value of liquid crystal thermography in the diagnosis of spinal root compression syndromes. Orthop Clin North Am 14:271, 1983.
45. Pochaczevsky R, Wexler CE, Myers PH, et al: Liquid crystal thermography of the spine and extremities. J Neurosurg 56:386, 1982.
46. Purcell-Jones G, Pither CE, Justins DM: Paravertebral somatic nerve block: A clinical, radiographic, and computed tomographic study in chronic pain patients. Anesth Analg 68:32, 1989.
47. Raj PP, Ramamurthy S: Differential nerve block studies. In Raj PP (ed): Practical Management of Pain. St. Louis, Mosby-Year Book, 1986, pp 173-177.
48. Sabbahi MA, Khalil M: Segmental H-reflex studies in upper and lower limbs of patients with radiculopathy. Arch Phys Med Rehabil 71:223, 1990.
49. Schmid U, Hess C, Ludin H: Somatosensory evoked potentials following nerve and segmental stimulation do not confirm cervical radiculopathy with sensory deficit. J Neurol Neurosurg Psychiatry 51:182, 1988.
50. Schoichet RP: Sodium Amytal in the diagnosis of chronic pain. Can Psychiatr Assoc J 23:219, 1978.
51. Schuchmann JA: Evaluation of H-reflex latency in radiculopathy. Arch Phys Med Rehabil 58:560, 1976.
52. Seyal M, Palma G, Sandhu L, et al: Spinal somatosensory evoked potentials following segmental stimulation: A direct measure of dorsal root function. Electroencephalogr Clin Neurophysiol 69:390, 1988.
53. Shea PA, Woods WW, Weden DH: Electromyography in diagnosis of nerve root compression syndrome. Arch Neurol Psychiatry 64:93, 1950.
54. Siivola J, Sulg I, Heiskari M: Somatosensory evoked potentials in diagnostics of cervical spondylosis and herniated disc. Electroencephalogr Clin Neurophysiol 52:276, 1981.
55. Sloan TB: Anesthesia during spinal surgery with electrophysiological monitoring. Semin Spine Surg 9:302 -308, 1997.
56. So YT, Aminoff MJ, Olney RK: The role of thermography in the evaluation of lumbosacral radiculopathy. Neurology 39:1154, 1989.
57. So YT, Olney RK, Aminoff MJ: A comparison of thermography and electromyography in the diagnosis of cervical radiculopathy. Muscle Nerve 13:1032, 1990.
58. Stark RJ, Kennard C, Swash M: Hand wasting in spondylotic high cord compression: An electromyographic study. Ann Neurol 9:58, 1981.
59. Thomas D, Cullum D, Siahamis G, Langlois S: Infrared thermographic imaging, magnetic resonance imaging, CT scan and myelography in low back pain. Br J Rheumatol 29:268, 1990.
60. Uematsu S, Edwin DH, Jankel WR, et al: Quantification of thermal asymmetry: I. Normal values and reproducibility. J Neurosurg 69:552, 1988.

61. Uematsu S, Edwin DH, Jankel WR, et al: Quantification of thermal asymmetry: II. Application in low-back pain and sciatica. J Neurosurg 69:556, 1988.
61a. Uematsu S, Haberman J, Pochaczevsky R, et al: A commentary on experimental methods, data interpretation and conclusion. Thermology 1:55, 1985.
61b. Uematsu S, Jankel WR, Edwin DH, et al: Quantification of thermal asymmetry. Part 2: Application in low back pain and sciatica. J Neurosurg 69:556, 1988.
62. Verdugo RJ, Ochoa JL: Use and misuse of conventional electrodiagnosis, quantitative sensory testing, thermography, and nerve blocks in the evaluation of painful neuropathic syndromes. Muscle Nerve 16:1056, 1993.
63. Verdugo RJ, Ochoa JL: Quantitative somatosensory thermotest: A key method for functional evaluation of small calibre afferent channels. Brain 115:893, 1992.
64. Waldman HJ: Evoked potentials. In Raj PP (ed): Practical Management of Pain, 2nd ed. St. Louis: Mosby-Year Book, 1992, pp 155-167.
65. Walk D, Fisher MA, Doundoulakis SH, et al: Somatosensory evoked potentials in the evaluation of lumbosacral radiculopathy. Neurology 42:1197, 1992.
66. Watson R, Waylonis GW: Paraspinal electromyographic abnormalities as a predictor of occult metastatic carcinoma. Arch Phys Med Rehabil 56:216, 1975.
67. Wilbourn AJ, Aminoff MJ: AAEM Minimonograph 32: The electrodiagnostic examination in patients with radiculopathies. Muscle Nerve 21:1612-1631, 1998.
68. Winnie AP, Collins VS: Differential neural blockade in pain syndrome of questionable etiology. Med Clin North Am 52:123, 1968.
69. York DH: Overview of neurophysiological monitoring of spinal cord function in relation to changes in the marketplace. Semin Spine Surg 9:295-301, 1997.

CHAPTER 9

A STANDARDIZED APPROACH TO THE DIAGNOSIS AND TREATMENT OF SPINAL PAIN

A patient with low back or neck pain presents to a physician with a set of symptoms and signs. At presentation, these clinical complaints are unassociated with any specific diagnosis. The task of the physician is to integrate patient complaints and physical findings into an accurate diagnosis and to prescribe appropriate therapy. The primary objective for the physician is to return patients to their normal level of function as quickly as possible. In this physician-patient interaction, there must be concern for the efficient and precise use of diagnostic studies and minimization of ineffectual medical and surgical treatments and monetary cost to the patient and society in general. Identification of the specific pain generators of the axial skeleton is not necessary, or possible, in all instances of spinal discomfort.

In most individuals, the back or neck problem improves whether anatomic abnormalities are identified or just suspected. As many as 85% of individuals with spinal disorders may have no identifiable cause for their pain.[15] Anatomic abnormalities are present in a substantial number of people who are asymptomatic. However, there remain a number of individuals with abnormalities who are symptomatic with disease associated with alterations from normal. The difficulty is our inability to detect those important abnormalities with currently available technology. The physician does not want to give a patient a chronic illness when the problem is transient. At the same time, there are individuals who present with low back or neck pain with significant medical disorders. The task of the physician is to separate these groups of patients. Attainment of this goal depends on the accuracy of the physician's decision-making process. The physician must use a combination of knowledge of medical literature that reports significant scientific findings and clinical experience to decide on the factors that are important for improving the lives of individuals with spinal dysfunction. This clinical acumen allows the physician to use the most helpful diagnostic and therapeutic measures at optimal times. For example, not every patient who presents with clinical findings of a herniated disc requires imaging with magnetic resonance (MR); only after initial treatment fails is this study appropriate. Although specific information is not available for every category of spinal pain, a large body of data is available to guide the handling of these patients, such as that presented in the previous chapters in this section.

Using the available knowledge, algorithms for the diagnosis and treatment of low back and neck pain have been designed (see the Low Back Pain and Neck Pain Algorithms immediately following their respective sections). The algorithms are a sequence of clinical decisions and thought processes found to be useful in approaching the universe of patients with lumbosacral and cervical spine problems. The algorithms follow well-delineated rules, established from the consensus of a broad segment of qualified physicians who diagnose and treat patients with low back or neck pain. The algorithms do not include all axial skeleton diagnoses, and there are exceptions to the rule. Not all patients fit easily into the categories to be discussed. Common sense helps the examining physician individualize the evaluation of the unusual patient. This protocol has been used in the evaluation of more than 5000 patients and has proved to be useful in the vast majority of those individuals.[27] The diagnostic process may also be presented in the format of a table (see Appendices A and B).

LOW BACK PAIN

A number of algorithmic approaches have been presented for the diagnosis and treatment of low back pain. Algorithms have come in different forms, trying to meet different needs.

The Pennsylvania Plan

The development of some algorithms has been based on the experience of a single institution. For example, "The Pennsylvania Plan" is based on the experience of Rothman and associates at Pennsylvania Hospital.[23] This algorithm concentrates on the mechanical disorders associated with alterations in the intervertebral disc and avoids discussion of medical causes of low back pain.

Quebec Task Force on Spinal Disorders

Another algorithm was published by the Quebec Task Force on spinal disorders. In 1983, this multidisciplinary group was established to formulate guidelines for the diagnosis and treatment of painful spinal disorders.[35] The algorithm was formulated in the context of occupation-related injury and disability. The data used for the algorithm were based on data from the Quebec Worker's Compensation Board and review of 469 publications in the medical literature. The report ranked scientific support for a variety of diagnostic measures and therapies for low back pain. In an effort to simplify diagnoses, the task force classified activity-related spinal disorders into 11 categories (Table 9-1). In addition, the categories were qualified by duration of symptoms and work status. The algorithm was formulated based on the scientific support and the classification system.

The first four categories of the classification system describe pain symptoms and radiation without associated specific pathologic changes that cause the symptoms. Categories 5 through 9 are associated with specific pathologic entities. Category 10 includes patients with no specific identifiable disease and chronic pain. The final category includes all individuals with medical causes for low back pain. The algorithm allows for the evaluation, using a few simple diagnostic tests, of individuals who are younger than 20 or older than 50 years of age and have experienced severe trauma, recurrent symptoms, neoplasm, fever, or a neurologic deficit. These tests include plain lumbar spine films and an "inflammatory screen" (blood test) that is not well defined for specific disorders. Most patients receive conservative therapy without diagnostic tests. Referral to consultants and more expensive diagnostic tests are reserved for individuals who do not improve after 7 weeks of therapy. Surgery is limited to those with specific radicular symptoms and is not indicated for back pain alone except for a small minority with severe lumbar spine instability. One of the strengths of this algorithm is the emphasis on a return to work as part of the treatment and measurement of outcome for patients with low back pain. The only therapies considered useful at the time of the formulation of the Quebec classification system in 1987 in randomized, controlled trials included bed rest for 2 days, back school for individuals in categories 1 through 4, and surgical decompression for patients with confirmed neural compression with radiculopathy. More recent studies have conflicted with the evidence-based findings of these older studies. For example, activity as tolerated has supplanted 2 days of bed rest as the preferred initial therapy for low back pain.

Although the Quebec Task Force algorithm is based on scientific literature and the outcomes of a large number of patients, it concentrates primarily on the evaluation of mechanical disorders. The medical causes of low back pain are briefly mentioned. The Quebec algorithm also has become outdated. Evidence-based medicine algorithms must be constantly updated with the results of contemporary studies. What may be considered the standard of care at a previous time may become hazardous when studied in a subgroup, in a larger population, or over a longer duration. The Women's Health Initiative study is an example of how evidence-based medicine can offer conflicting recommendations as it studies the use of estrogen/progesterone combination therapy for postmenopausal women.[48]

9-1 QUEBEC TASK FORCE CLASSIFICATION OF LOW BACK PAIN

1. Pain without radiation
   a, b, c, w or i
2. Pain + radiation to extremity, proximally
   a, b, c, w or i
3. Pain + radiation to extremity, distally
   a, b, c, w or i
4. Pain + radiation to lower limb neurologic
   a, b, c, w or i
5. Presumptive compression of a spinal nerve root on a simple roentgenogram (spinal instability or fracture)
6. Compression of a spinal nerve root confirmed by specific imaging techniques (CT, MR, myelogram), electromyography, or venography
7. Spinal stenosis
8. Postsurgical status 1 to 6 months after intervention
9. Postsurgical status > 6 months after intervention
10. Chronic pain syndrome
11. Other diagnoses

a, <7 days; b, 7 days to 7 weeks; c, >7 weeks; w, working; i, idle.
Modified from Spitzer WO, LeBlanc FE, Dupuis M, et al: Scientific approach to the assessment and management of activity-related spinal disorders: Report of the Quebec Task Force on Spinal Disorders. Spine 12:S17, 1987.

Agency for Health Care Policy and Research Acute Low Back Problem Monograph

In 1994, the AHCPR organized an evaluation of the extant medical literature concerning the diagnosis and treatment of acute low back pain.[4] The results of this review were published as a monograph. The recommendations of the publication were not meant to be used as guidelines; however, the report contained pathways that have been considered a guideline or algorithm for low back problems by a variety of groups. At the time of its publication, the AHCPR report was an accurate reflection of the knowledge concerning low back pain. However, the 1994 report has limitations that have appeared over time. Reviews of the report have illustrated the added expense associated with some report recommendations (e.g., radiographs for individuals older than 50 years of age).[36] The committee reviewed data in the literature up to 1994. A substantial number of articles reporting updated information have appeared in the subsequent period of time. A review of the guideline process suggests that recommendations should be reassessed for validity every 3 years.[34a] The Cochrane back review group has continued the review of articles pertaining to spine disease and has highlighted the limitations of the medical literature in regard to the number and design of clinical studies.[8] The Cochrane group has reported the relative value of therapies and diagnostic tests based on an ongoing review of the available evidence in the literature.

Low Back and Neck Pain: Comprehensive Diagnosis and Management Algorithms

The revised algorithms in this chapter incorporate some of the work-related issues associated with the Quebec algorithm while updating those factors important for the evaluation of patients with back pain associated with medical disorders. The specificity and sensitivity of historic, physical, and laboratory findings must be considered in deciding on those factors that are most helpful and cost effective in determining the diagnosis of a patient.[14] Historical data lack specificity in regard to a variety of disorders with similar clinical complaints. The reliability and reproducibility of physical findings are not of the degree that the cause of pain can be ascertained without doubt. Statistical probabilities are important in guiding evaluations, but they do not negate the importance of sound clinical judgment based on experience with patients with low back and neck pain. The algorithms are a balance between the available findings in medical literature and the requirements and limitations of evaluating individuals in a clinical, non-research setting.

Diagnostic and Treatment Protocol

The protocol is organized into the format of an algorithm (see "Low Back Pain Algorithm," pages 210–213). In *Webster's Dictionary* an algorithm is defined as "a set of rules for solving a particular problem in a finite number of steps."[43] This algorithm is an organized pattern of decision-making and thought processes that have proved useful in caring for patients with low back pain.

Each patient has an associated set of unique circumstances. There are, however, a number of common factors a physician should keep in mind when managing this population of patients. The primary objective for the physician is to return the patient with acute low back pain to regular activity as quickly as possible. In achieving this goal, the physician must be concerned with making efficient and precise use of diagnostic studies, avoiding ineffectual surgical procedures, and making therapy available at a reasonable cost to the patient and society. Although scientifically proven data demonstrating efficacy for every aspect of low back care are not available, there is a large body of information to guide physicians in handling these patients. The algorithm follows well-delineated rules established as the consensus of a broad segment of physicians.

Cauda Equina Compression

The protocol begins with the universe of patients who present with signs and symptoms of a low back problem. They will have undergone an initial medical history and physical examination. The first major decision is to rule in or out the presence of cauda equina compression (CEC) syndrome. Significant compression of the cauda equina or truly progressive motor weakness is the only major surgical emergency to be found in patients with an acute mechanical low back problem.[18]

The compression usually is due to extrinsic pressure on the caudal sac by a massive, centrally herniated disc. Epidural abscesses or tumor masses are other examples of disorders causing CEC. Other causes for acute-onset CEC syndrome include epidural hematoma and trauma. After surgery, patients who receive anticoagulants are at risk for development of epidural hematomas. The symptom complex includes low back pain, bilateral motor weakness of the lower extremities, bilateral sciatica, saddle anesthesia, and even frank paraplegia with bowel or bladder incontinence.

Once this diagnosis is suspected, the patient should undergo immediate MR, or computed tomography (CT)/myelography for those with contraindications for magnet exposure. If the radiographic test is positive, subsequent emergency surgical decompression is necessary. The major reason for prompt surgical intervention is to arrest the progression of neurologic loss.[34] The chance of actual return of neurologic function after surgery is unpredictable. Although the incidence of CEC syndrome in the total population of patients with low back pain is very low (less than 1%), it is the only entity affecting structures in the spine that requires immediate operative intervention.

Systemic Medical Illness

The patients who do not have a CEC syndrome should then be evaluated for acute, severe symptoms suggestive of underlying medical illness as the cause of their back pain.

Medical Emergencies. Patients with marked neurologic deficits, signs of severe systemic disease, and vascular collapse are frequently evaluated in emergency departments. Also, women with ectopic pregnancies may present to an emergency department with low back and pelvic pain. The emergency department physician plays a key role in the appropriate care of these patients. Thoughtful evaluation of these gravely ill patients with expedited admission to the hospital can be very important in the rare patient with life-threatening back disease.[30] Simple tests, such as determination of a human chorionic gonadotropin level or ultrasonography of the abdomen for ectopic pregnancy or expanding abdominal aneurysm, may be very helpful in determining which patients with low back pain have specific, life-threatening causes for their symptoms.

Systemic Disorders. These groups include individuals with constitutional symptoms of fever or weight loss suggestive of a tumor or infection. Patients with pain that is increased with recumbency may have a tumor of the spinal column or neural elements. Patients with prolonged morning stiffness may have a spondyloarthropathy. Acute severe, localized back pain is frequently associated with a vertebral crush fracture secondary to a systemic, generalized process (metabolic bone disease) or a local tumor. Patients with viscerogenic pain (e.g., renal colic, dyspepsia, pulsatile pain of an aneurysm) have symptoms associated with the organ system affected. Patients with a prior history of a neoplasm are at greater risk of having a medical cause for low back pain.

Medical evaluation, including laboratory and radiographic tests, of patients with low back pain should be initiated only if they have significant symptoms and signs of an underlying medical illness with initial presentation. Simple tests that may be helpful in patients with new-onset back pain who are 50 years of age or older and have another risk factor for a medical disorder (history of cancer) include plain roentgenography of the lumbar spine and erythrocyte sedimentation rate (ESR).[12,36] This allows for a cost-effective use of diagnostic tests for individuals at greatest risk for medical disorders. These patients need to be evaluated by the medical algorithm (see pages 212–213). If no definitive medical cause can be determined after the screening evaluation (including history and physical examinations), these individuals should start receiving initial conservative treatment for their symptoms.

Psychosocial Considerations. Another concern that may enter into the evaluation of patients with low back pain early in the algorithm is psychologic overlay affecting the presence and severity of pain. At the time of presentation to a physician, individuals may have experienced chronic pain in relationship to depression or a work-related injury. Patients with chronic pain frequently have no pathoanatomic cause for their symptoms.[20] Chronic pain is their disorder. The presence of continued back pain may be reinforced or perpetuated by social and psychologic factors. The concerns about the effects of pain on family relationships, income, job satisfaction, and employment status may add significant stress that tends to perpetuate pain.[3,25,42] Somatic amplification of symptoms may become an essential part of economic survival. Patients receiving workers' compensation respond less well to therapy than those not receiving compensation.[42] In patients with work-related back pain, job dissatisfaction plays a significant role in persistent low back pain resistant to therapy.[3]

In patients in whom psychologic factors or somatic amplification is suspected, components of the history (lack of response to all therapies) and positive "nonorganic" signs should identify patients with nonmechanical or nonmedical low back pain.[41] Two additional signs in addition to the Waddell signs include the production of back pain with movement of the cervical spine or limitation of motion of either shoulder producing low back pain.[26] In these patients, the use of screening tools for depression may be helpful. However, before a patient is branded as having a "nonorganic" problem, he or she should be evaluated by the process presented in this algorithm. If no specific abnormalities can be identified and psychologic factors are present, psychiatric evaluation is appropriate after the initial evaluation and response to therapy has been determined.

Conservative Therapy

The remaining patients who do not have a CEC syndrome or acute, severe medical illness should be started on a course of conservative (nonoperative) therapy regardless of the diagnosis at this stage. The specific diagnosis, whether a herniated disc or a simple back strain, is not important because the entire population with back pain is treated the same way with slight modifications. Some of these patients eventually will need an invasive procedure (epidural injection, surgery), but at this point there is no way to predict which individuals will respond to conservative therapy and which will not.

The early treatment of acute low back pain uses the tincture of time. The passage of time, the use of anti-inflammatory and muscle relaxant medications, and controlled physical activity are the modalities that have proved safest and most effective.[11] In a study by Cherkin and coworkers, the combination of nonsteroidal anti-inflammatory drugs (NSAIDs) and muscle relaxants had the best patient satisfaction at 1 week for the treatment of acute low back pain.[9] The vast majority of these patients will respond to this approach. In today's society, with its emphasis on quick solutions, many patients are pushed too rapidly toward more complex treatment, especially invasive treatment. Many return to regular exercise too early in the recuperative process. This "quick fix" has no place in the treatment of acute low back pain. In most cases, surgery does not return people to heavy work, and in the long run the best chance of getting a patient back to full activity is the nonoperative approach.

The physician should treat the patient conservatively and wait up to 6 weeks for a response. Most of these patients will improve within 2 to 10 days; a few will take longer.[13] Once the patient has achieved approximately 80% relief, he or she should be mobilized. A few of these patients will benefit from the help of a lightweight, flexible corset as they resume normal occupational activities. After becoming more comfortable and increasing his or her activity level, the patient should begin a program of back exercises and return to a normal lifestyle. The pathway along this section of the algorithm is a two-way street: should regression occur with exacerbation of symptoms, the physician can resort to more stringent conservative measures. The patient may require further controlled physical activity. Most patients with acute low back pain will proceed along this pathway, returning to their normal life patterns within 2 months of the onset of symptoms. Some will also benefit by attendance in a back school program.[24] Patients may also benefit from a work evaluation if physical conditions of employment place the individual at risk for recurrent back pain. This evaluation might include ergonomic review of the job site, work place modification, functional capacity examination, the possibility of work hardening for the patient, and vocational rehabilitation to find alternative employment if the individual is unable to complete the tasks associated with his or her initial job. In others, job satisfaction must be considered as the important factor that slows the return to work. All these factors should be considered in order to return patients to work without restrictions. The combination of controlled physical activity, medications, education, exercises, and work evaluation should be considered components of a conservative therapy protocol.

The vast majority in this initial group have nonradiating low back pain, termed *back strain.* The cause of back strain is not clear. There are several possibilities, including ligamentous or muscular strain, continuous mechanical stress from poor posture, or a small tear in the annulus fibrosus. Patients usually complain of pain in the low back, often localized to a single area. On physical examination, they demonstrate a decreased range of lumbar spine motion, tenderness to palpation over the involved area, and muscle contraction. Their roentgenographic examinations usually are normal, but if therapy is not rapidly successful, films should be obtained at 6 to 8 weeks to rule out other possible etiologic factors, such as an infection or tumor. The mainstay of successful treatment for back strain is controlled physical activity. Anti-inflammatory and muscle relaxant medications give patients symptomatic relief of their pain, allowing greater function, but do not hasten healing.[6]

After 6 weeks, patients in whom the initial treatment regimen fails are sorted into four groups. The first group is composed of people with pain localized to the low back. The second group includes those who complain mainly of leg pain, defined as pain radiating below the knee and commonly referred to as sciatica. Patients in the third group have anterior thigh pain, and those in the fourth group have posterior thigh pain. Each group follows a separate diagnostic path.

Localized Low Back Pain

The first group of patients will complain predominantly of low back pain despite 6 weeks of conservative care. This group should have their plain roentgenograms carefully examined for structural abnormalities. Flexion and extension views may be obtained, but a debate exists whether these views actually demonstrate spinal instability. Spondylolysis with or without spondylolisthesis is the most common structural abnormality to cause significant low back pain.

Spondylolysis/Spondylolisthesis. *Spondylolysis* can be defined as a break in the continuity of the pars interarticularis in the lamina.[32] Approximately 5% of the population have this defect, which is thought to be caused by a combination of genetic structural abnormalities and environmental stress (Fig. 9-1). If the defect permits displacement of one vertebra on another, it is termed *spondylolisthesis.* Most people with this defect are able to perform their activities of daily living with little discomfort. These patients usually will respond to nonoperative measures, including a thorough explanation of the problem, a back support, and exercises. In a small percentage of such cases, conservative treatment fails and fusion of the involved spinal segments becomes necessary (Fig 9-2).[31] This is one of the few times primary fusion of the lumbar spine is indicated in a nontraumatic situation, and it must be stressed that it is a relatively infrequent occurrence. Most patients with spondylolisthesis do not need surgery. Fusion surgery for spondylolisthesis is a successful operation in most circumstances. Patients with postoperative pain should be evaluated by the multioperated spine algorithm (see Fig. 20-5). Patients who fail to obtain pain relief with this portion of the algorithm should be treated with chronic pain therapy.

Lumbar Spondylosis. In addition to changes of spondylolysis, plain roentgenograms may show intervertebral disc changes in patients with low back pain. It is important to remember that decreased disc height and associated changes of the surrounding vertebral bodies (traction osteophytes) may be present in patients who are asymptomatic (Figs. 9-3 and 9-4). However, articular degeneration with facet joint sclerosis may be associated with decreased back motion and back pain. Osteoarthritis of the facet joints is the diagnosis most often associated with these roentgenographic changes (Fig. 9-5). In the patient with disc degeneration, other sources of back pain may need to be investigated before the physician ascribes the patient's pain to osteoarthritis of the spine. Acromegaly also causes degenerative changes of intervertebral discs, but these changes occur over a short period of time in comparison with those of primary osteoarthritis.

Disc Calcification. On occasion, disc calcifications are noted on plain roentgenograms in patients with low back pain. Disc calcification is associated with ochronosis, calcium pyrophosphate dihydrate disease, hemochromatosis, hyperparathyroidism, and acromegaly. Evaluation with specific laboratory tests will help discriminate among the disease entities that cause disc calcifications. In these diseases, once roentgenographic abnormalities are present, lumbosacral spine disease is progressive, even with effective therapy that rectifies hormonal imbalance or excessive iron stores. Soft tissue calcification can also occur in paraspinous structures that may overlap disc spaces. Lateral roentgenograms or CT evaluation can identify the location of the calcification (Fig. 9-6).

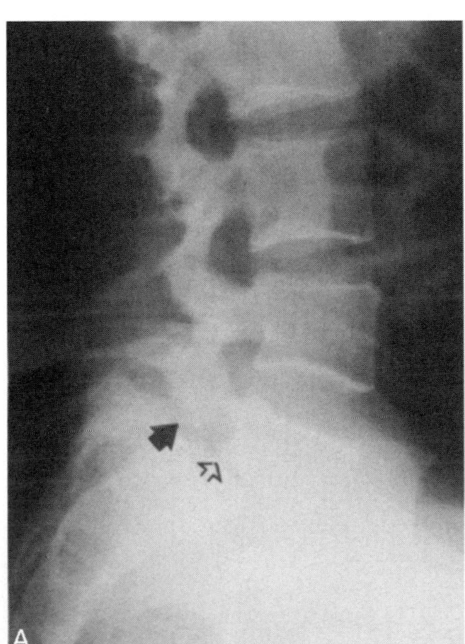

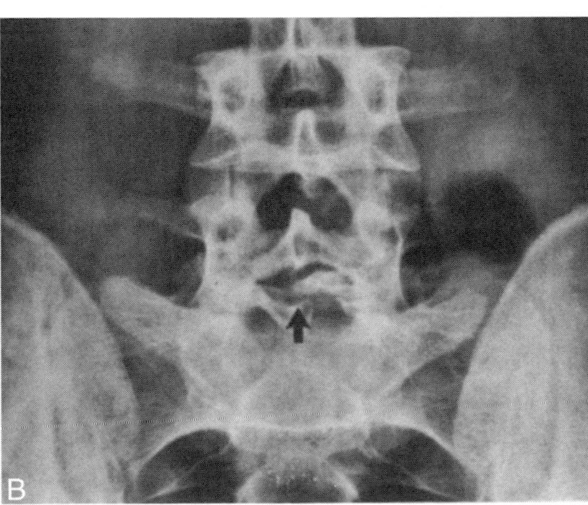

Figure 9-1 A 34-year-old man presented with low back pain that was exacerbated with extension. Conservative therapy was only mildly effective at decreasing low back pain. A plain lateral roentgenogram *(A)* reveals a grade 2 isthmic spondylolisthesis *(open black arrow).* The defect is present in the pars interarticularis *(black arrow).* The posteroanterior view *(B)* reveals a spina bifida occulta *(black arrow)* in addition to the spondylolisthesis. The patient responded to a change in his nonsteroidal therapy and an intensive flexion exercise program. *(A, From Borenstein DG: Low back pain. In Klippel JH, Dieppe P [eds]: Rheumatology. St. Louis, Mosby, 1994.)*

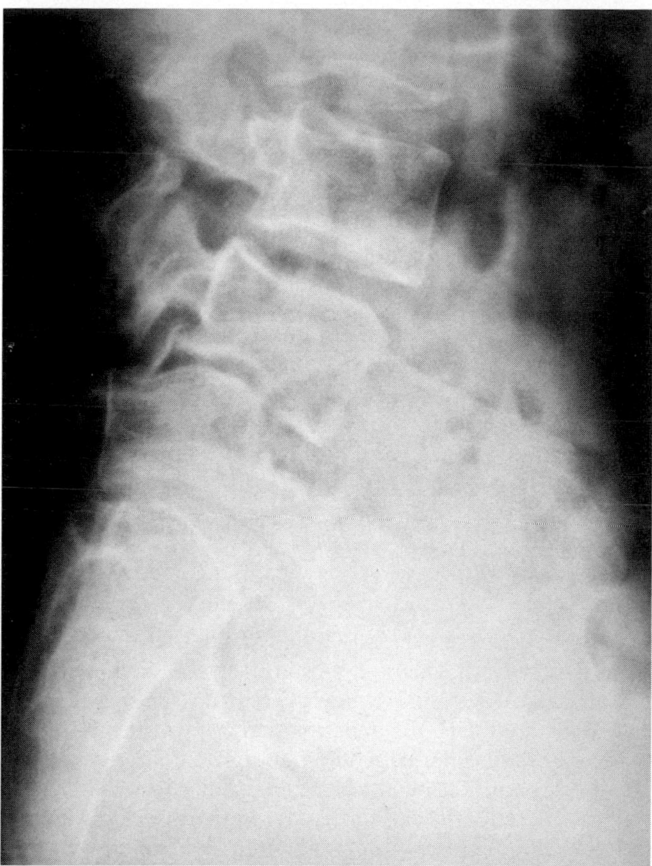

Figure 9-2 A 24-year-old-man presented with progressive low back pain approximately 8 years after a fusion for spondylolisthesis. He had a skiing accident and noticed increasing pain and motion. He now has pain after standing 5 minutes. The plain lateral roentgenogram reveals a grade 2 spondylolisthesis with remodeling of the inferior vertebral endplate. Evidence of the surgical fusion is absent. He is using exercises and NSAID therapy before undergoing additional surgery.

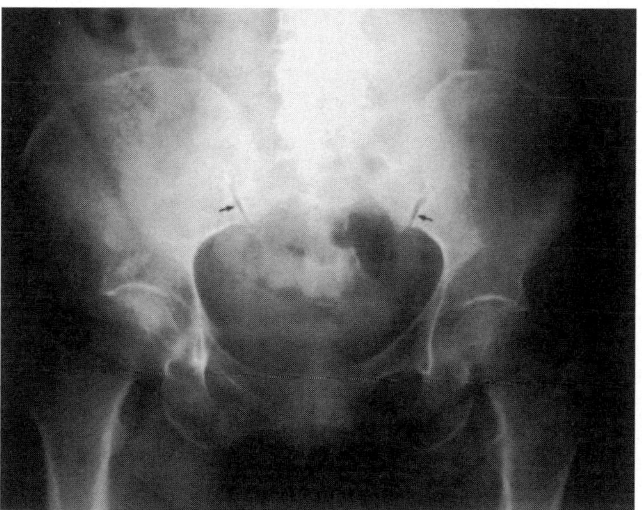

Figure 9-3 Posteroanterior view of the pelvis revealing vacuum phenomenon *(black arrows)* in both sacroiliac joints. The presence of vacuum signs is indicative of early degenerative changes in the joints. *(Courtesy of Anne Brower, MD.)*

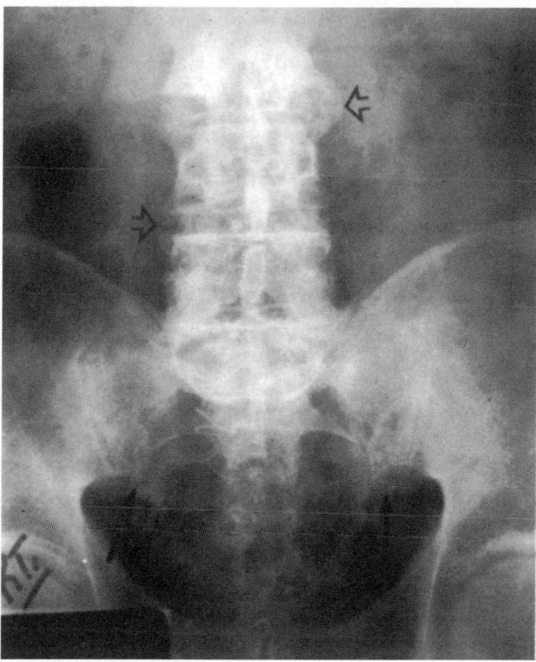

Figure 9-4 Posteroanterior view of the lumbar spine and pelvis revealing osteophyte formation in the lumbar spine *(open black arrows)* and the inferior border of the sacroiliac joints *(black arrows)*. *(Courtesy of Anne Brower, MD.)*

Injection Therapy. Patients who fail to respond to an initial course of conservative therapy may respond to a local injection of a combination of an anesthetic and a long-acting corticosteroid preparation into the area of maximal tenderness (trigger point injection).[21] If this is unsuccessful, the patient should undergo a thorough medical re-evaluation. This may be done by the physician who initially evaluated the patient. However, it may be in the patient's interest to be evaluated by another physician who has a different approach to the problem. Evaluation and treatment by two different physicians has proved helpful in patients who have experienced acute or chronic low back pain.[46]

Medical Re-evaluation. The back strain protocol includes a review of the patient's history and physical examination as well as specific diagnostic and therapeutic interventions if the patient fails to improve. Without roentgenographic findings of spine instability or disc calcification, the medical evaluation of the patient with low back pain limited to the back must start again with a review of the patient's history and physical examination. The time spent in the review of the patient's symptoms and signs is extremely important. The patient may have forgotten to list an important symptom during the initial evaluation, or the symptoms may have changed in character or intensity. Constitutional symptoms of weight loss or occasional fever may have appeared. The areas of pain that were ill defined have now localized to a vertebral body. The emergence of these symptoms and signs alerts the physician to a potential medical cause of the patient's back pain.

The histories of patients with medical low back pain may be divided according to symptoms into five groups (see "Medical Evaluation Algorithm for Low Back Pain," pages 212–213):

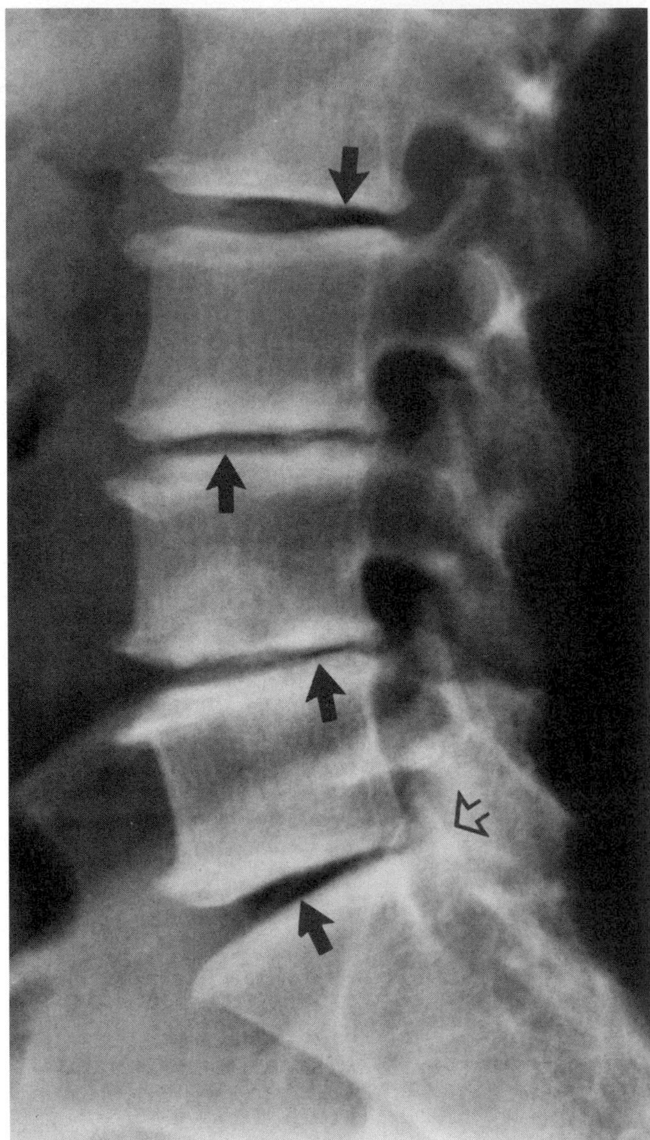

Figure 9-5 Plain lateral roentgenogram demonstrating disc space narrowing from L2-S1 associated with vacuum phenomena at all levels *(black arrows)* and facet joint narrowing *(open black arrow)*.

1. *Fever and/or weight loss.* Patients with a history of fever, weight loss, or other constitutional symptoms frequently will have an infection or tumor as the cause of pain. Occasionally, patients with a spondyloarthropathy will develop fever in association with their arthritis of the spine.
2. *Pain at night or with recumbency.* Patients who have a marked increase in back pain at night may have a benign or malignant neoplasm affecting tissues in or near the spinal column or cord. As opposed to patients with spondyloarthropathy, who develop increased pain at night after they have been recumbent in bed for hours, patients with malignancies have pain that is increased soon after they become recumbent.
3. *Morning stiffness.* Morning stiffness lasting for hours is a hallmark symptom of patients who have an inflammatory arthropathy of the spine. Patients with ankylosing spondylitis have great difficulty getting out of bed and are unable to "loosen up" until midday. Patients with osteoarthritis of the lumbosacral spine also have difficulty getting out of bed, but their stiffness rarely lasts more than 30 minutes.
4. *Acute, localized bone pain.* Patients who develop acute, localized bone pain with no or an insignificant history of trauma have sustained an acute fracture of a vertebra. In the absence of trauma, the development of vertebral fractures suggests decreased strength of bone structure secondary to diminished bone mineralization (osteopenia). Acute, localized bone pain may also be secondary to death of bone cells (avascular necrosis of bone). Tumors and granulomatous processes may replace bone calcium, resulting in abnormal bone architecture and pathologic fracture.
5. *Visceral pain.* Visceral pain occurs in patients with back pain who have symptoms of dysfunction in another organ system. Colicky back pain is suggestive of spasm in a hollow viscus, such as the ureter or cystic duct. Severe, tearing back pain associated with dizziness or syncope is very suggestive of an expanding abdominal aneurysm. Back pain that occurs at regular daily intervals and is associated with eating may be indicative of ulcer disease. Women who complain of back pain that is monthly and associated with their menstrual periods may have endometriosis.

The medical evaluation of each group of patients is different. It is helpful to identify the appropriate group of medical symptoms when first seeing the patient so that an appropriate evaluation is completed thoughtfully and expeditiously.

FEVER AND WEIGHT LOSS

The plain roentgenograms of patients with fever and weight loss should be reviewed. What seemed normal initially may not appear so in the face of constitutional symptoms. If the roentgenograms are unrevealing, a bone scan is indicated. The bone scan will identify areas of increased bone cell activity of any source. Therefore, it is a sensitive but nonspecific test. Patients with early osteomyelitis or tumor may have increased uptake on bone scan without any corresponding roentgenographic changes. More than 30% of bone mineral must be lost before the radiologist detects it on a plain roentgenogram. A negative bone scan does not eliminate the possibility of a tumor causing back pain. Multiple myeloma does not cause an osteoblastic response by bone, and there is no increased bone activity on bone scan. If the physician is suspicious of this possibility, a CT scan or MR image of the lumbar spine should be ordered along with serum protein tests to evaluate for myeloma (Figs. 9-7 and 9-8). If any of these tests are positive, the patient should undergo appropriate evaluation with cultures for infection or biopsy of the detected lesion when infection or tumor is suspected. The presence of diabetes, intravenous drug use, immunosuppression, vertebral surgery, leukocytosis, or elevated sedimentation rate is

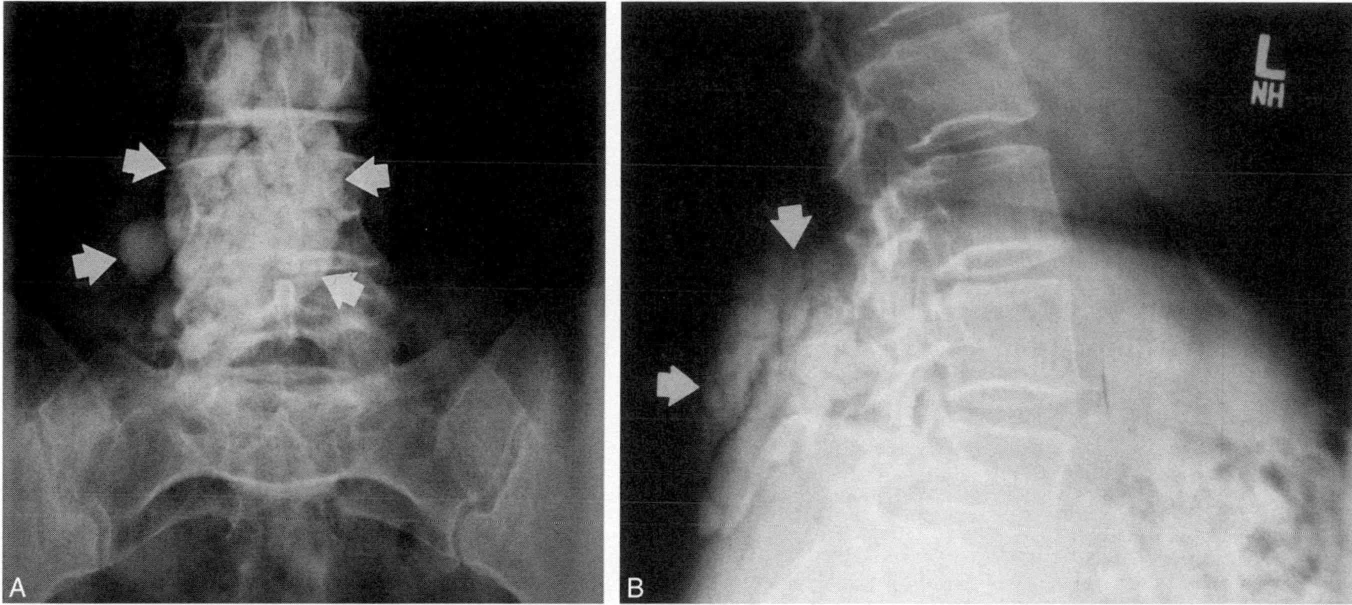

Figure 9-6 A 60-year-old woman has a 15-year history of systemic sclerosis. Over the past 2 years she has developed increasing low back pain. The examination of the lumbar region demonstrated the presence of a firm structure sensitive to palpation. Plain anteroposterior *(A)* and lateral *(B)* roentgenograms demonstrate a large, lobulated mass of calcium *(large white arrows)*. The pain is controlled with NSAIDs and occasional local injections of corticosteroids and anesthetics.

associated with a pyogenic infection of the spine.[10] Tuberculous osteomyelitis causes a prolonged clinical course, absence of fever, presence of spinal deformity, or epidural masses. Antibiotics are the treatment of choice for infections. Surgical excision is preferred if tumors, particularly of the benign variety, are accessible to total removal. Radiation therapy and chemotherapy are used occasionally with benign tumors but more commonly with malignant lesions. In postsurgical patients who develop fever, C-reactive protein (CRP), if available, or an ESR are useful tests to identify patients with infection. CRP is more sensitive than ESR for determination of individuals with postoperative infections.[33,37]

PAIN AT NIGHT OR WITH RECUMBENCY

Tumors of the spinal column or cord are of prime concern in the patient with nocturnal pain. After the re-evaluation of the patient's history and physical examination, the plain roentgenograms should be reviewed. If no abnormality is detected, the patient should undergo a bone scan. Bone scan is a sensitive test for detecting spinal column neoplasms but is not as useful for identifying spinal cord tumors. CT or MR scan is indicated if the bone scan is negative but multiple myeloma is suspected.

The alterations of bony architecture associated with spinal bone tumors are detectable by CT scan; however, subtle soft tissue changes may be missed by this technique. MR is a useful radiographic technique that does not use radiation or contrast dye to visualize the spinal cord. Extradural and intramedullary lesions are detectable by this technique (Fig. 9-9).

Patients with positive findings need a tissue diagnosis before therapy is instituted. If a primary source for the tumor other than the spinal column is detected, a tissue specimen for biopsy may be obtained from the most convenient location. Therapy is tailored to the specific neoplastic lesion. A combination of surgical, chemotherapeutic, and radiotherapeutic techniques may be effective at containing the growth of neoplasms.

MORNING STIFFNESS

Morning stiffness that lasts for hours in association with low back pain is a very common symptom of patients with a spondyloarthropathy. Occasionally, patients present with additional symptoms, such as iritis or keratodermia blennorrhagica, which help raise the suspicion of the possibility of a specific spondyloarthropathy. After completion of the examination for articular and extra-articular manifestations of disease, the physician should review the plain roentgenograms for early changes of spondyloarthropathy, including loss of lumbar lordosis, joint erosion in the lower one third of the sacroiliac joints, and squaring of the vertebral bodies (Fig. 9-10). If the plain views are normal, tilting the x-ray tube 30 degrees will line up the face of the sacroiliac joint in one plane (Ferguson view). This view is helpful in detecting early changes of sacroiliitis. A normal sacroiliac examination does not eliminate the possibility of a spondyloarthropathy causing the patient's symptoms. A bone scan can detect the pattern of joint involvement in other parts of the axial and peripheral skeleton. Areas of active inflammation over the axial and peripheral skeleton may be detected by this technique. A specific diagnosis is not established by the presence of increased scintigraphic activity (metastatic tumor is also "hot" on bone scan). Osteoarthritis also may be associated with widespread areas of increased uptake. However, the patient's symptoms, signs, and laboratory tests (e.g., normal ESR) should separate patients with osteoarthritis from those with inflammatory arthropathy (Fig. 9-11).

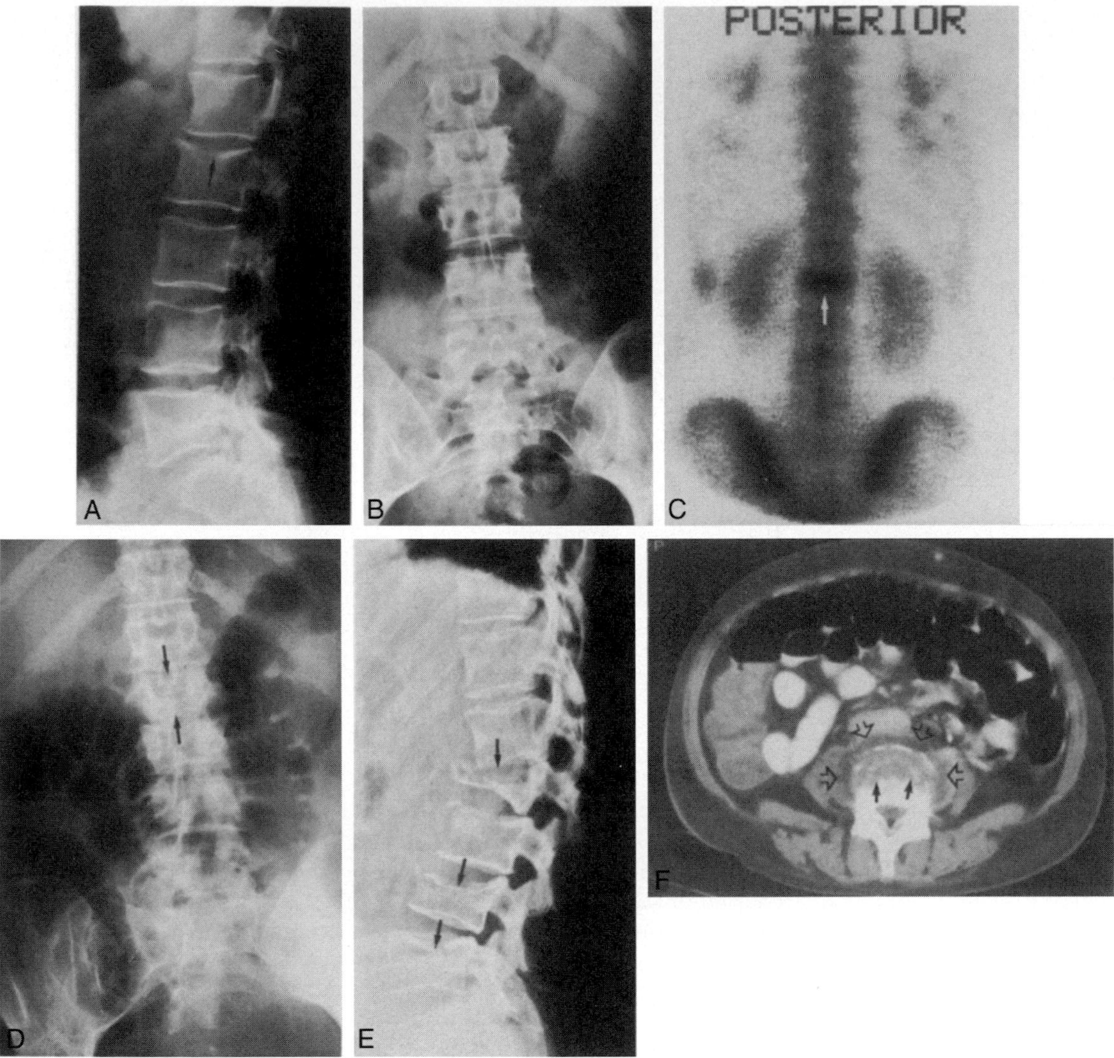

Figure 9-7 A 46-year-old woman with systemic lupus erythematosus manifested by severe skin and joint disease was treated with prednisone in doses ranging from 20 to 40 mg/day along with hydroxychloroquine, 400 mg/day. She developed abdominal pain in association with intermittent, low-grade fever. Plain posteroanterior *(A)* and lateral *(B)* roentgenograms of the lumbar spine revealed no specific abnormality except for slight indentation of the superior endplate of the L2 vertebral body *(black arrow)*. Localized back pain developed and she underwent bone scintiscan 2 weeks later. *C*, The scan revealed increased tracer in the L2 vertebral body *(white arrow)* compatible with compression fracture. Repeated blood cultures were negative for any growth. She received a 2-week course of antibiotics with some improvement in her abdominal pain. Over the next month, her back pain became more persistent and diffuse with increasing abdominal symptoms. She was readmitted to the hospital and repeat posteroanterior *(D)* and lateral *(E)* views of the lumbar spine at 2 months after her initial evaluation revealed marked destruction of the L2 vertebral body. Also affected were the endplates of L4 and L5 vertebral bodies *(black arrows)*. *F*, CT scan of the L2 vertebra revealed marked destruction of the body of the vertebra *(black arrows)* with an associated soft tissue abscess *(open black arrows)*. The abscess extended from the L2 to L5 vertebral level. The patient died of sepsis despite maximum antibiotic therapy. *(F, From Borenstein DG: Low back pain. In Klippel JH, Dieppe P [eds]: Rheumatology. St. Louis, Mosby, 1994.)*

Patients with spondyloarthropathy are usually treated with a combination of NSAIDs along with physical therapy. Etanercept is indicated for the therapy of ankylosing spondylitis.[8a] Occasionally, patients with specific forms of spondyloarthropathy (Whipple's disease, hidradenitis suppurativa) may require antibiotics as part of their treatment regimen.

Acute Localized Bone Pain

Acute localized bone pain is usually associated with either fracture or expansion of bone. Any process that increases mineral loss from bone (osteoporosis, osteomalacia, hyperparathyroidism), causes bone death (hemoglobinopathy), or replaces bone with abnormal cells (tumor, sarcoidosis) will weaken the bone to the point where fracture may occur spontaneously or with minimal trauma. Patients with acute fractures experience acute onset of pain in the area of the back that corresponds to the fractured bone. Palpation over bone during the physical examination may localize the specific vertebra affected. After the physical examination elicits localized bone pain, review of the plain roentgenogram in the painful area may help to identify abnormalities in affected skeletal structures that were initially thought to be normal. Bone scan is useful to detect increased bone activity soon after a fracture at a time when the plain roentgenogram is unremarkable. CT scan may

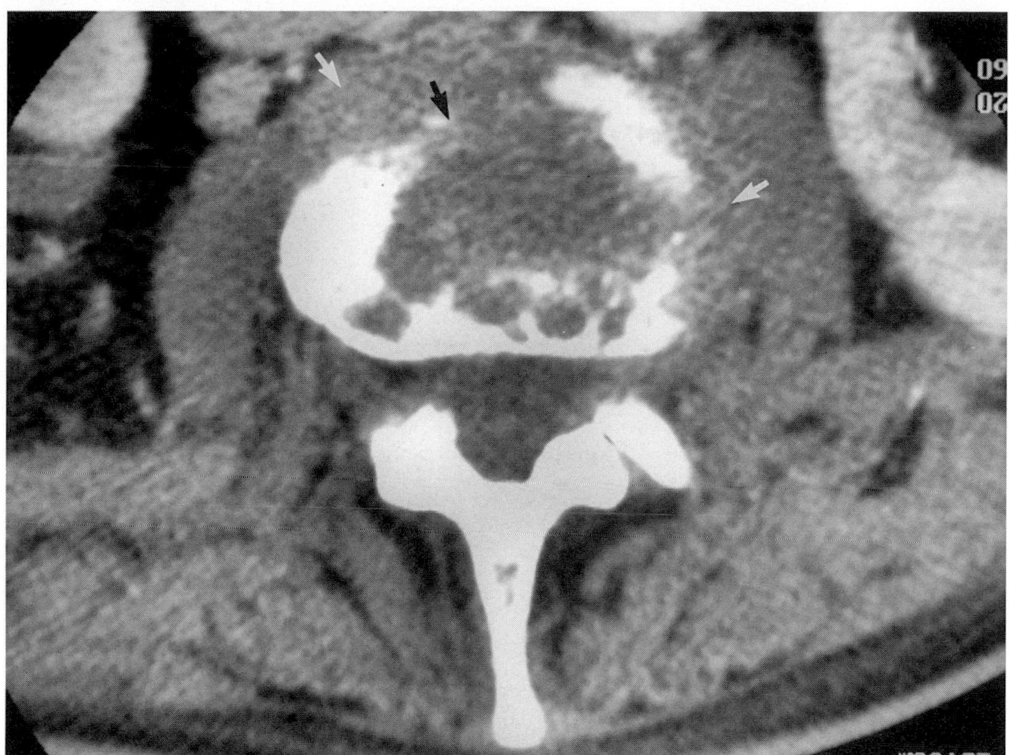

Figure 9-8 Discitis. A 68-year-old man developed intestinal obstruction requiring a colostomy and a prolonged course of antibiotics. He had increasing back pain that was not treated for months. The lesion was diagnosed as *Candida* discitis by a percutaneous aspiration. CT axial view demonstrates erosion of vertebral body *(black arrow)* and involvement of surrounding soft tissues *(white arrows)*.

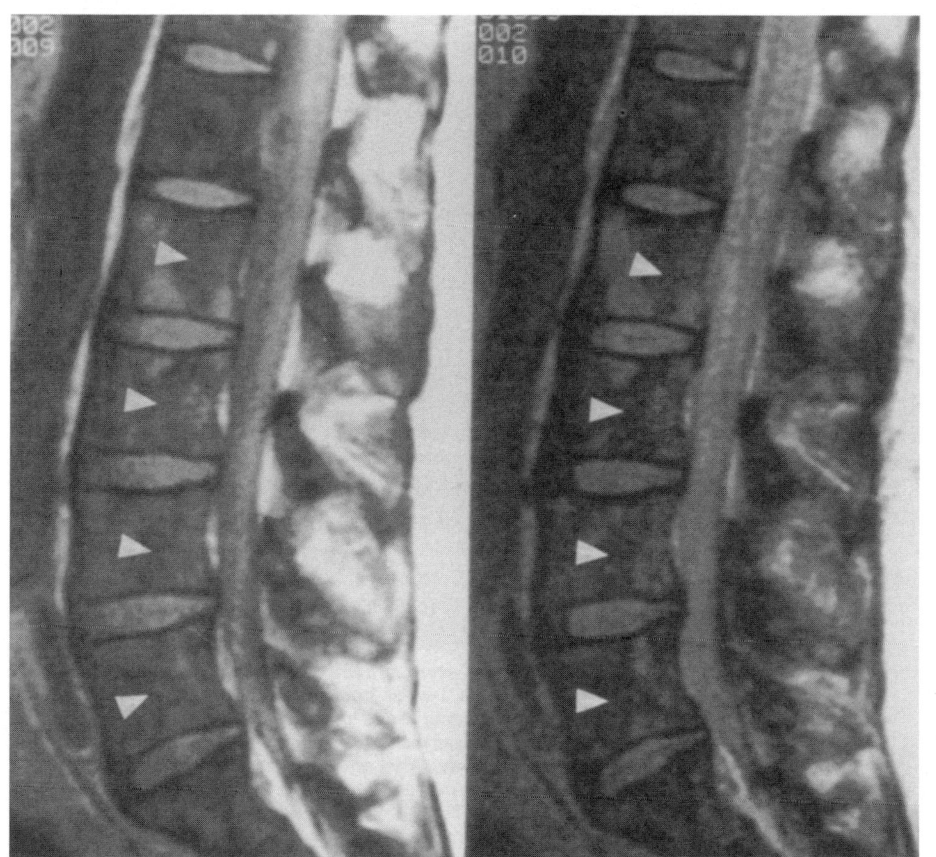

Figure 9-9 A 52-year-old man presented with right-sided back pain that did not radiate to the legs initially. He was treated with conservative therapy for 6 weeks. His pain increased to include the left side of his back and right hip and became persistent. He had to sleep in a chair at night. His hematocrit fell to 29%. MR image of the lumbar spine reveals on proton density *(left)* and T2-weighted sequence *(right)* decreased signal intensity in multiple vertebral bodies indicative of diffuse marrow replacement *(white arrows)*. A diagnosis of prostate cancer was made with biopsy of the prostate gland.

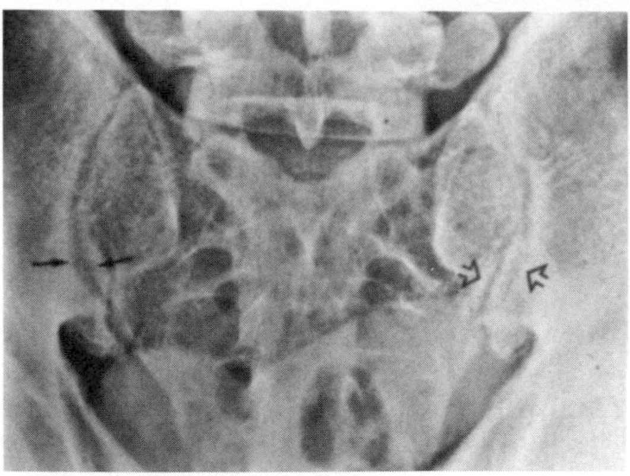

Figure 9-10 A 35-year-old man had a 5-year history of low back pain and morning stiffness. He previously had not sought medical care for back pain. A posteroanterior view of the sacroiliac joints revealed early joint margin erosions on both sides of the joints *(black arrows)* and sclerosis *(open black arrows)*. Bilateral sacroiliac joint disease was compatible with a diagnosis of ankylosing spondylitis. The patient responded to nonsteroidal drug therapy.

identify the location of a fracture, undetected by a plain roentgenogram, that is localized by increased tracer on bone scan. Finding an abnormality tells the clinician that a pathologic process is present but is not sufficient to define the specific cause of the bony change. MR may detect alterations in intravertebral bone marrow indicative of an inflammatory process, such as an infection, or a process that has replaced normal bone marrow (Fig. 9-12). Additional evaluation is necessary. Screening tests that are helpful in detecting systemic illnesses include an ESR along with a complete blood cell count. Abnormalities in any of these tests should heighten the physician's suspicion of a systemic illness causing the patient's symptoms. The differential diagnosis of the diseases associated with this symptom complex is quite broad. Further evaluation of these patients must be tailored to the specific situation. For example, evaluation for sickle cell anemia and sarcoidosis would be more appropriate in a black patient than in a white patient. An acid phosphatase determination is more appropriate in an older man than in a young woman.

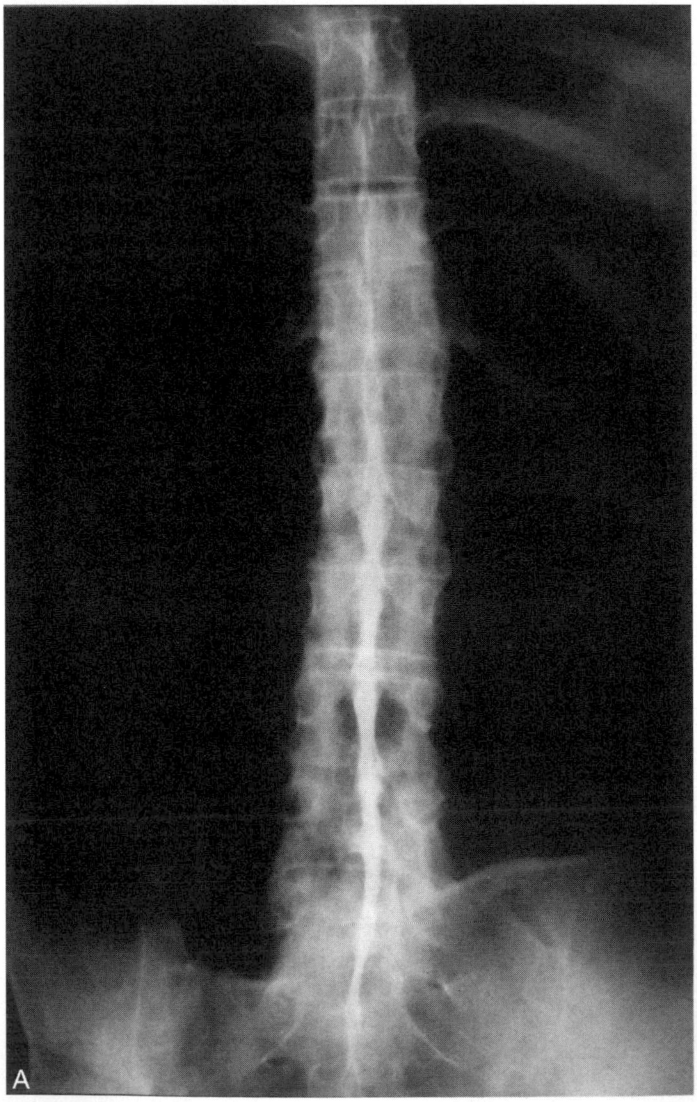

Figure 9-11 A 54-year-old woman had a 20-year history of ankylosing spondylitis. Anteroposterior *(A)* and lateral *(B)* roentgenograms demonstrate bilateral fused sacroiliac joints and calcification of the interspinous ligaments. The lateral view shows syndesmophytes, squaring of vertebral bodies, and apophyseal joint fusion.

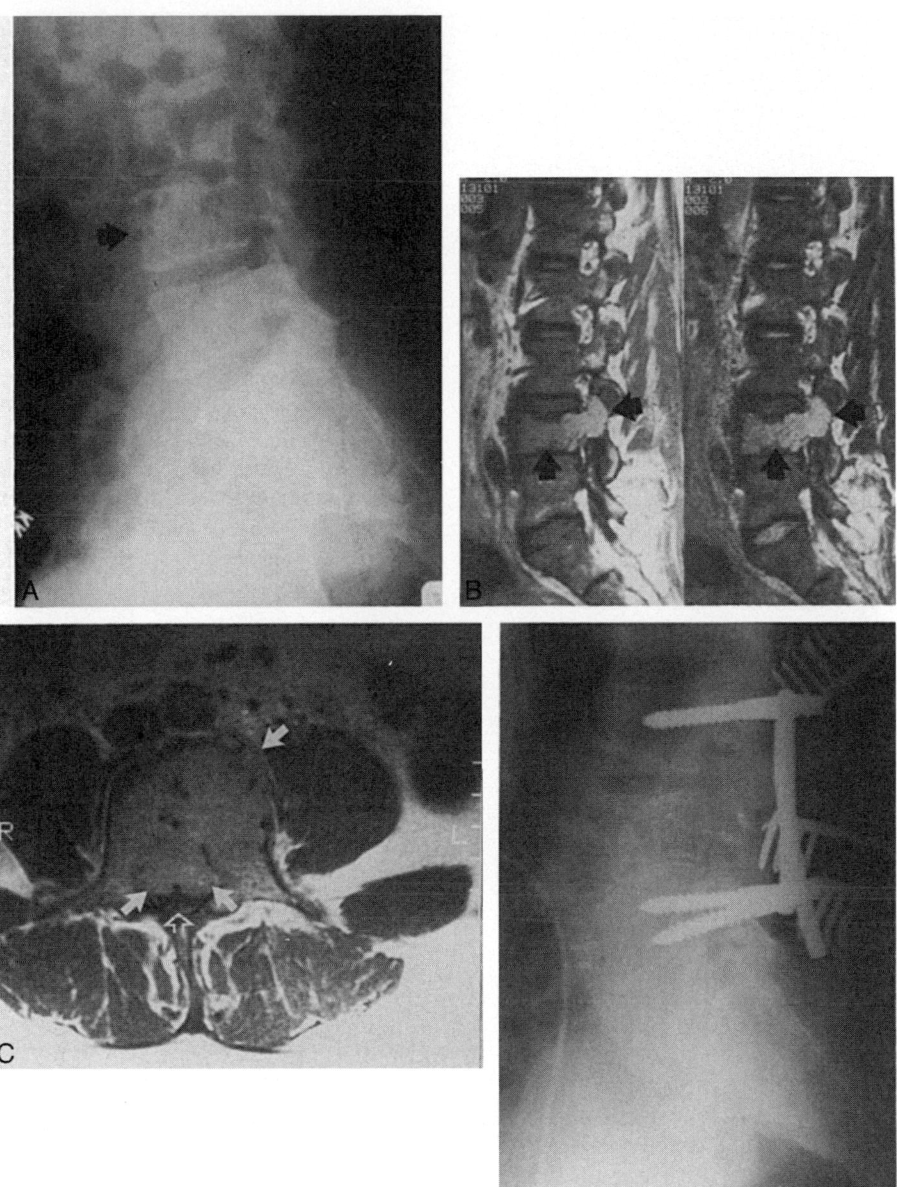

Figure 9-12 A 43-year-old man described the onset of left-sided low back pain after participating in a session of karate exercises. His examination revealed decreased range of motion of the lumbar spine without any neurologic deficits. He was treated with conservative therapy and was told to return in 2 weeks. During that period he had an increase in pain directly over the spine with radiation into the right anterior thigh. Lateral roentgenogram of the lumbar spine *(A)* reveals a loss of trabecular markings and integrity of the anterior vertebral body border *(black arrow)*. *B*, MR of a sagittal proton density *(left)* and T2-weighted image *(right)* reveals increased signal intensity involving the body and pedicle of the L4 vertebra *(black arrows)*. *C*, MR of an axial T2-weighted image reveals increased signal in the vertebral body with expansion beyond the vertebral body anteriorly and posteriorly *(white arrows)* with compression of the thecal sac. Marginal room remains in the canal for the cauda equina *(open white arrow)*. *D*, Postoperative lateral roentgenogram of the lumbar spine. The plasmacytoma was removed with decompression of the spinal canal. Rods were placed to stabilize the spine to prevent neurologic damage. The patient was discharged from the hospital 10 days after his surgery with normal neurologic function and only mild postoperative back pain. *(B, C, and D, From Borenstein DG: Progressive low back pain. In Klippel JH, Dieppe P [eds]: Rheumatology. St. Louis, Mosby, 1994.)*

The diagnostic evaluation and therapeutic regimen for each disease process are reviewed in Section III.

If the laboratory evaluation of the patient is entirely normal and decreased bone mineral is noted on roentgenograms, the patient's diagnosis is osteopenia, most likely osteoporosis (Fig. 9-13). These individuals should undergo a bone mineral density determination (i.e., DEXA) to measure their degree of osteoporosis. The therapy for osteoporosis involves increased activity and calcium supplements, along with vitamin D, bisphosphonates, selective estrogen receptor modulator (SERM), nasal or injectable calcitonin, or parathormone injections in the appropriate patient.[16,29]

VISCERAL PAIN

Patients with visceral pain have back pain in association with symptoms of gastrointestinal or genitourinary disease. These patients have symptoms of dyspepsia, abdominal pain, or change in bowel habits. They may have hematuria, polyuria, or flank pain (Fig. 9-14). Patients with visceral pain may have colicky, severe tearing, or episodic low back pain.

Colicky Pain. Patients with colicky pain have spasm in a hollow viscus. Two structures in the abdomen that cause colicky back pain associated with obstruction are the ureters and the cystic duct. Patients with colicky back pain should undergo urinalysis, ultrasonography, or intravenous pyelography. If these tests are normal and the patient continues to have colicky pain, a gallbladder scan or ultrasound of the gallbladder may help document decreased function and the presence of gallstones.

Tearing Pain. Patients with severe tearing pain may be particularly problematic. Severe tearing pain may be a sign of an expanding abdominal aneurysm. If these patients

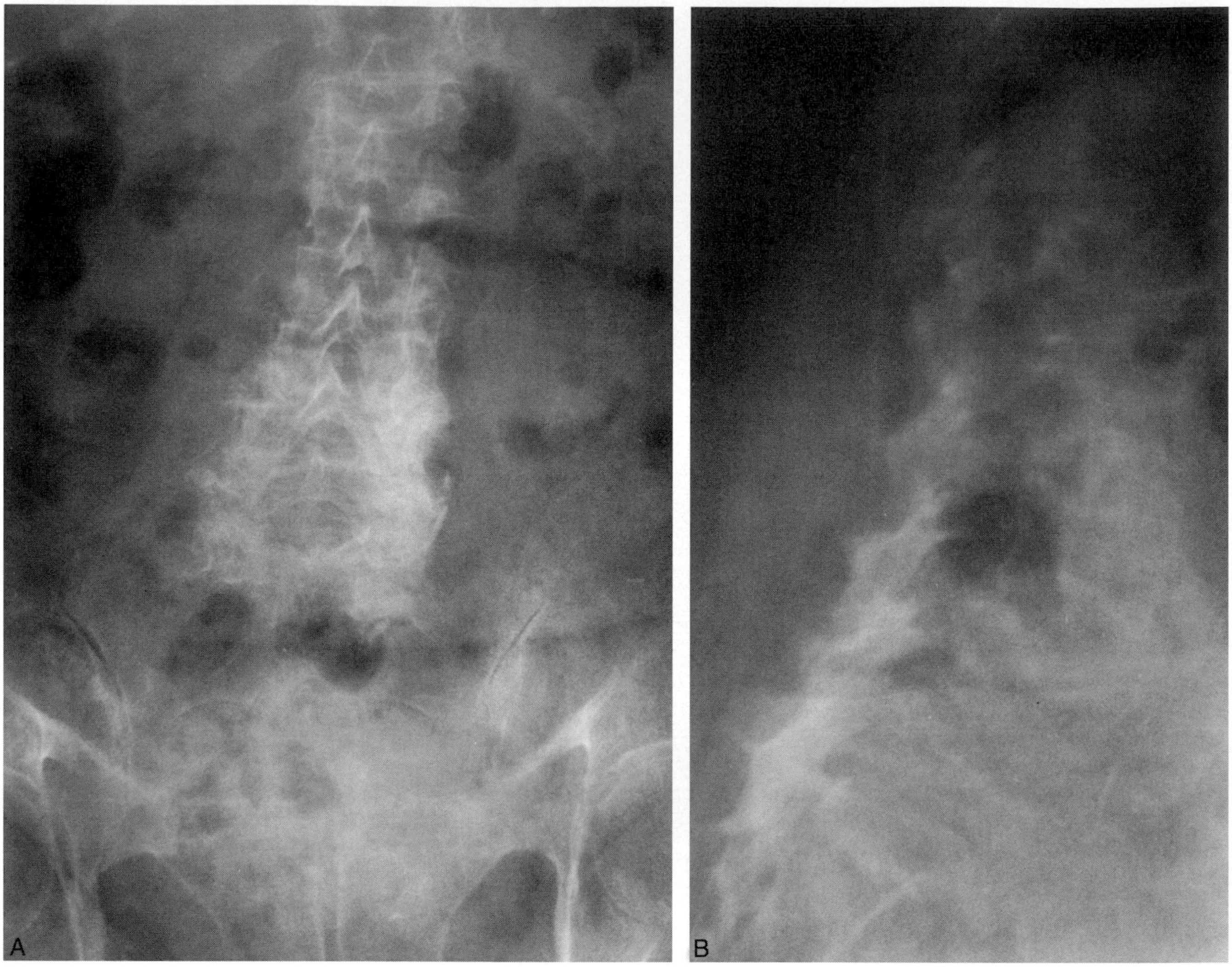

A B

Figure 9-13 A 75-year-old woman had a diagnosis of giant cell arteritis and received large doses of corticosteroids. She developed repeated episodes of acute low back pain. Anteroposterior *(A)* and lateral *(B)* roentgenograms reveal marked, generalized osteoporosis with compression fractures of all the vertebral bodies. The sacrum lacks definition because of severe osteoporosis.

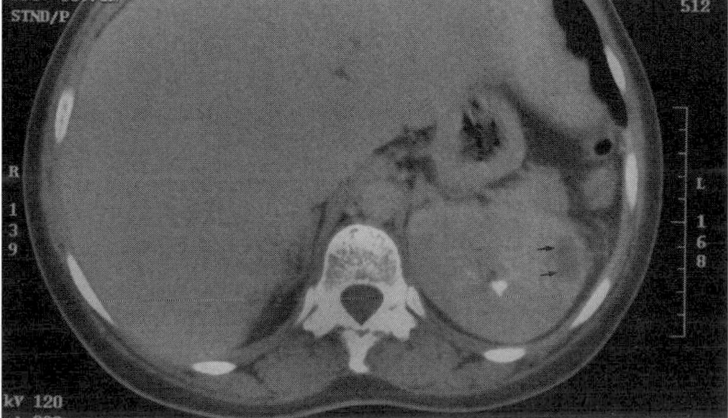

Figure 9-14 A 36-year-old drug abuser was admitted to the hospital for increasing low back and flank pain in the setting of fever and pyuria. A CT of the abdomen revealed a hypodense area in the kidney *(black arrows)* compatible with a renal abscess.

complain of syncope or are hypotensive, they must be evaluated for an aneurysm on an emergency basis. Their hematocrit can be checked as blood is drawn for typing and cross-match for possible transfusion. Patients with an aneurysm may be evaluated with ultrasonography, depending on their hemodynamic status. Patients with an expanding aneurysm usually require vascular surgery to repair the aortic defect. Patients who are candidates for surgical correction of expanding aneurysms should undergo CT scan if hemodynamically stable. The timing of surgery depends on a number of factors, including the size and location of the aneurysm. The surgeon and the evaluating physician work together to determine the time for surgery to maximize the potential for a good outcome.

Episodic Pain. Patients with visceral pain may have a recurrence of pain on a regular basis. The frequency may be daily, associated with eating (gastrointestinal, pancreatitis, peptic ulcer disease), or monthly, associated with menstrual periods (endometriosis). These patients have a history of low back pain that is not particularly modified by changes of position. Examination of the abdomen demonstrates tenderness with palpation that may be localized to the right upper quadrant (ulcer disease), epigastrium (pancreas), or lower quadrants (uterus and ovaries). Careful gynecologic examination demonstrates masses, nodules, or adhesions, which suggest the presence of an inflammatory intrapelvic process. Serum tests for pancreatic injury (amylase, trypsin) may identify those individuals with gastrointestinal-associated back pain. Rectal examination may identify abnormalities in the colon associated with defecation that may cause low back or sacral pain (Fig. 9-15).

Therapy for these entities is directed at decreasing inflammation in the affected organ system. Hormonal therapy is effective in endometriosis, whereas anti-ulcer (proton pump inhibitors/antibiotics) therapy is helpful in patients with peptic ulcer disease, including *Helicobacter pylori* infection.

Proximal Muscle/Tender Point Pain. If patients do not fit into any of the five categories, they should be evaluated for muscle stiffness and pain. Patients who are older than 50 years of age with proximal stiffness, particularly in the morning, may have polymyalgia rheumatica. Younger patients also may have muscle pain. In contrast to the diffuse areas of pain in polymyalgia rheumatica, local areas of tenderness are problematic in patients with fibromyalgia. "Tender points" are found in characteristic locations in certain muscles and tendons. There are no diagnostic tests for these diseases. The diagnosis is a clinical one. One laboratory test that is helpful in distinguishing between these two entities is measurement of the ESR. Polymyalgia rheumatica is associated with an elevated sedimentation rate whereas fibromyalgia is not. If a patient has not had a sedimentation rate test in the evaluation, the test should be done. Therapy for the two illnesses is quite different. Polymyalgia rheumatica is treated with low-dose corticosteroids (prednisone, 15 mg/day). Fibromyalgia is treated with mild aerobic exercise, injections, moderate doses of tricyclic antidepressants, and cognitive-behavioral therapies.

Some patients will go through the entire medical evaluation without any detectable abnormalities. A surreptitious illness may be present that has not progressed to the point of detectability by the physician's diagnostic tests. These patients need to be watched carefully while they continue therapy for localized low back pain as part of the back strain protocol. Re-evaluation is indicated if these patients complain of any new symptoms. A repeat ESR is a cost-effective method to identify those individuals who require close scrutiny. The development of an elevation in the ESR suggests an inflammatory process that has gone undetected. The presence of an elevated ESR helps separate those individuals with a systemic inflammatory disease from those with a mechanical process.

Psychosocial Evaluation. If the medical work-up is unrevealing, the patient should undergo a thorough psychosocial evaluation in an attempt to explain the failure of the previous treatment. This is predicated on the knowledge and belief that a patient's disability is related not only to his pathologic anatomy but also to his perception of pain and his mental stability in relation to his social environment. It is quite common to see a patient with a frank herniated disc continue working, regarding the disability as only a minor problem, while at the other end of the spectrum the hysterical patient takes to bed at the slightest twinge of low back discomfort.

Drug habituation, depression, alcoholism, and other psychiatric problems are seen frequently in association with back pain. If the evaluation suggests any of these problems, proper measures should be instituted. There are a small but significant number of ambulatory patients addicted to commonly prescribed medications who use back pain as an excuse to obtain these drugs. Narcotics and tranquilizers,

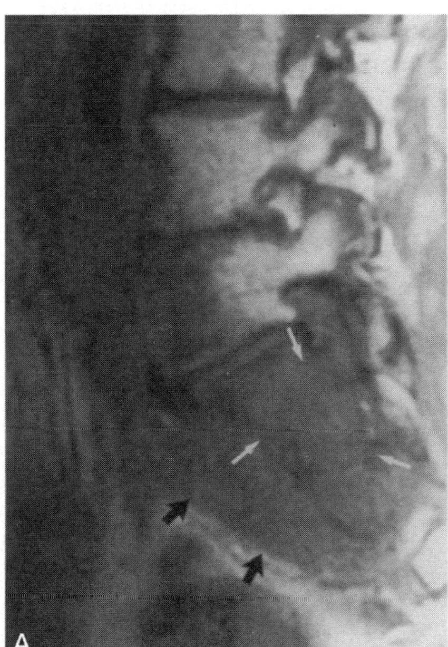

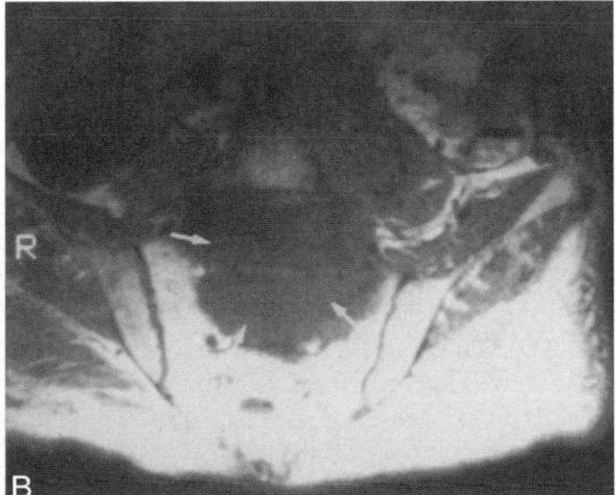

Figure 9-15 A 59-year-man had a history of bladder transitional cell carcinoma. He had a cystectomy and ileal loop placed and experienced resolution of colicky low back pain. Approximately 2 years later, he experienced increasing back pain and difficulty defecating. MR of the lumbar spine revealed on proton density sagittal *(A)* and coronal T1-weighted *(B)* views decreased signal intensity in the sacrum compatible with diffuse metastatic disease *(white arrows)*. Anterior soft tissue mass is also present *(black arrows)*. He died of metastatic disease within 1 year of the MR examination.

alone or in combination, are common offenders. Narcotics cause physical dependence, whereas tranquilizers have the potential for habituation and depression. Because the complaint of low back pain may be a manifestation of depression, it is counterproductive to treat such patients with agents that may exacerbate depression.

Patient Education. Those patients who do not show evidence of a systemic medical problem or psychiatric difficulties are referred to "low back school."[17] This concept has as its basis the belief that patients with low back pain, given proper education and understanding of their disease, often can return to a productive and functional life. Ergonomics, the proper and efficient use of the body in work and recreation, is stressed, particularly as it relates to the spine. Back school need not be an expensive proposition. It can be as simple as a one-time classroom session with a review of back problems and a demonstration of exercises with patient participation. This type of educational process has proved very effective. It is most important, however, that a patient be thoroughly screened before referral to this type of facility. One does not want to be in the position of treating a metastatic tumor in a classroom.

Chronic Pain Therapy. Individuals who continue to experience pain after 12 weeks of evaluation and therapy are considered to have chronic pain. Recent investigations have suggested that defining pain as acute, subacute, or chronic may not be a helpful classification in the identification of those individuals with the potential for improvement.[40] The pain intensity, disability, and depression experienced by an individual is a better determinant of potential for improvement than the duration of pain. Decreasing pain intensity and the perception of disability and depression are key factors in patient improvement at any point in a treatment program.

Chronic pain therapy may include a number of treatment modalities: medications, exercise, transcutaneous electrical nerve stimulation (TENS), and cognitive-behavioral therapy.[39] A single therapy is rarely effective for individuals with chronic pain. The combination of two or more of these therapies simultaneously is more effective at modifying pain while the patient increases physical function. Patients require a combination of drug therapies to improve function while experiencing chronic pain. An NSAID, a muscle relaxant, or a low-dose tricyclic antidepressant is frequently chosen. The use of additional medications (e.g., chronic narcotic therapy, anti-epilepsy agents, gabapentin) is necessitated by the degree of progress to reach a functional level of activity. Postsurgical patients who continue to experience chronic pain are those who require more combinations of therapies (e.g., sustained-release narcotics, antidepressants, alpha-adrenergic receptor antagonists) for relief. Some patients remain resistant to therapy. These individuals may benefit from a referral to a multidisciplinary pain clinic that offers expertise in a number of specialties of medical care that treat pain as a disease.

Sciatica (Leg Pain below the Knee)

The next group of patients consists of those with sciatica, which is defined in this instance as pain radiating below the knee. These people usually experience their symptoms secondary to mechanical pressure and inflammation of the nerve roots that originate between L4–L5 (L5 nerve root) and L5–S1 (S1 nerve root). Pain, numbness, and tingling can then travel down the leg along the anatomic course of the particular nerve involved. The cause of the mechanical pressure can be soft tissue (herniated disc), bone, or a combination of the two.

At this juncture, these patients have had up to 6 weeks of controlled physical activity and anti-inflammatory medication, including a course of low-dose corticosteroids, but still have persistent leg pain. The next therapeutic step is an epidural corticosteroid injection.[44] This may be performed on an outpatient basis. The anti-inflammatory medication (corticosteroid) is injected directly into the epidural space, close to the location of the actual compression of the nerve root. Epidural injections are usually prescribed after visualization of the lumbar spine by MR or CT scan. If symptoms and signs are classic for nerve impingement, the epidural injection may be given without radiographic tests. If the patient does not improve, radiographic evaluation of the lumbar spine is essential. Epidural injections have proved 40% effective in relieving leg pain. The maximum benefit from a single injection is achieved within 2 weeks. The injection may have to be repeated one or two times, and another 4 to 6 weeks should pass before its success or failure is determined. It should be pointed out that there are alternative conservative treatments available (e.g., traction, passive physical therapy, and manipulation). The efficacy of each is discussed in Section IV. Unfortunately, many of these methods in general have not stood the test of scientific scrutiny, so they should not become a part of the treatment program.[19]

If epidural corticosteroids are effective in alleviating the patient's leg pain or sciatica, the patient starts on a program of exercises and is encouraged to return promptly to a normal lifestyle. Heavy work (lifting more than 50 pounds regularly) is not recommended because these patients will be prone to recurrences of disc herniation. Those who have sustained a disc herniation should be placed on some type of restricted work. This treatment pathway usually will be completed in less than 3 months, and most patients with sciatica will not have to undergo any major invasive treatment. Thus, a radiculopathy in and of itself is not a contraindication to nonoperative therapy.

Should the epidural corticosteroid injections prove ineffective and 3 months have passed since the onset of pain, some type of invasive treatment should be considered. The patient group at this point is divided into those with probable herniated discs and those with symptoms secondary to spinal stenosis.

Herniated Disc. Patients with herniated discs have symptoms secondary to the nucleus pulposus herniating through the annulus fibrosus and causing pressure and inflammation of an individual nerve root. As already mentioned, the L5 and S1 nerve roots are those most commonly involved. The pain will radiate along the anatomic pathway of the nerves that travel below the knee and into the foot. The highest incidence of this entity occurs in the fourth decade of life but also can be seen in older patients.

The physician must now carefully re-evaluate the patient for a neurologic deficit and for a positive tension sign (straight leg–raising test). For those with either a neurologic deficit or positive tension sign along with continued leg pain, an MR or CT scan should be obtained. MR is preferred as the initial study because of better visualization of soft tissue structures (intervertebral discs) with adequate imaging of bony structures (Fig. 9-16). If MR or CT is clearly positive and correlates with the clinical findings, myelography need not be performed, because the test is invasive. If there is any question about the radiographic findings of the MR or CT, a metrizamide myelogram should be obtained.

Surgical Intervention. There is repeated documentation that for surgery to be effective for the treatment of a herniated disc, the surgeon must find unequivocal preoperative evidence of nerve root compression.[38] Thus, the more precise the preoperative diagnosis, the better the outcome. Mechanical nerve root compression must be firmly substantiated not only by neurologic examination but also by radiographic data before discectomy. There is no place for "exploratory" back surgery. If the patient has neither a neurologic deficit nor a positive straight leg–raising test, regardless of radiographic findings, there is not enough evidence of nerve root compression to undertake surgery. Twenty-five percent of asymptomatic patients have positive myelograms, and 35% have positive CT scans.[47] A similar proportion of patients have MR findings for anatomic abnormalities that are unassociated with symptoms.[5] MR images have no predictive value on the development of back or leg pain.[7] Normal patients also may have equivocal electromyographic findings. These patients without objective findings are the ones who have poor results and have given back surgery such a bad reputation.

If there are no objective findings of radiculopathy, the physician should avoid surgery and proceed to a psychosocial evaluation. Exceptions should be few and far between. When sympathy for the patient's complaints outweighs the objective evaluation, treatment is fraught with difficulties. Of those who meet these specific criteria for lumbar laminectomy, 95% can expect good to excellent results.[22]

Spinal Stenosis. The second group of patients whose symptoms are based on mechanical pressure on the neural elements are those with spinal stenosis.[45] Spinal stenosis is a narrowing of the spinal canal secondary to increased bone formation, a natural occurrence with age. Patients older than 60 years of age are most affected by spinal stenosis. If the spinal canal is small to start with and then decreases farther, pressure develops on the nerve, which may cause radiation of pain into the legs. These patients may or may not have a positive neurologic examination or straight leg–raising test. Ambulation may result in mechanical irritation, poor excursion of the spinal nerves due to entrapment, edema, and neural ischemia. Accordingly, if these patients ambulate until their symptoms are reproduced, such as with a "stress test," the initially negative neurologic and tension signs may become positive. A stress test may include walking up some stairs or walking for a distance in the office.

The diagnosis of spinal stenosis usually can be made from the plain roentgenograms, which will demonstrate facet degeneration, disc degeneration, and decreased interpedicular and sagittal canal diameter. Myelography, CT, or MR will better define the involved areas than plain films (Fig. 9-17) and may be helpful in delineating the extent of surgery required for decompression. If symptoms are severe and there is radiographic evidence of spinal stenosis, surgery is appropriate. Age alone is not a deterrent to surgery. Many elderly people who are in good health except for a narrow spinal canal will benefit greatly from adequate decompression of the lumbar spine (Fig 9-18).[1,2] Patients who have continued pain after surgery for a herniated intervertebral disc or spinal stenosis should be evaluated by the multioperated spine algorithm (see Fig. 20-5).

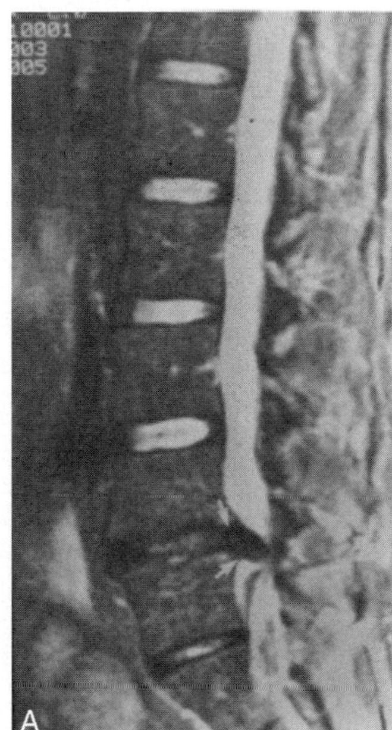

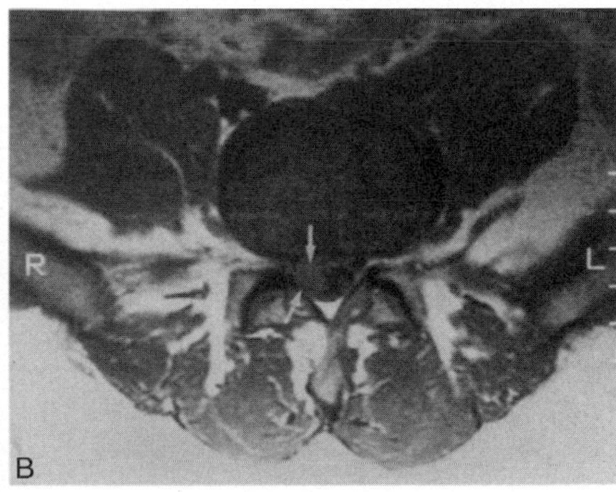

Figure 9-16 A 37-year-old man developed back pain after a piece of furniture fell on him while at work. He had back pain for about 2 years when he developed radicular right leg pain. MR of the lumbar spine revealed on T2-weighted sagittal *(A)* and T1-weighted axial *(B)* images a large herniated nucleus pulposus at the L5-S1 level *(white arrows)*. His leg pain resolved after three epidural corticosteroid injections.

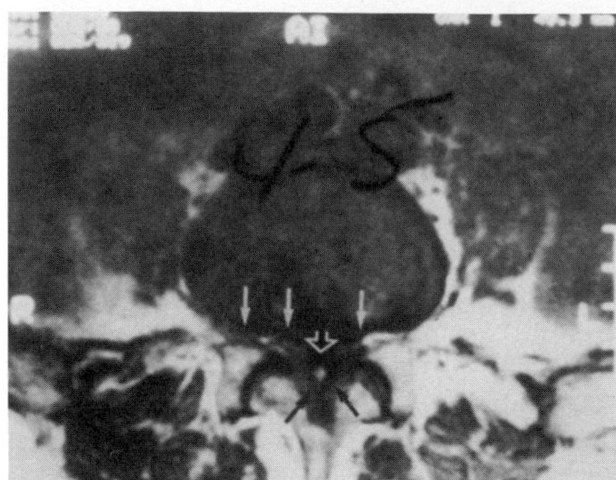

Figure 9-17 A 78-year-old woman developed increasing low back and leg pain associated with walking. She had a partial response to nonsteroidal therapy. MR was obtained in anticipation of lumbar epidural corticosteroid injection. The lumbar spine axial view revealed marked spinal stenosis with osteophytes, bulging disc *(white arrows)*, and ligamentum flavum hypertrophy *(black arrows)* compressing the cauda equina *(open white arrow)*. She responded to epidural injections and refused decompression surgery. *(From Borenstein DG: Low back pain. In Klippel J, Dieppe P [eds]: Rheumatology. St. Louis, Mosby, 1994.)*

Patients who fail to obtain pain relief with this algorithm should be treated with chronic pain therapy.

Anterior Thigh Pain

A small percentage of patients will have pain that radiates from the back into the anterior thigh. This pain usually is relieved by rest and anti-inflammatory medications. If, after 6 weeks of treatment, the discomfort persists, a work-up should be initiated to search for underlying pathologic changes. Several entities must be considered.

Inguinal Hernia. An inguinal hernia causes anterior thigh pain. Occasionally, hernia patients may experience pain in the lateral aspect of the low back. Careful physical examination is essential to identify those individuals with a direct or an indirect inguinal hernia.

Hip Arthritis. Hip arthritis causes pain that classically radiates to the groin. However, the peripheral nerves that supply the hip joint also innervate muscles in the low back and anterior thigh. Hip disease may present as lateral low back and anterior thigh pain. Once again, a careful physical examination will identify those individuals with decreased hip motion that may re-create their back pain. Roentgenograms of the hip demonstrate joint disease (Fig. 9-19).

Aneurysm. An abdominal aneurysm may cause pain that radiates into the anterior thigh. Ultrasonography is a useful technique for visualization of the abdominal aorta and determining its integrity. CT scan is necessary if surgical intervention is contemplated.

Kidney Disorders. Kidney disease should also be considered in a patient with anterior thigh pain. Stones in the kidney may cause pain that radiates from the back into the genitalia or anterior thigh. A urinalysis will reveal hematuria. An intravenous pyelogram (IVP) may be considered to evaluate the urinary tract.

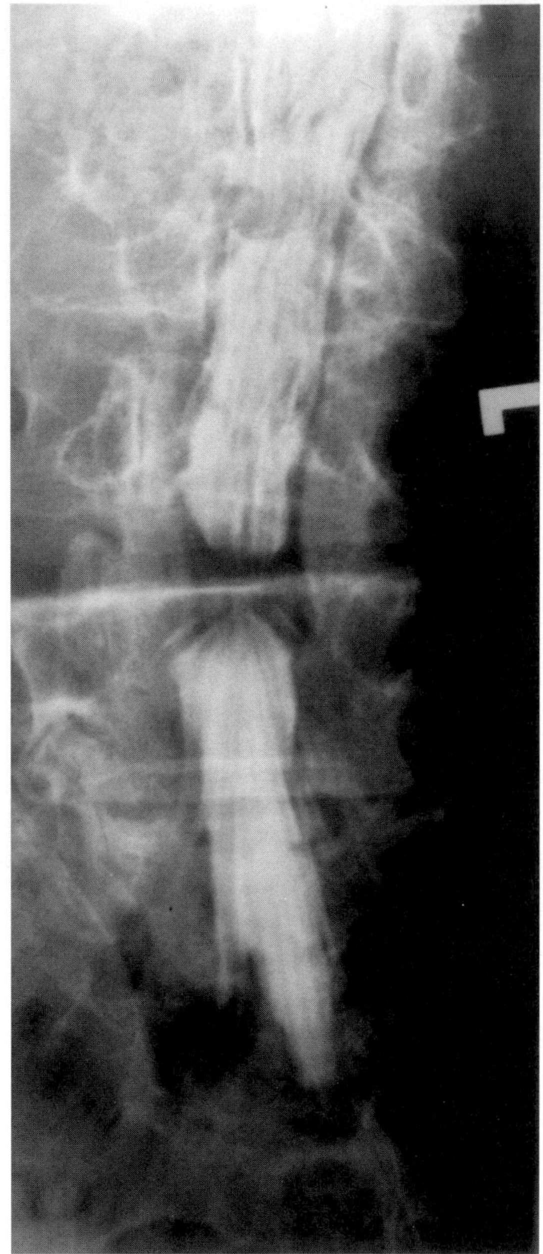

Figure 9-18 An 80-year-old man developed increasing neurogenic claudication and underwent a successful decompressive laminectomy extending from L2 to S1. He had good resolution of his leg pain. One year later he developed a recurrence of his leg pain. He has a pacemaker so a myelogram was performed instead of MR. The myelogram demonstrates severe central canal stenosis at the L4-L5 level. He had a second operation to remove scar tissue that was successful, with decreased leg pain.

Femoral Neuropathy. Peripheral neuropathy, most commonly caused by diabetes, also can present initially as back pain with radiation to the anterior thigh. An elevation in the fasting blood sugar level should raise the possibility of glucose intolerance. Raised values on a formal oral glucose tolerance test confirm the diagnosis. Patients with femoral neuropathy associated with diabetes may experience improvement in their symptoms with normalization of their glucose concentrations.

Retroperitoneal Disorders. Retroperitoneal processes secondary to expanding structures cause back and anterior

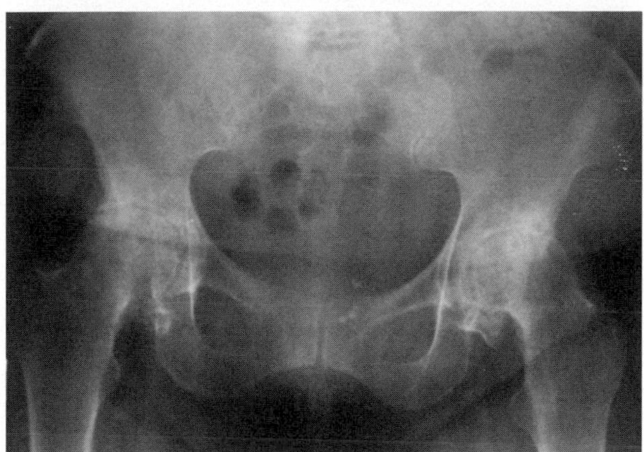

Figure 9-19 A 64-year-old woman had a history of right-sided low back pain with radiation into the anterior thigh. An evaluation of her lumbar spine, including MR, was unrevealing. Physical examination of her hips revealed marked decrease in range of motion. A posteroanterior view of the pelvis revealed severe joint space narrowing along with sclerosis and subchondral cysts. She underwent right hip joint arthroplasty with resolution of her back and leg pain. She has refused left joint replacement. Two years after her operation she remains ambulatory without significant left hip pain on maximum nonsteroidal therapy.

thigh pain. Retroperitoneal tumors cause symptoms including anterior thigh pain as well as back pain. Expanding structures in the retroperitoneum either compress or stretch the splanchnic nerves, which contain visceral afferents that share a common origin with those cutaneous nerves that innervate the anterior thigh. MR evaluation of the retroperitoneum is indicated if retroperitoneal tumors are suspected.

L3–L4 Disc Herniation. Patients with an L3–L4 disc herniation may experience anterior thigh weakness, sensory loss, or, to a lesser degree, pain. Radiographic evaluation of the spinal canal, including CT scan or MR image, can identify these individuals with a herniated disc.

If any of the entities just listed are discovered, the patient is treated accordingly. If no physical cause can be found for the anterior thigh pain, the patient is treated for recalcitrant back strain by following the algorithm.

Posterior Thigh Pain

The final group of patients will complain of back pain with radiation into the buttocks and posterior thigh. Most of them will be relieved of their symptoms with 6 weeks of conservative therapy. However, if their pain persists after the initial treatment period, they are considered to have back strain and are given a local injection of corticosteroids and local anesthetic in the area of maximum tenderness. If the injection is unsuccessful, the next decision point is to distinguish between referred and radicular pain.

Referred Pain. Referred pain is pain in mesodermal tissues of the same embryologic origin. The muscles, tendons, and ligaments of the buttocks, the sacroiliac joints, and the posterior thigh have the same embryologic origin as those of the low back. When the low back is injured, pain may be referred to the posterior thigh, where it is perceived by the patient. Referred pain cannot be cured with a surgical procedure.

Radicular Pain. Radicular pain is caused by compression of an inflamed nerve root along the anatomic course of the nerve. A herniated disc or spinal stenosis in the high lumbar area (e.g., at the L2–3 or L3–4 interspace) could cause radiation of pain into the posterolateral thigh. An MR is used in this situation. If it is normal, the patient is considered to have referred pain and the diagnosis of back strain. If either test is abnormal, the patient is diagnosed as having mechanical root compression from either a herniated disc or spinal stenosis. Epidural corticosteroids should be tried first; if these do not give adequate relief, MR imaging of the lumbar spine concentrating on the upper lumbar disc levels is indicated (Fig. 9-20). If the patient has an identifiable lesion and a lack of response to therapy, surgical intervention is recommended. Patients who have continued pain after surgery for a herniated intervertebral disc should be evaluated by the

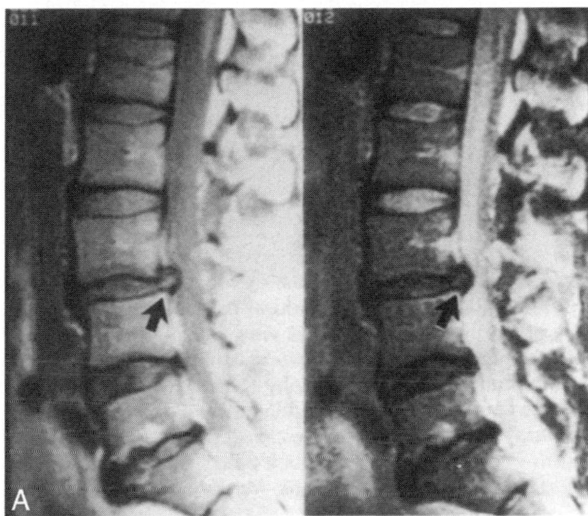

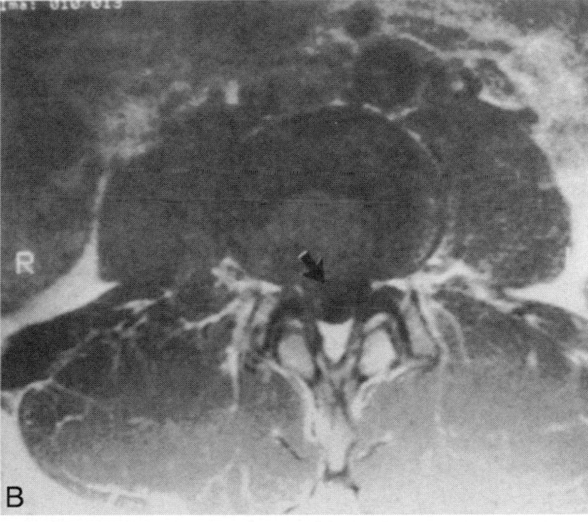

Figure 9-20 A 37-year-old man with a history of localized testicular carcinoma presented with right lateral thigh pain. Pain was localized to the trochanteric area initially but spread to the knee after an extended bicycle trip. Local trochanteric injection was helpful in decreasing the local pain but did not help the leg pain. MR of the lumbar spine reveals on proton density *(A, left side)* and T2-weighted sagittal *(A)* and T1-weighted axial *(B)* views a large posterolateral L3-L4 herniation *(black arrows)*. The disc is impinging the right L3 and L4 nerve roots. A slight anterior spondylolisthesis of 3 mm of L3 on L4 is present. Also noted is degenerative disc signal at L4-L5 and L5-S1. Subsequently, the patient underwent hemilaminectomy and discectomy at L3-L4 and foraminotomies at L5-S1. Postoperatively, the posterolateral leg pain to the knee improved. Subsequently, he developed a second primary testicular tumor with metastatic disease. He is currently receiving radiation and chemotherapy.

multioperated spine algorithm (see Fig. 20-5). Patients who fail to obtain pain relief with this algorithm should be treated with chronic pain therapy.

This group of patients is very difficult to evaluate. The most common mistake is the performance of surgery on people thought to have radicular pain who actually have referred pain. Again, referred pain is not responsive to surgery.

Summary

In the majority of cases, the diagnosis and management of low back pain is not necessarily a mystery. Fifteen percent to 20% of patients with low back pain have a specific pathoanatomic diagnosis.[28] The "Low Back Pain" algorithm on pages 210–211 presents a series of easy-to-follow and clearly defined decision-making processes to identify those patients with specific diagnoses. The "Medical Evaluation Algorithm for Low Back Pain" on pages 212–213 also offers therapies appropriate to the condition and the point in time of the condition's evolution. Use of this algorithm provides patients with the most helpful, expeditious evaluation and does not subject them to procedures that are useless technical exercises.

Additional aids for differential diagnosis may be found in Appendix A at the end of the book, which includes a truth table of differential diagnoses of low back pain and clinical data associated with specific disease entities that cause back pain.

References

Introduction/Low Back Pain

1. Airaksinen O, Herno A, Turunen V, et al: Surgical outcome of 438 patients treated surgically for lumbar spine stenosis. Spine 22:2278-2282, 1997.
2. Atlas SJ, Keller RB, Robson D, et al: Surgical and nonsurgical management of lumbar spinal stenosis: four-year outcomes from the Maine Lumbar Spine Study. Spine 25:556-562, 2000.
3. Bigos SJ, Battie MC, Spengler DM, et al: A prospective study of work perceptions and psychological factors affecting the report of back injury. Spine 16:1-6, 1991.
4. Bigos S, Bowyer O, Braen G, et al: Acute Low Back Problems in Adults. Clinical Practice Guideline No.14. AHCPR Publication No. 95-0642. Rockville, MD: Agency for Health Care Policy and Research, Public Health Service, U.S. Department of Health and Human Services, December 1994.
5. Boden SD, Davis DO, Dina TS, et al: Abnormal magnetic-resonance scans of the lumbar spine in asymptomatic subjects: A prospective investigation. J Bone Joint Surg 72S:403, 1990.
6. Borenstein DG, Korn S: Efficacy of a low-dose regimen of cyclobenzaprine hydrochloride in acute skeletal muscle spasm: Results of two placebo-controlled trials. Clin Ther 25:1056-1073, 2003.
7. Borenstein DG, O'Mara JW, Boden SD, et al: The value of magnetic resonance imaging of the lumbar spine to predict low-back pain in asymptomatic subjects: A seven-year follow-up study. J Bone Joint Surg 83A:1306-1311, 2001.
8. Bouter LM, Pennick V, Bombardier C, et al: Cochrane back review group. Spine 1215-1218, 2003.

8a. Brandt J, Khariouzov A, Listing J, et al: Six-month results of a double-blind, placebo-controlled trial of etanercept treatment in patients with active ankylosing spondylitis. Arthritis Rheum 48:1667-1675, 2003.

9. Cherkin DC, Wheeler KJ, Barlow W, et al: Medication use of low back pain in primary care. Spine 23:607-614, 1998.
10. Colmenero JD, Jimenez-Mejias ME, Sanchez-Lora FJ, et al: Pyogenic, tuberculous, and brucellar vertebral osteomyelitis: A descriptive and comparative study of 219 cases. Ann Rheum Dis 56:709-715, 1997.
11. Deyo RA: Conservative therapy for low back pain: Distinguishing useful from useless therapy. JAMA 250:1057, 1983.
12. Deyo RA, Diehl AK: Cancer as a cause of back pain: Frequency, clinical presentation, and diagnostic strategies. J Gen Intern Med 3:230, 1988.
13. Deyo RA, Diehl AK, Rosenthal M: How many days of bed rest for acute low back pain? A randomized clinical trial. N Engl J Med 315:1064, 1986.
14. Deyo RA, Rainville J, Kent DL: What can the history and physical examination tell us about low back pain? JAMA 268:760, 1992.
15. Deyo R, Weinstein J: Low back pain. N Engl J Med 344:363-370, 2001.
16. Eastell R: Treatment of postmenopausal osteoporosis. N Engl J Med 338:736-746, 1998.
17. Fisk JR, Dimonte P, Courington SM: Back schools: Past, present, and future. Clin Orthop 179:18, 1983.
18. Floman Y, Wiesel SW, Rothman RH: Cauda equina syndrome presenting as a herniated lumbar disk. Clin Orthop 147:234, 1980.
19. Frymoyer JW: Back pain and sciatica. N Engl J Med 318:291, 1988.
20. Gatchel RJ, Mayer TG, Capra P, et al: Quantification of lumbar function: VI. The use of psychological measures in guiding physical functional restoration. Spine 11:36, 1986.
21. Garvey TA, Marks MR, Wiesel SW: A prospective, randomized, double-blind evaluation of trigger-point injection therapy for low-back pain. Spine 14:962, 1989.
22. Hakelius A: Long term follow-up on sciatica. Acta Orthop Scand (Suppl) 129:33, 1972.
23. Holmes HE, Rothman RH: The Pennsylvania plan: An algorithm for the management of lumbar degenerative disc disease. Spine 4:156, 1979.
24. Hurri H: The Swedish back school in chronic low back pain: I. Benefits. Scand J Rehab Med 21:33, 1989.
25. Korbon GA, DeGood DE, Schroeder ME, et al: The development of a somatic amplification rating scale for low-back pain. Spine 12:787, 1987.
26. Kummel BMP: Nonorganic signs of significance in low back pain. Spine 21:1077-1081, 1996.
27. Lonstein MB, Wiesel SW: Standardized approaches to the evaluation and treatment of industrial low back pain. Spine State Art Rev 2:147, 1987.
28. Nachemsom AL: Advances in low-back pain. Clin Orthop 200:266, 1985.
29. Neer RM, Arnaud CD, Zanchetta JR, et al: Effect of parathyroid hormone (1-34) on fractures and bone mineral density in postmenopausal women with osteoporosis. N Engl J Med 344:1434-1441, 2001.
30. Neidre A: Low back pain: Evaluation and treatment in the emergency department setting. Emerg Med Clin North Am 2:441, 1984.
31. Rothman RH: Indications for lumbar fusion. Clin Neurosurg 71:215, 1973.
32. Rothman RH, Simeone FA: The Spine, 2nd ed. Philadelphia, WB Saunders, 1982.
33. Schulitz KP, Assheuer J: Discitis after procedures on the intervertebral disc. Spine 19:1172-1177, 1994.
34. Shapiro S: Medical realities of cauda equina syndrome secondary to lumbar disc herniation. Spine 25:348-352, 2000.

34a. Shekelle PG, Ortiz E, Rhodes S, et al: Validity of the Agency for Healthcare Research and Quality clinical practice guidelines: How quickly do guidelines become outdated? JAMA 286:1461-1467, 2001.

35. Spitzer WO, LeBlanc FE, Dupuis M, et al: Scientific approach to the assessment and management of activity-related spinal disorders: Report of the Quebec Task Force on spinal disorders. Spine 12:S1, 1987.
36. Suarez-Almazor ME, Belseck E, Russell AS, et al: Use of lumbar radiographs for the early diagnosis of low back pain: Proposed guidelines would increase utilization. JAMA 277:1782-1786, 1997.
37. Thelander U, Larsson S: Quantification of C-reactive protein levels and erythrocyte sedimentation rate after spinal surgery. Spine 17:400, 1992.
38. Tile M: The role of surgery in nerve root compression. Spine 9:57, 1984.
39. Turner JA, Romano JM: Cognitive-behavioral therapy for chronic pain. In Loeser JD (ed): Bonica's Management of Pain, 3rd ed. Philadelphia, Lippincott Williams & Wilkins, 2001, pp 1751-1758.
40. Von Korff M, Deyo RA, Cherkin D, et al: Back pain in primary care: Outcomes at 1 year. Spine 18:855, 1993.

41. Waddell G, McCulloch JA, Kummell E, et al: Nonorganic physical signs in low back pain. Spine 5:117, 1980.
42. Walsh NE, Dumitru D: The influence of compensation on recovery from low back pain. Spine State Art Rev 2:109, 1987.
43. Webster's Dictionary. Springfield, MA, F & C Merriam Co, 1982.
44. White AH, Derby R, Wynne G: Epidural injections for the diagnosis and treatment of low back pain. Spine 5:78, 1980.
45. Wiesel SW, Bernini PH, Roth RH: The Aging Lumbar Spine. Philadelphia, WB Saunders, 1983.
46. Wiesel SW, Feffer HL, Borenstein DG: Evaluation and outcome of low back pain of unknown etiology. Spine 13:679, 1988.
47. Wiesel SW, Tsourmas N, Feffer HL, et al: A study of computer-assisted tomography: I. The incidence of positive CAT scans in an asymptomatic group of patients (1984 Volvo Award in Clinical Sciences). Spine 9:549, 1984.
48. Writing group for the Women's Health Initiative Investigators: Risks and benefits of estrogen plus progestin in healthy postmenopausal women: Principal results from the Women's Health Initiative randomized controlled trial. JAMA 288:321-333, 2002.

LOW BACK PAIN (LBP) ALGORITHM

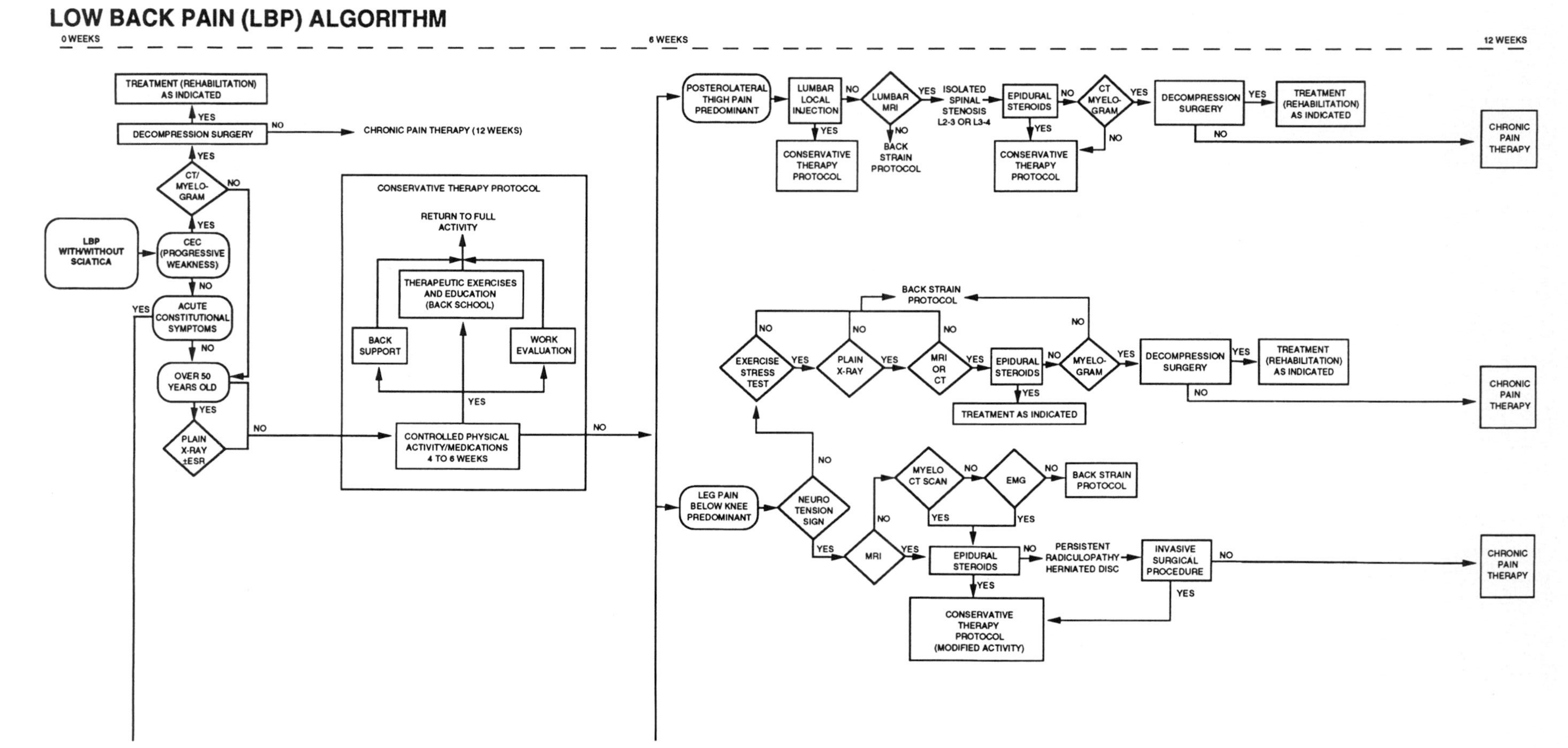

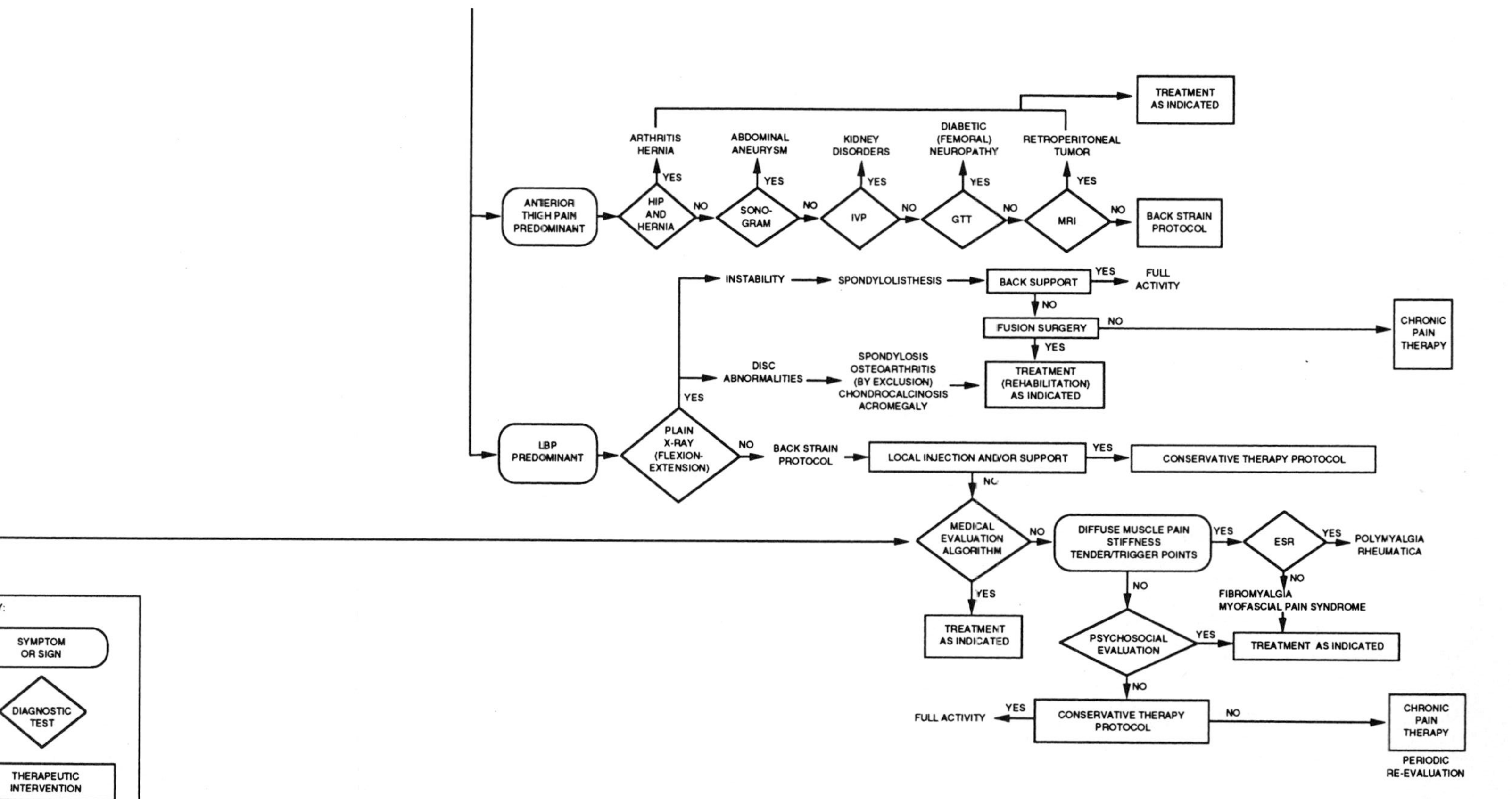
ANTERIOR THIGH PAIN PREDOMINANT
HIP AND HERNIA
YES
ARTHRITIS HERNIA
NO
SONO-GRAM
YES
ABDOMINAL ANEURYSM
NO
IVP
YES
KIDNEY DISORDERS
NO
GTT
YES
DIABETIC (FEMORAL) NEUROPATHY
NO
MRI
YES
RETROPERITONEAL TUMOR
TREATMENT AS INDICATED
NO
BACK STRAIN PROTOCOL
LBP PREDOMINANT
PLAIN X-RAY (FLEXION-EXTENSION)
YES
INSTABILITY
SPONDYLOLISTHESIS
BACK SUPPORT
YES
FULL ACTIVITY
NO
FUSION SURGERY
NO
CHRONIC PAIN THERAPY
YES
TREATMENT (REHABILITATION) AS INDICATED
DISC ABNORMALITIES
SPONDYLOSIS OSTEOARTHRITIS (BY EXCLUSION) CHONDROCALCINOSIS ACROMEGALY
NO
BACK STRAIN PROTOCOL
LOCAL INJECTION AND/OR SUPPORT
YES
CONSERVATIVE THERAPY PROTOCOL
NO
MEDICAL EVALUATION ALGORITHM
YES
TREATMENT AS INDICATED
NO
DIFFUSE MUSCLE PAIN STIFFNESS TENDER/TRIGGER POINTS
YES
ESR
YES
POLYMYALGIA RHEUMATICA
NO
FIBROMYALGIA MYOFASCIAL PAIN SYNDROME
TREATMENT AS INDICATED
NO
PSYCHOSOCIAL EVALUATION
YES
TREATMENT AS INDICATED
NO
CONSERVATIVE THERAPY PROTOCOL
YES
FULL ACTIVITY
NO
CHRONIC PAIN THERAPY
PERIODIC RE-EVALUATION
KEY:
SYMPTOM OR SIGN
DIAGNOSTIC TEST
THERAPEUTIC INTERVENTION

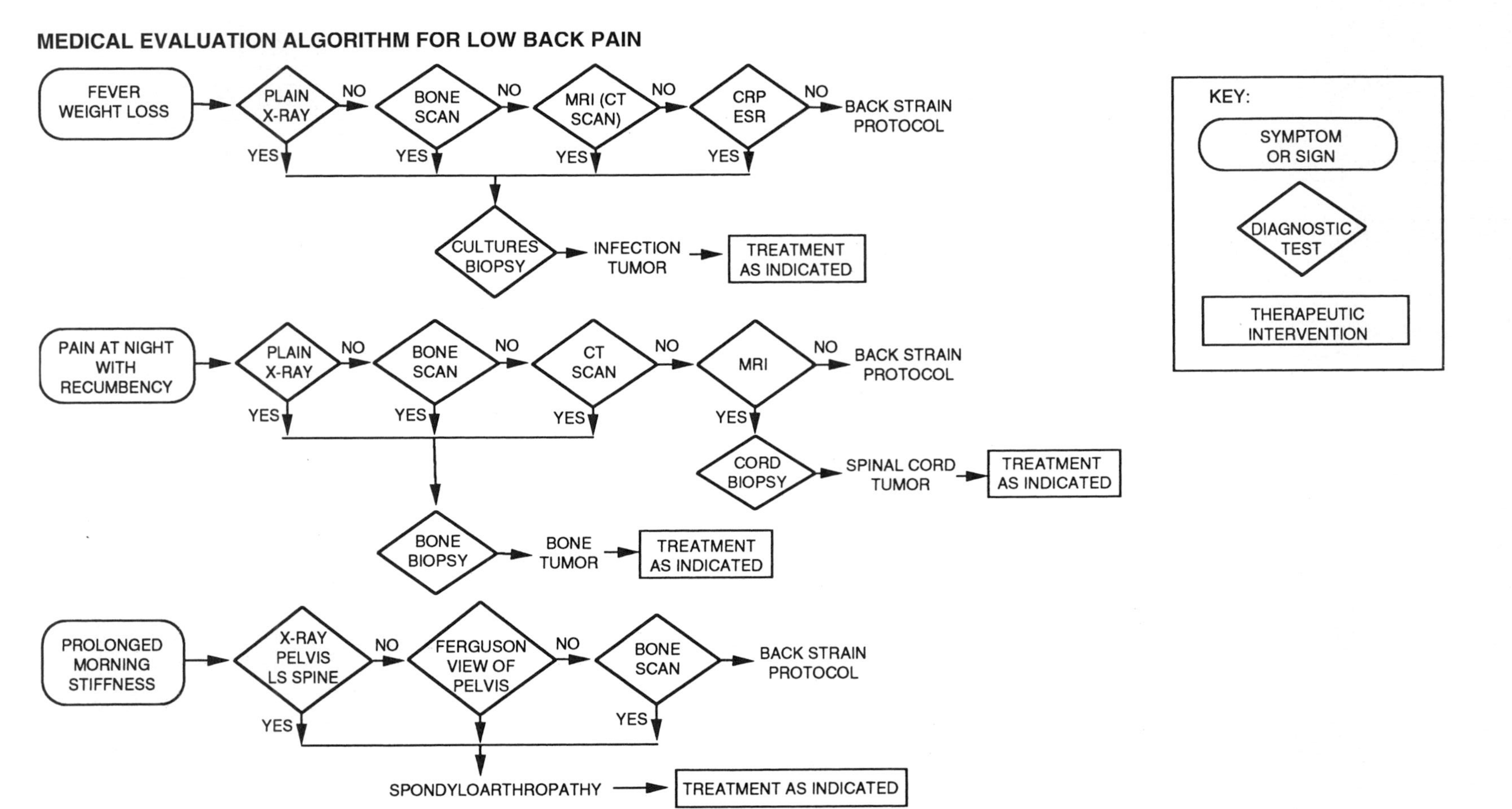
MEDICAL EVALUATION ALGORITHM FOR LOW BACK PAIN
FEVER WEIGHT LOSS
PLAIN X-RAY
NO
YES
BONE SCAN
NO
YES
MRI (CT SCAN)
NO
YES
CRP ESR
NO
YES
BACK STRAIN PROTOCOL
CULTURES BIOPSY
INFECTION TUMOR
TREATMENT AS INDICATED
PAIN AT NIGHT WITH RECUMBENCY
PLAIN X-RAY
NO
YES
BONE SCAN
NO
YES
CT SCAN
NO
YES
MRI
NO
YES
BACK STRAIN PROTOCOL
CORD BIOPSY
SPINAL CORD TUMOR
TREATMENT AS INDICATED
BONE BIOPSY
BONE TUMOR
TREATMENT AS INDICATED
PROLONGED MORNING STIFFNESS
X-RAY PELVIS LS SPINE
NO
YES
FERGUSON VIEW OF PELVIS
NO
BONE SCAN
YES
BACK STRAIN PROTOCOL
SPONDYLOARTHROPATHY
TREATMENT AS INDICATED
KEY:
SYMPTOM OR SIGN
DIAGNOSTIC TEST
THERAPEUTIC INTERVENTION

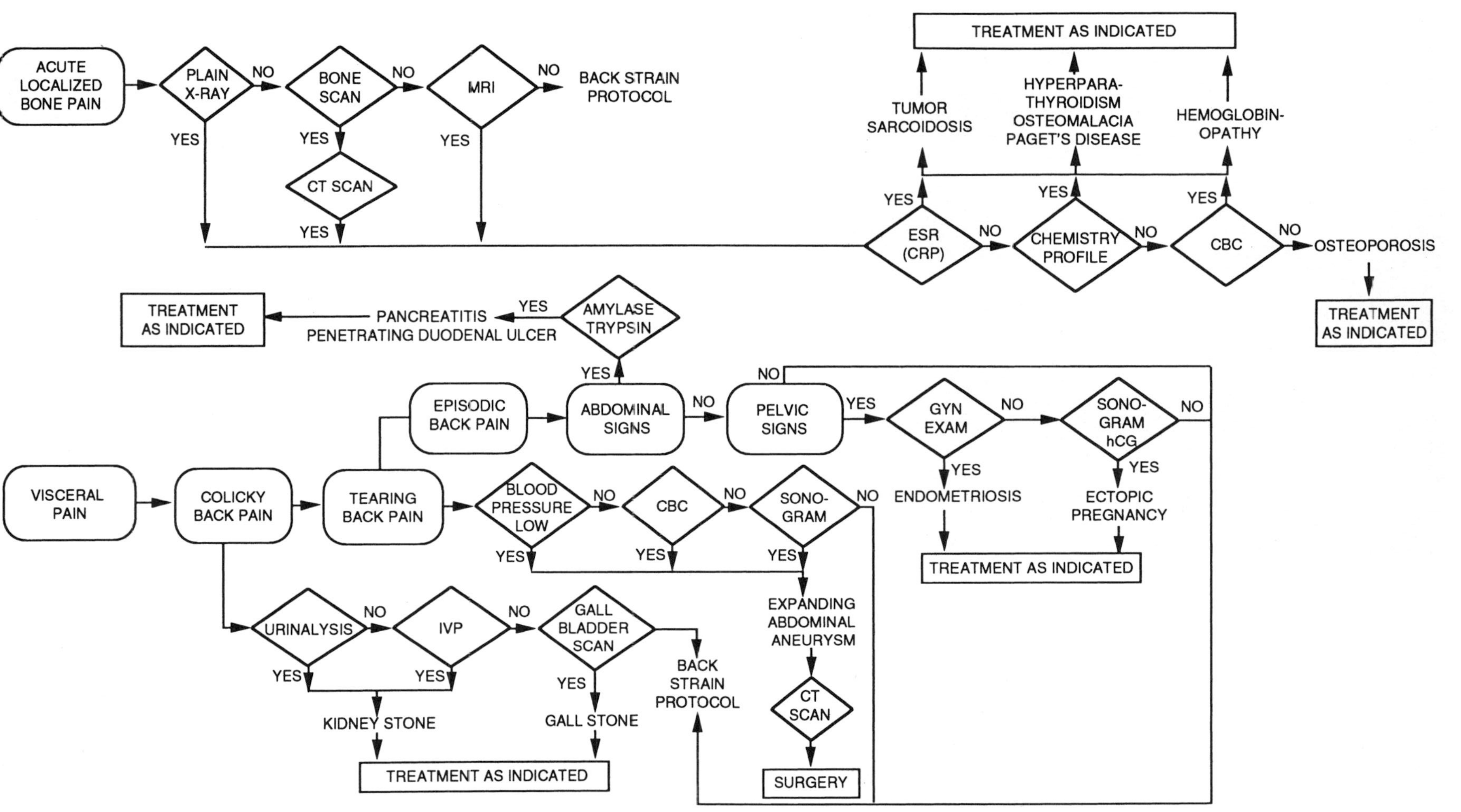

ACUTE LOCALIZED BONE PAIN
PLAIN X-RAY
NO
YES
BONE SCAN
NO
YES
CT SCAN
YES
MRI
NO
YES
BACK STRAIN PROTOCOL
TREATMENT AS INDICATED
TUMOR SARCOIDOSIS
HYPERPARA-THYROIDISM OSTEOMALACIA PAGET'S DISEASE
HEMOGLOBIN-OPATHY
YES
ESR (CRP)
NO
YES
CHEMISTRY PROFILE
NO
YES
CBC
NO
OSTEOPOROSIS
TREATMENT AS INDICATED
TREATMENT AS INDICATED
PANCREATITIS
PENETRATING DUODENAL ULCER
YES
AMYLASE TRYPSIN
YES
EPISODIC BACK PAIN
ABDOMINAL SIGNS
NO
PELVIC SIGNS
NO
YES
GYN EXAM
NO
YES
ENDOMETRIOSIS
SONO-GRAM hCG
NO
YES
ECTOPIC PREGNANCY
TREATMENT AS INDICATED
VISCERAL PAIN
COLICKY BACK PAIN
TEARING BACK PAIN
BLOOD PRESSURE LOW
NO
YES
CBC
NO
YES
SONO-GRAM
NO
YES
EXPANDING ABDOMINAL ANEURYSM
CT SCAN
SURGERY
URINALYSIS
NO
YES
IVP
NO
YES
KIDNEY STONE
GALL BLADDER SCAN
YES
GALL STONE
BACK STRAIN PROTOCOL
TREATMENT AS INDICATED

NECK PAIN

Diagnostic and Treatment Protocol

The diagnostic and treatment protocol begins with the evaluation of patients who are initially seen for neck pain with or without arm or shoulder pain. Patients with major trauma to the cervical spine, including fractures and dislocations, are not included because these individuals are treated primarily in emergency departments that have specific neck trauma protocols. After an initial medical history and physical examination are completed, and on the assumption that the patient's symptoms are originating from the cervical spine, the first major decision is to rule in or out the presence of cervical myelopathy.

Cervical Myelopathy

Cervical myelopathy occurs secondary to compression of the neural elements (spinal cord and nerve roots) in the cervical spinal canal.[4,11] Progressive and profound neurologic deficits, including weakness, spasticity, and gait abnormalities, are clinical manifestations of myelopathy. The etiology of the compression is usually a combination of osteoarthritis associated with osteophytes and degenerative disc disease that leads to a decrease in the volume of the spinal canal. If the canal becomes too small, the spinal cord may be compromised, resulting in neurologic dysfunction. Individuals with developmentally small spinal canals are at increased risk of manifesting spinal cord compression.

The character and severity of the problem depend on the size, location, and duration of the lesion. Ventrolateral lesions encroach on the nerve roots and lateral aspects of the spinal cord, producing all the manifestations of nerve root compression. The main radicular signs are weakness with loss of tone and volume of the muscles in the upper extremity. Pressure on the spinal cord may produce pyramidal tract signs and spasticity in the lower extremities. The most frequent presentation of myelopathy is a combination of arm and leg dysfunction.[1]

Midline lesions intrude on the central aspect of the anterior spinal cord. They generally do not produce signs of nerve root compression. Both lower extremities are usually involved, and the most common problem relates initially to gait disturbances. As the problem progresses, bowel and bladder control may be affected.

Although the natural history of cervical spondylitic myelopathy is one of gradual progression, severe myelopathy rarely develops in patients who do not demonstrate it when they first present to the physician. Once the diagnosis of cervical myelopathy is made, surgical intervention should be considered quickly. The best results are attained in patients with one or two motor units involved and with a myelopathy of relatively short duration. A cervical CT/myelogram or MR image should be obtained to define the neural compression precisely, and an adequate surgical decompression should be performed as soon as possible to achieve the best results (Fig. 9-21).[12,13] After surgical intervention, many individuals require rehabilitation to return to an improved functional status.

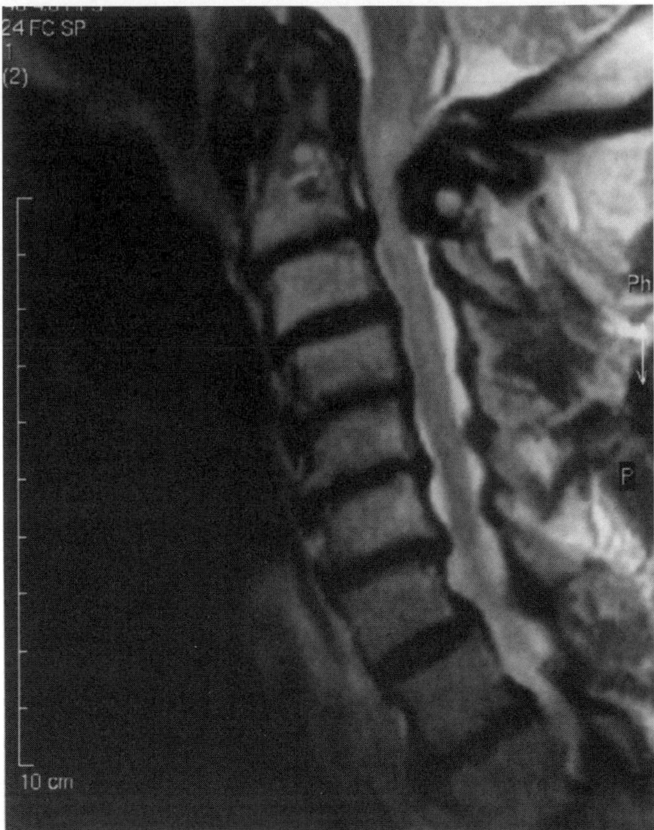

Figure 9-21 A 72-year-old man complained of increasing tingling in his hands and feet. He had an unstable gait and a positive Babinski sign. An MR sagittal view demonstrates spinal cord narrowing at the C2-C3 level.

Systemic Medical Illness

The patients who do not have cervical myelopathy should be evaluated for acute, severe symptoms suggestive of an underlying systemic medical illness as the cause of their neck pain. These individuals should be asked five questions that identify patients at increased risk of medical causes of neck pain. These groups include individuals with constitutional symptoms of fever or weight loss suggestive of an infection or tumor. Patients with pain that is increased with recumbency or at night may have a spinal cord infiltrative process or a tumor of the vertebral column. Patients with prolonged morning stiffness may have spondyloarthropathy. Localized cervical bone pain may be secondary to a systemic process that replaces bone (Paget's disease) or a local tumor (osteoblastoma). Patients with viscerogenic pain (angina, thoracic outlet syndrome, and esophageal disorders) have symptoms that affect structures beyond the cervical spine and recur in a regular pattern. Patients with constitutional symptoms should receive a medical evaluation that is specific for the corresponding symptom or sign. Patients with acute neck pain who are older than 60 years of age (malignant tumor) or younger than 15 years of age (benign bone tumor) should be considered for plain roentgenograms of the cervical spine and determination of ESR. These tests have a greater probability of showing abnormalities in this group of patients. If the test results are unrevealing, patients should be treated with conservative therapy for 3 to 6 weeks.

Conservative Therapy

After a cervical myelopathy and acute systemic medical disorders have been ruled out, the remainder of patients with neck pain, who constitute the majority, should be started on a course of medical (nonoperative) management. Initially, a specific diagnosis, such as a herniated disc, cervical spondylosis, or neck strain, is not required to start therapy because the entire group is treated in a similar fashion.

Short-term immobilization is useful in therapy for acute episodes and exacerbations in patients with chronic cervical intervertebral disc disease. Collars are needed in a small proportion of patients. A soft felt collar should fit properly and usually provides comfort for the patient. The collar initially should be worn continuously day and night. The patient must understand that the collar protects the neck from awkward positions and movements during sleep and is therefore important. Soft collars play a lesser role in conservative management of patients with other causes of neck pain, such as whiplash and osteoarthritis. The time in a collar is decreased as rapidly as tolerated so that motion of the cervical spine is gradually increased to its baseline status.[15] The other major component of the initial treatment program is drug therapy. Anti-inflammatory drugs, analgesics, and muscle relaxants usually improve patient comfort and should supplement appropriate position of the cervical spine.[2] Medication is used in conjunction with gradual mobilization.

Most patients respond to this short-term stabilization and pharmacotherapy in the first 10 days. The patients who improve should be encouraged to increase their activities gradually and begin a program of exercises directed at strengthening the paravertebral musculature rather than at increasing the range of motion. For patients with intervertebral disc problems, use of the soft collar is decreased over the next 2 to 3 weeks. The unimproved group of patients with disc herniation should continue with full-time collar immobilization and anti-inflammatory medication.

Injection Therapy. If there is not a significant improvement in symptoms in 3 to 4 weeks in patients with local neck pain, a local injection into the area of maximum tenderness in the paravertebral musculature and trapezii should be considered. Marked relief of symptoms is often achieved dramatically by infiltration of these trigger points with a combination of 3 to 5 mL of lidocaine (Xylocaine) and 12 mg of a corticosteroid betamethasone preparation.

Cervical Traction. For patients with cervical disc herniation and radiculopathy, a trial of cervical traction may be instituted if the trigger point injections and medical therapy are not successful at 4 to 5 weeks after the onset of symptoms. Patients are trained during physical therapy to apply traction to the cervical spine. They can continue to use the traction device with light weights at home. Isometric strengthening exercises should be instituted as the patient returns to full activity.

The remaining patients should be treated conservatively for up to 6 weeks. The majority of patients with cervical spine disorders get better and return to a normal life pattern within 2 months. If the initial conservative treatment fails, symptomatic patients may be separated into two groups. The first group consists of patients with neck pain as a predominant complaint, with or without interscapular radiation. The second group consists of those who complain primarily of arm pain (brachialgia).

NECK PAIN PREDOMINANT

If no symptomatic improvement is achieved after 6 weeks of medical nonoperative therapy, plain roentgenograms, including lateral flexion-extension motion films, should be taken and carefully examined. Roentgenograms before this point are usually not helpful because of the lack of significant differences between symptomatic and asymptomatic patients, except in individuals older than 60 years of age or younger than 15 years of age.[7] Nonspecific radiographic degenerative changes in the cervical spine are almost universal by age 60. Careful examination of roentgenograms in older individuals is necessary to be sure that lesions, in addition to spondylosis, are identified.

NECK PAIN INTERSCAPULAR PREDOMINANT

Patients with neck pain with radiation to the interscapular area have muscle tension in the trapezius muscles or instability in the cervical spine. In the lower cervical spine (C3-C7), instability is defined as horizontal translation of one vertebra on another of more than 3.5 mm or as an angulatory difference of adjacent vertebrae of more than 11 degrees.[17] Some patients may have objective evidence of instability on the motion films. A series of flexion and extension roentgenograms of the cervical spine should be obtained. The radiographs may demonstrate abnormal movement of the vertebral bodies (Fig. 9-22). The majority of patients with degenerative (nontraumatic) instability respond to a thorough explanation of the problem and to nonsteroidal anti-inflammatory drugs (NSAIDs), muscle relaxants, exercises, and the intermittent use of a cervical collar. Activity limitation may be all that is required to maintain function and limit pain in these individuals if the instability is mild. Those with persistent pain with progressive listhesis require segmental spinal fusion. If they do not improve with these interventions, these individuals are candidates for a chronic pain program.

Cervical Spondylosis. Other patients who complain mainly of neck pain show degenerative abnormalities on their plain films. The roentgenographic findings include loss of height of the intervertebral disc space, osteophyte formation, secondary encroachment of the intervertebral foramina, and osteoarthritic changes in the zygapophyseal joints.[6] The diagnostic difficulty is not in identifying these abnormalities but in determining their clinical significance. Degeneration in the cervical spine can be a normal part of aging. Many asymptomatic patients show roentgenographic, myelographic, and MR evidence of abnormal degenerative disease.[8] The most significant finding relevant to symptomatology is narrowing of the intervertebral disc space, particularly at C5–6 and C6–7 (Fig. 9-23). Changes at the zygapophyseal joints, foramina, and posterior articular processes do not correlate well with clinical symptoms. These patients should be treated with anti-inflammatory medications, cervical support, and trigger point injections as required. In the quiescent stages, they should be placed on isometric exercises. Finally, they should be re-examined periodically because some may develop myelopathy.

The majority of patients with neck pain have normal roentgenograms. The preliminary diagnosis for this group

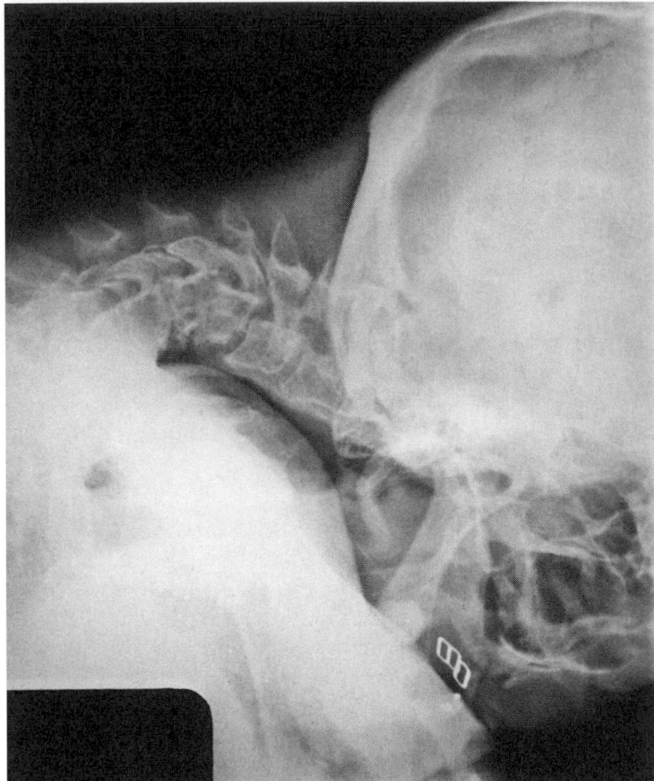

Figure 9-22 A 77-year-old woman presented with an 8-year history of progressive neck and shoulder blade pain. The patient has hypermobility syndrome and an eating disorder. She was concerned about her weight (112 pounds) and became anorectic. She lost increasing amount of muscle mass, including the paracervical muscles. She developed increasing curvature of the neck with inability to lift her head. She wears a soft collar intermittently. Plain lateral roentgenogram demonstrates marked kyphosis with anterolisthesis of C3 on C4 and C4 on C5. Disc space narrowing and osteophyte formation is noted at the lower cervical levels.

is neck strain.[9] However, in the absence of objective findings as well as failure to improve with appropriate medical nonoperative management, other problems must be considered.

Medical Re-evaluation

Without radiographic findings of degenerative spine disease, the evaluation of the patient with neck pain limited to the neck must start again with a review of the patient's history and physical examination. Symptoms may have appeared or changed in intensity since the initial evaluation. The histories of patients with neck pain may be divided according to symptoms into five groups (see the "Medical Evaluation for Neck Pain" algorithm, pages 225–226): fever and weight loss, pain at night or with recumbency, morning stiffness, acute localized bone pain, and visceral pain. The medical evaluation of each group differs. It is helpful to identify the patient's symptoms at the initial visit so that a specific evaluation can be completed thoughtfully and expeditiously.

Fever and Weight Loss

Patients with neck pain and fever should be evaluated for any change in mental status or severe headache. These individuals should have their cerebrospinal fluid (CSF) examined for inflammatory cells, increased protein, or decreased glucose concentration compatible with meningitis. These patients require immediate broad-spectrum antibiotic therapy while cultures are incubated from the CSF examination. Antibiotic therapy is altered as the causative organism is determined and antibiotic sensitivity is identified. Plain roentgenograms of the patients with fever and weight loss should be reviewed for alterations in bone integrity. Because a significant portion of bone cal-

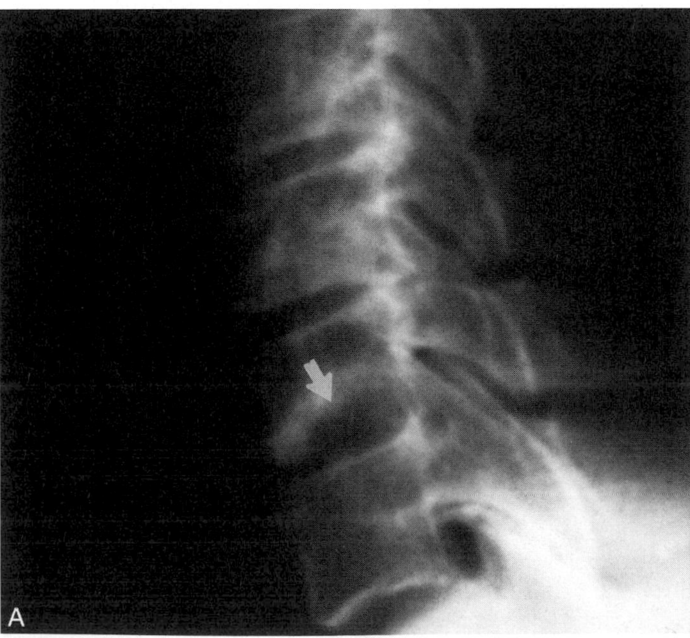

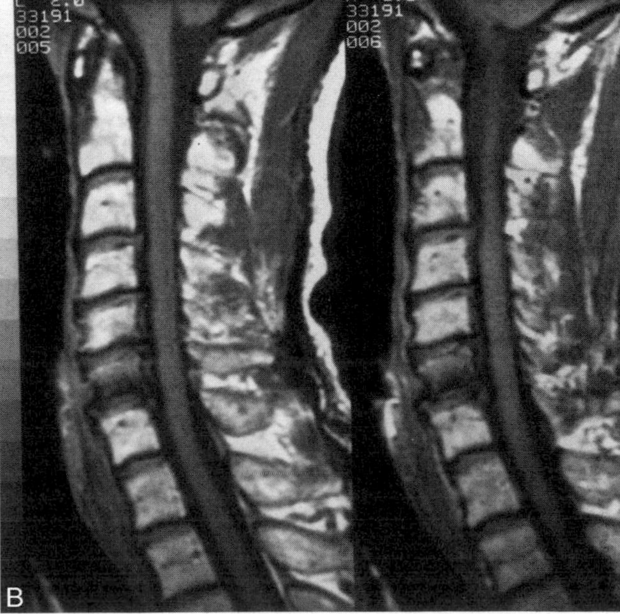

Figure 9-23 A 48-year-old HIV-positive man presented with 3 months of increasing neck pain. Plain lateral roentgenogram *(A)* demonstrated erosion of the C6 vertebral endplate along with disc space narrowing. Sagittal MR *(B)* demonstrated infiltration of the disc space. The patient underwent a biopsy that was negative for all organisms. The final diagnosis was cervical spondylosis with disc degeneration.

cium must be lost before lesions are identified, bone scan is a useful screening test to discover increased bone cell activity. A normal bone scan does not eliminate the possibility of a tumor. An MR image or CT scan identifies the patients with a destructive lesion without osteoblastic response (multiple myeloma) (Fig. 9-24). These radiographs locate the lesion for appropriate biopsy and culture. Determining ESR or C-reactive protein identifies those individuals with an inflammatory lesion of the cervical spine. Antibiotics are the treatment of choice for osteomyelitis and discitis. Surgical excision is preferred if tumors, particularly benign lesions, are accessible for total removal. In postsurgical patients who develop fever, determining CRP or ESR is useful to identify infections. CRP is the more sensitive indicator.[16]

Pain at Night or with Recumbency

Infiltrative lesions of the spinal cord and tumors of the spinal column are associated with nocturnal increase in pain. Patients with neurologic signs and nocturnal or recumbency pain should undergo MR evaluation of the central nervous system. The presence of multiple lesions compatible with plaques is compatible with a demyelinating disease such as multiple sclerosis. A spinal cord tumor appears as a single mass lesion. Such a lesion requires biopsy for diagnosis. Those patients without neurologic signs and nocturnal pain may have a bone tumor as the cause of symptoms. A plain roentgenogram of the cervical spine should be reviewed for the presence of benign or malignant tumors. Benign tumors tend to involve the posterior elements of vertebrae, and malignant tumors affect

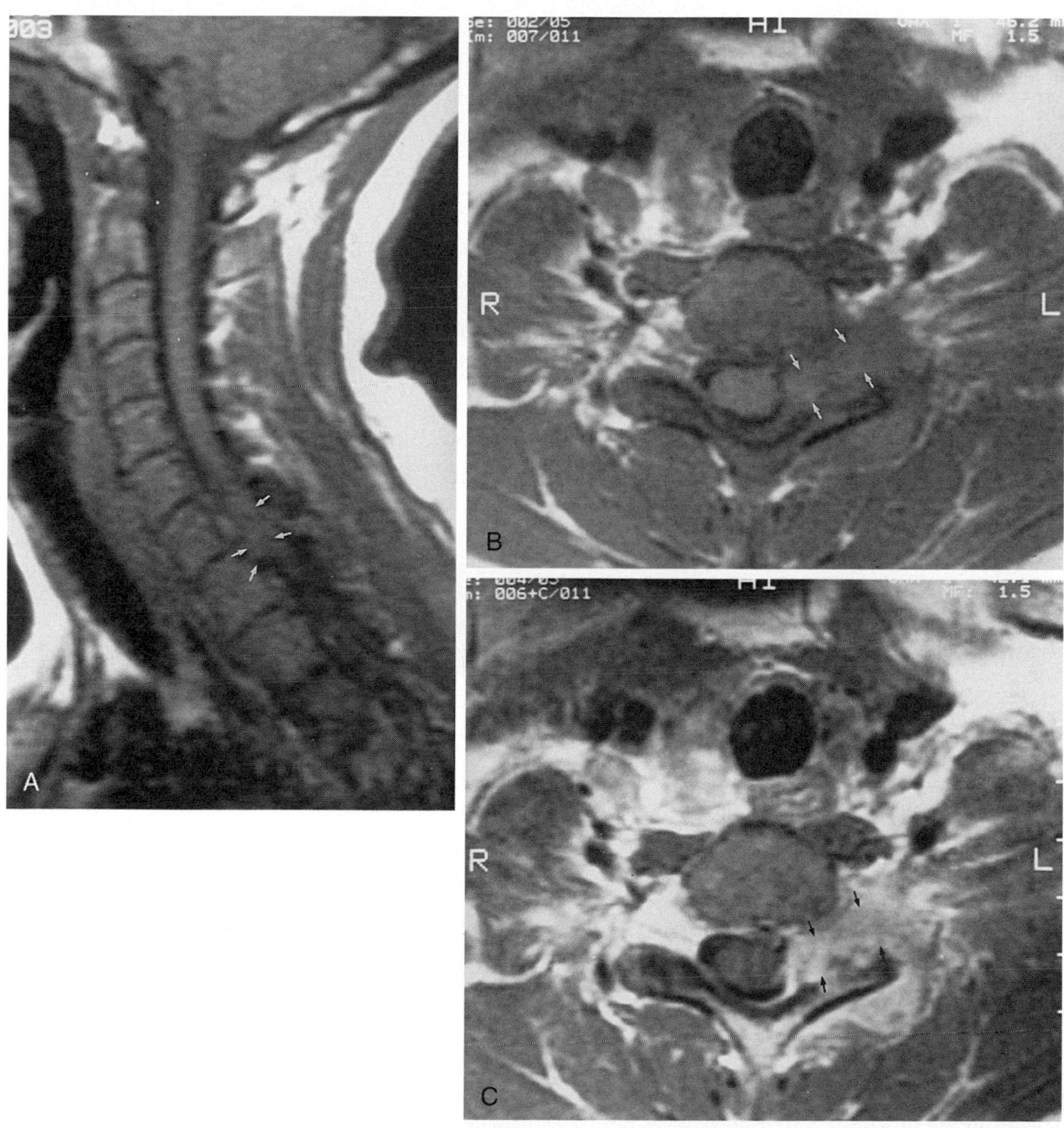

Figure 9-24 A 35-year-old hospital ward clerk with a history of sarcoidosis developed increasing nocturnal neck and left arm pain in an ulnar distribution within the setting of fever, anemia, elevated erythrocyte sedimentation rate, and positive fluorescent antinuclear antibodies. MR of the cervical spine reveals on a T1-weighted sagittal image *(A)* a mass lesion at the C8-T1 interspace *(arrows)*. T1-weighted axial image *(B)* reveals a mass lesion filling the left neural foramen *(arrows)* that enhances with gadolinium contrast media *(arrows)* in *(C)*.

Continued

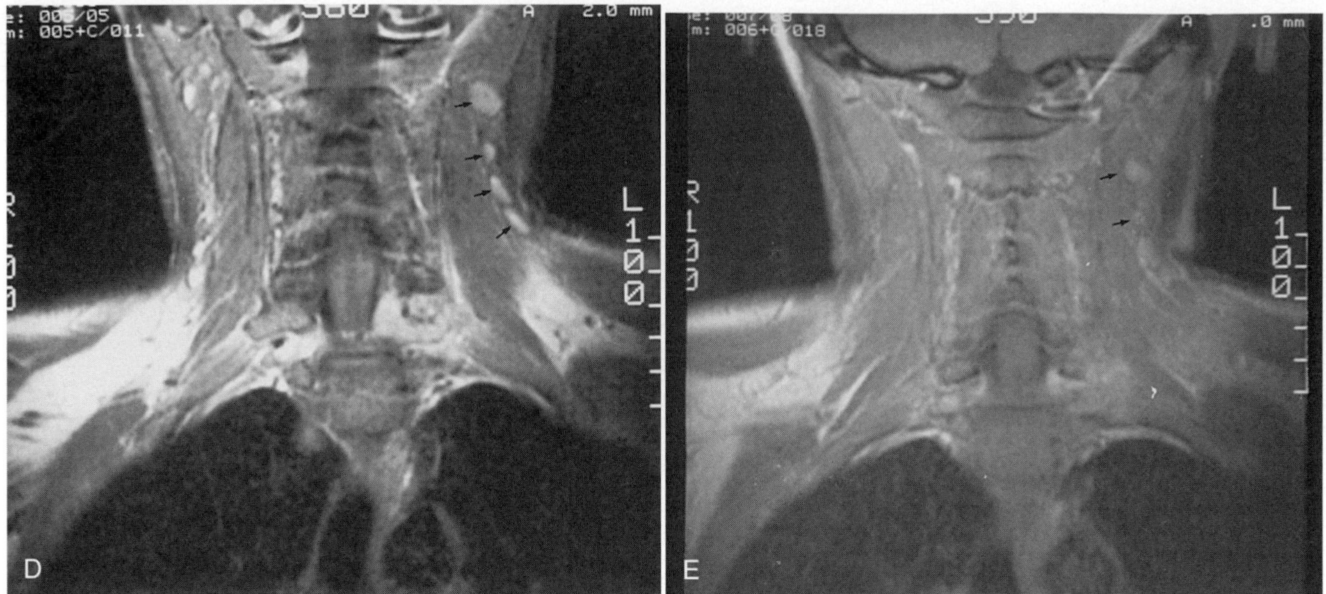

Figure 9-24, cont'd MR T1-weighted contrast coronal view *(D)* reveals enhancement of left cervical lymph glands *(arrows)*. Biopsy of the mass lesion revealed caseating granulomas, and culture grew *Mycobacterium tuberculosis*. The patient received five antituberculous drugs. After 5 months of therapy with resolution of neck and arm pain, T1-weighted contrast coronal view *(E)* reveals resolution of the enhancement of cervical lymph nodes *(arrows)*.

vertebral bodies. Plain roentgenograms may be unable to detect lesions because inadequate calcium has been lost. Bone scan is a more sensitive test in detecting increased bone turnover. A CT scan is better than an MR image for bone detail in identifying bone tumors (Fig 9-25). These lesions require biopsy and lesion-specific therapy.

Morning Stiffness

Morning stiffness of the neck lasting for hours is a common symptom of patients with spondyloarthropathy or rheumatoid arthritis. Patients with this symptom should have a flexion-extension view of the cervical spine to detect subluxation (Fig. 9-26). On occasion, a patient with rheumatoid arthritis may have mild peripheral joint disease and more significant cervical spine involvement. A positive rheumatoid factor may identify these unusual patients. Women with spondyloarthropathy may have neck disease without significant low back pain. Occasional patients with spondyloarthropathy do not have back pain despite the presence of sacroiliitis. Therefore, Ferguson's view of the pelvis is a useful test to identify the presence of sacroiliitis if neck films are unrevealing for squaring of vertebral bodies or syndesmophytes. Patients with spondyloarthropathy with increased neck pain require radiographic evaluation to eliminate the possibility of fracture (Fig. 9-27). A bone scan and ESR are useful tests to identify those individuals with inflammatory polyarthritis. If the bone scan is normal and the ESR is abnormal and the patient is 60 years or age or older, a diagnosis of polymyalgia rheumatica should be considered. Patients with polyarthritis are treated with NSAIDs and stabilization of the cervical spine. Patients with polymyalgia rheumatica are treated daily with low-dose corticosteroids.

Acute Localized Bone Pain

Acute localized bone pain is usually associated with either fracture or expansion of bone. Any condition that replaces bone with abnormal cells (tumor or sarcoidosis) or increases mineral loss from bone (hyperparathyroidism) weakens bone to the point at which fracture may occur spontaneously or with minimal trauma. Patients with acute fractures experience acute onset of pain in the area of the neck that corresponds to the fractured bone. Physical examination will identify the maximum point of tenderness. A plain roentgenogram should be reviewed with special attention to the painful area to identify a fracture. A bone scan is useful in detecting increased bone activity soon after a fracture when a plain roentgenogram is normal. A CT scan is capable of detecting fractures that are located by a bone scan. If the bone scan is normal, MR can identify the presence of malignant or inflammatory cells that do not stimulate osteoblasts (myeloma). An ESR test and chemistry profile can detect inflammatory and metabolic abnormalities associated with alteration of bony architecture. The diagnostic evaluation and therapeutic regimen for each disease are reviewed in Section III.

Visceral Pain

Patients with visceral pain have neck pain secondary to disorders in the cardiovascular, gastrointestinal, or neurologic systems. Patients may complain of neck and arm pain that occurs with exertion. If chest pain occurs in conjunction with arm pain, evaluation for coronary artery disease is indicated. These patients should have an electrocardiogram and a stress test. If these tests show abnormalities, referral to a cardiologist for angina therapy is required. If the exertional pain is

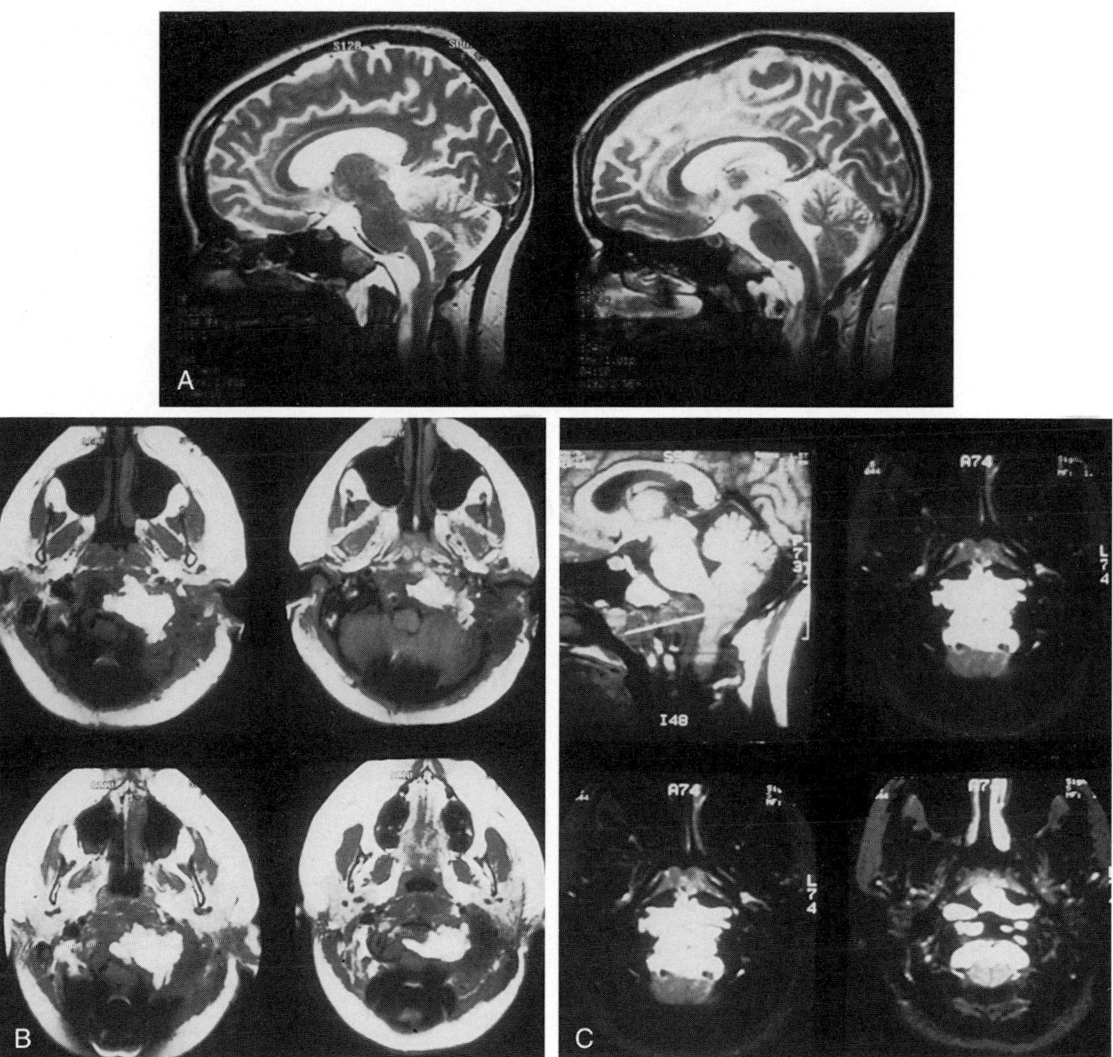

Figure 9-25 A 15-year-old woman had 18 months of persistent neck pain with recent onset of headache and disequilibrium. A T2-weighted sagittal magnetic resonance scan *(A)* reveals a mass lesion affecting the clivus and atlas, with posterior displacement of the brainstem. CT *(B)* reveals replacement of clival bone. Postoperative CT *(C)* reveals a decrease in the size of the mass with decompression of the brain stem. Pathologic examination of the mass revealed cells compatible with a chordoma. *(Courtesy of Laligam N. Sekhar, MD, and Donald Wright, MD.)*

limited to the arm alone, an evaluation for thoracic outlet syndrome is indicated. Adson's test identifies those patients with scalenus anterior syndrome; the hyperabduction test identifies compression of the neurovascular bundle between the costocoracoid membrane and the pectoralis minor. These individuals may improve with postural exercises.

If the arm pain is persistent, a chest roentgenogram with particular attention to the apices is indicated. Pancoast's tumors invade the inferior portions of the brachial plexus. These patients have malignant lesions that require palliative radiation therapy. Episodic neck or arm pain may be secondary to a transient ischemic attack. These individuals should have Doppler ultrasonography to evaluate vascular narrowing. An angiogram identifies constriction or dissection of the carotid or vertebral arteries. Therapy may include drugs to prevent thrombosis or surgical correction of the lesion.

Esophageal disorders should be considered if neck pain occurs in association with eating. Lesions in the posterior esophagus may affect the prevertebral space, causing neck pain. Spinal structures may constrict the esophagus (Fig 9-28). An esophagogram identifies abnormalities of function as well as stricture. Esophagoscopy may be required to identify mucosal abnormalities.

Patients with multiorgan system abnormalities in addition to neck pain should be asked about exposure to tick bites. If these individuals have erythema migrans, or Bell's palsy, a diagnosis of Lyme disease should be considered. The diagnosis of Lyme disease is considered in the patient with tick exposure and appropriate clinical symptoms and signs. Positive Lyme antibody titers are confirmatory but not diagnostic. Oral antibiotic therapy for 4 weeks is adequate for many patients with Lyme disease.

Proximal Muscle/Tender Point Pain. If the medical evaluation is normal, the patient should be evaluated for the presence of tender points or trigger points. An elevated ESR and muscle tenderness suggest a diagnosis of polymyalgia rheumatica. A normal ESR is compatible with fibromyalgia (tender points) or myofascial syndrome

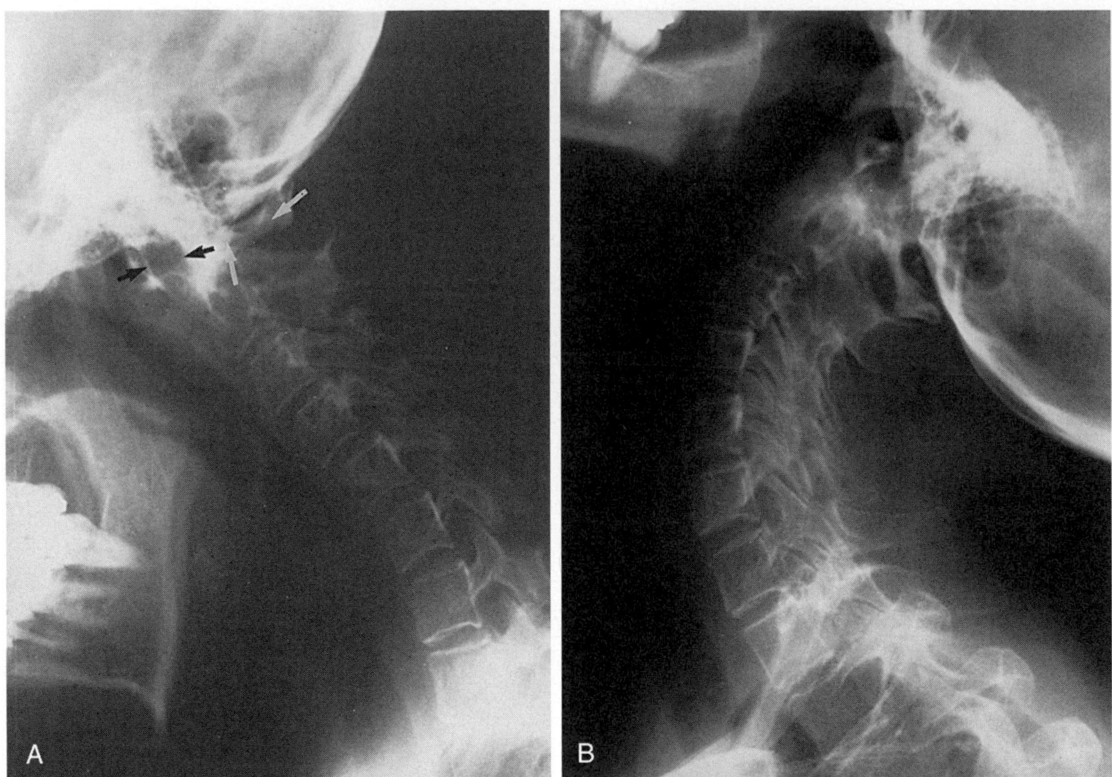

Figure 9-26 A 30-year-old woman with rheumatoid arthritis for 10 years complained of increased neck discomfort without any neurologic deficit. Flexion *(A)* and extension *(B)* views of the cervical spine demonstrate atlantoaxial subluxation with anterior measurement of 10 mm *(black arrows)* and posterior measurement of 15 mm *(white arrows)*. Flexion view reveals minimal anterior subluxation at the C3-C4 and C5-C6 levels. The patient is being followed for the appearance of headache or neurologic symptoms that would require evaluation for stabilization.

(trigger points). Patients with fibromyalgia improve with aerobic exercise and antidepressants; myofascial patients may benefit from injection at the maximum point of tenderness with a combination of an anesthetic and a corticosteroid.

Psychosocial/Occupational Evaluation. If the patient does not have muscle tenderness, he or she should have a complete psychosocial evaluation and receive treatment when appropriate for depression or substance dependence, which are frequently seen in association with neck pain. Patients who experience a variety of social problems (marital discord, job dissatisfaction, financial uncertainties) may manifest these difficulties as chronic neck pain. Identification of these social problems or psychiatric diagnoses can identify those individuals who require therapeutic interventions beyond those of usual conservative management.

Occasionally, it is difficult to distinguish those patients who have a true neck problem from those individuals using their neck pain as an excuse to miss work and collect compensation or because of pending litigation. The outcome of treatment of cervical disc disease can be adversely affected by litigation. Frequently with hyperextension neck injuries there are no objective findings to substantiate the subjective complaints. The best solution to this dilemma in the compensation setting is to recommend an independent medical examination early in the course of treatment. In general, compensation and noncompensation patients respond to therapy in similar ways.[14] Patients should be encouraged to remain functional in spite of pain and other symptoms.[3]

Chronic Pain Therapy. If the psychosocial evaluation proves normal, the patient is considered to have chronic neck pain. These patients require encouragement, patience, and education. They especially need to be encouraged to complete a regular exercise regimen for the neck and an aerobic exercise program. Medical therapy will need to be expanded to involve different categories of medications such as an NSAID and muscle relaxant the patient had not received previously. Many respond to antidepressant drugs, including tricyclic agents. The patients may require a selective serotonin reuptake inhibitor if they manifest symptoms and signs of depression. Long-acting narcotic therapy may be considered for the appropriate patient. Regardless, these patients need to be periodically re-evaluated to avoid missing any new problems.

Arm Pain Predominant (Brachialgia)

Compression Syndromes. Extrinsic pressure on the vascular structures or peripheral nerves is the most likely imitator of brachialgia and must be ruled out. Problems in the chest and shoulder must also be considered. A careful physical examination, including Adson's test, shoulder evaluation, and a test for Tinel's sign at the ulnar and carpal tunnels, should be conducted. If these test results are equivocal, appropriate radiographs and an electromyogram (EMG) should be obtained.

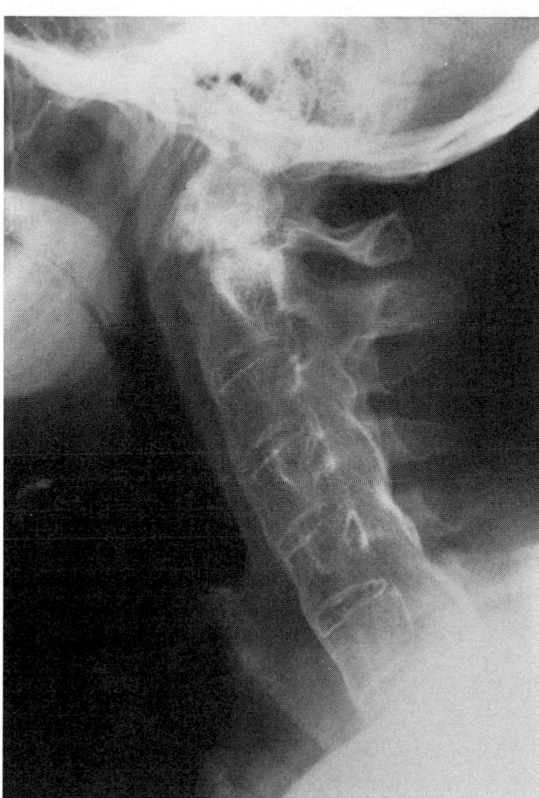

Figure 9-27 A 67-year-old man with a 20-year history of ankylosing spondylitis had increased neck pain without increased movement. Lateral view of the cervical spine reveals anterior and posterior syndesmophytes, fusion of zygapophyseal joints, and no evidence of fracture. Neck pain improved with an increase in nonsteroidal therapy and the addition of a muscle relaxant.

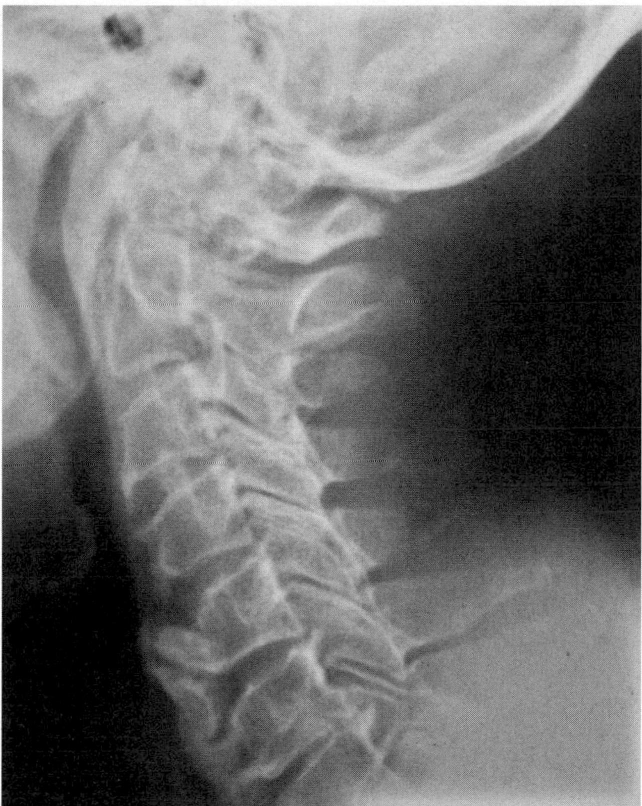

Figure 9-28 A 70-year-old man presented with increasing neck stiffness and difficulty swallowing certain foods. Plain roentgenogram lateral view reveals large anterior ligament calcifications at C5 and C6 levels constricting anterior soft tissue structures, compatible with diffuse idiopathic skeletal hyperostosis.

In addition to spinal nerve root encroachment, diseases that directly affect the brachial plexus may result in a variety of upper extremity symptoms that must be distinguished from cervical root syndromes. Although trauma is the most common cause of brachial plexus injury, compression by vascular structure, cervical ribs, muscular or fibrous bands, or tumors may result in a plexus neuropathy. Apical carcinoma of the lung may encroach on the brachial plexus and may be seen in Horner's syndrome.

Herniated Disc. The patients with arm pain predominant (brachialgia) refractory to nonoperative management may have symptoms due to mechanical pressure from a herniated disc or hypertrophic bone and secondary inflammation of the involved nerve roots.[5] The single best imaging test to confirm the diagnosis is MR. If the MR image is equivocal, a CT myelogram is then recommended. If the patient's pain, neurologic deficit, and imaging study abnormalities correlate, surgical decompression of the involved nerve root or spinal cord has an excellent success rate.[10]

Peripheral nerve compression occasionally manifests patterns of arm pain that exceed the expected regional involvement of the specific peripheral nerve. Although peripheral nerve entrapment can usually be identified by motor and sensory loss pattern and by EMG studies, these peripheral lesions may coexist with cervical root compression. The double-crush hypothesis maintains that axons compressed in one region may become more susceptible to impairment at a distant site.

If there is unequivocal evidence of nerve root compression (neurologic deficit, abnormal EMG, and abnormal CT myelogram or MR image) consistent with the physical findings, surgical decompression should be considered. Some studies suggest that patients with radicular symptoms seem to do better with surgery. Although conservative management of patients with radicular symptoms has shown that this problem rarely progresses to cervical myelopathy, persistent symptoms are common.

Patients who have no specific diagnosis and have pain that is resistant to a 12-week trial of medical nonoperative therapy are considered to have chronic neck pain. The primary goal for therapy with chronic neck pain is maximum function, not pain relief. Patients with chronic pain require multimodality therapy. Exercises, NSAIDs, tricyclic antidepressants, physical interventions (heat or cold), and psychological support are among the modalities to be considered for patients with chronic pain. These patients should be consistently encouraged to maximize their function and to return to some form of work. The appearance of new symptoms or marked exacerbation of preexisting complaints should be re-evaluated.

Summary

The "Neck Pain" algorithm on pages 222–223 presents a series of easy-to-follow and clearly defined decision-making processes to identify those patients with specific diagnoses.

Text continues on page 226

NECK PAIN ALGORITHM

0 WEEKS

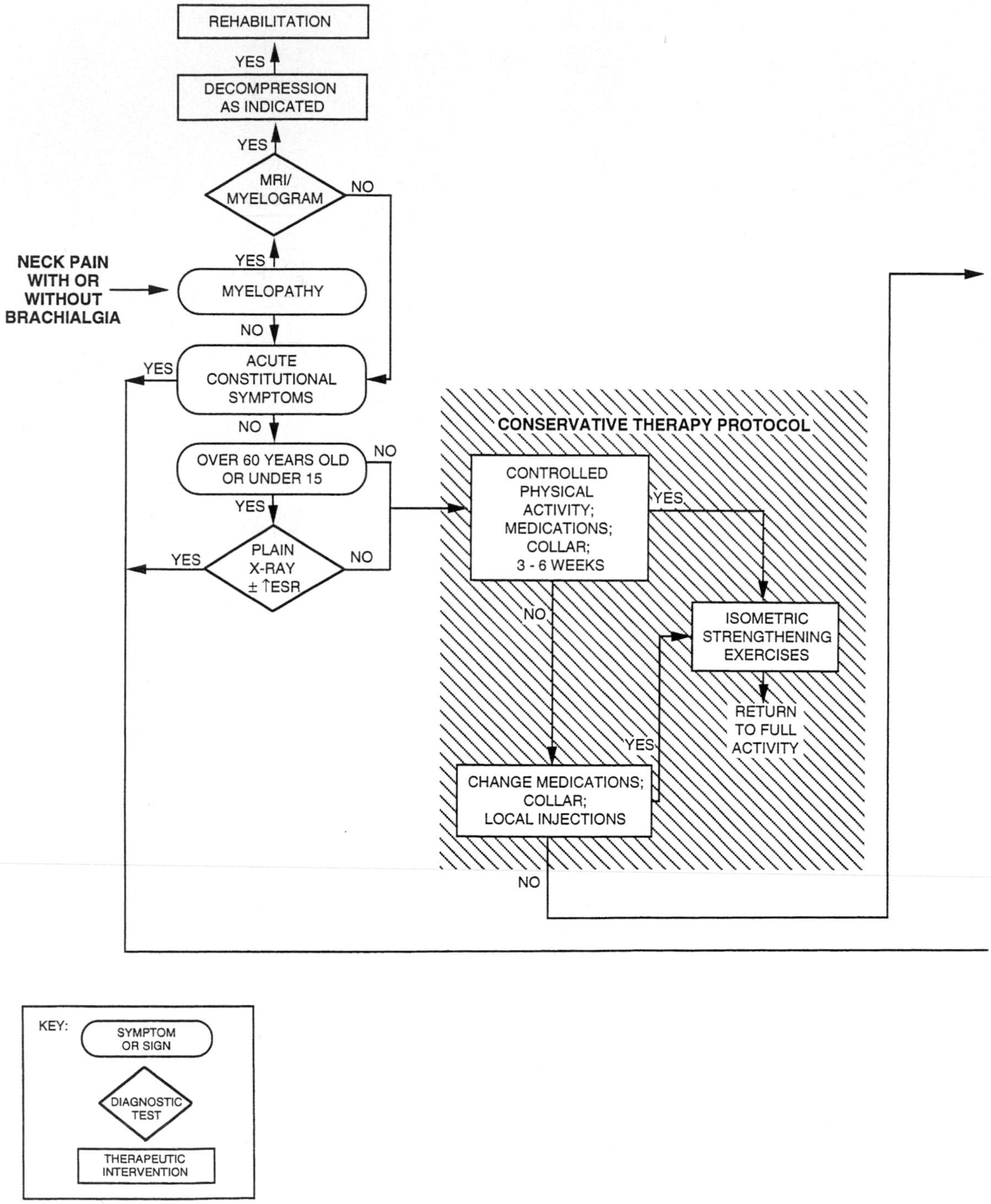

REHABILITATION

YES

DECOMPRESSION AS INDICATED

YES

MRI/ MYELOGRAM

NO

NECK PAIN WITH OR WITHOUT BRACHIALGIA

YES

MYELOPATHY

NO

YES

ACUTE CONSTITUTIONAL SYMPTOMS

NO

OVER 60 YEARS OLD OR UNDER 15

NO

YES

YES

PLAIN X-RAY ± ↑ESR

NO

CONSERVATIVE THERAPY PROTOCOL

CONTROLLED PHYSICAL ACTIVITY; MEDICATIONS; COLLAR; 3 - 6 WEEKS

YES

NO

ISOMETRIC STRENGTHENING EXERCISES

RETURN TO FULL ACTIVITY

YES

CHANGE MEDICATIONS; COLLAR; LOCAL INJECTIONS

NO

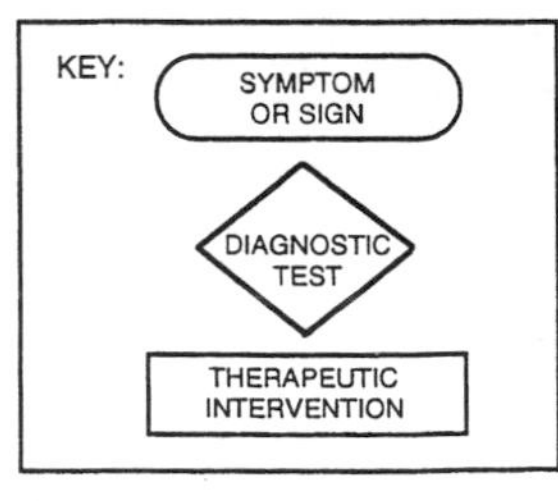

A

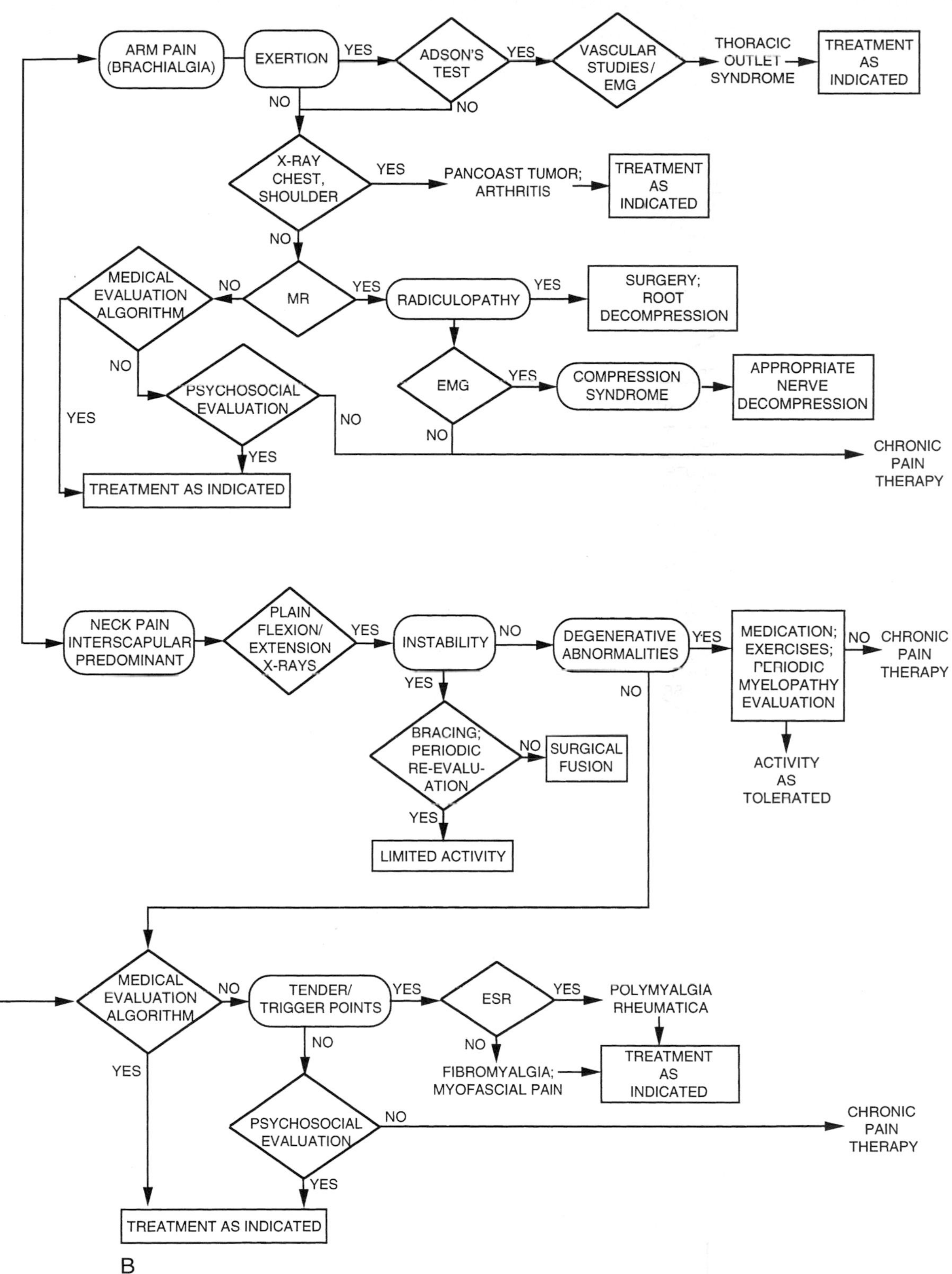
6 WEEKS
12 WEEKS
ARM PAIN (BRACHIALGIA)
EXERTION
YES
ADSON'S TEST
YES
VASCULAR STUDIES/ EMG
THORACIC OUTLET SYNDROME
TREATMENT AS INDICATED
NO
NO
X-RAY CHEST, SHOULDER
YES
PANCOAST TUMOR; ARTHRITIS
TREATMENT AS INDICATED
NO
MEDICAL EVALUATION ALGORITHM
NO
MR
YES
RADICULOPATHY
YES
SURGERY; ROOT DECOMPRESSION
NO
PSYCHOSOCIAL EVALUATION
EMG
YES
COMPRESSION SYNDROME
APPROPRIATE NERVE DECOMPRESSION
YES
NO
NO
YES
CHRONIC PAIN THERAPY
TREATMENT AS INDICATED
NECK PAIN INTERSCAPULAR PREDOMINANT
PLAIN FLEXION/ EXTENSION X-RAYS
YES
INSTABILITY
NO
DEGENERATIVE ABNORMALITIES
YES
MEDICATION; EXERCISES; PERIODIC MYELOPATHY EVALUATION
NO
CHRONIC PAIN THERAPY
YES
NO
BRACING; PERIODIC RE-EVALU-ATION
NO
SURGICAL FUSION
ACTIVITY AS TOLERATED
YES
LIMITED ACTIVITY
MEDICAL EVALUATION ALGORITHM
NO
TENDER/ TRIGGER POINTS
YES
ESR
YES
POLYMYALGIA RHEUMATICA
NO
NO
FIBROMYALGIA; MYOFASCIAL PAIN
TREATMENT AS INDICATED
YES
PSYCHOSOCIAL EVALUATION
NO
CHRONIC PAIN THERAPY
YES
TREATMENT AS INDICATED
B

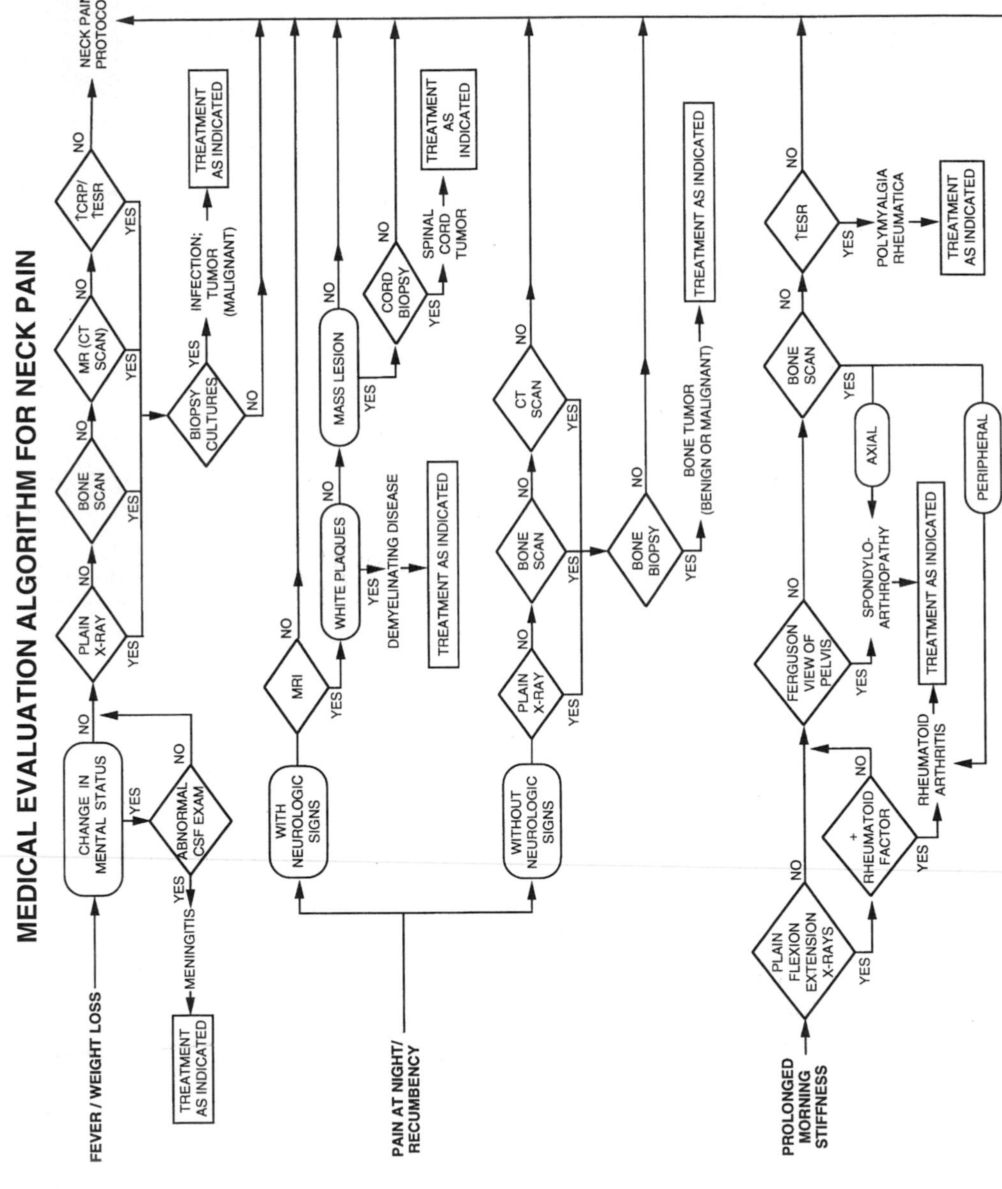
MEDICAL EVALUATION ALGORITHM FOR NECK PAIN
FEVER / WEIGHT LOSS
CHANGE IN MENTAL STATUS
YES
ABNORMAL CSF EXAM
YES
MENINGITIS
TREATMENT AS INDICATED
NO
NO
PLAIN X-RAY
YES
NO
BONE SCAN
YES
NO
MR (CT SCAN)
YES
NO
↑CRP/ ↑ESR
YES
NO
NECK PAIN PROTOCOL
BIOPSY CULTURES
YES
INFECTION; TUMOR (MALIGNANT)
TREATMENT AS INDICATED
NO
PAIN AT NIGHT/ RECUMBENCY
WITH NEUROLOGIC SIGNS
MRI
YES
NO
WHITE PLAQUES
YES
DEMYELINATING DISEASE
TREATMENT AS INDICATED
NO
MASS LESION
YES
NO
CORD BIOPSY
YES
SPINAL CORD TUMOR
TREATMENT AS INDICATED
NO
WITHOUT NEUROLOGIC SIGNS
PLAIN X-RAY
YES
NO
BONE SCAN
YES
NO
CT SCAN
YES
NO
BONE BIOPSY
YES
BONE TUMOR (BENIGN OR MALIGNANT)
TREATMENT AS INDICATED
NO
PROLONGED MORNING STIFFNESS
PLAIN FLEXION EXTENSION X-RAYS
YES
+ RHEUMATOID FACTOR
YES
RHEUMATOID ARTHRITIS
NO
NO
FERGUSON VIEW OF PELVIS
YES
SPONDYLO-ARTHROPATHY
TREATMENT AS INDICATED
NO
BONE SCAN
YES
AXIAL
PERIPHERAL
NO
↑ESR
YES
POLYMYALGIA RHEUMATICA
TREATMENT AS INDICATED
NO

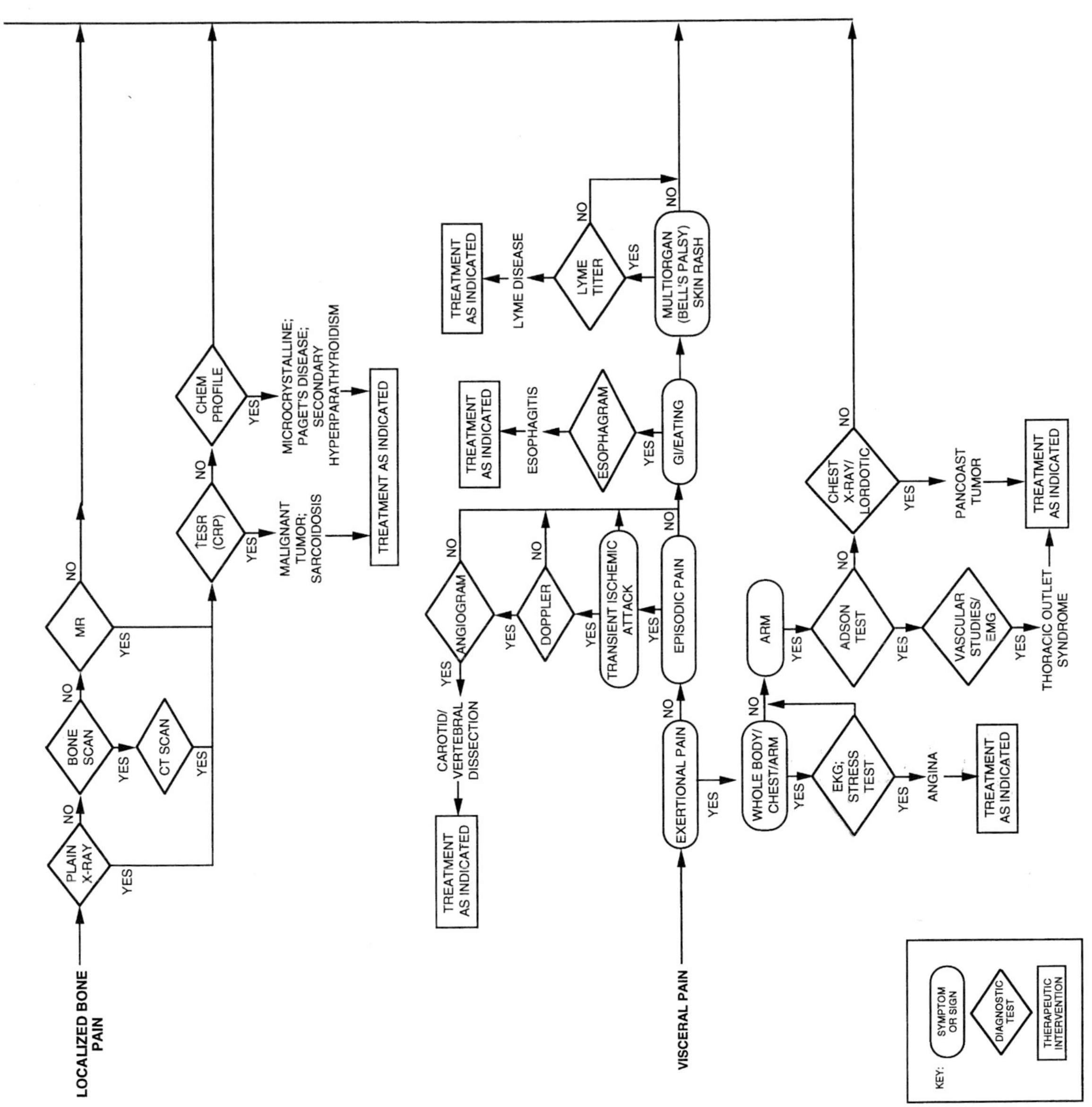
LOCALIZED BONE PAIN
PLAIN X-RAY
BONE SCAN
CT SCAN
MR
TESR (CRP)
CHEM PROFILE
MALIGNANT TUMOR; SARCOIDOSIS
MICROCRYSTALLINE; PAGET'S DISEASE; SECONDARY HYPERPARATHYROIDISM
TREATMENT AS INDICATED
VISCERAL PAIN
EXERTIONAL PAIN
EPISODIC PAIN
GI/EATING
MULTIORGAN (BELL'S PALSY) SKIN RASH
LYME TITER
LYME DISEASE
ESOPHAGRAM
ESOPHAGITIS
TRANSIENT ISCHEMIC ATTACK
DOPPLER
ANGIOGRAM
CAROTID/ VERTEBRAL DISSECTION
WHOLE BODY/ CHEST/ARM
EKG; STRESS TEST
ANGINA
ARM
ADSON TEST
CHEST X-RAY/ LORDOTIC
PANCOAST TUMOR
VASCULAR STUDIES/ EMG
THORACIC OUTLET SYNDROME
YES
NO
KEY:
SYMPTOM OR SIGN
DIAGNOSTIC TEST
THERAPEUTIC INTERVENTION

The "Medical Evaluation Algorithm for Neck Pain" on pages 224–225 also offers therapies appropriate to the condition and the point in time of the condition's evolution. Use of this algorithm provides patients with the most helpful, expeditious evaluation and does not subject them to procedures that are useless technical exercises.

An additional aid for differential diagnosis is in Appendix B, which includes a table of differential diagnoses of neck pain and clinical data associated with specific disease entities that cause neck pain.

References

Neck Pain

1. Bernhardt M, Hynes RA, Blume HW, White AA III: Cervical spondylotic myelopathy. J Bone Joint Surg 75:119, 1993.
2. Borenstein DG, Korn S: Efficacy of a low-dose regimen of cyclobenzaprine hydrochloride in acute skeletal muscle spasm: Results of two placebo-controlled trials. Clin Ther 25:1056-1073, 2003.
3. Carette S: Whiplash injury and chronic neck pain. N Engl J Med 330:1083, 1994.
4. Clark CR: Cervical spondylitic myelopathy: History and physical findings. Spine 13:847, 1988.
5. Dillin W, Booth R, Cuckler J, et al: Cervical radiculopathy: A review. Spine 11:988, 1986.
6. Friedenberg ZB, Miller WT: Degenerative disease of the cervical spine. J Bone Joint Surg 45:1171, 1963.
7. Gore DR: Roentgenographic findings in the cervical spine in asymptomatic persons: A ten-year follow-up. Spine 26:2463-2466, 2001.
8. Gore DR, Sepic SB, Gardner GM: Roentgenographic findings of the cervical spine in asymptomatic people. Spine 11:521, 1986.
9. Greenfield J, Ilfeld FW: Acute cervical strain. Clin Orthop 122:196, 1977.
10. Heckmann JG, Lang CJ, Zobelein I, et al: Herniated cervical intervertebral discs with radiculopathy: An outcome study of conservatively or surgically treated patients. J Spinal Dis 12:396-401, 1999.
11. LaRocca H: Cervical spondylitic myelopathy: Natural history. Spine 13:854, 1988.
12. Sampath P, Bendebba M, David JD, et al: Outcome of patients treated for cervical myelopathy: A prospective, multicenter study with independent clinical review. Spine 25:670-676, 2000.
13. Shafaie FF, Wippold FJ 2nd, Gado M, et al: Comparison of computed tomography myelography and magnetic resonance imaging in the evaluation of cervical spondylotic myelopathy and radiculopathy. Spine 24:1781-1985, 1999.
14. Shapiro AP, Roth RS: The effect of litigation on recovery of whiplash. Spine 7:531, 1993.
15. Spitzer WO, Skovron ML, Salmi LR, et al: Scientific monograph of the Quebec Task Force on whiplash-associated disorders: Redefining "whiplash" and its management. Spine 20:1, 1995.
16. Thelander U, Larsson S: Quantification of C-reactive protein levels and erythrocyte sedimentation rate after spinal surgery. Spine 17:400, 1992.
17. White AA, Panjabi MM, Posner I, et al: Spinal stability: Evaluation and treatment. Am Acad Orthop Surg Instruct Course Lect 30:457-483, 1981.

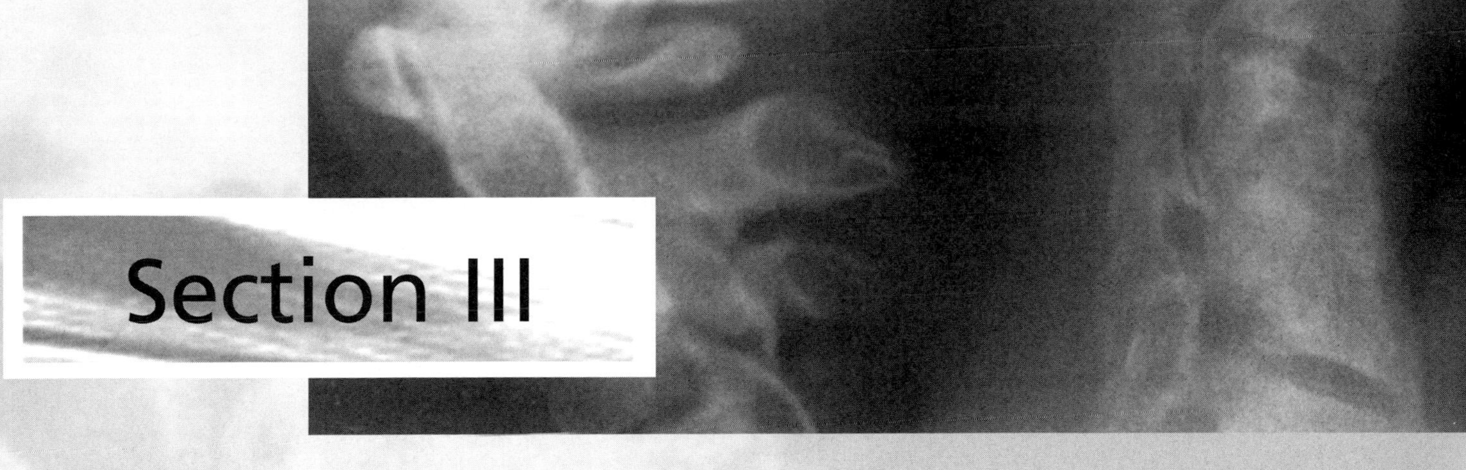

Section III

Diseases Associated with Spinal Pain

Section III is a review of the illnesses associated with spinal pain. The discussion of each illness opens with a capsule summary that lists the frequency, location, and quality of spinal pain; the associated symptoms, signs, laboratory data, and radiographic findings; and the forms of therapy that are effective. The specifics of therapy are contained in the body of the associated chapter and in Section IV.

The frequency of spinal pain associated with each illness is quantified by the terms *very common*, *common*, *uncommon*, and *rare*. The percentage of patients with spinal pain associated with each term is as follows:

Very common—76% or greater
Common—51% to 75%
Uncommon—26% to 50%
Rare—25% or less

Each chapter contains data concerning the prevalence, pathogenesis, clinical history, physical examination, laboratory data, radiographic evaluation, differential diagnosis, therapy, and prognosis for each disease.

The emphasis of each chapter is geared toward a review of spinal pain as it pertains to each illness. The chapter should not be considered a complete listing of all clinical characteristics associated with each disease. Factors that help the clinician recognize the underlying cause of the patient's spinal pain and make the appropriate diagnosis are listed.

The section is divided into chapters according to the following primary disease processes:

Mechanical disorders
Rheumatologic disorders
Infections
Tumor and infiltrative lesions
Endocrinologic and heritable disorders
Hematologic disorders
Neurologic and psychiatric disorders
Referred pain
Miscellaneous disorders

Discussions of diseases that are only very rarely associated with spinal pain and are not included in the major subheadings of these chapters may be found in the differential diagnosis section under each subheading. For example, hemochromatosis is included in the differential diagnosis of microcrystalline diseases.

Referred pain, though not in itself a primary disease process, is another major source of patients' complaints of spinal pain. The chapter on referred pain includes disorders of vascular, genitourinary, and gastrointestinal origin that are associated with spinal pain.

CHAPTER 10

MECHANICAL DISORDERS OF THE SPINE

Mechanical disorders of the spine are the most common cause of low back and neck pain. Mechanical spinal pain may be defined as pain secondary to overuse of a normal anatomic structure (muscle strain) or pain secondary to injury or deformity of an anatomic structure (herniated nucleus pulposus). Mechanical disorders are local disorders of the spine. That is, the processes that cause pain are limited to the structures of the spine. Mechanical disorders are truly musculoskeletal diseases. Systemic complications with involvement of other organ systems (except the nervous system) are not associated with mechanical disorders. The presence of systemic illness (e.g., fever, weight loss, or anemia) should make the clinician look for a disease other than a mechanical disorder as the cause of the patient's symptoms and signs.

Mechanical disorders are characteristically exacerbated by certain activities and relieved by others. The pattern of alleviating and aggravating factors helps localize the disorder to particular portions of the spine; for example, flexion exacerbates disc disease but alleviates facet joint disease. The physical examination helps identify individuals with neurologic dysfunction and significant muscle damage, but it is not sufficient to pinpoint the exact location of the injury. Laboratory data in the form of electrophysiologic tests can confirm the clinical suspicion of nerve impingement. Through radiologic evaluation of a patient with a mechanical disorder, the physician may be able to identify anatomic alterations in the spine but not necessarily correlate those changes with the patient's symptoms. The physician must take all the clinical data together and formulate a working diagnosis that is reasonable based on the collected information.

Mechanical disorders, for the most part, are self-limited in duration such that the majority of these patients will improve, given enough time. The physician does not want to intervene and cause the patient harm (inappropriate surgery) or overlook the possibility of a serious complication associated with a mechanical disorder (cauda equina syndrome or cervical myelopathy). Common sense is what is needed in the evaluation and treatment of these patients. The vast majority of patients will improve with controlled physical activity, nonaddictive nonsteroidal anti-inflammatory drugs, and, in appropriate patients, muscle relaxants. Surgical intervention is reserved for patients who have not shown improvement with conservative therapy and who have undeniable symptoms and signs associated with a mechanical disorder that is correctable by surgical intervention.

LOW BACK/NECK (SPINAL) STRAIN

CAPSULE SUMMARY

	LOW BACK	NECK
Frequency of spinal pain	Very common	Very common
Location of spinal pain	Low back, buttock, posterior thigh	Neck, between scapulae, top of shoulders
Quality of spinal pain	Ache, spasm—intermittent	Ache, spasm—sharp twinges
Symptoms and signs	Pain increased with activity, increased muscle tension	Pain increased with any motion of the neck, headache, decreased range of motion
Laboratory tests	None	None
Radiographic findings	None	None
Treatment	Controlled physical activity, medications	Controlled physical activity, neck collar, medications

PREVALENCE AND PATHOGENESIS

Epidemiology

Spinal strain can be defined as nonradiating low back or neck pain associated with a mechanical stress or a prolonged abnormal position (sleeping with a twisted spine).[23] The exact number of patients with spinal strain is difficult to determine. Most people with spinal pain (90%) have it on a mechanical basis.[65] Of patients with mechanical low back pain, back strain may account for 60% to 70% of abnormalities. Almost 85% of neck pain results from acute or repetitive neck injuries or chronic stress and strain.[49]

Pathogenesis

Lumbar Spine

The cause of spinal strain is not always clear but may be related to ligamentous or muscular strain secondary to either a specific traumatic episode or continuous mechanical stress. It is important to remember that the lumbosacral spine has two major biomechanical functions: It supports the upper part of the body in a balanced, upright position while allowing locomotion. In a static, upright position, maintenance of erect posture is achieved through a balance in the expansile pressure of the intervertebral discs, the stretch placed on the anterior and posterior longitudinal and facet joint ligaments, and the sustained involuntary tone generated by the surrounding lumbosacral and abdominal muscles. Balance of the spine is also related to the reciprocal physiologic curves in the cervical, thoracic, and lumbosacral areas of the vertebral column. The balance in curvature results in an individual's posture. Proper alignment is also influenced by structures in the pelvis and lower extremities, including the hip joint capsule and the hamstring and gluteus maximus muscles. An individual's posture is good if it can be maintained for extended periods in an effortless, nonfatiguing fashion.

Movement of the lumbar spine is associated with a lumbar pelvic rhythm that results in simultaneous reversal of the lumbar lordosis and rotation of the hips. During flexion and extension of the lumbar spine, tension is produced in the paraspinous, hamstring, and gluteal muscles; the fasciae that surround the muscles; and the ligaments that support the vertebral bodies and discs. In addition to the normal stress placed on these structures with lowering and raising of the torso, the stress on these anatomic structures is increased to an even greater degree when an individual is required to lift a heavy object. With lateral bending, paraspinous muscle activity increases on both sides of the spine, but primarily on the side toward the lateral flexion. During axial rotation of the spine, the erector spinae muscles on the ipsilateral side and the rotator and multifidus muscles on the contralateral side are active. Lateral bending is accomplished by contraction of the abdominal wall oblique muscles in conjunction with the ipsilateral quadratus lumborum and psoas major.

Low back pain that is associated with back strain may be related to anatomic structures that are tonically contracted in the resting position. Low back pain may also occur during motion if the stress is greater than the supporting structures can sustain or if the components of the lumbosacral spine are structurally abnormal.[15]

Pain related to posture (static position) is thought to be caused by an increase in the lumbosacral angle that results in accentuation of the lumbar lordosis (hyperlordosis). Some authorities have suggested that as much as 75% of all postural back pain is related to hyperlordosis.[15] The increased angle of the L5 and S1 vertebrae increases the shear forces on the disc, thereby resulting in approximation of the articular surfaces of the facet joints and modifying their function to that of weight-bearing units. This alteration irritates the synovial membrane and joint capsule. Hyperlordosis also increases stress on the supporting ligaments of the spine. Lumbar lordosis while standing is 50% greater on average than lumbar lordosis while sitting.[60] Sitting with a lumbar support reverses this loss of lordosis. Extension of the spine in younger individuals may increase to such a degree that the spinous processes approximate and form a pseudarthrosis (syndrome of Baastrup). In hyperextension, not only may the facet joints and spinous processes be stressed, but also the nerve root or recurrent nerve may be irritated (Fig. 10-1). Patients with recurrent nerve irritation may have low back pain only, whereas nerve root irritation is associated with radiation of pain to the leg, as seen with spinal stenosis.

It should be noted, however, that not all patients with increased lumbar lordosis have back pain. One study found that the degree of lumbar lordosis as determined by radiographs was no different for individuals with and without low back pain.[40] Until this controversy is resolved, hyperlordosis should be considered as a source of symptoms only after other causes of back pain have been eliminated from the physician's differential diagnostic list.

Low back pain may also occur during motion of the lumbosacral spine or with physical stress (weight) that is greater than the forces that can be supported by the muscular and ligamentous structures. The lumbar spine is required to support forces many times body weight. When

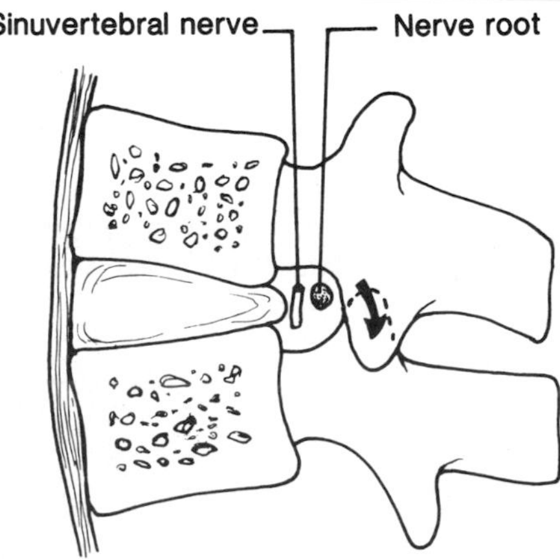

Figure 10-1 Nerve impingement with lumbosacral hyperextension. Extension approximates the articular surfaces of the facet joints *(arrow)* and narrows the neural foramen. Extension also causes the nucleus pulposus to move posteriorly with resultant stretching of the annular fibers. Pain may result from stretching of the annular fibers (back pain) or from compression of the sinuvertebral nerve (back pain), nerve root (radicular pain), or facet joint (back and radicular pain).

lifting an object, an individual initially contracts the appropriate muscles. If the force is too great to be resisted by the muscle or if the muscle is fatigued, the stress is transferred to the ligaments. Intradiscal pressure increases, and if sufficiently strong, the force is passed on to the facet joints, which are not normally weight-bearing articulations. If the force is of sufficient magnitude, damage can occur in the muscle fibers, tendons, ligaments, annulus fibrosus, or facet joints.

If the lumbosacral spine or surrounding structures are anatomically abnormal, "normal" motion may result in strain pain. For example, patients with scoliosis have asymmetric orientation of their facet joints. The position of the facet joints does not allow free movement. The joint surfaces may be impacted to a greater degree in this orientation of the spine than the joint surfaces found in a straight spine. Supporting structures may shorten in response to the curved configuration of the spine. Normal motion may be met with restriction because of limited excursion of the ligaments and muscles. Tight hamstrings may limit full flexion of the lumbar spine and thereby result in greater stretching forces being placed on the interspinous ligaments. In patients with normal hamstring motion but limited lumbar flexion, bending over will cause strain on the stretched posterior longitudinal ligaments and "tight" paraspinous muscles.

Damage may occur in the lumbosacral spinal structures if the amount of force generated does not match the stress placed on the spine. Through experience, an individual will gauge the amount of energy needed to complete a task, such as lifting a box. If the box is empty, a smaller amount of force is needed to lift the box. If the box is full and heavy, a greater amount of force is required. If a great amount of force is generated in anticipation of a box being heavy when in fact it is empty, the extra force that has been generated may be dissipated through excessive movement of the spine, which may exceed the usual limits imposed by the joint capsule and ligaments and result in tissue damage. On the other hand, if only a few muscle groups are recruited to lift an "empty" box when it is full, the force generated by the muscles will be inadequate to lift the object, and the muscles will be damaged.[62] These scenarios may be further complicated if the lumbar spine is in a mechanically disadvantaged position (rotated, fully flexed). In such positions, the fibers of the annulus fibrosus are strained and may tear and cause fissures to occur. Disruption of these annular fibers leads to degeneration of the disc and may be associated with the production of pain.[32] The pain associated with annular tears may account for the history of frequent episodes of low back discomfort in patients who eventually rupture a nucleus pulposus.

A great deal of controversy surrounds the concept of skeletal muscle as the cause of low back pain. Evidence has been presented suggesting that low back spasm is a myth.[52] The lack of electromyographic evidence of increased muscle activity is used to support the argument that increased muscle contraction does not occur.[41] The presence of muscle edema is suggested as a reason for the physical changes in the muscle noted on physical examination.[53]

Studies have demonstrated significant abnormalities in paraspinal muscle function. Dynamometry and postural endurance testing have revealed paraspinal weakness and excess fatigability in patients with low back pain.[8,19] Muscle wasting and weakness can arise rapidly as a result of reduced motor unit recruitment because of fear of pain or reflex inhibition. Hides and co-workers used real-time ultrasound imaging to measure the cross-sectional area of the multifidus muscle in patients with acute low back pain.[46] Twenty-six patients who had an initial episode of back pain with a mean duration of 12.1 days (range, 1 to 56) were examined. Unilateral muscle mass loss at a single lumbar level on the symptomatic side was identified in 24 patients. No correlation was found between the degree of asymmetry and the severity of symptoms, and localized areas of muscle atrophy could not be explained by disuse. Inhibition of movement by a long loop reflex may explain the acute development of muscle mass asymmetry. Muscle imbalance predisposes to mechanical disruption, which can perpetuate the mechanical disadvantage. The endurance of back muscles related to a task is a more useful predictor of the incidence of back pain than is the absolute strength of these muscles.[69]

Others have suggested that back strain is a manifestation of anxiety and is psychosomatic in origin.[72] Varying degrees of anxiety cause regional ischemia and altered states of muscle contractility and spasm mediated through the autonomic nervous system. However, review of a number of studies demonstrates no increased prevalence of neurotic symptoms in patients with back pain versus those without back pain.[21] Recruitment of other paraspinous muscles occurs with the development of back pain. This recruitment of muscles is further exacerbated by the increase in body weight that accompanies inactivity.[64]

The classification of muscle strain depends on the severity of the injury and the nature of the hematoma.[51] Mild (first degree) strain causes a tear in a few muscle fibers, minor swelling, and pain with minimal loss of strength or movement. A moderate (second degree) strain results in greater muscle fiber damage with loss of strength, but structural integrity is preserved. A severe (third degree) strain is associated with a complete tear through the muscle belly, and such tears result in total loss of function.

In summary, muscle pain in patients with low back pain may be caused by four different mechanisms[2]:

1. Pain may be associated with muscle strain that is related to muscle disruption from indirect trauma, such as excessive stretch or tension. An animal model of muscle strain reveals improved function by the seventh day after injury. A source of continued risk for recurrent injury is inelastic scar tissue.
2. Another possible source of muscle pain is muscle fatigue associated with overuse. Fatigue has a metabolic component that is manifested as increased concentrations of lactic acid, a byproduct of anaerobic metabolism. High loads requiring maximal effort of muscles causes ultrastructural damage to muscle with a delayed inflammatory response.[67] These alterations in muscle fibers cause the release of inflammatory mediators associated with edema and pain receptor stimulation that results in pain.
3. Muscle spasm is associated with persistent muscle contraction. The absence of blood flow with an accumulation of metabolic byproducts may stimulate

pain receptors within blood vessels. Studies involving integrated electromyography demonstrate the increased central recruitment of paraspinal muscles.[19]

4. Paraspinous muscles become deconditioned after injury. Radiographic evaluation of cross-sectional views of patients with back pain demonstrate decreased muscle mass in the paraspinous and psoas muscles.[20] Decreased muscle mass results in decreased muscle power, which puts individuals at risk for persistent muscle injury. Determination of the cause of muscle pain in patients with low back pain has implications for the choice of appropriate therapy.

Cervical Spine

The major biomechanical function of the cervical spine is to support the skull and provide movement in flexion, extension, and rotation. Injury to the anatomic structures (facet joints, muscles, and ligaments) that provide these motions can easily occur because the supporting structures are relatively unprotected. Except for a traumatic injury to a particular structure, the specific abnormality in neck strain can almost never be identified.

Trauma to cervical muscles that results in strain may occur from mere elongation of muscle fibers with subsequent edema to rupture of muscle and secondary hemorrhage.[16] The response of the muscle to injury is contraction with reflex recruitment of surrounding muscles for protection. This protective spasm is an autonomic reflex. The contracted state decreases blood flow and produces relative anaerobic conditions in the injured muscle. The buildup of byproducts of anaerobic metabolism causes nociceptive nerves to signal pain messages to the central nervous system.

The contracted state may occur secondary to environmental trauma, posture, or increased muscle tension. Early muscle contraction is a necessary component of the healing process.[36] Environmental trauma (whiplash and subluxation) is discussed later in this chapter. Normal posture is effortless and painless. Abnormal forward posture of the head results in chronic strain on the posterior structures of the neck, including the paracervical muscles. The position of the head results in drooping of the shoulders and a decrease in vital lung capacity. Postural tension is related to tonic isometric contraction of the extensor neck muscles. A variety of activities of daily living may result in chronic abnormal postures, such as prolonged use of a computer with a screen below eye level, a faulty sitting position, or the use of bifocal glasses.

Tension in muscles is controlled by the interaction of spindle organs, the Golgi tendon organs, and extrafusal nerve fibers. The Golgi organs, or neurotendinous endings, are large myelinated group IB afferent axons that lie in the musculotendinous junction and are stimulated by tension applied to the tendon during muscle contraction or, to a lesser extent, by passive stretching. The sensory endings are arranged in series with the muscle extrafusal fibers. Stimulation of these Golgi nerves results in inhibition of alpha motor neuron discharges to the corresponding muscle.[82] Muscle spindles have up to eight muscle fibers in a fluid-containing connective tissue capsule and are present in voluntary muscles. The contractile portion of the intrafusal muscle fibers is supplied with gamma efferent nerves, and the noncontractile portion is supplied with group IA afferent nerves (annulospiral endings) and group II flower-spray nerve endings that are arranged in parallel with the extrafusal fibers. Both types of nerves are tonic receptors that are depolarized by stretch. Stretching of extrafusal fibers applies tension to the spindle afferents, whereas extrafusal contraction relaxes the spindle fibers.

A balance exists between muscle tension and impulses from the Golgi apparatus stimulated by tendon stretch and activity of the spindle fibers. This system coordinates muscular length, rate of contraction, tension, and relaxation of opposing muscles. This sensor feedback system allows for the generation of appropriate muscle power for the physical task. When the muscle is contracted, the Golgi organ is stimulated and the spindle system is unstimulated. When the muscle is stretched, nerve impulses from the Golgi organs and spindle system are generated. With contraction of the extrafusal fibers, the intrafusal fibers (spindle system) record the change in muscle length and the Golgi organs record muscle force and tension. The gamma neurons that set the tension of the spindle fibers also affect the system. Increased stimulation of gamma fibers affects the sensory fibers such that the sensitivity of the muscle to tension is increased. Passive stretching of the muscle when obtaining a tendon reflex produces afferent discharges that result in alpha neuron stimulation; such stimulation causes the muscle to contract to regain its original length, a monosynaptic reflex. In contrast, persistent muscle stretch produces stimulation of all afferent receptors; such stimulation results in a polysynaptic reflex in which alterations in gamma fiber stimulation and tonic or continuous muscle contraction are elicited.[82] Postural tone is the state of partial contraction of muscles needed to maintain a particular posture of the body, including the neck. The extent of gamma fiber stimulation sets the level of tone in the skeletal muscle system. With increased tone, the skeletal muscle may demonstrate rigidity or spasticity. Coordinating systems in the spinal cord and the cerebral cortex influence the set-point of the balance between the two systems. Nerves from the reticulospinal tract have an inhibitory effect on the stretch reflex. Multisynaptic reflex arcs from the cerebellum, basal ganglia, and brain stem influence the level of excitability of the reticulospinal tract. Control of muscle tone is a multifactorial process. Thought processes in the cerebral cortex can be manifested as alterations in the function of other components of the nervous system, and such alterations can result in stress and increased muscle tone.[82]

Between contractions the muscle is able to relax. Relaxation is important for maintenance of muscle function. Relaxation allows for restoration of internal blood flow, removal of metabolic byproducts, and influx of nutrients. Ischemia and pain develop in chronically contracted muscles. In addition to direct effects on the paracervical muscles, sustained muscle contraction may cause sustained intervertebral disc compression. Disc degeneration may result from persistent contraction because the intervertebral discs are less able to imbibe nutrients when contracted.

Muscles may undergo isotonic or isometric contractions. Isotonic contractions occur with the same tension through the range of motion of the muscle while moving a constant load. Isometric contractions occur with increased tension without shortening of the muscle. Most contractions are hybrids that involve both load bearing and shortening. Eccentric contractions occur when muscles are stretched while generating tension. Walking downstairs requires eccentric contractions.

A variety of factors extraneous to muscles affect muscle tension. Factors such as fatigue, pain, anger, emotional stress, anxiety, and depression affect the level of muscle tension.[49] Spasm in the cervical muscles can cause pain in the occipital area that may radiate to the temples and frontal area.[59] Discrepancies exist between electromyography studies measuring the degree of muscle contraction and the degree of pain.[82] A cycle of pain and spasm may result in persistence of symptoms from relatively insignificant events. During the evaluation it may be difficult to ascertain whether pain or spasm was the initiating factor causing the patient's symptoms and signs.[3]

Sarcopenia

Sarcopenia is an involuntary decrease in muscle mass with aging that results in loss of strength and function.[80] Approximately 1% of muscle mass is lost each year after 50 years of age. The lower protein stores in the body are related to an inability to mobilize amino acids to produce new proteins essential for function of the immune system and other organs.[71] The rate of muscle protein synthesis in older people is similar to that in younger individuals, which suggests that adequate nutritional support, aggressive physical therapy, and exercise programs are essential to preserve function in older individuals.[47] In older individuals, spinal strain can develop in weaker muscles. Exercise must be encouraged in older individuals to maintain muscle strength so that the difficulties associated with sarcopenia are limited.[31] Sarcopenia puts elderly individuals at risk for increased spinal dysfunction and pain because of associated muscle wasting.

CLINICAL HISTORY

Lumbar Spine

Patients with muscle strain have back pain as their main complaint. The pain can be limited to a small local area or can cover a diffuse area of the lumbosacral spine, but it does not radiate to the lower extremities. At times, pain may be referred to the buttocks or posterior of the thigh because the mesenchymal structures in the lower back, buttock, and posterior thigh regions all originate from the same embryonic tissue. Such referral of pain does not necessarily connote any mechanical compression of the neural elements and should not be called sciatica.

The patient may experience pain simultaneously with an injury. Subsequently, the pain increases in intensity and distribution after a few hours. The change in pain is associated with increasing edema in the injured structure, along with reflex contraction of the surrounding muscles and subsequent limitation of motion. The patient may be able to continue to be active for a few hours. However, marked pain and stiffness occur the next day after sleeping. Flexion or extension of the spine may cause pain. Pain occurs with the motion that contracts the injured muscle. Certain motions may be painless, whereas others cause incapacitating pain. In general, muscle strain will be increased with activity and relieved with rest.

Cervical Spine

Pain is the most common initial symptom, although the associated complaint of headache is not unusual. The pain is usually located in the middle to lower part of the posterior aspect of the neck. The area of pain can be limited to a small local point (unilateral) or can cover a diffuse area (bilateral). The pain may not radiate to the arms but may radiate toward the shoulders. A history of injury is rarely obtained, but the pain may commence after a night's awkward sleep, turning the head rapidly, or coughing or sneezing.

The pain associated with a neck sprain is most often a dull, aching pain that is exacerbated by neck motion. Such pain is usually abated by rest or immobilization. The pain may be referred to other mesenchymal structures derived from a similar sclerotome during embryogenesis. Common referred pain patterns include the scapular area, the posterior of the shoulder, the occipital area, or the anterior chest wall (cervical angina pectoris). These referred pain patterns do not indicate a true radicular pain pattern and are not generally mechanical (nerve compression) in origin.

PHYSICAL EXAMINATION

Lumbar Spine

Muscle strain results from overuse or overstretching of a muscle. On physical examination, any active motion of the involved muscle against resistance will cause pain. In one study of 429 patients with low back pain, 56 (13%) had contracted muscles on physical examination.[61] If a patient stands and is asked to bend laterally against resistance, thereby resulting in muscle contraction without motion, the patient will complain of discomfort in the damaged muscle. The damaged muscle is tender on palpation. Passive stretching of the muscle will also cause pain. For example, backward bending against resistance will be instantaneously painful with muscle contraction, whereas forward flexion will become painful only after excursion is sufficient to stretch the muscle in a patient with erector spinae damage. The muscle has increased contraction and firmness in comparison to the surrounding muscles under normal tension.

Ensink and colleagues measured lumbar spine motion in 29 chronic back pain patients in the morning and afternoon.[30] Total lumbar range of motion increased significantly during the course of the day. Flexion was increased to the greatest degree during the day, whereas extension was independent of the time of measurement. The measurements were not affected by the gender, age, height, or weight of the patients.

Localized back pain also develops in patients with ligamentous sprains (disruption of the attachment of ligaments to bone). Patients with supraspinous ligament sprains do not have pain with active or passive extension, but they experience pain when the damaged ligament and its attachment to bone are stressed with flexion. The diagnosis of other ligamentous sprains is more difficult because these structures are deep inside the back. Passive movements that put stress on the involved ligament will cause back pain, but identifying the specific location of injury is difficult.

Not infrequently, patients with muscle or ligamentous strain will experience low back pain in an area lateral to the fourth and fifth lumbar vertebrae and medial to the posterior iliac crest. This area of pain also spreads down to the sacrum. This area, referred to as the "multifidus triangle," contains a number of tissues, including facet joints, the transversus ligament, the quadratus lumborum and multifidus muscles, the iliolumbar ligament, and the dorsolumbar fascia, which may be sources of low back pain.[5] The greatest portion of stress placed on the lumbosacral spine is concentrated in this area, thus making it a common location for tissue injury.

The usual physical findings are limited to local tenderness over the involved area with limited motion; however, the attacks will vary in intensity and can conveniently be divided into three categories: mild, moderate, and severe. The mild category is associated with subjective pain without objective findings, and patients are usually able to return to customary activity in less than a week. The moderate category is characterized by a limited range of spinal motion and paravertebral muscle spasm, as well as pain, and patients frequently resume full activity in less than 2 weeks. The severe category of pain may cause patients to tilt forward or list to one side. These patients have trouble ambulating and can take up to 3 weeks to recover full function.

Cervical Spine

Physical examination of patients with neck strain generally reveals nothing more than a locally tender area or areas just lateral to the spine. The intensity of pain is variable, and the loss of cervical motion correlates directly with the intensity of the pain. The presence of true spasm, defined as a continuous muscle contraction, is rare except in severe cases in which the head may be tilted to one side (torticollis). Muscles most commonly affected include the sternocleidomastoid and the trapezius. Active motion of the cervical spine against any type of resistance causes an increase in pain. Slow passive movement of the neck may allow for a greater arc of motion than determined during the active motion portion of the examination.

Other than the abnormalities already described, the remainder of the physical examination is normal in patients with spinal muscle strain. Specifically, the neurologic examination is normal in these individuals.

LABORATORY DATA

Laboratory test results are entirely normal in patients with spinal strain.

RADIOGRAPHIC EVALUATION

Lumbar Spine

Low back strain does not cause or result from abnormalities that can be seen on radiographic evaluation of the lumbosacral spine. Thus, if the physician feels confident of the diagnosis of mechanical low back strain, a radiographic study during the initial evaluation is not necessary.[24]

Congenital abnormalities of the lumbar spine are a frequent finding noted in about 5% of individuals in a normal population. The most common congenital abnormality is spina bifida occulta, which is found most frequently at the first sacral vertebra (Fig. 10-2). Another abnormality is sacralization, or incorporation of the transverse process of the fifth lumbar vertebra into the sacrum (Fig. 10-3).[78] A sixth lumbar vertebra in addition to the normal number of five is also occasionally seen with lumbarization of the spine (Fig. 10-4). Most congenital abnormalities are asymptomatic, and most frequently, a congenital abnormality is recognized as a serendipitous event on a roentgenogram taken for another purpose (intravenous pyelogram, flat plate of the abdomen).

Theoretically, congenital abnormalities may be thought of as causing mechanical imbalances in the spine that may be associated with pain. The loss of a spinous process with spina bifida results in loss of the bony attachment for the interspinous ligaments and paraspinous muscles and fascia. Sacralization of the fifth lumbar vertebra or lumbarization of the first sacral vertebra, particularly if unilateral, may cause an imbalance in motion that limits rotation and increases stress above the fused component. In the vast majority of patients, the fusions are extremely firm and are not associated with symptoms. Low back pain

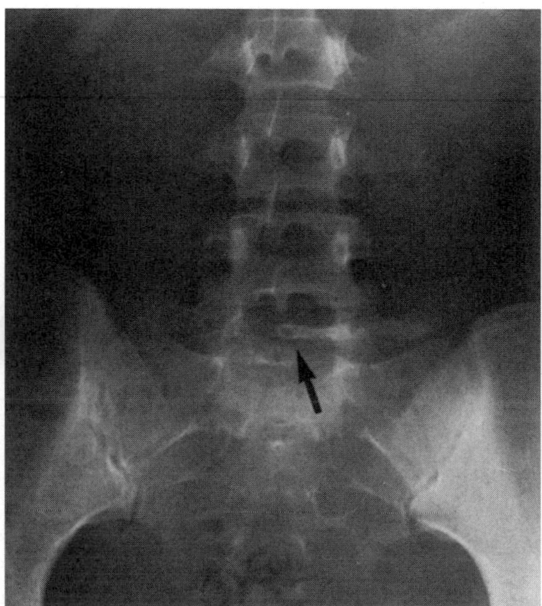

Figure 10-2 Anteroposterior view of the lumbosacral spine of a 22-year-old asymptomatic woman with a congenital abnormality of the L5 vertebral body, including spina bifida occulta *(arrow)*.

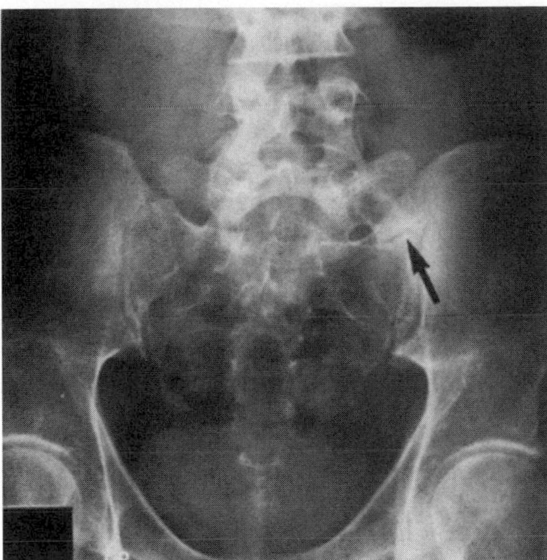

Figure 10-3 Anteroposterior view of the lumbosacral spine of a 28-year-old man with systemic lupus erythematosus and abdominal pain of peritoneal origin. The roentgenogram revealed sacralization of the left part of the L5 vertebra with the formation of a pseudarthrosis *(arrow)*.

should be ascribed to congenital abnormalities only after all other causes of back pain have been eliminated as possibilities.[55]

Cervical Spine

The radiographic evaluation of patients with neck strain is normal. On occasion, the muscle spasm may be great enough to cause some straightening of the normal lordosis of the cervical spine (Fig. 10-5). Such straightening is a nonspecific finding and only indicates significant muscle spasm secondary to pain. The presence of straightening of the cervical spine may be related as frequently to the positioning of the patient as to the presence of acute or chronic neck pain.[43] Thus, if the physician feels confident of the diagnosis of mechanical neck strain, a roentgenographic evaluation during the initial evaluation is not necessary. However, if the pain has not markedly resolved after 2 weeks or if other physical findings develop, a cervical spine roentgenogram should be obtained to rule out other serious etiologies such as neoplasia and instability.

Unlike the situation in the lumbar spine, congenital abnormalities are rare in the neck. The most common is block vertebrae, in which two bodies are congenitally fused together. The term *Klippel-Feil syndrome* is used to identify all patients with congenital fusion of the cervical vertebrae that involve two segments, block vertebrae, or the entire cervical spine.[44] Individuals with extensive fusion have a recognizably abnormal appearance and severe disability during childhood. These individuals also have anomalies in other parts of the body, including renal defects, scoliosis, Sprengel's deformity (undescended scapula), and facial anomalies (Apert's syndrome).[74] On physical examination they have a short neck, low hairline, and limited range of motion of the neck. Individuals with an autosomal dominant trait may have another form of Klippel-Feil syndrome associated with cervical fusion (block vertebrae) and segmental abnormalities in the thoracic and lumbar spine. Patients with the most benign form of Klippel-Feil syndrome are those with fusion of a single segment.[9] Theoretically, this abnormality could cause instability (increased motion) above or below the

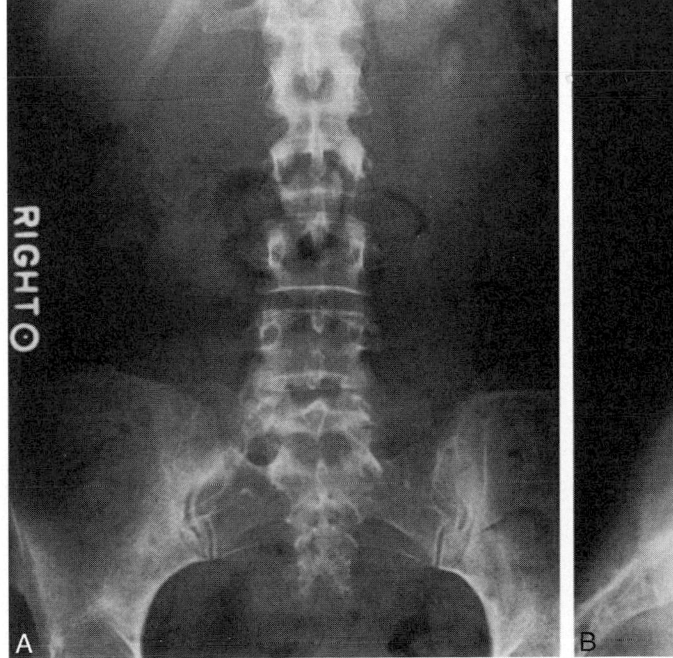

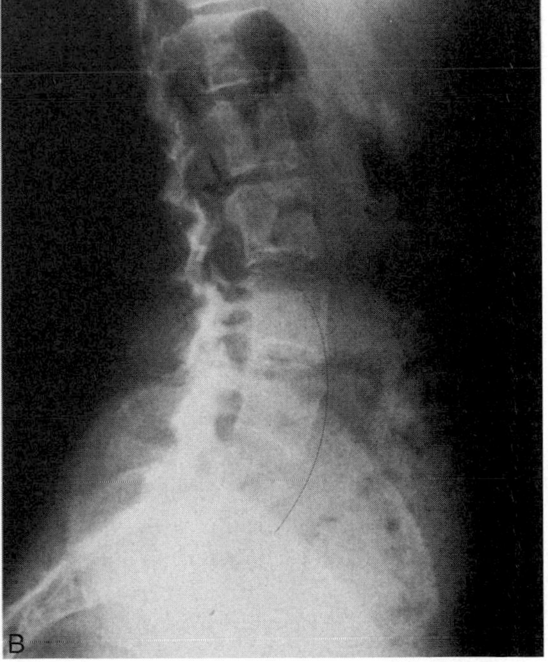

Figure 10-4 Anteroposterior *(A)* and lateral *(B)* views of the lumbosacral spine of a 48-year-old woman. The patient has six lumbar vertebrae. A chest roentgenogram was obtained to verify the presence of 12 thoracic vertebrae.

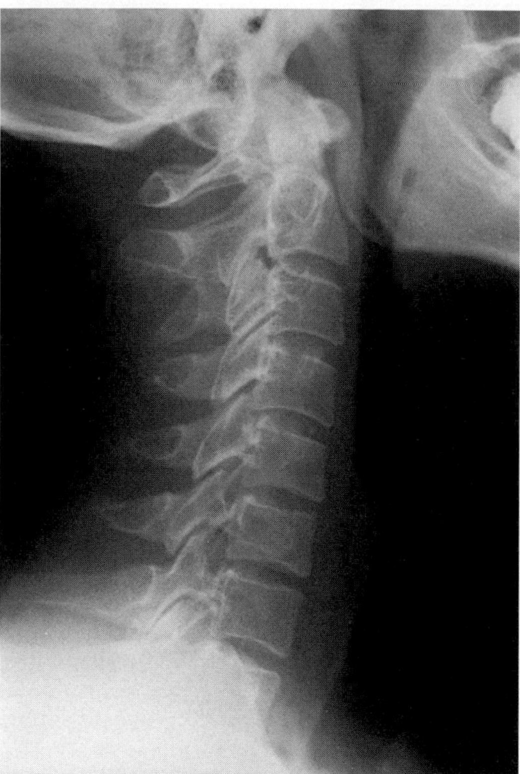

Figure 10-5 Neck strain in a 35-year-old computer analyst with a 4-month history of neck pain and muscle contraction of the trapezius and paracervical muscles. The lateral view of the cervical spine demonstrates straightening of the cervical spine with loss of lordosis and normal intervertebral disc spaces.

fused vertebrae because of increased stress. Although lateral flexion and extension x-ray films should be taken to determine the extent of motion, an associated problem is rarely present (Table 10-1).[3,31,36,43,47,71,80,82]

Other congenital abnormalities may be confused with fracture on roentgenograms or may predispose to clinical symptoms because of anatomic relationships that increase the risk of damage from minor trauma. For example, a pathologic process may be simulated by accessory ossicles around the odontoid; by overlying shadows from the pinna or teeth; by the Mach effect from overlapping shadows of the posterior arch of C1, the tongue, or the occiput; or by the persistence of odontoid synchondrosis.[54,56]

10-1 CONGENITAL ABNORMALITIES OF THE CERVICAL SPINE

CRANIO-OCCIPITAL DEFECTS	INCREASED RISK OF INJURY
Basilar impression[22]	Sharp clivoaxial angle
Hypoplasia of the occiput[73]	Atlanto-occipital subluxation
Occipitalization of the atlas[7]	Constriction of the foramen magnum
ATLANTOAXIAL DEFECT	Arnold-Chiari malformation (cerebellar tonsil ectopy)
Os odontoideum[33]	
Aplasia—arch of the atlas[28]	**ATLANTOAXIAL INSTABILITY**
Aplasia—arch of the axis[39]	
Laxity—transverse atlantal ligament[44]	**MYELOPATHY**
LOWER CERVICAL SPINE	
Klippel-Feil syndrome[45]	
Spondylolisthesis[17]	
Spina bifida[74]	

DIFFERENTIAL DIAGNOSIS

Lumbar Spine

The diagnosis of back strain is based on a history of localized low back pain associated with a traumatic event and a compatible physical examination demonstrating localized pain, muscle spasm, and a normal neurologic examination. The symptoms of back strain may be components of the list of complaints mentioned by patients with a wide variety of disease processes, including spondyloarthropathies and benign tumors of the lumbar spine. Muscle spasm is a reflex that occurs in response to bone or joint inflammation. The age of the patient, the presence of constitutional symptoms, or the persistence of pain should alert the physician to an alternative cause other than muscle strain (Table 10-2). In many circumstances, congenital abnormalities (spinal bifida) are not associated with any back pain. However, an articulation between the L5 transverse process and the sacrum may be a source of pain. Injection into the articulation may result in prolonged pain relief and should be considered if alternative diagnoses are not evident.[4]

Trauma

Trauma to the lumbosacral spine may also be associated with localized low back pain.[14] In a functional sense, there is little difference between apparent bone injuries and associated soft tissue disruptions. The functional effect of a sprain of the interspinous ligament is no different from that of a fracture or avulsion of a spinous process. Similarly, tearing of muscular attachments to the transverse process is functionally no different from an avulsion of that transverse process manifested as a fracture. The degree of trauma to the spine that is associated with a muscle strain or sprain may limit motion but does not cause any instability. Trauma to the spine that results in facet dislocations, severe compression fractures, or Chance fractures (seat belt injury) may cause instability of the spine and damage neural elements. Treatment of patients with these injuries requires the expertise of a trained spine surgeon.

Leg-Length Discrepancies

Patients with leg-length discrepancies may complain of low back pain associated with muscular contraction. Patients may have low back pain, greater trochanteric bursitis, or degenerative hip disease. The pelvic obliquity resulting from a discrepancy in leg length may contribute to muscle pain and eventual degenerative changes in the lumbar spine. Measuring the length of the legs with the patient in a supine position can determine the degree of leg-length inequality. A simple heel lift can provide symp-

10-2 MECHANICAL LOW BACK PAIN

	Muscle Strain	Herniated Nucleus Pulposus	Osteoarthritis	Spinal Stenosis	Spondylolisthesis	Scoliosis
Age (yr)	20–40	30–50	>50	>60	20	30
Pain pattern						
Location	Back (unilateral)	Back/leg (unilateral)	Back (unilateral)	Leg (bilateral)	Back	Back
Onset	Acute	Acute (previous episodes)	Insidious	Insidious	Insidious	Insidious
Standing	↑	↓	↑	↑	↑	↑
Sitting	↓	↑	↓	↓	↓	↓
Bending	↑	↑	↓	↓	↑	↑
Straight leg	–	+	–	+ (stress)	–	–
Plain radiograph	–	–	+	+	+	+

↑, increased; ↓, decreased; +, present; –, absent.

tomatic relief of low back pain in a patient with significant leg-length inequality.[70]

Cervical Spine

The diagnosis of neck strain is based on a history of localized neck pain and a compatible physical examination demonstrating localized pain, muscle spasm, and a normal neurologic examination. The symptoms of neck strain, however, may be components of the list of complaints mentioned by patients with a wide variety of disease processes, including spondyloarthropathies and tumors. Muscle spasm is a reflex that occurs in response to bone or joint inflammation and is a very nonspecific finding. The age of the patient, the presence of constitutional symptoms, or the persistence of pain should alert the physician to a cause other than a strain.

Trauma

Trauma to the cervical spine can result in major neural damage with paralysis. If a history of significant trauma is obtained, a thorough evaluation including x-ray films should be performed. Because of the significant consequences of potential damage to the spinal cord, it is recommended that the expertise of an orthopedic surgeon or neurosurgeon be sought for the evaluation of patients with cervical spine trauma.

A variety of mechanical disorders cause neck and arm pain. These disorders may be differentiated by factors that exacerbate and alleviate neck and arm symptoms (Table 10-3).

Torticollis

Torticollis is associated with severe muscle contracture of the neck. The neck is fixed in side flexion with the chin rotated away from the painful side. Torticollis can be congenital or acquired. Congenital torticollis is associated with anatomic or neurologic abnormalities, including Klippel-Feil syndrome, atlantoaxial subluxation, congenital absence of the cervical muscles, Arnold-Chiari malformation, and syringomyelia.[57] Acquired torticollis may occur in the setting of trauma, muscle injury, fracture, or atlantoaxial subluxation; infection such as upper respiratory infection, cervical adenitis, osteomyelitis, and fasciitis; postinfectious states, influenza, or diphtheria; neoplasm; scar; vascular abnormalities with compression; drugs such as phenothiazines; nerve disorders; syringomyelia; dystonia; or a herniated disc.[38,75] Spasmodic torticollis occurs equally in both sexes in the fourth or fifth decades and may be considered a form of segmental dystonia. Early in the course of the movement, the tilt may be corrected with pressure on the chin. When the process becomes chronic, the contracture becomes painful with tonic spasm of the sternocleidomastoid and secondary cervical osteoarthritis. Evaluation of patients with torticollis includes radiography, computed

10-3 MECHANICAL NECK PAIN

	Neck Strain	Herniated Nucleus Pulposus	Osteoarthritis	Myelopathy	Whiplash
Age (yr)	20–40	30–50	>50	>60	30–40
Pain pattern					
Location	Neck	Neck/arm	Neck	Arm/leg	Neck
Onset	Acute	Acute	Insidious	Insidious	Acute
Flexion	+	+	–	–	+
Extension	–	+/–	+	+	+
Plain radiograph	–	–	+	+	–

+, present; –, absent.

tomography (CT), or magnetic resonance (MR) imaging to determine the presence of anatomic abnormalities associated with congenital or acquired torticollis. Therapy for torticollis includes local trigger point injections (lidocaine and corticosteroids), cooling spray and stretching, range-of-motion exercises, or drug therapy (benztropine, amantadine, and haloperidol).[38] In severe cases, injection of botulinum toxin is warranted.[50] Surgical denervation is indicated in patients resistant to all medical therapy.[29] In patients with spasmodic torticollis who respond to botulinum toxin therapy, selective peripheral denervation of the posterior branches of the cervical roots may be helpful, as it was for 76% of the patients reported by Braun and Richter.[13] Torticollis is occasionally associated with psychopathology (hysteria). These individuals require biofeedback or psychotherapy. Patients with spasmodic torticollis of any etiology require therapy. In a study of 116 patients, only 14 (12%) had a spontaneous remission.[76]

Temporomandibular Joint

Abnormalities in the temporomandibular joint may be confused with neck strain and vice versa.[10] De Wijer and colleagues completed a study to determine clinical findings that differentiated between the two entities. Patients with temporomandibular joint disorders had pain maximally over the masticatory muscles, difficulty opening their mouth, jaw clicking, tinnitus, or dullness in the ears. Patients with cervical disorders have maximal pain in the neck and pain referred to the shoulders, as well as restricted mobility of the neck or aggravation of neck pain on movement.[26]

TREATMENT

Lumbar Spine

Therapy for back strain includes controlled physical activity, nonsteroidal anti-inflammatory drugs (NSAIDs), muscle relaxants, and physical therapy. Back strain is improved with controlled activity.[84] A period as short as 2 days has been shown to be effective in relieving back pain.[25] Continuing bed rest for 7 days did not appreciably decrease pain or hasten return to work. Malmivarra and colleagues studied 186 patient with acute low back pain treated by bed rest for 2 days, back extension and lateral bending exercises, or regular activity as tolerated.[63] At 3 and 12 weeks, individuals assigned to ordinary activity had the best outcome. Convincing the patient to limit excessive activities is a primary goal of therapy. Controlled physical activity allows the injured tissues to rest, thereby permitting a greater opportunity for healing without reinjury. The time spent by the physician explaining to the patient the rationale for controlled physical activity is worth the effort. Bed rest is kept to a minimum. Increasing evidence supports the use of active exercise early in the course of back strain to maximize function. As soon as the very acute pain is diminished, patients should be encouraged to increase physical activity. A physical therapist may be used if patients require encouragement to remain mobile.[81]

Non-narcotic analgesics in the form of NSAIDs are helpful in making patients comfortable while their injury heals. Nonsteroidal drugs with a rapid onset of action are most helpful in patients with acute pain. These drugs may be continued until the patients' symptoms have resolved. NSAIDs are helpful as part of early treatment after a muscle injury. NSAIDs have no adverse effects on the tensile or contractile properties of an injured muscle as it heals.[68] Muscle relaxants may be of use in a patient who has palpable spasms on physical examination or has difficulty sleeping at night because of muscle pain. In a study of 1445 patients (66% with back pain and 34% with neck pain), a low dose (5 mg) of cyclobenzaprine was more effective in improving pain and spasm than placebo was.[11] The 5 mg-dose was as effective as the 10-mg dose, without fewer toxicities. Nonaddictive analgesics and muscle relaxants are preferred. The combination of an NSAID with a muscle relaxant is better than an NSAID alone in improving pain relief in low back pain patients with muscle spasm on physical examination.[12] Cherkin and colleagues conducted a longitudinal observational study of the efficacy of medications at 7 days for the treatment of acute low back pain in 219 patients.[18] The drugs prescribed included none (21%), NSAIDs (69%), muscle relaxants (35%), narcotics (12%), and acetaminophen (4%). Those receiving medications had less severe symptoms after 1 week than did patients who did not take medications. Patients receiving a muscle relaxant and NSAIDs had the best self-reported outcome. The combination of an NSAID and a muscle relaxant produces good results in patients with limited range of motion and muscle pain related to muscle contraction.

Physical therapy modalities in the form of cold (ice massage) initially or heat (warm bath) subsequently may decrease pain and diminish spasm. Patients with very localized pain and severe spasm limiting mobility may benefit from injection of a local anesthetic with or without the addition of a corticosteroid preparation. The injection relieves pain and blocks reflex spasm. These injections should be given to compliant patients who will limit their activity during the natural course of healing. Increased activity may cause additional damage to musculoligamentous structures, which may not be recognized by the patient because the protective mechanism of pain has been blocked by the injection. These injections are indicated after 2 to 4 weeks of rest and medication without significant improvement. In a study of 31 patients with chronic low back pain, 11 of 15 who received 200 U of botulinum toxin A had greater than 50% improvement in pain at 8 weeks as compared with 4 of 16 who had a placebo injection.[34] The long-term effects of the injections were not determined. Another study of 33 patients who received either 50 or 100 U of botulinum toxin A found no difference in response.[83] This form of injection therapy cannot be considered a usual form of therapy for spinal pain until long-term follow-up studies are completed. Pressure over the maximal point of tenderness also may be effective in decreasing muscle spasm and pain.[37] Braces are reserved for patients who must remain active while healing continues. Braces may be recommended for subacute or chronic low back pain. A variety of therapies, including traction, manipulation, and facet injection, have been proposed for idiopathic low back pain. Scientific evidence to support the efficacy of many of these modalities is lacking, however.[66] (For additional information on therapy, see Section IV.)

Cervical Spine

The mainstay of treatment of neck strain includes controlled physical activity. Encouraging motion as tolerated allows tissues to heal while maintaining function. Some patients will experience increased pain with motion and will feel more comfortable with external support. Immobilization in a soft cervical orthosis should be limited. It is important that the patient wear the collar primarily at night. During sleep, the neck is at greatest risk of undergoing abnormal movements or assuming unnatural positions. The orthosis should be removed increasingly during the day as the patient improves. The chance of weakening neck muscles is minimized if the collar is used in conjunction with cervical strengthening exercises.[77] Convincing the patient to limit activities is a primary objective of therapy. Patients should refrain from their exercise routines during this initial phase of healing. Decreased activity allows the injured tissues to heal. Patients are encouraged to discontinue use of the cervical orthosis as they improve. Increasing physical activities are encouraged as the pain and limitation of motion are diminished.

Non-narcotic analgesics in the form of NSAIDs are helpful in making patients comfortable. These drugs may be continued until the patient's symptoms have resolved. Muscle relaxants may be beneficial in patients who have palpable spasm on physical examination or have difficulty sleeping at night. For example, cyclobenzaprine in a dose of 5 mg up to three times a day is able to decrease pain and spasm in neck strain patients when compared with placebo.[11] Physical therapy modalities may take the form of cold (ice) initially or heat (warm bath) subsequently. Intermittent lightweight cervical traction may decrease pain and diminish spasm. Patients with localized pain and severe spasm limiting mobility may benefit from injection of an anesthetic with or without the addition of corticosteroids. The injection relieves pain and blocks reflex spasm. Such injections are indicated after 2 to 4 weeks of rest and medication without significant improvement. Finally, once the patient starts to improve, a course of isometric exercises should begin. Neck pain and mobility are improved with physiotherapy.[58] Modification of the position of the patient while at work may help decrease neck pain. Relief of chronic muscle contraction is associated with pain relief.[42]

The course of patients with neck strain is one of progressive improvement with complete resolution of the symptoms over a period of several weeks. Recovery is total without any lasting impairment. A small percentage of patients may continue to experience neck pain in spite of adequate treatment. Pain may continue for months or years. These patients must be evaluated and treated in a manner that takes into account the special difficulties of individuals with chronic pain. The goal of therapy is to maximize function of the cervical spine. These patients may receive drugs, physical therapy, psychiatric support, and vocational rehabilitation as part of their therapeutic regimen. Injection therapy is an option for patients resistant to drug therapy. Botulinum toxin has been used for cervical dystonia (torticollis).

Ylinen and colleagues demonstrated the importance of strength training as a component of therapy for chronic nonspecific neck pain.[85] A total of 180 female office workers with chronic nonspecific neck pain were randomly assigned to two training groups or a control group. The endurance training group performed dynamic neck exercises. The strength training group performed high-intensity isometric neck strengthening and stabilization exercises with an elastic band. Both training groups performed dynamic exercises with dumbbells for the shoulders and upper extremities. All groups were advised to complete three sessions of aerobic and stretching exercises per week. The control group received written information about the same stretching exercises, which were prescribed three times a week for 30 minutes. At 12 months, the strengthening group had 110% improved flexion, 76% improved rotation, and 69% improved extension. The endurance training group had 28%, 29%, and 16% improvement, respectively. The control group had 10%, 10%, and 7% improvement, respectively. Neck pain and disability improved significantly in comparison to controls ($P < 0.001$). This study supports the inclusion of a neck strengthening program for chronic neck pain patients.

The positive effects of manipulation or mobilization of the cervical spine are marginal. Few studies with adequate design exist to be of significance. The effects were of short duration, measured in weeks.[48] In addition, manipulation of the cervical spine is associated with significant complications.[1]

PROGNOSIS

Lumbar Spine

The course of patients with back strain is one of gradual improvement over a 2-week period. Almost 90% are cured in a 2-month period.[27] Recovery is total, without any lasting impairment.

Ten percent of patients may continue to experience low back pain associated with muscle strain. Pain may continue for months or years. This group of patients accounts for 70% to 80% of the cost associated with low back pain.[35] These patients are experiencing chronic low back pain, which must be evaluated and treated in a manner that takes into account the special difficulties of individuals with chronic pain. The goal of therapy in these individuals is to maximize function of the lumbosacral spine. These patients may receive drugs, physical therapy, psychiatric support, and vocational rehabilitation as part of their therapeutic program.

Another important consideration in patients with low back strain is the likelihood of recurrence. The first episode of back pain is usually the briefest and least severe. However, the vast majority of individuals with an episode of back pain are at risk for another episode that will be more severe and of greater duration.[79] Of patients with occupationally related acute episodes of low back pain, 60% will have recurrent symptoms within 1 year.[6] The risk for an additional episode of back pain lessens after 2 years. The rate may be as high as 50% to 60% within 3 to 5 years.[79] These patients may have symptoms resistant to therapies that are beneficial in the management of acute back pain and may therefore require modifications in their work environment to limit the stress placed on the lumbosacral spine.

Cervical Spine

The course of patients with neck strain is one of progressive improvement with complete resolution of the symptoms over a period of several weeks. Recovery is total without any lasting impairment. A small percentage of patients may continue to experience neck pain in spite of adequate treatment, and the pain may persist for months or years. These patients must be evaluated and treated in a manner that takes into account the special difficulties of individuals with chronic pain. The goal of therapy is to maximize function of the cervical spine. These patients may receive drugs, physical therapy, psychiatric support, and vocational rehabilitation as part of their therapeutic regimen.

References

Low Back/Neck (Spinal) Strain

1. Aker PD, Gross AR, Goldsmith CH, et al: Conservative management of mechanical neck pain: Systematic overview and meta-analysis. BMJ 313:1291-1296, 1996.
2. Andersson GBJ: Evaluation of muscle function. In Frymoyer JW, Ducker TB, Hadler NM, et al (eds): The Adult Spine: Principles and Practice. New York, Raven Press, 1991, pp 241-274.
3. Ashton-Miller JA, McGlashen KM, Herzenberg JE, Stohler CS: Cervical muscle myoelectric response to acute experimental sternocleidomastoid pain. Spine 15:1006, 1990.
4. Avimadje M, Goupille P, Jeannou J, et al: Can an anomalous lumbosacral or lumbo-iliac articulation cause low back pain? A retrospective study of 12 cases. Rev Rhum Engl Ed 66:35-39, 1999.
5. Bauwens P, Cayer AB: The "multifidus triangle" syndrome as a cause of recurrent low back pain. BMJ 2:1306, 1955.
6. Berquist-Ullman M, Larsson U: Acute low back pain in industry: A controlled prospective study with special reference to therapy and confounding factors. Acta Orthop Scand Suppl 170:1, 1977.
7. Bharucha EP, Dastur HM: Craniovertebral anomalies: A report on 40 cases. Brain 87:469, 1964.
8. Biering-Sorensoen F: Physical measurements as risk indicators for low back trouble over a one year period. Spine 9:106, 1984.
9. Bland JH: Congenital anomalies. In Bland JH (ed): Disorders of the Cervical Spine, 2nd ed. Philadelphia, WB Saunders, 1994, pp 417-431.
10. Bokduk N, Lord SM: Cervical spine disorders. Curr Opin Rheumatol 10:110-115, 1998.
11. Borenstein DG, Korn S: Efficacy of a low-dose regimen of cyclobenzaprine hydrochloride in acute skeletal muscle spasm: Results of two placebo-controlled trials. Clin Ther 25:1056-1073, 2003.
12. Borenstein DG, Lacks SL, Wiesel S: Cyclobenzaprine and naproxen versus naproxen alone in the treatment of acute low back pain and muscle spasm. Clin Ther 12:125, 1990.
13. Braun V, Richter H: Selective peripheral denervation for the treatment of spasmodic torticollis. Neurosurgery 35:58, 1994.
14. Bucholz RW, Gill K: Classification of injuries to the thoracolumbar spine. Orthop Clin North Am 17:67, 1986.
15. Cailliet R: Low Back Pain Syndrome, 3rd ed. Philadelphia, FA Davis, 1981, pp 53-68.
16. Cailliet R: Neck and Arm Pain, 3rd ed. Philadelphia, FA Davis, 1991, pp 55-80.
17. Charlton DP, Gehweileer JA, Morgan CL, et al: Spondylolysis and spondylolisthesis of the cervical spine. Skeletal Radiol 3:79, 1978.
18. Cherkin DC, Wheeler KJ, Barlow W, et al: Medication use for low back pain in primary care. Spine 23:607-614, 1998.
19. Cooper RG: Understanding paraspinal muscle dysfunction in low back pain: A way forward. Ann Rheum Dis 52:413, 1993.
20. Cooper RG, Forbes W StC, Jayson MIV: Radiographic demonstration of paraspinal muscle wasting in patients with chronic low back pain. Br J Rheumatol 31:398, 1992.
21. Cypress BK: Characteristics of physician visits for back symptoms: A national perspective. Am J Public Health 73:389, 1983.
22. DeBarros MC, Farias W, Ataide L, Lins S: Basilar impression and Arnold-Chiari malformation: A study of 66 cases. J Neurol Neurosurg Psychiatry 31:596, 1968.
23. DePalma AP, Rothman RH: The Intervertebral Disc. Philadelphia, WB Saunders, 1970, pp 58-92.
24. Deyo RA, Diehl AK: Lumbar spine films in primary care: Current use and selective ordering criteria. J Gen Intern Med 1:20, 1986.
25. Deyo RA, Diehl AK, Rosenthal M: How many days of bed rest for acute low back pain? N Engl J Med 315:1064, 1986.
26. de Wijer A, de Leeuw JRJ, Steenks MH, et al: Temporomandibular and cervical spine disorders: Self-reported signs and symptoms. Spine 21:1638-1646, 1996.
27. Dillane JB, Fry J, Kalton G: Acute back syndrome: A study from general practice. BMJ 3:82, 1966.
28. Dubousett J: Torticollis in children caused by congenital anomalies of the atlas. J Bone Joint Surg Am 68-A:178, 1986.
29. Duvoisin RC: Spasmodic torticollis: The role of surgical denervation. Mayo Clin Proc 66:433, 1991.
30. Ensink F, Saur PMM, Frese K, et al: Lumbar range of motion: Influence of time of day and individual factors on measurement. Spine 21:1339-1343, 1996.
31. Evans WJ: Effects of exercise on senescent muscle. Clin Orthop 403(suppl):S211-S220, 2002
32. Farfan HF, Cossette JW, Robertson GW, et al: Effects of torsion on lumbar intervertebral joints: The role of torsion in the production of disc degeneration. J Bone Joint Surg Am 52-A:468, 1970.
33. Fielding JW, Hensinger RN, Hawkins RJ: Os odontoideum. J Bone Joint Surg Am 62-A:376, 1980.
34. Foster L, Clapp L, Erickson M, et al: Botulinum toxin A and chronic low back pain: A randomized, double-blind study. Neurology 56:1290-1293, 2001.
35. Frymoyer JW: Back pain and sciatica. N Engl J Med 318:291, 1988.
36. Garrett WE: Muscle strain injuries. Am J Sports Med 24(suppl): S2-S8, 1996.
37. Garvey TA, Marks MR, Wiesel SW: A prospective, randomized, double-blind evaluation of trigger-point injection therapy for low back pain. Spine 14:962, 1989.
38. Gilbert RL, Warfield CA: Neck pain. In Warfield CA (ed): Principles and Practice of Pain Management. New York, McGraw-Hill, 1994, pp 109-121.
39. Hanson EC, Shook JE, Wiesseman GJ, Wood VE: Congenital pedicle defects of the axis vertebra: Report of a case. Spine 15:236, 1990.
40. Hansson T, Bigos S, Beecher P, Wortley M: The lumbar lordosis in acute and chronic low-back pain. Spine 10:154, 1985.
41. Harell A, Mead S, Mueller E: The problem of spasm in skeletal muscle: A clinical and laboratory study. JAMA 143:640, 1950.
42. Harms-Ringdahl K, Ekholm J: Intensity and character of pain and muscular activity levels elicited by maintained extreme flexion position of the lower-cervical–upper-thoracic spine. Scand J Rehabil Med 18:117, 1986.
43. Helliwell PS, Evans PF, Wright V: The straight cervical spine: Does it indicate muscle spasm? J Bone Joint Surg Br 76-B:103, 1994.
44. Hensinger RN: Congenital anomalies of the cervical spine. Clin Orthop 264:16, 1991.
45. Hensinger RN, Lang JR, MacEwen GD: The Klippel-Feil syndrome: A constellation of related anomalies. J Bone Joint Surg Am 56-A:1246, 1974.
46. Hides JA, Stokes MJ, Saide M, et al: Evidence of lumbar multifidus muscle wasting ipsilateral to symptoms in patients with acute/subacute low back pain. Spine 19:165-172, 1994.
47. Hurley BF, Roth SM: Strength training in the elderly: Effects on risk factor for age-related diseases. Sports Med 30:249-268, 2000.

48. Hurwitz EL, Aker PD, Adams AH, et al: Manipulation and mobilization of the cervical spine: A systematic review of the literature Spine 21:1746-1759, 1996.
49. Jackson R: Cervical trauma: Not just another pain in the neck. Geriatrics 37:123, 1982.
50. Jankovic J, Brin MF: Therapeutic uses of botulinum toxin. N Engl J Med 324:1186, 1991.
51. Jarvinen TAH, Kaariainen M, Jarvinen M, et al: Muscle strain injuries. Curr Opin Rheumatol 12:155-161, 2000.
52. Johnson EW: The myth of skeletal muscle spasm. Am J Phys Med Rehabil 68:1, 1989.
53. Johnson EW: Editor's reply. Am J Phys Med Rehabil 68:256, 1989.
54. Keats TE: Atlas of Normal Roentgen Variants that May Simulate Disease, 5th ed. St Louis, Mosby–Year Book, 1992, pp 143-229.
55. Keim HA, Durning RP: A new modified classification of transitional lumbosacral vertebrae and an analysis of Bertolotti's symptom-complex. Orthop Rev 11(2):17, 1982.
56. Kim KS, Rogers LF, Regenbogen V: Pitfalls in plain film diagnosis of cervical spine injuries: False positive interpretation. Surg Neurol 25:381, 1986.
57. Kiwak K: Establishing an etiology for torticollis. Postgrad Med 75:129, 1984.
58. Koes BW, Bouter LM, van Mameren H, et al: The effectiveness of manual therapy, physiotherapy, and treatment by the general practitioner for nonspecific back and neck complaints: A randomized clinical trial. Spine 17:28, 1992.
59. Kunkel RS: Muscle contraction (tension) headache. Clin J Pain 5:39, 1989.
60. Lord MJ, Small JM, Dinsay JM, et al: Lumbar lordosis: Effects of sitting and standing. Spine 22:2571-2574, 1997.
61. Magora A: Investigation of the relation between low back pain and occupation. Scand J Rehabil Med 7:146, 1975.
62. Magora A: Investigation of the relation between low back pain and occupation: IV. Physical requirements: Bending, rotation, reaching, and sudden maximal effort. Scand J Rehabil Med 5:186, 1973.
63. Malmivarra A, Hakkinen U, Aro T, et al: The treatment of acute low back pain: Bed rest, exercises, or ordinary activity? N Engl J Med 332:351-355, 1995.
64. Marras WS, Davis KG, Ferguson SA, et al: Spine loading characteristics of patients with low back pain compared with asymptomatic individuals. Spine 26:2566-2574, 2001.
65. Nachemson A: The lumbar spine—an orthopaedic challenge. Spine 1:59, 1976.
66. Nachemson AL: Newest knowledge of low back pain: A critical look. Clin Orthop 279:8, 1992.
67. Newham DJ: The consequences of eccentric contractions and their relation to delayed onset muscle pain. Eur J Appl Physiol 57:353, 1988.
68. Obremsky WT, Seaber AV, Ribbeck BM, et al: Biochemical and histological assessment of a controlled muscle strain injury treated with piroxicam. Am J Sports Med 22:172-176, 1994.
69. Parnianpour M, Nordin MA, Kahanovitz N, Frankel V: The triaxial coupling of torque generation of trunk muscles during isometric exertions and effect of fatiguing isoinertial movements on the motor output and movement. Spine 13:982, 1988.
70. Rothenberg RJ: Rheumatic disease aspects of leg length inequality. Semin Arthritis Rheum 17:196, 1988.
71. Roubenoff R, Castaneda C: Sarcopenia—understanding the dynamics of aging muscle. JAMA 286:1230-1231, 2001
72. Sarno JE: Etiology of neck and back pain: An autonomic myoneuralgia? J Nerv Ment Dis 169:55, 1981.
73. Sherk HH: Lesions of the atlas and axis. Clin Orthop 109:33, 1975.
74. Sherk HH, Whitaker LA, Pasquariello PS: Facial malformations and spinal anomalies: A predictable relationship. Spine 7:526, 1982.
75. Shima F, Fukui M, Matsubara T, Kitamura K: Spasmodic torticollis caused by vascular compression of the spinal accessory root. Surg Neurol 26:431, 1986.
76. Shoen RP: Soft tissue cervical spine syndromes. In Bland JH (ed): Disorders of the Cervical Spine, 2nd ed. Philadelphia, WB Saunders, 1994, pp 365-372.
77. Swezey RL: Chronic neck pain. Rheum Dis Clin North Am 22:411-437, 1996
78. Timmi PG, Wieser C, Zinn W. The transitional vertebra of the lumbosacral spine. Rheumatol Rehabil 16:180, 1977.
79. Troup JDG, Martin JW, Lloyd DCEF: Backpain in industry: A prospective study. Spine 6:61, 1981.
80. Volpi E, Sheffield-Moore M, Rasmussen BB, et al: Basal muscle amino acid kinetics and protein synthesis in healthy young and older men. JAMA 286:1206-1212, 2001.
81. Waddell G: Simple low back pain: Rest or active exercise? Ann Rheum Dis 52:317, 1993.
82. Walton J: Brain's Diseases of the Nervous System, 9th ed. New York: Oxford University Press, 1985, pp 27-29.
83. Wheeler AH, Goolkasian P, Gretz SS: A randomized, double-blind, prospective pilot study of botulinum toxin injection for refractory, unilateral, cervicothoracic, paraspinal, myofascial pain syndrome. Spine 23:1662-1667, 1998.
84. Wiesel SW, Cuckler JM, Deluca F, et al: An objective analysis of conservative therapy. Spine 5:324, 1980.
85. Ylinen J, Takala E, Nykanen M, et al: Active neck muscle training in the treatment of chronic neck pain in women: A randomized controlled trial. JAMA 289:2509-2516, 2003

ACUTE HERNIATED NUCLEUS PULPOSUS

CAPSULE SUMMARY

	LOW BACK	NECK
Frequency of spinal pain	Very common	Very common
Location of spinal pain	Low back to lower leg	Neck to distal arm and hand
Quality of spinal pain	Sharp, shooting, burning paresthesias in lower leg	Sharp, shooting, burning paresthesias in hand
Symptoms and signs	Positive straight leg–raising test, weakness, asymmetric reflexes	Positive compression test, weakness in arms and hands, asymmetric reflexes
Laboratory tests	None	None
Radiographic findings	CT, MR, myelogram—disc herniation; MR is most sensitive test	CT, MR, myelogram—disc herniation; MR is most sensitive test
Treatment	Controlled activity, medications, surgical excision of disc for conservative therapy failures	Controlled activity, medications, surgical excision of disc for conservative therapy failures

PREVALENCE AND PATHOGENESIS

A herniated disc can be defined as herniation of the nucleus pulposus through the fibers of the annulus fibrosus.[74] Most disc ruptures occur during the third and fourth decades of life while the nucleus pulposus is still gelatinous. The time of the day that a herniation occurs may relate to diurnal alterations in spinal anatomy. A cadaveric study of the lumbar spine demonstrated changes in disc height, water content, swelling pressure, compressive stiffness, bulging, loading of apophyseal joints, and forward and backward bending properties when loaded with compressive force. The most likely time of day associated with increased force on the disc is the morning.[1] In the lumbar region, perforations usually arise through a defect just lateral to the posterior midline, where the posterior longitudinal ligament is weakest.

Epidemiology

Lumbar Spine

Symptomatic lumbar disc herniation occurs during the lifetime of approximately 2% of the general population.[52] Approximately 80% of the population will experience significant back pain during the course of a herniated disc. The groups at greatest risk for herniation of intervertebral discs are younger individuals (mean age of 35 years).[56,80] True sciatica actually develops in only 35% of patients with disc herniation. Not infrequently, sciatica develops 6 to 10 years after the onset of low back pain. The period of localized back pain may correspond to repeated damage to annular fibers that irritates the sinuvertebral nerve but does not result in disc herniation.

Cervical Spine

The average annual incidence of cervical radiculopathy is less than 0.1 per 1000 individuals. Pure soft disc herniations are less common than hard disc abnormalities (spondylosis) as a cause of radicular arm pain.[27]

In a study of 395 patients with nerve root abnormalities, radiculopathy occurred in the cervical and lumbar spine in 93 (24%) and 302 (76%), respectively.[121]

Pathogenesis

Alterations in intervertebral disc biomechanics and biochemistry over time have a detrimental effect on disc function. The disc is less able to work as a spacer between vertebral bodies or as a universal joint. Biomechanical, biochemical, nutritional, immunologic, and nociceptive factors that predispose the intervertebral disc to dysfunction are reviewed in Chapter 3.

Lumbar Spine

The two most common levels for disc herniation are L4–L5 and L5–S1, which account for 98% of lesions; pathology can occur at L2–L3 and L3–L4 but is relatively uncommon.[103] Overall, 90% of disc herniations are at the L4–L5 and L5–S1 levels. Less than 10% of herniations occur at higher lumbar levels. Disc herniations at L5–S1 will usually compromise the first sacral nerve root, a lesion at the L4–L5 level will most often compress the fifth lumbar root, and herniation at L3–L4 more frequently involves the fourth lumbar root. It should be appreciated that variations in root configuration as well as in the position of the herniation itself can modify these relationships. Thus, an L4–L5 disc rupture can at times affect the first sacral as well as the fifth lumbar root, and in extreme lateral herniations, the nerve exiting at the same level as the disc will be involved.[27] These far lateral lumbar disk herniations may not be recognized for a number of months.[14]

Disc herniation may also develop in older patients. Disc tissue that causes compression in elderly patients is composed of the annulus fibrosus and portions of the cartilaginous endplate (hard disc). The cartilage is avulsed from the vertebral body.[39] Tanaka and co-workers completed a pathologic study of disc herniation in the elderly.[109] A study of 88 discs from cadavers with a mean age of 77.6 years revealed cartilaginous endplate rupture with the attached annulus as the most characteristic form of disc herniation in 51.1% of specimens. The most severely degenerated disc levels were more closely associated with endplate rupture. The clinical correlate of these findings contradicts the axiom that disc herniation does not develop in the elderly because of desiccation of the nucleus pulposus. Nerve impingement can develop in the elderly on the basis of annular and endplate disruption.

A question exists concerning the relative importance of restriction of motion by the annulus fibrosus versus the facet joints in preventing disc herniation. Krismer and colleagues performed a cadaver study in which they measured the rotational movement of six spinal motion segments with an intact disc, with a disc having desiccated annular fibers angled in one direction, and after bilateral facetectomy.[65] Rotational motion was greater with section of the annular fibers than with bilateral facetectomy. This study suggests that in normal intervertebral discs, annular fibers restrict axial rotation more than the facet joints do. The initiating event in the process of degeneration of the lumbar motion segment is loss of integrity of the annular fibers. With greater rotational forces, the facet joints degenerate secondarily.

Moore and co-workers completed a histologic examination of herniated material, determined the degree of neovascularization of the fragmented specimens, and correlated clinical symptoms with the degree of neovascularization.[78] Of a total of 120 surgical specimens analyzed, the nucleus pulposus was present in 98%. Nuclear tissue was present alone (34%), with the annulus (14%), with the endplate (29%), or with both (19%). Annular components were always attached to herniated nuclear material. Neovascular repair enabling resorption was present in 89% of specimens, but no correlation could be made with the clinical spectrum of symptoms or the duration of back or leg pain.

It is important to realize that not everyone with a herniated disc has significant discomfort. A large herniation in a capacious canal may not be clinically apparent because of the absence of compression of the neural elements. On the other hand, a minor protrusion in a small canal may be crippling because of a lack of room to accommodate both the disc and the nerve root.[59]

Resolution of some of the compressive effects on neural structures requires resorption of the nucleus pulposus. Disc resorption is part of the natural healing process associated with disc herniation. The enhanced ability to resorb discs has the potential for resolving clinical symptoms more rapidly. Resorption of herniated disc material is associated with a marked increase in infiltrating macrophages and the production of matrix metalloproteinases (MMPs) 3 and 7. In a murine model, Haro and co-workers investigated the role of MMPs in disc resorption.[40] MMP-7 is required for release of tumor necrosis factor (TNF) from macrophages. Generation of TNF is essential for induction of MMP-3 from chondrocytes, which is required for generation of the macrophage chemoattractant necessary for macrophage infiltration. Theoretically, manipulation of MMP may result in increased macrophage infiltration and more rapid disc resorption. Also important in the resolution of disc herniation is the ability of phagocytic cells to remove damaged tissue. Nerlich and associates identified the origins of phagocytic cells in degenerated intervertebral discs.[82] The investigation identified cells that are transformed local cells rather than invaded macrophages. Degenerative discs contain the cells that add to their continued dissolution.

Cervical Spine

In the early 1940s, a number of reports appeared in which cervical intervertebral disc herniation with radiculopathy was described.[73,97,104] There is a direct correlation between the anatomy of the cervical spine and the location and pathophysiology of disc lesions.[31] The eight cervical nerve roots exit via intervertebral foramina that are bordered anteromedially by the intervertebral disc and posterolaterally by the zygapophyseal joint. The foramina are largest at C2–C3 and decrease in size until C6–C7. The nerve root occupies 25% to 33% of the volume of the foramen. The C1 root exits between the occiput and the atlas (C1). All lower roots exit above their corresponding cervical vertebrae (the C6 root at the C5–C6 interspace), except C8, which exits between C7 and T1. A differential growth rate affects the relationship of the spinal cord and nerve roots and the cervical spine. The lower cervical vertebrae are at the same level as the next lower cord segment.[31] The C5–C6 interspace is opposite the C7 cord level, where the C7 nerve root arises and the C6 root exits. Careful dissection of the cervical spine with a surgical microscope has confirmed the high incidence of intradural connections between the dorsal rootlets of the C5, C6, and C7 segments. This anatomic characteristic of the cervical spinal cord may play a role in the absence of symptoms that can be ascribed to a single spinal nerve level.[110] The sinuvertebral nerve is the primary innervation of the intervertebral disc.[9] It originates from both the ventral primary ramus (somatic) and the gray rami communicantes (autonomic) at each segmental level. The nerve runs back into the neural foramen and branches to supply innervation to structures in a variety of patterns, including one segment above and below the foramen, multiple levels above and below, and on the contralateral side.[38] Nerve fibers supply the periosteum of the pedicle, the vertebral body, the epidural veins, the dura mater, and the annulus fibrosus.[22] Innervation of the annulus runs parallel and perpendicular to the fibers of the annulus fibrosus. The nerves are most numerous in the middle third of the disc. The nerve receptors have Pacini's corpuscles, Golgi's tendon organs, and free nerve endings.[72] These nerve endings mediate proprioception, tension, and pain.

Most acute disc herniations occur posterolaterally and in patients around the fourth decade of life, when the nucleus is still gelatinous. The most common areas of disc herniation are C6–C7 and C5–C6. The C7 nerve root is affected in 37% to 75.6% of individuals with cervical radiculopathy reported in large studies.[45,68,84,122] The same studies reported a 15.8% to 48% frequency of C6 radiculopathy. C7–T1 and C3–C4 disc herniations are infrequent (less than 15%). Disc herniation of C2–C3 is rare. Patients with upper cervical disc protrusions in the C2–C3 region have symptoms that include suboccipital pain, loss of hand dexterity, and paresthesias over the face and unilateral arm.[23] Unlike lumbar herniated discs, cervical herniated discs may cause myelopathy in addition to radicular pain because of the spinal cord in the cervical region.[47] The uncovertebral prominences play a role in the location of ruptured disc material. Pure nerve root compression occurs if extruded disc material enters the nerve root canal. The uncovertebral joint tends to guide extruded disc material medially, where cord compression may also occur.

Disc herniation usually affects the nerve root numbered most caudally for the given disc level; for example, the C3–C4 disc affects the fourth cervical nerve root; C4–C5, the fifth cervical nerve root; C5–C6, the sixth cervical nerve root; C6–C7, the seventh cervical nerve root; and C7–T1, the eighth cervical nerve root. Individual disc herniations do not involve other roots but more commonly present some evidence of upper motor neuron findings secondary to spinal cord compression.

Not every herniated disc is symptomatic. The development of symptoms depends on the reserve capacity of the spinal canal, the presence of inflammation, the size of the herniation, and the presence of concomitant disease such as osteophyte formation. In disc rupture, protrusion of nuclear material results in tension on the annular fibers and compression of the dura or nerve root causing pain. Also important is the smaller size of the sagittal diameter, the intervertebral foramen, and the cross-sectional area of the bony cervical spinal canal. Individuals in whom a cervical herniated disc causes motor dysfunction have a smaller spinal canal.[26] Complete paraplegia may also be a complication of cervical disc herniation if the spinal canal is stenotic.[107]

Cervical radiculopathy has been divided into two categories according to the hardness of the disc lesion. Individuals usually younger than 45 years have soft disc lesions associated with herniation of the nucleus pulposus and subsequent nerve root or cord compression. Hard disc lesions, produced by disc calcification or osteophytes, occur in individuals older than 45 years. Soft disc lesions resolve more frequently than hard disc lesions. Hard discs are more closely associated with cord compression.

Inflammatory Mediators

Compression of a nerve root by a herniated disc explains only part of the pathophysiology of radicular pain.[37] A number of inflammatory mediators are released when an intervertebral disc herniates. A sample of these mediators includes prostaglandins, leukotrienes, nitric oxide, and proinflammatory cytokines, including interleukin-1-alpha, interleukin-6, and TNF-alpha. Leakage of these factors may produce excitation of the nerve root and enhancement of pain-producing substances (bradykinin). These factors are released early in the course of the herniation and are transient. The intervertebral disc cells are capable of producing nitric oxide, interleukins, and MMPs. Degenerative disc cells make smaller amounts of these factors than normal, nondegenerative disc cells do.[53] Chronic disc herniations fail to demonstrate the same degree of inflammation.

Another factor that may increase nerve root inflammation independent of compression is disruption of the blood-nerve barrier. Kobayashi and colleagues developed an animal model of nerve root compression for histologic evaluation of the blood-nerve barrier.[60] Gadolinium-diethylenetriamine pentaacetic acid (Gd-DTPA)–enhanced MR imaging of these damaged roots revealed increased uptake of contrast. In a clinical study of 50 patients with lumbar disc herniation, 42% underwent Gd-DTPA enhancement of the unaffected roots at the same level. The increased uptake is indicative of a breakdown of the blood-nerve barrier that is associated with intraradicular edema in symptomatic nerve roots.

Infectious Etiologies

Stirling and colleagues proposed that the inflammation involving the nerve root in patients with sciatica may be caused by microbial infection.[105] The infection is caused by low-virulence gram-positive microorganisms. An enzyme-linked immunosorbent assay (ELISA) was used to identify antibody to lipid S antigen from gram-positive organisms (*Propionibacterium acnes*, coagulase-negative staphylococci, *Corynebacterium propinquum*). In a group of 140 patients with sciatica, 43 (31%) had a positive ELISA test for lipid S antibody. In addition, positive bacterial cultures developed over a 7-day incubation period in 19 of 36 patients who underwent discectomy. Microorganisms were not detected in any Gram-stained section examined by direct microscopy, thus suggesting that they are present in low numbers. Discectomy samples from 14 control patients with other spinal disorders (scoliosis, trauma, myeloma) were culture negative. Low-virulence organisms are present in a minority of patients with radiculopathy. The majority of patients with sciatica are not infected. The presence of antibodies to lipid S is indicative of exposure to the associated organisms but is not specific for the site of colonization. These organisms are found in other locations (skin) that may be the cause of an antibody response. Just as with *Helicobacter pylori*, the presence of organisms in a location that they do not belong should not be dismissed. However, until more compelling data are amassed, antibiotics are not indicated for the treatment of radiculopathy.

CLINICAL HISTORY

Lumbar Spine

Clinically, the patient's major complaint is a sharp, lancinating pain. In many cases there may be a previous history of intermittent episodes of localized low back pain. The pain not only is present in the back but also radiates down the leg in the anatomic distribution of the affected nerve root. It will usually be described as deep and sharp and progressing from above downward in the involved leg. Its onset may be insidious or sudden and associated with a tearing or snapping sensation in the spine. Occasionally, when sciatica develops, the back pain may resolve because once the annulus has ruptured, it may no longer be under tension. Disc herniation occurs with sudden physical effort when the trunk is flexed or rotated. On occasion, patients with L4–L5 disc herniation have groin pain. In a study of 512 lumbar disc patients, 4.1% had groin pain.[123]

Finally, the sciatica may vary in intensity; it may be so severe that patients will be unable to ambulate and they will feel that their back is "locked." On the other hand, the pain may be limited to a dull ache that increases in intensity with ambulation. Pain is worsened in the flexed position and relieved by extension of the lumbar spine. Characteristically, patients with herniated discs have increased pain with sitting, driving, walking, coughing, sneezing, or straining.

Cervical Spine

Arm pain, not neck pain, is the patient's major complaint. The pain is often perceived as starting in the neck area and then radiating from this point down the shoulder, arm, and forearm and usually into the hand. The onset of the radicular pain is often gradual, although it can be sudden and occur in association with a tearing or snapping sensation. As time passes, the magnitude of the arm pain clearly exceeds that of the neck or shoulder pain. The arm pain may also be variable in intensity and preclude any use of the arm; it may range from severe pain to a dull, cramping ache in the arm muscles. The pain is usually severe enough to awaken the patient at night. Additionally, a patient may complain of associated headaches as well as muscle spasm, which can radiate from the cervical spine to below the scapulae. The pain may also radiate to the chest and mimic angina (pseudoangina) or to the breast.[12,66] Symptoms such as back pain, leg pain, leg weakness, gait disturbance, or incontinence suggest compression of the spinal cord.

PHYSICAL EXAMINATION

Lumbar Spine

Physical examination will demonstrate a decrease in range of motion of the lumbosacral spine, and patients may list to one side as they try to bend forward. The side of the disc herniation corresponds to the location of the scoliotic list. However, the specific level or degree of herniation does not correlate with the degree of list.[106] On ambulation, patients walk with an antalgic gait in which they hold the involved leg flexed so that they put as little weight as possible on the extremity.

Neurologic Examination

The neurologic examination is very important and may yield objective evidence of nerve root compression. It should be realized that in some cases, nerve root compression can cause pain but enough room is left for the root to function normally with no objective deficit. In addition, a nerve deficit may have little temporal relevance because it may be related to a previous attack at a different level. Compression of individual spinal nerve roots results in alterations in motor, sensory, and reflex function (see Table 5-1).

When the first sacral root is compressed, the patient may have gastrocnemius-soleus weakness and be unable to repeatedly raise up on the toes of that foot. Atrophy of the calf may be apparent, and the ankle (Achilles) reflex is often diminished or absent. Sensory loss, if present, is usually confined to the posterior aspect of the calf and the lateral side of the foot (see Fig. 3-14).

Involvement of the fifth lumbar nerve root can lead to weakness in extension of the great toe and, in a few cases, weakness of the everters and dorsiflexors of the foot. A sensory deficit can appear over the anterior of the leg and the dorsomedial aspect of the foot down to the great toe (see Fig. 3-13). Primary reflex changes do not generally occur, but on occasion, a diminution in the posterior tibial reflex can be elicited. There must be asymmetry in obtaining this reflex for it to have any clinical significance.

With compression of the fourth lumbar nerve root, the quadriceps muscle is affected; the patient may note weakness in knee extension, which is often associated with instability. Atrophy of the thigh musculature can be marked. Sensory loss may be apparent over the anteromedial aspect of the thigh, and the patellar tendon reflex can be diminished (see Fig. 3-12).

Sensory deficit on physical examination is used to identify the level of spinal nerve root compression. Nitta and co-workers identified the areas of sensory deficit associated with nerve blocks at three lumbar levels, L4, L5, and S1.[83] A total of 71 patients received 86 lumbar spinal nerve blocks. Characteristic areas of numbness were noted on the medial side of the lower part of the leg in 88% of L4 injections, the dorsum of the first digit in 82% of L5 injections, and the lateral aspect of the fifth digit in 83% of S1 injections. A continuous band of numbness was noted in the upper part of the thigh and buttock in 42% of L4, 44% of L5, and 92% of S1 injections. This investigation points out the fact that dermatomes may vary in a significant minority of patients and that L4 and L5 lesions may be associated with buttock and thigh dysesthesia.

Far lateral disc herniations constitute about 7% to 12% of all lumbar disc herniations.[32] The disc is far lateral or extraforaminal in location. The herniations occur at L3–L4 and L4–L5 in equal numbers, with sparing of L5–S1. The important difference in regard to the physical examination is the nerve root affected. Far lateral discs affect the superiorly situated nerve root. For example, an L4–L5 far lateral disc herniation affects the L4 nerve root.

Nerve root sensitivity can be elicited by any method that creates tension. The straight leg–raising (SLR) test is the one most commonly used. This test is performed with the patient supine. One of the examiner's hands is used to stabilize the pelvis while the other slowly raises the leg by the heel with the knee kept fully extended. The test is considered positive only if pain develops in the leg below the knee or if the patient's radicular symptomatology is reproduced. Back pain alone does not indicate a positive test. As noted in Chapter 5, many variations of this test have been described, and all can be useful as long as they are performed and interpreted correctly. One study correlated the location of the pain and the position of protrusion of the disc. Central protrusions cause back pain, lateral protrusions cause leg pain, and intermediate protrusions cause pain in both locations.[99] Although the SLR test is used as an important sign of nerve compression, the validity of the physical finding as an accurate reflection of an anatomic abnormality is not clear. Deville and co-workers reported on studies evaluating the SLR and the crossed SLR tests for the diagnosis of disc herniation with surgical confirmation.[28] The diagnostic accuracy of the SLR test is limited by its low specificity. Other tests are required to document the cause of radicular pain.

Cervical Spine

Physical examination of the neck usually shows some limitation of motion, and on occasion the patient may tilt the head in a cocked-robin position (torticollis) toward the side of the herniated cervical disc. Extension of the spine often exacerbates the pain as the intervertebral foramina are narrowed further (Spurling's sign). Axial compression, the Valsalva maneuver, and coughing may also exacerbate or re-create the pain pattern. Wainner and colleagues reported the clinical examination signs that identified patients with cervical radiculopathy.[114] The best test for differentiating radiculopathy and compartment neuropathy was the upper limb tension test, which re-creates the pain with scapula depression, shoulder abduction, forearm supination, wrist and finger extension, shoulder lateral rotation, and elbow extension.

Neurologic Examination

A neurologic examination that shows abnormalities is the most helpful aspect of the diagnostic work-up, although the examination may remain normal despite a chronic radicular pattern. Even when a deficit exists, it may not be temporally related to the present symptoms but to a previous attack at a different level. To be significant, the examination must show objective signs of reflex diminution, motor weakness, or atrophy. Manual muscle testing has greater specificity than reflex or sensory abnormalities do.[122] The presence of atrophy helps document the location of the lesion, as well as its chronicity. The presence of subjective sensory changes is often difficult to interpret and requires a coherent and cooperative patient to be of clinical value. Paresthesias are poorly localized because a number of nerve roots may result in a similar pain distribution. Slipman and co-workers administered cervical nerve blocks that demonstrated the distribution of sensory symptoms outside the classic dermatomal distribution.[101] The presence of sensory changes alone is not usually sufficient to confirm the presence and location of a disc herniation.

Compression of individual spinal nerve roots results in alterations in motor, sensory, and reflex function (Table 10-4). When the third cervical nerve root is compressed, no reflex change or motor weakness can be identified. The pain radiates to the back of the neck and toward the mastoid process and pinna of the ear.

Involvement of the fourth cervical nerve root leads to no readily detectable reflex changes or motor weakness. The pain radiates to the back of the neck and the superior aspect of the scapula. Occasionally, the pain radiates to the anterior chest wall. The pain is often exacerbated by neck extension.

Unlike the third and fourth cervical nerve roots, the fifth through eighth cervical nerve roots have motor functions. Compression of the fifth cervical nerve root is characterized by weakness of shoulder abduction, usually above 90 degrees, and weakness of shoulder extension. The biceps reflexes are often depressed and the pain radiates from the side of the neck to the top of the shoulder. Decreased sensation is often noted in the lateral aspect of the deltoid, which represents the autonomous innervation area of the axillary nerve.

Involvement of the sixth cervical nerve root produces biceps muscle weakness as well as a diminished brachioradialis reflex. The pain again radiates from the neck down the lateral aspect of the arm and forearm to the radial side of hand (index finger, long finger, and thumb). Numbness occurs occasionally in the tip of the index finger, the autonomous area of the sixth cervical nerve root.

Compression of the seventh cervical nerve root produces reflex changes in the triceps jerk test with associated loss of strength in the triceps muscles, which extend the elbow. The pain from this lesion radiates from the lateral aspect of the neck down the middle of the area to the middle finger. Sensory changes occur often in the tip of the middle finger, the autonomous area for the seventh nerve. Patients should also be tested for scapular winging, which may occur with C6 or C7 radiculopathy.[69]

Finally, involvement of the eighth cervical nerve root by a herniated C7–T1 disc produces significant weakness of the intrinsic musculature of the hand. Such involvement can lead to rapid atrophy of the interosseous muscles because of the small size of these muscles. Loss of the interossei leads to significant loss of fine hand motion. No reflexes are easily found, although the flexor carpi ulnaris reflex may be decreased. The radicular pain from the eighth cervical nerve root radiates to the ulnar border of the hand and the ring and little fingers. The tip of the little finger often demonstrates diminished sensation.

Nerve root sensitivity can be elicited by a method that increases tension on the nerve root. Radicular arm pain is often increased by the Valsalva maneuver or by directly compressing the head. Radicular pain secondary to a herniated cervical disc may be relieved by abduction of the affected arm.[4] Although these signs are helpful when present, their absence alone does not rule out a nerve root lesion.

Heckmann and co-workers reported a study of 119 consecutive patients with cervical intervertebral disc herniation and radiculopathy.[42] In this group 88.3% had acute symptoms and 11.7% had subacute or chronic symptoms. The common symptoms and signs associated with this group with cervical radiculopathy included brachialgia (98.3%), neck pain (93.3%), sensory deficits (88.3%), reflex abnormalities (61.7%), and motor weakness (51.7%).

LABORATORY DATA

Medical screening laboratory tests (blood counts, chemistry panels, erythrocyte sedimentation rate [ESR]) are normal in patients with a herniated disc.

Electrodiagnostic Testing

Electromyography (EMG) is an electronic extension of the physical examination. The primary use of EMG is to diagnose radiculopathy in cases of questionable neurologic origin. EMG findings may be positive in patients with nerve root impingement. Evidence of positive waves, giant

10-4 MOTOR, SENSORY, AND REFLEX DISTRIBUTION OF CERVICAL ROOTS

Interspace	Root	Motor Weakness	Sensory	Reflexes
C4–C5	C5	Deltoid, biceps Shoulder abduction External rotation	Axillary patch, proximal part of arm	Biceps (brachioradialis)
C5–C6	C6	Biceps, wrist extensors Elbow flexion (scapular winging)	Thumb, index finger	Brachioradialis
C6–C7	C7	Triceps Elbow extension Wrist and finger extension, pronation	Long finger, ring finger	Triceps
C7–T1	C8	Finger flexors Wrist flexors Thumb opposition Finger abduction	Little finger Hypothenar Medial part of forearm	Finger flexors

potentials, and insertional irritability suggests radiculopathy associated with significant nerve root impingement.[119] The EMG findings become much more significant in the presence of historical and physical findings consistent with herniation of a disc. Lower extremity somatosensory evoked potentials may be more sensitive than EMG in detecting abnormalities in patients who have sensory abnormalities alone.[115]

The degree of EMG abnormalities corresponds with the extent of nerve impingement. EMG findings associated with motor and sensory loss include higher thresholds, lower average amplitudes, and elongation of latency. Severe motor weakness for more than 6 months, a negative SLR test, and older age were considered to be poor prognostic factors for motor recovery.[71]

In the cervical spine, EMG and myelography correlate with the level of disc herniation in 77% to 90% of cases studied.[70,81] Although it is 80% to 90% accurate in establishing cervical radiculopathy as the cause of pain, false-negative results do occur. If cervical radiculopathy affects the sensory root only, EMG will be unable to demonstrate an abnormality. A false-negative examination also occurs if a patient with acute symptoms is examined early (4 to 28 days from the onset of symptoms). A normal study should be repeated in 2 to 3 weeks if symptoms persist.

RADIOGRAPHIC EVALUATION

Lumbar Spine

Roentgenograms

Plain roentgenograms may be entirely normal in a patient with symptoms and signs of nerve root impingement.

Computed Tomography

Radiographic evaluation by CT scan may demonstrate disc bulging but may not correlate with the level of nerve damage (Fig. 10-6).

Myelography

Myelographic evaluation is better for identifying the exact level of nerve root impingement (Fig. 10-7).[41,44,89]

Magnetic Resonance

MR imaging also allows visualization of soft tissues, including discs in the lumbar spine (Fig. 10-8).[76] Herniated discs are easily detected with MR evaluation (Figs. 10-9 and 10-10). MR imaging is a sensitive technique for the detection of far lateral and anterior disc herniations. Migratory fragments of discs that may be missed by other techniques are detectable by MR.[86] Contrast-enhanced MR imaging may also be able to detect inflammation of nerve roots by the uptake of contrast in neural structures in which the blood-brain barrier has been altered.[51] MR imaging has become the radiographic technique of choice for detecting the presence of a herniated intervertebral disc. However, the radiographic finding of a herniation only becomes important in the clinical setting of a patient who has historical and physical findings of radiculopathy. Boden and co-workers described MR abnormalities that are present in individuals who are asymptomatic.[7] Jensen and colleagues repeated this study by completing MR evaluations in 98 asymptomatic individuals.[50] Only 36% of these people (mean age, 42.3 years) had normal results. Fifty-two percent had a disc bulge at one level, 27% had a protrusion, and 1% had an extrusion. An abnormality at two levels or more was noted in 38%.

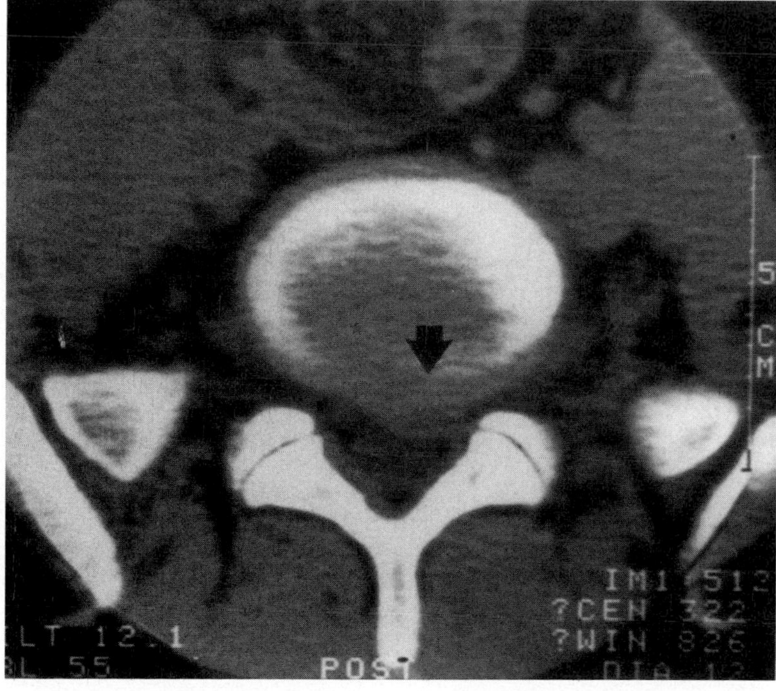

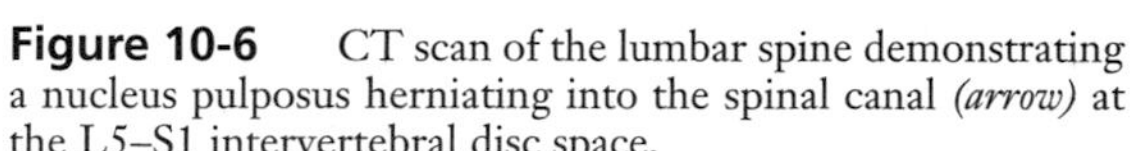
Figure 10-6 CT scan of the lumbar spine demonstrating a nucleus pulposus herniating into the spinal canal *(arrow)* at the L5–S1 intervertebral disc space.

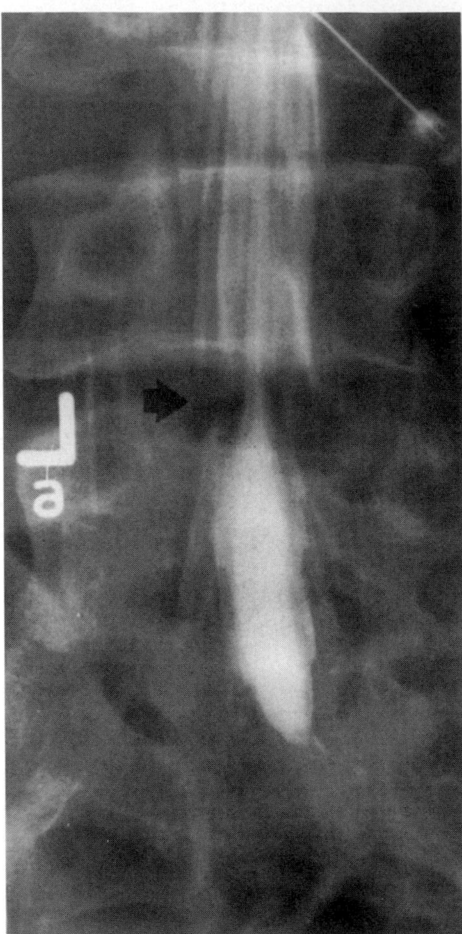

Figure 10-7 Lumbar myelogram with water-soluble dye demonstrating a large herniated nucleus pulposus (cutoff of the nerve root sleeves) at the L4–L5 intervertebral disc space *(arrow)*.

Boos and co-workers reported a prospective study of 46 patients with sciatica who required discectomy and 46 age-, sex-, and risk factor–matched asymptomatic volunteers.[10] Each group was evaluated by MR imaging and by psychosocial and work perception profiles. The goal of the study was to determine the best discriminating variables for the MR, work perception, and psychological categories to determine individuals with symptomatic disc disease. Disc herniation was present in 96% of the patient group and 76% of the asymptomatic group. The only key morphologic difference between both groups was the presence of neural compromise (83% versus 22%). Concerning work and psychosocial factors, mental stress, depression, and marriage were associated with increased symptoms. Risk factors such as heavy lifting, twisting, bending, vibration, and sedentary activity resulted in morphologic alterations but not symptoms of back pain. This study reinforces the previously reported finding of no correlation between the clinical symptom of radiculopathy and the radiographic presence of disc herniation in the absence of neural compression.

Borenstein and colleagues reported on a 7-year follow-up study of 50 asymptomatic patients with low back pain who underwent MR evaluation. In the original study of 67 patients, 31% of the test subjects had an identifiable abnormality. Of the 50 subjects who completed a questionnaire, 42% had back pain. Of these 21 individuals, 12 had normal findings, 5 had a herniated disc, 3 had stenosis, and 1 had disc degeneration. MR imaging was not predictive of the clinical symptoms associated with disc herniation.[13] Boos and co-workers completed a similar study of 46 asymptomatic individuals monitored for a 5-year period. Physical job characteristics were more powerful than MR abnormalities in predicting the need for low back pain–related therapy.[11] MR imaging with contrast is a

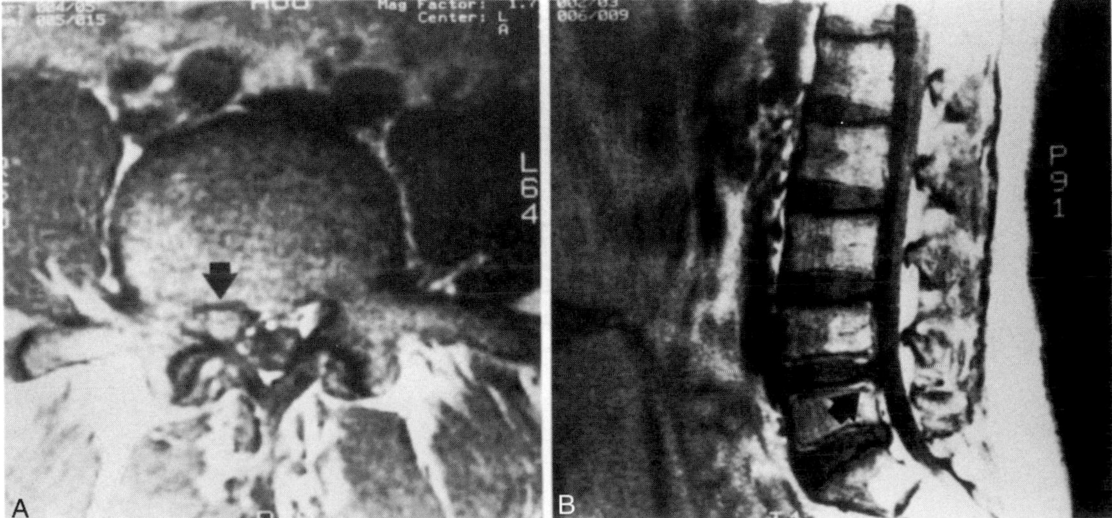

Figure 10-8 MR imaging of the lumbar spine: coronal *(A)* and sagittal *(B)* views. The scan demonstrated a herniated disc with protrusion into the spinal canal *(arrows)*.

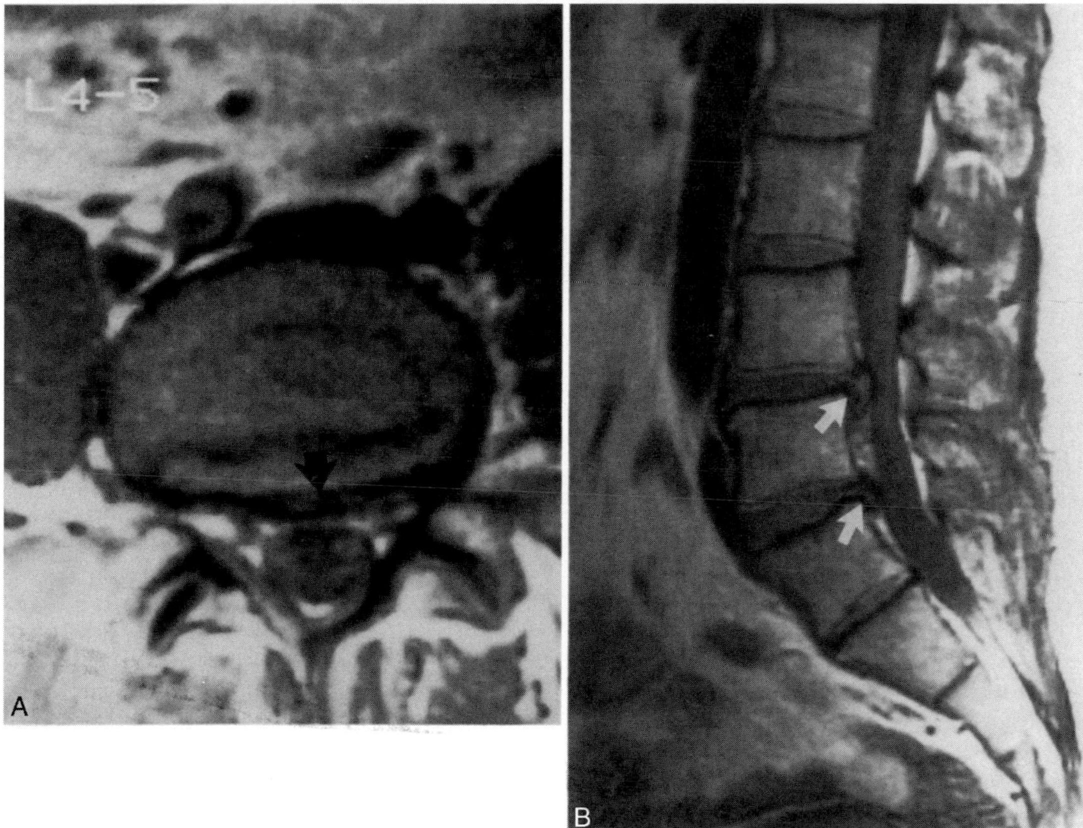

Figure 10-9 MR imaging of the lumbar spine: coronal *(A)* and sagittal *(B)* views of a 40-year-old man with chronic pain localized to the low back region. Radicular symptoms developed as well. The MR scan demonstrates a large herniated disc at the L4–L5 intervertebral disc space *(black arrow)*. The sagittal view reveals disc herniations at two disc levels *(white arrows)*.

sensitive technique for distinguishing between epidural scars and recurrent herniated discs in postoperative patients.[17,46]

Comparative Studies

A study by Albeck and associates compared myelography, CT, and MR imaging for detection of lumbar disc herniations confirmed at surgery.[2] In a study of 80 patients, MR and CT supplied greater diagnostic information than myelography did. MR is better at imaging soft tissue structures, whereas CT is superior for imaging bony structures. Myelography offers no advantages for the detection of lumbar intervertebral disc herniation.

Cervical Spine

Roentgenograms

Plain roentgenograms may be entirely normal in patients with an acute herniated cervical disc. Conversely, 70% of asymptomatic women and 95% of asymptomatic men between the ages of 60 and 65 years have evidence of degenerative disc disease on plain roentgenograms.[36] Views to be obtained include anteroposterior, lateral, flexion, and extension. Oblique views are optional because they increase the cost and radiation exposure without supplying significant additional information.[31] Plain roentgenograms may be used as an initial screening test for individuals who have failed conservative therapy, have sustained trauma to the cervical spine, or are 60 years or older with new symptoms of neck pain.

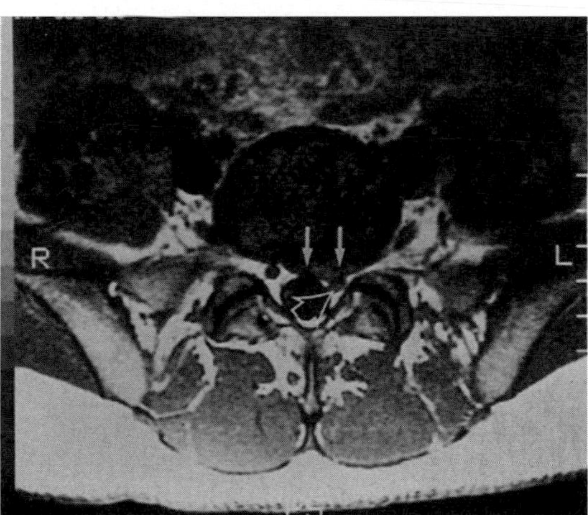

Figure 10-10 MR image of the lumbar spine. An axial view of the lumbar spine demonstrates a broad-based disc herniation *(small white arrows)* with impingement of the corresponding nerve root posteriorly *(black arrow)*. The patient had left radicular pain with a positive straight leg–raising test. His radiculopathy responded to conservative management.

Myelography

Additional radiographic studies are indicated for individuals who have myelopathic signs or progressive neurologic deficits, for those who have failed treatment, and for patients who are being considered for surgical intervention. Myelography identifies neural compression indirectly by changes in the contour of structures outlined by water-soluble contrast agents such as iohexol and iopamidol. This invasive procedure requires the introduction of dye through a lateral cisternal puncture at C1–C2. Myelography is able to visualize the entire length of the cervical spine and identify unsuspected abnormalities.[102] Myelography is useful for identifying the exact level of nerve root impingement. In a study of 53 patients with surgical confirmation of nerve compression, myelography accurately identified disc abnormalities in 85% of them.[5] Diagnostic inaccuracies occur as a result of small central disc protrusions and bone spurs. Cervical myelograms have been shown to be abnormal in 21% of asymptomatic individuals without neck or arm pain.[44]

Computed Tomography

CT permits direct visualization of compression of neural structures and is therefore more precise than myelography. Advantages of CT over myelography include better visualization of lateral abnormalities such as foraminal stenosis and abnormalities caudal to the myelographic block, less radiation exposure, and no hospitalization. From a surgical perspective, CT is best at distinguishing soft disc compression from hard bony compression.[25] Disadvantages of CT include the length of time to complete the study and changes in spinal configuration between motion segments. Myelographic dye may be injected and CT images obtained. A combination of the two studies gives excellent differentiation of bone and soft tissue lesions and allows direct demonstration of the spinal cord and the spinal canal dimensions. The CT-myelogram is accurate in 96% of cervical lesions.

Magnetic Resonance

MR imaging allows excellent visualization of soft tissues, including herniated discs in the cervical spine (Fig. 10-11). The test is noninvasive. In a study of 34 patients with cervical lesions, MR imaging predicted 88% of the surgically proven lesions versus 81% for myelography-CT, 58% for myelography, and 50% for CT alone.[15] Not all disc abnormalities detected by MR imaging are symptomatic. In a study of 63 asymptomatic individuals, 19% had MR abnormalities, including disc protrusion, that were identified by independent readings by three neuroradiologists.[7] This study highlights the importance of the correlation of clinical symptoms and signs with radiographic abnormalities. Exploratory MR imaging provides a significant opportunity to find anatomic abnormalities that have no correlation with clinical symptoms. MR imaging is the radiographic technique of choice for the evaluation of cervical radiculopathy to confirm the presence of anatomic changes that explain clinical findings. MR acquisition techniques (magnetization transfer) that allow for better delineation of disc herniation, foraminal stenosis, and intrinsic cord lesions continue to improve.[35]

MR findings have greater predictive value in the assessment of cervical radiculopathy than electrodiagnos-

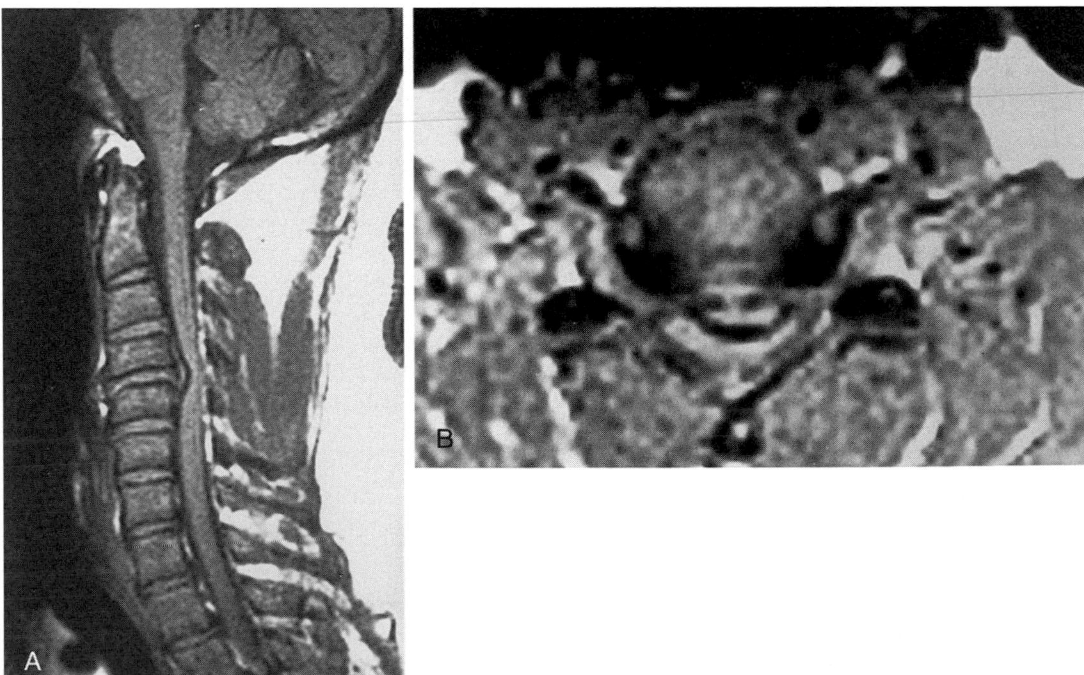

Figure 10-11 Herniated cervical disc in a 35-year-old man with left upper arm pain and decreased biceps reflex. MR scan of the cervical spine. *A*, A sagittal T1-weighted image demonstrates a large disc herniation compressing the spinal cord. The spinal cord is reduced to a 3-mm anteroposterior diameter. *B*, An axial T1-weighted image demonstrates central disc material compressing the spinal cord.

tic testing does.[3] The sensitivity of MR and electrodiagnostic testing for diagnosing cervical radiculopathy was 93% and 42%, respectively, in a study of 48 patients who underwent preoperative evaluation.

DIFFERENTIAL DIAGNOSIS

Lumbar Spine

The initial diagnosis of a herniated disc is ordinarily made on the basis of the history and physical examination (see Table 10-2). Plain radiographs of the lumbosacral spine will rarely add to the diagnosis but should be obtained to help rule out other causes of pain such as infection or tumor. Other tests such as MR, CT, and myelography are confirmatory by nature and can be misleading when used as screening tests.

Spinal Stenosis

Patients with spinal stenosis may also suffer from back pain that radiates to the lower extremities.[113] Patients with spinal stenosis tend to be older than those in whom herniated discs develop. Characteristically, patients with spinal stenosis experience lower extremity pain (pseudoclaudication) after walking for an unspecified distance. They also complain of pain that is exacerbated by standing or extending the spine. Radiographic evaluation is usually helpful in differentiating individuals with disc herniation from those with bony hypertrophy associated with spinal stenosis. In a study of 1293 patients, lateral spinal stenosis and herniated intervertebral discs coexisted in 17.7% of individuals. Radicular pain may be caused by more than one pathologic process in an individual.[6]

Facet Syndrome

Facet syndrome is another cause of low back pain that may be associated with radiation of pain to structures outside the confines of the lumbosacral spine.[77] Degeneration of articular structures in the facet joint causes pain to develop. In most circumstances, the pain is localized over the area of the affected joint and is aggravated by extension of the spine (standing). A deep, ill-defined, aching discomfort may also be noted in the sacroiliac joint, the buttocks, and the legs. The areas of sclerotome affected show the same embryonic origin as the degenerated facet joint. A direct association between facet joint disease and production of pain is questioned by some investigators. Many individuals with arthritic changes in their facet joints visible on radiographic evaluation experience no symptoms. Patients with pain secondary to facet joint disease may have relief of symptoms with apophyseal injection of a long-acting local anesthetic.[33] The true role of facet joint disease in the production of back and leg pain remains to be determined.

Other mechanical causes of sciatica include congenital abnormalities of the lumbar nerve roots, external compression of the sciatic nerve (wallet in a back pants pocket), and muscular compression of the nerve (piriformis syndrome). In rare circumstances, cervical or thoracic cord compression can mimic the clinical signs and symptoms of lumbar radiculopathy. A cervical or thoracic lesion should be considered if the lumbar spine is clear of abnormalities.[49] Medical causes of sciatica (neural tumors or infections, for example) are usually associated with systemic symptoms in addition to nerve pain in a sciatic distribution.

Cervical Spine

No diagnostic criteria exist for the clinical diagnosis of a herniated cervical disc.[114] The provisional diagnosis of a herniated cervical disc is made by the history and physical examination. Individuals who frequently lift heavy objects on the job, smoke, or often dive from a diving board are at increased risk for cervical disc herniation.[57] Interventional radiologists and cardiologists are at risk for cervical and multilevel disc disease. In a survey of 714 cardiologists, orthopedic surgeons, and rheumatologists, interventional cardiologists reported more neck and back pain, more days lost from work, and a higher incidence of cervical disc herniation and multiple-level disc disease (all $P < 0.01$).[92] The plain roentgenogram is usually nondiagnostic, although occasionally disc space narrowing at the suspected interspace or foraminal narrowing on oblique films is seen. The value of roentgenograms is to exclude other causes of neck and arm pain, such as infection and tumor. MR imaging and CT-myelography are the best confirmatory examinations for disc herniation.

Cervical disc herniations may affect structures other than nerve roots. Disc herniation may cause vessel compression (vertebral artery) associated with vertebrobasilar artery insufficiency and be manifested as blurred vision and dizziness.[16] Nerve root compression secondary to disc herniation may be mimicked by anomalous vessels. Expansion of vertebral arteries in transverse foramina may compress contiguous nerve roots.[29]

Other mechanical causes of arm pain should be excluded. The most common is some form of compression on a peripheral nerve. Such compression can occur at the elbow, forearm, or wrist. An example is compression of the median nerve by the carpal ligament leading to carpal tunnel syndrome. The best diagnostic test to rule out these peripheral neuropathies is EMG. Excessive traction on the arm secondary to heavy weights may cause radicular pain without disc compression of nerve roots.[67] Spinal cord abnormalities must be considered if signs of myelopathy are present in conjunction with radiculopathy. Spinal cord lesions such as syringomyelia are identified by MR imaging, and motor neuron disease is identified by EMG. Multiple sclerosis should be considered in a patient with radiculopathy if the physical signs indicate lesions above the foramen magnum (optic neuritis).[88] In very rare circumstances, lesions of the parietal lobe corresponding to the arm can mimic the findings of cervical radiculopathy.[24]

TREATMENT

Natural History

Komori and colleagues reported a study of repeat MR scans completed at an interval of 150 days in 77 patients with disc herniation treated by nonsurgical therapy.[61] Clinical improvement occurred in 50% of the patients at follow-up before MR-detected improvement in disc herniation. Sequestrated discs that migrated from the source disc had a greater decrease in size in the extruded portion than the protruded portion. In seven patients, the migrating portion of the disc was totally resorbed.

In a subsequent study, Komori and co-workers studied the use of contrast-enhanced MR imaging in predicting the outcome of conservative management of herniated intervertebral discs.[62] Forty-eight patients with historical and physical findings of lumbar radiculopathy underwent two or more gadolinium-enhanced MR evaluations at a mean interval of 191 days. Discs were classified as extruded (disc stalk < disc height at that level) or migrated (disk stalk > disc height). Contrast-enhanced MR imaging revealed greater uptake at initial and follow-up studies in migrating discs than extruded discs. A greater degree of enhancement, with involvement within the migrating piece, correlated with improvement in radiculopathy. In 22 cases of migrating discs with enhancement, 9 disc fragments disappeared and 7 were markedly decreased. Of the 22 patients, 17 had good outcomes. Five patients had no change in enhancement of the migrated fragment. Of these five patients, three required surgery. For the extruded discs of 26 patients, 20 had initial enhancement, with 15 showing enlargement on repeat study. Of these 15 individuals, 8 had some decrease in disc size and 7 had no change. In this total group of 15, 13 had a good ($n = 11$) or excellent ($n = 2$) outcome. In those with no increased enhancement ($n = 5$) or no initial enhancement ($n = 6$), nine had a poor outcome.

Mochida and associates replicated the natural history Komori study in patients with cervical disc herniation.[75] Thirty-eight patients with cervical radiculopathy underwent MR imaging on more than one occasion. Regression of the intervertebral disc herniation occurred in 40% of individuals. The location and type of disc herniation played a role in the subsequent resorption. Sequestrated discs exposed to vasculature in the epidural space were more likely to recede in size than subligamentous herniations were. The authors suggest that nonsurgical treatment is appropriate for sequestrated discs even in the setting of motor weakness. Bush and co-workers also reported a group of patients with cervical radiculopathy who had resolution of disc herniations.[18] MR scans were repeated at 12 months in patients who were asymptomatic at 6 months. Twelve of 13 patients had total resolution of the disc herniation. One patient with a herniation that had not regressed suffered from persistent minor symptoms.

Nonoperative Therapy

Treatment for most patients with a herniated disc is nonoperative inasmuch as 80% of them will respond to conservative therapy when monitored over a period of 5 years.[117] The efficacy of nonoperative treatment, however, depends on a healthy relationship between a capable physician and a well-informed patient. If patients have insight into the rationale for the prescribed treatment and follow instructions, the chances for success are greatly increased.

Controlled Physical Activity

The primary element in the nonoperative treatment of acute disease is controlled physical activity.[118] For the first several days in the acute situation, bed rest may be necessary and can usually be accomplished at home. The semi-Fowler position with hips and knees comfortably flexed is ideal because it keeps intradiscal pressure down and reduces nerve root tension. After the first few days, the patient should be gradually mobilized. Walking should be encouraged, whereas sitting is prohibited because it causes excessive pressure on the nerve root.

NSAIDs/Corticosteroids

Drug therapy is another important part of the treatment, and three categories of pharmacologic agents are commonly used: anti-inflammatory drugs, analgesics, and muscle relaxants or tranquilizers. Inasmuch as symptoms of low back pain and sciatica result from an inflammatory reaction, as well as mechanical compression, anti-inflammatory medications are indicated. Adequate doses of aspirin have been found to work quite well, although other nonsteroidal anti-inflammatory drugs (NSAIDs) are frequently used. The patient's pain will generally be relieved once the inflammation is brought under control. Residual numbness or tingling in the involved extremity may be present but is usually tolerable. Some patients who fail to respond to anti-inflammatory medication may get dramatic relief from a short course of systemic steroids administered in decreasing dosages over a period of weeks. The initial dose of corticosteroid is 20 mg/day of prednisone. Prednisone is continued with the other nonsteroidal medications. The dose is maintained at 20 mg while the patient is monitored for resolution of radiculopathy. The prednisone is gradually tapered over weeks as the signs of radiculopathy resolve (pain, numbness). If the patient has no response to the prednisone, use of the medication is discontinued at the end of 6 weeks.

Dyck and co-workers used intravenous methylprednisolone for lumbosacral radiculopathy.[30] In 11 nondiabetic patients with lumbar radiculopathy, 10 received infusions of intravenous methylprednisolone (1 g/wk) for 16 weeks and 1 received the equivalent dosage of oral prednisone. This dose of steroids was effective in all 11 patients. The concern is the long-term effects of such a large dose of corticosteroids. The toxicity is likely to outweigh the benefits with large, prolonged doses of methylprednisolone.

Analgesics

Analgesic medication is administered to control pain if it is severe. Codeine is recommended for home use. If codeine does not work, hospitalization should be considered so that a stronger analgesic medication such as morphine sulfate can be strictly controlled. Long-term use of narcotics for these patients should be modified as the radiculopathy resolves.

Muscle Relaxants

Muscle relaxants are used in patients with uncontrolled muscle contraction associated with nerve impingement.

The mechanism of action of these agents is unknown. Most agents, other than diazepam, do not act directly on muscle fibers but act on the central nervous system by diminishing reflex contractions. The beneficial effects of this group of drugs were thought to be related to their tranquilizing properties. In a study reported by Borenstein and Korn, the efficacy of cyclobenzaprine at 5 mg was not associated with the presence or absence of somnolence.[13a] In patients with severe muscle spasm, muscle relaxants do appear to be effective. It should be remembered, however, that the use of diazepam for muscle spasm should be discouraged. When used on a chronic basis, diazepam may become a depressant. Diazepam will only add to the psychological problems of patients with chronic pain. If other muscle relaxants without depressant properties are used from the outset, the problems related to depression, tolerance, and addiction can be prevented.

Injection Therapy

Epidural corticosteroid injections are useful for patients with radiculopathy.[13b] Injections should be considered for patients with radiculopathy who are not responding to modified activities, NSAID therapy, and muscle relaxants. Carette and co-workers studied the efficacy of epidural corticosteroid injections for sciatica secondary to herniated nucleus pulposus.[19] Over a 40-month period, 78 patients with sciatica and a herniated disc received three epidural injections consisting of 80 mg of methylprednisolone acetate, and 80 control patients received 1 mL of saline. At 3 weeks, the Oswestry disability score improved in the steroid group in comparison to controls. The corticosteroid patients also had greater improvement in finger-to-floor distance and sensory deficits. At 6 weeks, leg pain was less in the steroid group. At 3 months, no significant differences were found between the groups. The rate of withdrawal from the study was 5% in the steroid group and 14% in the control group. At 12 months, the cumulative probability of having back surgery was 25.8% in the corticosteroid group versus 24.8% with placebo. The surgery rates in this study were greater than the 10% to 15% usually reported in the literature. This increased surgery rate suggests that the patients in this study had more severe disease than the average patient with disc herniation and radiculopathy.

Nerve root injections are another form of nonoperative therapy for lumbar radicular pain. Riew and associates reviewed the benefits of up to four injections of bupivacaine and betamethasone or bupivacaine alone in the decision to proceed with operative treatment of lumbar radiculopathy.[90] Of the 27 who received bupivacaine alone, 9 elected to forego surgery. Of the 28 who received both drugs in their injections, 20 elected to forego surgery. The difference in operative rates between the two groups was significant ($P < 0.004$). The benefits lasted up to 28 months. In a study of 48 patients, fluoroscopically guided transforaminal corticosteroid injections had a success rate of 84% versus 48% in those receiving trigger point injections.[111] The benefits lasted up to 16 months after injection.

Tumor Necrosis Factor Inhibitors

TNF inhibitors show promise as therapy for patients with radiculopathy secondary to a herniated disc. In animal models of disc herniation and spinal nerve inflammation, TNF is located at the site of nerve damage.[48] TNF is produced by nucleus pulposus cells. Exogenous TNF produces neuropathologic alterations (wallerian degeneration of nerve fibers, macrophage recruitment to phagocytize the debris, and splitting of the myelin sheath) similar to those induced by herniated nucleus pulposus.[85] Etanercept, a TNF inhibitor, has reversed disc-induced porcine nerve conduction block by reversing edema and thrombosis.[85] With this background in mind, Karppinen and co-authors reported on a 3-month follow-up study of 10 patients with disc herniation and radiculopathy treated with a single infusion of 3 mg/kg of infliximab.[55] At 2 weeks, the open-label study demonstrated that 60% of the patients were painless versus 16% of historical controls. The differences were sustained at 3 months. By 1 month, every patient in the infliximab group returned to work. In an abstract presentation at 1 year, the beneficial effects of the single effusion continued.[63] Only 1 of the 10 patients underwent a decompression operation. This study is an open-label investigation without appropriate controls. A double-blind, placebo-controlled trial is under way to determine the true efficacy of TNF inhibitors. Treatment of sciatica will be significantly modified if a single infusion is effective in decreasing pain and improving function as measured by return to work.

Surgical Intervention

Surgical intervention is reserved for patients in whom conservative therapy fails. Patients with radicular pain, abnormal physical findings, and confirmatory radiographic tests are candidates for surgical intervention. The indications for surgery are listed in Chapter 20.

Cauda Equina Syndrome

Cauda equina syndrome is associated with compression of the spinal nerve roots that supply neurologic function to the bladder and bowel. Rapid diagnosis and decompression of this abnormality are essential to prevent permanent neurologic dysfunction. In a study of 44 patients with urologic problems of retention, incontinence, or saddle anesthesia, the syndrome developed in 39 in less than 24 hours.[98] MR imaging in 23 patients or CT in 21 patients identified nerve compression with massive disc herniation. Surgery was performed in 20 patients within 48 hours, whereas 24 patients underwent surgery after 48 hours, with a mean delay of 9 days. Delay in surgery beyond 48 hours was associated with persistent severe motor deficit, persistent sciatica, and sexual dysfunction. Cauda equina requires emergency diagnosis and surgical decompression within a 48-hour period to decrease the risk of permanent neurologic sequelae. Kennedy and co-workers also described a group of patients with cauda equina syndrome.[58] Patients with a poor outcome were those who had perineal sensory loss and urinary dysfunction. The 14 of 19 patients who had a good outcome after surgical decompression had the operation within 14 hours, whereas those with a poor outcome underwent surgery within 30 hours. Cauda equina lesions can cause neural impingement.[120] Many of these lesions are neoplasms (benign and malignant), such as ependymomas, nerve sheath tumors, meningiomas, and lipomas. A variety of symptoms were seen, including bilateral lower extremity weakness and tenderness. No specific relationship exists between pathologic diagnosis and symptoms.

Cervical Spine

Treatment of most patients with a herniated cervical disc is nonoperative because most respond to conservative treatment for 2 to 3 months. The efficacy of the nonoperative approach depends heavily on the physician-patient relationship. If a patient is well informed, insightful, and willing to follow instructions, the chances for a successful nonoperative outcome are greatly improved.

The cornerstone of management of a herniated cervical disc is rest and immobilization. The use of a cervical orthosis greatly increases the likelihood that the patient will rest. Initially, the patient should remain at home resting in bed except for necessary trips to the bathroom.[20] Controlled physical activity should be maintained for at least 2 weeks, and the patient should wear the cervical orthosis at all times. The Philadelphia collar is a plastic collar that offers greater support for individuals with cervical radiculopathy. Careful fitting is required in the suboccipital, submental, and sternal areas to maximize inhibition of lower cervical motion.[108] After the acute pain begins to abate, the patient should gradually increase activity and decrease use of the orthosis. Most people are able to return to work in a month in a light-duty capacity.

NSAIDs

Drug therapy is an important adjunct to controlled physical activity and immobilization. Anti-inflammatory medications, analgesics, and muscle relaxants have been used in the acute management of these patients. Because it is commonly believed that radicular pain is in part secondary to inflammation of the nerve root, the use of aspirin or other NSAIDs is appropriate.[93] All these medications have gastrointestinal side effects but are generally well tolerated for brief periods. If NSAIDs are required for longer periods, medications such as prostaglandin analogues are available to protect the gastrointestinal tract in individuals who have had a previous history of gastric ulcers. Oral systemic corticosteroids administered in a tapering dosage for 7 days may provide relief in more refractory cases but should not be used routinely.[31]

Injection Therapy

A trigger point injection may give dramatic relief of referred muscle pain. Epidural corticosteroid injections have been shown to improve cervical radicular pain. In a study of 16 patients, improvement of pain occurred in 12, with improvement in neurologic signs developing in 6 of the same patients.[116] Cervical epidural injections are most beneficial in individuals with radicular pain as opposed to those with axial pain.[34] Epidural corticosteroid injections may also be helpful in decreasing pain in patients with cervical radicular pain lasting 12 months or longer.[21] A lateral approach to injection therapy may likewise be effective for cervical radiculopathy. In radiculopathy patients who fail other therapies, the lateral percutaneous approach under fluoroscopic guidance is a method to inject periradicular corticosteroids. Improvement can be documented by 14 days and may be sustained for 6 months.[112]

Analgesic medication is only rarely needed if the patient is compliant and approaches full bed rest with nearly total immobility; however, if the pain is severe enough, a brief course of oral codeine may be prescribed. If the patient is resistant to oral narcotic therapy, inpatient hospitalization for intramuscular narcotics may be required in rare circumstances. Muscle relaxants and benzodiazepines have tranquilizing and central nervous system depressant properties. As such, they have at best a limited role in the management of patients with an acute herniated disc. Although it is true that benzodiazepines help the patient relax and ensure rest, the potential for an additive effect on the patient's psychosocial problems is not worth the long-term risk for the short-term gain.

Cervical traction is used to distract the interspace associated with disc herniation. Weights of up to 50 pounds are applied for periods of up to 60 seconds with the head flexed. Traction instruction is usually given by a physical therapist, and the traction may be applied by the patient at home. Traction is used for 15-minute sessions up to three times a day for 4 to 6 weeks. Although the efficacy of traction has not been proved, it is commonly used and thought to be of benefit.[31]

Surgical therapy for cervical herniation is appropriate for patients who have failed nonoperative therapy. Sampath and co-workers reported on 246 patients with radiculopathy.[96] Of 155 patients, 51 (33%) underwent surgery. Of the patients who underwent surgery, 26% had persistent excruciating pain. Surgical therapy is helpful in a large number of patients, but a significant minority will have persistent symptoms. Patients who undergo surgery may obtain more rapid resolution of symptoms. However, at 12 months, patients treated with physiotherapy or cervical collars will have similar improvement.[87]

PROGNOSIS

Eighty percent of those who follow the aforementioned regimen will be markedly improved.[79] Although noninvasive treatment of a herniated disc can be quite gratifying, it generally takes a significant period of controlled physical activity to improve. Patients must be aware of the time constraints from the onset of therapy to understand the rationale of the measures used.

Lumbar Spine

A prospective study of 11 patients with disc extrusions and radiculopathy monitored the course of symptoms from 8 to 77 months. The extruded portion of the disc is resorbed without any need for surgical removal. All 11 patients had a decrease in neural impingement.[94] Surgical therapy is required for only a very small number of individuals with a herniated disc.

Davis reported on a 32-year experience in 984 patients who underwent surgical decompression for herniated lumbar discs.[25a] The mean follow-up period was 10.8 years. Back pain with sciatica was the primary symptom in 81% of the patients. Herniated discs at L4–L5 and L5–S1 occurred with equal frequency (47%). In 89% of patients, the outcome was good as measured by economic and functional status. The recurrence rate of disc herniation was 6%, with about 33% occurring within the first postoperative year. Complications, primarily wound infection, developed in 4% of patients, without any operative deaths. The poor outcome in over 50% was associated with pending workers' compensation or liability claims.

Silvers and colleagues reported on the clinical characteristics and surgical outcome of 15 patients younger than 21 years who had herniated lumbar discs.[100] The physical findings of neurologic deficits were not as predominant as detected in older individuals with herniated discs. Surgical intervention in these individuals who failed nonoperative therapy was successful in decreasing leg pain in 85% and back pain in 75% after 10.5 years of follow-up. Discectomy without fusion is a reasonable choice of therapy with no increased risk for young patients who fail nonoperative therapy.

Cervical Spine

The majority of patients respond to nonoperative treatment. Even patients with MR-documented herniated cervical discs may have regression of the disc with conservative therapy.[64] Once these patients improve, they should be maintained on a graduated isometric neck exercise program. Saal and co-authors reported on the benefits of nonsurgical therapy in 26 consecutive patients with herniated cervical discs.[95] Management included traction, specific physical therapeutic exercises, NSAIDs, and patient education. Twenty patients responded well to the nonoperative therapy. Only two patients underwent cervical spine surgery. One in five patients fail conservative measures and require a surgical procedure. If performed with good surgical technique and for the correct clinical indications, surgery is successful in more than 90% of patients. Anterior discectomy with fusion results in excellent outcomes in 94% of patients.[43]

In the 60 patients reported by Heckmann and coworkers, 39 (65%) underwent nonoperative therapy (COG, conservative therapy) and 21 (35%) had surgical intervention (SOG, surgery) for a herniated cervical disc.[42] Brachialgia was essentially improved in 100% of the COG patients and 95.1% of the SOG patients. Sensory deficits remitted markedly in 97% of the COG and 75% of the SOG patients. Reflex abnormalities normalized in 59.2% of the COG and 53.3% of the SOG patients. Motor weakness improved in 94% of the COG and 50% of the SOG patients. Neck pain improved in only 36.1% of the COG and 20% of the SOG patients. In a self-rating scale, 89.7% had full function in the COG group whereas 66.7% had similar function in the SOG group. The patients who received surgical therapy had more severe and long-lasting neurologic disturbances at evaluation. Nonoperative therapy is appropriate and effective for a significant proportion of patients with cervical radiculopathy.

Surgical therapy for cervical disc herniation may have a better outcome than surgery for lumbar disc herniation in the setting of workers' compensation. In a study at the Portsmouth Naval Base from 1993 to 1995, 269 individuals underwent cervical operations and were monitored for application for disability.[54] The control for the lumbar surgeries was taken from historical records from the same naval base. Only 16% (43/269) of cervical patients received disability, whereas 24.7% (86/348) of lumbar patients had a poor result. Individuals with multilevel surgery and revision operations at the same level requested discharge more frequently.

Postdiscectomy Infections

Postdiscectomy infection is a rare, but difficult diagnostic problem. The findings on MR scan may be helpful in differentiating patients with postoperative healing versus infection. A report by Boden and co-workers suggested that the triad of intervertebral disc space and annular and vertebral body enhancement with gadolinium-enhanced MR imaging was associated with disc space infection.[8] Ross and colleagues evaluated preoperative and postoperative MR scans in 94 lumbar discectomy patients.[91] Of the 94 patients, 19 (20%) had postoperative intervertebral disc enhancement characterized by linear enhancement manifested as two thin bands paralleling the endplates. Endplate enhancement occurred in seven (37%) patients with disc enhancement. No relationship between disc enhancement and clinical symptoms was found. The report by Ross and co-authors suggests that the triad of enhancement is important only for a diagnosis of infectious discitis in the appropriate clinical setting of increased low back pain, fever, leukocytosis, or an elevated ESR or C-reactive protein.

References

Acute Herniated Nucleus Pulposus

1. Adams MA, Dolan P, Hutton WC, Porter RW: Diurnal changes in spinal mechanics and their clinical significance. J Bone Joint Surg Br 72-B:266, 1990.
2. Albeck MJ, Hilden J, Kjaer L, et al: A controlled comparison of myelography, computed tomography, and magnetic resonance imaging in clinically suspected lumbar disc herniation. Spine 20:443-448, 1995.
3. Ashkan K, Johnston P, Moore AJ: A comparison of magnetic resonance imaging and neurophysiological studies in the assessment of cervical radiculopathy. Br J Neurosurg 16:146-148, 2002.
4. Beatty RM, Fowler FD, Hanson EJ Jr: The abducted arm as a sign of ruptured cervical disc. Neurosurgery 21:731, 1987.
5. Bell GR, Ross JS: The accuracy of imaging studies of the degenerative cervical spine: Myelography, myelo-computed tomography, and magnetic resonance imaging. Semin Spine Surg 7:9, 1995.
6. Bernard TN Jr, Kirkaldy-Willis WH: Recognizing specific characteristics of nonspecific low back pain. Clin Orthop 217:266, 1987.

7. Boden SD, Davis DO, Dina TS, et al: Abnormal magnetic-resonance scans of the lumbar spine in asymptomatic subjects: A prospective investigation. J Bone Joint Surg Am 72-A:403, 1990.
8. Boden SD, Davis DO, Dina TS, et al: Postoperative discitis: Distinguishing early MR imaging findings from normal postoperative disk changes. Radiology 184:765-771, 1992.
9. Bogduk N, Windsor M, Inglis A: The innervation of the cervical intervertebral discs. Spine 13:2, 1988.
10. Boos N, Rieder R, Schade V, et al: The diagnostic accuracy of magnetic resonance imaging, work perception, and psychological factors in identifying symptomatic disc herniation. Spine 24:2613-2625, 1995.
11. Boos N, Semmer N, Elfering A, et al: Natural history of individuals with asymptomatic disc abnormalities in magnetic resonance imaging: Predictors of low back pain–related medical consultation and work incapacity. Spine 25:1484-1492, 2000.
12. Booth RE Jr, Rothman RH: Cervical angina. Spine 1:28, 1976.
13. Borenstein DG, O'Mara JW, Boden SD, et al: The value of magnetic resonance imaging of the lumbar spine to predict low back pain in asymptomatic subjects: A seven-year follow-up study. J Bone Joint Surg Am 83-A:1306-1311, 2001
13a. Borenstein DG, Korn S: Efficacy of a low-dose regimen of cyclobenzaprine hydrochloride in acute skeletal muscle spasm: Results of two placebo-controlled trials. Clin Ther 25:1056-1073, 2003.
13b. Borenstein D: Are epidural corticosteroid injections effective for sciatica? Curr Prac Med 1:19-21, 1998.
14. Broom MJ: Foraminal and extraforaminal lumbar disk herniations. Clin Orthop 289:118, 1993.
15. Brown BM, Schwartz RH, Frank E, Blank NK: Preoperative evaluation of cervical radiculopathy and myelopathy by surface-coil MR imaging. AJNR Am J Neuroradiol 9:859, 1988.
16. Budway RJ, Senter HJ: Cervical disc rupture causing vertebrobasilar insufficiency. Neurosurgery 33:745, 1993.
17. Bundschuh CV, Stein L, Slusser JH, et al: Distinguishing between scar and recurrent herniated disk in postoperative patients: Value of contrast-enhanced CT and MR imaging. AJNR Am J Neuroradiol 11:949, 1990.
18. Bush K, Chaudhuri R, Hillier S, et al: The pathomorphologic changes that accompany the resolution of cervical radiculopathy. A prospective study with repeat magnetic resonance imaging. Spine 22:183-186, 1997.
19. Carette S, LeClaire R, Marcoux S et al: Epidural corticosteroid injections for sciatica due to herniated nucleus pulposus. N Engl J Med 336:1634-1640, 1997.
20. Carlsson C, Nachemson A: Surgical treatment of neck pain. In Nachemson AL, Jonsson E (eds): Neck And Back Pain: The Scientific Evidence of Causes, Diagnosis, and Treatment. Philadelphia, Lippincott Williams & Wilkins, 2000, p 355.
21. Castagnera L, Maurette P, Pointillart V, et al: Long-term results of cervical epidural steroid injection with and without morphine in chronic cervical radicular pain. Pain 58:239, 1994.
22. Chabot MC, Montgomery DM: The pathophysiology of axial and radicular neck pain. Semin Spine Surg 7:2, 1995.
23. Chen TY: The clinical presentation of uppermost cervical disc protrusion. Spine 25:439-442, 2000.
24. Clar SA, Cianca JC: Intracranial tumor masquerading as cervical radiculopathy: A case study. Arch Phys Med Rehabil 79:1301-1302, 1998.
25. Coin CG: Cervical disc degeneration and herniation: Diagnosis by computerized tomography. South Med J 77:979, 1984.
25a. Davis RA: A long-term outcome analysis of 984 surgically treated herniated lumbar discs. J Neurosurg 80:415-421, 1994.
26. Debois V, Herz R, Berghmans D, et al: Soft cervical disc herniation: Influence of cervical spinal canal measurements on development of neurologic symptoms. Spine 24:1996-2002, 1999.
27. DePalma A, Rothman RH: The Intervertebral Disc. Philadelphia, WB Saunders, 1970.
28. Deville WLJM, van der Windt DAWM, Dzaferagic A, et al: The test of Lasegue: Systematic review of the accuracy in diagnosing herniated disc. Spine 25:1140-1147, 2000.
29. Duthel R, Tudor C, Motuo-Fotso M, Brunon J: Cervical root compression by a loop of the vertebral artery: Case report. Neurosurgery 35:140, 1994.
30. Dyck PJ, Norell JE, Dyck PJ: Methylprednisolone may improve lumbosacral radiculoplexus neuropathy. Can J Neurol Sci 28:224-227, 2001.
31. Ellenberg MR, Honet JC, Treanor WJ: Cervical radiculopathy. Arch Phys Med Rehabil 75:342, 1994.
32. Epstein NE: Foraminal and far lateral lumbar disc herniation: Surgical alternatives and outcome measures. Spinal Cord 40:491-500, 2002.
33. Fairbank JCT, Park WM, McCall IW, O'Brien JP: Apophyseal injection of local anesthetic as a diagnostic aid in primary low-back pain. Spine 6:598, 1981.
34. Ferrante FM, Wilson SP, Iacobo C, et al: Clinical classification as a predictor of therapeutic outcome after cervical epidural steroid injection. Spine 18:730, 1993.
35. Finelli DA, Hurst GC, Karaman BA, et al: Use of magnetization transfer for improved contrast on gradient-echo MR images of the cervical spine. Radiology 193:165, 1994.
36. Gore DR, Sepic SB, Gardner GM: Roentgenographic findings of the cervical spine in asymptomatic people. Spine 11:521, 1986.
37. Goupille P, Jayson MI, Valat JP, et al: The role of inflammation in disk herniation–associated radiculopathy. Semin Arthritis Rheum 28:60-71, 1998.
38. Groen GJ, Baljet B, Drukker J: Nerves and nerve plexuses of the human vertebral column. Am J Anat 188:282, 1990.
39. Harada Y, Nakahara S: A pathologic study of lumbar disc herniation in the elderly. Spine 14:1020, 1989.
40. Haro H, Crawford HC, Fingleton B, et al: Matrix metalloproteinase-7–dependent release of tumor necrosis factor alpha in a model of herniated disc resorption. J Clin Invest 105:143-150, 2000.
41. Haughton VM, Eldevik OP, Magnaes B, Amundsen P: A prospective companion of computed tomography and myelography in diagnosis of herniated lumbar disks. Radiology 142:103, 1982.
42. Heckmann JG, Lang CJ, Zobelein I, et al: Herniated cervical intervertebral discs with radiculopathy: An outcome study of conservatively or surgically treated patients. J Spinal Disord 12:396-401, 1999.
43. Herkowitz HN, Kurz LT, Overholt DP: Surgical management of cervical soft disc herniation: A comparison between the anterior and posterior approach. Spine 15:1026, 1990.
44. Hitselberger WE, Witten RM: Abnormal myelograms in asymptomatic patients. J Neurosurg 28:204, 1968.
45. Honet JC, Puri K: Cervical radiculitis: Treatment and results in 82 patients. Arch Phys Med Rehabil 57:12, 1976.
46. Hueftle MG, Modic MT, Ross JS, et al: Lumbar spine: Postoperative MR imaging with Gd-DTPA. Radiology 167:817, 1988.
47. Hunt WE, Miller CA: Management of cervical radiculopathy. Clin Neurosurg 33:485, 1986.
48. Igarashi T, Kikuchi S, Shubajev V, Myers RR: 2000 Volvo Award winner in basic science studies: Exogenous tumor necrosis factor-alpha mimics nucleus pulposus–induced neuropathology: Molecular, histologic, and behavioural comparisons in rats. Spine 25: 2975-2980, 2000.
49. Ito T, Homma T, Uchiyama S: Sciatica caused by cervical and thoracic spinal cord compression. Spine 24:1265-1267, 1999.
50. Jensen MC, Brant-Zawadzki MN, Obuchowski N, et al: Magnetic resonance imaging of the lumbar spine in people without back pain. N Engl J Med 331:69-73, 1994.
51. Jinkins JR: MR of enhancing nerve roots in the unoperated lumbosacral spine. AJNR Am J Neuroradiol 14:193, 1993.
52. Johnson MG, Errico TJ: Lumbar disc herniation. In Fardon DF, Garfin SR (eds): Orthopaedic Knowledge Update: Spine 2. Rosemont, IL, American Academy of Orthopaedic Surgeons, 2002, pp 323-332.
53. Kang JD, Stefanovic-Racic M, McIntyre LA, et al: Toward a biochemical understanding of human intervertebral disc degeneration and herniation. Contributions of nitric oxide, interleukins, prostaglandin E_2, and matrix metalloproteinases. Spine 22:1065-1073, 1997.
54. Kaptain GJ, Shaffrey CI, Alden TD, et al: Secondary gain influences the outcome of lumbar but not cervical disc surgery. Surg Neurol 52:217-223, 1999.
55. Karppinen J, Korhonen T, Malmivaara A, et al: Tumor necrosis factor-α monoclonal antibody, infliximab, used to manage severe sciatica. Spine 28:750-753, 2003.
56. Kelsey JL: An epidemiological study of acute herniated lumbar intervertebral disc. Rheumatol Rehabil 14:144, 1975.
57. Kelsey JL, Githens PB, Walter SD, et al: An epidemiological study of acute prolapsed cervical intervertebral disc. J Bone Joint Surg Am 66-A:907, 1984.

58. Kennedy JG, Soffe KE, McGrath A, et al: Predictors of outcome in cauda equina syndrome. Eur Spine J 8:317-322, 1999.
59. Kirkaldy-Willis WH: The relationship of structural pathology to the nerve root. Spine 9:49, 1984.
60. Kobayashi S, Yoshizawa H, Hachiya Y, et al: Vasogenic edema induced by compression injury to the spinal nerve root: Distribution of intravenously injected protein tracers and gadolinium-enhanced magnetic resonance imaging. Spine 18:1410-1424, 1993.
61. Komori H, Shinomiya K, Nakai O, et al: The natural history of herniated nucleus pulposus with radiculopathy. Spine 21:225-229, 1996.
62. Komori H, Okawa A, Haro H, et al: Contrast-enhanced magnetic resonance imaging in conservative management of lumbar disc herniation. Spine 22:67-73, 1998.
63. Korhonrn T, Karppinen J, Malmivarra A, et al: Efficacy of infliximab for disc herniation–induced sciatica: One-year follow-up. Paper presented at the 30th Annual Meeting of the International Society for the Study of the Lumbar Spine, 2003, #14, Vancouver, British Columbia, Canada.
64. Krieger AJ, Maniker AH: MRI-documented regression of a herniated cervical nucleus pulposus: A case report. Surg Neurol 37:457, 1992.
65. Krismer M, Haid C, Rabi W: The contribution of annulus fibers to torque resistance. Spine 21:2551-2557, 1996.
66. LaBan MM, Meerschaert JR, Taylor RS: Breast pain: A symptom of cervical radiculopathy. Arch Phys Med Rehabil 60:315, 1979.
67. LaBan MM, Braker AM, Meerschaert JR: Airport induced "cervical traction" radiculopathy: The OJ syndrome. Arch Phys Med Rehabil 70:845, 1989.
68. Lundsford LD, Bissonette DJ, Jannetta PJ, et al: Anterior surgery for cervical disc disease. Part 1: Treatment of lateral cervical disc herniation in 253 cases. J Neurosurg 53:1, 1980.
69. Makin GJV, Brown WF, Ebers GC: C7 radiculopathy: Importance of scapular winging in clinical diagnosis. J Neurol Neurosurg Psychiatry 49:640, 1986.
70. Marinacci AA: A correlation between the operative findings in cervical herniated discs with the electromyograms and opaque myelograms. Bull Los Angeles Neurol Soc 30:118-130, 1965.
71. Matsui H, Kanamori M, Kawaguchi Y, et al: Clinical and electrophysiologic characteristics of compressed lumbar nerve roots. Spine 22:2100-2105, 1997.
72. Mendel T, Wink CS, Zimny ML: Neural elements in human cervical intervertebral discs. Spine 17:132, 1992.
73. Michelsen JJ, Mixter WJ: Pain and disability of shoulder and arm due to herniation of the nucleus pulposus of cervical intervertebral disks. N Engl J Med 231:279, 1944.
74. Mixter WJ, Barr JS: Rupture of the intervertebral disc with involvement of the spinal canal. N Engl J Med 211:210, 1934.
75. Mochida K, Komori H, Okawa A, et al: Regression of cervical disc herniation observed on magnetic resonance images. Spine 23: 990-995, 1998.
76. Modic MT, Masaryk T, Boumphrey F, et al: Lumbar herniated disk disease and canal stenosis: Prospective evaluation by surface coil MR, CT, and myelography. AJNR Am J Neuroradiol 7:709, 1986.
77. Mooney V, Robertson J: The facet syndrome. Clin Orthop 115:149, 1976.
78. Moore RJ, Vernon-Roberts B, Fraser RD, et al: The origin and fate of herniated lumbar intervertebral disc tissue. Spine 21:2149-2155, 1996.
79. Nachemson AL: Newest knowledge of low back pain: A critical look. Clin Orthop 279:8, 1992.
80. Nachemson AL: The lumbar spine: An orthopaedic challenge. Spine 1:59, 1976.
81. Negrin P, Lelli S, Fardin P: Contribution of electromyography to the diagnosis, treatment and prognosis of cervical disc disease: A study of 114 patients. Electromyogr Clin Neurophysiol 31:173, 1991.
82. Nerlich AG, Weiler C, Zipperer J, et al: Immunolocalization of phagocytic cells in normal and degenerated intervertebral discs. Spine 27:2482-2490, 2002.
83. Nitta H, Tajima T, Sugiyama H, et al: Study of dermatomes by means of selective lumbar spine nerve block. 18:1782-1786, 1993.
84. Odom GL, Finney W, Woodhall B: Cervical disk lesions. JAMA 166:23, 1958.
85. Olmarker K, Rydevik B: Selective inhibition of tumor necrosis factor-alpha prevents nucleus pulposus–induced thrombus formation, intraneural edema, and reduction of nerve conduction velocity: Possible implications of future pharmacologic treatment strategies of sciatica. Spine 26:863-869, 2001.
86. Osborn AG, Hood RS, Sherry RG, et al: CT/MR spectrum of far lateral and anterior lumbosacral disk herniations. AJNR Am J Neuroradiol 9:775, 1988.
87. Persson LC, Moritz U, Brandt L, et al: Cervical radiculopathy: Pain, muscle weakness and sensory loss in patients with cervical radiculopathy treated with surgery, physiotherapy or cervical collar: A prospective, controlled study. Eur Spine J 6:256-266, 1997.
88. Ramirez-Lassepas M, Tulloch JW, Quinones MR, Snyder BD: Acute radicular pain as a presenting symptom in multiple sclerosis. Arch Neurol 49:255, 1992.
89. Raskin SP, Keating JW: Recognition of lumbar disc disease: Comparison of myelography and computed tomography. AJR Am J Roentgenol 139:349, 1982.
90. Riew KD, Yin Y, Gilula L, et al: The effect of nerve-root injections on the need for operative treatment of lumbar radicular pain. A prospective, randomized, controlled, double-blind study. J Bone Joint Surg Am 82-A:1589-1593, 2000.
91. Ross JS, Zepp R, Modic MT: The postoperative lumbar spine: Enhanced MR evaluation of the intervertebral disk. AJNR Am J Neuroradiol 17:323-331,1996.
92. Ross AM, Segal J, Borenstein D, et al: Prevalence of spinal disc disease among interventional cardiologists. Am J Cardiol 79:68-70, 1997.
93. Rubin D: Cervical radiculitis: Diagnosis and treatment. Arch Phys Med Rehabil 41:580, 1960.
94. Saal JA, Saal JS, Herzog RJ: The natural history of lumbar intervertebral disc extrusions treated nonoperatively. Spine 15:683, 1990.
95. Saal JS, Saal JA, Yurth EF: Nonoperative management of herniated cervical intervertebral disc with radiculopathy. Spine 21:1877-1883, 1996.
96. Sampath P, Bendebba M, Davis JD, et al: Outcome in patients with cervical radiculopathy. Prospective, multicenter study with independent clinical review. Spine 24:591-597, 1999.
97. Semmes RE, Murphey MF: The syndrome of unilateral rupture of the sixth cervical intervertebral disk with compression of the seventh cervical nerve root: A report of four cases with symptoms simulating coronary disease. JAMA 121:1209, 1943.
98. Shapiro S: Medical realities of cauda equina syndrome secondary to lumbar disc herniation. Spine 25:348-352, 2000.
99. Shiqing X, Quanzhi Z, Dehao F: Significance of the straight-leg-raising test in the diagnosis and clinical evaluation of lower lumbar intervertebral disc protrusion. J Bone Joint Surg Am 69-A:517, 1987.
100. Silvers HR, Lewis PJ, Clabeaux DE, et al: Lumbar disc excisions in patients under the age of 21 years. Spine 19:2387-2392, 1994.
101. Slipman CW, Plastaras CT, Palmitier RA, et al: Symptom provocation of fluoroscopically guided cervical nerve root stimulation: Are dynatomal maps identical to dermatomal maps? Spine 23:2235-2242, 1998.
102. Sobel DF, Barkovich AJ, Munderloh SH: Metrizamide myelography and postmyelographic computed tomography: Comparative adequacy in the cervical spine. AJNR Am J Neuroradiol 45:385, 1984.
103. Spangforth EV: The lumbar disk herniation: A computer-aided analysis of 2,504 operations. Acta Orthop Scand Suppl 142:1, 1972.
104. Spurling RG, Scoville WB: Lateral rupture of the cervical intervertebral discs: A common cause of shoulder and arm pain. Surg Gynecol Obstet 78:350, 1944.
105. Stirling A, Worthington T, Rafiq M, et al: Association between sciatica and *Propionibacterium acnes*. Lancet 357:2024-2025, 2001.
106. Suk KS, Lee HM, Moon SH, et al: Lumbosacral scoliotic list by lumbar disc herniation. Spine 26:667-671, 2001.
107. Suzuki T, Abe E, Murai H, et al: Nontraumatic acute complete paraplegia resulting from cervical disc herniations: A case report. Spine 28:E125-E128, 2003.
108. Swezey RL: Chronic neck pain. Rheum Dis Clin North Am 22:411-437, 1996.
109. Tanaka N, Fujimoto Y, An HS, et al: The anatomic relation among the nerve roots, intervertebral foramina, and intervertebral discs of the cervical spine. Spine 25:286-291, 2000.

110. Tanaka M, Nakahara S, Inoue H: A pathologic study of discs in the elderly. Spine 18:1456-1462, 1993.
111. Vad VB, Bhat AL, Lutz GE, et al: Transforaminal epidural steroid injections in lumbosacral radiculopathy: A prospective randomized study. Spine 27:11-16, 2002.
112. Vallee JN, Feydy A, Carlier RY, et al: Chronic cervical radiculopathy: Lateral-approach periradicular corticosteroid injection. Radiology 218:886-892, 2001.
113. Verbiest H: Pathomorphologic aspects of developmental lumbar stenosis. Orthop Clin North Am 1:177, 1975.
114. Wainner RS, Fritz JM, Irrgang JJ, et al: Reliability and diagnostic accuracy of the clinical examination and patient self-report measures for cervical radiculopathy. Spine 28:52-56, 2003.
115. Walk D, Fisher MA, Doundoulakis SH, Hemmati M: Somatosensory evoked potentials in the evaluation of lumbosacral radiculopathy. Neurology 42:1197, 1992.
116. Warfield CA, Biber MP, Crews DA, Dwarakanath GK: Epidural steroid injection as a treatment for cervical radiculitis. Clin J Pain 4:201, 1988.
117. Weber H: Lumbar disc herniation: A prospective study of prognostic factors including a controlled trial. J Oslo City Hosp 28:36, 1978.
118. Wiesel SW: Lumbar spine: Acute lumbar radicular syndromes. In Orthopaedic Knowledge Update, 2: Home Study Syllabus. Park Ridge, IL, American Academy of Orthopaedic Surgeons, 1987, pp 313, 323.
119. Wilbourn AJ, Aminoff MJ: The electrophysiologic examination in patients with radiculopathies. Muscle Nerve 11:1099, 1988.
120. Wippold FJ, Smirniotopoulos JG, Pilgram TK: Lesions of the cauda equina: A clinical and pathology review from the Armed Forces Institute of Pathology. Clin Neurol Neurosurg 99:229-234, 1997.
121. Woertgen C, Holzschuh M, Rothoerl RD, et al: Clinical signs in patients with brachialgia and sciatica: A comparative study. Surg Neurol 49:210-214, 1998.
122. Yoss RE, Corbin KB, McCarthy CS, Love JG: Significance of symptoms and signs of localization of involved root in cervical disc protrusion. Neurology 7:673, 1957.
123. Yukawa Y, Kato F, Kajino G, et al: Groin pain associated with lower lumbar disc herniation. Spine 22:1736-1740, 1997.

LUMBAR SPONDYLOSIS/CERVICAL SPONDYLOSIS OSTEOARTHRITIS

CAPSULE SUMMARY

	LOW BACK	NECK
Frequency of spinal pain	Very common	Very common
Location of spinal pain	Low back to thigh	Neck, between scapulae, top of shoulders
Quality of spinal pain	Ache	Ache
Symptoms and signs	Pain with standing and walking	Pain increased with activity, especially rotation of the neck
Laboratory tests	None	None
Radiographic findings	Osteophytes on plain roentgenograms, CT scan, myelogram, MR	Osteophytes and decreased disc space height on plain roentgenograms and MR
Treatment	Medications	Medications, controlled physical activity

PREVALENCE AND PATHOGENESIS

Osteoarthritis (degenerative joint disease) is a chronic, noninflammatory joint disease characterized by slowly developing joint pain, stiffness, deformity, and limitation of motion. The lumbosacral and cervical spine are only one of the many areas of the skeleton that are affected by this process. Lumbar and cervical spondylosis was formerly known as lumbar and cervical degenerative disc disease.[3]

Epidemiology

Osteoarthritis is the most common joint disease, and its prevalence is increasing with the age of the population. In an evaluation of 400 spine specimens, Nathan found 100% involvement of anterior osteophytes in individuals 40 years and older.[37] The severity of involvement increases with age. Osteoarthritis is almost universally present in individuals older than 75 years.[27] Both men and women are affected by this illness. Among individuals younger than 45 years, more men have the disease, whereas the disease develops in women to a greater degree than in men after 55 years of age.[26] The location of frequent involvement corresponds to areas of maximal activity. In the cervical area, the C5–C6 area is maximally affected. In the cervical spine, the inferior border of the vertebral body is more commonly affected, in contrast to the superior border in the lumbar spine.[37]

Pathogenesis

The etiology of osteoarthritis is multifactorial. Genetic, biochemical, and biomechanical factors play a role. Familial aggregation of generalized osteoarthritis, including involvement of the lumbar spine, has been reported. Thirty-six percent of relatives of men with generalized osteoarthritis and 49% of relatives of women with the disorder had the disease, as compared with expected values of 17% and 26%, respectively, for the same age group in the general population.[26]

Biochemical Factors

Biochemical and metabolic alterations in cartilage play a role in the pathogenesis of osteoarthritis. The proteoglycans present in cartilage matrix develop an altered composition over time. Glycosaminoglycans, which are a component of proteoglycans, act as sponges in the cartilage. They absorb water. The shock absorbency of cartilage is proportional to its proteoglycan content and ability to bind water. In osteoarthritis, the proteoglycan content is reduced, along with a relative reduction in keratan sulfate and an increase in chondroitin sulfate (both glycosaminoglycans).[33] Proteoglycans containing abnormal proportions of keratan and chondroitin sulfate form smaller subunits that retard glycosaminoglycan aggregation. The result of these alterations on the biochemical characteristics of osteoarthritic cartilage is retention of excess water in cartilage. In this state, the shock absorbency of cartilage is diminished, and the collagen matrix of cartilage is disrupted.[34,52] Growth factors, including fibroblast, transforming, and insulin-like factors, have a role in the repair of damaged cartilage. Investigation of how growth factor synthesis is regulated in traumatized articular cartilage would be beneficial to understanding the underlying mechanisms central to the pathogenesis of osteoarthritis.[32]

Significant biochemical alterations also occur in the intervertebral disc. Nerlich and colleagues completed an investigation to determine the age-related changes in human lumbar intervertebral discs.[38] The investigation determined the modification of distribution patterns of collagen types I, II, III, IV, V, VI, IX, and X, along with the production of *N*-(carboxymethyl)lysine (CML) as a biomarker of oxidative stress. A total of 229 sagittal lumbar motion segments from 47 individuals from fetal to 86 years of age were studied with macroscopic, histologic, and immunohistochemical techniques. CML modification of extracellular collagen was first observed in the nucleus pulposus of a 13-year-old. CML deposition increased with age and was accentuated in areas of macroscopic and histologic disc degeneration. CML deposition was followed by alterations in the collagen-type pattern: an initial increase in nuclear collagen types II, III, and VI and subsequent loss of collagen II, manufacture of collagen I, and persistence of collagen III and VI. The phenotypic expression of disc cells is modified in the pericellular matrix, with early expression of basement membrane collagen type IV in adolescents changing to type X hypertrophic cartilage collagen in mature adults with increasing disc degeneration. This important study confirmed the notion that disc degeneration starts in the second decade of life. Modifications of collagen production occur over time with associated modification of disc anatomy. The increased levels of CML staining in association with degenerative alterations suggest that cumulative oxidative stress may contribute to these alterations.

Gruber and Hanley compared the affects of aging and degeneration on disc cell function and matrix production.[17] The study analyzed the immunohistochemical distribution of types I, II, II, and VI collagen; the distribution of apoptotic disc cells; and the presence of tartrate-resistant acid phosphatase. The study demonstrated a high incidence of apoptotic disc cells in surgical specimens and controls. Surviving cells are not synthetically inactive but are producing inappropriate matrix products. The cells form a barrier that affects individuals' cell production and intercellular communication. Modifications of these factors may prevent disc cell senescence.

Biomechanical Factors

Biomechanical factors may play a role in the development of osteoarthritis. Investigators have suggested that stiffening of subchondral bone associated with microfractures results in disruption of articular cartilage.[43] Lotz and co-workers reported on the detrimental effects of sustained loading on intervertebral discs.[30] Included among the alterations are disorganization of the annulus fibrosus, an increase in apoptosis and associated loss of cellularity, and downregulation of collagen II and aggrecan gene expression. The response to these alterations is a modification of the cellular phenotype of cells that are altered from the natural state.

Genetic Factors

A variety of genetic and environmental influences have the potential to determine the rapidity and extent of disc dissolution. Battie and associates reviewed the occupational and leisure time physical loading, driving, and smoking histories of 114 male identical twin pairs.[2] The degree of disc degeneration was determined by measuring disc height, decreased signal intensity of the nucleus pulposus, and disc bulging by digital MR imaging. Heavier lifetime occupational and leisure loading was associated with greater disc degeneration of the upper lumbar discs. In the lower lumbar discs, leisure time heavy loading was the sole factor associated with increased disc degeneration. Driving, years of aerobic exercise, and smoking had no significant effect on the degree of disc changes. The general concordance of disc degeneration in twins points to a strong genetic influence on degeneration in comparison to environmental factors. Simmons and colleagues reported on the family members of individuals who underwent surgery for degenerative lumbar disc disease versus a control group admitted for nonspinal orthopedic procedures.[48] In a group of 65 patients who were surgically treated for degenerative disc disease, 44.6% were noted to have a positive family history, whereas 25.4% of patients in the control group had a positive family history. Spinal surgery was performed in 18.5% and 4.5% of the relatives of those with disc disease and the control group, respectively. This study is evidence for the genetic predisposition of families to disc degeneration.[48]

Harreby and colleagues reported the results of a study investigating the value of radiologic abnormalities of the thoracic and lumbar spine in predicting low back pain in a prospective cohort study of 640 schoolchildren monitored for 25 years.[18] During the initial radiographic evaluation, 13% had abnormalities, primarily Scheuermann's changes (irregular endplates, wedge vertebrae). No correlation was noted between the radiographic findings and the 11% of adolescents with back pain. Of the 83% of the original group who completed a self-administered questionnaire, 84% had experienced low back pain as adults. The two risk factors most closely associated with low back pain as an adult was a familial history and low back pain during the growth period as an adolescent.

Richardson and co-workers studied familial factors in the development of lumbar disc pain.[46] Questionnaires that reliably identified discogenic pain were administered to immediate relatives of patients with surgically proven lumbar disc herniation or repetitive upper extremity overuse (control group). The groups were investigated for demographic factors and physical activities known to increase the occurrence of lumbar disc injury. Of 60 disc patients, 16 (27%) had discogenic pain, whereas only 1 of 41 (2%) upper extremity subjects had similar symptoms. Disc surgery was documented in 7 (12%) of the disc patients and none of the control group. A family history and repetitive lifting were the only variables associated with discogenic pain. This study supports the role of genetic factors in the development of disc degeneration.

Whether a genetic, biochemical, or biomechanical abnormality, osteoarthritis causes degeneration of articular cartilage. As the cartilage is worn away, chondrocytes attempt to replace the cartilage. Degradation is more rapid than repair, and erosion of the articular surface evolves. In response to abnormal mechanical stress on joint surfaces, bony appendages (osteophytes) appear. In the lumbar spine, the location of osteoarthritis is primarily in the facet joints.

Lumbar Spine

In the first few decades of life, the gross appearance of the spine and its components will remain basically unchanged. The intervertebral discs will maintain their full height, with a thickened, laminated annulus fibrosus and a tense nucleus pulposus. The vertebrae are completely ossified except for their apophyseal rings and are essentially square in shape. The facets are well defined, with smooth capsules and normal articular cartilage. The ligamenta flava are only a few millimeters thick, and the space available for the neural elements within the canal and the foramina is capacious. Symptoms are unusual even though some developmentally and congenitally narrow canals have much less space available even early in life.

In some individuals, the final pathologic end stage of disc degeneration is fibrous ankylosis between two adjacent vertebrae along with osteophyte formation and marked narrowing of the disc space. If this phenomenon is stable, the patient may be relatively free of symptoms or will be aware of only a sense of stiffness in the spine.

As the spine ages, one can also encounter postural alterations with a reduction in lordosis. This change is an attempt by the body to decompress the degenerated articular facets by maintaining a flexed rather than an extended posture; however, such postural alterations can lead to chronic muscle tension and become symptomatic. This flexed position also provides more room for the sensitive neural elements that are dynamically compressed in extension.

Although most of the changes described in the motor segment units progress from decade to decade, there is a wide range in the rate of deterioration. It is important to understand that these anatomic alterations do not necessarily dictate the symptoms, define the disability, or determine the prognosis. As the spine ages, these phenomena appear to be tolerated to some degree by all.

The role of exercise in the development of spondylosis is an area of concern. Videman and colleagues conducted an important study to investigate the role of exercise in the development of lumbosacral spondylosis.[53] A questionnaire concerning back pain and disease was returned by 937 elite athletes, including 650 members of the Finnish Olympic teams from 1920 to 1965, and by 620 age-matched control subjects who were members of the military. The Finnish health system allowed documentation of hospital discharge diagnoses and the pension status of the study participants. A subset of athletes, including 24 long-distance runners, 26 soccer players, 19 weightlifters, and 25 shooters, underwent MR evaluation of the lumbar spine. Back pain was less common in all former athletes than controls (29.3% versus 51.7%). MR degenerative findings throughout the lumbar spine were greater in weightlifters than other athletes. Soccer players had greater degenerative disease in the lower segments of the lumbar spine than other athletes did. Athletes who complained of back pain had a significantly higher level of disc degeneration than did those who experienced back pain less than twice a year. Runners had no increased level of degeneration when compared with control subjects. The clinical implication of this study is that exercise over long periods is associated with less back pain despite the presence of spondylosis.

Cervical Spine

Cervical spondylosis is believed to be the direct result of age-related changes in the intervertebral disc.[8] Such changes include desiccation of the nucleus pulposus, loss of annular elasticity, and narrowing of the disc space with or without disc protrusion or rupture. In turn, fibers of the annulus fibrosus produce periosteal traction through the anterior and posterior longitudinal ligaments, thereby inducing bone formation at the insertion of Sharpey's fibers.[24] Loss of vascular supply to the area may also contribute to degeneration. In the early stage of disc degeneration, the involved segment becomes unstable, and movement of the surrounding vertebrae becomes excessive and irregular. The segment becomes vulnerable to local trauma with damage to the surrounding ligaments and corresponding facet joints. Once initiated, the early damage is amplified over time with increasing instability and associated tissue damage. The result is secondary changes, including overriding of facet joints, increased motion of the spinal segments, osteophyte formation in the uncovertebral and zygapophyseal joints, local inflammation of synovial joints, and microfractures. These macroscopic and microscopic changes can result in various clinical syndromes (spondylosis, ankylosis, central or foraminal spinal stenosis, radiculopathy, myelopathy, spinal segmental instability).

As humans assumed an erect posture, the cervical spine evolved to achieve a remarkable degree of mobility and flexibility. Although subjected to loads of less magnitude than the lumbar spine, the cervical spine manifests degenerative changes of aging with exceptional regularity. It may be because of this remarkable mobility that degenerative changes are so consistently seen during the process of aging. The radiographic and pathologic consequences of the aging process begin to be manifested in the third decade of life. Because the natural history of cervical spondylosis parallels the aging process, it is often difficult to determine whether these morphologic changes are a result of the aging process or disease states. Indeed, the anatomic and radiographic expression of cervical spondylosis becomes significant only when etiologically related to distinct clinical syndromes.

Cervical spondylosis may be manifested in several ways: cervical spondylosis alone, cervical spondylosis with radiculopathy, cervical spondylosis with myelopathy, and cervical spondylosis with myeloradiculopathy. Cervical radiculopathy caused by a soft herniated nucleus pulposus is discussed in the preceding section. Cervical spondylosis alone is presented in this section and with myelopathy in the following section.

CLINICAL HISTORY

Lumbar Spine

Patients with degenerative disease of the lumbosacral spine may complain of a broad variety of symptoms. Many patients with degenerative discs and osteoarthritis of the facet joints may be totally asymptomatic. Some may have mild discomfort in the low back region, whereas others may have radiating leg pain with an inability to walk. Patients with osteoarthritis of the facet joints have pain primarily over the joints in the lower part of the back. Patients may have morning stiffness of short duration (30 minutes or less). Any body movements that compress the joints (extension) exacerbate symptoms of dull, aching pain. Patients may also be aware of decreased motion of the spine.

Any positions that flex the lumbar spine are associated with resolution of symptoms. Characteristically, patients with spinal stenosis are able to ride a bicycle without difficulty. Walking up an incline or stairs does not cause symptoms, whereas walking down an incline or stairs (extension of the spine) does cause symptoms to appear.

Forty-two individuals with low back pain occurring immediately on sitting and relieved by standing up were evaluated by motion radiographs for spinal instability and compared with 32 controls by Maigne and colleagues.[31] Low back pain that occurred immediately on sitting and was relieved by standing up was statistically associated with instability or marked anterior loss of disc space in flexion. Dynamic radiographs may be indicated to document an unstable segment in individuals with this complement of clinical symptoms.

Cervical Spine

The usual patient with symptomatic cervical spondylosis is older than 40 years and complains of neck ache with an occasional associated headache.[40] Headache that is suboccipital with radiation to the base of the neck or vertex is reported in about one third of patients.[19] Osteoarthritis in the atlantoaxial central or atlantoaxial lateral joints may be associated with severe headaches in individuals older than 40 years.[49,56] The pain in the neck is poorly localized and exacerbated with movement. Not infrequently, however, these patients have very few neck pain symptoms but instead have referred pain patterns—shoulder area, suboccipital area, occipital headaches, interscapular areas, and anterior chest wall—or other vague symptoms suggestive of anatomic disturbances affecting vascular structures or the sympathetic nervous system, such as blurring of vision, vertigo, and tinnitus. In one study, suboccipital headache was particularly associated with atlantoaxial osteoarthritis.[57] About 15% of patients have vertigo or tinnitus, and 5% have vertebrobasilar vascular insufficiency with syncope.[4] Arthritis in the cervical zygapophyseal joints causes referred pain in the occiput (C2–C3), upper part of the neck (C3–C4), base of the neck (C4–C5), trapezius (C5–C6), or scapula (C6–C7).[10] In patients with predominantly referred pain, a history of neck pain is usually elicited.

PHYSICAL EXAMINATION

Lumbar Spine

The physical findings associated with osteoarthritis of the lumbar spine may be unimpressive. Patients may have mild decreases in range of motion, particularly with extension.

Cervical Spine

Physical examination of a patient with cervical spondylosis is often associated with a dearth of objective findings. The patient usually has some limitation in neck motion associated with midline tenderness. Not infrequently, palpation of the referred pain areas also produces local tenderness and should not be confused with local disease. The neurologic examination is normal.

LABORATORY DATA

Laboratory evaluation of patients with lumbar or cervical spondylosis and osteoarthritis is usually normal. Patients with degenerative joint disease of the cervical spine may experience greater paracervical muscle fatigue as measured by electromyography than control subjects do.[15]

RADIOGRAPHIC EVALUATION

Lumbar Spine

Roentgenograms

Plain roentgenograms are very helpful in visualizing osteoarthritis. Disc spaces increase in size from the L1–L2 interspace to L4–L5. The L5–S1 interspace has a variable size. However, a parallel position of the endplates of L5 and S1 is evidence of degeneration in that interspace.

Roentgenograms will reveal intervertebral disc degeneration with loss of disc space height, traction osteophytes, decreased interpedicular distance, decreased sagittal canal diameter, and facet degeneration (Fig. 10-12).

Claw and traction osteophytes are two abnormalities on the anterior aspect of the vertebral body commonly observed on conventional radiographs of patients with

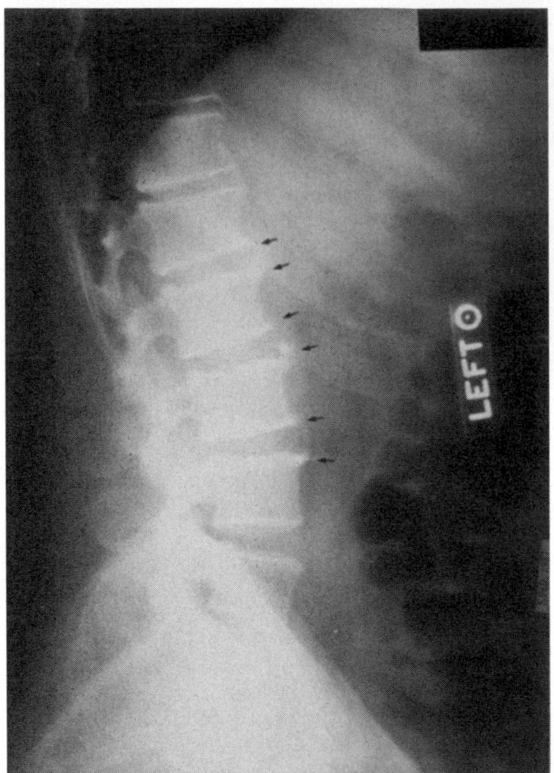

Figure 10-12 Lateral view illustrating traction osteophytes *(arrows)* at multiple levels associated with disc degeneration. Note that the osteophytes are horizontally oriented and emerge slightly above or below the disc space. A claw osteophyte is noted at the fourth *arrow* from the top, whereas a traction osteophyte is located at the fifth *arrow* from the top.

osteoarthritis of the lumbar spine.[42] A traction osteophyte is horizontally oriented and arises from the margins of two adjacent vertebral bodies. A claw osteophyte is triangular and curved at its tip. A traction osteophyte may be indicative of disc degeneration and an unstable discovertebral junction. These osteophytes form at the osseous site of attachment of the outer annular fibers to the anterior vertebral surface. With maturing of the lesion and less instability, periosteal deposition of bone converts a traction osteophyte to a claw osteophyte. These osteophytes may coexist in the same vertebral body and are indicative of progression of the same pathologic process affecting the lumbar spine.

Van Tulder and co-workers completed a systematic review of studies examining the relationship of nonspecific low back pain and anatomic abnormalities detected on lumbar spine roentgenograms.[51] A total of 194 papers were scored for methodologic quality, with 35 meeting the inclusion criteria. Degeneration in the form of disc space narrowing, sclerosis, and osteophytes was associated with nonspecific low back pain with an odds ratio ranging from 1.2 to 3.3. Spondylolysis, spondylolisthesis, spina bifida, transitional vertebrae, and Scheuermann's disease were not associated with the presence of low back pain.

Bone Scintigraphy

A technetium bone scan may supplement the physical examination and plain roentgenograms in assessing the extent and severity of osteoarthritis.[9] The technetium bisphosphonate and phosphate agents preferentially chemabsorb to hydroxyapatite crystals, particularly newly formed crystals in new bone. Increased uptake occurs in areas of subchondral sclerosis. Specialized techniques are helpful in screening bone abnormalities in the lumbar spine, including osteophytes (Fig. 10-13).[41]

Computed Tomography

CT is also a useful technique to identify the presence of facet joint disease along with disc degeneration. A CT scan can identify the trefoil configuration of the spinal canal along with the reduction in dimensions of the bony canal (Fig. 10-14). High-resolution CT scans may be reformatted to reconstruct three-dimensional views of the lumbar spine.[9]

Magnetic Resonance

In an MR study, Toyone and colleagues described the endplate and vertebral bone marrow changes associated with degenerative lumbar disc disease.[50] On T1-weighted images, decreased signal intensity was associated with thickened bony trabeculae and loss of fatty bone marrow. These individuals had hypermobility at the corresponding intervertebral space, with 73% (27 of 37) having low back pain. Increased signal intensity was associated with fatty replacement of bone marrow. These patients had stable lumbar spine segments, with 11% (4 of 37) having low back pain. These alterations in bone marrow content imaged by MR may be indicative of unstable segments of the lumbar spine that may be sources of back pain. Serial images of these individuals may be able to show whether hypermobile segments become stabilized over time with modification of the bone marrow content. MR evaluation of disc disease has no prognostic value with regard to the development or resolution of back pain.[35]

The position of the patient when undergoing MR evaluation may have significance when correlating functional anatomic alterations with clinical symptoms. Weishaupt and co-workers reported on positional MR scans taken in the seated flexed and extended position in 30 individuals with disc abnormalities but no neural compression.[55] Nerve root contact occurred in 34 of 152 instances in the supine position, in 62 instances in the seated flexed position, and in 45 instances in the seated extended position. Nerve root deviation decreased from 10 to 8 instances in the seated flexed position but increased from 10 to 13 instances in the extended position. Position pain score differences were related to changes in foraminal size, but not to differences in nerve root compromise. Positional MR demonstrated minor neural compromise more consistently than conventional MR did. An MR image in the seated extended posture may be necessary to detect the narrowing of the neural foramen that may be the source of neural pain not visualized with MR imaging in the supine position.

Cervical Spine

Roentgenograms

Roentgenograms (anteroposterior, lateral, oblique) of the cervical spine in cervical spondylosis show a continuum of

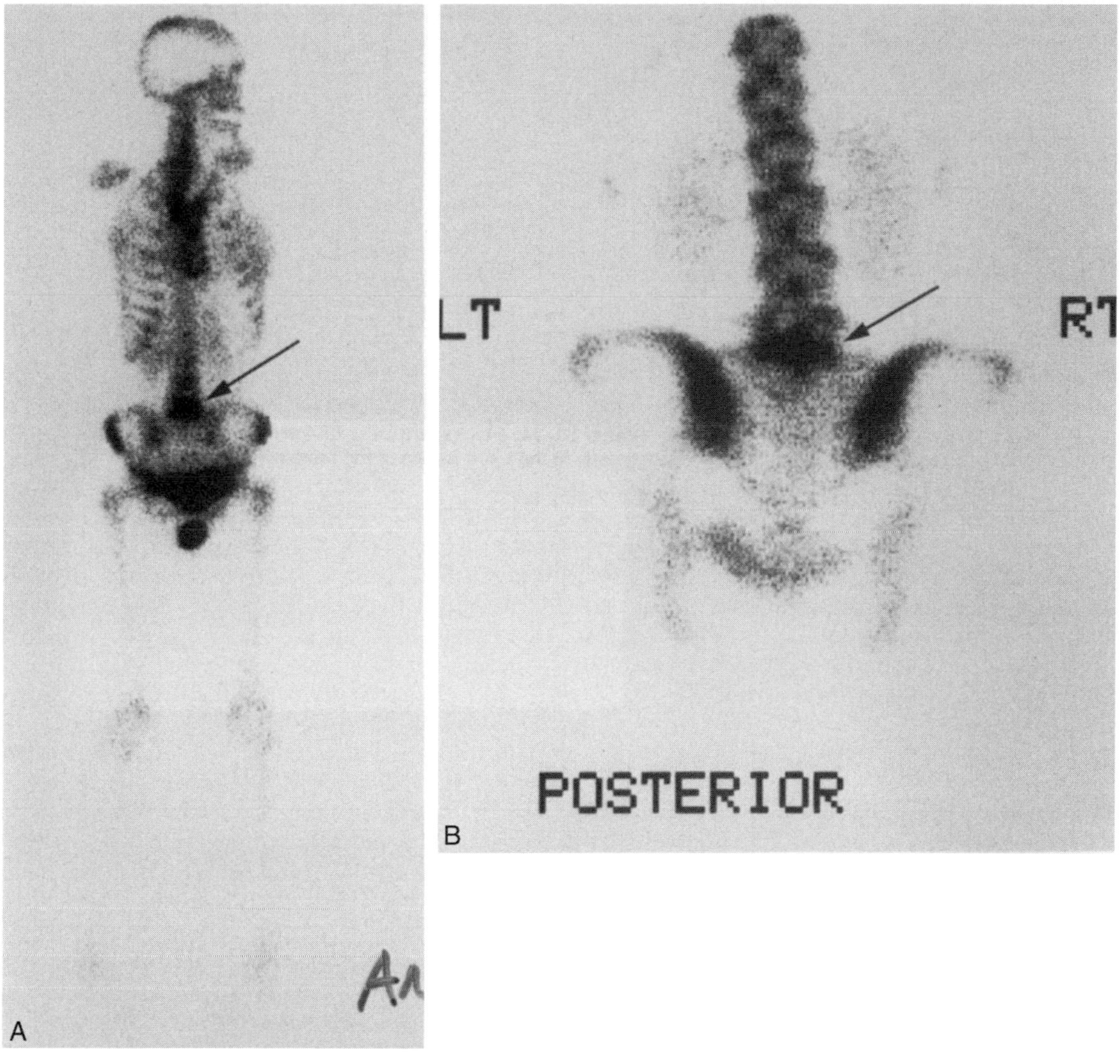

Figure 10-13 ^{99m}Tc-MDP bone scan of a 42-year-old woman with low back pain for 4 years. The bone scan was obtained to investigate possible generalized bone disease. *A*, The bone scan reveals increased uptake in the lumbar spine on the whole body view *(arrow)*. *B*, A posterior spot view demonstrates increased linear tracer uptake within the L5–S1 region compatible with degenerative disease.

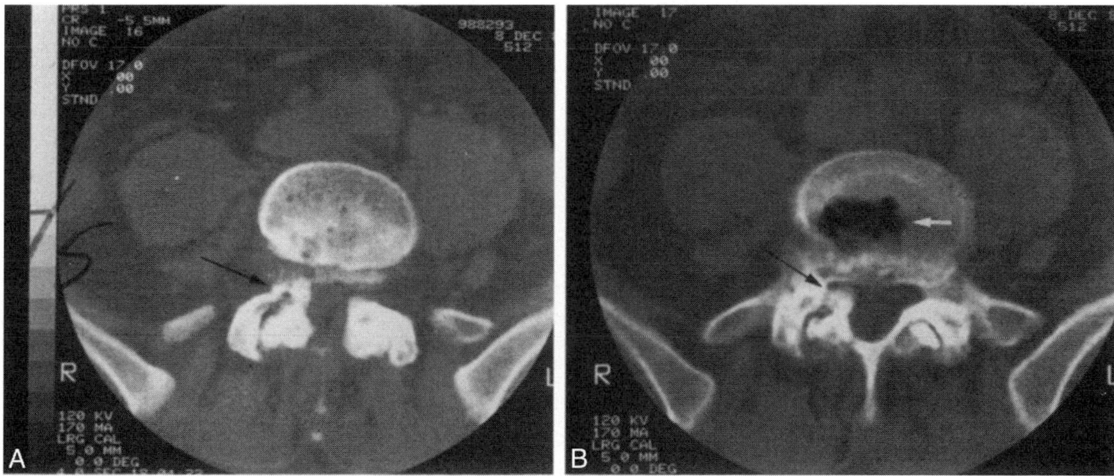

Figure 10-14 CT scan of a 68-year-old man with back pain that is exacerbated with standing. Cross-sectional views demonstrate a vacuum phenomenon in the intervertebral disc *(white arrow)* and facet hypertrophy (most prominent on the right) that has resulted in canal stenosis at multiple levels *(black arrows)*. The patient's symptoms responded to epidural steroid injections.

abnormalities. Initially, loss of disc hydration results in loss of disc height and the development of vacuum phenomena secondary to gas (nitrogen) forming in the nuclear clefts.[44] Reactive sclerosis of the endplates and the occasional appearance of Schmorl's nodules represent intraosseous disc displacements. Subsequent to these early changes, osteophytes with osteoarthritis of the apophyseal joints, foraminal narrowing, or segmental instability with degenerative spondylolisthesis may occur. Bony ankylosis occurs in advanced disease. Involvement of the uncovertebral processes results in hypertrophy of the ridges along with the development of osteophytes that may project into the foraminal space or the spinal canal and cause nerve impingement. *Spondylosis deformans* is the term used to designate bone production in the spine associated with more advanced degenerative disease (Fig. 10-15). Roentgenographic evidence of cervical spine disease occurs in more than 70% of individuals older than 70 years.[12] As previously discussed, these findings do not correlate with symptoms.[11,13,15a,16] However, patients with degenerative joint disease of the cervical spine may experience greater paracervical muscle fatigue as measured by electromyography than control subjects do.[15] In large part, the roentgenogram serves to rule out other more serious causes of neck and referred pain such as tumors.

Computed Tomography

CT imaging in cervical spondylosis reveals degenerative changes associated with bony fragmentation, sclerosis, cystic formation of the endplates, and hypertrophy of the facet joints.[47] Hypertrophic encroachment of the central and foraminal canals is visualized. However, disc evaluation is not optimal, and observations of the cervical cord are not ideal.

CT-myelography combines injection of dye into the spinal canal with CT. This test is able to determine levels of stenosis in the foraminal canal and central canal. However, the test is unable to determine the cause of cervical radiculopathy in a number of patients.[21] CT-myelography has limitations in that it is an invasive procedure, intramedullary lesions are not identified, and a high dose of ionizing radiation is required.

Magnetic Resonance

Further diagnostic testing in the form of MR imaging is not usually warranted unless greater detail of bony or soft tissue structures is required. In a population of 89 asymptomatic individuals, MR imaging identified degenerative cervical discs in 62% of individuals 40 years or older. No abnormalities were seen in those younger than 30 years.[28]

Discography

Controversy continues to surround the use of discography as a means to determine degenerative discs that are sources of low back pain. A controlled, prospective study reported on the accuracy of discography in detecting symptomatic intervertebral discs.[54] Discography revealed abnormal findings in 13 of 20 discs in symptomatic individuals. In asymptomatic individuals, the discogram was abnormal in 17%. A similar proportion (26%) was noted in a study by Holt.[20] Positive discographic findings are more closely associated with individuals with abnormal psychological profiles; such patients have significantly higher rates of positive disc injections than do either asymptomatic volunteers or symptomatic subjects with normal psychological screening.[7] Discography is not reliable and cannot be recommended as a specific test for the diagnosis of low back pain. The pain produced during provocative lumbar discography is strongly influenced by the subject's emotional and psychological state, chronic pain behavior, and ongoing compensation claims, regardless of whether the patient has any back pain illness. Pain production is related

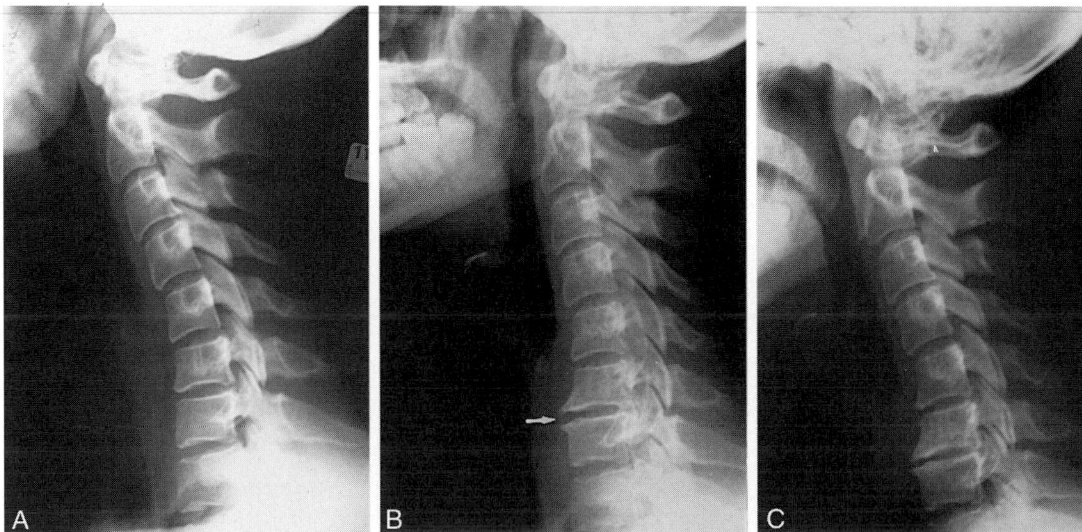

Figure 10-15 Cervical spondylosis. A 33-year-old physician was involved in a motor vehicle accident and suffered left neck and trapezial pain. Lateral view of the cervical spine. *A*, 4/11/89: Reversal of the normal cervical lordosis with angulation at the C5–C6 level. *B*, 1/16/92: Straightening of the cervical spine with narrowing at the C6–C7 level and anterior osteophytes *(arrow)*. *C*, 11/18/93: Further disc space narrowing and enlargement of osteophytes.

to penetration of the dye through the outer annulus and cannot reliably be used to confirm the location of the pain source.[6] Discography is associated with complications, including epidural abscess.[25]

DIFFERENTIAL DIAGNOSIS

The diagnosis of osteoarthritis is suggested by the patient's age and a clinical history of back or neck pain of long duration that increases with mechanical stress, and the diagnosis is documented by characteristic changes on radiographic evaluation of the lumbosacral or cervical spine. The diagnosis of osteoarthritis is one made by exclusion of other possible diagnoses. The radiographic changes of osteoarthritis, including loss of disc height and the presence of traction osteophytes, occur as patients age. These changes are not necessarily associated with back or neck pain.[14] The majority of patients with symptomatic osteoarthritis are in the same age group as most patients with tumors of the axial skeleton. The physician must feel confident about excluding the possibility of a more ominous cause of back or neck pain before ascribing the patient's complaints to osteoarthritis of the spine.

Facet Syndrome

Facet syndrome must also be considered in the differential diagnosis of patients who have low back pain with lumbar spine extension. Pain may be localized over a single apophyseal joint early in the osteoarthritic process. As the process progresses, the apophyseal joint becomes increasingly irritated with referred pain to the buttock and posterior of the thigh. Patients with facet syndrome have referred pain to the leg with extension of the spine and ipsilateral side bending. Pain may also occur with rotation of the spine. Abnormal neurologic signs are seldom detected on physical examination. Injection of local anesthetics produces variable results, with long-term relief in up to 60%.[36] Facet joint blocks are not always helpful in reducing pain. In one study, the diagnosis of facet syndrome could be confirmed in only 29% of referred patients.[23] No particular clinical finding could be identified that was specifically associated with a good response to injection. Another study of 109 patients with unilateral low back pain found improvement to be equal in the analgesic and placebo injection groups.[29] Similar outcome was also found in patients who received methylprednisolone injections and placebo recipients.[5] Another important point concerning facet joint injection is the lack of correlation between the response to injection and the outcome of posterior lumbar fusion. The clinical entity of facet joint syndrome and thus its appropriate treatment remain in question.[22]

TREATMENT

Lumbar Spine

The majority of patients with osteoarthritis of the lumbosacral spine can be treated nonsurgically. Nonsteroidal anti-inflammatory drugs are helpful in controlling symptoms. The toxicity of gastric irritation may be of greater concern in patients with osteoarthritis because the group of people with this ailment are older. Gastric upset may occur more commonly in an older patient population. Medications may be given to protect the gastric mucosa in patients who are at risk for significant morbidity or mortality from gastrointestinal bleeding. Lumbosacral corsets are helpful in reminding the patient to avoid excessive spinal movement.

Revel and co-workers assessed the efficacy of single–facet joint anesthesia versus saline in the treatment of painful facet joints.[45] The study identified clinical criteria that are predictive of significant relief of spinal pain after injection. Forty-three patients who had back pain with five of seven criteria associated with facet joint pain were compared with 37 people who met fewer than five criteria. The criteria included pain not exacerbated by coughing, forward flexion, rising from flexion, hyperextension, and extension-rotation; age older than 65 years; and pain relieved by recumbency. Lidocaine provided greater pain relief than saline did in back pain patients. The criteria identified 92% of patients responding to injections and 80% of those not responding to lidocaine.

Cervical Spine

Cervical spondylosis alone is treated by nonoperative measures. The mainstay of therapy for acute pain superimposed on the chronic problem is rest (controlled physical activity) and immobilization in a neck brace. In addition, oral nonsteroidal anti-inflammatory drugs are beneficial. Often, these medications need to be administered on a chronic basis. The same drugs may be given intermittently to patients who have pain only with acute exacerbations. Trigger point injections with local anesthetics (lidocaine) and corticosteroids (triamcinolone) may be therapeutic in patients with associated muscle pain. Referred pain in the shoulder and trapezius may be improved with zygapophyseal joint injections.[1] These injections are indicated only if other components of conservative therapy are ineffective. Once the pain abates, the immobilization (usually a soft cervical collar) should be discontinued and the patient maintained with a series of cervical isometric exercises. Further counseling about sleeping position, automobile driving, and work is in order. Manipulation and traction are rarely needed and may in fact be deleterious to the patient.

Gene Therapy

Nishida and associates cultured nucleus pulposus cells and infected them with replication-defective, *lacZ* gene–encoding adenoviruses.[39] The *lacZ* gene was detected by the expression of beta-galactosidase visualized by light microscopy. The viruses were then injected into the intervertebral discs of rabbits. A number of cells exhibited galactosidase staining, with no decrease in expression noted at 12 weeks. No cytotoxicity was detected, and the virus vectors were found only in the injected discs. This gene transfer technique may become a useful way to alter the disc environment with growth factors in individuals who have a greater risk (genetic predisposition) for disc degeneration.

PROGNOSIS

Most patients with osteoarthritis of the axial skeleton have a relapsing course with recurrent episodes of back or neck pain. Most of these patients respond to medical and physical therapy and do not require surgical intervention. The severity can vary and treatment is an ongoing process. The natural history of osteoarthritis is continued gradual deterioration of spinal structures.

References

Lumbar/Cervical Spondylosis (Osteoarthritis)

1. Aprill C, Dwyer A, Bogduk N: Cervical zygapophyseal joint pain patterns II: A clinical evaluation. Spine 15:458, 1990.
2. Battie MC, Videman T, Gibbons LE, et al: Determinants of lumbar disc determination: A study relating lifetime exposures and magnetic resonance imaging findings in identical twins. Spine 20:2601-2612, 1995.
3. Bohlman HH: Cervical spondylosis with moderate to severe myelopathy. Spine 2:151-162, 1977.
4. Brain L: Some unresolved problems of cervical spondylosis. BMJ 1:771, 1963.
5. Carette S, Marcoux S, Truchon R, et al.: A controlled trial of corticosteroid injections into facet joints for chronic low back pain. N Engl J Med 325:1002, 1991.
6. Carragee EJ: Is lumbar discography a determinate of discogenic low back pain: Provocative discography reconsidered. Curr Rev Pain 4:301-308, 2000.
7. Carragee EJ, Chen Y, Tanner C, et al: Provocative discography in patients after limited lumbar discectomy: A controlled, randomized study of pain response in symptomatic and asymptomatic subjects. Spine 25:3065-3071, 2000.
8. DePalma AF, Rothman RH, Levitt RL, et al: The natural history of severe cervical disc degeneration. Acta Orthop Scand 43:392, 1972.
9. Durrault RG, Lander PH: Imaging of the facet joints. Radiol Clin North Am 28:1033, 1990.
10. Dwyer A, Aprill C, Bogduk N: Cervical zygapophyseal joint pain patterns I: A study in normal volunteers. Spine 15:453, 1990.
11. Edward WC, LaRocca SH: The developmental segmental sagittal diameter in combined cervical and lumbar spondylosis. Spine 10:43, 1985.
12. Fenlin J: Pathology of degenerative disease of the cervical spine: Symposium on disease of the intervertebral disc. Orthop Clin North Am 2:371, 1971.
13. Friedenberg ZB, Miller WT: Degeneration disc disease of the cervical spine. J Bone Joint Surg Am 45-A:1171, 1963.
14. Frymoyer JW, Newberg A, Pope MH, et al: Spine radiographs in patients with low-back pain: An epidemiological study in men. J Bone Joint Surg Am 66-A:1048, 1984.
15. Gogia PP, Sabbahi MA: Electromyographic analysis of neck muscle fatigue in patients with osteoarthritis of the cervical spine. Spine 19:502, 1994.

15a. Gore DR: Roentgenographic findings in the cervical spine in asymptomatic persons: A ten-year follow-up. Spine 26:2463-2466, 2001.

16. Gore DR, Sepic SB, Gardner GM: Roentgenographic findings of the cervical spine in asymptomatic people. Spine 11:521, 1986.
17. Gruber HE, Hanley EN Jr: Analysis of aging and degeneration of the human intervertebral disc: Comparison of surgical specimens with normal controls. Spine 23:751-757, 1998.
18. Harreby M, Neergaard K, Hesselsoe G, et al: Are radiologic changes in the thoracic and lumbar spine of adolescents risk factors for low back pain in adults? A 25-year prospective cohort study of 640 school children. Spine 21:2298-2302, 1995.
19. Heller JG: The syndromes of degenerative cervical disease. Orthop Clin North Am 23:381, 1992.
20. Holt EP Jr: The question of lumbar discography. J Bone Joint Surg Am 50-A:720, 1968.
21. Houser OW, Onofrio BM, Miller GM, et al: Cervical neural foraminal canal stenosis: Computerized tomographic myelography diagnosis. J Neurosurg 79:84-88, 1993.
22. Jackson RP: The facet syndrome: Myth or reality? Clin Orthop 279:110, 1992.
23. Jackson RP, Jacobs RR, Montesano PX: Facet joint injection in low back pain: A prospective statistical study. Spine 13:966, 1988.
24. Jones MD, Pais MJ, Omiya B: Bony overgrowths and abnormal calcifications about the spine. Radiol Clin North Am 26:1213, 1988.
25. Junila J, Niinimaki T, Tervonen O: Epidural abscess after lumbar discography: A case report. Spine 22:2191-2193, 1997.
26. Kellgren JH, Lawrence JA, Bier F: Genetic factors in generalized osteoarthritis. Ann Rheum Dis 22:237, 1963.
27. Lawrence JS, Bremner JM, Bier F: Osteoarthrosis. Prevalence in the population and relationship between symptoms and x-ray changes. Ann Rheum Dis 25:1, 1966.
28. Lehto IJ, Tertti MO, Komu ME, et al: Age-related MRI changes at 0.1 T in cervical discs in asymptomatic subjects. Neuroradiology 36:49, 1994.
29. Lilius G, Laasonen EM, Myllynen P, et al: Lumbar facet joint syndrome: A randomised clinical trial. J Bone Joint Surg Br 71-B:681, 1989.
30. Lotz JC, Colliou OK, Chin JR, et al: Compression-induced degeneration of the intervertebral disc: An in vivo mouse model and finite-element study. Spine 23:2493-2506, 1998.
31. Maigne J, Lapeyre E, Morvan G, et al: Pain immediately upon sitting down and relieved by standing up is often associated with radiologic lumbar instability or marked anterior loss of disc space. Spine 28:1327-1334, 2003.
32. Malemud CJ: The role of growth factors in cartilage metabolism. Rheum Dis Clin North Am 19:569, 1993.
33. Mankin HJ: The reaction of articular cartilage to injury and osteoarthritis. N Engl J Med 291:1285, 1335, 1974.
34. Mankin HJ, Thrasher ZA: Water content and binding in normal and osteoarthritic human cartilage. J Bone Joint Surg Am 57-A:76, 1975.
35. Modic MT: Degenerative disc disease: Role of imaging. Semin Spine Surg 13:258-267, 2001.
36. Moran R, O'Connell D, Walsh MG: The diagnostic value of facet joint injections. Spine 13:1407, 1988.
37. Nathan H: Osteophytes of the vertebral column. J Bone Joint Surg Am 44-A:243, 1962.
38. Nerlich AG, Schleicher ED, Boos N: 1997 Volvo award winner in basic science studies: Immunologic markers for age-related changes of human lumbar intervertebral discs. Spine 22:2781-2795, 1997.
39. Nishida K, Kang JD, Suh J, et al: Adenovirus-mediated gene transfer to nucleus pulposus cells: Implications for the treatment of intervertebral disc degeneration. Spine 23:2447-2443, 1998.
40. Nurick S: The natural history and the results of surgical treatment of the spinal cord disorder associated with cervical spondylosis. Brain 95:101, 1972.
41. Papanicolaou N, Wilkinson RH, Emans JB, et al: Bone scintigraphy and radiography in young athletes with low back pain. AJR Am J Roentgenol 145:1039, 1985.
42. Pate D, Goobar J, Resnick D, et al.: Traction osteophytes of the lumbar spine: Radiographic-pathologic correlation. Radiology 166:843, 1988.
43. Radin EL, Paul IL, Rose RM: Role of mechanical fractures in the pathogenesis of primary osteoarthritis. Lancet 1:519, 1976.
44. Rahim KA, Stambough JL: Radiographic evaluation of the degenerative cervical spine. Orthop Clin North Am 23:395, 1992.
45. Revel M, Poiraudeau S, Auleley GR, et al: Capacity of the clinical picture to characterize low back pain relieved by facet joint anesthesia: Proposed criteria to identify patients with painful facet joints. Spine 23:1972-1977, 1998.
46. Richardson JK, Chung T, Schultz S, et al: A familial predisposition toward lumbar disc injury. Spine 22:1487-1493, 1997.
47. Schwartz AJ: Imaging of degenerative cervical disease. Spine St Art Rev 14:545-569, 2000.
48. Simmons ED Jr, Guntupalli M, Kowalski JM, et al: Familial predisposition for degenerative disc disease: A case-control study. Spine 21:1527-1529, 1996.

49. Star MJ, Curd JG, Thorne RP: Atlantoaxial lateral mass osteoarthritis: A frequently overlooked cause of severe occipitocervical pain. Spine 17:71, 1992.
50. Toyone T, Takahashi K, Kitahara H, et al: Vertebral bone-marrow change in degenerative lumbar disc disease: An MRI study of 74 patients with low back pain. J Bone Joint Surg Br 76-B:757-764, 1994.
51. Van Tulder MW, Assendelft WJJ, Koes BW, et al: Spinal radiographic findings and nonspecific low back pain: A systematic review of observational studies. Spine 22:427-434, 1997.
52. Venn MF, Maroudas A: Chemical composition and swelling of normal and osteoarthritic femoral head cartilage. I. Chemical composition. Ann Rheum Dis 36:121, 1977.
53. Videman T, Sarna S, Battie MC, et al: The long-term effects of physical loading and exercise lifestyles on back-related symptoms, disability, and spinal pathology among men. Spine 20:699-709, 1995.
54. Walsh TR, Weinstein JN, Spratt KF, et al: Lumbar discography in normal subjects: A controlled, prospective study. J Bone Joint Surg Am 72-A:1081, 1990.
55. Weishaupt D, Schmid MR, Zanetti MR et al: Positional MR imaging of the lumbar spine: Does it demonstrate nerve root compression not visible at conventional MR imaging? Radiology 215:247-253, 2000.
56. Zapletal J, Hekster REM, Straver JS, Wilmink JT: Atlanto-odontoid osteoarthritis: Appearance and prevalence at computed tomography. Spine 20:49, 1995.
57. Zapletal J, Hekster REM, Straver JS, et al: Relationship between atlanto-odontoid osteoarthritis and idiopathic suboccipital neck pain. Spine 21:2747-2751, 1996.

LUMBAR SPINAL STENOSIS

CAPSULE SUMMARY

	LOW BACK	NECK
Frequency of spinal pain	Uncommon	Not applicable (NA)
Location of spinal pain	Buttock, leg	NA
Quality of spinal pain	Ache	NA
Symptoms and signs	Difficulty walking	NA
Laboratory tests	None	NA
Radiographic findings	Plain roentgenograms display degenerative changes, MR reveals compression of spinal roots	NA
Treatment	Surgery, epidural injections	NA

PREVALENCE AND PATHOGENESIS

Spinal stenosis is narrowing of the spinal canal secondary to modifications that occur over time. These modifications can be related to degenerative, congenital, traumatic, postsurgical, or metabolic abnormalities.

Epidemiology

The prevalence of lumbar spinal stenosis increases with aging of the population. The prevalence of the disorders depends on the definition of canal narrowing. Midsagittal narrowing to less than 10.0 mm is pathologic.[23]

Clinical recognition of the syndrome is age related, with few cases diagnosed in patients younger than 50 years. Between 20% and 25% of asymptomatic individuals older than 40 years have marked narrowing of the lumbar spinal canal as documented by myelography, CT, or MR.[10,26,56]

Pathogenesis

The lumbar spinal canal is bounded anteriorly by the lumbar discs, vertebral bodies, and posterior longitudinal ligament; laterally by the laminae and facet joints; and posteriorly by the ligamentum flavum. The nerve root canals through which spinal nerves exit the spinal canal are bounded anteriorly by the posterior surface of discs and vertebral bodies, posteriorly by the facet joints and pars interarticularis, and medially by the central vertebral canal. Stenosis develops when relative narrowing of the dimensions of the lumbar spinal canal occur as a result of either congenital or acquired factors. The midsagittal diameter of the spinal canal is narrowest at the bodies of the second, third, and fourth lumbar vertebrae and widens at the level of the fifth lumbar vertebra.

Congenital spinal abnormalities are related to interpedicular narrowing such as that observed in achondroplasia, whereas acquired lumbar spinal stenosis is usually the result of spondylotic change and tends to cause midsagittal narrowing. Most cases of lumbar spinal stenosis syndrome are the result of both congenital and acquired narrowing of the lumbar spinal canal. Antenatal factors can have an effect on the diameter of the spinal canal of the fetus in utero. The L3 canal level is most sensitive to antenatal factors. Short gestational age had the greatest effect on the development of a small canal. Other factors include small placental weight, greater maternal age, primiparity, low socioeconomic class, and low birth weight.[42]

The degenerative changes that occur in the facet joints in association with alterations in intervertebral disc and soft tissue structures decrease the size of the spinal canal. The interaction of the two facet joints and the intervertebral articulation has been conceptualized into the "triple-joint complex" pathogenesis of spinal stenosis.[21] Narrowing of the spinal canal, whether on a congenital, developmental, or degenerative basis, is referred to as spinal stenosis. If the decrease in the spinal canal volume or neural foramen is severe, mechanical pressure on neural structures may occur.

Major changes occur in the lumbar spine between the third and fifth decades of life. The first manifestations of aging develop in the intervertebral discs. In the early years, the nucleus loses its vigor and the annulus fissures and degenerates. The first stage of lumbar stenosis is degeneration of the intervertebral disc. In an evaluation of 330 discs and 390 facet joints by MR and CT, degenerative disc alterations on MR occurred in the absence of facet joint changes on CT, whereas facet joint changes in the absence of disc alterations did not occur.[14] The resulting biomechanical insufficiency inevitably results in transfer of stress posteriorly to the facet joints and ligaments, which are ill suited to assume compressive, tensile, and shear loads. Capsular strain, hypermobility, and degenerative changes develop. These changes are often manifested radiologically by traction spurs, which form anteriorly, 1 to 2 mm from the disc. The ligamentum flavum is compelled to assume unnatural tensile loads in spite of having become redundant as the total spine length decreases with disc degeneration. The vertebrae themselves also tend to collapse and spread, thereby further compromising the space available for the neural elements. Disc degeneration in and of itself may not be a painful process. Patients with disc degeneration may be asymptomatic until alterations in facet joint alignment result in the onset of articular pain. This stage of the illness may be characterized by pain localized to an area just lateral to the midline, over an apophyseal joint, and exacerbated by extension of the spine without radicular radiation of pain.

Patients in their 40s and older can show the hypermobile endplate changes of the aging process. Degeneration of both the facet joints (osteoarthritis) and the intervertebral discs leads to narrowing of the spinal canal. The canal is rimmed by large osteophytes that have developed as a result of the excessive load on the now incompetent intervertebral disc. The facets are hypertrophic and deformed by osteophytic spurs that are encased within the joint capsule. The ligamentum flavum becomes redundant and, in combination with the aforementioned changes, encroaches on the spinal canal and foramina. Although such distortion of the spinal canal occurs to some degree in all active people, not everyone suffers significant disability. The symptoms that a person will have depend on the original size of the canal; if the spinal canal is small, the changes caused by aging of the disc and facet joints can lead to an absolute stenosis with compression of the neural elements. If, however, the spinal canal is large to begin with, the aging process will lead to only asymptomatic relative spinal stenosis without neural compression.[6]

Neural foraminal narrowing in a vertical dimension occurs secondary to disc space narrowing, posterior bulging of the intervertebral discs, retropulsion of the annulus fibrosus, and the formation of osteophytes around vertebral endplates. Movement of the spine will decrease the volume of the neural foramen and spinal canal. In extension and rotation, significant encroachment of the neural foramen takes place. In extension, the discs bulge posteriorly and the apophyseal joints are subluxed anteriorly.

If a disc herniation occurs in a spinal canal that is relatively small, compression of the neural elements will result. The patient will experience not only symptoms of low back pain, as mediated through the sinuvertebral nerve supply to the outer margin of the annulus, but also symptoms of radiating pain in the distribution of the compressed neural elements. In pure terms, this condition can be thought of as a relative spinal stenosis because the herniated nucleus pulposus is occupying space in an already small spinal canal. On the other hand, a similar-sized disc herniation in a large spinal canal may cause no symptoms at all because the neural elements have enough room to escape pressure. Thus, symptoms in this age group result from a combination of the disc herniation itself and the volume of the canal with which the person was born.

The pathogenesis of the symptoms of spinal stenosis remains undetermined. Some authors suggest that the symptoms associated with pseudoclaudication (leg pain) stem from compression of vascular structures, which results in diminished blood flow to the nerve roots. The compression may affect arteries, capillaries, or veins. Initially, the vascular abnormalities may result in no permanent change. However, over time, venous obstruction causes hypoxia associated with perineural fibrosis, which results in more persistent symptoms.[29] Baker and co-workers used a porcine animal model of spinal stenosis to study the vascular basis of neurogenic claudication.[8] Polyethylene balloons were placed over spinal roots to produce single or double areas of nerve compression. Blood flow to the nerve roots was monitored with laser Doppler probes. The function of the corresponding nerve roots was determined through measurement of the electromyographic activity of stimulated motor fibers proximal to areas of compression. Single-site compression did not affect blood flow, whereas double-site compression significantly decreased flow by 75% from the resting state. Proximal stimulation of the nerve root resulted in increased blood flow that was not sustained during prolonged compression. With the loss of blood flow, the corresponding motor nerve function was diminished. This model of neurogenic claudication suggests that venous pooling between two sites of blockage is responsible for impairment of the vasodilation response to exercise that culminates in impaired nerve function and radicular pain. Others believe that the symptoms are related directly to mechanical compression of neural structures.[30] In later stages of this disorder, increasing radicular pain develops with walking. The distance associated with the onset of radicular pain shortens with increasing severity of stenosis. The process may progress to the point that just standing upright without ambulation causes leg pain.

CLINICAL HISTORY

As the degenerative process continues, patients complain of symptoms associated with spinal stenosis, most commonly pseudoclaudication.[23] Pseudoclaudication is associated with pain in the buttock, thigh, or leg that develops with standing or walking and is relieved by rest, in the presence of adequate blood flow to the lower extremities. Many patients have leg pain with standing alone (94% in one study), in clear distinction to vascular claudication. Walking a distance as short as 200 yards may also bring on pain. Many patients may have bilateral leg pain. A majority of patients have back pain in combination with leg pain. However, it is important to remember that a small group of patients will have leg pain only, without any associated back pain. At times, similar symptoms can occur while lying down and are relieved only by walking around. In addition to pain, patients may also complain of numbness, paresthesias, and weakness in the lower extremities. Many patients will experience various combinations of these symptoms.[23]

Neurogenic claudication is relieved by lying down, sitting, or flexing at the waist. Patients with lumbar spinal stenosis assume a simian posture while walking or go to the grocery store to use the shopping carts. Such pseudoclaudication typically affects multiple dermatomes and is difficult to ascribe to a single nerve root lesion. Bilateral symptoms occur in 40% of spinal stenosis patients.

An internationally accepted classification of the anatomic state and its clinical syndrome known as lumbar spinal stenosis has been devised, and the production of symptoms attributed to these changes can be either localized or generalized in origin. It is important to realize, however, that structural changes in the spinal and foraminal canals that are exaggerated with posture are anatomic changes and not absolute determinants of pain. The symptoms manifested may vary significantly among patients with similar pathomorphologic changes because of the temporal framework in which the neural compression has occurred, the susceptibility of the nerves involved, and the unique functional demands and pain tolerance of each patient.

PHYSICAL EXAMINATION

Patients with spinal stenosis associated with persistent nerve impingement have objective signs of muscle weakness, atrophy, and asymmetric reflexes.[32] In patients in whom intermittent symptoms develop with standing or walking, neurologic changes will occur only after the patient is stressed. The following stress tests can be used in an outpatient clinic: after a neurologic examination has been performed, the patient is asked to walk until symptoms occur or a distance of 300 feet has been achieved. A repeat examination is then performed, and in some cases the second examination will reveal a neurologic deficit that was not present after the first examination.

Sciatica caused by lumbar spinal stenosis is distinct from the sciatica that typically follows herniation of the nucleus pulposus. Objective neurologic signs are absent. A positive straight leg–raising test is present in only 10% of cases of sciatica attributable to lumbar spinal stenosis. Ankle jerks are absent in 40%, knee jerks are absent in 10%, and a small percentage have sensory loss or weakness.[23,31]

Katz and co-workers studied 93 patients with low back pain to determine any characteristic historical and physical findings that would differentiate spinal stenosis.[34] Spinal stenosis was confirmed in 38 of 43 patients (88%) with imaging studies. Historical findings associated with stenosis were greater age, severe lower extremity pain, and absence of pain when seated. Physical findings included a wide-based gait, abnormal Romberg test, thigh pain after 30 seconds of lumbar extension, and neuromuscular deficits.

The presence or absence of lower extremity reflexes may not be a reliable sign of nerve compression. Bowditch and colleagues evaluated ankle reflexes in 1076 adult orthopedic patients with an age range of 16 to 99 years and no history of spinal (sciatica) or medical disorders (diabetes, peripheral neuropathy) associated with absent ankle jerks.[13] The 543 men and 533 women who were eligible patients were stratified by decade into nine groups. The earliest significant bilateral loss of ankle reflex occurred in the group between 51 and 60 years of age, with loss detected in 8%; in contrast, in those 61 to 70 years old, loss of the ankle reflex occurred in 30%. Unilateral loss of reflex increased with age, but never exceeded 10% of patients. Bilateral loss of ankle reflex will "hide" asymmetric pathology as the patient ages. Unilateral loss of an ankle reflex is a significant neurologic sign irrespective of age.

Bowel and bladder sphincter disturbance can develop but is relatively uncommon. Some men are unable to void in the standing position but are able to do so while sitting, a cauda equina equivalent of neurogenic claudication. The presence of bladder disturbance is an indication for surgery to stabilize the deficit and allow for the potential for recovery of bladder function.[15] Intermittent priapism is a rare manifestation of spinal stenosis in men.[44]

LABORATORY DATA

Laboratory evaluation of patients with lumbar spinal stenosis is usually normal. Any abnormality in the erythrocyte sedimentation rate or C-reactive protein suggests an alternative diagnosis to a mechanical cause of neurogenic claudication.

Electromyography (EMG) may be abnormal in some patients with persistent symptoms. Of 37 patients with surgically proven spinal stenosis, 34 had an abnormality on EMG with evidence of one or more radiculopathies.[23] The abnormalities can be difficult to interpret, with one study demonstrating that 11 of 36 patients with stenosis had EMG abnormalities at levels higher than those expected based on myelography.[50] The abnormal findings include changes associated with radiculopathies (positive waves, giant potentials).[23] Other neurophysiologic findings of spinal stenosis include bilateral and multisegmental neurogenic EMG abnormalities in the legs.[31] Much of the usefulness of EMG lies in excluding peripheral neuropathy and peripheral nerve entrapment syndromes.[47] Somatosensory potentials may also be helpful preoperatively in identifying the level of cord compression and intraoperatively to assess the adequacy of neural decompression.[36]

RADIOGRAPHIC EVALUATION

Roentgenograms

Roentgenograms usually demonstrate abnormalities of lumbar spondylosis but are not diagnostic of spinal canal narrowing. However, normal roentgenograms are an unusual finding. Roentgenographic abnormalities associated with lumbar spinal stenosis include narrowing of intervertebral disc spaces, facet joint osteoarthritis, and degenerative spondylolisthesis, particularly at L4–L5.[49] These features are common in asymptomatic older individuals, and their predictive value is limited. Measurements of interpedicular diameter and midsagittal measurements are of questionable clinical significance.

The intervertebral disc anteriorly and the two facet joints posteriorly form a triangle with the neural elements in the center. These three structures are sometimes referred to as the "triple-joint complex," and their degeneration leads to loss of volume (area) in the triangle. As stated earlier, if the loss is severe enough, compression of neural elements will take place (Fig. 10-16). The diagnosis of spinal stenosis depends less on absolute measurement of the size of the canal but rather on the configuration of the canal and the relative amount of space at various levels of the spine.[49]

Computed Tomography

CT scans visualize structures localized to a single level and can demonstrate articular facet hypertrophy, enlargement of laminae, hyperplasia and ossification of the ligamentum flavum, and disc prolapse. The technique allows visualization of the osseous margins and shape of the lumbar spinal canal. CT scans provide better visualization of the lateral recesses and nerve root exit canals than myelography does and shows the spinal canal below the level of a myelographic block. A trefoil shape of the lumbar canal is typical of those with severe lumbar spinal stenosis. The presence of normal epidural fat makes significant nerve root compression unlikely.

Myelography

Myelography is best suited for showing central lumbar spinal stenosis than stenosis isolated to the lateral recesses. Demonstration of obstruction to dye flow can be dependent on posture, with compression of the dural sac by the ligamentum flavum and disc being more severe in an extended posture. Myelography can also be extended to allow visualization of the conus medullaris and the lower thoracic levels. Myelography is frequently combined with CT for a better definition of the lateral recesses and nerve root canals than provided by CT or myelography alone.

Myelography will demonstrate subtotal or total obstruction of the column of dye in the lumbar region in patients with spinal stenosis. The L4 and L5 vertebral body levels are the ones most commonly affected (Fig. 10-17).

Myelography is a dynamic study characterized by movement of the water-soluble dye up and down the spinal canal. The radiologist is able to actually visualize the locations in the spine that are the most severely compressed. Myelography continues as one of the diagnostic tests for spinal stenosis (CT and MR are static tests).[2]

Magnetic Resonance

The role of MR continues to advance with the development of this radiographic technique (Figs. 10-18 and 10-19). Three-dimensional imaging has been developed for MR. Different three-dimensional techniques are capable of providing visualization of cerebrospinal fluid with either high or low signal intensity; thus, cerebrospinal

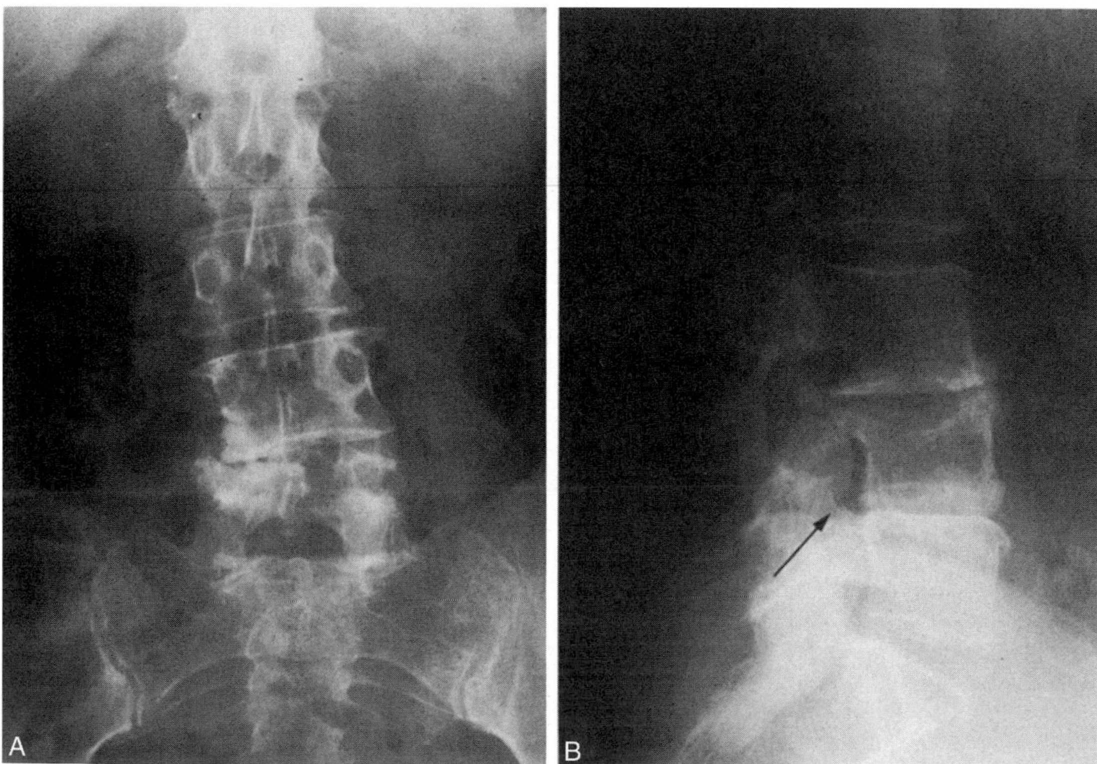

Figure 10-16 Anteroposterior *(A)* and lateral *(B)* views of the lumbar spine in a patient with spinal stenosis at the L4–L5 segment. A loss of area in the neural foramen is noted on the lateral view *(arrow)*.

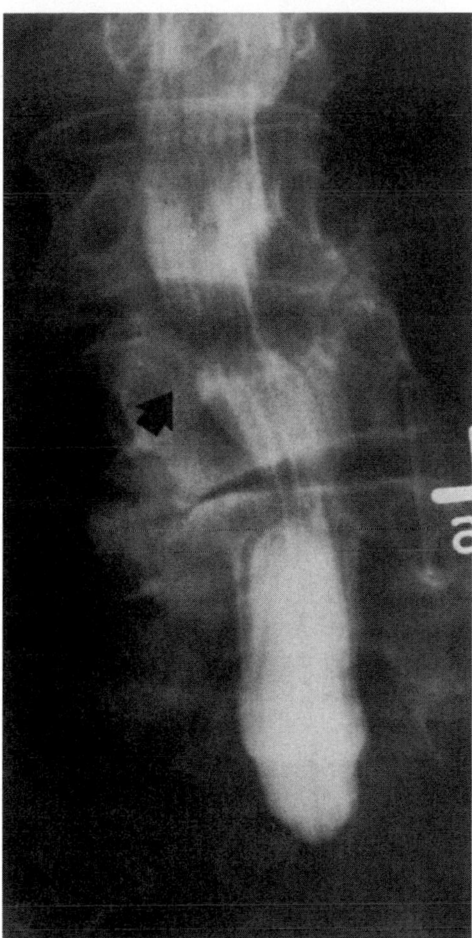

Figure 10-17 Myelogram of a 64-year-old patient with significant stenosis in the L3–L4 region of the lumbar spine *(arrow)*.

fluid may act as its own contrast agent and permit myelographic images without any need for the injection of dye. Further development of this technique may result in images that are as good as a myelogram but without the necessity of injecting dye.[46]

Scientific data to support the accuracy of one radiographic technique over another in the diagnosis of spinal stenosis are lacking.[37] A number of published studies have had methodologic flaws that limit their usefulness as proof of the sensitivity and specificity for making the diagnosis of spinal stenosis.[37] At this time, the choice of technique depends on the issues of cost, reimbursement, access to equipment, and skill of the radiologist. Determination of the most accurate technique will evolve as larger, more rigorous studies are published and with improvements in imaging accuracy.[44a]

At present, MR is the modality of choice for imaging lumbar spinal stenosis. MR is noninvasive and allows for superior resolution of soft tissue and bone. Contrast is not necessary unless patients have previously undergone back surgery. CT-myelography has a secondary role, mainly because of its invasive nature.[57]

DIFFERENTIAL DIAGNOSIS

Lumbar spinal stenosis is a clinical diagnosis characterized by specific historical and physical findings and confirmed, but not diagnosed by radiographic techniques showing compression of nerve roots. Pseudoclaudication syndrome, or pain in the calf, occurs in stenosis patients, but it is not necessary to establish a diagnosis of lumbar spinal stenosis.

Spinal stenosis may be caused by a number of processes that decrease space in the spinal canal for the neural

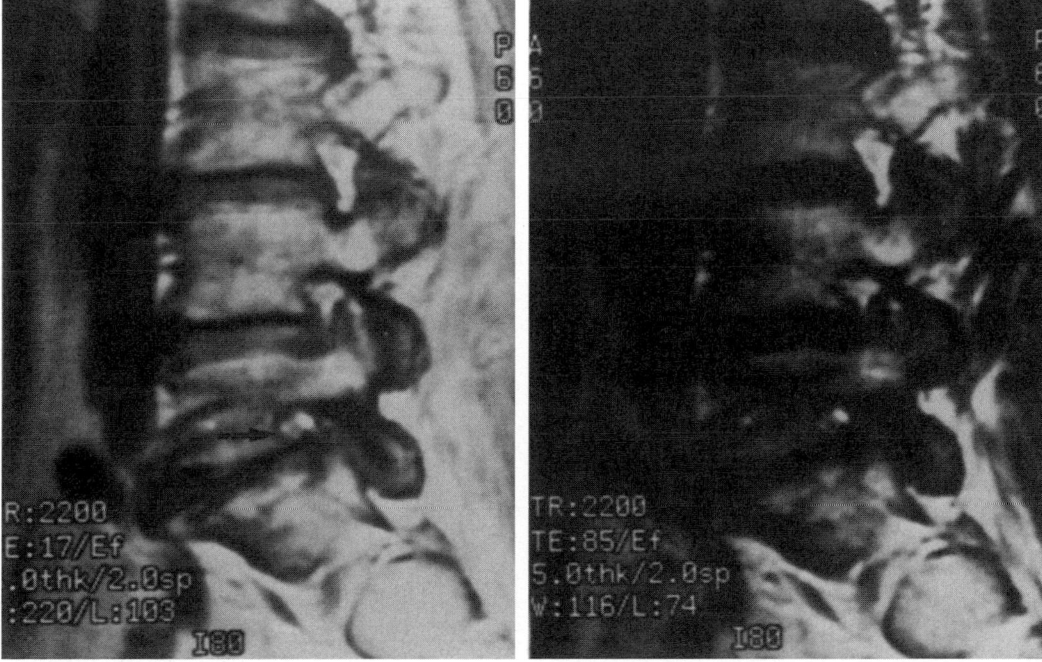

Figure 10-18 MR image of the lumbar spine. The sagittal view of a T2-weighted image demonstrates foraminal narrowing at the L5–S1 interspace *(black arrow)* with associated intervertebral disc degeneration.

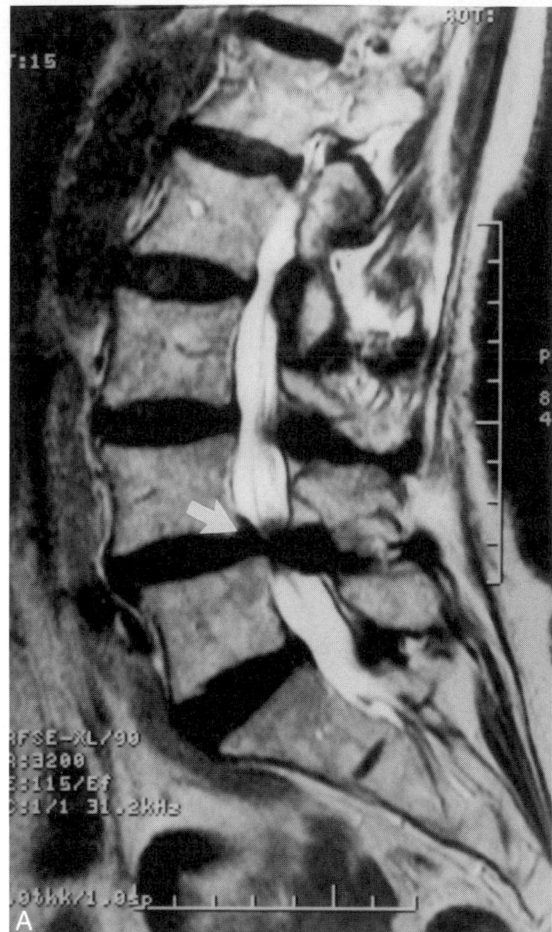

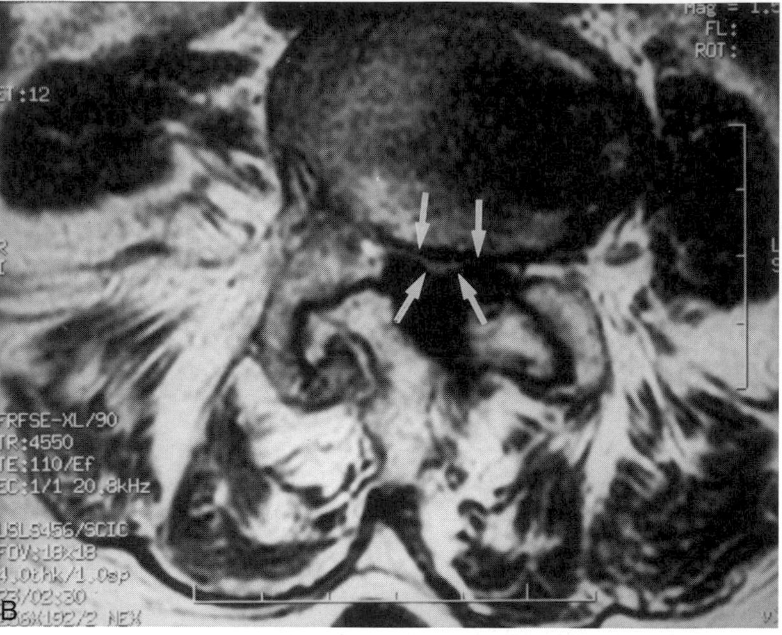

Figure 10-19 MR images of the lumbar spine of a 92-year-old woman with leg numbness and difficulty ambulating. Sagittal *(A)* and axial *(B)* views demonstrate severe stenosis at L4–L5 *(white arrows)* caused by facet joint osteophytes, a protruding intervertebral disc, and redundant ligamentum flavum.

elements.[40] The classification of spinal stenosis includes developmental and acquired forms (Table 10-5). Degenerative causes are responsible for lumbar spinal stenosis in the vast majority of individuals. A variety of medical disorders can cause stenosis, including calcium pyrophosphate crystal deposition, acromegaly, amyloid deposition, Paget's disease, and intradural spinal tumors.[16,27,39,53] The neurogenic and vascular types of claudication do have different associated symptoms and signs (Table 10-6).[9] Patients may have both neurogenic and vascular claudication simultaneously. The alternate cause of claudication should be investigated if partial improvement occurs with decompressive laminectomy or vascular surgery.[17]

Lateral Recess Stenosis

The lumbar spinal canal has three primary shapes: oval, triangular, and trefoil. The trefoil shape has a smaller area contiguous to the lateral recess. The exit area from the lumbar spinal canal can be divided into three zones[5]: zone 1 is the lateral recess under the articular process medial to the pedicle, zone 2 is the portion of the nerve root canal covered by the pedicle (foraminal), and zone 3 is the area lateral to the pedicle (extraforaminal). Verbiest defined the narrow lateral recess as the part of the vertebral canal giving access to the intervertebral foramen.[55] Narrowing of the trefoil lumbar canal can entrap the L5 or S1 nerve roots. These individuals experience neurogenic pain that may not be relieved with sitting. The lateral recess may become stenotic with hypertrophy of the superior articular process in the subarticular zone and the medial aspect of the pedicle. Foraminal stenosis occurs with vertical settling of the pedicle or foraminal disc herniation.[4] Symptoms are persistent and not modified by position. Kanamiya and co-workers reported on the different symptoms associated with lateral recess syndrome caused by bony overgrowth versus disc herniation.[33] In individuals with a herniated disc, low back pain developed initially and then lower leg pain. Bony lateral recess stenosis is associated with lower leg pain exclusively. Flexion and extension movements exacerbate symptoms associated with a herniated disc. Therapies used for other types of lumbar spinal stenosis can be tried, but are not usually effective. These individuals require surgical intervention to obtain relief. Partial facetectomy is a procedure that is associated with significant improvement in leg pain at 5-year follow-up.[48] Nerve impingement may also occur secondary to intraspinal synovial cysts (Fig. 10-20).

Tumoral Calcinosis

Dystrophic calcinosis can develop in the spinal canal in both the lumbar and cervical regions.[18,38] This disorder may be associated with hereditary disorders of calcium metabolism or could be a consequence of renal dialysis. In areas

10-5 CLASSIFICATION OF LUMBAR SPINAL STENOSIS

A. Congenital/developmental
  1. Idiopathic
  2. Genetic/metabolic
     Achondroplasia
     Morquio's syndrome
     Hypophosphatemic vitamin D–resistant rickets
  3. Other
     Down syndrome
     Scoliosis
B. Acquired
  1. Degenerative
     Spondylosis
     Isolated intervertebral disc resorption
     Lateral nerve entrapment
     Spondylolisthesis
     Adult scoliosis
     Calcification of the ligamentum flavum
     Intraspinal synovial cysts
     Spinal dysraphism
  2. Metabolic/endocrine
     Osteoporosis with fracture
     Acromegaly
     Calcium pyrophosphate dihydrate crystal deposition disease
     Renal osteodystrophy
     Hypoparathyroidism
     Epidural lipomatosis
  3. Postoperative
     Postlaminectomy
     Postfusion
     Postdiscectomy
  4. Traumatic
     Fracture
  5. Miscellaneous
     Paget's disease
     Diffuse idiopathic skeletal hyperostosis
     Fluorosis
     Conjoined origin of lumbosacral nerve roots
     Amyloid

Modified from Moreland LW, Lopez-Mendez A, Larcon GS: Spinal stenosis: A comprehensive review of the literature. Semin Arthritis Rheum 19:127, 1989.

other than the axial skeleton, the lesions are painless and discovered by chance. Involvement of the spine is rare but can cause confusion with other space-occupying processes. Patients exhibit leg, back, or neck pain. Radicular symptoms are present if a nerve root is compressed. Spinal cord involvement in the cervical spine may be manifested as paraparesis and sensory deficits. The lesions may not be apparent on plain roentgenograms but are discovered on MR images (Fig. 10-21). The MR changes can be misinterpreted as extruded discs, cysts, infections, or neoplasms. Histologic examination of surgical specimens reveals masses of calcium hydroxyapatite surrounded by a foreign body giant cell reaction. In rare circumstances, calcium pyrophosphate hydroxyhydrate crystals are admixed with hydroxyapatite crystals. In a group of 21 patients with this disorder, 9 underwent surgical decompression. This disorder is unusual but should be considered in patients with extensive calcification in unusual spinal locations.

10-6 NEUROGENIC VERSUS VASCULAR CLAUDICATION

Evaluation	Neurogenic	Vascular
Walking distance	Variable	Fixed
Palliative factors	Sitting/bending	Standing
Provocative factors	Walking/standing	Walking
Walking uphill	Painless	Painful
Bicycle test	Painless	Painful
Pulses	Present	Absent
Skin	Normal	Atrophic
Weakness	Occasional	Rare
Back pain	Common	Rare
Back motion	Limited	Normal
Pain character	Numbness, aching Proximal to distal	Cramping Distal to proximal
Atrophy	Occasional	Rare

Modified from Bell GR: Office evaluation of patients with spinal stenosis. Semin Spine Surg 11:191-194, 1999.

TREATMENT

The majority of patients with osteoarthritis and stenosis of the lumbosacral spine can be treated nonsurgically.[43,51] Nonsteroidal anti-inflammatory drugs are helpful in controlling symptoms. The toxicity of gastric irritation may be of greater concern in patients with osteoarthritis because individuals with this ailment are older. Gastric upset may occur more commonly in an older patient population. Medications may be given to protect the gastric mucosa in patients who are at risk for significant morbidity or mortality from gastrointestinal bleeding. Cyclooxygenase-2 (COX-2) inhibitors have equal efficacy but less gastrointestinal toxicity than combination COX-1/COX-2 inhibitors do. Lumbosacral corsets are helpful in reminding the patient to avoid excessive spinal movement. Functional rehabilitation involving activity modification, flexion exercises, postural training, stationary bicycle, and aquatic-based programs have shown benefit in decreasing symptoms and maintaining function.[45] Short courses of oral corticosteroids (methylprednisolone acetate [Medrol Dosepak]) are used on rare occasion in patients with severe symptoms of spinal stenosis who do not respond to nonsteroidal drugs. Oral corticosteroids must be given in low doses. The potential risk of large doses of corticosteroids, including osteoporosis and hypertension, must be weighed against the potential benefit that would only come with steroid use. Patients can respond to chronic, low-dose corticosteroids at the 5- to 10-mg level. A therapeutic trial for a specified period is undertaken. Patients who experience significant improvement in function (increased walking distance, diminished pain) are maintained on a low dose. Those who have no benefit are quickly tapered off corticosteroids.

Epidural corticosteroids should be considered before oral corticosteroids are given if the patient is amenable to injection therapy.[12] Patients may require a course of three injections before they report relief of symptoms. Patients may also benefit for an extended period from a single injection. The total dose of epidural corticosteroids is limited to 240 mg of methylprednisolone for a 6-month period. I have recommended that patients receive one injection and delay a subsequent injection until the recurrence of symptoms. In this way, patients may receive an injection every 2 months and maintain an improved level of function. The duration of benefit is variable. Some patients may have relief of symptoms that lasts months. With the return of symptoms, another course of injections may be given. Most patients who have responded to

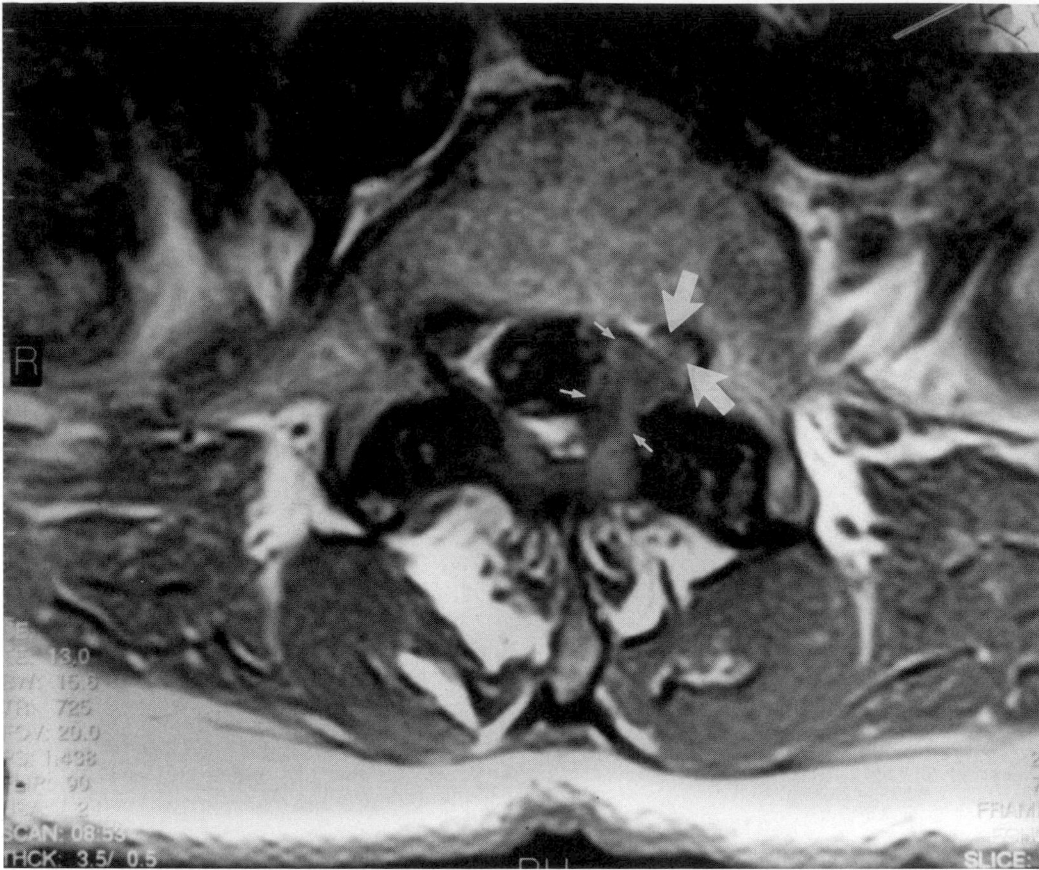

Figure 10-20 MR scan of a 49-year-old woman with increasing left L5 radicular pain. An axial view at the L4–L5 level reveals a synovial cyst *(small white arrows)* encroaching into the spinal canal with compression of the exiting nerve root *(big white arrows)*. Over a 12-month period a repeat MR scan documented resolution of the cyst after epidural injections.

injections have been controlled with two courses of therapy per year. In a study of 249 patients with back pain lasting 3 months or longer, those who did not benefit 1 year after epidural injection had pain that interfered with activities, were unemployed because of pain, had a normal straight leg–raising test, and had pain not decreased by medication.[28] Fluoroscopically guided lumbar transforaminal epidural steroid injections are helpful for unilateral leg pain associated with spinal stenosis. In a group of 34 patients, 75% had a successful long-term outcome with at least a 50% reduction in pain. Sixty-four percent of patients had improved walking and standing tolerance.[11] Calcitonin also has been helpful in controlling symptoms of spinal stenosis.[19] Patients realizing the greatest degree of pain relief were those with moderate pain and walking capacity of more than 200 m.[20] The use of injection therapy for spinal stenosis remains controversial.[44b] Operative therapy for spinal stenosis is reserved for patients who are totally incapacitated by their condition (see Chapter 20).

Surgery

Leg pain, not back pain, is most successfully relieved with an operation. Severe stenosis responds to a greater degree than mild stenosis does. The guiding principle for spinal stenosis surgery is obtaining adequate decompression without causing instability.[52] Older patients should not be excluded from surgical decompression. A complex group of data need to be analyzed to determine the appropriate time, location, and technique for surgical intervention. A stepwise approach to the problem can help with the decision making.[54]

Herno and colleagues reported the results of surgery for spinal stenosis in 311 patients.[24] The first operation in 251 spinal stenosis patients resulted in an excellent to good outcome in 67%. Severe myelographic changes correlated significantly with a good outcome in this group. Repeat operations had a similar good outcome in only 46% of 66 patients. Individuals who were older than 50 years and had no coexistent medical disorders had a greater opportunity for a good outcome. The first decompression operation is the best operation for success in spinal stenosis patients.

Herno and co-workers also completed a 10-year follow-up study to correlate the success of surgical decompression for spinal stenosis and clinical outcome in 56 patients.[25] Stenosis recurred in 73% of patients. Function, as measured by the Oswestry disability questionnaire and treadmill test, was matched against the degree of stenosis, disc degeneration, facet joint arthropathy, and spondylolisthesis. The patient's perception of improvement correlated with Oswestry scores and walking capacity. Degenerative

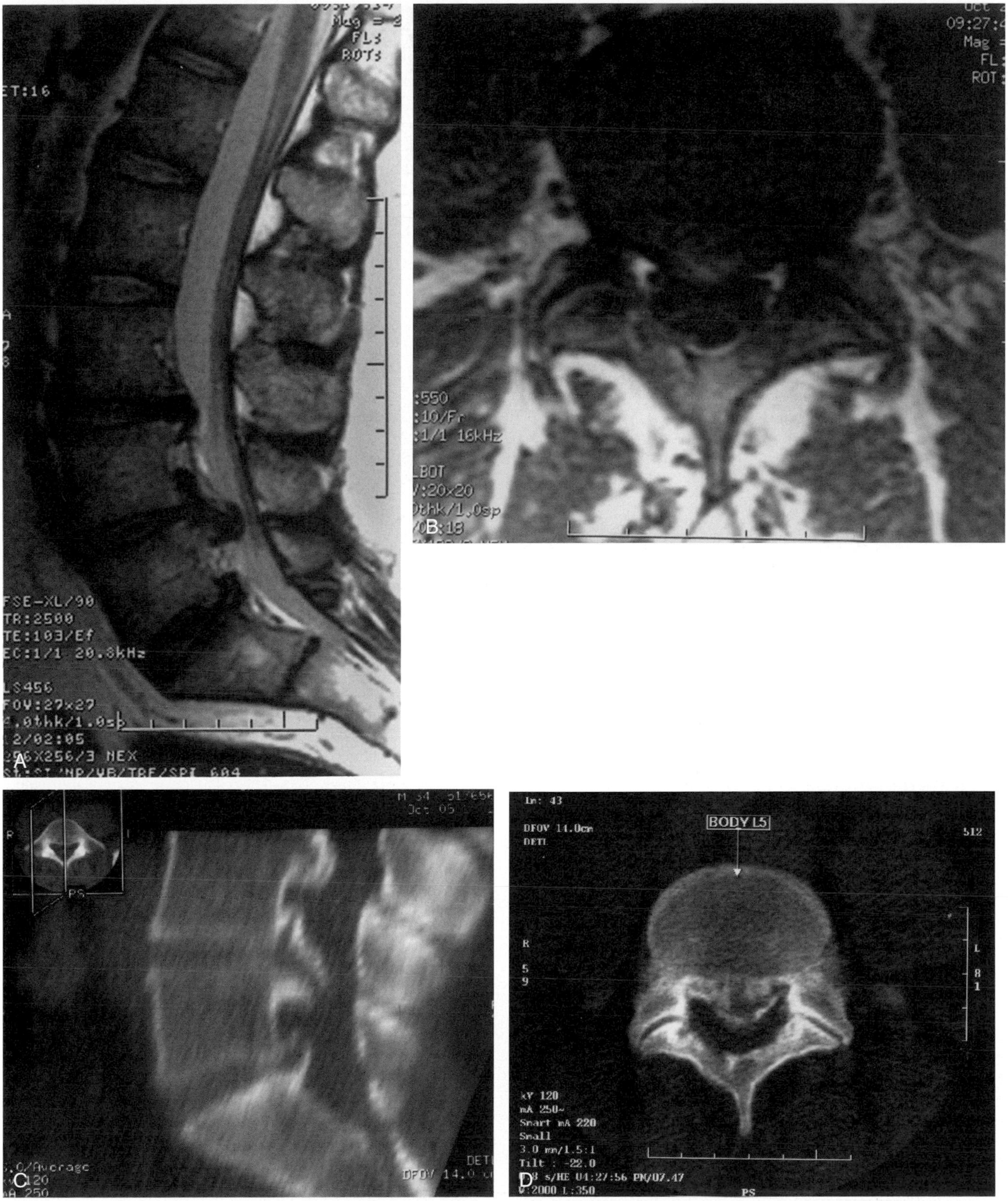

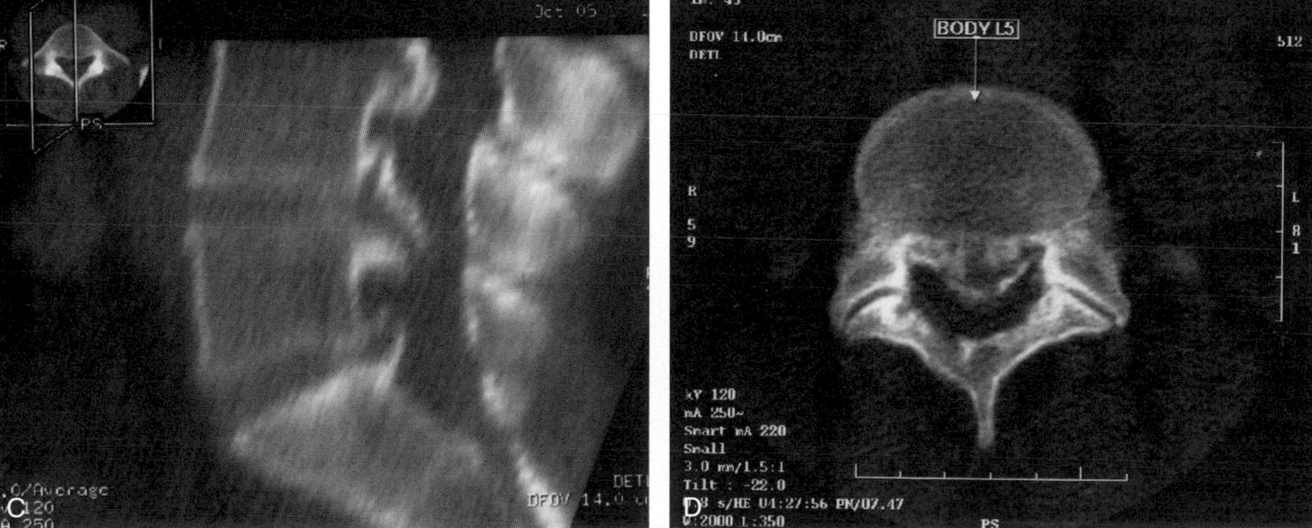

Figure 10-21 A 34-year-old man with increasing low back and leg pain. A sagittal MR scan *(A)* reveals calcified outgrowths at L3–L4, L4–L5, and L5–S1. An axial view *(B)* at L4–L5 demonstrates the extent of the encroachment into the spinal canal. A sagittal CT scan *(C)* reveals the form of the bony prominences. An axial view *(D)* at L5 highlights the inner composition of the bony exostosis.

findings had a greater effect on patients' walking capacity than stenotic findings did.

The presence of preoperative scoliosis is associated with an unfavorable outcome after decompression for degenerative lumbar spinal stenosis. However, an increase in olisthesis after surgery was associated with less leg pain and improved walking capacity at 6 and 24 months.[22]

PROGNOSIS

A 4-year prospective study of spinal stenosis reported that conservative, nonsurgical therapy was effective in decreasing or controlling the symptoms of spinal stenosis.[41] The natural course of lumbar stenosis is improvement in symptoms. A study of 32 patients who did not receive therapy revealed decreased symptoms in 15%, no change in 70%, and worsening in 15%. No severe deterioration requiring surgery occurred during the study period.

In a 7- to 10-year outcome study, Katz and co-workers described a 75% approval rating of 88 spinal stenosis patients after surgery.[35] Of the original cohort of 88, 20 were deceased and 20 had undergone a reoperation. Of the 55 patients with an average follow-up of 8.1 years who responded to a standardized questionnaire, 33% had severe back pain and 53% were unable to walk two blocks. Despite these results, 75% were satisfied with their surgery and would undergo the procedure again. An important consideration regarding the general function of patients was a limitation in functional status directly related to spinal symptoms despite a high prevalence of co-morbid conditions. This study reported the outcome of stenosis surgery at 10 years but did not have an adequate number of patients to determine the necessity of spinal fusion for spinal stenosis and the risk factors for repeat surgery. In contrast, Airaksinen and colleagues found that a combination of extraspinal and spinal disorders, including diabetes, hip arthritis, and fracture of the lumbar spine, was associated with a poor outcome in a cohort of 438 Finnish patients with spinal stenosis evaluated 4.3 years after surgery.[1] The proportion of good to excellent outcomes was 62%. The ability to work before or after surgery and a history of no previous back surgery were predictive of a good outcome. The age of the patient did not otherwise affect the outcome of surgical decompression.

Amundsen and co-workers reported on a cohort of 100 spinal stenosis patients treated surgically or with conservative therapy on a random basis and monitored for a 10-year period.[3] Patients with severe sciatica (19) received surgical therapy, those with moderate symptoms (31) underwent surgery or medical therapy, and those with mild symptoms (50) received medical therapy. At 4 years, 80% of the surgery patients and 50% of the medical patients had fair or excellent outcomes. Patients treated medically initially had a good response to delayed surgery, similar to individuals who underwent surgery during the initial phase of the study. Individuals with multilevel stenosis did not have a poorer outcome independent of the therapeutic option.

Atlas and colleagues reported their 4-year assessment of this same cohort of spinal stenosis patients regarding leg and back pain, functional status, and satisfaction with therapy.[7] Outcome data were available on 119 patients, 67 treated surgically and 52 nonsurgically. The surgically treated patients had more severe symptoms and worse function at baseline and better outcomes at the 4-year evaluation. Improvement in leg and back pain was reported by 70% of surgical and 52% of nonsurgical patients. Satisfaction with the current status was mentioned by 63% of surgical and 42% of nonsurgical patients. The benefits of surgery declined over the 4-year study but were still superior to nonsurgical therapy, which remained stable over the study period.

The results of studies of lumbar spinal stenosis suggest that initial conservative therapy is appropriate. Delayed surgery does not diminish the possibility of a favorable outcome, particularly in patients who believe that their health is excellent and who do not have any cardiovascular co-morbidities.

References

Lumbar Spinal Stenosis

1. Airaksinen O, Herno A, Turunen V, et al: Surgical outcome of 438 patients treated surgically for lumbar spinal stenosis. Spine 22:2278-2282, 1997.
2. Alam F, Moss SG, Schweitzer ME: Imaging of degenerative disease of the lumbar spine and related conditions. Semin Spine Surg 11:76-96, 1999.
3. Amundsen T, Weber H, Nordal HJ, et al: Lumbar spinal stenosis: Conservative or surgical management? A prospective 10-year study. Spine 25:1424-1436, 2000.
4. An HS, Butler JP: Lumbar spinal stenosis: Historical perspectives, classification, and pathoanatomy. Semin Spine Surg 11:184-190, 1999.
5. Andersson GBJ, McNeill TW: Definition and classification of lumbar spinal stenosis. In Andersson GBJ, McNeill TW (eds): Lumbar Spinal Stenosis. St Louis, Mosby–Year Book, 1992, pp 9-15.
6. Arnoldi CC, Brodsky AE, Cauchoix J, et al: Lumbar spinal stenosis and nerve root entrapment syndrome: Definition and classification. Clin Orthop 115:4, 1976.
7. Atlas SJ, Keller RB, Robson D, et al: Surgical and nonsurgical management of lumbar spinal stenosis: Four-year outcomes from the Main Lumbar Spine Study. Spine 25:556-562, 2000.
8. Baker AR, Collins TA, Porter RW, et al: Laser Doppler study of porcine cauda equina blood flow: The effect of electrical stimulation of rootlets during single and double site, low pressure compression of the cauda equina. Spine 20:660-664, 1995.
9. Bell GR: Office evaluation of patients with spinal stenosis. Semin Spine Surg 11:191-194, 1999.
10. Boden SD, Davis DO, Dina TS, et al: Abnormal magnetic-resonance scans of the lumbar spine in asymptomatic subjects: A prospective investigation. J Bone Joint Surg Am 72-A:403, 1990.
11. Botwin KP, Gruber RD, Bouchlas CG, et al: Fluoroscopically guided lumbar transforaminal epidural steroid injections in degenerative lumbar stenosis: An outcome study. Am J Phys Med Rehabil 81:898-905, 2002.
12. Botwin KP, Gruber RD: Lumbar epidural steroid injections in the patient with lumbar spinal stenosis. Phys Med Rehabil Clin N Am 14:121-141, 2003.
13. Bowditch MG, Sanderson P, Livesey JP: The significance of an absent ankle reflex. J Bone Joint Surg Br 78-B:276-279, 1996.
14. Butler D, Trafimow JH, Andersson GBJ, et al: Discs degenerate before facets. Spine 15:111, 1990.
15. Deen HG, Zimmerman RS, Swanson SK, et al: Assessment of bladder function after lumbar decompressive surgery for spinal stenosis: A prospective study. J Neurosurg 80:971-974, 1994.
16. Delamarter RB, Sherman JE, Carr J: Lumbar spinal stenosis secondary to calcium pyrophosphate crystal deposition (pseudogout). Clin Orthop 289:127, 1993.
17. Dodge LD, Bohlman HH, Rhodes RS: Concurrent lumbar spinal stenosis and peripheral vascular disease: A report of nine patients. Clin Orthop 230:141, 1988.
18. Durant DM, Riley LH III, Burger PC, et al: Tumoral calcinosis of the spine: A study of 21 cases. Spine 26:1673-1679, 2001.
19. Eskola A, Alaranta H, Pohjolainen T, et al: Calcitonin treatment in lumbar stenosis: Clinical observations. Calcif Tissue Int 45:372, 1989.
20. Eskola A, Pohjolainen T, Alaranta H, et al: Calcitonin treatment in lumbar spinal stenosis: A randomized, placebo-controlled, double-blind, cross-order study with one-year follow-up. Calcif Tissue Int 50:400, 1992.

21. Farfan HS: Mechanical Disorders of the Low Back. Philadelphia, Lea & Febiger, 1973.
22. Frazier DD, Lipson SJ, Fossel AH, Katz JN: Associations between spinal deformity and outcomes after decompression for spinal stenosis. Spine 22:2025-2029, 1997.
23. Hall S, Bartleson JD, Onofrio BM, et al: Lumbar spinal stenosis: Clinical features, diagnostic procedures and results of treatment in 68 patients. Ann Intern Med 103:271-275, 1985.
24. Herno A, Airaksinen O, Saari T, Sihoven T: Surgical results of lumbar spinal stenosis: A comparison of patients with or without previous back surgery. Spine 20:964-969, 1995.
25. Herno A, Patanen K, Talaslahti T, et al: Long-term clinical and magnetic resonance imaging follow-up assessment of patients with lumbar spinal stenosis after laminectomy. Spine 24:1533-1537, 1999.
26. Hitselberger WE, Witten RM: Abnormal myelograms in asymptomatic patients. J Neurosurg 28:204, 1968.
27. Honig S, Murali R: Spinal cord claudication from amyloid deposition. J Rheumatol 19:1988, 1992.
28. Jamison RN, VadeBoncouer T, Ferrante FM: Low back pain patients unresponsive to an epidural steroid injection: Identifying predictive factors. Clin J Pain 7:311-317, 1991.
29. Jayson MIV: The role of vascular damage and fibrosis in the pathogenesis of nerve root damage. Clin Orthop 279:40, 1992.
30. Jellinger K, Neumayer E: Claudication of the spinal canal and cauda equina. In Vinken PJ, Bruyn GW (eds): Handbook of Clinical Neurology, Vol 12. Vascular Diseases of the Nervous System. Amsterdam, North-Holland Publishing, 1972, pp 507-547.
31. Johnsson K, Rosen I, Uden A: Neurophysiologic investigation of patients with spinal stenosis. Spine 12:483, 1987.
32. Jonsson B, Stromqvist B: Symptoms and signs in degeneration of the lumbar spine: A prospective consecutive study of 300 operated patients. J Bone Joint Surg Br 75-B:381-385, 1993.
33. Kanamiya T, Kida H, Seki M, et al: Effect of lumbar disc herniation on clinical symptoms of lateral recess syndrome. Clin Orthop 398:131-135, 2002.
34. Katz JN, Dalgas M, Stucki G, et al: Degenerative lumbar spinal stenosis: Diagnostic value of the history and physical examination. Arthritis Rheum 38:1236-1241, 1995.
35. Katz JN, Lipson SJ, Chang LC, et al: Seven- to 10-year outcome of decompressive surgery for degenerative lumbar spinal stenosis. Spine 21:92-98, 1996.
36. Keim HA, Hajdu M, Gonzalez EG, et al: Somatosensory evoked potentials as an aid in the diagnosis and intraoperative management of spinal stenosis. Spine 10:338, 1985.
37. Kent DL, Haynor DR, Larson EB, Deyo RA: Diagnosis of lumbar spinal stenosis in adults: A metaanalysis of the accuracy of CT, MR, and myelography. AJR Am J Roengenol 158:1135, 1992.
38. Matsukado K, Amano T, Itou O, et al: Tumoral calcinosis in the upper cervical spine causing progressive radiculomyelopathy—case report. Neurol Med Chir 41:41-414, 2001.
39. McGuire RA, Brown MD, Green BA: Intradural spinal tumors and spinal stenosis: Report of two cases. Spine 12:1062, 1987.
40. Moreland LW, Lopez-Mendez A, Alarcon GS: Spinal stenosis: A comprehensive review of the literature. Semin Arthritis Rheum 19:127, 1989.
41. Onel D, Sari H, Donmerz C: Lumbar spinal stenosis: Clinical/radiologic therapeutic evaluation in 145 patients. Spine 18:291, 1993.
42. Papp T, Porter RW, Craig CE, et al: Significant antenatal factors in the development of lumbar spinal stenosis. Spine 22:1805-1810, 1997.
43. Postacchini F: Management of lumbar spinal stenosis. J Bone Joint Surg Br 78-B:154-164, 1996.
44. Ram Z, Findler G, Spiegelman R, et al: Intermittent priapism in spinal canal stenosis. Spine 12:377-378, 1987.
44a. Richmond BJ, Ghodadra T: Imaging of spinal stenosis. Phys Med Rehabil Clin N Am 14:41-56, 2003.
44b. Rydevik BL, Cohen DB, Kostuik JP: Spine epidural steroids for patients with lumbar spinal stenosis. Spine 22:2313-2317, 1997.
45. Rittenberg JD, Ross AE: Functional rehabilitation for degenerative lumbar spinal stenosis. Phys Med Rehabil Clin N Am 14:111-120, 2003.
46. Ross JS, Modic MT: Current assessment of spinal degenerative disease with magnetic resonance imaging. Clin Orthop 279:68, 1992.
47. Saal JA, Dillingham MF, Gamburd RS, Fanton GS: The pseudoradicular syndrome: Lower extremity peripheral nerve entrapment masquerading as lumbar radiculopathy. Spine 13:926-930, 1988.
48. Sanderson PL, Getty CJ: Long-term results of partial undercutting facetectomy for lumbar lateral recess stenosis. Spine 21:1352-1356, 1996.
49. Schonstrom NS, Bolender NF, Spengler DM: The pathomorphology of spinal stenosis as seen on CT scans of the lumbar spine. Spine 10:806, 1985.
50. Seppalainen AM, Alaranta H, Soini J: Electromyography in the diagnosis of lumbar spinal stenosis. Electromyogr Clin Neurophysiol 21:55-66, 1981.
51. Shakil MS, Vaccaro AR, Albert TJ, et al: Efficacy of conservative treatment of lumbar spinal stenosis. Semin Spine Surg 11:229-233, 1999.
52. Stambough JL: Principles of decompression for lumbar spinal stenosis. Semin Spine Surg 11:244-252, 1999.
53. Templin CR, Stambough JL: Uncommon causes of spinal stenosis. Semin Spine Surg 11:215-218, 1999.
54. Velan GJ, Curroer BL, Yaszemski MJ: Decision making in the evaluation and management of acquired spinal stenosis: An algorithmic approach. Semin Spine Surg 11:195-208, 1999.
55. Verbiest H: Fallacies of the present definition, nomenclature and classification of the stenoses of the lumbar vertebral canal. Spine 1:217-225, 1976.
56. Wiesel SW, Tsourmas N, Feffer HL, et al: A study of computer-assisted tomography. I. The incidence of positive CAT scans in an asymptomatic group of patients. Spine 9:549, 1984.
57. Wolfe RM, Wiesel S, Boden SD: Lumbar spinal stenosis: Neurodiagnostic evaluation including myelography. Semin Spine Surg 11:219-228, 1999.

CERVICAL MYELOPATHY

Capsule Summary

	Low Back	Neck
Frequency of spinal pain	Not applicable (NA)	Uncommon
Location of spinal pain	NA	Neck, head, between scapulae
Quality of spinal pain	NA	Ache
Symptoms and signs	NA	Headaches, difficulty walking associated with clumsiness and weakness of arms
Laboratory tests	NA	None
Radiographic findings	NA	Plain roentgenograms demonstrate degenerative changes, MR reveals compression of the spinal cord
Treatment	NA	Surgery, epidural injections

PREVALENCE AND PATHOGENESIS

When the secondary bony changes of cervical spondylosis encroach on the spinal cord, a pathologic process called myelopathy develops. When it involves both the spinal cord and nerve roots, it is called myeloradiculopathy. Radiculopathy, regardless of its etiology, causes shoulder or arm pain.[5,6,37]

Epidemiology

Myelopathy is the most serious and difficult sequela of cervical spondylosis to treat effectively. Brain and colleagues were the first to describe the syndrome in 1952.[6] Myelopathy develops in less than 5% of patients with cervical spondylosis, and they usually range in age from 40 to 60 years. Cervical spondylotic myelopathy (CSM) is the most common cause of spinal cord dysfunction in individuals older than 55 years.[4]

Pathogenesis

The changes of myelopathy are most often gradual and associated with posterior osteophyte formation (called spondylitic bone or hard disc) and spinal canal narrowing (spinal stenosis). The pathogenesis of this condition begins extrinsic to the spinal cord. Deterioration of the intervertebral disc results in reactive hyperostosis. Osteophytes project posteriorly into the spinal canal and compress the spinal cord and its vascular supply. Other potential sources of osteophytes are the uncovertebral and zygapophyseal joints. The onset of symptoms may occur in the static and dynamic states. The size of the canal is the important static component. Congenital narrowing of the canal increases the risk of myelopathy.[19] Stenosis has been associated with a midsagittal (anteroposterior) diameter of 10 mm or less. Space-occupying bodies such as the foreshortened and thickened ligamentum flavum and posterior longitudinal ligament, bulging of disc material, and loss of cervical lordosis add to the risk of static stenosis. Dynamic stenosis may occur as a result of segment instability causing compression of different portions of the spinal cord with flexion or extension.

Compression of the spinal cord results in a consistent pattern of nerve degeneration in the posterior and lateral white matter columns.[27,39] The anterior columns are relatively spared. Pressure on the spinal cord causes a blockage of axoplasmic flow, distortion of the tissue of the cord, and stretching of the intrinsic transverse terminations of the anterior spinal artery.[4] Persistent pressure causes demyelination. Pressure on the anterior spinal artery in the lower cervical region is another mechanism of tissue damage.[11] Acute myelopathy is most often the result of a central soft disc herniation producing a high-grade block.

CLINICAL HISTORY

The clinical picture of CSM varies considerably. The onset of symptoms is usually after 50 years of age, and males are more often affected. Its onset is usually insidious, although occasionally a history of trauma is elicited. The natural history is that of initial deterioration followed by a plateau period lasting several months. The resulting clinical picture is often one of an incomplete spinal lesion with a patchy distribution of deficits. Disability varies with the number of vertebrae involved and the degree of involvement at each level.

CSM may be divided into five distinct clinical syndromes (Table 10-7). The lateral syndrome is associated with radicular pain. The medial syndrome causes myelopathy associated with long-tract signs. The combined syndrome includes both radicular and myelopathic signs and is the most common manifestation of CSM. The least common syndrome is vascular and is associated with variable symptoms and signs related to ischemia of the spinal cord. The anterior syndrome is associated with painless upper extremity weakness. This syndrome occurs secondary to pressure affecting only the anterior horns containing motor neurons in the spinal cord.

The characteristic stooped, wide-based, and somewhat jerky gait of the aged summarizes the chronic effects of cervical spondylosis with myelopathy on ambulation. The spinal cord changes may develop at single or multiple levels and as such are not manifested in a standard manner. A typical clinical finding of chronic myelopathy begins with the gradual onset of a peculiar sensation in the hands associated with clumsiness and weakness. The patient may also note lower extremity symptoms that may antedate the upper extremity findings, including difficulty walking, peculiar sensations, leg weakness, and spontaneous leg movements indicative of hyperreflexia, spasticity, and clonus. Older patients may describe leg stiffness, shuffling

10-7 CERVICAL SPONDYLOTIC MYELOPATHY CLINICAL SYNDROMES

Syndrome	Pain	Extremity Involvement	Gait Abnormality	Location
Lateral (radicular)	Yes	Arm	Occasional	Unilateral
Medial (myelopathic)	No	Leg	Yes	Bilateral
Combined	Occasional	Both	Yes	Unilateral/upper Bilateral/lower
Vascular	No	Both	Yes	Bilateral
Anterior (weakness in arms)	No	Arm	No	Unilateral

Modified from Bernhardt M, Hytes RA, Blume HW, White AA III: Cervical spondylotic myelopathy. J Bone Joint Surg Am 75:119, 1993.

of their feet, and an associated fear of falling. The upper extremity findings may start out unilaterally and include hyperreflexia, a brisk Hoffmann sign, and muscle atrophy (especially the hand muscles). Neck pain per se is not a prominent feature of myelopathy. In a study of 199 patients with CSM, radicular pain and paresthetic pain were reported in 39% and 34% of patients, respectively. In contrast, 98% reported spasticity.[10] Sensory changes can evolve at these levels and are often a less reliable index of spinal cord disease. Bladder incontinence is uncommon.

PHYSICAL EXAMINATION

For clinicians treating patients with CSM, the most critical problem is identification of the level (or levels) responsible for the clinical symptoms. The patient's gait should be observed, and the extent of motor disability, which may vary from mild to severe, should be ascertained. Pyramidal tract weakness and atrophy are more frequently seen in the lower extremities and are the most common abnormal physical signs. The usual clinical findings in the lower extremities are spasticity and weakness. Weakness and wasting of the upper extremities and hands along with fasciculations may also be the result of a combined CSM syndrome that includes myelopathy and radiculopathy. Hands that are clumsy and numb may be caused by a myelopathic lesion in the upper cervical cord at C3–C5.[16] Decreased adduction and extension of the ulnar digits and an inability to open and close the hand quickly may have their source in a lesion affecting the pyramidal tract at or above the C7 cord level.[17,29] A diminished or absent upper extremity deep tendon reflex, often the triceps reflex, can indicate compressive radiculopathy superimposed on spondylitic myelopathy.

Sensory deficits in spinothalamic (pain and temperature) and posterior column (vibration and proprioception) function should be documented. Alterations in sensation may include numbness, loss of temperature on the contralateral side, loss of proprioception, or decreased dermatomal sensation.[8] Usually, patients do not have any gross impairment of sensation; rather, a patchy decrease in light touch and pinprick is noted. Hyperreflexia, clonus, and a positive Babinski sign are seen in the lower extremities. Hoffmann's sign and hyperreflexia may be observed in the upper extremities.

The physical findings may be confusing when cervical and lumbar spinal stenosis coexist.[14] Lumbar compression may hide upper motor neuron signs. Both upper and lower extremity reflexes should be tested in stenosis patients. Abnormal physical findings in the lower extremities may be elicited by having the patient assume an extended, upright position or by walking. The finding of jaw hyperreflexia suggests a lesion above the foramen magnum or a systemic process such as hyperthyroidism.

LABORATORY DATA

Serum laboratory tests are normal in patients with CSM. Patients with CSM may have abnormalities in somatosensory and motor evoked potentials. Change in the position of the neck may result in abnormal somatosensory potentials.[42] An experienced electromyographer may have greater success in identifying these abnormalities in complicated patients.

RADIOGRAPHIC EXAMINATION

Roentgenograms

Roentgenographic evaluation may include anteroposterior, lateral, flexion-extension, atlanto-occipital, and oblique views. Roentgenograms of the cervical spine in these patients often reveal advanced degenerative disease, including spinal canal narrowing with prominent posterior osteophytosis, variable foraminal narrowing, disc space narrowing, facet joint arthrosis, and instability (Fig. 10-22). These findings are usually more prominent in the lower cervical spine. Lumbar disc disease frequently

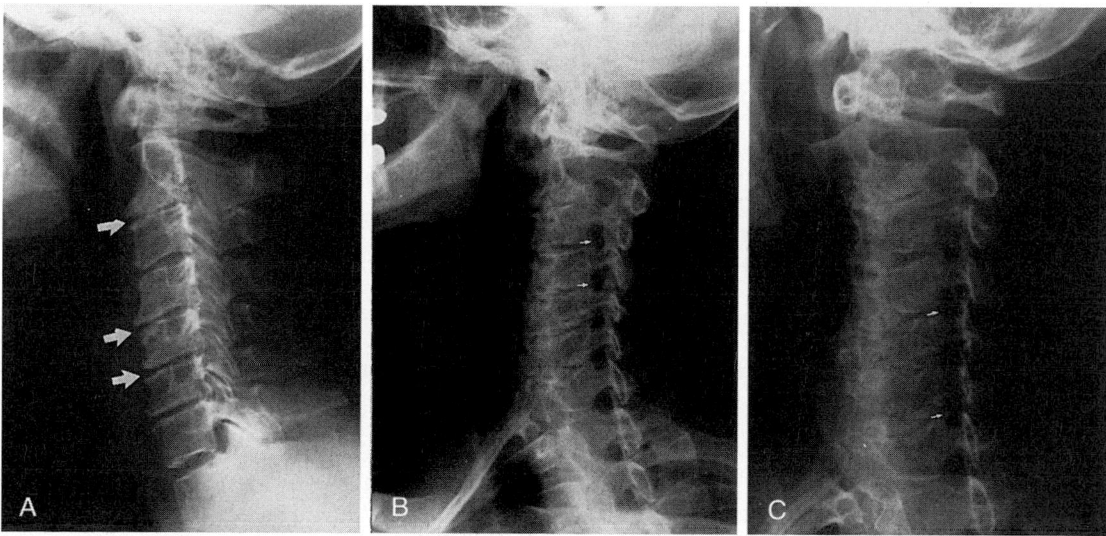

Figure 10-22 Cervical spondylosis in a 64-year-old woman with generalized osteoarthritis and decreased motion of the cervical spine without neurologic signs. A lateral view, *A*, and oblique views, *B* and *C*, reveal loss of lordosis, diffuse narrowing of disc spaces C2–C7 *(large arrows)*, and moderate encroachment by osteophytes of the neural foramina *(small arrows)*.

coexists in the setting of cervical spondylosis.[18] Congenital canal narrowing may be detected if the ratio of Pavlov is 0.8 or less.[31] This ratio is determined by dividing the anteroposterior diameter of the canal by the anteroposterior diameter of the corresponding vertebral body. The ratio is usually 1.0. Although plain roentgenograms are able to detect bony alterations in the vertebrae, the technique is unable to determine the extent of damage to soft tissues in the cervical spine. Other radiographic techniques such as myelography, CT, or MR imaging are required.

Myelography

Myelography is a diagnostic technique that introduces dye into the spinal canal to determine whether posterior or anterior defects are compressing the neural elements. Posterior defects are secondary to facet arthrosis and buckling of the ligamentum flavum. Anterior defects are secondary to changes in the posterior longitudinal ligaments and intervertebral discs.[32]

Computed Tomography

CT is superior to MR imaging for the identification of osteophytes. CT-myelography is useful for distinguishing disc tissue from osteophytes.[7]

Magnetic Resonance

MR imaging is the noninvasive examination of choice for evaluation of CSM. The spinal cord is visualized in the sagittal and axial planes. MR imaging is able to detect the extent of spinal cord compression and alterations in the spinal cord proper (Fig. 10-23).[26] The degree of reformation of the spinal cord can be considerable (Fig. 10-24).

Shafaie and co-workers completed a study matching the concordance of CT-myelography and MR for findings of CSM.[35] Different anatomic abnormalities are detected by each technique. For most parameters of interpretation in the differentiation of disc and bony pathology, CT-myelography and MR are complementary studies. Bartlett and colleagues also studied the relative sensitivity of two-dimensional MR at 1.5 and 0.5 T versus CT-myelography in the assessment of cord and root compression.[3] In a study of 23 patients with cervical spondylosis, high field strength MR is superior to midfield strength MR, but the MR 4-mm sections are inadequate for presurgical assessment of root compression. Further investigation will be needed to determine whether white cerebrospinal fluid volume sequences of gadolinium-enhanced studies can replace CT-myelography. Both studies may be required before surgical intervention.

DIFFERENTIAL DIAGNOSIS

The diagnosis of CSM is based on the clinical symptoms and signs and is confirmed by abnormalities detected on MR or CT evaluation. A variety of disorders that affect the spinal cord, peripheral nerves, and skeletal muscles or that cause narrowing of the spinal canal need to be considered in patients with myelopathic symptoms. The most common problem is an intradural tumor (primary or metastatic) compressing the spinal cord. Other disorders to be considered include multiple sclerosis, cerebrovascular disease, hydrocephalus (normal pressure), intracranial tumor, syringomyelia, amyotrophic lateral sclerosis, Arnold-Chiari malformation, vascular ischemia of the cord, tabes dorsalis, myopathies, and neuropathies. Vascular space-occupying lesions may cause compressive symptoms.[2] Many of these abnormalities may be detected by MR evaluation of the head and spine.[1] MR imaging may also identify the effects of radiation therapy on the spinal cord resulting in myelopathic syndrome.[40] Syphilis can be diagnosed by serologic tests. Peripheral neuropathies and myopathies can be identified by electromyography and by muscle and nerve biopsy. Disorders that increase bone growth may also cause stenosis. For example, cervical myelopathy may develop in acromegalic patients.[25] Ossification of the posterior longitudinal ligament or ligamenta flava may cause compression.[30] In addition, chest and shoulder abnormalities need to be excluded.

TREATMENT

Patients with CSM may improve in 50% of instances with nonoperative therapy.[21] Other studies have reported greater disability in individuals who do not undergo surgical decompression.[33,36] Conservative therapy should be attempted in individuals without severe neurologic compromise or those who are poor surgical risks. Conservative therapy includes immobilization with a firm cervicothoracic orthosis, intermittent bed rest, nonsteroidal anti-inflammatory drugs, muscle relaxants, epidural corticosteroid injections, and physical therapy.[4] Individuals with a soft cervical disc herniation and mild myelopathy symptoms may improve with nonoperative therapy. Matsumoto and colleagues reported on 27 patients with soft cervical disc herniation who were treated for 6 months with cervical bracing and restriction of daily activities.[24] Of the 27, 10 underwent surgical decompression because of neurologic deterioration. In the 17 patients treated nonoperatively, 10 had repeat MR scans revealing resorption of the extruded herniated disc. This study suggests that close observation is appropriate for patients with myelopathy when a structure causing compression can be resorbed spontaneously.

In general, myelopathy is a surgical disease. However, myelopathy is not an absolute indication for surgical decompression. The goal of surgery in a myelopathic patient is to decompress the spinal canal to prevent further spinal cord compression and vascular compromise. If the myelopathy is progressive despite a trial of conservative treatment, surgery is clearly indicated. In rare circumstances, prompt surgical decompression is indicated for individuals with a rapid onset of myelopathic symptoms and signs associated with spinal cord compression.[41] These indications may vary slightly from surgeon to surgeon because of the lack of absolute or definitive clinical data. Surgical therapy works best in the early stages of disease. Elderly patients with long-standing disease and profound

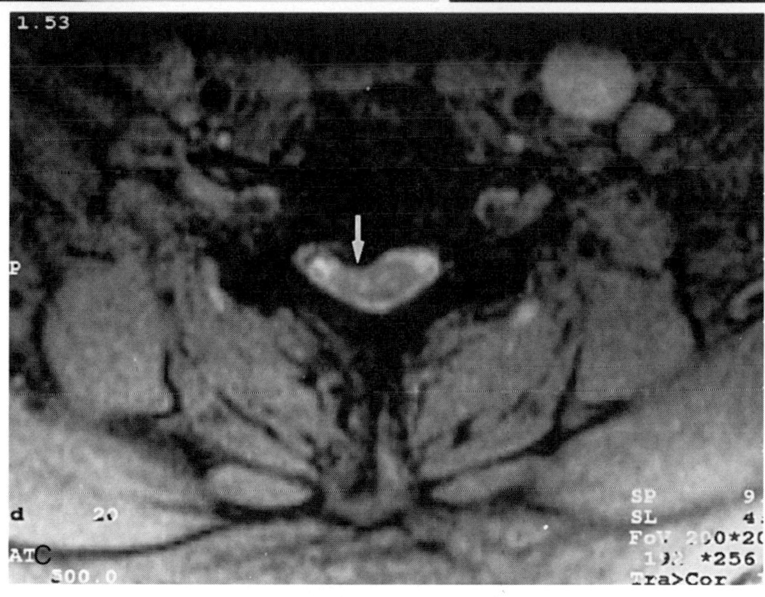

Figure 10-23 Cervical spondylotic myelopathy. A 65-year-old woman had bilateral carpal tunnel syndrome documented by electromyography, along with right shoulder pain and arm heaviness. *A*, A lateral view of the cervical spine reveals cervical spondylosis with anterior osteophytes at C4–C6. MR T1-weighted sagittal, *B*, and axial, *C*, views reveal diffuse spondylosis with a spondylitic bar at C4–C5 causing moderate canal stenosis *(arrow)*.

neurologic deficits are poor candidates. A number of surgical procedures are available for decompression of neural elements. Among these procedures are anterior cervical discectomy with interbody arthrodesis, anterior cervical corpectomy and strut graft arthrodesis, posterior cervical laminectomy, and posterior cervical laminaplasty.[20] Each procedure has its potential benefits and complications. Anterior decompression is recommended for anterior compression at one or two levels. Emery and colleagues reported on the results of anterior decompression and arthrodesis in 108 patients with CSM.[12] Thirty-eight of 82 patients who had a preoperative gait abnormality achieved a normal gait, 33 demonstrated improvement in gait, 6 had no change, 4 had improvement and later deterioration, and 1 worsened. Motor deficits were also improved. Pseudarthrosis occurred in 16 patients, 13 of whom underwent multilevel procedures. Pain was associated with pseudarthrosis. The posterior approach is indicated for

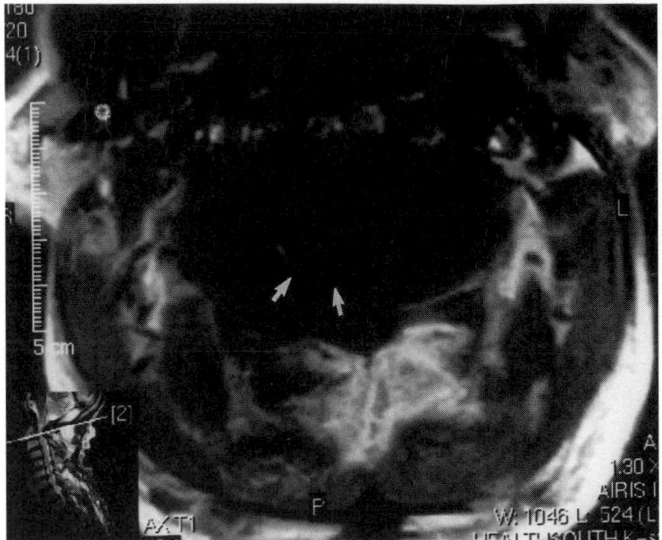

Figure 10-24 Cervical spondylotic myelopathy. A 72-year-old man complained of increasing tingling in his hands and feet. He had an unstable gait and a positive Babinski sign. An axial MR scan at C2–C3 reveals marked narrowing of the spinal canal and significant flattening of the spinal cord *(white arrows)*.

compression at multiple levels. An experienced spine surgeon should be able to choose the appropriate procedure for the specific clinical characteristics of the patient.

Fouyas and co-workers reviewed randomized controlled trials of surgical therapy for improved outcomes in 49 cervical myelopathy patients.[15] In general, in patients with mild functional deficits associated with cervical myelopathy, no significant difference between the groups was observed at 1 year. In contrast, Engsberg reported the benefits of surgical decompression for spasticity, strength, and gait in a patient with cervical myelopathy.[13] Arm spasticity, elbow strength, and gait speed were significantly improved at 6 months in comparison to presurgical functional levels. The age of the patient should not preclude surgery, if indicated. Patients older than 75 years are able to achieve improved activities of daily living after surgical decompression.[23]

PROGNOSIS

The natural history of CSM was described by Clarke and Robinson in 120 patients.[9] Most patients have progressive deterioration between episodes of increased symptoms. Twenty percent of patients had slow progression without remission and 5% had a rapid onset with long periods of no progression. Another study of 44 patients described only 5 of 15 patients with symptoms for 10 years or longer who had improvement.[22] Symon and Lavender reported that only 18% of patients had improvement from the time of initial evaluation.[36]

Patients with congenital narrowing of the spinal canal are at risk for transient neurapraxia in the absence of spondylosis. Transient quadriplegia with hyperflexion or hyperextension of the neck may develop in these patients. These people are usually athletes who undergo direct pressure on the head. Such patients should be evaluated for the presence of spinal stenosis, which would preclude participation in contact sports.[38]

Patients with overt signs of myelopathy have a guarded future. Surgery may bring some relief, but they will continue to have intermittent difficulty. Okada and colleagues reported that a shorter duration of disease, a greater preoperative spinal cord area, and normal intramedullary signal intensity on MR evaluation were associated with a better surgical outcome in CSM patients.[28] Sampath and co-workers reported on a prospective study for the treatment of cervical myelopathy completed by the Cervical Spine Research Society.[34] Sixty-two of the 503 patients entered for cervical spondylosis had myelopathy. Of individuals with follow-up data, 20 underwent surgery and 23 continued with medical therapy. Surgically treated patients had improvement in functional status, pain relief, and neurologic impairment. Medically treated patients experienced worsening of their neurologic symptoms and physical functioning.

References

Cervical Myelopathy

1. Arlien-Soborg P, Kjaer L, Praestholm J: Myelography, CT, and MRI of the spinal canal in patients with myelopathy: A prospective study. Acta Neurol Scand 87:95, 1993.
2. Atkinson JLD, Miller GM, Krauss WE, et al: Clinical and radiographic features of dural arteriovenous fistula, a treatable cause of myelopathy. Mayo Clin Proc 76:1120-1130, 2001.
3. Bartlett RJ, Hill CA, Devlin R, et al: Two-dimensional MRI at 1.5 and 0.5 T versus CT myelography in the diagnosis of cervical radiculopathy. Neuroradiology 38:142-147, 1996.
4. Bernhardt M, Hynes RA, Blume HW, White AA III: Cervical spondylotic myelopathy. J Bone Joint Surg Am 75-A:119, 1993.
5. Bohlman HH: Cervical spondylosis with moderate to severe myelopathy. Spine 2:151-162, 1977.
6. Brain WR, Northfield D, Wilkinson M: The neurological manifestations of cervical spondylosis. Brain 75:187-225, 1952.
7. Brown BM, Schwartz RH, Frank E, Blank NK: Preoperative evaluation of cervical radiculopathy and myelopathy by surface-coil MR imaging. AJR Am J Roentgenol 151:1205, 1988.
8. Clark CR: Cervical spondylotic myelopathy: History and physical findings. Spine 13:847, 1988.
9. Clarke E, Robinson PK: Cervical myelopathy: A complication of cervical spondylosis. Brain 79:483, 1956.
10. Crandall PH, Batzdorf U: Cervical spondylotic myelopathy. J Neurosurg 25:57, 1966.
11. Doppman JL: The mechanism of ischemia in anteroposterior compression of the spinal cord. Invest Radiol 10:543, 1975.
12. Emery SE, Bohlman HH, Bolesta MJ, et al: Anterior cervical decompression and arthrodesis for the treatment of cervical spondylotic myelopathy: Two to seventeen-year follow-up. J Bone Joint Surg Am 80-A:941-951, 1998.
13. Engsberg JR, Lauryssen C, Ross SA, et al: Spasticity, strength, and gait changes after surgery for cervical spondylotic myelopathy: A case report. Spine 28:E136-E139, 2003.
14. Epstein NE, Epstein JA, Carras R, et al: Coexisting cervical and lumbar spinal stenosis: Diagnosis and management. Neurosurgery 15:489, 1984.
15. Fouyas IP, Statham PF, Sandercock PA: Cochrane review on the role of surgery in cervical spondylotic radiculomyelopathy. Spine 27:736-747, 2002.
16. Good DC, Couch JR, Wacaser L: Numb, clumsy hands and high cervical spondylosis. Surg Neurol 22:285, 1984.
17. Heller JG: The syndromes of degenerative cervical disease. Orthop Clin North Am 23:381, 1992.
18. Jacobs B, Ghelman B, Marchisello P: Coexistence of cervical and lumbar disc disease. Spine 15:1261, 1990.

19. Kessler JT: Congenital narrowing of the cervical spinal canal. J Neurol Neurosurg Psychiatry 38:1218, 1975.
20. Kurz LT, Herkowitz HN: Surgical management of myelopathy. Orthop Clin North Am 23:495, 1992.
21. LaRocca H: Cervical spondylotic myelopathy: Natural history. Spine 13:854, 1988.
22. Lees F, Turner JWA: Natural history and prognosis of cervical spondylosis. BMJ 2:1607, 1963.
23. Matsuda Y, Shibata T, Oki S, et al: Outcomes of surgical treatment for cervical myelopathy in patients more than 75 years of age. Spine 24:529-534, 1999.
24. Matsumoto M, Chiba K, Ishikawa M, et al: Relationships between outcomes of conservative treatment and magnetic resonance imaging findings in patients with mild cervical myelopathy caused by soft disc herniations. Spine 26:1592-1598, 2001.
25. Mikawa Y, Watanabe R, Nishishita Y: Cervical myelopathy in acromegaly. Spine 17:1542, 1992.
26. Nagata K, Kiyonaga K, Ohashi T, et al: Clinical value of magnetic resonance imaging for cervical myelopathy. Spine 15:1088, 1990.
27. Nurick S: The pathogenesis of the spinal cord disorder associated with cervical spondylosis. Brain 95:87, 1972.
28. Okada Y, Ikata T, Yamada H, et al: Magnetic resonance imaging study on the results of surgery for cervical compression myelopathy. Spine 18:2024, 1993.
29. Ono K, Ebara S, Fuji T, et al.: Myelopathy hand: New clinical signs of cervical cord damage. J Bone Joint Surg Br 69-B:215, 1987.
30. Pascal-Mousselard H, Smadja D, Cabre P, et al: Ossification of the ligamenta flava with severe myelopathy in a black patient. A case report. Spine 23:1607-1608, 1998.
31. Pavlov H, Torg JS, Robie B, Jahre C: Cervical spinal stenosis: Determination with vertebral body ratio method. Radiology 164:771, 1987.
32. Penning L, Wilmink JT, van Woerden HH, Knol E: CT myelographic findings in degenerative disorders of the cervical spine: Clinical significance. AJR Am J Roentgenol 146:793, 1986.
33. Phillips DG: Surgical treatment of myelopathy with cervical spondylosis. J Neurol Neurosurg Psychiatry 36:879, 1973.
34. Sampath P, Bendebba M, David JD, et al: Outcome of patients treated for cervical myelopathy: A prospective, multicenter study with independent clinical review. Spine 25:670-676, 2000.
35. Shafaie FF, Wippold FJ II, Gado M, et al: Comparison of computed tomography myelography and magnetic resonance imaging in the evaluation of cervical spondylotic myelopathy and radiculopathy. Spine 24:1781-1985, 1999.
36. Symon L, Lavender P: The surgical treatment of cervical spondylotic myelopathy. Neurology 17:117, 1967.
37. The Cervical Spine Research Society: The Cervical Spine. Philadelphia, JB Lippincott, 1989, pp 388-430.
38. Torg JS, Pavlov H, Genuario SE, et al: Neuropraxia of the cervical spinal cord with transient quadriplegia. J Bone Joint Surg Am 68-A:1354, 1986.
39. Veidlinger OF, Colwill JC, Smyth HS, et al: Cervical myelopathy and its relationship to cervical stenosis. Spine 6:550, 1981.
40. Wang P, Shen W, Jan J: MR imaging in radiation myelopathy. AJNR Am J Neuroradiol 13:1049, 1992.
41. Wilberger JE Jr, Chedid MK: Acute cervical spondylytic myelopathy. Neurosurgery 22:145, 1988.
42. Yiannikas C, Shahani BT, Young RR: Short-latency somatosensory-evoked potentials from radial, median, ulnar, and peroneal nerve stimulation in the assessment of cervical spondylosis: Comparison with conventional electromyography. Arch Neurol 43:1264, 1986.

CERVICAL HYPEREXTENSION INJURIES (WHIPLASH)

CAPSULE SUMMARY

	LOW BACK	NECK
Frequency of spinal pain	Not applicable (NA)	Very common
Location of spinal pain	NA	Neck, head, between scapulae, shoulders
Quality of spinal pain	NA	Ache, soreness
Symptoms and signs	NA	Headaches, neck pain with movement of the head
Laboratory tests	NA	Normal
Radiographic findings	NA	Loss of lordosis
Treatment	NA	Medications, physical therapy

PREVALENCE AND PATHOGENESIS

Epidemiology

The prevalence of whiplash injury has not been measured prospectively. Of individuals involved in a rear-end motor vehicle accident (MVA), neck pain develops in approximately 20%.[47] In data collected by the Quebec Task Force on Whiplash-Associated Disorders, the incidence rate was 131 whiplash injuries per 100,000 vehicles per year in 1987.[45] In Australia, an annual incidence rate of 80 per 100,000 has been reported.[2] In a study of 1551 subjects with whiplash injury, the frequency of individuals who continued to have pain at 1 year was 3%.[18]

The frequency of low back pain in the setting of MVAs has not been studied as well as whiplash injuries. In Saskatchewan, Canada, the 6-month incidence of low back pain associated with MVAs was 256 per 100,000 adults. When a no-fault insurance system was instituted, the frequency of reported episodes decreased to 175 per 100,000 adults.[10]

Pathogenesis

Whiplash-type injuries were first recognized in World War I pilots in airplanes without head supports who were catapulted on takeoff. In 1928, Crowe introduced the term *whiplash* to describe hyperextension injuries from an indirect force.[13] In 1953, Gay and Abbott redefined whiplash injury,[16] and the term has been used extensively in the medical literature and as a diagnostic code for insurance reimbursement.

Mechanism of Injury

Hyperextension injuries of the neck occur most often when the driver of a stationary car is struck from behind by another vehicle.[27] The driver is usually relaxed and unaware of the impending collision. The sudden acceleration of the struck vehicle pushes the back of the car seat against the driver's torso. This force pushes the driver's torso (shoulders) forward while the head remains static but moves posteriorly, thereby causing hyperextension of the neck. This process occurs quickly after impact. If no headrest is present, the driver's head is hyperextended past the normal limit of stretch of the soft tissues of the neck. This injury is called whiplash because of the hyperextension of the head. Neck pain may also be the result of lateral and frontal collisions. Whiplash is an acceleration-deceleration mechanism of energy transfer to the neck. The impact may result in bony or soft tissue injuries, which in turn may lead to a variety of clinical manifestations.[45] The sternocleidomastoid, scalene, and longus colli muscles may be mildly or severely stretched or, at worst, torn. Tears of the longus colli muscles might involve injury to the sympathetic trunk unilaterally or bilaterally and result in Horner's syndrome, nausea, or dizziness. Further hyperextension may injure the esophagus and result in temporary dysphagia and injury to the larynx causing hoarseness. Tears in the anterior longitudinal ligament may cause hematoma formation with resultant cervical radiculopathy (arm pain) and injury to the intervertebral disc. In the recoil forward flexion that occurs when the car stops accelerating, the head is thrown forward. This forward flexion of the head is generally limited by the chin striking the chest and does not usually cause significant injury. However, if the head is thrown forward and strikes the steering wheel or the windshield, a head injury can occur. If the head is in slight rotation, additional stress is placed on the capsules of the zygapophyseal joints, intervertebral discs, and alar ligaments. In MVAs, the neck is subject to forced flexion, extension, and lateral flexion, as well as shear forces parallel to the direction of impact. Muscles do not have time to react to protect the structures of the neck. A variety of potential injuries corresponding to the type of injury may occur.[2] Autopsy studies have detected injuries to the cervical intervertebral discs. Clefts in the cartilage plates of the intervertebral discs of neck trauma patients are distinctly different from those associated with spondylosis.[49]

Disc abnormalities, including herniation, can develop in individuals with whiplash injuries.[35] Arm pain compatible with radiculopathy developed later in these individuals in the course of the injury. These patients benefited from MR evaluation as opposed to those with localized pain associated with whiplash.

Zygapophyseal Joints

The role of cervical zygapophyseal joint pain as a component of whiplash syndrome was studied by Lord and colleagues.[24] Sixty-eight patients with whiplash-related neck pain received active and placebo injections into specific facet joints. Individuals with headaches received injections into the C2–C3 facet joints. Those with lower neck and shoulder pain received injections in the lower cervical facet joints (C5–C6 most common). Overall, 31 of the 52 patients completing the study had cervical facet joint pain at C2–C3 or at lower levels, for a prevalence of 60%. This study demonstrated the clinical importance of facet joint pain in whiplash injuries.

Late Whiplash Syndrome

Whether MVAs result in whiplash injuries with chronic symptoms (late whiplash injury) has not been definitively resolved. A retrospective and prospective study from Lithuania reported a frequency of late whiplash injuries similar to the frequency of neck pain in a matched population, 4% versus 6%, respectively.[29,42] Men (78%) were more frequently affected than women. The authors suggested that the absence of injury compensation and meager awareness of whiplash syndrome were the reasons for the paucity of subjects. A number of criticisms were raised regarding the study. A study by Cote and colleagues reported twice as many women as men having neck pain.[12] In addition, women appear to be at greater risk for whiplash injuries.[18] The absence of women from the Lithuania study could in part explain the findings. Another important factor is the presence of neck pain before the MVA. Berglund and co-authors reported a greater persistence of whiplash symptoms after an MVA in those with a history of neck pain than in a control group without neck pain. At 7 years, those with accident-related persistent neck pain had a 2.7% risk for continued neck pain versus a 1.3% risk for those without initial pain.[4] Physicians may have greater resistance to late whiplash syndrome than the general public. In a study of 149 physicians and 207 nonphysicians, 64% had been in an MVA, with 39% suffering acute whiplash.[51] About 31% of the physicians and 46% of the nonphysicians had acute pain. Symptoms for physicians was measured in weeks, whereas nonphysicians had symptoms for over 1 year. Physicians took no more than 1 week off, whereas the nonphysicians took more than 6 months. Ward clerks were more likely to be out of work than the paramedical staff. Occupational factors and knowledge may play a significant role in the development of chronic symptoms and the amount of work absence.

Compensation Effects

Another important factor in the resolution of whiplash symptoms may be the availability of compensation for pain and suffering. In Saskatchewan, Canada, data were available before and after the institution of a no-fault MVA insurance system.[9] The median time from the date of injury to closure of the claim went from 433 days to 194 days. The intensity of neck pain, the level of physical functioning, and the presence of depression were all affected by closure of the cases.

CLINICAL HISTORY

Usually, the driver is often unaware of having been injured. The driver suffers little discomfort at the scene of the accident and often does not wish to go to the hospital. Later, 12 to 14 hours after the accident, the driver begins to feel stiffness in the neck. Pain at the base of the neck increases and is made worse by head and neck movements. Soon, any movement of the head or neck causes excruciating pain. Headaches are the second most common symptom associated with whiplash injury.[26] The anterior cervical muscles are often tender to touch. The patient may have pain on opening the mouth or chewing, hoarseness, or difficulty swallowing and seeks medical care. Other symptoms associated with whiplash injuries include visual disturbances manifested as accommodative problems and oculomotor dysfunction mediated through increased sympathetic tone.[21] Dizziness may occur secondary to damage to the vestibular apparatus, with perilymph fistulas causing dysequilibrium.[11] Paresthesias in the arms, particularly in the ulnar nerve distribution, may develop in whiplash patients. One proposed mechanism of injury is compression of the lower nerve roots of the inferior portion of the brachial plexus as it passes under the scalene muscles, a form of thoracic outlet syndrome.[8] Other patients may have dysesthesias of the face below the ear associated with traction injuries to the great auricular nerve and superficial branches of the cervical plexus as they are stretched while winding around the sternocleidomastoid muscle. Cognitive functions such as concentration, memory, and attention span are decreased in whiplash patients.[36]

The frequency of temporomandibular joint symptoms in whiplash injuries is unknown.[50] It is controversial whether the source of pain is related to internal derangement of the joint or to myofascial pain in the masseter muscle. Clicking occurs with talking or chewing.

Psychological factors have been suggested as playing a role in the symptom complex and delaying the resolution of whiplash injuries.[30] However, recent studies have refuted this notion because of a lack of correlation between psychological stress and personality traits with the outcome of a whiplash injury.[37] The psychological stress that whiplash patients experience is similar to that associated with chronic pain of any source.[28] The primary reason for psychological dysfunction in association with whiplash injuries is the trauma itself. Patients with whiplash do complain of impaired cognitive functioning (processing information, learning, memory, and speaking). Radanov and Dvorak concluded that higher cognitive functions were not disturbed after whiplash.[38] Taylor and co-workers conducted neuropsychological tests on a group of patients with whiplash, with head injuries, and with chronic pain but no head injuries.[48] No differences between the groups were found. Patients with whiplash are not cognitively impaired. They may have chronic pain, depression, and anxiety that may affect concentration.[22]

PHYSICAL EXAMINATION

The physical examination must be detailed and complete to rule out other significant problems. If the patient has only a hyperextension injury, the neurologic examination is normal. The only finding, which is subjective, is decreased range of motion and, on occasion, persistent muscle contraction.

Dall'Alba and co-authors reported on the range of motion of whiplash patients versus asymptomatic controls. Range of motion was reduced in all primary movements in patients with whiplash-associated disorders. Sagittal plane movements were the most frequently affected. Asymptomatic individuals could be differentiated from those with whiplash injuries by the range of motion.[14]

Patients with whiplash injuries have certain degrees of physical and psychological stress that are difficult to falsify. Wallis and Bogduk completed a study to determine whether individuals, for a fee, who were pain free could recreate the findings of a whiplash patient on a psychological examination.[52] The test results were compared with those of a group of 132 whiplash patients who completed the psychological test. Forty visual arts students completed the study. The "actors" overestimated the degree of distress and the level of pain measured by a visual analogue pain scale, but were correct on description of the pain. This paper suggests that whiplash patients undergo psychological stress that cannot be fabricated.

LABORATORY DATA

Laboratory test results are normal for patients with a hyperextension neck injury.

RADIOGRAPHIC EVALUATION

Imaging of the cervical spine is not required because an individual sustained a whiplash injury. The technique required depends on the clinical symptoms associated with the event.[15]

Roentgenograms

Plain roentgenograms are the screening modality of choice for individuals with an MVA injury, and on the lateral view they may demonstrate some loss of the normal lordotic curve because of muscle spasm. A recent study suggests that loss of lordosis is not a specific finding in whiplash patients and may occur in normal individuals.[20] Otherwise, no characteristic abnormalities are found on plain roentgenograms or other examinations such as MR imaging.

Magnetic Resonance

The association of clinical symptoms and signs and abnormalities on MR scans in patients with hyperextension injuries is poor.[33]

Ronnen and co-workers studied 100 patients who had MR scans within 3 weeks of trauma.[40] The MR scans demonstrated no specific abnormalities if plain roentgenograms were normal. MR imaging has no role in individuals who have normal plain roentgenograms and a normal neurologic examination.

DIFFERENTIAL DIAGNOSIS

Considering other abnormalities to account for the patient's complaints is the most important aspect of the diagnostic process for the treating physician. One does not want to be in the situation of treating a patient for a hyperextension injury when in fact a significant traumatic abnormality such as a subdural hematoma can account for the patient's symptom complex.

Each patient requires a thorough examination with particular attention given to neurologic function. Abrasions on the forehead suggest forward flexion of the head resulting from an impact on the steering wheel or windshield. A dilated pupil might suggest Horner's syndrome secondary to injury to the sympathetic chain along the longus colli muscles or be a sign of significant intracranial injury if the patient's level of consciousness is altered. Point tenderness in front of the ear is suggestive of injury to the temporomandibular joint, and tenderness to palpation in the suboccipital area suggests impact of the head on the back of the seat.

The Quebec Task Force on Whiplash-Associated Disorders proposed a classification of whiplash injuries (Table 10-8). A complete neurologic examination is crucial to differentiate the extent of damage. Any evidence of an objective neurologic deficit merits immediate diagnostic tests to determine the cause. Although by definition, hyperextension cervical injury causes damage only to the soft tissue structures of the neck, plain roentgenograms of the cervical spine should be obtained in all instances of neurologic dysfunction.[2] Unsuspected fracture-dislocations of the cervical spine, facet fractures, odontoid fractures, or spinous process fractures might otherwise be missed in a neurologically intact patient. The Quebec study suggests that patients with grade II or greater injuries should have plain roentgenograms of the cervical spine.[45] Cervical spondylosis is demonstrated on plain roentgenograms as well. Of course, if objective neurologic deficits are present, further diagnostic aids are necessary, including CT of the head or spine, myelography, or MR imaging.

Hartling and associates evaluated the prognostic value of the Quebec Task Force classification ratings.[19] In a study of 446 patients entered over a 2-year period, patients were classified by the Quebec system. Patients were monitored over a period of 24 months. Individuals with increasing grades had a greater risk for long-term symptoms, including increased point tenderness and limited range of motion.

TREATMENT

A great deal of controversy is involved in the treatment of whiplash injuries because few scientific studies have been conducted that demonstrate definite efficacy of a number of treatment modalities.[45] A reasonable medical routine, inasmuch as most patients have no neurologic deficit, is based on the premise of resting the involved injured soft tissues.[17] Soft cervical collars have been used with the thought that they relieve muscle spasm and prevent quick movements of the head. Collars were worn for no more than 2 to 4 weeks lest the recovering muscles start weakening from nonuse.[32] Recommendations from the Quebec Task Force suggest restricting the use of collars to a minimal period. They suggest that prolonged use of a collar is detrimental.[45] Cervical soft collars do not limit motion of the cervical spine. Other braces such as the Philadelphia collar or four-poster brace are needed to restrict neck motion significantly.

Rosenfeld and colleagues reported on a study of 97 whiplash patients treated within 96 hours with a program of gentle active rotational movements repeated up to 10 times in each direction in each waking hour, active treatment at 2 weeks, or a standard treatment of rest, a soft cervical collar, and gradual return to activity commencing 2 weeks after injury.[41] Active therapy was best given immediately for the greatest benefit. Standard therapy was better given later to reduce neck pain and increase cervical flexion. Initial therapy for whiplash should be encouragement to commence movement. In a study involving 201 patients, Borchgrevink and co-workers reported on the benefit of two different regimens implemented during the first 14 days after an MVA: instruction to remain active as tolerated versus immobilization for the first 14 days after the neck sprain injury.[6] Review of the medical literature by Peeters and co-workers also suggests the benefit of active interventions for whiplash injury.[31]

Heat is helpful and should be applied via a heating pad, hot showers, or hot tub soaks. If the neck pain is severe, a short period of bed rest may be necessary. Mild analgesics, nonsteroidal anti-inflammatory drugs, and muscle relaxants are helpful and are generally indicated. Narcotic analgesics should be avoided if at all possible. Activity should be encouraged as determined by the severity of the symptoms. Generally, driving should be avoided for the acute symptomatic period. After approximately 2 weeks of this regimen, significant improvement should be noted. If not, 2 more weeks of continued conservative care with the addition of some light home cervical traction should be instituted. If symptoms persist 4 weeks after injury, further testing is necessary before emotional overlay complicates the clinical course of the patient. If headaches persist, a cranial CT scan should be obtained.

10-8 CLASSIFICATION OF WHIPLASH-ASSOCIATED DISORDERS

Grade	Neck Pain, Stiffness, Tenderness	Physical Signs	Musculoskeletal Signs	Neurologic Signs	Fracture-Dislocation
0	–	–	–	–	–
I	+	–	–	–	–
II	+	+	+	–	–
III	+	+	+/–	+	–
IV	+	+	–	+/–	+

Modified from Spitzer WO, Skovron ML, Salmi LR, et al: Scientific monograph of the Quebec Task Force on Whiplash-Associated Disorders: Redefining "whiplash" and its management. Spine 20:1, 1995.

If normal at 4 weeks, the patient can be assured that no intracranial abnormality is present. If arm or shoulder pain persists, a spine CT scan or MR image should be performed. If these tests are normal, the patient can be assured that no compression of neural structures is present and be strongly encouraged to increase activities.

Manual therapy has not been shown to be of greater benefit than placebo in the treatment of neck pain.[23] Corticosteroid injections of the cervical facet joints are not helpful in patients with chronic whiplash pain.[3] However, Pettersson and Toolanen reported on the benefits of high-dose intravenous methylprednisolone started within 8 hours of the MVA.[34] In a study of 20 patients receiving steroids and 20 controls, the actively treated patients had fewer disabling symptoms and sick days. The authors agree that the number of patients in the study was small. Is the toxicity of the therapy worth the beneficial effect? Additional studies are required before this therapy can be recommended.

Lord and co-workers reported the benefits of percutaneous radiofrequency neurotomy for facet joint pain associated with whiplash injuries.[25] Twenty-four patients who had complete relief of pain with confirmatory diagnostic injections were included. Median time before pain returned to at least 50% of the preoperative level was 263 days in the active group and 8 days in the control group. Five patients in the active treatment group and one patient in the control group were pain free. This kind of therapy can provide lasting relief.

Treatment of whiplash is directed at the elimination of pain. No specific treatments have been demonstrated to improve any of the other components (dizziness, visual disturbances, or cognitive dysfunction) associated with whiplash. The assumption is that the improvement in pain will result in a similar effect on other components of the illness. Proof of therapeutic efficacy in eliminating these nonpain symptoms is limited.[5]

PROGNOSIS

Most whiplash injuries resolve over a period of up to 12 weeks. The majority of individuals, particularly those with lower-grade lesions, improve rapidly from 7 to 14 days. Patients with finger paresthesias have a greater likelihood of persistent neck pain for 6 months.[37] Patients with preinjury headaches are at risk for persistent headache at 6 months.[39] For individuals with persistent neck pain, few experience significant improvement in symptoms that are present for a period of 2 years.[2] Conflicting information exists regarding the role of litigation in prolonging symptoms in patients with whiplash injuries. The Canada study suggested that no-fault insurance shortened the period that individuals were symptomatic. Other studies have reported that chronicity is independent of litigation. Compensation and noncompensation patients respond to therapy in similar ways.[43] Compensation may play a role in the chronicity of symptoms, depending on the study population.

Between 80% and 90% of whiplash victims recover from their injury.[1] However, whiplash symptoms may persist for an extended period. Individuals with degenerative disc disease and impaired neck motion have a poorer prognosis. In a study by Squires and colleagues, 40 patients were monitored for 15.5 years after a whiplash injury.[46] Twenty-eight (70%) continued to complain of neck pain related to the MVA. Women and older patients with more degenerative disc disease had a worse outcome. Evidence of a psychological disturbance was found in 52% of these symptomatic patients. Little clinical improvement occurs 1 to 2 years after the initiating event.[44]

Buitenhuis and associates completed a prospective study investigating factors affecting the prognosis of whiplash injuries. In this Dutch study of 242 individuals, 40% of men and 50% of women had neck pain at 12 months. Individuals who sought social support as a coping mechanism and shared concerns with others had a shorter duration of neck pain. Those who were active in their care and avoided a palliative coping style also had a shorter duration of pain. Attention to the early social interactions and coping style used in the initial treatment of whiplash can contribute to the prevention of the late whiplash syndrome.[7]

References

Cervical Hyperextension Injuries (Whiplash)

1. Barnsley L, Lord SM, Bogduk N: The pathophysiology of whiplash. Spine St Art Rev 12:209-242, 1998
2. Barnsley L, Lord S, Bogduk N: Whiplash injury. Pain 58:283, 1994.
3. Barnsley L, Lord SM, Wallis BJ, Bogduk N: Lack of effect of intra-articular corticosteroids for chronic pain in cervical zygapophyseal joints. N Engl J Med 330:1047, 1994.
4. Berglund A, Alfredsson L, Jensen I, et al: The association between exposure to a rear-end collision and future health complaints. J Clin Epidemiol 54:851-856, 2001.
5. Bogduk N: Treatment of whiplash injuries. Spine St Art Rev 12:469-483, 1998.
6. Borchgrevink GE, Kaasa A, McDonagh, et al: Acute treatment of whiplash neck sprain injuries: A randomized trial of treatment during the first 14 days after a car accident. Spine 23:25-31, 1998.
7. Buitenhuis J, Spanjer J, Fidler V: Recovery from acute whiplash: The role of coping styles. Spine 28:896-901, 2003.
8. Capistrant TD: Thoracic outlet syndrome in whiplash injury. Ann Surg 185:175, 1977.
9. Cassidy JD, Carroll LJ, Cote P, et al: Effect of eliminating compensation for pain and suffering on the outcome of insurance claims for whiplash injury. N Engl J Med 342:1179-1186, 2000.
10. Cassidy JD, Carroll L, Cote P, et al: Low back pain after traffic collisions: A population-based cohort study. Spine 28:1002-1009, 2003.
11. Chester JB Jr: Whiplash, postural control, and inner ear. Spine 16:716, 1991.
12. Cote P, Cassidy JD, Carroll L: The factors associated with neck pain and its related disability in the Saskatchewan population. Spine 25:1109-1117, 2000.
13. Crowe HE: Injuries to the cervical spine. Paper presented at a meeting of the Western Orthopaedic Association, 1928, San Francisco.
14. Dall'Alba PT, Sterling MM, Treleaven JM, et al: Cervical range of motion discriminates between asymptomatic persons and those with whiplash. Spine 26:2090-2094, 2001.
15. Fortin JD, Weber EC: Imaging of whiplash injuries. Spine St Art Rev 12:419-435, 1998.
16. Gay JR, Abbott KH: Common whiplash injuries of the neck. JAMA 152:1698, 1953.
17. Greenfield J, Ilfeld FW: Acute cervical strain: Evaluation and short-term prognostic factors. Clin Orthop 122:196, 1977.
18. Harder S, Veilleux M, Suissa S: The effect of socio-demographic and crash-related factors on the prognosis of whiplash. J Clin Epidemiol 51:377-384, 1998.
19. Hartling L, Brison RJ, Ardern C, Pickett W: Prognostic value of the Quebec classification of whiplash-associated disorders. Spine 26:36-41, 2001.

20. Helliwell PS, Evans PF, Wright V: The straight cervical spine: Does it indicate muscle spasm? J Bone Joint Surg Br 76-B:103, 1994.
21. Hildingsson C, Wenngren BI, Toolanen G: Eye motility dysfunction after soft-tissue injury of the cervical spine. Acta Orthop Scand 64:129, 1993.
22. Katz RT, Deluca J, Smith SL: Minor traumatic brain injury following whiplash. Spine St Art Rev 12:395-408, 1998.
23. Koes BW, Bouter LM, Mameren H, et al: The effectiveness of manual therapy, physiotherapy, and treatment by the general practitioner for nonspecific back and neck complaints: A randomized clinical trial. Spine 17:28, 1992.
24. Lord SM, Barnsley L, Wallis BJ, et al: Chronic cervical zygapophysial joint pain after whiplash: A placebo-controlled prevalence study. Spine 21:1737-1745, 1996.
25. Lord SM, Barnsley L, Wallis BJ, et al: Percutaneous radio-frequency neurotomy for chronic cervical zygapophyseal-joint pain. N Engl J Med 335:1721-1726, 1996.
26. Maimaris C, Barnes MR, Allen MJ: "Whiplash injuries" of the neck: A retrospective study. Injury 19:393, 1988.
27. McNab I, McCulloch J: Neck Ache and Shoulder Pain. Baltimore, Williams & Wilkins, 1994, pp 140-159.
28. Merskey H: Psychological consequences of whiplash injuries. Spine 7:471, 1993.
29. Obelieniene D, Schrader H, Bovim G, et al: Pain after whiplash: A prospective controlled inception cohort study. J Neurol Neurosurg Psychiatry 66:279-283, 1999.
30. Pearce JM: Whiplash injury: A reappraisal. J Neurol Neurosurg Psychiatry 52:1329, 1989.
31. Peeters GG, Verhagen AP, de Bie RA et al: The efficacy of conservative treatment in patients with whiplash injury: A systematic review of clinical trials. Spine 26:E64-E74, 2001.
32. Pennie BH, Agambar LJ: Whiplash injuries: A trial of early management. J Bone Joint Surg Br 72-B:277, 1990.
33. Pettersson K, Hildingsson C, Toolanen G, et al: MRI and neurology in acute whiplash trauma: No correlation in prospective examination of 39 cases. Acta Orthop Scand 65:525, 1994.
34. Pettersson K, Toolanen G: High-dose methylprednisolone prevents extensive sick leave after whiplash injury: A prospective, randomized, double-blind study. Spine 23:984-989, 1998.
35. Pettersson K, Hildingsson C, Toolanen G, et al: Disc pathology after whiplash injury: A prospective magnetic resonance imaging and clinical investigation. Spine 22:283-288, 1997.
36. Radanov BP, Di Stefano G, Schnidrig A, et al: Cognitive functioning after common whiplash: A controlled follow-up study. Arch Neurol 50:87, 1993.
37. Radanov BP, Stefano G, Schnidrig A, Ballinari P: Role of psychological stress in recovery from common whiplash. Lancet 338:712, 1991.
38. Radanov BP, Dvorak J: Spine update: Impaired cognitive functioning after whiplash injury of the cervical spine. Spine 21:393-397, 1996.
39. Radanov BP, Sturzenegger M, Di Stefano G, et al: Factors influencing recovery from headache after common whiplash. BMJ 307:652, 1993.
40. Ronnen HR, de Korte PJ, Brink PRG, et al: Acute whiplash injury: Is there a role for MR imaging?—a prospective study of 100 patients. Radiology 201:93-96, 1996.
41. Rosenfeld M, Gunnarsson R, Borenstein P: Early intervention in whiplash-associated disorders: Comparison of two treatment protocols. Spine 25:1782-1787, 2000.
42. Schrader H, Obelieniene D, Bovim G, et al: Natural evolution of late whiplash syndrome outside the medicolegal context. Lancet 347:1207-1211, 1996.
43. Shapiro AP, Roth RS: The effect of litigation on recovery of whiplash. Spine 7:531, 1993.
44. Smith J, Everett CR: Prognosis after whiplash-related injury. Spine St Art Rev 12:287-300, 1998.
45. Spitzer WO, Skovron ML, Salmi LR, et al: Scientific monograph of the Quebec Task Force on Whiplash-Associated Disorders: Redefining "whiplash" and its management. Spine 20:1, 1995.
46. Squires B, Gargan MF, Bannister GC: Soft-tissue injuries of the cervical spine. 15-year follow-up. J Bone Joint Surg Br 78-B:955-957, 1996
47. States JD, Korn MW, Masengill JB: The enigma of whiplash injuries. N Y State J Med 70:2971, 1970.
48. Taylor AE, Cox CA, Mailis A: Persistent neuropsychological deficits following whiplash: Evidence for chronic mild traumatic brain injury? Arch Phys Med Rehabil 77:529-535, 1996.
49. Taylor JR, Twomey LT: Acute injuries to cervical joints: An autopsy study of neck sprain. Spine 18:1115, 1993.
50. Teasel RW, Shapiro AP: The clinical picture of whiplash injuries. Spine St Art Rev 12:257-270, 1998.
51. Virani SN, Ferrari R, Russell AC: Physician resistance to the late whiplash syndrome. J Rheumatol 28:2096-2099, 2001.
52. Wallis BJ, Bogduk N: Faking a profile: Can naïve subjects simulate whiplash responses? Pain 66:223-227, 1996.

SPONDYLOLYSIS/SPONDYLOLISTHESIS

CAPSULE SUMMARY

	LOW BACK	NECK
Frequency of spinal pain	Common	Not applicable (NA)
Location of spinal pain	Low back, posterior thigh, lower leg	NA
Quality of spinal pain	Ache	NA
Symptoms and signs	Pain increased with activity, lumbar "stepoff"	NA
Laboratory tests	Normal	NA
Radiographic findings	Lateral roentgenogram—pars abnormality on plain roentgenogram	NA
Treatment	Controlled activity, medications, bracing, surgical fusion	NA

PREVALENCE AND PATHOGENESIS

Spondylolisthesis is a spinal condition in which all or part of a vertebra has slipped on another. The word is derived from the Greek *spondylos* meaning "vertebra" and *olisthesis* meaning "to slip." Five major types of this condition are recognized, and the etiology of each is different (Table 10-9).[46]

Type I, dysplastic spondylolisthesis, is secondary to a congenital defect of either the superior sacral or inferior L5 facets or both, with gradual slipping of the L5 vertebra. Type II, isthmic or spondylolytic, in which the lesion is in the isthmus or pars interarticularis, has the greatest clinical importance in persons younger than 50 years. If a defect in the pars interarticularis can be identified but no slippage has occurred, the condition is termed *spondylolysis*. If one vertebra has slipped forward on the other (horizontal translation), it is referred to as *spondylolisthesis*. Type II spondylolisthesis occurs secondary to a lytic process (fatigue fracture of the

10-9 TYPES OF SPONDYLOLISTHESIS

I. Dysplastic—the upper sacrum or arch of L5 permits the listhesis to occur
II. Isthmic—the lesion is in the pars interarticularis
Three types can be recognized
  a. Lytic—fatigue fracture of the pars
  b. Elongated but intact pars
  c. Acute fracture
III. Degenerative—resulting from long-standing intersegmental instability
IV. Traumatic—resulting from fractures in other areas of the bony hook and pars
V. Pathologic—generalized or localized bone disease

From Wiesel SW, Bernini P, Rothman RH: The Aging Lumbar Spine. Philadelphia, WB Saunders, 1982.

pars interarticularis), elongation (attenuation) of an intact pars, or an acute fracture. Type III, or degenerative spondylolisthesis, occurs secondary to degeneration of the lumbar facet joints, with alteration in the joint plane allowing forward or backward displacement. Degenerative spondylolisthesis is most common in older populations. No pars defect is present, and the vertebral body slippage is never greater than 30% (Table 10-10). Type IV, traumatic spondylolisthesis, is associated with acute fracture of a posterior element (pedicle, lamina, or facets) other than the pars interarticularis. Type V, pathologic spondylolisthesis, occurs because of a structural weakness of the bone secondary to a disease process such as a tumor.

Epidemiology

Spondylolisthesis is a very common cause of back pain in young individuals. Macnab, after studying 1000 patients with back pain, concluded that spondylolisthesis is the most likely cause of pain in patients younger than 26 years but rarely the sole cause of complaints after the age of 40.[25] Isthmic spondylolisthesis affects 5% to 7% of the U.S. population, with a higher proportion of whites affected than blacks.[7,13]

Pathogenesis

The etiology of the defect in spondylolysis is not clear. Although a hereditary component may be present, the lesion is seldom seen in patients younger than 5 years and is found in 5% of people older than 7. The most attractive explanation is that although these children inherit a potential deficiency in the pars, they are not born with any identifiable defect. Between the ages of 5 and 7, however, they become more active and a stress fracture develops in the inherently weakened pars.[47] Some investigators have suggested that patients with spondylolysis have an increased incidence of sacral spina bifida. These abnormalities are found more commonly in patients with dysplastic and isthmic spondylolisthesis than in the general population.[48] Young individuals involved in regular sports activities are at risk for structural abnormalities, including spondylolysis. In a study of young athletes, back pain was reported most frequently in male gymnasts, whereas radiologic abnormalities occurred most frequently in wrestlers. Patients with the most severe back pain had radiographic evidence of spondylolysis, scoliosis, reduced disc height, Schmorl's nodes, or changes in vertebral body configuration.[42]

Degenerative spondylolisthesis occurs as a result of alterations in the articular orientation of the apophyseal joint. One risk factor for greater degenerative spondylolisthesis in women is pregnancy. Multiparous women have a higher incidence of L4–L5 degenerative spondylolisthesis than age-matched nulliparous women and men do.[35]

Questions remain concerning the natural history of this disorder. In adults, the lesion is considered to be stable, with progression a rare occurrence. Floman reported on 18 patients (32 to 55 years of age) with isthmic spondylolisthesis and incapacitating back or leg pain monitored for 6 years.[12] Serial decubitus lateral radiographs documented slip progression calculated as a percentage of vertebral body length. Documented slip progression ranged from 9% to 30% (average, 14.6%) and occurred over a 2- to 20-year period (average duration, 6.8 years). Slip progression commences after the third decade of life and coincides with marked disk degeneration at the olisthetic level. The development of disc vacuum phenomena and vertebral osteophytes corresponds to the development of clinical symptoms of spinal instability and spinal stenosis. Bilateral lateral fusion with pedicle screw fixation and decompression was successful in 11 of 14 patients who underwent surgery, with 12 obtaining resolution of back and leg pain. Four patients who did not undergo surgery continued to have a limited ability to stand or walk for prolonged periods. In rare circumstances, the progression from spondylolysis to spondylolisthesis may be rapid.[41]

Beutler and co-workers reported on a 45-year follow-up evaluation of 500 first-grade children studied to determine the natural history of spondylolysis and spondylolisthesis, independent of pain.[2] Of this group, 30 subjects were found to have a unilateral (n = 8) or bilateral (n = 22) pars interarticularis defect. Three unilateral lysis defects healed over a 15- to 20-year period. Individuals with unilateral pars defects had no further slippage or disability. Patients with bilateral L5 pars defects had a clinical course similar to that of the general population. Progression of slippage slows with each decade to the age of 50 years. Slippage exceeding 15% was always associated with moderate to severe disc degeneration. This finding is similar to that of Floman.[12] Back pain was documented once in all the study patients during childhood and

10-10 COMPARISON OF ISTHMIC AND DEGENERATIVE SPONDYLOLISTHESIS

	Isthmic	Degenerative
Spine level	L5	L4
Sex	Male	Female
Age at onset	Under 20	Over 40
Race	White	Black
Sacralization	1%	22%

Modified from Rosenberg N: Degenerative spondylolisthesis. Paper presented at the meeting of the American Orthopedic Association, June 26, 1973, Hot Springs, VA. (Published in Wiltse LL: Spondylolisthesis and its treatment: Conservative treatment, fusion with and without reduction. In Ruge D, Wiltse LL [eds]: Spinal Disorders. Philadelphia, Lea & Febiger, 1977.)

adolescence. Back pain increased as the study population aged. In general, spondylolisthesis has a benign course for the first 50 years of life.

CLINICAL HISTORY

The most common clinical manifestation of spondylolisthesis is low back pain. Although the cause of this type of back pain in adults has been studied extensively, its origin is not clear. There is no clear understanding of how this lesion develops in so many patients between the ages of 5 and 7 but causes no back complaints until perhaps the age of 35, when a sudden twisting or lifting motion will precipitate an acute episode of back and leg pain. The pain is improved with extension of the spine and exacerbated with flexion. The degree of slippage does not necessarily correlate with the degree of pain experienced by the patient.

A large number of patients with significant degrees of slippage will go through life with no discomfort, whereas other patients with a minimal degree of slip will have significant pain.

Fifty percent of patients will normally associate an injury with the onset of the symptoms. The physician should be aware that it is possible to sustain an acute fracture of the pars, but such a fracture is a very rare occurrence. When a case involving a fracture is suspected, a bone scan taken within 3 months of the injury can document the fracture. If the defect is long-standing, it will not be apparent on scintiscan.[47]

Besides back pain, these patients may also complain of leg pain. Leg pain occurs because of the frequent buildup of a fibrocartilaginous mass at the site of the defect, which can cause pain by irritating the nerve root as it exits the neural foramen.

Once symptoms begin, the patient usually has constant low-grade back discomfort that is aggravated by activity and relieved by rest. During some periods the pain is more intense, but unless the picture is complicated by severe leg pain, total incapacitation is rare. Patients are seldom aware of any sensory or motor deficit. At this point it should be re-emphasized that in some people even severe displacement is asymptomatic and gives rise to no disability. It is not uncommon to detect a previously unrecognized spondylolisthesis on a routine gastrointestinal radiologic study of a 50-year-old patient.

Patients with degenerative spondylolisthesis, spinal stenosis, and congestive heart failure may experience increased nocturnal back and leg pain. The proposed mechanism of pain production is increased venous volume and pressure in Batson's plexus. Improved cardiac function has the potential to lessen the lumbar pain.[22]

PHYSICAL EXAMINATION

The physical findings of spondylolisthesis are fairly characteristic. In the absence of any radicular pain, the patient exhibits no postural scoliosis, but usually has an exaggeration of the lumbar curve and a palpable "stepoff." The slip is generally apparent once it reaches three quarters of a vertebral body. A dimple may also be present at the site of the abnormality. Anteriorly, a transverse crease may be found at the level of the umbilicus. Occasionally, mild muscle spasm is demonstrable, and in most instances, some local tenderness can be elicited. Although range of motion is usually complete, some pain can be expected on hyperextension. Usually, the neurologic examination is normal.

Hamstring tightness is commonly found in symptomatic patients with spondylolysis or spondylolisthesis.[13] The mechanism of muscle tightness is not clear. Originally thought to be related to nerve root irritation, hamstring tightness is more closely associated with an attempt to stabilize the unstable L5–S1 junction.[33,44] Patients with severe tightness assume a typical position consisting of flexion of the hips and knees, a backward-tilted pelvis, and flattening of the lumbar lordosis. These patients may have a stiff-legged gait with short strides referred to as a "pelvic waddle."[31]

The single-leg standing hyperextension test (stork test) may identify injury to a posterior element.[20] The patient balances on the ipsilateral leg and then extends the lumbar spine. The test is positive when the pain localizes to the site of spondylolysis.

In general, no specific symptoms or signs can be used to differentiate chronic low back pain associated with spondylolisthesis from other causes.[29]

LABORATORY DATA

Laboratory test results are normal in patients with spondylolysis and spondylolisthesis.

RADIOGRAPHIC EXAMINATION

Plain roentgenograms of the lumbar spine in any projection are usually adequate to localize the abnormality if the lesion is large enough. If the lesion is unilateral, as seen in 20% of patients, it may be visible only on an oblique view of the lumbar spine.[13] Recognizing the "collar on the Scottie dog's neck" helps identify the local lesion. Patients with a dysplastic pars have an elongated interarticular region along with altered pedicles.

Forward subluxation of the body (spondylolisthesis) is best visualized on the lateral roentgenogram. The amount of slippage is graded by the system of Meyerding (Fig. 10-25).[28] The top of the sacrum is divided into four parallel quarters, posterior to anterior. Slippage of 25% or less of the sacrum is grade I, whereas movement of 75% or more of the sacrum is grade IV (Figs. 10-26 and 10-27). The subluxation occurs most commonly at the L5 level in isthmic spondylolisthesis but may occur at any of the lumbar vertebrae, particularly with other types of spondylolisthesis (Fig. 10-28).

In some patients, static views of the lumbar spine may be unremarkable, but the suspicion of spondylolisthesis is high. In these patients, flexion and extension views of the lumbosacral junction may be obtained to evaluate the presence of excessive motion. Measurement of dynamic vertebral translation, defined as a change in relative position from flexion to extension, is preferred over static displacement on a single view. Normal lumbar vertebral levels

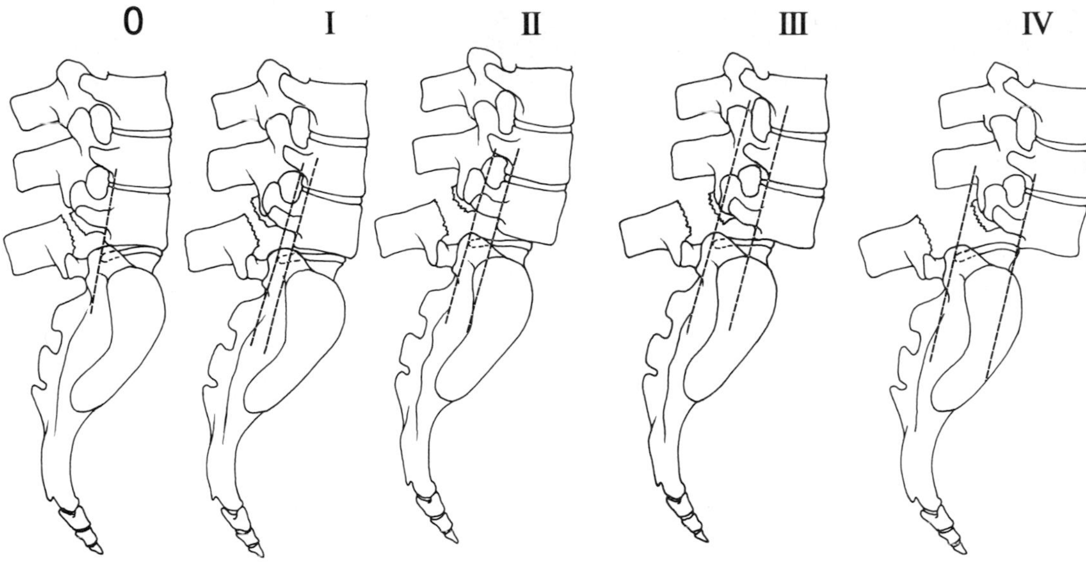

Figure 10-25 Grading system for spondylolisthesis.

should have less than 3.0 mm of dynamic anteroposterior translation.[3]

Other radiographic techniques, including CT and myelography, are rarely indicated. Advances in bone scintigraphy in the form of single-photon emission computed tomography (SPECT) allow for the identification of lesions not imaged by planar bone scan. SPECT is able to detect fractures in the pars interarticularis, transverse process, and vertebral body not detected by plain bone scan.[10,34] A false-positive rate of 15% has been noted with SPECT scans.[6] These lesions are usually detectable by thin-cut CT. MR evaluation of individuals older than 25 years with spondylolisthesis has demonstrated advanced degenerative disc disease at the level of the spondylolysis or spondylolisthesis when compared with controls.[43] MR imaging is able to detect entrapment and direct impingement of the spinal nerve roots associated with spondylolisthesis.[17] It is able to identify the presence of spondylolisthesis but may poorly delineate bone fragments around the defect, or it may detect alterations in the pars interarticularis (osteoblastic metastases, sclerosis of the neck of the pars) that may be confused

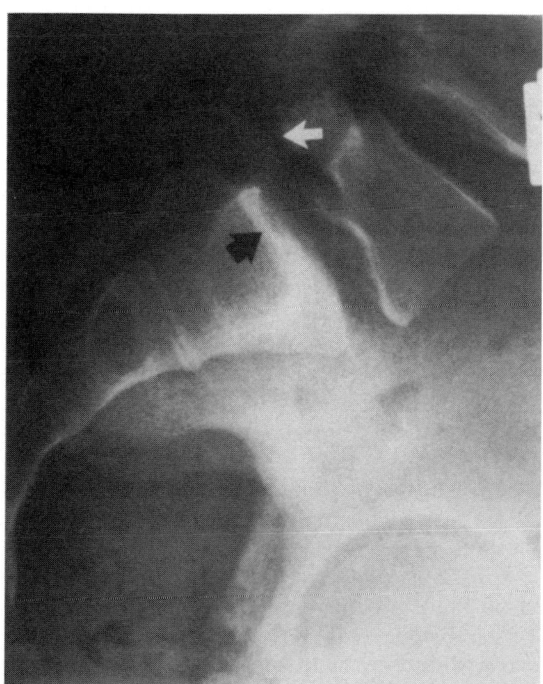

Figure 10-26 Lateral spot view of the lumbosacral junction. Grade I spondylolisthesis is present with 25% slippage of the superior vertebral body *(black arrow)*. This view demonstrates type II spondylolisthesis with a pars defect *(white arrow)*.

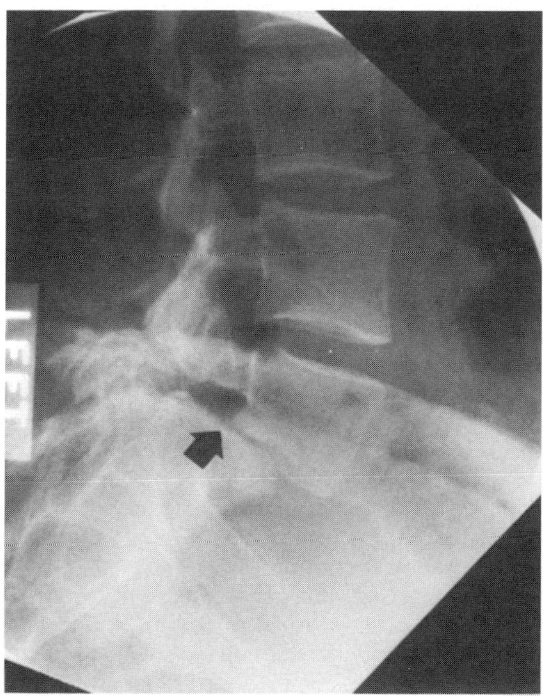

Figure 10-27 Lateral spot view of the lumbosacral junction. Grade II spondylolisthesis is seen with 50% slippage of the vertebral body.

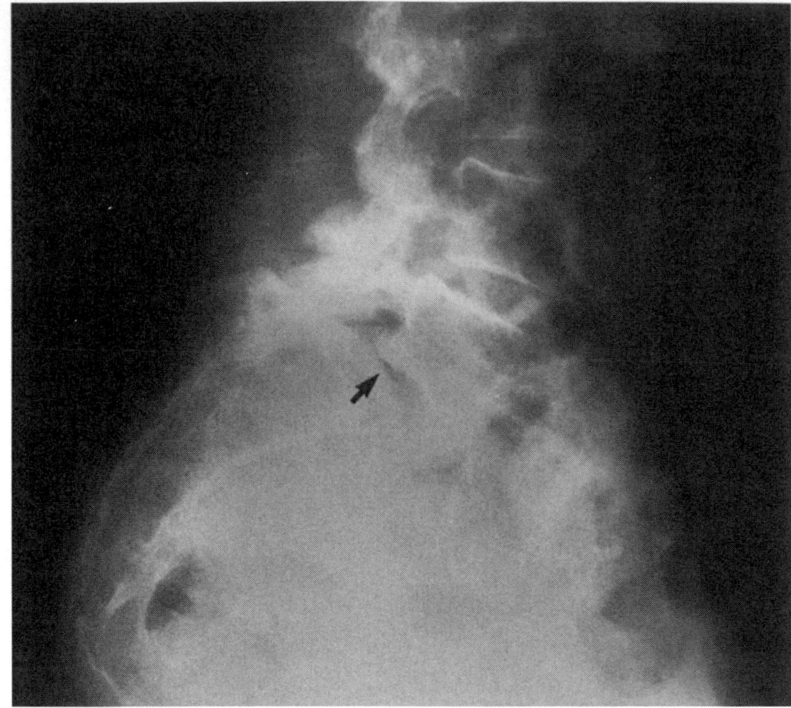

Figure 10-28 An 82-year-old woman was evaluated for low back pain of 2 months' duration. The pain is constant, exacerbated by anterior flexion, and relieved by lying supine. A lateral view of the lumbosacral spine reveals grade II degenerative spondylolisthesis at the L5–S1 interspace. A vacuum phenomenon is also present at the same interspace *(arrow)*.

with spondylolisthesis.[14,18] Although MR may identify spondylolysis without radiation exposure, the benefits of this procedure over other radiographic techniques has not been tested.[16,39]

Changes of degenerative spondylolisthesis are most common at the L4–L5 interspace.[11] Stress on the lumbar spine may be maximal at L4. Comparison of the anatomic structure of L4 and L5 may explain the increased stress on this vertebra. The L4 vertebra has relatively small transverse processes, less ligamentous support, and more mobility. This excess stress results in advanced degenerative changes in the facet joints at this level of the spine. The facets at the L4–L5 level are directed more sagittally than those of the L5–S1 joints and therefore allow more anterior motion. In the presence of degenerative changes, the normal limitation of movement of a facet on the one in front becomes deficient and permits forward displacement of L4. Slippage is never greater than 30% of the anteroposterior diameter of L5 because the spinous process of L4 hooks up on the body of the next lower vertebra. Radiographic findings associated with degenerative spondylolisthesis include signs of facet joint osteoarthritis—joint space narrowing, sclerosis, osteophytes, intervertebral disc space narrowing, vacuum phenomenon, and vertebral body sclerosis.

Motion roentgenograms may not be helpful in identifying the unstable segment causing back pain. A recent study reported no statistical difference between the amount of motion at symptomatic segments and that at nonsymptomatic segments in patients with degenerative instability.[40] An interventional open MR study of lumbar spondylolisthesis patients demonstrated no difference in mobility in those with and without back pain.[27]

In extreme degeneration of intervertebral discs, retrolisthesis may occur. With decreased disc height, the excess motion that occurs in adjacent vertebral bodies allows posterior motion.[45] The L1 and L2 vertebrae seem to be more commonly affected by this process. It is important to measure the anteroposterior diameter of adjacent vertebral bodies when diagnosing retrolisthesis. One of the vertebral bodies may be smaller in diameter and give a false impression of abnormal motion.

DIFFERENTIAL DIAGNOSIS

The diagnosis of spondylolysis is confirmed by the discovery of a pars defect on a lateral roentgenogram and spondylolisthesis by the forward position of one vertebral body on another on flexion and extension views of the lumbosacral spine (see Table 10-2).[23] Fractures of the spine may cause abnormal motion of the lumbar spine. However, these fractures rarely occur spontaneously and are more common in the setting of significant trauma to the lumbosacral spine.

It is important to remember that in adolescents and young adults, spondylolysis is usually asymptomatic. If back pain is present, a search should be made for other causes of back discomfort, including disc space infection, spinal cord tumor, osteoid osteoma, or early spondyloarthropathy. Disc herniation rarely occurs in this setting.

TREATMENT

Nonoperative treatment of adults with spondylolisthesis is much the same as that used for backache of other causes. Nonoperative management is indicated in all patients with spondylolisthesis who have slippage of less than 50% and are asymptomatic. When the symptoms are acute, rest is indicated. If leg pain is a significant problem, anti-inflammatory medication can be quite beneficial. Exercises should be started once the patient is in remission, and the patient is usually advised to wear a corset during occasional strenuous activity. Brace therapy may be helpful in decreasing symptoms in patients with spondylolisthesis. In a study of 28 patients who used antilordotic braces over a period of 25 months, those with spondylolisthesis had a significant reduction in lumbar lordosis and sacral inclination. At the conclusion of the period of brace treatment, all patients were pain free and none had demonstrated a significant increase in slippage.[1] In patients with positive bone scintiscans in the area of the pars defect, a trial of bracing may be successful in improving the pars defect.[38] Flexion or extension exercises may be indicated for symptomatic spondylolisthesis. In a study of 48 patients with spondylolisthesis treated by flexion or extension exercises, after 3 years of therapy 62% of patients treated with flexion exercises had improvement whereas 0% of patients treated with extension exercises improved.[37] Flexion exercises are more effective than extension exercises for the treatment of spondylolisthesis.

Surgery in the form of fusion of the unstable segment is indicated only to relieve pain, not to prevent slippage. Not infrequently, patients whose spondylolisthesis progresses beyond grade II need surgical intervention to decrease symptoms.[8] Surgical therapy may include spinal fusion for patients with low back symptoms and decompression with fusion for those with nerve root compression.[19] Considerations for surgical intervention include persistent or recurrent leg pain despite a 3-month trial of medical therapy, progressive neurologic deficit, reduction in quality of life, and imaging that confirms the clinical findings.[15] Surgical fusion of isthmic spondylolisthesis can increase the functional outcome of patients who do not improve with nonoperative therapy.[24]

In a comparison of treatment modalities, surgical intervention with posterolateral fusion resulted in greater pain relief and better function than exercises did in 111 patients with isthmic spondylolisthesis.[30] The 2-year follow-up period limits determination of the long-term benefits of fusion surgery. In addition, a different stabilizing exercise program might have shown a better outcome with conservative management.[32] Surgical techniques that result in solid fusions are necessary to reduce rates of pseudarthrosis.[21] In patients treated by decompression, autogenous iliac crest bone grafting, fusion of the intertransverse process, and segmental instrumentation, a 5-year follow-up reported a low complication rate and 77% satisfaction with the operation.[4]

PROGNOSIS

Identification of adolescents who are at risk for symptomatically significant spondylolisthesis remains difficult. The source of pain in spondylolysis and spondylolisthesis remains to be determined. Individuals with an acute pars fracture may heal, but the number of individuals who heal spontaneously is unknown. Athletes with spondylolysis may be asymptomatic. Adolescents with slippage greater than 50% are at risk for progression of the disease according to some studies.[5] Patients in whom the diagnosis is made at a younger age have a flattened lumbar lordosis, demonstrate minimal slippage at initial evaluation, have spina bifida, are male, and progress to spondylolisthesis. Patients with these findings should undergo serial evaluations. In most studies of young patients with isthmic lumbar spondylolisthesis, radiologic progression of slippage is rare and occurs slowly.[9] In a study of 272 children and adolescents, 190 patients who underwent posterolateral surgical fusion had a similar amount of progression as those treated nonsurgically.[36] In a study of 40 patients with degenerative spondylolisthesis, progression of slippage was noted in 30%. No progression occurred in patients after restabilization of the spine, progression being characterized by narrowing of the intervertebral disc, spur formation, subcartilaginous sclerosis, or ossification of ligaments. No correlation was found between clinical symptoms and progression of the slippage.[26]

Once patients experience symptoms secondary to spondylolisthesis, it is unreasonable to expect them to perform heavy work or participate in high-performance athletics. These individuals should be restricted from activities generally involving heavy lifting or repetitive bending. Surgical outcomes are good in patients who undergo fusion to relieve pain. The operation will not return people to strenuous activity and should not be undertaken with that expectation in mind.

References

Spondylolysis/Spondylolisthesis

1. Bell DF, Ehrlich MG, Zaleske DJ: Brace treatment for symptomatic spondylolisthesis. Clin Orthop 236:192, 1988.
2. Beutler WJ, Frederickson BE, Murtland A, et al: The natural history of spondylolysis and spondylolisthesis: 45-year follow-up evaluation. Spine 28:1027-1035, 2003.
3. Boden SD, Wiesel SW: Lumbosacral segmental motion in normal individuals: Have we been measuring instability properly? Spine 15:571, 1990.
4. Booth KC, Bridwell KH, Eisenberg BA, et al: Minimum 5-year results of degenerative spondylolisthesis treated with decompression and instrumented posterior fusion. Spine 24:1721-1727, 1999.
5. Bovall DW, Bradford DS, Moe JH, Winter RB: Management of severe spondylolisthesis (grade III and IV) in children and adolescents. J Bone Joint Surg Am 61-A:479, 1979.
6. Congeni J, McCulloch J, Swanson K: Lumbar spondylolysis: A study of natural progression in athletes. Am J Sports Med 25:248-253, 1997.
7. Connolly PJ, Fredrickson BE: Surgical management of isthmic and dysplastic spondylolisthesis and spondylolysis. In Fardon DF, Garfin SR (eds): Orthopaedic Knowledge Update: Spine 2. Rosemont, IL, American Academy of Orthopaedic Surgeons, 2002, pp 353-360.
8. Dandy DJ, Shannon MJ: Lumbosacral subluxation (group I spondylolisthesis). J Bone Joint Surg Br 53-B:578, 1971.
9. Danielson BI, Frennered AK, Irstam LKH: Radiologic progression of isthmic lumbar spondylolisthesis in young patients. Spine 16:422, 1991.
10. Dutton JA, Hughes SP, Peters AM: SPECT in the management of patients with back pain and spondylolysis. Clin Nucl Med 25:93-96, 2000.
11. Fitzgerald JAW, Newman PH: Degenerative spondylolisthesis. J Bone Joint Surg Br 58-B:184, 1976.
12. Floman Y: Progression of lumbosacral isthmic spondylolisthesis in adults. Spine 25:342-347, 2000.
13. Fredrickson BE, Baker D, McHolick WJ, et al: The natural history of spondylolysis and spondylolisthesis. J Bone Joint Surg Am 66-A:699-707, 1984.

14. Grenier N, Kressel HY, Schiebler ML, Grossman RI: Isthmic spondylolysis of the lumbar spine: MR imaging at 1.5 T. Radiology 170:489, 1989.
15. Herkowitz HN, Abraham DJ: Degenerative lumbar spondylolisthesis. Semin Spine Surg 11:28-33, 1999.
16. Hollenberg GM, Beattie PF, Meyers SP, et al: Stress reaction of the lumbar pars interarticularis and development of a new MRI classification system. Spine 27:181-186, 2002.
17. Jinkins JR, Matthes JC, Sner RN, et al: Spondylolysis, spondylolisthesis, and associated nerve root entrapment in the lumbosacral spine: MR evaluation. AJR Am J Roentgenol 152:327, 1989.
18. Johnson DW, Farnum GN, Latchaw RE, Erba SM: MR imaging of the pars interarticularis. AJR Am J Roentgenol 152:327, 1989.
19. Johnson LP, Nasca RJ, Dunham WK: Surgical management of isthmic spondylolisthesis. Spine 13:93, 1988.
20. Keene JS: Low back pain in the athlete: From spondylogenic injury during recreation or competition. Postgrad Med 74:209-217, 1983.
21. Kim DH, Albert TJ: Update on use of instrumentation in lumbar spine disorders. Best Pract Res Clin Rheumatol 16:123-140, 2002.
22. Laban MM, Wesolowski DP: Night pain associated with diminished cardiopulmonary compliance: A concomitant of lumbar spinal stenosis and degenerative spondylolisthesis. Am J Phys Med Rehabil 67:155, 1988.
23. Laurent LE: Spondylolisthesis. Acta Orthop Scand Suppl 35:20, 1958.
24. L'heureux EA Jr, Perra JH, Pinto MR, et al: Functional outcome analysis including preoperative and postoperative SF-36 for surgically treated adult isthmic spondylolisthesis. Spine 28:1269-1274, 2003.
25. Macnab I: Spondylolisthesis with an intact neural arch—the so-called pseudospondylolisthesis. J Bone Joint Surg Br 32-B:325, 1950.
26. Matsunaga S, Sakou T, Morizono Y, et al: Natural history of degenerative spondylolisthesis: Pathogenesis and natural course of the slippage. Spine 15:1204, 1990.
27. McGregor AH, Anderton L, Gedroyc WMW, et al: The use of interventional open MRI to assess the kinematics of the lumbar spine in patients with spondylolisthesis. Spine 27:1582-1586, 2002.
28. Meyerding HW: Low backache and sciatic pain associated with spondylolisthesis and protruded intervertebral disc. J Bone Joint Surg 23:461, 1941.
29. Moller H, Sundin A, Hedlund R, et al: Symptoms, signs, and functional disability in adult spondylolisthesis. Spine 25:683-689, 2000.
30. Moller H, Hedlund R: Surgery versus conservative management in adult isthmic spondylolisthesis: A prospective randomized study. I. Spine 25:1711-1715, 2000.
31. Newman PH: A clinical syndrome associated with severe lumbosacral subluxation. J Bone Joint Surg Br 47-B:472, 1965.
32. O'Sullivan PB, Phyty GDM, Twomey LT, et al: Evaluation of specific stabilizing exercise in the treatment of chronic low back pain with radiologic diagnosis of spondylolysis or spondylolisthesis. Spine 22:2959-2967, 1997.
33. Phalen GS, Dickson JA: Spondylolisthesis and tight hamstrings. J Bone Joint Surg Am 43-A:5095, 1961.
34. Ryan PJ, Evans PA, Gibson T, Fogelman I: Chronic low back pain: Comparison of bone SPECT with radiography and CT. Radiology 182:849, 1992.
35. Sanderson PL, Fraser RD: The influence of pregnancy on the development of degenerative spondylolisthesis. J Bone Joint Surg Br 78-B:951-954, 1996.
36. Seitsalo S, Osterman K, Hyvarinen H, et al: Progression of spondylolisthesis in children and adolescents: A long-term follow-up of 272 patients. Spine 16:417, 1991.
37. Sinaki M, Lutness MP, Ilstrup DM, et al: Lumbar spondylolisthesis: Retrospective comparison and three-year follow-up of two conservative treatment programs. Arch Phys Med Rehabil 70:594, 1989.
38. Southern EP, An HS: Classification, diagnosis, radiographs, natural history, and conservative treatment of spondylolisthesis. Semin Spine Surg 11:1-13, 1999.
39. Standaert CJ, Herring SA: Spondylolysis: A critical review. Br J Sports Med 34:415-422, 2000.
40. Stokes IAF, Frymoyer JW: Segmental motion and instability. Spine 12:688, 1987.
41. Stone AT, Tribus CB: Acute progression of spondylolysis to isthmic spondylolisthesis in an adult. Spine 27:E370-E372, 2002.
42. Sward L, Hellstrom M, Jacobsson B, Peterson L: Back pain and radiologic changes in the thoracolumbar spine of athletes. Spine 15:124, 1990.
43. Szypryt EP, Twining P, Mulholland RC, Worthington BS: The prevalence of disc degeneration associated with neural arch defects of the lumbar spine assessed by magnetic resonance imaging. Spine 14:977, 1989.
44. Turner RH, Bianco AJ Jr: Spondylolysis and spondylolisthesis in children and teenagers. J Bone Joint Surg Am 53:1298, 1971.
45. Willis TA: Lumbosacral retrodisplacement. AJR Am J Roentgenol 90:1263, 1963.
46. Wiltse LL, Newman PH, Macnab I: Classification of spondylolisthesis. Clin Orthop 117:23, 1976.
47. Wiltse LL, Widell EH Jr, Jackson DW: Fatigue fractures: The basic lesion in isthmic spondylolisthesis. J Bone Joint Surg Am 57-A:17, 1975.
48. Wynne-Davies R, Scott JHS: Inheritance and spondylolisthesis: A radiographic family survey. J Bone Joint Surg Br 61-B:301, 1979.

ADULT SCOLIOSIS

Capsule Summary

	Low Back	Neck
Frequency of spinal pain	Uncommon	Not applicable (NA)
Location of spinal pain	Lumbar curve	NA
Quality of spinal pain	Ache	NA
Symptoms and signs	Lumbar curvature	NA
Laboratory tests	None	NA
Radiographic findings	Curvature on plain roentgenogram	NA
Treatment	Medications, physical therapy, braces, surgery	NA

PREVALENCE AND PATHOGENESIS

Scoliosis is lateral curvature of the spine. The term is usually applied to curves in excess of 10 degrees. The normal spine does curve in the lateral plane and should be straight (no lateral deviation) when viewed from the front or back. Many patients with lumbar or thoracolumbar curves are asymptomatic. It is thought by some that the incidence of low back pain in patients with scoliosis is no higher than that in the general population. However, others believe that pain is indirectly associated with scoliosis and that the larger the curve, the more severe the pain is likely to be. Scoliotic curves may be either structural (fixed), characterized by fixed rotation on forward bending, or compensatory (functional), tending to maintain body alignment of the head over the pelvis and normal position on forward bending. When the apex of the curve is from L2 to L4, the curve is termed *lumbar*. When the apex is at L5 or the sacrum, the curve is termed *lumbosacral*. Kyphoscoliosis is lateral curvature of the spine associated with either increased posterior or decreased anterior angulation in the sagittal plane in excess of the accepted normal curve for that area. Kyphoscoliosis affects both the thoracic and the lumbar spine.

The major categories of adult scoliosis include individuals younger than 40 years with spinal deformity beginning in adolescence but no degenerative alterations of the spine, individuals older than 40 years with spinal deformity and degenerative changes, and elderly individuals with no preexisting curvature in whom scoliosis develops as a component of osteoarthritis of the thoracolumbar spine.[5] Adult degenerative scoliosis affects the L2–L3 or L3–L4 levels most frequently. The curves are shorter than those associated with adolescent scoliosis.

The Scoliosis Research Society has proposed three-dimensional terminology for spinal deformity. Deformity can be divided into local (vertebra), regional (curve), spinal (entire spine), and global (entire body) components.[30]

Epidemiology

Studies of adults have recognized scoliosis in 3.9% to 7.5% of all individuals.[16,24,32] In a study of postpartum radiographs, 5% had curves measuring 10 to 19 degrees and 2% had curves greater than 20 degrees.[31] Kostuik and Bentivoglio reviewed 5000 intravenous pyelograms of adults and reported scoliosis greater than 10 degrees in 3.9%.[16] A female-to-male ratio of 1:1 is associated with curves under 10 degrees, whereas a female-to-male ratio of 5.4:1 is observed in those with curves greater than 20 degrees.[3] The prevalence of scoliosis does increase with age.

Pathogenesis

The causes of adolescent scoliosis are unknown. A variety of abnormalities have been implicated, including genetic predisposition; disorders of bone, muscle, or cartilage growth; and neuromuscular dysfunction. Monozygous twins have a higher concordance rate than dizygous twins do for the development of adolescent scoliosis.[15] No single mechanism has been identified. Idiopathic scoliosis aggregates within families. However, no specific genetic propensity has been identified.[18] Any etiologic mechanism will have to explain the higher prevalence in girls and the development during growth spurts. Melatonin, a product of the pineal gland, has been implicated in the orderly development of the spine. Decreased levels have been detected in adolescents with progressive scoliosis.[8,17]

In 1973, the Scoliosis Research Society developed a classification of spine deformity. The major categories include idiopathic, neuromuscular, congenital, neurofibromatosis, mesenchymal disorders, rheumatoid disease, trauma, extraspinal contractures, osteochondrodystrophies, infection of bone, metabolic disorders, disorders related to the lumbosacral joint, and tumors (Table 10-11). Nonstructural (compensatory) forms of scoliosis include those related to postural, hysterical, nerve root, inflammatory, leg-length, and hip abnormalities. By far the largest group of cases of scoliosis are idiopathic, with over 90% falling in this category.[9]

CLINICAL HISTORY

An adult patient with scoliosis is typically a woman between the ages of 20 and 40, although some patients may be initially seen as late as at 80 years of age.[4] The patient is asymptomatic at first, but a feeling of tiredness at the end of the day gradually develops in the lumbar area. The pain of scoliosis is mechanical in nature and is probably caused by disc or facet joint degeneration. In some instances, the pain is radicular and secondary to nerve root compression on the concave side of the lumbar curve. In severe cases, impingement of the ribs on the iliac crest may cause severe pain (Fig 10-29).

Patients will state that the pain becomes worse the longer they are ambulatory and that the symptoms are relieved rapidly by lying down.[35] The site of the pain is at or just below the apex of the curve. As time passes, the pain occurs more frequently and is more severe. Certain movements or physical activities cause increased pain, thus suggesting the possibility of a mechanically unstable segment contributing to the dysfunction.[1]

Progression of the curve usually coexists with increased pain. In the lumbar spine, a curve over 40 degrees will generally lead to a constant rate of progression of 1 degree per year. The rate may increase to an even greater extent with pregnancy. Under 40 degrees in a skeletally mature individual, the curve will remain stable. The lumbar component of thoracolumbar scoliosis tends to progress more rapidly than the coronal portion of the curve.

In taking the history of adolescents, the physician should inquire about the family history and connective tissue, neuromuscular, and traumatic disorders. Positive responses to these inquiries help identify individuals who have specific reasons for the development of scoliosis (neurofibromatosis, Marfan's syndrome, muscular dystrophy) and do not belong in the idiopathic group. For example, spinal deformity is noted in 10% of individuals with neurofibromatosis.[2] The family history may give some insight into the prognosis if a close relative has had progression with severe deformity.

Patients may complain of pain with certain motions of the spine. Patients with scoliosis do not have parallel facet joints. The planes of the facets are at an angle. The soft tissues on the concave side of the curve tend to shorten, thereby resulting in mechanical restriction of motion. With spinal flexion past a certain degree, the ligamentous and capsular tissues are stretched, and pain occurs. In addition, extension of the spine may cause impingement of the asymmetric facet joints and, as a result, low back pain.

PHYSICAL EXAMINATION

The patient should be undraped except for underwear. Specific examination should be performed to identify

10-11 CLASSIFICATION OF SCOLIOSIS

STRUCTURAL SCOLIOSIS

I. Idiopathic
  A. Infantile (0–3 yr)
    1. Resolving
    2. Progressive
  B. Juvenile (3–10 yr)
  C. Adolescent (>10 yr)
II. Neuromuscular
  A. Neuropathic
    1. Upper motor neuron
      a. Cerebral palsy
      b. Spinocerebellar degeneration
        i. Friedreich's disease
        ii. Charcot-Marie-Tooth disease
        iii. Roussy-Lévy disease
      c. Syringomyelia
      d. Spinal cord tumor
      e. Spinal cord trauma
      f. Other
    2. Lower motor neuron
      a. Poliomyelitis
      b. Other viral myelitides
      c. Traumatic
      d. Spinal muscular atrophy
        i. Werdnig-Hoffmann
        ii. Kugelberg-Welander
      e. Myelomeningocele (paralytic)
    3. Dysautonomia (Riley-Day)
    4. Other
  B. Myopathic
    1. Arthrogryposis
    2. Muscular dystrophy
      a. Duchenne (pseudohypertrophic)
      b. Limb-girdle
      c. Facioscapulohumeral
    3. Fiber type disproportion
    4. Congenital hypotonia
    5. Myotonia dystrophica
    6. Other
III. Congenital
  A. Failure of formation
    1. Wedge vertebra
    2. Hemivertebra
  B. Failure of segmentation
    1. Unilateral (unsegmented bar)
    2. Bilateral
  C. Mixed
IV. Neurofibromatosis
V. Mesenchymal disorders
  A. Marfan's
  B. Ehlers-Danlos
  C. Others
VI. Rheumatoid disease
VII. Trauma
  A. Fracture
  B. Surgical
    1. Postlaminectomy
    2. Post-thoracoplasty
  C. Irradiation
VIII. Extraspinal contractures
  A. Postempyema
  B. Post-burns
IX. Osteochondrodystrophies
  A. Diastrophic dwarfism
  B. Mucopolysaccharidoses (e.g., Morquio's syndrome)
  C. Spondyloepiphyseal dysplasia
  D. Multiple epiphyseal dysplasia
  E. Other
X. Infection of bone
  A. Acute
  B. Chronic
XI. Metabolic disorders
  A. Rickets
  B. Osteogenesis imperfecta
  C. Homocystinuria
  D. Others
XII. Related to lumbosacral joint
  A. Spondylolysis and spondylolisthesis
  B. Congenital anomalies of lumbosacral region
XIII. Tumors
  A. Vertebral column
    1. Osteoid osteoma
    2. Histiocytosis X
    3. Other
  B. Spinal cord (see neuromuscular)

NONSTRUCTURAL SCOLIOSIS

I. Postural scoliosis
II. Hysterical scoliosis
III. Nerve root irritation
  A. Herniation of nucleus pulposus
  B. Tumors
IV. Inflammatory (e.g., appendicitis)
V. Related to leg-length discrepancy
VI. Related to contractures about the hip

From Bradford DS, Moe JH, Winter RB: Scoliosis and kyphosis. In Rothman RH, Simeone FA (eds): The Spine, 2nd ed. Philadelphia, WB Saunders, 1982.

scapular asymmetry and unilateral prominence, waist asymmetry, the shoulder level, and asymmetry in the distance between the arms and the torso. As the patient bends over, prominence of one side of the rib cage is noted. From the rear, the distance right or left from the gluteal cleft to a line drawn from C7 to the ground is a measurement of spinal imbalance. An inability to bend side to side may be secondary to intraspinal lesions such as a tumor, herniated disc, or osteoid osteoma, as well as scoliosis.

Lumbar scoliosis frequently involves the L1 vertebral body. Tilting of the lumbar spine at this level is associated with pelvic obliquity (unequal heights of the iliac wings), which is noted on physical examination.

A complete neurologic examination is useful to detect individuals who may be experiencing signs of nerve root compression. Muscle fatigue after exercise may be indicative of spinal stenosis associated with scoliosis. Pulmonary evaluation is also appropriate for individuals with more severe curvature.

LABORATORY DATA

Laboratory test results are normal in patients with idiopathic adult scoliosis.

RADIOGRAPHIC EVALUATION

Roentgenographic evaluation of scoliosis may be obtained with an erect full-length anteroposterior and lateral view of the thoracolumbar spine. The anteroposterior view is

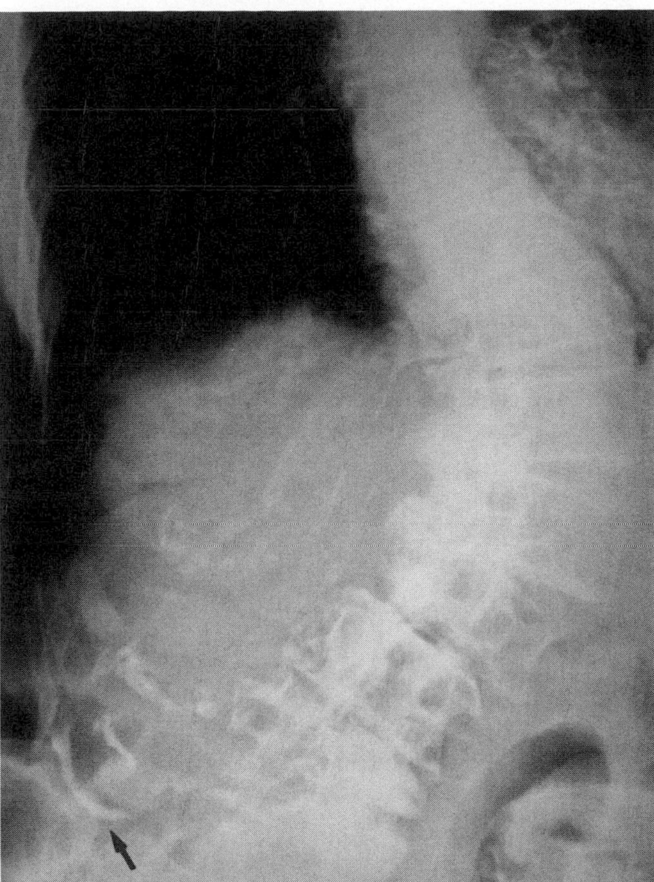

Figure 10-29 An 83-year-old woman was evaluated for increasing low back and flank pain. An anteroposterior view of a plain roentgenogram demonstrates degenerative scoliosis starting at T8 with the apex of the curve at L3 with a rotatory component. The tips of the lower ribs descend below the iliac wing *(black arrow)*.

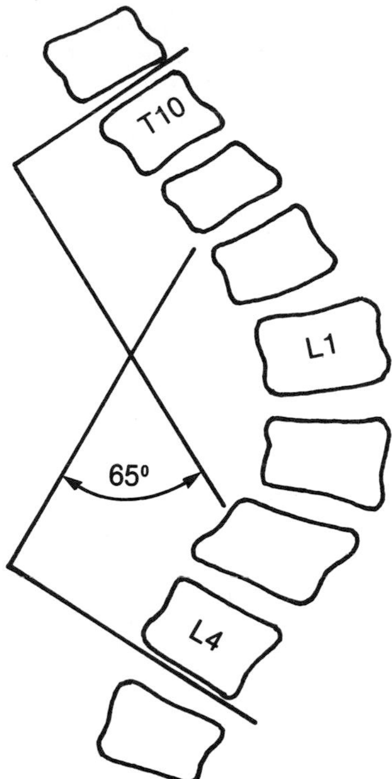

Figure 10-30 Cobb's method for measurement of spinal curvature. Lines are drawn along the superior end-vertebra at the uppermost extension of the vertebra and along the lower border of the inferior end-vertebra. The angle formed by the intersecting lines drawn perpendicular to the endplates is Cobb's angle.

used to measure the degree of curvature of the spine, whereas the lateral view detects the presence of spondylolisthesis. Additional projections may be obtained to assess spinal flexibility. They should be performed in a standardized manner so that progressive curvature can be measured. Different traction views are recommended for some patients with severe curves to determine curve flexibility.[25]

Cobb's method is used to measure spine curvature (Fig. 10-30). The vertebrae forming the ends of the curve are those that are most severely tilted toward its concavity. Lines are drawn along the upper border of the superior end-vertebra and along the lower border of the inferior end-vertebra. Perpendiculars are erected from each of these lines and are extended so that they intersect. Cobb's angle is the angle formed by the intersection of these two perpendicular lines.[6] The severity of rotation of the vertebrae associated with scoliosis may be determined by the method of Nash and Moe, in which rotatory scoliosis is graded by the location of the pedicle on the concave side of the scoliosis. In grades 1 and 2, the convex pedicle is visible on the anteroposterior view. In grades 3 and 4, the convex pedicle has twisted out of view (Fig. 10-31).[21] The use of other radiographic techniques, such as bone scintigraphy, spiral CT with myelography, and MR, is lim-

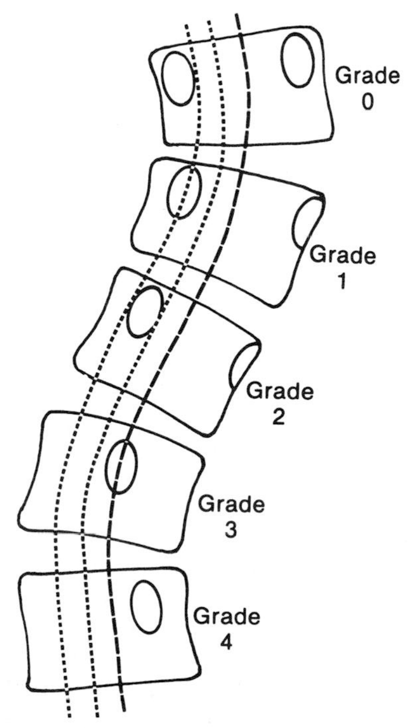

Figure 10-31 Grading of rotatory scoliosis.

ited to individuals with neurologic dysfunction or those who are to undergo surgery. Radiographic studies of patients with neurologic dysfunction may identify a tumor or an area of nerve impingement.

To diagnose progression of scoliosis, a definite increase in curvature greater than 5 degrees must be seen on roentgenographic evaluation. The initial film taken in adulthood must be compared with the most current films to show progression.

DIFFERENTIAL DIAGNOSIS

The diagnosis of adult scoliosis is suspected during the physical examination and is confirmed by measurement of the lumbar spine angulation observed on roentgenographic examination (see Table 10-2). The curve is significant in an adult if it is greater than 40 degrees. Spinal angulation of less than 40 degrees does not progress and rarely causes symptoms. Monitoring of adolescent idiopathic scoliosis over a period of 40 years has shown that 68% of patients had progression of curvature after skeletal maturity.[33] Although the vast majority of individuals will have an idiopathic or degenerative form of adult scoliosis, in some adults spinal curvature will develop as a result of specific medical or mechanical abnormalities. In patients with an osteoid osteoma, a reversible form of scoliosis may develop secondary to muscle contraction.[11] Patients with osteomalacia of long duration are subject to weakening of bones, which may result in spinal curvature.[29]

Leg-Length Disparity

Leg-length disparity is a correctable, but frequently overlooked cause of adult scoliosis.[12] Patients with this type of scoliosis frequently complain of pain on standing or walking that starts within 30 minutes of commencing the activity and resolves quickly on sitting down. Placing a lift in the shoe on the short leg, which partially corrects the length discrepancy, helps improve the scoliosis and relieves symptoms. Recognition of this abnormality and correction by equalization of leg length is worthwhile even if the individual has not recognized the leg-length discrepancy for a number of years.[27]

TREATMENT

Treatment in a young adult is directed toward prevention of future problems. If the curve is under 40 degrees in the lumbar spine and the pain is not severe, nonoperative treatment can be initiated. Such treatment includes analgesics and anti-inflammatory medication, local facet injections, physical therapy, and braces.[36] The Milwaukee brace is a mainstay of nonoperative therapy in young individuals and is used to prevent progression of spinal curvature.[19] For the most part this form of bracing is rarely effective in the adult population. Recent reviews have questioned the efficacy of bracing. For example, young adults do not wear braces for the prescribed periods.[10] If discomfort cannot be controlled or the curve is progressive, surgery is indicated. The aim of surgery is to straighten the spine as much as safely possible and to stabilize it in a corrected position.

Indications for surgery in an adult scoliosis patient younger than 40 years include thoracic curves greater than 50 degrees or a deformity unacceptable to the patient. In older adults, indications for surgery include curve progression with imbalance, radicular pain associated with nerve impingement, or pulmonary compromise.[7]

In an older adult, treatment is directed toward correction of existing problems. Besides pain and curve progression, an older adult is more likely to have compression of neural elements because of the degenerative changes associated with adult scoliosis of longer duration. The goal is to keep these patients functional. In most patients with a lumbar curve under 40 degrees, this goal is possible without surgery. An operative procedure is indicated for unremitting pain, curve progression, or uncontrolled radiculopathy. With the newer internal fixation devices available (e.g., Harrington rods and pedicle fixation), scoliosis surgery in the adult lumbar spine can be quite rewarding and result in spine stabilization and reduction of symptoms (Fig. 10-32).[13] Improvement may be measured not only by pain relief but also by restored function.[28]

Selection of the appropriate patient for corrective surgery is complicated. Patients may need to undergo electrodiagnostic testing consisting of diagnostic injections to determine the neural levels impaired by the scoliosis. The nutritional status of patients must be monitored to limit surgical complications.[14]

PROGNOSIS

Most patients with adult scoliosis do not require therapy because their curvature is mild and nonprogressive. A follow-up study of 444 patients with late-onset idiopathic scoliosis reported an increased frequency of back pain in comparison to age-matched controls but no significant difference in physical function.[34] Patients with progressive curvature are subject to persistent pain at the apex of the curve, which may respond to medical therapy. In patients with even greater curvature, neurologic deficits and pulmonary insufficiency may develop, particularly with thoracic scoliosis.[22]

Untreated severe scoliosis is associated with major disability and death. In adults, the pain may become progressive and severe as increasing degenerative changes occur in the facet joints and intervertebral discs. Respiratory insufficiency may limit stamina and work potential in those with double curvature (thoracolumbar scoliosis).

Premature death may also be a complication of severe scoliosis. Nachemson reported mortality from cardiorespiratory causes to be twice that of the normal population at age 40 in 130 nontreated scoliosis patients of all types.[20] Once again, this increased mortality occurs in patients with double curvature.

Early surgical intervention is appropriate for individuals with spinal deformity and respiratory insufficiency. In a study by Rizzi and colleagues, 16 patients with respiratory insufficiency (vital capacity, <60%; PaO_2, 80 mm Hg; or $PaCO_2$, >45 mm Hg) underwent scoliosis surgery.[26] The 16 patients with a good outcome had a mean age of

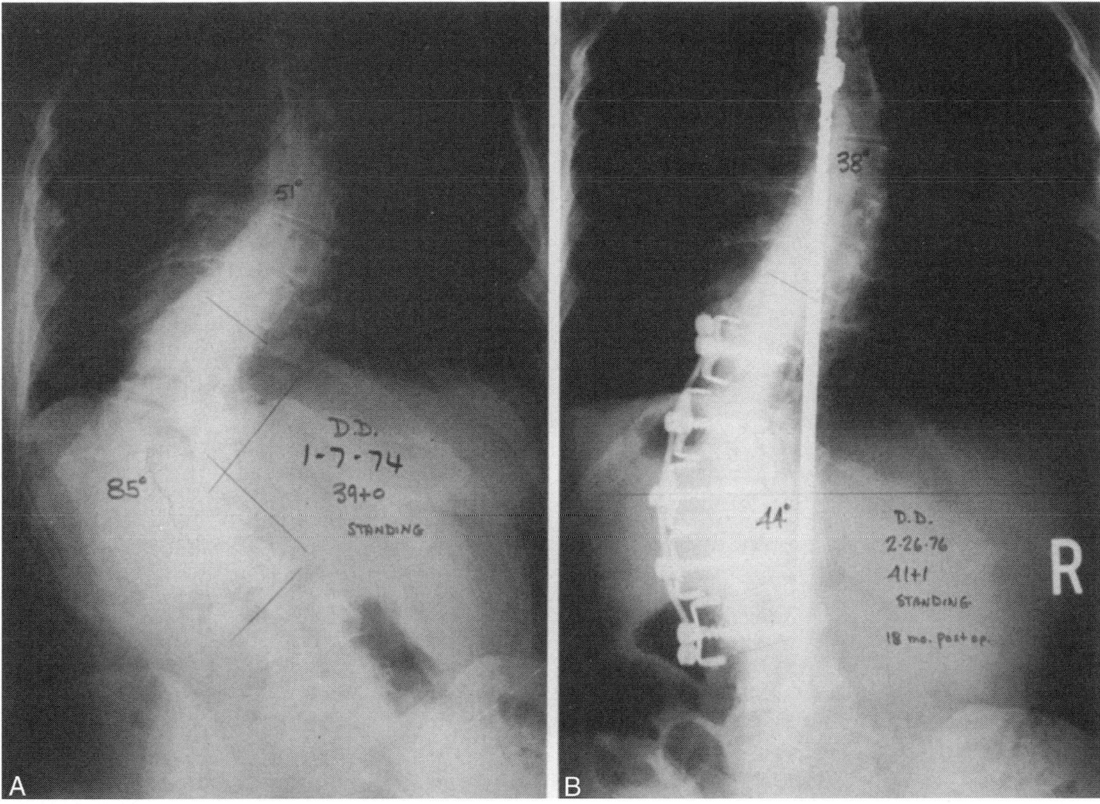

Figure 10-32 *A*, D.D., a 39-year-old woman with progressive and painful idiopathic curvatures. The lumbar curve was the more progressive and more painful of the two curves. *B*, The same patient, 18 months after anterior Dwyer instrumentation, followed by fusion of the lumbar curve, posterior Harrington instrumentation, and fusion of both curves. Almost all her pain is gone. *(From Rothman RH, Simeone FA [eds]: The Spine, 2nd ed. Philadelphia, WB Saunders, 1982.)*

35 years with a 47% correction of kyphosis and a 40% correction of scoliosis with corrective surgery. These patients had an 8% improvement in forced vital capacity, a 10-mm Hg increase in PaO_2, and a 6% decrease in $PaCO_2$. In the eight patients with a poor outcome, the mean age was 45 years, and the degree of improvement of kyphosis and scoliosis was 26% and 37%, respectively. Seven of these patients died in the first postoperative year because of progressive respiratory failure or surgical complications.

Surgical intervention in the form of fusion or rods can halt further progression of spine curvature and relieve pain. Surgery is not without its complications, including pseudarthrosis, infection, and curvature above the area of fusion. The location of the fusion and the configuration of the stabilizing device may result in complications after surgery. Patients older than 30 years with fusions at L3 or lower undergo more secondary surgeries for pseudarthrosis, discectomy for disc herniation caudal to the fusion, and decompression for spinal stenosis. These individuals may also experience more back pain and interference with activities of daily living and have a greater requirement for regular pain medication.[23] Careful consideration must be given to the selection of surgical candidates. Scoliosis surgery is best performed by physicians who have had extensive experience with the complexity of the surgical procedures and the special needs of patients with this mechanical abnormality.

References

Adult Scoliosis

1. Aebi M, Marchesi DG: The degenerative adult scoliosis: Classification and indication for treatment. Spine St Art Rev 12: 73-84, 1998.
2. Akbarnia BA, Gabriel KR, Beckman E, Chalk D: Prevalence of scoliosis in neurofibromatosis. Spine 17(suppl):S244, 1992.
3. Armour EF, Seimon LP, Margulies J: What every physician should know about scoliosis: Strategies for early detection. Spine St Art Rev 12:193-197, 1998.
4. Balderston RA: Adult scoliosis: Patient evaluation and operative considerations that differ from adolescent. Semin Spine Surg 9: 164-168, 1997.
5. Boachi-Adjei O, Gupta MC: Adult scoliosis and deformity In Fardon DF, Garfin SR (eds): Orthopaedic Knowledge Update: Spine 2. Rosemont, IL, American Academy of Orthopaedic Surgeons, 2002, pp 377-391.
6. Bradford DS, Moe JH, Winter RB: Scoliosis and kyphosis. In Rothman RH, Simeone FA (eds): The Spine, 2nd ed. Philadelphia, WB Saunders, 1982, pp 316-439.
7. Bradford DS, Tay B, Hu S: Adult scoliosis: Surgical indications, operative management, complications, and outcomes. Spine 24:2617-2629, 1999.
8. Burwell RG, Dangerfield PH: Adolescent idiopathic scoliosis: Hypotheses of causation. Spine St Art Rev 14:319-333, 2000
9. Cobb JR: Outline for the study of scoliosis. Am Acad Orthop Surgeons Lect 5:261, 1948.
10. Dickson RA: Spinal deformity—adolescent idiopathic scoliosis: Nonoperative treatment. Spine 24:2601-2606, 1999.
11. Freiberger RH: Osteoid osteoma of the spine: A cause of backache and scoliosis in children and young adults. Radiology 75:232, 1960.

12. Gofton JP: Persistent low back pain and leg length disparity. J Rheumatol 12:747, 1985.
13. Harrington PR: An eleven year clinical investigation of Harrington instrumentation, a preliminary report on 578 cases. Orthop Clin North Am 3:113, 1972.
14. Hu SS, Fontaine F, Kelly B, et al: Nutritional depletion in staged spinal reconstructive surgery: The effect of total parenteral nutrition. Spine 23:1401-1405, 1998.
15. Kessling KL, Reinker KA: Scoliosis in twins: A meta-analysis of the literature and report of six cases. Spine 22:2009-2015, 1997.
16. Kostuik JP, Bentivoglio J: The incidence of low back pain in adult scoliosis. Spine 6:268-273, 1981.
17. Machida M: Cause of idiopathic scoliosis. Spine 24:2576-2583, 1999.
18. Miller NH: Cause and natural history of adolescent idiopathic scoliosis. Orthop Clin North Am 30:343-352, 1999.
19. Moe JH: Indication for Milwaukee brace nonoperative treatment in idiopathic scoliosis. Clin Orthop 93:38, 1973.
20. Nachemson A: A long-term follow-up study of non-treated scoliosis. Acta Orthop Scand 39:466, 1968.
21. Nash CL, Moe JH: A study of vertebral rotation. J Bone Joint Surg Am 51-A:223, 1969.
22. Nilsonne U, Lundgren KD: Long-term prognosis in idiopathic scoliosis. Acta Orthop Scand 39:456, 1968.
23. Paonessa KJ, Engler GL: Back pain and disability after Harrington rod fusion to the lumbar spine for scoliosis. Spine 17(suppl):S249, 1992.
24. Perennou D, Marcelli C, Herisson C, et al: Adult lumbar scoliosis. Epidemiologic aspects in a low-back pain population. Spine 19: 123-128, 1996.
25. Polly DW Jr, Sturm PF: Traction versus supine side bending. Which technique best determines curve flexibility? Spine 23: 804-808, 1998.
26. Rizzi PE, Winter RB, Lonstein JE, et al: Adult spinal deformity and respiratory failure: surgical results in 35 patients. Spine 22:2517-2531, 1997.
27. Rothenberg RJ: Rheumatic disease aspects of leg length inequality. Semin Arthritis Rheum 17:196, 1988.
28. Shapiro GS, Taira G, Boachie-Adjei O: Results of surgical treatment of adult idiopathic scoliosis with low back pain and spinal stenosis: A study of long-term clinical radiographic outcomes. Spine 28:358-363, 2003.
29. Steinbach HL, Noetzli M: Roentgen appearance of the skeleton in osteomalacia and rickets. AJR Am J Roentgenol 91:955, 1964.
30. Stokes IAF (chair): Scoliosis Research Society working group on 3-D terminology of spinal deformity: Three-dimensional terminology of spinal deformity. Spine 19:236-248, 1994.
31. Strayer LM III: The incidence of scoliosis in the postpartum female on Cape Cod. J Bone Joint Surg Am 55-A:436, 1973.
32. Vanderpool DW, James JIP, Wynne-Davies R: Scoliosis in the elderly. J Bone Joint Surg Am 51-A:446, 1969.
33. Weinstein SL, Ponsetti IV: Curve progression in idiopathic scoliosis. J Bone Joint Surg Am 65-A:447-455, 1983.
34. Weinstein L, Weinstein SL, Dolan LA, Spratt KF, et al: Health and function of patients with untreated idiopathic scoliosis: A 50-year natural history study. JAMA 289:559-567, 2003.
35. Winter RB, Lonstein JE, Denis F: Pain patterns in adult scoliosis. Orthop Clin North Am 19:339-345, 1988.
36. Wood KB: Nonsurgical treatment of adult scoliosis. Semin Spine Surg 10:361-366, 1998.

CHAPTER 11

RHEUMATOLOGIC DISORDERS OF THE SPINE

Rheumatologic disorders of the axial skeleton are common causes of spinal pain. These disorders affect the bones, joints, ligaments, tendons, and muscles that are anatomic components of the spine. Whereas mechanical disorders, such as muscle strain, disease of the intervertebral discs, and osteoarthritis of the spine, are frequent causes of spinal pain, a number of other inflammatory and noninflammatory disorders are associated with pain in the axial skeleton. The most important rheumatic disorders that cause inflammation of the joints of the axial skeleton are the seronegative spondyloarthropathies and rheumatoid arthritis. The spondyloarthropathies are characterized by involvement of the sacroiliac joints, peripheral large-joint disease, and the absence of rheumatoid factor. The seronegative spondyloarthropathies include ankylosing spondylitis, reactive arthritis, psoriatic arthritis, enteropathic arthritis, familial Mediterranean fever, Behçet's syndrome, Whipple's disease, and arthritis associated with hidradenitis suppurativa. They are closely associated with genetic factors that predispose patients to these illnesses. Environmental factors play a role as triggers of the inflammatory response in genetically predisposed individuals, but these factors have only partially been identified. Bacterial infection is associated with the onset of reactive arthritis. The role of trauma as an environmental trigger in ankylosing spondylitis, reactive arthritis, and psoriatic arthritis remains controversial.

Rheumatoid arthritis, a disease that causes chronic inflammation of the synovial lining of the joints, affects the cervical spine at the atlantoaxial junction and the subaxial apophyseal joints. These changes occur in patients with diffuse disease of long duration. Cervical spine involvement in rheumatoid arthritis is associated with a wide range of symptoms and signs, from mild neck pain and headaches to severe neurologic dysfunction consisting of radiculopathy, paresthesias, incontinence, quadriplegia, and sudden death.

In the seronegative spondyloarthropathies and rheumatoid arthritis, joint pain is most severe in the morning and improves with activity. Physical examination demonstrates localized tenderness on palpation and limitation in all planes of motion of the axial skeleton. Laboratory abnormalities are consistent with systemic inflammatory disease but are nonspecific, except for the presence of rheumatoid factor in 80% of patients with rheumatoid arthritis. Radiographic evaluation is very useful in identifying characteristic joint space narrowing, sclerosis, and fusion in the sacroiliac joints, vertebral body squaring, and ligamentous calcification, which may help in the differential diagnosis of a patient with axial skeletal pain.

Noninflammatory lesions affecting bone in the lumbosacral spine include osteochondritis (Scheuermann's disease) and osteitis condensans ilii. Diffuse idiopathic skeletal hyperostosis may involve the entire spine. Muscle syndromes associated with low back and neck pain include polymyalgia rheumatica and fibromyalgia.

In addition to drug therapy, treatment of these rheumatologic disorders involves a number of therapeutic modalities that include patient education and physical and occupational therapies. Although these illnesses have no cures, medical therapy can be effective in controlling symptoms and slowing progression. New therapy in the form of tumor necrosis factor-alpha and interleukin-1 inhibitors offers the potential to prevent joint inflammation and destruction to a greater degree than with previous therapies.

The prognosis and course of these rheumatic conditions are rarely related to the extent of spine disease alone. Occasionally, atlantoaxial subluxation secondary to rheumatoid arthritis or the spondyloarthropathies may result in catastrophic neurologic dysfunction. In most circumstances, the status of disease in other areas of the musculoskeletal system and the severity of constitutional symptoms have a greater effect on the patient's daily existence.

ANKYLOSING SPONDYLITIS

See page 302 for Capsule Summary.

PREVALENCE AND PATHOGENESIS

Ankylosing spondylitis (AS) (Greek *ankylos*, bent; *spondylos*, vertebra) is a chronic inflammatory disease characterized by a variable symptomatic course and progressive involvement of the sacroiliac and axial skeletal joints. It is the

CAPSULE SUMMARY

	LOW BACK	NECK
Frequency of spinal pain	Common	Common
Location of spinal pain	Lumbar spine	Cervical spine
Quality of spinal pain	Ache	Ache
Symptoms and signs	Morning stiffness, decreased back motion	Morning stiffness, decreased neck motion
Laboratory tests	Increased erythrocyte sedimentation rate	Increased erythrocyte sedimentation rate
Radiographic findings	Squaring of vertebral bodies on plain roentgenograms	Squaring of vertebral bodies on plain roentgenograms
Treatment	Range-of-motion exercises, NSAIDs, muscle relaxants, tumor necrosis factor antagonists	Range-of-motion exercises, NSAIDs, muscle relaxants, tumor necrosis factor antagonists

prototype of the seronegative spondyloarthropathies. This disease complex is characterized by axial skeletal arthritis, absence of rheumatoid factor in serum (seronegative), lack of rheumatoid nodules, and the presence of a tissue factor on host cells, human leukocyte antigen B27 (HLA-B27). AS is a disease of antiquity in that it has been found in the remains of mummies from Egypt and was known to Hippocrates.[190] A reappraisal of skeletal remains from the period of the Egyptian dynasties to the 19th century suggests that AS may not have been as common as once suspected. Forestier's disease (diffuse idiopathic skeletal hyperostosis [DISH]), reactive arthritis, or psoriatic spondylitis may have occurred more commonly.[184] During that period and to the present, AS has had many names, including rheumatoid spondylitis, Marie-Strümpell disease, von Bechterew's disease, and rheumatoid variant.

Epidemiology

AS affects about 1% to 2% of whites, a number equal to the prevalence of rheumatoid arthritis.[24,91,111] Some studies have suggested that 6.7% of white adults in certain populations may have AS.[127] The prevalence of disease relates to the penetrance of HLA-B27 in the population. A strikingly high association between HLA-B27 and AS has been demonstrated. HLA-B27 is present in more than 90% of white patients with AS versus 7% to 8% in a normal white population.[195] Eskimos, who have a prevalence of HLA-B27 of 25% to 40%, have 4% rates of AS; in contrast, it is rare in Japanese persons, who have an HLA-B27 penetrance of less than 1%.[24,115,126,194] Other ethnic groups such as the Haida and Pima Indians have a large proportion of people affected by AS in association with an increased prevalence of HLA-B27. In the North American white population, which has a 7% prevalence of HLA-B27, the frequency of AS is 0.2%.[142] Any spondyloarthropathy may occur in 13.6% to 20.0% of HLA-B27–positive individuals.[24,39] In randomly chosen cohorts of white individuals possessing HLA-B27, AS developed in approximately 2% to 6%. HLA-B27 is present in 50% of American blacks with AS, with a prevalence of 4% in the normal black population.[85] African blacks do not have the HLA-B27 antigen, and AS rarely develops. A positive family history of AS or a related spondyloarthropathy increases the risk to as high as 30% in HLA-B27–positive first-degree relatives versus 1% to 4% in HLA-B27–positive control subjects.[181]

Initially, the male-to-female ratio was thought to be 10:1, but more recent studies have demonstrated the ratio to be in the range of 3:1.[39] Women tend to be less symptomatic and have less severe disease, which may explain their small representation in earlier studies. Women may also initially have cervical spine disease more often, with minimal lumbar symptoms. In addition, the specificity of criteria necessary for the diagnosis of AS has an effect on the number of people who have the disease. The overall pattern of illness may be similar in men and women.[92]

Genetics

HLA STRUCTURE

HLAs are cell surface markers that are present on all nucleated mammalian cells. The portion of the short arm of the sixth chromosome of humans that determines expression of HLA is the major histocompatibility complex (MHC); this complex is associated with control of the immune response of the host (Fig. 11-1). In the MHC region are loci that code for the A, B, C, and D HLA antigens. A, B, and C loci are class I antigens that are serologically (antibody) defined. The antigen consists of two polypeptide chains: a large glycosylated chain that carries antigenic specificity and a small chain (beta$_2$-microglobulin) (Fig. 11-2). Each locus has many alleles (HLA-A: 263 alleles; HLA-B: 521 alleles; HLA-C: 125 alleles).[68] MHC class I genes are expressed on all nucleated cells. The heavy chain is divided into five distinct regions: three extracellular domains, a transmembrane region, and a cytoplasmic domain. The two outermost domains (alpha 1 and 2) form the peptide-binding groove. The membrane-proximal domain unites with beta$_2$-microglobulin to stabilize the molecule on the cell surface. The remaining domains function in anchoring the molecule to the cell surface and in signal transduction to cytoplasm. The binding site or groove is the location for attachment of antigen that is presented to the T-cell receptor for processing as an antigen.[27] The peptide-binding groove is composed of six pockets (A to F) that work to anchor the peptide in the

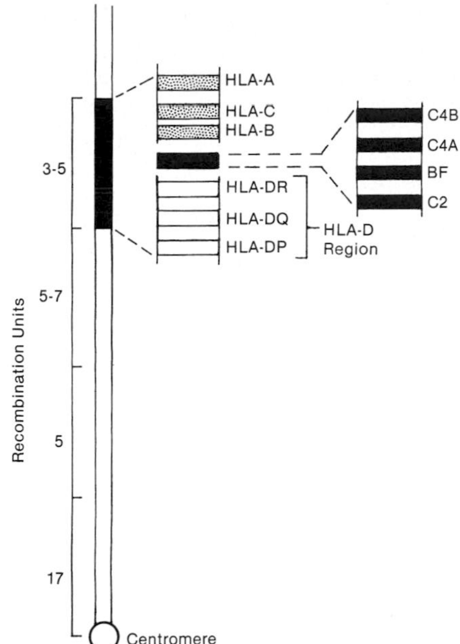

Figure 11-1 The short arm of the sixth chromosome of humans containing the histocompatibility locus (HLA). Included in this area are the A, B, C, and D loci. The D locus includes three alleles (DR, DQ, and DP). Interposed between the B and D loci is genetic material that codes for some of the complement components (C4b, C4A, BF, C2).

groove and optimize presentation of antigen to the T-cell receptor (Fig. 11-3). The floor of the antigen-binding site is formed by the beta strands, and the margins are formed by alpha helices.

The D locus, or class II antigens, are determined by interaction with specific lymphocytes (mixed lymphocyte reaction). The class II antigen consists of two membrane-inserted, glycosylated polypeptides that are noncovalently bound (see Fig. 11-2). Humans have at least three sets of genes for class II molecules: HLA-DR, HLA-DP, and HLA-DQ. Different alleles exist for each class II molecule. MHC class II antigens are expressed on cells that present antigens to CD4+ T lymphocytes. Class II molecules have an alpha and beta chain. Each chain has two domains: a transmembrane segment and an intracytoplasmic tail. Investigators have identified specific antigens associated with each locus.

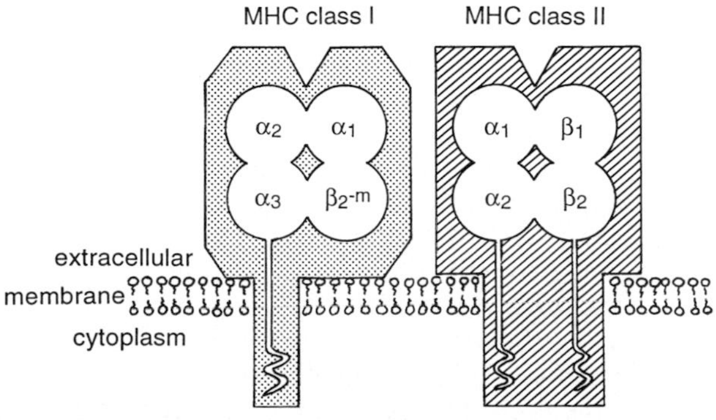

Figure 11-2 Major histocompatibility complex (MHC) class I molecules consist of a single alpha chain forming three domains along with beta-microglobulin, which acts as a stabilizer for the alpha chain. MHC class II molecules consist of two separate alpha and beta chains that form four extracellular domains.

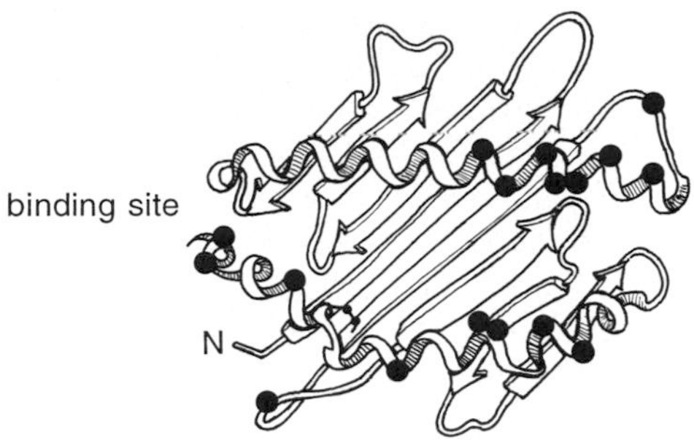

Figure 11-3 Structure of the major histocompatibility complex class I peptide-binding groove. The alpha 1 and 2 domains of the polypeptide chain form a beta-pleated sheet platform and two alpha helices that form the walls of groove into which the antigen peptides can bind. The *filled circles* correspond to residues critical in defining serologic epitopes on the alpha 1 and 2 domains.

HLA-B27

The HLA-B27 "B" pocket of the binding groove is unique. The B pocket accommodates the side chain of residue 2 (P2) of the bound peptide. The HLA-B27 B pocket preferentially binds peptides that have arginine at P2. Each of the binding pockets contributes to the overall binding. However, the C-terminal peptide residue in pocket F and the P2 residue in pocket B are the main anchors. Optimal residues at one position may compensate for suboptimal residues at another position.[140] Certain residues are highly variable and are associated with the subtypes of HLA-B27.[14]

HLA-B27 represents a family of 25 different subtypes or alleles that encode 23 proteins. HLA-B*2701 to HLA-B*2723 have a varied racial and ethnic distribution throughout the world.[181] The B27 subtypes differ from one another by one or more amino acid substitutions that affect the alpha 1 and 2 domains. The various B27 alleles differ from each other by one to six amino acids scattered throughout the peptide-binding groove of the class I molecule. HLA-B2705 is the most widespread B27 subtype and is associated with AS and other spondyloarthropathies. The sequence variation of the B27 subtypes and their pattern of worldwide distribution suggest that B*2705 might be the ancestral subtype from which the others have evolved.[3] Approximately 90% of B27-positive individuals of northern European extraction have B*2705.[128] The subtypes associated with AS and the related spondyloarthropathies include B*2701, B*2702, B*2704, B*2705, and B*2707.[128] B*2701 is a rare subtype found in white, Asian, and black populations. B*2702 is present in 10% of individuals of northern European extraction, 20% of Spanish Europeans, and 55% of Semitic B27-positive populations. B*2703 is found only in American blacks.[110] B*2704 is a predominant subtype in Chinese and Japanese individuals. B*2707 is a predominant form in India. B*2706 (southeast Asia) and B*2709 (Sardinia) are not associated with disease and have a substitution at residue 116.[129] Residue 116 is positioned at the floor of the peptide-binding cleft and is important in formation of the F pocket. There is only a 30% difference in peptide repertoires of the associated and nonassociated subtypes. The key to the difference in susceptibility may not be the subtype itself but the antigenic properties of the peptide specific to each subtype. The cytotoxic T-cell responses elicited in the context of each subtype are different.[96] Additional studies are being reported in regard to identification of the HLA-B27 subtypes associated with the various spondyloarthropathies.[148] Currently, the HLA-B27 subtypes are similar between groups.

Genetic Susceptibility

Additional evidence for certain subclasses of B27-positive individuals being at increased risk for AS arises from the observation that spondylitis is more common in B27-positive relatives of spondylitics than in B27-positive relatives of healthy B27 control subjects. Susceptibility may be related to the B27 epitope or to the presence of additional or linked genes that increase susceptibility.[40,64,67] Because genetic information in the MHC region other than class I antigen (complement components—class III antigens) does not increase susceptibility to spondylitis, additional genetic information that predisposes to spondylitis is probably distant from the B27 locus.[95] Over 90% of susceptibility to the disease is related to genetics. The environmental factors that contribute to the illness are common.

However, genetic factors alone do not result in expression of the disease. Many individuals who have HLA-B27 have no evidence of a spondyloarthropathy. Identical twins who have HLA-B27 may be discordant for AS. One twin may have AS, whereas the other may be normal or have symptoms and signs of a form of spondyloarthropathy other than AS.[112]

Other genes within the MHC appear to further enhance the risk for or modify the clinical expression of AS, including HLA-B60, tumor necrosis factor (TNF), HLA-DRB1 and HLA-DR8, and low-molecular-weight proteasome genes. Recent studies of twins and siblings with AS suggest that HLA-B27 and other MHC genes account for less than 50% of the genetic contribution to this disease.[31] Chromosomes 1, 2, 6, 9, 10, 16, and 19 contain genes that add to disease susceptibility.[32] The strongest linkage observed outside the MHC is on chromosome 16q.[30]

Pathogenesis

The pathogenesis of AS is unknown. In the past, infection, trauma, and heredity were thought to be involved. A genetic predisposition to AS and to the seronegative spondyloarthropathies in general does exist.

The mechanism by which HLA-B27 antigen results in spondylitis is not known. Hypotheses proposed to explain this occurrence have included B27 as a receptor site for infectious agents, B27 as a marker for an immune response gene that determines susceptibility to an environmental trigger, and B27 as a factor that induces tolerance to cross-reactive foreign antigens.[36,80] The persistence of HLA-B27 as a genetic trait may be related to its ability to control viral infections. Khare and colleagues suggest that the HLA-B27 molecule is one of the best class I molecules in generating viral-specific immunity. The evolutionary advantage would explain the penetrance of the gene in a wide geographic area, as well as the generation of multiple subtypes to protect against new viral mutations.[133]

A genetically determined host response to an environmental factor in genetically susceptible individuals seems to be the most likely basis for the pathogenesis of the spondyloarthropathies. That B27 is not sufficient for the development of AS is supported by the fact that disease does not develop in all individuals with B27, that even in a homogeneous form B27 does not cause disease, and that a small number of AS patients do not have B27. Recent studies in animals suggest that the HLA-B27 molecule plays a role in the pathogenesis of spondylitis. In transgenic rats made to express high levels of B27, an illness similar to AS develops.[103] The environmental component that may play a role in disease pathogenesis may be intestinal flora. Manifestations of AS do not develop in transgenic rats that are free of bacteria, whereas the disease subsequently develops in those exposed to bacteria. This model provides direct evidence for participation of the HLA-B27 molecule and environmental factors in disease pathogenesis.[210]

HLA-B27 has a unique structure that may contribute to the pathogenesis of AS. HLA-B27 has an unpaired cysteine residue (CYS67) in the extracellular alpha 1 domain, and free HLA-B27 heavy chains can form a stable disulfide-bonded heavy chain homodimer (HC-B27) on the cell surface.[2] This dimer may be pathogenic. In addition, studies have documented HLA-B27 heavy chain misfolding during assembly.[50] Such misfolding can influence intracellular signaling pathways. Accumulation of HLA-B27 may result in a stress response in the endoplasmic reticulum that leads to the production and activation of nuclear factor κB,[96] which can stimulate the synthesis of proinflammatory cytokines such as TNF-alpha in mononuclear cells.

Though not frequently mentioned in the context of spondylitis, DR antigens may play a role in the appearance of certain disease manifestations. Miehle and associates reported an increased prevalence of peripheral joint arthritis in HLA-DR4–positive patients with AS.[158]

Trauma

The role of incidental trauma to the spine in the initiation of the inflammatory process of AS is unknown. Patients with AS may initially have radicular arm or leg pain that is thought to be secondary to a herniated cervical or lumbar disc, respectively. Some of these patients have had laminectomies, and then classic changes of AS later developed in the axial skeleton. One of the potential complications of total hip joint replacement in a patient with AS is myositis ossificans, or calcification of the soft tissues surrounding a joint. It may be possible that in patients predisposed to this disease, significant tissue injury to the spine or peripheral joints can result in an inflammatory process that promotes tissue calcification and joint ankylosis.[179]

The difficulty substantiating the role of spinal trauma and the development of AS is illustrated by two histories. In a case of fraternal twin brothers, one was asymptomatic with no evidence of AS. In the other brother, who was asymptomatic before a fall at work, low back pain developed. He underwent a decompression procedure (laminectomy) for a suspected herniated lumbar disc. Subsequently, progressive fusion of the lumbar, thoracic, and cervical spine and peripheral arthritis of the hip developed. In another case, an Egyptian soldier who had symptoms of low back pain compatible with AS was wounded with shrapnel in the lumbar spine and thighs. He was immobilized for an extended period and experienced marked limitation of axial skeletal motion, including the cervical spine. Radiographic evaluation demonstrated increased spondylitic changes in his entire axial skeleton. Did significant tissue damage to the axial skeleton or peripheral joints in patients with active AS result in an exacerbation of symptoms and progression of disease in the injured area? Would AS have developed to the same extent in the absence of spinal surgery or tissue injury? Jacoby and colleagues reported their experience with five patients in whom spondylitic symptoms developed after trauma. Radiographic evaluation of these patients revealed disease already present at the time of the injury.[118] They suggest that trauma does not cause spondylitis but brings the patient to medical attention.

Infectious Agents

Infective agents have also been proposed as initiators of the inflammatory process that causes AS. *Klebsiella pneumoniae* has been singled out as the most likely pathogen.[79] Immunologic abnormalities specific to individuals with HLA-B27 have been described.[207] Certain bacteria *(Klebsiella, Shigella, Yersinia)* cause alterations in lymphocyte responses in patients who are B27 M_1 or M_2 positive.[198,215] However, findings demonstrating increased colonization of the gut and heightened lymphocyte sensitivity to *Klebsiella* in AS patients have not been borne out in other investigations.[65,222] Increased sensitivity of lymphocytes from B27-positive patients has also not been found with exposure to *K. pneumoniae* nitrogenase or *Yersinia* outer membrane proteins.[138]

The complete role of the HLA-B27 molecule in the pathogenesis of AS and related spondyloarthropathies remains to be determined. HLA-B27 has the potential to affect the pathogenesis of the illness in multiple ways. Infection with arthrogenic microorganisms produces proteins that bind to HLA-B27, and such binding triggers an immune response by CD8+ T cells. Bacterial products may also be disseminated to distant tissues such as synovium and thereby result in persistent inflammation. Alternatively, HLA-B27 receptor sites may recognize bacterial proteins and respond by induction of autoreactivity to host tissues that share identical epitopes. HLA-B27 may select a clone of T cells that specifically react with microbial antigens.[42,147]

Enthesitis

Enthesitis is the hallmark that distinguishes the spondyloarthropathies from other forms of arthritis. Investigators have proposed that all the alterations in the musculoskeletal system associated with AS are a direct result of enthesitis.[26] An enthesis is an insertion of a tendon, ligament, capsule, or fascia into bone.[78] Entheses come in two forms. Fibrous entheses are dense fibrous tissue linking tendon and ligament to bone. They are found at the metaphyses and diaphyses of long bones. Fibrocartilage entheses have fibrocartilage in a transition zone near the bony interface. The fibrocartilage anchors the tendon to bone.[96] An enthesis is a dynamic structure that undergoes constant modification in response to applied stress. This area is a target for inflammation. Although entheses are primarily affected in the spondyloarthropathies, inflammation of these structures is insufficient to explain the alterations that occur in joints (sacroiliac). Synovitis plays an important role. However, synovitis may be a secondary event after the initiation of enthesitis.[155]

AS is a disease of the synovial and cartilaginous joints of the axial skeleton, including the sacroiliac joints, spinal apophyseal joints, and symphysis pubis. The large appendicular joints—the hips, shoulders, knees, elbows, and ankles—are also affected in 30% of patients. The inflammatory process is characterized by chondritis (inflammation of cartilage) or osteitis (inflammation of bone) at the junction of cartilage and bone in the spine. An inflammatory granulation tissue forms and erodes the margins of the vertebral body. As opposed to rheumatoid arthritis, which is associated with osteoporosis as an early manifestation of disease, the inflammation of AS is characterized by ankylosis of the joints and ossification of the ligaments surrounding the vertebrae (syndesmophytes) and other musculotendinous structures such as the heels and pelvis. Magnetic resonance (MR) imaging is able to detect the extent of enthesitis in peripheral locations such as the Achilles tendon.[171]

The histopathology of AS differs from that of rheumatoid arthritis.[8] AS synovitis is characterized by overexpression of CD163 by activated macrophages. Lymphoid aggregates are less frequent in AS than in rheumatoid arthritis, and CD3+, CD4+, and CD20+ lymphocytes are also expressed at lower levels in AS. Vascularity is greater in AS. Both entities have a high concentration of TNF-alpha, including dense cellular infiltrates in the sacroiliac joints.[23] AS patients have a higher ratio of immunosuppressive cytokines, such as interleukin-4 (IL-4) and IL-10, to proinflammatory cytokines, such as TNF-alpha and interferon-gamma. This higher proportion of immunosuppressive cytokines leads to a blunted T helper type 1 (TH1) cell response in spondyloarthropathy patients. The tendency to form new bone is associated with an elevated level of transforming growth factor-beta in ligaments and entheses.

CLINICAL HISTORY

The classic AS patient is a man 15 to 40 years of age with intermittent dull low back pain and stiffness slowly progressing for months.[168] AS rarely occurs in individuals older than 50 years. Patients with spondyloarthropathy commencing after the age of 50 are more likely to have a non-AS spinal inflammatory disorder such as psoriatic spondylitis.[41] Back pain, which occurs throughout the disease in 90% to 95% of patients, is greatest in the morning and is increased by periods of inactivity. Patients may have difficulty sleeping because of pain and stiffness; they may awaken at night and find it necessary to leave bed and move about for a few minutes before returning to sleep.[225] Fatigue can be a major symptom and correlates with the level of disease activity, functional ability, global well-being, and mental health status.[220] The back pain improves with exercise. The mode of onset is variable, with pain developing in a majority of patients in the lumbosacral region. In a small number, the peripheral joints (hips, knees, and shoulders) are initially involved, but occasionally, acute iridocyclitis (eye inflammation) or heel pain may be the first manifestation of disease. Rarely, ankylosis of the spine may develop without any back pain.[113] Occasionally, individuals older than 50 years may have mild symptoms despite extensive spinal involvement.[149] Conversely, the back pain may be severe, with radiation to the lower extremities mimicking acute lumbar disc herniation. Patients have symptoms related to the piriformis syndrome.[173] The belly of the piriformis muscle crosses over the sciatic nerve. Inflammation in the sacroiliac joint, where the muscle attaches, results in muscle spasm and nerve compression. No abnormal, persistent neurologic signs are associated with the sciatic pain. The symptoms are reversible with medical therapy that relieves joint inflammation. This symptom complex of radicular pain is referred to as pseudosciatica.

The usual patient has a moderate degree of intermittent aching pain localized to the lumbosacral area. Paraspinal musculoskeletal spasm may also contribute to the discomfort. With progression of the disease, pain develops in the dorsal and cervical spine and rib joints.

Spinal involvement is manifested by flattening of the lumbar spine and loss of the normal lordosis. Thoracic spine disease causes decreased motion at the costovertebral joints, reduced chest expansion, and impaired pulmonary function. Thoracic disease may cause discal wedging that results in hyperkyphosis.[81] In 81% of patients the initial symptoms are back pain; back stiffness; thigh, hip, or groin pain; and sciatica. Pain in the peripheral joints is the initial complaint in 13%, pain in the chest in 2%, and generalized aches in 1%.[106]

Cervical spine disease in AS occurs less frequently than lumbosacral involvement and at a later time in the course of the illness. Studies of large groups of AS patients report cervical spine involvement to range from 0% to 53.9%.[106,107,144] Cervical involvement occurs about 5 to 8 years after onset of the illness in the lumbosacral spine.[164] Studies of different populations have demonstrated increased frequency of cervical spine disease in both women and men when the sexes are compared.[93,178] A number of reasons may explain the underestimation of AS in women.[90] Women do not have radiographs taken as often as men. They have a more benign course. Peripheral arthritis occurs more commonly in women, thus suggesting an alternative diagnosis (rheumatoid arthritis). The disease has a slower progression in women. Women have cervical spine disease characteristic of AS with little lumbar spine involvement.[38] The primary symptom of cervical spine disease is neck stiffness and pain, but intermittent episodes of torticollis may develop. Involvement of the cervical spine causes the head to protrude forward, thus making it difficult to look straight ahead.

Peripheral joint arthritis (hips, knees, ankles, shoulders, and elbows) occurs in 30% of patients within the first 10 years of disease.[43] Joint disease first appears as pain and stiffness. The inflammatory process may proceed to joint space narrowing and contractures. Fixed flexion contractures of the hips give rise to difficulty walking and cause a rigid gait. Hip disease is the most frequent factor limiting mobility rather than spinal stiffness. In fact, peripheral joint disease, particularly of the hips, when it appears in the first 10 years of disease, is associated with greater disease activity and more extensive restriction of spinal motion.[29]

Ankylosis may also occur in cartilaginous joints such as the symphysis pubic, sternomanubrial, and costosternal joints. Erosions of the plantar surface of the calcaneus at the attachment of the plantar fascia result in an enthesitis (inflammation of an enthesis—attachment of tendon to bone).[9] This inflammation causes fasciitis and a periosteal reaction that results in heel pain and the formation of heel spurs. Achilles tendinitis is another enthesitis associated with heel pain and AS.

Osteoporosis

AS causes significant changes in the spine over time. First, although the disease is associated with calcification of ligaments and joints, the vertebrae become osteoporotic. Osteoporosis is a process in which loss of bone calcium occurs. Osteoporotic bones are weaker and are at greater risk of fracture.[116] Dual-energy x-ray absorptiometric (DEXA) studies of AS have revealed variable levels of bone mineral density (BMD) that depend on the duration of disease. In mild early AS, men and women may have reduced BMD, with normal levels reported in disease of longer duration.[166] Osteoporosis in the early stage of the illness may be a result of proinflammatory cytokines.[97] Other studies using DEXA, single-photon absorptiometry, and quantitative computed tomography (CT) report lower BMD in more extensive disease.[143] Mineralization defects are a probable cause of the low bone mass. Osteoid volume and thickness are greater in AS patients than controls.[208] These findings indicate that the reduced bone mass in AS is mainly due to depression in bone formation rather than an increase in bone resorption.

Neurologic Complications

Atlantoaxial Subluxation

Neurologic complications of AS are secondary to nerve impingement or trauma to the spinal cord. In a study of 33 patients with AS and neurologic complications, cervical abnormalities were the most common cause of neurologic compromise.[77] Atlantoaxial subluxation occurs in the setting of AS but less often than in rheumatoid arthritis.[153,197,200] In a study of 103 AS patients, 21% had atlantoaxial subluxation. Vertical subluxation is a rare complication. About a third of patients have progression of the subluxation. Five of the 22 subluxation patients required surgical fusion.[176] In rare instances, symptoms of atlantoaxial subluxation may be the initial manifestation of AS.[102] Significant instability may occur without symptoms in rheumatoid arthritis because of generalized ligamentous laxity and erosion of bone. AS patients have symptoms and signs of nerve impingement more frequently in the setting of instability secondary to the immobilized state of the calcified structures surrounding the spine. Patients with peripheral joint disease are at greater risk of C1–C2 subluxation (6 of 17 AS patients in one study), thus implying a generalized synovitis affecting a wide range of joints, including those at the atlantoaxial junction.[205] Symptoms of subluxation with impingement of the upper nerve roots include severe neck pain radiating to the occipital and mastoid areas. Spinal cord compression is associated with myelopathic symptoms, including sensory deficits, spasticity, paresis, and incontinence.

Spinal Fracture

The other change is the loss of normal flexibility because of ankylosis of the spinal joints and ligaments. The spine in this ankylosed state is much more brittle and is prone to fracture, even with minimal trauma. The most common location for fracture is the cervical spine, although dorsal and lumbar spine fractures have also been described.[28,117] The occurrence of traumatic cervical spine injury is 3.5 times greater in AS patients than in the normal population.[56] The frequency of AS as the cause of spinal cord injury is 0.3% to 0.5%.[16,74,99,229] The lower cervical spine (C6–C7) is the most frequent location of fracture, and it is often associated with a fall. Spinal fractures can occur after trivial trauma and are easily overlooked (Fig 11-4).[72,212] Patients who sustain fractures may complain of nothing more than localized pain and decreased or increased spinal motion, but severe sensory and motor function loss corresponding to the location of the lesion may develop. The onset of neurologic dysfunction may be delayed for weeks after the initial trauma.[28] In AS patients, an unexpected increase in neck pain or neck motion or the appearance of neurologic symptoms with or without a history of recent trauma is an indication for radiographic evaluation of the axial spine because multiple fractures may occur.[172] The diagnosis of fracture may be delayed because of the difficulty of detecting fractures in osteoporotic bone with plain

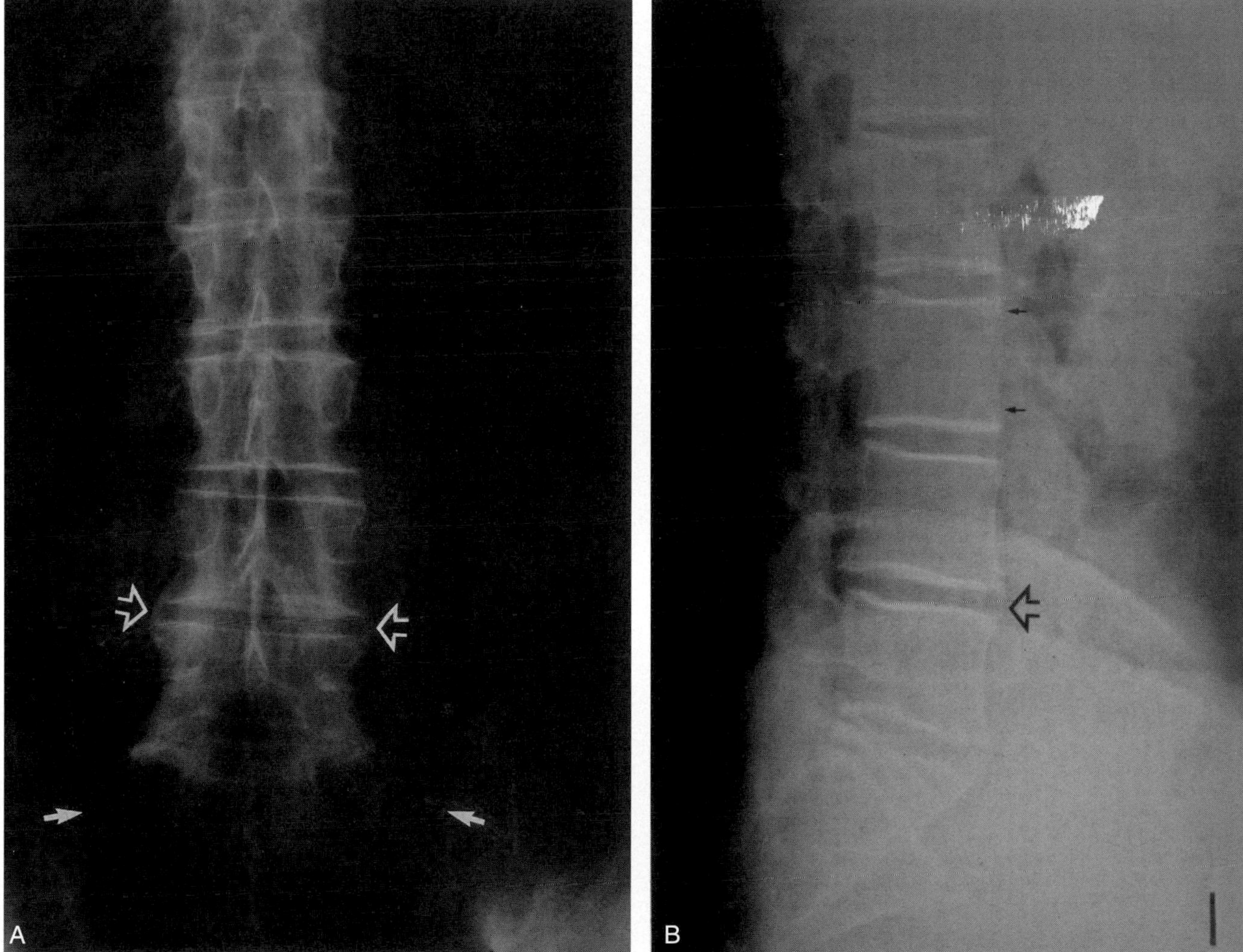

Figure 11-4 Ankylosing spondylitis (AS). *A*, Anteroposterior view of the pelvis and lumbar spine with fusion of the sacroiliac joints *(white arrows)* and syndesmophytes *(open white arrows)*. *B*, Lateral view with squaring of the vertebral bodies *(black arrows)* and syndesmophytes *(open black arrow)* in a 38-year-old man with AS associated with back and neck immobility. He had an accident in which he hit his head against a fence and suffered increasing neck pain. Ten days later, sudden paralysis developed in his arms and legs.

Continued

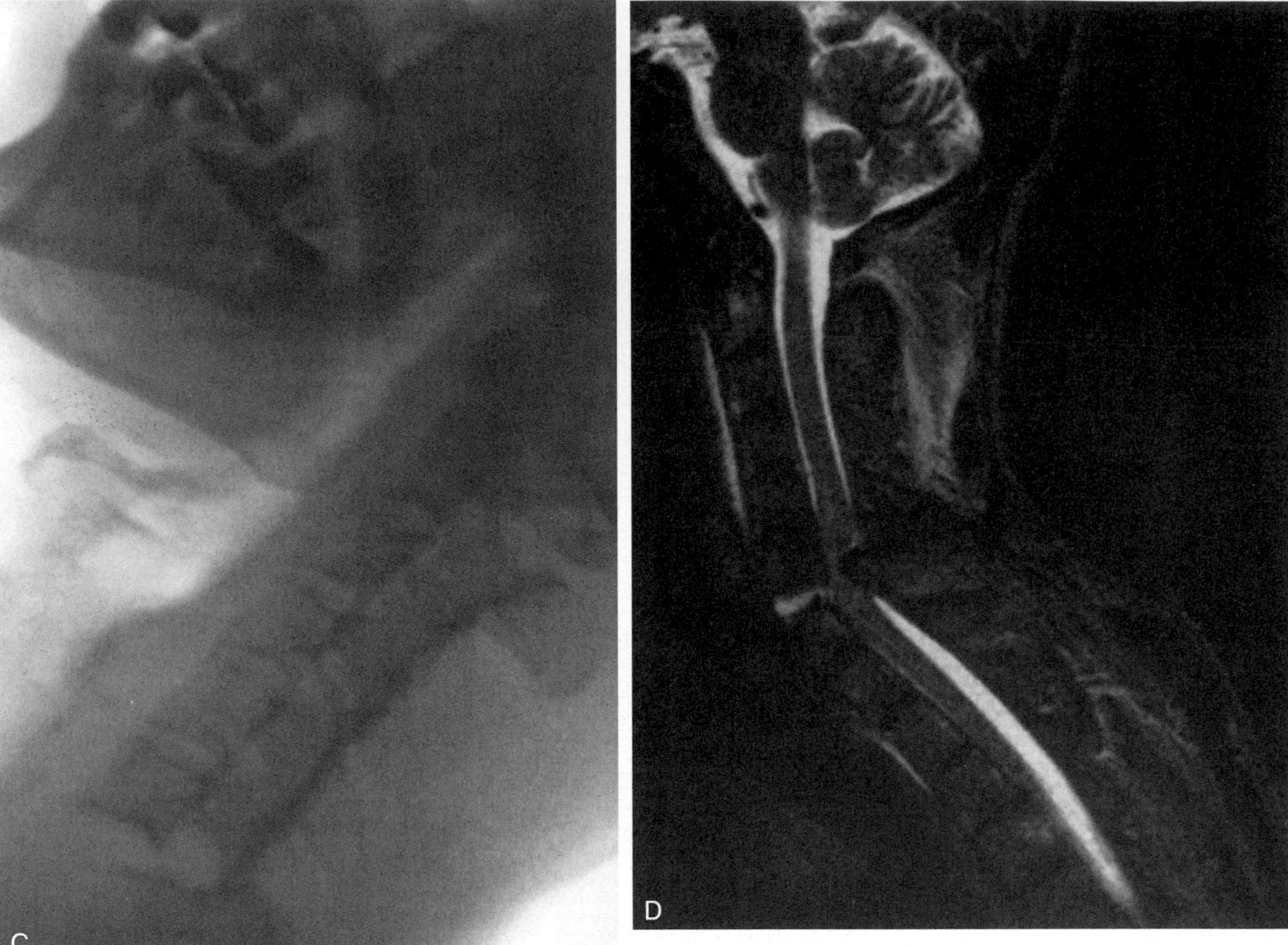

Figure 11-4, cont'd *C*, Fluoroscopic image of the cervical spine showing fracture and subluxation at C6–C7. *D*, MR image of the cervical fracture and spinal cord injury.

roentgenograms. MR evaluation of these patients may identify the location of the fracture.[117] Radiographic evaluation, including MR imaging, is helpful in detecting the rare disc herniation or epidural hematoma associated with a fracture. An MR image may be difficult to obtain in AS patients because the shape of their spine does not allow entry into the gantry to perform an optimal scan. Therapy usually consists of external fixation with a brace when neurologic symptoms are minimal, but surgical decompression and fusion are required for severe neurologic abnormalities such as paraplegia.[189] Fractures that mend with external bracing or with surgical fusion heal with normal bone formation. Neurologic deficits may persist despite surgical intervention in as many as 85.7% of patients.[73,189] A mortality rate of 35% to 50% may be found, particularly in AS patients who are elderly, who have complete cord lesions, or in whom pulmonary complications develop after fracture.[74,116,223,229]

Spondylodiscitis

Another complication of long-standing AS is spondylodiscitis, a destructive lesion of the disc and its surrounding vertebral bodies.[46,58,61,224] This lesion is associated with a new onset of localized pain in the spine, which uncharacteristically for an AS patient is improved with bed rest. The cause of these lesions may be localized inflammation or minor trauma. An MR study revealed increased activity in the central portion of the vertebral endplate, thus confirming this area as an enthesis.[151] Enthesitis may be a mechanism that facilitates spondylodiscitis. In one study, AS patients who performed heavy manual labor were at greater risk for this abnormality than those who had sedentary occupations.[58] In most cases, external immobilization was effective in controlling symptoms, and surgical fusion was reserved for the more severely affected patients.

Cauda Equina Syndrome

In the lumbar spine, spinal stenosis was present in one patient. In patients with long-standing AS in whom new leg pain or urinary or bowel incontinence develops, impingement of the nerves at the caudal end of the spinal cord, the cauda equina, may be developing.[108,192] As the impingement progresses, sensory loss in the perineum develops along with thigh and leg weakness. The advent of more sensitive radiographic techniques has allowed a better understanding of the pathogenesis of this complication of AS.[100,160,213] The inflammation affecting ligaments causes dorsal meningeal inflammation, with subsequent arachnoid adhesions (arachnoiditis) resulting in erosion of the lamina. The hydrostatic pressure of cerebrospinal fluid adds to the modification of bony architecture. Nerve root injury is related to arachnoiditis in association with adhesion formation and tethering of the nerve roots. MR imaging is able to detect the formation of diverticula and erosions of the laminae.[83] No effective therapy is available, although surgical intervention has been attempted in spondylitic patients in whom cauda equina syndrome develops secondary to degenerative processes (e.g., DISH).[188]

Extra-articular Manifestations

Ocular

AS is also associated with many nonarticular abnormalities. Constitutional manifestations of disease, such as fever, fatigue, and weight loss, are seen in a small number of patients with active disease, particularly those with peripheral joint manifestations. Iritis, or inflammation of the anterior uveal tract of the eye, may be the initial complaint of 25% of patients with AS and is present in up to 40% over the course of the disease. It is generally unilateral and recurrent and is most often independent of the severity of the joint disease. Iritis is normally treated with topical corticosteroids along with the occasional use of systemic corticosteroids. Mild visual loss may be associated with iritis, but blindness is rare. Iritis is associated with HLA-B27 positivity in 50% of individuals with the ocular disorder independent of the presence of AS.[70]

Cardiovascular

Cardiac involvement occurs in 10% of patients with a disease duration of 30 years or longer. The fibrosing lesion causes the aortic valve and proximal root to thicken. Aortic disease may be more common in patients with peripheral arthritis.[87] Mild features include tachycardia, conduction defects, and pericarditis. AS causes cardiac conduction disturbances in men, particularly bradyarrhythmias.[12] In a study of patients with pacemakers, 8.5% of 223 men had evidence of sacroiliitis and spondylitis.[13] Isolated aortic insufficiency and heart blocks occur in the setting of HLA-B27 positivity with or without arthritis. Echocardiography may detect cardiac abnormalities in some patients without clinical signs.[185] The most serious cardiac abnormality is proximal aortitis, which results in aortic valve insufficiency, heart failure, and death.[34] Prosthetic valve replacement may forestall cardiac deterioration.

Pulmonary

Pulmonary involvement is manifested as decreased chest expansion, which limits lung capacity, particularly in severely kyphotic individuals. In a review of 26 patients with an average duration of AS of 18.5 years, 70% had either interstitial lung disease, bronchiectasis, emphysema, mycetoma, or apical fibrosis.[45] High-resolution CT was needed to detect these abnormalities because they were not visible on plain roentgenograms. Plain roentgenograms were abnormal in only four and did not reveal interstitial fibrosis. The fibrotic process affects the apical segments of the lung as a late and rare complication.[6,187]

Renal

Renal abnormalities do occur in AS patients. Microscopic hematuria and albuminuria may appear in 35% of patients.[221] Deposition of amyloid, a protein-like material found in a number of visceral organs and diagnosed by abdominal fat pad or rectal biopsy, is a rare complication of AS.[53] Secondary amyloidosis occurs in 7% of AS patients and is associated with nephropathy manifested as proteinuria.[98]

Another form of proteinuria associated with AS patients is IgA nephropathy. AS patients have increased IgA levels. IgA levels correlate with elevation in the erythrocyte sedimentation rate (ESR) and C-reactive protein (CRP). One hypothesis explaining the increased levels of IgA implicated the presence of bacterial peptides in AS patients, causing mucosal stimulation of antibody production. However, IgA formation has been documented in bone marrow and joints, thus suggesting systemic production of the antibody.[174,182] This finding suggests that the IgA abnormality in AS patients is faulty catabolism of the antibody. Failure of removal of IgA results in deposition in the kidney. Investigators have proposed that increased IgA might be a "protective" mechanism to prevent joint inflammation.[165] IgA nephropathy results in proteinuria and renal impairment.[139] The incidence of renal failure is low.

PHYSICAL EXAMINATION

A careful musculoskeletal examination, particularly of the lumbosacral spine, is necessary to detect the early findings of limitation of motion of the axial skeleton, which is especially noticeable with lateral bending or hyperextension. Percussion over the sacroiliac joints elicits pain in most circumstances. Other tests that may be helpful in identifying sacroiliac joint dysfunction place stress on the joint. Tests to be considered include the Faber maneuver, the Gaenslen test (pressure on a hyperextended thigh with the contralateral hip flexed), the Yoeman test (hyperextension of the thigh in a prone patient), and distraction of the pelvic wings anteriorly and posteriorly.

Measurements of spinal motion, including the Schober test (lumbar spine motion), lateral bending of the lumbosacral spine with the occiput to the wall (cervical spine motion), and chest expansion, are important in ascertaining the limitations of motion and monitoring progression of the disease (Fig. 11-5). The paraspinous muscles may be tender to palpation and in spasm, thereby resulting in limitation of back motion. Finger-to-floor measurements should be obtained but are performed more to determine flexibility, which is more closely associated with hip motion than with back mobility. Rotation may be checked with the patient seated. Seating fixes the pelvis

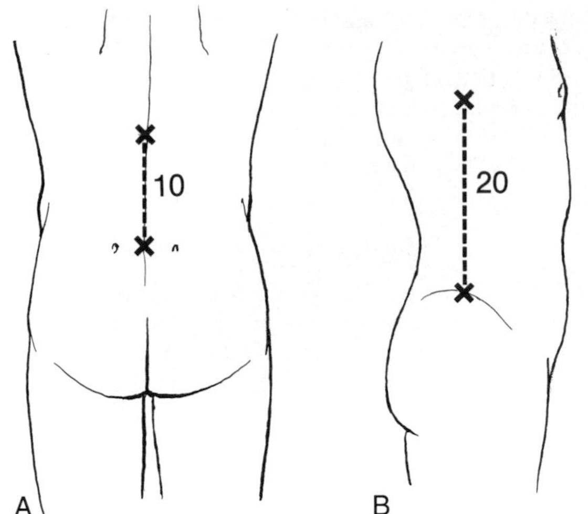

Figure 11-5 Measurement of anterior spinal flexion *(A)* and right and left lateral flexion *(B)*.

and thus limits pelvic rotation. Chest expansion is measured at the fourth intercostal space in men and below the breasts in women. Patients raise their hands over their head and are asked to take a deep inspiration. Normal expansion is 2.5 cm or greater. Cervical spine evaluation includes measurement of all planes of motion. Peripheral joint examination is also indicated. Careful hip examination is necessary to determine the potential loss of function associated with simultaneous arthritis of the back and hip.[106] Examination of the eyes, heart, lungs, and nervous system may uncover unsuspected extra-articular disease.

LABORATORY DATA

Laboratory results are nonspecific and add little to the diagnosis of AS. Only 15% of patients have mild anemia. The ESR is increased in 80% of patients with active disease.[123] Patients with normal sedimentation rates and active arthritis may have elevated levels of CRP.[167,203] Rheumatoid factor and antinuclear antibody are characteristically absent.

Histocompatibility testing (for HLA) is positive in 90% of AS patients but is also positive in an increased percentage of patients with other spondyloarthropathies (reactive arthritis, psoriatic spondylitis, and spondylitis with inflammatory bowel disease). It is not a diagnostic test for AS. HLA testing may be useful in a young patient with early disease for whom the differential diagnosis may be narrowed by the presence of HLA-B27.[131] The presence of HLA-B27 homozygosity was evaluated in 100 patients with AS.[206] Homozygosity was associated with more severe disease but did not impart a greater risk for spondylitis in the families of patients with AS. HLA-B27–negative patients are older at disease onset, have a negative family history, and have less extra-articular disease (iritis or cardiac conduction abnormalities).[141]

RADIOGRAPHIC EVALUATION

Roentgenograms

Characteristic changes of AS in the sacroiliac joints and lumbosacral spine are helpful in making a diagnosis but may be difficult to determine in the early stages of the disease.[154] The disease affects synovial and cartilaginous joints, as well as sites of tendon and ligament attachment to bone (enthesis). Areas of the skeleton most frequently affected include the sacroiliac, apophyseal, discovertebral, and costovertebral joints.

The disease affects the sacroiliac joints initially and then appears in the upper lumbar and thoracolumbar areas.[135,186] Subsequently, in ascending order, the lower lumbar, thoracic, and cervical spine is involved. The radiographic progression of disease may be halted at any stage, although sacroiliitis alone is a rare finding except in some women with spondylitis or men in the early stage of disease (Fig. 11-6).[178,225] The combination of roentgenographic findings of sacroiliitis and cervical spondylitis without lumbar or thoracic involvement occurs more commonly in women than men.[178] In the peripheral skeleton, the hip and shoulder (glenohumeral) joints are most commonly affected, followed by the knees, hands, wrists, and feet, including the heels.[63,82,177]

Evaluation of the sacroiliac joints is difficult on a conventional anteroposterior supine view of the pelvis because of bony overlap and the oblique orientation of the joint. A Ferguson projection of the pelvis (x-ray tube tilted 15 to 30 degrees in a cephalad direction) provides a useful view of the anterior portion of the joint, the initial area of inflammation in sacroiliitis. Radiographic evaluation of the sacroiliac joints is based on five observations: (1) distribution, (2) subchondral mineralization, (3) cystic or erosive bony change, (4) joint width, and (5) osteophyte formation.[51] Comparison of the symmetry of involvement must include the same areas of the joint (superior—fibrous, inferior—synovial) and the iliac (thinner cartilage) and sacral (thicker cartilage) sides of the joint.

Sacroiliitis in AS is a bilateral, symmetrical process. Early sacroiliitis appears in the inferior portion of the joint on the iliac side of the articulation. Patchy periarticular osteopenia appears along with areas of subchondral bony sclerosis. During the next stage, the articular space becomes "pseudowidened" secondary to joint surface erosions. With continued inflammation, the area of sclerosis expands and is joined by proliferative bony changes that cross the joint space. In the final stages of sacroiliitis, complete ankylosis with total obliteration of the joint space occurs. Ligamentous structures surrounding the sacroiliac joint may also calcify. The radiographic changes associated with sacroiliitis may be graded from 0 (normal) to 5 (complete ankylosis) (Table 11-1).[55]

It is important to realize that the inflammatory process associated with sacroiliitis does not always result in ankylosis. The inflammatory process may diminish and the joint may undergo healing along with some resolution of the alterations associated with early disease (Fig. 11-7).[6]

Abnormalities also occur in the lumbar, thoracic, and cervical spine. Classic AS causes vertebral column disease

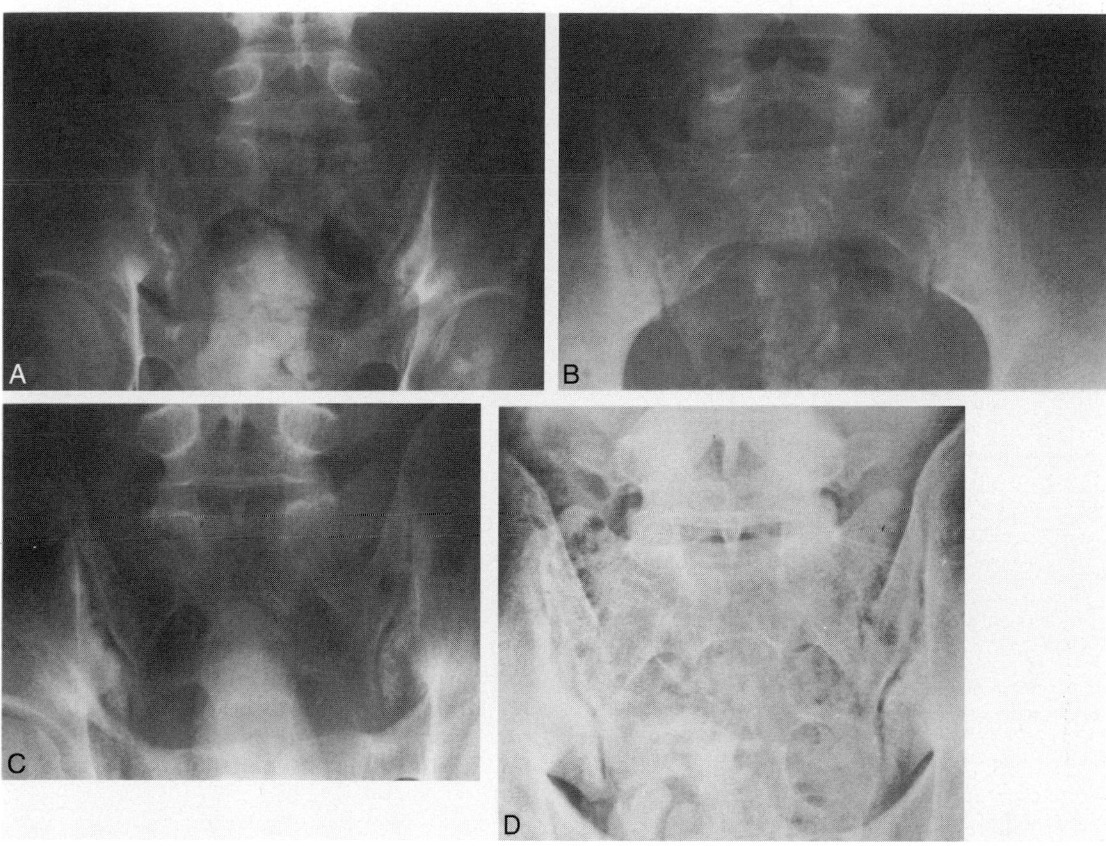

Figure 11-6 Serial views of the pelvis of a 30-year-old man with ankylosing spondylitis. *A*, 3/80—Sclerosis is noted primarily on the iliac sides of both sacroiliac joints with cystic erosions of the joint space. *B*, 10/83—Bilateral involvement with greater sclerosis in the right sacroiliac joint. *C*, 10/86—The degree of joint involvement has diminished, with less sclerosis and greater definition of the joint margins. *D*, 10/88—The joint space remains intact with continuing resolution of the erosions.

in association with sacroiliac disease. The occurrence of spondylitis without sacroiliitis in AS is an extremely rare finding.[47] This pattern of involvement is much more common in reactive arthritis or psoriatic spondylitis.

In the lumbar spine, osteitis affecting the anterior corners of vertebral bodies is an early finding. The inflammation associated with osteitis results in loss of the normal concavity of the anterior vertebral surface, and such loss gives rise to a "squared" body (Fig. 11-8). As the inflammation heals, reactive sclerosis, or "whitening," appears in the anterior portion of the vertebral bodies. A simple method to assess vertebral squaring involves drawing a vertical line joining the upper and lower margins of each lumbar vertebral body at the junction of the vertebral endplate and the anterior surface of the vertebral body. The distance between this line and the anterior aspect of the vertebral body at its most concave point is then measured. This distance is the concavity measurement. The reference range for vertebral concavity is 1.1 to 4 mm based on measurements from 255 lumbar vertebrae. Squaring is associated with changes of 1 mm or less. This method may be helpful in monitoring the course of the illness over time.[175]

11-1 RADIOGRAPHIC GRADING OF SACROILIITIS

Grade	Criteria
0	Normal—normal width, sharp joint margins
1	Suspicious changes—radiologist is uncertain whether grade 2 changes are present
2	Definite early changes—pseudowidening with erosion or sclerosis on both sides of the joint
3	Unequivocal abnormality—erosions; sclerosis; widening, narrowing, or partial ankylosis
4	Severe abnormalities—narrowed joint space, ankylosis
5	Ankylosis of body joints with regression of surrounding sclerosis

Adapted from Dale K: Radiographic grading of sacroiliitis in Bechterew's syndrome and allied disorders. Scand J Rheumatol Suppl 32:92, 1979.

While osteopenia of the bony structures appears, calcification of the disc and ligamentous structures emerges. Thin, vertically oriented calcifications of the annulus fibrosus and anterior and posterior longitudinal ligaments are termed *syndesmophytes*. *Bamboo spine* is the term used to describe the spine of a patient with AS and extensive syndesmophytes encasing the axial skeleton (Fig. 11-9).[54] Osteoporosis has been documented in AS patients by quantitative CT.[57]

The discovertebral junction may be affected centrally, peripherally, or in combination.[46] Central erosions cause irregularity of the superior and inferior vertebral margins with surrounding sclerosis. Peripheral lesions cause erosions in the noncartilaginous portion of the junction. Radiographic findings include anterior or posterior bony erosion. Combined lesions affecting the central and peripheral portion of the discovertebral junction may

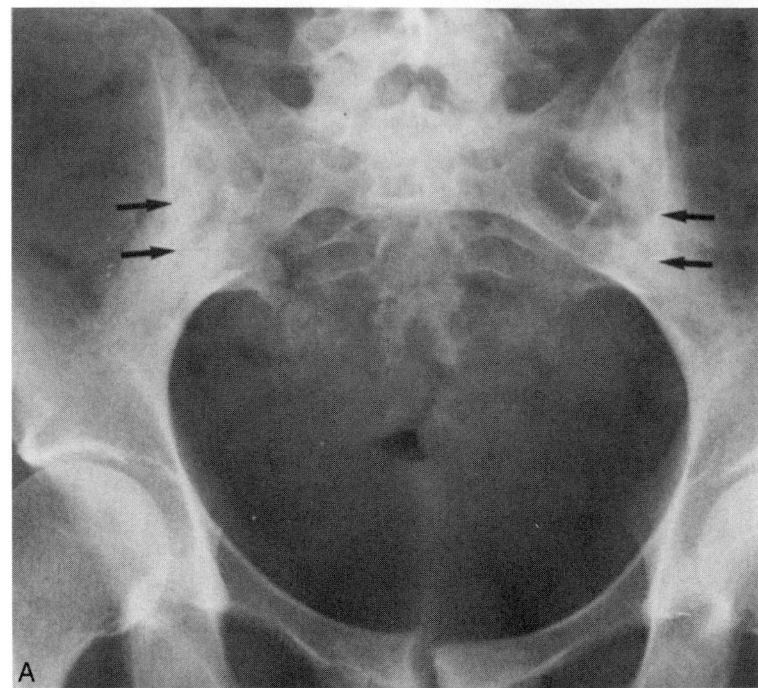

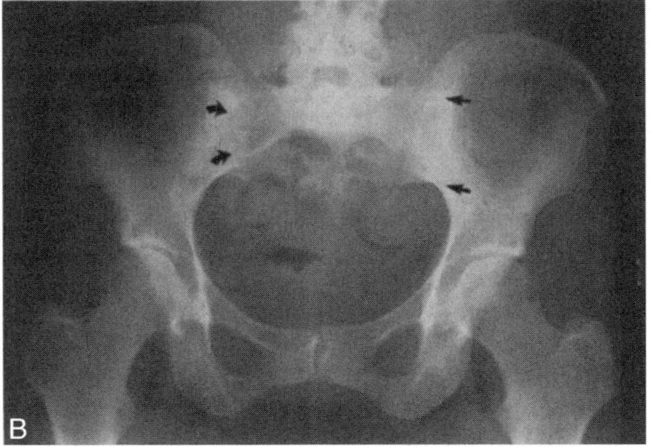

Figure 11-7 Ankylosing spondylitis, anteroposterior view of the pelvis. *A,* A 44-year-old woman with persistent back pain since the age of 14 and recurrent iritis. Bilateral sacroiliitis is noted along with fusion of those joints *(arrows)*. *B,* 10/91—Seven years later, the left sacroiliac joint is obliterated *(black straight arrows)*. The right sacroiliac is barely visible *(curved black arrows)*.

cause ballooning of the disc space ("fish vertebrae") or narrowing of the disc space (spinal pseudarthrosis).[152,202] This latter finding occurs most commonly in patients with AS of long duration who sustain trauma to the spine. In the cervical spine, discovertebral erosion may occur without apophyseal joint disease and before the appearance of syndesmophytes.[180] Intervertebral disc narrowing and bony sclerosis in vertebral bodies may be accompanying findings.

The apophyseal joints are also affected in the illness. As the disease progresses, fusion of the apophyseal joints occurs. Radiographs of the spine may demonstrate loss of the joint space and complete fusion of the joints. Cervical spine ankylosis may be particularly severe. Complete obliteration of the articular spaces between the posterior elements of C2 through C7 results in a column of solid bone (Fig. 11-10).[180] In patients with complete ankylosis of the apophyseal joints and syndesmophytes, extensive bony resorption of the anterior surface of the lower cervical vertebrae may develop late in the course of the illness. Bone under the ligaments connecting the spinous processes may also be eroded in the setting of apophyseal joint ankylosis.

The C1–C2 joints may become eroded and subluxed. Synovial tissue around the dens may cause erosion of the odontoid process.[153] Further damage to the surrounding ligaments results in instability that is measured by movement of the odontoid process from the posterior aspect of the atlas with flexion and extension views of the cervical spine. Widening of the space is indicative of dynamic subluxation. No change in the distance between the atlas and axis suggests a fixed subluxation. In addition to atlantoaxial subluxation, migration of the odontoid into the foramen magnum and rotary subluxation may occur.[10,145,146] Subaxial subluxation is more characteristic of rheumatoid arthritis than AS.

Scintigraphy

The use of other radiographic techniques in the diagnosis of AS is of marginal additional benefit. They have been

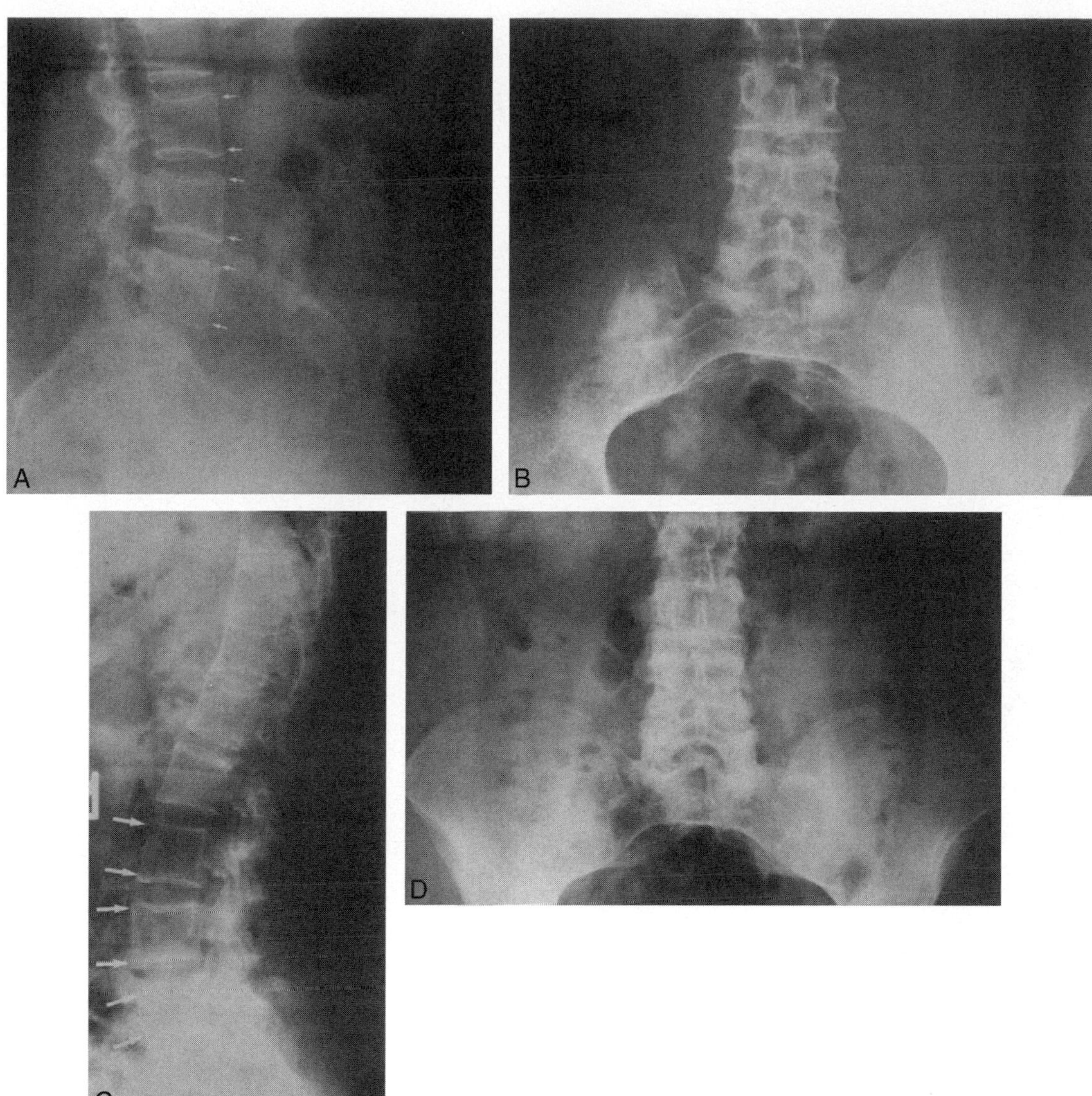

Figure 11-8 Ankylosing spondylitis. *A*, Lateral view of lumbar spine. Squaring of the L3, L4, and L5 vertebral bodies with loss of the concave contour is apparent *(arrows)*. *B*, An anteroposterior (AP) view of the pelvis reveals fusion of both sacroiliac joints. The extent of disease in the sacroiliac joints does not predict the degree of involvement in other areas of the axial skeleton. *C*, 10/90—Five years later, squaring of vertebral bodies has stabilized *(arrows)*. Syndesmophytes have not developed. *D*, An AP view of the pelvis reveals obliteration of the sacroiliac joints.

used primarily for the evaluation of sacroiliitis. Scintigraphic evaluation by bone scan may demonstrate increased activity over the sacroiliac joints in early disease before any detectable radiographic changes in the spinal joints.[191] However, quantitative scintigraphy is insufficiently discriminatory to be of consistent help clinically in differentiating spondylitis patients from normal individuals and from patients with other causes of back pain.[69] Scintigraphy also may not be adequately sensitive to monitor the course of the illness over time.[211]

Computed Tomography

CT of the sacroiliac joint has been reported to be more sensitive and equally specific in the recognition of sacroiliitis when compared with conventional roentgenography.[44] However, CT should not be used for routine evaluation of the sacroiliac joints. The test should be reserved for patients with normal or equivocal roentgenographs in whom a diagnosis of spondyloarthropathy is suspected.[136] CT scan detects erosions on both sides of the joint that are frequently missed by plain roentgenograms.[75]

Magnetic Resonance

A number of MR studies have been reported in which alterations in the sacroiliac joints are demonstrated that are not noted on plain roentgenograms.[1] MR scan was better able to identify erosions, abnormalities of articular cartilage, and subchondral bone marrow. MR is able to localize early spondylitis in discal structures and vertebral edges.[25] MR scanning with fat saturation or contrast-enhanced

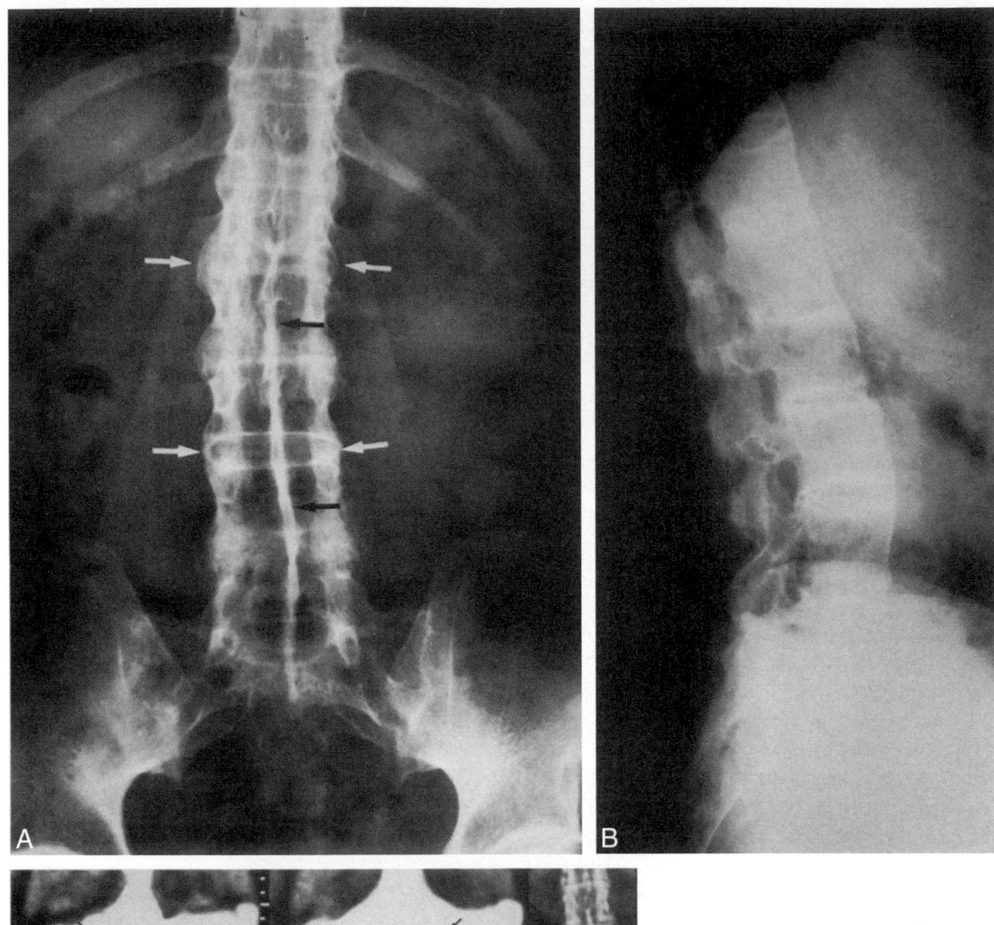

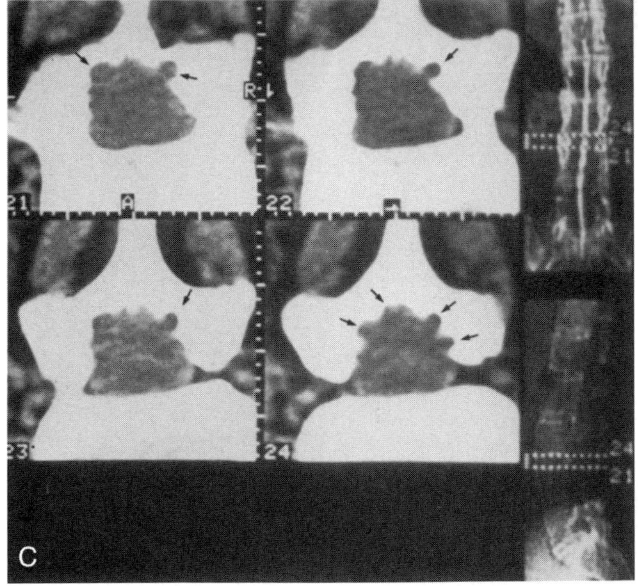

Figure 11-9 Ankylosing spondylitis. *A*, Bamboo spine with syndesmophytes involving the entire spine *(arrows)*. The interspinous ligaments have calcified *(black arrows)*, and the sacroiliac joints are fused. *B*, A lateral view reveals thin, vertically oriented syndesmophytes and preservation of the intervertebral disc spaces. *C*, CT scan of the L3 vertebra of a 53-year-old man in whom cauda equina symptoms developed. The view reveals scalloping of the laminae of the vertebra. These erosions are secondary to dural ectasia or dural diverticula *(arrows)*. At 60 years of age, bilateral leg weakness, increasing incontinence, and sensory deficits have developed, as well as severe Parkinson's disease. He must use a motorized scooter for ambulation.

images is able to detect early inflammatory lesions in the sacroiliac joints and lumbar spine.[17] The ability of MR to detect early lesions may have implications for monitoring therapy that may slow the progression of disease. MR scan detects abnormalities of the spinal cord in patients with severe disease (Fig. 11-11), including those with pseudarthroses (Fig. 11-12).[59] MR is a good choice for young women with suspected sacroiliitis as a means of decreasing x-ray exposure.[22]

Scintigraphic, CT, or MR evaluation of the cervical spine would be useful in the setting of spinal fracture or subluxation to determine the location of fracture and the status of the spinal cord (see Fig. 11-12). From a diagnostic and clinical perspective, plain roentgenograms provide adequate information at a reasonable cost. Plain roentgenograms remain the usual radiographic technique for the diagnosis of AS.

DIFFERENTIAL DIAGNOSIS

Two sets of diagnostic criteria exist for AS. The Rome clinical criteria, used in studies of AS, include bilateral sacroiliitis on radiologic examination and low back pain for

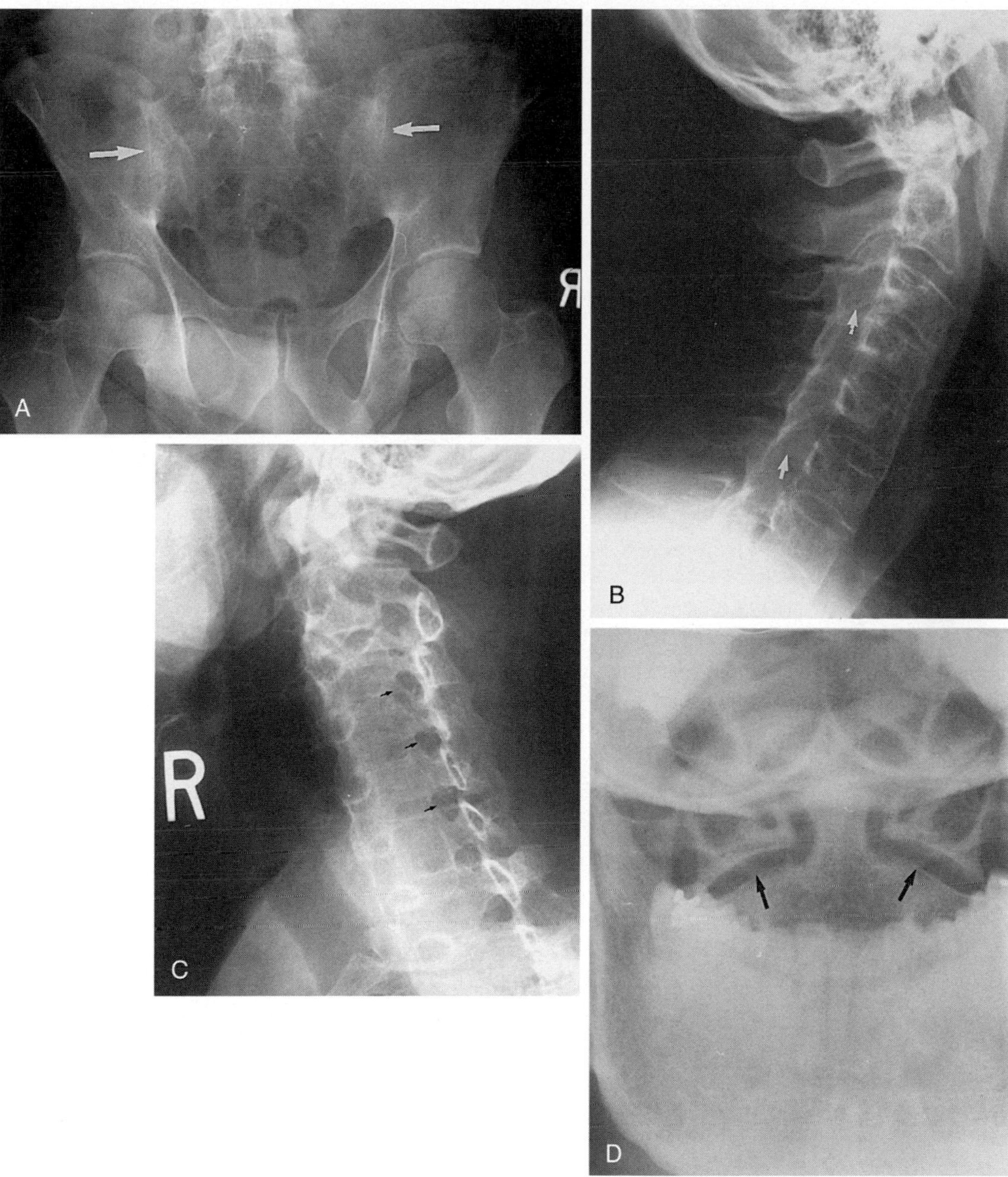

Figure 11-10 Ankylosing spondylitis in a 42-year-old man with a 20-year history of the disease. *A*, An anteroposterior view of the pelvis reveals bilateral sacroiliitis with fusion of these joints *(arrows)*. *B*, Lateral view of the cervical spine. Anterior and posterior syndesmophytes are present from C3 to C7, in addition to apophyseal joint fusion from C3 to C7 *(arrows)*. *C*, Oblique view of the cervical spine. Maintenance of the space for the neural foramina is noted *(arrows)*. *D*, Open-mouth view of the C1–C2 articulation. Despite severe disease in other portions of the cervical spine, the atlantoaxial articulations are intact *(arrows)*.

more than 3 months that is not relieved by rest, pain in the thoracic spine, limited motion in the lumbar spine, and limited chest expansion or iritis.[122] When these criteria proved to lack sensitivity in identifying patients with spondylitis, the Rome criteria were modified at a New York symposium in 1966 (Table 11-2). These criteria included a grading system for radiographs of the sacroiliac joints, in addition to limited spine motion, limited chest expansion, and back pain.[11] Although these criteria are used mostly for studies of patient populations, they are helpful in the office setting. The criteria are not ideal for population surveys because radiographic sacroiliitis may not be present to the extent to satisfy the criteria, thereby missing early disease.[162] Some of the measures of decreased mobility and chest expansion are imprecise. In the office setting, a physician makes the diagnosis of AS when the patient is a young male with bilateral sacroiliac pain, lumbar spine stiffness improves with activity, recurring radicular pain alternates side to side, the patient has a history of iritis and radiologic changes of spondylitis, and the HLA-B27 status is determined. However, in the early stages of the disease, clinical symptoms may be mild or

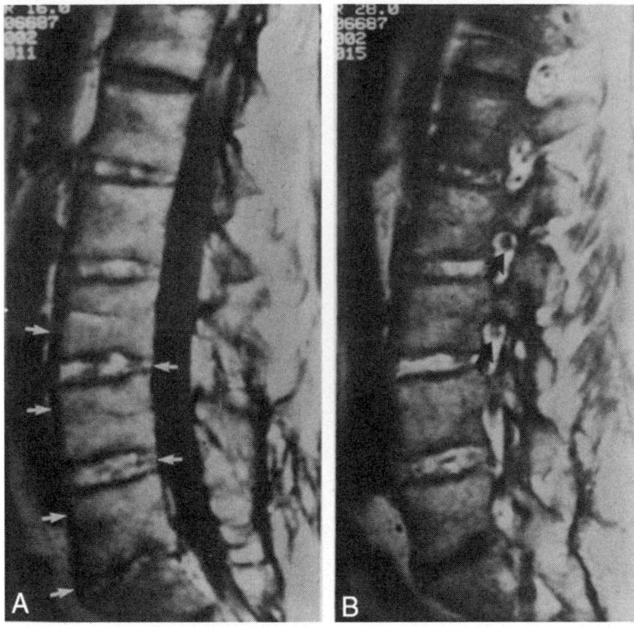

Figure 11-11 Ankylosing spondylitis in a 67-year-old man with a 20-year history of the disease. He has no range of motion in his axial skeleton and has a right hip replacement. *A*, T1-weighted, midline sagittal MR image with increased signal as a result of calcification in well-maintained intervertebral discs. Syndesmophytes are present anteriorly and posteriorly *(white arrows)*. *B*, T1-weighted parasagittal MR image with intact neural foramina (nerve root = *black arrow*).

atypical and radiologic changes nonexistent, thereby preventing early diagnosis. It has been suggested that individual characteristics of the illness be weighted to allow better codification of the diagnosis.[161] Others have also pointed out that the diagnostic criteria are too restrictive for certain patients with early disease or undifferentiated spondyloarthropathy. The European Spondyloarthropathy Study Group has developed a preliminary classification system for spondyloarthropathy in general (Table 11-3).[132]

Although spondyloarthropathies are a common inflammatory musculoskeletal disorder, this group of illnesses is frequently overlooked by nonrheumatologists.[134] The delay in diagnosis from the onset of symptoms to referral to a rheumatologist ranged from 6 to 264 months. Individuals whose condition is misdiagnosed by primary care physicians have mild to moderate disease, with atypical manifestations, and are women.[19]

The differential diagnosis of spinal pain in a young patient includes other spondyloarthropathies, herniated intervertebral disc, rheumatoid arthritis, osteoarthritis, fibromyalgia, infection, and tumors. Characteristics of these specific diseases are listed in Table 11-4. The course of AS may be complicated by other common arthritic diseases. AS and rheumatoid arthritis have developed in the same patient. The hosts (AS in men, rheumatoid arthritis in women) and disease patterns are different, thus suggesting that the diseases are unassociated.[48] Reactive arthritis

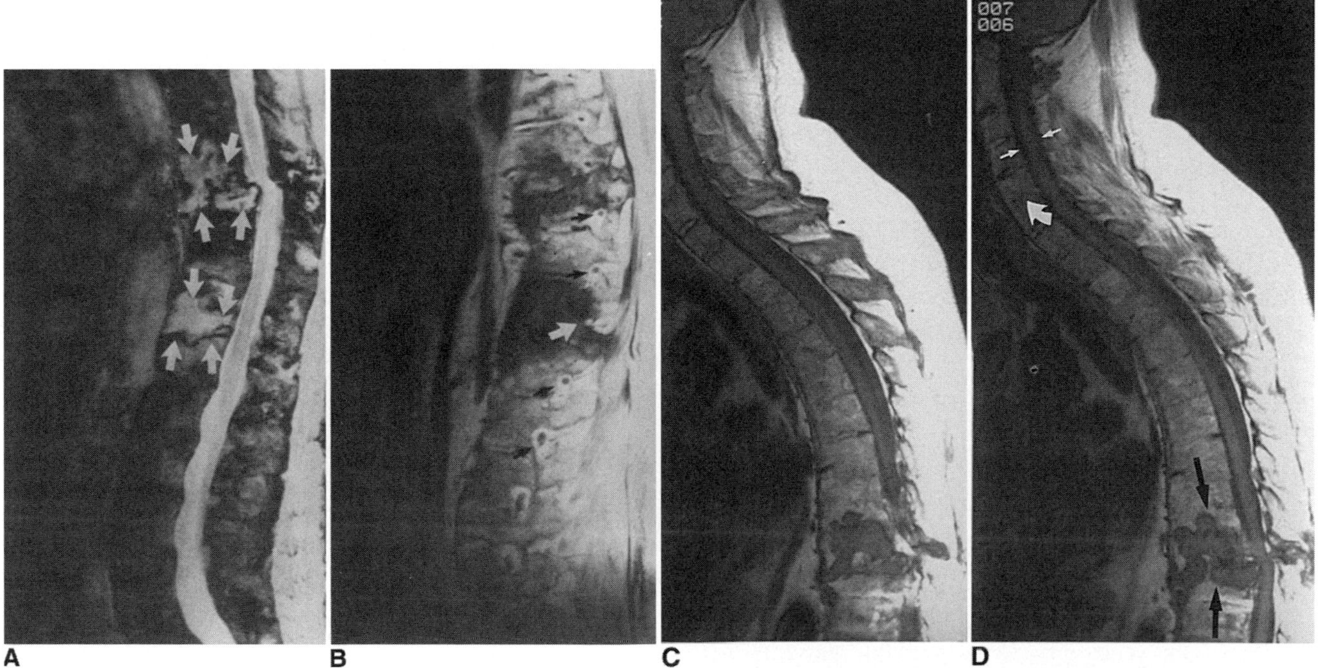

Figure 11-12 Ankylosing spondylitis (AS) in a 62-year-old man with a 30-year history of severe AS. He had a history of thoracic spine pain associated with a pseudarthrosis at the T8 level. The patient had a falling accident with an onset of radicular pain in an L1 distribution. *A*, T2-weighted sagittal MR image demonstrating two levels with pseudarthrosis *(white arrows)*. *B*, T1-weighted image demonstrating intact neural foramina *(black arrows)*. The L1 foramen is obliterated with inflammatory tissue associated with the pseudarthrosis *(white arrow)*. Paraplegia developed and the patient died of a respiratory infection. C and D, In the same patient with AS, a T1-weighted sagittal MR image of the cervical spine reveals pseudarthrosis in the thoracic spine with compression of the thoracic spinal cord *(black arrows)*. The cervical spine is ankylosed, with calcification of the anterior and posterior longitudinal ligaments and fusion of intervertebral disc spaces *(curved white arrow)*. The spinal canal has adequate room for the cervical spinal cord with cerebrospinal fluid anterior and posterior to the cord *(small white arrows)*.

11-2 CLINICAL CRITERIA FOR ANKYLOSING SPONDYLITIS

ROME CRITERIA[122]

A. Clinical Criteria

1. Low back pain and stiffness more than 3 months not relieved by rest
2. Pain and stiffness in the thoracic region
3. Limited motion in the lumbar spine
4. Limited chest expansion
5. History of evidence of iritis or its sequelae

B. Radiologic Criterion

1. Radiograph showing bilateral sacroiliac changes characteristic of ankylosing spondylitis

Diagnosis: Criterion B + 1 clinical criterion
or
4 clinical criteria in the absence of radiologic sacroiliitis

NEW YORK CRITERIA[11]

A. Clinical Criteria

1. Limitation of motion of the lumbar spine in anterior flexion, lateral flexion, and extension
2. History of or presence of pain at the dorsolumbar junction or in the lumbar spine
3. Limitation of chest expansion to 1 inch or less

B. Radiologic Criteria (Sacroiliitis)

Grade 3—unequivocal abnormality, moderate or advanced sacroiliitis with one or more erosions, sclerosis, widening, narrowing, or partial ankylosis
Grade 4—severe abnormality, total ankylosis

Diagnosis: Definite—Grade 3-4 bilateral sacroiliitis + 1 clinical criterion
or
Grade 3-4 unilateral or grade 2 bilateral sacroiliitis with clinical criterion 1 or 2 and 3
Probable—Grade 3-4 bilateral sacroiliitis alone

secondary to *Yersinia enterocolitica* has been reported to cause atlantoaxial arthritis in a patient with AS.[94]

Diffuse Idiopathic Skeletal Hyperostosis

Another disease that may occur in the setting of spondylitis is DISH. Patients with AS and DISH should be easily differentiated by careful radiographic evaluation.[228] DISH may cause alterations in the sacroiliac joints.[62] CT scan of the sacroiliac joints differentiates hyperostotic joint changes from those associated with joint erosion and fusion. Also of note is the occurrence of fracture in patients with DISH, as well as those with AS.[4] Convergence of two common diseases in the same host, a middle-aged man, is likely. The occurrence of simultaneous AS and DISH of the cervical spine has been reported (Fig. 11-13).[227]

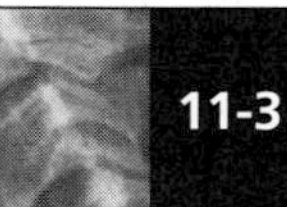

11-3 EUROPEAN SPONDYLOARTHROPATHY STUDY GROUP CRITERIA FOR SPONDYLOARTHROPATHY

Inflammatory spinal pain or synovitis
  Asymmetric
  Predominantly in the lower extremities
And 1 of the following:
  Positive family history
  Psoriasis
  Inflammatory bowel disease*
  Alternate buttock pain†
  Enthesopathy
Adding
  Sacroiliitis‡

*Sensitivity, 77%.
†Specificity, 89%.
‡Sensitivity, 86%; specificity, 87%.

TREATMENT

The goals of therapy, as with other forms of inflammatory arthritis, are to control pain and stiffness, reduce inflammation, maintain function, and prevent deformity with avoidance of undue toxicity. The International Assessment in AS (ASAS) group has established a core set of domains to monitor the course of the spondyloarthropathies (Table 11-5).[156a] This outcome measurement tool will allow for the identification of responders and nonresponders to new therapies, including biologic agents.

Education and Exercise

Patients require a comprehensive program of education, physiotherapy, medications, and other measures. Patients are educated about their disease. They are told what they can reasonably expect from treatment and are encouraged to continue with as normal a lifestyle as possible. Unsupervised recreational exercise for 30 minutes per day along with back exercises 5 days a week has a beneficial effect on pain and function.[214] Patients are taught proper posture and mobilizing and breathing exercises to prevent the tendency to stoop forward and lose chest motion. The importance of a firm upright chair for sitting and a hard mattress with no pillows for sleeping is stressed. Physical therapy with range-of-motion exercises may improve neck movement.[170] The physician gives encouragement and support to patients to adapt their lives to their disease. The use of braces, splints, and corsets should be avoided. Occasionally, patients may find neck braces helpful while driving, but their use must be limited to time in the car. Individuals with limited neck motion benefit from wide rear-view mirrors to make driving safer. Transcutaneous nerve stimulators, in addition to nonnarcotic analgesics, are useful in reducing pain in patients with a partial response to nonsteroidal drugs. Physiotherapy and patient education can result in an improved range of motion and function that lasts for months.[219]

When the physician cannot give patients adequate time to quell their concern, additional support should be arranged for patients in the form of a social worker, psychiatrist, or vocational counselor. The genetic implications of the disease are placed in perspective. Offspring have a 10% risk of AS if a parent is HLA-B27 positive. In addition, the importance of self-help groups, such as the Spondylitis Association of America in Sherman Oaks, California, cannot be underestimated. These organizations offer medical literature, exercises, and other resources that are useful to AS patients. An updated Web site offers the most current information about the spondyloarthopathies.[167a] These interventions improve function and decrease health care costs.[130]

11-4 DIFFERENTIAL DIAGNOSIS OF ANKYLOSING SPONDYLITIS

	Ankylosing Spondylitis	Psoriatic Arthritis	Enteropathic Arthritis	Reactive Arthritis	Herniated Nucleus Pulposus	Osteitis Condensans Ilii	Osteoarthritis of the Spine	Rheumatoid Arthritis	Fibromyalgia	Infection	Tumors
Sex	Male	=	=	=	=	Female	=	Female	Female	=	=
Age at onset	15-40	30-40	15-45	Any age	20-40	30-40	40-50	20-60	30-50	Any age	Young—benign Older—malignant
Manifestation	Back pain	Extremity arthritis Psoriasis Back pain	Abdominal pain	GI, GU infection	Radicular pain	Back pain	Back pain	Peripheral arthritis	Generalized fatigue	Acute, severe unilateral back pain	Slowly progressive, insidious pain
Sacroiliitis	Symmetrical	Asymmetric	Symmetrical	Symmetrical	—	Asymmetric	—	Symmetrical	—	Asymmetric	Asymmetric
Axial skeleton	+	+/–	+	+/–	–	–	+	(Cervical spine)	–	–	–
Peripheral joints	Lower	Upper	Lower	Lower	—	—	Lower	Upper and lower	—	—	—
Enthesopathy	+	+	–	+/–	–	–	–	–	–	–	–
Erythrocyte sedimentation rate	Elevated	Elevated	Elevated	Elevated	Normal	Normal	Normal	Elevated	Normal	Elevated	Elevated (malignant)
Rheumatoid factor	—	—	—	—	—	—	—	80%			
HLA-B27	90%	60%	50%	90%	8%	8%	8%	8%	8%	8%	8%
Course	Continuous	Continuous	Continuous	Self-limited or continuous	Episodic	Self-limited	Relapsing	Continuous	Continuous	Episodic	Continuous
Therapy	NSAIDs Exercise TNF	NSAIDs Methotrexate TNF	NSAIDs Corticosteroids Antibiotics TNF	NSAIDs Antibiotics	NSAIDs Epidural corticosteroids Surgery	Bed rest Bracing NSAIDs	NSAIDs	NSAIDs Methotrexate TNF	Tricyclic antidepressants NSAIDs Exercise CBT	Antibiotics Bracing	En bloc excision Chemotherapy Radiation therapy
Disability	Hip	Lower extremity	Hip	—	Neurologic dysfunction	—	Neurologic dysfunction	Generalized joint deformities (sacroiliitis late in disease)	Muscle pain	Neurologic dysfunction	Local invasion—benign Metastases—malignant

CBT, Cognitive-behavioral therapy; NSAIDs, nonsteroidal anti-inflammatory drugs; TNF, tumor necrosis factor inhibitors.

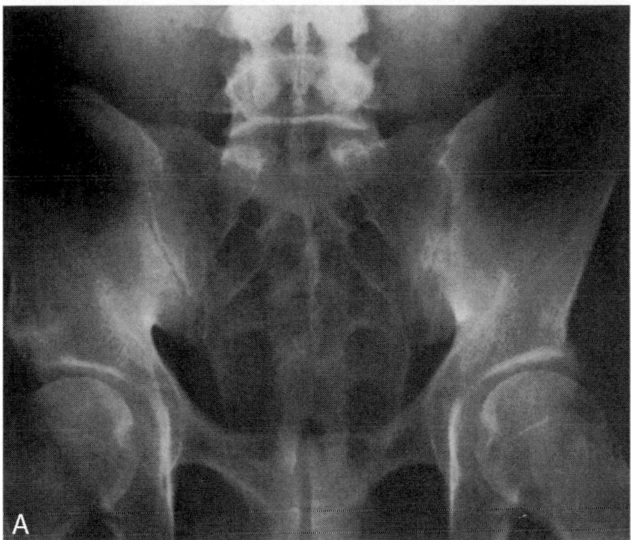

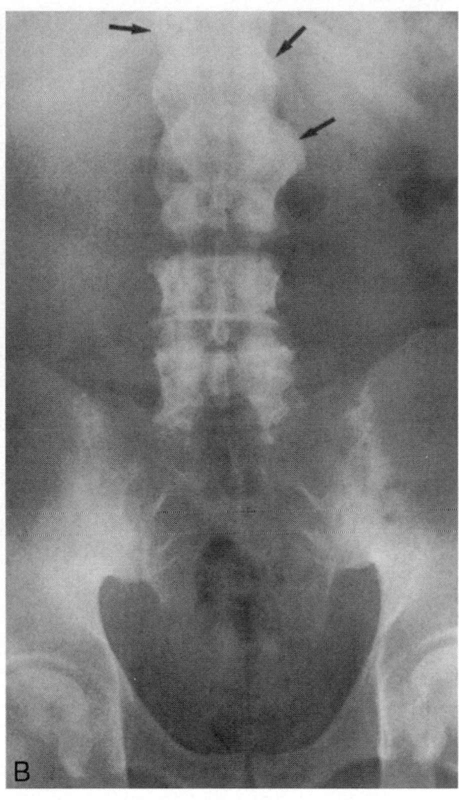

Figure 11-13 Ankylosing spondylitis and diffuse idiopathic skeletal hyperostosis (DISH) in a 37-year-old man with a 17-year history of back pain. *A*, An anteroposterior (AP) view of the pelvis reveals mild bilateral sacroiliitis with sclerosis and early joint erosions. *B*, An AP view of the entire lumbosacral spine demonstrates large bony calcifications that flowed from the thoracic area to the first three lumbar vertebrae *(arrows)*. L4 and L5 were spared. These flowing calcifications are characteristic of DISH.

Medications

Nonsteroidal Anti-inflammatory Drugs

Medications to control pain and inflammation are useful in patients with AS.[84] In a patient with mild spinal or peripheral joint disease, aspirin may be somewhat effective. However, in a patient with more severe disease, aspirin is usually ineffective. If salicylates are used, anti-inflammatory salicylate serum concentrations (20 to 25 mg/dL) should be maintained. Other nonsteroidal anti-inflammatory drugs (NSAIDs) that have been demonstrated to be effective in AS are indomethacin and phenylbutazone. These drugs are effective in controlling spinal and peripheral joint disease but are associated with potentially serious side effects.[76] In a retrospective radiographic study, phenylbutazone decreased the rate of progression of axial skeletal disease in AS.[15] Phenylbutazone is not available from pharmaceutical manufacturers and is not used for therapy for AS patients. A follow-up study of 14 patients with AS who took indomethacin for 18 years reported a beneficial effect for the majority, including remission in 28% of patients.[35] NSAIDs such as ibuprofen, tolmetin, fenoprofen, piroxicam, diclofenac, etodolac, flurbiprofen, ketoprofen, sulindac, and mefenamic acid also may be effective in AS.[89,199] Sulindac has been compared with indomethacin and has comparable efficacy and a tolerance advantage of a twice-a-day dose regimen.[37] This drug has Food and Drug Administration (FDA) approval for use in AS. Naproxen also has FDA approval, and studies have shown efficacy of the drug in the treatment of AS patients.[5] As mentioned, other NSAIDs may be useful for control of joint symptoms but are not approved by the FDA for use in patients with spondylitis. NSAIDs are effective in decreasing pain and improving movement but have not been proved to slow the progression of disease. The

11-5 ASSESSMENT IN ANKYLOSING SPONDYLITIS (ASAS) WORKING GROUP OUTCOME MEASURES

Domain	Instrument
Function	BASFI or Dougados Functional Index
Pain	VAS, last week, spine at night, caused by AS; VAS, last week, caused by AS
Spine mobility	Chest expansion and modified Schober and occiput-to-wall distances
Patient global	VAS, last week
Stiffness	Duration of motion stiffness, spine, last week
Peripheral joints and entheses	Number of swollen joints (44-joint count) Validated enthesis index
Acute phase reactants	ESR
Radiograph spine	AP + lateral lumbar and lateral cervical spine and x-ray of pelvis (SI joints and hips)
Radiograph hips	Pelvis
Fatigue	VAS, fatigue

AP, anteroposterior; AS, ankylosing spondylitis; BASFI, Bath Ankylosing Spondylitis Functional Index; ESR, erythrocyte sedimentation rate; SI, sacroiliacs; VAS, Visual Analogue Scale.

benefits of NSAIDs must be balanced against their potential toxicity.[157]

Cyclooxygenase Inhibitors

Cyclooxygenase-2 (COX-2) inhibitors are a class of NSAIDs that have efficacy equal to that of combined COX-1/COX-2 inhibitors (aspirin, naproxen) but with less gastrointestinal toxicity. COX-2 inhibitors are effective in osteoarthritis and rheumatoid arthritis. AS patients were reported to be responsive to celecoxib, a COX-2 inhibitor, in a 6-week controlled study.[60] Studies reporting the efficacy of other COX-2 inhibitors (etoricoxib) have appeared in abstract form.[156]

Muscle Relaxants

Severe muscle spasm with associated limited motion may develop in patients with acute AS and hinder their return to normal, daily activities. In these patients, the addition of a muscle relaxant to an NSAID helps decrease muscle pain and muscle spasm and improve back motion. Muscle relaxants such as cyclobenzaprine at low dosage levels (10 mg/day) are helpful while limiting possible drug toxicity. The sleepiness associated with muscle relaxants with long half-lives can be limited by giving the medication 2 hours before bedtime. Recent studies report a lower frequency of sedation with a smaller dose of cyclobenzaprine used for short duration.[18a]

Corticosteroids

Systemic corticosteroids are rarely needed and are ineffective for the spinal articular disease of AS. For the occasional patient with continued joint symptoms while receiving maximal doses of NSAIDs, adding small doses of corticosteroids (5 mg of prednisone per day) may prove to be useful. Larger doses of corticosteroids cause appreciably more toxicity without an increased benefit. Occasionally, systemic corticosteroids are needed to control persistent iritis. Intra-articular injection of a long-acting steroid preparation is indicated if a patient has peripheral joint disease with persistent effusions. Injections in the sacroiliac joints are ineffective in relieving pain.[105]

Pulse intravenous methylprednisolone has resulted in improvement in patients who failed to respond to nonsteroidal drugs. The use of intravenous pulses yielded dramatic responses lasting 14 months.[159] In another study, pulse methylprednisolone was helpful, but improvement in spinal motion lasted only 2 months.[183]

Disease-Modifying Antirheumatic Drugs

The number of placebo-controlled trials studying disease-modifying antirheumatic drugs in AS is limited.[218] Drugs that ameliorate peripheral arthritis have no effect on axial disease. In addition, consensus regarding measurement tools to determine improvement in AS has only recently been reached.[217]

Intramuscular gold salt injections or oral gold is not indicated for the axial skeletal disease of AS, but such agents may be helpful in the rare patient with peripheral joint disease who demonstrates persistent synovitis and joint destruction. Antimalarials have not been used on a regular basis in AS patients. Immunosuppressive medications, primarily methotrexate, have been used for AS in only a small number of patients with some success, particularly for peripheral arthritis.[71,104] In a 1-year open-label study, methotrexate was effective at a 12.5-mg weekly dose in 53% of AS patients with peripheral arthritis.[193] Methotrexate is ineffective in late-stage, severe disease. Azathioprine is ineffective and is associated with toxicity. Leflunomide, a pyrimidine inhibitor effective in rheumatoid arthritis, has not been assessed in AS. A double-blind, placebo-controlled trial of penicillamine in AS detected no significant difference between the test drug and placebo in clinical and laboratory indices.[204]

Sulfasalazine is effective for peripheral arthritis in AS patients.[49] It may improve spinal mobility while reducing ESR and CRP levels.[169] The drug is well tolerated with few toxicities. The daily dose is up to 30 to 40 mg/kg.

Bisphosphonates

Bisphosphonates are synthetic analogues of pyrophosphate and impair resorption of bone, thereby resulting in improved BMD. Pathologic examination of the sacroiliac joints reveals subchondral bone marrow inflammation in AS patients. In vitro observations have reported anti-inflammatory properties of bisphosphonates mediated by decreasing cytokine production, independent of their effects on bone metabolism.[101] Open-label trials of monthly intravenous pamidronate infusions have reported efficacy in AS patients. In a placebo-controlled trial of NSAID-resistant AS patients, the effects of intravenous pamidronate therapy, 60 mg monthly, were better than 10 mg monthly for 6 months. The benefits took months to appear.[150] However, a lack of decline in ESR and CRP indicated that inflammation was not suppressed by pamidronate in these AS patients. Oral bisphosphonates do not have therapeutic effects. The role of bisphosphonates in the treatment of AS remains to be determined.

Anti–Tumor Necrosis Factor-Alpha Inhibitors

TNF is an inflammatory cytokine associated with the inflammatory process that results in the phenotypic expression of AS. Anti-TNF therapies are available in the form of infliximab, etanercept, and adulimimab, drugs that inhibit the inflammatory effects of TNF. Infusion of intravenous infliximab in a dose of 5 mg/kg at 0, 2, and 6 weeks in a placebo-controlled trial resulted in improvement in axial symptoms and signs, enthesitis, and peripheral arthritis.[216] Open-label extension of studies for as long as 54 weeks has documented persistent improvement with infliximab infusions at 6-week intervals.[21] In a 12-week infliximab (5 mg/kg) versus placebo study, 40% of the group with AS receiving active treatment had regression of spinal inflammation, versus 6% of the group receiving placebo, as measured by MR.[55a] In a placebo-controlled, 4-month study of 40 AS patients treated with 25 mg of etanercept, 80% of patients receiving active drug experienced an improvement in morning stiffness, enthesitis, quality of life, ESR, or CRP.[86] In a 6-month trial of etanercept versus placebo, 56% of patients with AS receiving active therapy improved, compared with 6% of patients receiving placebo. A relapse occurred within weeks of cessation of therapy.[20a] Etanercept is approved by the U.S. Food and Drug Administration for the treatment of AS. The full benefits of anti-TNF therapy in AS remains to be determined. The efficacy of these agents in disease of long duration is less certain. These agents are expensive, and their availability is limited. Toxicities are associated with their use, including activation of latent tuberculosis. The therapeutic effect of TNF inhibitors may be related to the increase in TH1 cytokines (interferon-gamma and IL-2) to levels comparable to those in healthy controls, along with normalization of lymphocyte number. These findings suggest that TNF blockade reverses the state of anergy of TH1 cells with no significant effect on TH2 cells.[96] Repeated infusions of infliximab remain effective in AS over a 12-month period.[137]

Thalidomide is a synthetic derivative of glutamic acid with an infamous history of causing phocomelia in children. This agent has immunomodulatory effects that are not fully understood. One potential mechanism is inhibition of TNF-alpha. Open-label studies have been reported in the treatment of patients with severe AS. Approximately 68% of AS patients treated with thalidomide reported improvement.[114]

Radiation Therapy

Radiation therapy was used frequently in patients with AS up to the 1960s, and it was effective in controlling pain and stiffness in the lumbosacral spine.[33] The effects of this therapy, however, were transient and did not prevent progression of the disease. In addition, long-term follow-up studies on these patients demonstrated increased mortality secondary to leukemia. A Canadian study has shown decreased survival of men who received spinal radiation therapy after a 27-year follow-up period.[121] The therapy has been abandoned except for the rarest of patients who are intolerant of all other treatment. Local radiation therapy may be considered for a patient with spondylodiscitis who fails all other therapies.[52] This treatment is of historical interest for the remaining patients who were exposed to radiation therapy in the 1960s. These individuals need careful monitoring of their hematologic status.

Surgical Therapies

Orthopedic appliances, such as a heel cup for plantar fasciitis or a temporary spinal brace to prevent forward flexion, are useful in appropriate patients. In patients with fixed flexion deformities of the hip, total joint replacement relieves pain and increases mobility.[226] Surgical procedures on the spine, such as lumbar spine osteotomy, are limited to patients who have such a degree of forward flexion that it prevents them from looking up from the ground.[196] This operation has multiple potential complications and is viewed as a procedure of last resort. Bradford and colleagues reported a good outcome of spinal osteotomy in 20 of 21 patients, including 2 with progressive paraplegia.[20] Minimally invasive procedures and improved fixation devices have improved the surgical outcomes of patients with AS. These operations can be performed for correction of cervical, thoracic, or lumbar deformities that are associated with a poor quality of life.[66] These interventions are major procedures that should be undertaken by spine surgeons with expertise in the care of patients with inflammatory arthropathies of the spine. Fractures of the cervical spine must be stabilized with appropriate plating. Stabilization may be accomplished without the need for a halo vest.[209]

PROGNOSIS

The general course of AS is benign and is characterized by exacerbations and remissions. Many patients with AS may have sacroiliitis with mild involvement of the lumbosacral spine. Limitation of lumbosacral motion may be mild. The disease can become quiescent at any time. Patients in whom total fusion of the spine eventually develops may feel better because ankylosis of the spinal joints is associated with decreased pain. In a study of 1492 patients for 2 years, the frequency of patients with a total remission of disease was less than 2%.[124]

The effect of HLA-B27 homozygosity on the course and severity of AS has been controversial. It has been suggested that homozygosity for HLA-B27 increases both the risk and the severity of AS and may be associated with severe peripheral arthritis along with axial disease.[7,120] Other investigators have been unable to confirm this finding.[163,201] Suarez-Almazor and Russell reported their experience of the effect of homozygosity on the severity of disease and familial penetrance of spondylitis in association with HLA-B27.[206] HLA-B27 was associated with statistically significantly more severe disease in homozygous patients but was not associated with earlier onset of disease or an increased risk of spondylitis in family members.

In AS, a worse prognosis is expected with peripheral joint disease, young age at onset, an elevated ESR, and poor response to NSAIDs.[125] The prognosis of men and women with AS has been reported to be different.[109,119] Women were said to have a milder course, more peripheral disease, and less radiographic change in the axial skeleton. Gran and colleagues compared 44 women and 82 men with AS and found no difference between the sexes with respect to age at onset, initial symptoms, work performance, restriction of spinal motion, and peripheral joint involvement.[93]

Most studies report that the majority of patients remain functional and employed over the duration of the disease.[43] The disease may flare over the course of the illness. Prolonged sick leaves may occur, with depression developing in approximately 33%.[214] In a study of Dutch AS workers, 15.7% of males and 16.9% of females were disabled from work.[18] The prime predictor of more severe dysfunction is the presence of peripheral joint involvement, particularly in the hips, and such involvement usually appears within the first 10 years of disease. Severe spinal restriction develops in a majority of these patients. Patients with fixed flexion contractures of the hips and ankylosis of the spine are severely limited in their functional capacity; however, total hip joint replacement may improve their mobility. Patients with spinal rigidity but normal hip function have minimal disability, but they should avoid heavy labor such as lifting objects heavier than 40 pounds.

References

Ankylosing Spondylitis

1. Ahlstrom H, Feltelius N, Nyman R, et al: Magnetic resonance imaging of sacroiliac joint inflammation. Arthritis Rheum 33:1763, 1990.
2. Allen RL, O'Callaghan CA, McMichael AJ, et al: Cutting edge: HLA-B27 can form a novel beta 2-microglobulin–free heavy chain homodimer structure. J Immunol 162:5045-5048, 1999.
3. Alvarez L, Lopez de Castro JA: HLA-B27 and immunogenetics of spondyloarthropathies. Curr Opin Rheumatol 12:248-253, 2000.
4. Anas PP: Case records of the Massachusetts General Hospital. N Engl J Med 321:1178, 1989.
5. Ansell BM, Major G, Liyanage G, et al: A comparative study of butacote and Naprosyn in ankylosing spondylitis. Ann Rheum Dis 37:436, 1978.
6. Applerouth D, Gottlieb NL: Pulmonary manifestations of ankylosing spondylitis. J Rheumatol 2:446, 1975.
7. Arnett FC, Schacter BZ, Hochberg M, et al: Homozygosity for HLA-B27: Impact on rheumatic disease expression in two families. Arthritis Rheum 20:797, 1977.
8. Baeten D, Demetter P, Cuvelier C, et al: Comparative study of the synovial histology in rheumatoid arthritis, spondyloarthropathy, and osteoarthritis: Influence of disease duration and activity. Ann Rheum Dis 59:945-953, 2000.
9. Ball J: Enthesopathy of rheumatoid and ankylosing spondylitis. Ann Rheum Dis 30:213, 1971.
10. Baron M, Tator CH, Little H: Hangman's fracture in ankylosing spondylitis preceded by vertical subluxation of the axis. Arthritis Rheum 23:850, 1980.
11. Bennett PH, Wood PHN: Population studies of the rheumatic diseases: Proceedings of the 3rd International Symposium, New York, 1966. Amsterdam, Excerpta Medica, 1968, p 456.
12. Bergfeldt L: HLA-B27–associated cardiac disease. Ann Intern Med 127:621-629, 1997.
13. Bergfeldt L, Edhag O, Vedin H, Vallin H: Ankylosing spondylitis: An important cause of severe disturbances of the cardiac conduction system. Prevalence among 223 pacemaker-treated men. Am J Med 73:187, 1982.
14. Bjorkman PJ, Saper MA, Samraoui B, et al: Structure of the human class I histocompatibility antigen, HLA-A2. Nature 329:506, 1987.
15. Boersma JW: Retardation of ossification of the lumbar vertebral column in ankylosing spondylitis by means of phenylbutazone. Scand J Rheumatol 5:60, 1976.
16. Bohlman HH: Acute fractures and dislocations of the cervical spine: An analysis of three hundred hospitalized patients and review of the literature. J Bone Joint Surg Am 61-A:1119-1142, 1979.
17. Bollow M, Enzweiler C, Taupitz M, et al: Use of contrast enhanced magnetic resonance imaging to detect spinal inflammation in patients with spondyloarthritides. Clin Exp Rheumatol 20(suppl 28):S167-S174, 2002.
18. Boonen A, Chorus A, Miedema H, et al: Employment, work disability, and work days lost in patients with ankylosing spondylitis: A cross sectional study of Dutch patients. Ann Rheum Dis 60:353-358, 2001.

18a. Borenstein D, Korn S: Efficacy of a low-dose regimen of cyclobenzaprine hydrochloride in acute skeletal muscle spasm: Results of two placebo-controlled trials. Clin Ther 25:1056-1073, 2003.

19. Boyer GS, Templin DW, Bowler A, et al: A comparison of patients with spondyloarthropathy seen in specialty clinics with those identified in a communitywide epidemiologic study. Arch Intern Med 157:2111-2117, 1997.
20. Bradford DS, Schumacher WL, et al: Ankylosing spondylitis: Experience in surgical management of 21 patients. Spine 12:238, 1987.

20a. Brandt J, Khariouzov A, Listing J, et al: Six-month results of a double-blind, placebo-controlled trial of etanercept treatment in patients with active ankylosing spondylitis. Arthritis Rheum 48:1667-1675, 2003.

21. Brandt J, Sieper J, Braun J: Infliximab in the treatment of active and severe ankylosing spondylitis. Clin Exp Rheumatol 20(suppl 28):S106-S110, 2002.
22. Braun J, Bollow M: The Diagnostic Imaging in Rheumatology Study Group of the Berlin Regional Rheumatology Center. J Clin Rheumatol 6:339-349, 2000.
23. Braun J, Bollow M, Neure L, et al: Use of immunohistologic and in situ hybridization techniques in the examination of sacroiliac joint biopsy specimens from patients with ankylosing spondylitis. Arthritis Rheum 38:499, 1995.
24. Braun J, Bollow M, Remlinger G, et al: Prevalence of spondyloarthropathies in HLA-B27 positive and negative blood donors. Arthritis Rheum 41:58-67, 1998.
25. Braun J, Bollow M, Sieper J: Radiologic diagnosis and pathology of the spondyloarthropathies. Rheum Clin North Am 24:697-735, 1998.
26. Braun J, Khan MA, Siepper J: Enthesitis and ankylosis in spondyloarthropathy: What is the target of the immune response? Ann Rheum Dis 59:985-994, 2000.
27. Breur-Vriesendorp BS, Vingerhoed J, Kuijpers KC, et al: Effect of a Tyr-to-His point-mutation at position 59 in the alpha-1 helix of the HLA-B27 class-I molecule on allospecific and virus-specific cytotoxic T-lymphocyte recognition. Scand J Rheumatol Suppl 87:36, 1990.
28. Broom MJ, Raycroft JF: Complications of fractures of the cervical spine in ankylosing spondylitis. Spine 13:763, 1988.
29. Brophy S, Calin A: Ankylosing spondylitis: Interaction between genes, joints, age at onset, and disease expression. J Rheumatol 28:2283-2288, 2001
30. Brown MA, Crane A, Wordsworth BP: Genetic aspects of susceptibility, severity, and clinical expression in ankylosing spondylitis. Curr Opin Rheumatol 14:354-360, 2002.
31. Brown MA, Kennedy GL, MacGregor AJ, et al: Sussceptibility to ankylosing spondylitis in twins—the role of genes, HLA, and the environment. Arthritis Rheum 40:1823-1828, 1997.
32. Brown MA, Pile KD, Kennedy LG, et al: A genome-wide screen for susceptibility loci in ankylosing spondylitis. Arthritis Rheum 41:588-595, 1998.
33. Brown WMC, Doll R: Mortality from cancer and other causes after radiotherapy for ankylosing spondylitis. BMJ 2:1327, 1965.
34. Bulkey BH, Roberts WC: Ankylosing spondylitis and aortic regurgitation: Description of the characteristic cardiovascular lesion from study of eight necropsy patients. Circulation 48:1014, 1973.
35. Calabro JJ: Appraisal of efficacy and tolerability of Indocin (indomethacin, MSD) in acute gout and moderate to severe ankylosing spondylitis. Semin Arthritis Rheum 12(suppl 1):112, 1982.
36. Calin A: The relationship between genetics and environment in the pathogenesis of rheumatic diseases. West J Med 131:205, 1979.
37. Calin A, Britton M: Sulindac in ankylosing spondylitis: Double-blind evaluation of sulindac and indomethacin. JAMA 242:1885, 1979.
38. Calin A, Elswood J: The relationship between pelvic, spinal and hip involvement in ankylosing spondylitis: One disease process or several? Br J Rheumatol 27:393, 1988.
39. Calin A, Fries JF: Striking prevalence of ankylosing spondylitis in "healthy" W27 positive males and females: A controlled study. N Engl J Med 293:835, 1975.
40. Calin A, Marder A, Becks E, Burns T: Genetic differences between B27 positive patients with ankylosing spondylitis and B27 positive healthy controls. Arthritis Rheum 26:1460, 1983.
41. Caplanne D, Tubach F, Le Parc JM: Late onset spondyloarthropathy: Clinical and biological comparison with early onset patients. Ann Rheum Dis 56:176-179, 1997.
42. Careless DJ, Inman RD: Etiopathogenesis of reactive arthritis and ankylosing spondylitis. Curr Opin Rheumatol 7:290, 1995.
43. Carette S, Graham D, Little H, et al: The natural disease course of ankylosing spondylitis. Arthritis Rheum 26:186, 1983.
44. Carrera GF, Foley WD, Kozin F, et al: CT of sacroiliitis. AJR Am J Roentgenol 136:41, 1981.
45. Casserly IP, Fenlon HM, Breatnach, et al: Lung findings on high-resolution computed tomography in idiopathic ankylosing

spondylitis: Correlation with clinical findings, pulmonary function testing and plain radiography. Br J Rheumatol 36:677-682, 1997.
46. Cawley MID, Chalmers TM, Kellgren JH, Ball J: Destructive lesions of vertebral bodies in ankylosing spondylitis. Ann Rheum Dis 31:345, 1972.
47. Cheatum DE: "Ankylosing spondylitis" without sacroiliitis in a woman without the HLA-B27 antigen. J Rheumatol 3:420, 1976.
48. Clayman MD, Reinertsen JL: Ankylosing spondylitis with subsequent development of rheumatoid arthritis, Sjögren's syndrome, and rheumatoid vasculitis. Arthritis Rheum 21:383, 1978.
49. Clegg DO, Reda DJ, Abdellatif M, et al: Comparison of sulfasalazine and placebo for the treatment of axial and peripheral articular manifestations of the seronegative spondyloarthropathies. Arthritis Rheum 42:2325-2329, 1999.
50. Colbert RA: HLA-B27 misfolding and spondyloarthropathies: Not so groovy after all? J Rheumatol 27:1107-1109, 2000.
51. Cone RD, Resnick D: Roentgenographic evaluation of the sacroiliac joints. Orthop Rev 12:95, 1983.
52. Creemers MCW, van Riel PLCM, Franssen MJAM, et al: Second-line treatment in seronegative spondyloarthropathies. Semin Arthritis Rheum 24:71, 1994.
53. Cruickshank B: Pathology of ankylosing spondylitis. Clin Orthop 74:43, 1971.
54. Dale K: Radiographic changes of the spine in Bechterew's syndrome and allied disorders. Scand J Rheumatol Suppl 32:103, 1979.
55. Dale K: Radiographic grading of sacroiliitis in Bechterew's syndrome and allied disorders. Scand J Rheumatol Suppl 32:92, 1979.
55a. De Keyser F, Baeten D, Van den Bosch F, et al: Infliximab in patients who have spondyloarthropathy: Clinical efficacy, safety, and biological immunomodulation. Rheum Dis Clin North Am 29:463-479, 2003.
56. Detwiler KN, Loftus CM, Godersky JC, et al: Management of cervical spine injuries in patients with ankylosing spondylitis. J Neurosurg 72:210, 1990.
57. Devogelaer JP, Maldague B, Malghem J, et al: Appendicular and vertebral bone mass in ankylosing spondylitis. Arthritis Rheum 35:1062, 1992.
58. Dihlmann W, Delling G: Discovertebral destructive lesions (so-called Andersson lesions) associated with ankylosing spondylitis. Skeletal Radiol 3:10, 1978.
59. Docherty P, Mitchell MJ, MacMillan L, et al: Magnetic resonance imaging in the detection of sacroiliitis. J Rheumatol 19:393, 1992.
60. Dougados M, Behier JM, Jolchine I, et al: Efficacy of celecoxib, a cyclooxygenase 2–specific inhibitor, in the treatment of ankylosing spondylitis: A six-week controlled study with comparison against placebo and against a conventional non-steroidal anti-inflammatory drug. Arthritis Rheum 44:180-185, 2001.
61. Dunn N, Preston B, Jones KL: Unexplained acute backache in longstanding ankylosing spondylitis. BMJ 291:1632, 1985.
62. Durback MA, Edelstein G, Schumacher HR Jr: Abnormalities of the sacroiliac joints in diffuse idiopathic skeletal hyperostosis: Demonstration by computed tomography. J Rheumatol 15:1506, 1988.
63. Dwosh IL, Resnick D, Becker MA: Hip involvement in ankylosing spondylitis. Arthritis Rheum 19:683, 1976.
64. Ebringer A, Shipley M (eds): Pathogenesis of HLA-B27–associated disease. Br J Rheumatol 2(suppl):1, 1983.
65. Edmonds J, Macauley D, Tyndall A, et al: Lymphocytotoxicity of anti-*Klebsiella* antisera in ankylosing spondylitis and related arthropathies: Patient and family studies. Arthritis Rheum 24:1, 1981.
66. El Saghir H, Boehm H: Surgical options in the treatment of spinal disorders in ankylosing spondylitis. Clin Exp Rheumatol 20(suppl 28):S101-S105, 2002.
67. Engleman EG, Calin A, Grumet FC: Analysis of HLA-B27 antigen with monoclonal antibodies. J Rheumatol Suppl 10:59, 1983.
68. Engleman EG, Rosenbaum JT: HLA and disease: An overview. In Calin A (ed): Spondyloarthropathies. Orlando, FL, Grune & Stratton, 1984, pp 279-296.
69. Esdaile JM, Rosenthall L, Terkeltaub R, Kloiber R: Prospective evaluation of sacroiliac scintigraphy in chronic inflammatory back pain. Arthritis Rheum 23:998, 1980.
70. Feltkamp TEW, Ringrose JH: Acute anterior uveitis and spondyloarthropathies. Curr Opin Rheumatol 10:314-318, 1998.
71. Ferraz MB, da Silva HC, Altra E: Low dose methotrexate with leucovorin rescue in ankylosing spondylitis. J Rheumatol 18:146, 1991.
72. Finkelstein JA, Chapman JR, Mirza S: Occult vertebral fractures in ankylosing spondylitis. Spinal Cord 37:444-447, 1999.
73. Foo D, Rossier AB: Post-traumatic spinal epidural hematoma. Neurosurgery 11:25, 1982.
74. Foo D, Sarkarati M, Marcelino V: Cervical spinal cord injury complicating ankylosing spondylitis. Paraplegia 23:358, 1985.
75. Forrester DM: Imaging of the sacroiliac joint. Radiol Clin North Am 28:1054, 1990.
76. Fowler P: Phenylbutazone and indomethacin. Clin Rheum Dis 1:267, 1975.
77. Fox MW, Onofrio BM, Kilgore JE: Neurological complications of ankylosing spondylitis. J Neurosurg 78:781, 1993.
78. Francois RJ, Braun J, Khan MA: Entheses and enthesitis: A histopathologic review and relevance to spondyloarthropathies. Curr Opin Rheumatol 13:255-264, 2001.
79. Geczy AF, Alexander K, Bashir HV, et al: HLA-B27, *Klebsiella*, and ankylosing spondylitis: Bacteriologic and chemical studies. Immunol Rev 70:23, 1983.
80. Geczy AF, Prendergast JK, Sullivan JS, et al: HLA-B27, molecular mimicry and ankylosing spondylitis: Popular misconceptions. Ann Rheum Dis 46:171, 1987.
81. Geusens P, Vosse D, van der Heijde D, et al: High prevalence of thoracic vertebral deformities and discal wedging in ankylosing spondylitis patients with hyperkyphosis. J Rheumatol 28:1856-1861, 2001.
82. Ginsburg WW, Cohen MD: Peripheral arthritis in ankylosing spondylitis: A review of 209 patients followed up for more than 20 years. Mayo Clin Proc 58:593, 1983.
83. Ginsburg WW, Cohen MD, Miller GM, et al: Posterior vertebral body erosion by arachnoid diverticula in cauda equina syndrome: An unusual manifestation of ankylosing spondylitis. J Rheumatol 24:1417-1420, 1997.
84. Godfrey RG, Calabro JJ, Mills D, Matty BA: A double blind crossover trial of aspirin, indomethacin and phenylbutazone in ankylosing spondylitis [Abstract]. Arthritis Rheum 15:110, 1972.
85. Good AE, Kawaniski H, Schultz JS: HLA-B27 in blacks with ankylosing spondylitis or Reiter's disease. N Engl J Med 294:166, 1976.
86. Gorman JD, Sack KE, David JC Jr: Treatment of ankylosing spondylitis by inhibition of tumor necrosis factor alpha. N Engl J Med 346:1349-356, 2002.
87. Graham DC, Smythe HA: The carditis and aortitis of ankylosing spondylitis. Bull Rheum Dis 9:171, 1958.
89. Gran JT, Husby G: Ankylosing spondylitis: Current drug treatment. Drugs 44:585, 1992.
90. Gran JT, Husby G: Ankylosing spondylitis in women. Semin Arthritis Rheum 19:303, 1990.
91. Gran JT, Husby F, Hordvik M: Prevalence of ankylosing spondylitis in males and females in a young middle-aged population of Tromso, Northern Norway. Ann Rheum Dis 44:359, 1985.
92. Gran JT, Ostensen M: Spondyloarthritides in females. Ballieres Clin Rheumatol 12:695-715, 1998.
93. Gran JT, Ostensen M, Husby G: A clinical comparison between males and females with ankylosing spondylitis. J Rheumatol 12:126, 1985.
94. Gran JT, Paulsen AQ, Gaskjenn H, Schulz T: Reactive arthritis of the cervical spine due to *Yersinia enterocolitica* in patients with pre-existing ankylosing spondylitis. Scand J Rheumatol 21:95, 1992.
95. Gran JT, Teiberg P, Olaissen B, et al: HLA-B27 and allotypes of complement components in ankylosing spondylitis. J Rheumatol 11:324, 1984.
96. Granfors K, Marker-Hermann E, de Keyser F, et al: The cutting edge of spondyloarthropathy research in the millennium. Arthritis Rheum 46:606-613, 2002.
97. Gratacos J, Collado A, Pons F, et al: Significant loss of bone mass in patients with early, active ankylosing spondylitis: A followup study. Arthritis Rheum 42:2319-2324, 1999.
98. Gratocos J, Orella C, Sanmarti R, et al: Secondary amyloidosis in ankylosing spondylitis: A systemic survey of 137 patients using abdominal fat aspiration. J Rheumatol 24:912-915, 1997.
99. Guttmann L: Traumatic paraplegia and tetraplegia in ankylosing spondylitis. Paraplegia 4:188, 1966.
100. Haddad FS, Sachdev JS, Bellapravalu M: Neuropathic bladder in ankylosing spondylitis with spinal diverticula. Urology 35:313, 1990.
101. Haibel H, Braun J, Maksymowych WP: Bisphosphonates—Targeting bone in the treatment of spondyloarthritis. Clin Exp Rheumatol 20(suppl 280: S162-S166, 2002.

102. Hamilton MG, MacRae ME: Atlantoaxial dislocation as the presenting symptom of ankylosing spondylitis. Spine 18:2344, 1993.
103. Hammer RE, Maika SD, Richardson JA, et al: Spontaneous inflammatory disease in transgenic rats expressing HLA-B27 and human beta 2m: An animal model of HLA-B27–associated human disorders. Cell 63:1099, 1990.
104. Handler RP: Favorable results using methotrexate in the treatment of patients with ankylosing spondylitis. Arthritis Rheum 32:234, 1989.
105. Hanly JG, Mitchell M, MacMillan L, et al: Efficacy of sacroiliac corticosteroid injections in patients with inflammatory spondyloarthropathy: Results of a 6 month controlled study. J Rheumatol 27:719-722, 2000.
106. Hart FD, MacLagen NF: Ankylosing spondylitis: A review of 184 cases. Ann Rheum Dis 34:87, 1975.
107. Hart FD, Robinson KC: Ankylosing spondylitis in women. Ann Rheum Dis 18:15, 1959.
108. Hassan I: Cauda equina syndrome in ankylosing spondylitis: A report of six cases. J Neurol Neurosurg Psychiatry 39:1172, 1976.
109. Hill HFH, Hill AGS, Bodmer JG: Clinical diagnosis of ankylosing spondylitis in women and relation to presence of HLA-B27. Ann Rheum Dis 35:267, 1976.
110. Hill AVS, Kwiatkowski D, Greenwood BM, et al: HLA class I typing by PCR: HLA-B27 and an African B27 subtype. Lancet 337:640, 1991.
111. Hochberg MC: Epidemiology. In Calin A (ed): Spondyloarthropathies. Orlando, FL, Grune & Stratton, 1984, pp 21-42.
112. Hochberg MC, Bias WB, Arnett FC Jr: Family studies in HLA-B27 associated arthritis. Medicine (Baltimore) 57:463, 1978.
113. Hochberg MC, Borenstein DG, Arnett FC: The absence of back pain in classical ankylosing spondylitis. Johns Hopkins Med J 143:181, 1978.
114. Huang F, Wei JCC, Breban M: Thalidomide in ankylosing spondylitis. Clin Exp Rheumatol 20(suppl 28):S158-S161, 2002.
115. Hukuda S, Minami M, Saito T, et al: Spondyloarthropathies in Japan: Nationwide questionnaire survey performed by the Japan Ankylosing Spondylitis Society. J Rheumatol 28:554-559, 2001.
116. Hunter T, Dubo H: Spinal fractures complicating ankylosing spondylitis. Ann Intern Med 88:546, 1978.
117. Iplikcioglu AC, Bayar MA, Kokes F, et al: Magnetic resonance imaging in cervical trauma associated with ankylosing spondylitis: Report of two cases. J Trauma 36:412, 1994.
118. Jacoby RK, Newell RLM, Hickling P: Ankylosing spondylitis and trauma: The medicolegal implications. A comparative study of patients with nonspecific back pain. Ann Rheum Dis 44:307, 1985.
119. Jeannet M, Saudan Y, Bitter T: HLA-27 in female patients with ankylosing spondylitis. Tissue Antigens 6:262, 1975.
120. Kahn MA, Kushner I, Braun WE, et al: HLA-B27 homozygosity in ankylosing spondylitis: Relationship to risk and severity. Tissue Antigens 11:434, 1978.
121. Kaprove RE, Little AH, Graham DC, Rosen PS: Ankylosing spondylitis: Survival in men with and without radiotherapy. Arthritis Rheum 23:57, 1980.
122. Kellgren JH: Diagnostic criteria for population studies. Bull Rheum Dis 13:291, 1962.
123. Kendal MJ, Lawrence DS, Shuttleworth GR, Whitefield AGW: Hematology and biochemistry of ankylosing spondylitis. BMJ 2:235, 1973.
124. Kennedy LG, Edmunds L, Calin A: The natural history of ankylosing spondylitis: Does it burn out? J Rheumatol 20:688, 1993.
125. Kerr HE, Sturrock RD: Clinical aspects, outcome assessment, disease course, and extra-articular features of spondyloarthropathies. Curr Opin Rheumatol 11:235-237, 1999.
126. Khan MA: A worldwide overview: The Epidemiology of HLA-B27 and associated spondyloarthropathies. In Calin A, Taurog J (eds): Spondyloarthropathies. Oxford, Oxford University Press, 1998, pp 17-27.
127. Khan MA: An overview of clinical spectrum and heterogeneity of spondyloarthropathies. Rheum Dis Clin North Am 18:1, 1992.
128. Khan MA: HLA-B27 and its subtypes in world populations. Curr Opin Rheumatol 7:263, 1995.
129. Khan MA: HLA-B27 polymorphism and association with disease. J Rheumatol 27:1257-1259, 2000.
130. Khan M: Update on spondyloarthropathies. Ann Intern Med 136:896-907, 2002.
131. Khan MA, Khan MK: Diagnostic value of HLA-B27 testing in ankylosing spondylitis and Reiter's syndrome. Ann Intern Med 906:70, 1982.
132. Khan MA, van der Linden SM: A wider spectrum of spondyloarthropathies. Semin Arthritis Rheum 20:107, 1990.
133. Khare SD, Luthra HS, David CS: HLA-B27 and other predisposing factors in spondyloarthropathies. Curr Opin Rheumatol 10:282-291, 1998.
134. Kidd BL, Cawley MID: Delay in diagnosis of spondylarthritis. Br J Rheumatol 27:230, 1988.
135. Kinsella TD, MacDonald FR, Johnson LG: Ankylosing spondylitis: A late re-evaluation of 92 cases. Can Med Assoc J 95:1, 1966.
136. Kozin F, Carrera GF, Ryan LM, et al: Computed tomography in the diagnosis of sacroiliitis. Arthritis Rheum 24:1479, 1981.
137. Kruithof E, van den Bosch F, Baeten D, et al: Repeated infusions of infliximab, a chimeric anti-TNFα monoclonal antibody, in patients with active spondyloarthropathy: One year followup. Ann Rheum Dis 61:207-212, 2002.
138. Lahesmaa R, Skurnik M, Gransfors K, et al: Molecular mimicry in the pathogenesis of spondyloarthropathies: A critical appraisal of cross-reactivity between microbial antigens and HLA-B27. Br J Rheumatol 31:221, 1992.
139. Lai KN, Li PKT, Hawkins B, et al: IgA nephropathy associated with ankylosing spondylitis: Occurrence in women as well as in men. Ann Rheum Dis 48:435, 1989.
140. Lamas JR, Paradela A, Roncal F, et al: Modulation at multiple anchor positions of the peptide specificity of HLA-B27 subtypes differentially associated with ankylosing spondylitis. Arthritis Rheum 42:1975-1985, 1999.
141. Lau CS, Burgos-Vargas R, Louthrenoo W, et al: Features of spondyloarthritis around the world. Rheum Dis Clin North Am 24:753-770, 1998.
142. Lawrence RC, Helmick CG, Arnett FC, et al: Estimates of the prevalence of arthritis and selected musculoskeletal disorders in the United states. Arthritis Rheum 41:58-67, 1998.
143. Lee YSL, Schlotzhauer T, Ott SM, et al: Skeletal status of men with early and late ankylosing spondylitis. Am J Med 103:233-241, 1997.
144. Lehtinen K: 76 patients with ankylosing spondylitis seen after 30 years of disease. Scand J Rheumatol 12:5, 1983.
145. Leventhal MR, Maguire JK Jr, Christian CA: Atlantoaxial rotary subluxation in ankylosing spondylitis: A case report. Spine 15:1374, 1990.
146. Little H, Swinson DR, Cruickshank B: Upward subluxation of the axis in ankylosing spondylitis. Am J Med 60:279, 1976.
147. Lopez de Castro JA: Structural polymorphism and function of HLA-B27. Curr Opin Rheumatol 7:270, 1995.
148. Maclean IL, Iqball S, Woo P, et al: HLA-B27 subtypes in the spondyloarthropathies. Clin Exp Immunol 91:214, 1993.
149. Mader R: Atypical clinical presentations of ankylosing spondylitis. Semin Arthritis Rheum 29:191-196, 1999.
150. Maksymowych WP, Jhangri GS, Fitzgerald AA, et al: A six-month randomized, controlled, double-blind, dose-response comparison of intravenous pamidronate (60 mg versus 10 mg) in the treatment of nonsteroidal anti-inflammatory drug–refractory ankylosing spondylitis. Arthritis Rheum 46:766-773, 2002.
151. Marc V, Dromer C, LeGuennec P, et al: Magnetic resonance imaging and axial involvement in spondyloarthropathies: Delineation of the spinal entheses. Rev Rheum Engl Ed 64: 465-473, 1997.
152. Martel W: Spinal pseudoarthrosis: A complication of ankylosing spondylitis. Arthritis Rheum 21:485, 1978.
153. Martel W: The occipito-atlanto-axial joints in rheumatoid arthritis and ankylosing spondylitis. AJR Am J Roentgenol 86:223, 1961.
154. McEwen C, DiTata D, Ling GC, et al: Ankylosing spondylitis and spondylitis accompanying ulcerative colitis, regional enteritis, psoriasis, and Reiter's disease: A comparative study. Arthritis Rheum 14:291, 1971.
155. McGonagle D, Gibbon W, Emery P: Classification of inflammatory arthritis by enthesitis. Lancet 352:1137-1140, 1998.
156. Melian A, van der Heijde D, James MK, et al: Etoricoxib in the treatment of ankylosing spondylitis. Arthritis Rheum 346 (suppl):S432, 2002.
156a. Micheli-Richard C, van der Heijde D, Dougados M: Spondyloarthropathy for practicing rheumatologists: Diagnosis, indication

for disease-controlling antirheumatic therapy, and evaluation of the response. Rheum Dis Clin North Am 29:449-462, 2003.
157. Miceli-Richard C, Dougados M: NSAIDs in ankylosing spondylitis. Clin Exp Rheumatol 20(suppl 28):S65-S66, 2002.
158. Miehle W, Schattenkirchner M, Albert D, Bunge M: HLA-DR4 in ankylosing spondylitis with different patterns of joint involvement. Ann Rheum Dis 44:39, 1985.
159. Mintz G, Enriquez RD, Mercado U, et al: Intravenous methylprednisolone pulse therapy in severe ankylosing spondylitis. Arthritis Rheum 24:734, 1981.
160. Mitchell MJ, Sartoris DJ, Moody D, et al: Cauda equina syndrome complicating ankylosing spondylitis. Radiology 175:521, 1990.
161. Moll JM: Criteria for ankylosing spondylitis: Facts and fallacies. Br J Rheumatol 27(suppl):34, 1988.
162. Moll JMH, Wright V: New York clinical criteria for ankylosing spondylitis. Ann Rheum Dis 32:354, 1973.
163. Moller P, Berg K: Family studies in Bechterew's syndrome (ankylosing spondylitis). III: Genetics. Clin Genet 24:73, 1983.
164. Moller P, Vinje O, Kass E: How does Bechterew's syndrome (ankylosing spondylitis) start? Scand J Rheumatol 12:289, 1983.
165. Montenegro V, Monteiro RC: Elevation of serum IgA in spondyloarthropathies and IgA nephropathy and its pathogenic role. Curr Opin Rheumatol 11:265-272, 1999.
166. Mullaji AB, Upadyay SS, Ho EKW: Bone mineral density in ankylosing spondylitis. J Bone Joint Surg Br 76-B:660-665, 1997.
167. Nashel DJ, Petrone DL, Ulmer CC, Sliwinsi AJ: C-reactive protein: A marker for disease activity in ankylosing spondylitis and Reiter's syndrome. J Rheumatol 13:364, 1986.
167a. Newman PA, Bruckel JC: Spondylitis Association of America: The member-directed, nonprofit health organization addressing the needs of ankylosing spondylitis patients. Rheum Dis Clin North Am 29:561-574, 2003.
168. Neustadt DH: Ankylosing spondylitis. Postgrad Med 61:124, 1977.
169. Nissila M, Lehtinen K, Leirsalo-Repo M, et al: Sulfasalazine in the treatment of ankylosing spondylitis. A twenty-six-week, placebo-controlled trial. Arthritis Rheum 31:1111-1116, 1988.
170. O'Driscoll SL, Jayson MIV, Baddeley H: Neck movements in ankylosing spondylitis and their responses to physiotherapy. Ann Rheum Dis 37:64, 1978.
171. Olivieri I, Barozzi L, Padula A: Enthesiopathy: Clinical manifestations, imaging and treatment. Ballieres Clin Rheumatol 12:665-681, 1998.
172. Osgood CP, Abbasy M, Mathews T: Multiple spine fractures in ankylosing spondylitis. J Trauma 15:163, 1975.
173. Pace JB, Nagle D: Piriformis syndrome. West J Med 124:435, 1976.
174. Peeters A, Daha M, Smeets TJM, et al: Bone marrow IgA, and IgA subclass synthesis in ankylosing spondylitis. J Rheumatol 19:751-753, 1992.
175. Ralston SH, Urquhart GDK, Brzeski M, et al: A new method for the radiological assessment of vertebral squaring in ankylosing spondylitis. Ann Rheum Dis 51:330, 1992.
176. Ramos-Remus C, Gomez-Vargas A, Hernandez-Chavez A, et al: Two year follow-up of anterior and vertical atlantoaxial subluxations in ankylosing spondylitis. J Rheumatol 24:507-510, 1997.
177. Resnick D: Patterns of peripheral joint disease in ankylosing spondylitis. Radiology 110:523, 1974.
178. Resnick D, Dwosh IL, Goergen TG, et al: Clinical and radiographic abnormalities in ankylosing spondylitis: A comparison of men and women. Radiology 119:293, 1978.
179. Resnick D, Dwosh IL, Goergen TG, et al: Clinical and radiographic "reankylosis" following hip surgery in ankylosing spondylitis. AJR Am J Roentgenol 126:1181, 1976.
180. Resnick D, Niwayama G: Ankylosing spondylitis. In Resnick D (ed): Diagnosis of Bone and Joint Disorders, 3rd ed. Philadelphia, WB Saunders, 1995, pp 1008-1074.
181. Reveille JD, Ball EJ, Khan MA: HLA-B27 and genetic predisposing factors in spondyloarthropathies. Curr Opin Rheumatol 13:265-272, 2001.
182. Revell PA, Mayston V: Histopathology of the synovial membrane of peripheral joints in ankylosing spondylitis. Ann Rheum Dis 41:579-586, 1982.
183. Richter MB: Management of the seronegative spondyloarthropathies. Clin Rheum Dis 11:147, 1985.
184. Rogers J, Watt I, Dieppe P: Paleopathology of spinal osteophytosis, vertebral ankylosis, ankylosing spondylitis and vertebral hyperostosis. Ann Rheum Dis 44:113, 1985.
185. Roldan CA, Chavez J, Wiest PW, et al: Aortic root disease and valve disease associated with ankylosing spondylitis. J Am Coll Cardiol 32:1397, 1998.
186. Rosen PS, Graham DC: Ankylosing (Strümpell-Marie) spondylitis (a clinical review of 128 cases). AIR 5:158, 1962.
187. Rosenow EC III, Strimlan CV, Muhm JR, Ferguson RH: Pleuropulmonary manifestations of ankylosing spondylitis. Mayo Clin Proc 52:641, 1977.
188. Rotes-Querol J, Tolosa E, Rosello R, Granados J: Progressive cauda equina syndrome and extensive calcification/ossification of the lumbosacral meninges. Ann Rheum Dis 44:227, 1985.
189. Rowed DW: Management of cervical spinal cord injury in ankylosing spondylitis: The intervertebral disc as a cause of cord compression. J Neurosurg 77:241, 1992.
190. Ruffer A: Arthritis deformans and spondylitis in ancient Egypt. J Pathol 22:159, 1918.
191. Russell AS, Lentle BC, Percy JS: Investigation of sacroiliac disease: Comparative evaluation of radiological and radionuclide techniques. J Rheumatol 2:45, 1975.
192. Russell ML, Gordon DA, Orgryzlo MA, McPhedran RS: The cauda equina syndrome of ankylosing spondylitis. Ann Intern Med 78:551, 1973.
193. Sampalo-Barros PD, Costallat LTL, Bertolo MB, et al: Methotrexate in the treatment of ankylosing spondylitis. Scand J Rheumatol 29:160-163, 2000.
194. Saraux A, Guedes C, Allain J, et al: Prevalence of rheumatoid arthritis and spondyloarthropathy in Brittany, France. Societe de Rheumatologie de l'Ouest. J Rheumatol 26:2622-2267, 1999.
195. Schlosstein L, Terasaki PI, Bluestone R, Pearson CM: High association of an HL antigen, W27, with ankylosing spondylitis. N Engl J Med 288:704, 1973.
196. Scudese VA, Calabro JJ: Vertebral wedge osteotomy: Correction of rheumatoid (ankylosing) spondylitis. JAMA 186:627, 1963.
197. Sharp J, Purser DW: Spontaneous atlanto-axial dislocation in ankylosing spondylitis and rheumatoid arthritis. Ann Rheum Dis 20:47, 1961.
198. Sheldon PJ, Pell PA: Lymphocyte proliferative responses to bacterial antigens in B-27 associated arthropathies. J Rheumatol 24:11, 1985.
199. Simon LS, Mills JA: Nonsteroidal anti-inflammatory drugs. N Engl J Med 302:1179, 1237, 1980.
200. Sorin S, Askari A, Moskowitz RW: Atlantoaxial subluxation as a complication of early ankylosing spondylitis. Arthritis Rheum 22:273, 1979.
201. Spencer DG, Dick HM, Dick WC: Ankylosing spondylitis: The role of HLA-B27 homozygosity. Tissue Antigens 14:379, 1979.
202. Spencer DG, Park WM, Dick HM, et al: Radiological manifestations in 200 patients with ankylosing spondylitis: Correlation with clinical features and HLA-B27. J Rheumatol 6:305, 1979.
203. Spoorenberg A, van der Heijde, de Klerk E, et al: Relative value of erythrocyte sedimentation rate and C-reactive protein in assessment of disease activity in ankylosing spondylitis. J Rheumatol 26:980-984, 1999.
204. Steven MM, Morrison M, Sturrock RD: Penicillamine in ankylosing spondylitis: A double blind placebo controlled trial. J Rheumatol 12:735, 1985.
205. Suarez-Almazor ME, Russell AS: Anterior atlanto-axial subluxation in patients with spondyloarthropathies: Association with peripheral disease. J Rheumatol 15:973, 1988.
206. Suarez-Almazor ME, Russell AS: B27 homozygosity and ankylosing spondylitis. J Rheumatol 14:302, 1987.
207. Sullivan JS, Geczy AF: The modification of HLA-B27–positive lymphocytes by the culture filtrate of *Klebsiella* K43 BTS 1 is a metabolically active process. Clin Exp Immunol 62:672, 1985.
208. Szejnfeld VL, Monier-Faugere MC, Bognar BJ, et al: Systemic osteopenia and mineralization defect in patients with ankylosing spondylitis. J Rheumatol 24:683-688, 1997.
209. Taggard DA, Traynelis VC: Management of cervical spinal fractures in ankylosing spondylitis with posterior fixation. Arthritis Rheum 25:2035-2039, 2000.
210. Taurog JD, Richardson JA, Croft JT, et al: The germfree state prevents development of gut and joint inflammatory disease in HLA-B27 transgenic rats. J Exp Med 180:2359, 1994.

211. Taylor HG, Gadd R, Beswick EJ, et al: Quantitative radioisotope scanning in ankylosing spondylitis: A clinical, laboratory and computerized tomographic study. Scand J Rheumatol 20:274, 1991.
212. Tico N, Ramon S, Garcia-Ortun F, et al: Traumatic spinal cord injury complicating ankylosing spondylitis. Spinal Cord 36:349-352, 1998.
213. Tullous MW, Skerhut HEI, Story JL, et al: Cauda equina syndrome of long-standing ankylosing spondylitis: Case report and review of the literature. J Neurosurg 873:441, 1990.
214. Uhrin Z, Kuzis, Ward MM: Exercise and changes in health status in patients with ankylosing spondylitis. Arch Intern Med 160:2969-2975, 2000.
215. Van Bohemen GG, Grumet FC, Zanen HC: Identification of HLA-B27 M_1 and M_2 cross-reactive antigens in *Klebsiella*, *Shigella*, and *Yersinia*. Immunology 52:607, 1984.
216. Van den Bosch F, Kruithof E, Baeten D, et al: Randomized double-blind comparison of chimeric monoclonal antibody to tumor necrosis factor alpha (infliximab) versus placebo in active spondyloarthropathy. Arthritis Rheum 46:755-765, 2002.
217. Van der Heijde, van der Linden S, Dougados M, et al: Ankylosing spondylitis: Plenary discussion and results of voting on selection of domains and some specific instruments. J Rheumatol 26:1003-1005, 1999.
218. Van der Horst-Bruinsma IE, Clegg DO, Dijkmans BAC: Treatment of ankylosing spondylitis with disease modifying antirheumatic drugs. Clin Exp Rheumatol 20(suppl 28):S67-S70, 2002.
219. van der Linden S, van Tubergen A, Hidding A: Physiotherapy in ankylosing spondylitis. Clin Exp Rheumatol 20(suppl 28)S60-S64, 2002.
220. Van Tubergen A, Coenen J, Landewe R, et al: Assessment of fatigue in patients with ankylosing spondylitis: A psychometric analysis. Arthritis Rheum 47:8, 2002.
221. Vilar MJP, Cury SE, Ferraz MB, et al: Renal abnormalities in ankylosing spondylitis. Scand J Rheumatol 26:19-23, 1997.
222. Warren RE, Brewerton DA: Faecal carriage of *Klebsiella* by patients with ankylosing spondylitis and rheumatoid arthritis. Ann Rheum Dis 39:37, 1980.
223. Weinstein PR, Karpman RR, Gall EP, et al: Spinal cord injury, spinal fracture, and spinal stenosis in ankylosing spondylitis. J Neurosurg 57:609, 1982.
224. Wholey MH, Pugh DG, Bickel WH: Localized destructive lesions in rheumatoid spondylitis. Radiology 74:54, 1960.
225. Wilkinson M, Bywaters EGL: Clinical features and course of ankylosing spondylitis as seen in a follow-up of 222 hospital referred cases. Ann Rheum Dis 17:209, 1958.
226. William F, Taylor AR, Arden GP, Edwards DH: Arthroplasty of the hip in ankylosing spondylitis. J Bone Joint Surg Br 59-B:393, 1977.
227. Williamson PK, Reginato AJ: Diffuse idiopathic skeletal hyperostosis of the cervical spine in a patient with ankylosing spondylitis. Arthritis Rheum 27:570, 1984.
228. Yagan R, Khan MA: Confusion of roentgenographic differential diagnosis of ankylosing hyperostosis (Forestier's disease) and ankylosing spondylitis. Spine St Art Rev 4:561, 1990.
229. Young JS, Cheshire DJE, Pierce JA, et al: Cervical ankylosis with acute spinal cord injury. Paraplegia 15:133, 1977.

PSORIATIC ARTHRITIS

CAPSULE SUMMARY

	LOW BACK	NECK
Frequency of spinal pain	Rare	Uncommon
Location of spinal pain	Sacroiliac joints and lumbar spine	Cervical spine
Quality of spinal pain	Ache	Ache
Symptoms and signs	Morning stiffness, rash with plaques, back tenderness, decreased motion	Morning stiffness, rash with plaques, neck tenderness, decreased motion
Laboratory tests	Increased erythrocyte sedimentation rate	Increased erythrocyte sedimentation rate
Radiographic findings	Nonmarginal syndesmophytes on plain roentgenogram, with or without sacroiliitis	Nonmarginal syndesmophytes on plain roentgenogram, with or without sacroiliitis
Treatment	Topical drugs, NSAIDs, methotrexate, tumor necrosis factor inhibitors	Topical drugs, NSAIDs, methotrexate, tumor necrosis factor inhibitors

PREVALENCE AND PATHOGENESIS

Patients with psoriasis and a characteristic pattern of joint disease have psoriatic arthritis (PsA). The French physicians Bazin and Bourdillon in the last century were the first to name the disease and describe it in detail.[12,17] In the United States, there was hesitancy in ascribing joint disease to psoriasis. Many physicians thought that two common diseases—psoriasis and rheumatoid arthritis (RA)—were occurring in patients simultaneously. More recent studies, however, have clearly demonstrated the association of psoriasis and arthritis.[122] Moll has suggested a working definition of the disease to include three components: psoriasis (skin or nail), inflammatory arthritis (peripheral or axial), and a negative test for rheumatoid factor.[77] However, the disease should be considered as a range, with components developing gradually. Some patients have inflammatory arthritis compatible with psoriatic disease before the appearance of skin lesions. Like reactive arthritis, incomplete forms of the disease are relevant to the clinical disease.

Epidemiology

Precise data concerning the prevalence of psoriasis are not available. Many patients with mild disease may never be seen by physicians. Therefore, only estimates of prevalence have been made; such estimates suggest that 1% to 3% of the population is affected by psoriasis. Psoriasis does, however, occur more commonly in people from temperate climate zones. The prevalence of psoriasis in the United States and Japan is similar. People from eastern and northern Africa are also similarly affected. Psoriasis is rare in southern and western Africa, as reflected by the low percentage of American blacks affected, most of whom originated from western Africa. Psoriatic arthritis occurs in 5% to 7% of individuals with psoriasis and in 0.1% of the general population.[7,55,111] Others have suggested a higher prevalence of arthritis—20% to 34%—in patients with psoriasis.[102,107,110] An epidemiologic study in Olmstead County, Minnesota, reported that 6.25% of psoriasis patients have arthritis.[105] Psoriasis and PsA occur with equal frequency in both sexes. In a study of 220 patients with PsA, 47% were men and 53% were women.[50]

Pathogenesis

The basic abnormality that results in increased metabolic activity of the skin is unknown. Some investigators believe that this abnormality resides in the most superficial layers of the skin (epidermis), whereas others believe that the inner layers of the skin (dermis) are the source of the increased metabolic activity. A psoriatic diathesis exists in patients who are at risk for disease. Abnormalities in protein synthesis, blood flow, and metabolism are present in normal-appearing skin, hair, and nails in these individuals. Experiments have shown a hyperproliferative effect on normal keratinocytes by psoriatic skin fibroblasts. These cells undergo unrestrained growth, which reflects the condition of the skin in vivo.[96]

Genetic Susceptibility

A genetic predisposition for the development of psoriasis and PsA does exist. Although a positive family history is obtained in about a third of patients with psoriasis, a definite pattern of inheritance has not been established. PsA occurs more frequently in family members than in unrelated controls.[78] Psoriasis is more concordant in monozygotic twins than dizygotic twins. The concordance in monozygotic twins is 35% to 70% versus 12% to 20% for dizygotic twins.[56] The skin disease of psoriasis has also been associated with HLA-B13, HLA-Bw17, HLA-Cw6, and HLA-DRw6.[73] Population studies have identified HLA-B13, HLA-B17, HLA-B37, HLA-Cw6, and HLA-DR7 as haplotypes associated with psoriasis.[42] Genetic factors also play a role in PsA. Patients with peripheral PsA have an increased frequency of HLA-Bw38, HLA-DR4, and HLA-DR7.[34] Others investigators have reported HLA-Bw57, HLA-Bw39, HLA-Bw6, and HLA-Bw7 associated with peripheral arthropathy.[13] Other reported haplotypes associated with PsA include HLA-B39 and HLA-DRB1*0402.[48,75] Psoriatic spondylitis is associated with an increased frequency of HLA-B27.[19]

The major psoriasis susceptibility gene resides on chromosome 6 near the HLA-C locus.[9,44] A non-HLA gene within the major histocompatibility complex (MHC) locus is associated with an increased susceptibility for psoriasis.[2] The HLA-Cw*0602 allele is increased in patients with PsA and is associated with an earlier age of onset of psoriasis.[45] The class I MHC chain–related gene A *(MICA)* adds to the susceptibility for psoriasis. The trinucleotide repeat polymorphism MICA-A9, which associates with the MICA-002 allele, is significantly higher in PsA patients, independent of Cw*0602. Patients with Cw*0602 and MICA-A9 have additional susceptibility to PsA.[101]

Patients with PsA versus psoriasis alone show an increased frequency of HLA-B7 and HLA-B27 and a lower frequency of HLA-DR7 and HLA-Cw7.[43] The frequency of HLA-B27 in PsA is not as high as in AS or reactive arthritis. Some patients with psoriatic spondylitis are HLA-B27 negative.

Immunologic Factors

The synovial joints in psoriasis patients may be more liable to damage because of an enzyme deficiency in synovial fluid.[113] Psoriatic synovium has fewer macrophages, a greater number of blood vessels, and less expression of endothelial adhesion molecule-1 than rheumatoid synovium does.[89] Arthroscopic evaluation of PsA knee joints demonstrates a combination of vessel dilation and increased tortuosity of capillary loops throughout the joint. RA vessels are straight-branching vessels limited to the capsule, synovium, and pannus.[38] Psoriatic synovium makes more tumor necrosis factor-alpha (TNF-alpha), interleukin-1 beta (IL-1 beta), IL-2, IL-10, and interferon-gamma and less IL-4 and IL-5 than RA synovium does.[90] Genetic control of cell growth may be impaired in psoriasis patients. The oncogene c-*myc* is expressed to a greater degree in the skin and synovium of psoriasis patients than in normal cells. The greater turnover of skin and synovial cells may be directly related to the role of oncogenes in cell proliferation.[12] The decline in the number of CD4+ cells may also play a role in the development of arthritis in light of the expression of more severe disease in individuals infected with human immunodeficiency virus (HIV).[5] CD8+ T cells are predominant in PsA in comparison to RA. Other immunologic abnormalities associated with psoriasis include increased levels of complement activation fragments, decreased T-cell subpopulations, lipoxygenase products, and local release of cytokines, including interferon-gamma.[80,94,95,115] TNF-alpha, IL-1, IL-6, and IL-8 are increased in psoriatic synovial fluid.

Environmental Factors

Other environmental factors, including infection with *Staphylococcus aureus* and *Clostridium perfringens* and delayed hypersensitivity, have also been suggested as important in the development of PsA.[65,70] Ribosomal RNA from group A streptococci is a common finding in the peripheral blood and joint fluid of PsA patients.[116] The question is whether the presence of streptococci is a primary or secondary event in the progression of psoriasis. Psoriatic skin plaques are easily infected.

Trauma

Like ankylosing spondylitis (AS) and reactive arthritis, PsA may develop after exposure to a number of environmental factors. Trauma has been reported by a number of investigators as the initiator of arthritis or osteolysis (bone loss) in psoriasis.[66,82,100,118] Chronic arthritis has developed after trauma to normal joints in patients with psoriasis uncomplicated by arthritis. In a comparison of environmental events immediately preceding the onset of arthritis, 12 patients (9%) with PsA versus 2 patients (1%) with RA had an acute traumatic event, including surgery, articular trauma, abortion, myocardial infarction, thrombophlebitis, or drug exposure.[25] Other authors have also described anecdotal accounts of trauma initiating PsA.[98] Synovial joints in psoriasis patients may be more liable to damage owing to an enzyme deficiency of synovial fluid.[25]

CLINICAL HISTORY

PsA has more than one clinical form, and this variability initially caused confusion in description of the illness (Table 11-6).[3,61,79] Classic PsA is described as involving only the distal interphalangeal (DIP) joints, along with associated nail disease. This pattern occurs in 5% of patients. The most common form of the disease, which affects 70% of patients with PsA, is an asymmetric oligoarthritis; a few large or small joints are involved. Dactylitis, or diffuse swelling of a digit, is most closely associated with this form of the disease. Skin activity and joint symptoms do not correlate—patients with little skin activity may experience continued joint pain and stiffness. As opposed to RA, the clinical appearance of an involved joint does not necessarily correlate with patient symptoms. Patients with severely affected joints may be asymptomatic. Symmetrical polyarthritis, which affects the small joints of the hands and feet and resembles RA, occurs in 15% of patients. Arthritis mutilans, characterized by extensive destruction of bone in the hands, is found in 5% of patients. Spondylitis with or without peripheral joint disease occurs in 5% of patients. HLA-B27 is more common in individuals with axial disease. In one study, axial disease was associated with an occurrence of HLA-B27 of 43% versus 11% for peripheral arthritis.[71]

In one report, clinical forms of PsA were simplified to three major types—asymmetric oligoarticular arthritis (54%), symmetrical arthritis (25%), and spondyloarthritis (21%).[61] DIP involvement occurred most commonly in the asymmetric oligoarthritis group and rarely in the spondyloarthropathy group. Arthritis mutilans occurred rarely in all groups.

Other large studies have reported on the subsets of PsA patients. These groups of patients are listed in Table 11-6.[3,114] The largest subset in all the studies is the group with asymmetric oligoarthritis. Spondyloarthropathy is found in a minority of patients ranging from 5% to 23% of those with PsA.

Patients in whom axial skeletal disease, sacroiliitis, or spondylitis develops are usually men who have an onset of psoriasis later in life.[64] Patients in whom PsA first develops before the age of 20 may be more susceptible to the development of arthritis mutilans. Low back pain indistinguishable from the pain associated with the other spondyloarthropathies is present in the vast majority of patients with axial skeletal disease. These patients may have back pain or peripheral joint symptoms as their initial complaint. Asymmetric or symmetrical peripheral joint involvement may antedate the development of axial skeletal disease. The number of psoriatic patients with involvement of the cervical spine varies from 45% to 70% of individuals.[60,97] The variation depends on the definition of involvement, characterized as clinical symptoms or radiographic abnormalities. In one study, 40% and, in another, 45% of PsA patients had symptoms of inflammatory cervical spine disease, including neck pain or prolonged stiffness.[60,97] Similar to a minority of patients with AS, psoriatic spondylitis patients may have no axial skeletal pain despite radiographic abnormalities. In a study of 70 individuals with psoriatic spondylitis, 20% were asymptomatic despite radiographic sacroiliitis or other abnormalities associated with psoriasis.[86]

The typical patient with the symmetrical or asymmetric form of PsA is a man or woman 35 to 45 years of age. Patients with more severe disease have an onset of symptoms at an earlier age manifested as inflammation in a few joints or diffuse swelling of an entire digit (dactylitis). Psoriasis antedates the arthritis in the majority of patients (Table 11-7).[91] From 10% to 20% of patients have characteristic arthritis before the appearance of psoriatic lesions. Patients with severe skin involvement are more susceptible to the development of arthritis.[67] However, even patients with minimal skin involvement still have some risk of joint disease. Patients with active peripheral PsA may be more likely to have moderate skin disease of the plaque type.[23] Nail involvement, characterized by pitting, horizontal ridging, onycholysis (opacification of the nail bed), and discoloration, occurs in 80% of patients with PsA, in contrast to a 30% incidence in patients with uncomplicated psoriasis. The activity of skin and nail disease does not necessarily correlate with joint symptoms because any of the forms of psoriatic skin disease, whether guttate, pustular, seborrheic, or others, may be associated with joint involvement.[32,123] Isolated spinal hyperostosis is a rare extracutaneous manifestation of psoriasis vulgaris.[88]

11-6 CLASSIFICATION OF PSORIATIC ARTHRITIS

Form	Incidence (%)
Asymmetric oligoarthritis	70
Symmetrical "rheumatoid arthritis–like"	15
Distal interphalangeal predominant	5
Arthritis mutilans	5
Psoriatic spondylitis	5

11-7 ONSET OF PSORIATIC ARTHRITIS

Sequence	Percentage of Cases
Psoriasis before arthritis	70
Psoriasis simultaneous with arthritis	20
Arthritis before psoriasis	10

Extra-articular Manifestations

Although constitutional symptoms of fever, anorexia, and weight loss are rare in patients with PsA, fatigue and morning stiffness are common. Ocular involvement includes conjunctivitis in 20%, iritis in 10%, and scleritis in 2% of patients with PsA.[63] Iritis is more commonly seen in patients with axial skeletal disease. In a 10-year study, 18% of PsA patients had iritis. Iritis occurred in patients with bilateral sacroiliitis, syndesmophytes, and HLA-DR13.[85] Cardiac complications, such as the aortic insufficiency as seen in AS, are rare and usually associated with spondylitis.[93]

PHYSICAL EXAMINATION

An extensive examination of the skin is an essential part of the investigation of a patient with suspected PsA. The diagnosis of psoriasis is not difficult to make when the patient has the characteristic erythematous, raised, circumscribed, dry scaling lesions over the elbows, knees, and scalp and pitting of the nails. Skin lesions may be hidden in the scalp, gluteal folds, perineum, rectum, or umbilicus and may remain undetected unless a complete skin examination is performed. Nails are examined for the presence of pitting, ridges, opacification, and hyperkeratosis.[51]

A complete musculoskeletal examination is essential for determining the extent of joint involvement. Patients may be asymptomatic in a specific joint, although physical examination demonstrates decreased function. The skin over affected joints may have a bluish tinge, in contrast to the skin color associated with RA.[59] Patients may have dactylitis of a toe and may be unaware of the change until pointed out by the physician. PsA patients may also have distal extremity swelling and pitting edema. In a study of 183 PsA patients and 366 controls, distal swelling was identified in 21% of PsA patients but in only 4.9% of controls. In 20% of this group, distal swelling was the initial manifestation of PsA.[21]

Examination of the axial skeleton should be completed even in an asymptomatic patient. Loss of spinal motion may be a manifestation of axial skeletal disease. Sacroiliac involvement may be unilateral or bilateral. Percussion over the sacroiliac joints can elicit symptoms over the affected side. Spondylitis may develop in the absence of sacroiliitis and is characterized by maximal tenderness with percussion over the spine above the sacrum. In the cervical spine, limitation of motion is a primary manifestation of neck involvement. Patients may have radiographic evidence of cervical spine arthritis with normal movement of the neck.[97]

LABORATORY DATA

The findings of anemia, mild leukocytosis, and an elevated erythrocyte sedimentation rate occur in a minority of patients.[8] C-reactive protein, an acute phase reactant, may be elevated. C-reactive protein is a marker of clinical disease activity and may be persistently elevated in those with extensive joint destruction.[112] An elevated uric acid level, hyperuricemia, is detected in 20% of patients. This abnormality may be secondary to an increased metabolic rate and protein breakdown in patients with extensive skin involvement. Secondary gout may develop in these patients. Psoriatic synovial fluid is inflammatory but has no diagnostic features. Rheumatoid factor and antinuclear antibody are usually absent; if present, they occur at the same frequency as found in age-matched controls. HLA-B27 is detected in approximately 35% to 60% of patients with axial skeletal disease.[18] In one study, patients with sacroiliitis and spondylitis were 90% positive for HLA-B27, and in another study, patients with spondylitis and normal sacroiliac joints were 43% positive.[19,64] In a study of 180 patients, 85% of those with bilateral sacroiliitis and 22% of those with asymmetric sacroiliitis were B27 positive.[3] Peripheral joint disease is associated with HLA-B38 and HLA-B39, and psoriasis alone is associated with HLA-B13, HLA-B17, and HLA-Cw6.[31,35]

RADIOGRAPHIC EVALUATION

Roentgenograms

Whereas the radiologic features of PsA and RA may be similar, certain features of the DIP and proximal interphalangeal (PIP) joints in PsA are distinctive.[6,121] The joint involvement is oligoarticular with erosive changes in the DIP joint and terminal phalanx, especially the big toe. The "pencil-in-cup" deformity, or osteolysis of the proximal phalanx and widening of the distal phalanx, is characteristic of PsA. Periosteal reaction occurs along the shafts of the long bones, as opposed to the periosteal changes in reactive arthritis, which are localized to the metatarsal and phalanges of the feet and hands.

Axial skeletal involvement was first emphasized by Dixon and Lience.[27] Up to 25% of patients have sacroiliac involvement manifested as sacroiliitis, which can be unilateral or bilateral.[54,69,72] Symmetrical involvement, from side to side and in the severity of disease, predominates over asymmetric disease. Sacroiliitis may occur without spondylitis (Fig. 11-14). Roentgenographic characteristics of sacroiliitis include erosions and sclerosis predominantly in the ilium, along with joint widening. Joint ankylosis occurs less commonly than in AS. Sacroiliitis with psoriasis has no roentgenographic changes that can be considered specific for the disease.[76] Spondylitis is characterized by asymmetric involvement of the vertebral bodies and nonmarginal syndesmophytes (Fig. 11-15). Spondylitis with normal sacroiliac joints may show up radiographically. Rare patients have been described with axial skeletal disease that mirrors the involvement characteristic of AS. Paravertebral ossification separated from the vertebral body may occur in the thoracolumbar region.[20] Squaring of vertebral bodies, osteitis of bone, and facet joint ankylosis occur less frequently in psoriatic spondylitis than in AS.[81] Progression of spinal disease occurs in a random rather than orderly fashion; it ascends the spine as commonly noted in AS.

In psoriatic spondylitis, the cervical spine is affected less frequently than the lumbar spine.[84] Cervical spine disease may occur in the absence of sacroiliitis or lumbar spondylitis.[97] Alterations in the cervical spine include joint

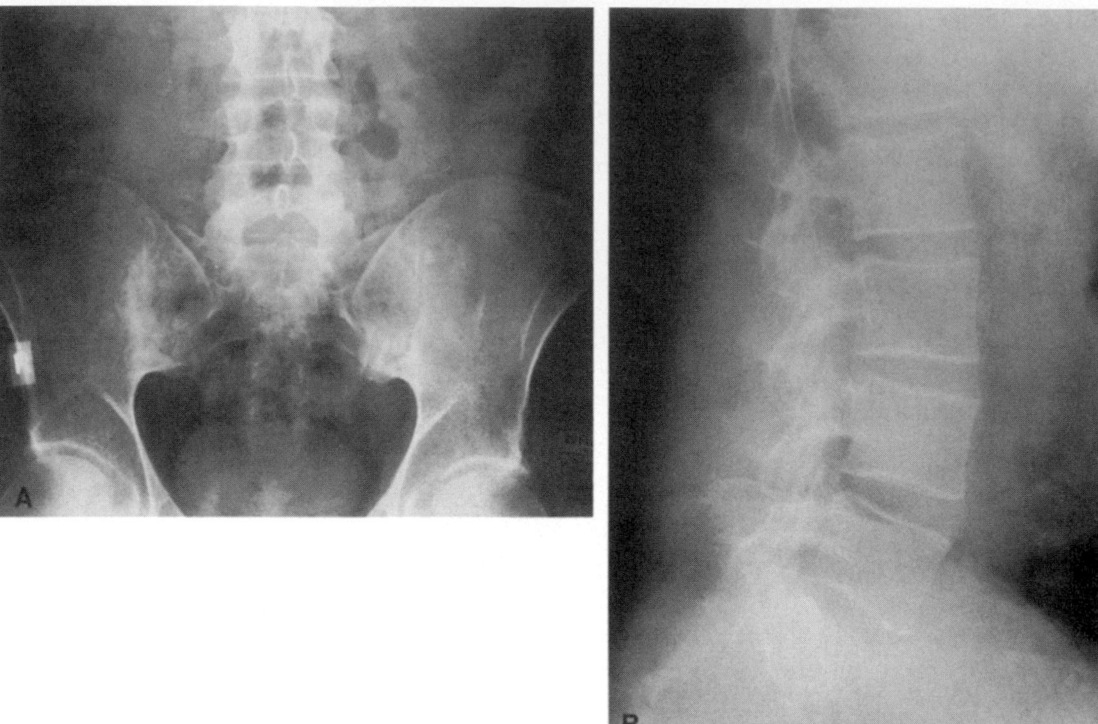

Figure 11-14 Psoriatic arthritis in a 36-year-old man with psoriasis, chronic back pain of 10 years' duration, and negative HLA-B27 antigen. *A*, An anteroposterior view of the pelvis reveals sacroiliac joint space narrowing, erosions, and sclerosis more prominent on the right than on the left. *B*, A lateral view of the lumbar spine is unremarkable, with no changes of spondylitis.

space sclerosis and narrowing and anterior ligamentous calcification.[62] This form of involvement follows the pattern of the spondyloarthropathies characterized by ankylosis and calcification (Fig. 11-16). These patients may have nonmarginal or marginal syndesmophytes. Another group of patients has disease characterized by erosions and subluxations in the absence of ligamentous calcifications, more reminiscent of the alterations associated with RA (see Fig. 11-16).[60] The "rheumatoid-like" group has subaxial subluxations and/or instability at the atlantoaxial joint.[16] Subluxations may occur without spinal cord compression.[97]

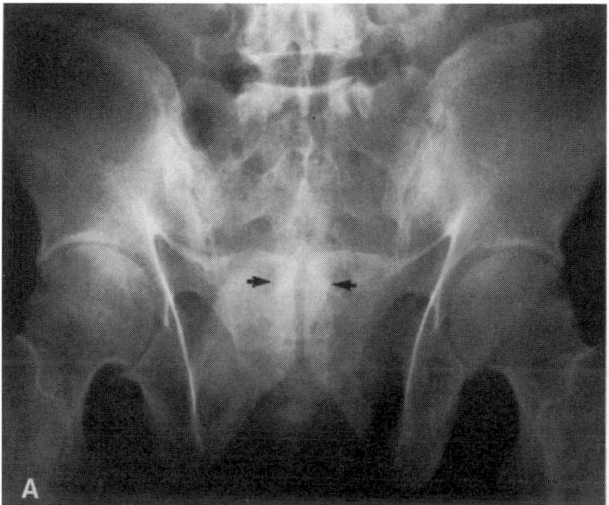

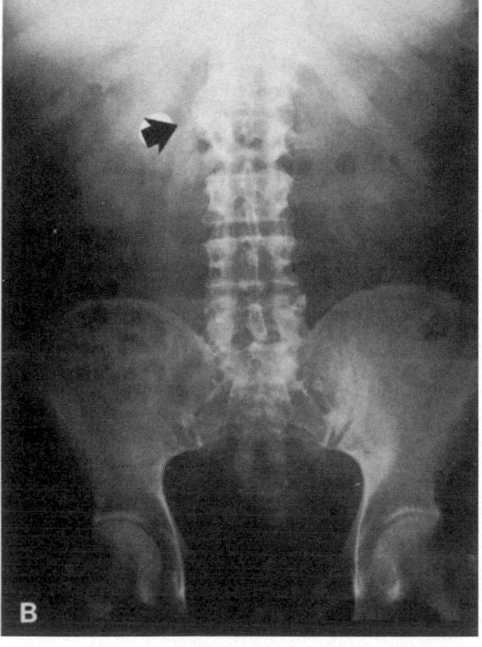

Figure 11-15 Psoriatic arthritis in a 55-year-old man with a 34-year history of the disease. *A*, A Ferguson view of the pelvis reveals bilateral sacroiliitis along with erosion and reactive sclerosis of the symphysis pubis *(arrows)*. *B*, An anteroposterior view of the lumbosacral spine demonstrates a large nonmarginal syndesmophyte connecting L1 and L2 *(arrow)*.

Scintigraphy, Computed Tomography, and Magnetic Resonance

As with the other spondyloarthropathies, a scintiscan may demonstrate increased activity over the sacroiliac joints or axial skeleton before radiographic changes are detectable.[10] Other radiographic techniques, CT or MR imaging, do not reveal specific abnormalities that help differentiate PsA patients from others. CT or MR imaging may be of value in patients with cervical spine arthritis and neurologic symptoms compatible with myelopathy or radiculopathy. These radiographic techniques can identify the occasional patient with psoriatic spondylitis and neural compression.

DIFFERENTIAL DIAGNOSIS

The diagnosis of PsA is easily made when the patient has the characteristic skin lesions and joint changes. The diagnosis is more difficult in a patient who has joint symptoms before the appearance of skin lesions. In addition, the diagnosis may be missed if the examining physician does not complete a careful search for hidden psoriatic skin lesions.[52] Although PsA can be differentiated from other spondyloarthropathies, specific diagnostic and classification criteria for PsA have not been validated.[39]

The differential diagnosis for such a patient should include reactive arthritis, gout, erosive osteoarthritis, and RA.[41] Reactive arthritis may be differentiated by urethritis, predominantly lower extremity involvement, and periosteal changes. Acute gout is confirmed by the detection of monosodium urate crystals in synovial fluid. Erosive osteoarthritis occurs in postmenopausal women and is characterized by inflammation of the DIP and PIP joints and radiographic findings of osteophytes, sclerosis, and cysts in these joints. The erythrocyte sedimentation rate remains normal. The clinical appearance of symmetrical polyarthritis in PsA and RA is similar. The absence of rheumatoid nodules and rheumatoid factor and the presence of DIP involvement and periostitis help differentiate a patient with PsA from one with RA (see Table 11-4).

TREATMENT

The goals of therapy are maintenance and improvement of function through a reduction in inflammation. Therapy includes patient education, nonsteroidal anti-inflammatory drugs (NSAIDs), immunosuppressives, biologic agents, and physical therapy.[74a]

Skin Care

The importance of appropriate skin care must be stressed. Whereas in the past no correlation between improvement in skin and joint symptoms could be demonstrated, a study reported improvement of nonspondylitic PsA in patients who responded to photochemotherapy for their skin disease.[83] A variety of topical therapies are available for control of localized skin disease. Topical therapies include emollients, salicylic acid, corticosteroids, tar shampoos, anthralin, vitamin D analogues, and retinoids. These remedies are particularly effective for the vast majority of individuals who have less than 5% of their body surface involved with psoriatic lesions.[117]

Medications

Nonsteroidal Anti-inflammatory Drugs

NSAIDs are useful in controlling pain and stiffness in the peripheral and axial joints. NSAIDs are given in maximal doses tolerated by patients to better control the inflammation associated with their joint disease (indomethacin, 150 mg/day, naproxen, 1500 mg/day, and sulindac, 400 mg/day). The drugs should be given for 4 to 6 weeks before deciding on the efficacy of the agent. A series of NSAIDs should be tried before deciding on the inefficacy of this group of drugs in an individual patient. The primary toxicity of NSAIDs is gastrointestinal. These agents do not increase the severity of psoriatic skin disease.[104] NSAIDs do not alter the progression of axial skeletal joint disease. However, they are helpful in decreasing joint stiffness and pain, thereby allowing greater spine motion. This benefit of joint motion should not be overlooked in the treatment of spondylitis patients. NSAIDs may allow greater ease in activities of daily living and may therefore improve patient comfort on a recurring basis.

Cyclooxygenase Inhibitors

Cyclooxygenase-2 (COX-2) inhibitors are a class of NSAIDs that have efficacy equal to that of combined COX-1 and COX-2 inhibitors (aspirin, naproxen) and less gastrointestinal toxicity. COX-2 inhibitors are effective in osteoarthritis and RA, as has been documented in double-blind, placebo-controlled trials. Similar benefits for PsA have not been systematically proved. Clinical experience suggests that PsA patients have similar benefits as other patients with polyarthritis.

Corticosteroids

Systemic corticosteroids are rarely used for skin or joint disease because a rebound phenomenon appears when use of the drug is discontinued.[57] Intra-articular corticosteroids are useful in patients with psoriatic monarthritis and persistent effusion, usually of the knee. Immunosuppressives and corticosteroids are more effective for control of peripheral arthritis than for axial skeletal disease.

Disease-Modifying Antirheumatic Drugs

Drugs with rash as a potential toxicity have been contraindicated in the past; however, recent studies have demonstrated the efficacy and lack of skin toxicity for hydroxychloroquine and gold salts.[29,61,99] These drugs are given in the same dose and frequency as used for RA patients and are most helpful in patients with refractory peripheral arthritis. Sulfasalazine has been studied for the treatment of PsA. Patients receiving the drug have had modest improvement, but with gastrointestinal and

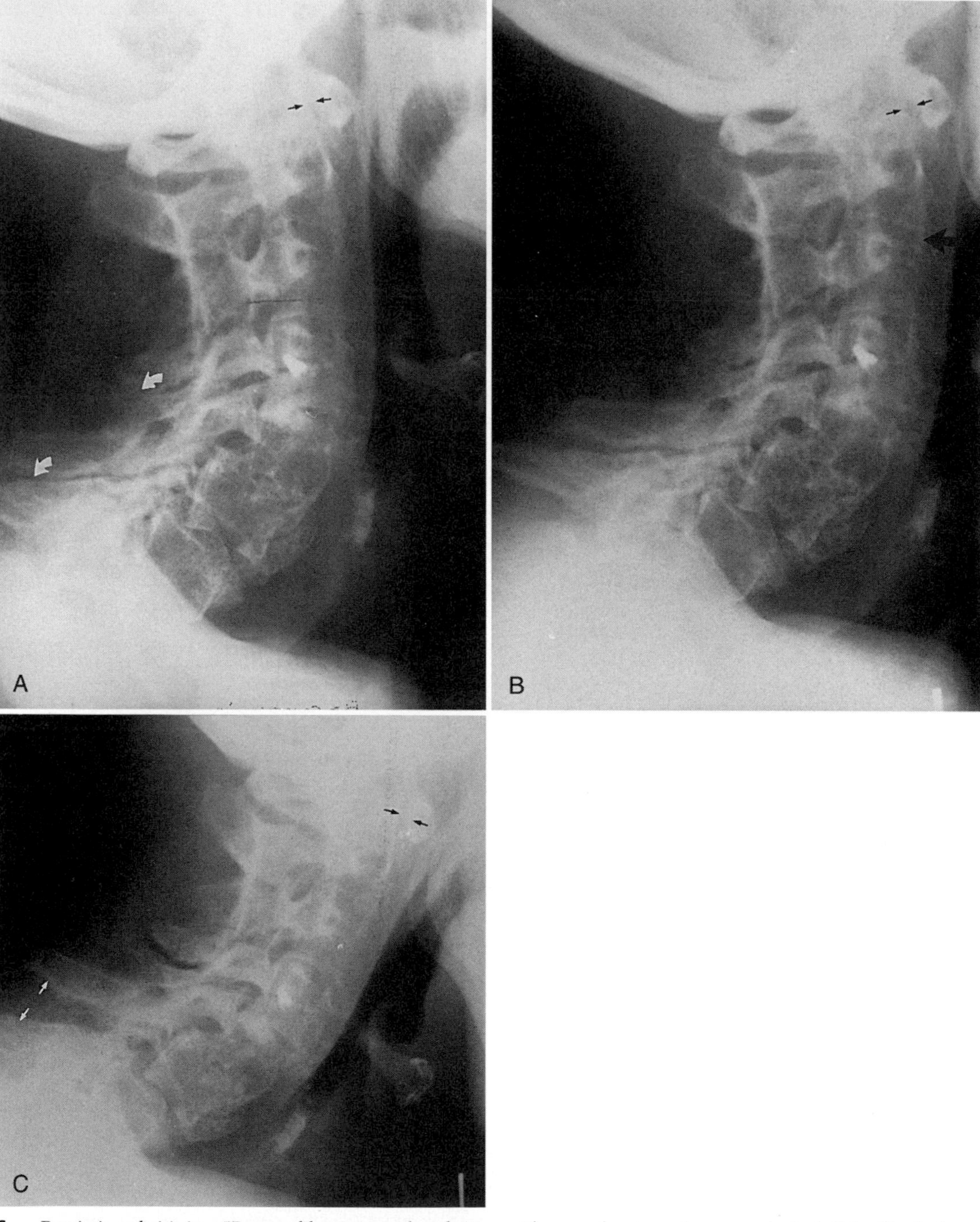

Figure 11-16 Psoriatic arthritis in a 57-year-old woman with arthritis mutilans, neck pain, and no neurologic deficits. She had seronegative polyarthritis for 20 years before a psoriatic rash appeared. *A*, Lateral view of the cervical spine, extension; *B*, neutral; *C*, flexion. Anterior syndesmophytes are present in *B* from C2 to C5 *(large black arrow)*. Fusion is present between the spinous process of C3–C4. Pseudoarticulation and erosion of the spinous processes of C4–C5 and C6–C7 can be seen in *A (curved white arrows)*. Atlantoaxial subluxation of 4 mm remains the same in all views *(small black arrows)*. Anterior subluxation with total loss of intervertebral disc space is noted at the C5–C6 interspace. The C6–C7 interspace is subluxed and mobile. With flexion of the neck, C6 moves forward on C7, and the distance between the spinous processes widens in *C (small white arrows)*. The triangular metal item is the tip of a knife remaining from a physical assault. At 61 years of age, she had increasing difficulty with walking and balance. Myelopathic symptoms with lower extremity paralysis developed. Decompression of the cervical spine was accomplished, but the patient expired during the postoperative period.

cutaneous toxicity. In general, sulfasalazine has not been recommended for PsA patients.[26]

In patients with severe and extensive skin disease and destructive arthritis, immunosuppressive therapy with methotrexate, 6-mercaptopurine, and azathioprine is indicated.[11,15,30] The drug 6-mercaptopurine is associated with excessive toxicity and has been supplanted by methotrexate for the treatment of PsA. Methotrexate is usually given orally (2.5 mg every 12 hours or as a single dose) for a total dose of 7.5 mg. It is given once a week to limit toxicity. Liver fibrosis is the most common serious side effect of methotrexate. Liver biopsy has been recommended in the past when the patient received 2 g of medicine.[92] However, the complications of liver biopsy outweigh the benefits associated with identifying the rare individual with liver fibrosis caused by methotrexate therapy. A cost analysis of liver biopsy did not demonstrate a definite benefit unless the risk of cirrhosis was high.[14] Only a few rheumatologists in Canada obtain liver biopsies before or after a cumulative dose of methotrexate.[24] Liver biopsy should be reserved for individuals with elevated liver function test results or complications such as hepatitis and ethanolism because such patients are at increased risk for cirrhosis.[14]

Methotrexate has been shown to be a safe, effective agent for the treatment of PsA. A multicenter study demonstrated methotrexate to be helpful in patients with psoriasis, as compared with control subjects, for improvement of skin lesions and subjective physician assessment.[119] A study of 40 patients documented control of peripheral arthritis and skin and nail disease in a majority of PsA patients.[36] These drugs have the potential for liver toxicity and leukopenia. Patients receiving this drug were monitored closely on a monthly basis.

Retinoids (vitamin A) have been associated with improvement in PsA,[37] but maintenance therapy was required to prevent relapse. Of interest is the observation that less psoralen treatment was needed to achieve a clinical response when it was used in conjunction with retinoids. The need for less psoralen for control of psoriasis may decrease the incidence of squamous cell cancer of the skin, which is noted in patients taking psoralens for an average of 5.7 years.[106]

Cyclosporine has been used in the treatment of PsA patients. The response to joint and skin disease was modest, but the renal toxicity was persistent. In addition, this drug is expensive when compared with other agents. The drug should be limited to only the most severely affected and to drug-resistant psoriatic patients.[28]

Anti–Tumor Necrosis Factor-Alpha Inhibitors

TNF is an inflammatory cytokine associated with the destructive process that results in the phenotypic expression of PsA. Anti-TNF therapies are available in the form of infliximab, etanercept, and adulimimab, and these drugs inhibit the inflammatory effects of TNF. Etanercept has been approved by the Food and Drug Administration as being safe and effective for the treatment of PsA. Etanercept, 25 mg subcutaneously twice a week for 24 weeks, has shown efficacy in 59% of PsA patients versus 15% of controls.[74] Infliximab has also demonstrated greater efficacy than placebo in PsA.[4] An effective dose was 5 mg/kg intravenously given at weeks 0, 2 and 6. Infliximab is also effective for control of cutaneous disease, particularly severe plaque-type disease.[22] The beneficial effects of the therapy can be sustained for 54 weeks with continued infusions. TNF inhibitors are associated with significant toxicity, including reactivation of tuberculosis and other bacterial infections. HIV infection can exacerbate the severity of psoriatic skin and joint disease. Psoriasis can improve dramatically with etanercept administered subcutaneously. However, the therapy can result in the development of frequent polymicrobial infections that require discontinuation of etanercept to resolve the infections.[1]

PROGNOSIS

The course of PsA is unpredictable.[91] Destructive, disabling disease develops in approximately 20% of patients.[40] The extent of radiologic damage may be similar in PsA and RA.[87] A survey found that women in whom symmetrical large- and small-joint disease developed had more destructive arthritis.[61] Progression of PsA is related to the number of actively inflamed and swollen joints and the number of medications taken before the patient's first physician visit.[47] In one large study, 97% of psoriatic patients were able to work at their jobs and missed less than 12 months of work during a minimum of a 10-year follow-up period.[91] Other groups of PsA patients have reported more severe impairments, similar to the disability and quality-of-life difficulties experienced by RA patients.[58,108] These studies point out the heterogeneous nature of PsA. In some patients the disease is mild. In others, PsA is as destructive and devastating as any form of generalized inflammatory arthritis. The frequency of remission is limited to a small minority of patients, 17% in one study.[49]

Varying degrees of restriction of spinal motion develop in patients with psoriatic spondylitis. No consistent correlation has been found between the severity of peripheral joint disease and axial skeletal disease. A study of patients with AS, psoriatic spondylitis, and enteropathic spondylitis found the psoriatic patients to be most severely affected.[33] Another study found AS patients to be more severely affected.[103] Other studies have demonstrated radiographic progression of spondylitis without an increase in symptoms or decreased spinal mobility.[53] The results of these studies leave the physician to monitor each patient to identify an individual course. PsA may not be as benign a disease as previously thought. Patients with a longer duration of disease or those with HLA-B39 and HLA-DR4 and radiocarpal erosions may be at increased risk for psoriatic spondyloarthropathy involving the cervical spine.[60,97] Atlantoaxial subluxation with evidence of cervical myelopathy may develop in patients with PsA on rare occasion.[68] Greater respect should be given to the destructive potential of this disorder. Patients with psoriatic spondylitis and fusion of the cervical spine have a risk similar to that of AS patients. Fracture after minor trauma may be overlooked for an extended period.[109] Patients with this disease should be treated earlier and more aggressively.[40] Patients with PsA and more active and severe disease at initial evaluation have increased mortality in comparison to the general population.[46,120]

References

Psoriatic Arthritis

1. Aboulafia DM, Bundow D, Wilske K, et al: Etanercept for the treatment of human immunodeficiency virus–associated psoriatic arthritis. Mayo Clin Proc 75:1093-1098, 2000.
2. Allen MH, Veal C, Faassen A, et al: A non-HLA gene within the MHC in psoriasis. Lancet 353:1589-1590, 1999.
3. Alonso JCT, Perez AR, Castrillo AMA, et al: Psoriatic arthritis (PA): A clinical, immunological and radiological study of 180 patients. Br J Rheumatol 30:245, 1991.

4. Antoni C, Manger B: Infliximab for psoriasis and psoriatic arthritis. Clin Exp Rheumatol 20(suppl 28):S122-S125, 2002.
5. Arnett FC, Reveille JD, Duvic M: Psoriasis and psoriatic arthritis associated with human immunodeficiency virus infection. Rheum Dis Clin North Am 17:59, 1991.
6. Avila R, Pugh DG, Slocumb CH, Winkelman RK: Psoriatic arthritis: A roentgenographic study. Radiology 75:691, 1960.
7. Baker H: Epidemiological aspects of psoriasis and arthritis. Br J Dermatol 78:249, 1966.
8. Baker H, Golding DH, Thompson M: Psoriasis and arthritis. Ann Intern Med 58:909, 1963.
9. Balendran N, Clough RL, Arguello JR, et al: Characterization of the major susceptibility region for psoriasis at chromosome 6p21.3. J Invest Dermatol 113:322-328, 1999.
10. Barraclough D, Russell AS, Percy JS: Psoriatic spondylitis: A clinical radiological and scintiscan survey. J Rheumatol 4:282, 1977.
11. Baum J, Hurd E, Lewis D, et al: Treatment of psoriatic arthritis with 6-mercaptopurine. Arthritis Rheum 16:139, 1973.
12. Bazin P: Leçons Theoriques et Cliniques sur les Affections Cutane es de Nature Arthritique et Darteux. Paris, Delahaye, 1860, pp 154-161.
13. Beaulieu AD, Roy R, Mathon G, et al: Psoriatic arthritis: Risk factors for patients with psoriasis—a study based on histocompatibility antigen frequencies. J Rheumatol 10:633, 1983.
14. Bergquist SR, Felson DT, Prashker MJ, Freedberg KA: The cost-effectiveness of liver biopsy in rheumatoid arthritis patients treated with methotrexate. Arthritis Rheum 38:326, 1995.
15. Black RL, O'Brien WM, Van Scott EJ, et al: Methotrexate therapy in psoriatic arthritis: Double-blind study in 21 patients. JAMA 189:743, 1964.
16. Blau R, Kaufman RL: Erosive and subluxing cervical spine disease in patients with psoriatic arthritis. J Rheumatol 14:111, 1987.
17. Bourdillon C: Psoriasis et Arthropathies. Paris, These, 1888.
18. Brewerton DA, Coffrey M, Nicholls A, et al: HLA-B27 and arthropathies associated with ulcerative colitis and psoriasis. Lancet 1:956, 1974.
19. Buckley WR, Raleigh RL: Psoriasis with acro-osteolysis. N Engl J Med 261:539, 1959.
20. Bywaters EGL, Dixon ASJ: Paravertebral ossification in psoriatic arthritis. Ann Rheum Dis 24:313, 1965.
21. Cantini F, Salvarani C, Olivieri I, et al: Distal extremity swelling with pitting edema in psoriatic arthritis: A case-control study. Clin Exp Rheumatol 19:291-296, 2001.
22. Chaudhari U, Romano P, Mulcahy LD, et al: Efficacy and safety of infliximab monotherapy for plaque-type psoriasis: A randomized trial. Lancet 357:1842-1847, 2001.
23. Cohen MR, Reda DJ, Clegg DO: Baseline relationships between psoriasis and psoriatic arthritis: Analysis of 221 patients with active psoriatic arthritis. J Rheumatol 26:1752-1756, 1999.
24. Collins D, Bellamy N, Campbell J: A Canadian survey of current methotrexate prescribing practices in rheumatoid arthritis. J Rheumatol 21:1220, 1994.
25. Cotton DWK, Mier PD: An hypothesis on the aetiology of psoriasis. Br J Dermatol 76:519, 1969.
26. Cuellar ML, Citera G, Espinoza LR: Treatment of psoriatic arthritis. Baillieres Clin Rheumatol 8:483, 1994.
27. Dixon AS, Lience E: Sacroiliac joint in adult rheumatoid arthritis and psoriatic arthropathy. Ann Rheum Dis 20:247, 1961.
28. Donnelly S, Doyle DV: Cyclosporin A (CyA)—long-term assessment of tolerability in psoriatic arthritis. Br J Dermatol 3(suppl):25, 1992.
29. Dorwart BB, Gall EP, Schumacher HR, Krauser RE: Chrysotherapy in psoriatic arthritis: Efficacy and toxicity compared to rheumatoid arthritis. Arthritis Rheum 21:513, 1978.
30. DuVivier A, Munro DD, Verbov J: Treatment of psoriasis with azathioprine. BMJ 1:49, 1974.
31. Eastmond CJ: Genetics and HLA antigens. Baillieres Clin Rheumatol 8:263, 1994.
32. Eastmoral CJ, Wright V: Nail dystrophy of psoriatic arthritis. Ann Rheum Dis 38:226, 1979.
33. Edmunds L, Elswood J, Kennedy LG, et al: Primary ankylosing spondylitis, psoriatic and enteropathic spondyloarthropathy: A controlled analysis. J Rheumatol 118:696, 1991.
34. Espinoza LR, Vasey FB, Gaylord SW, et al: Histocompatibility typing in the seronegative spondyloarthropathies: A survey. Semin Arthritis Rheum 11:375, 1982.
35. Espinoza LR, Vasey FB, Oh JH, et al: Association between HLA-Bw38 and peripheral psoriatic arthritis. Arthritis Rheum 21:72, 1978.
36. Espinoza LR, Zaraoui L, Espinoza CG, et al: Psoriatic arthritis: Clinical response and side effects to methotrexate therapy. J Rheumatol 19:872, 1992.
37. Farber EM, Abel EA, Charuworn A: Recent advances in the treatment of psoriasis. J Am Acad Dermatol 8:311, 1983.
38. Fioco L, Cozzi L, Chieco-Bianchi F, et al: Vascular changes in psoriatic knee joint synovitis. J Rheumatol 28:2480-2486, 2001.
39. Gladman DD: Current concepts in psoriatic arthritis. Curr Opin Rheumatol 14:361-366, 2002.
40. Gladman DD: Natural history of psoriatic arthritis. Baillieres Clin Rheumatol 8:379-394, 1994.
41. Gladman DD: Psoriatic arthritis. Rheum Dis Clin North Am 24:829-844, 1998.
42. Gladman DD: Psoriatic arthritis: Recent advances in pathogenesis and treatment. Rheum Dis Clin North Am 18:247, 1992.
43. Gladman DD, Anhorn KA, Schachter RK, et al: HLA antigens in psoriatic arthritis. J Rheumatol 13:586-592, 1986.
44. Gladman DD, Cheung C, Ng CM, et al: HLA-C locus alleles in patients with psoriatic arthritis (PsA). Hum Immunol 60:259-261, 1999.
45. Gladman DD, Farewell VT, Hustead J, et al: Mortality studies in psoriatic arthritis. Results from a single center. II. Prognostic indicators for mortality. Arthritis Rheum 41:1103-1048, 1998.
46. Gladman DD, Farewell VT, Kopciuk K, et al: HLA antigens and progression in psoriatic arthritis. J Rheumatol 25:730 -733 1998.
47. Gladman DD, Farewell VT, Nadeau C: Clinical indicators of progression in psoriatic arthritis (PSA): Multivariate relative risk model. J Rheumatol 22:675-679, 1995.
48. Gladman DD, Farewell VT, Rahman P, et al: HLA-DRB1*04 alleles in psoriatic arthritis: Comparison with rheumatoid arthritis and healthy controls. Hum Immunol 62:1239-1244, 2001.
49. Gladman DD, Hing ENT, Schentag CT, et al: Remission in psoriatic arthritis. J Rheumatol 28:1045-1048, 2001.
50. Gladman DD, Shuckett R, Russell ML, et al: Psoriatic arthritis (PSA): An analysis of 220 patients. Q J Med 238:127, 1987.
51. Goodfield M: Skin lesions in psoriasis. Baillieres Clin Rheumatol 8:295, 1994.
52. Gorter S, Der Heijde DM, van Der LS, et al: Psoriatic arthritis: Performance of rheumatologists in daily practice. Ann Rheum Dis 61:219-224, 2002.
53. Hanly JG, Russell ML, Gladman DD: Psoriatic spondyloarthropathy: A long-term prospective study. Ann Rheum Dis 47:386, 1988.
54. Harvie JN, Lester RS, Little AH: Sacroiliitis in severe psoriasis. AJR Am J Roentgenol 127:579, 1976.
55. Hellgren L: Association between rheumatoid arthritis and psoriasis in total populations. Acta Rheum Scand 15:316, 1969.
56. Hohler T, Marker-Hermann E: Psoriatic arthritis: Clinical aspects, genetics, and the role of T cells. Curr Opin Rheumatol 13:273-279, 2001.
57. Hollander JL, Brown EM, Jessar RA, et al: The effect of triamcinolone on psoriatic arthritis: A two-year study. Arthritis Rheum 2:513, 1959.
58. Hustead JA, Gladman DD, Farewell VT, et al: Health-related quality of life of patients with psoriatic arthritis: Comparison with patients with rheumatoid arthritis. Arthritis Rheum 45:151-158, 2001.
59. Jajic I: Blue coloured skin in psoriatic arthritis. Clin Rheumatol 20:304-305, 2001.
60. Jenkinson T, Armas J, Evison G, et al: The cervical spine in psoriatic arthritis: A clinical and radiological study. Br J Rheumatol 33:255, 1994.
61. Kammer GM, Soter WA, Gibson DJ, Schur PH: Psoriatic arthritis: A clinical, immunologic and HLA study of 100 patients. Semin Arthritis Rheum 9:75, 1979.
62. Kaplan D, Plotz CM, Nathanson L, Frank L: Cervical spine in psoriasis and in psoriatic arthritis. Ann Rheum Dis 23:50, 1964.
63. Lambert JR, Wright V: Eye inflammation in psoriatic arthritis. Ann Rheum Dis 35:354, 1976.
64. Lambert JR, Wright V: Psoriatic spondylitis: A clinical radiological description of the spine in psoriatic arthritis. Q J Med 46:411, 1977.
65. Landau JW, Gross BG, Newcomer VD, Wright ET: Immunologic response of patients with psoriasis. Arch Dermatol 91:607, 1965.
66. Langevitz P, Buskila D, Gladman DD: Arthritis precipitated by physical trauma. J Rheumatol 17:695, 1990.

67. Leczinsky CG: The incidence of arthropathy in a ten-year series of psoriasis cases. Acta Derm Venereol 28:483, 1948.
68. Lee S, Lui T: Psoriatic arthritis with C1-C2 subluxation as a neurosurgical complication. Surg Neurol 26:428, 1986.
69. Maldonado-Cocco JA, Porrini A, Garcia-Morteo O: Prevalence of sacroiliitis and ankylosing spondylitis in psoriasis patients. J Rheumatol 5:311, 1978.
70. Mansson I, Olhagen B: Intestinal *Clostridium perfringens* in rheumatoid arthritis and other connective tissue disorders: Studies of fecal flora, serum antitoxin levels, and skin hypersensitivity. Acta Rheum Scand 12:167, 1966.
71. Marsal S, Armadans-Gil L, Martinez M, et al: Clinical, radiographic and HLA association as markers for different patterns of psoriatic arthritis. Rheumatology 38:332-337, 1999.
72. McEwen C, DiTata D, Lingg C, et al: Ankylosing spondylitis and spondylitis accompanying ulcerative colitis, regional enteritis, psoriasis and Reiter's disease: A comparative study. Arthritis Rheum 14:291, 1971.
73. McKendry RJR, Sengar DPS, DesGroseilliers JP, Dunne JV: Frequency of HLA antigens in patients with psoriasis or psoriatic arthritis. Can Med Assoc J 130:411, 1984.
74. Mease P: Psoriatic arthritis: The role of TNF inhibition and the effect of its inhibition with etanercept. Clin Exp Rheumatol 20(suppl 28):S116-S121, 2002.
74a. Mease PJ: Current treatment of psoriatic arthritis. Rheum Dis Clin North Am 29:495-511, 2003.
75. Metzger AL, Morris RI, Bluestone R, Teraski PI: HLA-W27 in psoriatic arthropathy. Arthritis Rheum 18:111, 1975.
76. Molin L: Sacroiliitis in psoriasis. Scand J Rheumatol Suppl 32:133, 1979.
77. Moll JMH: The place of psoriatic arthritis in the spondarthritides. Baillieres Clin Rheumatol 8:465, 1994.
78. Moll JMH, Wright V: Familial occurrence of psoriatic arthritis. Ann Rheum Dis 32:181, 1973.
79. Moll JMH, Wright V: Psoriatic arthritis. Semin Arthritis Rheum 3:55, 1973.
80. O'Connell PG, Gerber LH, Digiovanna JJ, Peck GL: Arthritis in patients with psoriasis treated with gamma-interferon. J Rheumatol 19:80, 1992.
81. Oriente P, Biondi-Oriente C, Scarpa R: Clinical manifestations. Baillieres Clin Rheumatol 8:277, 1994.
82. Pages M, Lassoued S, Fournile B, et al: Psoriatic arthritis precipitated by physical trauma: Destructive arthritis or associated with reflex sympathetic dystrophy? J Rheumatol 19:185, 1992.
83. Perlman SG, Gerber LH, Roberts RM, et al: Photochemotherapy and psoriatic arthritis: A prospective study. Ann Intern Med 91:717, 1979.
84. Porter GG: Plain radiology and other imaging techniques. Baillieres Clin Rheumatol 8:465, 1994.
85. Queiro R, Belzunegui J, Gonzalez C, et al: Clinically asymptomatic axial disease in psoriatic spondyloarthropathy: A retrospective study. Clin Rheumatol 21:10-13, 2002.
86. Queiro R, Torre JC, Belzunegui J, et al: Clinical features and predictive factors in psoriatic-related uveitis. Semin Arthritis Rheum 31:264-270, 2002.
87. Rahman P, Nguyen E, Cheung C, et al: Comparison of radiological severity in psoriatic arthritis and rheumatoid arthritis. J Rheumatol 28:1041-1044, 2001.
88. Rahman P, Alderdice C, Curtis B, et al: Spinal hyperostosis—a rare skeletal manifestation of psoriasis vulgaris. J Rheumatol 27:2513-2515, 2000.
89. Reveille JD: The interplay of nature versus nurture in predisposition to the rheumatic diseases. Rheum Dis Clin North Am 19:15, 1993.
90. Ritchlin C, Haas-Smith SA, Hicks D, et al: Patterns of cytokine production in psoriatic synodium. J Rheumatol 25:1544-1552, 1998.
91. Roberts MET, Wright V, Hill AGS, Mehra AC: Psoriatic arthritis: Follow-up study. Ann Rheum Dis 35:206, 1976.
92. Roenigk HH, Auerbach RM, Mailbach HI, Weinstein GD: Methotrexate guidelines revised. J Am Acad Dermatol 6:145, 1982.
93. Roller DH, Muna WF, Ross AM: Psoriasis, sacroiliitis and aortitis. Chest 75:641, 1979.
94. Rosenberg EW, Noah PW, Wyatt RJ, et al: Complement activation in psoriasis. Clin Exp Dermatol 15:16, 1990.
95. Rubins AY, Merson AG: Subpopulations of T lymphocytes in psoriasis patients and their changes during immunotherapy. J Am Acad Dermatol 17:972, 1987.
96. Saiag P, Coulomb B, Lebreton C, et al: Psoriatic fibroblasts induce hyperproliferation of normal keratinocytes in a skin equivalent model in vitro. Science 230:669, 1985.
97. Salvarani C, Macchioni P, Cremonesi W, et al: The cervical spine in patients with psoriatic arthritis: A clinical, radiological and immunogenetic study. Ann Rheum Dis 51:73, 1992.
98. Sandorfi N, Freundlich B: Psoriatic and seronegative inflammatory arthropathy associated with a traumatic onset: 4 cases and a review of the literature. J Rheumatol 24:187, 1997.
99. Sayers ME, Mazanec DJ: Use of antimalarial drugs for the treatment of psoriatic arthritis. Am J Med 93:474, 1992.
100. Scarpa R, Del Puente A, di Girolamo C, et al: Interplay between environmental factors, articular involvement, and HLA-B27 in patients with psoriatic arthritis. Ann Rheum Dis 51:78, 1992.
101. Scarpa R, Mathieu A: Psoriatic arthritis: Evolving concepts. Curr Opin Rheumatol 12:274-280, 2000.
102. Scarpa R, Oriente P, Pucino A, et al: Psoriatic arthritis in psoriatic patients. Br J Rheumatol 23:246, 1984.
103. Scarpa R, Oriente P, Pucino A, et al: The clinical spectrum of psoriatic spondylitis. Br J Rheumatol 27:133, 1988.
104. Scarpa R, Pucino A, Iocco M, et al: The management of 138 psoriatic arthritis patients. Acta Derm Venereol 146:199, 1989.
105. Shbeeb M, Uramoto KM, Gibson LE, et al: Epidemiology of psoriatic arthritis in Olmstead County, Minnesota, USA, 1982-1991. J Rheumatol 27:1247-1250, 2000.
106. Skern RS, Laud N, Melski J, et al: Cutaneous squamous cell carcinoma in patients treated with PUVA. N Engl J Med 310:1156, 1984.
107. Smiley JD: Psoriatic arthritis. Bull Rheum Dis 44:1, 1995.
108. Sokoll KB, Helliwell PS: Comparison of disability and quality of life in rheumatoid and psoriatic arthritis. J Rheumatol 28:1842-1846, 2001.
109. Sosner J, Fast A, Kahan BS: Odontoid fracture and C1-C2 subluxation in psoriatic cervical spondyloarthropathy. Spine 21:519-521, 1996.
110. Stern RS: The epidemiology of joint complaints in patients with psoriasis. J Rheumatol 12:315, 1985.
111. Taylor WJ: Epidemiology of psoriatic arthritis. Curr Opin Rheumatol 14:98-103, 2002.
112. Troughton PR, Morgan AW: Laboratory findings and pathology of psoriatic arthritis. Baillieres Clin Rheumatol 8:439, 1994.
113. Veale D, Yanni G, Rogers S, et al: Reduced synovial membrane macrophage numbers, ELAM-1 expression, and lining layer hyperplasia in psoriatic arthritis as compared with RA. Arthritis Rheum 36:893, 1993.
114. Veale D, Rogers S, Fitzgerald O: Classification of clinical subsets in psoriatic arthritis. Br J Rheumatol 33:133, 1994.
115. Voorhees JJ: Leukotrienes and other lipoxygenase products in the pathogenesis and therapy of psoriasis and other dermatoses. Arch Dermatol 119:541, 1983.
116. Wang G, Vasey FB, Mahfood JP, et al: V2 regions of 16S ribosomal RNA used as a molecular marker for the species identification of streptococci in peripheral blood and synovial fluid from patients with psoriatic arthritis. Arthritis Rheum 42:2055-2059, 1999.
117. Whitman PM: Topical therapies for localized psoriasis. Mayo Clin Proc 76:943-949, 2001.
118. Williams KA, Scott JT: Influence of trauma on the development of chronic inflammatory polyarthritis. Ann Rheum Dis 26:532, 1967.
119. Willkens RF, Williams JH, Ward JR, et al: Randomized, double-blind, placebo-controlled trial of low-dose pulse methotrexate in psoriatic arthritis. Arthritis Rheum 27:376, 1984.
120. Wong K, Gladman DD, Hustead J, et al: Mortality studies in psoriatic arthritis. Results from a single center. I. Risk and causes of death. Arthritis Rheum 40:1868-1872, 1997.
121. Wright V: Psoriatic arthritis: A comparative study of rheumatoid arthritis and arthritis associated with psoriasis. Ann Rheum Dis 20:123, 1961.
122. Wright V: Rheumatism and psoriasis: A re-evaluation. Am J Med 27:454, 1959.
123. Wright V, Roberts MD, Hill AGS: Dermatologic manifestations in psoriatic arthritis: A follow-up study. Acta Derm Venereol 59:235, 1979.

REACTIVE ARTHRITIS

CAPSULE SUMMARY

	LOW BACK	NECK
Frequency of spinal pain	Very common	Rare
Location of spinal pain	Sacroiliac joints and lumbar spine	Cervical spine
Quality of spinal pain	Ache	Ache
Symptoms and signs	Morning stiffness, conjunctivitis, urethritis, decreased spinal motion	Morning stiffness, conjunctivitis, urethritis, decreased spinal motion
Laboratory tests	Increased erythrocyte sedimentation rate	Increased erythrocyte sedimentation rate
Radiographic findings	Sacroiliitis and/or spondylitis on plain roentgenogram	Spondylitis on plain roentgenogram
Treatment	Exercises, NSAIDs, antibiotics	Exercises, NSAIDs, antibiotics

PREVALENCE AND PATHOGENESIS

Reactive arthritis is a disease associated with an infectious agent causing aseptic inflammation in joints and other organs. This disorder has been associated with the triad of urethritis (inflammation of the lower urinary tract), arthritis, and conjunctivitis. This triad of disease manifestations has been named *Reiter's syndrome*. which is a form of reactive arthritis. However, Reiter's syndrome is no longer the preferred name for this entity. The name has been changed because Hans Reiter was not the first physician to describe this triad. Hans Reiter has also been associated with Nazi medical experiments. Some physicians in the medical community have questioned the propriety of having a medical syndrome associated with this individual.[100]

Reactive arthritis is the most common cause of arthritis in young men and primarily affects the lower extremity joints and the low back region. Involvement of the cervical spine is rare. The disease results from the interaction of an environmental factor, usually a specific infection, and a genetically predisposed host. The course of the disease, though usually benign, may be chronic and remitting and result in significant disability.

Many physicians, including Hippocrates, have written about the apparent relationship between venereal and gastrointestinal infections and the development of arthritis. In 1916, Fiessinger and Leroy, as well as Reiter, described young soldiers with an acute febrile illness that included conjunctivitis, urethritis, and polyarthritis appearing after a dysenteric illness.[32,82] However, the triad and the term Reiter's syndrome were not associated until Bauer and Engleman in 1942 referred to the findings of urethritis, conjunctivitis, and arthritis in World War II soldiers as Reiter's disease.[12]

Epidemiology

Reactive arthritis occurs throughout the world and has no racial or ethnic predilection. The syndrome develops in approximately 1% of patients with the common infection nongonococcal urethritis.[26] Others suggest that reactive arthritis develops in about 3% of individuals with nonspecific urethritis.[46] The syndrome develops in 0.2% to 15% of all patients with enteric infections secondary to *Shigella*, *Salmonella*, *Campylobacter*, and *Yersinia*.[73] In a recent epidemic of *Salmonella* infection in Finland, reactive arthritis was diagnosed in 6.9% of exposed individuals.[63] In another example, reactive arthritis developed in 19 of 260 (7.3%) individuals infected with *Salmonella typhimurium*.[44] In an outbreak of *Salmonella enteritidis* in Sweden, reactive arthritis developed in 15% of those infected.[5]

The male-to-female ratio in venereal infection is in the range of 10:1, and the ratio is 1:1 in large outbreaks secondary to enteric infection. The ratio may also be 1:1 in patients with no antecedent infection or in those in whom the urogenital symptoms may be a manifestation of the disease instead of a primary infection.[72,105] In one study, the incidence was 3.5 per 100,000 men younger than 50 years.[69]

Pathogenesis

The etiology of reactive arthritis is unknown. However, the relationship of the environment to genetics is crucial in the pathogenesis of the illness.[19] Initiation of the disease is thought to be related to dysenteric (epidemic) or venereal (endemic) infections. The joint inflammation associated with reactive arthritis can be due to a variety of mechanisms.[95] Organisms may be arthrotropic and cause a septic process in a joint. Alternatively, organisms may be expired but elicit a cytokine respone. The foreign antigen may persist in the affected joint. In another scenario, the organism may persist intracellularly in cells that are incapable of mechanisms to kill the organism. The molecular mimicry theory hypothesizes that host and pathogen antigens are so similar that the inflammatory response directed at the pathogen results in host damage. Pathogens enter the body through mucosal surfaces protected by IgA. These mechanisms suggest that an impaired immune system that is incapable of removing pathogenic antigens is at risk for development of this arthropathy.

The postdysenteric form of reactive arthritis follows infections by *Shigella dysenteriae* and *Shigella flexneri*,

S. enteritidis, *Yersinia enterocolitica*, and *Campylobacter jejuni*.[40,45,54,78,96,99] Bacterial components of gram-negative organisms associated with reactive arthritis are arthrogenic. DNA from the organism may not be required to elicit an inflammatory response. For example, these organisms possess common antigens, such as lipopolysaccharide (LPS). LPS has been detected in the inflamed joints of patients with reactive arthritis. Intracellular LPS stimulates lymphocytes to produce cytokines and thereby results in inflammation.[59] Peripheral blood mononuclear cells (PBMCs) may carry enteric pathogens to the joint. The lower extremity distribution of reactive arthritis may be related to the recruitment of PBMCs to more traumatized, weight-bearing joints.[95] DNA from *Salmonella* and *Campylobacter* may be present in joints.[90]

The relationship of sexually acquired genital infections with *Chlamydia trachomatis* and *Ureaplasma urealyticum* and the development of joint disease is not clearly established.[44] Although the evidence for *Ureaplasma* is weak, increasing evidence in the medical literature has connected the pathogenesis of reactive arthritis with *Chlamydia* infection.[80] *Chlamydia*-induced arthritis is associated with nonreplicative, but live bacteria that persist in the joint.[104] Outer membrane protein 2 from *Chlamydia* is implicated in the development of joint inflammation.[77] The organism induces the release of proinflammatory cytokines, which perpetuate synovial inflammation.[52a]

The distinction of urethritis as an initiating event and as an integral manifestation of the syndrome is a difficult one to make. Patients with enteric infections contract urethritis without urethral infection.[78] *C. trachomatis* is cultured in 50% to 69% of patients with reactive arthritis at the onset of joint disease.[48,51] Patients with reactive arthritis may also a have higher prevalence and titer of antichlamydial antibodies and may demonstrate higher lymphocyte transformation stimulation indices than control subjects do.[62] No correlation was found between reactive arthritis and *Mycoplasma hominis* or *U. urealyticum* infection by the same authors.[62] The role of *Neisseria gonorrhoeae* in reactive arthritis is not clear because 40% of patients with gonococcal infection also have chlamydial infection simultaneously.[42]

Trauma

Reactive arthritis may develop in patients who deny enteric or venereal infection. Some of these patients can correlate the onset of their disease with an episode of joint trauma.[10] The trauma is associated with swelling, stiffness, and pain in the traumatized joint, followed by the emergence of additional joint symptoms, urethritis, conjunctivitis, or cutaneous lesions. Another possible manifestation of a response to trauma in these patients is the presence of bony bridging or nonmarginal syndesmophytes in the spine in the absence of sacroiliitis or axial symptoms.[20,24] However, no scientific evidence has substantiated the role of trauma as an initiator of reactive arthritis.

Genetic Susceptibility

Characteristic of the spondyloarthropathies in general, reactive arthritis is associated with HLA-B27. From 60% to 80% of whites are positive for HLA-B27. In blacks, the prevalence of HLA-B27 has varied from 15% to 75%.[7,39,50] A majority of those who are negative for this antigen have HLA-B antigens that cross-react with B27, including B7, Bw22, B40, and Bw42.[7] HLA-B27 and related antigens may be linked to genes controlling the cellular immune response to certain infectious agents, and these genes cause an abnormal immune response. Alternatively, the HLA-B27 antigen may cross-react immunologically with certain infectious agents (molecular mimicry).[65]

HLA-B27 may increase the intracellular survival of organisms.[95] HLA-B27–positive cells produce more of the proinflammatory cytokine MCP-1 than HLA-B27–negative cells do. HLA-B27 may also have an effect on the production of heat shock protein 60 from pathogens, and this protein may have cross-reactivity with human heat shock proteins.[77]

Despite its association with reactive arthritis, the HLA-B27 haplotype is not the only determinant of disease expression; in only a minority of HLA-B27–positive individuals does reactive arthritis develop after exposure to infectious agents. In addition, HLA-B27 is associated with a wide range of diseases that cause spondyloarthropathy. There may be genetic material closely linked to HLA-B27 that actually determines the expression of reactive arthritis or other spondyloarthropathies.[83]

Evaluation of the HLA molecule reveals an antigen-binding groove that appears to serve the function of capturing appropriate corresponding antigen and presenting it to the T-cell receptors of CD8+ cytotoxic cells. An explanation for the variability of HLA-B27 being associated with a variety of arthritides might be the variability in key amino acid residues that affect the form of the binding site. HLA-B27 has been divided into six subtypes, including B*2701 through B*2706. Different subtypes are associated with particular ethnic groups and susceptibility for spondyloarthropathy.[49]

CLINICAL HISTORY

The classic picture of a patient with reactive arthritis is a young man about 25 years old in whom urethritis and mild conjunctivitis develop, followed by the onset of a predominantly lower extremity oligoarthritis. The symptoms of urethritis are usually mild and consist of a mucopurulent discharge and dysuria. Acute or chronic prostatitis may also develop in men. Women may have vaginitis or cervicitis, although many with these manifestations of genitourinary tract involvement in reactive arthritis may be asymptomatic. This paucity of symptoms from the genitourinary tract may in part explain the infrequency of the diagnosis of reactive arthritis in women.[72] Urethritis occurs in both epidemic and endemic forms of the disease. Urethral inflammation may occur as a result of a mechanism other than local infection. Up to 93% of patients with reactive arthritis have genitourinary symptoms during the course of their illness.[34]

The conjunctivitis is usually mild and is manifested as erythema (redness) and crusting of the lids. Conjunctival inflammation is usually bilateral and gradually resolves in a few days, but it may recur spontaneously. Acute iritis occurs in 20% of reactive arthritis patients and is marked by severe pain, photophobia, and scleral injection. Iritis may occur more commonly with recurring disease.

Arthritis may develop 1 to 3 weeks after the initial infection. In many patients, arthritis is the only manifestation of disease.[8] The term *reactive arthritis* is used for patients in whom only the arthritis of reactive arthritis develops after an enteric or genitourinary infection. The weight-bearing joints—knees, ankles, and feet—are most frequently affected in an asymmetric manner. A minority of patients have persistent monarthritis as their only articular abnormality. The involved joints are acutely inflamed, with large effusions developing in some joints.

Back pain is a frequent symptom of patients with reactive arthritis. During the acute course, pain in the lumbosacral region may develop in 31% to 92% of patients.[34,79,87] The pain is of an aching quality and is improved with activity. Occasionally, the pain will radiate to the posterior of the thighs but rarely below the knees; it may be unilateral. This finding corresponds to the asymmetric involvement of the sacroiliac joints and contrasts with the symmetrical involvement of ankylosing spondylitis (AS).[87] Sacroiliitis is the cause of back pain in a majority of patients who, as determined by increased activity over the sacroiliac joints on scintiscan, are in the acute phase of the disease.[88] Radiographic evidence of sacroiliitis is usually restricted to patients with severe disease. In retrospective studies, sacroiliitis can be detected radiographically in 9% of patients in the acute phase of illness and in up to 71% of patients who have had disease activity longer than 5 years.[26] Spondylitis affecting the lumbar, thoracic, and cervical spine occurs less commonly than sacroiliitis, with up to 23% of patients who have severe disease showing such involvement.[38]

Cervical Spine

Neck pain is a rare symptom in patients with reactive arthritis. Most studies of reactive arthritis do not include patients with neck symptoms. Cervical spine disease occurs in 2.2% to 2.4% of patients with reactive arthritis.[61,73,91] In a study of 153 men and 119 women, cervical spine disease occurred in 2.5% and 5.0% of patients with reactive arthritis, respectively.[105] On occasion, torticollis, indicative of cervical spine involvement, may develop in patients with reactive arthritis.[74]

Enthesitis

Another musculoskeletal manifestation of reactive arthritis is inflammation of the insertion of tendons and fascia. This anatomic structure is called an enthesis, and a process that results in inflammation of an enthesis is an enthesopathy. Enthesopathy occurs in 40% of patients with reactive arthritis.[5] Heel pain, or "lover's heel," secondary to inflammation of the plantar fascia, is a common finding.[11] Other manifestations of enthesopathy in patients with reactive arthritis are Achilles tendinitis, chest wall pain, dactylitis or "sausage digit," and low back pain with no evidence of active sacroiliitis.

Cutaneous

Though not part of the classic triad of the disease, mucocutaneous lesions are characteristic of reactive arthritis. Keratoderma blennorrhagicum is a rash characterized by waxy, macular lesions that become vesicular and scaly. They are found predominantly on the palms and soles. Histologically, they are indistinguishable from pustular psoriasis. Keratoderma that appears on the glans penis is referred to as circinate balanitis. The lesion is painless and occurs in up to 31% of patients. Oral ulcers occur on the palate, tongue, buccal mucosa, and lips. These lesions are shallow and painless and develop in 33% of patients. Nail involvement is characterized by opacification and hyperkeratosis, but not pitting.

Extra-articular

Gastrointestinal abnormalities may include acute diarrhea that precedes arthritis by a month or more. In patients with postdysenteric reactive arthritis, the severity and duration of diarrhea correlate with the severity and duration of arthritis. The causative organisms may have disappeared from the gut before arthritis appears. *Salmonella* is the organism that can be recovered from stool most frequently. Chronic diarrhea is an unusual manifestation of reactive arthritis.

Constitutional symptoms occur in about a third of patients and are characterized by fever, anorexia, weight loss, and fatigue. Cardiac complications, including heart block and aortic regurgitation, occur as a late manifestation of disease in 2% of patients.[86] Neurologic disease develops in 1% of patients and is associated with peripheral neuropathy, hemiplegia, and cranial nerve abnormalities.[37] Amyloidosis is also a rare and late complication of reactive arthritis.[70]

PHYSICAL EXAMINATION

Physical examination should include all organ systems that may be involved in the disease process. Many of the manifestations of reactive arthritis may be overlooked by patients. Important findings such as oral ulcers, circinate balanitis, and limitation of axial motion may be missed if not sought by the physician. Conjunctivitis is manifested by erythema of the conjunctivae and crusting of the lids. Urethritis may be detected only by "milking" the urethra before urination for the presence of a mucopurulent discharge.

A complete musculoskeletal examination should include both the upper and lower extremities, as well as the axial skeleton. Men tend to have involvement in the knees, ankles, and feet, and women have more upper extremity disease.[72] The usual patient has six or fewer joints affected. Percussion tenderness over the sacroiliac joints may be unilateral and correlate with asymmetric involvement in reactive arthritis. The mobility of the lumbosacral and cervical spine should be measured in all planes of motion. Patients with cervical spine involvement may have straightening of the neck. The paracervical muscles should be palpated for increased tension. A search for evidence of enthesopathy, heel pain, or tenderness of the Achilles tendon is also required.

An examination of the oropharynx, genitals, palms, soles, and nails covers the areas that are associated with the mucocutaneous lesions of reactive arthritis.

LABORATORY DATA

Laboratory results are nonspecific and not helpful in making the diagnosis of reactive arthritis. A mild anemia of chronic disease, an elevated white blood cell count (leukocytosis), and an elevated platelet count (thrombocytosis) are demonstrated in about a third of patients.[10] The erythrocyte sedimentation rate is increased in 70% to 80% of patients, but it does not follow the course of the disease. The C-reactive protein level is elevated, particularly in patients with reactive arthritis.[53,71] Stool cultures can be positive during an outbreak of gastroenteritis but are negative when the arthritis commences. Rheumatoid factor and antinuclear antibodies are not present in this illness. HLA-B27 or one of the cross-reactive antigens is found in 80% of patients. HLA-B27 positivity is helpful in differentiating reactive arthritis from rheumatoid arthritis (such differentiation is more easily achieved by clinical examination). The test, however, is not helpful in differentiating reactive arthritis from the other spondyloarthropathies. Histocompatibility testing should not be regarded as a routine diagnostic test. Testing may be most helpful early in the course of an arthropathy, when no typical extra-articular features are present.[18] Analysis of synovial fluid demonstrates an inflammatory fluid with no specific abnormalities.

Detection of bacterial antigens is an active area of research but is not essential for the diagnosis of reactive arthritis. Culture-proven *Chlamydia* infection is found in about one in three individuals with sexually transmitted disease. *C. trachomatis* can be detected by microimmunofluorescence with specific antisera on urethral or cervical swabs. Synovial lymphocyte proliferation in response to a variety of organisms associated with reactive arthritis has been documented in patients by culture of body fluids without growth.[93,94] These proliferation assays are research tests and should not be used for therapeutic decisions. Culture of stool is rarely successful in patients with reactive arthritis and should be performed only if a specific organism is suspected. Serologic tests may detect antibody elevations but are not as useful as culture.[103]

RADIOGRAPHIC EVALUATION

Roentgenograms

In patients who do not manifest the complete triad of reactive arthritis, roentgenographic changes are helpful in confirming the diagnosis.[61] Joint destruction is most severe in the feet; the hips and shoulders are usually spared. The radiologic correlate of the enthesopathy of reactive arthritis is periosteal new bone formation at the attachments of the plantar fascia and Achilles tendon into the calcaneus. The incidence of sacroiliac disease increases with disease chronicity and may be more common in postvenereal HLA-B27–positive patients.[88] Sacroiliac involvement may mimic AS (symmetrical disease) or may be asymmetric in the severity of joint changes (Figs 11-17 and 11-18). Unilateral sacroiliac disease occurs early in the disease process.[75] Bone erosion is more common on the iliac than sacral side of the joint. Variable amounts of sclerosis are associated with erosions. Widening of the joint (erosion), then narrowing (fusion), is the progression of radiographic changes. Fusion of the joints occurs less frequently than in AS. Sacroiliitis may be detected in 5% to 10% of individuals early in the illness and in up to 60% with prolonged illness.

Spondylitis is discontinuous in its involvement of the axial skeleton (skip lesions) and is characterized by nonmarginal bony bridging of vertebral bodies (Fig 11-19). These vertebral hyperostoses are markedly thickened in

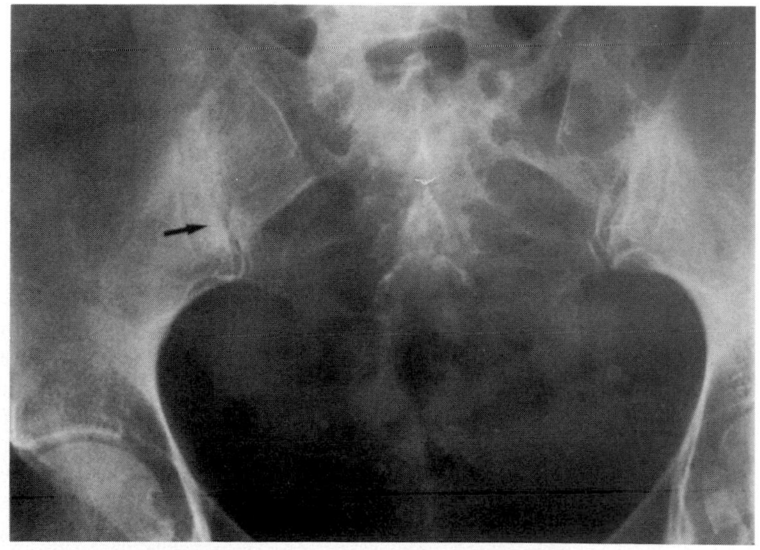

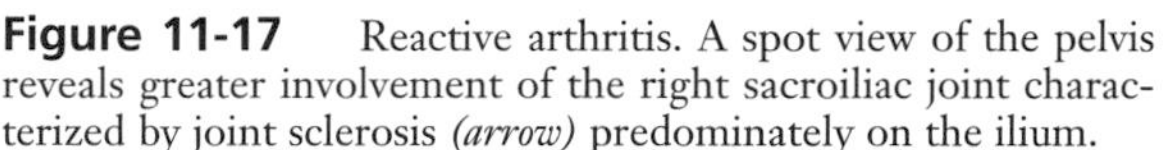

Figure 11-17 Reactive arthritis. A spot view of the pelvis reveals greater involvement of the right sacroiliac joint characterized by joint sclerosis *(arrow)* predominately on the ilium.

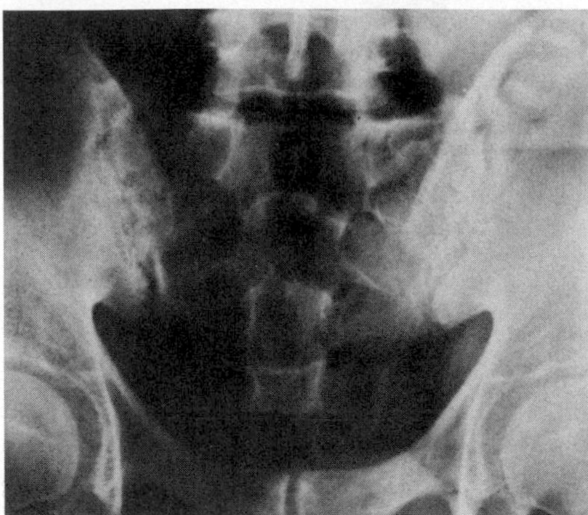

Figure 11-18 Reactive arthritis. A 42-year-old man was evaluated for left knee pain and persistent effusion that had been present for many years. Back pain developed after 6 years of knee pain. A Ferguson view of the pelvis demonstrates bilateral sacroiliitis with more joint narrowing and sclerosis on the left.

comparison to the thin syndesmophytes of AS. Cervical spine disease is associated with hyperostoses at the anteroinferior corners of one or more cervical vertebrae.[61] Extensive syndesmophytes may be present in the cervical spine, without similar lesions in the thoracic or lumbar spine.[91] Atlantoaxial subluxation is a rare complication of reactive arthritis (Fig. 11-20).[52,55] In rare circumstances, reactive arthritis may have atlantoaxial subluxation as an initial manifestation.[68] Patients in whom a nonreducible rotational head tilt develops may have involvement of the craniocervical junction.[41]

Paravertebral ossification may appear about the lower three thoracic and upper three lumbar vertebrae.[23] This roentgenographic finding may antedate the appearance of sacroiliac or peripheral joint alterations.[97] Paravertebral ossification may be the source of nonmarginal syndesmophytes. Ossification may skip areas of the spine as opposed to the continuous vertebral involvement in AS. In addition, typical thin syndesmophytes similar to those of AS may also develop in patients with reactive arthritis. The apophyseal joints may fuse, but the frequency of this finding is less than in classic AS.[33]

Whether spinal disease should be considered a complication of reactive arthritis or a manifestation of HLA-B27 disease is unclear. The difference in the appearance of spondylitis in reactive arthritis and AS suggests that the spondylitic process is dissimilar in the two conditions. The fact that spinal disease is often asymmetric and has skip areas and little squaring of vertebral bodies, along with the finding of increased spinal involvement with severe, long-standing reactive arthritis, suggests that the process is related to reactive arthritis itself rather than HLA-B27. Spondylitis in reactive arthritis occurs in an older age group than noted with AS.

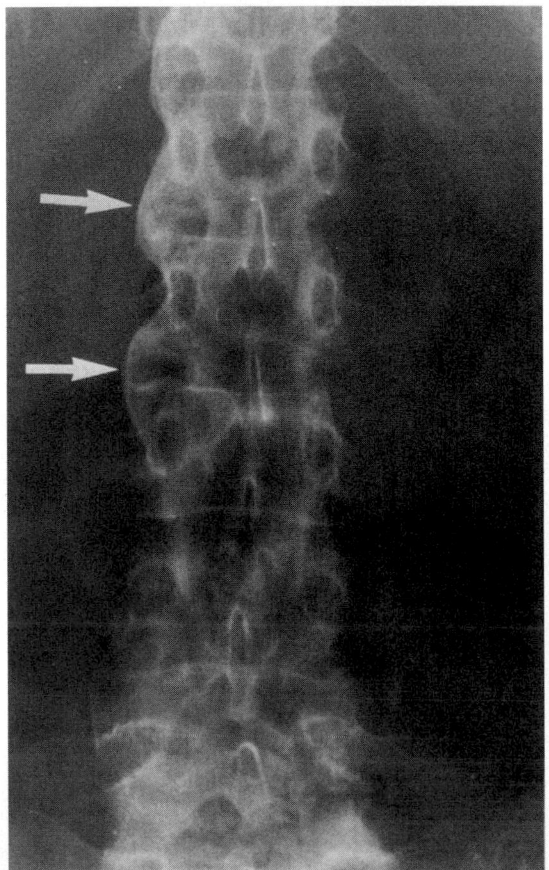

Figure 11-19 Reactive arthritis. A 35-year-old man with midline back pain has asymmetric nonmarginal syndesmophytes on the right side (more common on the nonaortic side) of the lumbar spine *(arrows)*. A similar pattern may be seen with psoriatic spondylitis. *(Courtesy of Anne Brower, MD.)*

Scintigraphy, Computed Tomography, Magnetic Resonance

Increased uptake of tracer on bone scintigraphy can identify inflammatory involvement of the sacroiliac joint but is a nonspecific finding. Enthesopathic lesions can be visualized at an early stage by focal uptake of ^{99m}Tc-methylene diphosphonate (MDP).[58] CT scan may also be useful to identify inflammatory alterations when changes on plain roentgenographs are minimal.[3]

DIFFERENTIAL DIAGNOSIS

Preliminary criteria for the diagnosis of acute reactive arthritis have recently been reported by the American Rheumatism Association, now the American College of Rheumatology.[101] Patients with reactive arthritis were distinguished from patients with other spondyloarthropathies and gonococcal arthritis by an episode of peripheral arthritis of more than 1 month's duration occurring in association with urethritis, cervicitis, or both. Amor and colleagues have proposed a set of clinical factors for diagnosing spondyloarthropathies, including reactive arthritis (Table 11-8).[6] Ahvonen and associates introduced the term *reactive arthritis* to describe the nonpurulent joint inflammation associated with *Y. enterocolitica* and *Yersinia pseudotuberculosis* enteric infection.[2] Reactive arthritis refers to an inflammatory joint disease that follows an infection elsewhere in the body without microbial invasion of the synovial space.[81] The reasons for the development of arthropathy alone in reactive arthritis instead of the full range of the triad after exposure to infectious agents are

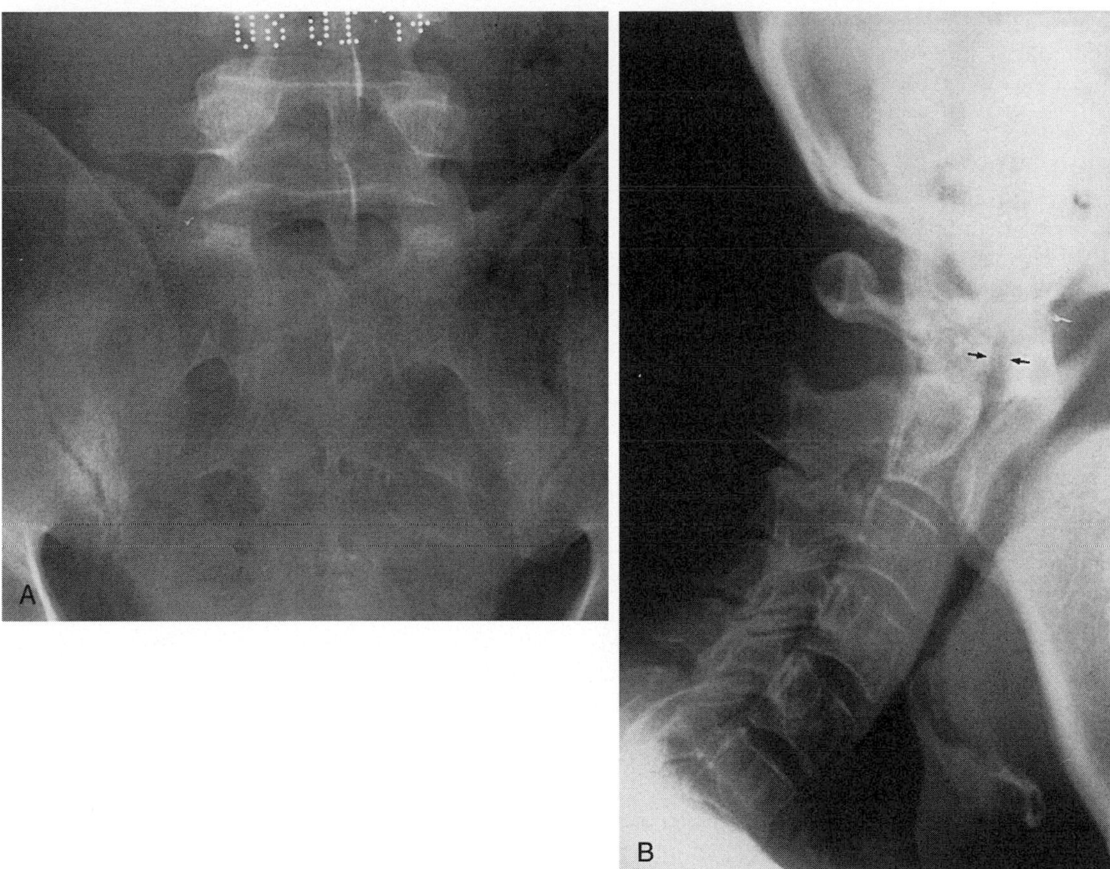

Figure 11-20 Reactive arthritis in a 26-year-old man with neck pain. *A*, A spot view of the pelvis reveals greater involvement of the right sacroiliac joint characterized by joint sclerosis and erosion. *B*, A lateral view of the cervical spine reveals atlantoaxial subluxation of 10 mm *(arrows)*. *(Courtesy of Anne Brower, MD.)*

11-8 AMOR CRITERIA FOR DIAGNOSING SPONDYLOARTHROPATHY*

A. Clinical symptoms or past history of
   1. Lumbar or dorsal pain during the night or morning stiffness of the lumbar or dorsal spine (1)
   2. Asymmetric oligoarthritis (2)
   3. Buttock pain (1)
      If alternately affecting the right or the left buttock (2)
   4. Dactylitis (2)
   5. Heel pain (2)
   6. Iritis (2)
   7. Nongonococcal urethritis or cervicitis accompanying or within 1 month before the onset of arthritis (1)
   8. Acute diarrhea accompanying or within 1 month before the onset of arthritis (1)
   9. Presence of a history of psoriasis and/or balanitis and/or inflammatory bowel disease (ulcerative colitis, Crohn's disease) (2)

B. Radiologic finding
   10. Sacroiliitis (grade >2 if bilateral; grade >3 if unilateral) (3)

C. Genetic background
   11. Presence of HLA-B27 and/or family history of ankylosing spondylitis, reactive arthritis, uveitis, psoriasis, or chronic enterocolopathies (2)

D. Response to treatment
   12. Improvement of rheumatic complaints with NSAIDs in <48 hours or relapse of the pain in <48 hours if NSAIDs are discontinued (2)

*Diagnosis of spondyloarthropathy—6 points or greater. Points—1, 2, or 3—in parentheses.

unknown.[4] The infectious agents include *Salmonella*,[40] *Shigella*,[78] *Yersinia*,[45] and *Campylobacter*[54]; parasites, including *Giardia*,[14,35] *Chlamydia*,[48] *Neisseria gonorrhoeae*,[84] and streptococci[43]; and nonspecific chronic urogenital infections.[76,98] About 80% of patients with reactive arthritis are HLA-B27 positive.[1,57] Like epidemic Reiter's syndrome, young men and women are affected equally. The onset and pattern of disease of reactive arthritis are similar to that of Reiter's syndrome. Back pain develops in approximately 30% of patients with reactive arthritis.[57] These patients are HLA-B27 positive and are also at greater risk for the development of radiographic evidence of sacroiliitis. Patients with arthritis alone respond to the same therapy that is effective for the clinical triad. At a 5-year follow-up, one third of patients with reactive arthritis may continue to have back pain and show evidence of sacroiliitis.[57,60]

The differential diagnosis of a patient with spinal pain and no other manifestation of reactive arthritis is the same as that presented for AS. This differential diagnosis includes the other spondyloarthropathies, herniated intervertebral disc, diffuse idiopathic skeletal hyperostosis, and tumors (see Table 11-4). In a patient in whom acute monarticular disease develops after sexual intercourse, the diagnosis of infectious arthritis secondary to *N. gonnorrhoeae* must not be overlooked.[64] Bacterial culture of the urethra, rectum, pharynx, and synovial fluid is necessary to detect the presence of the bacterium. Examination of synovial fluid for bacterial fatty acids, particularly succinic acid, helps differentiate individuals with septic arthritis from those with effusions secondary to reactive arthritis.[15]

Human Immunodeficiency Virus

Human immunodeficiency virus (HIV) infection was first recognized during the early 1980s.[92] The disease is characterized by fever, weight loss, anorexia, lymphadenopathy, multiple infections, and Kaposi's sarcoma. HIV is an RNA retrovirus with high affinity for the CD4 receptor that is expressed preferentially on helper/inducer T lymphocytes. Killing of these cells by the virus results in dysfunction of the surveillance role of the immune system. Absence of this function leads to opportunistic infections and malignancies. Many organ systems are affected by the immune dysfunction and the persistent infections.[89] When compared with other organ systems, the musculoskeletal system is spared. In a study of 556 patients with HIV infection, only 11% had musculoskeletal disorders and 0.5% had reactive arthritis.[31] Other reports document the prevalence of reactive arthritis to be between 2.1% and 10.8% of HIV patients.[27] Reactive arthritis was the first distinct rheumatologic disorder described in association with HIV infection.[102] HIV-associated reactive arthritis occurs more frequently in homosexuals than intravenous drug abusers who contract the infection. Reactive arthritis may precede or follow the onset of acquired immunodeficiency syndrome (AIDS). The usual articular symptoms are asymmetric oligoarthritis of the large joints, enthesopathy, and skin lesions.[47] Fever, weight loss, and generalized lymphadenopathy may develop. The disorder may progress to severe, persistent joint pain with severe enthesopathy and rash. Interestingly, involvement of the cervical spine in patients with axial skeletal disease is greater in reactive arthritis patients with HIV infection than in those without HIV.[31,85] Cervical spine disease includes straightening of the neck with evidence of sclerosis and apophyseal joint narrowing on roentgenograms. The thoracic and lumbar spine may be affected in the presence or absence of sacroiliitis. Radiographic alterations of the spine occur, and 66% of patients are HLA-B27 positive. Therapy directed at controlling arthritis has the potential to exacerbate the underlying immunodeficiency.[85] Patients may respond to nonsteroidal anti-inflammatory drugs (NSAIDs). For the 20% who remain resistant to therapy, sulfasalazine is effective.[107] Patients in whom reactive arthritis develops are severely ill. Debate remains regarding the association of AIDS and reactive arthritis. Some reports have suggested a clear association,[29] but other studies have suggested that the increased risk is from risky behavior associated with AIDS (bowel infections) and not from the virus itself.[21]

TREATMENT

The therapeutic regimen includes patient education, medications, and physical therapy. Patients are confused by the association of reactive arthritis and sexual relations. Many are likely to have guilt or anxiety over sexual intercourse. The fact that urethritis may recur without any obvious cause must be made clear to the patient.

Acute joint symptoms are treated symptomatically with NSAIDs and the modalities of physical therapy. The drugs that are most effective for reactive arthritis are reviewed in the section "Enteropathic Arthritis." The joint and enthesopathic manifestations of reactive arthritis appear to respond better to indomethacin or the other newer NSAIDs than to aspirin. Treatment is continued as long as the patient remains symptomatic. The effect of these agents on the long-term course of the disease is unknown. In patients with decreased range of motion of the spine associated with reactive arthritis, NSAIDs are useful to decrease pain. The addition of muscle relaxants in these patients can also be helpful in improving the component of immobility secondary to the muscle tightness and spasm associated with arthritis or enthesopathy. Local corticosteroid injections relieve focal synovitis in accessible joints. Oral corticosteroids are less effective in this polyarthritis than in rheumatoid arthritis.

Antibiotics

The role of antibiotic therapy in the acute phase of reactive arthritis remains controversial. A study demonstrated that antibiotic therapy did not influence the appearance of reactive arthritis in patients with nonspecific urethritis.[48] Antibiotics may not be effective for *Chlamydia*-associated reactive arthritis.[13] A double-blind, placebo-controlled study of 3 months' duration to evaluate treatment with a lysine conjugate of tetracycline showed that those with *Chlamydia*-associated reactive arthritis recovered more rapidly than those with post-*Yersinia* arthritis.[56] Ciprofloxacin for 3 months had little effect on the course of reactive arthritis when compared with placebo.[106]

Disease-Modifying Antirheumatic Drugs

A recent review studied the role of second-line agents (gold, sulfasalazine, methotrexate, and azathioprine) in the treatment of spondyloarthropathies, including reactive arthritis.[25] Gold salt therapy may be helpful in patients with progressive, destructive peripheral joint disease.

Sulfasalazine has been reported to improve spine pain and swollen joints in patients with reactive arthritis. The usual dose of sulfasalazine is 2 g/day in divided doses. The dose may be increased to 3 g in divided doses.[22] The benefits of sulfasalazine may be of short duration.[28] The immunosuppressive methotrexate is reserved for patients with uncontrolled progression of joint disease and unresponsive, extensive skin involvement.[30] The dose of methotrexate used ranges from 7.5 to 50 mg weekly. Most individuals have a beneficial response consisting of improved joint symptoms without toxicity. Azathioprine has been shown to be effective in controlling the activity of intractable reactive arthritis in a placebo-controlled crossover study.[17] Corticosteroids are used as drops for iritis and as long-acting preparations for intra-articular injection. Systemic corticosteroids have less of an effect in reactive arthritis than they do in rheumatoid arthritis and are rarely used.

Anti–Tumor Necrosis Factor-Alpha Inhibitors

Tumor necrosis factor (TNF) is an inflammatory cytokine associated with the destructive process that results in the phenotypic expression of reactive arthritis. Anti-TNF therapies are available in the form of infliximab, etanercept, and adulimimab, which inhibit the inflammatory effects of TNF. TNF levels are increased with organisms in the synovial space.[67] A faulty TNF response may increase susceptibility to reactive arthritis. Because TNF is necessary for microbial elimination, anti-TNF therapy may increase the persistence of organisms. A small group of reactive arthritis patients experienced improved global function, including improvement in joint swelling, in a 6-month trial of etanercept, 25 mg subcutaneously twice weekly.[16] A question remains about the long-term effects of anti-TNF therapy on arthritis with bacterial DNA resident in joints. An exacerbation of arthritis may potentially develop in such individuals. Ongoing evaluation of these reactive arthritis patients is necessary to determine the full benefits and detriments of this therapy in this group of patients.

PROGNOSIS

Reactive arthritis has no cure, and the course of the illness is unpredictable. About 30% to 40% of patients have a self-limited illness lasting 3 months to 1 year. Another 30% to 50% have a relapsing pattern of illness with periods of complete remission. Chronic, unremitting disease associated with significant disability develops in the final 10% to 25%.[34,36] Measuring the C-reactive protein level may be a better method for monitoring the activity of disease than the erythrocyte sedimentation rate in reactive arthritis, in addition to looking for clinical parameters (such as morning stiffness and joint swelling).[71] Patients in whom significant disability develops from reactive arthritis typically have painful or deformed feet or visual loss from iritis. A 5-year follow-up study of 131 consecutive patients with Reiter's syndrome revealed that 83% of the patients had some disease activity.[34] Fifty-one percent of patients had continued low back pain, and 45% had persistent foot or heel pain. Thirty-four percent of patients had disease activity that interfered with their job; 26% had to change jobs or were unemployed. Heel involvement at the time of diagnosis was the finding most closely associated with a poor functional outcome. The presence of HLA-B27 did not correlate with functional outcome; however, a report from Finland suggested that the HLA-B27 status of the patient was associated with disease severity.[57] Patients who were HLA-B27 positive had more frequent back pain and mucocutaneous and genitourinary symptoms. They also had a longer duration of disease and more frequent chronic low back pain and sacroiliitis. Chronic joint symptoms continued in 68% of 140 reactive arthritis patients studied, and 41% had chronic back pain. Most patients were able to lead normal lives, although 16% of the group had chronic destructive peripheral arthritis. Another report suggested that homozygosity for HLA-B27 may also be associated with more severe disease.[9]

In contrast, a study of 55 reactive arthritis patients monitored for 9.3 years showed a 40% incidence of sacroiliitis. Sacroiliitis was rarely associated with spondylitis, 33 patients had mild limitation of back motion, and only 1 patient was functionally impaired by back disease.[66] The patients with sacroiliitis had more iritis, a prolonged disease duration, and HLA-B27 positivity.

Seven predictive factors present during the first 2 years of reactive arthritis may be associated with more severe disease—hip arthritis (4), erythrocyte sedimentation rate greater than 30 mm/hr (3), poor effect of NSAIDs (3), limitation of lumbar movement (3), dactylitis (2), oligoarthritis (1), and onset younger than 16 years (1). A sum of the numbers in parentheses of 7 or more predicts a severe course, whereas a sum of 3 or less has a benign course.[6]

Reactive arthritis is no longer considered a benign disease. Most patients do not have significant impairment secondary to spinal disease. Impairment is more closely associated with disease in other locations in the skeleton and in other organ systems. Early treatment with NSAIDs, physical therapy, and appropriate shoes may have beneficial effects on patient function. Newer anti-TNF therapies may hold promise for greater control of the illness, but at a risk of exacerbation in those with persistent infection. Unfortunately, even aggressive therapy is unable to prevent disease activity and progressive disability in many reactive arthritis patients.

References

Reactive Arthritis

1. Aho K, Ahvonen P, Lassus A, et al: HLA-27 in reactive arthritis: A study of *Yersinia* arthritis and Reiter's disease. Arthritis Rheum 17:521, 1974.
2. Ahvonen P, Sievers K, Aho K: Arthritis associated with *Yersinia enterocolitica* infection. Acta Rheum Scand 15:232, 1969.
3. Aliabadi P, Nikpoor N: Imaging evaluation of sacroiliitis. Rheum Dis Clin North Am 17:809, 1991.
4. Amor B: Reiter's syndrome and reactive arthritis. Clin Rheumatol 2:315, 1983.
5. Amor B: Reiter's syndrome: Diagnosis and clinical features. Rheum Dis Clin North Am 24:677-695, 1998.
6. Amor B, Silva-Santos R, Nahal R, et al: Predictive factors for the longterm outcome of spondyloarthropathies. J Rheumatol 21:1883-1887 1994.
7. Arnett FC, Hochberg MD, Bias WB: Cross-reactive HLA antigens in B27-negative Reiter's syndrome and sacroiliitis. Johns Hopkins Med J 141:193, 1977.
8. Arnett FC, McClusky E, Schacter BZ, Lordon RE: Incomplete Reiter's syndrome: Discriminating features and HLA-W27 in diagnosis. Ann Intern Med 84:8, 1976.
9. Arnett FC, Schacter BZ, Hochberg MC, et al: Homozygosity for HLA-B27: Impact on rheumatic disease expression in two families. Arthritis Rheum 20:797, 1977.
10. Arnett FC Jr: Reiter's syndrome. Johns Hopkins Med J 150:39, 1982.
11. Ball J: Enthesopathy of rheumatoid and ankylosing spondylitis. Ann Rheum Dis 30:213, 1971.
12. Bauer W, Engleman EP: A syndrome of unknown etiology characterized by urethritis, conjunctivitis, and arthritis (so-called Reiter's disease). Trans Assoc Am Physicians 57:307, 1942.
13. Beutler AM, Hudson AP, Whittum-Hudson JA, et al: Chlamydia trachomatis can persist in joint tissue after antibiotic treatment in chronic Reiter's syndrome/reactive arthritis. J Clin Rheumatol 3:125-130, 1997
14. Bocanegra TS, Espinoza LR, Bridgeford PH, et al: Reactive arthritis induced by parasitic infestation. Ann Intern Med 94:207, 1981.

15. Borenstein DG, Gibbs CA, Jacobs RP: Gas-liquid chromatographic analysis of synovial fluid. Arthritis Rheum 25:947, 1982.
16. Brandt J, Haibel H, Reddig J, et al: Successful short term treatment of severe undifferentiated spondyloarthropathy with the anti-tumor necrosis factor-α monoclonal antibody infliximab. J Rheumatol 29:118-122, 2002.
17. Calin A: A placebo-controlled, crossover study of azathioprine in Reiter's syndrome. Ann Rheum Dis 45:653, 1986.
18. Calin A: HLA-B27: To type or not to type? Ann Intern Med 92:208, 1980.
19. Calin A: The relationship between genetics and environment in the pathogenesis of rheumatic diseases (medical progress). West J Med 131:205, 1979.
20. Calin A, Fries JF: Striking prevalence of ankylosing spondylitis in "healthy" W27-positive males and females: A controlled study. N Engl J Med 293:835, 1975.
21. Clark MR, Solinger AM, Hochberg MC: Human immunodeficiency virus is not associated with Reiter's syndrome: Data from three large cohort studies. Rheum Dis Clin North Am 18:267, 1992.
22. Clegg CO, Reda DJ, Weisman MH, et al: Comparison of sulfasalazine and placebo in the treatment of reactive arthritis (Reiter's syndrome). Arthritis Rheum 39:2021-2027, 1996.
23. Cliff JM: Spinal bony bridging and carditis in Reiter's disease. Ann Rheum Dis 30:171, 1971.
24. Cohen LM, Mittal KK, Schmid FR, et al: Increased risk for spondylitis stigmata in apparently healthy HLA-W27 men. Ann Intern Med 84:1, 1976.
25. Creemers MCW, van Riel PLCM, Franssen MJAM, et al: Second-line treatment in seronegative spondyloarthropathies. Semin Arthritis Rheum 24:71, 1994.
26. Csonka GW: The course of Reiter's syndrome. BMJ 1:1088, 1958.
27. Cuellar ML: HIV infection–associated inflammatory musculoskeletal disorders. Rheum Dis Clin North Am 24:403-421, 1998.
28. Egsmose C, Hansen TM, Andersen LS, et al: Limited effect of sulphasalazine treatment in reactive arthritis: A randomized double blind placebo controlled trial. Ann Rheum Dis 56:32-36, 1997.
29. Espinoza LR, Jara LJ, Espinoza CG, et al: There is an association between human immunodeficiency virus infection and spondyloarthropathies. Rheum Dis Clin North Am 18:257, 1992.
30. Farber GA, Forshner JG, O'Quinn SE: Reiter's syndrome: Treatment with methotrexate. JAMA 200:171, 1967.
31. Fernandez SM, Cardenal A, Balsa A, et al: Rheumatic manifestations in 556 patients with human immunodeficiency virus infection. Semin Arthritis Rheum 21:30, 1991.
32. Fiessinger N, Leroy E: Contribution a l'etude d'une epidemic de dysenterie dans le somme. Bull Soc Med Hop Paris, 40:2030, 1916.
33. Ford DK: Natural history of arthritis following venereal urethritis. Ann Rheum Dis 12:177, 1953.
34. Fox R, Calin A, Gerber RC, Gibson D: The chronicity of symptoms and disability in Reiter's syndrome: An analysis of 131 consecutive patients. Ann Intern Med 91:190, 1979.
35. Goobar JP: Joint symptoms in giardiasis. Lancet 1:1010, 1977.
36. Good AE: Involvement of the back in Reiter's syndrome: Follow-up study of thirty-four cases. Ann Intern Med 57:44, 1962.
37. Good AE: Reiter's disease: A review with special attention to cardiovascular and neurologic sequelae. Semin Arthritis Rheum 3:253, 1974.
38. Good AE: Reiter's syndrome: Long-term follow-up in relation to development of ankylosing spondylitis. Ann Rheum Dis 38:39, 1979.
39. Good AE, Kawaniski H, Schultz JS: HLA-B27 in blacks with ankylosing spondylitis or Reiter's disease. N Engl J Med 294:166, 1976.
40. Good AE, Schultz JS: Reiter's syndrome following *Shigella flexneri* 2a. Arthritis Rheum 20:100, 1977.
41. Halla JT, Bliznak J, Hardin JG: Involvement of the craniocervical junction in Reiter's syndrome. J Rheumatol 15:1722, 1988.
42. Holmes KK, Handsfield HH, Wang SP, et al: Etiology of nongonococcal arthritis. N Engl J Med 292:1199, 1975.
43. Hubbard WN, Hughes GRV: Streptococci and reactive arthritis. Ann Rheum Dis 41:435, 1982.
44. Inman RD, Johnston MEA, Hodge M, et al: Post-dysenteric reactive arthritis: A clinical and immunogenetic study following an outbreak of salmonellosis. Arthritis Rheum 31:1377, 1988.
45. Jones RAK: Reiter's disease after *Salmonella typhimurium* enteritis. BMJ 1:1391, 1977.
46. Keat AC, Maini RN, Nkwazi GC, et al: Role of *Chlamydia trachomatis* and HLA-B27 in sexually acquired reactive arthritis. BMJ 1:605, 1978.
47. Keat A, Rowe I: Reiter's syndrome and associated arthritides. Rheum Dis Clin North Am 17:25, 1991.
48. Keat AC, Thomas BJ, Taylor-Robinson D, et al: Evidence of *Chlamydia trachomatis* infection in sexually acquired reactive arthritis. Ann Rheum Dis 39:431, 1980.
49. Khan MA: An overview of clinical spectrum and heterogeneity of spondyloarthropathies. Rheum Dis Clin North Am 18:1, 1992.
50. Khan MA, Askari AD, Braun WE, Aponte CJ: Low association of HLA-B27 with Reiter's syndrome in blacks. Ann Intern Med 90:202, 1979.
51. Kousa M, Saikku P, Richmond S, Lassus A: Frequent association of chlamydial infection with Reiter's syndrome. Sex Transm Dis 5:57, 1978.
52. Kransdorf MJ, Wehrle PA, Moser RP Jr: Atlantoaxial subluxation in Reiter's syndrome: A report of three cases and review of the literature. Spine 13:12, 1988.
52a. Kuipers JG, Zeidler H, Kohler L: How does Chlamydia cause arthritis? Rheum Dis Clin North Am 29:613-629, 2003.
53. Kvien TK, Glennas A, Melby K, et al: Reactive arthritis: Incidence, triggering agents, and clinical presentation. J Rheumatol 21:115, 1994.
54. Laitenen O, Leirisalo M, Skylv G: Relation between HLA-B27 and clinical features in patients with *Yersinia* arthritis. Arthritis Rheum 20:121, 1977.
55. Latchaw RE, Meyer GW: Reiter disease with atlanto-axial subluxation. Radiology 126:303, 1978.
56. Lauhio A, Leirisalo-Repo M, Lahdevirta J, et al: Double-blind, placebo-controlled study of three-month treatment with lymecycline in reactive arthritis, with special reference to *Chlamydia* arthritis. Arthritis Rheum 34:6, 1991.
57. Leirisalo M, Skylv G, Kousa M, et al: Follow-up study on patients with Reiter's disease and reactive arthritis, with special reference to HLA-B27. Arthritis Rheum 25:249, 1982.
58. Lin WY, Wang SJ, Lang JL, et al: Bone scintigraphy in evaluation of heel pain in Reiter's disease compared with radiography and clinical examination. Scand J Rheumatol 24:18-21, 1995.
59. Liu Y, Penttinen MA, Granfors K: Insights into the role of infection in the spondyloarthropathies. Curr Rheumatol Rep 3:428-434, 2001.
60. Marsal L, Winblad S, Wollheim FA: *Yersinia enterocolitica* arthritis in southern Sweden: A four-year follow-up study. BMJ 283:101, 1981.
61. Martel W, Braunstein EM, Borlaza G, et al: Radiologic features of Reiter's disease. Radiology 132:1, 1979.
62. Martin DH, Pollock S, Kuo C, et al: *Chlamydia trachomatis* infections in men with Reiter's syndrome. Ann Intern Med 100:207, 1984.
63. Mattila L, Leirisalo-Repo M, Koskimies S, et al: Reactive arthritis following an outbreak of *Salmonella* infection in Finland. Br J Rheumatol 33:1136, 1994.
64. McCord WC, Nies KM, Louie JS: Acute venereal arthritis: Comparative study of acute Reiter's syndrome and acute gonococcal arthritis. Arch Intern Med 137:858, 1977.
65. McDevitt HO, Bodmer WF: HLA, immune response genes and disease. Lancet 1:1269, 1974.
66. McGuigan LE, Hart HH, Gow PJ, et al: The functional significance of sacroiliitis and ankylosing spondylitis in Reiter's syndrome. Clin Exp Rheumatol 3:311, 1985.
67. Meade R, Hsia E, Kitumnuaypong T, et al: TNF involvement and anti-TNF therapy of reactive and unclassified arthritis. Clin Exp Rheumatol 20(6 suppl 28)S130-134, 2002.
68. Melsom RD, Benjamin JC, Barnes CG: Spontaneous atlantoaxial subluxation: An unusual presenting manifestation of Reiter's syndrome. Ann Rheum Dis 48:170, 1989.
69. Michet CJ, Machado EBV, Ballard DJ, et al: Epidemiology of Reiter's syndrome in Rochester, Minnesota: 1950-1980. Arthritis Rheum 31:428, 1988.
70. Miller LD, Brown EC, Arnett FC: Amyloidosis in Reiter's syndrome. J Rheumatol 6:225, 1979.
71. Nashel DJ, Petrone DL, Ulmer CC, Sliwinski AJ: C-reactive protein: A marker for disease activity in ankylosing spondylitis and Reiter's syndrome. J Rheumatol 13:364, 1986.
72. Neuwelt CM, Borenstein DG, Jacobs RP: Reiter's syndrome: A male and female disease. J Rheumatol 9:268, 1982.

73. Noer HR: An "experimental" epidemic of Reiter's syndrome. JAMA 198:693, 1966.
74. Oates JK, Hancock JAH: Neurological symptoms and lesions occurring in the course of Reiter's disease. Am J Med Sci 238:79, 1959.
75. Oates JK, Young AC: Sacroiliitis in Reiter's disease. BMJ 1:1013, 1959.
76. Olhagen B: Postinfective or reactive arthritis. Scand J Rheumatol 9:193, 1980.
77. Pacheo-Tena C, Zhand X, Stone M, et al: Innate immunity in host-microbial interactions: Beyond B27 in the spondyloarthropathies. Curr Opin Rheumatol 14:373-382, 2002.
78. Paronen I: Reiter's disease: A study of 344 cases observed in Finland. Acta Med Scand Suppl 212:1, 1948.
79. Popert AJ, Gill AJ, Laird SM: A prospective study of Reiter's syndrome: An interim report on the first 82 cases. Br J Vener Dis 40:160, 1964.
80. Rahman MU, Hudson AP, Schumacher HR Jr: *Chlamydia* and Reiter's syndrome (reactive arthritis). Rheum Dis Clin North Am 18:67, 1992.
81. Reactive arthritis [Editorial]. BMJ 281:311, 1980.
82. Reiter H: Über eine bisher unerkannte Spirochaeteninfektion (Spirochaetosis arthritica). Dtsch Med Wochenschr 42:1535, 1916.
83. Reveille JD, McDaniel DO, Barger BO, et al: Restriction fragment length polymorphism (RFLP) analysis in familial ankylosing spondylitis: Independent segregation of a 9.2 kb PVU II RFLP from B27 haplotypes [Abstract]. Arthritis Rheum 30(suppl):S36, 1987.
84. Rosenthal L, Olhagen B, Ek S: Aseptic arthritis after gonorrhea. Ann Rheum Dis 39:141, 1980.
85. Rowe IF, Forster SM, Seifert MH, et al: Rheumatological lesion in individuals with human immunodeficiency virus infection. Q J Med 73:1167, 1989.
86. Ruppert GB, Lindsay J, Barth WF: Cardiac conduction abnormalities in Reiter's syndrome. Am J Med 73:335, 1982.
87. Russell AS, Davis P, Percy JS, Lentle GC: The sacroiliitis of acute Reiter's syndrome. J Rheumatol 4:293, 1977.
88. Russell AS, Lentle BC, Percy JS: Investigation of sacroiliac disease: Comparative evaluation of radiological and radionuclide techniques. J Rheumatol 2:45, 1975.
89. Sande MA, Volberding PA: The Medical Management of AIDS, 3rd ed. Philadelphia, WB Saunders, 1992, p 525.
90. Schumacher HR: Reactive arthritis. Rheum Dis Clin North Am 24:261-273, 1998.
91. Sholkoff SD, Glickman MG, Steinbach HL: Roentgenology of Reiter's syndrome. Radiology 97:497, 1970.
92. Siegal FP, Lopez C, Hammer GS, et al: Severe acquired immunodeficiency in male homosexuals, manifested by chronic perianal ulcerative herpes simplex lesions. N Engl J Med 305:1439, 1981.
93. Sieper J, Braun J, Wu P, et al: The possible role of *Shigella* in sporadic enteric reactive arthritis. Br J Rheumatol 32:582, 1993.
94. Sieper J, Kingsley G, Palacios-Boix A, et al: Synovial T lymphocyte specific immune response to *Chlamydia trachomatis* in Reiter's disease. Arthritis Rheum 34:588, 1991.
95. Sigal L. Update on reactive arthritis. Bull Rheum Dis 50(4):1-4, 2001.
96. Solem JH, Lassen J: Reiter's disease following *Yersinia enterocolitica* infection. Scand J Infect Dis 8:83, 1971.
97. Sundaram M, Patton JT: Paravertebral ossification in psoriasis and Reiter's disease. Br J Radiol 48:628, 1975.
98. Szanto E, Hagenfeldt K: Sacro-iliitis and salpingitis. Scand J Rheumatol 8:129, 1979.
99. Van de Putte LBA, Berden JHM, Boerbooms AM, et al: Reactive arthritis after *Campylobacter jejuni* enteritis. J Rheumatol 7:531, 1980.
100. Wallace DJ, Weisman M. Should a war criminal be rewarded with eponymous distinction? The double life of Hans Reiter (1881-1969). J Clin Rheumatol 6:49-54, 2000.
101. Willkens RF, Arnett FC, Bitter T, et al: Reiter's syndrome: Evaluation of preliminary criteria for definite disease. Bull Rheum Dis 32:31, 1982.
102. Winchster R, Bernstein DH, Fischer HD, et al: The co-occurrence of Reiter's syndrome and acquired immunodeficiency. Ann Intern Med 106:19, 1987.
103. Wollenhaupt J, Schnarr S, Kuipers JG: Bacterial antigens in reactive arthritis and spondarthritis. Rational use of laboratory testing in diagnosis and follow-up. Balliere's Clin Rheumatol 12:627-647, 1998.
104. Wollenhaupt J, Zeidler H: Undifferentiated arthritis and reactive arthritis. Curr Opin Rheumatol 10:306-313, 1998.
105. Yli-Kerttua UI: Clinical characteristics in male and female uroarthritis or Reiter's syndrome. Clin Rheumatol 3:351, 1984.
106. Yli-Kerttula T, Luukkainen R, Yli-Kerttula U, et al: Effect of a three month course of ciprofloxacin on the outcome of reactive arthritis. Ann Rheum Dis 59:565-570, 2000.
107. Youssef PP, Bertouch JV, Jones PD: Successful treatment of human immunodeficiency virus–associated Reiter's syndrome with sulfasalazine. Arthritis Rheum 35:723-1992.

ENTEROPATHIC ARTHRITIS

CAPSULE SUMMARY

	LOW BACK	NECK
Frequency of spinal pain	Rare	Rare
Location of spinal pain	Sacroiliac joints	Cervical spine
Quality of spinal pain	Ache	Ache
Symptoms and signs	Morning stiffness, abdominal pain or cramps	Morning stiffness, abdominal pain or cramps
Laboratory tests	Increased erythrocyte sedimentation rate, blood in stool	Increased erythrocyte sedimentation rate, blood in stool
Radiographic findings	Syndesmophytes on plain roentgenogram	Syndesmophytes on plain roentgenogram
Treatment	Exercises, NSAIDs, biologicals	Exercises, NSAIDs, biologicals

PREVALENCE AND PATHOGENESIS

Ulcerative colitis and Crohn's disease are inflammatory bowel diseases (IBDs). Ulcerative colitis is limited to the colon, whereas Crohn's disease, or regional enteritis, may involve any part of the gastrointestinal tract. Inflammation of the gut results in numerous gastrointestinal symptoms, including abdominal pain, fever, and weight loss. These inflammatory diseases are also associated with extraintestinal manifestations, including arthritis. Articular involvement in these IBDs includes both the peripheral and axial skeletal joints. Peripheral arthritis is generally nondeforming and follows the activity of the underlying bowel disease; axial skeletal disease is similar to ankylosing spondylitis and follows a course independent of the activity of bowel inflammation.

The association of arthritis and ulcerative colitis was first elucidated by Bargen in the 1920s.[6] Crohn's disease was described by Crohn and colleagues in 1932.[11] The association of arthritis and Crohn's disease was commented on by Van Patter and colleagues and by Steinberg and Storey in the 1950s.[76,82]

Epidemiology

Ulcerative colitis occurs four times more commonly in whites than nonwhites and more commonly in Jews than non-Jews. In a white population, the annual incidence of disease is up to 10 per 100,000 people.[37,50] Symptomatic ulcerative colitis usually occurs from 25 to 45 years of age, and the disease is more common in women than men.

Crohn's disease occurs in all races and is distributed worldwide. In the United States, the annual incidence of the disease is 4 per 100,000 people.[50] The disease appears most often from 15 to 35 years of age. Men and women are equally affected, and patients from urban backgrounds and with high levels of education are at greater risk.

The frequency of peripheral arthritis is 11% in ulcerative colitis and 20% in Crohn's disease.[28,29] Spondylitis occurs in 3% to 4% of both diseases, and radiographic sacroiliitis occurs in 10%.[1,18] A study in Norway reported that the frequency of spondylitis was 2.6% in ulcerative colitis and 6% in Crohn's disease [61] Women and men are equally affected by Crohn's disease; women are affected half as often as men in ulcerative colitis with spondylitis. In a study of 1459 patients from the Oxford Inflammatory Bowel Disease Clinic, arthritis was reported in 6% of ulcerative colitis patients and 10% of Crohn's disease patients.[59] In a study from Belgium, the prevalence of a history of swollen joints was 29%.[15]

Pathogenesis

The etiology of both these inflammatory bowel diseases is unknown.[37] Specific infections with bacteria, overproduction of enzymes, vascular disorders, and hypersensitivity to foods are a few of the unproven theories suggested as possible causes.

Genetic Susceptibility

No specific HLA genetic predisposition for these illnesses has been discovered, although they may have a familial predilection.[2,63] Studies have suggested that first-degree relatives of an affected patient have a risk of IBD that is 4 to 20 times higher than that in the general population. The absolute risk for first-degree relatives is 7%.[60,80] After screening families with IBD, an area of linkage on chromosome 16, designated *IBD1*, was associated with Crohn's disease, but not ulcerative colitis. The gene on chromosome 16 encodes for a cytoplasmic protein, NOD2.[56] *NOD2* is a capsase activation and recruitment domain that produces proteins mediating apoptosis.[20] NOD2 is expressed by macrophages as a pattern recognition receptor for bacterial lipopolysaccharides. NOD2 affects nuclear factor κB (NFκB), a factor that signals gene transcription. NFκB activates the production of multiple inflammatory cytokines, including tumor necrosis factor (TNF). Crohn's disease patients have reduced macrophage activation in response to lipopolysaccharide. Other loci on other chromosomes (3, 7, 12) have also been identified to increase the risk for IBD.[71]

The axial arthritis of IBD may be a hereditary accompaniment of the disease and not a manifestation of the activity of bowel disease itself. Familial aggregation of spondylitis and sacroiliitis in relatives of patients with IBD has been reported.[30,44] Both non–HLA-related factors and HLA-B27 may play a role. Enlow and colleagues reported an incidence of HLA-B27 of 30% in patients with axial arthritis and IBD.[21] In the same study, when relatives of the HLA-B27–negative spondylitis patients were studied, four were found to have axial arthritis without IBD. No specific HLA haplotype was associated with axial arthropathy. This study suggests that both HLA-B27 and non-HLA genetic determinants predispose to axial arthropathy in patients with IBD. In patients with enteropathic spondylitis, HLA-B27 is positive in 50% to 75% of patients.[85] Although no association is reported between the bowel disease activity and axial arthritis, Mielants and Veys have described silent inflammatory gut disease identified at colonoscopy.[48] Patients with chronic spondyloarthropathy in association with peripheral arthritis have a higher frequency of IBD than do patients with axial skeletal disease alone. Crohn's disease in an early stage is the cause of bowel lesions in 26% of these patients with chronic axial and peripheral arthritis.[39]

Mucosal Barrier

The pathogenesis of peripheral and axial arthritis may be different. Peripheral arthritis may evolve as a complication of active bowel disease. Hypothetically, endogenous or exogenous antigens may be absorbed through the bowel wall and initiate an immune response (antigen-antibody complexes) that would collect in peripheral joints and cause synovitis. This scheme has clinical correlations in the close association of the activity of bowel disease and peripheral arthritis and the association of peripheral arthritis and other extraintestinal manifestations of disease, including erythema nodosum and iritis.[32] A decrease in breakdown of the mucosal barrier may decrease the risk for IBD. Early appendectomy decreases the risk for ulcerative colitis.[3] A similar immune complex mechanism may also explain the arthritis associated with another bowel abnormality, intestinal bypass arthritis.[75,84] Polyarthritis, including peripheral arthritis, and spondylitis have been linked to ileal pouch surgery after proctocolectomy. The development of arthritis after bowel surgery suggests the role of exposure to bowel antigens in the development of joint disease.[5]

The integrity of the mucosal barrier is compromised in IBD.[72] Bacteria enter the mucosa and activate macrophages that produce a variety of inflammatory cytokines such as TNF, interleukin-1, and interleukin-6.[66]

Activation of TH1 lymphocytes produces other inflammatory mediators, including prostaglandins, and nitric oxide. Recruitment of inflammatory cells is also enhanced by the expression of adhesion molecules in the local microvasculature. Patients with IBD lose tolerance to their own bacterial flora, which is reversed when IBD comes under control.[19]

The role of gut inflammation in the development of spondyloarthropathies, in general, remains an active area of research. European investigators documented gut inflammation in 66% of spondyloarthropathy patients by ileocolonoscopy. The acute form of inflammation resembled acute bacterial enterocolitis with preservation of mucosal architecture. The chronic form of inflammation resembled Crohn's disease. When the second ileocolonoscopies were performed, remission of joint inflammation was associated with resolution of gut inflammation. Some patients with spondyloarthropathy may have a subclinical form of Crohn's disease in which joint symptoms are the only clinical manifestation.[14,74]

CLINICAL HISTORY

The early symptoms of ulcerative colitis are frequent bowel movements with blood or mucus. Mild disease is associated with some abdominal pain and a few bowel movements per day. Severe disease is characterized by fatigue, weight loss, fever, and extracolonic involvement. Crohn's disease is frequently an indolent illness characterized by generalized fatigue, mild nonbloody diarrhea, anorexia, weight loss, and cramping lower abdominal pain. Patients may have symptoms for years before the diagnosis is made.

Articular involvement in these IBDs is divided into two forms: peripheral and spondylitic. In ulcerative colitis, peripheral arthritis starts as an acute monarticular or oligoarticular arthritis affecting the knee, ankle, elbow, proximal phalangeal, wrist, or shoulder joints in patients with active bowel disease.[87] The attacks are painful and sometimes associated with effusions. They subside after 6 to 8 weeks and are nondeforming.[62] Joint symptoms follow the activity of the bowel disease. Recurrences are common.[13] Patients with arthritis frequently demonstrate other extracolonic manifestations of ulcerative colitis, such as erythema nodosum, pyoderma gangrenosum, and uveitis, as well as extensive and chronic bowel disease with pseudopolyps and perianal disease.[47]

The peripheral joint involvement in Crohn's disease is similar in onset and distribution to that of ulcerative colitis.[4] However, the correlation of bowel inflammation and joint symptoms may continue while gastrointestinal complaints subside. The lack of association is probably secondary to the more scattered nature of Crohn's disease throughout the gut as opposed to the colonic involvement of ulcerative colitis and the difficulty in ascertaining complete remission of the illness.[30] In a prospective study of 123 patients with spondyloarthropathy, Crohn's disease developed in 8 (6%) 2 to 9 years after joint symptoms appeared.[49] Patients with colonic involvement and Crohn's disease may be at greater risk for peripheral arthritis.[55] On rare occasion, the peripheral arthritis may mimic the distribution of rheumatoid arthritis in the absence of rheumatoid factor.[10]

The axial skeletal involvement in ulcerative colitis and Crohn's disease is similar. Three groups of patients with IBD and spondylitis have been described by Dekher-Saeys and colleagues.[17] In about a third of patients, spondylitis antedates the bowel disease. This interval may be as long as 10 to 20 years.[1] Seventy percent were HLA-B27 positive, 68% had radiographic changes of spondylitis, and 25% had iritis. An association between sacroiliitis and iritis in ulcerative colitis was also reported by Wright and colleagues.[86] Bowel symptoms developed in a fourth of the patients before the onset of spondylitis. Thirteen percent were HLA-B27 positive, 36% had radiographic changes of spondylitis, and none had iritis. These patients had severe disease of the gut. The remaining patients had a simultaneous onset of gut and spine disease. The spondylitis of IBD has a course totally independent of that of the bowel disease. The clinical and radiographic findings are similar to those of ankylosing spondylitis, including involvement of the shoulders and hips, although some have suggested that it is a milder disease and has an increased proportion of women with spondylitis.[46] Patients with spondylitis complain of aching low back pain with stiffness that is maximal in the early morning, similar to ankylosing spondylitis.[7] As in uncomplicated ankylosing spondylitis, the development of cervical spine stiffness and pain is a manifestation of disease progression to generalized spondylitis. In a study of classic ankylosing spondylitis, only 7.6% of patients had an initial complaint of neck pain.[26] Neck pain occurs in patients after the disease has been present for a number of years. In a study lasting 15 years, cervical spine disease developed in 33% of enteropathic arthritis patients.[46] Occasional patients with Crohn's disease have been reported with severe back pain, limitation of lumbar motion, and decreased chest expansion, even though they have no radiographic changes of spondylitis. In these patients, improvement in bowel disease was associated with improved musculoskeletal function.[17] This form of arthritis is a secondary phenomenon of the activity of Crohn's disease. Other musculoskeletal complications of IBD include clubbing and periostitis, avascular necrosis of bone, septic arthritis of the hips, and granulomatous inflammation of synovium, bone, and muscle.[43,53]

PHYSICAL EXAMINATION

The general physical examination concentrates on the abdomen and gastrointestinal tract, including inspection of the oropharynx, perineum, and rectum. Examination for extraintestinal disease such as aphthous ulcers, iritis, erythema nodosum, and pyoderma gangrenosum is indicated. The musculoskeletal examination must include both peripheral joints and the axial skeleton. Patients with spondyloarthropathy may have decreased motion of the spine in all planes and tenderness to percussion over the sacroiliac joints. In rare circumstances, chest expansion is diminished. Patients with more extensive disease have limitation of motion of the cervical spine. Straightening is the main postural abnormality.[46] Occiput-to-wall measurements document the immobility of the entire axial skeleton, including the cervical spine. In a small number of patients, peripheral and axial skeletal disease may coexist.

LABORATORY DATA

Usual laboratory test results such as a decreased hematocrit level, increased white blood cell (WBC) count, an extreme platelet count (thrombocytosis of 700,000 to 1,000,000/mm^3), hypoalbuminemia, and hypokalemia are abnormal but nonspecific. The inflammatory findings of an increased WBC count with poor mucin clot in synovial fluid is also nondiagnostic. Rheumatoid factor and antinuclear antibodies are absent. Perinuclear (p)-cytoplasmic antibodies (ANCAs) have been reported in 70% of patients with ulcerative colitis.[66] p-ANCA is directed against lactoferrin autoantigens. Crohn's disease is associated with antibodies to *Saccharomyces cerevesiae* in over 50% of patients.[64,83] No specific HLA antigen has been associated with ulcerative colitis, Crohn's disease, or peripheral joint disease. Approximately 50% of patients with symptomatic spondylitis and IBD are HLA-B27 positive.[51]

RADIOGRAPHIC EVALUATION

Roentgenograms

Roentgenograms of peripheral joints demonstrate soft tissue swelling and occasionally joint effusions.[8,9,47] Findings of joint destruction, joint space narrowing, erosions, and periosteal proliferation are rare.[24] The roentgenographic changes of spondylitis in IBD are indistinguishable from those of classic ankylosing spondylitis (Fig. 11-21).[88] On occasion, asymmetric sacroiliitis has been reported.[31] Findings include squaring of vertebral bodies, erosions, widening and fusion of the sacroiliac joints, symmetrical involvement of the sacroiliac joints, and marginal syndesmophytes involving the lumbar, thoracic, or cervical spine (Fig. 11-22).[46] No correlation between colonic disease and spondylitis could be ascertained in a study of patients with Crohn's disease.[52] Asymptomatic roentgenographic sacroiliitis is demonstrated in up to 15% of patients with IBD. In contrast to classic ankylosing spondylitis, this condition has no association with HLA-B27, and women and men have equal involvement.[33] Scintigraphic evaluation of the sacroiliac joints in patients with IBD has detected increased uptake of radiotracer in 52%.[12] The clinical significance of these findings remains to be determined.

Bone Scintigraphy, Computed Tomography, Magnetic Resonance

Bone scintigraphy may identify all areas of the osseous system that are inflamed. Increased activity is a sensitive, but nonspecific finding in inflammatory arthritis. CT can identify erosions and sclerosis in the sacroiliac joints, but at the expense of increased x-ray exposure.[58] MR images may identify areas of subchondral edema as early findings of inflammation in the sacroiliac joints and vertebral bodies.

The clinical diagnosis of IBD is suspected in an individual with diarrhea, rectal bleeding, abdominal cramps, abdominal pain, perianal fistula or abscess, and an abdominal mass along with erythema nodosum, iritis, or arthritis. Radiographic evaluation of ulcerative colitis reveals mucosa ulceration, edema, and varying lengths of bowel. Crohn's disease causes deep ulcerations with strictures, fistulization, loop separation, and a mass effect in a discontinuous pattern that may involve the small intestine as well as the colon.

DIFFERENTIAL DIAGNOSIS

A specific diagnosis of ulcerative colitis or Crohn's disease is made from the histologic examination of biopsy material from the gut. The inflammatory abnormalities of ulcerative colitis are limited to the superficial layers of the gut, mucosa, and submucosa. The most characteristic findings in ulcerative colitis are atrophy of the mucosal glands and inflammatory cells in the crypts of the colon causing crypt abscesses with no skip areas. Crohn's disease is characterized by transluminal granulomatous inflammation. Whereas biopsy material yields supportive evidence for one or the other illness, the final differentiation rests heavily on the history, clinical course, and barium contrast studies of the gut. The differential diagnosis for the bowel disease includes infectious colitis, diverticulitis, pseudomembranous colitis, and ischemic colitis. Infectious agents associated with colitis include *Shigella*, *Salmonella*, *Campylobacter fetus*, *Yersinia enterocolitica*, cytomegalovirus, amebiasis, and histoplasmosis.

Culture of an early-morning stool specimen is an important part of the evaluation of a patient with chronic diarrhea. Special stains of biopsy material may detect an unsuspected organism. Diverticulitis causes localized pain, fever, and diarrhea. Radiographic studies help identify the localized nature of the disorder caused by infection of a colonic diverticulum. In patients who receive oral or parenteral antibiotics, a nonbloody, watery diarrhea may develop up to 4 weeks later that on endoscopic examination is associated with a yellowish white pseudomembrane on the colonic surfaces. Stool cultures that grow *Clostridium difficile* or reveal *C. difficile* toxin virtually ensure the diagnosis of pseudomembranous colitis. The abrupt onset of abdominal cramps with bleeding in a patient 60 years or older with preexisting atherosclerotic cardiovascular disease suggests an ischemic insult to the bowel. An abdominal flat plate film may demonstrate scalloping ("thumbprinting") of the wall. This finding is consistent with ischemic colitis. Of the various entities included in the preceding differential diagnosis of IBD, bacterial infection of the gut is the only condition associated with spondyloarthropathy (reactive arthritis).[57] See the preceding section, "Reactive Arthritis."

The diagnosis of enteropathic arthritis is not difficult to make in a patient with ulcerative colitis or Crohn's disease and nondeforming peripheral arthritis. Because peripheral arthritis develops in most patients after the onset of gastrointestinal symptoms, the possibilities for the cause of their arthritis are limited. The real difficulty arises in patients with back symptoms before the onset of bowel disease; their differential diagnosis encompasses the other

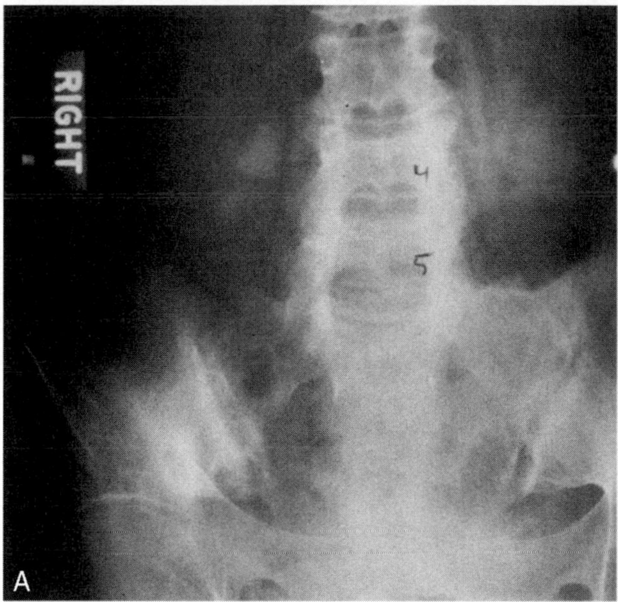

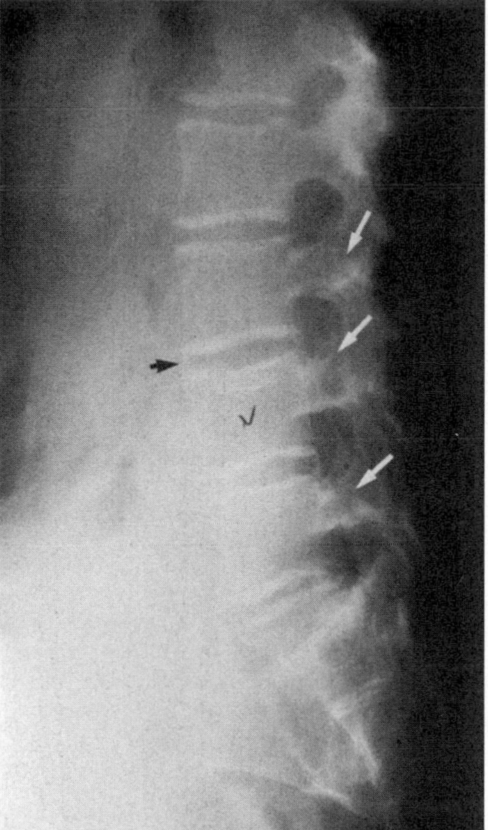

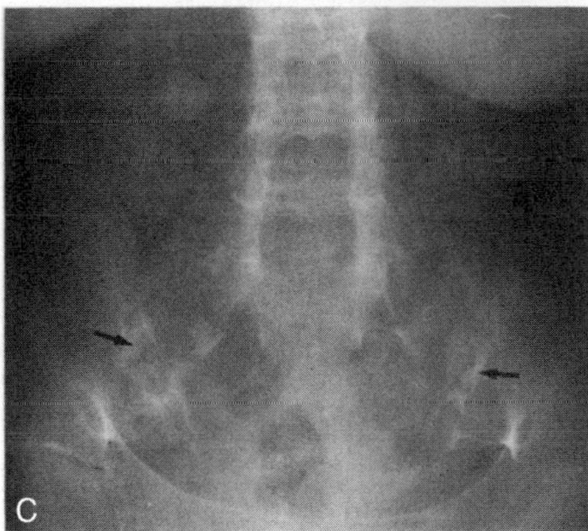

Figure 11-21 Crohn's disease. A 25-year-old woman with a 9-year history of Crohn's disease had been experiencing lower back pain and stiffness for 4 years. The patient had a chest expansion of 2 cm and no movement of the lumbar spine with flexion. *A*, An anteroposterior (AP) view of the pelvis reveals bilateral symmetrical sacroiliac joint abnormalities characterized by erosion and sclerosis. *B*, A lateral view of the lumbar spine demonstrates loss of lumbar lordosis, fusion of the facet joints *(white arrows)*, and early syndesmophyte formation *(black arrow)*. *C*, Five years later, an AP view of pelvis on 7/3/90 revealed progressive joint erosion *(black arrows)* and generalized osteoporosis.

spondyloarthropathies, including ankylosing spondylitis and reactive arthritis. The lower frequency of HLA-B27 may help differentiate enteropathic arthritis from ankylosing spondylitis. The absence of conjunctivitis, urethritis, and periostitis, particularly in the heels, may help distinguish it from reactive arthritis.

A patient with enteropathic spondyloarthropathy commonly has back pain in the absence of gastrointestinal symptoms. The finding of morning stiffness should raise the suspicion of a spondyloarthropathy. The factors that help make the diagnosis of enteropathic spondyloarthropathy are the pattern of peripheral arthritis if present (upper extremity disease uncommon in ankylosing spondylitis and reactive arthritis; bilateral ankle arthritis uncommon in psoriatic disease), erythema nodosum, and iritis.

Intestinal Bypass Surgery

Patients who have undergone intestinal bypass surgery for morbid obesity may be disposed to polyarthritis as a complication of this procedure. The majority of patients are women in whom polyarthritis most commonly develops after jejunocolostomy, probably secondary to a systemic

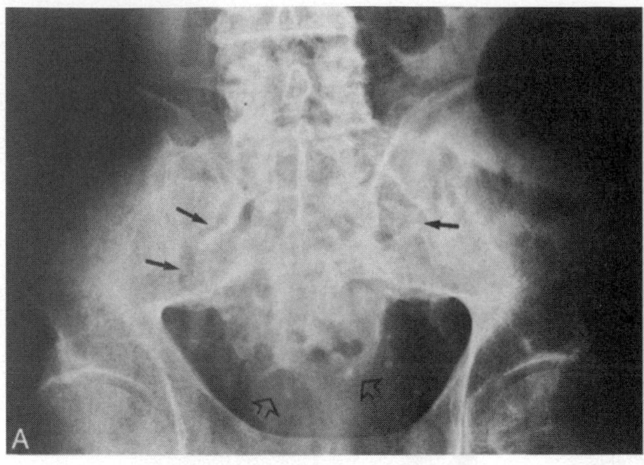

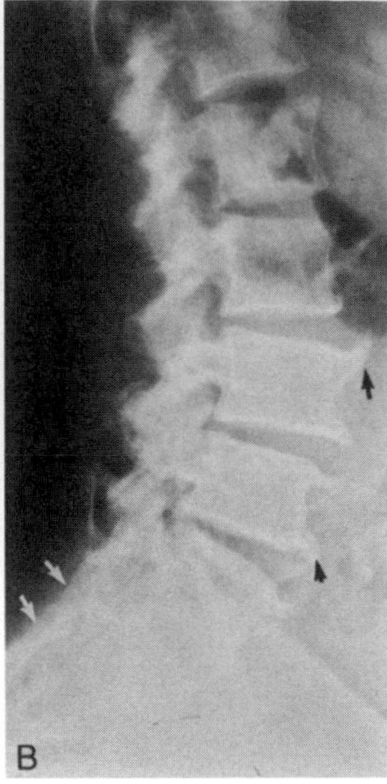

Figure 11-22 Crohn's disease in a 56-year-old man with a long history of the disease and alcoholism. Crohn's disease was manifested by rectal fistulas associated with sacral osteomyelitis. *A,* An anteroposterior view of the pelvis reveals bilateral sacroiliitis *(black arrows)* and erosion of the inferior section of the sacrum *(open black arrows)*. *B,* A lateral view reveals traction osteophytes *(black arrows)* (manifestation of intervertebral disc degeneration) and bony erosion of the dorsal portion of the sacrum *(white arrows)* (compatible with sacral osteomyelitis).

reaction to bacterial products.[73,84] The arthritis affects the knees, hands, feet, wrists, elbows, and hips. Involvement of the axial skeleton, particularly the sacroiliac joints, has only rarely been reported.[70] Radiographs of these patients reveal erosions, sclerosis, and articular space narrowing at the sacroiliac joint and syndesmophytes of the spine. HLA-B27 may be detected in patients with axial joint involvement. Nonsteroidal anti-inflammatory drugs (NSAIDs) may be somewhat helpful in controlling the joint pain. Patients with severe symptoms unresponsive to drugs may obtain improvement with revision of the bypass.[38]

TREATMENT

The therapeutic program for peripheral joint disease may also include NSAIDs, intra-articular injections of corticosteroids, and physical therapy. No evidence of increased gastrointestinal adverse effects with NSAIDs has been detected in these patients with IBD. Initially, lower therapeutic doses of the NSAIDs may be tried to test drug tolerability. An increased dosage can be used if the patient tolerates the medicine but experiences inadequate relief of symptoms. If a patient has a good response to an NSAID but gastrointestinal symptoms develop, medications to control those symptoms may be added to the patient's therapeutic program. In rare circumstances, NSAIDs have been implicated as factors causing an exacerbation of IBD.[25,36]

Therapy for enteropathic spondylitis is similar to that for classic ankylosing spondylitis. The program includes patient education, NSAIDs, and physical therapy. Control of bowel disease does not necessarily correlate with improvement in axial skeletal symptoms. In ulcerative colitis, colectomy should not be performed with the expectation that the spondylitic symptoms will resolve.

Colectomized patients with ulcerative colitis do not have recurrences of peripheral joint disease.[87] Surgery is not nearly as effective in Crohn's disease because the disease may have a more extensive distribution through the gastrointestinal tract.

Treatment of peripheral arthritis must be directed toward control of the underlying bowel disease. Therapy might include sulfasalazine (Azulfidine, 4 to 6 g/day), metronidazole, corticosteroid enemas, oral corticosteroids, and colectomy for patients with severe ulcerative colitis.[65,67,77] A variety of therapies have been developed for the treatment of Crohn's disease. Newer forms of sulfasalazine that contain only the active moiety 5-aminosalicylic acid, such as olsalazine and mesalamine, have fewer side effects and may be given orally or as a suppository.[35] These drugs may be used for the treatment of mild, initial attacks or for the prophylaxis of recurrent attacks of ulcerative colitis.[34,68] In active, severe disease, the combination of sulfasalazine and corticosteroids is effective in 90% of patients.[69] Although antibiotics may be of limited utility in ulcerative colitis, these drugs have efficacy in Crohn's disease. Metronidazole at doses up to 750 mg three times daily is necessary to treat perianal fistulas.[78] Corticosteroids are effective when given orally or rectally.[40] Budesonide is an oral form of steroid that is released in the ileum. This form of corticosteroid may decrease bowel inflammation with less risk of systemic side effects.[27]

Immunosuppressives

Occasionally, immunosuppressive drugs in the form of azathioprine or mercaptopurine are needed to control severe Crohn's disease. Mercaptopurine is given in doses of 50 mg/day, whereas azathioprine is administered in doses of 1 mg/kg. Clinical effect may take months to appear because of the slow-acting nature of the drug.[41,45]

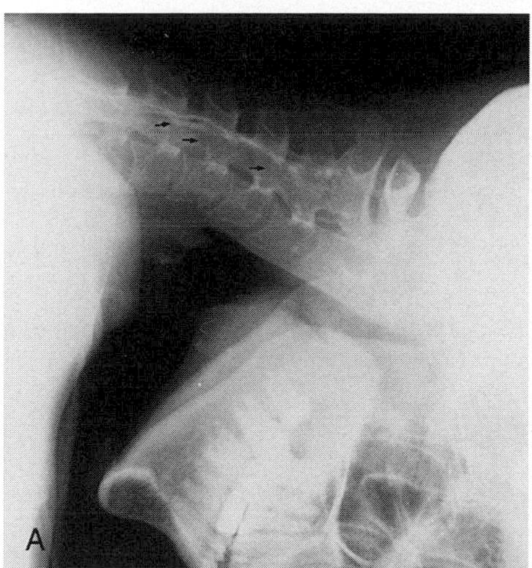

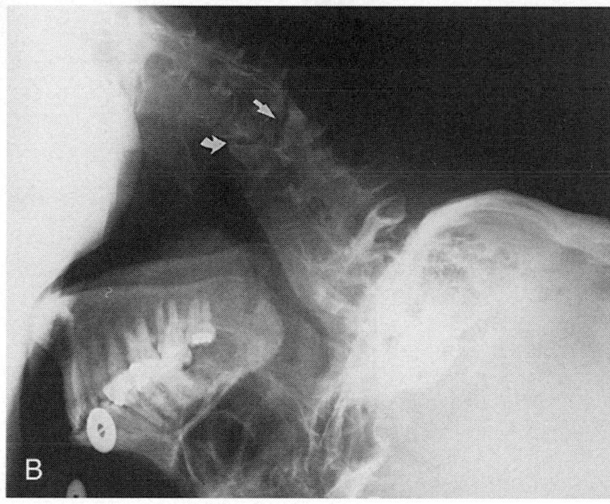

Figure 11-23 Crohn's disease. A 30-year-old woman with a 14-year history of Crohn's disease had been experiencing spine pain and stiffness for 9 years. The patient had a chest expansion of 2 cm and no movement of the lumbar spine with flexion. Fusion of the sacroiliac joints and the apophyseal joint was prominent. Cervical spine disease resulted in neck pain and gradual neck flexion, with the woman's chin coming to rest on her chest wall. She was to undergo vertebral osteotomy when she sustained a spontaneous fracture of the cervical spine without any neurologic deficits. She was placed in a halo cast and healed in a more functional position. *A*, 7/3/90—A lateral view of the cervical spine reveals fusion of all the facet joints *(arrows)* and space between the mandible and chest wall. *B*, 2/26/91—A lateral view of the cervical spine shows fracture through the C4–C5 interspace *(straight arrow)* and anterior subluxation *(curved arrow)*.

Individuals with genetic variants of thiopurine *S*-methyltransferase are at greater risk for life-threatening bone marrow suppression from azathioprine. Methotrexate is helpful for steroid-dependent Crohn's disease to maintain remission at doses of 15 mg/wk.[23] Other immunosuppressive agents used for IBD include cyclosporine and mycophenolate mofetil.[66]

Anti–Tumor Necrosis Factor-Alpha Inhibitors

The anti-TNF agent infliximab is effective in the treatment of patients with severe Crohn's disease, including those with fistulas. Infliximab binds to precursor cell surface TNF, and such binding leads to monocyte apoptosis. A single infusion of infliximab may result in a significant reduction in disease activity in two thirds of patients with moderate disease.[79] The effect may be sustained for weeks to months. Patients who renew production of TNF have a shorter duration of response to infliximab.[54] The benefits of infliximab for the treatment of ulcerative colitis remain uncertain.[66] In small groups of patients with enteropathic arthritis and peripheral and axial involvement, infliximab improved both bowel and joint disease.[81] Etanercept may be effective for joint inflammation but may not control bowel disease.[32a] However, large groups of patients with enteropathic arthritis have not been treated in a study to determine the true effect of anti-TNF therapy.

Other biologic therapies attack different portions of the inflammatory cascade. Such therapies include agents affecting levels of cytokines (TNF inhibitors, NFκB inhibitors, and interleukins). Adhesion molecules and integrins are also immunologic factors that are future targets of therapy in Crohn's disease. Initial trials involving these therapies have been completed. However, further double-blind trials will need to be conducted to determine the clinical efficacy of these agents.[16]

PROGNOSIS

The ultimate course and outcome of these patients depend on the severity of their bowel disease. Patients with severe ulcerative colitis have a mortality rate of 10% to 20% over a 5-year period. Patients with a severe initial attack, continuous clinical activity, involvement of the entire colon, and disease for 10 years or longer have a higher risk for cancer of the colon.[22] These patients may require colectomy. Although Crohn's disease is associated with frequent recurrences, the overall mortality rate of 5% for the first 5 years of disease is much less than in ulcerative colitis.[42]

Patients with peripheral enteropathic arthritis have nondeforming disease of short duration. These patients experience little disability from the arthritis and are able to work. The disability associated with enteropathic spondylitis is similar to that of ankylosing spondylitis in severely affected patients. The association of hip disease and spondylitis results in a marked decrease in mobility. Patients with spinal rigidity are at risk for fracture (Fig. 11-23). These patients should not perform heavy labor associated with lifting.

References

Enteropathic Arthritis

1. Acheson ED: An association between ulcerative colitis, regional enteritis and ankylosing spondylitis. Q J Med 29:489, 1960.
2. Almy TP, Sherlock P: Genetic aspects of ulcerative colitis and regional enteritis. Gastroenterology 51:757, 1966.
3. Andersson RE, Olaison G, Tysk C, et al: Appendectomy and protection against ulcerative colitis. N Engl J Med 344:808-814, 2001.

4. Ansell BM, Wigley RAD: Arthritic manifestations in regional enteritis. Ann Rheum Dis 23:64, 1964.
5. Axon JMC, Hawley PR, Huskisson EC: Ileal pouch arthritis. Br J Rheumatol 32:586, 1993.
6. Bargen JA: Complications and sequelae of chronic ulcerative colitis. Ann Intern Med 3:335, 1929.
7. Bowen GE, Kirsner JB: The arthritis of ulcerative colitis and regional enteritis ("intestinal arthritis"). Med Clin North Am 49:17, 1965.
8. Bywaters EGL, Ansell BM: Arthritis associated with ulcerative colitis: A clinical and pathological study. Ann Rheum Dis 17:169, 1958.
9. Clark RL, Muhletaler CA, Margulies SI: Colitic arthritis: Clinical and radiographic manifestations. Radiology 101:585, 1971.
10. Cornes JS, Stecher M: Primary Crohn's disease of the colon and rectum. Gut 2:189, 1961.
11. Crohn BB, Ginzburg L, Oppenheimer GD: Regional ileitis: A pathologic and clinical entity. JAMA 99:1323, 1932.
12. Davis P, Thomson ABR, Lentle B: Quantitative sacroiliac scintigraphy in patients with Crohn's disease. Arthritis Rheum 21:234, 1978.
13. De Keyser F, Baeten D, Van den Bosch F, et al: Gut inflammation and spondyloarthropathies. Curr Rheumatol Rep 4:525-532, 2002.
14. De Keyser F, Elewaut D, de Vos M, et al: Bowel inflammation and the spondyloarthropathies. Rheum Dis Clin North Am 24:785-813, 1998.
15. De Vlam K, De Vos M, Mielants H, et al: Spondyloarthropathy is underestimated in inflammatory bowel disease: Prevalence and HLA association. J Rheumatol 27:2860-2865, 2000.
16. De Vos M: Standard and innovative therapy of inflammatory bowel diseases. Clin Exp Rheumatol 20(suppl 28):S95-S100, 2002.
17. Dekher-Saeys BJ, Meuwissen SGM, van den Berg-Loonen EM, et al: Clinical characteristics and results of histocompatibility typing (HLA-B27) in 50 patients with both ankylosing spondylitis and inflammatory bowel disease. Ann Rheum Dis 37:36, 1978.
18. Dekher-Saeys BJ, Meuwissen SGM, van den Berg-Loonen EM, et al: Prevalence of peripheral arthritis, sacroiliitis and ankylosing spondylitis in patients suffering from inflammatory bowel disease. Ann Rheum Dis 37:33, 1978.
19. Duchmann R, Kaiser I, Hermann E, et al: Tolerance exists towards resident intestinal flora but is broken in active inflammatory bowel disease. Clin Exp Immunol 102:448-455, 1995.
20. Elson CO: Genes, microbes, and T cells—new therapeutic targets in Crohn's disease. N Engl J Med 346:614-616, 2002.
21. Enlow RW, Bias WB, Arnett FC: The spondylitis of inflammatory bowel disease: Evidence for a non–HLA-linked axial arthropathy. Arthritis Rheum 23:1359, 1980.
22. Farmer RG, Hawk WA, Turnbull RB Jr: Carcinoma associated with mucosal ulcerative colitis, and with transmural colitis and enteritis (Crohn's disease). Cancer 28:289, 1971.
23. Feagan BG, Fedorak RN, Irvine EJ, et al: A comparison of methotrexate with placebo for the maintenance of remission in Crohn's disease. N Engl J Med 342:1627-1632, 2000.
24. Frayha R, Stevens MB, Bayless TM: Destructive monoarthritis and granulomatous synovitis as the presenting manifestations of Crohn's disease. Johns Hopkins Med J 137:151, 1975.
25. Gran JT, Husby G: Ankylosing spondylitis: Current drug treatment. Drugs 44:585, 1992.
26. Gran JT, Ostensen M, Husby G: A clinical comparison between males and females with ankylosing spondylitis. J Rheumatol 12:126, 1985.
27. Greenberg GR, Feagan BG, Martin F, et al: Oral budesonide as maintenance treatment for Crohn's disease: A placebo-controlled, dose-ranging study. Canadian Inflammatory Bowel Disease Study Group. Gastroenterology 110:45-51, 1996.
28. Greenstein AJ, Janowitz HD, Sachar DB: The extra-intestinal complications of Crohn's disease and ulcerative colitis: A study of 700 patients. Medicine (Baltimore) 55:401, 1976.
29. Haslock F, Wright V: The musculoskeletal complications of Crohn's disease. Medicine (Baltimore) 52:217, 1973.
30. Haslock I: Arthritis and Crohn's disease: A family study. Ann Rheum Dis 32:479, 1973.
31. Helliwell PS, Hickling P, Wricht V: Do the radiological changes of classical ankylosing spondylitis differ from the changes found in the spondylitis associated with inflammatory bowel disease? Ann Rheum Dis 57:135-140, 1998.
32. Hochberg MC, Feinstein RS, Moser RL, Ryan MJ: Colitic arthritis. Johns Hopkins Med J 151:173, 1982.
32a. Holden W, Orchard T, Wordsworth P: Enteropathic arthritis. Rheum Dis Clin North Am 29:513-530, 2003.
33. Hyla JF, Franck WA, Davis JS: Lack of association of HLA-B27 with radiographic sacroiliitis in inflammatory bowel disease. J Rheumatol 3:196, 1976.
34. Ireland A, Mason CH, Jewell DP: Controlled trial comparing olsalazine and sulfasalazine for the maintenance treatment of ulcerative colitis. Gut 29:835, 1988.
35. Jarnerot G: Newer 5-aminosalicylic acid–based drugs in chronic inflammatory bowel disease. Drugs 37:76, 1989.
36. Kaufmann HJ, Taubin HL: Nonsteroidal anti-inflammatory drugs activate quiescent inflammatory bowel disease. Ann Intern Med 107:513, 1988.
37. Kirsner JB, Shorter RG: Recent developments in non-specific inflammatory bowel disease. N Engl J Med 306:837, 1982.
38. Leff RD, Aldo-Benson MA, Madura JA: The effect of revision of the intestinal bypass on post-intestinal bypass arthritis. Arthritis Rheum 26:678, 1983.
39. Leirisalo-Repo M, Turunen U, Stenman S, et al: High frequency of silent inflammatory bowel disease in spondyloarthropathy. Arthritis Rheum 37:23, 1994.
40. Linn FV, Peppercorn MA: Drug therapy for inflammatory bowel disease. I. Am J Surg 164:85, 1992.
41. Linn FV, Peppercorn MA: Drug therapy for inflammatory bowel disease. II. Am J Surg 164:178, 1992.
42. Lock MR, Farmer RG, Fazio VW, et al: Recurrence and reoperation for Crohn's disease: The role of disease in prognosis. N Engl J Med 304:1586, 1981.
43. London D, Fitton JM: Acute septic arthritis complicating Crohn's disease. Br J Surg 57:536, 1970.
44. Macrae I, Wright V: A family study of ulcerative colitis. Ann Rheum Dis 32:16, 1973.
45. Marsh JW, Vehe KL, White HM: Immunosuppressants. Gastroenterol Clin North Am 21:679, 1992.
46. McEwen C, DiTata D, Lingg C, et al: Ankylosing spondylitis and spondylitis accompanying ulcerative colitis, regional enteritis, psoriasis and Reiter's disease: A comparative study. Arthritis Rheum 14:291, 1971.
47. McEwen C, Lingg C, Kirsner JB, Spencer JA: Arthritis accompanying ulcerative colitis. Am J Med 33:923, 1962.
48. Mielants H, Veys EM: The gut in the spondyloarthropathies. J Rheumatol 17:7, 1990.
49. Mielants H, Veys EM, Cuvelier C, et al: the evolution of spondyloarthropathies: Relation to gut histology. Part 1. Clinical aspects. J Rheumatol 22:2266-2272, 1995.
50. Monk M, Mendeloff AI, Siegel CI, Lilienfeld A: An epidemiological study of ulcerative colitis and regional enteritis among adults in Baltimore: Hospital incidence and prevalence, 1960 to 1963. Gastroenterology 53:198, 1967.
51. Morris RI, Metzger AL, Bluestone R, Terasaki PI: HLA-w27—a useful discriminator in the arthropathies of inflammatory bowel disease. N Engl J Med 290:1117, 1974.
52. Mueller CE, Seeger JF, Martel W: Ankylosing spondylitis and regional enteritis. Radiology 112:579, 1974.
53. Neale G, Kelsall AR, Doyle FH: Crohn's disease and diffuse symmetrical periostitis. Gut 9:383, 1968.
54. Nikolaus S, Raedler A, Kuhbacher T, et al: Mechanisms in failure of infliximab for Crohn's disease. Lancet 356:1475-1479, 2000.
55. Norton KI, Eichenfield AH, Rosh JR, et al: Atypical arthropathy associated with Crohn's disease. Am J Gastroenterol 88:948, 1993.
56. Ogura Y, Bonen DK, Inohara N, et al: A frameshift mutation in NOD2 associated with susceptibility to Crohn's disease. Nature 411:603-606, 2001.
57. Olhagen B: Postinfective or reactive arthritis. Scand J Rheumatol 9:193, 1980.
58. Oostveen JCM, van de Laar MAFJ: Magnetic resonance imaging in rheumatic disorders of the spine and sacroiliac joints. Semin Arthritis Rheum 30:52-69, 2000.
59. Orchard TR, Wordsworth BP, Jewell DP: Peripheral arthropathies in inflammatory bowel disease: Their articular distribution and natural history. Gut 42:387-391, 1998.
60. Orholm M, Munkholm P, Langholz E, et al: Familial occurrence of inflammatory bowel disease. N Engl J Med 324:84-88, 1991.
61. Palm O, Moum B, Ongre A, et al: The prevalence of ankylosing spondylitis and other spondyloarthropathies among patients with inflammatory bowel disease: A population study (the IBSEN study). J Rheumatol 29:511-515, 2002.

62. Palumbo PJ, Ward LE, Sauer WG, Scudamore HH: Musculoskeletal manifestations of inflammatory bowel disease: Ulcerative and granulomatous colitis and ulcerative proctitis. Mayo Clin Proc 48:411, 1973.
63. Paulley JW: Ulcerative colitis: A study of 173 cases. Gastroenterology 16:566, 1950.
64. Peeters M, Joossens, Vermeire S, et al: Diagnostic value of anti–*Saccharomyces cerevisiae* and antineutrophil cytoplasmic autoantibodies in inflammatory bowel disease. Am J Gastroenterol 96:730-734, 2001.
65. Peppercorn MA: Sulfasalazine: Pharmacology, clinical use, toxicity, and related new-drug development. Ann Intern Med 101:377, 1984.
66. Podolsky DK: Inflammatory bowel disease. N Engl J Med 347:417-429, 2002.
67. Present DW, Korelitz BI, Wise HN, et al: Treatment of Crohn's disease with 6-mercaptopurine: A long-term randomized double-blind study. N Engl J Med 302:981, 1980.
68. Rao SS, Dundas SA, Hildsworth CD, et al: Olsalazine or sulfasalazine in first attacks of ulcerative colitis: A double-blind study. Gut 30:675, 1989.
69. Rijk MC, Hogezand RA, van Lier HJ, et al: Sulphasalazine and prednisone compared with sulfasalazine for treating active Crohn's disease: A double-blind, randomized multicenter trial. Ann Intern Med 114:445, 1991.
70. Rose E, Espinoza LR, Osterland CK: Intestinal bypass arthritis: Association with circulating immune complexes. J Rheumatol 4:129, 1977.
71. Satsangi J, Parkes M, Louis E, et al: Two stage genome-wide search in inflammatory bowel disease provides evidence for susceptibility loci on chromosomes 3, 7, and 12. Nat Genet 14:199-202, 1996.
72. Schmitz H, Barmeyer C, Fromm M, et al: Altered tight junction structure contributes to the impaired epithelial barrier function in ulcerative colitis. Gastroenterology 116:301-309, 1999.
73. Shagrin JW, Frame B, Duncan H: Polyarthritis in obese patients with intestinal bypass. Ann Intern Med 75:377, 1971.
74. Smale S, Natt RS, Orchard TR, et al: Inflammatory bowel disease and spondyloarthropathy. Arthritis Rheum 44:2728-2736, 2001.
75. Stein HB, Schlappner OLA, Boyko W, et al: The intestinal bypass arthritis-dermatitis syndrome. Arthritis Rheum 24:684, 1981.
76. Steinberg VL, Storey G: Ankylosing spondylitis and chronic inflammatory lesions of the intestines. BMJ 2:1157, 1957.
77. Summers RW, Switz DM, Session JT, et al: National Cooperative Crohn's Disease Study: Results of drug treatment. Gastroenterology 77:847, 1979.
78. Sutherland L, Singleton J, Sessions J, et al: Double blind, placebo controlled trial of metronidazole in Crohn's disease. Gut 32:1071-1075, 1991
79. Targan SR, Hanauer SB, van Deventer SJH, et al: A short-term study of chimeric monoclonal antibody cA2 to tumor necrosis factor α for Crohn's disease. N Engl J Med 337:1029-1035, 1997.
80. Tysk C, Lindberg E, Jarnerot G, et al: Ulcerative colitis and Crohn's disease in an unselected population of monozygotic and dizygotic twins: A study of heritability and the influence of smoking. Gut 29:990-996, 1988.
81. Van den Bosch F, Kruithof E, De Vos M, et al: Crohn's disease associated with spondyloarthropathy: Effect of TNF-α blockade with infliximab on the articular symptoms. Lancet 356:1821-1822, 2000.
82. Van Patter WN, Bargen JA, Dockerty MB, et al: Regional enteritis. Gastroenterology 26:347, 1954.
83. Vermeire S, Joossens S, Peeters M, et al: Comparative study of ASCA (Anti–*Saccharomyces cerevisiae* antibody) assays in inflammatory bowel disease. Gastroenterology 120:827-833, 2001.
84. Wands JR, Lamont JT, Mann E, Isselbacher KJ: Arthritis associated with intestinal-bypass procedure for morbid obesity: Complement activation and characterization of circulating cryoproteins. N Engl J Med 294:121, 1976.
85. Weiner SR, Clarke J, Taggart NA, et al: Rheumatic manifestations of bowel disease. Semin Arthritis Rheum 20:353, 1991.
86. Wright R, Lumsden K, Luntz MH, et al: Abnormalities of the sacro-iliac joints and uveitis in ulcerative colitis. Q J Med 134:229, 1965.
87. Wright V, Watkinson G: The arthritis of ulcerative colitis. BMJ 2:670, 1965.
88. Zvaifler NJ, Martel W: Spondylitis in chronic ulcerative colitis. Arthritis Rheum 3:76, 1960.

BEHÇET'S SYNDROME

CAPSULE SUMMARY

	LOW BACK	NECK
Frequency of spinal pain	Rare	Not applicable (NA)
Location of spinal pain	Sacroiliac joints	NA
Quality of spinal pain	Ache	NA
Symptoms and signs	Morning stiffness, oral and genital ulcers, iritis, meningitis	NA
Laboratory tests	Increased erythrocyte sedimentation rate	NA
Radiographic findings	Sacroiliitis on plain roentgenogram	NA
Treatment	Corticosteroids, thalidomide, colchicine	NA

PREVALENCE AND PATHOGENESIS

Behçet's syndrome is a chronic relapsing systemic disease characterized by the triad of oral and genital ulcers and iritis. Additional features of the disease include vasculitis with aneurysms, erythema nodosum, meningoencephalitis, and arthritis with sacroiliitis. The disability associated with Behçet's syndrome is most commonly loss of vision secondary to iritis and neurologic impairment secondary to meningoencephalitis and stroke. The disease was first described by Hulusi Behçet, a Turkish dermatologist, in 1937.[3] The triad of this syndrome has also been referred to as the mucocutaneous ocular syndrome.[42]

Epidemiology

Behçet's syndrome occurs most frequently in people from eastern Asia to the Mediterranean countries (the ancient silk road) and Japan.[4,38] The disease is most common in Turkey, with a prevalence of 37 per 10,000 population.[43] The prevalence in Japan is approximately

1 in 7500.[33] In Olmsted County, Minnesota, the prevalence is 1 in 25,000.[34] The disease affects men more commonly than women, except in North America, where a study demonstrated an increased frequency in women.[35]

Pathogenesis

The etiology of Behçet's syndrome is unknown, although a number of immunologic abnormalities of a cellular and humoral variety have been described. Polymorphonuclear neutrophils (PMNs) exhibit increased motility and endothelial adhesion.[14] PMNs are primed for activation with increased phosphorylation of intracellular proteins. PMNs have increased superoxide production and exhibit increased production of lysosomal enzymes. This PMN activation is manifested clinically by pustular acne, pathergy, and hypopyon.

Lymphocyte function is abnormal in Behçet's syndrome. Patients with Behçet's syndrome have relative increases in the CD8/CD4 ratio, with reduced numbers of suppressor T cells. Some increase in B-cell number and activation occurs in association with an increased concentration of immunoglobulins and the formation of immune complexes.[23,28,35,47] However, Behçet's syndrome is not associated with autoantibodies and is not characterized as an autoimmune disease, as systemic lupus erythematosus is.[54] Increased levels of cytokines associated with TH1 and TH2 responses have been reported.[14] No single pattern of immune dysfunction has been associated with the illness.

Bacterial antigens that have cross-reactivity with human peptides may play a pathogenic role. Heat shock proteins (HSPs) are scavengers of intracellular proteins under denaturing stress conditions such as infection, trauma, and hypoxia. Sequence homology (50%) exists between mycobacterial and human HSPs. T cells responsive to bacterial HSP may stimulate autoreactive T cells by cross-reactivity mechanisms and thereby result in the activation of Behçet's syndrome.[24] Recent studies have suggested that antibodies directed at HSPs from streptococcal species, particularly *Streptococcus sanguis*, are present in higher titer in Behçet's patients than in normal controls.[26]

Genetic Susceptibility

Genetic factors may play a significant role in Japanese and Turkish patients.[36] HLA-B51 is the haplotype that is most frequently associated with Behçet's disease.[1,5] HLA-B51 has been linked to earlier development of ocular and vessel disease. An association between B51 and retinal disease may exist in the presence of retinal S antigen. A portion of the S antigen has homology with HLA-B molecules such as B51 and B27. CD4+ T cells may become activated when this antigen is exposed.[14] HLA-B27 positivity is seen in patients with sacroiliitis.[6] HLA-B12 is found in a few patients with mucocutaneous involvement.[25] The genetic susceptibility to Behçet's syndrome is multifactorial. The HLA-B contribution to development of the illness is estimated to be 20% or less.[18]

CLINICAL HISTORY

The typical patient is 30 years old and has multiple, painful oral ulcers that resolve over weeks. Genital ulcers, which are also painful, occur over the vulva, penis, or scrotum and are present in 80% of patients. Eye lesions, predominantly unilateral or bilateral iritis, occur in 66% of patients and may be manifested as blurred vision with little ocular pain. Iritis may lead to blindness in these patients.[10] Skin manifestations, including ulceration, vasculitis, erythema nodosum, erythema multiforme, and the formation of pustules after the trauma of venipuncture (pathergy), occur in a majority of patients.[7] Central nervous system involvement is noted in 24% of patients. A multitude of neurologic manifestations have been described, including meningoencephalitis characterized by fever, headache, stiff neck, cerebrovascular accident or stroke, hemiparesis, seizures, loss of speech, and profound confusion.[39] Neurologic involvement is a bad prognostic sign, with a mortality rate of 31% to 41% in two studies.[52,53] Vascular disease is associated with thrombophlebitis and arterial aneurysm. Between 7% and 37% of patients experience venous occlusions.[31] Gastrointestinal involvement includes colonic disease similar to ulcerative colitis.[7]

Articular involvement occurs in a majority of patients with Behçet's syndrome.[29,58] Joint involvement has ranged from 18% to 64% in different studies.[2] The four patterns of involvement include relapsing, remittent, remittent-progressive, and progressive. Most arthritic attacks last less than 2 months.[31] Peripheral arthritis is usually polyarticular and involves the knees, ankles, wrists, or elbows. Monarticular disease occurs in the knees or ankles but is less common. Joint symptoms frequently occur after the onset of oral ulcerations.[46] The arthritis is asymmetric, recurrent, and nondeforming. Axial skeletal disease consisting of back pain and sacroiliitis has been reported in a small proportion of patients with Behçet's syndrome.[11,13,40] In one study, 10 of 79 patients demonstrated radiographic changes of marked sacroiliitis. Other studies have not found an increased prevalence of sacroiliitis.[27] Spondylitis also has been described with the disease.[53] Debate exists concerning the classification of Behçet's syndrome as a spondyloarthropathy.

PHYSICAL EXAMINATION

Examination of the oropharynx and genitourinary system is essential in Behçet's syndrome. Ophthalmologic examination is frequently necessary to demonstrate iritis, which may be mildly symptomatic. A complete neurologic examination is also indicated to document any abnormalities in mentation or neurologic function.

Examination of the back reveals tenderness to percussion over the sacroiliac joints in patients with sacroiliitis. Range of motion of the lumbar spine may be diminished in these individuals.

LABORATORY DATA

Laboratory results are nonspecific in Behçet's syndrome. With active disease, the erythrocyte sedimentation rate and C-reactive protein are elevated along with an increase in peripheral white blood cells. Synovial fluid is inflammatory in type, with an increase in white cells from 80,000 to 250,000, normal glucose, and poor mucin clotting.[58]

Pathology

Pathologic evaluation of synovial tissue from Behçet's patients demonstrates dense granulation tissue filled with inflammatory cells, including neutrophils, lymphocytes, and macrophages. Vasculitis is a frequent pathologic finding. Cellular infiltration occurs in a perivascular distribution, sometimes with leukocytoclastic vasculitis with endothelial swelling and fibrinoid necrosis of the vessel walls in association with thrombosis.[9] Inflammatory cells are also noted in the vasa vasorum of blood vessels associated with aneurysmal dilation.

RADIOGRAPHIC EVALUATION

Roentgenograms

Bone and joint findings are usually mild and characterized by osteoporosis and soft tissue swelling. Osseous erosions and joint space narrowing are rarely encountered.[51] Sacroiliitis, both unilateral and bilateral, has been noted in patients with Behçet's syndrome along with the rarer occurrence of spondylitis (Fig. 11-24).[13] Sacroiliitis is characterized by subchondral erosions and reactive sclerosis.[41] Patients who are HLA-B27 positive may be at greater risk for sacroiliitis and spondylitis. In patients with inflammatory disease of the bowel, sacroiliitis similar to that seen with ulcerative colitis or Crohn's disease may develop.[7,15]

Computed Tomography

Some radiographic studies of sacroiliitis in patients with Behçet's syndrome have suggested that sacroiliitis is not increased in frequency in comparison to controls.[8] However, CT evaluation of the sacroiliac joints of Behçet's patients may increase the sensitivity of detecting the presence of sacroiliitis that may be missed by plain roentgenograms.[37]

DIFFERENTIAL DIAGNOSIS

The diagnosis of Behçet's syndrome is based on clinical features because of the lack of pathognomonic laboratory findings. Diagnostic criteria that have been suggested include oral ulcers, genital ulcers, iritis, and skin lesions as a major group and gastrointestinal, vascular, musculoskeletal, and central nervous system lesions and family history as a minor group.[45] The diagnosis is difficult to make because the different manifestations of the illness may take years to appear. The diagnosis should be considered in a patient with recurrent oral ulcerations and one other manifestation of the disease. The differential diagnosis is very small when a patient has multisystem involvement with Behçet's syndrome. In patients with disease in a single organ system, the differential diagnosis is directed toward diseases that affect that organ system. For example, the differential diagnosis of oral ulcers would include herpes simplex infection; gastrointestinal disease, ulcerative colitis or Crohn's disease; and aseptic meningitis and Mollaret's meningitis. In patients with oral ulcers, back pain, and lower extremity arthritis, the diagnosis of reactive arthritis must be excluded. Patients with reactive arthritis usually have painless oral ulcerations. Five sets of diagnostic criteria exist for the diagnosis for Behçet's disease,[49] but a

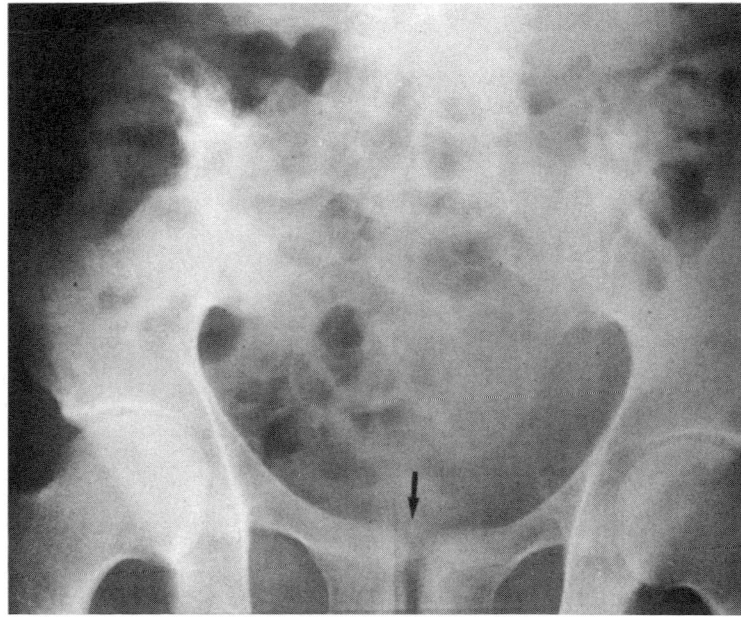

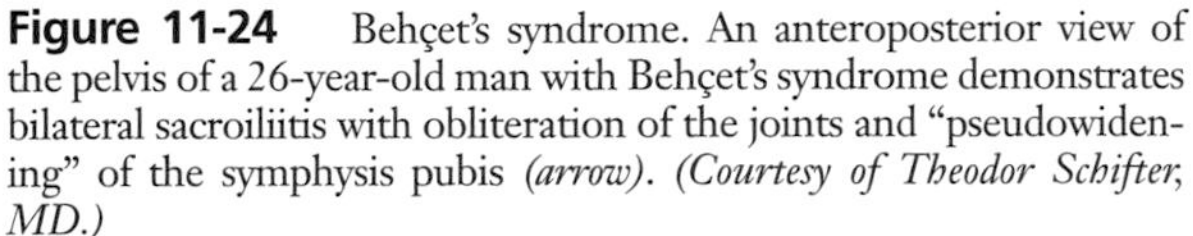

Figure 11-24 Behçet's syndrome. An anteroposterior view of the pelvis of a 26-year-old man with Behçet's syndrome demonstrates bilateral sacroiliitis with obliteration of the joints and "pseudowidening" of the symphysis pubis *(arrow)*. *(Courtesy of Theodor Schifter, MD.)*

simplification of the criteria has been proposed. These new criteria are oral ulcerations in combination with any two other manifestations, including genital ulceration, typical defined eye lesions, typical defined skin lesions, or a positive pathergy test.[48] Pathergy does not occur as commonly in northern European and North American patients. Possible alternative diagnostic entities suggested include cerebral vasculitis, recurrent phlebitis, arteritis, synovitis, aseptic meningitis, and bowel ulceration.[17]

TREATMENT

No specific therapy has been demonstrated to be effective in controlling the manifestations of Behçet's syndrome on a continued basis, but a number of medications are being studied for a variety of manifestations of Behçet's disease.[55] Systemic corticosteroids suppress skin and joint inflammation. They are less effective on oral and genital ulcers and iritis. Colchicine, 0.6 mg twice or three times daily, is effective for the treatment of genital lesions in women, but not men.[57] Colchicine is effective in reducing the development of arthralgias.[55] The eye disease in Behçet's syndrome is responsive to azathioprine at a dose of 2.5 mg/kg/day.[56] Cyclosporine (5 mg/kg/day) acts more rapidly than azathioprine does in the treatment of eye disease. However, the toxicity of cyclosporine (nephrotoxicity, neurotoxicity) limits its utility for long-term use.[30]

Immunosuppressives/Tumor Necrosis Factor Inhibitors

Cytotoxic drugs, particularly chlorambucil, are reserved for patients with severe iritis and central nervous system dysfunction.[20] Chlorambucil's toxicity (sterility, neoplasms) limits its utility. Cyclophosphamide (1 g/m^2 monthly by intravenous pulse) is effective for ocular, mucocutaneous, and vascular disease. Methotrexate, up to 25 mg/wk, is indicated for iritis and arthritis.[22] Other experimental treatments used in uncontrolled trials that have produced some benefit have included levamisole, thalidomide (200 mg/day), and interferon alfa-2b (5 million U three times per week).[12,19,21,32,59] Tumor necrosis factor inhibitors in the form of infliximab have been used in individual patients with a variety of manifestations of Behçet's syndrome.[50] Orogenital ulcerations and refractory ocular and gastrointestinal lesions responded to a variety of infusion regimens.[44] Whether this form of therapy will be effective in other forms of the illness remains to be proved in clinical trials.

PROGNOSIS

Behçet's syndrome is characterized by frequent attacks early in the course of the illness. After 3 to 7 years, the frequency of attacks decreases. The disease is rarely disabling when the illness is limited to ulcerations, skin disease, and arthritis. Blindness is a major disability in patients with iritis. Severe ocular disease is more characteristic of Japanese patients with Behçet's syndrome than it is of patients from other geographic areas.[45] Central nervous system disease is associated with increased mortality. Death may be secondary to cranial nerve involvement, paraplegia, or encephalitis. For those with neurologic involvement, the mortality rate is 20% at 7 years.[31] Vascular disease is a late complication of Behçet's syndrome and is associated with severe disease. Patients with arterial disease are at risk for the development of aneurysms and rupture leading to death.[16]

References

Behçet's Syndrome

1. Arber N, Klein T, Meiner Z, et al: Close association of HLA-B51 and B52 in Israeli patients with Behçet's syndrome. Ann Rheum Dis 50:351, 1991.
2. Arbesfeld SJ, Kurban AK: Behçet's disease: New perspectives on an enigmatic syndrome. J Am Acad Dermatol 19:767, 1988.
3. Behçet H: Über rezidivierende, aphthöse durch ein Virus verursachte Geschwüre am Mund, am Auge und an den Genitalien. Dermatol Wochenschr 105:1152, 1937.
4. Chajek T, Fainam M: Behçet's syndrome: Report of 41 cases and a review of the literature. Medicine (Baltimore) 54:179, 1975.
5. Chajek-Shaul T, Pisanty S, Knobler H, et al: HLA-B51 may serve as an immunogenetic marker for a subgroup of patients with Behçet's syndrome. Am J Med 83:666, 1987.
6. Chamberlain MA: Behçet's disease. Ann Rheum Dis 34(suppl):53, 1975.
7. Chamberlain MA: Behçet's syndrome in 32 patients in Yorkshire. Ann Rheum Dis 36:491, 1977.
8. Chamberlain MA, Robertson RJ: A controlled study of sacroiliitis in Behçet's disease. Br J Rheumatol 32:693, 1993.
9. Chambers JC, Haskard DO, Kooner JS: Vascular endothelial function and oxidative stress mechanisms in patients with Behçet's syndrome. J Am Coll Cardiol 37:517-520, 2001.
10. Colvard DM, Robertson DM, O'Duffy JD: The ocular manifestations of Behçet's disease. Arch Ophthalmol 95:1813, 1977.
11. Cooper DA, Penny R: Behçet's syndrome: Clinical immunological and therapeutic evaluation of 17 patients. Aust N Z J Med 4:585, 1974.
12. DeMerieux P, Spitler LE, Paulus HE: Treatment of Behçet's syndrome with levamisole. Arthritis Rheum 24:64, 1981.
13. Dilsen AN: Sacroiliitis and ankylosing spondylitis in Behçet's disease [Abstract]. Scand J Rheum Suppl 8:20, 1975.
14. Direskeneli H: Behçet's disease: Infectious aetiology, new autoantigens, and HLA-B51. Ann Rheum Dis 60:996-1002, 2001.
15. Empey DW, Hale JE: Rectal and colonic ulceration in Behçet's syndrome. Proc R Soc Med 65:163, 1972.
16. Enoch BA, Castillo-Olivares JL, Khoo TCL, et al: Major vascular complications in Behçet's syndrome. Postgrad Med J 44:453, 1968.
17. Ferraz MB, Walter SD, Heymann R, et al: Sensitivity and specificity of different diagnostic criteria for Behçet's disease according to the latent class approach. Br J Rheumatol 34:932-935, 1995.
18. Gul A, Hajer AH, Worthington J, et al: Evidence for linkage of the HLA-B locus in Behçet's disease, obtained using the transmission disequilibrium test. Arthritis Rheum 44:239-240, 2001.
19. Hamuryudan V, Mat C, Saip S, et al: Thalidomide in the treatment of the mucocutaneous lesions of the Behçet syndrome. A randomized, double-blind, placebo-controlled trial. Ann Intern Med 128:443-450, 1998.
20. James DG: Behçet's syndrome [Editorial]. N Engl J Med 301:431, 1979.
21. Jenkins JS, Allen BR, Maurice PDL, et al: Thalidomide in severe orogenital ulceration. Lancet 2:1424, 1984.
22. Kaklamani VG, Kaklamanis PG: Treatment of Behçet's disease—an update. Semin Arthritis Rheum 30:299-312, 2001.
23. Lehner T: Behçet's syndrome and autoimmunity. BMJ 1:465, 1967.
24. Lehner T: The role of heat shock protein, microbial and autoimmune agents in the aetiology of Behçet's disease. Int Rev Immunol 14:21-32, 1997.
25. Lehner T, Batchelor JR, Challacombe SJ, Kennedy L: An immunogenetic basis for the tissue involvement in Behçet's syndrome. Immunology 37:895, 1979.

26. Lehner T, Lavery E, Smith R, et al: Association between the 65-kilodalton heat shock protein, *Streptococcus sanguis*, and the corresponding antibodies in Behçet's syndrome. Infect Immun 59:1434, 1991.
27. Maghraoui AE, Tabache E, Bezz A: A controlled study of sacroiliitis in Behçet's disease. Clin Rheumatol 20:189-191, 2001.
28. Marquardt JL, Snyderman R, Oppenheim JJ: Depression of lymphocyte transformation and exacerbation of Behçet's syndrome by ingestion of English walnuts. Cell Immunol 9:263, 1973.
29. Mason RM, Barnes CG: Behçet's syndrome with arthritis. Ann Rheum Dis 28:95, 1969.
30. Masuda K, Urayama A, Kogune M: Double-masked trial of cyclosporin versus colchicine and long-term open study of cyclosporin in Behçet's syndrome. Lancet 1:1093, 1989.
31. Meador R, Ehrlich G, Von Feldt JM: Behçet's disease: Immunopathologic and therapeutic aspects. Curr Rheumatol Rep 4:47-54, 2002.
32. Nussenblatt RB, Palestine AG, Chan C, et al: Effectiveness of cyclosporin therapy for Behçet's disease. Arthritis Rheum 28:671, 1985.
33. O'Duffy JD, Lehner T, Barnes CG: Summary of the Third International Conference on Behçet's disease, Tokyo, Japan, October 23-24, 1981. J Rheumatol 10:154, 1983.
34. O'Duffy JD: Behçet's disease. In Kelley WN, Harris ED Jr, Ruddy S, Sledge CB (eds): Textbook of Rheumatology, 2nd ed. Philadelphia, WB Saunders, 1985, pp 1174-1178.
35. O'Duffy JD, Carney JA, Deadhar S: Behçet's syndrome: Report of 10 cases, 3 with new manifestations. Ann Intern Med 75:561, 1971.
36. Ohno S, Nakarayama E, Sugiura S, et al: Specific histocompatibility antigens associated with Behçet's syndrome. Am J Ophthalmol 80:636, 1975.
37. Olivieri I, Gemignani G, Camerini E, et al: Computed tomography of the sacroiliac joints in four patients with Behçet's syndrome: Confirmation of sacroiliitis. Br J Rheumatol 29:264, 1990.
38. Oshima Y, Shimizu T, Yokakari R, et al: Clinical studies on Behçet's syndrome. Ann Rheum Dis 22:36, 1963.
39. Pallis CA, Fudge BJ: The neurological complications of Behçet's syndrome. Arch Neurol Psychiatry 75:1, 1956.
40. Perkins ES: Behçet's disease. Ophthalmological aspects. Proc R Soc Med 54:106, 1961.
41. Resnick D: Periodic, relapsing and recurrent disorders. In Resnick D, Niwayama G (eds): Diagnosis of Bone and Joint Disorders, 2nd ed. Philadelphia, WB Saunders, 1988, pp 1252-1264.
42. Robinson HM Jr, McCrumb FR Jr: Comparative analysis of the mucocutaneous-ocular syndromes: Report of eleven cases and review of the literature. Arch Derm Syph 61:539, 1950.
43. Sakane T, Takeno M, Suzuki N, et al: Behçet's disease. N Engl J Med 341:1284-1291, 1999.
44. Sfikakis PP, Theodossiadis PG, Katsiari CG, et al: Effect of infliximab on sight-threatening panuveitis in Behçet's disease. Lancet 358:295-296, 2001.
45. Shimizu R, Ehrlich GE, Inaba G, Hayashi K: Behçet disease (Behçet syndrome). Semin Arthritis Rheum 8:223, 1979.
46. Strachen RW, Wigzell FW: Polyarthritis in Behçet's multiple symptom complex. Ann Rheum Dis 22:26, 1963.
47. Suh CH, Park YB, Song J, et al: Oligoclonal B lymphocyte expansion in the synovium of a patient with Behçet's disease. Arthritis Rheum 44:1707-1712, 2001.
48. The International Study Group for Behçet's Disease: Criteria for diagnosis of Behçet's disease. Lancet 335:1078, 1990.
49. The International Study Group for Behçet's Disease:. Evaluation of diagnostic (classification) criteria in Behçet's disease—towards internationally agreed criteria. Br J Rheumatol 31:299, 1992.
50. Tutuncu Z, Morgan GJ, Kavanaugh A: Anti-TNF therapy for other inflammatory conditions. Clin Exp Rheumatol 20(suppl 28):S146-S151, 2002.
51. Vernon-Roberts B, Barnes CG, Revell PA: Synovial pathology in Behçet's syndrome. Ann Rheum Dis 37:139, 1978.
52. Wolff SM, Schotland DL, Phillips LL: Involvement of nervous system in Behçet's syndrome. Arch Neurol 12:315, 1965.
53. Wright VA, Chamberlain MA, O'Duffy JD: Behçet's syndrome. Bull Rheum Dis 29:972, 1978-1979.
54. Yazici H: Behçet's syndrome: Where do we stand? Am J Med 112:75-76, 2002.
55. Yazici H, Barnes CG: Practical treatment recommendations for pharmacotherapy of Behçet's syndrome. Drugs 42:796, 1991.
56. Yazici H, Pazarli H, Barnes CG, et al: A controlled trial of azathioprine in Behçet's syndrome. N Engl J Med 322:281, 1990.
57. Yurdakul S, Mat C, Ozyazgan Y, et al: A double blind trial of colchicines in Behçet's syndrome. Arthritis Rheum 44:2686-2692, 2001.
58. Zizic TM, Stevens MB: The arthropathy of Behçet's disease. Johns Hopkins Med J 136:243, 1975.
59. Zouboulis CC, Orfanos CE: Treatment of Adamantiades-Behçet disease with systemic interferon alfa. Arch Dermatol 134:1010-1016, 1998.

WHIPPLE'S DISEASE

CAPSULE SUMMARY

	LOW BACK	NECK
Frequency of spinal pain	Rare	Not applicable (NA)
Location of spinal pain	Sacroiliac joint and lumbar spine	NA
Quality of spinal pain	Ache	NA
Symptoms and signs	Weight loss, diarrhea, arthralgias, lymphadenopathy, hypotension	NA
Laboratory tests	Anemia, abnormal intestinal absorption tests	NA
Radiographic findings	Sacroiliitis on plain roentgenogram	NA
Treatment	Procaine penicillin G, streptomycin, trimethoprim-sulfamethoxazole	NA

PREVALENCE AND PATHOGENESIS

Whipple's disease (WD), or intestinal lipodystrophy, was first described by G. H. Whipple in 1907 and characterized by multiorgan system dysfunction.[36] Abnormalities of the musculoskeletal, gastrointestinal, cardiovascular, pulmonary, and nervous systems characterize the illness.

Epidemiology

WD is a rare illness, with approximately 741 cases reported in the world literature as of 1988.[8] The disease occurs most commonly in white men of European ancestry between the ages of 40 and 60. The male-to-female ratio is 10:1. Familial clustering of the disease has been reported.[28]

Pathogenesis

WD has an infectious etiology, and the organism that causes the disease has been identified by the use of molecular genetic techniques[31] The organism is a gram-positive actinomycete, *Tropheryma whippelii*. The inflammation caused by these bacteria is granulomatous and manifested by macrophages filled with periodic acid–Schiff (PAS)-positive organisms in biopsy specimens. Uptake of the bacillus is widespread, with absence of a vigorous inflammatory response. Patients with WD have decreased reactivity to mitogens but normal levels of immunoglobulins, indicative of a specific defect in cell-mediated immunity.[31] Antigen presentation by major histocompatibility complex class II receptors is diminished on the intestinal epithelial cells of patients with active disease but normalizes with treatment. These findings are evidence of immune downregulation by the organism.[11] The organisms are able to accumulate in massive amounts as a result of underlying host immune deficiency and the secondary downregulation induced by the organism. No information is currently available to identify this organism as a rare member of the normal human microbial flora or a rare organism in the environment.[9]

CLINICAL HISTORY

Musculoskeletal symptoms, arthralgias, joint pain without inflammation, and arthritis occur as the earliest manifestations of disease in a majority of patients.[23] A study of 52 WD patients reported 67% with articular disease.[10] Arthritis may antedate other manifestations of disease by as long as 20 to 35 years.[6] Peripheral joint involvement is marked by a migratory, oligoarticular or polyarticular arthritis affecting the knees, ankles, elbows, or fingers.[4] The joint disease is episodic and recurrent and rarely causes damage to articular structures, although cases of joint destruction have been reported.[1] Back pain and axial skeletal involvement, spondylitis or sacroiliitis, may occur in up to 19% of patients.[19] Sacroiliitis may be unilateral or bilateral.[27] Many patients with axial skeletal arthritis have concomitant peripheral joint disease. Axial joint involvement may occur in the setting of a prolonged period of appendicular joint disease.[32]

The classic triad of malabsorption, diarrhea, and weight loss occurs at unspecified intervals after the onset of joint symptoms. In some patients, arthritic complaints remit after the onset of intestinal symptoms.[17] Some of the other protean manifestations of this illness include hypotension, lymphadenopathy, hyperpigmentation, fever, peripheral edema, and central nervous system (CNS) dysfunction, including headache, diplopia, depression, confusion, and personality change.[14,23] Also reported is myopathy associated with infiltration of PAS-positive material, which responds to antibiotic therapy.[34]

Cervical Myelopathy

A rare, but serious manifestation of WD is cervical myelopathy with involvement of the cervical spinal cord. Patients have neck pain, limb paresthesias, paraparesis, or sphincter dysfunction. These manifestations may appear without other characteristic findings of WD in other organ systems. Other CNS findings may also be lacking. These patients present a difficult differential diagnosis that may be clarified only by evaluation of biopsy specimens.[5,25] Thoracic spinal cord disease has also been reported.[16]

PHYSICAL EXAMINATION

Patients may be febrile with hyperpigmented skin and lymphadenopathy. The abdominal examination may be normal. Later in the course of the illness, abdominal distention secondary to ascites and adenopathy may appear. Patients with axial skeletal disease have tenderness over the spine with limitation in all planes of motion. The peripheral joints may be normal.

LABORATORY DATA

The hematologic findings are nonspecific, with anemia developing in 90% of patients. Intestinal absorption studies consisting of serum carotene, 5-hour D-xylose absorption, and 72-hour fecal fat demonstrate values consistent with malabsorption. Synovial fluid analysis shows an inflammatory exudate with a white blood cell count up to 36,000. Rheumatoid factor and antinuclear antibody are absent. The frequency of HLA-B27 in WD patients has varied from 8% to 28% , depending on the study population.[2,7] In an Italian population with WD, no association was noted between HLA-B27 and spondyloarthropathy.[26]

Pathology

The synovial tissue from biopsy specimens is hyperplastic, with PAS-positive bodies in synoviocytes.[18] Immunohistologic techniques are available to detect Whipple bacillus in a variety of tissues, including lymph nodes.[22]

RADIOGRAPHIC EXAMINATION

Radiographic findings are infrequent in patients with peripheral joint disease, but rare instances of joint destruction and ankylosis have been reported.[1] Patients with spondylitis have changes in the sacroiliac joints and lumbar spine similar to those of ankylosing spondylitis.[3,20]

DIFFERENTIAL DIAGNOSIS

The diagnosis of WD is made by mucosal biopsy of the jejunum of the small intestine. The biopsy is accomplished by an oral route. The histologic material is stained with PAS to demonstrate the bacteria-like structures in granulomas. Identification of *T. whippelii* is possible with the use of polymerase chain reaction (PCR) primers and oligonucleotide probes, which identify the organism without the need for culture of body tissues.[29,35] PCR has identified *T. whippelii* in tissue taken from a patient with spondylodiscitis.[24] The organism has been cultivated, but cultivation is difficult to accomplish.[30] The differential diagnosis includes the other spondyloarthropathies, particularly reactive arthritis and enteropathic arthritis, Addison's disease, and lymphoma.

The presence of urethritis and/or conjunctivitis occurs in a large proportion of reactive arthritis patients. Biopsy of the small or large bowel in patients with inflammatory bowel disease will be positive for crypt abscesses in ulcerative colitis or for transmural inflammation in Crohn's disease. Addison's disease is associated with hyperpigmentation. Decreased response to adrenocorticotropic hormone will help identify patients with Addison's disease. Lymphoma is diagnosed by lymph node biopsy.

TREATMENT

Prolonged antibiotic therapy with tetracycline has a favorable effect on the disease process.[12] Joint pain, diarrhea, and lymphadenopathy resolve within a few months. Relapses have occurred in the CNS approximately 2 years after the cessation of tetracycline therapy. These relapses probably occurred because of the persistence of organisms in the CNS and inadequate penetration of tetracycline into the CNS to eradicate the organisms. An antibiotic regimen that will cross the blood-brain barrier includes parenterally administered procaine penicillin G, 1.2 million U/day, and streptomycin, 1 g/day, followed by a 1-year regimen of orally administered trimethoprim-sulfamethoxazole. Trimethoprim-sulfamethoxazole induced remission in 92% of patients versus 59% treated with tetracycline.[13] Antibiotic therapy does have a beneficial effect on the gastric mucosa that has been documented by endoscopic observation.[15] The effect of antibiotic therapy on the progression of spondylitis is unknown.

The response to treatment can be monitored by following the hematocrit, weight, and resolution of constitutional symptoms. After treatment, repeat PCR evaluation of small bowel biopsy material is useful to document resolution of the infection. In one series of small bowel biopsies after treatment, none of 5 patients who were PCR negative had a relapse as opposed to 12 of 17 who were PCR positive.[29]

PROGNOSIS

Early diagnosis is essential to a favorable outcome of this treatable illness. Patients may be ill for a number of years before it is correctly diagnosed. Antibiotic therapy has a beneficial effect on the manifestations of this illness. The joint disease is nondeforming and does not cause disability, but axial skeletal involvement is associated with some limitation of motion. Occasionally, severe manifestations, such as CNS disease, do occur in patients who are receiving continuous antibiotic therapy.[21] Individuals with CNS relapse may require higher levels or chronic intravenous delivery of ceftriaxone.[33]

References

Whipple's Disease

1. Ayoub WT, Davis DE, Toreetti D, Viozzi FJ: Bone destruction and ankylosis in Whipple's disease. J Rheumatol, 9:930, 1982.
2. Bai JC, Mota AH, Maurino E, et al: Class I and class II HLA antigens in a homogeneous Argentinian population with Whipple's disease: Lack of association with HLA-B27. Am J Gastroenterol 86:992, 1991.
3. Canoso JJ, Saini M, Hermos JA: Whipple's disease and ankylosing spondylitis simultaneous occurrence in HLA-B27 positive male. J Rheumatol 5:79, 1978.
4. Caughey DE, Bywaters EGL: The arthritis of Whipple's syndrome. Ann Rheum Dis 22:327, 1963.
5. Clarke CE, Falope ZF, Abdelhadi HA, et al: Cervical myelopathy caused by Whipple's disease. Neurology 50:1505-1506, 1998.
6. DeLuca RF, Silver TS, Rogers AI: Whipple disease: Occurrence in a 76-year-old man with a 20-year prodrome of arthritis. JAMA 233:59, 1975.
7. Dobbins WO III: HLA antigens in Whipple's disease. Arthritis Rheum 30:102, 1987.
8. Dobbins WO: Whipple's disease. Mayo Clin Proc 63:623, 1988.
9. Donaldson RM Jr: Whipple's disease: Rare malady with uncommon potential. N Engl J Med 327:346, 1992.
10. Durand DV, Lecomte C, Cathebras P, et al: Whipple disease: Clinical review of 52 cases. Medicine (Baltimore) 76:170-184, 1997.
11. Ectors NL, Geboes KJ, De Vos RM, et al: Whipple's disease: A histological, immunocytochemical, and electron microscopic study of the small intestinal epithelium. J Pathol 172:73-79, 1994.
12. England MT, French JM, Brawson AB: Antibiotic control of diarrhea in Whipple's disease. A six year follow-up of a patient diagnosed by jejunal biopsy. Gastroenterology 39:219, 1960.
13. Feurle GE, Marth T: An evaluation of antimicrobial treatment for Whipple's disease. Tetracycline versus trimethoprim-sulfamethoxazole. Dig Dis Sci 39:1642-1648, 1994.
14. Fleming JL, Wiesner RH, Shorter RG: Whipple's disease: Clinical, biochemical, and histopathologic features and assessment of treatment in 29 patients. Mayo Clin Proc 63:539, 1988.
15. Geboes K, Ectors N, Heidbuchel H, et al: Whipple's disease: Endoscopic aspects before and after therapy. Gastroenterol Endosc 36:247, 1990.
16. Gerard A, Sarrot-Reynauld F, Liozon E, et al: Neurologic presentation of Whipple's disease. Medicine (Baltimore) 81:443-457, 2002.
17. Hargrove MD Jr, Verner JV, Smith AG, et al: Whipple's disease: Report of two cases with intestinal biopsy before and after treatment. Gastroenterology 39:619, 1960.
18. Hawkins CF, Farr M, Morris CJ, et al: Detection by electron microscope of rod-shaped organisms in synovial membrane from a patient with the arthritis of Whipple's disease. Ann Rheum Dis 35:502, 1976.
19. Kelley JJ, Weisiger BB: The arthritis of Whipple's disease. Arthritis Rheum 6:615, 1963.
20. Khan MA: Axial arthropathy in Whipple's disease. J Rheumatol 9:928, 1982.
21. Knox DL, Bayless TM, Pittman FE: Neurological disease in patients with treated Whipple's disease. Medicine (Baltimore) 55:467, 1976.
22. Lepidi H, Costedoat N, Piette J, et al: Immunohistological detection of *Tropheryma whipplei* (Whipple bacillus) in lymph nodes. Am J Med 113:334-336, 2002.
23. LeVine ME, Dobbins WO: Joint changes in Whipple's disease. Semin Arthritis Rheum 3:79, 1973.
24. Louie JS, Liebling MR: The polymerase chain reaction in infectious and post-infectious arthritis. Rheum Dis Clin North Am 24: 227-236, 1998.
25. Messori A, Di Bella P, Polonara G, et al: An unusual spinal presentation of Whipple's disease. AJNR Am J Neuroradiol 22:1004-1008, 2001.
26. Olivieri I, Brandi G, Padula A, et al: Lack of association with spondyloarthritis and HLA-B27 in Italian patients with Whipple's disease. J Rheumatol 28:1294-1297, 2001.
27. Puechal X: Whipple disease and arthritis. Curr Opin Rheumatol 13:74-79, 2001.

28. Puite RH, Tesluk H: Whipple's disease. Am J Med 19:383, 1955.
29. Ramzan NN, Loftus E Jr, Burgart LJ, et al: Diagnosis and monitoring of Whipple disease by polymerase chain reaction. Ann Intern Med 126:520-527, 1997.
30. Raoult D, Birg ML, LaScola B, et al: Cultivation of the bacillus of Whipple disease. N Engl J Med 342:620-625, 2000.
31. Relman DA, Schmidt TM, MacDermott RP, Falkow S: Identification of the uncultured bacillus of Whipple's disease. N Engl J Med 327:293, 1992.
32. Scheib JS, Quinet RJ: Whipple's disease with axial and peripheral joint destruction. South Med J 83, 684, 1990.
33. Schnider PJ, Reisinger EC, Berger T, et al: Treatment guidelines in central nervous system Whipple's disease. Ann Neurol 41:561-562, 1997.
34. Swash M, Schwartz MS, Vandenburg MJ, Pollock DJ: Myopathy in Whipple's disease. Gut 18:800, 1977.
35. Tasken K, Schulz T, Elgjo K, et al: Diagnostic utility of the polymerase chain reaction in 2 cases of suspected Whipple disease. Arch Intern Med 158:801-803, 1998.
36. Whipple GH: A hitherto undescribed disease characterized anatomically by deposits of fat and fatty acids in the intestinal and mesenteric lymphatic tissues. Bull Johns Hopkins Hosp 18:382, 1907.

FAMILIAL MEDITERRANEAN FEVER

CAPSULE SUMMARY

	LOW BACK	NECK
Frequency of spinal pain	Rare	Not applicable (NA)
Location of spinal pain	Sacroiliac joints	NA
Quality of spinal pain	Ache	NA
Symptoms and signs	Episodic abdominal pain	NA
Laboratory tests	Leukocytosis, increased erythrocyte sedimentation rate with attacks	NA
Radiographic findings	Sacroiliitis on plain roentgenogram	NA
Treatment	Colchicine, biologicals	NA

PREVALENCE AND PATHOGENESIS

Familial Mediterranean fever (FMF) is a hereditary disorder characterized by recurrent, brief episodes of fever, serosal inflammation (peritonitis or pleuritis), and arthritis. Back symptoms and sacroiliitis have been described in a minority of patients with this disorder. Major disability occurs in patients with FMF in whom persistent, destructive hip disease develops, and the disease can be fatal for those in whom amyloidosis and associated renal failure develop. FMF was first described in 1945 by Siegal,[28] and the term FMF was associated with the illness in the 1950s.[17] The disease has also been called benign paroxysmal peritonitis and recurrent polyserositis.

Epidemiology

The people most commonly affected are from eastern Mediterranean countries, including Sephardic Jews, Armenians, Turks, and some Arabs, but FMF may occur sporadically in other nationalities. Men are more frequently affected than women by a ratio of 3:2. Approximately 10,000 individuals worldwide have FMF.[10]

Pathogenesis

FMF is an autosomal recessive disorder. Large family studies suggest that the disease is transmitted by a single recessive gene, but no specific HLA antigen has been associated with the illness.[32] Investigation of both Armenians and non-Ashkenazi Jews have linked the gene for FMF to the alpha-globin complex on the short arm of chromosome 16.[24,27] The *MEFV* gene on chromosome 16 associated with FMF encodes a protein, pyrin or marenostrin, that contains 781 amino acids. MEFV is expressed by myeloid cells. Gene expression is increased with myeloid differentiation and inflammatory mediators such as interferon-gamma and tumor necrosis factor.[7] Pyrin is thought to be a regulator of neutrophil-mediated inflammation. The protein works inside the nucleus and functions as a transcriptional regulator of inflammation in granulocytes.[25] Pyrin mediates anti-inflammatory factors, including complement C5a inhibitor and lipocortin-1. Cytokines that are increased during attacks of FMF include interleukin-6.[12] More than 10 mutations in *MEFV* have been discovered, but 4 are associated with 85% of the mutations found in patients.[23] Two common missense mutations are *M694V* and *V726A*. The *M694V* mutation is a more severe phenotype and has a higher risk of amyloidosis.[15] These mutations result in proteins with one amino acid substitution that makes the protein inactive. The mutations originated in common ancestors who lived 2500 years ago in the Middle East.[34]

CLINICAL HISTORY

The disease is characterized by acute attacks of fever associated with peritonitis, pleuritis, or arthritis. The episodes of abdominal or chest pain are limited to a period of hours to days, whereas arthritis may persist much longer. Areas of painful erythema may also occur on the lower extremities below the knee. The onset of this illness is usually during childhood or adolescence.

The most frequent manifestation of FMF, which occurs in 95% of patients, is peritonitis. Severe abdominal pain with absent bowel sounds suggestive of an acute abdominal crisis develops. Not uncommonly, patients undergo a laparotomy that reveals no specific pathology. Within 24 to 48 hours, symptoms abate and leave patients in their usual state of health. Pleural pain with difficulty breathing and a minor effusion occurs in 40% of FMF patients. Recurrences of abdominal or pleural pain occur irregularly, with remissions lasting months to years. Factors that have been suggested as possible initiators of attacks include menstruation, stress, heavy activity, and exposure to cold.[26]

Sacroiliitis, frequently asymptomatic, is another manifestation of FMF, with 10% to 17% of patients having either unilateral or bilateral disease.[6,16] Another study found a smaller prevalence of sacroiliitis (0.004%) in a group of 3000 FMF patients. Patients who were symptomatic with chronic arthritis were investigated for spondyloarthropathy. Individuals with asymptomatic sacroiliitis were not included.[19] Sacroiliitis also has been described in children, in whom clinical symptoms of back pain are significant.[20] Lumbar spine changes consistent with spondylitis occur less commonly.

Articular manifestations of FMF occur in 75% of patients and are an initial feature in 33%.[16] The joints most commonly affected are the knee, ankle, hip, shoulder, and rarely, the sacroiliac.[13] The usual joint attack has an abrupt onset, with rapidly intensifying pain affecting a single joint. An effusion may accompany the development of joint pain, and the attacks may last from a few days to a month. Most episodes of joint pain and swelling are not associated with residual joint damage. Occasionally, a protracted episode of arthritis affecting a single joint, such as a knee or hip, may develop in patients with FMF, and this episode may last for a year or more.[16] Marked swelling and surrounding muscle atrophy develop in these joints. The sacroiliac joint is mostly affected when the arthritis becomes long-standing. Complete recovery of function may be expected in the patient, with resolution of a protracted attack of arthritis in the knee. The outcome of hip arthritis, however, is more ominous, with residual limitation of motion and pain being the issue. Hip joint destruction also may occur.

Amyloidosis is a complication of FMF that is fatal because of the deposition of amyloid in the kidneys. Nephrotic syndrome, characterized by proteinuria and peripheral edema, ensues and results in renal failure.[30] Most patients in whom amyloidosis develops die before they reach 40 years of age.[31]

PHYSICAL FINDINGS

Patients with FMF may have an entirely normal examination between attacks.[29] During attacks, examination of the abdomen, chest, skin, and joints, including the back, is essential. Examination of the lower extremities for peripheral edema is helpful in detecting the presence of nephrotic syndrome or an erysipelas-like erythema associated with acute attacks.

Patients with sacroiliitis on radiographs may have a normal lumbosacral spine examination. Others may demonstrate tenderness to percussion over the involved joints.

LABORATORY DATA

Laboratory findings are nonspecific in FMF.[20] During attacks, white blood cells may be markedly elevated along with increases in the erythrocyte sedimentation rate. Abnormal values quickly return to normal with resolution of the attack. Urinalysis may demonstrate protein and red blood cells indicative of renal amyloidosis. Rheumatoid factor and antinuclear antibody are absent. A number of studies have investigated the presence of autoantibodies in FMF patients versus controls.[3,33] Autoantibodies, including RNP, SSA/SSB, anti-DNA, and anticardiolipin, are not present in FMF patients. Synovial fluid may have increased white blood cells to 1 million, good mucin clot, increased protein, and normal or low glucose.[31] HLA testing does not demonstrate any increased frequency of any specific antigen.

RADIOGRAPHIC EVALUATION

Roentgenograms

Sacroiliac joint changes include loss of cortical definition and sclerosis on both sides of the joint, with or without erosions and fusions.[6] Involvement of the sacroiliac joints may be unilateral or bilateral, with an asymmetric severity of involvement (Fig. 11-25). Changes in the lumbar spine include bony bridging between the lumbar vertebrae.[16]

Soft tissue swelling and osteoporosis are seen in patients during brief attacks, but these changes are rapidly reversible with remission. Radiographic changes are more severe in patients with protracted attacks. When the knee is affected, osteoporosis may be widespread throughout the limb. On at least two occasions, resumption of weight bearing has resulted in fracture of the tibia or femur secondary to the osteoporosis.[31] Other findings include sclerosis, joint space narrowing, and erosions. Marked joint space narrowing is a common finding after protracted attacks in a hip.

DIFFERENTIAL DIAGNOSIS

Diagnostic criteria for FMF include recurrent short attacks of fever with peritonitis, pleuritis, arthritis, erythema, and absence of data suggesting an alternative diagnosis. A Mediterranean ancestry is a helpful piece of data when a patient has an initial attack. A recent report has suggested that FMF attacks can be provoked in patients by metaraminol infusion. Noradrenaline has been associated with the precipitation of attacks of FMF. Metaraminol acts competitively to displace noradrenaline. Attacks developed in 21 patients after receiving infusions. An equal number of controls did not have attacks. If confirmed, metaraminol infusion would become a useful diagnostic test.[1] This

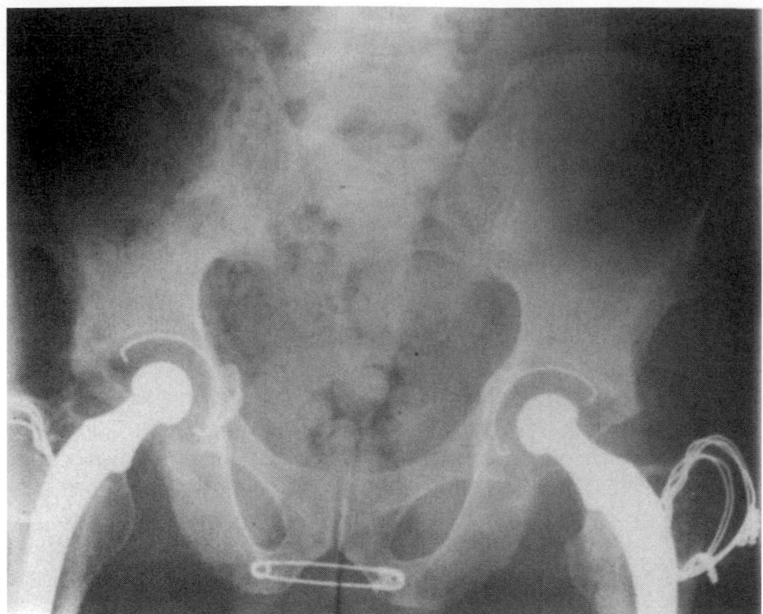

Figure 11-25 Familial Mediterranean fever (FMF). A 40-year-old man had active FMF since the age of 18. Bilateral hip arthritis required hip replacements at age 32. An anteroposterior view of the pelvis reveals bilateral sacroiliitis with asymmetric involvement, greater on the right than the left. *(Courtesy of Jacob Bar-Ziv, MD, and Theodor Schifter, MD.)*

finding also suggests that FMF may be the result of an inborn error of catecholamine metabolism. Dopamine beta-hydroxylase is the enzyme responsible for the conversion of dopamine to noradrenaline. This enzyme has been found to be elevated in patients with FMF without treatment with colchicine.[2] Attempts at reproducing these findings in other populations of patients with FMF have not produced the same results.[8] Measurement of this enzyme cannot be recommended as a diagnostic test for FMF. Genetic testing is available for identifying common mutations of the *MEFV* gene. However, 45% of individuals with FMF in the United States had mutations that were not identifiable.[25] Therefore, the current genetic tests do not identify all the mutations associated with FMF. Consequently, the diagnosis should rest on clinical criteria.[21]

Other hereditary periodic febrile illnesses include tumor necrosis factor receptor–associated periodic syndrome (TRAPS) and hyper-IgD syndrome.[10,18] These disorders have different patterns of attacks or laboratory findings (elevated IgD levels) that help differentiate them.

Sacroiliac joint involvement is similar to that associated with the seronegative spondyloarthropathies. Abdominal symptoms differentiate FMF from ankylosing spondylitis, reactive arthritis, and psoriatic arthritis. Diarrhea develops in patients with inflammatory bowel disease, whereas FMF patients have normal bowel habits, even during attacks. Crohn's disease can occur in patients with FMF. The onset of Crohn's disease occurs later than in patients without FMF. FMF patients with Crohn's disease have more frequent abdominal attacks. Amyloidosis also develops more frequently in these patients.[11]

The absence of HLA-B27 in FMF patients suggests that the pathogenesis of the lumbosacral spine changes is different from that of the HLA-B27–positive spondyloarthropathies. The sacroiliitis of FMF patients is not related to a second disease, ankylosing spondylitis, but rather to some unspecified mechanism associated with FMF.

TREATMENT

An effective treatment of FMF is colchicine. A regimen of colchicine (0.6 mg orally twice a day) helps in both ameliorating the attacks and reducing their frequency.[9] Colchicine may work through its potent inhibitory effect on leukocyte chemotaxis.[5] Colchicine was also shown to be beneficial in preventing amyloidosis in patients with FMF.[35] Articular involvement is less responsive to colchicine than the acute attacks of polyserositis are. Colchicine has been used for extended periods to prevent attacks without significant toxicity.[4] Non-narcotic analgesics are useful in controlling pain. Bed rest, anti-inflammatory drugs, and corticosteroids may not provide any benefit for the joint disease in FMF.[31] Prolonged immobilization may aggravate the osteoporosis and muscle atrophy. Joint replacement may be necessary for advanced disease of the hip. Therapy for renal failure is necessary for patients in whom renal amyloidosis develops.

PROGNOSIS

The major morbidity from FMF, other than the frequency of acute attacks, is protracted disease of the hip. In one study, severe limitation of motion and pain developed in 16 of 18 affected hips.[31] Eight of these patients required joint arthroplasty and had a good outcome.

The major cause of mortality from FMF is amyloidosis and renal failure.[22] This complication may be more common in patients in Israel than the United States. Studies suggest that daily colchicine therapy may prevent the development or progression of amyloidosis in these patients, although not all patients, particularly those of European ethnicity, respond to colchicine therapy.[14,35]

References

Familial Mediterranean Fever

1. Barakat MH, El-Khawad AO, Gumaa KA, et al: Metaraminol provocative test: A specific diagnostic test for familial Mediterranean fever. Lancet 1:656, 1984.
2. Barakat MH, Gumaa KA, Malhas LN, et al: Plasma dopamine beta-hydroxylase: Rapid diagnostic test for recurrent hereditary polyserositis. Lancet 2:1280, 1988.
3. Ben-Chetrit E, Levy M: Autoantibodies in familial Mediterranean fever (recurrent polyserositis). Br J Rheumatol. 29:459, 1990.
4. Ben-Chetrit E, Levy M: Colchicine prophylaxis in familial Mediterranean fever: Reappraisal after 15 years. Semin Arthritis Rheum 20:241, 1991.
5. Ben-Chetrit E, Levy M: Colchicine: 1998 update. Semin Arthritis Rheum 28:48-59, 1998.
6. Brodey PA, Wolff SM: Radiographic changes in the sacroiliac joints in familial Mediterranean fever. Radiology 114:331, 1975.
7. Centola M, Wood G, Frucht DM, et al: The gene for familial Mediterranean fever, MEFV, is expressed in early leukocyte development and is regulated in response to inflammatory mediators. Blood 95:3223-3231, 2000.
8. Courillon-Mallet A, Cauet N, Dervichian M, et al: Plasma dopamine beta-hydroxylase activity in familial Mediterranean fever. Isr J Med Sci 28:427, 1992.
9. Dinarello CA, Wolff SM, Goldfinger SE, et al: Colchicine therapy for familial Mediterranean fever: A double-blind trial. N Engl J Med 291:934, 1974.
10. Drenth JPH, van der Meer JWM: Hereditary periodic fever. N Engl J Med 345:1748-1757, 2001.
11. Fiddler HH, Chowers Y, Lidar M, et al: Crohn disease in patients with familial Mediterranean fever. Medicine (Baltimore) 81: 411-416, 2002.
12. Gang N, Drenth JPH, Langevitz O, et al: Activation of the cytokine network in familial Mediterranean fever. J Rheumatol 26:890-897, 1999.
13. Garcia-Gonzalez A, Weisman MH: The arthritis of familial Mediterranean fever. Semin Arthritis Rheum 22:139, 1992.
14. Gertz MA, Petitt RM, Perrault J, Kyle RA: Autosomal dominant familial Mediterranean fever–like syndrome with amyloidosis. Mayo Clin Proc 62:1095, 1987.
15. Grateau G: The relation between familial Mediterranean fever and amyloidosis. Curr Opin Rheumatol 12:61-64, 2000.
16. Heller H, Gafni J, Michaeli D, et al: The arthritis of familial Mediterranean fever. Arthritis Rheum 9:1, 1966.
17. Heller H, Sohar E, Kariv I, Sherf L: Familial Mediterranean fever. Harefuah 48:91, 1955.
18. Hull KM, Drewe E, Aksentijevich I, et al: The TNF receptor–associated periodic syndrome (TRAPS): Emerging concepts of an autoinflammatory disorder. Medicine (Baltimore) 81:349-368, 2002.
19. Langevitz P, Livneh A, Zemer D, et al: Seronegative spondyloarthropathy in familial Mediterranean fever. Semin Arthritis Rheum 27:67-72, 1997.
20. Lehman TJA, Hanson V, Kornreich H, et al: HLA-B27–negative sacroiliitis: A manifestation of familial Mediterranean fever in childhood. Pediatrics 61:423, 1978.
21. Livneh A, Langevitz P, Zemer D, et al: Criteria for the diagnosis of familial Mediterranean fever. Arthritis Rheum 40:1879-1885, 1997.
22. Meyerhoff J: Familial Mediterranean fever: Report of a large family, review of the literature and discussion of the frequency of amyloidosis. Medicine (Baltimore) 59:66, 1980.
23. Ozen S: Vasculopathy, Behçet's syndrome, and familial Mediterranean fever. Curr Opin Rheumatol 11:393-398, 1999.
24. Pras E, Aksentijevich I, Gruberg L, et al: Mapping of a gene causing familial Mediterranean fever to the short arm of chromosome 16. N Engl J Med 326:1508, 1992.
25. Samuels J, Aksentijevich I, Torosyan Y, et al: FMF at the Millennium: Clinical spectrum, ancient mutation, and a survey of 100 American referrals to the National Institutes of Health. Medicine (Baltimore) 77:268-297, 1998.
26. Schwartz J: Periodic peritonitis, onset simultaneously with menstruation. Ann Intern Med 53:407, 1960.
27. Shohat M, Bu X, Sholat T, et al: The gene for familial Mediterranean fever in both Armenians and non-Ashkenazi Jews is linked to the alpha-globin complex on 16p: Evidence for locus homogeneity. Am J Hum Genet 51:1349, 1992.
28. Siegal S: Benign paroxysmal peritonitis. Ann Intern Med 23:1, 1945.
29. Siegal S: Familial paroxysmal peritonitis: Analysis of fifty cases. Am J Med 36:893, 1964.
30. Sohar E, Gafni J, Pras M, Heller H: Familial Mediterranean fever: A survey of 470 cases and review of the literature. Am J Med 43:227, 1967.
31. Sohar E, Pras M, Gafni J: Familial Mediterranean fever and its articular manifestations. Clin Rheum Dis 1:195, 1975.
32. Sohar E, Pras M, Heller J, Heller H: Genetics of familial Mediterranean fever. A disorder with recessive inheritance in non-Ashkenazi Jews and Armenians. Arch Intern Med 107:529, 1961.
33. Swissa M, Schul V, Korish S, et al: Determination of autoantibodies in patients with familial Mediterranean fever and their first degree relatives. J Rheumatol 18:606-608, 1991.
34. The International FMF consortium: Ancient missense mutations in a new member of the RoRet gene family are likely to cause familial Mediterranean fever. Cell 90:797-807, 1997.
35. Zemer D, Pras M, Sohar E, et al: Colchicine in the prevention and treatment of the amyloidosis of familial Mediterranean fever. N Engl J Med 314:1001, 1986.

HIDRADENITIS SUPPURATIVA

CAPSULE SUMMARY

	LOW BACK	NECK
Frequency of spinal pain	Rare	Not applicable (NA)
Location of spinal pain	Sacroiliac joints, lumbar spine	NA
Quality of spinal pain	Ache	NA
Symptoms and signs	Skin disease, lymphadenopathy, acne conglobata	NA
Laboratory tests	Anemia, increased erythrocyte sedimentation rate with attacks	NA
Radiographic findings	Unilateral or bilateral sacroiliitis on plain roentgenogram	NA
Treatment	Antibiotics, incision and drainage	NA

PREVALENCE AND PATHOGENESIS

Hidradenitis suppurativa (HS) and acne conglobata (AC) are chronic suppurative disorders of the skin that are associated with peripheral and axial skeletal arthritis, similar to the seronegative spondyloarthropathies.[19] In 1854, the French surgeon Aristide Verneuil first associated hidradenitis with sweat glands.[15]

Epidemiology

These skin diseases are relatively uncommon conditions, and their exact prevalence is unknown. HS is predominantly a disease of women.

Pathogenesis

The cause of HS remains an area of debate. One mechanism involves the occlusion of hair follicles, not apocrine glands. Such closure results from a defect in the terminal follicular epithelium.[24] Early lesions first demonstrate occlusion of follicles, with stasis and destruction of apocrine glands being a secondary phenomenon.[3] Others have described HS as an initial infection of the apocrine sweat glands located in the axillae and inguinal regions. The disease is characterized by the development of recurrent inflammatory suppurative nodules and sinus tracts. AC is a form of acne in which large abscesses and interconnecting sinuses develop in the skin; they form cysts similar to those of HS. AC is not associated with signs of an acute illness and ulcerating lesions. The third component of the follicular occlusion triad is dissecting cellulitis of the scalp. The musculoskeletal abnormalities associated with the follicular occlusion triad can be differentiated from those associated with acne fulminans, another severe form of acne. Acne fulminans is manifested by ulcerative, crusting lesions causing deep dermal involvement in the setting of an acute severe illness and is usually associated with arthritis above the lumbosacral spine.[13]

The etiology of the arthritis associated with these skin conditions is unknown. Chronic cutaneous superinfections are components of the inflammatory process in HS and AC. The joint disease that develops in these patients may be a reactive arthritis secondary to chronic infection, similar to the arthritis that develops in patients after a genitourinary or enteric infection; however, as opposed to other patients with reactive arthritis, patients with HS or AC and arthritis do not have an increased frequency of HLA-B27 positivity.[13]

A number of factors suggest that this arthritis is a manifestation of chronic infection of the skin. The infections produce large quantities of bacterial products that are antigenic. These bacterial cellular fragments may cross-react with joint tissues or may be transported to joints where they lodge in synovial structures and elicit an inflammatory response, or a combination of both mechanisms. The initiating factor may be molecular mimicry of bacterial products, and the phlogistic characteristics of these products sustain the inflammation in the joint. The partial response of arthritic patients with this condition to antibiotics suggests that bacterial infection plays a role in the pathogenesis of this process.[10]

CLINICAL HISTORY

The typical patient is 32 years of age and black.[13,19] Most have both HS and AC. The skin disease is axillary and vulvar in women and perianal in men. In the majority of patients, the skin disease precedes the onset of arthritis by 1 to 20 years. Peripheral arthritis affects the knees, elbows, wrists, and ankles most commonly, but the small joints of the hands and feet may also be involved.[23] Attacks of arthritis last from weeks to months. Axial skeletal disease of the cervical and thoracic spine occurs less often. Joint symptoms frequently mirror the activity of the skin disease.[8,14]

PHYSICAL EXAMINATION

Skin examination is essential to document the extent and activity of the cutaneous disease. Musculoskeletal examination may show swelling, effusion, and warmth in the peripheral joints, along with limitation of spinal movement and tenderness to percussion over the sacroiliac joints. The ankles and joints of the feet are most frequently affected. Peripheral joint involvement is symmetrical in 60% of patients.[13]

LABORATORY DATA

Mild anemia occurs in a majority of patients along with occasional leukocytosis. The erythrocyte sedimentation rate is usually elevated. Rheumatoid factor and antinuclear antibody are not present, and cultures of skin lesions are frequently sterile. These diseases are not associated with an increased frequency of HLA-B27 or its cross-reactive antigens.

RADIOGRAPHIC EVALUATION

Roentgenograms

Roentgenographic findings in patients with peripheral arthritis include swelling, periarticular osteoporosis, periosteal new bone formation, and joint space erosions of finger joints. Axial skeletal abnormalities include sacroiliitis with narrowing, sclerosis, erosion, and fusion; the abnormalities are unilateral in most circumstances. Axial skeletal disease is associated with squaring of vertebral bodies, ligamentous calcification, and asymmetric syndesmophytes (Fig. 11-26). Sacroiliitis occurs in up to 80% of patients with the follicular occlusion triad.[13] The asymmetric syndesmophytes occur in any portion of the axial skeleton and have characteristics similar to those associated with reactive arthritis and psoriatic spondyloarthropathy.[5] Asymmetric sacroiliitis has also been described in a white patient with acne fulminans.[17]

DIFFERENTIAL DIAGNOSIS

The diagnosis of HS or AC is based on the appearance and distribution of the skin lesions. These lesions must be differentiated from other suppurative infections of the skin, including Bartholin abscesses and actinomycosis.

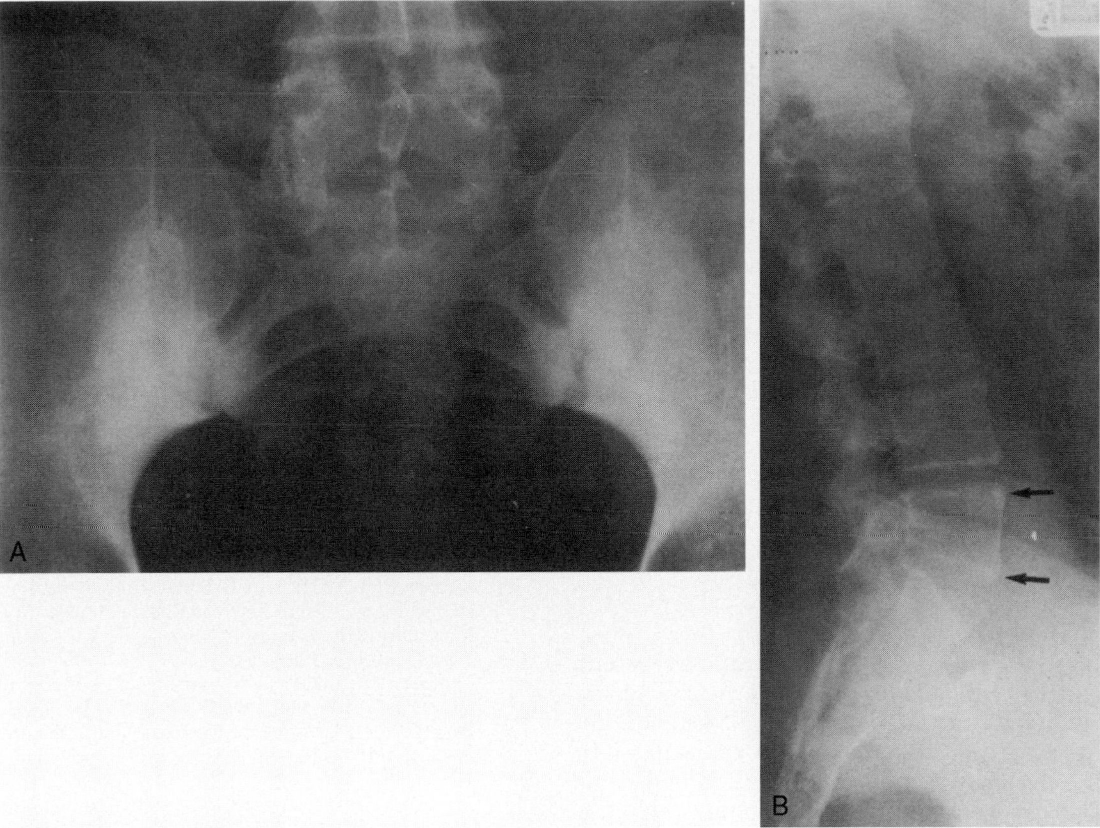

Figure 11-26 Hidradenitis suppurativa. A 24-year-old man had an 8-year history of hidradenitis suppurativa, acne conglobata, and dissecting cellulitis of the scalp, which responded to intermittent courses of antibiotics. The patient complained of bilateral back pain localized over the sacroiliac joints. *A*, A spot view of the pelvis reveals bilateral sacroiliac joint involvement manifested by joint narrowing on the right and widening on the left, along with extensive periarticular sclerosis. *B*, A lateral view of the lumbar spine demonstrates early changes of spondylitis manifested by osseous erosion and sclerosis of the vertebral body, which produced whitening of the corners of the L5 vertebra *(arrows)* along with early straightening of the anterior border.

The associated arthritis must be differentiated from the other seronegative spondyloarthropathies (see the section "Reactive Arthritis" earlier in this chapter).

SAPHO Syndrome

SAPHO is an acronym for a syndrome including *s*ynovitis, severe *a*cne, palmoplantar *p*ustulosis, *h*yperostosis, and *o*steitis.[22] This disorder has characteristics of spondyloarthritis but is HLA-B27 negative.[9] It causes hyperostosis of the bones and joints of the anterior chest wall. This hyperostosis affects the sternoclavicular areas along with the ribs. Skin disease is not always present, and the sacroiliac joints may be spared while the cervical spine undergoes loss of disc space and bony sclerosis.[20] The local area of involvement is swollen and painful. Skin lesions may be mild and characterized by scaling of the palms, psoriasis of the scalp, macular rash, or acne vulgaris. The erythrocyte sedimentation rate is normal or slightly raised. Radiographic abnormalities include expansion of the anterior ribs and clavicle. In the cervical spine, disc spaces are fused, with irregular vertebral body endplates. Therapy with nonsteroidals has modest efficacy. Intravenous infusion of pamidronate (single dose of 30 mg) may result in quick relief of pain that may last for months.[20] Individual patients with SAPHO syndrome who have demonstrated increased levels of tumor necrosis factor in bone biopsy specimens have responded to etanercept injections or infliximab infusions over a 9-month period.[21]

Vitamin A Derivatives

Synthetic vitamin A derivatives, including isotretinoin, are used to treat severe acne; however, isotretinoin causes a number of side effects, such as skeletal hyperostosis.[7,12] The location of the hyperostosis includes the axial skeleton, and skeletal changes more frequently affect the cervical and thoracic spine. Small horizontal spurs extending from the anterior margin of the vertebral body develop. The sacroiliac joints are not affected.[7] The presence of these radiographic changes does not correlate with musculoskeletal signs or symptoms.[13] No consistent correlation has been found between cessation of isotretinoin therapy and resolution of the hyperostosis, although improvement has been reported in some patients.[4]

TREATMENT

Therapy for HS includes antibiotics and incision and drainage of skin tracts. Topical clindamycin (1% lotion twice daily for 3 months) has been shown to be effective in a randomized clinical trial and was as potent as oral tetracycline.[11] Antibiotic therapy with tetracycline is worthwhile on a long-term basis in some cases. Occasionally, corticosteroids or low-dose x-ray therapy is given to patients with persistent skin disease. AC is effectively treated with corticosteroids, but such drugs are limited in utility because of side effects. Severe disease often requires the addition of retinoids, including isotretinoin. Isotretinoin (1 to 2 mg/kg/day in divided doses) is effective in the early stages of the illness.[2] Joint disease is responsive to nonsteroidal anti-inflammatory drugs, but rarely, corticosteroids are needed for control of the joint symptoms. Surgery is required for severe, extensive disease. Different techniques, such as local excision, en bloc excision, and laser excision, have different success rates in regard to control of recurrences.[6,16] Surgery for control of active skin disease may improve the joint disease. Effective control frequently requires a combination of medical and surgical interventions.

PROGNOSIS

Both skin diseases tend to be chronic and recurrent. They cause disfigurement in their severe forms but not physical disability. In rare circumstances, HS can be complicated by squamous cell carcinoma of the skin.[1] The joint disease associated with HS and AC is associated with loss of range of motion in affected joints.[18] No significant disability has been reported; however, patients with severe axial skeletal and hip disease may be at the same risk for disability as those with other spondyloarthropathies.

References

Hidradenitis Suppurativa

1. Black SB, Woods JE: Squamous cell carcinoma complicating hidradenitis suppurativa. J Surg Oncol 19:25-26, 1982.
2. Boer J, van Gemert MJ: Long-term results of isotretinoin in the treatment of 68 patients with hidradenitis suppurativa. J Am Acad Dermatol 40:73-76, 1999.
3. Boer J, Welevreden EF: Hidradenitis suppurativa or acne inversa. A clinicopathological study of early lesions. Br J Dermatol 135: 721-725, 1996.
4. Carey BM, Parkin GJS, Cunliffe WJ, Pritlove J: Skeletal toxicity with isotretinoin therapy: A clinico-radiological evaluation. Br J Dermatol 119:609, 1988.
5. Ellis BI, Shier CK, Leisen JJC, et al: Acne-associated spondyloarthropathy: Radiographic feature. Radiology 162:541, 1987.
6. Finley EM, Ratz JL: Treatment of hidradenitis suppurativa with carbon dioxide laser excision and second-intention healing. J Am Acad Dermatol 34:465-469, 1996.
7. Gerber LH, Helfgott RK, Gross EG, et al: Vertebral abnormalities associated with synthetic retinoid use. J Am Acad Dermatol 10:817, 1984.
8. Golding DN: Acne and joint disease. J R Soc Med 78(suppl 10): 19, 1985.
9. Hayem G, Bouchaud-Chabot A, Banali K, et al: SAPHO syndrome: A long-term followup study of 120 cases. Semin Arthritis Rheum 29:159-171, 1999.
10. Hellmann DB: Spondyloarthropathy with hidradenitis suppurativa. JAMA 267:2363, 1992.
11. Jemec GB, Wendelboe P: Topical clindamycin versus systemic tetracycline in the treatment of hidradenitis suppurativa. J Am Acad Dermatol 39:971-974, 1998.
12. Kilcoyne RF, Cope R, Cunningham W, et al: Minimal spinal hyperostosis with low-dose isotretinoin therapy. Invest Radiol 21:41, 1986.
13. Knitzer RH, Needleman BW: Musculoskeletal syndromes associated with acne. Semin Arthritis Rheum 20:247: 1991.
14. McKendry RJR, Hamdy H: Acne, arthritis, sacroiliitis. Can Med Assoc J 128:156, 1983.
15. Nijhawan PK, Elkin PL: 59-year-old man with right hip pain. Mayo Clin Proc 73:541-544, 1998.
16. Parks RW, Parks TG: Pathogenesis, clinical features and management of hidradenitis suppurativa. Ann R Coll Surg Engl 79:83-89, 1997.
17. Piazza I, Giunta G: Lytic bone lesions and polyarthritis associated with acne fulminans. Br J Rheumatol 30:387, 1991.
18. Rosner IA, Burg CG, Wisnieski JJ, et al: The clinical spectrum of the arthropathy associated with hidradenitis suppurativa and acne conglobata. J Rheumatol 20:684, 1993.
19. Rosner IA, Richter DE, Huettner TL, et al: Spondyloarthropathy associated with hidradenitis suppurativa and acne conglobata. Ann Intern Med 97:520, 1982.
20. Van Doornum S, Barraclough D, McColl G, et al: SAPHO: Rare or just not recognized. Semin Arthritis Rheum 30:7077, 2000.
21. Wagner AD, Andresen J, Jendro MC, et al: Sustained response to tumor necrosis factor α–blocking agents in two patients with SAPHO syndrome. Arthritis Rheum 46:1965-1968, 2002.
22. Winchester R: Psoriatic arthritis and the spectrum of syndromes related to the SAPHO (synovitis, acne, pustulosis, hyperostosis, and osteitis) syndrome. Curr Opin Rheumatol 11:251-256, 1999.
23. Windom RE, Sanford JP, Ziff M: Acne conglobata and arthritis. Arthritis Rheum 4:632, 1961.
24. Yu CC, Cook MG: Hiadrenitis suppurativa: A disease of follicular epithelium, rather than apocrine glands. Br J Dermatol 122: 763-769, 1990.

RHEUMATOID ARTHRITIS

Capsule Summary

	Low Back	Neck
Frequency of spinal pain	Rare	Very common
Location of spinal pain	Diffuse	Cervical spine, occiput
Quality of spinal pain	Ache	Ache
Symptoms and signs	Joint disease of long duration, lumbosacral spine tenderness	Joint disease of long duration, cervical spine tenderness
Laboratory tests	Anemia, rheumatoid factor	Anemia, rheumatoid factor
Radiographic findings	Unilateral or bilateral sacroiliitis without reactive sclerosis	Atlantoaxial subluxation, subaxial subluxation
Treatment	NSAIDs, DMARDs, corticosteroids, biologicals	NSAIDs, DMARDs, corticosteroids, biologicals

PREVALENCE AND PATHOGENESIS

Rheumatoid arthritis (RA) is a chronic, systemic inflammatory disease that causes pain, heat, swelling, and destruction in synovial joints. The joints characteristically affected by RA are the small joints of the hands and feet, wrists, elbows, hips, knees, ankles, and cervical spine. A majority of RA patients have cervical spine disease manifested as neck pain, headaches, or arm numbness. Signs of cervical spine disease include decreased neck motion with stiffness, undue prominence of the spinous process of the axis (C2), and neurologic dysfunction, including paresthesias, spasticity, incontinence, and quadriplegia. The diagnosis of RA is made in the setting of a history of persistent joint inflammation in the appropriate joints and the presence of specific serum antibodies (rheumatoid factor). The degree of cervical spine destruction in RA does not always correlate with patient complaints and is detected by radiographic evaluation. RA of the cervical spine responds to the same therapy that is effective for the peripheral joints. Surgical intervention with stabilization of the cervical spine is required for persistent neurologic abnormalities.

Epidemiology

The prevalence of RA is approximately 1% to 3% of the U.S. population.[114] RA is found in all racial and ethnic groups. The condition occurs in all age groups but is most common in those between 40 and 70 years of age.[86] The male-to-female ratio is approximately 1:3. Symptoms of cervical spine disease occur in 40% to 80% of RA patients.[37,134] Radiographic evidence of cervical spine involvement is found in up to 86% of RA patients, whereas neurologic symptoms from cervical spine disease occur less frequently, in 10% of patients with radiographic changes.[12,16] Cervical spine disease usually occurs in the setting of active peripheral disease; however, on occasion, neck symptoms may be the initial or predominant symptom without clinical signs of RA in other locations.[13,14]

The lumbar spine is rarely involved in the rheumatoid process. Patients in whom low back pain develops secondary to RA have long-standing, extensive disease in the usual joint locations associated with the illness. RA of the lumbosacral spine may be associated with apophyseal joint erosions and secondary intervertebral disc narrowing. Involvement of the sacroiliac joint is characterized by narrowing of the joint space without erosions or bony sclerosis. RA of the lumbosacral spine responds to the same therapy that is effective for joint disease in other locations. One study suggested that 5% of men and 3% of women with RA may have lumbar spine involvement.[85] Another study reported that 4% of men and 5% of women had pronounced involvement of the sacroiliac joints.[55] In a study of RA patients with low back pain, 17% had sacroiliitis on radiographic evaluation.[65] These patients were almost evenly split between unilateral and bilateral disease.

Pathogenesis

The causes of RA are probably multifactorial and mediated through environmental and genetic factors. The combination of these factors produces an imbalance in immune function that results in inflammation of the synovial joints.[12,142]

Overview

RA is a chronic immune-mediated disease whose initiation and perpetuation are dependent on the T-lymphocyte response to unknown antigens.[117] A possible environmental factor that may initiate RA is a virus.[138] After an initial flurry of scientific interest in associating the presence of Epstein-Barr virus (EBV) as a source of infection in RA, subsequent investigations have not found convincing evidence of a cause-and-effect relationship between the two processes.[40] Cross-reactivity may exist between EBV nuclear antigens and autoantigens, including collagen, actin, and cytokeratin, and synovial membrane antigens.[6] Cellular immunity is altered in RA. T-cell stimulation produces lymphokines (interferon-gamma) that activate macrophages to release monokines (interleukin-1 [IL-1]), tumor necrosis factor-alpha (TNF-alpha), granulocyte-macrophage colony-stimulating factor, and other growth factors. Fibroblasts and endothelial cells proliferate, new blood vessels form, and osteoclasts are stimulated to erode bone. Increased numbers of CD4+ lymphocytes that activate B lymphocytes to produce immunoglobulin are frequently found in synovium from RA patients.[152] Many of the B and T lymphocytes and monocytes in rheumatoid synovium express histocompatibility antigens (DR and DQ), thus indicating increased cellular activity of these cells.[69] Lymphocytes from RA patients demonstrate sensitivity to the collagen present in the joints and eyes (types II and III).[149] Collagen and chondrocytes may present antigens that help perpetuate the illness.[3,79] Activation of macrophages results in the production of monokines. These factors attract additional lymphocytes and neutrophils. T lymphocytes accumulate in the synovial membrane. Helper-inducer T lymphocytes adhere better to the endothelial adhesive proteins than suppressor-inducer subsets do and gain access more easily to the extracellular matrix of the synovial membrane. There is a relative absence of suppressor-inducer T cells. Angiogenesis factors result in the growth of new capillaries. Activated metalloproteinases, including procollagenase and progelatinase, are released by synovial cells and cause tissue destruction. Arachidonic acid metabolites are produced and affect components of the inflammatory response.

Genetic Susceptibility

Genetic factors play a role in development of the illness as demonstrated by the increased risk for RA in monozygotic twins versus dizygotic twins (12% to 15% versus 4%).[1,136] Approximately 60% of the predisposition to RA can be ascribed to genetic factors.[92] At the initiation of RA, unspecified environmental antigens are presented to antigen-presenting cells bearing major histocompatibility complex class II antigens.[110] The haplotypes associated with RA include HLA-DR4 and HLA-DR1.[62] Subtypes of DR4 associated with RA include DRB*0401, DRB*0404/08, and DRB1*0405.[156] In the white population, the presence of HLA-DR4 confers a relative risk of 3.5 for RA. Non-HLA genetic factors also predispose to the development of RA but require additional study.[93] The appropriately presented antigen located in the peptide-binding groove formed by the HLA molecule activates lymphocytes, which attract macrophages into synovium.

Cytokines

A wide variety of cytokines are produced in RA synovium (Table 11-9).[140] Different cytokines have proinflammatory and anti-inflammatory effects. In RA, macrophages produce excessive amounts of proinflammatory cytokines, including TNF-alpha and IL-1.[155] These cytokines play a key role in the development of inflammation in RA. TNF controls the production of other proinflammatory cytokines, including IL-8 and IL-12, and the expression of adhesion molecules, prostaglandins, and metalloproteinases. IL-1 causes bone destruction by enhancing proteoglycan degradation and bone resorption. Anti-inflammatory cytokines are also produced but do not have adequate potency to dampen the inflammatory response. Transforming growth factor-beta, interferon-beta, IL-4, and IL-10 are examples of cytokines with anti-inflammatory properties. Other means of controlling inflammation include soluble receptors that adhere to cytokines before attachment to cells (TNF) or receptor antagonists that inactivate receptor function (IL-1). This immune-mediated process becomes self-perpetuating even if the initiating factor is removed.[63] The end result of this unbalanced immune process is a systemic illness with immune cells localizing in synovial tissue, proliferating, and producing soluble factors that are inflammatory and destructive to joint tissue.

Synovial Inflammation

RA causes inflammation that is centered in the synovial membrane. The joints that are affected by the inflammation associated with RA are lined by a thin tissue layer, the synovial membrane, which produces synovial fluid that nourishes the cartilage and lubricates the joint. Synovial membrane is not limited to joints alone but is found in many parts of the musculoskeletal system associated with motion, such as tendons, bursae, and ligaments. The inflammation associated with RA causes hypertrophy of this membrane along with the production of humoral factors that cause destruction of cartilage and bone cells. Some of the factors that cause damage include superoxide radicals, nitric oxide, disordered apoptosis, and activators of osteoclasts (receptor activator of nuclear factor κB ligand and osteoprotegrin ligand) .[54,140] The end result of this inflammatory process, if left unchecked, is a destroyed joint with thinning cartilage, eroded bone, and disrupted supporting structures.

11-9 CYTOKINES ASSOCIATED WITH RHEUMATOID ARTHRITIS

Cytokine	Activity
Interleukin-1	Activates T cells, metalloproteinases—destroys cartilage
Interleukin-2	Stimulates proliferation of T cells and other cytokines
Interleukin-4	Anti-inflammatory, decreases TH1 cytokines, stimulates B-cell antibody production
Interleukin-6	B-cell differentiation, acute phase reactants
Interleukin-8	Neutrophil chemotactic factor
Interleukin-10	Anti-inflammatory, inhibits interferon-induced expression of class II human leukocyte antigens
Interleukin-12	Activates natural killer and TH1 cells
Tumor necrosis factor-α	Enhances intercellular adhesion molecules, class II expression on antigen-presenting cells
Interferon-γ	Enhances intercellular adhesion molecules, class II expression on antigen-presenting cells
Transforming growth factor-β	Enhances production of tissue inhibitor of metalloproteinase; suppresses production of tumor necrosis factor-α, interleukin-1, interleukin-6, and neutrophil chemoattractant; causes late-stage fibrosis

Modified from Smith JB, Haynes MK: Rheumatoid arthritis—a molecular understanding. Ann Intern Med 136:908-922, 2002.

Cervical Subluxation

In the cervical spine, structures lined with synovial membrane may be involved in RA. These structures include the atlantoaxial joint. This joint connects the atlas (C1) with the axis (C2) and is responsible for rotation of the skull on the cervical spine. Synovial tissue is located between the atlas and axis and between the ligaments and atlas (see Fig. 1-9). Other synovial joints include the zygapophyseal and uncovertebral. Bursae are also lined with synovial membrane and are found in the C1–C2 region and the interspinous ligaments.[29]

RA causes disease in the cervical spine by inducing chronic inflammatory changes in the atlanto-occipital, atlantoaxial, zygapophyseal, and uncovertebral joints, along with the discs and ligamentous and bursal structures. At the level of the atlantoaxial joint, synovial inflammation of the bursae and ligaments results in laxity of the transverse ligament that holds the atlas and axis together. Normally, the distance between the bones does not exceed 2.5 to 3 mm in adults.[68] Relaxation of the supporting ligaments results in excess motion of the axis in relation to the atlas, or atlantoaxial subluxation.[99] Luxation of the atlantoaxial joint may occur anteriorly, posteriorly, superiorly or vertically, or laterally.[28,50,124,144] Biomechanical models have demonstrated that the addition of mechanical stress to inflammation causes the erosive manifestations of RA at the C1–C2 complex.[123] Anterior subluxation is the most common form, found in up to 49% of patients, and results from insufficiency of the transverse ligament or fracture of the odontoid.[127] Posterior subluxation occurs when C1 moves posteriorly on C2; it results from erosion or fracture of the odontoid and occurs in 7% of patients. Vertical or superior subluxation is caused by destruction of the lateral atlantoaxial joints around the foramen magnum and is found in 38% of patients. Lateral subluxation occurs in 20% and results from erosion of the lateral mass and odontoid.[109] Abnormal motion of this joint in any direction may lead to compression of the cervical spinal cord or medulla oblongata and result in the development of neurologic symptoms and signs of myelopathy, including paresthesias, muscle weakness, reflex changes, spasticity, and incontinence.[95,104] The vertebral arteries may be compressed during subluxation of the atlantoaxial joint by the odontoid process of the axis and the posterior arch of the atlas. The vertebral arteries are compressed as they travel through the foramina in the transverse processes of C1 and C2. Vertebral artery compression may cause tetraplegia, coma, or sudden death.[45,170] Subluxation may occur in multiple directions in an individual.[161] Autopsy evaluation of RA patients with paralysis reveals spinal cords with mechanical neural compression; marked physical distortion, flattening, and destruction of the cord; and vascular compression causing ischemic damage to the cord with necrosis of the lateral columns in the watershed regions supplied by the anterior and posterior spinal arteries.[41]

The initial disorder occurs at C1–C2 in isolated anterior subluxation. It progresses to C1–C2 instability with superior migration of the odontoid. In the final stages, the anterior C1–C2 subluxation may stabilize with superior migration alone. This stable form of subluxation occurs with the development of erosion and collapse of the lateral facet joints.[75] Cervical subluxations occur by the second year after the diagnosis of RA in 10% of subluxation patients.[116]

Subluxation may occur between cervical vertebrae below the atlantoaxial joint. Common levels include C3–C4 and C4–C5. Inflammation in the zygapophyseal joints and surrounding bursae undermines the stability of these joints and results in excessive motion and angulation of the cervical spine.[169] The intervertebral discs may be invaded by growing synovial tissue with resultant disc space narrowing.[13] The reported frequency of subaxial subluxation ranges from 7% to 29% in RA patients.[58]

Myelopathy may also occur in patients without atlantoaxial or cervical spine subluxation. In these patients, synovitis from the zygapophyseal joints along with intervertebral disc lesions may compromise the blood supply to the spinal cord through stenosis of vertebral vessels that feed the anterior spinal artery. Ischemic myelopathy is the result.[45] Sudden death may also be a consequence of thrombosis of the vertebral vessels.[157]

The neurologic impairments from C1–C2 disease tend to be more severe than subluxations in other portions of the cervical spine. Cerebrospinal fluid flow may be impaired with the development of hydrocephalus or syringomyelia.[170] The types of neurologic deficits may vary, depending on the specific tracts affected in the spinal cord. For example, cruciate paralysis occurs with compression of the upper corticospinal tract decussation in the center of the spinal cord without affecting the uncrossed tract supplying the lower extremities. The clinical result is bilateral weakness in the upper extremities and normal strength in the lower extremities.[11] Compression of the lateral aspect of the pyramidal decussation results in paresis of the ipsilateral arm and contralateral leg.[170]

CLINICAL HISTORY

Patients with RA suffer from joint pain, heat, swelling, and tenderness. The joint involvement is additive and symmetrical. The joints at greatest risk of being affected by the disease process include the proximal interphalangeal, metacarpal-carpal, wrist, elbow, hip, knee, ankle, and metatarsophalangeal joints. In the axial skeleton, the cervical spine is most frequently affected. Patients have joint pain and stiffness, most severe in the morning. Activity improves the symptoms. This phenomenon, stiffness of a joint with rest, occurs frequently with active disease. As a component of systemic inflammation, afternoon fatigue, anorexia, and weight loss are common complaints.

The cervical spine is the most commonly affected component of the axial skeleton. Neck movement frequently precipitates or aggravates neck pain that is aching and deep in quality. Atlantoaxial disease is experienced in the upper part of the cervical spine, and pain radiates over the occiput to the temporal and frontal regions with increasing disease of the C1–C2 joint. Occipital headaches are frequently associated with active rheumatoid involvement of the cervical spine. Other symptoms of C1–C2 subluxation include a sensation of the head falling forward with flexion of the neck, loss of consciousness or syncope, incontinence, dysphagia, vertigo, convulsions, hemiplegia, dysarthria, nystagmus, and peripheral paresthesias.[61] Peripheral joint erosion is a harbinger of C1–C2 subluxation. Cervical subluxation develops in patients who have joint erosions of the hands and feet, serum rheumatoid factor, and subcutaneous nodules.[166,167]

The pain associated with RA in the subaxial segments of the cervical spine is located in the lateral aspects of the neck and clavicles (C3–C4) and over the shoulders (C5–C6). Neurologic symptoms include paresthesias and numbness. The paresthesias have a burning quality that may be attributed to an entrapment neuropathy (carpal tunnel syndrome) but are sufficiently different to not be confused with joint pain. Patients with sensory symptoms alone may have their symptoms ascribed to arthritis, thereby delaying the diagnosis of cervical myelopathy.[95]

The appearance of spasticity, gait disturbance, muscular weakness, and incontinence (urinary or fecal) indicates significant compression of the spinal cord. Symptoms suggesting vertebrobasilar artery insufficiency include visual disturbances, dizziness, paresthesias of the face, ataxia, and dysarthria.[71,102]

Patients with severe, generalized RA may have neck symptoms with cervical subluxation. However, marked subluxation may develop with little peripheral arthritis.[13] Similarly, the extent of cervical subluxation may not be closely correlated with the extent of neck pain or neurologic dysfunction. This lack of correlation may occur because there is adequate room at the C1–C2 level (the most capacious portion of the spinal canal) to allow the spinal cord to slip laterally around the odontoid and escape compression.[16]

Patients with RA of the lumbosacral spine usually have a history of extensive involvement of long duration. Low back pain appears along with increased synovitis in the peripheral joints. The pain may be localized to the low back region or may radiate to the thighs.[139] The sacroiliac joints are asymptomatic or mildly symptomatic.[55]

In a questionnaire study of 503 RA patients, 221 complained of back pain, with 167 having pain lasting 3 months or longer. Most patients complained of more than one area of low back pain. The character of the pain was dull in 80% of patients. Pain radiated to the thigh in 27% and to the lower part of the leg in 10%. Pain was increased by certain positions, including flexion (50%) and sitting (52%), and with exercise (52%). In contrast to mechanical etiologies of back pain, pain was not exacerbated by inspiration (10%), cough (13%), and extension of the back (13%). Relief of pain was obtained by rest (75%), physiotherapy (28%), and analgesics (28%). A small minority had the combination of nocturnal pain, aggravation with rest, and relief with exercise.[65]

PHYSICAL EXAMINATION

Physical examination of an RA patient with cervical spine disease reveals diffuse peripheral joint involvement characterized by heat, swelling, bogginess, tenderness, and loss of motion. Nodules over the extensor surfaces are noted in 20% of RA patients. Examination of the cervical spine may show tenderness with palpation over the bony skeleton and limitation of all spinal movements. Pseudoaneurysm of the vertebral artery may be manifested as a pulsatile mass.[48] Inspection may show fixation of the head tilted down and to one side. This lateral tilt is caused by asymmetric destruction of the lateral atlantoaxial joints. The normal cervical lordosis may also be absent. With the neck flexed, the spinous process of the axis may be prominent in the midline of the neck of patients with atlantoaxial subluxation. Palpation of the posterior of the pharynx during flexion may reveal abnormal separation of the anterior arch of the atlas from the body of the axis. Anteroposterior laxity may also be detected by applying pressure on the forehead while palpating the spinous process of the axis. In a patient with subluxation, the flexed head glides backward as the subluxation is reduced. This test is not frequently used, however, for fear of causing neurologic symptoms. Patients with subaxial subluxation may demonstrate abnormalities in the upper extremities. For example, compression of the C6–C8 segments causes distinctive numb, clumsy hands and tactile agnosia.[33]

Neurologic abnormalities may include loss of sensation and weakness of the muscles of the upper or lower extremities. Abnormal Babinski signs may occur but are uncommon. Vertigo, nystagmus, dysphagia, or coma is present in the occasional patient with vertebral artery compression. Vertical subluxation may affect the medulla oblongata and cranial nerves. Abnormal neurologic signs in these patients may include internuclear ophthalmoplegia, facial diplegia, downbeat nystagmus, spastic quadriparesis, sleep apnea, loss of pinprick and light touch sensation in the trigeminal nerve distribution, and dysfunction of cranial nerves IX, X, and XII.[170] In general, neurologic abnormalities are seen in approximately 7% of RA patients.[37]

Examination of the lumbar spine may show tenderness with palpation over the bony skeleton and limitation of all spinal movement. A number of patients may not demonstrate a significant decrease in back motion despite considerable damage in the peripheral joints. Neurologic examination, including the straight leg–raising test, is normal.

LABORATORY DATA

Abnormal laboratory findings include anemia, an elevated erythrocyte sedimentation rate, and increases in serum globulin levels. Thrombocytosis is found in patients with active RA. Rheumatoid factors (antibodies directed against host antibodies) are present in 80% of patients with RA, and antinuclear antibodies are present in 30%. C-reactive protein, an acute phase reactant, may be helpful when obtained in a serial manner to predict individuals who are at increased risk for joint deterioration and as a measure of response to therapy.[115] Individuals with persistent elevations in C-reactive protein are at risk for progressive cervical spine subluxations.[51] Synovial fluid analysis demonstrates an inflammatory fluid characterized by poor viscosity, increased number of white blood cells, decreased glucose level, and increased protein level.

Pathology

Histologic examination of the synovium from affected joints demonstrates an inflammatory, hyperplastic tissue characterized by mononuclear cell infiltration, synovial cell proliferation, fibrin deposition, and necrosis. Examination of cervical spine apophyseal joints from autopsied RA patients has shown similar hyperplastic changes consistent with the synovial alterations associated with inflammatory disease in peripheral joints.[13]

Somatosensory evoked potentials are useful in detecting spinal cord impingement in patients with subluxation and severe arthritis. Neurologic signs may be difficult to elicit in patients with joint destruction. Somatosensory potentials may localize an area of cord impingement that may not be conclusively documented by physical examination or radiographs.[72]

RADIOGRAPHIC EVALUATION

Characteristic roentgenographic changes of RA in the peripheral joints include soft tissue swelling, bony erosion without reactive sclerotic bone, joint space narrowing, and periarticular osteopenia. Roentgenographic evaluation of the cervical spine includes anteroposterior, lateral with flexion and extension, oblique, and open-mouth frontal projections.

The roentgenographic criteria for the diagnosis of RA cervical spine disease as proposed by Bland and colleagues are (1) atlantoaxial subluxation of 2.5 mm or greater; (2) multiple subluxation of C2–C3, C3–C4, C4–C5, and C5–C6; (3) narrow disc spaces with little or no osteophytosis; (4) erosion of vertebrae, especially the vertebral plates; (5) odontoid, small, pointed, eroded loss of cortex; (6) basilar impression; (7) apophyseal joint erosion, blurred facets; (8) cervical spine osteoporosis; (9) wide space (more than 5 mm) between the posterior arch of the atlas and the spinous process of the axis (flexion to extension); and (10) secondary osteosclerosis in the atlantoaxial-occipital complex, which may indicate local degenerative change.[17]

Anterior subluxation is the most common form of cervical spine derangement, but its frequency varies in RA patients. This variability may be related to not taking all the roentgenographic views (flexion) necessary to observe subluxation or to difficulty in observing the anterior edge of the odontoid process. Anterior subluxation is present in

25% of all RA patients and in 70% of RA patients with neck pain.[97,101] In postmortem studies, anterior subluxation is noted in 46% of RA patients.[15] The normal distance between the odontoid and atlas is 2.5 and 3.0 mm in women and men, respectively, as measured from the posteroinferior aspect of the tubercle of C1 to the nearest point on the odontoid (Fig. 11-27).[80] The posterior atlanto-odontoid interval is the remaining distance between the posterior surface of the odontoid process and the anterior edge of the posterior ring of the atlas. RA patients with a posterior interval of more than 14 mm did not have neurologic deficits. The mechanism of spinal cord compression with anterior subluxation has been studied by cineradiography.[118] During flexion, the atlas slowly separates anteriorly from the axis. With increasing displacement, the spinal canal is narrowed by the posterior arch of the atlas. In extension, subluxation persists as long as the head is below the horizontal. The atlas slides backward and rests against the dens (producing a clicking sensation when motion is abrupt) when the horizontal plane is reached.

Posterior subluxation occurs in 6.7% of RA patients.[162] The atlas must be partially destroyed or malformed or the odontoid eroded, fractured, or congenitally absent for posterior subluxation to occur. Posterior subluxation may also occur if the atlas "jumps" over the axis and rests in a dorsal position.[88,146] Vertebrobasilar artery insufficiency associated with neurologic dysfunction is a manifestation of this form of subluxation.

Vertical subluxation of the dens through the foramen magnum into the posterior fossa occurs in 5% to 35% of RA patients.[47,108,162] Upward translocation occurs when the bony and ligamentous integrity of the atlanto-occipital articulations is disrupted. Disease of the occipital condyles, lateral masses of the atlas, and lateral articulations of the axis results in bony erosions or collapse.[98] The extent of vertical migration may be measured by a number of methods (Fig. 11-28).[106] McRae's line defines the true foramen magnum and is constructed by drawing a line between its anterior margin (basion) and posterior margin (opisthion). The tip of the dens is below this line. Other lines have been described because the basion may be difficult to observe on lateral roentgenograms of the cervical spine. Chamberlain's line is drawn from the hard palate to the opisthion. The odontoid tip should not be more than 3 mm above this line. McGregor's line extends from the

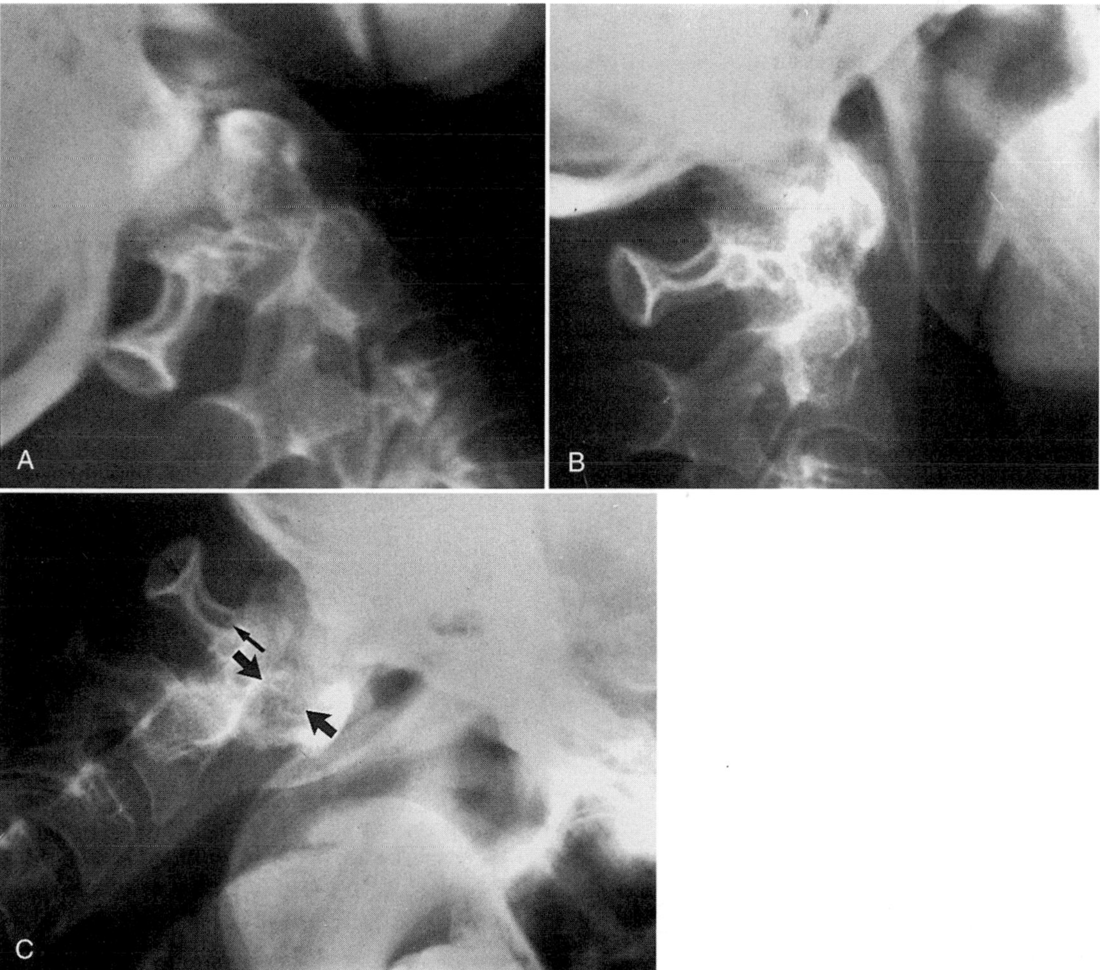

Figure 11-27 Rheumatoid arthritis as seen on a lateral view of the cervical spine of a 46-year-old woman with neck pain and a 12-year history of seropositive disease. *A*, Extension position; *B*, neutral position; *C*, flexion view. The series of views reveals a dynamic 10-mm atlantoaxial subluxation *(large black arrows)* and a posterior atlanto-odontoid interval of 14 mm *(small black arrow)*.

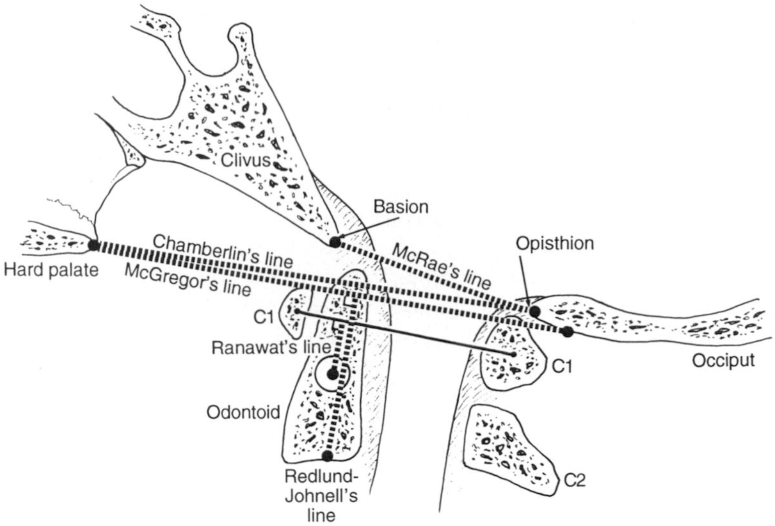

Figure 11-28 Vertical subluxation. Lines are drawn at the base of the skull to determine subluxation of the dens into the foramen magnum.

posterior margin of the hard palate to the most caudal point of the occiput. The dens should not project more than 4.5 mm above this line. These methods are based on the position of the tip of the odontoid. Because the location of the odontoid tip may be difficult to determine as a result of bony erosion, two alternative methods for determining vertical subluxation were devised. Ranawat's line is constructed by determining the coronal axis of C1 by connecting the center of the anterior arch of C1 with its posterior ring. The sclerotic ring in the center of C2 identifies the pedicle. The vertical distance along the dens axis is measured. In men the distance is 17 ± 2 mm, and in women the distance is 15 ± 2 mm. Any distance less than 13 mm is indicative of superior migration.[80] The Redlund-Johnell line is determined by the vertical distance between the inferior border of the axis and McGregor's line.[126]

Rotatory-lateral subluxation occurs in up to 30% of RA patients.[58] Erosion of the lateral apophyseal joints allows for a rotational head tilt.[57] The open-mouth view may demonstrate narrowing of the atlanto-occipital and atlantoaxial joints, as well as erosion of the odontoid. Subluxation occurs when the lateral masses of the atlas are displaced more than 2 mm with respect to those of the axis. Bony erosion is the most important factor in the development of severe lateral subluxation.[20]

In addition to changes in the upper cervical spine, radiographic abnormalities, including subaxial subluxation, apophyseal joint narrowing, and disc space narrowing, occur in the lower cervical spine. Subaxial subluxation develops in up to 29% of RA patients.[106] Subaxial subluxation is present in patients with more than 3.5 mm of malalignment. The stability of flexion and extension of the lower cervical spine depends on the integrity of the anterior and posterior longitudinal ligaments. Greater than 3.5 mm of malalignment is indicative of a mechanically unstable spine.[164] Multiple subluxations may occur and produce a "staircase" appearance on lateral radiographs.[106] Anterior subluxation is more frequent than posterior subluxation. Subaxial subluxation is most notable on a lateral flexion view of the cervical spine (Fig 11-29). Apophyseal joint disease includes narrowing, erosions, and sclerosis. Disc destruction in the cervical spine is associated with disc space narrowing and is caused by extension of erosive disease from the uncovertebral joints or by ongoing trauma to the vertebral endplates secondary to instability. The final stage of apophyseal disease is fibrous ankylosis of one or more levels, which may rarely simulate the appearance of ankylosing spondylitis (AS).[168]

Radiographic examination of patients with lumbar spine RA demonstrates apophyseal joint erosion without sclerosis, secondary disc space narrowing with bony

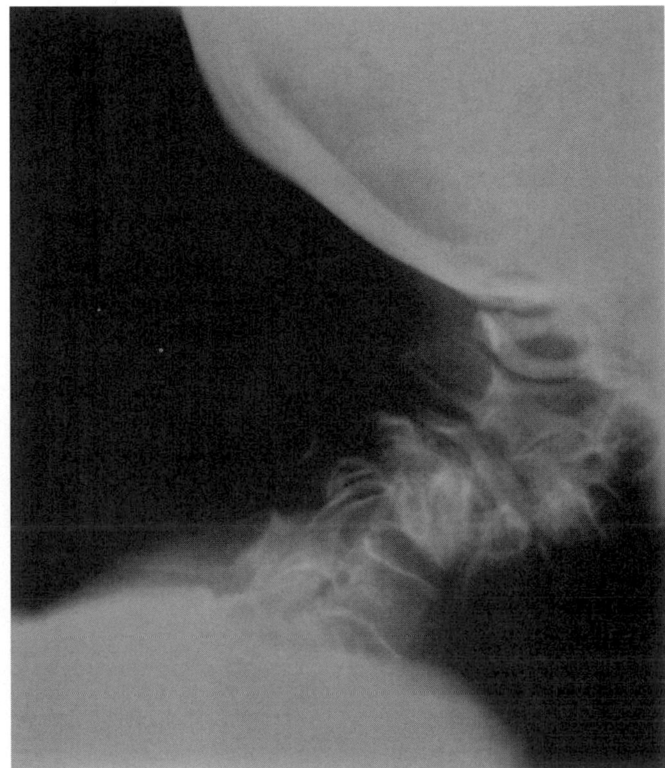

Figure 11-29 Rheumatoid arthritis. A lateral view of the cervical spine in a patient with severe seropositive disease demonstrates severe subaxial subluxation of C3 on C4. *(Courtesy of Herbert Baraf, MD.)*

destruction as a result of rheumatoid nodules, and malalignment.[42,110,120,128,134] Some of the alteration in vertebral body configuration may be related to the presence of rheumatoid nodules.[66] The apophyseal joints are frequently affected in RA. However, unlike in AS, joint fusion is rare.[65] Osteoporosis secondary to the illness or corticosteroid therapy is also a frequent finding in the spine of RA patients. Disc space narrowing, without osteophytosis, was commonly found in RA patients when compared with age-matched controls.[65] Sacroiliac joint changes include asymmetric involvement with mild narrowing, iliac erosions, minimal sclerosis, and fibrous fusion.[7] Involvement of the sacroiliac joints with RA may be unilateral or bilateral. Ankylosis, if it develops, is not as sturdy as that associated with AS, and the site of the joint cleft usually persists as a linear density on roentgenographic images of the joint. The sacroiliac margins above the synovial part of the joints are not affected.[96] On occasion, dislocation of the sacroiliac joint may be noted in RA patients.[52] As many as 35% of patients with long-standing disease may have sacroiliac changes.[135]

Patients with RA may also have a spondyloarthropathy such as AS or psoriatic arthritis. In these patients, differentiation of radiographic findings may be difficult. Unless diagnostic criteria are followed carefully, an increased incidence of sacroiliac disease may be attributed to RA in surveys of patients with radiographic abnormalities in the lumbosacral spine, when in fact the accompanying disease process may be the source of the joint alterations.[12]

Computed Tomography

CT is a useful radiographic technique for detecting the extent of bony destruction of structures that may not be easily visualized with plain roentgenograms. CT scan detects the position of an eroded odontoid process that may not be seen on roentgenograms taken in the open-mouth projection.[163] CT also demonstrates the posterior obliteration of subarachnoid space that marks individuals at risk for progressive myelopathy.[125] In a comparison of plain roentgenograms and CT, Braunstein and colleagues reported on the usefulness of plain roentgenograms as the initial examination of choice.[23] CT visualized the transverse ligament but did not provide significant additional information. Others believe that CT images offer views of the spinal canal, spinal cord, and neural foramina that are useful in detecting the extent and severity of disease.[73]

Magnetic Resonance

MR imaging is a noninvasive method that is useful in detecting soft tissue abnormalities in the cervical spine of RA patients. MR imaging allows direct visualization of the spinal cord at sites of bony or soft tissue compression (Fig. 11-30).[2,24,122] It is able to detect pannus around the odontoid and alterations in the substance of the spinal cord.[44,76] MR imaging may also be useful in documenting the response of pannus to therapy or the status of the spinal cord in the postoperative state.[84] When compared with CT and plain roentgenograms, MR imaging versus plain roentgenograms demonstrated cytic lesions, odontoid erosions, and vertical atlantoaxial subluxations more often, showed anterior subluxations as often, and visualized lateral subluxations less often.[113]

DIFFERENTIAL DIAGNOSIS

RA is a clinical diagnosis based on the history of joint pain, the distribution of joint involvement, and characteristic laboratory abnormalities (rheumatoid factor). Criteria for the classification of RA were published by the American College of Rheumatology (Table 11-10).[5] In the setting of generalized, active disease, the finding of neck pain associated with multiple abnormalities, including atlantoaxial subluxation, apophyseal joint erosion without sclerosis, disc space narrowing without osteophytes, and multiple subluxations, is most appropriately attributed to RA. The cervical spine abnormalities of AS, psoriatic arthritis, reactive arthritis, enteropathic arthritis, osteoarthritis, and diffuse idiopathic skeletal hyperostosis are associated with new bone formation or ligamentous calcification, which differentiates them from RA. Occasionally, atlantoaxial subluxation may occur alone in the setting of little peripheral disease. In these

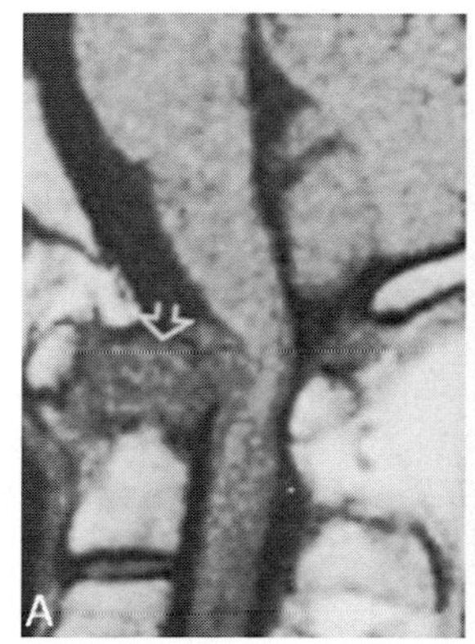

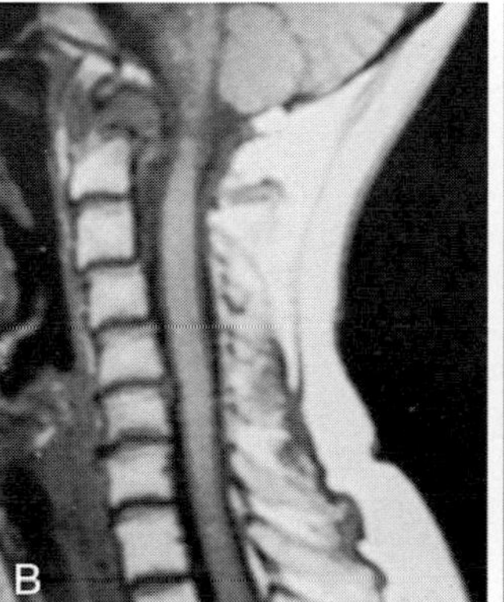

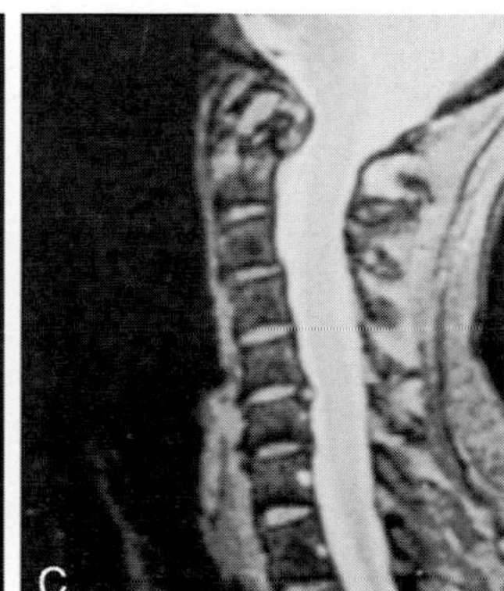

Figure 11-30 MR imaging in rheumatoid arthritis: evaluation of spinal involvement. Periodontoid disease. *A*, A sagittal T1-weighted spin echo MR image (TR/TE 450/30) of the upper cervical spine reveals a mass of intermediate signal intensity *(arrow)* that is eroding the odontoid process and causing cord compression. *B*, Sagittal T1-weighted spin echo (TR/TE 600/11) and multiplanar gradient recalled image. *C*, Sagittal T1-weighted spin echo (TR/TE 600/11) MR image shows similar involvement in a different patient. Note the high signal intensity around the odontoid process. *(A, From Neuhold A, et al: Medicamundi 32:38, 1987; B, from Resnick D: Rheumatoid arthritis. In Resnick D [ed]: Diagnosis of Bone and Joint Disorders, 3rd ed. Philadelphia, WB Saunders, 1995, p 952; and C, courtesy of C. Gundry, MD, Minneapolis, MN.)*

11-10 AMERICAN RHEUMATISM ASSOCIATION 1987 REVISED CRITERIA FOR THE CLASSIFICATION OF RHEUMATOID ARTHRITIS

Criterion	Definition
1. Morning stiffness	Morning stiffness in and around the joints lasting at least 1 hour before maximal improvement
2. Arthritis of three or more joint areas	At least three joint areas simultaneously have soft tissue swelling or fluid (not bony overgrowth)
3. Arthritis of hand joints	At least one area swollen (as defined above) in a wrist, metacarpophalangeal (MCP), or proximal interphalangeal (PIP) joint.
4. Symmetrical arthritis	Simultaneous involvement of PIP, MCP, or metatarsophalangeal joints is acceptable without absolute symmetry
5. Rheumatoid nodules	Subcutaneous nodules over bony prominences, extensor surfaces, or juxta-articular regions, observed by a physician
6. Serum rheumatoid factor	Demonstration of abnormal amounts of serum rheumatoid factor by any method for which the result has been positive in less than 5% of normal control subjects
7. Radiographic changes	Radiographic change typical of rheumatoid arthritis on posteroanterior hand and wrist radiographs; must include erosions or unequivocal bony decalcification localized in or most marked adjacent to the involved joints (osteoarthritis changes alone do not qualify)

For classification purposes, a patient is said to have rheumatoid arthritis if at least four of seven criteria have been satisfied. Criteria 1 through 4 must have been present for at least 6 weeks. Patients with two clinical diagnoses are not excluded. Designation as classic, definite, or probable rheumatoid arthritis is not to be made.

From Arnett FC, Edworthy SM, Block DA, et al.: The American Rheumatism Association 1987 revised criteria for the classification of rheumatoid arthritis. Arthritis Rheum 31:315, 1988.

circumstances, other disease processes that may cause subluxation include AS, psoriatic arthritis, reactive arthritis, trauma, and local infection.

Multicentric Reticulohistiocytosis

Multicentric reticulohistiocytosis, or lipoid dermatoarthritis, is a rare disorder of adults characterized by the presence of histiocytic nodules in the skin and severe, mutilating arthritis. A variety of lipids, including triglycerides, cholesterol esters, and phospholipids, are stored in histiocytes, which coalesce to form granulomas and produce enzymes that destroy joint and other tissue structures.[83] In 70% of patients, the first sign of the disease is a symmetrical polyarthritis that simulates the peripheral arthritis of rheumatoid disease.[46] The lumbosacral spine is affected less frequently. Pigmented skin nodules develop over the fingers, face, neck, and chest and are not associated with RA.[9] Patients with reticulohistiocytosis do not usually have rheumatoid factor. Radiologic abnormalities noted in the hands include circumscribed bone erosions, widened joint spaces, minimal periosteal reaction, and periarticular osteopenia,.[53] Sacroiliac joint abnormalities include erosion and obliteration with bony ankylosis of the articular space.[53,70] The process may be bilateral, but the lack of bony sclerosis helps differentiate this disease from AS. Therapy for this illness includes anti-inflammatory drugs. Corticosteroids and immunosuppressives, including cyclophosphamide, are used in patients with continued destructive disease.[60]

Relapsing Polychondritis

Relapsing polychondritis is a rare disease characterized by inflammation of cartilaginous structures; it is associated with peripheral arthritis that mimics RA. Patients with polychondritis produce antibodies against type II collagen.[49] Acute swelling of cartilaginous structures (ears, nose) develops, as well as swelling of the hand joints.[112] Between 12% and 30% of patients with relapsing polychondritis may have axial skeletal complaints.[103] Radiographic findings in the hands are usually those of a nondeforming, nonerosive arthropathy. On occasion, sacroiliac joint abnormalities are noted. These abnormalities include unilateral or bilateral involvement, which may be asymmetric in regard to the severity of disease. Relapsing polychondritis may also be complicated by a spondyloarthropathy that resembles AS or Reiter's syndrome.[119] Abnormalities include absence of spondylitis, sacroiliac joint thinning, erosion, and surrounding sclerosis.[22] Therapy for relapsing polychondritis is high-dose prednisone (40 to 60 mg/day). Corticosteroids are usually effective for control of the joint disease associated with polychondritis.

TREATMENT

Treatment of RA has undergone a paradigm shift with the advent of new drug therapies directed at control of the factors that mediate the immunologic destruction of joints.[34,86] Previous management involved an initial conservative approach with few medications prescribed until definite erosions were documented. Treatment for control of generalized RA included a regimen of patient education, physical therapy, nonsteroidal anti-inflammatory drugs (NSAIDs), remittive agents (gold, salts, penicillamine, or hydroxychloroquine), corticosteroids, and immunosuppressive agents (methotrexate).[63] Treatment was organized into a therapeutic pyramid based on the use of less toxic therapies for all patients. Drugs of greater toxicity were added with increasing clinical activity of disease. A reassessment of the treatment regimen was proposed.[165] This regimen initiated therapy with a multitude of drugs that were more toxic than NSAIDs because it was thought that the increased morbidity and mortality rates of RA require aggressive initial therapy. The difficulty was the absence of new medicines to better control the disorder. The advent of new agents has offered the opportunity to be more aggressive in preventing lesions before disability occurs.

The American College of Rheumatology has reviewed the available therapies and has proposed new options for the treatment of RA.[4] These new guidelines include data supporting the use of biologic agents in the treatment of RA.

Education

Therapy is directed at the control of pain and stiffness, reduction of inflammation, maintenance of function, and prevention of deformity. Patients are educated about their disease so that they may be active participants in their care. They are encouraged to continue with as normal a lifestyle as possible. Physical therapy provides temperature modalities (heat or cold) that relieve pain, exercises that maintain muscle strength, and assistive devices (canes, crutches, and splints) that promote normal function and ambulation.

Medications

Nonsteroidal Anti-inflammatory Drugs

Medications to control pain and inflammation are useful in patients with RA. Aspirin is a very effective agent for RA if given in adequate doses to reach a serum concentration of 20 to 25 mg/dL. For patients who are unable to take the number of tablets necessary to reach that serum level, who are intolerant of the drug, or on whom it has no effect, other NSAIDs are useful in controlling symptoms. Such agents include ibuprofen, tolmetin, fenoprofen, naproxen, indomethacin, piroxicam, sulindac, mefenamic acid, ketoprofen, etodolac, diclofenac, nabumetone, oxaprozin, and meloxicam. The choice of agent is dependent on a number of factors, including drug half-life, formulation, dose range, and tolerability.[26]

Cyclooxygenase Inhibitors

Cyclooxygenase-2 (COX-2) inhibitors are a class of NSAIDs that have efficacy equal to that of combined COX-1/COX-2 inhibitors (aspirin, naproxen), but with less gastrointestinal toxicity. COX-2 inhibitors are effective in RA.[21,137]

Disease-Modifying Antirheumatic Drugs

Patients who continue to have joint inflammation or who demonstrate joint damage (joint space narrowing, bony erosions, or cysts) despite adequate nonsteroidal therapy are candidates for remittive therapy. Remittive agents such as hydroxychloroquine, gold salts, and penicillamine have an onset of action that is delayed in comparison to NSAIDs. Hydroxychloroquine has a moderate, disease-suppressive action with few adverse reactions at doses of 400 mg/day or less.[147] Injectable gold salts (50 mg/wk) alter the natural history of RA.[31] The manufacture of some gold salts has been halted, and this therapeutic option will not be available in the future. The combination of D-penicillamine (125 to 750 mg/day) and sulfasalazine (2 g/day) has been reported to have a beneficial effect on the inflammation associated with RA.[145] The toxicities of penicillamine have limited its use.

Methotrexate at doses of 7.5 to 15 mg/wk is effective in decreasing the inflammation of RA and may also slow progression of the disease.[133] Methotrexate may be given all at once during the week. It is effective over a long duration of therapy.[132] In a study using methotrexate, 587 RA patients were monitored for 70 months; 76% of the patients took methotrexate for that period.[27] The drug remained effective in a majority of patients for the duration of the study. In another long-term study of 132 months, methotrexate remained an effective agent for 10 of the original 26 individuals who remained on the drug regimen.[160] Patients who have a stable course may be able to take methotrexate every second week and maintain control of joint inflammation.[82]

Leflunomide is an oral pyrimidine inhibitor used for the treatment of RA.[81] After ingestion, leflunomide is converted into the active metabolite A77 1726. Binding of this agent to the enzyme dihydroorotate dehydrogenase in the intramitochondrial pyrimidine biosynthetic pathway results in decreased levels of pyrimidine nucleotides. Lefluonomide is effective in the treatment of RA in a fashion similar to methotrexate.[143] The dose is 100 mg for 3 days, then 20 or 10 mg as tolerated. Toxicities include abnormal liver function test results and diarrhea. Leflunomide and methotrexate can be used together. These patients need to be monitored closely for potential hepatotoxicity.[86]

Corticosteroids

Systemic corticosteroids are effective in controlling the inflammatory components of RA. Corticosteroids are the most powerful and predictable remedy inducing immediate relief of joint inflammation in RA.[64] At low doses, corticosteroids may have a modest effect on reducing the rate of radiologically detected joint destruction.[78] A prospective trial demonstrated disease-modifying properties of 10 mg of prednisone over a 2-year period.[153] Corticosteroids are also associated with a wide range of toxicities, from hypertension and diabetes to cataracts and osteonecrosis of bone. Glucocorticoid-induced osteoporosis is a significant complication of this therapy.[90,130] Intra-articular corticosteroid injections are used when a single joint remains active in the face of general control of the arthritic process.

Anti–Tumor Necrosis Factor-Alpha Inhibitors

Anti-TNF therapies are available in the form of infliximab, etanercept, and adulimimab; these agents inhibit the inflammatory effects of TNF and are efficacious in the treatment of RA.

Infliximab is a partially humanized mouse monoclonal antibody directed against TNF-alpha. It is administered intravenously. Infliximab is added to methotrexate to limit the production of neutralizing antibodies to the mouse component of the agent. In a 30-week trial, infliximab plus methotrexate was more effective than methotrexate alone in patients with active RA.[94] In a 54-week study, infliximab, 3 mg or 10 mg/kg of body weight, and a stable dose of methotrexate prevented radiographic progression to a greater degree than methotrexate alone did.[87]

Etanercept is a recombinant form of the p75 TNF receptor fusion protein. Etanercept, 25 mg, is administered by subcutaneous injection twice weekly. It is more effective than placebo in limiting joint activity in RA.[107] Etanercept is also effective and safe when added to methotrexate.[159] The drug is effective over a 12-month period.[10]

Adulimimab is a fully human monoclonal TNF-alpha antibody given by subcutaneous injection every 2 weeks at a dose of 40 mg. This anti-TNF agent is effective with methotrexate in decreasing joint activity.[158]

The concern with anti-TNF therapies is toxicity. Blocking TNF does increase the risk for serious infection. TNF helps maintain containment of organisms in granulomas. Inhibition of TNF has been associated with the reactivation of tuberculosis.[8,77]

Anakinra is a recombinant, nonglycosylated form of human IL-1 receptor antagonist. This agent works by competitively inhibiting IL-1 from binding to its receptor site. Anakinra is given as a daily subcutaneous 100-mg injection. Anakinra in combination with methotrexate has been demonstrated to be effective in improving RA.[25,36]

Immunosuppressive Agents

Immunosuppressives are associated with severe toxicity (aplastic anemia and cancer), which limits their benefit to severely affected patients. Only a small number of patients with RA require this therapy. Some of the immunosuppressives used in RA include azathioprine, chlorambucil, cyclophosphamide, and cyclosporine.[32,43,91,154] A combination of cyclosporine and methotrexate may be effective for the treatment of patients with severe disease.[150]

Experimental therapy for RA includes the use of total lymph node irradiation, monoclonal antibodies, and antibiotics (minocycline). Studies investigating these agents are not conclusive in demonstrating their long-term beneficial effect on the course of RA.[67,141,148]

Cervical Spine Therapy

Conservative treatment of RA cervical spine disease is supportive. Early aggressive medical management is important to prevent joint destruction. Early disease-modifying antirheumatic drug (DMARD) therapy results in better outcomes. Combination therapy administered early in the course of RA can limit the development of atlantoaxial and vertical subluxation. Sulfasalazine, methotrexate, hydroxychloroquine, and prednisolone were more effective than a single DMARD with prednisolone in preventing cervical subluxation.[111] Soft cervical collars offer comfort but do not protect against progressive subluxation. Rigid collars can limit anterior subluxation but do not allow reduction of the subluxation in extension. Rigid collars are poorly tolerated by RA patients with temporomandibular disease.[74]

Spinal Surgical Intervention

The role of surgery in the treatment of RA patients with cervical spine disease, particularly those who are asymptomatic, is very controversial. Myelopathic signs occur in up to 33% of patients.[106] Balanced against the potential for neurologic dysfunction is a mortality rate of 15% and a successful fusion rate of only 50%.[108] If neurologic function progresses to paralysis, the success of surgery to improve function is significantly compromised, and surgical mortality increases.[171] Boden and colleagues reviewed the 20-year course of 73 RA patients with cervical spine disease.[19] Paralysis developed in 42 of these patients. The posterior atlanto-odontoid interval and the diameter of the subaxial sagittal spinal canal were the measurements most closely associated with progression to paralysis. Patients with less than a 10-mm posterior atlanto-odontoid interval had no recovery after correction of atlantoaxial subluxation. Patients with vertical and atlantoaxial subluxation had neurologic recovery if the atlanto-odontoid interval was 13 mm. Good results with repair of subaxial subluxation required a diameter of 14 mm.

Surgical intervention is indicated in RA patients with intractable pain and neurologic deficit or evidence of increased signal intensity within the spinal cord on T2-weighted MR sequences. Patients with isolated atlantoaxial subluxations and no neurologic deficit can be observed. Other forms of subluxation must be evaluated with concern regarding neural impingement and adequate space in the spinal canal.[127]

When surgical therapy is required for atlantoaxial subluxation, reducible atlantoaxial subluxations are managed by posterior arthrodesis (Fig 11-31).[35] Posterior arthrodesis stabilizes the joint, and stabilization results in the resorption of pannus.[56] Irreducible subluxation may require a transoral approach for decompression and posterior fusion.[39] Vertical subluxation with any evidence of cord compression requires surgical correction because of the high mortality associated with this lesion. These

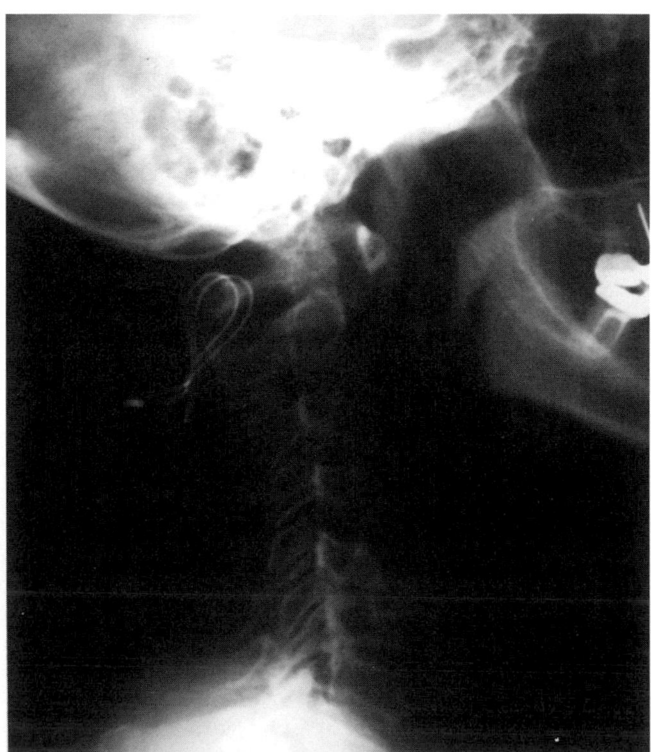

Figure 11-31 Rheumatoid arthritis visualized on a lateral view of the cervical spine in a 56-year-old woman with over 20 years of disease. Increasing neck pain and dysesthesias developed in her arms. She had significant dynamic subluxations. Her C1–C2 spinous processes were wired together, and she has had resolution of her symptoms for the subsequent 5 years.

patients require tong traction to reduce subluxation, transoral anterior decompression, and occipitocervical fusion to prevent recurrent cranial settling.[18,106] Patients with subaxial subluxation and compression should undergo reduction of the subluxation because granulation tissue may result in increased neural compression. One approach is that of posterior stabilization of the subluxed segment.[89] Other approaches are anterior decompression and fusion.[131] Common complications of RA cervical spine surgery include death (5% to 10%), infection, wound dehiscence, nonunion (5% to 20%), wire breakage and loss of reduction, and subluxation at the level below the fused segment.[38] Good outcomes occur when surgical intervention is undertaken before severe myelopathy is present.

PROGNOSIS

The course of RA cannot be predicted at the time of onset. Some patients have disease that is associated with joint destruction and resistance to therapy. Patients who are older with seropositive generalized disease and nodules are at greater risk for the development of cervical spine disease. Subluxation does not develop in all patients. In a 5- to 14-year follow-up study, 25% of patients had an increase in subluxation, 50% had no change, and 25% had improvement.[134] In a 5-year study of 106 RA patients, the prevalence of cervical spine subluxation increased from 43% to 70%.[121] In subaxial disease, myelopathy was associated with narrowing of the canal, destruction of spinous processes, axial shortening, younger age of the patient, longer duration of disease, higher dose of corticosteroids, and higher stage of disease.[169] Sudden death remains a complication of RA cervical spine disease, particularly in those with vertical subluxation.[105] Individuals with subluxation had eight times the mortality as RA patients without subluxation.[129] Improved surgical outcomes for cervical myelopathy are related to early intervention for clinical symptoms.[59] Occipitocervical fusion for myelopathy has been associated with improvement over a 10-year period and maintenance of ambulation for a mean of 7.5 years.[100] Van Asselt and associates reported a 73% survival rate 2 years after surgery for myelopathy.[151] Individuals with quadriparesis and very poor functional capacity have greater mortality.

A practical consideration in the preoperative care of RA patients is the need for cervical spine roentgenograms. In 128 RA patients with no symptoms of cervical cord compression who underwent elective orthopedic surgery, unsuspected C1–C2 disease was detected in 5.5%. Findings on roentgenograms had little effect on the type of anesthesia given at the time of surgery. Alternative methods of anesthesia without the need for hyperextension of the neck were used without complication. Communication between the physician and anesthesiologist may negate the need for cervical spine roentgenograms in RA patients who are asymptomatic with regard to the cervical spine.[30]

Patients with long-term disease are at risk for lumbar spine involvement. Although lumbar spinal disease occurs in patients with a more active process, these particular symptoms are responsive to therapeutic measures. Patients with RA are not disabled specifically because of lumbar spine involvement. However, patients with lumbar spine disease have extensive generalized involvement, which usually affects their functional status and ability to function in a job.

References

Rheumatoid Arthritis

1. Aho K, Koskenvuo M, Tuominen J, et al: Occurrence of rheumatoid arthritis in a nationwide series of twins. J Rheumatol 13:899-902, 1986.
2. Aisen AM, Martel W, Ellis JH, McCune WJ: Cervical spine involvement in rheumatoid arthritis: Magnetic resonance imaging. Radiology 165:159, 1987.
3. Alasalameh S, Mollenhauer J, Hain N, et al: Cellular immune response toward human articular chondrocytes. Arthritis Rheum 33:1477, 1990.
4. American College of Rheumatology Subcommittee on Rheumatoid Arthritis guidelines: Guidelines for the management of rheumatoid arthritis: 2002 update. Arthritis Rheum 46:328-346, 2002.
5. Arnett FC, Edworthy SM, Block DA, et al: The American Rheumatism Association 1987 revised criteria for the classification of rheumatoid arthritis. Arthritis Rheum 31:315, 1988.
6. Baboonian C, Venables PJW, Williams DG, et al: Cross-reaction of antibodies to a glycine-alanine repeat sequence of Epstein-Barr virus nuclear antigen-1 with collagen, cytokeratin, and actin. Ann Rheum Dis 50:772, 1991.
7. Baggenstoss AH, Bidkel WH, Ward LE: Rheumatoid granulomatous nodules as destructive lesions of vertebrae. J Bone Joint Surg Am 34-A:601, 1952.
8. Baghai M, Osmon DR, Wolk DM, et al: Fatal sepsis in a patient with rheumatoid arthritis treated with etarnercept. Mayo Clin Proc 76:653-656, 2001.
9. Barrow MV, Holubar K: Multicentric reticulohistiocytosis: A review of 33 patients. Medicine (Baltimore) 48:287, 1969.
10. Bathon JM, Martin RW, Fleischmann RM, et al: A comparison of etanercept and methotrexate in patients with early rheumatoid arthritis. N Engl J Med 343:1586-1593, 2000.
11. Bell HS: Paralysis of both arms from injury of the upper portion of the pyramidal decussation: "Cruciate paralysis." J Neurosurg 33:376, 1970.
12. Bernhard G: Extra-articular rheumatoid arthritis: Clinical features and treatment overview. In Utsinger PD, Zvaifler NJ, Ehrlich GE (eds): Rheumatoid Arthritis: Etiology, Diagnosis, Management. Philadelphia, JB Lippincott, 1985, p 337.
13. Bland JH: Rheumatoid arthritis of the cervical spine. Bull Rheum Dis 18:471, 1967.
14. Bland JH: Rheumatoid arthritis of the cervical spine. J Rheumatol 1:319, 1974.
15. Bland JH: Rheumatoid subluxation of the cervical spine. J Rheumatol 17:134, 1990.
16. Bland JH, Davis PH, London MG, et al: Rheumatoid arthritis of the cervical spine. Arch Intern Med 112:892, 1963.
17. Bland JH, Van Buskirk FW, Tampas JP, et al: A study of roentgenologic criteria for rheumatoid arthritis of the cervical spine. AJR Am J Roentgenol 95:949, 1965.
18. Boden SD: Rheumatoid arthritis of the cervical spine: Surgical decision making based on predictors of paralysis and recovery. Spine 19:2275, 1994.
19. Boden SD, Dodge LD, Bohlman HH, Rechtine GR: Rheumatoid arthritis of the cervical spine: A long-term analysis with predictors of paralysis and recovery. J Bone Joint Surg Am 75-A:1282, 1993.
20. Bogduk N, Major GAC, Carter J: Lateral subluxation of the atlas in rheumatoid arthritis: A case report and post-mortem study. Ann Rheum Dis 43:341, 1984.
21. Bombardier C, Laine L, Reicin A, et al: Comparison of upper gastrointestinal toxicity of rofecoxib and naproxen in patients with rheumatoid arthritis. N Engl J Med 343:1520-1528, 2000.
22. Braunstein EM, Martel W, Stillwell E, Kay D: Radiologic aspects of the arthropathy of relapsing polychondritis. Clin Radiol 30:441, 1979.
23. Braunstein EM, Weissman BN, Seltzer SE, et al: Computed tomography and conventional radiographs of the craniocervical region in rheumatoid arthritis: A comparison. Arthritis Rheum 27:26, 1984.

24. Breedveld FC, Algra PR, Veilvoye CJ, Cats A: Magnetic resonance imaging in the evaluation of patients with rheumatoid arthritis and subluxations of the cervical spine. Arthritis Rheum 30:624, 1987.
25. Bresnihan B, Alvaro-Gracia JM, Cobby M, et al: Treatment of rheumatoid arthritis with recombinant human interleukin-1 receptor antagonist. Arthritis Rheum 41:2196-2204, 1998.
26. Brooks PM, Day RO: Nonsteroidal anti-inflammatory drugs—differences and similarities. N Engl J Med 324:1716, 1991.
27. Buchbinder R, Hall S, Sambrook PN, et al: Methotrexate therapy in rheumatoid arthritis: A life table review of 587 patients treated in community practice. J Rheumatol 20:639, 1993.
28. Burry HC, Tweed JM, Robinson RG, Howes R: Lateral subluxation of the atlanto-axial joint in rheumatoid arthritis. Ann Rheum Dis 37:525, 1978.
29. Bywaters EGL: Rheumatoid and other disease of the cervical interspinous bursae, and changes in the spinous processes. Ann Rheum Dis 41:360, 1982.
30. Campbell RSD, Wou P, Watt I: A continuing role for preoperative cervical spine radiography in rheumatoid arthritis? Clin Radiol 50:157, 1995.
31. Capell HA, Lewis D, Carey J: A three-year follow-up of patients allocated to placebo, or oral or injectable gold therapy for rheumatoid arthritis. Ann Rheum Dis 45:705, 1986.
32. Cash JM, Klippel JH: Second-line drug therapy for rheumatoid arthritis. N Engl J Med 330:1368, 1994.
33. Chang MH, Liao KK, Cheung SC, et al: “Numb, clumsy hands” and tactile agnosia secondary to high cervical spondylotic myelopathy: A clinical and electrophysiological correlation. Acta Neurol Scand 86:622, 1992.
34. Choy EHS, Panayi GS: Cytokine pathways and joint inflammation in rheumatoid arthritis. N Engl J Med 344:907-916, 2001.
35. Clark CR, Goetz DD, Menezes AH: Arthrodesis of the cervical spine in rheumatoid arthritis. J Bone Joint Surg Am 71-A:381, 1989.
36. Cohen S, Hurd E, Cush J, et al: Treatment of rheumatoid arthritis with anakinra: A recombinant human interleukin-1 receptor antagonist, in combination with methotrexate: Results of a twenty-four-week, multicenter, randomized, double-blind, placebo-controlled trial. Arthritis Rheum 46:614-624, 2002.
37. Colon PW, Isdale IC, Rose BS: Rheumatoid arthritis of the cervical spine: An analysis of 333 cases. Ann Rheum Dis 25:120, 1966.
38. Conaty JP, Mongan ES: Cervical fusion in rheumatoid arthritis. J Bone Joint Surg Am 63-A:1218, 1991.
39. Crockard HA, Pozo JL, Ransford HO, et al: One-stage transoral anterior decompression and posterior stabilization in cervical myelopathy complicating rheumatoid arthritis. J Bone Joint Surg Br 67-B:498, 1985.
40. Decker JL: Rheumatoid arthritis: Evolving concept of pathogenesis and treatment. Ann Intern Med 101:810, 1984.
41. Delamarter RB, Bohlman HH: Postmortem osseous and neuropathologic analysis of the rheumatoid cervical spine. Spine 19:2267, 1994.
42. Dixon ASJ, Lience E: Sacro-iliac joint in adult rheumatoid arthritis and psoriatic arthropathy. Ann Rheum Dis 20:247, 1961.
43. Dougados M, Duchesne L, Awada H, et al: Assessment of efficacy and acceptability of low dose cyclosporine in patients with rheumatoid arthritis. Ann Rheum Dis 48:550, 1989.
44. Dvorak J, Grob D, Baumgartner H, et al: Functional evaluation of the spinal cord by magnetic resonance imaging in patients with rheumatoid arthritis and instability of upper cervical spine. Spine 14:1057, 1989.
45. Editorial: Rheumatoid atlantoaxial subluxation. BMJ 2:200, 1951.
46. Ehrlich GE, Young I, Rosherry SZ, Katz WA: Multicentric reticulo-histiocytosis (lipoid dermatoarthritis): A multi-system disorder. Am J Med 52:830, 1972.
47. El-Khoury GY, Wener MH, Menezes AH, et al: Cranial settling in rheumatoid arthritis. Radiology 137:637, 1980.
48. Fedele FA, Ho G Jr, Dorman BA: Pseudoaneurysm of the vertebral artery: A complication of rheumatoid cervical spine disease. Arthritis Rheum 29:136, 1986.
49. Foidart JM, Abe S, Martin GR, et al: Antibodies to type II collagen in relapsing polychondritis. N Engl J Med 299:1203, 1978.
50. Frigaard E: Posterior atlanto-axial subluxation in rheumatoid arthritis. Scand J Rheumatol 7:65, 1978.
51. Fujiwara K, Fujimoto M, Owaki H, et al: Cervical lesions related to the systemic progression in rheumatoid arthritis. Spine 23: 2052-2056, 1998.
52. Gersoff WK, Burkus JK: Dislocation of the sacroiliac joint associated with rheumatoid arthritis. A case report. Clin Orthop 209:219, 1986.
53. Gold RH, Metzger AL, Miria JM, et al: Multicentric reticulohistiocytosis (lipoid dermatoarthritis): An erosive polyarthritis with distinctive clinical, roentgenographic and pathologic features. AJR Am J Roentgenol 124:610, 1975.
54. Goldring SR, Gravallese EM: Pathogenesis of bone lesions in rheumatoid arthritis. Curr Rheumatol Rep 4:226-231, 2002.
55. Graudal H, de Carvalho A, Lassen L: The course of sacroiliac involvement in rheumatoid arthritis. Scand J Rheumatol Suppl 32:34, 1979.
56. Grob D, Wursch R, Grauer W, et al: Atlantoaxial fusion and retrodental pannus in rheumatoid arthritis. Spine 22:1580-1584, 1997.
57. Halla JT, Fallahi S, Hardin JG: Nonreducible rotational head tilt and lateral mass collapse. Arthritis Rheum 25:1316, 1982.
58. Halla JT, Hardin JG, Vitek J, et al: Involvement of the cervical spine in rheumatoid arthritis. Arthritis Rheum 32:652, 1989.
59. Hamilton JD, Gordon, M, McInnes IB, et al: Improved medical and surgical management of cervical spine disease in patients with rheumatoid arthritis over 10 years. Ann Rheum Dis 59:434-438, 2000.
60. Hanauer LB: Reticulohistiocytosis: Remission after cyclophosphamide therapy. Arthritis Rheum 15:636, 1972.
61. Harris ED Jr: Clinical features of rheumatoid arthritis. In Kelley WN, Harris ED Jr, Ruddy S, Sledge CB (eds): Textbook of Rheumatology, 4th ed. Philadelphia, WB Saunders, 1995, pp 874-911.
62. Harris ED Jr: Excitement in synovium: The rapid evolution of understanding of rheumatoid arthritis and expectations for therapy. J Rheumatol 19(suppl 32):3, 1992.
63. Harris ED Jr: Rheumatoid arthritis: Pathophysiology and implications for therapy. N Engl J Med 322:1277, 1990.
64. Harris ED Jr, Emkey RD, Nichols JE, et al: Low dose prednisone therapy in rheumatoid arthritis: A double-blind study. J Rheumatol 10:713, 1983.
65. Helliwell PS, Zebouni LNP, Porter G, et al: A clinical and radiological study of back pain in rheumatoid arthritis. Br J Rheumatol 32:16, 1993.
66. Heywood AWB, Meyers OL: Rheumatoid arthritis of the thoracic and lumbar spine. J Bone Joint Surg Br 68-B:362, 1986.
67. Horneff G, Burmester GR, Emrich F, et al: Treatment of rheumatoid arthritis with an anti-CD4 monoclonal antibody. Arthritis Rheum 32:523, 1989.
68. Jackson H: Diagnosis of minimal atlanto-axial subluxation. Br J Radiol 23:672, 1950.
69. Janossy G, Panayi G, Duke O, et al: Rheumatoid arthritis: A disease of lymphocyte/macrophage immunoregulation. Lancet 2:839, 1981.
70. Johnson HM, Tilden IL: Reticulohistiocytic granulomas of skin associated with arthritis mutilans: Report of a case followed fourteen years. Arch Dermatol 75:405, 1957.
71. Jones MW, Kaufmann JCE: Vertebrobasilar artery insufficiency in rheumatoid atlantoaxial subluxation. J Neurol Neurosurg Psychiatry 39:122, 1976.
72. Katz LM, Emsellem HA, Borenstein DG: Evaluation of cervical spine inflammatory arthritis with somatosensory evoked potentials. J Rheumatol 17:508, 1990.
73. Kaufman RL, Glenn WV Jr: Rheumatoid cervical myelopathy: Evaluation by computerized tomography with multiplanar reconstruction. J Rheumatol 10:33, 1983.
74. Kauppi M, Anttila P: A stiff collar can restrict atlantoaxial instability in rheumatoid atlantoaxial subluxations. Br J Rheumatol 35:771-774, 1996.
75. Kauppi M, Sakaguchi M, Konttinen YT, et al: Pathogenetic mechanisms and prevalence of the stable atlantoaxial subluxations in rheumatoid arthritis. J Rheumatol 23:831-834, 1996.
76. Kawaida H, Sakou T, Morizono Y, et al: Magnetic resonance imaging of upper cervical disorders in rheumatoid arthritis. Spine 14:1144, 1989.
77. Keane J, Gershon S, Wise RP, et al: Tuberculosis associated with infliximab, a tumor necrosis factor α–neutralizing agent. N Engl J Med 345:1098-1104, 2001.

78. Kirwan JR: The effect of glucocorticoids on joint destruction in rheumatoid arthritis. N Engl J Med 333:142, 1995.
79. Klimiuk PS, Clague RB, Grennan DM, et al: Autoimmunity to native type II collagen: A distinct genetic subset of rheumatoid arthritis. J Rheumatol 12:865, 1985.
80. Komusi T, Munro T, Harth M: Radiologic review: The rheumatoid cervical spine. Semin Arthritis Rheum 14:187, 1985.
81. Kremer JM: Rational use of new and existing disease-modifying agents in rheumatoid arthritis. Ann Intern Med 134:695-706, 2001.
82. Kremer JM, Davies JMS, Rynes RI, et al: Every-other-week methotrexate in patients with rheumatoid arthritis: A double-blind, placebo-controlled prospective study. Arthritis Rheum 38:601, 1995.
83. Krey PR, Comerford FR, Cohen AS: Multicentric reticulohistiocytosis. Fine structural analysis of the synovium and synovial fluid cells. Arthritis Rheum 17:615, 1974.
84. Larsson EM, Holtas S, Zygmunt S: Pre- and postoperative MR imaging of the craniocervical junction in rheumatoid arthritis. AJR Am J Roentgenol 152:561, 1989.
85. Lawrence JS, Sharp J, Ball J, Bier F: Rheumatoid arthritis of the lumbar spine. Ann Rheum Dis 23:205, 1964.
86. Lee DM, Weinblatt ME: Rheumatoid arthritis. Lancet 358:903-911, 2001.
87. Lipsky PE, van der Heijde DMFM, St Clair EW, et al: Infliximab and methotrexate in the treatment of rheumatoid arthritis. N Engl J Med 343:1594-1602, 2000.
88. Lipson SJ: Cervical myelopathy and posterior atlanto-axial subluxation in patients with rheumatoid arthritis. J Bone Joint Surg Am 67-A:593, 1985.
89. Lipson SJ: Rheumatoid arthritis in the cervical spine. Clin Orthop 239:121, 1989.
90. Lukert BP, Raisz LG: Glucocorticoid-induced osteoporosis: Pathogenesis and management. Ann Intern Med 112:352, 1990.
91. Luqmani RA, Palmer RG, Bacon PA: Azathioprine, cyclophosphamide and chlorambucil. Clin Rheumatol 4:595, 1990.
92. MacGregor AJ, Sneider H, Rigby AS, et al: Characterizing the quantitative genetic contribution to rheumatoid arthritis using data from twins. Arthrits Rheum 43:30-37, 2000.
93. MacKay K, Eyre S, Myersrough A, et al: Whole-genome linkage analysis of RA susceptibility loci in 252 affected sibling pairs in the United Kingdom. Arthritis Rheum 46:632-639, 2002.
94. Maini R, St Clair EW, Breedveld F, et al: Infliximab (chimeric anti–tumor necrosis factor α monoclonal antibody) versus placebo in rheumatoid arthritis patients receiving concomitant methotrexate: A randomized phase III trial. Lancet 354:1932-1939, 1999.
95. Marks JS, Sharp J: Rheumatoid cervical myelopathy. Q J Med 199:307, 1981.
96. Martel W: Radiologic differential diagnosis of ankylosing spondylitis (Bechterew's syndrome). Scand J Rheumatol Suppl 32:141, 1979.
97. Martel W: The occipito-atlanto-axial joints in rheumatoid arthritis and ankylosing spondylitis. AJR Am J Roentgenol 86:223, 1961.
98. Martel W, Page JW: Cervical vertebral erosions and subluxation in rheumatoid arthritis and ankylosing spondylitis. Arthritis Rheum 3:546, 1960.
99. Mathews JA: Atlanto-axial subluxation in rheumatoid arthritis: A five-year follow-up study. Ann Rheum Dis 33:526, 1974.
100. Matsunaga S, Ijiri K, Koga H: Results of a longer than 10-year follow-up of patients with rheumatoid arthritis treated by occipitocervical fusion. Spine 25:1749-1753, 2000.
101. Matthews JA: Atlanto-axial subluxation in rheumatoid arthritis. Ann Rheum Dis 28:260, 1969.
102. Mayer JW, Messner RP, Kaplan RJ: Brain stem compression in rheumatoid arthritis. JAMA 236:2094, 1976.
103. McAdam LP, O'Hanlan MA, Bluestone R, Pearson CM: Relapsing polychondritis: Prospective study of 23 patients and review of the literature. Medicine (Baltimore) 55:193, 1976.
104. Meijers KAE, van Beusekom GT, Luyendijk W, et al: Dislocation of the cervical spine with cord compression in rheumatoid arthritis. J Bone Joint Surg Br 56-B:668, 1974.
105. Mikulowski P, Wollheim FA, Rotmil P, Olsen I: Sudden death in rheumatoid arthritis with atlanto-axial dislocation. Acta Med Scand 198:445, 1975.
106. More J, Sen C: Neurological management of the rheumatoid cervical spine. Mt Sinai J Med 61:257, 1994.
107. Moreland LW, Schiff MH, Baumgartner SW, et al: Etanercept therapy in rheumatoid arthritis: A randomized controlled trial. Ann Intern Med 130:478-486, 1999.
108. Morizono Y, Sakou T, Kawaida H: Upper cervical involvement in rheumatoid arthritis. Spine 12:721, 1987.
109. Nakano KK: Neurologic complications of rheumatoid arthritis. Orthop Clin North Am 6:861, 1975.
110. Nepom GT, Byers P, Seyfried C, et al: HLA genes associated with rheumatoid arthritis: Identification of susceptibility alleles using specific oligonucleotide probes. Arthritis Rheum 32:15, 1989.
111. Neva MH, Kauppi MJ, Kautiainen H, et al: combination drug therapy retards the development of rheumatoid atlantoaxial subluxations. Arthritis Rheum 43:2397-2401, 2000.
112. O'Hanlan M, McAdam LP, Bluestone R, Pearson CM: The arthropathy of relapsing polychondritis. Arthritis Rheum 19:191, 1976.
113. Oostveen JCM, Roozeboom AR, van de Laar AFJ, et al: Functional turbo spin echo magnetic resonance imaging versus tomography for evaluating cervical spine involvement in rheumatoid arthritis. Spine 23:1237-1244, 1998.
114. O'Sullivan JB, Cathcart ES: The prevalence of rheumatoid arthritis: Follow-up evaluation of the effect of criteria on rates in Sudbury, Massachusetts. Ann Intern Med 76:573, 1972.
115. Otterness IG: The value of C-reactive protein measurement in rheumatoid arthritis. Semin Arthritis Rheum 24:91, 1994.
116. Paimela L, Laasonen L, Kankaanpaa E, et al: Progression of cervical spine changes in patients with early rheumatoid arthritis. J Rheumatol 24:1280-1284, 1997.
117. Panayi GS: The immunopathogenesis of rheumatoid arthritis. Br J Rheumatol 32(suppl 1):4, 1993.
118. Park W, O'Neill M, McCall IW: The radiology of rheumatoid involvement of the cervical spine. Skeletal Radiol 4:1, 1979.
119. Pazirandeh M, Ziran BH, Khandelwal BK, et al: Relapsing polychondritis and spondyloarthropathies. J Rheumatol 15:630, 1988.
120. Pearson ME, Kosco M, Huffer W, et al: Rheumatoid nodules of the spine: Case report and review of the literature. Arthritis Rheum 30:709, 1987.
121. Pellicci PM, Ranawat CS, Tsairis P, Bryan WJ: A prospective study of the progression of rheumatoid arthritis of the cervical spine. J Bone Joint Surg Am 63-A:342, 1981.
122. Pettersson H, Larsson EM, Holtos A, et al: Magnetic resonance imaging of the cervical spine in rheumatoid arthritis. AJNR Am J Neuroradiol 9:573, 1988.
123. Puttlitz CM, Goel VK, Clark CR et al: Biomechanical rationale for the pathology of rheumatoid arthritis in the craniovertebral junction. Spine 25:1607-1616, 2000.
124. Rana NA, Hancock DO, Taylor AR, Hill AGS: Upward translocation of the dens in rheumatoid arthritis. J Bone Joint Surg Br 55-B:471, 1973.
125. Raskin RJ, Schnapf DJ, Wolf CR, et al: Computerized tomography in evaluation of atlantoaxial subluxation in rheumatoid arthritis. Arthritis Rheum 10:33, 1983.
126. Redlund-Johnell I, Pettersson H: Radiographic measurements of the cranio-vertebral region. Acta Radiol 25:23, 1984.
127. Reiter MF, Boden SD: Inflammatory disorders of the cervical spine. Spine 23:2755-2766, 1998.
128. Resnick D: Thoracolumbar spine abnormalities in rheumatoid arthritis. Ann Rheum Dis 37:389, 1978.
129. Riise T, Jacobsen BK, Gran JT: High mortality in patients with rheumatoid arthritis and atlantoaxial subluxations. J Rheumatol 28:2425-2429, 2001.
130. Saag KG: Glucocorticoid use in rheumatoid arthritis. Curr Rheumatol Rep 4:218-225, 2002.
131. Santavirta S, Konittinen YT, Sandelin J, et al: Operations for the unstable cervical spine in rheumatoid arthritis: Sixteen cases of subaxial subluxation. Acta Orthop Scand 61:106, 1990.
132. Sany J, Anaya JM, Lussiez V, et al: Treatment of rheumatoid arthritis with methotrexate: A prospective open long-term study of 191 cases. J Rheumatol 18:1323, 1991.
133. Scully CJ, Anderson CJ, Cannon GW: Long-term methotrexate therapy for rheumatoid arthritis. Semin Arthritis Rheum 20:317, 1991.

134. Sharp J, Purser DW, Lawrence JS: Rheumatoid arthritis of the cervical spine in the adult. Ann Rheum Dis 17:303, 1958.
135. Sievers K, Laine V: The sacro-iliac joint in adult rheumatoid arthritis in adult females. Acta Rheumatol Scand 9:222, 1963.
136. Silman AJ, MacGregor AJ, Thompson W, et al: Twin concordance rates for rheumatoid arthritis: Results from a nationwide study. Br J Rheumatol 32:903-907, 2000.
137. Silverstein FE, Faich G, Goldstein JL, et al: Gastrointestinal toxicity with celecoxib vs nonsteroidal anti-inflammatory drugs for osteoarthritis and rheumatoid arthritis: the CLASS study: A randomized controlled trial. JAMA 284:1247-1255, 2000.
138. Simpson RW, McGinty L, Simon L, et al: Association of parvoviruses with rheumatoid arthritis of humans. Science 223:1425, 1984.
139. Sims-Williams H, Jayson MIV, Baddeley H: Rheumatoid involvement of the lumbar spine. Ann Rheum Dis 36:524, 1977.
140. Smith JB, Haynes MK: Rheumatoid arthritis-A molecular understanding. Ann Intern Med 136:908-922, 2002.
141. Soden M, Hassan J, Scott DL, et al: Lymphoid irradiation in intractable rheumatoid arthritis. Arthritis Rheum 32:523, 1989.
142. Stastny P: Immunogenetic factors in rheumatoid arthritis. Clin Rheum Dis 3:315, 1977.
143. Strand V, Cohen S, Schiff M, et al: Treatment of active rheumatoid arthritis with leflunomide compared with placebo and methotrexate. Arch Intern Med 159:2542-2550, 1999.
144. Swinson DR, Hamilton EBD, Mathews JA, Yatres DAH: Vertical subluxation of the axis in rheumatoid arthritis. Ann Rheum Dis 31:359, 1972.
145. Taggart AJ, Hill J, Asbury C, et al: Sulphasalazine alone or in combination with D-penicillamine in rheumatoid arthritis. Br J Rheumatol 26:32, 1987.
146. Teigland J, Magnaes B: Rheumatoid backward dislocation of the atlas with compression of the spinal cord. Scand J Rheumatol 9:253, 1980.
147. Tett SE, Cutler D, Day RO: Antimalarials in rheumatic diseases. Clin Rheumatol 4:467, 1990.
148. Tilley BC, Alarcon GS, Heyse SP, et al: Minocycline in rheumatoid arthritis: A 48-week, double-blind, placebo-controlled trial. Ann Intern Med 122:81, 1995.
149. Trentham DE, Dynesius RA, Rocklin RE, David JR: Cellular sensitivity to collagen in rheumatoid arthritis. N Engl J Med 299:327, 1978.
150. Tugwell P, Pincus T, Yocum D, et al: Combination therapy with cyclosporine and methotrexate in severe rheumatoid arthritis. N Engl J Med 333:137, 1995.
151. Van Asselt KM, Lems WF, Bongartz EB, et al: Outcome of cervical spine surgery in patients with rheumatoid arthritis. Ann Rheum Dis 60:448-452, 2001.
152. Van Boxel JA, Paget SA: Predominantly T-cell infiltrate in rheumatoid synovial membranes. N Engl J Med 293:517, 1975.
153. Van Everdingen AA, Jacobs JWG, van Reesema DRS, et al: Low-dose prednisone therapy for patients with early active rheumatoid arthritis: Clinical efficacy, disease-modifying properties, and side effects. Ann Intern Med 136:1-12, 2002.
154. van Rijthoven AW, Dijkmans BA, The HS, et al: Comparison of cyclosporine and D-penicillamine for rheumatoid arthritis: A randomized, double-blind, multicenter study. J Rheumatol 18:815, 1991.
155. Vervoordeldonk MJBM, Tak PP: Cytokines in rheumatoid arthritis. Cur Rheumatol Rep 4:208-217, 2002.
156. Walport MJ, Ollier WER, Silman AJ: Immunogenetics of rheumatoid arthritis and the Arthritis and Rheumatism Council's national repository. Br J Rheumatol 31:701, 1992.
157. Webb F, Hickman J, Brew D: Death from vertebral artery thrombosis in rheumatoid arthritis. BMJ 2:537, 1968.
158. Weinblatt ME, Keystone EC, Furst DE, et al: Adalimumab, a fully human anti–tumor necrosis factor alpha monoclonal antibody, for the treatment of rheumatoid arthritis in patients taking concomitant methotrexate: the ARMADA trial. Arthritis Rheum 48:35-45, 2003.
159. Weinblatt ME, Kremer JM, Bankhurst AD, et al: A trial of etanercept, a recombinant tumor necrosis factor:Fc fusion protein in patients with rheumatoid arthritis receiving methotrexate. N Engl J Med 340:253-259, 1999.
160. Weinblatt ME, Maier AL, Fraser PA, et al: Longterm prospective study of methotrexate in rheumatoid arthritis: Conclusion after 132 months of therapy. J Rheumatol 25:238-242, 1998.
161. Weiner S, Bassett L, Spiegel T: Superior, posterior, and lateral displacement of C1 in rheumatoid arthritis. Arthritis Rheum 25:1378, 1982.
162. Weissman BNW, Aliabadi P, Weinfield MS, et al: Prognostic features of atlanto-axial subluxation in rheumatoid arthritis patients. Radiology 144:745, 1982.
163. Westmark KD, Weissman BN: Complications of axial arthropathies. Orthop Clin North Am 21:423, 1990.
164. White AA III, Johnson RM, Panjabi MM, et al: Biomechanical analysis of clinical stability in the cervical spine. Clin Orthop 109:737, 1978.
165. Wilske KR, Healey LA: Remodeling the pyramid, a concept whose time has come. J Rheumatol 16:565, 1989.
166. Winfield J, Young A, Williams P, et al: Prospective study of the radiological changes in hands, feet, and cervical spine in adult rheumatoid disease. Ann Rheum Dis 42:613, 1983.
167. Wolfe BK, O'Keefe D, Mitchell DM, et al: Rheumatoid arthritis of the cervical spine: Early and progressive radiographic features. Radiology 165:145, 1987.
168. Wong RL, Wilson AJ, Ingenito FS, et al: Apophyseal joint ankylosis of the cervical spine in adult-onset rheumatoid arthritis. Arthritis Rheum 28:958, 1985.
169. Yonezawa T, Tsuji H, Matsui H, Hirano N: Subaxial lesions in rheumatoid arthritis: Radiographic factors suggestive of lower cervical myelopathy. Spine 20:208, 1995.
170. Zeidman SM, Ducker TB: Rheumatoid arthritis: Neuroanatomy, compression, and grading of deficits. Spine 19:2259, 1994.
171. Zoma A, Sturrock RD, Fisher WD, et al: Surgical stabilization of the rheumatoid cervical spine: A review of indications and results. J Bone Joint Surg Br 69-B:8-12, 1987.

VERTEBRAL OSTEOCHONDRITIS

CAPSULE SUMMARY

	LOW BACK	NECK
Frequency of spinal pain	Common	Not applicable (NA)
Location of spinal pain	Midline, thoracolumbar junction	NA
Quality of spinal pain	Ache	NA
Symptoms and signs	Increased kyphosis, percussion tenderness	NA
Laboratory tests	None	NA
Radiographic findings	Vertebral body wedging, irregular endplates on plain roentgenograms	NA
Treatment	Exercises, bracing	NA

PREVALENCE AND PATHOGENESIS

Vertebral osteochondritis (Scheuermann's disease) is a condition associated with an irregularity in ossification and endochondral growth, with pathologic changes developing at the junction of the vertebral body and intervertebral disc. This abnormality results in increasing wedging of vertebral bodies and progressive forward flexion of the spine (kyphosis). Vertebral osteochondritis primarily affects the thoracic spine in teenagers; however, a similar process has also been described as affecting the lumbar spine.[15] If left untreated, the illness may result in progressive kyphosis, persistent back pain, and signs of spinal cord compression. Scheuermann's disease, juvenile kyphosis, and osteochondritis deformans juvenilis dorsi are other names used interchangeably for this illness. Scheuermann first demonstrated the radiographic changes of wedged vertebrae in this disease in 1920.[23]

Epidemiology

The prevalence of vertebral osteochondritis has been reported to vary from 0.4% to 8.3% of the general population, depending on whether the diagnosis was based on radiographic or clinical criteria.[17] The male-to-female ratio is 1:2 for thoracic involvement, whereas the exact opposite ratio may be seen in disease of the lumbar spine.[7,10] The overall prevalence is equal between the sexes.[32]

Pathogenesis

The pathogenesis of vertebral osteochondritis is unknown. In the past, Scheuermann suggested that the wedge deformities associated with this illness are secondary to avascular necrosis of bone. Histologic examination of tissue from vertebral osteochondritic lesions has not revealed any evidence of bone necrosis.[8] Schmorl suggested, instead, that disc material is extruded through the endplates into the cancellous bone of the body.[25] Alexander has postulated a similar mechanism.[1] Basically, during a period of rapid growth when the vertebral endplates are weakened, increased dynamic load through compression or shear forces causes disc material to move into vertebral bodies and results in an alteration in vertebral growth. The hereditary nature of the illness (increased familial occurrence) suggests a genetic predisposition to weakened vertebral endplates.[14] A study in Russian families revealed a pattern of familial aggregation consistent with dominant inheritance of a major allele.[3] Additional evidence for a genetic etiology of this disorder is the occurrence of this disease in monozygotic twins.[13] Other disease processes that result from compression forces (e.g., spondylolysis, intervertebral disc degeneration) are also associated with vertebral osteochondritis.[20] The radiographic abnormalities of intraosseous radiolucent areas and irregular contour of vertebral bodies fit into this pathogenetic schema. A cadaveric study of 103 spinal columns with Scheuermann's disease demonstrated anterior extension of the vertebral bodies and the highest incidence of Schmorl's nodes at the vertebra with the greatest wedging, T8.[26] The location and the histologic and radiographic characteristics of the lesions suggested a mechanical disorder. In the setting of late adolescence, when posterior and posterolateral endplate growth is nearly complete, increased pressure from forward posture results in disruption of endochondral ossification in the anterior endplate and, as a consequence, anterior wedging and other manifestations of this illness.

Other possibilities seem unlikely. Scheuermann suggested that heavy labor at a young age may be associated with the development of vertebral osteochondritis.[24] However, vertebral osteochondritis usually occurs in young individuals with no history of heavy labor or trauma. Therefore, the effect of heavy labor on the development of vertebral osteochondritis in the thoracic spine is unknown. In the lumbar spine, athletically active adolescent males and those doing heavy lifting are at greater risk for thoracolumbar abnormalities.[32] Endocrinologic dysfunction has not been detected in enough patients to be of pathogenetic importance. Although Scheuermann's disease has been associated with osteoporosis, recent studies have demonstrated no significant difference in bone mineralization in patients with this illness and controls.[12,16]

CLINICAL HISTORY

Thoracic vertebral osteochondritis may initially be manifested in three ways. Patients may complain of back pain, may demonstrate increasing kyphosis, or may be discovered to have vertebral osteochondritis by chance on a radiograph of the spine. Between 20% and 60% of patients have back pain, and the pain is concentrated over the area of kyphosis. The pain may radiate down the back and is usually relieved with bed rest and exacerbated with activity.

Vertebral osteochondritis of the lumbar spine may occur independently or in conjunction with disease in the thoracic spine. The main symptoms of lumbar involvement include local pain and tenderness gradually increasing over weeks, radiation of pain to the hip, paravertebral muscle spasm, and limitation of back motion.

PHYSICAL EXAMINATION

Physical findings include a kyphotic deformity occasionally associated with scoliosis. The kyphosis occurs in the thoracic (75%), thoracolumbar (20%), and lumbar (5%) regions. Thoracic kyphosis is frequently associated with increased lumbar and cervical lordosis. Pain on palpation over the affected portion of the axial skeleton is not unusual, and patients complain of paravertebral muscle spasm and tightness of the hamstrings. When viewed from the side in the forward-bending position (the Adam test), the deformity is sharply angulated; in contrast, postural kyphosis is manifested as a uniform rounding of the entire spine.[18] Rarely, neurologic signs of cord compression may be elicited.[5,21] Thoracic disc herniation is described in patients with Scheuermann's disease.[11,28,34]

LABORATORY DATA

Laboratory parameters such as hematocrit, white blood count, erythrocyte sedimentation rate, blood studies, rheumatoid factor, and antinuclear antibody are normal.

RADIOGRAPHIC EVALUATION

Roentgenograms

Roentgenographic abnormalities of vertebral osteochondritis include wedging of vertebral bodies, Schmorl's nodules (invasion of the vertebral body by an intervertebral disc), irregular endplates, and increased kyphosis. Lumbar spine changes are similar (Fig. 11-32). In adult patients, the healed lesion results in characteristic roentgenographic changes, including increased anteroposterior diameter of a vertebral body, disc space narrowing, loss of normal spine curvature, large Schmorl's nodules, and persistence of a separate fragment of bone anterosuperior to the front edge of a vertebral body (limbus vertebra). Over time, ossification of contiguous portions of the anterior aspects of intervertebral discs can lead to synostosis of neighboring vertebral bodies.[9] In younger patients with lumbar Scheuermann's disease, vertebral endplate irregularities, anterior Schmorl's nodes, and disc space narrowing may be identified without the 5-degree wedging of three consecutive vertebrae.[4] Some of these adolescents with lumbar involvement have a history of acute vertical compression injury associated with severe back pain and endplate fracture. About one in three will also have scoliosis.

Part of the difficulty in determining thoracic kyphosis is the normal range of angulation. The Scoliosis Research Society has defined the normal range as being between 20 and 40 degrees in adlolescents.[30] The angle increases with age. In addition, determination of kyphosis by Cobb's method is not precise. Significant interobserver differences are common.[29]

DIFFERENTIAL DIAGNOSIS

The diagnosis of thoracic vertebral osteochondritis is easily made when three contiguous vertebral bodies are wedged by 5 degrees or more[27]; however, this criterion eliminates patients with fewer affected vertebrae or those with vertebral irregularity without wedging. No specific criteria have been suggested for lumbar involvement. Therefore, the diagnosis of vertebral osteochondritis should be suspected in a patient with characteristic radiographic changes of one or more thoracic or lumbar vertebrae. The lack of any constitutional symptoms such as fever, weight loss, and loss of appetite, as well as the absence of abnormal laboratory tests, helps differentiate vertebral osteochondritis in its early stages from infections (e.g., tuberculosis), neoplasm, hyperparathyroidism, Paget's disease, and rheumatoid arthritis.

TREATMENT

Five indications for treatment include pain, progressive deformity, neurologic compromise, cardiopulmonary compromise, and cosmesis.[30] Neurologic compromise and cardiopulmonary compromise (kyphosis >100 degrees) require surgical intervention. Treatment is directed at preventing deformity during the patient's rapid growth years and avoiding the development of poor body posture,

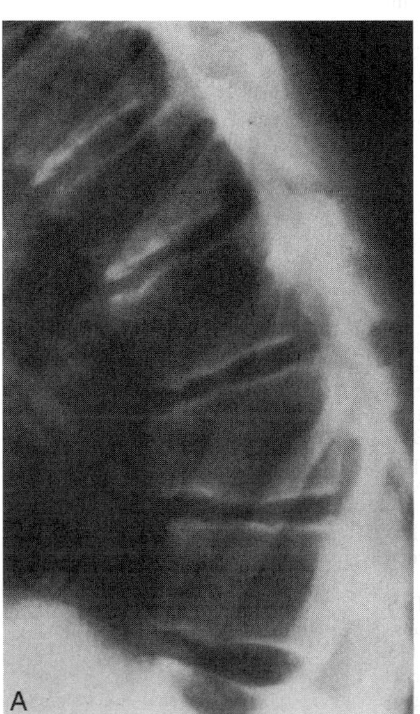

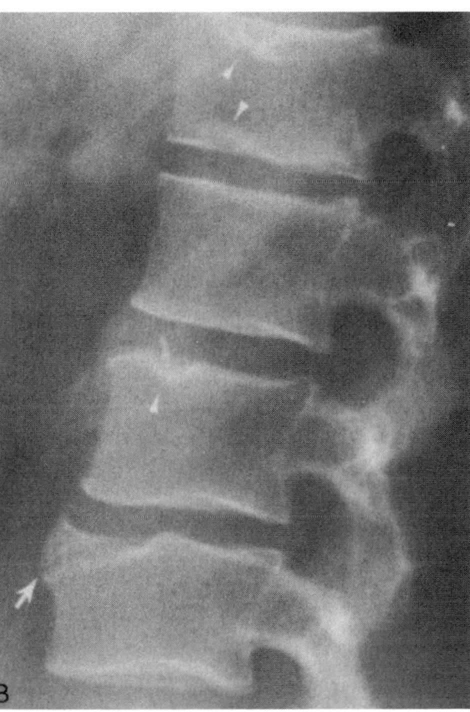

Figure 11-32 Vertebral osteochondritis (Scheuermann's disease). *A*, Thoracic spine. Findings include irregularity of the vertebral contour, reactive sclerosis, intervertebral disc space narrowing, anterior vertebral wedging, and kyphosis. *B*, Lumbar spine. Observe the cartilaginous nodes *(arrowheads)* creating surface irregularity, radiolucent areas, and reactive sclerosis. Anterior discal herniation *(arrow)* has produced an irregular anterosuperior corner of a vertebral body, the limbus vertebra. *(A and B, From Resnick D, Niwayama G: Diagnosis of Bone and Joint Disorders. Philadelphia, WB Saunders, 1988.)*

associated back pain, and neurologic deficits as an adult. If the patient has mild, reversible kyphosis, bed rest and daily exercises to strengthen the back extensor muscles are usually adequate to prevent further deformity and limit pain. However, progression of kyphosis or radiographic changes of vertebral wedging require body casting or a Milwaukee brace. Patients who have thoracic kyphosis with an apex above T7 are best managed with a Milwaukee brace. Those with thoracolumbar kyphosis are best managed with an underarm orthosis that has anterior infraclavicular outriggers.[18] Milwaukee brace treatment, continued until growth is complete, has been effective in preventing the deformity in 40% of patients with vertebral osteochondritis.[7] A more recent follow-up study of patients treated with bracing reported a 69% improvement with reduced kyphosis and anterior vertebral wedging.[22]

Surgical intervention is reserved for patients with severe kyphosis, intolerable back pain, visceral compromise (respiratory insufficiency), or progressive neurologic deficit.[2] A combination of anterior and posterior spinal fusion was helpful in decreasing pain and deformity in 24 patients reported by Bradford and co-authors.[6] Other surgical techniques using a variety of rod instrumentation have been associated with improvement in vertebral deformity.[17] Discography has been used to identify symptomatic levels to be fused.[33]

PROGNOSIS

In patients with greater than 70 degrees of kyphosis, increasing curvature may develop after skeletal maturation is complete. Curvature of this degree can be associated with a marked increase in lumbar lordosis and persistent low back pain. Severe deformities also present a greater risk of neurologic compromise.

Lumbar spine osteochondritis may be associated with premature degeneration of the intervertebral discs.[10] Butler has suggested that vertebral osteochondritis that results in loss of normal lumbar lordosis and mobility of the upper lumbar discs may make the lower lumbar discs more vulnerable to degeneration and protrusion. He believes that the low back pain in middle-aged adults with this disorder is secondary to osteochondritis and disc degeneration that occurred in their youth. In a study of 67 patients who were monitored for an average of 32 years, pulmonary dysfunction in the form of restrictive lung disease occurred in those with kyphotic angles greater than 100 degrees of curvature and with the apex of the curve between the first and eighth segments.[19] The limitations of the 67 patients were relatively minor with regard to physical functioning at work. From a social standpoint, those with curves greater than 85 degrees were more likely to be single than married. In general, Scheuermann's kyphosis was considered a benign disorder. Surgical intervention is associated with significant complications and should be limited as a form of treatment for these patients. Transient paraparesis is an example of a complication associated with surgical treatment of Scheuermann's kyphosis.[31]

References

Vertebral Osteochondritis

1. Alexander CT: Scheuermann's disease. A traumatic spondylodystrophy? Skeletal Radiol 1:209, 1977.
2. Ali RM, Green DW, Patel TC: Scheuermann's kyphosis. Curr Opin Orthop 11:131-136, 2000.
3. Axenovich TI, Zaidman AM, Zorkoltseva IV, et al: Segregation analysis of Scheuermann disease in nine families from Siberia. Am J Med Genet 100:275-279, 2001.
4. Blumenthal SL, Roach J, Herring JA: Lumbar Scheuermann's: A clinical series and classification. Spine 12:929, 1987.
5. Bradford DS: Neurological complications in Scheuermann's disease: A case report and review of the literature. J Bone Joint Surg Am 51-A:567, 1969.
6. Bradford DS, Ahmed KB, Moe JH, et al: The surgical management of patients with Scheuermann's disease. J Bone Joint Surg Am 62-A:705, 1980.
7. Bradford DS, Moe JH, Montalvo FJ, Winter RB: Scheuermann's kyphosis and roundback deformity: Results of Milwaukee brace treatment. J Bone Joint Surg Am 56-A:740, 1974.
8. Bradford DS, Moe JH: Scheuermann's juvenile kyphosis: A histologic study. Clin Orthop 110:45, 1975.
9. Butler RW: Spontaneous anterior fusion of vertebral bodies. J Bone Joint Surg Br 53-B:230, 1971.
10. Butler RW: The nature and significance of vertebral osteochondritis. Proc R Soc Med 48:895, 1955.
11. Chiu KY, Luk KD: Cord compression caused by multiple disc herniations and intraspinal cyst in Scheuermann's disease. Spine 20:1075-1079, 1995.
12. Gilsanz V, Gibbens DT, Carlson M, King J: Vertebral bone density in Scheuermann's disease. J Bone Joint Surg Am 71-A:894, 1989.
13. Graat HCA, van Rhijn LW, Schrander-Stumpel CTRM, et al: Classical Scheuermann disease in male monozygotic twins: Further support for the genetic etiology hypothesis. Spine 27:E485-E487, 2002.
14. Halal F, Gledhill RB, Fraser FC: Dominant inheritance of Scheuermann's juvenile kyphosis. Am J Dis Child 132:1105, 1978.
15. Lamb DW: Localized osteochondritis of the lumbar spine. J Bone Joint Surg Br 36-B:591, 1954.
16. Lopez RA, Burke SW, Levine DB, Schneider R: Osteoporosis in Scheuermann's disease. Spine 13:1099, 1988.
17. Lowe TG: Scheuermann's disease. J Bone Joint Surg Am 72:940, 1990.
18. Lowe TG: Scheuermann's disease. Orthop Clin North Am 30:475-484, 1999.
19. Murray PM, Weinstein SL, Spratt KF: The natural history and long-term follow-up of Scheuermann kyphosis. J Bone Joint Surg Am 75-A:236, 1993.
20. Ogilvie JW, Sherman J: Spondylolysis in Scheuermann's disease. Spine 12:251, 1987.
21. Ryan MD, Taylo TKF: Acute spinal cord compression in Scheuermann's disease. J Bone Joint Surg Br 64-B:409, 1982.
22. Sachs B, Bradford D, Winter R, et al: Scheuermann kyphosis: Follow-up of Milwaukee-brace treatment. J Bone Joint Surg Am 69-A:50, 1987.
23. Scheuermann HW: Kyfosis dorsalis juvenile. Ugeskr Laeger 82:385, 1920.
24. Scheuermann HW: Kyphosis Juvenilis (Scheuermann's Krankheit). Fortschr Geb Rontgenstr 53:1, 1936.
25. Schmorl G: Die Pathogenese der juvenilen Kyphose. Fortschr Geb Rontgenstr 41:359, 1930.
26. Scoles PV, Latimer BM, DiGiovanni BF, et al: Vertebral alterations in Scheuermann's kyphosis. Spine 16:509, 1991.
27. Sorenson KH: Scheuermann's Juvenile Kyphosis. Munksgaard, Copenhagen, 1964.
28. Stambough JL, VanLoveren HR, Cheeks ML: Spinal cord compression in Scheuermann's kyphosis: Case report. Neurosurgery 30:127-130, 1992.
29. Stotts Ak, Smith JT, Santora SD, et al: Measurement of spinal kyphosis: Implications for the management of Scheuermann's kyphosis. Spine 27:2143-2146, 2002.
30. Tribus CB: Scheuermann's kyphosis in adolescents and adults: Diagnosis and management. J Am Acad Orthop Surg 6:36-43, 1998.

31. Tribus CB: Transient paraparesis: A complication of the surgical management of Scheuermann's kyphosis secondary to thoracic stenosis. Spine 26:1086-1089, 2001.
32. Wenger DR, Frick SL: Scheuermann kyphosis. Spine 24:2630-2639, 1999.
33. Winter RB, Schellhas KB: Painful adult thoracic Scheuermann's disease. Diagnosis by discography and treatment by combined arthrodesis. Am J Orthop 25:783-786, 1996.
34. Yablon JS, Kasdon DL, Levine H: Thoracic cord compression in Scheuermann's disease. Spine 13:896-898, 1988.

OSTEITIS CONDENSANS ILII

CAPSULE SUMMARY

	LOW BACK	NECK
Frequency of spinal pain	Uncommon	Not applicable (NA)
Location of spinal pain	Sacroiliac joints	NA
Quality of spinal pain	Dull ache	NA
Symptoms and signs	Postpartum onset, percussion tenderness	NA
Laboratory tests	None	NA
Radiographic findings	Triangular area of sclerosis on iliac side of sacroiliac joint on plain roentgenogram	NA
Treatment	Exercises	NA

PREVALENCE AND PATHOGENESIS

Osteitis condensans ilii is a disease characterized by mild back pain and unilateral or bilateral bony sclerosis of the lower ilium with sparing of the sacral portion of the sacroiliac joints. The illness is not progressive and is not associated with functional disability. The major difficulty with osteitis condensans ilii is that it is frequently confused with ankylosing spondylitis (AS).

Epidemiology

The prevalence of osteitis condensans ilii has been estimated to be 1.6% in the Japanese and 3% in Scandinavians.[4,12] The usual patient is a woman 30 to 40 years of age. The ratio of women to men is 9:1 or greater.

Pathogenesis

The pathogenesis of osteitis condensans ilii is unknown. Urinary tract infections, inflammatory diseases of the sacroiliac joint, and abnormal mechanical stresses have been suggested as possible etiologies of this illness. Urinary tract infections may reach the ilium via nutrient arteries and result in reactive sclerosis.[13] The absence of a history of urinary tract infection in many individuals makes this mechanism unlikely. Others have suggested that osteitis condensans ilii is a subset of AS.[11] One study reported that AS subsequently developed in a third of a population of women with osteitis. However, histocompatibility testing for HLA-B27 has not documented an increased incidence of this antigen in osteitis patients.[8] In addition, part of the confusion of differentiating osteitis condensans ilii and AS is the milder form of the latter illness in women.[7] Careful review of the clinical symptoms and radiographic findings of the two groups of patients demonstrates the clear-cut differences that exist between the two illnesses (Table 11-11).

A more likely cause of osteitis condensans ilii is mechanical stress across the sacroiliac joint in association with pregnancy and diastasis of the symphysis pubis. Autopsy studies have suggested that a normal physiologic zone of hyperostosis on the anterior iliac margin of the sacroiliac joint may become exaggerated in response to abnormal stress.[2] Abnormal stress is placed across the sacroiliac joints during pregnancy.[8] However, this fact alone would not explain the occasional man with osteitis or a woman in whom osteitis develops without having been pregnant. Therefore, the mechanical stress that causes osteitis condensans ilii must be commonly, but not exclusively associated with pregnancy. Diastasis of the symphysis pubis may explain this clinical occurrence. Diastasis of the pubis occurs frequently during pregnancy secondary to relaxin, a product of the corpus of pregnancy that allows greater laxity of the supporting structures (ligaments) of the pelvis.[9] Patients may actually notice movement or a "popping" sensation in the sacroiliac joints and pubis. Diastasis may occur in as many as 1 in 600 deliveries.[10] Diastasis is not exclusively related to pregnancy but may occur secondary to trauma. Individuals with diastasis related to trauma, both men and women, may be at risk for osteitis condensans ilii.

CLINICAL HISTORY

The major symptom of osteitis condensans ilii is low back pain, which occurs in 30% of patients. The pain is dull and

11-11 SACROILIAC JOINT SCLEROSIS

	Osteitis Condensans Ilii	Ankylosing Spondylitis	Osteoarthritis	Metastatic Tumor (Prostate)
Age	30-40	20-40	60	60
Sex	Women greater than men	Men greater than women	Equal	Men
Distribution	Bilateral or unilateral	Bilateral	Bilateral or unilateral	Unilateral
Erosions	Absent	Common	Absent	Uncommon
Osteophytes	Rare	Rare	Common	Absent
Ligamentous calcification	Absent	Common	Rare	Absent
Intra-articular bony ankylosis	Absent	Common	Rare	Absent

localized to one or the other side of the midline, with radiation to the buttock on occasion. The pain is not exacerbated by coughing, sneezing, or straining at stool but may be increased with menstruation. Not uncommonly, women notice the onset of pain during pregnancy or the postpartum period. Morning stiffness is usually mild and lasts less than an hour. The episodes of pain may have a duration of weeks to months. The disease may then go into complete or partial remission, which may last for years. A small proportion of patients may complain of fibrositic symptoms characterized by widespread musculoskeletal aching and local point tenderness.[1]

PHYSICAL EXAMINATION

Physical examination may demonstrate tenderness on percussion of the sacroiliac joint, pain with sacroiliac joint motion, and mild limitation of motion. The rest of the physical examination is normal.

LABORATORY DATA

Laboratory values are generally normal in patients with osteitis condensans ilii. The hematocrit, white blood count, platelets, urinalysis, and chemistry studies are normal. Rheumatoid factor and antinuclear antibody are negative.

RADIOGRAPHIC EVALUATION

Radiographic findings include an area of triangular sclerosis on the iliac aspect of the sacroiliac joint. The bony sclerosis is not associated with joint erosions or extensive involvement of the sacrum (Figs. 11-33 and 11-34). The

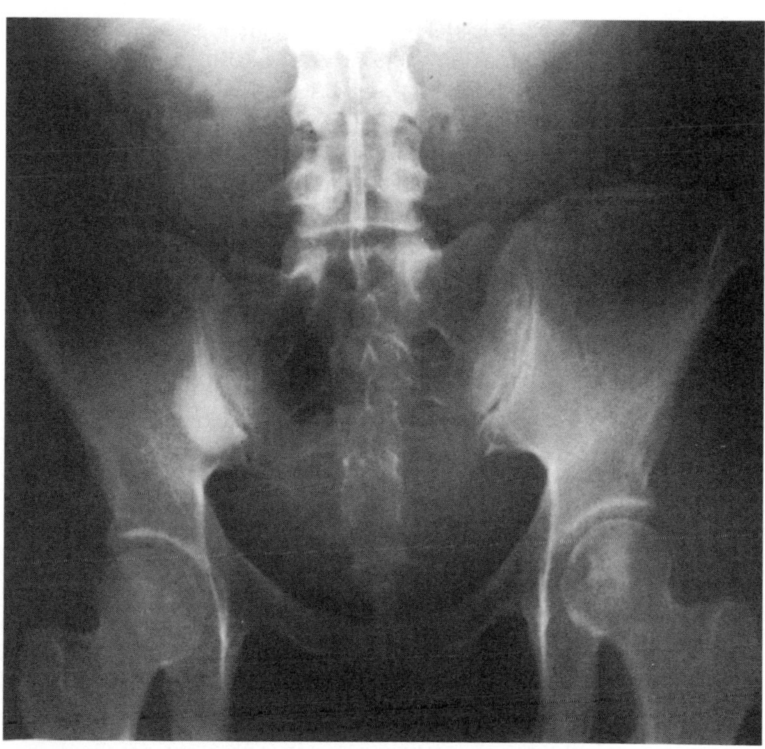

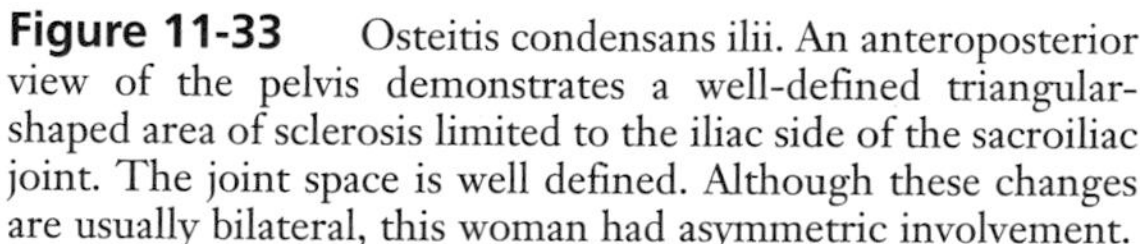

Figure 11-33 Osteitis condensans ilii. An anteroposterior view of the pelvis demonstrates a well-defined triangular-shaped area of sclerosis limited to the iliac side of the sacroiliac joint. The joint space is well defined. Although these changes are usually bilateral, this woman had asymmetric involvement.

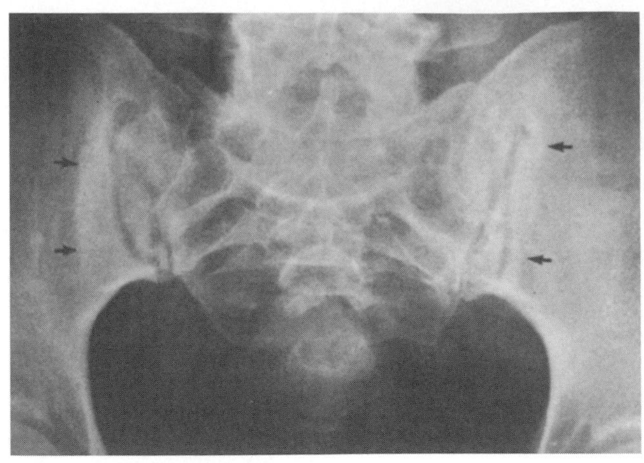

Figure 11-34 Osteitis condensans ilii. An anteroposterior view of the pelvis of a 57-year-old woman demonstrates bilateral sclerosis of the iliac portions of the sacroiliac joints *(black arrows)*. The woman was asymptomatic with regard to low back pain.

radiographic changes may resolve over time. There are no characteristic abnormalities in other portions of the lumbar, thoracic, or cervical spine.[4]

DIFFERENTIAL DIAGNOSIS

The diagnosis of osteitis condensans ilii is based on the presence of radiographic changes on the iliac side of the sacroiliac joint and the absence of findings consistent with spondylitis. Patients with spondyloarthropathy have more persistent low back pain associated with more stiffness and limitation of motion. The radiographic changes of spondyloarthropathy are characterized by erosion on both sides of the sacroiliac joints (see Table 11-11).[14] CT may be helpful in differentiating the presence of sclerosis with joint space abnormalities from bony sclerosis alone.[5] Other processes that might cause confusion in diagnosis include septic arthritis with bacteria or tuberculosis, Paget's disease, or tumor. The clinical features of these illnesses and the associated radiographic changes help distinguish the specific diseases.

Septic arthritis secondary to tuberculosis or bacterial infection causes changes on both sides of the joint. Paget's disease is associated with lytic and blastic changes on roentgenograms and increased serum alkaline phosphatase. Osteoblastic tumors metastatic to the ilium will increase in size on a rapid basis. The rapid rate of growth helps differentiate tumors from osteitis condensans ilii. Patients with metastatic lesions to the ilium and sclerosis that resembles osteitis condensans ilii frequently have persistent, progressive back pain that would be out of character for patients with primary osteitis.[6]

TREATMENT

The majority of patients benefit from a conservative regimen of a firm mattress for sleeping, local wet or dry heat, and exercise. Nonsteroidal anti-inflammatory drugs are rarely required. Surgical intervention for pelvic instability is reserved for patients with severe symptoms. Internal fixation of the sacroiliac joint and symphysis pubis may be necessary.[3]

PROGNOSIS

The course of osteitis condensans ilii is benign. In many circumstances the radiographic changes may reverse to normal.[12] Low back pain may persist for months but is responsive to therapy. The low back pain of osteitis condensans ilii does not cause decreased motion of the lumbosacral spine. This illness is not associated with disability, and patients are able to continue to work even though they experience symptoms of the illness.

References

Osteitis Condensans Ilii

1. DeBosset P, Gordon DA, Smythe HA, et al: Comparison of osteitis condensans ilii and ankylosing spondylitis in female patients: Clinical, radiological and HLA typing characteristics. J Chronic Dis 31:171, 1978.
2. Dihlmann W: Diagnostic Radiology of the Sacroiliac Joints. New York, Georg Thieme Verlag, 1980, p 104.
3. Jenkins DH, Young MH: The operative treatment of sacroiliac subluxation and disruption of the symphysis pubis. Injury 10:139, 1978.
4. Numaguchi Y: Osteitis condensans ilii, including its resolution. Radiology 98:1, 1971.
5. Olivieri I, Gemignani G, Camerini E, et al: Differential diagnosis between osteitis condensans ilii and sacroiliitis. J Rheumatol 17:1504, 1990.
6. Parhami N, DiGiacomo R, Jouzevicius JL: Metastatic bone lesions of leiomyosarcoma mimicking osteitis condensans ilii. J Rheumatol 15:1035, 1988.
7. Resnick D, Dwosh I, Goergen TG, et al: Clinical and radiographic abnormalities in ankylosing spondylitis. A comparison of men and women. Radiology 119:293, 1976.
8. Singal DP, deBosset P, Gordon DA, et al: HLA antigens in osteitis condensans ilii and ankylosing spondylitis. J Rheumatol 4(suppl 3):105, 1977.
9. Szlachter BN, Quagliarello J, Jewelewicz R, et al: Relaxin in normal and pathogenic pregnancies. Obstet Gynecol 59:167, 1982.
10. Taylor RW, Sonson RD: Separation of the pubic symphysis. An underrecognized peripartum complication. J Reprod Med 31:203, 1986.
11. Thompson M: Osteitis condensans ilii and its differentiation from ankylosing spondylitis. Ann Rheum Dis 13:147, 1954.
12. Wassman K: Osteitis condensans ilii. Acta Med Scand 151:151, 1955.
13. Wells J: Osteitis condensans ilii. AJR Am J Roentgenol 76:1141, 1956.
14. Withrington RH, Sturge RA, Mitchell N: Osteitis condensans ilii or sacro-iliitis? Scand J Rheumatol 14:163, 1985.

DIFFUSE IDIOPATHIC SKELETAL HYPEROSTOSIS

CAPSULE SUMMARY

	LOW BACK	NECK
Frequency of spinal pain	Common	Common
Location of spinal pain	Thoracolumbar spine	Cervical spine
Quality of spinal pain	Ache	Ache
Symptoms and signs	Decreased back motion	Dysphagia, decreased neck motion
Laboratory tests	None	None
Radiographic findings	Flowing calcification of the anterolateral aspect of four contiguous vertebral bodies on plain roentgenogram	Flowing calcification of the anterolateral aspect of four contiguous vertebral bodies on plain roentgenogram
Treatment	NSAIDs, range-of-motion exercises	NSAIDs, range-of-motion exercises

PREVALENCE AND PATHOGENESIS

Diffuse idiopathic skeletal hyperostosis (DISH) is a disease characterized clinically by spinal stiffness and pain and radiographically by exuberant calcification of spinal and extraspinal structures. Despite impressive radiographic abnormalities, patients rarely have significant loss of function or disability from the illness except for the rare individual who has difficulty swallowing (dysphagia) secondary to cervical spine involvement. This disease has been known by many different names, including spondylitis ossificans ligamentosa, vertebral osteophytosis, ankylosing hyperostosis of Forestier and Rotes-Querol, and Forestier's disease. DISH was suggested in 1975 by Resnick and Niwayama as a more appropriate name in light of the diffuse bone growth that develops in both spinal and extraspinal locations.[64]

Epidemiology

DISH is a common entity found in 6% to 28% of autopsy populations.[5,65,80] The usual patient is a man 48 to 85 years old.[79] The prevalence increases with age. A study of 2364 individuals from the University of Minnesota Hospital and Hennepin County Medical Center reported an overall prevalence of DISH of 25% in men older than 50 years and 15% in women of similar age. The prevalence climbed to 28% and 26% in men and women older than 80 years, respectively.[82] The ratio of men to women is 2:1.[14] The prevalence rate increases in both sexes with weight and age.[16,78] The disease occurs most commonly in whites and rarely in blacks, Asians, and Native Americans. DISH has been described in populations from all continents except Antarctica.

Pathogenesis

The etiology of DISH is unknown. In one study, occupational stress or spinal trauma was reported in 57% of patients with this condition.[64] The patients usually had occupations that required a moderate degree of physical activity, including construction, ranching, and roofing. Other people in the same study had no history of occupational or accidental trauma. Endocrinologic abnormalities associated with bony hyperostosis, acromegaly, and hypoparathyroidism have been suggested as causes of DISH. No abnormalities in growth hormone (acromegaly) or parathormone (hypoparathyroidism) have been found.[79] Diabetes mellitus occurs in 30% of patients with the disease; however, this frequency of diabetes mellitus may be related to the age of the population rather than being a true association of the two disorders.[64] Impaired glucose tolerance occurs in DISH patients to a greater degree than in control subjects.[15] The level of glucose intolerance does not correlate with the extent of bony overgrowth. In addition, elevated concentrations of insulin have been measured in DISH patients when compared with control subjects.[35] Insulin may be acting as a growth-like factor for new bone formation. The systemic exposure from insulin would be compatible with the distribution of DISH lesions throughout the skeleton. A study of 131 individuals with DISH versus 131 with spondylosis reported greater body mass index, hyperuricemia, and hyperglycemia in the DISH patients.[29] Levels of endogenous retinoic acids are elevated in DISH patients in comparison to control subjects.[53] The elevation in 13-*cis*- and all-*trans*-retinoic acid and associated bone growth may be similar to the increased concentration of retinoids found in patients with hyperostosis who use these agents for the treatment of psoriasis and acne.

A specific genetic predisposition to the development of DISH has not been identified. HLA-B27 positivity was found in 34% of DISH patients in one study,[68] but a subsequent study found no significant association with HLA antigens.[72] Until further data are obtained to the contrary, DISH should not be classified with the HLA-B27–positive, seronegative spondyloarthropathies (ankylosing spondylitis and reactive arthritis).

CLINICAL HISTORY

The principal musculoskeletal complaint in 80% of patients is spinal stiffness.[64] The duration of spinal stiffness before diagnosis may be 10 to 20 years, with onset when the patient is 40 to 50 years of age. Morning stiffness dissipates within an hour, only to recur in the late evening.[14] Symptoms may increase with inclement weather. Immobility increases symptoms as well. Individuals may be stiff without spinal pain. Spinal osteophytes may be present without any spinal pain. Back pain in the thoracolumbar spine occurs in 57% of patients as their initial complaint.[64] The back pain is usually mild, intermittent, and rarely radiating. In one study, 67% of DISH patients had lumbar spine pain.[22] In some study populations with DISH, back pain occurs at the same frequency as in age-matched controls.[67]

A minority of patients have cervical spinal pain as the initial complaint. Neck pain is a complaint of more than 50% of patients with DISH during the course of the illness.[22] Subsequently, cervical stiffness may become the prominent symptom.[73] Dysphagia is seen in 17% to 28% of patients.[79] It may be an initial complaint of patients with cervical anterior osteophytes.[41] Dysphagia occurs secondary to constriction of the esophagus by anteriorly located cervical osteophytes.[18] Osteophytes adjacent to the location of esophageal fixation near the cricoid cartilage (C5–C6) are those most closely associated with esophageal compression and dysphagia.[62] The intensity of dysphagia can be variable, from mild to severe, and it may be associated with exclusion of solids from the diet and significant loss of weight.[66] Patients with DISH and anterior osteophytes may also be at risk for aspiration and pneumonia.[81] The symptoms of aspiration pneumonia may develop over a period of months before diagnosis.[4] Stridor may also be a manifestation of impingement of osteophytes on the upper airways.[52] Intubation may be difficult in patients with DISH of the cervical spine.[9] Procedures involving the upper airway or esophagus may result in damage to these structures if the diagnosis of DISH is not recognized.[36]

Extraspinal manifestations of DISH occur in 37% of patients. In 20%, extraspinal pain was the initial or predominant complaint. The most common extraspinal skeletal areas that are symptomatic secondary to an enthesopathy include the shoulders, knees, elbows, and heels.

PHYSICAL EXAMINATION

Physical examination usually reveals little limitation of motion in the cervical and lumbar spine.[28] Occasionally, a slight decrease in cervical or lumbar lordosis may be present.[64] A small accentuation in dorsal kyphosis may be noted. A minority of patients are tender to percussion over the cervical spine or sacroiliac joints.[79] On palpation of the neck, bilateral fullness may be appreciated lateral to the trachea.[31] Neurologic signs from spinal cord compression may develop in rare patients secondary to DISH.[2] Patients with extraspinal disease may have diminished range of motion and pain on palpation over affected areas. Areas that may show abnormalities include the hips, subtalar joints, shoulders, knees, elbows, heels, and ankle joints.

LABORATORY DATA

Laboratory parameters are essentially normal in patients with DISH.[72] Occasionally, a mildly elevated erythrocyte sedimentation rate (ESR) is noted. Because patients with the disease are elderly, laboratory abnormalities may be secondary to another illness affecting the patient. Therefore, elevations in fasting and 2-hour postprandial glucose are probably secondary to impending diabetes rather than DISH.

Pathology

Pathologic evaluation of the axial skeleton is not necessary for the diagnosis of DISH. However, pathologic findings do correlate with the radiographic characteristics of DISH. These findings include fibrous tissue separating anterior calcification and the annulus fibrosus of the intervertebral disc, normal disc height, close proximity of anterior calcifications without fusion, and widespread osteoporosis in most circumstances.[80]

The location for initiation of the process that results in DISH is the enthesis, or the attachment of tendon to bone. The earliest changes are connective tissue proliferation followed by fibrocartilaginous metaplasia. Chondrocytes develop and produce proteoglycans, with subsequent ossification. Ossification preferentially occurs close to an enthesis.[16] The source of pain in patients with DISH is not clear. Pain may result from the enthesopathy or be secondary to the abnormal biomechanical stress placed across a skeletal structure. Of the two, the latter is more likely because many DISH lesions are asymptomatic.

RADIOGRAPHIC EVALUATION

Roentgenograms

The diagnosis of DISH is a radiographic one. It is made, not uncommonly, in asymptomatic people who happen to have characteristic bony changes in the thoracic spine on a chest radiograph (Fig.11-35). The three criteria for spinal involvement include flowing calcification along the anterolateral aspect of four contiguous vertebral bodies, preservation of intervertebral disc height, and absence of apophyseal joint bony ankylosis and sacroiliac joint sclerosis, erosion, or fusion.[65] These criteria help differentiate DISH from spondylosis deformans, intervertebral disc degeneration, and ankylosing spondylitis. The fact that the posterior spinal elements are not affected permits almost

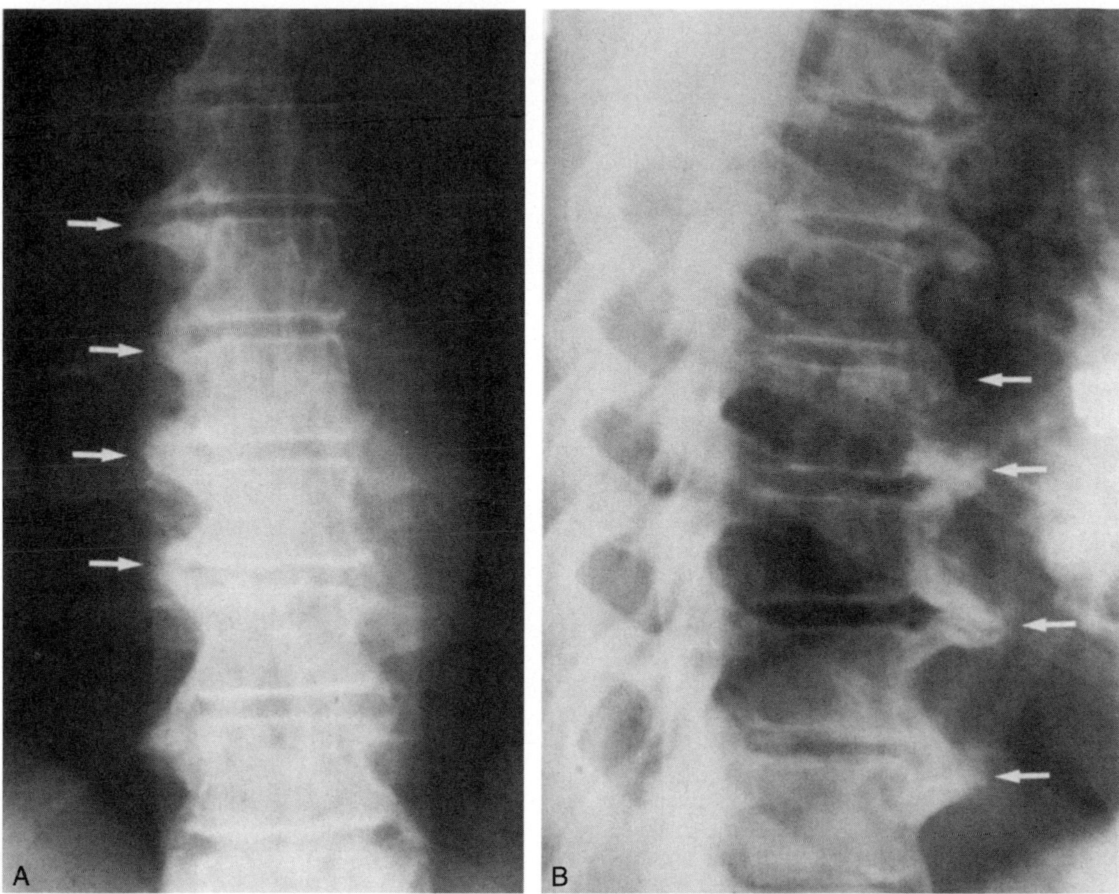

Figure 11-35 Diffuse idiopathic skeletal hyperostosis. Anteroposterior (*A*) and lateral (*B*) views of the thoracic spine demonstrate anterior, contiguous flowing ossification involving multiple vertebral bodies *(arrows)*. The radiolucency of the disc space has expanded into the flowing ossification and created a Y or T configuration. *(A and B, Courtesy of Anne Brower, MD.)*

normal range of motion on physical examination. Roentgenographic abnormalities are seen most frequently in the thoracic and lumbar spine (Fig.11-36).[64] Cervical spine lesions also develop in a majority of patients.

In the lumbar spine, the upper vertebrae (first through third) are most commonly affected. Calcification occurs initially along the anterior aspect of the vertebral body. Bony excrescences are located in an anterosuperior position near the disc margin and extend upward across the intervertebral disc space. The excrescences are thick relative to syndesmophytes. Careful observation will identify a thin radiolucent line that separates the vertebral body proper from the anterior calcification. The right-sided predilection of DISH in the thoracic spine is not continued in the lumbar spine, where bilateral or left-sided involvement is frequently seen.[62]

In the cervical spine, the lower vertebrae (C4–C7) are most commonly affected (Fig. 11-37).[74] Calcification occurs initially along the anterior aspect of the vertebral body (Fig. 11-38). A flowing pattern, like candle wax, may result from interruption of the column by radiolucent disc extensions at the intervertebral discs. An ossicle, a small triangular bony fragment, may form anterior to the intervertebral disc. Anterior calcifications may reach sufficient size to impinge on the anterior soft tissue structures of the throat, including the esophagus (Fig. 11-39). A thin radiolucent line that separates the vertebral body proper and the anterior calcification occurs less commonly in the cervical spine than the thoracic or lumbar spine. In contrast to other locations in the axial skeleton, posterior vertebral abnormalities, including osteophytes of the posterior vertebral bodies, and ligament calcification occur in the cervical spine.[46] Hyperostosis may also affect midline structures, including the atlantoaxial joint and the base of the occiput.[62] The stylohyoid ligament may become ossified in patients with DISH. These patients with Eagle's syndrome may complain of throat pain, dysphagia, otalgia, and a foreign body sensation.[10] These symptoms are similar to the classic syndrome associated with tonsillectomy. The carotid syndrome is caused by irritation of the sympathetic nerves within the wall of the carotid artery. Individuals with this form of Eagle's syndrome have pain along the carotid artery, temporomandibular pain, glossopharyngeal neuralgia, or facial pain in addition to the classic symptoms.[20] Atlantoaxial subluxation is a rare event in DISH patients. Subluxation may occur secondary to the excessive force placed on mobile segments when lower portions of the cervical spine are fused as a result of DISH.[7,49]

Extraspinal radiographic changes include bony proliferation or "whiskering," ligamentous calcification, and

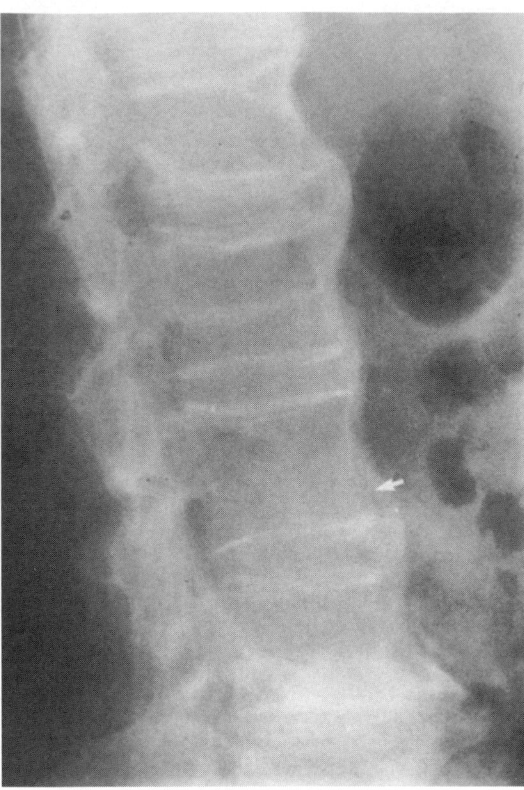

Figure 11-36 Diffuse idiopathic skeletal hyperostosis of the lumbar spine associated with "flowing" anterior ligament calcification involving five lumbar vertebrae. Notice the clear area separating the vertebral body and ligamentous calcification *(arrow)*. Characteristic of the process, the disc spaces are spared. *(Courtesy of Anne Brower, MD.)*

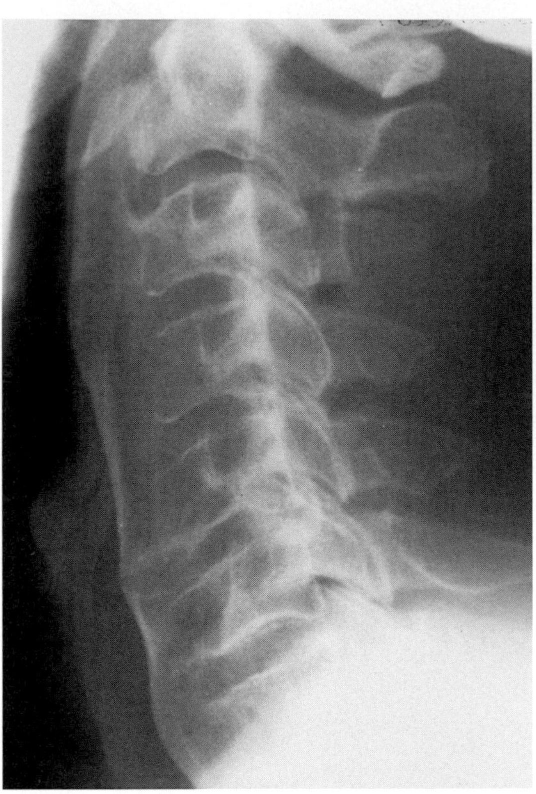

Figure 11-38 Diffuse idiopathic skeletal hyperostosis. A lateral view of the cervical spine reveals "flowing" anterior calcification extending from C2 to C7. *(Courtesy of Anne Brower, MD.)*

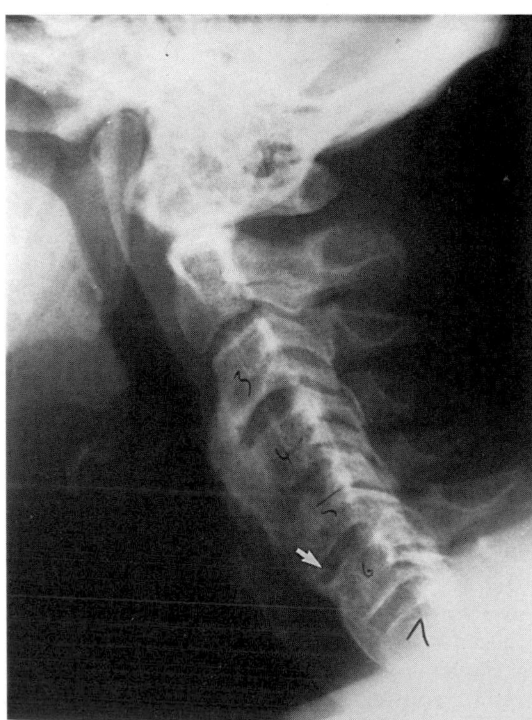

Figure 11-37 Diffuse idiopathic skeletal hyperostosis. A lateral view of the cervical spine reveals "flowing" anterior ligament calcification involving C3–C7. Notice the radiolucent extension at the level of the intervertebral disc *(arrow)*.

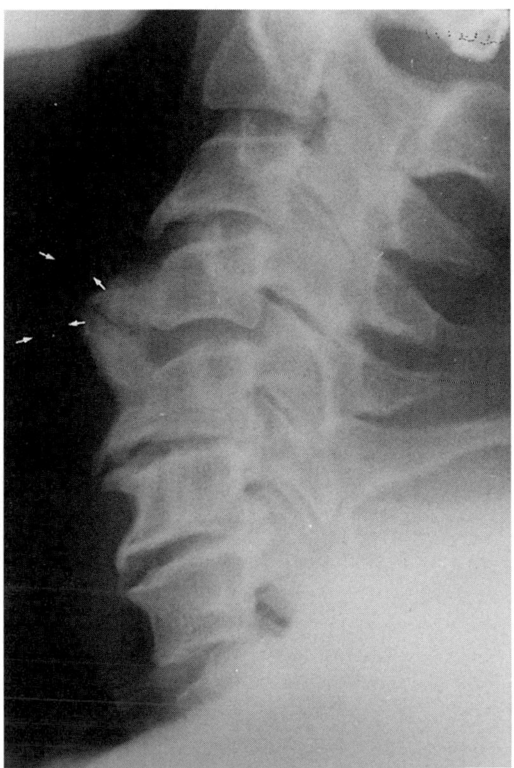

Figure 11-39 Diffuse idiopathic skeletal hyperostosis in a 65-year-old woman with dysphagia. A lateral view of the cervical spine shows a large anterior bony projection at the C4–C5 level. The soft tissues and hollow viscus anterior to this bony projection are constricted *(arrows)*. *(Courtesy of Anne Brower, MD.)*

para-articular osteophytes.[14] Common locations for these changes are in the pelvis, heels, feet, patellae, elbows, shoulders, and wrists. In the pelvis, the iliolumbar, sacrotuberous, and sacroiliac ligaments and iliopsoas tendon were locations for calcification. The calcification of ligaments was different from the pattern of pelvic involvement associated with spondylosis deformans, thus suggesting that DISH is a distinct entity independent of spondylosis deformans.[21]

Information concerning the presence of DISH may be serendipitously obtained from abdominal CT scans performed for other diagnostic purposes. Degenerative alterations in the sacroiliac joints are most easily observed with CT. In a study of 100 abdominal CT scans in patients 55 years or older, patients with DISH had more severe degenerative changes in the sacroiliac joints.[41] Some of the alterations noted in the sacroiliac joints include large bridging osteophytes at the anterior aspects of the joint.[62]

A comprehensive scoring system is available to evaluate the extent of involvement of the skeleton with DISH. The system is more accurate for summary measurements than for any single determination.[39]

Magnetic Resonance

MR imaging is useful for evaluation of fractures that may complicate the course of DISH. Fractures occur in the vertebral bodies and may bleed. The intravertebral fluid collections are well delineated, with linear borders that allow distinction from infections or neoplasms.[34]

DIFFERENTIAL DIAGNOSIS

The diagnosis of DISH is based on the presence of characteristic radiographic changes and an absence of clinical abnormalities suggestive of another illness. Resnick and Niwayama proposed the following criteria for the diagnosis of DISH[64]:

1. Flowing calcification and ossification along the anterolateral aspect of four contiguous vertebral bodies with or without associated localized pointed excrescences at the intervening vertebral body–intervertebral disc junctions
2. Relative preservation of intervertebral disc height in the involved vertebral segment and the absence of radiographic evidence of degenerative disc disease
3. Absence of apophyseal joint bony ankylosis and sacroiliac joint erosion, sclerosis, or intra-articular osseous fusion

Bony outgrowths of the spine have a number of causes, including spondyloarthropathies, acromegaly, hypoparathyroidism, fluorosis, ochronosis, neuropathic arthropathy, and trauma. Specific abnormalities associated with each of these entities, which are reviewed in other sections of this chapter, help differentiate these diseases from DISH.

Spondyloarthropathies are frequently associated with sacroiliac and cervical spine disease. The syndesmophytes associated with ankylosing spondylitis are thin and vertically oriented. These patients with ankylosing spondylitis are young and have prolonged morning stiffness that improves with activity during the day. The simultaneous presence of DISH and other diseases does occur. For example, a patient with a diagnosis of DISH and ankylosing spondylitis has been reported (Fig. 11-40).[83] Patients may have DISH of the cervical spine and spondylitis of the lumbosacral spine. Currently, eight patients have been reported in the medical literature with coexistent DISH and ankylosing spondylitis. Only four of these patients are HLA-B27 positive.[37]

Acromegaly is associated with posterior scalloping of the vertebral body and increased intervertebral disc space height in the thoracic and lumbar spine. In the cervical spine, elongation and widening of the vertebral bodies are observed. These alterations in vertebral bodies and disc spaces are similar to those associated with spondylosis deformans. Osteophytes may bridge the intervertebral disc space. Patients with DISH do not have soft tissue hypertrophy or joint space enlargement.[33] In patients with hypoparathyroidism, osteophytes develop with preservation of the intervertebral disc spaces. Hypoparathyroidism is associated with hypocalcemia and tetany, conditions not found in patients with DISH. Fluorosis causes generalized bone sclerosis to a greater extent than DISH does.[71] Ochronotic involvement of the vertebral column is manifested as loss of disc height and calcifications.[45] Neuropathic arthropathy causes disorganization and destruction of bone in conjunction with bone formation. Trauma causes callus formation in localized areas of the spine.

Spondylosis is not the same illness as DISH. In a study of 56 DISH patients, 43 spondylosis patients, and 43 healthy controls, DISH patients had more upper extremity pain, enthesitis of the patella and heel, dysphagia, and greater reduction in neck rotation and thoracic movements.[38]

Sternocostoclavicular Hyperostosis

Sternocostoclavicular hyperostosis (SCCH) is one of the illnesses associated with the SAPHO syndrome (*s*ynovitis, *a*cne, *p*ustules, *h*yperostosis, *o*steitis). SCCH is a rare syndrome, is found most commonly in Japan, and is characterized by hyperostosis and soft tissue ossification between the clavicle and anterior part of the upper ribs.[58] Men who are 30 to 50 years of age are at greatest risk for this illness. Swelling, tenderness, erythema, and pain are prominent over the anterior chest wall. Patients with cervical spine disease have pain in the neck with radiation to the shoulders.[56] Physical examination of the cervical spine reveals varying degrees of limited motion, depending on the extent of spinal involvement. Swelling over the clavicles or sternum may be prominent. Pustulosis palmaris et plantaris, a cutaneous disorder affecting the palms and soles, is associated with SCCH in up to 50% of patients.[70] Laboratory abnormalities are nonspecific, compatible with an inflammatory state. The ESR remains increased during the course of the illness. The radiographic abnormalities associated with SCCH may occur without disease in other portions of the axial skeleton. In contrast to the frequent occurrence of clinical symptoms, the radiologic signs of

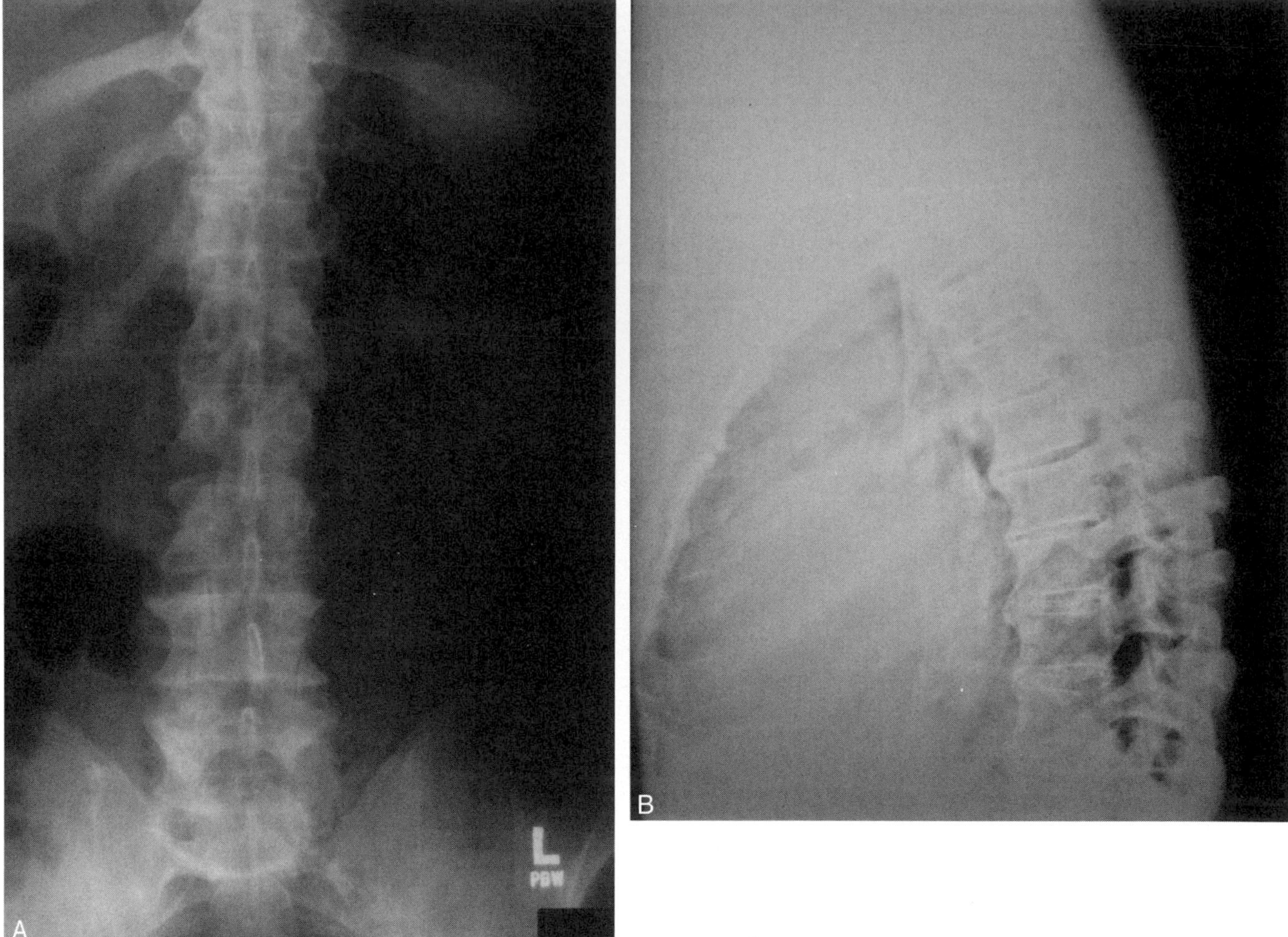

Figure 11-40 Diffuse idiopathic skeletal hyperostosis (DISH) in a 62-year-old man with chronic back pain. An anteroposterior *(A)* view reveals bilateral sacroiliitis with fusion. A lateral *(B)* view of the thoracic spine demonstrates flowing osteophytes compatible with DISH. The patient was HLA-B27 positive.

disease progression take several years to become detectable. SCCH has characteristics that resemble ankylosing spondylitis, DISH, and psoriatic spondylitis. New bone formation in the cervical spine is occasionally exuberant; it predominately occurs in the anterior aspect of the vertebral bodies and intervertebral discs and leads to obliteration of the anterior vertebral surface (Fig. 11-41).[63] Other roentgenographic findings of the cervical spine include ossification of the anterior and posterior longitudinal ligaments, ankylosis of the apophyseal joint, atlantoaxial subluxation, endplate erosions, and sclerosis of vertebral bodies.[8,12,59] In addition, hyperostosis of the sternum, manubriosternal junction, clavicle, or upper ribs is encountered. Bone scintigraphy is helpful in documenting increased activity in joints that may be difficult to visualize on plain roentgenograms.[55] *Arthro-osteitis* is the term used to describe this illness if spinal and extraspinal abnormalities are present in the absence of anterior chest involvement.[63] The use of CT to identify retrosternal proliferation of soft tissue is valuable because this finding helps differentiate SCCH from other benign hyperostotic processes.[17] The alteration in intervertebral discs and vertebral endplates may resemble an infectious process. Biopsy of these discal lesions usually reveals nonspecific chronic inflammation with scar formation.[17] Treatment of the disease includes nonsteroidal anti-inflammatory drugs (NSAIDs) and antibiotics.[8] The course of the disease is protracted, with periods of remission and exacerbation. The disease starts as an enthesopathy that ends decades later with total ankylosis of affected structures.

Ossification of the Posterior Longitudinal Ligament

Ossification of the posterior longitudinal ligament (OPLL) is a disease of unknown etiology that results in calcification of the posterior longitudinal ligament, particularly in the cervical spine. Terayama and colleagues are credited with naming the disease.[75] The disease is found most frequently in the Japanese,[27] in whom the incidence has been reported to be 1% to 2% of the population with cervical spine symptoms.[43,77] OPLL may affect people of other Asian or non-Asian nationalities.[23,40] It occurs in a

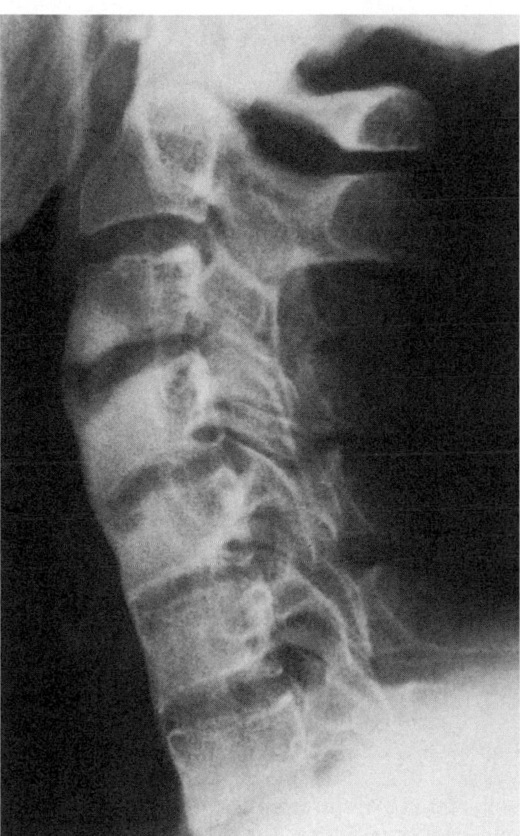

Figure 11-41 Sternocostoclavicular hyperostosis. Observe the hyperostotic changes involving the anterior portion of the third and seventh cervical vertebral bodies and the development of syndesmophytes. *(Courtesy of C. Resnick, MD, Baltimore.)*

male-to-female ratio of 2:1.[57] A genetic predisposition for OPLL on chromosome 6p may exist in Japanese patients.[24] Bone morphogenetic proteins and transforming growth factor-beta are increased and result in matrix hyperplasia and ossification of the spinal ligaments.[48]

Most patients with the disease are 50 to 60 years of age. The onset of disease is insidious. Twenty percent of patients may have an acute onset associated with minor trauma caused by slipping or a fall.[77] Ono and colleagues divided 166 symptomatic OPLL patients with musculoskeletal and neurologic abnormalities into three groups: myelopathy with motor and sensory signs in the lower extremities (56%), segmental signs with motor and sensory signs in the upper extremities (16%), and cervicobrachialgia manifested by pain in the neck, shoulder, and arm (28%).[46] The combination of sensory and motor signs in the upper extremity may be so severe that it affects daily living habits. Gait disturbances occur in 25% and an inability to ambulate in 10%.[77] Myelopathic findings were observed when the thickness of the calcification exceeded 30% to 60% of the sagittal diameter of the cervical spinal canal. The presence of such findings may also be affected by the rapidity of compression.[13] Acute quadriparesis has been reported in OPLL patients.[54] Physical examination may reveal decreased neck motion and stiffness along with neurologic signs corresponding to areas of nerve compression. Laboratory findings include an elevated ESR but are nonspecific. Pathologic findings include cortical bone with haversian canals and immature bone marrow. Proposed mechanisms of ligamentous calcification have included proliferation of cartilage cells in the ligament, mucoid degeneration of the ligament, and coalescence of hydroxyapatite crystals to form calcifying masses.[57] Ossification starts on the dural side of the ligament and progresses in a posteroanterior direction to involve the deep layers of the ligament. In the final stage, the ligament becomes fused with the vertebral body and dura. OPLL is a radiologic diagnosis.[27] On lateral roentgenograms, a dense ossified strip 1 to 5 mm long is evident along the posterior margin of the vertebral bodies and intervertebral discs. The ossification may be continuous or segmental. A thin radiolucent zone separates the vertebral body and the layer of ossification. The intervertebral discs and apophyseal joints are spared, although anterior osteophytes are common. The midcervical region (C3–C5) is the most frequently affected spinal level. The thoracic and lumbar ligaments are affected in 10% of OPLL patients.[77] Thoracic and lumbar lesions may be identified in people who do not have cervical spine disease.[47] Anterior calcifications may be indicative of DISH. Resnick and colleagues reported OPLL in 50% of DISH patients.[60] Other investigators have also reported the simultaneous occurrence of these two illnesses (Fig. 11-42).[19,40] DISH may be present in 40% of OPLL patients.[3] CT is able to detect the size and location of the ossified ligament to a greater extent than plain roentgenograms can. Nose and colleagues reported that midline lesions were associated with myelopathy and that lateral lesions were associated with radiculopathy when viewed with CT myelography.[44] MR evaluation allows for detection of marrow in the ossified ligament and determination of the status of the spinal cord in regard to compression.[50] Conservative treatment of OPLL consists of rest, traction, and bracing and is effective in 70% of patients.[30] Indications for surgical intervention include persistent neurologic impairment, intractable pain, and risk of additional cord damage. Surgical techniques may approach the calcification from an anterior or posterior direction, but they may not stop postoperative progression of calcification.[26] The surgical approach needs to match the component of OPLL or DISH that is causing symptoms.[11] Japanese and non-Japanese patients have similar clinical characteristics and respond to therapy in the same manner.[76]

TREATMENT

Treatment is directed at relieving pain and maximizing function. In patients with spinal pain and stiffness, NSAIDs may be helpful. Exercise programs are designed to encourage maximal range of motion throughout the axial skeleton. Local injections of lidocaine and corticosteroid are used for pain relief in areas of bony overgrowth, such as the heel.

Patients with severe dysphagia may require removal of the offending hyperostosis.[31] Postoperative swallowing studies can document return of normal function of the epiglottis and elimination of aspiration.[1] A possible complication of the surgical excision of exostoses is recurrence

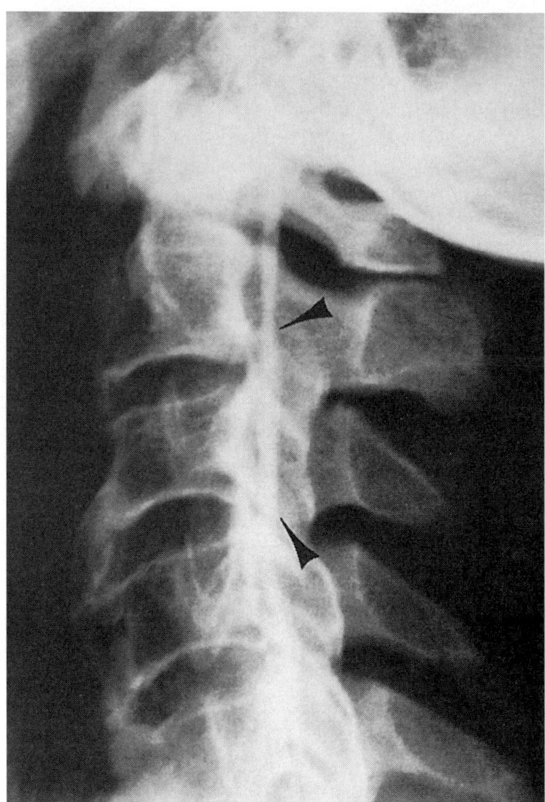

Figure 11-42 Coexistent ossification of the posterior longitudinal ligament and diffuse idiopathic skeletal hyperostosis (DISH). Extensive posterior ligamentous ossification *(arrows)* is combined with the anterior vertebral changes typical of DISH. *(From Resnick D: Calcification and ossification of the posterior spinal ligaments and tissues. In Resnick D [ed]: Diagnosis of Bone and Joint Disorders, 3rd ed. Philadelphia, WB Saunders, 1995, p 1503.)*

of bony overgrowth. Postoperative heterotopic ossification has developed in some patients with DISH who have undergone hip joint replacement.[61] Procedures for removal of osteophytes are successful in most circumstances. In a series of 19 patients, only 2 had a poor outcome, 1 with unrecognized esophageal cancer and another with postoperative apnea.[69]

PROGNOSIS

The course of DISH is usually benign. Confusion in diagnosis may occur in patients who are initially evaluated in their 40s for spinal pain but have no physical findings or early radiographic changes. The differential diagnosis for such patients requires investigation for a number of illnesses that affect the axial skeleton. Patients with DISH have a slow, progressive course. They may have aching back or neck pain and stiffness for an extended period measured in years, but rarely do they have any limitations in activities or morbidity from the disease.

Lumbar Spine

Symptoms of spinal stenosis may develop in patients with DISH. Ligamentous and capsular calcifications cause canal stenosis secondary to DISH. Hyperostotic stenosis differs from the simple degenerative changes associated with osteoarthritic alterations of the spine. The hyperostotic narrowing of the canal may be associated with neural compression.[32]

The course of patients with DISH may be complicated by other disease processes. For example, erosion in an area of hyperostosis in the lumbar spine may develop in patients with DISH. The erosive process may be secondary to an expanding abdominal aneurysm.[6]

Cervical Spine

Patients with DISH are at risk for fracture through ankylosed segments. Fracture occurs most commonly in the cervical spine.[25] Fractures may also occur, though less frequently, in the upper lumbar spine.[34] Neurologic dysfunction develops immediately or on a delayed basis in patients with fractures.[51] Most fractures occur through vertebral bodies in the midportion of the ankylosed segment. Less commonly, fractures may occur through discs at levels above or below the ankylosed segment. This pattern is in contrast to fractures associated with ankylosing spondylitis, which occur through discs—the weakest part of the ankylosed spine. The trauma that causes a fracture may be minimal.[25] Flexion injuries result in greater neurologic deficits than extension injuries do because of the positional alterations in the size of the spinal canal.[42] Spinal fractures resulted in quadriplegia in 7 of 15 DISH patients in one study. Only 3 of 15 patients did not have any neurologic damage after a fracture. Fractures heal with early stabilization. Death is a potential result of fracture if the fracture is not recognized.

References

Diffuse Idiopathic Skeletal Hyperostosis

1. Akhtar S, O'Flynn PE, Kelly A, et al: The management of dysphagia in skeletal hyperostosis. J Laryngol Otol 114:154-157, 2000.
2. Algenhat JP, Hallet M, Kido DK: Spinal cord compression in diffuse idiopathic skeletal hyperostosis. Radiology 142:119, 1982.
3. Arlet PJ, Pujol M, Buc A, et al: Role de l'hyperostose vertebrale dans les myelopathies cervicales. Rev Rhum Mal Osteoartic 43:167, 1976.
4. Babores M, Finnerty JP: Aspiration pneumonia secondary to giant cervical osteophyte formation (diffuse idiopathic skeletal hyperostosis or Forrestier's disease). Chest 114:1481-1482, 1998.
5. Boachie-Adjei O, Bullough PG: Incidence of ankylosing hyperostosis of the spine (Forestier's disease) at autopsy. Spine 12:739, 1987.
6. Chaiton A, Fam A, Charles B: Disappearing lumbar hyperostosis in a patient with Forestier's disease: An ominous sign. Arthritis Rheum 22:799, 1979.
7. Chiba H, Annen S, Shimada T, et al: Atlantoaxial subluxations complicated by diffuse idiopathic skeletal hyperostosis. Spine 17:1414-1417, 1992.
8. Chigira M, Maehara S, Nagase M, et al: Sternocostoclavicular hyperostosis: A report of nineteen cases with special reference to etiology and treatment. J Bone Joint Surg Am 68-A:103, 1986.
9. Crosby ET, Grahovac S: Diffuse idiopathic skeletal hyperostosis: A unique cause of difficult intubation. Can J Anaesth 40:54, 1993.
10. Eagle W: Elongated styloid process: Further observations and a new syndrome. Arch Otolaryngol 47:630, 1948.
11. Epstein NE: Simultaneous cervical diffuse idiopathic skeletal hyperostosis and ossification of the posterior longitudinal ligament resulting in dysphagia or myelopathy in two geriatric North Americans. Surg Neurol 53:427-431, 2000.

12. Fallet GH, Arroyo J, Vischer TL: Sternocostoclavicular hyperostosis: Case report with a 31-year follow-up. Arthritis Rheum 26:784, 1983.
13. Firooznia H, Rafii M, Golimbu C, et al: Computed tomography of calcification and ossification of posterior longitudinal ligament of the spine. J Comput Assist Tomogr 8:317, 1984.
14. Forestier J, Lagier R: Ankylosing hyperostosis of the spine. Clin Orthop 74:65, 1971.
15. Forgacs SS: Diabetes mellitus and rheumatic disease. Clin Rheum Dis 12:729, 1986.
16. Fornasier VL, Littlejohn GO, Urowitz MB, et al: Spinal entheseal new bone formation: The early changes of diffuse idiopathic skeletal hyperostosis. J Rheumatol 10:939, 1983.
17. Fritz P, Baldauf G, Wilke H, Reitter I: Sternocostoclavicular hyperostosis: its progression and radiological features: A study of 12 cases. Ann Rheum Dis 51:658, 1992.
18. Granville L, Musson N, Altman R, et al: Anterior cervical osteophytes as a cause of pharyngeal stage dysphagia. J Am Geriatr Soc 46:1003-1007, 1998.
19. Griffiths ID, Fitzjohn TP: Cervical myelopathy, ossification of the posterior longitudinal ligament, and diffuse idiopathic skeletal hyperostosis: Problems in investigation. Ann Rheum Dis 46:166, 1987.
20. Guo B, Javisidha S, Sartoris DJ, et al: Correlation between ossification of the stylohyoid ligament and osteophytes of the cervical spine. J Rheumatol 24:1575-1781, 1997.
21. Haller J, Resnick D, Miller CW, et al: Diffuse idiopathic skeletal hyperostosis: Diagnostic significance of radiographic abnormalities of the pelvis. Radiology 172:835, 1989.
22. Harris J, Carter AR, Glick EN, Storey GO: Ankylosing hyperostosis: I. Clinical and radiological features. Ann Rheum Dis 33:210, 1974.
23. Harsh GR IV, Sypert GW, Weinstein PR, et al: Cervical spine stenosis secondary to ossification of the posterior longitudinal ligament in non-Orientals. J Neurosurg 67:349, 1987.
24. Havelka S, Vesela M, Pavelkova A, et al: Are DISH and OPLL genetically related? Ann Rheum Dis 60:902-903, 2001.
25. Hendrix RW, Melany M, Miller F, Rogers LF: Fracture of the spine in patients with ankylosis due to diffuse idiopathic skeletal hyperostosis: Clinical and imaging findings. AJR Am J Roentgenol 162:899, 1994.
26. Hirabayashi K, Miyakawa J, Satomi K, et al: Operative results and postoperative progression of ossification among patients with ossification of cervical posterior longitudinal ligament. Spine 6:354, 1981.
27. Jones MD, Pais MJ, Omiya B: Bony overgrowths and abnormal calcification about the spine. Radiol Clin North Am 26:1213, 1988.
28. Julkunen H, Heinonen OP, Pyorala K: Hyperostoses of the spine in an adult population: Its relationship to hyperglycemia and obesity. Ann Rheum Dis 30:605, 1971.
29. Kiss C, Szilagyi M, Paksy A, et al: Risk factors for diffuse idiopathic skeletal hyperostosis: A case-control study. Rheumatology 41: 27-30, 2002.
30. Klara PM, McDonnell DE: Ossification of the posterior longitudinal ligament in Caucasians: Diagnosis and surgical intervention. Neurosurgery 19:212, 1986.
31. Kritzer RO, Parker WD: DISH: A cause of anterior cervical osteophyte-induced dysphagia. Spine 13:130, 1988.
32. Kurihara A, Tanaka Y, Tsumura N, et al: Hyperostotic lumbar spinal stenosis: A review of 12 surgically treated cases with roentgenographic survey of ossification of the yellow ligament at the lumbar spine. Spine 12:1308, 1988.
33. Lang EK, Bessler WT: Roentgenologic features of acromegaly. AJR Am J Roentgenol 86:321, 1961.
34. Le Hir PX, Sautet A, Le Gars L, et al: Hyperextension vertebral body fractures in diffuse idiopathic skeletal hyperostosis: A cause of intravertebral fluidlike collections on MR imaging. AJR Am J Roentgenol 173:1679-1683, 1999.
35. Littlejohn GO, Smythe HA: Marked hyperinsulinemia after glucose challenge in patients with diffuse idiopathic skeletal hyperostosis. J Rheumatol 8:965, 1981.
36. Mader R: Clinical manifestations of diffuse idiopathic skeletal hyperostosis of the cervical spine. Semin Arthritis Rheum 32:130-135, 2002.
37. Maertens M, Mielants H, Verstraete K, et al: Simultaneous occurrence of diffuse idiopathic skeletal hyperostosis and ankylosing spondylitis in the same patient. J Rheumatol 19:1978, 1992.
38. Mata S, Chhem RK, Fortin PR, et al: Comprehensive radiographic evaluation of diffuse idiopathic skeletal hyperostosis: Development and interrater reliability of a scoring system. Semin Arthritis Rheum 28:88-96, 1998.
39. Mata S, Fortin PR, Fitzcharles M, et al: A controlled study of diffuse idiopathic skeletal hyperostosis: Clinical features and functional state. Medicine (Baltimore) 76:104-117, 1997.
40. McAfee PC, Regan JJ, Bohlman HH: Cervical cord compression from ossification of the posterior longitudinal ligament in non-Orientals. J Bone Joint Surg Br 69-B:569, 1987.
41. Meeks LW, Renshaw TS: Vertebral osteophytosis and dysphagia. J Bone Joint Surg Am 55-A:197, 1973.
42. Meyer PR: Diffuse idiopathic skeletal hyperostosis in the cervical spin. Clin Orthop 359:49-57, 1999.
43. Nahanshi T, Mannen T, Toyokura Y: Asymptomatic ossification of the posterior longitudinal ligament of the cervical spine: Incidence and roentgenographic findings. J Neurol Sci 19:375, 1973.
44. Nose T, Egashira T, Enomoto T, et al: Ossification of the posterior longitudinal ligament: A clinico-radiological study of 74 cases. J Neurol Neurosurg Psychiatry 50:321, 1987.
45. O'Brien WM, Banfield WG, Sokoloff L: Studies on the pathogenesis of ochronotic arthropathy. Arthritis Rheum 4:137, 1961.
46. Ono K, Ota H, Tada K, et al: Ossified posterior longitudinal ligament: A clinicopathologic study. Spine 2:126, 1977.
47. Ono M, Russell WJ, Kudo S, et al: Ossification of the thoracic posterior longitudinal ligament in a fixed population: Radiological and neurological manifestations. Radiology 143:469, 1982.
48. Ono K, Yoenobu K, Miyamoto S, et al: Pathology of ossification of the posterior longitudinal ligament and ligamentum flavum. Clin Orthop 359:18-26, 1999.
49. Oostveen JCM, van de Laar MAFJ, Tuynman FHB: Anterior atlantoaxial subluxations in a patient with diffuse idiopathic skeletal hyperostosis. J Rheumatol 23:1441-1444, 1996.
50. Otake S, Matusi M, Nishizawa S, et al: Ossification of the posterior longitudinal ligament: MR evaluation. AJNR Am J Neuroradiol 13:1059, 1992.
51. Paley D, Schwartz M, Cooper P, et al: Fractures of the spine in diffuse idiopathic skeletal hyperostosis. Clin Orthop 267:22, 1991.
52. Papakostas K, Thakar A, Nandapalan V, et al: An unusual case of stridor due to osteophytes of the cervical spine (Forestier's disease). J Laryngol Otol 113:65-67, 1999.
53. Periquet B, Lambert W, Garcia J, et al: Increased concentrations of endogenous 13-*cis*- and all-*trans*-retinoic acids in diffuse idiopathic skeletal hyperostosis as demonstrated by HPLC. Clin Chim Acta 203:57, 1991.
54. Pouchot J, Watts CS, Esdaile JM, Hill RO: Sudden quadriplegia complicating ossification of the posterior longitudinal ligament and diffuse idiopathic skeletal hyperostosis. Arthritis Rheum 30:1069, 1987.
55. Prevo RL, Rasker JJ, Kruijsen MWM: Sternocostoclavicular hyperostosis or pustulotic arthro-osteitis. J Rheumatol 16:1602, 1989.
56. Resnick CS, Ammann AM: Cervical spine involvement in sternocostoclavicular hyperostosis. Spine 10:846, 1985.
57. Resnick D: Calcification and ossification of the posterior spinal ligaments and tissues. In Resnick D (ed): Diagnosis of Bone and Joint Disorders, 3rd ed. Philadelphia, WB Saunders, 1995, pp 1496-1507.
58. Resnick D: Hyperostosis and ossification in the cervical spine. Arthritis Rheum 27:564, 1984.
59. Resnick D: Sternocostoclavicular hyperostosis. AJR Am J Roentgenol: 135:1278, 1980.
60. Resnick D, Guerra J Jr, Robinson CA, et al: Association of DISH and calcification and ossification of the PLL. AJR Am J Roentgenol 131:1049, 1978.
61. Resnick D, Linovitz RJ, Feingold ML: Postoperative heterotopic ossification in patients with ankylosing hyperostosis of the spine (Forestier's disease). J Rheumatol 3:313, 1976.
62. Resnick D, Niwayama G: Diffuse idiopathic skeletal hyperostosis (DISH): Ankylosing hyperostosis of Forrestier and Rotes-Querol. In Resnick D (ed): Diagnosis of Bone and Joint Disorders, 3rd ed. Philadelphia, WB Saunders, 1995, pp 1463-1495.
63. Resnick D, Niwayama G: Enostosis, hyperostosis, and periostitis. In Resnick D (ed): Diagnosis of Bone and Joint Disorders, 3rd ed. Philadelphia, WB Saunders, 1995, pp 4396-4466.
64. Resnick D, Niwayama G: Radiographic and pathologic features of spinal involvement in diffuse idiopathic skeletal hyperostosis (DISH). Radiology 119:559, 1976.
65. Resnick D, Shaul SR, Robins JM: Diffuse idiopathic skeletal hyperostosis (DISH): Forestier's disease with extraspinal manifestations. Radiology 115:513, 1975.

66. Rotes-Querol J: Clinical manifestations of diffuse idiopathic skeletal hyperostosis (DISH). Br J Rheumatol 35:1193-1196, 1996.
67. Schlapbach P, Beyeler C, Gerber NJ, et al: Diffuse idiopathic skeletal hyperostosis (DISH) of the spine: A cause of back pain: A controlled study. Br J Rheumatol 28:299, 1989.
68. Shapiro RF, Utsinger PD, Wiesner KB, et al: The association of HLA-B27 with Forestier's disease (vertebral ankylosing hyperostosis). J Rheumatol 3:4, 1976.
69. Sobol S, Rigual N: Anterolateral extrapharyngeal approach for cervical osteophyte-induced dysphagia. Ann Otol Rhinol Laryngol 93:498, 1984.
70. Sonozaki H, Kawashima M, Hongo O, et al: Incidence of arthro-osteitis in patients with pustulosis palmaris. Ann Rheum Dis 40:554, 1981.
71. Soriano M, Manchon F: Radiological aspects of a new type of bone fluorosis, periostitis deformans. Radiology 87:1089, 1966.
72. Spagnola AM, Bennet PH, Terasaki PI: Vertebral ankylosing hyperostosis (Forestier's disease) and HLA antigens in Pima Indians. Arthritis Rheum 21:467, 1978.
73. Spilberg I, Lieberman DM: Ankylosing hyperostosis of the cervical spine. Arthritis Rheum 15:208, 1972.
74. Suzuki K, Ishida Y, Ohmori K: Long term follow-up of diffuse idiopathic skeletal hyperostosis in the cervical spine: Analysis of progression of ossification. Neuroradiology 33:427, 1991.
75. Terayama K, Maruyama S, Miyashita R, et al: Ossification of the posterior longitudinal ligament of the cervical spine (Jpn). Jpn Orthop Surg (Tokyo) 15:1083, 1964.
76. Trojan DA, Pouchot J, Pokrupa R, et al: Diagnosis and treatment of ossification of the posterior longitudinal ligament: Report of eight cases and literature review. Am J Med 92:296, 1992.
77. Tsuyama N: Ossification of the posterior longitudinal ligament of the spine. Clin Orthop 184:71, 1984.
78. Utsinger PD: Diffuse idiopathic skeletal hyperostosis. Clin Rheum Dis 11:325, 1985.
79. Utsinger PD, Resnick D, Shapiro R: Diffuse skeletal abnormalities in Forestier disease. Arch Intern Med 136:763, 1976.
80. Vernon-Roberts B, Pirie CJ, Trenwith V: Pathology of the dorsal spine in ankylosing hyperostosis. Ann Rheum Dis 33:281, 1974.
81. Warnick C, Sherman MS, Lesser RW: Aspiration pneumonia due to diffuse cervical hyperostosis. Chest 98:763, 1990.
82. Weinfeld RM, Olson PN, Maki DD, et al: The prevalence of diffuse idiopathic skeletal hyperostosis (DISH) in two large American Midwest metropolitan hospital populations. Skeletal Radiol 26:222-225, 1997.
83. Williamson PK, Reginato AJ: Diffuse idiopathic skeletal hyperostosis of the cervical spine in a patient with ankylosing spondylitis. Arthritis Rheum 27:570, 1984.

POLYMYALGIA RHEUMATICA

Capsule Summary

	Low Back	Neck
Frequency of spinal pain	Uncommon	Very common
Location of spinal pain	Buttocks, upper thighs	Paracervical muscles, shoulders
Quality of spinal pain	Diffuse ache with stiffness	Diffuse ache with stiffness
Symptoms and signs	Morning stiffness, normal strength, diffuse muscle pain in proximal musculature	Morning stiffness, normal strength, diffuse muscle pain in proximal musculature
Laboratory tests	Increased erythrocyte sedimentation rate, anemia	Increased erythrocyte sedimentation rate, anemia
Radiographic findings	None	None
Treatment	Corticosteroids, 15-25 mg daily initially, decreasing doses with improvement	Corticosteroids, 15-25 mg daily initially, decreasing doses with improvement

PREVALENCE AND PATHOGENESIS

Polymyalgia rheumatica (PMR) is a clinical syndrome characterized by severe stiffness, tenderness, and aching of the proximal musculature of the upper and lower extremities. Patients who are 50 years or older are most commonly affected by this syndrome, and they have an elevated erythrocyte sedimentation rate (ESR) as the primary abnormal laboratory finding. No pathognomonic abnormality is available to help physicians diagnose this disease; therefore, other diseases that may be associated with proximal muscle pain must be eliminated before a diagnosis of PMR is made.

Epidemiology

The incidence of PMR depends to a great extent on the patient population studied. In one population study of whites older than 50 years, the incidence of PMR was 19.8 per 100,000 people 50 to 59 years of age; it rose to 112.2 per 100,000 people 70 to 79 years of age. In the total population, the incidence rate was 11 per 100,000 population.[16] A follow-up study completed in Olmstead County, Minnesota, from 1970 to 1991 found the prevalence of PMR in people older than 50 years to be 6 per 1000 with an incidence of 52.5 per 100,000.[66] The frequency may be as common as 1 case for every 133 people older than 50 years.[66] The prevalence of the disease increases in older age groups, with the majority of patients being 60 years or older.[57] The male-to-female ratio is 1:4. The Olmstead County study found a ratio of 39.9% men and 61.7% women.[66] The illness rarely develops in blacks.[4] However, reports of giant cell arteritis (GCA) occurring in blacks have appeared in the literature.[6] In general, the incidence of GCA is increasing.[64]

Pathogenesis

The pathogenesis of PMR is unknown.[42] No familial predisposition has been shown, although occasional familial cases appear in the literature.[64] The haplotypes HLA-DRB1*04 and HLA-DRB1*01 are associated with increased susceptibility to PMR and GCA.[39] Efforts to prove a viral etiology have not been successful.[51] An increased prevalence of antibodies against parainfluenza virus type 1 is reported in PMR and GCA patients.[26] Others have found an association between parvovirus B19 infection and the development of GCA.[67] A report of PMR developing in a married couple simultaneously is supportive of an environmental pathogenesis.[28] In addition, seasonal clustering associated with onset of the disease during the summer months (May to August) suggests a temporal or environmental mechanism of initiation.[18]

Some have suggested that PMR is an arthritic condition affecting the axial joints.[10,19] The joints primarily affected include the sternoclavicular and humeroscapular. Synovitis has been demonstrated in these joints on bone scan. However, the relatively small proportion of patients with PMR and synovitis and the distribution of involved joints (relative absence in hip joints) make this mechanism unlikely. Additional studies supporting the presence or absence of joint disease in PMR patients have been reported. Investigations of PMR patients, including radiographic studies and necropsy, have been unable to demonstrate synovitis in these patients.[10,19] Nonetheless, clinical reports have presented data describing patients with synovitis that may be confused with rheumatoid arthritis in whom classic PMR developed. However, synovitis in the form of bilateral subacromial and subdeltoid bursitis visualized by MR imaging or ultrasonography is present in a majority of PMR patients.[12] Studies supporting an increased presence of haplotype DR4 in PMR patients provide additional evidence for a relationship between PMR and rheumatoid arthritis. HLA-DR4 is found to be increased in PMR patients in comparison to control subjects.[17,63]

Immunologic mechanisms, including circulating immune complexes, cell-mediated immunity, and shifts in the lymphocyte population, have been studied in patients with PMR. No consistent correlation of the quantity or composition of immune complexes or the status of lymphocyte numbers or function with disease pathogenesis has been clearly found.[14,60,61] Additional studies have demonstrated alterations in lymphocyte distribution and elevated levels of a variety of cytokines, including interleukin-6, interleukin-2 receptors, and intercellular adhesion molecule type 1.[21,53,69] However, no consistent correlation of normalization of these abnormalities with clinical improvement during an extended period has been reported.

Weyand and Goronzy presented a model of pathogenesis for GCA and PMR that involves the differential production of cytokines that result in phenotypic expression of the corresponding illness.[74,75] Antigen in the adventitia is recognized by T cells that enter the artery from the vasa vasorum, undergo clonal expansion, and produce interferon-gamma. Macrophages are attracted and form giant cells. In the adventitia, macrophages produce interleukin-1 and interleukin-6, whereas in the media and intima, macrophages produce metalloproteinases and nitric oxide. Repair of the artery results in degradation of the internal elastic lamina and occlusion of the lumen. Cytokine production in patients with GCA and PMR is associated with higher concentrations of interleukin-2 mRNA. Patients with ischemic symptoms have interferon-gamma mRNA and interleukin-1 beta mRNA.

A new area of study has been investigation of muscle from PMR patients by electron microscopy. The mitochondria in affected muscle are abnormal. In one study, 71% contained crystals that may impair their metabolic activity.[29]

Barber in 1957 was the first to propose the name *polymyalgia rheumatica* for the clinical syndrome.[2] PMR has had numerous names, including senile rheumatic gout, polymyalgia arteritica, and anarthritic rheumatoid disease.

CLINICAL HISTORY

The classic PMR patient is a woman older than 50 years with symmetrical pain and stiffness in the muscles of the neck and shoulder girdle.[31] Shoulder pain is the initial symptom in 70% to 90% of patients. Discomfort in the low back region, pelvic girdle, and thighs is also commonly experienced in 50% to 70% of patients. The pain starts initially in the shoulders and neck more commonly than in the low back area or pelvis. The pain is worse in the morning, such that getting out of bed is difficult. Activity decreases the pain as the day progresses. Symptoms reappear when the patient becomes inactive. The onset of symptoms may be abrupt or gradual. Constitutional symptoms may also be present, including fever, malaise, fatigue, anorexia, weight loss, and depression. In about a third of patients, a history of a prodromal viral illness may be elicited.

PHYSICAL EXAMINATION

Physical examination demonstrates muscle tenderness on palpation and muscle pain with motion, but atrophy and weakness are not present. Although active range of motion of joints may be limited by pain, passive motion is normal. Neck or low back motion is not limited. Occasionally, joint swelling may be seen, particularly in the sternoclavicular area.[55] Distal manifestations include asymmetric peripheral arthritis in the knees and wrists, carpal tunnel syndrome, and swelling and pitting edema of the dorsum of the hands and feet.

LABORATORY DATA

The characteristic laboratory finding is an increased ESR, and it is present in almost every case of PMR.[4] ESR is more sensitive than C-reactive protein (CRP) for the diagnosis of disease in PMR patients.[47] CRP is a more sensitive indicator of active disease.[11] A small proportion (7% to 22.5%) of PMR and GCA patients will have a normal ESR at time of diagnosis.[62,68]

Hypochromic anemia may also develop in patients with active disease.[33] Increases in leukocytes and platelets may be more closely related to GCA, which may accompany PMR, than to PMR itself.[5] Chemical studies are usually normal except for about a third of patients with abnormal liver function test results, particularly alkaline phosphatase.[73] Tests for rheumatoid factor and antinuclear antibody are generally negative, or these elements are present in the same proportion as found in normal age-matched control subjects. Antimitochondrial antibodies have been reported in a minority of patients with PMR.[70] Their clinical significance remains in doubt. Muscle enzyme levels are normal. Anticardiolipin antibodies, IgG or IgM, are elevated in only 27% of PMR patients, whereas 80% of GCA patients have antibodies. GCA patients with both antibodies may be at risk for more severe vascular complications.[27]

11-12 DIAGNOSTIC CRITERIA FOR POLYMYALGIA RHEUMATICA*

Age ≥50 years
Bilateral aching of the neck, shoulders, or pelvic girdle
Morning stiffness >1 hour
ESR >40 mm/hr
Rapid response to prednisone (<20 mg/day)
Exclusion of other diagnoses

*All criteria need to be fulfilled.
From Healy LA: Long-term follow-up of polymyalgia rheumatica: Evidence for synovitis. Semin Arthritis Rheum 13:322-328, 1984.

Pathology

Pathologic examination of muscle biopsy specimens from PMR patients is unremarkable.[9] Synovial biopsy demonstrates nonspecific inflammation of the synovium.[15,34] The diagnosis of GCA is made by identification of giant cells in a histologic section of a biopsied temporal artery. The biopsy may be positive in 50% of patients at onset.[25]

RADIOGRAPHIC EVALUATION

Plain roentgenograms demonstrate typical changes in the skeleton that might be expected in patients of this age group. PMR is not associated with any specific radiographic abnormality, but technetium pertechnetate scans may demonstrate increased uptake in the shoulder joints.[58] MR imaging demonstrates bursitis of the subacromial, subdeltoid, and iliopectineal bursae and synovitis of the hip in a proportion of patients with PMR.[65] Sacroiliitis and osteitis pubis are reported in individuals with PMR.[13] A direct relationship between PMR and spondyloarthropathy has not been proved.

DIFFERENTIAL DIAGNOSIS

Bird and colleagues suggested seven criteria for the diagnosis of PMR[7]: (1) bilateral shoulder pain and stiffness, (2) onset of illness of less than 2 weeks' duration, (3) initial ESR greater than 40 mm/hr, (4) duration of morning stiffness exceeding 1 hour, (5) 65 years or older, (6) depression or weight loss, and (7) bilateral tenderness of the upper part of the arm. The diagnosis of PMR is probable if three or more criteria are met. Other diagnostic criteria have been proposed for PMR by Healy (Table 11-12).[40]

PMR is a diagnosis made after a number of other diseases with similar symptoms are excluded. Other conditions associated with proximal muscle pain include viral infections, subacute bacterial endocarditis, malignancy, osteoarthritis, rheumatoid arthritis, polymyositis, GCA, fibromyalgia, thyroid dysfunction, and parathyroid dysfunction. A complete history, physical examination, and laboratory evaluation can usually differentiate these diseases. In some instances in which the clinical symptoms or laboratory abnormalities are not absolutely characteristic, a tentative diagnosis of PMR is made and therapy is initiated. These patients are then continuously observed to be sure that another illness is not causing their muscle symptoms. When other diseases have been excluded and a patient demonstrates shoulder pain of a month's duration, is 50 years or older, has an increased ESR, and responds to corticosteroid therapy, a diagnosis of PMR can be made.

The diagnosis of PMR should not be considered until at least 6 weeks after the onset of symptoms. Viral syndromes frequently resolve in this period. Subacute bacterial endocarditis causes cardiac abnormalities (murmur or change in heart size) that are not associated with PMR. Malignancy does not usually respond to the dose of corticosteroid that is effective for PMR. For example, patients with renal cell carcinoma and lymphoma have had PMR symptoms that are resistant to therapy.[56,71] Osteoarthritis causes symptoms that are maximal at the end of the day, and it is associated with a normal ESR. Rheumatoid arthritis affects more joints in the peripheral skeleton than is usually noted in PMR. In the initial state of rheumatoid arthritis in an elderly patient, symptoms of arthritis and muscle pain may be difficult to differentiate from those associated with PMR. The presence of rheumatoid nodules may be helpful in these circumstances. In one study, PMR patients were differentiated from rheumatoid arthritis patients by the presence of upper arm tenderness, the lack of rheumatoid factor, and normal ceruloplasmin levels.[38] Fibromyalgia causes muscle pain in specific locations and has a normal ESR. Signs of thyroid disease (tachycardia and hyperreflexia) and parathyroid disease (polyuria and ulcer disease) should help differentiate these endocrine abnormalities from PMR.

Patients with GCA, an inflammation of blood vessels, frequently have symptoms of PMR.[37] However, in addition to symptoms of PMR, these patients also have symptoms of headache, pain in the jaw with chewing (jaw claudication), and visual changes, including scotoma, or blindness. The major complication of GCA is blindness caused by occlusion of the artery that supplies the retina. The diagnosis of GCA is suspected in a patient with PMR who has headache, visual symptoms, or jaw claudication, and the diagnosis is confirmed by biopsy of the temporal artery. Almost all GCA patients have an ESR that is markedly increased. In rare circumstances, the ESR may be normal or minimally increased. Thrombocytosis is a risk factor for permanent visual loss.[52] This unusual manifestation may occur when patients have received low-dose corticosteroids, which may suppress the ESR without controlling the disease.[76] Another complication of GCA is the formation of aneurysms and occlusion in large vessels. For example, thoracic aortic aneurysm occurs late in the course of the illness. These occlusive episodes can cause infarction of the spinal cord with associated neurologic dysfunction.[32]

Polymyositis

Polymyositis is an inflammatory disease of muscle associated with muscle weakness. Muscle pain occurs in 50% of patients with polymyositis. Muscle weakness and pain occur in the shoulder and pelvic girdle, but low back pain can rarely be an associated symptom. A muscle biopsy showing inflammatory changes helps differentiate polymyositis from PMR.[8] The presence of increased serum creatine kinase concentrations should also raise suspicion for the diagnosis of polymyositis. Polymyositis may be associated with tumors such as gastric or ovarian cancer. PMR may also be associated with tumors, particularly myelodysplastic syndromes.[46]

TREATMENT

The generally accepted treatment of PMR is daily corticosteroids. Patients with PMR respond rapidly to corticosteroids with dramatic relief of symptoms. The prompt response is regarded as additional confirmation of the diagnosis. The use of steroids may also help improve the vasculitis that may be associated with GCA. However, the doses needed to control GCA are higher, and GCA has been reported to develop in patients while taking corticosteroids for PMR.[43,44,59]

The dose of corticosteroid is usually 15 mg of prednisone every morning. Many patients have a remarkable diminution of symptoms within 24 to 48 hours.[22] If the patient remains symptomatic, an increase to 25 mg is in order. Doses of 10 mg or less per day of prednisolone are inadequate to control symptoms at the onset.[48] If patients remain symptomatic at this dosage, splitting the dose in the morning and evening may be helpful while limiting any further increase in prednisone dosage. Alternate-day therapy is not usually effective.[48] Intramuscular injections of depot methylprednisolone have also been used to control PMR disease activity. An injection of 120 mg every 3 weeks followed by monthly injections resulted in disease control without suppression of the adrenal gland.[20,54]

The patient's response to therapy is monitored by normalization of the ESR. The CRP level may fall more rapidly with therapy and may be a better test acutely if it is available from a convenient clinical laboratory.[54] CRP is most helpful in monitoring response to therapy during the early stages of the illness. Subsequently, ESR is a more sensitive measure of disease activity. As the ESR or CRP normalizes, the prednisone dose may be tapered slowly. Initially, the dose may be reduced by 2.5 mg until 7.5 mg is reached. The usual time between reductions is 1 month. Once 7.5 mg is reached, the reductions are 1 mg in magnitude. The goal is to wean the patient from corticosteroids by the end of a year, if possible.

Approximately 30% of patients who discontinue steroids before a 2-year period of therapy has concluded are at risk for relapse.[30] A patient with an exacerbation of symptoms has an associated rise in ESR. The prednisone dose should be raised to that patient's initial dosage level. The level can be tapered quickly once symptoms are controlled. After an exacerbation of symptoms, the maintenance dose of prednisone should be kept at a higher level (10 mg) and the pace of tapering slowed to 1 mg every 2 to 3 months. In a study of 210 patients with PMR and GCA, the mean duration of treatment was 27.5 months for PMR and 30.9 months for GCA.[24] In rare circumstances, PMR patients may require corticosteroids for 5 to 7 years.[35] Return of hypothalamic-pituitary-adrenal axis function does not require alternate-day corticosteroid therapy. Patients whose condition is controlled with the equivalent of 5 mg of prednisone have return of function despite daily doses of medicine. The cumulative dose does not affect return of function.[50]

Corticosteroids have many toxicities, including osteopenia, which may be particularly troublesome in elderly women. These same women are the individuals at greatest risk for PMR. Nonsteroidal anti-inflammatory drugs (NSAIDs) may be useful in diminishing symptoms in PMR patients. They may act as steroid-sparing agents. However, in general, NSAIDs are helpful only in patients with mild disease whose diagnosis may be called into question. Deflazacort, another form of corticosteroid, is effective in controlling the disease activity of PMR without the toxicity associated with prednisone. Cortisol secretion is not suppressed and calcium excretion is increased by deflazacort.[36] A very rare, but potentially serious manifestation of corticosteroid toxicity is epidural lipomatosis.[72] A patient with epidural lipomatosis is at risk for neurologic deficits from neural compression. Immunosuppressive drugs, particularly azathioprine, have been used to decrease the steroid dependence of patients with PMR,[23] especially those with compression fractures secondary to chronic corticosteroid use. The immunosuppressives are not benign drugs and increase a patient's risk for infection or malignancy. Immunosuppressives should be used only after other alternative therapies have been tried.[3]

Patients with GCA require high-dose (60 mg or more) corticosteroids to control disease. These higher doses are necessary to diminish the risk of blindness developing.[43] The frequency of steroid toxicity may be as high as 66%, if weight gain is included as a side effect, with doses of prednisolone of 30 mg/day or greater.[49] Methotrexate has been used with corticosteroids and is an effective combination therapy for GCA.[45]

PROGNOSIS

The course of PMR is usually benign. In one study of 76 patients, most patients were able to have their disease controlled with a mean prednisone dosage of 22.8 mg/day.[1] Ayoub and colleagues suggest that patients with PMR may be divided into two groups.[1] The first group has limited disease that lasts about 2 years. The second group has disease that is active for 3 to 4 years. These patients require higher doses for a longer period.[1] No specific characteristic could be ascertained that helps predict the classification of individual patients.

References

Polymyalgia Rheumatica

1. Ayoub WT, Franklin CM, Torretti D: Polymyalgia rheumatica: Duration of therapy and long-term outcome. Am J Med 79:309, 1985.
2. Barber HS: Myalgic syndrome with constitutional effects: Polymyalgia rheumatica. Ann Rheum Dis 16:230, 1957.
3. Barilla-LaBarca M, Lenshow DJ, Brasington RD Jr: Polymylagia rheumatica/temporal arteritis: Recent advances. Curr Rheumatol Rep 4:39-46, 2002.
4. Bell W, Klinefelter HF: Polymyalgia rheumatica. Johns Hopkins Med J 121:175, 1967.
5. Bengtsson BA, Malmvall BE: Giant cell arteritis. Acta Med Scand Suppl 658:1, 1982.
6. Bielroy L, Ogunkoya A, Frohman LP: Temporal arthritis in blacks. Am J Med 86:707, 1989.
7. Bird HA, Esselinck W, Dixon A, et al: An evaluation of criteria for polymyalgia rheumatica. Ann Rheum Dis 38:434, 1979.
8. Bohan A, Peter JB, Bowman RL, Pearson CM: A computer-assisted analysis of 153 patients with polymyositis and dermatomyositis. Medicine (Baltimore) 56:255, 1977.
9. Brooke MH, Kaplan H: Muscle pathology in rheumatoid arthritis, polymyalgia rheumatica and polymyositis: A histochemical study. Arch Pathol 94:101, 1972.
10. Bruk MI: Articular and vascular manifestations of polymyalgia rheumatica. Ann Rheum Dis 26:103, 1967.
11. Cantini F, Salvarani C, Olivieri I, et al: Erythrocyte sedimentation rate and C-reactive protein in the evaluation of disease activity and severity in polymyalgia rheumatica: A prospective follow-up study. Semin Arthritis Rheum 30:17-24, 2000.
12. Cantini F, Salvarani C, Olivieri I, et al: Inflamed shoulder structures in polymyalgia rheumatica: A case-control study. J Rheumatol 28:1049-1055, 2001.
13. Carter JD, Vasey FB, Kanik S, et al: Polymyalgia rheumatica and temporal arteritis with sacroiliitis and osteitis pubis. J Clin Rheumatol 7:261-264, 2001.
14. Chelazzi G, Broggini M: Abnormalities of peripheral blood T lymphocyte subsets in polymyalgia rheumatica. Clin Exp Rheumatol 2:333, 1984.
15. Chou C, Schumacher HR Jr: Clinical and pathologic studies of synovitis in polymyalgia rheumatica. Arthritis Rheum 27:1107, 1984.
16. Chuang TY, Hunder GG, Ilbtrup DM, Kurland LT: Polymyalgia rheumatica: A 10-year epidemiologic and clinical study. Ann Intern Med 97:672, 1982.
17. Cid MC, Ercilla G, Vilaseca J, et al: Polymylagia rheumatica: A syndrome associated with HLA-DR4 antigen. Arthritis Rheum 31:678, 1988.
18. Cimmino MA, Caporali R, Montecucco CM, et al: A seasonal pattern in the onset of polymyalgia rheumatica. Ann Rheum Dis 49:521, 1990.
19. Coomes EN, Sharp J: Polymyalgia rheumatica—a misnomer? Lancet 2:1328, 1961.
20. Dasgupta B, Gray J, Fernandes I, et al: Treatment of polymyalgia rheumatica with intramuscular injection of depot methylprednisolone. Ann Rheum Dis 50:942, 1991.
21. Dasgupta D, Panayi GS: Interleukin-6 in serum of patients with polymyalgia rheumatica and giant cell arteritis. Br J Rheumatol 29:456, 1990.
22. Davison S, Spiera H: Concepts and treatment in polymyalgia rheumatica. J Mt Sinai Hosp N Y 35:473, 1968.
23. De Silva M, Hazelman BL: Azathioprine in giant cell arteritis–polymyalgia rheumatica: A double-blind study. Ann Rheum Dis 45:136, 1986.
24. Delecoueillerie G, Joly P, Cohen de Lara A, et al: Polymyalgia rheumatica and temporal arteritis: A retrospective analysis of prognostic features and different corticosteroid regimens (1-year survey of 210 patients). Ann Rheum Dis 47:733, 1989.
25. Docken WP: Case 23-2002. N Engl J Med 347:272-278, 2002.
26. Duhaut P, Bosshard S, Calvert A, et al: Giant cell arteritis, polymyalgia rheumatica, and viral hypothesis: A multicenter, prospective case-control study. J Rheumatol 26:361-369, 1999.
27. Espinoza LR, Jara LJ, Silveira LH, et al: Anticardiolipin antibodies in polymyalgia rheumatica–giant cell arteritis: Association with severe vascular complications. Am J Med 90:474, 1991.
28. Faerk KK: Simultaneous occurrence of polymyalgia rheumatica in a married couple. J Intern Med 231:621, 1992.
29. Fassbender R, Simmling-Annefeld M: Ultrastructural examination of the skeletal muscles in polymyalgia rheumatica. J Pathol 137:181, 1982.
30. Fauchald P, Rygvold O, Ystsese B: Temporal arteritis and polymyalgia rheumatica: Clinical and biopsy findings. Ann Intern Med 77:845, 1972.
31. Fernandez-Herlihy L: Polymyalgia rheumatica. Semin Arthritis Rheum 1:236, 1971.
32. Fruchter O, Ben-Ami H, Schapira D, et al: Giant cell arteritis complicated by spinal cord infarction: A therapeutic dilemma. J Rheumatol 29:1556-1558, 2002.
33. Gordon I: Polymyalgia rheumatica: A clinical study of 21 cases. Q J Med 29:473, 1960.
34. Gordon I, Rennie AM, Branwood AW: Polymyalgia rheumatica: Biopsy studies. Ann Rheum Dis 23:447, 1964.
35. Gran JT: Current therapy of polymyalgia rheumatica. Scand J Rheumatol 28:269-272, 1999.
36. Gray RE, Doherty GM, Galloway J, et al: A double-blind study of deflazacort and prednisone in patients with chronic inflammatory disorders. Arthritis Rheum 34:287, 1991.
37. Hamilton CR, Shelley WM, Tumulty PA: Giant cell arteritis including temporal arteritis and polymyalgia rheumatica. Medicine (Baltimore) 50:1, 1971.
38. Hantzschel H, Bird HA, Seidel W, et al: Polymyalgia rheumatica and rheumatoid arthritis of the elderly: A clinical, laboratory, and scintigraphic comparison. Ann Rheum Dis 50:619, 1991.
39. Haworth S, Ridgeway J, Stewart I, et al: Polymylagia rheumatica is associated with both HLA-DRB1*0401 and DRB1*0404. Br J Rheumatol 35:632-635, 1996.
40. Healy LA: Long term follow up of polymyalgia rheumatica: Evidence for synovitis. Semin Arthritis Rheum 13:322-328, 1984.
41. Healy LA, Parker F, Wilske KR: Polymyalgia rheumatica and giant cell arteritis. Arthritis Rheum 14:138, 1971.
42. Hunder GG: Giant cell arteritis and polymyalgia rheumatism. In Kelley WN, Harris ED, Ruddy S Jr, Sledge CB (eds): Textbook of Rheumatology, 4th ed. Philadelphia, WB Saunders, 1993, pp 1103-1112.
43. Hunder GG, Allen GL: Giant cell arteritis: A review. Bull Rheum Dis 29:980, 1978.
44. Hunder GG, Sheps SG, Allen GI, Joyce JW: Daily and alternate-day corticosteroid regimens in treatment of giant cell arteritis: Comparison in prospective study. Ann Intern Med 82:613, 1975.
45. Jover JA, Hernandez-Garcia C, Morado IC, et al: Combined treatment of giant-cell arteritis with methotrexate and prednisone. A randomized, double-blind, placebo-controlled trial. Ann Intern Med 134:106-114, 2001.
46. Kohli M, Bennett RM: An association of polymyalgia rheumatica with myelodysplastic syndromes. J Rheumatol 21:1357, 1994.
47. Kyle V, Cawston TE, Hazelman BL: Erythrocyte sedimentation rate and C-reactive protein in the assessment of polymyalgia rheumatica/giant cell arteritis on presentation and during followup. Ann Rheum Dis 48:667, 1989.
48. Kyle V, Hazelman BL: Treatment of polymyalgia rheumatica and giant cell arteritis: I. steroid regimens in the first two months. Ann Rheum Dis 48:658, 1991.
49. Kyle V, Hazelman BL: Treatment of polymyalgia rheumatica and giant cell arteritis: II. relation between steroid dose and steroid-associated side effects. Ann Rheum Dis 48:662, 1989.
50. LaRochelle GE, LaRochelle AG, Ratner RE, et al: Recovery of the hypothalamic-pituitary-adrenal (HPA) axis in patients with rheumatic disease receiving low-dose prednisone. Am J Med 95:258, 1993.
51. Liang M, Greenberg H, Pincus T, Robinson WS: Hepatitis B antibodies in polymyalgia rheumatica. Lancet 1:43, 1976.
52. Liozon E, Hermann F, Ly K, et al: Risk factors for visual loss in giant cell (temporal) arteritis: A prospective study of 174 patients. Am J Med 111:211-217, 2001.
53. Macchioni P, Boiardi L, Meliconi R, et al: Elevated soluble intercellular adhesion molecule 1 in the serum of patients with polymyalgia rheumatica: Influence of steroid treatment. J Rheumatol 21:1860, 1994.
54. Mallya RK, Hind CR, Berry H, Pepys MB: Serum C-reactive protein in polymyalgia rheumatica: A prospective serial study. Arthritis Rheum 28:383, 1985.

55. Miller LD, Stevens MB: Skeletal manifestations of polymyalgia rheumatica. JAMA 240:27, 1978.
56. Montanaro M, Bizarri F: Non-Hodgkin's lymphoma and subsequent acute lymphoblastic leukemia in a patient with polymyalgia rheumatica. Br J Rheumatol 31:277, 1992.
57. Mowat AG, Hazelman BL: Polymyalgia rheumatica: A clinical study with particular reference to arterial disease. J Rheumatol 1:190, 1974.
58. O'Duffy JD, Wahner HW, Hunder GG: Joint imaging in polymyalgia rheumatica. Mayo Clin Proc 51:519, 1976.
59. Papadakis MA, Schwartz ND: Temporal arteritis after normalization of erythrocyte sedimentation rate in polymyalgia rheumatica. Arch Intern Med 146:2283, 1986.
60. Papaioannou CC, Hunder CG, McDuffie FC: Cellular immunity in polymyalgia rheumatica and giant cell arteritis: Lack of response to muscles or artery homogenates. Arthritis Rheum 22:740, 1979.
61. Park JR, Jones JG, Harkiss GD, Hazelman BL: Circulating immune complexes in polymyalgia and giant cell arteritis. Ann Rheum Dis 40:360, 1981.
62. Proven A, Gabriel SE, O'Fallon WM, Hunder GG: Polymyalgia rheumatica with low erythrocyte sedimentation rate at diagnosis. J Rheumatol 26:1333-1337, 1999.
63. Sakhas LI, Loqueman N, Panayi GS, et al: Immunogenetics of polymyalgia rheumatica. Br J Rheumatol 29:331, 1990.
64. Salvanari C, Cantini F, Boiardi L, et al: Polymyalgia rheumatica and giant-cell arteritis. N Engl J Med 347:261-271, 2002.
65. Salvarani C, Cantini F, Olivieri I, et al: Proximal bursitis in active polymyalgia rheumatica. Ann Intern Med 127:27-31, 1997.
66. Salvarani C, Gabriel SE, O'Fallon WM, Hunder GG: Epidemiology of polymyalgia rheumatica in Olmstead County, Minnesota, 1970-1991. Arthritis Rheum 38:369, 1995.
67. Salvanari C, Gabriel SE, O'Fallon WM, et al: The incidence of giant cell arteritis in Olmstead County, Minnesota: Apparent fluctuations in a cyclic pattern. Ann Intern Med 123:192-194, 1995.
68. Salvarani C, Hunder GG: Giant cell arteritis with low erythrocyte sedimentation rate: Frequency of occurrence in a population-based study. Arthritis Rheum 45:140-145, 2001.
69. Salvarini C, Macchioni P, Boiardi L, et al: Soluble interleukin-2 receptors in polymyalgia rheumatica/giant cell arteritis: Clinical and laboratory correlations. J Rheumatol 19:1100, 1992.
70. Sattar MA, Cawley MID, Hamblin TJ, Robertson JC: Polymyalgia rheumatica and antimitochondrial antibodies. Ann Rheum Dis 43:264, 1984.
71. Sidhom DA, Basalaev M, Sigal LH: Renal cell carcinoma presenting as polymyalgia rheumatica: Resolution after nephrectomy. Arch Intern Med 153:2043, 1993.
72. Tabron J: Epidural lipomatosis as a cause of spinal cord compression in polymyalgia rheumatica. J Rheumatol 18:286, 1991.
73. Von Knorring J, Wasastjerna C: Liver involvement in polymyalgia rheumatica. Scand J Rheumatol 8:197, 1976.
74. Weyand CM, Goronzy JJ: Arterial wall injury in giant cell arteritis. Arthritis Rheum 42:844-853, 1999.
75. Weyand CM, Goronzy JJ: The pathogenesis of giant cell arteritis. Bull Rheum Dis 51(8):1-9, 2002.
76. Wise CM, Agudelo CA, Shelley WM, Tumulty PA: Giant cell arteritis with low erythrocyte sedimentation rate: A review of five cases. Arthritis Rheum 34:1571, 1991.

FIBROMYALGIA

CAPSULE SUMMARY

	LOW BACK	NECK
Frequency of spinal pain	Common	Very common
Location of spinal pain	Buttocks	Paracervical muscles, occiput
Quality of spinal pain	General ache, sharp pain with pressure over tender points	General ache, sharp pain with pressure over tender points
Symptoms and signs	Generalized fatigue, muscle soreness, multiple tender points	Generalized fatigue, muscle soreness, multiple tender points
Laboratory tests	None	None
Radiographic findings	None	None
Treatment	Rest, aerobic exercise, antidepressants, NSAIDs	Rest, aerobic exercise, antidepressants, NSAIDs

PREVALENCE AND PATHOGENESIS

Fibromyalgia (FM) is a soft tissue, pain amplification syndrome. It is characterized by chronic pain in discrete tender point areas and specific sleep disturbance that occurs in a perfectionist, compulsive individual. FM is not associated with any structural abnormalities of muscle, bone, or cartilage. However, the persistent pain and chronic fatigue associated with the syndrome prevent patients from achieving their full potential.

The concept of FM has evolved over many years. The central theme of the disease has been the tender point or fibrositic nodule, which was first described in 1824 by Balfour.[4] These areas were only tender with pressure, in contrast to trigger points, which were soft tissue regions that spontaneously caused radiating pain.[45] Myofascial pain syndromes were defined as muscle disorders with symptoms that were amplified by abnormalities in the central nervous system (CNS).[76] Subsequently, Gowers introduced the term *fibrositis*, although no inflammatory alterations could be identified in muscle.[34] More recently, a specific set of symptoms and signs have become associated with FM.[85] Although some authors do not believe that FM is a distinct entity, this disease has been reported by other rheumatologists to have a prevalence in the United States of 3 to 6 million.[37,79]

Epidemiology

The prevalence and incidence of FM are unknown; however, many primary care physicians believe FM to be a common disease, with more than 10 million Americans affected.[75] FM is 10 times more common in women than men. In the United States, the prevalence is approximately 2% and increases with age.[48] In the family practice setting, 2.1% of patients have FM.[39] In rheumatology practices, the syndrome is present in 12% to 20% of new patients.[84,97] The syndrome occurs most commonly in white women at a mean age of 29 years, or 34 years if all patients with other rheumatic conditions are excluded.[97] The prevalence was reported to be 2% in a general community population, 3.4% in women, and 0.5% in men with a mean age of 59 years.[87] The syndrome has also been found in other populations in Europe, Africa, and Asia.[14,27]

Pathogenesis

Central Nervous System

Pain Processing

The exact etiology of the disease is unknown. The hypothesis that best explains the clinical symptoms is that of a disorder of central pain signaling, with the CNS functioning in an overly sensitive manner to nociceptive and non-nociceptive stimuli. Patients with FM perceive various sensory stimuli (heat, pressure) as painful at lower levels of physical stimulation than controls do.[9,29,46] FM patients may experience "wind-up" in the CNS. Repetitious stimulation of a peripheral nerve results in a progressive increase in magnitude of the electrical response in the CNS. The biochemical equivalent of "wind-up" is activation of *N*-methyl-D-aspartate (NMDA) receptors. These receptors mediate chronic pain. This augmented sensory processing is called non-nociceptive pain. Characteristics of non-nociceptive pain include poor correlation with tissue pathology, hyperalgesia, allodynia, and expansion of receptive fields.[9] Modification of pain transmission also occurs in the cerebral cortex. Different areas of the brain are activated in response to pain as determined by regional brain blood flow using functional MR imaging. FM patients have more brain activation than controls do when similar pressure is applied.[35]

Sleep Abnormalities

Moldofsky and colleagues suggested that specific disturbances in sleep may result in the development of FM.[59] The abnormality in sleep is the superimposition of light stages of sleep, characterized by alpha waves on the electroencephalogram, on deep stages of sleep, characterized by delta waves (non–rapid eye movement sleep). In a second study, Moldofsky and Scarisbrick produced FM symptoms in healthy volunteers when their deep sleep was interrupted by loud noises for 3 days.[58] Phasic alpha activity simultaneous with delta activity is the sleep pattern most closely associated with the clinical manifestations of FM.[63] Sleep disturbances are frequent complaints of patients with FM.[16,56] FM may be a disorder of nonrestorative sleep in which a disorder of serotonin metabolism results in musculoskeletal pain. Chlorpromazine, a drug that increases delta sleep, decreased patients' pain and tender points in one study.[56] However, the role of sleep in the pathogenesis of FM remains in question because other studies have not been able to reproduce the findings of Moldofsky and other groups of patients (those with depression) have similar sleep disturbances without pain.[30,57,82]

Abnormalities in sleep are thought to disorder the processing of painful stimuli by the CNS.[93] The CNS is capable of modifying the way it processes a variety of impulses (neuronal plasticity).[26] These abnormalities can lower pain thresholds. Substance P levels in the CNS (not in serum) are higher in FM patients than in control subjects.[62,78]

Neuroendocrine/Autonomic Nervous System Abnormalities

Other measures of CNS dysfunction include an abnormal cortisol response, decreased somatomedin C levels, and decreased serotonin levels.[10,54,67] For example, women with FM have a reduced sympathetic nervous system response to hypoglycemia.[2] The sensitivity of tender points and secondary manifestations of FM are related to autonomic system activity and may be modified by sympathetic inhibition.[6] Individuals with FM have orthostatic hypotension.[51] FM patients also have increased supine resting heart rates.[23] Irritable bowel syndrome is present in 32% of FM patients.[73] These abnormalities are not exclusive to FM and may be of secondary importance and not the mechanism causing the disease. Abnormalities in the promoter region of the serotonin transporter gene are found in FM patients.[61,22] Individuals with these gene abnormalities have greater depression and psychological stress.

Muscle Metabolism

Fowler and Kraft suggested that patients with FM have increased muscle tone.[28] When performing a standardized task, they have 50% more electrical activity on the electromyogram than normal control subjects do. In a study of fatigue characteristics as measured by surface integrated electromyographic activity, FM patients had findings similar to those of control subjects.[74] Individuals with increased muscle tension and abnormal sleep patterns may be at risk for FM. Muscle metabolism may be disordered in patients with FM. A decrease in levels of adenosine triphosphate, adenosine diphosphate, and phosphoryl creatine and an increase in levels of adenosine monophosphate and creatine were found in the trapezius muscle of patients with FM. These findings suggest that the source of pain in patients with FM may be local tissue hypoxia.[8] Other studies have reported similar results in FM and control patients in regard to generation of muscle force and lactate production during exercise.[38] This similarity in findings suggests that muscle deconditioning is a phenomenon caused by pain and inactivity.

Trauma

Smythe has suggested that trauma in a single incident or repeated episodes may be a cause of FM.[72] In an anxious, perfectionist-type person, trauma in areas of increased sensitivity may result in perpetuation of pain long after the injury and associated pain that should have subsided. For example, cervical FM may develop in cab drivers, and FM of the back may develop in bus drivers. The association of trauma and FM remains a conjecture because no prospective study has been completed that demonstrates this relationship. A 10-year follow-up study of patients who were traumatized as a result of motor vehicle accidents, work injuries, surgery, or sports injuries revealed that 56 of 67 (83%) had 11 or more tender points. Other symptoms were similar to those of primary FM patients.[80] The relationship between trauma in the workplace and FM remains to be determined.[13,50]

Psychiatric Disturbance

FM was also thought to be a psychogenic disorder and was classified with psychogenic rheumatism.[68] Most recent studies have shown no increased prevalence of psychological disorders in patients with FM in comparison to normal control subjects.[20] The majority of patients with FM do not have any psychiatric disorder.[32] Some of the psychiatric difficulties associated with these patients may be related to chronic pain and dysfunction.[55]

CLINICAL HISTORY

Patients with FM complain of generalized aching pain associated with profound stiffness and fatigue. Areas of pain are confined to articular and periarticular structures, including ligaments, tendons, muscles, and bony prominences. The pain may be unremitting, with durations of 20 years or longer. Generalized stiffness is most notable in the morning and usually lasts up to an hour. A smaller percentage of patients have evening stiffness, and some patients have daylong stiffness. Fatigue is also a prominent feature of patients with FM. Characteristically, these patients arise in the morning feeling exhausted after a restless sleep. Some patients complain of unrelenting fatigue. Other clinical features include polyarthralgias, occasionally associated with hand swelling, numbness, headaches, and anxiety.

Cold or humid weather, overactivity, total inactivity, and poor sleep exacerbate FM. Patients with FM have increased symptoms with changes in barometric pressure.[36] Factors that improve symptoms include moderate activity, warm dry weather, and massage.

FM also occurs in older patients, who have clinical findings similar to those of younger patients. In a study of 31 older patients with FM, only 17% had the disease diagnosed before referral to a rheumatologist. A significant number of these patients were treated inappropriately with corticosteroids.[96] In a spine center setting, 12% of 125 referred patients had FM. The diagnosis was not recognized by the majority of physicians who referred these patients. These patients had clinical symptoms and signs of FM when examined for the disease.[12]

PHYSICAL EXAMINATION

Physical examination demonstrates specific areas that are tender on palpation. These areas are referred to as tender points and are localized to certain anatomic sites. The most commonly affected areas include the upper border of the trapezius, the medial part of the knees, the lateral border of the elbows, the posterior iliac crest, and the lumbar spine. Pressure over the area results in a pattern of local pain (Fig. 11-43). There is no tenderness outside the local area. In one study, patients had 4 to 33 tender points.[97] Usually, patients with primary FM have 12 or more discrete areas. The exact location that differentiates patients with FM from control subjects continues to be evaluated. Some locations that may be useful include the anterior shoulder, anterior chest, posterior scapula, and medial knee areas.[69]

Patients with FM may have fibrositic nodules located about the sacrum and posterior iliac crest. The nodules are mobile, firm, and tender on palpation. Results of biopsy of these nodules demonstrate fibrofatty tissue without inflammation. Other than the finding of tender points and nodules, the physical examination is normal, with full range of motion of the cervical and lumbosacral spine.

LABORATORY DATA

Laboratory parameters are normal. Blood studies, hematologic parameters, the erythrocyte sedimentation rate, rheumatoid factor, and antinuclear antibody are all normal in primary FM. Among the findings that are normal are serum tryptophan levels, absence of autoantibodies, and distribution of human leukocyte antigens.[7,42,95] Assessment of the hypothalamic-pituitary-adrenal axis reveals low 24-hour urinary free cortisol, hyporesponsiveness of the adrenal gland to stimulation, and decreased levels of neuropeptide Y.[24] The clinical importance of these laboratory results has not been determined.

Pathology

Pathologic evaluation of muscle biopsy specimens is unrevealing on histoimmunochemical and ultrastructural

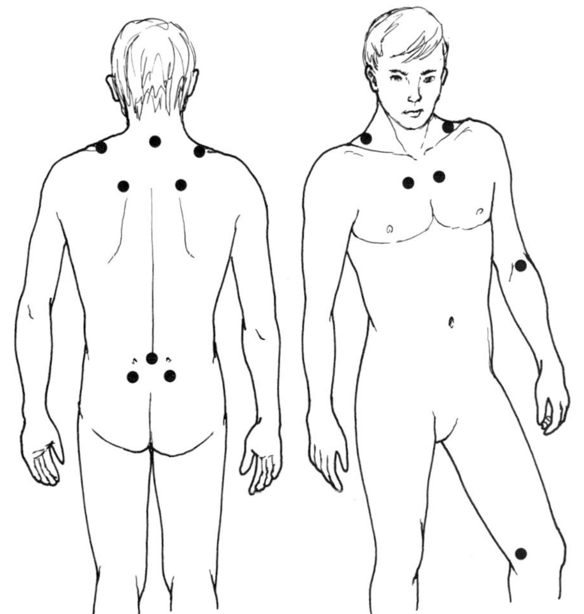

Figure 11-43 Diagram of common sites of tenderness on palpation in fibromyalgia patients.

studies. Biopsy may be important only to eliminate other disorders as the cause of muscle pain.[25]

RADIOGRAPHIC EVALUATION

Radiographic findings are normal in patients with FM. The results of bone scintiscans are no different in FM patients and control subjects.[94]

DIFFERENTIAL DIAGNOSIS

The diagnosis of primary FM is based on the presence of characteristic musculoskeletal abnormalities in the absence of stigmata of other diseases. Patients who have diffuse aching and fatigue of at least 3 months' duration, at least 12 tender points, and disturbed sleep patterns probably have FM. No specific physical or laboratory findings are pathognomonic for this disease. Therefore, the diagnosis of FM is one of exclusion, and these patients require constant re-evaluation. A variety of diagnostic criteria have been proposed for FM.[85,97] Goldenberg has divided the clinical characteristics of the disease into major and minor criteria (Table 11-13).[31] The presence of three major criteria and four of six minor criteria was necessary for the diagnosis of FM by Goldenberg's approach. In 1990, a committee of the American College of Rheumatology presented classification criteria for FM (Table 11-14).[89]

Repeat evaluation is necessary to detect early physical or laboratory findings indicative of an underlying disease process such as rheumatoid arthritis or a malignancy. Patients with an underlying disease and muscle pain have secondary FM. Other diseases associated with secondary FM include rheumatoid arthritis, osteoarthritis, spondyloarthropathies, connective tissue diseases, malignancies, hypothyroidism, hyperparathyroidism, chronic infections, and sarcoidosis.[5] FM also develops in patients infected with human immunodeficiency virus.[70] Characteristic physical findings, inflammatory joint signs, laboratory abnormalities, increased sedimentation rate, and positive rheumatoid factor help differentiate these diseases from primary FM.

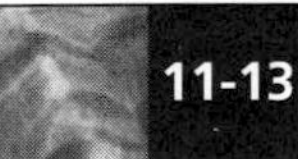

11-13 DIAGNOSTIC CRITERIA FOR FIBROMYALGIA

MAJOR CRITERIA

Chronic, generalized aches, pains, or stiffness (involving ≥3 anatomic sites for ≥3 mo)
Absence of other systemic condition to account for these symptoms
Multiple tender points at characteristic locations

MINOR CRITERIA

Disturbed sleep
Generalized fatigue or tiredness
Subjective swelling, numbness
Pain in neck, shoulders
Chronic headaches
Irritable bowel symptoms

Modified from Goldenberg DL: Fibromyalgia syndrome: An emerging but controversial condition. JAMA 257:2782, 1987.

11-14 AMERICAN COLLEGE OF RHEUMATOLOGY CLASSIFICATION CRITERIA FOR FIBROMYALGIA

1. History of widespread pain. Pain is on both sides of the body and above and below the waist. Low back pain is considered lower segment pain.
2. Pain in 11 of 18 tender points on digital palpation—4 kg of force should be applied with digital pressure. The site must be painful, not tender.

Widespread pain should be present for 3 months or more. A second clinical disorder does not exclude the diagnosis of fibromyalgia.

Modified from Wolfe F, Smythe HA, Yunus MB, et al: The American College of Rheumatology 1990 criteria for the classification of fibromyalgia: Report of the Multicenter Criteria Committee. Arthritis Rheum 33:160, 1990.

Psychogenic Rheumatism

FM must also be differentiated from psychogenic rheumatism, which is characterized by significant anxiety, depression, or neurosis.[65] Patients with psychogenic rheumatism have severe pain of a burning or cutting quality. The pain is excruciating in intensity and without any recognizable anatomic boundaries. Patients usually deny stiffness. On examination, they have a marked response to minimal pressure on palpation. Their areas of tenderness do not correspond to the tender points of FM. Laboratory evaluation of these patients is normal, and their complaints are resistant to all forms of therapy.

Chronic Fatigue Syndrome

Chronic fatigue syndrome is another disorder with a clinical spectrum that overlaps with FM. Patients with FM, chronic fatigue syndrome, and temporomandibular disorders share clinical symptoms.[1] This syndrome is associated with chronic fatigue that does not resolve with bed rest, no other complicating illness, mild fever, sore throat, painful lymph nodes, muscle weakness, headaches, arthralgias, and insomnia.[40] The severity of fatigue is greater in patients with chronic fatigue syndrome. In a review of patients with FM, only 20% fulfilled the criterion of fatigue.[60]

Myofascial Pain Syndrome

Myofascial pain syndrome (MPS) is a regional pain syndrome characterized by two major components: the first is a localized area of deep muscle tenderness (trigger point) that is accompanied by a palpable abnormality in muscle consistency (fibrositic nodule), and the second is a specific area of referred pain distant from the trigger point.[77] Muscles in patients with MPS have extreme tenderness on palpation, decreased flexibility, abnormal consistency, pain on contraction, and a localized "twitch response" to rapid snapping of the trigger point or fibrositic nodules. Pressure over a trigger point results in a dull, aching pain in a referral pattern that does not follow any characteristic myotomal structure. A trigger point may be a muscle region of increased energy consumption with an inadequate oxygen supply.[71] Neck pain is a common symptom in patients with MPS.[15] The neck muscles associated with MPS and their associated pain radiation are listed in Table 11-15. The muscles affected in the lumbar spine and legs are listed in Table 11-16. MPS and FM are not the same disease, although superficially they seem quite similar. MPS is a localized pain syndrome with sudden onset and trigger points with distant referred pain. FM is a diffuse pain syndrome with gradual onset, multiple tender points, and disturbed sleep. It is controversial whether MPS exists as a separate clinical entity. The characteristic clinical findings of MPS, including trigger points, may not be different in patients with MPS or FM or normal control subjects.[88] Therapy for MPS consists of injection of local anesthetic into trigger points along with the use of superficial cooling in association with muscle stretching. In patients with chronic MPS symptoms, local injection of botulinum toxin (which blocks the release of acetylcholine) has decreased pain for a small number.[19] Several clinical, psychological, and sociologic factors are associated with a poor response to trigger point injections. These factors (unemployment, constant pain, and poor coping ability) suggest that the pain associated with MPS goes beyond abnormal muscle physiology.[41]

TREATMENT

Treatment of FM requires a multifactorial approach.[33] In many circumstances, educating patients about their illness is reassuring and relieves some symptoms. Many patients are encouraged by having a specific diagnosis for their ailments. Their symptoms are no longer "in their head." They are told that their condition is not life-threatening, deforming, or degenerating, but that it causes chronic pain.

Rest and relaxation are important for patients who are overworked. Patients are encouraged to remain at work, but they should not become excessively fatigued.[97] Some patients require a change in their job status to lighter duty. Simple interventions in the environment, including chairs with cervical support, cervical pillows, a firm mattress, and a comfortable work position, may have a beneficial effect on pain. Range-of-motion and stretching exercises encourage improved muscle function. Patients are also encouraged to participate in an aerobic exercise program. Studies have demonstrated the benefit of cardiovascular training in reducing pain in FM patients.[53] The exercise program should also contain a home component so that patients become active participants in their own care.[64] Heat treatments are also useful. Drug therapy in the form of aspirin or other nonsteroidal anti-inflammatory drugs (NSAIDs) is helpful in reducing the pain associated with FM.[5] NSAIDs are preferred over acetaminophen for symptomatic relief.[90] Injection of tender points with a combination of an anesthetic agent and a long-acting corticosteroid is helpful in controlling localized pain.[47] Systemic corticosteroids are not used in patients with primary FM.[21] Non-narcotic analgesics, such as tramadol, may be helpful in decreasing pain in an attempt to improve physical function. Narcotics are also not indicated for this disease.

Tricyclic Antidepressants

With the thought that abnormal serotonin metabolism plays a role in the pathogenesis of FM, antidepressants and muscle relaxants that increase serotonin levels have been studied in controlled short-term, placebo-based drug trials. Cyclobenzaprine hydrochloride (Flexeril), a tricyclic muscle relaxant, produced significant improvement in pain, sleep, and tender points at dosages of 10 to 40 mg/day when compared with placebo.[11] Improvement was also seen in another study with another tricyclic drug, amitriptyline hydrochloride (Elavil), at a dose of 50 mg at bedtime.[18] Amitriptyline, when effective, results in decreased symptoms within 2 weeks of starting therapy.[44] A report of a controlled study of 208 patients undergoing a 6-month trial of cyclobenzaprine, amitriptyline, and placebo demonstrated no benefit of active drug versus placebo after the first few weeks of therapy.[17] Imipramine hydrochloride at 50 to 75 mg/day had no beneficial effect on the symptoms of FM.[92] Marginal benefit has been associated with aprazolam.[66] The antidepressant fluoxetine is not helpful in decreasing pain in FM patients.[86] Tizanidine at a dose of 2 to 4 mg at sleep may be helpful

11-15 PAIN LOCATION AND MUSCLES ASSOCIATED WITH MYOFASCIAL PAIN SYNDROME OF THE NECK

Muscle with Trigger Point	Physical Abnormality with Pain	Referred Pain Distribution
Trapezius	Active rotation of head toward opposite side, side bending	Upper posterolateral neck, scapulas
Levator scapulae	Decreased neck rotation	Base of neck, medial scapulas
Splenius capitis	Decreased neck flexion, rotation same side	Vertex of head
Splenius cervicis	Decreased neck flexion, rotation same side	Occiput, back of orbit, angle of neck
Semispinalis capitis/cervicis, multifidus	Decreased neck flexion, extension, rotation	Occiput, above orbit, angle of neck
Suboccipital	Decreased head flexion, rotation, side bending	Occiput, back of orbit

From Travell JG, Simons DG: Myofascial Pain and Dysfunction: The Trigger Point Manual: The Upper Extremities. Baltimore, Williams & Wilkins, 1983, p 713.

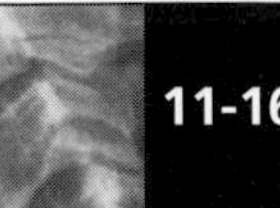

11-16 PAIN LOCATION AND MUSCLES ASSOCIATED WITH MYOFASCIAL PAIN SYNDROME

Muscle with Trigger Point	Referred Pain Distribution
Quadratus lumborum	Buttock, sacrum, abdominal wall
Iliopsoas	Paravertebral lumbar spine, anterior thigh
Pelvic floor (obturator internus, levator ani)	Sacrum, posterior thigh
Gluteus maximus	Sacrum, buttock
Gluteus medius	Sacrum, buttock, lateral thigh
Gluteus minimus	Buttock, lateral thigh, lateral calf
Piriformis	Buttock, posterior thigh

in individuals who are intolerant of tricyclics. A meta-analysis of antidepressant therapy for FM demonstrated beneficial effects. The largest improvement is associated with sleep quality, whereas more modest effects were found with stiffness and tenderness.[3]

The basic program of therapy for a patient with FM is a tricyclic agent along with patient education and controlled activity in a physical therapy program. The addition of an NSAID is optional, depending on the patient's muscle pain. Injection of tender points is useful if they are few in number.

All these modes of therapy do have a beneficial effect on the symptoms of FM; however, FM is a chronic disease that may be exacerbated by a number of factors, including increased tension, exposure to cold, and sleep disturbances. Compliance with a program is essential for long-term management. Appropriate rest, exercise, and stress management may control disease symptoms without the need to use medications or injections.

Men with FM may have sleep apnea as a cause of their chronic pain syndrome. These patients may benefit from therapy directed at improving their sleep apnea.[52]

PROGNOSIS

The course of FM is one of exacerbations and remissions. Patients have neck, low back, knee, and chest pain that hinders their ability to perform up to their potential. Wood, in a study of English workers, reported that nonarticular rheumatism, which included patients with FM, accounted for 10.9% of absences from work and corresponded to 10.5% of the days lost from work.[91] FM may go unrecognized for an extended period. In such circumstances, a person may be thought of as a malingerer who is unwilling to do a full day's work. FM is a chronic condition. In a 4-year follow-up study of FM patients, 97% continued to experience symptoms and 85% fulfilled the diagnostic criteria for FM.[49] In one study of over 500 FM patients treated by rheumatologists, the clinical symptoms of pain, insomnia, and anxiety were unchanged at 8-year follow-up.[83] FM patients treated by primary care physicians may have a better prognosis. In one study, 35% of FM patients had resolution of their symptoms at 2 years.[81] The difference may relate to the severity of symptoms in patients treated by rheumatologists. The disease is associated with functional disability and high levels of anxiety and depression despite therapy.[43]

Although FM is not disabling in the same sense as the spondyloarthropathies, it is associated with reduced productivity and absenteeism. Recognition of the disease and institution of appropriate therapy can have a beneficial effect on a patient's outlook and work performance.

References

Fibromyalgia

1. Aaron LA, Burke MM, Buchwald D: Overlapping conditions among patients with chronic fatigue syndrome, fibromyalgia, and temporomandibular disorder. Arch intern Med 160:221-227, 2000.
2. Adler GK, Kinsley BT, Hurwitz S, et al: Reduced hypothalamic-pituitary and sympathoadrenal responses to hypoglycemia in women with fibromyalgia syndrome. Am J Med 106:534-543, 1999.
3. Arnold LM, Keck PE Jr, Welge JA: Antidepressant treatment of fibromyalgia: A meta-analysis and review. Psychosomatics 41:104-113, 2000.
4. Balfour W: Observations with cases illustrative of a new, simple, and expeditious mode of curing rheumatism and sprains. Lond Med Phys J 51:446, 1824.
5. Beetham WP Jr: Diagnosis and management of fibrositis syndrome and psychogenic rheumatism. Med Clin North Am 63:433, 1979.
6. Bengtsson M, Bengtsson A, Jorfeldt L: Diagnostic epidural opioid blockade in primary fibromyalgia at rest and during exercise. Pain 39:171, 1989.
7. Bengtsson A, Ernerudh J, Vrethem M, et al: Absence of autoantibodies in primary fibromyalgia. J Rheumatol 17:1682, 1990.
8. Bengtsson A, Henriksson KG, Larsson J: Reduced high-energy phosphate levels in the painful muscle of patients with primary fibromyalgia. Arthritis Rheum 24:817, 1986.
9. Bennett RM: Emerging concepts in the neurobiology of chronic pain: Evidence of abnormal sensory processing in fibromyalgia. Mayo Clin Proc 74:385-398, 1999.
10. Bennett RM, Clark SR, Campbell SM, et al: Low levels of somatomedin C in patients with fibromyalgia syndrome: A possible link between sleep and muscle pain. Arthritis Rheum 35:550, 1992.
11. Bennett RM, Gatter RA, Campbell SM, et al: A comparison of cyclobenzaprine and placebo in the management of fibrositis: A double-blind controlled study. Arthritis Rheum 31:1535, 1988.
12. Borenstein D: Prevalence and treatment outcome of primary and secondary fibromyalgia in patients with spinal pain. Spine 20:796, 1995.
13. Buskila D: Fibromyalgia, chronic fatigue syndrome, and myofascial pain syndrome. Curr Opin Rheumatol 13:117-127, 2001.
14. Buskila D, Press J, Gedalia A, et al: Assessment of nonarticular tenderness and prevalence of fibromyalgia in children. J Rheumatol 20:368, 1993.
15. Campbell SM: Regional myofascial pain syndromes. Rheum Dis Clin North Am 15:31, 1989.
16. Campbell SM, Clark S, Tyndall EA, et al: Clinical characteristics of fibrositis: I. A "blinded" controlled study of symptoms and tender points. Arthritis Rheum 26:817, 1983.
17. Carette S, Bell MJ, Reynolds WJ, et al: Comparison of amitriptyline, cyclobenzaprine, and placebo in the treatment of fibromyalgia: A randomized, double-blind clinical trial. Arthritis Rheum 37:32, 1994.
18. Carette S, McCain GA, Bell DA, Fam AG: Evaluation of amitriptyline in primary fibrositis. Arthritis Rheum 29:655, 1986.
19. Cheshire WP, Abashian SW, Mann JD: Botulinum toxin in the treatment of myofascial pain syndrome. Pain 59:65, 1994.
20. Clark S, Campbell SM, Forehand ME, et al: Clinical characteristics of fibrositis. Arthritis Rheum 28:132, 1985.
21. Clark S, Tindall E, Bennett RM: A double-blind crossover trial of prednisone versus placebo in the treatment of fibrositis. J Rheumatol 12:980, 1985.
22. Cohen H, Buskila D, Neumann L, et al: Confirmation of an association between fibromyalgia and serotonin transporter promoter region (5-HTTLPR) polymorphism and relationship to anxiety-related personality traits. Arthritis Rheum 46:845-847, 2002.

23. Cohen H, Neumann L, Shore M, et al: Autonomic dysfunction in patients with fibromyalgia: Application of power spectral analysis of heart rate variability. Semin Arthritis Rheum 29:217-227, 2000.
24. Crofford LJ, Pillemer SR, Kalogera KT, et al: Hypothalamic-pituitary-adrenal axis perturbations in patients with fibromyalgia. Arthritis Rheum 37:1583, 1994.
25. Drewes A, Andreasen A, Schnider HD, et al: Pathology of skeletal muscle in fibromyalgia: A histo-immuno-chemical and ultrastructural study. Br J Rheumatol 32(suppl):479, 1993.
26. Dubner R: Hyperalgesia and expanded receptive fields. Pain 48:3, 1992.
27. Forseth KO, Gran JT: The prevalence of fibromyalgia among women aged 20-49 years in Arendal, Norway. Scand J Rheumatol 21:74, 1992.
28. Fowler RS Jr, Kraft GH: Tension perception in patients having pain associated with chronic muscle tension. Arch Phys Med Rehabil 55:28, 1974.
29. Gibson SJ, Littlejohn GO, Gorman MM, et al: Altered heat pain thresholds and cerebral event–related potentials following painful CO_2 laser stimulation in subjects with fibromyalgia syndrome. Pain 58:185-193, 1994.
30. Golden H, Weber SM, Bergen D: Sleep studies in patients with fibrositis syndrome. Arthritis Rheum 26:S32, 1983.
31. Goldenberg DL: Fibromyalgia syndrome: An emerging but controversial condition. JAMA 257:2782, 1987.
32. Goldenberg DL: Psychiatric and psychologic aspects of fibromyalgia syndrome. Rheum Dis Clin North Am 15:105, 1989.
33. Goldenberg DL: Treatment of fibromyalgia syndrome. Rheum Dis Clin North Am 15:61, 1989.
34. Gowers WR: Lumbago: its lessons and analogues. BMJ 1:117, 1904.
35. Gracely RH, Petzke F, Wolf JM, et al: Functional magnetic resonance imaging evidence of augmented pain processing in fibromyalgia. Arthritis Rheum 46:1333-1343, 2002.
36. Guedj D, Weinberger A: Effect of weather conditions on rheumatic patients. Ann Rheum Dis 49:158, 1990.
37. Hadler WM: Medical Management of the Regional Musculoskeletal Disease. New York, Grune & Stratton, 1985.
38. Hakkinen A, Hakkinen K, Hannonen P, et al: Force production capacity and acute neuromuscular responses to fatiguing loading in women with fibromyalgia are not different from those of healthy women. J Rheumatol 27:1277-1282, 2000.
39. Hartz A, Kirchdoerfer E: Undetected fibrositis in primary care practice. J Fam Pract 25:365, 1987.
40. Holmes GP, Kaplan JE, Gabtz NM, et al: Chronic fatigue syndrome: A working case definition. Ann Intern Med 108:387, 1988.
41. Hopwood MB, Abram SE: Factors associated with failure of trigger point injections. Clin J Pain 10:227, 1994.
42. Horven S, Stiles TC, Holst A, et al: HLA antigens in primary fibromyalgia syndrome. J Rheumatol 19:1269, 1992.
43. Hudson JI, Goldenberg DL, Pope HG, et al: Comorbidity of fibromyalgia with medical and psychiatric disorders. Am J Med 92:363, 1992.
44. Jaeschke R, Adachi J, Guyatt G, et al: Clinical usefulness of amitriptyline in fibromyalgia: The results of 23 N-of-1 randomized controlled trials. J Rheumatol 18:447-451, 1991.
45. Kellgren JH: Observations on referred pain arising from muscle. Clin Sci 3:175, 1938.
46. Kosek E, Ekholm J, Hansson P: Sensory dysfunction in fibromyalgia patients with implications for pathogenic mechanisms. Pain 68:375-383, 1996.
47. Kraus H: Triggerpoints. N Y State J Med 73:1310, 1973.
48. Lawrence RC, Helmick CG, Arnett FC, et al: Estimates of the prevalence of arthritis and selected musculoskeletal disorders in the United States. Arthritis Rheum 41:778-799, 1998.
49. Ledingham J, Doherty S, Doherty M: Primary fibromyalgia syndrome: An outcome study. Br J Rheumatol 32:139, 1993.
50. Littlejohn GO: Fibrositis/fibromyalgia syndrome in the workplace. Rheum Dis Clin North Am 15:45, 1989.
51. Martinez-Lavin M: Management of dysautonomia in fibromyalgia. Rheum Dis Clin North Am 28:379-387, 2002.
52. May KP, West SG, Baker MR, et al: Sleep apnea in male patients with the fibromyalgia syndrome. Am J Med 94:505, 1993.
53. McCain GA, Bell DA, Mai FM, et al: A controlled study of the effects of supervised cardiovascular fitness training program on the manifestations of primary fibromyalgia. Arthritis Rheum 31:1135, 1988.
54. McCain GA, Tilbe KS: Diurnal hormone variation in fibromyalgia syndrome: A comparison with rheumatoid arthritis. J Rheumatol Suppl 19:154, 1989.
55. Merskey H: Physical and psychological considerations in the classification of fibromyalgia. J Rheumatol Suppl 16:72, 1989.
56. Moldofsky A, Lue FA: The relationship of alpha and delta EEG frequencies to pain and mood in fibrositis patients treated with chlorpromazine and L-tryptophan. Electroencephalogr Clin Neurophysiol 50:71, 1980.
57. Moldofsky H: Workshop on sleep studies. Am J Med 81(suppl 3A):107, 1986.
58. Moldofsky H, Scarisbrick P: Induction of neurasthenic musculoskeletal pain syndrome by selective sleep stage deprivation. Psychosom Med 38:35, 1976.
59. Moldofsky H, Scarisbrick P, England R, Smythe H: Musculoskeletal symptoms and non-REM sleep disturbance in patients with “fibrositis syndrome” and healthy subjects. Psychosom Med 37:341, 1975.
60. Norregaard J, Bulow PM, Prescott E, et al: A four-year follow-up study in fibromyalgia: Relationship to chronic fatigue syndrome. Scand J Rheumatol 22:35, 1993.
61. Offenbaecher M, Bondy B, de Jonge S, et al: Possible association of fibromyalgia with a polymorphism in the serotonin transporter gene regulatory region. Arthritis Rheum 42:2482-2488, 1999.
62. Reynolds WJ, Chiu B, Inman RD: Plasma substance P levels in fibrositis. J Rheumatol 15:1802, 1988.
63. Roizenblatt S, Moldofsky H, Benedito-Silva AA, et al: Alpha sleep characteristics in fibromyalgia. Arthritis Rheum 44:222-230, 2001.
64. Rosen NB: Physical medicine and rehabilitation approaches to the management of myofascial pain and fibromyalgia syndromes. Baillieres Clin Rheumatol 8:881, 1994.
65. Rotes-Querol J: The syndromes of psychogenic rheumatism. Clin Rheum Dis 5:797, 1979.
66. Russell IJ, Fletcher EM, Michalek JE, et al: Treatment of primary fibrositis/fibromyalgia syndrome with ibuprofen and alprazolam: A double-blind, placebo-controlled study. Arthritis Rheum 34:552, 1991.
67. Russell IJ, Vaeroy H, Javors M, et al: Cerebrospinal fluid biogenic amine metabolites in fibromyalgia/fibrositis syndrome and rheumatoid arthritis. Arthritis Rheum 35:550, 1992.
68. Savage O: Management of rheumatic diseases in the armed forces. BMJ 2:336, 1942.
69. Simms RW, Goldenberg DL, Felson DT, et al: Tenderness in 75 anatomic sites: distinguishing fibromyalgia patients from controls. Arthritis Rheum 31:182, 1988.
70. Simms RW, Zerbini CA, Ferrante N, et al: Fibromyalgia syndrome in patients infected with human immunodeficiency virus: The Boston City Hospital clinical AIDS team. Am J Med 92:368, 1992.
71. Simons DG: Myofascial pain syndromes: Where are we? Where are we going? Arch Phys Med Rehabil 69:207, 1988.
72. Smythe HA: Non-articular rheumatism and psychogenic musculoskeletal syndromes. In McCarty DJ Jr (ed): Arthritis and Allied Conditions, 10th ed. Philadelphia, Lea & Febiger, 1985, pp 1083-1094.
73. Sperber AD, Atzmon Y, Neumann L, et al: Fibromyalgia in the irritable bowel syndrome: Studies of prevalence and clinical implications. Am J Gastroenterol 94:3541-3546, 1999.
74. Stokes MJ, Colter C, Klevstov A, et al: Normal paraspinal muscle electromyographic fatigue characteristics in patients with primary fibromyalgia. Br J Rheumatol 32:71, 1993.
75. The American Rheumatism Association Committee on Rheumatologic Practice: A description of rheumatology practice. Arthritis Rheum 20:1278, 1977.
76. Travell J, Ringler SH: The myofascial genesis of pain. Postgrad Med 11:425, 1952.
77. Travell JG, Simons DG: Myofascial Pain and Dysfunction. The Trigger Point Manual: The Upper Extremities, Vol 1. Baltimore, Williams & Wilkins, 1992.
78. Vaeroy H, Helle R, Forre O, et al: Elevated CSF levels of substance P and high incidence of Raynaud's phenomenon in patients with fibromyalgia: New features for diagnosis. Pain 32:21, 1988.
79. Wallace DJ: Systemic lupus erythematosus, rheumatology, and medical literature: Current trends. J Rheumatol 12:913, 1985.
80. Waylonis GW, Perkins RH: Post-traumatic fibromyalgia: A long-term follow-up. Am J Phys Med Rehabil 73:403, 1994.

81. White KP, Speechley M, Harth M, et al: Comparing self-reported function and work disability in 100 community cases of fibromyalgia syndrome versus controls in London, Ontario: The London Fibromyalgia Epidemiology Study. Arthritis Rheum 42:76-83, 1999.
82. Wittig R, Zorick FJ, Blumer D, et al: Disturbed sleep in patients complaining of chronic pain. J Nerv Ment Disord 170:429, 1982.
83. Wolfe F, Anderson J, Harkness D, et al: Health status and disease severity in fibromyalgia: Results of a six-center longitudinal study. Arthritis Rheum 40:1571-1579, 1997.
84. Wolfe F, Cathey MA: Prevalence of primary and secondary fibrositis. J Rheumatol 10:965, 1983.
85. Wolfe F, Cathey MA: The epidemiology of tender points: A prospective study of 1520 patients. J Rheumatol 12:1164, 1985.
86. Wolfe F, Cathey MA, Hawley DJ: A double-blind placebo-controlled trial of fluoxetine in fibromyalgia. Scand J Rheumatol 23:255, 1994.
87. Wolfe F, Ross K, Anderson J, et al: The prevalence and characteristics of fibromyalgia in the general population. Arthritis Rheum 38:19, 1995.
88. Wolfe F, Simons DG, Fricton J, et al: The fibromyalgia and myofascial pain syndromes: A preliminary study of tender points and trigger points in persons with fibromyalgia, myofascial pain syndrome, and no disease. J Rheumatol 19:944, 1992.
89. Wolfe F, Smythe HA, Yunus MB, et al: The American College of Rheumatology 1990 criteria for the classification of fibromyalgia: Report of the Multicenter Criteria Committee. Arthritis Rheum 33:160, 1990.
90. Wolfe F, Zhao S, Lane N: Preference for nonsteroidal anti-inflammatory drugs over acetaminophen by rheumatic disease patients: A survey of 1,799 patients with osteoarthritis, rheumatoid arthritis, and fibromyalgia. Arthritis Rheum 43:378-385, 2000.
91. Wood PHN: Rheumatic complaints. Br Med Bull 27:82, 1971.
92. Wysenbeek AJ, Mor F, Lurie Y, Weinberger A: Imipramine for the treatment of fibrositis: A therapeutic trial. Ann Rheum Dis 44:752, 1985.
93. Yunus MB: Toward a model of pathophysiology of fibromyalgia—aberrant central pain mechanism with peripheral modulation. J Rheumatol 19:846, 1992.
94. Yunus MB, Berg BC, Masi AT: Multiphase skeletal scintigraphy in primary fibromyalgia syndrome: A blinded study. J Rheumatol 16:1466, 1989.
95. Yunus MB, Dailey JW, Aldag JC, et al: Plasma tryptophan and other amino acids in primary fibromyalgia: A controlled study. J Rheumatol 19:90, 1992.
96. Yunus MB, Holt GS, Masi AT: Fibromyalgia syndrome among the elderly: Comparison with younger patients. J Am Geriatr Soc 36:987, 1988.
97. Yunus M, Masi AT, Calabro JJ, et al: Primary fibromyalgia (fibrositis): Clinical study of 50 patients with matched normal controls. Semin Arthritis Rheum 11:151, 1981.

CHAPTER 12

INFECTIONS OF THE SPINE

Infections of the spine are uncommon causes of low back or neck pain but they must be included in the differential diagnosis of the patient with systemic spinal pain. This is particularly important because the outcome of these infections is excellent if the disease processes are recognized early and treated appropriately. When spinal infections are not promptly recognized, however, they can lead to catastrophic complications, including spinal deformity and spinal cord compression with associated paralysis, incontinence, and, ultimately, death.

The clinical symptoms and course of spinal infections depend on the organism involved. Bacterial infections cause acute, toxic symptoms, whereas tuberculous and fungal diseases are more indolent in onset and course. The primary symptom of patients with spinal infection is spinal pain that tends to be localized over the anatomic structure involved. Infection of the meninges will cause severe neck pain and headache. Physical examination demonstrates decreased motion, muscle spasm, and percussion tenderness over the involved area. Results of common laboratory tests are not always present, and they are nonspecific. Radiographic abnormalities including vertebral body subchondral bone loss, disc space narrowing, and erosions of contiguous bony structures are helpful when present but often lag behind clinical symptoms by weeks to months. Patients may present with nondescript spinal pain ascribed to "degenerative disc disease" on plain roentgenograms, only to develop increasing low back or neck pain, neurologic dysfunction, and marked bony destruction on radiographic evaluation over a short period.

The definitive diagnosis of spinal infection requires identification of the offending organism by culturing aspirated or sampled material from the lesion. Treatment consists of antimicrobial drugs directed against the specific organism causing the infection, immobilization with bed rest to relieve pain, a cast if spinal instability is present, and surgical drainage of abscesses to relieve spinal cord compression. Patients who have a prompt diagnosis and appropriate antimicrobial therapy are able to combat the infection without residual disability. Significant disability from persistent pain, spinal instability, and spinal cord compression may occur when there has been a delay in diagnosing persistent osteomyelitis or epidural abscess. These patients require surgical decompression and stabilization.

Herpes zoster is a viral infection of dorsal root ganglia that causes severe pain in association with a rash. The diagnosis of this infection is easy in the presence of a dermatomal rash but quite difficult in the period before the rash appears. Postherpetic neuralgia, a complication of the infection, causes significant morbidity with persistent spinal pain, particularly in the elderly population.

Lyme disease is a spirochetal infection caused by *Borrelia burgdorferi*. Low back or neck pain is a manifestation associated with the early stage of the illness and the appearance of a characteristic rash, erythema migrans. In later stages of the illness, polyradiculitis affecting the upper or lower extremities may develop. The diagnosis of Lyme disease is established by a history of tick exposure, characteristic symptoms and signs, and confirmatory laboratory tests. The illness is treated by the use of oral or intravenous antibiotics.

VERTEBRAL OSTEOMYELITIS

See page 410 for Capsule Summary.

PREVALENCE AND PATHOGENESIS

Vertebral osteomyelitis is a disease process caused by the growth of a potentially wide variety of organisms in the bones that comprise the axial skeleton. These organisms include some of the following bacteria: *Staphylococcus aureus*, *Escherichia coli*, and *Brucella abortus*; mycobacteria: *Mycobacterium tuberculosis*; fungi: *Coccidioides immitis*; spirochetes: *Treponema pallidum*; and parasites: *Echinococcus granulosus*. Vertebral osteomyelitis develops most commonly from hematogenous spread through the bloodstream. The clinical symptoms and course depend on the infecting organism and the associated host inflammatory response. Bacterial infections are generally associated with an acute, toxic reaction, whereas granulomatous infections caused by tuberculous or fungal organisms are more indolent in onset and course. The diagnosis of vertebral osteomyelitis is frequently missed because patient symptoms are ascribed to more common causes of spinal pain, such as muscle strain, and radiographic changes lag behind the evolution of the infection.

Capsule Summary

	Low Back	Neck
Frequency of spinal pain	Very common	Very common
Location of spinal pain	Lumbar spine or sacrum—involved bone	Cervical spine, involved bone
Quality of spinal pain	Sharp ache, radicular with nerve compression	Sharp ache, radicular with nerve compression
Symptoms and signs	General malaise, percussion tenderness, fever	General malaise, percussion tenderness, fever
Laboratory tests	Leukocytosis, increased erythrocyte sedimentation rate	Leukocytosis, increased erythrocyte sedimentation rate
Radiographic findings	Subchondral bone loss on plain roentgenogram, soft tissue mass on CT scan, abnormal signal on MR imaging	Subchondral bone loss on plain roentgenogram, soft tissue mass on CT scan, abnormal signal on MR imaging
Treatment	Antibiotics, immobilization	Antibiotics, immobilization, fusion for instability

Epidemiology

Over a 10-year period, 348 cases of vertebral osteomyelitis were reported in the medical literature.[175] In a study from 1979, the incidence of vertebral osteomyelitis was estimated at 1 in 250,000 individuals.[46] The frequency is increasing since that time secondary to increasing illicit intravenous drug use, nosocomial infections secondary to implanted devices, and the aging of the population. Vertebral involvement has been found to account for 2% to 4% of all cases of osteomyelitis.[95] In one study, more than 52% of patients with vertebral osteomyelitis were 50 years of age or older.[149] Another article reviewed 397 vertebral osteomyelitis patients in the literature and reported the mean age of adults with the disease to be from 45 to 62 years.[156] Those in the seventh decade of life represented the single largest group. Another group between 20 to 40 years of age more recently identified includes those with human immunodeficiency virus (HIV) who develop opportunistic infections.[178] Tuberculosis remains a frequent cause of infection in Southeast Asia, sub-Saharan Africa, and eastern Europe.[48] The male-to-female ratio is 3:1.

The lumbar spine is the most frequently affected area of the spine, followed by the thoracic spine, with the sacrum and cervical spine affected in equal frequencies.[60] However, different studies do report different frequencies of involvement. The frequency of infections in one study was 48% in the lumbar spine, 35% in the thoracic spine, 7% in the cervical spine, and 5% both in the thoracolumbar and lumbosacral junctions.[149] In another study of 40 patients with vertebral osteomyelitis, 42.5% had lumbar infection, 30% had cervical osteomyelitis, and 27.5% had thoracic disease.[126] In another, the cervical vertebrae were involved in 27% of patients with vertebral osteomyelitis.[150]

In general, the cervical spine is a rare location for osteomyelitis of the spine. Approximately 8% of patients with vertebral osteomyelitis have cervical involvement (Table 12-1).[156] In intravenous drug users, the frequency of cervical vertebral osteomyelitis is increased.

Pathogenesis

Vertebral body bone is most frequently infected by hematogenous spread through the bloodstream. It is supplied by the paravertebral venous system and nutrient arteries.[12,182] The venous Batson's plexus is a network of valveless veins that lines the vertebral column, and the flow in this venous system is modified by changes in intra-abdominal pressure. Increased pressure tends to force blood from infected areas into the veins of the vertebral column. The presence of cellular bone marrow and the sluggish venous blood flow have been suggested as predisposing factors for bone infection.[2] Although genitourinary infections are more frequent in women than men, the incidence of vertebral osteomyelitis is higher in men. A possible explanation is the highly vascularized tissue around the longer urethra, which may develop metastatic infection

12-1 VERTEBRAL SITE OF PYOGENIC VERTEBRAL OSTEOMYELITIS (n = 396 patients)

Vertebral Site	No. of Patients	% of Patients
Cervical	32	8.0
Cervical thoracic	1	0.3
Thoracic	137	35.0
Thoracolumbar	31	8.0
Lumbar	168	42.0
Lumbosacral	26	7.0
Sacral	1	0.3

From Schwartz ST, Spiegel M, Ho G Jr: Bacterial vertebral osteomyelitis and epidural abscess. Semin Spine Surg 2:95, 1990.

after urologic manipulation.[149] Other potential hematogenous sources of infection include soft tissue infection, infective endocarditis, dental extraction, furunculosis, and intravenous drug abuse.[74,149]

On the other hand, the localization of early foci of osteomyelitis in vertebral bodies in the subchondral region corresponds to an area richly supplied by nutrient arteries.[182] The spread of infection from extraspinal foci is associated with the constitutional symptoms of septicemia. It is probable that both routes may be involved in individual patients.

Infection from contiguous sources, direct implantation by cisternal puncture or disc operations, is relatively rare compared with that caused by hematogenous spread. Occasional patients with vertebral osteomyelitis may have a history of prior trauma to the spine, but trauma usually does not play a role in the pathogenesis of hematogenous vertebral osteomyelitis.[60] Studies of patients with vertebral osteomyelitis and epidural abscess, however, report a significant percentage with a history of substantial trauma before the development of the infection.[9] Hematoma associated with trauma can become a culture medium for hematogenously spread organisms. The role of minor trauma, such as muscle strain, as a predisposing factor for vertebral osteomyelitis is uncertain. The importance of unrelated and coincident minor trauma may be overestimated in some patients with vertebral osteomyelitis, thus confusing the diagnosis and delaying the initiation of appropriate antibiotic therapy to the disadvantage of the patient. Injection into the jugular vein by heroin addicts is a form of trauma that is associated with the increased risk of cervical osteomyelitis.[52] Hematogenous or contiguous spread may be the mechanism of infection in patients who develop cervical osteomyelitis after endotracheal intubation, dental extraction, or esophagoscopy.[11,109,135]

Grisel's syndrome, spontaneous atlantoaxial subluxation in association with infection in neighboring soft tissue structures, may occur secondary to hematogenous spread from the pharyngovertebral veins to the periodontoidal venous plexus.[129] This syndrome occurs in children most often and is associated with infections in the throat, including pharyngitis, tonsillitis, alveolar periostitis, adenitis, and pharyngeal ulcers.[180] These people experience neck pain and torticollis.

Approximately 40% or more of patients with vertebral osteomyelitis have an unequivocal extraspinal primary source for infection.[146] The usual locations for these infections include the genitourinary tract, skin, and respiratory tract (Table 12-2).[156] Parenteral drug abusers also develop vertebral osteomyelitis, particularly with *Pseudomonas aeruginosa*.[92] Any person with a chronic disease that decreases host immunity, such as diabetes mellitus, chronic alcoholism, malignancy, and sickle cell anemia, is also at risk of developing vertebral osteomyelitis.[156] Other medical disorders and personal habits that predispose to the development of vertebral osteomyelitis include rheumatoid arthritis, HIV infection, malignancy, renal failure, smoking, and drug abuse.[3] Cervical vertebral osteomyelitis may be a complication of older people with cervical spondylosis who undergo manipulation by a chiropractor.[101]

The organisms gain entrance into the vertebral bodies in the subchondral area, which is richly supplied by nutrient arterioles on the anterior surface and by the main nutrient artery entering through the posterior vertebral nutrient foramen.[182] The infection may spread across the periphery of the disc to involve the adjacent vertebra or may rupture through the endplates into the disc. The posterior elements are affected less often and later in the course of the infection. The infection spreads through the disc material to reach the opposite endplate and vertebra. The disc material is quickly destroyed by bacterial enzymes. This is in contrast to tuberculous infection, which causes bony destruction but little damage to the intervertebral disc.[33] Infection of three or more vertebral bodies is quite rare. Involvement of the posterior elements of the vertebrae is unusual.

12-2 SOURCE OF INFECTION IN PYOGENIC VERTEBRAL OSTEOMYELITIS (n = 370 patients)

	No. of Patients	% of Patients with Source Identified
Source identified	188	
Genitourinary tract	87	46
Skin	35	19
Respiratory tract	27	14
Spinal surgery	16	9
Bowel	7	4
Intravenous drug abuse	6	3
Dental	4	2
Bacterial endocarditis	1	1
No source identified	182	

From Swartz ST, Spiegel M, Ho G Jr: Bacterial vertebral osteomyelitis and epidural abscess. Semin Spine Surg 2:95, 1990.

An infection of a vertebral body may extend beyond the bone into the soft tissues. Infections in the lumbar spine can produce a psoas abscess, which can become very large. The infection may also drain into the spinal canal, causing an epidural abscess, or penetrate the dura, causing a picture of meningitis.[9] Infections in the cervical spine can produce a retropharyngeal abscess that can become very large.[97] Paravertebral masses may cause draining sinuses. Inferior dissection along fascial planes may cause a mediastinitis. Bone destruction in the lumbar or cervical spine may cause instability, which may result in compression of the spinal cord or nerve roots.[71]

The most frequently encountered organism causing infection is *S. aureus* in up to 60% of cases (Table 12-3).[156] In rare circumstances, *Staphylococcus epidermidis* may cause vertebral osteomyelitis in immunocompetent people.[44] Other gram-positive organisms causing osteomyelitis include streptococci, including *Streptococcus pneumoniae*, and group B streptococci from the vaginal tract.[107] Group G streptococcal osteomyelitis of the spine has been reported in elderly individuals with malignancies.[68] Gram-negative organisms, including *E. coli*, *Pseudomonas*, *Klebsiella*, *Pasteurella*, and *Salmonella*, are relatively uncommon.[21] Other rare gram-negative organisms include *Proteus mirabilis* and polymicrobial infections, including *Bacteroides fragilis*.[27,53,140,150] Anaerobic organisms cause infection in 3% or less of patients.[79,156] Even more infrequent as causes

12-3 BACTERIOLOGY OF PYOGENIC VERTEBRAL OSTEOMYELITIS (n = 220 bacteria)

	No. of Cases	% of Bacterial Isolates
Gram-positive aerobic cocci	159	72
Staphylococcus aureus	139	63
Staphylococcus coagulase negative	5	2
Streptococcal species	15	7
Gram-negative aerobic bacilli	55	24
Escherichia coli	35	16
Proteus species	11	5
Pseudomonas species	3	1
Klebsiella species	3	1
Other*	3	1
Anaerobic bacteria†	6	3

**Serratia* species, *Enterobacter agglomerans*, *Eikenella corrodens*.
†*Corynebacterium diphtheriae*, *Bacteroides fragilis*, *Peptostreptococcus*, and *Propionibacterium*.
From Swartz ST, Spiegel M, Ho G Jr: Bacterial vertebral osteomyelitis and epidural abscess. Semin Spine Surg 2:95, 1990.

of infection are mycobacteria, fungi, spirochetes, and parasites. These frequencies of organisms causing infection depend on the local environment. In certain locations such as Europe and Africa, infections with brucellosis and mycobacterial organisms are more common.[32] In Africa, part of the reason for increased mycobacterial infection is related to the high prevalence of HIV infection in the population.[176]

CLINICAL HISTORY

The primary symptom of patients with vertebral osteomyelitis is spinal pain in a corresponding location. The pain may develop over 8 to 12 weeks before the diagnosis is established in patients.[146] A history of a recent primary infection, or an invasive diagnostic procedure, is common. The pain may be intermittent or constant, may be present at rest, and is exacerbated by motion. Local spine pain is present in 98% of patients with vertebral osteomyelitis, with radicular symptoms in 30%.[126] Dysphagia and persistent sore throat may be seen in about 11% of patients with cervical spine involvement.[149] Patients may also complain of neck stiffness associated with occipital headache. Pain may develop over 8 to 12 weeks before the diagnosis is established. Paralysis is an occasional complication of cervical vertebral osteomyelitis.[103] A significant proportion (9 of 15) of cervical spine osteomyelitis patients in one study developed neurologic deficits that deteriorated rapidly.[153]

Guri described the symptoms of four clinical syndromes of pyogenic vertebral osteomyelitis.[67] Pain may be intermittent or constant, may be present at rest, and is exacerbated by motion. The other three clinical syndromes include patients who may develop a hip joint syndrome characterized by acute pain in the hip with limited motion and flexion contracture. The patient with the abdominal syndrome presents with symptoms that are easily confused with those of appendicitis. Signs of acute meningitis, including positive Kernig and Brudzinski tests and positive straight leg–raising tests, are components of the meningeal syndrome. Paraplegia without back pain is a very rare occurrence.[106]

Bacterial Osteomyelitis

Patients with certain underlying illnesses may develop vertebral osteomyelitis secondary to specific organisms. *S. aureus* is associated with soft tissue infection, endocarditis, or infected intravenous lines. It is a cause of osteomyelitis in older individuals who have concomitant medical illnesses.[123] Pneumococci are associated with respiratory infection. Those with diabetes mellitus or chronic urinary tract infections develop vertebral osteomyelitis secondary to gram-negative bacteria.[60] Parenteral drug abusers develop *Pseudomonas* and *Candida* osteomyelitis.[151] Patients with sickle cell anemia may get *Salmonella* osteomyelitis. Fungal osteomyelitis secondary to *Candida* has been reported to complicate vertebral osteomyelitis previously infected with *Serratia marcescens*.[1]

Brucellar Osteomyelitis

Brucellosis, a disease caused by *Brucella*, affects patients who ingest unpasteurized milk products or, more commonly, since the advent of pasteurization, workers involved with meat processing.[184] The infection, which is passed from lower animals, cattle, or hogs to humans, occurs in government meat inspectors, veterinarians, farmers, stockyard workers, rendering-plant workers, and laboratory personnel. The *Brucella* organisms, *Brucella melitensis* (the most virulent), *Brucella suis*, *Brucella canis*, or *B. abortus*, penetrate the mucous membranes of the oropharynx or enter through breaks in the skin, traverse the lymph nodes, and enter the bloodstream where they spread to the reticuloendothelial system. The clinical manifestations of brucellosis vary and may be classified into asymptomatic or serologic, acute systemic or localized, and chronic or relapsing forms.[111] The most common complication is osseous, occurring in up to 70% of cases.[30,32,63] Patients with *Brucella* spondylitis are men, older than 50 years of age, with preexisting spine disease.[5] The lumbosacral spine is affected most often, with cervical spine disease a rare occurrence.[31,50,138,170] The range of involvement of the cervical spine is between 1% and 3% in large study populations from endemic areas.[88,90] The disease has an insidious onset with intermittent fever, chills, weakness, weight loss, and headache. Patients commonly complain of tenderness of pain over the vertebral bodies, which is worse with activity and relieved by rest.[88,90] Radiation of pain is associated with nerve root irritation of a mechanical or inflammatory nature.[90]

Postsurgical Osteomyelitis

The risk for spinal infection after standard discectomy is 1%. The risk increases to 2% when fusion is added and is 6% when instrumentation is required.[167] Postsurgical spinal infection is caused by *S. aureus* most commonly. *S. epidermidis* and other gram-positive and gram-negative organisms, including *P. aeruginosa*, are other potential organisms.

Mycobacterial Osteomyelitis

Elderly patients, alcoholics, and drug abusers are at greatest risk of developing vertebral osteomyelitis secondary to *M. tuberculosis*.[54] Before antibiotic therapy, children were most frequently affected, but more recent data from patients with skeletal tuberculosis in the United States show average ages of 40 to 51 years.[20,58] Skeletal tuberculosis occurs as a result of hematogenous spread from another source, usually pulmonary, during an acute infection or as a reactivation of a quiescent focus present in bone for many years after initial seeding.[25,62] From 50% to 60% of patients with skeletal tuberculosis have axial skeletal disease.[62] This may be explained in part by the affinity of this organism to relatively high oxygen concentrations that exist in the cancellous bone of the vertebral bodies. Involvement of the spine may be peridiscal, anterior, or central. With peridiscal involvement, tuberculous spondylitis begins in the subchondral area of the vertebral body adjacent to the intervertebral disc and the organism creates an inflammatory process characterized by the formation of granulomas and caseation necrosis of bone. Initially, only the vertebral body is affected; however, the infection can spread to involve contiguous structures, which may include the intervertebral disc, other vertebral bodies, and soft tissues such as muscle and ligaments, to form a paravertebral abscess, or it can spread to the spinal cord and meninges. Sparing of the disc is characteristic, as opposed to pyogenic infection. Anterior involvement involves spread beneath the anterior longitudinal ligament, with anterior erosion over a number of segments. Central involvement remains restricted to one segment.[16] The more extensive the destruction, the greater the potential for deformity of the axial skeleton with kyphoscoliosis and associated spinal cord compression.[157]

The clinical presentation of a patient with tuberculous spondylitis consists of pain over the involved vertebrae radiating into a buttock or lower extremity, low-grade fever, and weight loss of varying duration. Patients with more advanced disease may present with neurologic symptoms and angular deformities of the spine with loss of height. The onset of symptoms is gradual, and the time before presentation to a physician may be as long as 3 years.[64] Paraplegia may be the first manifestation of tuberculous spondylitis even before any deformity of the spine is apparent.[141] In contrast, heroin addicts may present with a more toxic picture associated with back pain, fever, night sweats, weight loss, and neurologic dysfunction of rapid evolution.[54]

Cervical involvement is a rare complication of tuberculous osteomyelitis. In a review of 1000 people with skeletal tuberculosis, cervical involvement was identified in 3.5%.[75] In people with tuberculosis, the cervical spine is affected in 0.03%.[47] Of special consideration with cervical involvement is the potential for cord compression in 40% of patients.[87]

The clinical presentation of a patient with tuberculous osteomyelitis consists of two primary forms. Younger children develop more diffuse and extensive involvement, the formation of the large abscesses, and a lower incidence of quadriplegia. The adult type is more localized and produces less pus but has a higher incidence of paraplegia.[183] In children, pain is found over the involved vertebrae associated with stiffness and with radiation into a shoulder or upper extremity. Low-grade fever and weight loss of varying duration may occur. Patients with more advanced disease may present with neurologic symptoms. Angular deformities of the neck with loss of height occurs less commonly than lesions in the thoracic spine unless three or more vertebral bodies are involved, because the weight of the head is borne through the articular processes rather than the vertebral body. However, when infection in the lower cervical spine spreads down to the upper dorsal region, forward subluxation or dislocation of the cervical spine may occur on the thoracic spine so that the undersurface of the lowest remaining cervical vertebra comes to rest on the anterior surface of the uppermost thoracic vertebra.[75] These lesions may heal with spontaneous fusion of the posterior apophyseal joints.

The second primary form affects adults. The disease is more localized and does not spread as extensively as it does in children. However, quadriplegia is a more common complication of the infection in adults. In a series of 40 patients, 13 of 16 older than 10 years of age with tuberculosis of the lower cervical spine had cord compression versus 4 of 24 younger than 10 years of age.[183] Possible explanations for the increased frequency of quadriplegia may include progressive narrowing of the spinal canal from degenerative disease, loss of flexibility, and inelasticity of the prevertebral fascia.[75] Tuberculous osteomyelitis in adults may spread over more than one intervertebral segment in the cervical spine.[104] This occurs as the infection lifts the supporting longitudinal ligaments and spreads to contiguous structures. The disease may also present as a lesion of a single intervertebral segment or a vertebral body. Solitary lesions are not uncommon in the upper and lower portions of the cervical spine, including the atlantoaxial area.[35,76,99]

The onset of symptoms is gradual, and the time before presentation to a physician may be as long as 3 years.[64] Paraplegia may be the first manifestation of tuberculous spondylitis even before any deformity of the spine is apparent.[141] General symptoms of malaise, fever, weight loss, night sweats, and fatigue precede the onset of spinal pain and stiffness. Pain in the lumbar spine may refer to the buttocks or upper thighs. Pain from lower neck involvement may refer to the shoulders and arms. Upper cervical spine disease may cause occipital or forehead referred pain. Pharyngeal symptoms may be present if an anterior abscess has formed in the retropharyngeal area. Heroin addicts may present with a more toxic picture associated with neck pain, fever, night sweats, weight loss, and neurologic dysfunction of rapid evolution.[54]

In regard to tuberculin skin testing, over 90% of immunocompetent patients with skeletal tuberculosis test positive. However, skin tests may be negative in a small proportion of immunocompetent and a larger proportion of immunocompromised individuals. Therefore, a negative skin test does not eliminate the possibility of tuberculosis as a cause of a vertebral infection.

Fungal Osteomyelitis

Infections secondary to *Actinomyces israelii*, *Nocardia asteroides*, and fungal organisms such as *C. immitis* are rare causes of vertebral osteomyelitis. Patients with *Actinomyces* infection of the spine may develop lesions from extension of adjacent abscesses or from hematogenous spread.[34,158] Actinomycosis may be the cause of anaerobic infection in patients with infected wounds of the face or pressure sores. The clinical course of these infections is similar to that of tuberculosis. These patients present with a history of constitutional symptoms over an extended period and complain of localized pain over the affected vertebral body.[96] *Nocardia*, an aerobic, gram-positive actinomycete, may cause hematogenous spread to vertebral bones in the patients with underlying immunodeficiency.[7] In patients with chronic obstructive pulmonary disease, vertebral *Aspergillus* osteomyelitis may occur without any other form of immunocompromise.[112] Cervical spine infection with *Nocardia* has been reported.[98] Coccidioidomycosis may affect the spine in 50% of the 0.5% of patients with disseminated disease,[113] and it may also infect the upper cervical spine.[143]

Spirochetal Osteomyelitis

Before the advent of penicillin, syphilis was a common cause of axial skeleton infection, but it is currently an extremely rare complication.[77,142] Syphilis may affect the axial skeleton by direct infection of bone or by the loss of normal sensation.[81] Both forms are a result of tertiary syphilis, which is the form of the disease that occurs after the initial infection (primary) and hematogenous spread (secondary) of the organism. Spinal pain is associated with arthritis in larger joints as well as other clinical manifestations of secondary syphilis. The growth of the organism in bone results in the formation of a gumma and bony destruction.[55] The cervical spine is the most frequently affected in the axial skeleton, but the disease also has been detected in the lumbar area.[15] The most common symptom is pain in the involved area, which is greatest at night and is accompanied with stiffness and loss of normal spinal curvatures. Patients may develop neurologic symptoms, including radicular pain secondary to nerve root impingement.[85] Patients with neurosyphilis, on the other hand, lose normal sensation; without this protective awareness, fractures and destruction of the bony skeleton result. This is called a neuropathic arthropathy or Charcot's disease. These patients feel little pain and are frequently symptom free. However, patients may have back pain with bone deformity. This is particularly true if patients develop nerve impingement secondary to spinal instability and collapse.[139] Patients with syphilis may also develop back pain on a muscular or osseous basis in the early stages of neurosyphilis.[145,177]

Parasitic Osteomyelitis

Echinococcus granulosus is a cestode worm of the dog.[4] Intermediate hosts for the ova of this worm are sheep, cattle, hogs, and humans. The ova attach to the intestinal mucosa and gain entrance to the bloodstream where they disseminate, particularly to the liver and occasionally to bone where they form cysts (hydatid disease). The skeleton is affected in about 3% of patients with hydatid disease, and 50% of those cases are found in the spine.[120] The disease produces a slowly destructive lesion of bone that, in the spine, erodes through the vertebral bodies and can rupture into the neural canal. The cysts then migrate up and down the canal. Patients with hydatid disease of the spine have symptoms that can last from a few weeks to 5 years. Pain is a common symptom associated with swelling. Occasionally painless paraplegia of sudden onset may be the presenting sign of disease. Patients may develop neurologic impingement from extraspinal hydatidosis that extends through the neural foramina.[70] Patients who develop paraplegia either die of the disease or are chronically disabled.[171]

PHYSICAL EXAMINATION

Physical findings in patients with vertebral osteomyelitis include a decreased range of motion, muscle spasm, and percussion tenderness over the involved bone. Patients with psoas muscle irritation may demonstrate decreased hip motion along with a flexion contracture. Those with thoracolumbar vertebral osteomyelitis may have abdominal tenderness on palpation. Patients with cervical osteomyelitis may have muscle spasm, torticollis, or Horner's syndrome.[133] They may also have tenderness over the midline and occiput, with pain exacerbation on head compression. An abscess anterior to the spine may be palpable near the throat. Some of the patients with bacterial vertebral osteomyelitis have a fever.[29,46] A body temperature of greater than 100°F was calculated at 52% of one series of vertebral osteomyelitis patients.[149] Neurologic abnormalities, including paraplegia, are reported in a number of series of patients with vertebral osteomyelitis.[56,60,65] In one study, patients who developed paralysis had a period from symptoms to diagnosis of 3 months and were diabetic or had a urinary tract infection.[103] Patients with the more indolent infections of tuberculosis and coccidioidomycosis usually have less fever but greater spinal deformity than those with pyogenic vertebral osteomyelitis.

LABORATORY DATA

The commonly ordered blood tests (complete blood cell count, erythrocyte sedimentation rate [ESR], and serum chemistries) yield results that are normal or nonspecific. The ESR is abnormal in the majority of patients with vertebral osteomyelitis, particularly during the acute phase.[29,60] In a study by Joughin and colleagues, the ESR was better than fever or leukocytosis as a marker of vertebral osteomyelitis.[82] The hematocrit level may be normal, and there is a normal or slightly elevated white blood cell count. A small but significant number of patients have normal ESR and white blood cell counts.[155]

In postsurgical patients, the C-reactive protein (CRP), ESR, and white blood cell count (WBC) are significantly higher for individuals with instrumentation than those without hardware. Individuals who had an infection developed an increase in CRP, ESR, and WBC 4 to 11 days after surgery.[167]

The most useful laboratory test for the diagnosis of vertebral osteomyelitis is the direct culture of blood and bone lesions. This may be abnormal in 50% of patients with acute osteomyelitis and negate the need for bone biopsy. In patients with normal blood cultures, bone aspiration or surgical biopsy produces material that on culture is often abnormal for the offending organism (Fig. 12-1).[25] *S. aureus* is the bacterium associated with vertebral osteomyelitis in up to 60% of patients.[46,65] Gram-negative organisms, *E. coli*, *Proteus*, and *Pseudomonas*, are often grown from elderly patients and parenteral drug abusers with vertebral osteomyelitis. When an infection in the cervical spine is secondary to penetrating trauma, cultures for multiple organisms are appropriate. In cases of stab wounds to the cervical spine, *Staphylococcus pyogenes* with *Bacteroides melaninogenicus* and *Streptococcus viridans* with *Candida albicans* have been identified on culture.[36] Cultures from peripheral sources of infection, such as urinary tract, skin, and respiratory tract, may be abnormal and should be obtained from the patient with suspected vertebral osteomyelitis. The diagnosis of brucellosis is associated with an abnormal bone culture or elevations in brucellar agglutinin titers of 1:32 or greater. Radioimmunoassay and enzyme-linked immunosorbent assay methods for *Brucella* antigens are also available.[130,159] In general, IgM antibodies are associated with acute brucellosis and IgG antibodies are associated with chronic infection.[122]

The purified protein derivative (PPD) test is usually positive for patients with tuberculous spondylitis, unless they are anergic secondary to miliary disease. The number of organisms in an infected spine is less than 1 million bacteria. Therefore, it is appropriate to culture both purulent material and biopsy specimens to improve the potential for a positive culture.[43] Histologic evidence of granulomas suggests tuberculous or fungal infection. The ESR is rarely elevated in tuberculous spondylitis. As far as fungal infections are concerned, antibody titers may be raised or skin tests may be reactive, but none of these tests is as specific as the growth of organisms from either aspirated material or biopsy specimens. The laboratory abnormalities of tertiary syphilis include the presence of antibodies to nontreponemal (Venereal Disease Research Laboratory test) and treponemal (fluorescent treponemal antibody absorption test) antigens. Spirochetal organisms are not usually found in tertiary lesions on histologic examination. The histologic changes include a granulomatous necrotizing process with a prominent obliterative endarteritis.

RADIOGRAPHIC EVALUATION

Roentgenograms

Radiographic changes follow the symptomatic onset of disease by 1 to 2 months (Table 12-4). The early abnormalities in pyogenic vertebral osteomyelitis include subchondral bone loss, narrowing of the disc space, and loss of definition of vertebral body. Continued dissemination of infection may produce soft tissue swelling associated with paravertebral abscesses (loss of psoas shadow). Once the lesion starts to heal, bony regeneration appears and is characterized by osteosclerosis, which may finally result in bony fusion across the disc space (Fig. 12-2). The lumbar vertebrae, particularly the first and second, are the vertebral bodies in the axial skeleton most commonly affected.[9,60,146] In the cervical spine, retropharyngeal swelling can lead to displacement and obliteration of contiguous prevertebral fat planes (Fig. 12-3).[164] Once the lesion starts to heal, bony regeneration appears and is characterized by osteosclerosis, which may finally result in bony fusion across the disc space. Conventional tomograms may be done to obtain better bony and soft tissue details than plain films.

12-4 TIMETABLE FOR RADIOGRAPHIC FINDINGS IN BACTERIAL VERTEBRAL OSTEOMYELITIS

Period	Time of Appearance	Observations
1	3-6 wk	Rarefaction of adjacent body endplates Widening of paraspinal lines Intervertebral space narrowing
2	6-10 wk	Lytic scalloping and destruction of vertebral body endplates Compression of vertebral body as a result of central osteolysis Paravertebral soft tissue mass (abscess)
3	8-12 wk	Reactive sclerosis
4	12-24 wk	New bone formation with bony bridging of disc spaces
5	24 wk and longer	Bony fusion of vertebral bodies

Brucellar spondylitis causes narrowing of the intervertebral disc space and destruction of the contiguous vertebrae, which may be associated with a large paravertebral abscess. Bone sclerosis with parrot-beak exostosis is a late roentgenographic sign and usually indicates the stage of healing.[90]

The vertebral body is more commonly affected than posterior elements in tuberculous spondylitis; they are affected in only 2% of spinal tuberculous cases. The infection causes erosion of the subchondral bone and invades the disc space. These changes occur much less rapidly with tuberculous spondylitis than with pyogenic spondylitis. The infection may also spread to soft tissue, forming paraspinal abscesses (Fig. 12-4). In this form, the anterior cortex of the vertebral body is destroyed. Severe angular deformities occur from marked destruction of vertebral bodies. Vertebral bodies may appear wedge-shaped whereas the disc spaces are preserved. The lesion may look like a vertebra plana and may be confused with eosinophilic granuloma. The reactive sclerosis characteristic of healing pyogenic vertebral osteomyelitis does not occur with tuberculous spondylitis. In many patients the disease is limited to two contiguous vertebrae, although four or more segments may be involved (Fig.12-5).

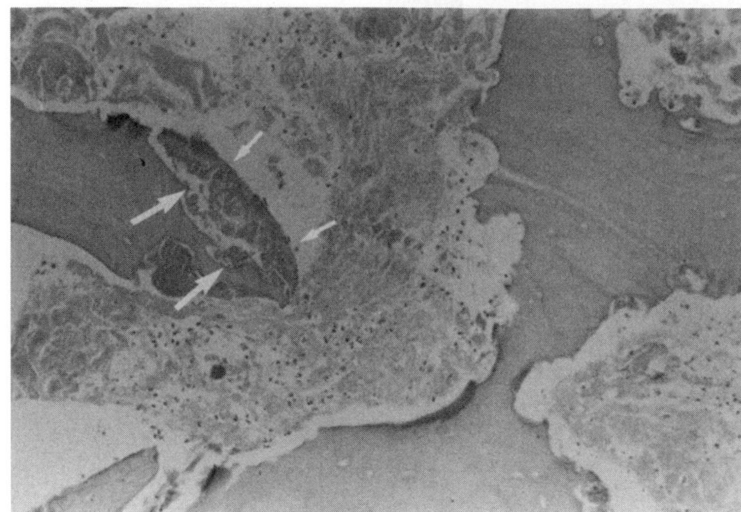

Figure 12-1 Osteomyelitis. Histologic section of acute osteomyelitis demonstrating necrotic bone, fibrin, acute inflammatory cells, and a collection of organisms *(arrows)*. *(Courtesy of Arnold Schwartz, MD.)*

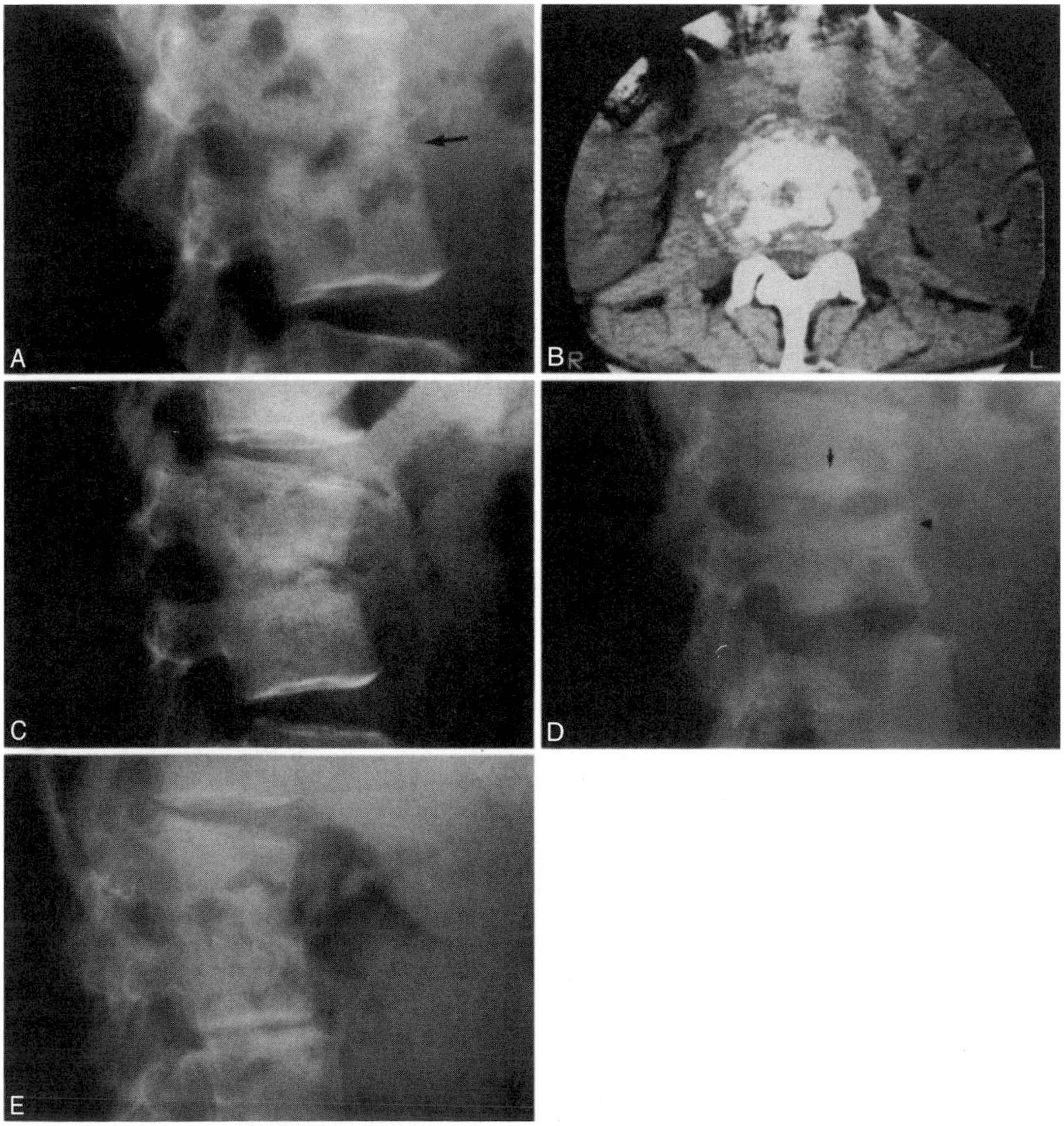

Figure 12-2 Serial roentgenograms of a 41-year-old man with staphylococcal osteomyelitis of the lumbar spine. *A*, 11/8/85. Erosion of the L2 and L3 endplates is associated with destruction of the intervertebral disc *(arrow)*. *B*, 11/20/85. CT scan reveals marked bony destruction associated with soft tissue extension of the infection. *C*, 11/27/85. Further collapse of the L2 vertebral body is seen with reactive sclerosis. *D*, 11/4/86. Reactive sclerosis is noted in the vertebral body *(arrow)* and osteophytes are forming *(arrowhead)* at the body margin. *E*, 1/13/87. Total fusion of the L2 and L3 vertebral bodies has occurred. The duration of infection from onset to total fusion was 12 to 14 months.

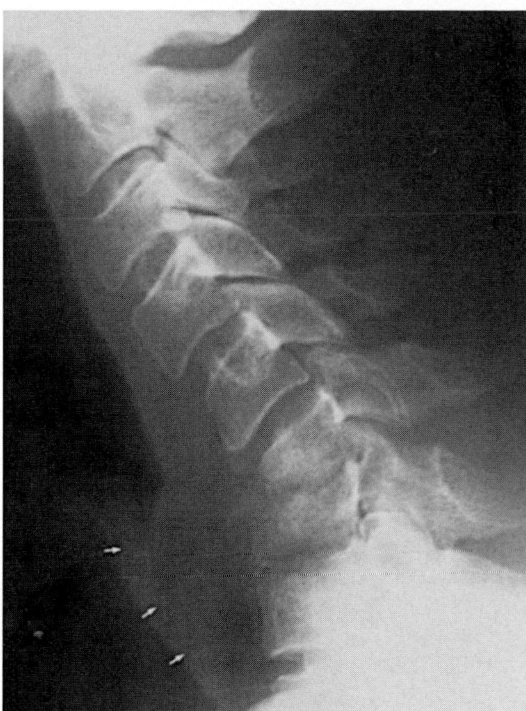

Figure 12-3 Vertebral osteomyelitis. A 41-year-old man presented with osteomyelitis involving C6 and C7. The infection has spread across the disc space, involving contiguous vertebral bodies. A soft tissue mass is noted anterior to the vertebral bodies *(arrows)*. *(Courtesy of Anne Brower, MD.)*

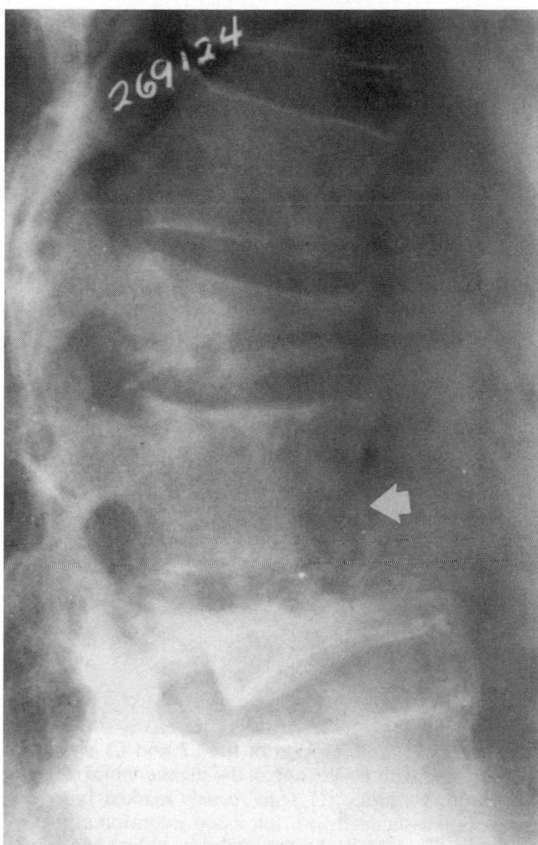

Figure 12-4 Tuberculous spondylitis resulting in vertebral and some discal destruction with collapsed vertebral bodies, loss of intervertebral disc height, reactive sclerosis, and anterior destruction. The *arrow* indicates subligamentous spread of infection. The multiple vertebral body involvement and the anterior destruction separate this process from pyogenic spondylitis. *(Courtesy of Anne Brower, MD.)*

Fungal infections of the spine spare the intervertebral discs, involve the anterior and posterior elements of the vertebral body, and rarely cause vertebral collapse, particularly with infections secondary to actinomycosis and coccidioidomycosis.[137] Actinomycosis causes lytic lesions of bone surrounded by a rim of sclerotic new bone. The disc is spared, although soft tissue abscesses may be present.[185] Coccidioidal spondylitis affects one or more vertebral bodies with paraspinal masses. This infection spares the discs and rarely causes vertebral collapse. The lesions are radiolucent and well demarcated. Periosteal new bone is seen, but sclerosis is infrequent.[40,69]

Cryptococcal involvement of the spine is unusual. The infection is related to direct implantation at skeletal sites, including the spine. Lesions are osteolytic with mild surrounding sclerosis and no periosteal reaction. The limited periostitis is characteristic of cryptococcosis.[108,119] Disseminated blastomycosis affects bones in 50% of patients and has a radiographic appearance resembling that of tuberculosis of the spine. When the thoracolumbar area is affected, the anterior vertebral body is eroded with soft tissue masses and paravertebral extension.[13] Aspergillosis is a very rare cause of vertebral infection. However, recent reports have described vertebral involvement similar to that seen with tuberculosis secondary to *Aspergillus fumigatus* infection of an aortic bypass graft.[19]

Radiographic changes in the spine may include marked destruction and dissolution of bone in Charcot's arthropathy of the spine (neuropathic) and may show lysis and sclerosis in bone from gummatous osseous lesions (spirochetal infection).[28,81] Periosteal changes may also be present.

In hydatid disease, the vertebral column is a common osseous location for this infection.[166] Hydatid disease is associated with single or multiple expansile osteolytic lesions containing altered trabeculae. Soft tissue calcification may also be seen, but periosteal new bone formation is unusual.[78]

Plain roentgenograms may be normal in patients with vertebral osteomyelitis. Plain roentgenograms might have the greatest opportunity to detect axial skeletal abnormalities in patients who are 50 years of age or older, have long duration of symptoms, and have point vertebral tenderness.[45] Others have suggested that younger people with risk factors, such as intravenous drug abuse, are appropriate candidates for plain roentgenographic evaluation.[24] Once again, good clinical judgment should guide the physician to the use of appropriate tests.

Scintigraphy

Bone scintigraphy demonstrates abnormalities in the area of infection at an earlier stage of disease than do plain roentgenograms.[80] A bone scan may also demonstrate areas of involvement other than the one that is symptomatic. Technetium-99m bone scans become abnormal within 72 hours of infection and have about a 75% specificity for the

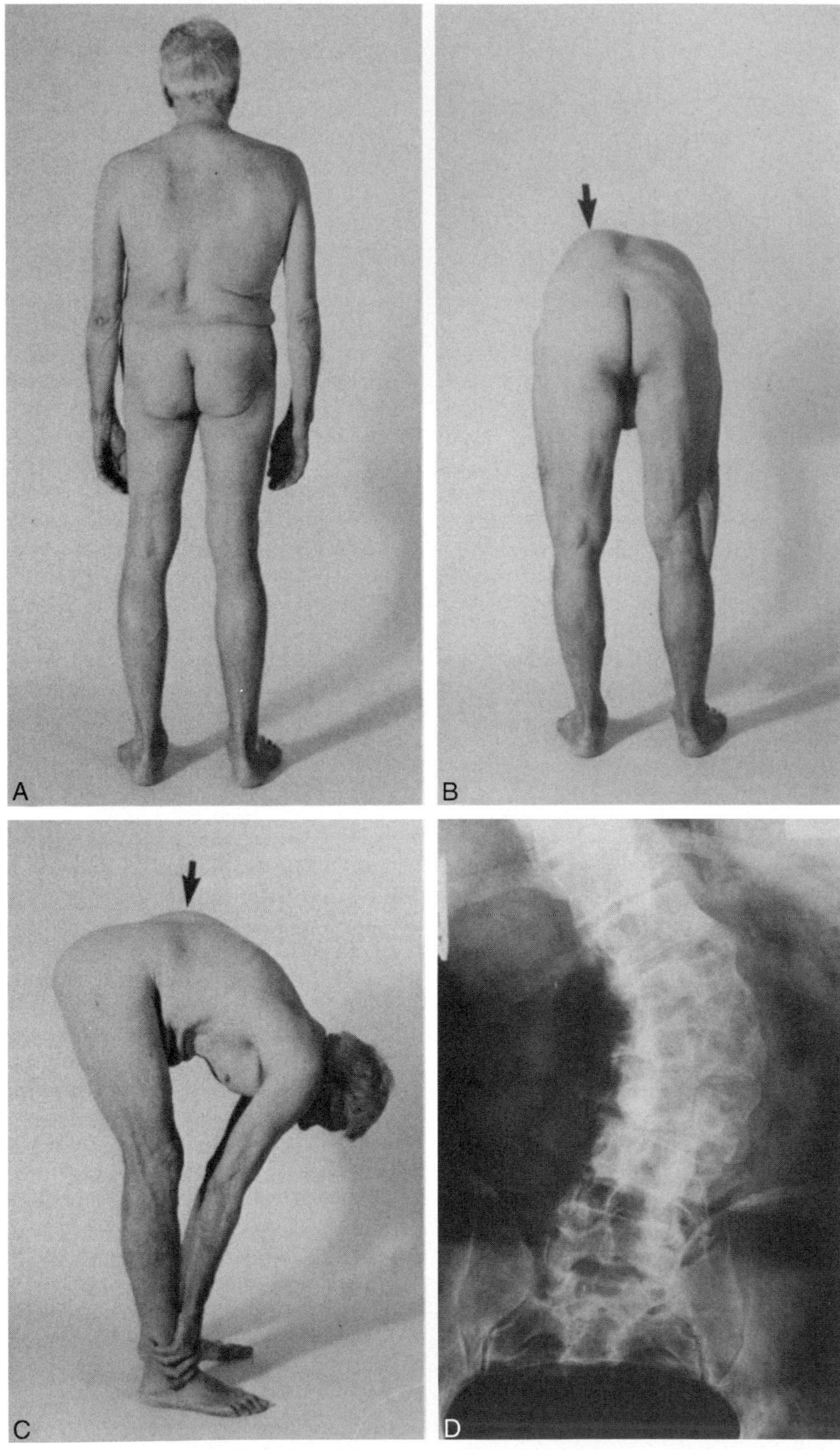

Figure 12-5 Tuberculous spondylitis. This 61-year-old man had miliary tuberculosis in 1966 and developed Pott's disease affecting his lumbar spine. *A*, In the upright position, the patient has a scoliosis centered in the lumbar area with convexity on the left. The right shoulder is higher than the left. In forward flexion, posterior (*B*) and lateral (*C*) views reveal a prominence in the left lumbar area compatible with a gibbus of the spine (*arrow*). *D*, Anteroposterior view of the lumbar spine taken on 4/4/90 demonstrates a rotatory scoliosis with vertebral body loss of the L1, L2, and L3 bodies with reactive osteophytes at the L4 and L5 levels. MR examination revealed fusion of L1-L2 and posterolateral disc herniations at the L2-L3 and L3-L4 levels with only mild spinal canal stenosis (not shown). The patient remains functional with a mild limp. *(D, From Borenstein DG: Low back pain. In Klippel J, Dieppe P [eds]: Rheumatology. St. Louis, CV Mosby, 1994.)*

diagnosis.[152] False-positive and false-negative results do occur, and increased uptake on bone scan may be caused by tumor, trauma, or arthritis. Normal bone scans may occur if the test is completed too early in the course of the disease.[154] The combination of technetium and indium scans can add specificity to the 90% sensitivity in the diagnosis of osteomyelitis.[161]

Single-photon emission computed tomography (SPECT) provides radionuclide images similar to those of CT scanning. SPECT scan detects the location of infections within the spinal elements by improving contrast resolution and by adding three-dimensional localization.[84]

Computed Tomography

Computed tomography (CT) may show bony changes before their appearance on routine radiographs (Fig. 12-6). The extent of soft tissue abscesses is also more easily visualized by this method.[52,86] CT may also be used to follow the course of illness after therapy is initiated. Difficulties in the CT diagnosis of vertebral osteomyelitis can occur when the radiographic features believed to be pathognomonic of specific disease entities, such as vertebral malignancy and severe degenerative disc disease, are present that may be confused with characteristics of osteomyelitis.[161]

Magnetic Resonance

The value of magnetic resonance (MR) imaging in the diagnosis of vertebral infections continues to grow.[117] MR imaging changes correspond to the extent of the inflammatory process and increased water content in production of exudates containing white blood cells and fibrin. Variations in marrow signal are also noted with decreased T1-weighted image and increased signal on T2-weighted image. Atypical T2-weighted images of isointense or hypointense vertebral bodies may be seen in 44% of patients with spinal infections.[39] MR imaging has a high sensitivity for inflammatory processes in soft tissue or bone. It has a sensitivity exceeding that of plain films and CT scan and approaches that of scintiscans.[116] It is abnormal when other radiographic techniques, such as scintigraphic and CT scans, are normal.[115]

In patients with bacterial vertebral osteomyelitis, MR imaging is able to determine the involvement of the vertebral bodies and intervening disc and the extent of the extraosseous infection into the surrounding soft tissues.[115] In a retrospective study of 103 individuals with pyogenic vertebral osteomyelitis, MR scan gave the correct diagnosis in 55% of individuals with less than 2 weeks of symptoms.[22] The presence of vertebral body signal changes without morphologic changes, marked signal increase in the intervertebral disc on T2-weighted and contrast medium–enhanced sequences, and soft tissue involvement without abscess formation have been suggested as findings specific for brucellar spondylitis.[127] The MR findings associated with tuberculous spondylitis that are different from bacterial vertebral osteomyelitis include the lack of abnormal signal of the intervertebral disc space, the involvement of the posterior elements rather than the endplates, and the presence of large paraspinal soft tissue masses (Fig. 12-7).[162] These findings are not specific for tuberculosis. Patients with fungal infection of the spine may also demonstrate similar MR findings, including preservation of disc height, destruction of posterior elements, and paravertebral masses.[37] Gadolinium-enhanced MR imaging has advantages over nonenhanced MR imaging in the evaluation of spinal infections.[136] Enhanced MR imaging detects the presence of epidural abscesses. This technique also localizes the portion of a lesion that is most active. MR may demonstrate progressive disease at a time when other clinical parameters document improvement. This may correlate to the advancement of bony abnormalities with healing. In contrast, paravertebral soft tissue abnormalities may resolve as the first indication of improvement.[61] An editorial by Kaiser suggests that MR imaging is the preferred method of diagnosing vertebral osteomyelitis but should not be utilized with or without contrast medium enhancement for monitoring improvement.[83]

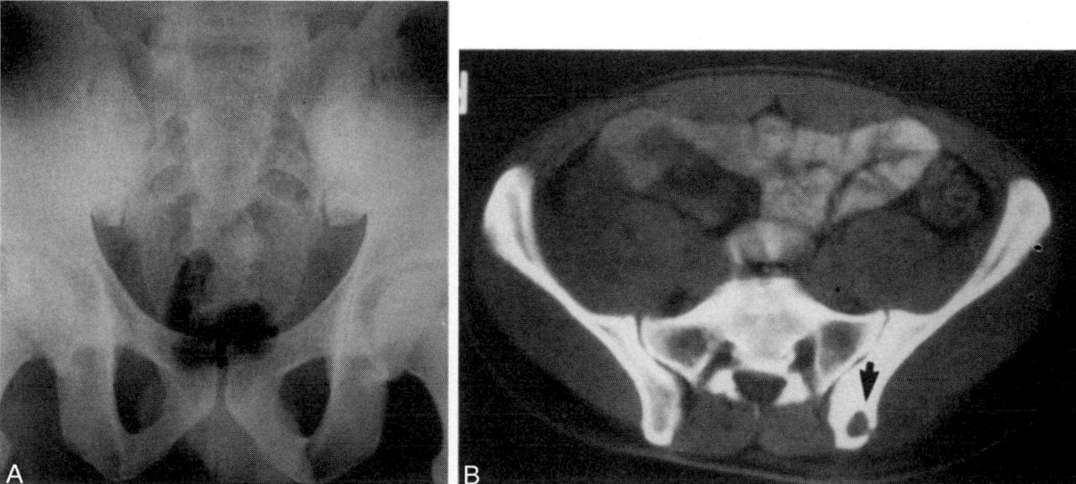

Figure 12-6 Osteomyelitis of the ilium. A 22-year-old man developed acute, severe pain over the left sacroiliac joint. *A*, Ferguson view of the pelvis revealed sclerosis of the iliac bone. The mineralization of the sacrum was difficult to determine. *B*, CT scan revealed a lytic area surrounded by reactive sclerosis limited to the left ilium *(arrow)*. Biopsy and culture of the area was positive for *Staphylococcus aureus*.

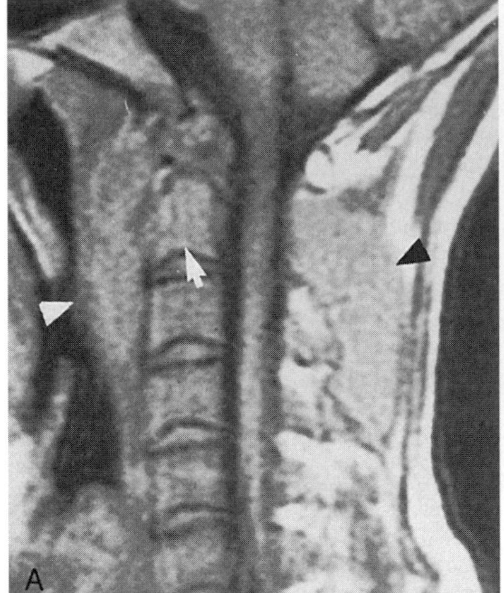

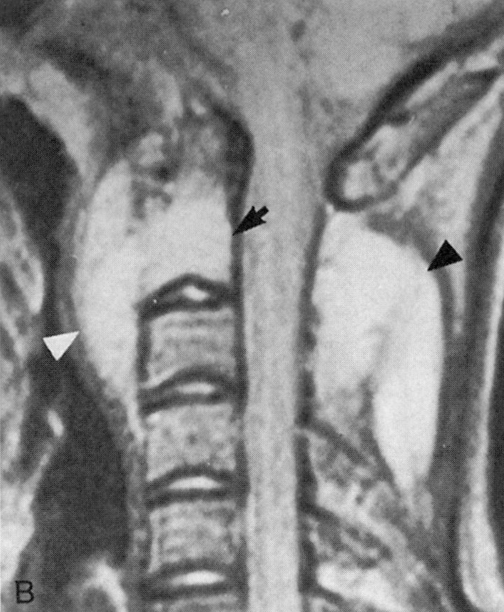

Figure 12-7 Tuberculous spondylitis: atlantoaxial destruction. In a 23-year-old man, sagittal T1-weighted (TR/TE 450/30) *(A)* and T2-weighted (TR/TE 1800/50) *(B)* spin-echo MR images reveal tuberculous involvement of the upper cervical spine. Findings include abnormalities of the axis *(arrows)* with anterior and posterior extension of the process *(arrowheads)*. *(A and B, Courtesy of T. Mattsson, MD, Riyadh, Saudi Arabia.)*

DIFFERENTIAL DIAGNOSIS

The definitive diagnosis of vertebral osteomyelitis is based on the recovery and identification of the causative organism from aspirated material or biopsy.[121] Clinical history, physical examination, and laboratory investigations are too nonspecific to ensure an accurate diagnosis.[93] A presumptive diagnosis may be accepted as indication for specific antibiotic therapy when the clinical and radiographic presentations are characteristic and abnormal blood cultures are obtained. When cultures are negative for growth, trochar aspiration from bone or needle aspiration from a retropharyngeal abscess may identify the source of the infection. Open vertebral biopsy may be required in the cervical spine because the chance for damage of the esophagus and vertebral artery with closed biopsy is real.[97] Osteomyelitis may occur in bones in the pelvis and may be associated with severe low back pain or abdominal pain.[179] Conditions confused with vertebral osteomyelitis include discitis, metastatic tumors, multiple myeloma, eosinophilic granuloma, aneurysmal bone cyst, giant cell tumor of bone, and sarcoidosis. MR evaluation may help differentiate infection from other pathologic processes, but culture evidence of the causative organism is required.[17] The appropriate diagnosis is reached by careful review of biopsy material. If in doubt, biopsy of the lesions of the vertebral body must be performed. In elderly individuals, the organism that causes osteomyelitis may differ from the one that causes a concomitant infection.[173] Only after biopsy is it possible to differentiate tuberculosis from sarcoidosis, myeloma, other tumors, and osteomyelitis.

On occasion more than one vertebral body is affected by osteomyelitis. Although in most instances simultaneous involvement occurs in contiguous vertebral bodies, involvement of distant vertebrae may occur. A bone scan showing two or more areas of increased uptake in the spine may be inappropriately attributed to metastases, compression fractures, or osteoarthritis.[46]

TREATMENT

Therapy for vertebral osteomyelitis includes antibiotics, bed rest, and immobilization. The goals for therapy for cervical osteomyelitis are eradication of the offending organism, minimization of instability or deformity, and preservation of neurologic function. In patients with retropharyngeal abscess and no vertebral deformity, needle aspiration suffices to obtain culture material and for drainage. However, patients with bony destruction and deformity require an open biopsy from an anterior approach that allows for adequate drainage and definitive reconstruction.[97]

Bacterial Therapy

The choice of antibiotic therapy is decided by the organism causing the infection and its sensitivity to specific agents. Gram-positive bacteria such as *Staphylococcus* require semisynthetic penicillin (nafcillin) since *S. aureus* has become resistant to penicillin. Methicillin-resistant *S. aureus* requires vancomycin therapy with the addition of rifampin or tetracycline to enhance bone penetration.[42] Gram-negative bacteria are sensitive to aminoglycosides or to third-generation cephalosporins such as ceftriaxone. Patients are treated for 4 to 6 weeks with parenteral antibiotics, followed by a course of oral antibiotics that may have a duration of as long as 6 months (Table 12-5). Others have suggested a shorter course of therapy of about 3 weeks to decrease the risk of antibiotic reactions.[131] In a study of 65 patients with vertebral osteomyelitis, 25% had relapse of

12-5 ANTIMICROBIAL THERAPY FOR ADULT VERTEBRAL OSTEOMYELITIS

Organism	Preferred Intravenous (IV) Therapy	Preferred Oral Therapy	Alternative Therapy
Staphylococcus aureus (methicillin sensitive)	Nafcillin, 2 g/4 h	Clindamycin, 300 mg/6 h	Clindamycin, 900 mg/8 h IV
S. aureus (methicillin resistant)	Vancomycin, 1 g/12 h	NA	NA
Streptococcus A	Penicillin G, 3 million U/4 h	Penicillin-VK, 500 mg/6 h + probenecid	Clindamycin, 900 mg/8 h IV
Streptococcus D (enterococci)	Ampicillin, 2 g/4 h + gentamicin, 1-1.5 mg/kg/8 h	NA	Vancomycin, 1 g/12 h IV + gentamicin, 1-1.5 mg/kg/8 h
Escherichia coli	Ceftriaxone, 1 g/24 h or cefazolin, 1 g/8 h	Trimethoprim/sulfamethoxazole DS 12 h Ciprofloxacin, 500 mg/12 h	Trimethoprim/sulfamethoxazole, 10 mg/kg/d 12 h IV Ciprofloxacin, 400 mg/12 h IV
Klebsiella pneumoniae	Ceftriaxone, 1 g/24 h	Trimethoprim/sulfamethoxazole DS 12 h Ciprofloxacin, 500 mg/12 h	Trimethoprim/sulfamethoxazole, 10 mg/kg/d 6 h IV Ciprofloxacin, 400 mg/12 h IV
Pseudomonas aeruginosa	Ceftazidime, 2 g/8 h IV or ciprofloxacin, 400 mg/12 h	Ciprofloxacin, 750 mg/12 h	Imipenem, 500 mg/6 h
Bacteroides	Metronidazole, 500 mg/6 h	Clindamycin, 300 mg/6 h	Clindamycin, 900 mg/8 h IV

Choice of antibiotic should be matched to organism sensitivities determined with culture. Antibiotics listed in this table may be used as initial therapy until sensitivity results are available.

Modified from Norden C, Gillespie WJ, Nade S: Infections in Bones and Joints. Boston, Blackwell Scientific, 1994, pp 211-230; Staubaugh LJ: Vertebral osteomyelitis. In Jauregui LE (ed): Diagnosis and Management of Bone Infections. New York, Marcel Dekker, 1995, pp 167-200; and Gary Simon, MD.

infection when treated for less than 28 days.[27] With more effective antibiotics, the need for prolonged therapy may be diminished. However, the correct duration of therapy depends on the results of ongoing studies and the clinical response of the individual patient with the infection. Bed rest is helpful in decreasing pain by limiting motion. Some patients require a collar as a temporary means to decrease neck pain. Some patients require plaster casts or braces when there is major bone destruction or instability of the lumbar spine.

Brucellosis may be treated with oral tetracycline (doxycycline) at a dose of 100 mg twice daily. Therapy should continue for 6 weeks. In severe cases, 1.0 g of streptomycin is injected per day for the first 14 to 21 days. Relapses occur between 3 to 6 months after completing therapy. Improvement in sanitation and handling of food products does result in a decrease in the incidence of brucellosis in populations at risk.[14]

Postsurgical Therapy

Irrigation and débridement is the first component of therapy. Empirical therapy, if cultures are negative, includes vancomycin for gram-positive organisms and a third- or fourth-generation cephalosporin (ceftazidime or cefepime) or fluoroquinolone.[42]

Mycobacterial Therapy

The current recommendation for treatment of tuberculosis in the United States is a first-line, three-drug regimen including isoniazid (300 mg/day), rifampin (600 mg/day), and pyrazinamide (up to 2 g/day) for 2 months. Two drugs (rifampin and isoniazid) are continued for an extended period. The duration of therapy has been given as 12 to 18 months.[160] Drug-resistant tuberculosis is becoming an increasingly frequent problem.[57] The importance of taking all the drugs in a regimen for the full treatment period cannot be underestimated. The emergence of multidrug-resistant organisms is a constant threat.[128] Additional drugs for longer periods are required to control these infections. Patients may require a regimen of five to seven drugs for control of the drug-resistant organism.[124] The actual duration of therapy depends on the clinical response of the patient with osseous tuberculosis.[10] Spinal tuberculosis can be treated successfully with medical therapy in most patients. Clinical indicators such as pain relief and weight gain are the best means of monitoring improvement. Radiographic progression may occur during the first 6 months as the lesions heal and is not an indication of treatment failure.[18] Surgical intervention is required for severe kyphosis or paraplegia.[118] Poor outcome is related to individuals older than 70 years of age who develop paraplegia from involvement of the central nervous system.[132]

Fungal Therapy

Fungal osteomyelitis requires parenteral amphotericin B therapy at a dose that the patient can tolerate without developing renal dysfunction. A total dose of 2.5 g is usually employed as the initial course of therapy. Bone lesions, however, may be resistant to chemotherapy and may require surgical débridement. Immobilization is required for these patients as well.

Spirochetal Therapy

Patients with tertiary syphilis without neurologic involvement are effectively treated with penicillin. Long-acting penicillin, benzathine penicillin G at 2.4 million units intramuscularly weekly for 3 weeks, is usually used. Patients who are allergic to penicillin may take tetracycline or erythromycin. Individuals with HIV infection require intravenous penicillin G therapy with between 3 to 4 million units every 4 hours for 10 to 14 days.

Parasitic Therapy

Hydatid disease has been resistant to most anthelmintic therapy. Mebendazole has shown some efficacy in preliminary studies. The dose of mebendazole is 1 g orally three times a day for 3 months. Definitive therapy requires surgical excision of cysts, with care being taken to remove them totally.[89] In patients with neurologic dysfunction and hydatid disease, anterior spinal decompression and fusion along with mebendazole therapy is associated with good neural recovery.[26] Albendazole (200-mg tablets) in a dose of 400 mg twice a day for 3 to 6 months is another effective therapy.[108a]

Surgical Therapy

Surgical procedures on the spine are needed in patients with vertebral osteomyelitis for abscess, spinal cord compression and neurologic defect, severe deformity, persistent symptoms and elevated ESR, and open biopsy to obtain culture material. Another indication for surgical intervention is the presence of spinal instability in association with osteomyelitis.[131] Common to all surgical approaches to vertebral osteomyelitis includes thorough débridement of all necrotic and infected tissues, the deliverance of adequate blood flow through débridement or soft tissue transfer, and the reestablishment of spinal stability.[172] Many surgeons use an anterior approach to reach the spine if multiple segments are affected. Laminectomy is not indicated in patients with vertebral osteomyelitis because the removal of bone results in increased spinal column instability, dislocation, and spinal cord compression.[91] A number of surgeons include interbody fusion along with anterior débridement as a means for obtaining neural decompression in combination with spinal stability.[51,103,105]

PROGNOSIS

The improvement in vertebral osteomyelitis may be monitored by following the decrease in a patient's symptoms, pain, and fever and the return of the ESR to normal. A study of 44 pyogenic vertebral osteomyelitis patients who had ESR before diagnosis and during the course of the illness demonstrated the variability of this measure of improvement. During the first month, over 50% of individuals (19 of 32) who had a cure of their infection without surgery had an ESR higher at 1 month than at baseline. A rapid fall in ESR was associated with resolution of the infection. Patients who were older than 60 years of age with immunocompromise were at greatest risk of failure. The ESR must not be the sole laboratory finding to determine the prognosis of the patient with vertebral osteomyelitis.[23]

With early diagnosis and appropriate therapy, vertebral osteomyelitis resolves with minimal disability in the patient.[169] The case-fatality rate in the antibiotic era is less than 5%.[165] Relapses may occur in 10% of individuals who receive inadequate type and duration of antibiotic. When the diagnosis is delayed and the infection spreads to involve the spinal cord by compression (resulting in epidural abscess and granulation tissue) or direct extension (meningitis), potentially life-threatening complications may occur.[9,64] Anterior decompression is not free of risks in that osteomyelitis and vertebral artery injury may be complications of the operation.[163]

Epidural Abscess

A number of large series have been published reviewing the clinical manifestations, diagnostic evaluation, treatment modalities, prognostic indicators, and final outcomes of 112 patients with epidural abscesses.[38,41,73] In one large series, epidural abscess occurred in 1.2 per 10,000 hospital admissions.[9] A lower rate of 0.8 cases per 10,000 admissions was noted in another study.[51] Epidural infection occurs more commonly in men in most studies. Predisposing disorders include diabetes mellitus, alcoholism, intravenous drug abuse, hemodialysis, and cirrhosis.[125,174] Although osteoarthritis of the spine is present in a number of patients with epidural abscess, the degenerative abnormalities are not a risk factor for infection.[156] Although the source of an epidural infection may be distant (dental abscess) or local (decubitus ulcer or mediastinum), most often it is unknown.[8,66] Individuals with endocarditis, particularly those with prosthetic valves, may develop epidural abscesses from unusual organisms *(Candida albicans)*.[102] The posterior epidural space in the lumbar area is a common location for the infection. The anatomic correlation for these observations is that the extradural space is expanded posteriorly and laterally below L1 as well as at T4–T9.[156] In a study of 45 patients the posterior epidural space in the cervical and cervicothoracic junction was the location for epidural abscess in 20% of cases.[41] Cervical epidural abscess is also described in occasional patients with osteomyelitis.[6,100,114] Organisms that have caused cervical epidural abscesses include *S. aureus* and *Brucella*.[134,181]

The clinical manifestations of this infection occur secondary to direct compression by the abscess or granulation tissue or from thrombosis of subarachnoid vessels. Spinal pain is common but not universally seen in all patients who are unable to report their pain. The progression of symptoms goes from local spinal pain to root pain, then weakness, and finally quadriparesis, or paraparesis. Neurologic findings appear with the onset of radicular symptoms. Spinal tenderness as well as fever, sweats, or rigors are present in the majority of patients. The course of symptoms may be days to several months.[49]

Laboratory data in the form of peripheral WBC and ESR are not helpful because they are normal or nonspecifically elevated. Low platelet count is associated with a poor prognosis.[168] Blood cultures are positive for the infecting organism 50% to 95% of the time, depending on the study group.[41,156] In a study of 23 cases of cervical epidural abscess, a bacteriologic agent was identified in 91% of patients.[144] *S. aureus* is the predominant pathogen. The diagnosis is established by culture of cerebrospinal fluid (CSF). CSF is abnormal in 97% of patients, including elevated protein concentrations, low glucose levels, or pleocytosis. CSF cultures may be positive for bacterial growth in the setting of a normal WBC.

Radiographic evaluation of the spine is helpful in identifying the location and extent of the abscess. Roentgenograms of the spine reveal vertebral changes of osteomyelitis in 44%.[41] Technetium bone scan may be abnormal in most patients, and gallium scan may miss the location of the abscess in about one third of patients. Scintiscans are abnormal if underlying osteomyelitis is present in the setting of the epidural abscess. CT with intrathecal contrast establishes the presence of spinal cord encroachment in a majority. MR imaging is superior to CT/myelogram in defining the extent of the lesion. MR imaging is able to determine the extent of the cervical abscess in the spinal canal, the extraspinal extent of the lesion, the presence of intramedullary infection, and the presence of osteomyelitis in the contiguous vertebral bodies.[94] The use of gadolinium contrast for MR helps to delineate lesions that may be equivocal with plain MR testing.[147,148] MR imaging is also able to document the response to therapy noninvasively.[147] In a study of 60 patients with epidural infection, 19 (32%) had cervical spine disease. MR imaging was able to locate the three vertebral bodies that showed abnormal bone marrow signal in the setting of epidural inflammation that extended an average of four levels. The most frequently involved levels in association with epidural abscess were C5 and C6. MR imaging documented spinal cord compression in 74% of the patients.[59]

Therapy includes the use of antibiotics and drainage of the abscess without causing instability of the spine. Speed in making the diagnosis is essential for obtaining a good outcome. Patients diagnosed within 36 hours of the onset of symptoms have minimal residual weakness. No recovery is observed in patients with paralysis for longer than 48 hours.[72] Mortality rates from epidural abscess range from 5% to 23%.[41,72] These patients are significantly older than the rest of the patients who survive. The presence of preoperative paraplegia or quadriplegia is a poor prognostic factor.[110] Morbidity remains a significant problem when the cervical spinal cord is affected and the diagnosis is delayed.

References

Vertebral Osteomyelitis

1. Ackerman G, Bayley JC: *Candida albicans* osteomyelitis in a vertebral body previously infected with *Serratia marcescens*. Spine 15:1362, 1990.
2. Adatepe MH, Parnell OM, Issacs GH, et al: Hematogenous pyogenic vertebral osteomyelitis: Diagnostic value of radionuclide bone imaging. J Nucl Med 27:1680, 1986.

3. Alamin TF, Hanley EN: Profiles of patients with spine infections. Semin Spine Surg 12:212-222, 2000.
4. Alldred AJ, Nisbet NW: Hydatid disease of bone in Australia. J Bone Joint Surg Br 46B:260, 1964.
5. Ariza J, Gudiol F, Valverde J, et al: *Brucella spondylitis:* A detailed analysis based on current findings. Rev Infect Dis 7:656, 1985.
6. Auten GM, Levy CS, Smith MA: *Haemophilus parainfluenzae* as a rare cause of epidural abscess: Case report and review. Rev Infect Dis 13:609, 1991.
7. Awad I, Bay JW, Petersen JM: Nocardial osteomyelitis of the spine with epidural cord compression: A case report. Neurosurgery 15:254, 1984.
8. Babington CK, Yung MD, James CK, et al: Aggressive thoracic actinomycosis complicated by vertebral osteomyelitis and epidural abscess leading to spinal cord compression. Spine 25:745-748, 2000.
9. Baker AS, Ojemann RG, Swartz MN, Richardson EP Jr: Spinal epidural abscess. N Engl J Med 293:463, 1975.
10. Barnes PF, Barrows SA: Tuberculosis in the 1990s. Ann Intern Med 119:400, 1993.
11. Barr RJ, Hannon DG, Adair IV, et al: Cervical osteomyelitis after rigid esophagoscopy: Brief report. J Bone Joint Surg Br 70B:147, 1988.
12. Batson OV: The function of the vertebral veins and their role in the spread of metastases. Ann Surg 112:138, 1940.
13. Baylin GJ, Wear JM: Blastomycosis and actinomycosis of spine. AJR Am J Roentgenol 69:395, 1953.
14. Belzunegui J, Del Val N, Intxausti JJ et al: Vertebral osteomyelitis in northern Spain: Report of 62 cases. Clin Exp Rheumatol 17:447-452, 1999.
15. Bingold AC: Luetic lumbar spondylosis. Proc R Soc Med 55:354, 1962.
16. Boachie-Adjei O, Squillante RG: Tuberculosis of the spine. Orthop Clin North Am 27:95-103, 1996.
17. Borges LF: Case records of the Massachusetts General Hospital. N Engl J Med 320:1610, 1989.
18. Boxer DI, Pratt C, Hine AL, et al: Radiological features during and following treatment of spinal tuberculosis. Br J Radiol 65:476-479, 1992.
19. Brandt SJ, Thompson RL, Wenzel RP: Mycotic pseudoaneurysm of an aortic bypass graft and contiguous vertebral osteomyelitis due to *Aspergillus fumigatus*. Am J Med 79:259, 1985.
20. Brashear HR Jr, Rendleman DA: Pott's paraplegia. South Med J 71:1379, 1978.
21. Byrne FD, Thrall TM, Wheat LJ: Hematogenous vertebral osteomyelitis: *Pasteurella multocida* as the causative agent. Arch Intern Med 139:1182, 1979.
22. Carragee EJ: The clinical use of magnetic resonance imaging in pyogenic vertebral osteomyelitis. Spine 22:780-785, 1997.
23. Carragee EJ, Kim D, van der Vlugt T, et al: The clinical use of erythrocyte sedimentation rate in pyogenic vertebral osteomyelitis. Spine 22:2089-2093, 1997.
24. Chandrasekar P: Low back pain and intravenous abusers. Arch Intern Med 150:1125, 1990.
25. Chapman M, Murray RO, Stoker DJ: Tuberculosis of the bones and joints. Semin Roentgenol 14:266, 1979.
26. Charles RW, Govender CS, Naidoo KS: Echinococcal infection of the spine with neural involvement. Spine 13:47, 1988.
27. Charles RW, Mody GM, Govender S: Pyogenic infection of the lumbar vertebral spine due to gas-forming organisms. Spine 14:541, 1989.
28. Cleveland M, Wilson HJ: Charcot disease of the spine: A report of two cases treated by spine fusion. J Bone Joint Surg Am 41A:336, 1959.
29. Collert S: Osteomyelitis of the spine. Acta Orthop Scand 48:283, 1977.
30. Colmenero JD, Jimenez-Mejias ME, Sanchez-Lora J, et al: Pyogenic tuberculous, and brucellar vertebral osteomyelitis: A descriptive and comparative study of 219 cases. Ann Rheum Dis 56:709-715, 1997.
31. Colmenero JD, Reguera JM, Fernandez-Nebro A, Cabrera-Franquelo F: Osteoarticular complications of brucellosis. Ann Rheum Dis 50:23, 1991.
32. Colmenero JD, Reguera JM, Martos F, et al: Complications associated with *Brucella melitensis* infection: A study of 530 cases. Medicine 75:195-211, 1996.
33. Compere EL, Garrison M: Correlation of pathologic and roentgenologic findings in tuberculosis and pyogenic infections of the vertebrae. Ann Surg 104:1038, 1936.
34. Cope VZ: Actinomycosis of bone with special reference to infection of the vertebral column. J Bone Joint Surg 330:205, 1951.
35. Corea JR, Tamimi TM: Tuberculosis of the arch of the atlas: Case report. Spine 12:608, 1987.
36. Craig JB: Cervical spine osteomyelitis with delayed onset tetraparesis after penetrating wounds of the neck. S Afr Med J 69:197, 1986.
37. Cure JK, Mirich DR: MR imaging in cryptococcal spondylitis. AJNR Am J Neuroradiol 12:1111, 1991.
38. Curling OD, Gower DJ, McWhorter JM: Changing concepts in spinal epidural abscess: A report of 29 cases. Neurosurgery 27:185, 1990.
39. Dagirmanjian A, Schils J, McHenry M, et al: MR imaging of vertebral osteomyelitis revisited. AJR Am J Roentgenol 167:1539-1543, 1996.
40. Dalinka MK, Greendyke WH: The spinal manifestations of coccidioidomycosis. J Can Assoc Radiol 22:93, 1971.
41. Darouiche RO, Hamill RJ, Greenberg SB, et al: Bacterial spinal epidural abscess: Review of 43 cases and literature survey. Medicine 71:369, 1992.
42. Datta SK, Kirkland TN: Microbiology and antimicrobial therapy of vertebral osteomyelitis. Semin Spine Surg 12:176-182, 2000.
43. David PT, Horowitz T: Skeletal tuberculosis: A review with patient presentations and discussion. Am J Med 48:77, 1970.
44. De Wit D, Mulla R, Cowie MR, et al: Vertebral osteomyelitis due to *Staphylococcus epidermidis*. Br J Rheumatol 32:339, 1993.
45. Deyo RA: Plain roentgenography for low-back pain: Finding needles in a haystack. Arch Intern Med 149:27, 1989.
46. Digby JM, Kersley JB: Pyogenic non-tuberculous spinal infection: An analysis of thirty cases. J Bone Joint Surg Br 61B:47, 1979.
47. Dobson J: Tuberculosis of the spine. J Bone Joint Surg 33B:517, 1951.
48. Dye C, Scheele S, Dolin P, et al: Global burden of tuberculosis: Estimated incidence, prevalence, and mortality by country. JAMA 282:677-686, 1999.
49. Eismont FJ, Montero C: Infections of the Spine. In Davidoff RA (ed): Handbook of the Spinal Cord. New York, Marcel Dekker, 1987, pp 411-449.
50. El-Desouki M: Skeletal brucellosis: Assessment with bone scintigraphy. Radiology 181:415, 1991.
51. Emery SE, Chan DPK, Woodward HR: Treatment of hematogenous pyogenic vertebral osteomyelitis with anterior débridement and primary bone grafting. Spine 14:284, 1989.
52. Endress C, Guyot DR, Fata J, Salciccioli G: Cervical osteomyelitis due to IV heroin use: Radiologic findings in 14 patients. AJR Am J Roentgenol 155:3333, 1990.
53. Feng J, Austin TW: Anaerobic vertebral osteomyelitis. Can Med Assoc J 145:132, 1991.
54. Forlenza SW, Axelrod JL, Grieco MH: Pott's disease in heroin addicts. JAMA 241:379, 1979.
55. Freedman E, Merschan I: Syphilitic spondylitis. AJR Am J Roentgenol 49:756, 1943.
56. Freehafer AA, Furey JG, Pierce DS: Pyogenic osteomyelitis of the spine: Resulting in spinal paralysis. J Bone Joint Surg Am 44A:710, 1962.
57. Freiden TR, Sterling T, Pascal-Mendez A, et al: The emergence of drug resistant tuberculosis in New York City. N Engl J Med 328:521, 1993.
58. Friedman B: Chemotherapy of tuberculosis of the spine. J Bone Joint Surg Am 48A:451, 1966.
59. Friedmand DP, Hillis JR: Cervical epidural spinal infection: MR imaging characteristics. AJR Am J Roentgenol 163:699, 1994.
60. Garcia A Jr, Grantham SA: Hematogenous pyogenic vertebral osteomyelitis. J Bone Joint Surg Am 42A:429, 1960.
61. Gilliams AR, Chaddha B, Carter AP: Appearances of the temporal evolution and resolution of infectious spondylitis. AJR Am J Roentgenol 166:903-907, 1996.
62. Goldblatt M, Cremin BJ: Osteoarticular tuberculosis: Its presentation in the coloured races. Clin Radiol 29:669, 1978.
63. Gonzalez-Gay MA, Garcia-Porrua C, Ibanez D, et al: Osteoarticular complications of brucellosis in an Atlantic area of Spain. J Rheumatol 26:141-145, 1999.

64. Gorse GJ, Pais MJ, Kusske JA, Cesario TC: Tuberculous spondylitis: A report of six cases and a review of the literature. Medicine 62:178, 1983.
65. Griffiths HED, Jones DM: Pyogenic infection of the spine: A review of twenty-eight cases. J Bone Joint Surg Br 53B:383, 1971.
66. Guerrero IC, Slap GB, MacGregor RB, et al: Anaerobic spinal epidural abscess. J Neurosurg 48:465, 1978.
67. Guri JP: Pyogenic osteomyelitis of the spine: Differential diagnosis through clinical roentgenographic observations. J Bone Joint Surg Am 28A:29, 1946.
68. Hall M, Williams A: Group G streptococcal osteomyelitis of the spine. Br J Rheumatol 32:342, 1993.
69. Halpern AA, Rinsky LA, Fountains S, Nagel DA: Coccidioidomycosis of the spine: Unusual roentgenographic presentation. Clin Orthop 140:78, 1979.
70. Hamdan TA, Al-Kaisy MA: Dumbbell hydatid cyst of the spine: Case report and review of the literature. Spine 25:1296-1299, 2000.
71. Heary RF, Hunt CD, Wolansky LJ: Rapid bony destruction with pyogenic vertebral osteomyelitis. Surg Neurol 41:34, 1994.
72. Heusner AP: Nontuberculous spinal epidural infections. N Engl J Med 239:845, 1948.
73. Hlavin ML, Kaminski HJ, Ross JS, Ganz E: Spinal epidural abscess: A ten-year perspective. Neurosurgery 27:177, 1990.
74. Holzman RS, Bishko F: Osteomyelitis in heroin addicts. Ann Intern Med 75:693, 1971.
75. Hsu LC, Yau ACMC: Tuberculosis. In Sherk HH, Dunn EJ, Eismont FJ, et al (eds): The Cervical Spine, 2nd ed. Philadelphia, JB Lippincott, 1989, pp 544-551.
76. Hsu LES, Leong JEY: Tuberculosis of the lower cervical spine (C2-C7). J Bone Joint Surg Br 66B:1, 1984.
77. Hunt JR: Syphilis of the vertebral column: Its symptomatology and neural complications. Am J Med Sci 148:164, 1914.
78. Hutchinson WF, Thompson WB, Derian PS: Osseous hydatid (echinococcus) disease. JAMA 182:81, 1962.
79. Incavo SJ, Muller DL, Krag MH, Gump D: Vertebral osteomyelitis caused by *Clostridium difficile*. Spine 13:111, 1988.
80. Jensen AG, Espersen F, Skinhoj P, et al: Bacteremic *Staphylococcus aureus* spondylitis. Arch Intern Med 158:509-517, 1998.
81. Johns D: Syphilitic disorders of the spine: Report of two cases. J Bone Joint Surg Br 52B:724, 1970.
82. Joughin E, McDougall C, Parfitt C, et al: Causes and clinical management of vertebral osteomyelitis in Saskatchewan. Spine 16:1049, 1991.
83. Kaiser JA: Point of view. Spine 22:785, 1997.
84. Kanmaz B, Collier BD, Liu Y, et al: SPET and three-phase planar bone scintigraphy in adult patients with chronic low back pain. Nucl Med Commun 19;13-21, 1998.
85. Karaharju EO, Hannuksela M: Possible syphilitic spondylitis. Acta Orthop Scand 44:289, 1973.
86. Kattapuram SV, Phillips WC, Boyd R: CT in pyogenic osteomyelitis of the spine. AJR Am J Roentgenol 140:1199, 1983.
87. Kauffman CP, Williams SK, Stimson EO, et al: Spinal granulomatous infection. Semin Spine Surg 12:192-202, 2000.
88. Keenan JD, Metz CW Jr: *Brucella* spondylitis: A brief review and case report. Clin Orthop 82:87, 1972.
89. Keller TM, Schweitzer JS, Helfend LK, et al: Treatment of progressive cervical spinal instability secondary to hydatid disease: A case report. Spine 22:915-919, 1997.
90. Kelley PJ, Martin WJ, Schirger A, Weed LA: Brucellosis of the bones and joints: Experience with 36 patients. JAMA 174:347, 1960.
91. Kemp HBS, Shaw NC: Laminectomy in paraplegia due to infective spondylosis. Br J Surg 61:66, 1974.
92. Kido D, Bryan D, Halpern M: Hematogenous osteomyelitis in drug addicts. AJR Am J Roentgenol 118:356, 1973.
93. Kornberg M, Rechtine GR, Dupuy TE: Unusual presentation of spinal osteomyelitis in a patient taking propylthiouracil: A case report. Spine 10:104, 1985.
94. Kricun R, Shoemaker EI, Chovanes GI, Stephens HW: Epidural abscess of the cervical spine: MR findings in five cases. AJR Am J Roentgenol 158:1145, 1992.
95. Kulowski J: Pyogenic osteomyelitis of the spine: An analysis and discussion of 102 cases. J Bone Joint Surg Am 18A:343, 1936.
96. Lane T, Goings S, Fraser D, et al: Disseminated actinomycosis with spinal cord compression: Report of two cases. Neurology 29:890, 1979.
97. LaRocca SH, Eismont FJ: Other infectious diseases. In Sherk HH, Dunn EJ, Eismont FJ, et al (eds): The Cervical Spine, 2nd ed. Philadelphia, JB Lippincott, 1989, pp 552-563.
98. Laurin JM, Resnick CS, Wheeler D, et al: Cervical osteomyelitis related to *Nocardia asteroides*. J Infect Dis 149:824, 1984.
99. Levin MF, Vellet AD, Munk PL, et al: Tuberculosis of the odontoid bone: A rare but treatable cause of quadriplegia. J Can Assoc Radiol 43:199, 1992.
100. Levy ML, Wieder BH, Schneider J, et al: Subdural empyema of the cervical spine: Clinicopathological correlates and magnetic resonance imaging. J Neurosurg 79:929, 1993.
101. Lewis M, Grundy D: Vertebral osteomyelitis following manipulation of spondylitic necks: A possible risk. Paraplegia 30:788, 1992.
102. Liang JD, Fang CT, Chen YC, et al: *Candida albicans* spinal epidural abscess secondary to prosthetic valve endocarditis. Diagn Microbiol Infect Dis 40:121-123, 2001.
103. Liebergall M, Chaimsky G, Lowe J, et al: Pyogenic vertebral osteomyelitis with paralysis: Prognosis and treatment. Clin Orthop 269:142, 1991.
104. Lifeso R: Atlanto-axial tuberculosis in adults. J Bone Joint Surg Br 69B:183, 1987.
105. Lifeso RM: Pyogenic spinal sepsis in adults. Spine 15:1265, 1990.
106. Ling CM: Pyogenic osteomyelitis of the spine. Orthop Rev 4:23, 1975.
107. Lischke JH, McCreight PHB: Maternal group B streptococcal vertebral osteomyelitis: An unusual complication of vaginal delivery. Obstet Gynecol 76:489, 1990.
108. Litvinoff J, Nelson M: Extradural lumbar cryptococcosis: Case report. J Neurosurg 49:921, 1978.
108a. Liu LX, Weller PF: Antiparasitic drugs N Engl J Med 334:1178, 1996.
109. Lloyd TV, Johnson JC: Infectious cervical spondylitis following traumatic endotracheal intubation. Spine 5:478, 1980.
110. Lu CH, Chang WN, Lui CC, et al: Adult spina epidural abscess: Clinical features and prognostic factors. Clin Neurol Neurosurg 104:306-310, 2002.
111. Maguire JH: Case 37–1986. N Engl J Med 315:748, 1986.
112. Martinez M, Lee AS, Hellinger WC, et al: Vertebral *Aspergillus* osteomyelitis and acute discitis in patients with chronic obstructive pulmonary disease. Mayo Clin Proc 74:579-583, 1999.
113. McGahan JP, Graves DS, Palmer PES: Coccidioidal spondylitis: Usual and unusual radiographic manifestations. Radiology 136:5, 1980.
114. McKnight P, Friedman J: Torticollis due to cervical epidural abscess and osteomyelitis. Neurology 42:696, 1992.
115. Meyers SP, Weiner SN: Diagnosis of hematogenous pyogenic vertebral osteomyelitis by magnetic resonance imaging. Arch Intern Med 151:683, 1991.
116. Modic MT, Feiglin DH, Piraino DW, et al: Vertebral osteomyelitis: Assessment using MR. Radiology 157:157, 1985.
117. Modic MT, Pelanze W, Feiglin DHI, Belbobek G: Magnetic resonance imaging of musculoskeletal infections. Radiol Clin North Am 24:247, 1986.
118. Moon M: Spine update: Tuberculosis of the spine: Controversies and a new challenge. Spine 22:1791-1797, 1997.
119. Morris E, Wolinsky E: Localized osseous cryptococcosis: A case report. J Bone Joint Surg Am 47A:1027, 1965.
120. Morshed AA: Hydatid disease of the spine. Neurochirurgia 20:211, 1977.
121. Musher DM, Thorsteinsson SB, Minuth JN, Luchi RJ: Vertebra osteomyelitis: Still a diagnostic pitfall. Arch Intern Med 136:105, 1976.
122. Neinstein LS, Goldenring J: *Brucella* sacroiliitis. Clin Pediatr 22:645, 1983.
123. Nolla JM, Ariza J, Gomez-Vaquero C, Fiter J, et al: Spontaneous pyogenic vertebral osteomyelitis in nondrug users. Semin Arthritis Rheum 31:271-278, 2002.
124. Norden C, Gillespie WJ, Nade S: Mycobacterial infections of the musculoskeletal system. In Norden C, Gillespie WJ, Nade S: Infections in Bones and Joints. Boston, Blackwell Scientific Publications, 1994, pp 211-230.
125. Obrador GT, Levenson DJ: Spinal epidural abscess in hemodialysis patients: Report of three cases and review of the literature. Am J Kidney Dis 27:75-83, 1996.

126. Osenbach RK, Hitchon PW, Menezes AH: Diagnosis and management of pyogenic vertebral osteomyelitis. Surg Neurol 33:266, 1990.
127. Ozaksoy D, Yucesoy K, Yucesoy M, et al: Brucellar spondylitis: MRI findings. Eur Spine J 10:529-533, 2001.
128. Pablos-Mendez A, Raviglione MC, Laszlo A: Global surveillance for antituberculosis-drug resistance. N Engl J Med 338:1641-1649, 1998.
129. Parke WW, Rothman RH, Brown MD: The pharyngovertebral veins: An anatomic rationale for Grisel's syndrome. J Bone Joint Surg Am 66A:568, 1984.
130. Parrett D, Neilsen KH, White RG: Radioimmunoassay of IgM, IgG, and IgA *Brucella* antibodies. Lancet 1:1075, 1977.
131. Patzakis MJ, Rao S, Wilkins J, et al: Analysis of 61 cases of vertebral osteomyelitis. Clin Orthop 264:178, 1991.
132. Pertuiset E, Beaudreuil J, Liote F, et al: Spinal tuberculosis in adults: A study of 103 cases in a developed country, 1980-1994. Medicine 78:309-320, 1999.
133. Piercy EA, Smith JW: Vertebral osteomyelitis. In Schlossberg D (ed): Orthopedic Infection. New York, Springer, 1988, pp 21-38.
134. Pina MA, Modrego PJ, Uroz JJ, et al: Brucellar spinal epidural abscess of cervical location: Report of four cases. Eur Neurol 45:249-253, 2001.
135. Pinckney LE, Currarino G, Higgenboten CL: Osteomyelitis of the cervical spine following dental extraction. Radiology 135:335, 1980.
136. Post MJ, Sze G, Quencer RM, et al: Gadolinium-enhanced MR in spinal infection. J Comput Assist Tomogr 14:721, 1990.
137. Pritchard DJ: Granulomatous infections of bones and joints. Orthop Clin North Am 6:1029, 1975.
138. Rajapakse CNA, Karin Al-Aska, Al-Orainey I, et al: Spinal brucellosis. Br J Rheumatol 26:28, 1987.
139. Ramani PS, Sengupta RP: Cauda equina compression due to tabetic arthropathy of the spine. J Neurol Neurosurg Psychiatry 36:260, 1973.
140. Redfern RM, Cottam SN, Phillipson AP: *Proteus* infection of the spine. Spine 13:439, 1988.
141. Reeder MM, Palmer PCS: The Radiology of Tropical Diseases with Epidemiological, Pathological, and Clinical Correlation. Baltimore, Williams & Wilkins, 1981.
142. Reginato AJ: Syphilitic arthritis and osteitis. Rheum Dis Clin North Am 19:379, 1993.
143. Resnick D, Niwayama G: Osteomyelitis, septic arthritis, and soft tissue infection: Organisms. In Resnick D (ed): Diagnosis of Bone and Joint Disorders, 3rd ed. Philadelphia, WB Saunders, 1995, pp 2448-2558.
144. Rigamonti D, Liem L, Wolf AL, et al: Epidural abscess in the cervical spine. Mt Sinai J Med 61:357, 1994.
145. Roberts PW: Syphilis as a cause of backache. NY State J Med 19:20, 1919.
146. Ross PM, Fleming JL: Vertebral body osteomyelitis: Spectrum and natural history: A retrospective analysis of 37 cases. Clin Orthop 118:190, 1976.
147. Sadato N, Numaguchi Y, Rigamonti D, et al: Spinal epidural abscess with gadolinium-enhanced MRI: Serial follow-up studies and clinical correlations. Neuroradiology 36:44, 1994.
148. Sandhu FS, Dillon WP: Spinal epidural abscess: Evaluation with contrast-enhanced MR imaging. AJNR Am J Neuroradiol 12:1087, 1992.
149. Sapico F, Montgomery JL: Pyogenic vertebral osteomyelitis: Report of nine cases and review of the literature. Rev Infect Dis 5:754, 1979.
150. Sapico FL, Montgomerie JZ: Vertebral osteomyelitis. Infect Dis Clin North Am 4:539, 1990.
151. Sapico FL, Montgomerie JZ: Vertebral osteomyelitis in intravenous drug abusers: Report of three cases and review of the literature. Rev Infect Dis 2:196, 1980.
152. Schauwecker DS: The scintigraphic diagnosis of osteomyelitis. AJR Am J Roentgenol 158:9, 1992.
153. Schimmer RC, Jeanneret C, Nunley PD, et al: Osteomyelitis of the cervical spine: A potentially dramatic disease. J Spinal Disord 15:110-117, 2002.
154. Schlaeffer F, Mikolich DJ, Mates SM: Technetium Tc 99m diphosphonate bone scan: False-normal findings in elderly patients with hematogenous vertebral osteomyelitis. Arch Intern Med 147:2024, 1987.
155. Schofferman L, Schofferman J, Zucherman J, et al: Occult infections causing persistent low-back pain. Spine 14:417, 1989.
156. Schwartz ST, Spiegel M, Ho G Jr: Bacterial vertebral osteomyelitis and epidural abscess. Semin Spine Surg 2:95, 1990.
157. Seddon HJ: Pott's paraplegia: Prognosis and treatment. Br J Surg 22:769, 1935.
158. Simpson WM, McIntosh CA: Actinomycosis of the vertebrae (actinomycotic Pott's disease). Arch Surg 14:1166, 1927.
159. Sippel JD, Masry NA, Farid Z: Diagnosis of human brucellosis with ELISA. Lancet 2:19, 1982.
160. Small PM, Fujiwara PI: Management of tuberculosis in the United States. N Engl J Med 345:189-200, 2001.
161. Smith AS, Blaser SI: Infectious and inflammatory processes of the spine. Radiol Clin North Am 29:809, 1991.
162. Smith AS, Weinstein MA, Mizushima A, et al: MR imaging characteristics of tuberculous spondylitis vs vertebral osteomyelitis. AJR Am J Roentgenol 153:399, 1989.
163. Smith MD, Emery SE, Dudley A, et al: Vertebral artery injury during anterior decompression of the cervical spine: A retrospective review of ten patients. J Bone Joint Surg Br 75B:410, 1993.
164. Stauffer RN: Pyogenic vertebral osteomyelitis. Orthop Clin North Am 6:1015, 1975.
165. Stausbaugh LJ: Vertebral osteomyelitis. In Jauregui LE (ed): Diagnosis and Management of Bone Infections. New York, Marcel Dekker, 1995, pp 167-200.
166. Stewart GR, Loewenthal J: Vertebral hydatidosis. Aust NZ J Surg 36:175, 1967.
167. Takahashi J, Ebara S, Kaminura M, et al: Early-phase enhanced inflammatory reaction after spinal instrumentation surgery. Spine 26:1698-1704, 2001.
168. Tang HJ, Lin HJ, Liu YC, et al: Spinal epidural abscess: Experience with 46 patients and evaluation of prognostic factors. J Infect 45:76-81, 2002.
169. Thacker AK, Radhakrishnan K, Maloo JC: Pyogenic cervical vertebral osteomyelitis. Br J Clin Prac 44:763, 1990.
170. Torres-Rojas J, Taddonio RF, Sanders CV: Spondylitis caused by *Brucella abortus*. South Med J 72:1166, 1979.
171. Unger HS, Schneider LH, Sher J: Paraplegia secondary to hydatid disease: Report of a case. J Bone Joint Surg Am 45A:1479, 1963.
172. Vaccaro AR, Harris BM: Presentation and treatment of pyogenic vertebral osteomyelitis. Semin Spine Surg 12:183-191, 2000.
173. Velan GJ, Leitner J, Gepstein R: Pyogenic osteomyelitis of the spine in the elderly: Three cases of a synchronous non-axial infection by a different pathogen. Spinal Cord 37:215-217, 1999.
174. Verdu A, Garcia-Granero E, Garcia-Fuster MJ, et al: Lumbar osteomyelitis and epidural abscess complicating recurrent pilonidal cyst: Report of a case. Dis Colon Rectum 43:1015-1017, 2000.
175. Waldvogel FA, Vasey H: Osteomyelitis: The past decade. N Engl J Med 303:360, 1980.
176. Watters DA: Surgery for tuberculosis before and after human immunodeficiency virus infection: A tropical perspective. Br J Surg 84:8-14, 1997.
177. Waught M: Syphilis as a cause of backache. BMJ 1:803, 1972.
178. Weinstein MA, Patel TC, Bell GR: Evaluation of the patient with spinal infection. Semin Spine Surg 12:160-175, 2000.
179. Weld PW: Osteomyelitis of the ilium masquerading as acute appendicitis. JAMA 173:634, 1960.
180. Wetzel FT, La Rocca H: Grisel's syndrome: A review. Clin Orthop 240:141, 1989.
181. Wiedau-Pazos M, Curio G, Grusser C: Epidural abscess of the cervical spine with osteomyelitis of the odontoid process. Spine 24:133-136, 1999.
182. Wiley AM, Trueta J: The vascular anatomy of the spine and its relationship to pyogenic vertebral osteomyelitis. J Bone Joint Surg Br 41B:796, 1959.
183. Wurtz R, Quader Z, Simon D, et al: Cervical tuberculous vertebral osteomyelitis: Case report and discussion of the literature. Clin Infect Dis 16:806, 1993.
184. Young EJ: Human brucellosis. Rev Infect Dis 5:821, 1983.
185. Young WB: Actinomycosis with involvement of the vertebral column: Case report and review of the literature. Clin Radiol 11:175, 1960.

INTERVERTEBRAL DISC SPACE INFECTION

CAPSULE SUMMARY

	LOW BACK	NECK
Frequency of spinal pain	Very common	Very common
Location of spinal pain	Disc space	Disc space
Quality of spinal pain	Sharp, severe	Sharp, severe
Symptoms and signs	Percussion tenderness, decreased motion	Percussion tenderness, decreased motion
Laboratory tests	Elevated erythrocyte sedimentation rate, culture of disc and blood	Elevated erythrocyte sedimentation rate, culture of disc and blood
Radiographic findings	Disc space narrowing on plain radiographs; MR for early infection	Disc space narrowing on plain radiographs; MR for early infection
Treatment	Antibiotics, immobilization	Antibiotics, immobilization

PREVALENCE AND PATHOGENESIS

Infection of the intervertebral disc (IVD) is an uncommon but potentially disabling cause of spinal pain. Although once thought to be exclusively a complication of vertebral osteomyelitis, IVD infection also can develop secondary to hematogenous invasion through the bloodstream and by direct penetration during disc surgery. A significant clinical feature of this illness is the long delay between the onset of symptoms of spinal pain, muscle spasm, and limitation of motion and the establishment of the diagnosis.

Epidemiology

IVD infection is uncommon in adults, occurring with an incidence of two patients per year at an orthopedic hospital.[25] Approximately 2.8% of patients who have lumbar disc surgery develop disc space infection.[51] IVD infection occurs more commonly in the lumbar spine compared with the frequency of infection in the cervical spine.[34] Men are more frequently affected, and the disease has been diagnosed in patients up to 63 years of age.

Pathogenesis

The pathogenesis of disc space infections in adults in the absence of a surgical or diagnostic procedure remains in doubt. In children, blood vessels supply the IVDs. Infection occurs secondary to hematogenous spread of organisms. Others have considered discitis in children a noninfectious disease, an inflammatory or traumatic disorder. The course in children is relatively benign.[5]

Although it is generally believed that the IVDs are avascular in adult life, a number of investigators have demonstrated some blood flow in adults.[62,72] While there is a decrease in the number of vessels that enter the nucleus pulposus with aging, an adequate circumferential supply is maintained from the periphery.[21] The blood supply to IVDs is greater in children, which may explain the increased frequency of disc space infection in the pediatric age group as compared with adults.[5]

There is evidence supporting the importance of both the venous and arterial systems in the development of disc infections. Patients with pelvic and urinary tract infections may develop involvement of disc spaces with the identical organism, and it is postulated that these organisms may spread by means of the vertebral venous plexus of Batson.[3,11,17] Batson's plexus is a network of veins that surrounds the vertebral column and is connected to the major veins that return blood to the heart and the inferior and superior vena cava. However, other investigators believe that the reversal of flow in the venous system, which would allow infected blood to enter Batson's plexus, does not occur under usual circumstances. Instead, they suggest hematogenous spread through the arterial system as the source of infection.[14,72] It is probable that either route may be involved in appropriate circumstances.

The IVDs are infected by hematogenous spread, most commonly through the bloodstream. A variety of infections of the skin, urinary tract, and soft tissues in compromised hosts have been associated with disc infection.[31] However, other mechanisms may play a role in some circumstances. Patients using corticosteroids for asthma or who are debilitated may develop atypical disc infections with fungal organisms such as *Aspergillus*.[27,59] A few patients have been reported to have developed IVD infection after trauma or heavy physical labor.[12,45] Trauma in the area of the IVD may result in the formation of a hematoma that is then infected by blood-borne organisms, but the likelihood of this occurrence is not great. In fact, most patients with IVD infections deny previous trauma.[25] Therefore, the association of this infection and trauma is unlikely. Patients who undergo operative procedures, needle biopsy, discography, or puncture of a disc during a lumbar puncture can develop infection by direct inoculation of the organism at the time of the procedure.[51] Epidural spinal anesthesia at the time of delivery has been associated with discitis.[2] In the cervical spine, IVD infection has been reported to occur spontaneously with cervical discography and subsequent to cerebral angiography.[6,29,43] Spinal infection associated with lumbar disc surgery occurs less than 1% of the time whether an anterior, posterior, or percutaneous route is used.[1] Others may develop disc space infection from organisms that arise from contiguous abscesses.[15]

Honan and colleagues reviewed a group of 68 adults with spontaneous infectious discitis: 16 individuals treated by the authors in a community hospital and 52 described in the medical literature.[23] In contrast to postoperative discitis, a variety of gram-positive and gram-negative organisms caused the infection. Patients with spontaneous infection had diabetes, vertebral fracture, or preexisting spinal trauma. Elevated erythrocyte sedimentation rate (ESR) (14 of 15 tested patients) and abnormal MRI results were the most sensitive diagnostic tests. Individuals with prolonged symptoms before diagnosis had discitis in the cervical and not the lumbar spine.

CLINICAL HISTORY

Patients with IVD infections of the spine have symptoms of localized spinal pain. In some, the onset of the pain is acute and very severe. In other patients, the pain may be more insidious and milder. The duration of pain before diagnosis ranges from 1 month to 2 years.[45] It becomes chronic and may be associated with radiation into the flanks, abdomen, testes, or lower extremities. In the neck, radiating pain affects the arms and hands. The pain is exacerbated by movement and relieved by absolute rest. Motion may initiate paroxysms of paravertebral muscle spasm, and the patients usually have great difficulty walking. Loss of motor strength or sensory symptoms in the upper and lower extremities suggests spinal cord compression with the development of epidural abscess.[29]

In one series, 77% of cases affected the lumbar disc, 15% the cervical spine, and 8% the thoracic spine.[45] In one group of patients, 3 of 13 had neurologic deficits at time of diagnosis. The two patients with lumbar infection had severe L5 root weakness and paraparesis.[45]

Discitis also may be a complication of invasive procedures including discography and discectomy. Patients who have postoperative infection develop a significant increase in back or neck pain after a period of initial relief with no significant increase in radicular pain. Radicular or myelopathic symptoms may appear as the infection spreads from the disc to the bone to the epidural space.

Prophylactic use of antibiotics before discectomy prevents infection. In a study of 1642 patients, 19 of 508 patients who did not receive antibiotic prophylaxis (3.7%) developed postoperative spondylodiscitis, whereas none of the 1134 patients who received antibiotic prophylaxis did.[57]

PHYSICAL EXAMINATION

Physical findings in patients with disc infection include localized tenderness on palpation, limitation of motion of the spine, and paravertebral muscle spasm. Fever is rarely present.[45] Patients prefer to remain motionless in bed. Examination of the skin, respiratory system, gastrointestinal system, and genitourinary system may demonstrate the primary source of infection. Neurologic examination may demonstrate evidence of myelopathy (spasticity, sensory level, hyperreflexia, and positive extensor response) in patients with spinal cord compression in the cervical area.[43]

LABORATORY DATA

The laboratory findings are nonspecific in disc space infections. The most commonly abnormal test is the ESR. It is elevated in up to 75% of patients.[25] The ESR is elevated in lumbar spine surgery patients for 2 to 4 weeks postoperatively. Rates remain elevated in patients with disc space infection for longer periods of time.[24] C-reactive protein (CRP) returns to normal more rapidly than ESR after uncomplicated lumbar spine surgery. A persistently elevated CRP may be associated with a postoperative infection.[69] A mild leukocytosis with a normal differential is also seen.[45] Individuals who are febrile, have an ESR above 25 mm/hr, and have a CRP greater than 2.0 mg after the fifth postoperative day are at risk of a disc infection.[60] Occasionally, blood cultures are positive during the acute phases of the illness,[45] but culture of fluid obtained by needle aspiration or at surgery is usually positive.[45,58] The most frequently cultured organism causing disc infection is *S. aureus*. Other gram-positive organisms include *S. epidermidis*[54] and streptococcal species, including *Streptococcus milleri*.[36] Gram-negative organisms also have been implicated, particularly *Pseudomonas aeruginosa*, in intravenous drug abusers.[58,61] *Enterobacter cloacae* and *E. coli* have been the source of infection in other immunocompromised patients, including the elderly and those with urosepsis.[52,63] Gram-negative organisms, including *Campylobacter fetus*, Group Ve-1, and *Kingella kingae*, have caused discitis in otherwise immunocompetent patients.[28,33,35] *Serratia* spondylodiscitis was caused by contaminated normal saline utilized for surgical lavage.[19] Anaerobic organisms have been implicated in rare circumstances,[47] as have fungal organisms.[49] The list of anaerobes and fungal organisms associated with discitis has been expanded to include *Eikenella corrodens* and *Aspergillus fumigatus*, respectively.[7,41,64]

Pathology

Histopathologic evaluation of disc tissue biopsy specimens demonstrates vascularization with or without granulation tissue, myxoid degeneration, and cellular necrosis. Adjacent to these areas is evidence of chronic osteomyelitis.[30]

RADIOGRAPHIC FINDINGS

Roentgenograms

The radiographic features of disc infection are distinctive and help to differentiate it from that of vertebral osteomyelitis; however, they may lag behind clinical symptoms by 6 weeks or more.[25] The earliest change is a decrease in the height of the affected IVD space (Fig. 12-8).

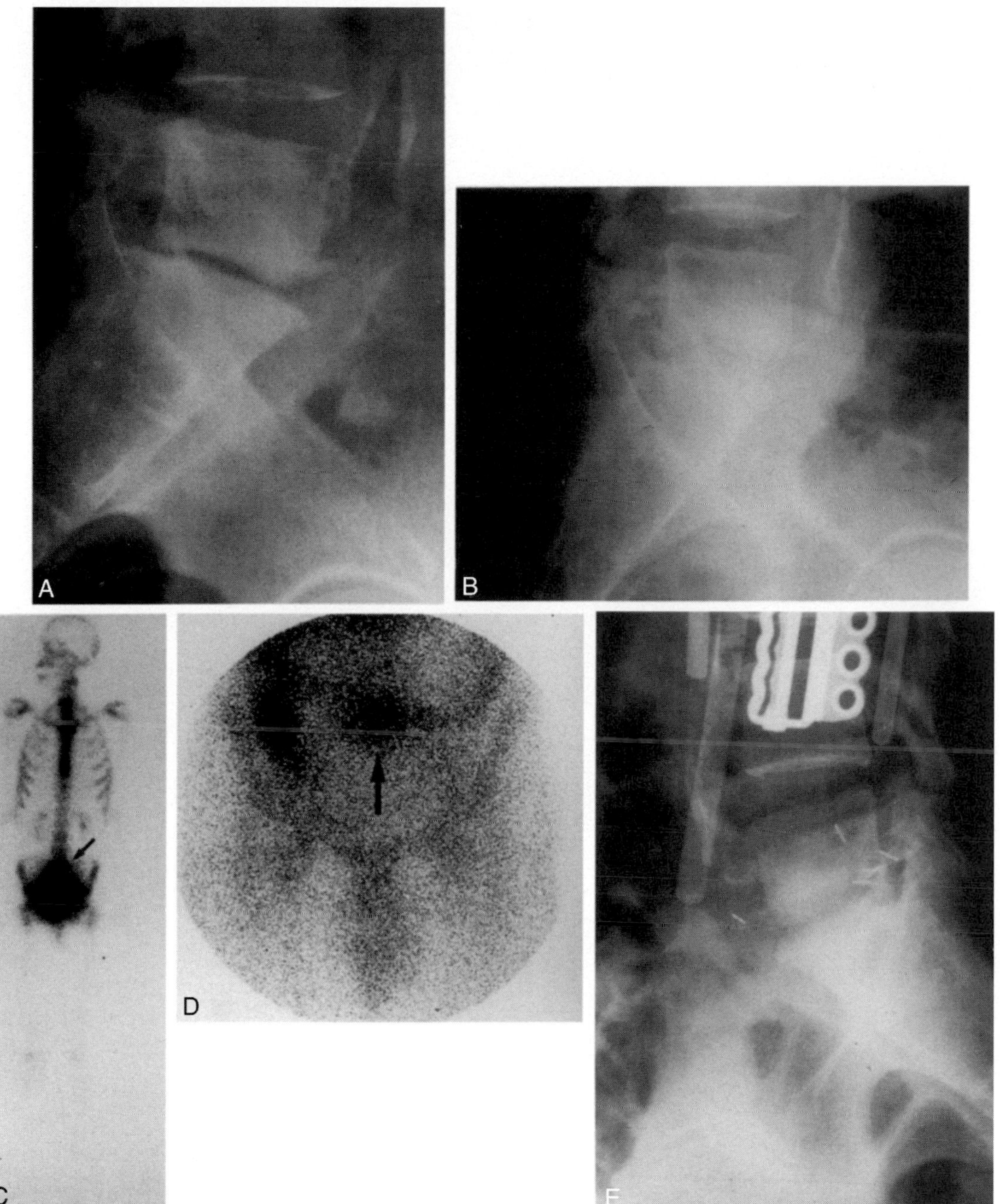

Figure 12-8 A 50-year-old man with a prior history of *S. aureus* endocarditis and drug abuse fell at work, striking his back. Roentgenograms were normal and the patient was given conservative therapy with a good response. Four months later the patient complained of severe, localized lower lumbar pain. Percussion tenderness over the L5 vertebra was painful. *A*, 2/17/86. Lateral roentgenogram reveals marked disc space narrowing with early sclerosis of surrounding endplates. *B*, 3/4/86. Continued disc space dissolution has occurred with reactive bony sclerosis. *C*, 3/7/86. Bone scan revealed markedly increased uptake in the L5 region *(arrow)*. *D*, 3/14/86. Gallium scan demonstrated increased uptake in the L5 vertebral area *(arrow)*. *E*, 3/22/86. The patient admitted to intravenous drug use. Blood cultures grew *Staphylococcus epidermidis*. Biopsy of the disc while the patient was on antibiotics obtained disc material that did not grow organisms on culture. The patient received antibiotics for staphylococcal infection and a lumbosacral brace. He was asymptomatic at time of discharge.

Two months after the appearance of disc space narrowing, reactive sclerosis of subchondral bone appears in the adjoining vertebral bodies. Subsequently, progressive irregularity of the vertebral endplates develops and indicates a local extension of the inflammatory process and an osteomyelitis (Fig. 12-9). At this juncture, the loss of vertebral bone may be associated with a "ballooning" of the IVD space.[25] This increase in apparent disc space is usually associated with involvement of the vertebral body posteriorly. Repair may occur at any stage of infection and is manifested by bony proliferation about the outside margin of the disc. The process may heal with bony ankylosis of the adjacent vertebral bodies across the affected disc space.

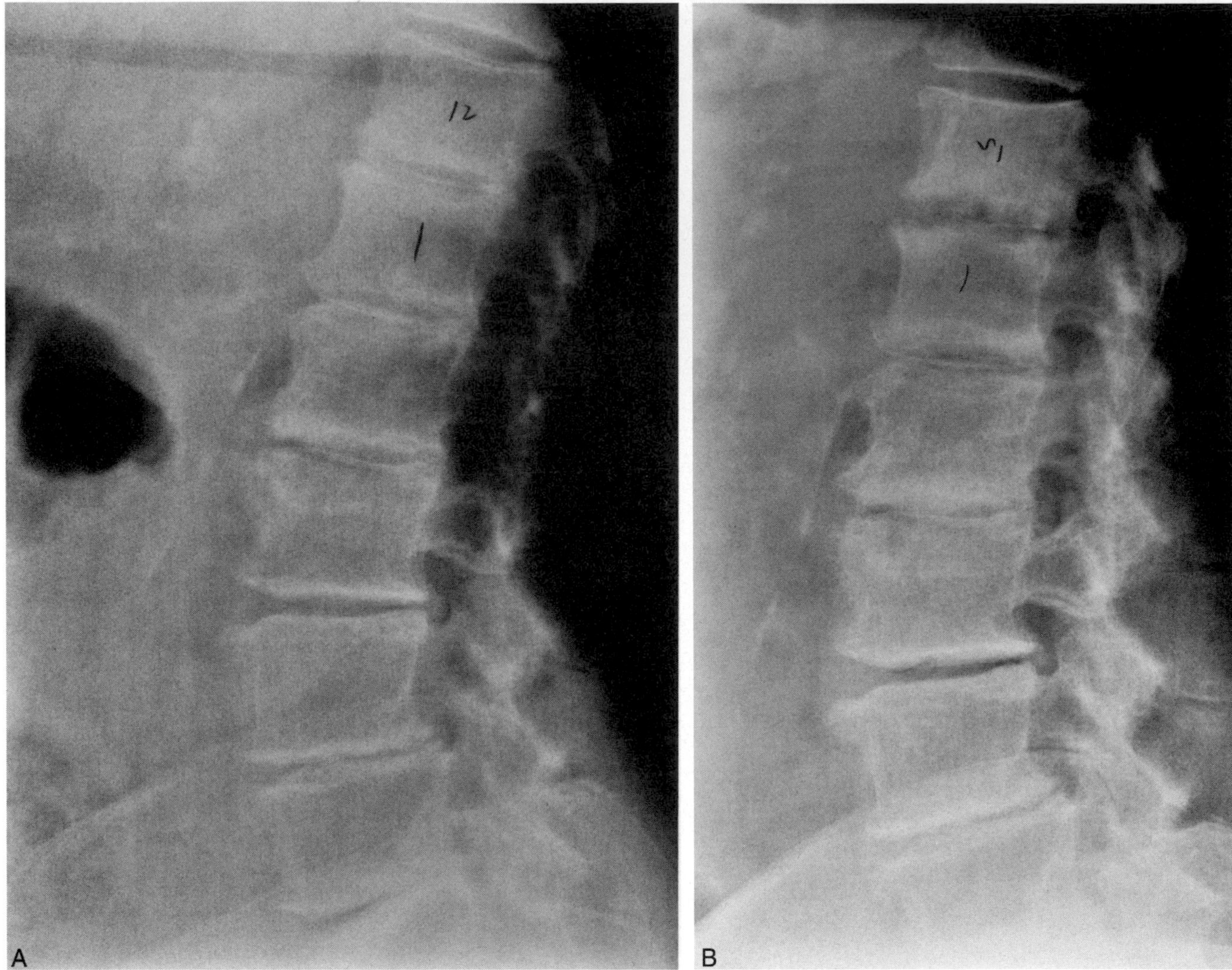

Figure 12-9 Discitis. A 74-year-old woman had a history of lumbar spondylosis and polymyalgia rheumatica treated with corticosteroids. She developed increasing upper back pain and weight loss. Lateral radiographic view *(A)* demonstrates generalized disc space narrowing with anterior osteophytes and intact endplates. Roentgenogram 12 months later *(B)* demonstrates endplate erosion at T12 and L1. She had streptococcal endocarditis that required a prolonged course of antibiotics.

Scintigraphy

Bone scintiscans are very useful in rapidly identifying increased bone activity in areas contiguous to infected discs. The bone scan may be positive in an area of infection that appears normal on plain radiographs.[42] Both ^{99m}Tc and ^{67}Ga citrate scans are more sensitive than plain roentgenograms in detecting early disc infections.[8,40] The use of single-photon emission computed tomography has increased the sensitivity of bone scintigraphy in the diagnosis of infectious processes in the axial skeleton. Indium leukocyte imaging has not proved to be adequately sensitive to be clinically useful in patients with IVD infections.[71]

Computed Tomography

CT is helpful in assessing bony alterations and soft tissue involvement to a greater extent than scintiscan. Sensitivity is increased if CT technique includes soft tissue and bone windows. CT findings consistent with discitis include disc narrowing and endplate erosion. CT is unable to detect early changes of discitis during the first 14 days of symptoms and cannot differentiate postoperative changes from infection.[10,39]

Magnetic Resonance

MR is a sensitive method for the early detection of inflammation in infected tissues. It is able to detect early disc infection before changes occur on plain roentgenograms (Figs. 12-10 and 12-11).[38] In the acute stage, the disc is hypodense in T1-weighted images and hyperdense in T2-weighted images.[32] MR with gadolinium enhancement is a useful test for the differentiation of normal postoperative healing changes from those related to septic discitis. Gadolinium-enhanced MR findings associated with infection include decreased signal intensity on T1-weighted

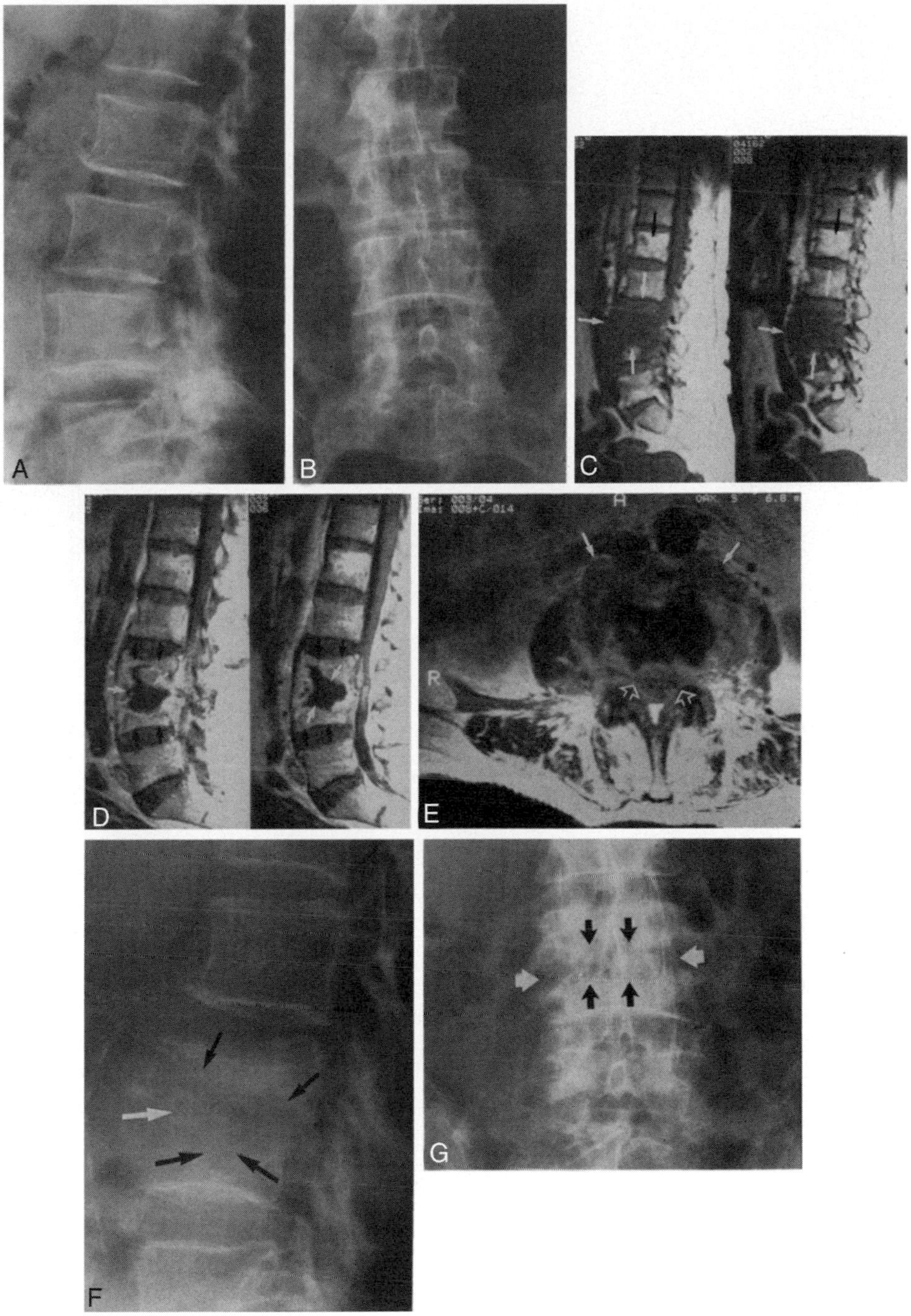

Figure 12-10 Discitis. An 86-year-old woman had an episode of *Escherichia coli* urosepsis treated with antibiotics in 9/91. Lateral *(A)* and anteroposterior *(B)* plain roentgenograms were taken on 9/28/91 demonstrating intact intervertebral disc spaces in the lumbar area with the presence of small osteophytes. She developed low back pain and, then, leg pain over a 6-week-period. On 11/2/91, she was readmitted to the hospital. Blood cultures were positive for *E. coli*. MR examination was done on 11/5/91. Sagittal T1-weighted images *(C)* reveal decreased signal in the area of the disc and the bodies of L3 and L4 *(white arrows)* compatible with inflammatory tissue. Hemangioma was the cause of increased signal in L1 *(black arrows)*. Sagittal *(D)* and axial *(E)* T1-weighted gadolinium images demonstrate enhancement of the superior portion of L3 and the inferior portion of L4 *(black arrows)* and an irregular, nonenhancing area *(white arrows)* involving the disc and surrounding vertebral bodies compatible with an infectious process. Paraspinous *(white arrows)* and epidural *(white open arrows)* extension is best seen on axial view *(E)*. Lateral *(F)* and anteroposterior *(G)* plain roentgenograms were taken on 11/28/91 and demonstrated vertebral body erosion *(black arrows)* and total dissolution of the intervertebral disc space *(white arrows)*. *(A–G, Courtesy of Bernardo Kotelanski, MD.)*

images in the bone marrow adjacent to the disc, increased signal intensity with loss of the intranuclear cleft in the disc space, and posterior annulus on T2-weighted sequences.[4] However, in the postoperative period, the MR differences are not great enough to conclude a definitive diagnosis of infection.[16] Van Goethem and colleagues suggest that the absence of Modic type I changes, of contrast enhancement of the disc, or of enhancing paravertebral soft tissue suggests the absence of an infection. In these circumstances, MR images are useful to exclude infection rather than to confirm the diagnosis.[70]

DIFFERENTIAL DIAGNOSIS

The diagnosis of IVD infection is often overlooked because of nonspecific symptoms and its relative infrequency as a cause of back pain compared with mechanical disorders and the spondyloarthropathies. Nonetheless, physicians should be aware of this treatable entity so that the appropriate diagnosis will be made in an expeditious manner. The definitive diagnosis of a disc infection depends on the aspiration or biopsy of the infected site with subsequent confirmation by culture of the causative

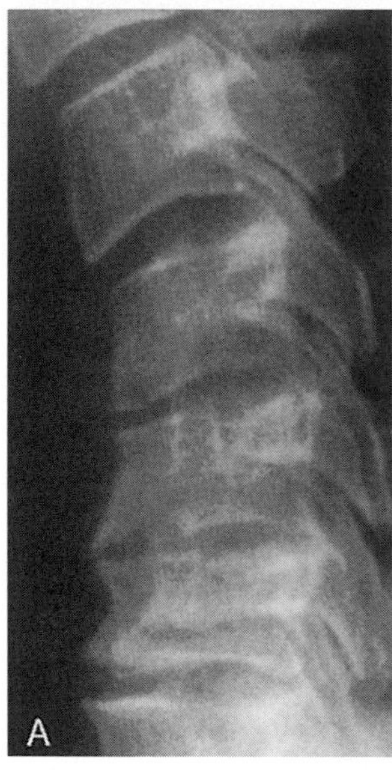

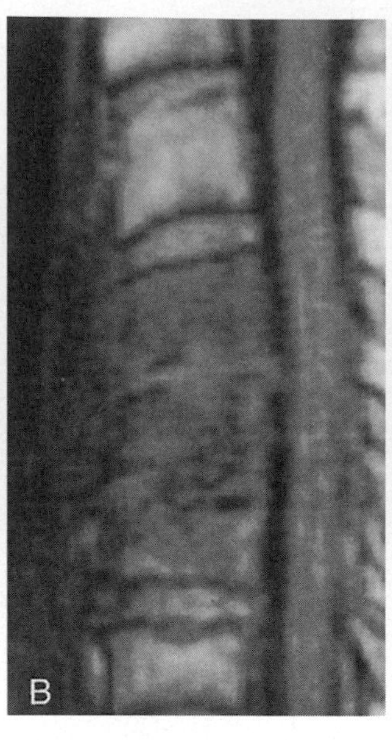

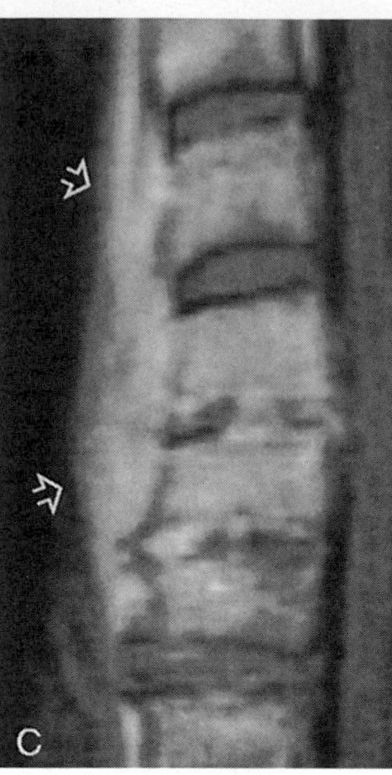

Figure 12-11 Spinal infection: MR imaging. Pyogenic spondylitis. This 40-year-old man developed infective spondylitis after multilevel cervical discography. *A*, Routine radiography shows narrowing of the intervertebral discs at the C4-C5 and the C5-C6 levels. Prevertebral soft tissue swelling was also evident. *B*, Sagittal T1-weighted (TR/TE 500/12) spin-echo MR image reveals low signal intensity of the marrow of the fourth, fifth, and sixth cervical vertebral bodies. *C*, After intravenous administration of gadolinium contrast agent, a sagittal T1-weighted (TR/TE 500/12) spin-echo MR image shows hyperintensity in the prevertebral soft tissues *(arrows)*. In comparison with the findings in *B*, the marrow involvement is less apparent. *(A–C, From Resnick D, Niwayama G: Osteomyelitis, septic arthritis, and soft tissue infection: Axial skeleton. In Resnick D [ed]: Diagnosis of Bone and Joint Disorders, 3rd ed. Philadelphia, WB Saunders, 1995, p 2434.)*

organism. Fine-needle aspiration is able to obtain adequate samples to culture the causative organisms.[50] A bone scan may help identify this entity in the patient who has normal roentgenograms.

Hadjipavlou and associates described their retrospective experience with 101 patients with primary, nonsurgical, pyogenic spinal infections.[20] Spondylodiscitis was the most common form of spinal infection in 96 of 202 patients. Infections occurred in the lumbar, thoracic, and cervical spine in 56%, 35%, and 9% of patients, respectively. The greatest risk for a spinal infection was the presence of a concurrent extraspinal infection (29.7%). Epidural abscess complicated spondylodiscitis in 35% of individuals, with the greatest risk of neurologic decompensation occurring in the thoracic and cervical lesions. The most common isolated organisms included *S. aureus* (62.7%), *Streptococcus* species (19.6%), and *S. epidermidis* (14.7%). Leukocyte counts were elevated in a minority (42.6%) of spondylodiscitis patients. Surgical intervention was required most frequently for neurologic dysfunction related to abscess formation. Complete resolution of paralysis after surgical decompression was limited to 23% of paralytic patients. Intravenous antibiotics for 6 weeks followed by 6 weeks of oral antibiotics are adequate for resolution of pyogenic spinal infections in the absence of neurologic abnormalities. Surgical patients had less residual back pain (5/19) than nonsurgical patients (18/28).[20]

The differential diagnosis of septic discitis and mechanical discitis is a problem in patients who have undergone invasive procedures (discography, discectomy) involving the intervertebral disc.[13,18] The frequency of discitis occurring after discography ranges from 1% to 4% of procedures.[46] Patients with septic discitis (culture positive or negative) have elevated ESR and CRP levels and evidence of large infiltrates of lymphoplasmacytic cells.[18] Patients who develop discitis postoperatively present with new onset of pain as early as 3 days and as late as 20 months after their surgery. The pain occurs after resolution of the preoperative pain and may be of a different quality and radiation. The organism that causes this infection is *S. epidermidis*, a skin contaminant, suggesting seeding at the time of operation.[67] The pain is severe and may be ascribed to a recurrent herniated disc or hysteria.[68] Diagnosis of discitis including postoperative infections may be confirmed by the use of an automated percutaneous biopsy.[44]

Other diseases that may be associated with IVD narrowing accompanied by lysis or sclerosis of adjacent vertebrae include osteomyelitis of a vertebral body, degenerative disease, calcium pyrophosphate dihydrate crystal deposition, neuroarthropathy, and trauma.[48] Sarcoidosis may cause similar changes on occasion. MR is able to detect the presence of sarcoid spondylodiscitis but cannot differentiate pyogenic from granulomatous inflammation. Biopsy of the disc space is required.[26] Patients with chronic renal failure may develop spinal erosive changes that simulate disc space infections. Disc changes range from superficial erosions at the anterosuperior and anteroinferior margins of the vertebral bodies to large resorptive defects mimicking disc infection.[66] These changes occur after 3 years on dialysis. Table 12-6 describes the characteristic alterations that help differentiate these possible diagnoses. Primary or metastatic tumor in the spine does not lead to significant loss of IVD space. An intact disc space with adjacent vertebral body lysis is more characteristic of a tumor than of infection. On occasion, myeloma and chordoma can extend across or around the IVD to involve contiguous vertebrae.[56] It is also possible for intraosseous disc herniation to occur secondary to vertebral body bone weakening secondary to invasion.[55]

TREATMENT

Therapy for IVD infections includes antibiotics and immobilization by bed rest, casts, or bracing. There is lit-

12-6 DIFFERENTIAL DIAGNOSIS OF SOME DISORDERS PRODUCING DISCAL NARROWING

Disease	Discovertebral Margin	Sclerosis	"Vacuum Phenomena"	Osteophytes	Other Findings
Infection	Poorly defined	Variable*	Absent (except with gas-forming organisms)[†]	Absent	Bone lysis, soft tissue mass
Rheumatoid arthritis	Poorly or well defined with "erosions"	Variable	Absent	Absent or mild	Apophyseal joint abnormalities, subluxation
Intervertebral osteochondrosis	Well defined	Prominent	Present	Variable	Cartilaginous nodes
Calcium pyrophosphate crystal deposition disease	Poorly or well defined	Prominent	Variable	Variable	Fragmentation, subluxation
Neuroarthropathy	Well defined	Prominent	Variable	Prominent	Disorganization, fragmentation, subluxation
Trauma	Well defined	Prominent	Variable	Prominent	Fracture, soft tissue mass
Sarcoidosis	Poorly or well defined	Variable	Absent	Absent	Soft tissue mass

*Usually evident in pyogenic infections and in tuberculosis in the black patient.
[†]Vacuum phenomena initially may be evident when intervertebral osteochondrosis also is present or, rarely, when a gas-forming microorganism is responsible for the infection.
Modified from Resnick D, Niwayama G (eds): Diagnosis of Bone and Joint Disorders, 3rd ed. Philadelphia, WB Saunders, 1995, p 2436.

tle agreement in the literature as to just what component of therapy is most effective. Some authors suggest bed rest and immobilization are adequate and antibiotics are not necessary[65]; however, most patients receive a 4- to 6-week course of antibiotic therapy.[45] The response to treatment is monitored by a relief of pain, return of the ESR to normal, and radiographic evidence of disc space restoration or bony ankylosis of adjacent vertebral bodies. Five French immunosuppressed patients with *Aspergillus* discitis were treated with itraconazole alone or in combination with flucytosine and amphotericin B. Surgical débridement was not necessary in these patients.[9] Patients with severe pain may benefit from epidural morphine injection if the use of oral or parenteral narcotics needs to be limited.[73] Surgical exploration is not indicated unless there are signs of spinal cord compression, spinal instability, or severe deformity. In patients who have concomitant illnesses, CT-guided percutaneous drainage is possible.[37] Surgical fusion is usually unnecessary. Patients who develop a disc space infection after lumbar disc surgery may be treated with immobilization and antibiotics; surgical exploration is usually unnecessary.[51] Patients with fungal discitis may require surgical decompression, although resolution of the fungal infection has been reported with amphotericin B therapy alone.[22] Surgical exploration is not indicated unless there are signs of spinal cord compression.[43]

PROGNOSIS

Most patients with disc infections have a benign course and fully recover without disability. Spinal bracing may be required for a year or longer until ankylosis of adjacent vertebral bodies occurs. Patients usually have full range of motion with healing and are asymptomatic.[45] In the cervical spine, spontaneous fusion occurs in 6 to 7 weeks after discitis secondary to discography.[18]

When discitis is suspected early and antibiotics are given in high doses until normalization of ESR, discitis resolves in a few weeks and no or mild vertebral erosion occurs. When antibiotic therapy is delayed or is inadequate in regard to the sensitivity of the organism, dosage, or duration, infection may last months and be associated with marked destruction of the vertebral bodies (Fig.12-12).[53]

The most serious complication of disc space infection was reported by Kemp.[25] In his group of 13 patients, three were hemiplegic, three were paraplegic, and all required surgical decompression. At operation, direct extension of inflammatory granulation tissue was identified growing posteriorly and involving the meninges and spinal cord. Cord damage was secondary to compression of the cord by edema, by inflammatory tissue, or from thrombosis of spinal cord vessels. Of the 6 patients with neurologic

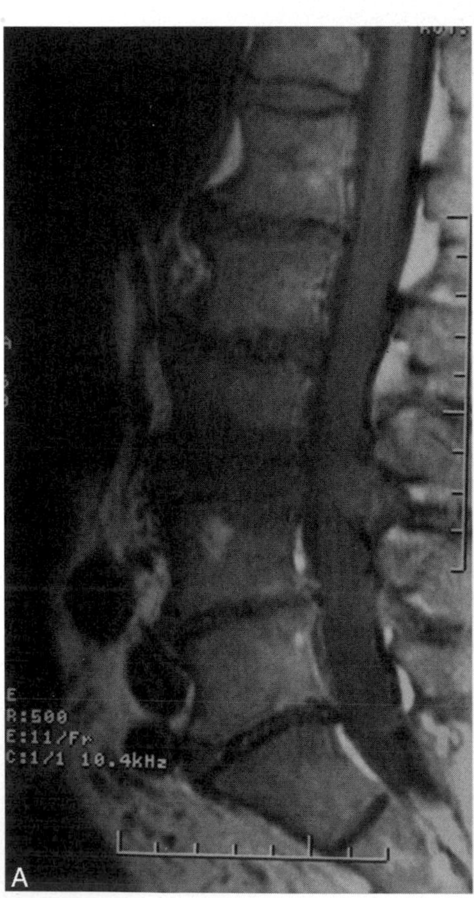

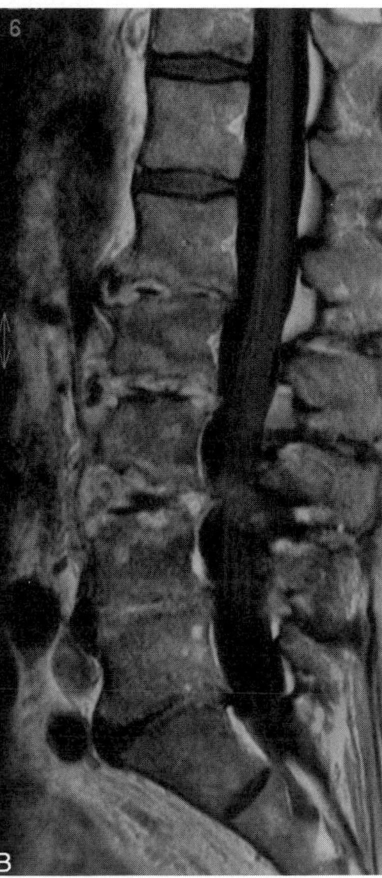

Figure 12-12 Discitis. A 68-year-old man developed intestinal obstruction requiring a colostomy and a prolonged course of antibiotics. He developed increasing back pain that was not treated for months. The lesion was diagnosed as candidal discitis, and a percutaneous aspiration was performed. *A*, MR scan sagittal view demonstrating multiple disc level involvement at L1-L2, L2-L3, and L4-L5. *B*, Two months into antifungal therapy an MR scan sagittal view demonstrates erosion of endplates and the extent of anterior soft tissue involvement.

symptoms, 2 had complete recovery, 2 had partial recovery, and 2 had no recovery after surgical decompression. The appearance of neurologic symptoms was rapid in these patients, although most of them had back pain for longer than 4 months. Accurate diagnosis and the prompt institution of appropriate therapy should prevent the emergence of this complication of disc infection.

References

Intervertebral Disc Space Infection

1. Abramovitz JN: Complications of surgery for discogenic disease of the spine. Neurosurg Clin North Am 4:167, 1993.
2. Bajwa ZH, Ho C, Grush A, et al: Discitis associated with pregnancy and spinal anesthesia. Anesth Analg 94:415-416, 2002.
3. Batson OV: The function of the vertebral veins and their role in the spread of metastasis. Ann Surg 112:138, 1940.
4. Boden SD, David DO, Dina T, et al: Postoperative diskitis: Distinguishing early MR imaging findings from normal postoperative disk space changes. Radiology 184:765, 1992.
5. Boston HC Jr, Bianco AJ Jr, Rhodes KH: Disc space infections in children. Orthop Clin North Am 6:953, 1975.
6. Cashion EL: Cervical intervertebral disc space infection following cerebral angiography. Neuroradiology 2:176, 1971.
7. Castelli C, Benazzo F, Minoli L, et al: *Aspergillus* infection of the L3-L4 disc space in an immunosuppressed heart transplant patient. Spine 15:1369, 1988.
8. Choong K, Monaghan P, McGuigan L, McLean R: Role of bone scintigraphy in the early diagnosis of discitis. Ann Rheum Dis 49:932, 1990.
9. Cortet B, Deprez X, Trili R, et al: *Aspergillus* discitis: A report of five cases. Rev Rheum [Engl] 60:38, 1993.
10. Dall BE, Rowe DE, Odette WG, Batts DH: Postoperative discitis: Diagnosis and management. Clin Orthop 224:138, 1987.
11. Doyle JR: Narrowing of the intervertebral disc space in children. J Bone Joint Surg Am 42A:1191, 1960.
12. Ettinger WH Jr, Arnett FC Jr, Stevens MB: Intervertebral disc space infections: Another low back syndrome of the young. Johns Hopkins Hosp Med J 141:23, 1977.
13. Fouquet B, Goupille P, Jattiot F, et al: Discitis after lumbar disc surgery: Features of "aseptic" and "septic" forms. Spine 17:356, 1992.
14. Ghormley RK, Bickel WH, Dickson DD: A study of acute infectious lesions of the intervertebral discs. South Med J 33:347, 1940.
15. Gordon EJ: Infection of disc space secondary to fistula from pelvic abscess. South Med J 70:114, 1977.
16. Grane P, Josephsson A, Seferlis A, et al: Septic and aseptic postoperative discitis in the lumbar spine: Evaluation by MR imaging. Acta Radiol 39:108-115, 1998.
17. Griffiths HED, Jones DM: Pyogenic infection of the spine. J Bone Joint Surg Br 53B:383, 1971.
18. Guyer RD, Collier R, Stith WJ, et al: Discitis after discography. Spine 13:1352, 1988.
19. Hadjipavlou AG, Gaitanis IN, Papadopoulos CA, et al: *Serratia* spondylodiscitis after elective lumbar spine surgery: A report of two cases. Spine 27:E507-512, 2002.
20. Hadjipavlou AG, Mader JT, Necessary JT, et al: Hematogenous pyogenic spinal infections and their surgical management. Spine 25:1668-1679, 2000.
21. Hassler O: The human intervertebral disc. Acta Orthop Scand 40:765, 1970.
22. Holmes PF, Osterman DW, Tullos HS: *Aspergillus* discitis: Report of two cases and review of the literature. Clin Orthop 226:240, 1988.
23. Honan M, White GW, Eisenberg GM: Spontaneous infectious discitis in adults. Am J Med 100:85-89, 1996.
24. Jonsson B, Soderholm R, Stromqvist B: Erythrocyte sedimentation rate after lumbar spine surgery. Spine 16:1049, 1991.
25. Kemp HBS, Jackson JW, Jeremiah JD, Hall AJ: Pyogenic infections occurring primarily in intervertebral discs. J Bone Joint Surg Br 55B:698, 1973.
26. Kenney CM III, Goldstein SJ: MRI of sarcoid spondylodiskitis. J Comput Assist Tomogr 16:660, 1992.
27. Lang EW, Pitts LH: Intervertebral disc space infection caused by *Aspergillus fumigatus*. Eur Spine J 5:207-209, 1996.
28. Levy DI, Bucci MN, Hoff JT: Discitis caused by the centers for Disease Control Microorganism Group Ve-1. Neurosurgery 25:655, 1989.
29. Lownie SP, Ferguson GG: Spinal subdural empyema complicating cervical discography. Spine 14:1415, 1989.
30. Lucio E, Adesokan A, Hadjipavlou AG, et al: Pyogenic spondylodiskitis: A radiologic/pathologic and culture correlation study. Arch Pathol Lab Med 124:712-716, 2000.
31. Lundstrom TS, Levine DP: Disk space infections. In Jauregui LE (ed): Diagnosis and Management of Bone Infections. New York, Marcel Dekker, 1995, pp 151-166.
32. Maiuri F, Iaconetta G, Gallicchio B, et al: Spondylodiscitis: Clinical and magnetic resonance diagnosis. Spine 22:1741-1746, 1997.
33. Mathieu E, Koeger A, Rozenberg S, Bourgeois P: *Campylobacter* spondylodiscitis and deficiency of cellular immunity. J Rheumatol 18:1929, 1991.
34. McCain GA, Harth M, Bell DA, et al: Septic discitis. J Rheumatol 8:100, 1981.
35. Meis JF, Sauerwein RW, Gyssens IC, et al: *Kingella kingae* intervertebral diskitis in an adult. Clin Infect Dis 15:530, 1992.
36. Meyes E, Flipo R, Van Bosterhaut B, et al: Septic *Streptococcus milleri* spondylodiscitis. J Rheumatol 17:1421, 1990.
37. Miltner O, Kisielinski K, Chalabi K, et al: Polysegmental spondylodiscitis and concomitant aortic aneurysm rupture: Case report with 3-year follow-up period. Spine 27:E423-427, 2002.
38. Morgenlander JC, Rozear MP: Disc space infection: A case report with MRI diagnosis. Am Fam Phys 42:984, 1990.
39. Nielsoen VAH, Iversen E, Ahlgren P: Postoperative discitis: Radiology of progress and healing. Acta Radiol 31:559, 1990.
40. Nolla-Sole JM, Mateo-Soria L, Rozadilla-Sacanell A, et al: Role of technetium-99m diphosphonate and gallium-67 citrate bone scanning in the early diagnosis of infectious spondylodiscitis: A comparative study. Ann Rheum Dis 51:665, 1992.
41. Noordeen MHH, Godfrey LW: Case report of an unusual cause of low back pain: Intervertebral diskitis caused by *Eikenella corrodens*. Clin Orthop 280:175, 1992.
42. Norris S, Ehrlich MG, Keim DE, et al: Early diagnosis of disc-space infection using gallium-67. J Nucl Med 19:384, 1978.
43. Oliff JFC, Gwyther SJ, Hart G: Case of the month: A case of postoperative paresis. Br J Radiol 63:819, 1990.
44. Onik G, Shang Y, Maroon JC: Automated percutaneous biopsy in postoperative diskitis: A new method. AJNR Am J Neuroradiol 11:391, 1990.
45. Onofrio BM: Intervertebral discitis: Incidence, diagnosis and management. Clin Neurosurg 27:481, 1980.
46. Osti OL, Fraser RD, Vernon-Roberts B: Discitis after discography. J Bone Joint Surg Br 72B:271, 1990.
47. Pate D, Katz A: Clostridia discitis: A case report. Arthritis Rheum 22:1039, 1979.
48. Patton JT: Differential diagnosis of inflammatory spondylitis. Skel Radiol 1:77, 1976.
49. Pennisi AK, Davis DO, Wiesel S, Moskovitz P: CT appearance of *Candida* diskitis. J Comput Assist Tom 9:1050, 1985.
50. Phadke DM, Lucas DR, Madan S: Fine-needle aspiration biopsy of vertebral and intervertebral disc lesions: Specimen adequacy, diagnostic utility, and pitfalls. Arch Pathol Lab Med 125:1463-1468, 2001.
51. Pilgaard S: Discitis (closed space infection) following removal of lumbar intervertebral disc. J Bone Joint Surg Am 51A:713, 1969.
52. Ponte CD, McDonald M: Septic discitis resulting from *Escherichia coli* urosepsis. J Fam Pract 34:767, 1992.
53. Postacchini F, Cinotti G: Iatrogenic lumbar discitis. J Bone Joint Surg Br 74B(Suppl 1):70, 1992.
54. Rawlings CE III, Wilkins RH, Gallis HA, et al: Postoperative intervertebral disc space infection. Neurosurgery 13:371, 1983.
55. Resnick D, Niwayama G: Intervertebral disc abnormalities associated with vertebral metastasis: Observations in patients and cadavers with prostate cancer. Invest Radiol 13:182, 1978.
56. Resnick D, Niwayama G: Osteomyelitis, septic arthritis, and soft-tissue infection: The axial skeleton. In Resnick D, Niwayama G (eds): Diagnosis of Bone and Joint Disorders. Philadelphia, WB Saunders, 1981, pp 2130-2153.
57. Rohde V, Meyer B, Schaller C, et al: Spondylodiscitis after lumbar discectomy: Incidence and a proposal for prophylaxis. Spine 23:615-620, 1998.

58. Scherbel AL, Gardner JW: Infections involving the intervertebral discs: Diagnosis and management. JAMA 174:370, 1960.
59. Schubert M, Schar G, Curt A, et al: *Aspergillus* spondylodiscitis in an immunocompetent paraplegic patient. Spinal Cord 36:800-803, 1998.
60. Schulitz KP, Assheuer J: Discitis after procedures on the intervertebral disc. Spine 1172-1177, 1994.
61. Selby RC, Pillary KV: Osteomyelitis and disc infection secondary to *Pseudomonas aeruginosa* in heroin addiction: Case report. J Neurosurg 37:463, 1972.
62. Smith NR: The intervertebral discs. Br J Surg 18:358, 1931.
63. Solans R, Simeon P, Cuenca R, et al: Infectious discitis caused by *Enterobacter cloacae*. Ann Rheum Dis 51:906, 1992.
64. Sugar AM: Case records of the Massachusetts General Hospital. N Engl J Med 324:754, 1991.
65. Sullivan CR: Diagnosis and treatment of pyogenic infections of the intervertebral disc. Surg Clin North Am 41:1077, 1961.
66. Sundaram M, Seelig R, Pohl D: Vertebral erosions in patients undergoing maintenance hemodialysis for chronic renal failure. AJR Am J Roentgenol 149:323, 1987.
67. Taylor TKF, Bye WA: Role of antibiotics in the management of postoperative disc space infections. Aust N Z J Surg 48:74, 1978.
68. Teplick JG, Haskin ME: Intravenous contrast-enhanced CT of the postoperative lumbar spine: Improved identification of recurrent disk herniation, scar, arachnoiditis, and diskitis. AJR Am J Roentgenol 143:845, 1984.
69. Thelander U, Larsson S: Quantitation of C-reactive levels and erythrocyte sedimentation rate after spinal surgery. Spine 17:400, 1992.
70. Van Goethem JW, Parizel PM, van den Hauwe L, et al: The value of MRI in the diagnosis of postoperative spondylodiscitis. Neuroradiology 42:580-585, 2000.
71. Whalen JL, Brown ML, McLeod R, Fitzgerald RH: Limitations of indium leukocyte imaging for the diagnosis of spine infections. Spine 16:193, 1991.
72. Wiley AM, Trueta J: The vascular anatomy of the spine and its relationship to pyogenic vertebral osteomyelitis. J Bone Joint Surg Br 41B:796, 1959.
73. Zampella EJ, Zeiger HE: Epidural morphine as an adjunct in the treatment of intervertebral disc infection. Spine 12:825, 1987.

PYOGENIC SACROILIITIS

Capsule Summary

	Low Back	Neck
Frequency of spinal pain	Very common	Not applicable (NA)
Location of spinal pain	Sacroiliac joint	NA
Quality of spinal pain	Severe, sharp	NA
Symptoms and signs	Buttock, thigh, or calf tenderness, unwillingness to walk on affected leg, Patrick's test positive	NA
Laboratory tests	Leukocytosis, blood cultures (positive in 50%)	NA
Radiographic findings	Blurred joint margins on plain roentgenographs. MR for early infection	NA
Treatment	Antibiotics, abscess drainage	NA

PREVALENCE AND PATHOGENESIS

Septic arthritis is a disease process caused by the direct invasion of a joint space by infectious agents, usually bacteria. Joints become infected by direct penetration, by spread from contiguous structures, or more often by hematogenous invasion through the bloodstream. Septic arthritis occurs more commonly in large peripheral joints (knees, shoulders) than in the lumbosacral spine; but when a joint of the axial skeleton is involved, the sacroiliac is the one most commonly affected. Facet joint infection is a rare event.

Epidemiology

Pyogenic sacroiliitis is an uncommon illness, accounting for 0.07% of hospital admissions in one study.[8] Approximately 80 patients with pyogenic sacroiliitis have been reported in the medical literature, although new cases continue to be reported, particularly with unusual organisms.[4,14,20,25,27] A recent article reviewed 166 patients with pyogenic sacroiliitis reported in the medical literature. This review excluded patients with sacroiliitis secondary to tuberculosis or brucellosis.[47] The disease occurs most commonly in young adult men. The range of ages is 20 to 66,[8] and the male-to-female ratio is 3:2.[14] The average age of patients with pyogenic sacroiliitis is 22 years.[47]

Pathogenesis

The initial factor that may result in joint infection is entry of organisms into the sacroiliac joint. Most commonly, infectious agents reach the sacroiliac joint by traveling through the bloodstream. They lodge in the vascular synovial membrane that lines the lower portion of the sacroiliac joint. The infectious agents grow in the synovium and invade the joint space. The organisms also might lodge in the ilium, the most frequently infected flat bone in the body, and grow into the sacroiliac joint. The relatively symmetrical involvement of ilium and sacrum in pyogenic sacroiliitis suggests that the joint is the initial area affected.[8] Once an infection is established in a joint, rapid destruction may occur because of both the direct toxic effects of products of organisms on joint structures and the host's inflammatory response to them.

Any factor, such as intravenous drug abuse, skin infections, bone and urinary tract infections, endocarditis, pregnancy, and bowel disease,[6,8,25] that promotes bloodborne infection or inhibits the normal defense mechanisms of the synovial joint predisposes the host to infection. Although the role of trauma in the pathogenesis of pyogenic sacroiliitis is unclear, buttock or hip injuries have been reported in patients before development of pyogenic sacroiliitis.[9,25] In one study in a rural population, 5 of 10 patients with pyogenic sacroiliitis had a history of pelvic trauma.[31] Most patients, however, deny a history of trauma, and its importance as a direct cause of infection is in question. In a significant number of patients, 41% in one review, no primary source of infection can be identified.[47] The histocompatibility typing associated with seronegative spondyloarthropathies, HLA-B27, is not associated with pyogenic sacroiliitis.[46]

Another mechanism of joint infection is contamination by local spread from a contiguous suppurative focus. Extension of a pelvic infectious process may cause disruption of the joint capsule or of the periosteum of the ilium or sacrum.[13] Infections spreading beneath the spinal ligaments may gain entry into the sacroiliac joints.[36] Another even more uncommon mechanism of joint infection is direct seeding of organisms into the joint during diagnostic or surgical procedures.

CLINICAL HISTORY

The typical patient with pyogenic sacroiliitis is a young man with fever who develops acute pain over the buttock.[14] Those who have subacute or chronic symptoms are frequently afebrile. The period of time between onset of symptoms and diagnosis may range from 12 to 20 days.[7] The pain is severe and may radiate to the low back, hip, thigh, abdomen, or calf.[8] Radiation of pain is related to irritation of the first two sacral, superior gluteal, and obturator nerves that cross anterior to the joint capsule. Abdominal pain associated with nausea and vomiting can confuse the diagnosis.[24,35] A normal appendix was surgically removed because of the clinical impression of appendicitis in one patient.[7] Patients also complain of severe leg pain that prevents them from bearing weight on the affected limb. Irritation of the iliopsoas muscle as it passes anterior to the sacroiliac joint may cause persistent hip flexion and result in pain on motion of the hip. Pyogenic sacroiliitis is usually unilateral, although bilateral disease can occur.

PHYSICAL EXAMINATION

Physical examination demonstrates tenderness over the sacroiliac joint and pain on compression of the joint. Hyperextension of the hip, Gaenslen's sign, stresses the sacroiliac joint capsule and causes pain in the buttock. Patrick's test, or the fabere sign—flexion, abduction, external rotation, and extension—of the hip, may be associated with sacroiliac joint pain. The test is done by placing the ankle of the affected side on the opposite knee and exerting downward pressure on the bent knee. If the maneuver is performed slowly, the hip may be taken through a full range of motion without producing sacroiliac pain. Therefore, the test should be done rapidly so that the sacroiliac joint will be stressed and become painful. Straight leg–raising may be limited, owing to stretching of inflamed sacral nerve roots over the anterior of the sacroiliac joint. A subgluteal abscess with swelling of the buttock and obliteration of the gluteal fold may also be seen. Infection may track along different fascial planes, presenting as masses in the inner thigh, posterior thigh, hip, lumbar spine, or abdomen.[2,24] Rectal examination is important to detect the presence of these lesions. Muscle spasm of the gluteal and lumbar paravertebral muscles may be severe. The severity of the spasm may cause severe pain and scoliosis of the lumbar spine.[25] Fever and chills may be seen in the patient with an acute onset of disease.[27]

LABORATORY FINDINGS

Laboratory results demonstrate mild anemia, leukocytosis, and elevation in the ESR. Blood cultures may be positive in up to 50% of patients, eliminating the need for joint aspiration. Arthrocentesis of the sacroiliac joint under general anesthesia with fluoroscopic guidance is the most effective method of diagnosing pyogenic sacroiliitis.[18] Closed-needle biopsy is of particular utility in patients with negative blood cultures.[37] Aspirations without fluoroscopy do not obtain adequate specimens.[14] CT scanning has also been used for aspiration of the sacroiliac joint.

S. aureus and *S. epidermidis* account for a majority of infections of the sacroiliac joint.[8] *P. aeruginosa* is frequently cultured from sacroiliac joints in parenteral drug abusers.[11] Aerobic and anaerobic streptococci may also be cultured.[27] A wide variety of organisms have been associated with pyogenic sacroiliitis, including *S. milleri*, *E. coli*, *Neisseria gonorrhoeae*, *P. mirabilis*, *Salmonella heidelberg*, and *Veillonella parvula*.[19,21,29,39,43,47] Unilateral sacroiliitis also has been associated with syphilis during its secondary phase.[40]

Brucellosis is an infectious disease most commonly diagnosed in individuals in the Middle East (an endemic area), those who consume raw milk, or those who attend infected animals. The most commonly affected joint is the sacroiliac joint. In a series of 214 patients, the sacroiliac joints were affected in 72.4%.[10] These individuals have low back pain with or without tenderness. Brucellar sacroiliitis has been reported in individuals who have emigrated to the United States.[1]

Tuberculosis also is associated with pyogenic sacroiliitis. Sacroiliac tuberculosis was a more common disease before the development of effective antituberculous antibiotic therapy. Strange reported 329 cases of sacroiliac tuberculosis.[44] The patients developed this complication as a manifestation of a generalized tubercular infection (Fig. 12-13). Sacroiliac joint involvement occurs in up to 9.7% of patients with skeletal tuberculosis. Patients have buttock pain and tenderness on direct palpation of the affected

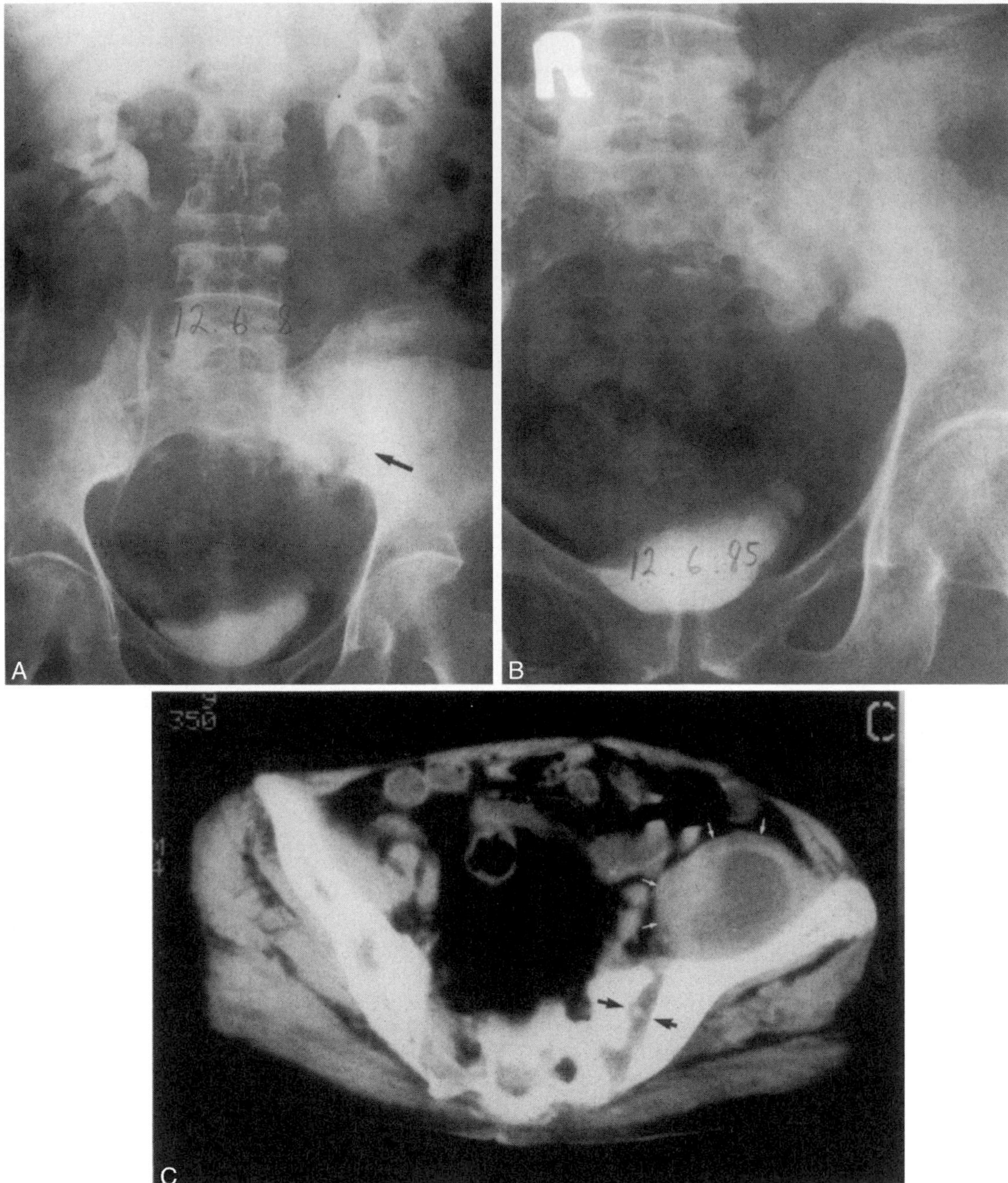

Figure 12-13 Tuberculous sacroiliitis in a 77-year-old man. *A*, Intravenous pyelography reveals marked sclerosis and widening of the left sacroiliac joint *(arrow)*. *B*, Close-up view of the left sacroiliac joint. *C*, CT scan of pelvis demonstrating erosion of the left sacroiliac joint *(black arrows)* and associated soft tissue abscess *(white arrows)*. *(A and B, Courtesy of Theodor Schifter, MD.)*

joint.[38] The onset of disease is insidious, the pain aching, and the course indolent. The diagnosis of tuberculous sacroiliitis may be confirmed by aspiration of fluid. The yield is improved by the simultaneous culture of synovial tissue. Therefore, open surgical biopsy may be required to confirm this diagnosis.[48] Closed biopsy may be adequate to yield tissue for culture and microscopic evaluation if open biopsy is too invasive.[38] Open biopsy also may be required from patients with fungal sacroiliitis as well, although aspiration may be adequate to obtain specimens that are subsequently positive on culture.[4]

RADIOGRAPHIC EVALUATION

Roentgenograms

The duration of symptoms before the appearance of radiographic changes in the sacroiliac joints in bacterial sacroiliitis is 2 weeks (Fig. 12-14).[8] The radiographic findings include blurring of joint margins, pseudowidening of the joint space, erosions, and reactive sclerosis. The lower ilium is affected first, because the fibrocartilage is thinner

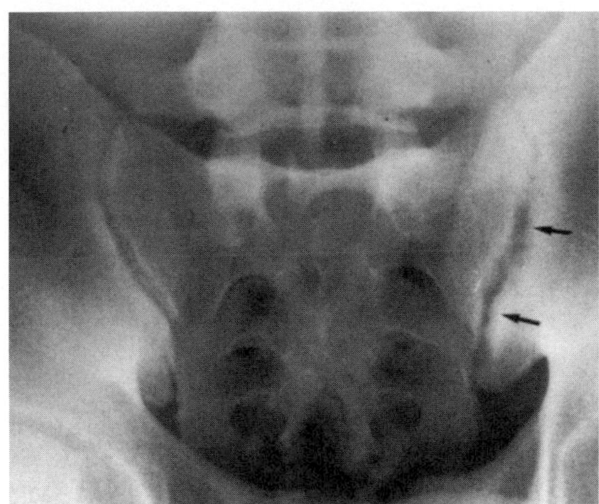

Figure 12-14 Pyogenic sacroiliitis. A 24-year-old man developed systemic lupus erythematosus requiring prednisone, 80 mg/day. The patient developed acute, severe, left-sided low back pain. The patient remained immobilized in bed because of pain. Aspiration of the sacroiliac joint yielded purulent fluid that grew *Staphylococcus aureus* on culture. The patient improved with 6 weeks of vancomycin therapy. A roentgenogram of the pelvis at 17 months after hospitalization reveals unilateral involvement *(arrows)* with joint widening, erosion, and reactive sclerosis of the left sacroiliac joint.

on the iliac side compared with the sacral side of the joint. Healing is associated with bony ankylosis.

Scintigraphy

Bone scintiscans are very useful in rapidly identifying increased joint activity associated with infection, and localization is possible within 2 days of symptoms.[3] Shielding of radioactivity in the urinary bladder may allow detection of minimal asymmetry in tracer uptake early in the course of the illness. The three-phase bone scan may be useful in differentiating osteomyelitis, septic arthritis, and cellulitis and consists of perfusion, blood pool, and delayed images. Blood pool is increased in all, whereas only osteomyelitis is associated with increased uptake on delayed bone images.[26] ^{99m}Tc methylene diphosphonate or gallium scintiscans are more sensitive than plain roentgenograms in intravenous drug abusers.[16]

Computed Tomography

CT may be more useful than plain radiographs in detection of early joint changes.[5] It may identify subtle joint space widening, osseous erosion, or increased density of periarticular fat.[30] CT is preferred for guidance of percutaneous needle arthrocentesis.[49]

Magnetic Resonance

MR is a sensitive radiographic technique for the detection of inflammatory conditions. A comparison of scintiscan, CT, and MR demonstrates a 100% sensitivity of MR compared with lesser sensitivities for the other techniques. MR demonstrated fluid in the sacroiliac joint, inflammation in bone marrow of the sacrum or ilium, and swelling in the iliopsoas muscle, along with tracking of fluid posterior to the psoas muscle.[22] MR also is able to identify joint erosions in patients with disease of longer duration.[33]

DIFFERENTIAL DIAGNOSIS

The diagnosis of pyogenic sacroiliitis is frequently missed, owing to a lack of physician awareness of this infection and the nonspecific low back symptoms of these patients, but it must be suspected in the appropriate host who presents with severe radiating low back pain. A bone scan will help localize the lesion to the sacroiliac joints. CT or MR may identify early changes of joint inflammation before plain roentgenograms are positive. Positive synovial fluid cultures from the sacroiliac joint confirm the diagnosis if blood cultures are negative. Biopsy is necessary if the diagnosis remains in doubt, cultures are negative, and granulomatous infection is being considered.

Other structures in the spine may become infected and confused with pyogenic sacroiliitis. The solid portion of the sacrum may become infected. This area of osteomyelitis is contiguous with the sacroiliac joint. The distribution and severity of pain may be similar. MR imaging is able to differentiate the location of the infection.[23]

Unilateral sacroiliac joint infection must be differentiated from appendicitis, septic arthritis of the hip, gluteal abscess, psoas abscess, pyelonephritis, intervertebral disc herniation, intraspinal tumors, and metastatic disease.[34] Osteomyelitis of the ilium may cause infection of a contiguous sacroiliac joint. The converse rarely occurs because of the tendency of primary infections of the sacroiliac joint to perforate the joint capsule anteriorly as opposed to invading surrounding bone.

Careful examination of the patient by physical and radiographic means should differentiate the patient with a local infection in the sacroiliac joint from those with infection in other areas in the axial skeleton and surrounding soft tissues. Cancer affecting bone usually has a more indolent course and multiple areas of involvement. Neoplasms of the sacrum include benign primary tumors, such as an aneurysmal bone cyst, osteoblastoma and giant cell tumor, and malignant primary tumors, which include sarcomas, chordomas, myeloproliferative tumors, and metastatic tumors.[28]

The rare occurrence of bilateral disease must be differentiated from the seronegative spondyloarthropathies, including ankylosing spondylitis, enteropathic arthritis, psoriatic arthritis, and reactive arthritis. These diseases have a much less explosive course. They are frequently associated with other systemic manifestations of disease (e.g., rash, urethritis, and iritis), which helps differentiate them from bilateral septic joint infection.

Facet Joint Pyogenic Arthritis

Facet joint infection is another form of pyogenic arthritis that is easily overlooked. The vertebral apophyseal joints become infected in rare circumstances. The infection occurs secondary to hematogenous spread to a lumbar joint in an individual usually 55 years of age.[32] Patients have localized back pain radiating into the buttock and lower extremity. Extension of the infection may cause extradural infection or epidural abscesses.[41] Epidural abscess complicates the clinical picture in 25% of patients, with 38% of those developing severe neurologic deficits. The ESR and the C-reactive protein level are elevated in all cases. Plain roentgenograms may not demonstrate an abnormality. Apophyseal joint infection should be considered if posterior elements of the vertebral bodies are affected. The abnormality may be suspected in individuals with unilateral abnormalities on bone single-photon emission CT, bone scintigraphy, or CT.[17,45] MR imaging is able to detect the location of the septic joint and the presence of any associated abscess.[42] Antibiotics alone are usually adequate for resolution of the infection in 71% of patients. A smaller number of patients require percutaneous drainage and have a better outcome than those receiving antibiotics alone.

TREATMENT

The therapy for septic arthritis of the sacroiliac joint consists of a high dose of parenteral antibiotics, which are chosen on the basis of susceptibility testing. The duration of the therapy is variable, but some studies have reported control of the infection in just days of antibiotic therapy.[8] Most studies have suggested that a minimum of 4 to 6 weeks of parenteral therapy is preferable,[14,25] but oral antibiotics may be used if adequate bactericidal levels of antibiotics against the patient's organism are achieved at 1:8 dilution. Surgical drainage is required for periarticular abscesses and the débridement of necrotic bone and cartilage. Immobilization in a spica cast is unnecessary.

Tuberculous infection of the sacroiliac joint requires triple-drug therapy. This regimen includes isoniazid, ethambutol, and rifampin or streptomycin for 3 months. Two drugs are usually continued for 18 months.[15] Others have used two drugs for shorter periods of time.[12] Fungal infection may require amphotericin B or oral 5-fluorocytosine, or both, for at least a 6-week course.[4]

PROGNOSIS

With early diagnosis and adequate antibiotic therapy, septic arthritis of the sacroiliac joint has a good outcome. With therapy, patients can expect resolution of symptoms of pain, limitation of motion, and fever. The ESR returns to normal. Many patients have no radiographic changes and return to normal function. Even patients who have fusion of the sacroiliac joint as a result of an infection should expect no functional disability.

References

Pyogenic Sacroiliitis

1. Abeles M, Mond CB: Sacroiliitis and brucellosis. J Rheumatol 16:136, 1989.
2. Avila L: Primary pyogenic infections of the sacroiliac articulation. J Bone Joint Surg 23:922, 1941.
3. Berghs H, Remans J, Drieskens L, et al: Diagnostic value of sacroiliac joint scintigraphy with ^{99m}technetium pyrophosphate in sacroiliitis. Ann Rheum Dis 37:190, 1978.
4. Brand C, Warren R, Luxton M, Barraclough D: Cryptococcal sacroiliitis: Case report. Ann Rheum Dis 44:126, 1985.
5. Carrera GF, Foley WD, Kozin F, et al: CT of sacroiliitis. AJR Am J Roentgenol 136:41, 1981.
6. Chandler FA: Pneumococcic infection of the sacroiliac joint complicating pregnancy. JAMA 101:114, 1933.
7. Coy JT, Wolf CR, Brower TD, Winter WG Jr: Pyogenic arthritis of the sacroiliac joint: Long-term follow-up. J Bone Joint Surg Am 58A:845, 1976.
8. Delbarre F, Rondier J, Delrieu F, et al: Pyogenic infection of the sacroiliac joint. J Bone Joint Surg Am 57A:819, 1975.
9. Dunn EJ, Bryan DM, Nugent JT, Robinson RA: Pyogenic infections of the sacroiliac joint. Clin Orthop 118:113, 1976.
10. El-Desouki M: Skeletal brucellosis: Assessment with bone scintigraphy. Radiology 181:415, 1991.
11. Gifford DB, Patzakis M, Ivler D, Swezey RL: Septic arthritis due to *Pseudomonas* in heroin addicts. J Bone Joint Surg Am 57A:631, 1975.
12. Goldberg J, Kovarsky J: Tuberculous sacroiliitis. South Med J 76:1175, 1983.
13. Goldstein MJ, Nasr K, Singer HC, Anderson JG: Osteomyelitis complicating regional enteritis. Gut 10:264, 1969.
14. Gordon G, Kabins SA: Pyogenic sacroiliitis. Am J Med 69:50, 1980.
15. Gorse GJ, Pais MJ, Kusske JA, Cesario TC: Tuberculous spondylitis: A report of six cases and a review of the literature. Medicine 62:178, 1978.
16. Guyot DR, Manoli A II, Kling GA: Pyogenic sacroiliitis in IV drug abusers. AJR Am J Roentgenol 149:1209, 1987.
17. Halpin DS, Gibson RD: Septic arthritis of a lumbar facet joint. J Bone Joint Surg Br 69B:457, 1987.
18. Hendrix RW, Lin PJP, Kane WJ: Simplified aspiration or injection technique for the sacroiliac joint. J Bone Joint Surg Am 64A: 1249, 1982.
19. Humphreys H, Keane CT, Marron P, Casey E: Infective sacroiliac arthritis and psoas abscess caused by *Streptococcus milleri*. J Infect 19:77, 1989.
20. Iczkovitz JM, Leek JC, Robbins DL: Pyogenic sacroiliitis. J Rheumatol 8:157, 1981.
21. Kerns SR, Dougherty K, Pope TL, Scheld WM: Septic sacroiliitis due to *Proteus mirabilis*. South Med J 83:589, 1990.
22. Klein MA, Winalski CS, Wax MR, Piwnica-Worms DR: MR imaging of septic sacroiliitis. J Comput Assist Tomogr 15:126, 1991.
23. Koh YD, Kim JO, Choi CH, et al: Pyogenic spondylitis in an S1-S2 immobile segment. Spine 26:588-589, 2001.
24. L'Episcopo JB: Suppurative arthritis of the sacroiliac joint. Ann Surg 104:289, 1936.
25. Lewkonia RM, Kinsella TD: Pyogenic sacroiliitis: Diagnosis and significance. J Rheumatol 8:153, 1981.
26. Lisbona R, Rosenthall L: Observation on the sequential use of ^{99m}Tc-phosphate complex and ^{67}Ga imaging in osteomyelitis and septic arthritis. Radiology 123:123, 1977.
27. Longoria RK, Carpenter JL: Anaerobic pyogenic sacroiliitis. South Med J 76:649, 1983.
28. Mansfield FL: Case records of the Massachusetts General Hospital. N Engl J Med 318:306, 1988.
29. Mayall BC, Rodgers-Wilson S, Veit F: Sacroiliac joint infection by *Salmonella heidelberg*. Med J Aust 151:600, 1989.
30. Mitchell M, Howard B, Haller J, et al: Septic arthritis. Radiol Clin North Am 26:1295, 1988.
31. Moyer RA, Bross JE, Harrington TM: Pyogenic sacroiliitis in a rural population. J Rheumatol 17:1364, 1990.
32. Muffoletto AJ, Ketonen LM, Mader JT, et al: Hematogenous pyogenic facet joint infection. Spine 26:1570-1576, 2001.
33. Murphey MD, Wetzel LH, Bramble JM, et al: Sacroiliitis: MR imaging findings. Radiology 180:239, 1991.
34. Murphy ME: Primary pyogenic infection of sacroiliac joint. NY State J Med 77:1309, 1977.
35. Norman GF: Sacroiliac disease and its relationship to lower abdominal pain. Am J Surg 116:54, 1968.
36. Oppenheimer A: Paravertebral abscesses associated with Strümpell-Marie diseases. J Bone Joint Surg 25:90, 1943.
37. Pouchot J, Vinceneux P: Usefulness of closed needle biopsy of sacroiliac joint in pyogenic sacroiliitis. J Rheumatol 18:1944, 1991.

38. Pouchot J, Vinceneux P, Barge J, et al: Tuberculosis of the sacroiliac joint: Clinical features, outcome, and evaluation of closed needle biopsy in 11 consecutive cases. Am J Med 84:622, 1988.
39. Pouchot J, Vinceneux P, Michon C, et al: Pyogenic sacroiliitis due to *Veillonella parvula*. Clin Infect Dis 15:175, 1992.
40. Reginato AJ, Ferreiro-Seoane JL, Falasca G: Unilateral sacroiliitis in secondary syphilis. J Rheumatol 15:717, 1988.
41. Roberts WA: Pyogenic vertebral osteomyelitis of a lumbar facet joint with associated epidural abscess: A case report with review of the literature. Spine 13:948, 1988.
42. Rombauts PA, Linden PM, Buyse AJ, et al: Septic arthritis of a lumbar facet joint caused by *Staphylococcus aureus*. Spine 25:1736-1738, 2000.
43. Sacks-Berg A, Strampfer MJ, Cunha BA: *Escherichia coli* sacroiliitis: Report of a case and review of the literature. Heart Lung 17:371, 1988.
44. Strange FGS: The prognosis in sacroiliac tuberculosis. Br J Surg 50:561, 1963.
45. Swayne LC, Dorsky S, Caruana V, Kaplan IL: Septic arthritis of a lumbar facet joint: Detection with bone SPECT imaging. J Nucl Med 30:1408, 1989.
46. Veys EM, Govaerts A, Coigne E, et al: HLA and infective sacroiliitis. Lancet 2:349, 1974.
47. Vyskocil JJ, McIlroy MA, Brennan TA, Wilson FM: Pyogenic infection of the sacroiliac joint: Case reports and review of the literature. Medicine 70:188, 1991.
48. Wallace R, Cohen AS: Tuberculous arthritis: A report of two cases with review of biopsy and synovial fluid findings. Am J Med 61:277, 1976.
49. Zimmermann B, Mikolich DJ, Lally EV: Septic sacroiliitis. Semin Arthritis Rheum 26:592-604, 1996.

MENINGITIS

CAPSULE SUMMARY

	LOW BACK	NECK
Frequency of spinal pain	Not applicable (NA)	Very common
Location of spinal pain	NA	Cervical spine, occiput
Quality of spinal pain	NA	Sharp ache
Symptoms and signs	NA	Fever, meningismus, mental status changes
Laboratory tests	NA	Leukocytosis, increased erythrocyte sedimentation rate, abnormal cerebrospinal fluid
Radiographic findings	NA	None
Treatment	NA	IV antibiotics

PREVALENCE AND PATHOGENESIS

Meningitis is an infection of the lining of the central nervous system (CNS), the meninges. It may be caused by the following bacteria: *Streptococcus pneumoniae*, *Neisseria meningitidis*, and *Haemophilus influenzae*; viruses: retrovirus, coxsackievirus, and echovirus; mycobacteria: *Mycobacterium tuberculosis*; fungi: *Coccidioides immitis*, *Cryptococcus neoformans*; spirochetes: *Treponema pallidum*; and protozoa: *Toxoplasma gondii*. Meningitis usually develops from hematogenous spread through the bloodstream from a distant, infected location to the choroid plexus; from septic emboli to small arteries; or by contiguous spread from local structures, such as the nasopharynx and mastoid bone. Recurrent episodes of meningitis suggest an opening of the CNS to the outside environment, such as a dural tear, a skull fracture, or an immunocompromised state.[10] The infection causes an exudation of cells and protein into the subarachnoid space. The meningeal reaction spreads through the CNS, involving the meninges covering the spinal cord as well as the brain. The clinical symptoms and course of the infection depend on the infecting organism and host inflammatory response. Bacterial and viral infections are characterized by constitutional symptoms including fever and change in mentation. Cerebral irritation results in headache, seizures, photophobia, and cranial nerve palsies. A more indolent course associated with gradual changes in mentation is more closely associated with tuberculous, fungal, spirochetal, and protozoal infections.

Epidemiology

Meningitis remains a significant health problem despite the use of bacterial and viral vaccines and antibodies. The yearly attack rate is 3 to 10 cases per 100,000 population in the United States.[41] Higher yearly attack rates are found in developing countries. A significant proportion of infections occurred in children younger than 12 years of age before *H. influenzae* type b vaccinations were available. Since 1995, *H. influenzae* infections have decreased in young children. In a study of bacterial meningitis, an estimate was made of 12,920 cases in 1986 and 5755 cases in 1995, a 55% reduction. The median age of these patients increased from 15 months in 1986 to 25 years in 1995 as a result of the decrease in *H. influenzae* infections.[43]

Pathogenesis

The diagnosis of bacterial or viral meningitis in the patient with acute symptoms is made without difficulty because of the high index of suspicion of the physician. The diagnosis of chronic meningitis is more difficult because symptoms and signs develop more gradually. The inflammatory response with bacterial infection results in the exudation of polymorphonuclear (PMN) leukocytes into the subarachnoid space. The cellular changes are accompanied by the seepage of proteins, which are usually excluded by the blood-brain barrier, into the meninges. The cerebrospinal fluid (CSF) becomes thick with the protein, eventually slowing the usual flow from the basal cisterns through Luschka's and Magendie's foramina to the lower spinal canal. Increasing CSF pressure, in an acute state, results in the clinical symptoms of meningismus and altered cerebral function.

The definitive diagnosis of meningitis is confirmed by culturing the offending organism from CSF obtained by lumbar puncture. The cornerstone of therapy for meningitis is antibiotics that are selected for their ability to kill the infecting organisms and their diffusing capacity across the meninges. When diagnosed expeditiously and treated aggressively, meningitis can be cured with no residual deficit. Delay in diagnosis is associated with increased neurologic morbidity and mortality.

Certain characteristics of the subarachnoid space allow for the development of meningitis.[50] In its normal state, the subarachnoid space contains lower concentrations of immunoglobulins and complement than the serum.[45] Organisms that gain entry into the subarachnoid space face less intense defense mechanisms than those present in the serum. Certain of these same factors may predispose certain individuals to infection with specific organisms. Otitis media, mastoiditis, and pneumonia predispose to *S. pneumoniae. Staphylococcus aureus* is associated with neurosurgical procedures, and *Staphylococcus epidermidis* may be associated with infected ventriculoperitoneal shunts.[7,42] Factors that may play a role include the patient's age, immunologic status, trauma, and exposure to carrier of an organism (*N. meningitidis*). For example, patients who lack the terminal components of the complement system are at increased risk of *N. meningitidis* infection.[39] Adult bacterial meningitis is caused by *S. pneumoniae*, *N. meningitidis*, and *H. influenzae* in more than 80% of the infections (Table 12-7).[54] Meningitis secondary to *H. influenzae* occurs less frequently than infection secondary to the other organisms. *H. influenzae* occurs in adults exposed to children with the infection.[51] Meningitis in children may be caused by additional organisms, including group B *Streptococcus*, *Escherichia coli*, and other coliform organisms.[40,44] *Listeria monocytogenes* is a gram-positive bacillus that causes 2% of meningitis in the United States. The most common hosts are neonates and immunocompromised adults. Most occurrences are associated with consumption of contaminated food, mostly dairy products.[54]

12-7 ORGANISMS CAUSING ADULT BACTERIAL MENINGITIS

Organism	Percentage
Streptococcus pneumoniae	30%-50%
Neisseria meningitidis	10%-35%
Staphylococcus aureus/epidermidis	5%-15%
Gram-negative bacilli	1%-10%
Streptococci	5%
Listeria	5%
Haemophilus influenzae	1%-3%

Modified from Wispelwey B, Tunkel AR, Scheld WM: Bacterial meningitis in adults. Infect Dis Clin North Am 4:645, 1990.

CLINICAL HISTORY

Bacterial Meningitis

The primary symptoms of patients with meningitis include head and neck pain along with neck stiffness (meningismus). Patients with bacterial meningitis usually have associated fever. Changes in mental status ranging from mild confusion to frank coma occur in a majority of patients. The onset of symptoms with bacterial meningitis is usually acute and develops over 24 to 36 hours. In a minority of patients, the progression of symptoms may occur over 3 to 5 days. The course of symptoms is from headache and neck stiffness to confusion, obtundation, and coma.

Aseptic (Viral) Meningitis

Of the 4000 cases of aseptic (nonbacterial) meningitis that occur each year in the United States, 25% have a defined cause.[33] Of these, echoviruses and coxsackieviruses are enteroviruses and are the most common cause of aseptic meningitis.[8] After the virus enters the body through the gastrointestinal or respiratory tract, it enters the meninges after a generalized viremia through the bloodstream. The incubation period for growth of the virus may range from a few days to several weeks. The patient develops fever, sore throat, and myalgias, followed by frontal headache, photophobia, neck pain, neck stiffness, and fever. Human immunodeficiency virus (HIV) can also cause an acute or chronic aseptic meningitis associated with headache, fever, meningismus, and cranial neuropathies. This infection may occur before the appearance of acquired immunodeficiency syndrome (AIDS).[32] Other forms of aseptic meningitis involve intracranial tumors, medications, and systemic illnesses (Table 12-8).

Tuberculous Meningitis

Tuberculous meningitis, once a disease of children, occurs more commonly in the elderly.[21] *M. tuberculosis* enters the body through the respiratory tract and grows in regional lymph nodes. Hematogenous seeding of the meninges may occur at that time. The infection may remain dormant for an extended period, only to become activated at a time of diminished host resistance to infection. The organisms grow in the meninges, which elicits an intense inflammatory reaction that is most prominent at the base

12-8 ACUTE ASEPTIC MENINGITIS

SYSTEMIC ILLNESSES
Systemic lupus erythematosus
Sjögren's syndrome
Rheumatoid arthritis
Polymyositis
Behçet's syndrome
Sarcoidosis
Vogt-Koyanagi-Harada syndrome

INTRACRANIAL TUMORS
Pharyngioma
Pituitary adenoma
Astrocytoma
Glioblastoma multiforme
Medulloblastoma
Ependymoma

MISCELLANEOUS
Post seizure
Post migraine
Serum sickness
Heavy metal poisoning
Recurrent benign meningitis (Mollaret's)

VIRUSES
Enteroviruses
Mumps
Herpes simplex
Lymphocytic choriomeningitis

MEDICATIONS
Trimethoprim-sulfamethoxazole
Ibuprofen
Sulindac
Naproxen
Tolmetin
Azathioprine
Isoniazid

PROCEDURE RELATED
Post neurosurgery
Spinal anesthesia
Intrathecal injections
Chymopapain injection

Modified from Connolly KJ, Hammer SM: The acute aseptic meningitis syndrome. Infect Dis Clin North Am 4:599, 1990.

of the brain. The inflammation in this location may result in inflammatory tissue that compresses cranial nerve blood vessels. This inflammation results in vessel thrombosis and infarction of tissue supplied by that vessel or in a blockage of the free flow of CSF around the brain, leading to increased intracranial pressure and hydrocephalus. Once the infection has started, the clinical manifestations of the infection progress throughout a 2- to 3-week period. Patients develop an insidious prodrome of malaise, lassitude, low-grade fever, and intermittent headache. During the next 2 to 3 weeks, the patient may experience protracted headache, neck pain, neck stiffness, fever, vomiting, and alterations in mental status. In untreated patients, seizures, coma, and death occur within 5 to 8 weeks.[28,34]

Fungal Meningitis

Fungal infection with *C. immitis* or *C. neoformans* causes similar symptoms as those of tuberculous meningitis.[14] Approximately 30% of patients with extrapulmonary *C. immitis* infection develop meningitis. The pulmonary infection is asymptomatic or self-limited. Other extrapulmonary sites of infection include the skin and musculoskeletal systems. Meningitis affects the base of the brain with a granulomatous inflammatory response that blocks the flow of CSF, resulting in hydrocephalus and cranial nerve palsies. The onset of these symptoms is gradual. Headache is the most prominent symptom of patients with fungal meningitis. Meningismus, personality changes, and fever are less prominent symptoms.[49]

Cryptococcal meningitis is an important and potentially life-threatening form of this infection.[11] *C. neoformans* is a ubiquitous yeastlike fungus found in association with pigeons, fruits, vegetables, and soil. In light of frequent exposure of humans to this fungus, natural resistance to this organism is substantial.[1] Cryptococcosis develops after inhalation and a mild pulmonary infection. Hematogenous dissemination results in an exposure of a number of organs and a predilection to the CNS.[49] The onset of disease is usually gradual, with intermittent episodes of persistent headache and fever. Headache is the most common symptom. The organism grows in the meninges and brain with a minimal inflammatory response. As the infection progresses over months, patients complain increasingly of impaired mentation, irritability, dizziness, weakness, and changes in vision. A stiff, painful neck is a frequent symptom but may be absent. If left untreated, both coccidioidal and cryptococcal meningitis may result in increasing neurologic deficits, coma, and death. Cryptococcal meningitis is a common manifestation of AIDS, affecting 6% to 66% of patients.[26,30] It may be the first opportunistic infection affecting AIDS patients.

Spirochetal Meningitis

T. pallidum is the spirochete that causes syphilis. Invasion of the CNS occurs during the primary and secondary stages of the illness when *T. pallidum* may be isolated from CSF.[31] *T. pallidum* gains entrance to the bloodstream during the primary stage of the infection after direct exposure of the genitourinary tract or oropharynx. During dissemination, or the secondary phase, meningitis and cranial nerve palsies may occur. However, the frequency of acute meningitis is only 1% to 2%. More commonly, dissemination is associated with vague symptoms, including headache, stiff neck, photophobia, and myalgias without fever. Progressive lesions associated with arteritis cause mental confusion, seizures, and focal deficits. If untreated, tertiary syphilis causes a wide range of neurologic dysfunctions, including general paresis, tabes dorsalis, space-occupying lesions (gummas), and meningovascular disease.[9] Patients with HIV infection may be at increased risk of following a more rapid course to symptomatic neurosyphilis.[22]

Parasite Meningitis

A more unusual form of meningitis is caused by the protozoan *T. gondii*. CNS toxoplasmosis occurs most commonly in the immunosuppressed host who has a lymphoreticular malignancy, has taken immunosuppressive drugs, or has a viral infection that impairs cellular immune function (AIDS).[48] Patients with CNS toxoplasmosis may present with an acute or subacute course, including headache, stiff neck, and seizures. If brain tissue is also infected (encephalitis), the patient may develop focal neurologic deficits that progress to cause changes in mentation as well as coma. Patients with AIDS frequently have intracranial mass lesions in association with their toxoplasmosis.

Toxoplasmosis may be the most frequent cause of that cerebral lesion in HIV patients.[35]

PHYSICAL EXAMINATION

The patient with meningitis may manifest abnormalities in a number of organ systems during the physical examination. Patients with meningitis of any cause are frequently febrile. Patients with meningeal irritation develop reflex contraction of neck muscles (nuchal rigidity), Kernig's sign (pain in the hamstrings with knee extension in the supine position), and Brudzinski's sign (involuntary flexion of the hips with neck flexion). These signs are abnormal in 50% of bacterial meningitis patients.[6] A maculopetechial or purpuric rash may be present in the patients with meningococcal meningitis or other bacterial infections. About 50% of meningococcal patients have a rash.[54] Echovirus may cause a maculopapular rash that appears on the face before other parts of the body are affected. Funduscopic examination may demonstrate papilledema (swelling of the head of the optic nerve), which is secondary to increased intracranial pressure. Infection of the middle ear (otitis media), a possible local source of infection, would be noted on examination of the ear. Chest examination may be positive for decreased breath sounds indicative of a pneumonic process secondary to bacteria (*S. pneumoniae*), mycobacteria (*M. tuberculosis*), or fungi (*C. immitis*). Murmurs on cardiac examination suggest endocarditis, which may be the source of the primary infection, including *S. aureus*.

The range of neurologic abnormalities is wide. Loss of mental function in the form of memory loss or inability to perform calculations occurs with all forms of meningitis. A change in mental status or coma is found in 50% or more of bacterial meningitis patients and is a strong indicator of this type of infection.[17]

Elderly patients with bacterial meningitis are frequently confused and have severe mental status changes in the setting of pneumonia. Confusion occurs in 92% with pneumococcal meningitis and in 78% with gram-negative bacillary meningitis.[3,19] Fever may be absent. Neck stiffness must be differentiated from that of osteoarthritis of the cervical spine.

Neurologic abnormalities are also associated with meningitis caused by other organisms, including *M. tuberculosis*, *C. immitis*, and *T. pallidum*.[5,23,25] Abnormalities of cranial nerves (eyes, facial, and tongue movements) occur most commonly in patients with granulomatous meningitis, which affects the base of the brain.

LABORATORY DATA

Nonspecific findings, such as elevation in peripheral white blood cells (WBCs) and erythrocyte sedimentation rate, are not helpful in making a diagnosis of meningitis but are useful in following the response of patients to therapy.

The diagnosis of meningitis is made by the examination of CSF, which is obtained by lumbar puncture. In most circumstances, a lumbar puncture can be completed without complication. Contraindications for this procedure are signs of increased intracranial pressure or skin infection overlying the needle entry point. Lumbar puncture in the presence of increased intracranial pressure may cause the brain to be pressed against the base of the skull, causing acute compression of the brain stem, which controls autonomic functions of the lungs and heart. Patients who "cone" develop cardiopulmonary arrest. Attempting an injection through an area of cellulitis may result in inoculating organisms into the CNS, causing meningitis or vertebral osteomyelitis.

The definitive diagnosis of meningitis is based on the growth of the offending organism from CSF or blood. Unfortunately, cultures take time to become positive, leaving the diagnosis of meningitis to be based on other characteristic changes in CSF. Bacterial meningitis causes WBC counts greater than 1000 cells/mm^3, a predominance of PMN leukocytes, a decreased glucose level that is less than 50% of the serum level, an elevated protein level of greater than 100 mg/dL, and positive Gram stain smear of organisms from a spun specimen in 80% of patients.[17,24] Gram's stain smear is positive in 90% of *S. pneumoniae* and *S. aureus*, 86% in *H. influenzae*, 75% in *N. meningitidis*, and 50% or less in other gram-negative organisms.[20] CSF cultures are positive for growth of the causative organism in the majority of patients if the samples are cultured promptly to minimize the loss of fastidious organisms such as *H. influenzae*, *N. meningitidis*, and anaerobes. The presence of bacteria in CSF may also be detected through identification of bacterial antigens with coagglutination and latex agglutination tests. These tests are less sensitive than CSF culture and are not a substitute for it.[55]

Viral meningitis causes less of a leukocytosis (less than 500 WBC/mm^3), predominantly lymphocytic in character, with normal glucose and slightly elevated protein levels.[29] CSF obtained early in the course of aseptic meningitis may reveal an increased number of PMN leukocytes. A repeat CSF examination is warranted because subsequent evaluations reveal a switch to a predominance of lymphocytes.[15] The measurement of CSF pressure is not associated with a specific form of meningitis. CSF protein concentrations are also nondiagnostic.

Tuberculous and fungal meningitis cause a CSF WBC count of less than 500 cells/mm^3, with a predominance of lymphocytes. Tuberculous meningitis causes a marked reduction in glucose and marked increase in protein levels. Organisms are rarely seen on smear. Culture may be positive in 78% of patients[20] but may require up to 8 weeks before growth is detected. The use of polymerase chain reaction (PCR) amplification tests can detect *M. tuberculosis* before the results obtained by culture. The variability of the sensitivity and specificity of the PCR tests do not allow confidence in the detection of the infection. In one study, 60% of 15 patients with definite disease had a positive test.[4] Fungal meningitis is associated with a slight reduction of glucose level, moderate increase in protein level, and, in the case of *Cryptococcus*, the presence of organisms by India ink examination. In toxoplasmosis, CSF examination may be normal or demonstrate mild WBC elevation with lymphocytes.

Other ancillary laboratory tests may detect the presence of pathogenic organisms in locations other than the CNS. Blood cultures detect bacteremia with *H. influenzae*, *S. pneumoniae*, and *N. meningitidis*, in 80%, 50%, and 40%

of patients, respectively.[46] Respiratory tract cultures are useful for organisms that are associated with pulmonary infections.

RADIOGRAPHIC EVALUATION

Radiographic examination is not useful in the diagnosis or management of uncomplicated meningitis.[53] CT in meningitis may detect widening of the subarachnoid space. Radiographic techniques are most useful in the patient with meningitis who has an associated abnormality such as a parameningeal focus of infection or brain abscess. CT can localize the space-occupying lesion in the patient with focal cerebral signs who does not respond to usual therapy. CT may demonstrate contrast medium enhancement of the leptomeninges, widening of the subarachnoid space, and patchy areas of diminished density in the brain.[52] In a study of tuberculous meningitis, CT evaluation demonstrated hydrocephalus, parenchymal enhancement, cerebral infarct, local or diffuse edema, or tuberculoma.[37] MR imaging may also be useful to document intracranial lesions that may be associated with meningeal infection.[27]

The need for a CT scan before a lumbar puncture can be determined by careful history and physical examination. In a prospective study of 111 patients evaluated in an emergency department, 2.7% had CT results that contraindicated a lumbar puncture.[18] The parameters associated with space-occupying lesions included altered mentation, papilledema, focal neurologic deficits, and overall clinical impression. The appropriate patients can be excluded who require a CT before lumbar puncture so that CSF can be obtained for culture and antibiotics can be instituted.

DIFFERENTIAL DIAGNOSIS

The diagnosis of meningitis is based on the results of cultures of CSF. The clinical course, CSF abnormalities, and with culture results help differentiate the various forms of meningitis (pyogenic vs. granulomatous vs. protozoan). Parameningeal infection, such as epidural abscess, subdural empyema, and brain abscess, may cause meningeal symptoms and neurologic signs. Radiographic evaluation should differentiate these entities from meningitis alone.

TREATMENT

The treatment of bacterial meningitis is with intravenous or intrathecal antibiotic that is bactericidal for the infecting organisms. Bacterial meningitis represents an infection in a location of impaired host defenses. Factors including inefficient surface phagocytosis in a body fluid, lack of immunoglobulin and complement, and opsonic and bactericidal activity require bactericidal antibiotics. A problem obtaining and maintaining adequate concentrations of antibiotic in CSF is the blood-brain barrier. The blood-brain barrier excludes proteins and antibiotics from the brain and CNS. When inflamed, the integrity of the blood-brain barrier is lost, allowing the ingress of antibiotics. Antibiotics are administered intravenously, in high, divided doses, every few hours (Table 12-9). Penicillin, nafcillin, ampicillin, cefotaxime, and ceftriaxone are antibiotics used with gram-positive and gram-negative infections. Some gram-negative meningitis requires aminoglycoside (gentamicin) therapy. Aminoglycosides do not cross the blood-brain barrier and require intrathecal administration (lumbar puncture, ventricular pump).[47]

The therapy for aseptic meningitis is symptomatic. There is no effective antiviral therapy that shortens the course of the infection. Recovery begins within days and is usually complete in a few weeks. Patients with HIV meningitis also have a self-limited illness that resolves without specific treatment in 4 weeks.[32]

Tuberculous meningitis requires three drug therapies, including isoniazid, rifampin, and ethambutol or pyrazinamide. This therapy must be continued for 12 months. Drug-resistant tuberculosis is becoming an increasingly frequent problem. Additional drugs for longer periods are required to control these infections. These patients may

12-9 ANTIBIOTIC THERAPY FOR BACTERIAL MENINGITIS

Organism	Antibiotic	Adult 24-Hour Dose	Alternate Therapy 24-Hour Dose
Streptococcus pneumoniae	Ceftriaxone ± vancomycin, 2 g IV	4 g	NA
Streptococcus groups A and B	Penicillin G	24 million U IV	Ceftriaxone, 4 g IV
Streptococcus group D (enterococci)	Penicillin G + gentamicin	24 million U IV + gentamicin IT	Vancomycin, 2 g IV + gentamicin IV and IT
Neisseria meningitidis	Penicillin G	24 million U IV	Ceftriaxone, 4 g IV
Haemophilus influenzae			
Beta-lactamase negative	Ampicillin IV	12 g	Ceftriaxone, 4 g IV
Beta-lactamase positive	Ceftriaxone	4 g IV	Chloramphenicol, 4 g IV
Staphylococcus aureus	Nafcillin	12 g IV	Vancomycin, 2 g IV
Gram negative	Ceftazidime	6-9 g IV	Gentamicin, 4-10 mg IT

Choice of antibiotic should be matched to organism sensitivities determined with culture. Antibiotics listed in this table may be used as initial therapy until sensitivity results are available.
IT, intrathecal; IV, intravenous.
Courtesy of Gary Simon, MD.

require five to seven drugs for periods up to 24 months. Patients with hydrocephalus, or cranial nerve dysfunction secondary to tuberculous meningitis, may benefit from a course of corticosteroids.[36]

Patients with fungal meningitis require amphotericin B therapy. Cryptococcal meningitis may be cured with intravenous therapy, which is given in increments of 20 to 30 mg/day up to a total of 2 to 3 g. Patients with HIV-related cryptococcal meningitis may require a 6-week course of amphotericin B and flucytosine, followed by long maintenance therapy.[9,12] In coccidioidal meningitis, amphotericin B therapy given by an intravenous route does not reach adequate levels in CSF.[16] Intrathecal administration is necessary for control of the infection.

Neurosyphilis requires treatment with intravenous penicillin. The recommended dose is 2 to 4 million units IV every 4 hours.[9] The infusion is continued for 10 to 14 days.

CNS toxoplasmosis requires prolonged therapy with pyrimethamine and sulfonamides. In adults, 25 mg of pyrimethamine is given daily along with four 1-g doses of sulfadiazine daily. Therapy must be continued for a minimum of 6 weeks.

PROGNOSIS

The course and outcome of meningitis depend on the agent that causes the infection and the immunologic status of the patient. Patients who have a compromised immune system are at risk of developing tuberculous or fungal meningitis and have a poorer prognosis than those patients who have an episode of aseptic, viral meningitis. Patients with bacterial meningitis will have a full recovery if the diagnosis is made expeditiously and appropriate therapy is given. Antibiotic therapy is given for 2 weeks, with the response to therapy monitored by the return of CSF abnormalities to normal. Patients with parameningeal foci of infection may not improve until the focus is drained. The mortality rate may vary between 18.6% to 25% with a complication rate of 50%.[13,38] Some of the complications associated with bacterial meningitis include cerebrovascular accidents, cerebral edema, and hydrocephalus.

In a study of community-acquired bacterial meningitis, three baseline clinical features, hypotension, altered mental status, and seizures were independently associated with adverse clinical outcomes. The administration of antibiotics before the development of these clinical features was associated with a better clinical result.[2]

Tuberculous meningitis is associated with a 20% mortality rate even in patients who receive drug therapy. The improvement with therapy may be slow, with survivors continuing with neurologic dysfunction.

Patients with fungal meningitis may have relapses of their disease despite receiving long courses of amphotericin B therapy. Patients who have a poor clinical outcome with cryptococcal meningitis have an underlying lymphoreticular malignancy, continued abnormal CSF white blood cells, or cryptococci on smear.[20]

CNS toxoplasmosis is uniformly fatal unless aggressively treated. Patients with AIDS or other immunocompromised states may have a poor outcome despite maximum therapy.

References

Meningitis

1. Armstrong D: Problems in management of opportunistic fungal diseases. Rev Infect Dis 11:S1591, 1989.
2. Aronin SI, Peduzzi P, Quagliarello VJ: Community-acquired bacterial meningitis: Risk stratification for adverse clinical outcome and effect of antibiotic timing. Ann Intern Med 129:862-869, 1998.
3. Behrman RE, Meyer BR, Mendelsohn MH, et al: Central nervous system infections in the elderly. Arch Intern Med 149:1596, 1989.
4. Bonington A, Strang JI, Klapper PE, et al: Use of Roche AMPLICOR *Mycobacterium tuberculosis* PCR in early diagnosis of tuberculous meningitis. J Clin Microbiol 36:1251-1254, 1998.
5. Bouza E, Dreyer JS, Hewitt WL, et al: Coccidioidal meningitis: An analysis of thirty-one cases and review of the literature. Medicine 60:139, 1981.
6. Carpenter RR, Petersdorf RG: The clinical spectrum of bacterial meningitis. Am J Med 33:262, 1962.
7. Chernick NL, Armstrong D, Posner JB: Central nervous system infections in patients with cancer. Medicine 52:563, 1973.
8. Connolly KJ, Hammer SM: The acute aseptic meningitis syndrome. Infect Dis Clin North Am 4:599, 1990.
9. Coyle PK, Dattwyler R: Spirochetal infection of the central nervous system. Infect Dis Clin North Am 4:731, 1990.
10. Critchley EMR: Meningitis disorders and myelopathies. In Critchley E, Eisen A (eds): Diseases of the Spinal Cord. London, Springer, 1992, pp 209-233.
11. Diamond RD, Bennett JE: Prognostic factors in cryptococcal meningitis: A study in 111 cases. Ann Intern Med 80:176, 1974.
12. Dismukes WE, Cloud G, Gallis HA, et al: Treatment of cryptococcal meningitis with combination amphotericin B and flucytosine for four as compared with six weeks. N Engl J Med 317:334, 1987.
13. Durand MI, Calderwood SB, Weber DJ, et al: Acute bacterial meningitis in adults. N Engl J Med 328:21-28, 1993.
14. Ellner JJ, Bennett JE: Chronic meningitis. Medicine 55:341, 1976.
15. Feigin RD, Shackelford PG: Value of repeat lumbar puncture in the differential diagnosis of meningitis. N Engl J Med 304:1278, 1973.
16. Galgiani JN, Ampel NM, Catanzaro A, et al: Practice guideline for the treatment of coccidioidomycosis. Infectious Diseases Society of America. Clin Infect Dis 30:658-661, 2000.
17. Geiseler PJ, Nelson KE, Levin S, et al: Community-acquired purulent meningitis: A review of 1216 cases during the antibiotic era, 1954-1976. Rev Infect Dis 2:725, 1980.
18. Gopal AK, Whitehouse JD, Simel DL, et al: Cranial computed tomography before lumbar puncture: A prospective clinical evaluation. Arch Intern Med 159:2681-2685, 1999.
19. Gorse GJ, Thrupp LD, Nudlenan KL, et al: Bacterial meningitis in the elderly. Arch Intern Med 144:1603, 1984.
20. Greenlee JE: Approach to diagnosis of meningitis: Cerebrospinal fluid evaluation. Infect Dis Clin North Am 4:583, 1990.
21. Hinman AR: Tuberculous meningitis at Cleveland Metropolitan General Hospital 1959 to 1963. Am Rev Respir Dis 95:670, 1967.
22. Johns DR, Tierney M, Felsenstein D: Alteration in the natural history of neurosyphilis by concurrent infection with the human immunodeficiency virus. N Engl J Med 316:1569, 1987.
23. Jordan KG: Modern neurosyphilis: critical analysis. West J Med 149:47, 1988.
24. Karandanis D, Shulman JA: Recent survey of infectious meningitis in adults: Review of laboratory findings in bacterial, tuberculous, and aseptic meningitis. South Med J 68:449, 1976.
25. Kennedy DH, Fallon RJ: Tuberculous meningitis. JAMA 241:64, 1979.
26. Kovacs JA, Kovacs AA, Polis M, et al: Cryptococcosis in the acquired immunodeficiency syndrome. Ann Intern Med 103:533, 1985.
27. Krol G, Becker R, Zimmerman R, et al: Contribution of MRI to the diagnosis of intracranial complications of acquired immune deficiency syndrome. Neuroradiology 86:99, 1985.
28. Leonard JM, Des Prez RM: Tuberculous meningitis. Infect Dis Clin North Am 4:769, 1990.

29. Lepow ML, Carver DH, Wright HT Jr, et al: A clinical, epidemiologic, and laboratory investigation of aseptic meningitis during the four-year period 1955-58. N Engl J Med 266:1181, 1962.
30. Levy RM, Bresden DE, Rosenblum ML: Neurological manifestations of acquired immunodeficiency syndrome (AIDS). J Neurosurg 62:475, 1985.
31. Lukehart SA, Hook EW, Baker-Zander SA, et al: Invasion of the central nervous system by *Treponema pallidum*: Implications of diagnosis and treatment. Ann Intern Med 109:855, 1988.
32. McArthur J: Neurologic manifestations of AIDS. Medicine 66:407, 1987.
33. Meyer HM, Johnson RT, Crawford IP, et al: Central nervous system syndromes of "viral" etiology: A study of 713 cases. Am J Med 29:334, 1960.
34. Molavi A, LeFrock JL: Tuberculous meningitis. Med Clin North Am 69:315, 1985.
35. Novia BA, Petito CK, Gold JWM: Cerebral toxoplasmosis complicating the acquired immune deficiency syndrome. Ann Neurol 19:224, 1985.
36. O'Toole RD, Thorton GF, Mukherjee MK, Nath RL: Dexamethasone in tuberculous meningitis: Relationship of cerebrospinal fluid effects to therapeutic effects to therapeutic efficacy. Ann Intern Med 70:39, 1969.
37. Ozates M, Kemaloglu S, Gurkan F, et al: CT of the brain in tuberculous meningitis: A review of 289 patients. Acta Radiol 41:13-17, 2000.
38. Pfister HW, Feiden W, Einhaupl KM: Spectrum of complications during bacterial meningitis in adults: Results of a prospective clinical study. Arch Neurol 50:575-581, 1993.
39. Ross SC, Densen P: Complement deficiency states and infection: Epidemiology, pathogenesis, and consequences of neisserial and other infections in an immune deficiency. Medicine 63:243, 1984.
40. Saez-Llorens X, McCracken GH Jr: Bacterial meningitis in neonates and children. Infect Dis Clin North Am 4:623, 1990.
41. Schlech WF III, Ward JI, Band JD, et al: Bacterial meningitis in the United States, 1978 through 1981: The National Bacterial Meningitis Surveillance Study. JAMA 253:1749, 1985.
42. Schoenbaum SC, Gardner P, Shillito J: Infections of cerebrospinal fluid shunts: Epidemiology, clinical manifestations, and therapy. J Infect Dis 131:543, 1975.
43. Schuchat A, Robinson K, Wenger JD, et al: Bacterial meningitis in the United States in 1995. N Engl J Med 337:970-976, 1997.
44. Shelton MM, Marks WA: Bacterial meningitis. Neurol Clin 8:605, 1990.
45. Smith H, Bannister B, O'Shea MJ: Cerebrospinal fluid immunoglobulins in meningitis. Lancet 1:591, 1973.
46. Swartz MN, Dodge PR: Bacterial meningitis: A review of selected aspects: I. General clinical features, special problems and unusual meningeal reactions mimicking bacterial meningitis. N Engl J Med 272:725, 1965.
47. Tauber MG, Sande MA: General principles of therapy of pyogenic meningitis. Infect Dis Clin North Am 4:661, 1990.
48. Townsend JJ, Wolinsky JS, Baunger JR, Johnson PC: Acquired toxoplasmosis: A neglected cause of treatable nervous system disease. Arch Neurol 32:335, 1975.
49. Treseler CB, Sugar AM: Fungal meningitis. Infect Dis Clin North Am 4:789, 1990.
50. Tunkel AR, Wispelwey B, Scheld WM: Pathogenesis and pathophysiology of meningitis. Infect Dis Clin North Am 4:555, 1990.
51. Ward JL, Fraser DW, Baraff LJ, et al: *Haemophilus influenzae* meningitis: A national study of secondary spread in household contact. N Engl J Med 301:122, 1979.
52. Weisberg LA: Cerebral computerized tomography in intracranial inflammatory disorders. Arch Neurol 37:137, 1980.
53. Weisberg LA: Computed tomography in the diagnosis of intracranial disease. Ann Intern Med 91:87, 1979.
54. Wispelwey B, Tunkel AR, Scheld WM: Bacterial meningitis in adults. Infect Dis Clin North Am 4:645, 1990.
55. Yogev R: Advances in diagnosis and treatment of childhood meningitis. Pediatr Infect Dis J 4:321, 1985.

HERPES ZOSTER

CAPSULE SUMMARY

	LOW BACK	NECK
Frequency of spinal pain	Very common	Very common
Location of spinal pain	Lumbar dermatomes	Cervical dermatomes
Quality of spinal pain	Burning, tingling, sharp, deep, boring	Burning, tingling, sharp, deep, boring
Symptoms and signs	Vesicular dermatomal rash, fever	Vesicular dermatomal rash, fever
Laboratory tests	Lymphocytosis, increased antibody response, lesional culture	Lymphocytosis, increased antibody response, lesional culture
Radiographic findings	None	None
Treatment	Antiviral agents, corticosteroids, analgesics, gabapentin	Antiviral agents, corticosteroids, analgesics, gabapentin

PREVALENCE AND PATHOGENESIS

Herpes zoster (HZ), or shingles, is a late complication of a varicella infection (chickenpox) during childhood. The disease is characterized by an erythematous, papular rash accompanied by pain in the distribution of a peripheral sensory nerve. Pain may antedate the skin lesions by 4 to 7 days and confuse the diagnosis. The process may resolve without any residual symptoms but, in older patients, the infection may result in scarring and persistent pain that is resistant to treatment. In some patients, the pain is severe enough to cause considerable disability.

Epidemiology

Over 90% of adults in the United States have serologic evidence of varicella-zoster virus (VZV) infection and are at risk for HZ.[7] HZ has increased incidence in patients older than 50 years of age. Hope-Simpson reported in a study of 182 HZ patients a rate of 2 to 3 cases per 1000 for patients 20 to 50 years of age, 5 cases per 1000 for patients 50 years of age, and more than 10 cases per 1000 for those 80 years of age.[23] In another study, HZ also occurred more frequently in an elderly population.[62] HZ occurs in 10% to 20% of the population.[55]

HZ also occurs more commonly in patients with impaired immune function. This may be particularly true in patients with diminished cell-mediated immunity to VZV; lesional interferon concentrations are decreased in those with more widespread disease.[52] HZ was associated with lymphoreticular malignancies, with VZV infection occurring in 25% of patients with Hodgkin's disease and 10% of non-Hodgkin's lymphoma patients during a 2-year study.[50] Patients who are receiving chemotherapy or radiation therapy may also have an increased risk of developing HZ. HZ occurs with higher frequency among persons who are seropositive for human immunodeficiency virus (HIV) than those who are seronegative. The relative incidence is 29.4 and 2.0 cases of HZ per 1000 person-years for HIV-positive and HIV-negative individuals, respectively.[3] However, people who are otherwise normal who develop HZ are not more likely to develop a malignancy than any other healthy person.[46] Often, there is no identifiable precipitating cause for the reactivation of the virus, although trauma to an area of skin may precede the appearance of lesions. HZ exhibits no sexual predilection and has no seasonal variation or relation to varicella epidemics. A study of 1019 HZ patients reported 60% women, with a mean age of 58 years, with a prevalence varying between 1.3 to 1.6 per 1000 per year.[20] This study also reported a statistically significant seasonal variation, with the lesions appearing most often in summer and least often in spring.[20] The frequency of HZ is two to four times more frequent in elderly whites as compared with blacks.[51]

Pathogenesis

VZV is one of eight herpesviruses that infect humans, which include herpes simplex virus, cytomegalovirus, and Epstein-Barr virus. These viruses contain deoxyribonucleic acid (DNA) in a viral capsid surrounded by an envelope that allows the VZV to gain entrance into the host cells. The VZV attaches to cells by binding to heparan sulfate proteoglycans.[33] The VZV can replicate itself only within host cells. It incorporates variable amounts of host membrane into its envelope, allowing it to lie dormant in a normal cell. Clinical expression of the disease occurs when immune surveillance diminishes, allowing the virus to emerge from its hiding place. The factors that initiate the resurgence of infection are not known, but advancing age and diminished immune competence play a role.

The initial infection with VZV is varicella (chickenpox), at which time patients develop a viremia with dissemination of the virus throughout the body. The termination of this illness corresponds with the development of both humoral and cellular immune mechanisms. The VZV is sequestered in the posterior spinal sensory ganglia in the spinal cord, where it remains dormant for an unspecified time. Subclinical activation occurs in immunocompetent and immunocompromised individuals throughout life, with infection limited by cellular immunity directed against VZV.[18] During a period of low host resistance, the viruses grow in a ganglion or nerve, resulting in skin lesions and pain. These patients are infectious and can transmit a varicella infection to previously unexposed people. Evidence suggests that zoster is a reactivation of a previous infection and is not the result of a new exposure: a varicella infection in a patient does not give HZ to someone who has previously had chickenpox.[39] Chickenpox generally confers lifelong protection against a subsequent viremia, but second infections have been documented.[33]

HZ starts in an individual with a history of chickenpox with replication of virus in the cell body of a cutaneous sensory neuron lying in the dorsal root ganglion. The entire viral genome is present in multiple ganglia in the entire neuraxis. The virus spreads within the sensory nerve centrally and peripherally. Histologic examination of the central nervous system reveals inflammation, hemorrhage, and necrosis in the dorsal root ganglion, the posterior horn, and, occasionally, the corresponding motor neuron in the adjacent anterior horn. (This finding correlates with the occasional patient with motor loss associated with herpes zoster lesions.) The large, myelinated sensory fibers are preferentially affected; this results in a decreased ratio of large position to small pain fibers, diminishing pain modulation at the spinal cord level. The virus travels down the sensory nerve to the skin, producing demyelination, cellular infiltration and subsequent scarring, and fibrosis of peripheral nerves. The virus reaches the skin and replicates in the lower epidermal layers with ballooning degeneration of cells and development of multinucleated giant cells and intranuclear inclusion bodies. Inflammation in the skin causes erythema, edema, vesicular eruptions, hemorrhage, and necrosis. Healing in the skin results in depigmentation, atrophy, and permanent scarring. The virus can be grown from early vesicles, but that is unlikely once the lesion becomes pustular and develops a crust.

In patients who are immunocompromised, HZ may cause damage to the spinal cord (myelitis) and brain (encephalitis).[12,25] These patients have symptoms and signs that extend beyond the dermatome that was initially affected.

CLINICAL HISTORY

HZ presents with a 4- to 28-day prodrome of constitutional symptoms including fever, malaise, chills, lethargy, and gastrointestinal symptoms, particularly in the elderly. The first local symptom is usually pain in the nerve segment, which is burning or shooting in character and is often associated with dysesthesias in the area of skin supplied by the affected nerve root. Within a week after the onset of pain, an eruption appears as a series of localized erythematous papules that develop into vesicles grouped together on an erythematous base and follow a segmental distribution (Fig. 12-15). The exanthem consist of grouped vesicles involving usually one, but occasionally up to three adjacent dermatomes.[33] This may occur in up to 20% of patients. Rarely, the pain may be followed by minimal erythema or

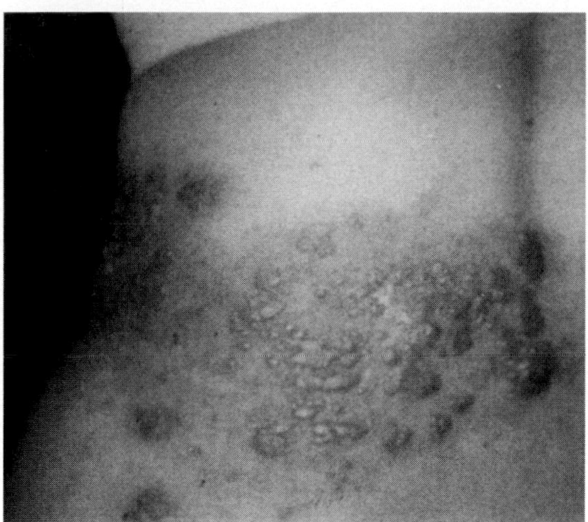

Figure 12-15 Herpes zoster. A 44-year-old woman with connective tissue disease on no medication developed severe, burning pain over the left side of her back. Four days after the onset of pain, the patient developed vesicular lesions in an T11 dermatomal pattern. The patient was treated with prednisone, 40 mg/day for 3 weeks. She had no postherpetic neuralgia and her skin healed with residual hyperpigmentation. Over the following 5 years, her skin hyperpigmentation has lessened and she has experienced no postherpetic pain.

no skin changes at all (zoster sine herpete).[5] In this situation, the central nervous system is damaged without producing skin ulcers. This form of the disease may cause extensive neurologic disease and may be fatal in patients who are immunocompromised.[13] Within days, the eruption fades and the vesicles dry with crusts, leaving small scars in the skin. The skin may become partially or completely analgesic. Pain usually resolves with the skin lesion; however, it may persist for years. This postherpetic neuralgia is more likely to occur in elderly patients.

The course of pain of HZ follows a characteristic pattern. Once the rash appears, pain of the prodrome period recedes. As the rash evolves, the sensory and pain disturbances disappear, especially in people younger than 40 years of age. In people older than 50 years of age, the pain is more pronounced and is usually associated with unpleasant dysesthesias, the most distressing of which is pressure sensitivity of the skin to any touch. When the rash is at its greatest extent, pain is minimal. As the rash crusts, pain recurs, usually with an intense, lancinating quality. Pain becomes constant, deep, and boring. The skin feels increasingly tightened. The course of the rash and the pain are clearly not synchronous. Patients with resolution of the rash but continued pain are considered to have postherpetic neuralgia. Healing occurs over a period of 2 to 4 weeks.

The frequency and severity of postherpetic neuralgia increase with age, with 35% of patients 60 years of age and 50% of patients older than 70 years of age developing HZ.[10] The symptoms may last weeks to years. Pain has an unrelenting, deep, boring quality that is intensified by paroxysms of lancinating pain. Patients try to keep clothes off the area to diminish the dysesthesias. Others may complain of a feeling of worms under the skin or ants crawling on the skin (formication). Patients may become clinically depressed because of the pain.

The dermatomes over the whole back are frequently affected. The thoracic spinal nerves are affected in 50% to 55% of cases, the cervical nerves in 15% to 24%, the lumbar and sacral nerves in 10% to 15%, and the cranial nerves in 10% to 15%.[20,61] The upper cervical segments (C2–C4) are more commonly affected than the lower segments.[61] The upper lumbar segments are also more commonly affected than the lower segments. The same segment may be involved with HZ on two or three occasions.[23] HZ infection is not associated with lumboradicular syndromes with or without a herniated disc.[57]

PHYSICAL EXAMINATION

The skin lesions may be found in any segmental sensory nerve distribution. They have a characteristic appearance that helps distinguish this lesion from other skin diseases and begin as an erythematous patch or indurated plaque. Scattered, grouped vesicles (1 to 3 mm) on an erythematous base are usual. The distal end of a skin dermatome is affected initially, and new lesions appear in a more central location for a week. The lesions tend to coalesce and form a linear array but remain unilateral and do not cross the midline. Occasionally, patients do develop bilateral disease and a few scattered extradermatomal vesicles. This is not necessarily a sign of disseminated disease associated with a worse prognosis.[26]

The vesicles initially clear, then grow cloudy, crust, and desquamate for 3 weeks. Once crusts appear, the lesions are no longer contagious. The lesions heal with postinflammatory hypopigmented macules or patches. If secondarily infected, lesions may have depressed scars. A number of areas of cutaneous lesions suggest disseminated disease.

In addition to cutaneous manifestations, patients with HZ may demonstrate other manifestations of neurologic dysfunction. Patients may have mild motor paresis in the motor nerve that corresponds to the spinal root level of the involved cutaneous nerve. The paresis is usually temporary.[57] Visceral involvement as well as autonomic nerve involvement occurs. Patients with cervical HZ may develop diaphragmatic paralysis and respiratory insufficiency.[54] Hoarseness secondary to spinal cord involvement may be a complication. Sacral HZ is sometimes associated with urinary retention and bladder paralysis. Cystoscopy reveals vesicles of the bladder neck, representing involvement of the autonomic supply of the bladder.[16] Other rare signs of central nervous system involvement include transverse myelitis, encephalitis, and cerebral vasculitis.[22,24] Patients with cervical HZ may develop brain stem infarction with associated hemiplegia.[67]

Physical examination may reveal fever and localized lymphadenopathy during the initial phase of disease. A nonimmunosuppressed patient with no known underlying disease who develops disseminated lesions warrants a careful physical examination for lymphadenopathy and splenomegaly and laboratory tests (complete blood cell count, renal function, and anergy panel) to screen for a hidden lymphoproliferative malignancy. People who are younger than age 50 years who develop HZ in a cervical or lumbar distribution should be examined for signs of acquired immunodeficiency syndrome. These people may have signs of other infections, including herpes simplex and candidiasis as well as oral hairy leukoplakia or lymphoma.[8]

LABORATORY DATA

Cerebrospinal fluid examination may demonstrate an increase in white blood cells in up to one third of patients with HZ. Viral cultures may be positive if fluid from acute vesicular lesions is cultured. Gel-precipitin techniques can also be used to demonstrate specific antigens in fluid and crusts of lesions. Viral culture is less sensitive than immunofluorescence staining or polymerase chain reaction analysis. HZ antibodies may show a fourfold rise during an infection.[68] Only 5% of adults have detectable titers of 1:640 or higher of VZV antibodies in the absence of infection. Antibodies are developed after vaccination for chickenpox. Antibody response to immunization with live attenuated varicella vaccine is typically lower than that achieved after natural VZV infection.[30]

Pathology

Dermal epithelial cells obtained from scraping the early lesions may show giant cells and intranuclear inclusion bodies. Tzanck test findings are compatible but not diagnostic of HZ infection because herpes simplex may show similar abnormalities.

RADIOGRAPHIC EVALUATION

Radiographs of the lumbar spine may demonstrate abnormalities such as fracture-dislocation, metastatic disease, or spinal tumor, which correspond to the location of the affected sensory root ganglion.

MR imaging of the cervical spinal cord may demonstrate enlargement of the cord with noncontiguous areas of increased intramedullary signal in HZ patients. These enhanced images may extend beyond the level of the involved dermatome. Gadolinium enhancement may highlight the dorsal root entry zone as well as the spinal cord. Repeat MR imaging may demonstrate a return of the spinal cord to normal size, but continued increased signal in the dorsal and intramedullary zones is suggestive of glial scarring.[15]

DIFFERENTIAL DIAGNOSIS

The diagnosis of HZ offers little difficulty when the characteristic pain and vesicular eruption are present. The diagnosis is more difficult in the pre-eruptive stage. HZ should be considered in patients with sudden onset of burning pain in a segmental distribution. Following these patients for a short time until the appearance of vesicles helps establish the correct diagnosis. Specific diagnosis of HZ can be made by viral culture or direct immunofluorescence assay. The direct immunofluorescence assay is more sensitive than viral cultures and has a lower cost and more rapid turnaround time.[9] Polymerase chain reaction techniques are useful for detecting HZ virus DNA in fluid and tissues.[19] HZ needs to be considered in the differential diagnosis of radiculopathy, even in the absence of rash.[6] Individuals with disorders with decreased immune surveillance (rheumatoid arthritis, systemic lupus erythematosus) are at risk of developing HZ that may mimic radiculopathy.[1,40]

Other skin lesions may be confused with HZ infection. Herpes simplex does not usually affect an entire dermatome like HZ. Culture of lesions should help make the distinction. Contact dermatitis may appear in a linear band but lacks the painful prodrome. It is pruritic as opposed to painful, may cross the midline, and does not cause paresthesias. Superficial pyoderma, like impetigo, has fewer lesions, is not linear, and has no associated paresthesias. The radiation of pain may be confused with muscle strain or a herniated intervertebral disc.[47] The appearance of the rash helps to differentiate the diagnosis in these individuals.

TREATMENT

The treatment of HZ is directed at decreasing viral replication and controlling pain. Antibiotic therapy is indicated only for patients who develop bacterial superinfection. Patients with vesicles are infectious and should limit contact with people who have not had varicella; they are no longer infectious once the lesions crust over.

The therapeutic goals are to limit segmental infection and prevent general dissemination, tissue injury, and postherpetic neuralgia (Table 12-10). The first two deal with limiting viral replication, and the second two deal with limiting inflammation that causes tissue injury.[45] HZ is a self-limited disease such that treatment must be tailored specifically to the patient's age and status of immune function. In healthy patients younger than 50 years of age, therapy may be limited to analgesics, mild sedatives, antipruritics, and antibacterial ointments. Some physicians consider antiviral therapy to be optional for younger patients with uncomplicated shingles, although therapy with

12-10 THERAPY FOR HERPES ZOSTER

Immunocompetent	
Younger than 50 yr	Analgesics, sedatives, topical antibacterial ointment for ulcerations
Older than 50 yr	Corticosteroids (60 mg/d for 3 wk)
	Valacyclovir 1000 mg three times daily for 1 wk
	Adenosine monophosphate (?)
Immunocompromised	Intravenous acyclovir, 500 mg/m², for 1 hr three times daily for 1 wk *or* oral valacyclovir 1000 mg three times daily for 1 wk *or* oral famciclovir 500 mg three times daily for 1 wk
Postherpetic neuralgia	Amitriptyline up to 100 mg daily, cutaneous nerve stimulation, local nerve blocks, capsaicin (?)

antiviral agents has minimal risk and is potentially beneficial.[21] In healthy patients older than 50 years of age, the goal is to prevent postherpetic neuralgia. Corticosteroids in short-course therapy have been shown to prevent the development of postherpetic pain in a significant percentage of patients.[14,28]

Antiviral Therapy

Antiviral therapy prevents the adsorption, penetration, uncoating, genome synthesis, and assembly of viral particles.[33] Drugs that interfere with viral thymidine kinase phosphorylation and targeted at viral DNA polymerase include acyclovir, valacyclovir, and famciclovir. Drugs targeted at viral DNA polymerase include vidarabine and foscarnet.

Acyclovir is converted to acyclovir triphosphate that competes with deoxyguanosine triphosphate for incorporation into viral DNA. Acyclovir results in chain termination because of an absence of a hydroxyl group. In placebo-controlled trials, acyclovir (800 mg five times daily) shortened the duration of viral shedding, halted the formation of new lesions more quickly, accelerated the rate of healing, and reduced the severity of acute pain.[64] Acyclovir is superior to placebo for the reduction of postherpetic neuralgia. Among patients of 50 years or older, the median time to resolution of postherpetic pain was 41 days, compared with 101 days in the placebo group. At 6 months the acyclovir group had 15% with persistent pain versus 35% in the placebo group.[70] A study of oral high-dose acyclovir in 205 immunocompetent patients older than 60 years of age demonstrated faster healing when the drug was given early in the course of the eruption.[37]

Valacyclovir is cleaved to acyclovir after absorption. It produces three to five times higher acyclovir levels than those achieved with oral acyclovir therapy. Valacyclovir shortens the median time to resolution of postherpetic neuralgia pain from 51 to 38 days (P=0.001) The proportion of patients with pain at 6 months was 25.7% in the acyclovir group and 19.3 in the valacyclovir group (P=0.02).[4]

Famciclovir acts similarly to acyclovir once in the cell but has a prolonged intracellular half-life. It shortens the median resolution of postherpetic neuralgia pain from 163 days in the placebo group to 63 days in the famciclovir group.[59]

Vidarabine, a purine analogue that blocks viral replication through its effects on viral DNA polymerase, when given within 3 days of the onset of rash, accelerates healing and decreases dissemination and postherpetic neuralgia when compared with control subjects.[65] The disadvantages of the drug include the need for 12-hour continuous intravenous infusion and renal toxicity. Vidarabine is utilized for acyclovir-resistant HZ infections, which occur most commonly in HIV-immunocompromised patients.

Foscarnet is a pyrophosphate analogue that blocks viral replication through direct inhibition of viral DNA polymerase. Like vidarabine, foscarnet requires intravenous administration and is nephrotoxic. Foscarnet is effective in HIV-immunocompromised hosts with acyclovir-resistant HZ infection.[49]

Of the antiviral agents, valacyclovir and famciclovir are preferred to acyclovir. The former have superior pharmacokinetic properties and have simpler dosing regimens. The dose of these agents needs to be reduced in patients with renal impairment.

Immunocompromised Host

Appropriate therapy for immunocompromised patients, young and old, is associated with greater potential toxicities. The therapy is instituted to prevent the dissemination of virus beyond the primary dermatome. Zoster immune globulin has not been shown to be better than serum gamma globulin for prevention of dissemination and postherpetic neuralgia in immunocompromised patients and has not been recommended for this purpose.[53]

Intravenous acyclovir has become the recommended therapy for immunocompromised patients. The recommended intravenous dosage of 500 mg/m^2 administered for 1 hour three times a week for 1 week at the earliest sign of the rash has reduced pain and dissemination and increased the rate of healing. Acyclovir is more selective an antiviral agent and has less host toxicity. Oral acyclovir is used in ambulatory patients. Foscarnet is another intravenous therapy with efficacy in AIDS patients with HZ.

The role of corticosteroids in the immunocompromised group is limited. Corticosteroids may promote dissemination and not prevent postherpetic pain. Therefore, they have not been recommended for this group of patients.

Postherpetic Neuralgia

Postherpetic neuralgia, once established, is a difficult problem to treat. Oral acyclovir is no better than placebo in relieving pain secondary to postherpetic neuralgia.[56] Therapy is directed at controlling pain not at killing virus. Some of the therapies that have been tried include amitriptyline (25 mg nightly, with maintenance doses of 100 mg), oral corticosteroids, intralesional triamcinolone, cutaneous nerve stimulation, anesthetic nerve blocks, and topical medications, including capsaicin and lidocaine.[60] Niv and colleagues have suggested that different components of postherpetic pain be treated with specific agents.[41] Burning pain may best respond to tricyclic antidepressants. Lancinating pain responds to anticonvulsant drugs (valproic acid). Dysesthetic pain responds to neuroleptic medication (fluphenazine). Patients with intact skin sensitivity respond to transcutaneous electrical nerve stimulator therapy. Patients with intact sensation may respond to dry needling to the level of the underlying muscle. The majority of the 97 consecutive patients treated with components of this conservative therapy had significant pain relief.[41] Epidural or sympathetic blockade in patients with herpes zoster for 28 days or less does not prevent the onset of postherpetic neuralgia.[42,71]

Corticosteroids

The use of oral corticosteroids remains an area of controversy. Some studies have demonstrated no definite improvement compared with placebo for postherpetic neuralgia.[44] Others have assessed corticosteroids in combination with acyclovir and have demonstrated a moderate but statistically significant acceleration in the rate of cutaneous healing and alleviation of acute pain.[69] In addition, quality of life was improved and the use of analgesics was diminished.[66] However, corticosteroids did not have an effect on the duration of postherpetic neuralgia. Patients at risk from corticosteroid toxicities (diabetes) may not experience an overall benefit. Antiviral medications should be used when corticosteroid therapy is initiated. In patients with severe, persistent postherpetic neuralgia resistant to other therapies, intrathecal injections of methylprednisolone and lidocaine may offer pain relief.[27]

Other Therapies

Antidepressants—amitriptyline and desipramine but not lorazepam—have been associated with relief of postherpetic pain.[29,34] Anticonvulsants have activity in the relief of neuropathic pain, such as postherpetic neuralgia.[58] Gabapentin is an effective agent in the relief of postherpetic neuralgia.[48] Therapy is initiated as a single 100-mg dose three times a day on the first day, 200 mg three times a day on the second day, and 300 mg three times a day on the third day. The dose may then be titrated to between 1800 and 3600 mg/day depending on pain relief. Treatment duration is 8 weeks. Topical capsaicin is more effective than the cream's vehicle for pain relief when applied daily for 6 weeks.[2] Lidocaine patch 5% is an effective therapy for decreasing postherpetic pain. The patch is placed for 12 hours and is then removed for 12 hours. The patch should be applied to skin without blisters. Efficacy has been maintained for a month or longer.[17] On a single-dose basis, 0.2 mg of clonidine has greater pain relief than 120 mg of codeine, 800 mg of ibuprofen, and placebo for postherpetic neuralgia.[35] Mexiletine, an oral lidocaine-like antiarrhythmic agent, has been helpful in the treatment of diabetic neuropathy.[11] Mexiletine, administered 450 to 900 mg in divided doses, has been effective in decreasing pain associated with peripheral nerve injuries.[71] This drug may also have the potential to be an effective agent for the treatment of neuralgia secondary to herpesvirus reactivation. Studies involving HZ patients need to be completed before the efficacy is documented. In general, many patients with neuralgia remain resistant to these therapies and continue with pain.

Varicella Vaccine

A live attenuated varicella vaccine is available for immunization of infants to adults who have not contracted chickenpox and are not pregnant. The virus remains local at the site of injection in immunocompetent individuals. This localization limits the spread of virus to distant organs, including the dorsal root ganglia. Although patients have developed HZ after varicella vaccine, the frequency of reinfection is less than that after natural infection.[63] In addition, vaccine administered to older individuals may boost cellular immunity to varicella virus and result in a decreased occurrence of HZ.[31,32] This hypothesis is being tested.[43]

PROGNOSIS

HZ is usually a disease of short duration resulting in little permanent disability; however, the patient who is older and has an underlying disease may be left with permanent residual effects. These may include postherpetic neuralgia, paralysis, and widespread dissemination. Postherpetic neuralgia is rare in patients younger than 40 years of age but occurs in up to 75% of patients older than 60 years of age.[28] Disseminated HZ with at least 20 or more vesicles outside the primary dermatome occurs up to 10 days after the onset of rash and affects up to 10% of HZ infections. Approximately 30% of these patients are immunocompromised, particularly those with lymphoproliferative malignancy, immunosuppressive therapy, and poor cell-mediated immunity.[36,38] Most patients have resolution of disseminated HZ without sequelae. However, the immunocompromised patient has a worse prognosis. Patients with cervical HZ may develop myelitis. These patients have more neurologic dysfunction that may not return to normal. These individuals are at risk for a worse prognosis.

Those patients left with persistent and intractable postherpetic pain may suffer significant disability. Available therapy to prevent this component of HZ infection or to manage its aftereffects needs to be improved.

References

Herpes Zoster

1. Antonelli MS, Moreland LW, Brick JE: Herpes zoster in patients with rheumatoid arthritis treated with weekly, low-dose methotrexate. Am J Med 90:295-298, 1991.
2. Bernstein JE, Korman NJ, Bickers DR, et al: Topical capsaicin treatment of chronic postherpetic neuralgia. J Am Acad Dermatol 21:265, 1989.
3. Buchbinder SP, Katz MH, Hessol NA, et al: Herpes zoster and human immunodeficiency virus infection. J Infect Dis 166:1153-1156, 1992.
4. Buetner KR, Friedman DJ, Forszpaniak C, et al: Valacyclovir compared with acyclovir for improved therapy for herpes zoster in immunocompetent adults. Antimicrob Agents Chemother 39:1546-1553, 1995.
5. Burgoon CF, Burgoon JS, Baldridge GD: The natural history of herpes zoster. JAMA 164:265, 1957.
6. Burkman KA, Gaines RW Jr, Kashani SR, Smith RD: Herpes zoster: A consideration in the differential diagnosis of radiculopathy. Arch Phys Med Rehabil 69:132, 1988.
7. Choo PW, Donahue JG, Manson JE, et al: The epidemiology of varicella and its complications. J Infect Dis 172:706-712, 1995.
8. Corey JP, Seligman I: Otolaryngology problems in the immune compromised patient: An evolving natural history. Otolaryngol Head Neck Surg 104:196, 1991.
9. Dahl H, Marcoccia J, Linde A: Antigen detection: The method of choice in comparison with virus isolation and serology for laboratory diagnosis of herpes zoster in human immunodeficiency virus–infected patient. J Clin Microbiol 35:345-349, 1997.
10. de Moragas JM, Kierland RR: The outcome of patients with herpes zoster. Arch Dermatol 75:193, 1957.
11. Dejgard A, Petersen P, Kastrup J: Mexiletine for the treatment of chronic painful diabetic neuropathy. Lancet 1:9, 1988.
12. Devinsky O, Cho E, Petito CK, Price RW: Herpes zoster myelitis. Brain 114:1181, 1991.

13. Dueland AN, Devlin M, Martin JR, et al: Fatal varicella-zoster virus meningoradiculitis without skin involvement. Ann Neurol 29:569, 1991.
14. Eaglestein WH, Katz R, Brown JA: The effects of early corticosteroid therapy on skin eruption and pain of herpes zoster. JAMA 211:1681, 1970.
15. Esposito MB, Arrington JA, Murtaugh FR, et al: MR of the spinal cord in a patient with herpes zoster. AJNR Am J Neuroradiol 14:203, 1993.
16. Frengley JF: Herpes zoster: A challenge in management. Primary Care 8:715, 1981.
17. Galer BS, Rowbotham MC, Perander J, et al: Topical lidocaine patch relieves postherpetic neuralgia more effectively than a vehicle topical patch: Results of an enriched enrollment study. Pain 80:533-538, 1999.
18. Gilden DH, Dueland AN, Devlin ME, et al: Varicella-zoster virus reactivation without rash. J Infect Dis 166:S30-S34, 1992.
19. Gilden DH, Kleinschmidt-DeMaster BK, LaGuardia JJ, et al: Neurologic complications of the reactivation of varicella-zoster virus. N Engl J Med 342:635-645, 2000.
20. Glynn C, Crockford G, Gavaghan D, et al: Epidemiology of shingles. J R Soc Med 83:617, 1990.
21. Gnann JW Jr, Whitley RJ: Herpes zoster. N Engl J Med 347: 340-346, 2002.
22. Hogan EL, Krigman MR: Herpes zoster myelitis: Evidence for viral invasion of the spinal cord. Arch Neurol 29:309, 1973.
23. Hope-Simpson RE: The nature of herpes zoster: A long-term study and a new hypothesis. Proc R Soc Med 58:9, 1965.
24. Horte B, Price RW, Jiminez D: Multifocal varicella-zoster virus leukoencephalitis temporally remote from herpes zoster. Ann Neurol 9:251, 1981.
25. Jemesek J, Greenberg SB, Taber L, et al: Herpes zoster-associated encephalitis: Clinicopathologic report of 12 cases and review of the literature. Medicine 52:81, 1983.
26. Juel-Jensen BE: Herpes simplex and zoster. BMJ 1:406, 1973.
27. Katoni N, Kushikata T, Hashimoto H, et al: Intrathecal methylprednisolone for intractable postherpetic neuralgia. N Engl J Med 343:1514-1519, 2000.
28. Keczkes K, Basheer AM: Do corticosteroids prevent post-herpetic neuralgia? Br J Dermatol 102:551, 1981.
29. Kishore-Kumar R, Max MB, Schafer SC, et al: Desipramine relieves postherpetic neuralgia. Clin Pharmacol Ther 47:305, 1990.
30. Krah DL: Assays for antibodies to varicella-zoster virus. Infect Dis Clin North Am 10:507-527, 1996.
31. Levin MJ, Barber D, Goldblatt E, et al: Use of a live attenuated varicella vaccine to boost varicella-specific immune responses in seropositive people 55 years of age and older duration of booster effect. J Infect Dis 178(Suppl 1):S109-S112, 1998.
32. Levin MJ, Murray M, Zerbe GO, et al: Immune responses of elderly persons 4 years after receiving a live attenuated varicella vaccine. J Infect Dis 170:522, 1994.
33. Liesegang TJ: Varicella zoster viral disease. Mayo Clin Proc 74:983-998, 1999.
34. Max MB, Schafer SC, Culnane M, et al: Amitriptyline, but not lorazepam, relieves postherpetic neuralgia. Neurology 38:1427, 1988.
35. Max MB, Schafer SC, Culnane M, et al: Association of pain relief with drug side effects in postherpetic neuralgia: A single-dose study of clonidine, codeine, ibuprofen, and placebo. Clin Pharmacol Ther 43:363, 1988.
36. Mazur W, Whitley R, Dolin R: Serum antibody levels as risk factors in the dissemination of herpes zoster. Arch Intern Med 139:1341, 1979.
37. McKendrick MW, McGill JI, White JE, Wood MJ: Oral acyclovir in acute herpes zoster. BMJ 293:1529, 1986.
38. Merselis J, Kaye D, Hook E: Disseminated herpes zoster: A report of 17 cases. Arch Intern Med 113:679, 1964.
39. Miller LH, Brunell PA: Zoster, reinfection or activation of latent virus? Observations on the antibody response. Am J Med 49:480, 1970.
40. Montori VM, Rho JP, Bauer BA: 37-year-old man with back pain. Mayo Clin Proc 74:923-926, 1999.
41. Niv D, Ben-Ari S, Rappaport A, et al: Postherpetic neuralgia: Clinical experience with a conservative treatment. Clin J Pain 5:295, 1989.
42. Nurmikko TJ, Rasanen A, Hakkinen V: Clinical and neurophysiological observations on acute herpes zoster. Clin J Pain 6:284, 1990.
43. Oxman MN: Immunization to reduce the frequency and severity of herpes zoster and its complications. Neurology 45(Suppl 8): S41-S46, 1995.
44. Post BT, Philbrick JT: Do corticosteroids prevent postherpetic neuralgia? J Am Acad Dermatol 18:605, 1988.
45. Price RW: Herpes zoster: An approach to systemic therapy. Med Clin North Am 66:1105, 1982.
46. Ragozzino MW, Melton LJ, Kurland LT, et al: Risk of cancer after herpes zoster: A population-based study. N Engl J Med 307:393, 1982.
47. Rash MR: Herpes zoster complicating a herniated-thoracic disc. Orthop Rev 11:91, 1982.
48. Rowbotham M, Harden N, Stacey B, et al: Gabapentin for the treatment of postherpetic neuralgia: A randomized controlled trial. JAMA 280:1837-1842, 1998.
49. Safrin S, Berger TG, Gilson I, et al: Foscarnet therapy in five patients with AIDS and acyclovir-resistant varicella-zoster virus infection. Ann Intern Med 115:19-21, 1991.
50. Schimpff S, Serpick A, Stoler B, et al: Varicella-zoster infection in patients with cancer. Ann Intern Med 76:241, 1972.
51. Schmader K George LK, Burchett BM, et al: Racial and psychological risk factors for herpes zoster in the elderly. J Infect Dis 178(Suppl 1):S67-70, 1998.
52. Stevens DA, Merigan TC: Interferon, antibody, and other host factors in herpes zoster. J Clin Invest 51:1170, 1972.
53. Stevens D, Merigan T: Zoster immune globulin prophylaxis of disseminated zoster in compromised hosts. Arch Intern Med 140:52, 1980.
54. Stowasser M, Cameron J, Oliver WA: Diaphragmatic paralysis following cervical herpes zoster. Med J Aust 153:555, 1990.
55. Strauss SE, Ostrove JM, Inchauspe G, et al: Varicella-zoster virus infections: Biology, natural history, treatment, and prevention. Ann Intern Med 108:221, 1988.
56. Surman OQ, Flynn T, Schooley RT, et al: A double-blind, placebo-controlled study of oral acyclovir in postherpetic neuralgia. Psychosomatics 31:287, 1990.
57. Thomas JE, Howard FM Jr: Segmental zoster paresis: A disease profile. Neurology 22:459, 1972.
58. Tremont-Lukats IW, Megeff C, Backonja M: Anticonvulsants for neuropathic pain syndromes: Mechanisms of action and place in therapy. Drugs 60:1029-1052, 2000.
59. Tyring SK, Beutner KR, Tucker BA, et al: Famciclovir for the treatment of acute herpes zoster: Effects on acute disease and postherpetic neuralgia: A randomized, double-blind, placebo-controlled trial. Ann Intern Med 123:89-96, 1995.
60. Watson CP, Evans RJ, Reed K, et al: Amitriptyline vs placebo in postherpetic neuralgia. Neurology 32:671, 1982.
61. Watson CPN: Postherpetic neuralgia. Neurol Clin 7:231, 1989.
62. Weller TH: Varicella and herpes zoster: Changing concepts of the natural history, control, and importance of a not-so-benign virus. N Engl J Med 309:1362, 1983.
63. White CJ: Varicella-zoster virus vaccine. Clin Infect Dis 24:753-761, 1997.
64. Whitley RJ, Gnann JW Jr: Acyclovir: A decade later. N Engl J Med 327:782, 1992.
65. Whitley RJ, Soong SJ, Dolin R, et al: NIAID collaborative antiviral study group: Early vidarabine therapy to control the complications of herpes zoster in immunocompromised patients. N Engl J Med 307:971, 1982.
66. Whitley RJ, Weiss H Gnann JW, et al: Acyclovir with and without prednisone for the treatment of herpes zoster: A randomized, placebo controlled trial. Ann Intern Med 125:376-383, 1996.
67. Willeit J, Schmutzhard E: Cervical herpes zoster and delayed brainstem infarction. Clin Neurol Neurosurg 93:245, 1991.
68. Williams V, Gershon A, Brunnel PA: Serologic response varicella-zoster membrane antigens measured by indirect immunofluorescence. J Infect Dis 130:669, 1974.
69. Wood MJ, Johnson RW, McKendrick MW, et al: A randomized trial of acyclovir for 7 days and 21 days with and without prednisone for treatment of acute herpes zoster. N Engl J Med 330:896-900, 1994.
70. Wood MJ, Kay R, Dworkin RH, et al: Oral acyclovir therapy accelerates pain resolution in patients with herpes zoster: A meta-analysis of placebo-controlled trials. Clin Infect Dis 22:341-347, 1996.
71. Yanagida H, Suwa K, Corssen G: No prophylactic effect of early sympathetic blockade on postherpetic neuralgia. Anesthesiology 66:73, 1987.

LYME DISEASE

CAPSULE SUMMARY

	LOW BACK	NECK
Frequency of spinal pain	Uncommon	Uncommon
Location of spinal pain	Lumbar spine	Cervical spine
Quality of spinal pain	Ache	Ache
Symptoms and signs	Erythema migrans, general malaise, back stiffness, radiculoneuritis	Erythema migrans, general malaise, neck stiffness, radiculoneuritis
Laboratory tests	Increased erythrocyte sedimentation rate, *Borrelia* antibodies, cerebrospinal fluid pleocytosis	Increased erythrocyte sedimentation rate, *Borrelia* antibodies, cerebrospinal fluid pleocytosis
Radiographic findings	None	None
Treatment	Antibiotics: oral for early disease, IV for late disease	Antibiotics: oral for early disease, IV for late disease

PREVALENCE AND PATHOGENESIS

Lyme disease is an infectious disease caused by the spirochete *Borrelia burgdorferi.* The organism was identified by Willie Burgdorfer and colleagues in 1982.[12] Three pathogenic species are associated with the illness. *B. burgdorferi* causes the disease in the United States, whereas *Borrelia afzelii* and *Borrelia garinii* cause the illness in Europe and Asia.[81] The organism is transmitted to humans by a tick vector. The clinical manifestations of the disease appear as the *Borrelia* disseminate through the organs of the body and the immune system mounts a cellular and humoral response to the organism. A generalized malaise mimicking a flulike state, including neck or low back pain and stiffness, occurs simultaneously with the appearance of a characteristic rash, erythema migrans (EM, formerly known as erythema chronicum migrans). In later stages of the disease, cardiac and neurologic manifestations become prominent. Polyradiculitis, including the upper and lower extremities, is associated with this stage of the disease. Chronic arthritis, chronic fatigue, and encephalomyelitis are potential manifestations of late disease. The diagnosis of Lyme disease is suspected in an individual exposed to ticks who develops an appropriate array of symptoms and signs and whose disease is confirmed by the presence of IgM or IgG antibodies to the *Borrelia* antigens. All stages of the disease are treated with antibiotics, which are most successful in the early stages.

Epidemiology

Lyme disease is the most common vector-transmitted disease in the United States.[61] Over 40,000 cases were reported to the Centers for Disease Control and Prevention from 1982 to 1991.[22] Currently, about 15,000 cases are reported each year in the United States.[56] The disease is endemic in three areas of the United States: the Northeast, from Maryland to Maine; the upper Midwest, in Minnesota and Wisconsin; and the West, primarily the coast of California and Oregon. Approximately 85% of human Lyme disease cases are reported from the endemic areas of the Northeast and Midwest.[13] The 10 states with 88% of the patients are New York, Connecticut, New Jersey, Pennsylvania, Rhode Island, Massachusetts, Maryland, Wisconsin, Minnesota, and California. These locations correspond to areas associated with large deer populations. Deer are the primary hosts for the deer tick, the vector for transmission of Lyme disease. The tick species responsible for transmitting *B. burgdorferi* to humans is restricted to the *Ixodes* genus.[27] In the East, *Ixodes scapularis* and, in the West, *Ixodes pacificus* are the tick vectors associated with Lyme disease. The populations of *I. scapularis* occurring in the Northeast and upper Midwest were formerly referred to as a separate third species, *Ixodes dammini,* because of important ecologic and behavioral attributes that differ from those of populations occurring in the middle and southern states.[27,55] The disease is not exclusively limited to these areas of the United States; cases have been reported in 46 of the contiguous states and Hawaii.[13] The geographic spread of the disease in individual states has increased.[83] The disease has also been reported in Europe (Germany, Austria, Slovenia, Sweden), Russia, Japan, China, and Australia. In Europe, the principal vector is *Ixodes racinus,* and in Asia, *Ixodes persulcatus.* The deer tick is also a vector for ehrlichiosis and babesiosis. Lyme disease affects people in all age groups. A significant number of children are affected up to the age of 9 years. Females and males are almost equally affected (53% and 47%, respectively).[22] The disease occurs primarily in whites, reflecting the exposure of this group to nonurban settings.

Pathogenesis

The disease is spread to the geographic areas by the tick vector. Other ticks and biting insects may be secondary vectors of infection. Other types of ticks and horseflies, deerflies, and mosquitoes have been reported to carry *B. burgdorferi*.[4,49] The tick has a four-stage, 2-year life cycle. The life cycle includes an egg, larval, nymphal, and adult stage of development. Each of the three motile stages feeds only once before molting into the next stage. The usual host for the larval and nymph stage is the white-footed mouse, *Peromyscus leucopus*. The mouse is the primary reservoir for *B. burgdorferi*. The *Borrelia* parasitize the mice without causing any illness. The host is disease free from the *Borrelia* for the remainder of its life.

The life cycle of the tick is a complex process. Eggs are deposited in the early summer. Larvae do not hatch until July. Larvae that feed before September molt to become nymphs. Those that do not feed will feed the following spring. Nymphs must feed again before they molt to become adults. Adult females attach to large vertebrates to feed and mate. After mating, the females are able to lay eggs to start a new cycle. White-tailed deer are the favorite host for the adult ticks. Each stage of the life cycle is a balance between death from the environment or survival with host contact. The balance between these two outcomes determines the number of ticks in any given geographic area. The frequency of Lyme disease infections relates, to a significant extent, to the size of the local deer population.

Larval and nymphal ticks feed on the infected mice and become colonized with *B. burgdorferi*. The ticks become vectors of the disease for humans when the ticks feed in a later developmental stage. The *B. burgdorferi* reside in the midgut of the tick. With attachment of the tick to a host, the organisms are mobilized to the salivary glands, where they infect the vertebrate.[11] This process requires approximately 24 hours to complete. Adult ticks do not transfer *B. burgdorferi* to their offspring. Larvae typically become infected with *Borrelia* by feeding on a reservoir host rather than from congenital transmission. The passage of *B. burgdorferi* between ticks and mice maintains the high rate of infection of the tick vectors in an endemic area.

The pathogenesis of Lyme disease is not entirely clear.[29] The currently accepted theory is that the organisms persist throughout the course of the disease. Organisms, although few in number, have been detected in affected organ systems long after the onset of the disease.[7,36] Further evidence for the persistence of organisms is the variety of new IgG antibodies that emerge over time with prolonged disease. Amplification of the B-cell response would be unlikely without a changing antigenic stimulus.[18] In addition, antibiotics have a beneficial effect on the course of the disease at all of its stages.[71] In regard to genetic predisposition to particular manifestations of the disease, people with histocompatibility typing DR4 are susceptible to chronic Lyme arthritis.[77]

The structure of *B. burgdorferi* is that of a typical spirochete. The organism contains a protoplasmic cylinder surrounded by a periplasm containing the flagella, which is surrounded by an outer membrane. Many of the outer membrane proteins are encoded by plasmid genes. The complete genome of B. *burgdorferi* has been sequenced.[72] The ability to produce a wide range of outer membrane proteins allows the organism to exist in arthropod and mammalian environments. The dissemination of the organisms through the human body may be facilitated by the ability to attach to host integrins, matrix glycosaminoglycans, and extracellular matrix proteins.[32] The spirochete initiates an immune response by binding to the CD14 molecule and toll-like receptor 2 on macrophages, resulting in the release of macrophage-derived cytokines.[34] However, the immune response may be ineffective with decreased levels of cytokines (decreased interferon-γ), resulting in persistence of the organisms.[51]

CLINICAL HISTORY

The clinical manifestations of Lyme disease may be dermatologic, cardiac, neurologic, or musculoskeletal during the course of the illness (Table 12-11). The disease is best described by a classification system that divides it into early and late infection. The affected organ systems manifest a variety of abnormalities, depending on the duration of the infection.

Early Disease

Early infection is characterized by the emergence of pathognomonic skin lesions, localized lymphadenopathy, and a flulike syndrome (Fig. 12-16). This stage corresponds to the local invasion of the skin and associated lymph nodes by the organisms, along with systemic response manifested by a flulike syndrome. EM is the most common and distinctive cutaneous manifestation of Lyme disease. It appears at the site of the tick bite and is identified in 60% to 80% of patients.[8,71] Skin lesions appear 2 to 28 days after the bite of an infected tick. The lesion starts as a single, expanding red macule and expands in an annular fashion. In the United States, most lesions of EM occur within 2 weeks of onset and lack central clearing.[53] The central area may clear, forming a target lesion. Central clearing may be a characteristic of EM, lasting 5 to 6 weeks. The skin lesion is usually asymptomatic but may be tender, warm, or pruritic and may become 15 cm or

12-11 CLINICAL STAGES OF LYME DISEASE

Localized	Disseminated	Persistent
Erythema migrans	Multiple annular lesions	Chronic arthritis
Local lymphadenopathy	Bell's palsy	Encephalomyelitis
	Meningitis	Chronic fatigue
	Radiculoneuritis	Acrodermatitis chronica atrophicans
	Atrioventricular nodal block	
	Migratory arthralgias	
	Severe fatigue	
	Generalized lymphadenopathy	

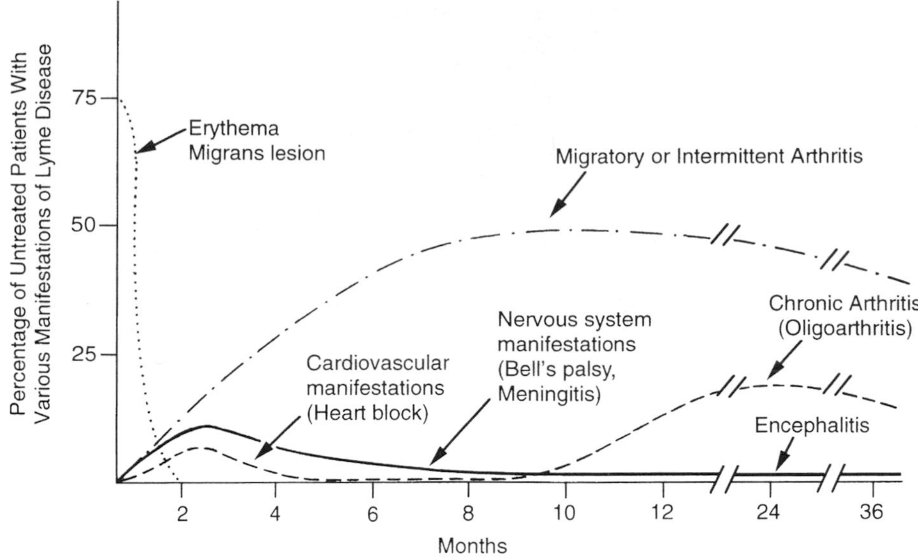

Figure 12-16 Lyme disease. Clinical course of organ system involvement.

larger. A small number (less than 5%) may have a vesicular center. The EM lesion is located at the site of attachment of the tick. Only 32% of patients may recall a tick bite. The lack of awareness may be related to the small size of the nymphal *I. scapularis* tick, the lack of local tenderness or pruritus, and areas that may be difficult to visualize.[53] *B. burgdorferi* may be isolated occasionally from skin biopsies obtained from the advancing front of the lesion but are rarely needed to identify the origin of the skin lesion.[79] Skin lesions appear most commonly on the trunk (38%), lower extremities (38%), upper extremities (11%), pelvic region (7%), and head and neck (6%).[9] Skin folds are preferred areas for tick attachment.

Constitutional. The flulike syndrome is characterized by fatigue, fever, chills, malaise, headache, stiff neck, and arthralgias. Neck stiffness or back pain occurs in approximately 26% of patients.[64,74] In another study, 42% developed stiff neck.[76] These constitutional symptoms may be the only clues to the diagnosis of Lyme disease when skin lesions are absent. Less common manifestations include malar rash, sore throat, nausea, and vomiting.

Cutaneous. As the *B. burgdorferi* organisms escape to the systemic circulation, the disseminated phase of early infection occurs. Additional organ systems are affected. Within a few weeks of disease onset, up to 48% of untreated patients develop multiple annular skin lesions.[10] Other studies have reported the incidence of secondary lesions in less than 25% of patients.[53] Hematogenous spread of the organisms causes these lesions, which resemble EM, to appear. The lesions may vary in number up to 20, are smaller than lesions of EM, and are less expansive. Secondary lesions may be evanescent, appear suddenly during an examination, and then fade. Lesions may become more prominent with heating associated with bathing.[53]

Cardiovascular. Cardiac manifestations of early disseminated disease appear 4 days to 7 months after the onset of disease.[75] Cardiac disease has been reported in 4% to 20% of Lyme disease patients. Heart block is the primary manifestation of cardiac involvement.[50] First-degree to complete heart blocks have been reported. Cardiac conduction abnormalities are temporary, lasting a few weeks. Temporary pacing is occasionally required for high-grade atrioventricular block. Atrial arrhythmias occur in association with Lyme pericarditis, and ventricular arrhythmias are associated with myocarditis.

Neurologic. Neurologic system involvement complicates early disseminated disease in 20% of patients.[65] Throughout the disease, 40% of symptomatic infections have neurologic involvement.[17] Neurologic symptoms and signs develop weeks to 12 months after the resolution of EM. Both the peripheral nervous system (PNS) and the central nervous system (CNS) may be involved. The manifestations of nervous system disease include one or more of six neurologic syndromes: lymphocytic meningitis, cranial nerve palsies, and radiculoneuritis (early infection); and encephalopathy, polyneuropathy, and meningoencephalomyelitis (late infection).[17,60] Lyme meningitis, the most common CNS manifestation of Lyme disease, is associated with severe headache, stiff neck, photophobia, nausea, vomiting, and irritability.[63] Meningitis is the result of direct invasion of the CNS by *B. burgdorferi.* Meningitis may be acute, relapsing, or chronic. Most patients describe a fluctuating, mild headache. Meningismus, in the form of a stiff neck, is minimal to mild.[58] Patients with meningitis may also have significant myalgias. Approximately 50% of patients with Lyme meningitis have associated encephalitis. Concentration deficits, emotional lability, and persistent fatigue are manifestations of encephalitis. A majority of patients, up to 80%, may develop facial (Bell's) palsy.[58] Other cranial nerves, including the third, fifth, and eighth, have also been affected. A minority of patients (31% to 44%) develop radiculoneuritis, usually in the setting of cranial neuropathy.[60,63] The PNS is also involved. Peripheral neuritis; sensory radiculitis; brachial, lumbar, or sacral plexitis; and sensorimotor radiculoneuritis may occur within the first months of the disease.[12,57] These neurologic disorders may present with a variety of symptoms and signs including burning pain, paresthesia, loss of reflexes, and focal motor weakness. Rarely does the neuropathy result in atrophy or marked weakness.[58] Upper extremity abnormalities are more common than lower extremity abnormalities. Involvement of the sensory and motor nerves of the lower extremities may occur in the setting of similar disease in the upper extremities. The patients with lower extremity disease have severe radicular pain, dysesthesias, sensory loss, leg weakness, and mononeuritis multiplex. Pain is the first symptom, followed within 4 weeks by motor weakness. Weakness begins gradually and may progress to mild atrophy of the muscle. Sensory loss follows pain in a similar period in 50% of patients.[65] The sensory loss is dermatomal in distribution in the upper extremities. In the lower extremities a symmetrical distal sensory loss may also occur. The occurrence simultaneously of radiculoneuritis and cerebrospinal fluid pleocytosis is common in Europe and is known as Bannwarth's syndrome or tick-borne meningopolyneuritis.[1]

Musculoskeletal. Musculoskeletal manifestations of early disease are primarily arthralgias and myalgias that occur within 8 weeks of infection.[80] Pain occurs in one or two sites at a time and migrates to other musculoskeletal structures. These locations may be affected for hours to days, with spontaneous resolution of symptoms lasting for months. Fatigue is the most common associated symptom. Subsequently, a majority of untreated patients develop intermittent episodes of frank arthritis 4 days to 2 years after disease onset.[80] The large joints, particularly the knee, become swollen and warm but not significantly painful. Other joints affected include the shoulder, ankle, elbow, temporomandibular, wrist, and hip.[73] The pattern of involvement is asymmetrical. Small joint involvement, independent of large joint disease, is unusual. The most frequently affected extra-articular locations as reported in 28 patients with Lyme disease are the back and neck in 32% and 21% of cases, respectively.[73] Periarticular involvement may occur, interspersed with episodes of arthritis in other locations of the musculoskeletal system. In most circumstances, only one periarticular structure is affected at a time, with pain lasting weeks to months in a given location.

Late Disease

Late infection manifestations occur as the organisms persist in organ systems infected during earlier stages. Acrodermatitis chronica atrophicans is the skin manifestation of persistent infection in Lyme borreliosis.[5] The lesion occurs predominantly in women from 40 to 70 years of age. It begins insidiously with bluish-red discoloration and swollen skin on an extremity, usually the lower leg or foot. The inflammatory stage of the lesion may persist for years. Subsequently, the skin in the involved area becomes atrophic and develops a wrinkled appearance. EM may have been present at the same site years earlier. *B. burgdorferi* may be cultured from these lesions as long as 10 years after their onset.[6]

Neurologic. A range of CNS and PNS abnormalities has been described in late disease that occurs more than 1 year after the onset of disease. These disease manifestations are uncommon. Patients with late symptomatic neurologic disease may have both an encephalopathy and polyneuropathy syndrome. The most clearly defined syndrome is progressive encephalomyelitis, which is characterized by spastic paresis, bladder dysfunction, ataxia, cranial nerve deficits, and dementia.[2] Late polyneuropathy may be manifested by sensory or motor abnormalities. Tingling paresthesias may occur in 50% of patients with late Lyme borreliosis.[46] The paresthesias are located distally in the arms, legs, or both and are asymmetrical and patchy in distribution. Radicular pain in the legs occurs in 25% of patients, with onset corresponding with the onset of paresthesias.[45] Median nerve entrapment (carpal tunnel syndrome) has been reported in up to 25% of patients with late symptomatic infections.[33] Other rare syndromes associated with Lyme disease include pseudotumor cerebri, strokelike syndromes, hallucinations, and myositis.[17]

Musculoskeletal. Monarticular or oligoarticular arthritis involving the knee is the most common musculoskeletal manifestation of late Lyme borreliosis.[80] Approximately 11% of untreated people with EM develop arthritis that persists for 1 year or longer. Synovitis appears 4 months to 4 years after EM. In addition to the knee, the shoulder or hip is affected. Joint involvement is a more frequent manifestation of illness in Europe than in the United States. The arthritis may persist for 4 years or longer or resolve spontaneously.[37] Figure 12-4 depicts the course of organ system involvement throughout time.

In about 10% of patients, particularly those with HLA-DRB1*0401, the arthritis in the knees persists for years despite antibiotic therapy.[72] The individuals who are resistant to antibiotic therapy versus those who respond are differentiated by their cellular and humoral immune response to OspA.[14] OspA antigens may be retained in the patients' dendritic cells in the absence of live organisms. Molecular mimicry exists between OspA and human lymphocyte function–associated antigen 1 (hLFA-1). hLFA-1 is an adhesion molecule expressed on T cells in synovium. The cross-reactivity between the proteins may perpetuate a synovitis in the absence of the organism, similar to the pathogenesis of reactive arthritis.[82]

PHYSICAL EXAMINATION

Physical findings in the initial stages of the disease include the presence of EM and regional lymphadenopathy. Musculoskeletal pain may occur at rest or with motion. The cervical or lumbar spine may be painful on palpation. Pain occurs in only one or two regions at a time. Episodes may resolve in hours to several days. This syndrome has been referred to as localized, intermittent musculoskeletal pain (LIMP).[40] Irregular pulse may be noticed in patients with cardiac involvement. Neurologic abnormalities may include cranial nerve dysfunction (Bell's palsy), sensory or motor nerve impairment (including brachial nerve), and mental confusion or impaired memory. Patients with late disease may have patches of atrophic skin, persistent monarticular arthritis, spastic paresis, or organic brain syndrome.

LABORATORY DATA

The commonly ordered screening blood tests, including complete blood cell count, erythrocyte sedimentation rate

(ESR), and serum chemistries, yield results that are normal or nonspecific during early disseminated disease.[62] The ESR is elevated in a majority of patients. A smaller proportion of patients have abnormal levels of immunoglobulins, cryoglobulins, liver enzymes, and microscopic hematuria.[42] In patients with neurologic involvement, the cerebrospinal fluid (CSF) is found to have a lymphocytic pleocytosis and elevated protein concentration.[65] CSF is invariably abnormal in Lyme meningitis and patients with acute radicular syndromes. Patients with PNS disease, encephalopathy, and cranial neuropathy frequently have normal CSF findings. Normal CSF tests do not rule out the possibility of *B. burgdorferi* infection of the nervous system.[17] Antibodies against *Borrelia* may be locally produced and detected in CSF. The most useful CSF test is the detection of antibody to *B. burgdorferi* by Western blot analysis. This test is able to differentiate individuals with false-positive enzyme-linked immunosorbent assay (ELISA) serum assays for antibody.[58] It is essential to compare serum with CSF antibody levels to estimate the amount of intrathecal production. Synovial fluid analysis reveals findings consistent with an inflammatory arthropathy, including leukocyte counts of 5000 to 100,000/mm^3 predominantly polymorphonuclear leukocytes, with elevated protein and normal glucose concentrations.[71] Culture of skin, blood, CSF, or synovial fluid rarely renders a positive result for *B. burgdorferi* and is rarely obtained in the clinical setting.[84]

Serologic Tests

Serologic tests are helpful in detecting the antibody response, including IgM and IgG antibodies, to epitopes on the surface structures of *B. burgdorferi.*[48] Within the first 2 to 4 weeks of infection, IgM antibodies directed against the flagellar antigen of *B. burgdorferi* appear. IgM antibodies peak after 6 to 8 weeks of disease. IgG antibodies appear over the next few weeks, corresponding with the gradual 4- to 6-month decrease in IgM antibody titer. Patients with persistent disease have IgG antibodies exclusively that remain indefinitely. Successful antibiotic therapy may result in a fall in IgG titer, but only throughout several months. Some patients have persistently elevated antibodies despite eradication of the organism. These antibodies are most effectively detected by the ELISA test. The ELISA test is more sensitive and reproducible than immunofluorescence assays. Most ELISA tests use extracts of sonicated whole *B. burgdorferi* as antigen. The ELISA test is associated with false-negative and false-positive results. False-negative results occur during the first few weeks of infection before antibodies develop or in individuals who receive an inadequate course of antibiotic therapy early in the course of the disease and remain infected with live organisms. False-positive results occur in patients with a variety of spirochetal illnesses, including gingivitis, syphilis, Rocky Mountain spotted fever, mononucleosis, and autoimmune disorders such as rheumatoid arthritis and systemic lupus erythematosus. Although poor reproducibility of results is a major concern in interpreting Lyme antibody titers, the standardization of ELISA tests along with a relative high titer level has helped to differentiate true positive tests from sources of background cross-reactivity. Patients with Lyme arthritis usually have higher *Borrelia*-specific antibody titers than patients with any other manifestation of the illness.[3]

Western blot analysis is an immunoblotting technique used to confirm ELISA results or to detect antibodies early in the clinical course of the disease that may not be detected by the ELISA method.[47] Western blot analysis is able to detect antibodies to a number of specific *Borrelia* antigens. Although the ELISA method and Western blot analyses are helpful, great diversity exists in the results of laboratories when testing the same samples.[15] These inconsistencies emphasize the utility of serologic tests as adjuncts in the clinical diagnosis of Lyme disease.

In rare circumstances, when the diagnosis of Lyme disease is suspected but serologic tests are inconclusive, T-lymphocyte assays for reactivity to *Borrelia*-specific antigens may be helpful.[19] The subset of patients with late Lyme disease who have negative or indeterminate antibody responses are the best candidates for the T-cell proliferative assay.[24] T cells from infected patients proliferate when exposed to whole organisms. This assay is time consuming and should be completed in patients who elicit a strong suspicion for the diagnosis without abnormal serologic tests.

A test that should be available soon for the diagnosis of Lyme disease uses polymerase chain reaction (PCR) technology.[66] PCR is able to detect the presence of a small amount of genomic DNA of *B. burgdorferi.* The PCR is superior to the ELISA or the Western blot analysis because it relies on the presence of the organism itself for a positive result. The PCR assay is very specific because particular parts of the *Borrelia* genome may be chosen for replication. The PCR of CSF of patients with Lyme meningitis is positive in about 50% of samples tested.[59] The 50% yield is consistent with the absence of *Borrelia* in organs other than the skin, and the perivascular location, and the absence in body fluids of the organisms in chronic infections.[58] The PCR has also been used for the rapid identification of *B. burgdorferi* in the serum. The PCR is three times more sensitive than culture for identifying *Borrelia* in serum for early diagnosis of Lyme disease.[30]

Pathology

Histopathologic evaluation of tissue biopsy specimens has the potential to identify the presence of organisms in affected organs.[25] The organisms are most easily identified in the skin when the organisms are most abundant before dissemination. Inflammatory infiltrates may be identified in a variety of tissue samples but are not specific enough in the absence of organisms to permit a specific diagnosis. For example, synovial biopsy specimens reveal histopathologic changes that are similar to rheumatoid arthritis and reactive arthritis.[26]

RADIOGRAPHIC EVALUATION

Radiographic findings of the axial skeleton are normal in patients with Lyme disease. Radiographic abnormalities, when they occur, are located in the peripheral joints, primarily the knee. Abnormalities include soft tissue swelling, loss of articular cartilage, chondrocalcinosis, and periarticular osseous erosions.[43]

Neuroimaging of the brain is abnormal in 25% of patients with neuroborreliosis. The most common finding is scattered white matter lesions that do not enhance on MR evaluation. These lesions are smaller than those associated with demyelinating diseases. Occasionally, MR imaging reveals enhancing lesions of cranial nerves and meninges.[54]

DIFFERENTIAL DIAGNOSIS

A case definition has been presented by the CDC for surveillance of Lyme disease (Table 12-12).[72] The definition is more stringent than needed for the clinical diagnosis of Lyme disease. The diagnosis of Lyme disease is based on the presentation of appropriate clinical symptoms in a patient who lives in or has visited an endemic area. The history of a tick bite is helpful but not essential for the diagnosis. Culture of the organism from skin or viewing it on histologic sections of biopsies from affected organs is usually unrevealing. Serologic tests are useful adjuncts in diagnosis, but abnormal findings may be present in people previously exposed to the organisms but who have cleared the infection. Basing a diagnosis solely on the presence of antibodies reactive to *B. burgdorferi* is to be discouraged.

The differential diagnosis as it affects spinal pain is related to the muscle pain syndromes and neurologic disorders that cause radiculopathy and plexopathy. Fibromyalgia has been associated with Lyme disease. Patients may develop tender points in the setting of Lyme disease.[23,68] More often, patients develop the LIMP syndrome confined to one or two joint areas in clear distinction of the multiple areas affected with fibromyalgia.

The differential diagnosis of radiculopathy includes mechanical, neoplastic, and autoimmune disorders. Patients with mechanical disorders describe radiating pain that is affected by body position. Assuming a comfortable position frequently relieves pain in patients with a mechanical cause of radiculopathy. Patients with neoplastic disorders frequently have associated systemic symptoms that are rapidly progressive and disabling. Autoimmune disorders, such as systemic lupus erythematosus and systemic vasculitis, are associated with characteristic abnormalities in a variety of organ systems (malar rash and nodose lesions). These abnormalities help separate those patients with autoimmune disorders who may have false-positive serologic tests for Lyme disease from patients infected with *B. burgdorferi.*

Other tick-borne illnesses, including ehrlichiosis and babesiosis, may occur separately or in combination with Lyme disease.[21,41] Ehrlichieae (an obligate intracellular bacteria) causes an illness associated with fever, myalgias, and headaches in 50% of patients. Rash occurs in a minority of patients. Stiff neck as a manifestation of neurologic involvement occurs occasionally. Tetracycline is an effective therapy for this organism.[28] Babesiosis is caused by a protozoa that infects red blood cells and causes hemolysis.[31] The vector for this organism is the Ixodid tick. Cattle are the main reservoir of the organisms. Immunodeficient patients are at greatest risk of significant infection. Doxycycline is one of the antibiotics given for this infection.

TREATMENT

The risk of tick bites can be reduced in endemic areas. Lyme disease starts in late May when tick nymphs start searching for hosts. About 25% of nymphs contain *Borrelia* but are responsible for 90% of Lyme disease patients.[27] The association between the nymphs and disease relates to their greater abundance, their small size, and the temporal coincidence of their peak feeding activity with human outdoor activity.[27] Therefore, starting in late spring, proper dress should be encouraged by covering the skin, including tucking trousers into socks to block attachment of ticks on the lower extremities. Clothes may be impregnated with

12-12 CASE DEFINITION OF LYME DISEASE FOR NATIONAL SURVEILLANCE

1. Erythema migrans observed by a physician. The skin lesion expands slowly over a period of days or weeks to form a large, round lesion, often with central clearing. To be counted for surveillance purposes, a solitary lesion must reach a size of at least 5 cm.
2. At minimum, one manifestation and laboratory finding of infection
   a. Nervous system: Lymphocytic meningitis, cranial neuritis, radiculoneuropathy, or, rarely, encephalomyelitis, alone or in combination: For encephalomyelitis to be counted for surveillance purposes, cerebrospinal fluid must contain production of antibody against *B. burgdorferi.*
   b. Cardiovascular system: Acute-onset, high-grade (second- or-third degree) atrioventricular conduction defects that resolve in days or weeks and are sometimes associated with myocarditis
   c. Musculoskeletal system: Recurrent, brief attacks (lasting weeks to months) of objectively confirmed joint swelling in one or a few joints, sometimes followed by chronic arthritis in one or a few joints
   d. Laboratory evidence: Isolation of *B. burgdorferi* from tissue or body fluid or detection of diagnostic levels of antibody against the spirochete by the two-test approach of enzyme-linked immunosorbent assay and Western blotting, interpreted according to the criteria of the Centers for Disease Control and Prevention and the Association of State and Territorial Public Health Laboratory Directors*

*In a person with acute disease of less than 1 month's duration, IgM and IgG antibody responses should be measured in serum samples obtained during the acute and convalescent phases. A Western blot for IgM antibodies is considered positive if at least two of the following three bands are present: 23, 39, and 41 kDa. A blot for IgG antibodies is considered positive if at least 5 of the following 10 bands are present: 18, 23, 28, 30, 39, 41, 45, 58, 66, and 93 kDa. Only the IgG response should be used to support the diagnosis after the first month of infection; after that time, IgM response alone is likely to represent a false-positive result.

Modified from Steere AC: Lyme disease. N Engl J Med 345:115-125, 2001.

N,N-diethylmetatoluamide or permethrin to deter ticks. However, exposure of the skin to these chemicals must be limited to decrease toxicities from these agents. During periods of feeding by the various forms of the tick from spring to late summer, individuals should be examined daily for the presence of ticks. The transmission of disease is diminished by the daily removal of ticks because the inoculation of *B. burgdorferi* requires 24 hours or longer.

Randomized studies have demonstrated that the probability of developing symptoms of Lyme disease after an *Ixodes* tick bite is low and equals the rate of toxicity of the antibiotics used to treat the illness.[16] In one study the prevention of Lyme disease with the administration of a single dose of doxycycline, 200 mg, given within 72 hours of a tick bite was reported. Individuals who received the antibiotic had more toxicities (30%) versus placebo (11%).[52] Despite this study, the consensus is that prophylactic antibiotics should not be given routinely for tick bites, unless a rash appears.

Antibiotic Therapy

Therapy for Lyme disease is based on antibiotics effective in eradicating *B. burgdorferi* from infected patients when clinical symptoms appear. *B. burgdorferi* is highly sensitive to tetracyclines, semisynthetic penicillins, and second- and third-generation cephalosporins. Erythromycin is an alternative agent but is less desirable than amoxicillin or doxycycline.[35] The choice of agent and its formulation, oral or intravenous, depend on the stage and organ involvement of the illness (Table 12-13).[69] The treatment of choice for early local disease including EM is doxycycline or tetracycline. Amoxicillin is used for children and pregnant women. Cefuroxime axetil is an alternative for those allergic to doxycycline and ampicillin. Erythromycin is less effective but is an alternative for patients allergic to penicillin. The duration of therapy is 14 to 21 days. If patients have early disseminated disease, therapy may be continued for 30 days. Patients with facial palsy or first-degree heart block can be treated with oral antibiotics.

Patients with evidence of meningitis, radiculitis, or complete heart block have been treated with intravenous antibiotics. No ideal antibiotic regimen has been determined. Intravenous antibiotics used to treat Lyme borreliosis include ceftriaxone and penicillin. Cefotaxime is also effective for disseminated disease. Therapy is continued for 14 to 28 days. Patients with Lyme arthritis are also treated with intravenous antibiotics. Although no controlled studies have been completed for persistent late infection including CNS or PNS disease, intravenous antibiotics are given for 28 days. The symptoms may not rapidly respond to the course of antibiotics. Clinical response may be delayed for as long as 6 to 8 months.[78] In a comparison of intravenous penicillin and ceftriaxone, ceftriaxone was significantly more effective with an 85% cure rate.[20] There is no scientific evidence supporting repeated courses of antibiotics for extended periods in the treatment of Lyme disease. Prolonged oral or intravenous antibiotic therapy for 90 days for Lyme disease patients with persistent musculoskeletal pain, neurocognitive dysfunction, or fatigue was no more effective than placebo.[39]

Major concern remains involving the use of parenteral antibiotic therapy for patients with nonspecific musculoskeletal pains and fatigue and a positive serologic test for Lyme disease. Lightfoot and co-workers suggest that costs and risks of intravenous antibiotic therapy outweigh the likelihood of improvement of nonspecific constitutional symptoms. Only when the value of patient anxiety about leaving a positive Lyme test untreated exceeds $3500 for empirical antibiotic therapy is treatment cost effective.[44]

12-13 ANTIBIOTIC THERAPY FOR LYME DISEASE

EARLY LOCAL INFECTION	
Erythema migrans	Tetracycline, 500 mg, four times daily for 10-30 days
	Doxycycline, 100 mg, twice daily for 10-30 days
Children	Amoxicillin, 500 mg, three times daily for 10-30 days
Penicillin allergic	Erythromycin, 500 mg, three times daily for 10-30 days
EARLY DISSEMINATED INFECTION	
Flu syndrome, Bell's palsy, first-degree heart block	Oral regimens
Meningitis, radiculopathy, complete heart block, arthritis	Ceftriaxone, 2 g IV, four times daily for 14 to 28 days *or* cefotaxime, 3 g IV, twice daily for 14 to 28 days
LATE PERSISTENT INFECTION	
	Benzylpenicillin, 5 million U IV, four times daily for 14 to 28 days

Vaccine

A vaccine for Lyme disease was tested and found to be effective.[70] The vaccine induced antibodies to OspA that neutralized the organism before traveling from the tick to the host. Although effective, the vaccine was not used and was removed from the market and is no longer available.

PROGNOSIS

The prognosis of patients with Lyme disease and spinal pain is excellent if these patients receive an appropriate course of antibiotics. They usually have no residual spinal pain or stiffness. Patients who have radiculopathy have neuroborreliosis. These patients may also respond to antibiotics but may require intravenous medicines to improve. Clinical awareness of the symptoms and signs of Lyme disease in patients who are exposed to ticks should result in the rapid identification of the patient at risk for this disease. This is the most important way to prevent the dissemination of the organisms resulting in more serious forms of this disease. This may prevent the development of chronic Lyme disease caused by the early dissemination of the *Borrelia* organisms to the nervous system.[38] Radiculoneuropathy and peripheral neuropathy may resolve slowly for 24 months. The slow recovery may correspond to the slow healing of axonal damage. Prolonged courses of antibiotics do not influence the rate of recovery. Although patients with Lyme disease may report increased difficulty in completing activities of daily living years after infection, the frequency of complaints is no different than age-matched controls without Lyme disease.[67]

References

Lyme Disease

1. Ackerman R, Horstrup P, Schmidt R: Tick-borne meningopolyneuritis (Garin-Boujadoux, Bannwarth). Yale J Biol Med 57:485, 1984.
2. Ackermann R, Rehse-Kupper B, Gollmer E, Schmidt R: Chronic neurologic manifestations of erythema migrans borreliosis. Ann N Y Acad Sci 539:16, 1988.
3. Akin E, McHugh GL, Flavell RA, et al: The immunoglobulin (IgG) antibody response to OspA and OspB correlates with severe and prolonged Lyme arthritis and the IgG response to P35 correlates with mild and brief arthritis. Infect Immun 67:173-181, 1999.
4. Anderson JF, Magnarelli LA: Avian and mammalian hosts for spirochete-infected ticks and insects in a Lyme disease focus in Connecticut. Yale J Biol Med 57:621, 1984.
5. Asbrink E, Hovmark A: Early and late cutaneous manifestations of *Ixodes*-borne borreliosis (erythema migrans borreliosis, Lyme borreliosis). Ann N Y Acad Sci 539:4, 1988.
6. Asbrink E, Hovmark A: Successful cultivation of spirochetes from skin lesions of patients with erythema chronicum migrans Afzelius and acrodermatitis chronica atrophicans. Acta Pathol Microbiol Immunol Scand 66:161, 1985.
7. Asbrink E, Hovmark A, Hederstedt B: The spirochetal etiology of acrodermatitis chronica atrophicans herxheimer. Acta Derm Venereol 64:506, 1984.
8. Berger BW: Cutaneous manifestations of Lyme borreliosis. Rheum Dis Clin North Am 15:627, 1989.
9. Berger BW: Dermatologic aspects. In Coyle PK (ed): Lyme Disease. St. Louis, Mosby–Year Book, 1993, pp 69-72.
10. Berger BW: Erythema chronicum migrans of Lyme disease. Arch Dermatol 120:1017, 1984.
11. Burgdorfer W: Vector/host relationships of Lyme disease spirochete *Borrelia burgdorferi*. Rheum Dis Clin North Am 15:775, 1989.
12. Burgdorfer W, Barbour AG, Hayes SF, et al: Lyme disease: A tick-borne spirochetosis? Science 216:1317, 1982.
13. Centers for Disease Control and Prevention: Lyme Disease—United States, 1993. MMWR Morb Mortal Wkly Rep 43:564, 1993.
14. Chen J, Field JA, Glickstein L, et al: Association of antibiotic treatment-resistant Lyme arthritis with T-cell responses to dominant epitopes of outer surface protein A of *Borrelia burgdorferi*. Arthritis Rheum 42:1813-1822, 1999.
15. Corpuz M, Hilton E, Lardis P, et al: Problems in the use of serologic tests for the diagnosis of Lyme disease. Arch Intern Med 151:1837, 1991.
16. Costello CM, Steere AC, Pinkerton RE, Feder HM: A prospective study of tick bites in an endemic area of Lyme disease. J Infect Dis 159:136, 1989.
17. Coyle PK: Neurologic complications of Lyme disease. Rheum Dis Clin North Am 19:993, 1993.
18. Craft JE, Fischer DF, Shimamoto GT, Steere AC: Antigens of *Borrelia burgdorferi* recognized during Lyme disease: Appearance of a new immunoglobulin M response and expansion of the immunoglobulin G response late in the illness. J Clin Invest 78:934, 1986.
19. Dattwyler RJ, Volkman DJ, Luft BJ, et al: Seronegative Lyme disease: Dissociation of specific T- and B-lymphocyte responses to *Borrelia burgdorferi*. N Engl J Med 319:1441, 1988.
20. Dattwyler RJ, Halperin JJ, Volkman DJ, et al: Treatment of late Lyme disease: Randomized comparison of ceftriaxone and penicillin. Lancet 2:1191, 1988.
21. DeMartino SJ, Carlyon JA, Fikrig E: Coinfection with *Borrelia burgdorferi* and the agent of human granulocytic ehrlichiosis. N Engl J Med 345:150-151, 2001.
22. Dennis DT: Epidemiology. In Coyle PK (ed): Lyme Disease. St. Louis, Mosby–Year Book, 1993, pp 27-37.
23. Dinerman H, Steere AC: Lyme disease associated with fibromyalgia. Ann Intern Med 117:281, 1992.
24. Dressler F, Yoshinari NH, Steere AC: The T-cell proliferative assay in the diagnosis of Lyme disease. Ann Intern Med 115:533, 1991.
25. Duray PH: Histopathology of human borreliosis. In Coyle PK (ed): Lyme Disease. St. Louis, Mosby–Year Book, 1993, pp 49-58.
26. Duray PH: The surgical pathology of human Lyme disease: An enlarging picture. Am J Surg Pathol 11:47, 1987.
27. Fish D: Environmental risk and presentation of Lyme disease. Am J Med 98 (suppl 4A):2S, 1995.
28. Fishbein DB, Dawson JE, Robinson LE: Human ehrlichiosis in the United States, 1985-1990. Ann Intern Med 120:736-743, 1994.
29. Garcia-Monco JC, Benach JL: The pathogenesis of Lyme disease. Rheum Dis Clin North Am 15:711, 1989.
30. Goodman JL, Bradley JF, Ross AE, et al: Bloodstream invasion in early Lyme disease: Results from a prospective, controlled, blinded study using the polymerase chain reaction. Am J Med 99:6, 1995.
31. Gorenflot A, Moubri K, Precigout E, et al: Human babesiosis. Ann Trop Med Parasitol 92:489-501, 1998.
32. Guo BP, Brown EL, Dorward DW, et al: Decorin-binding adhesions from *Borrelia burgdorferi*. Mol Microbiol 30:1003-1015, 1998.
33. Halperin JJ, Volkman DJ, Luft BJ, et al: CTS in Lyme borreliosis. Muscle Nerve 12:397, 1989.
34. Hirschfeld M, Kirschning CJ, Schwander R, et al: Inflammatory signaling by *Borrelia burgdorferi* lipoproteins is mediated by toll-like receptor 2. J Immunol 163:2382-2386, 1999.
35. Johnson RC, Kodner C, Russell M: In vitro and in vivo susceptibility of the Lyme disease spirochete *Borrelia burgdorferi* to four antimicrobial agents. Antimicrob Agents Chemother 31:164, 1987.
36. Johnston YE, Duray PH, Steere AC, et al: Lyme arthritis: Spirochetes found in synovial microangiopathic lesions. Am J Pathol 118:26, 1985.
37. Kaell AT, Bennett RS, Hamburger MI: Rheumatic manifestations. In Coyle PK (ed): Lyme Disease. St. Louis: Mosby–Year Book, 1993, pp 73-85.
38. Kalish RA, Kaplan RF, Taylor E, et al: Evaluation of study patients with Lyme disease, 10-20-year follow-up. J Infect Dis 183:453-460, 2001.
39. Klempner MS, Linden TH, Evans J, et al: Two controlled trials of antibiotic treatment in patients with persistent symptoms and a history of Lyme disease. N Engl J Med 345:85-92, 2001.
40. Kolstoe J, Messner RP: Lyme disease: Musculoskeletal manifestations. Rheum Dis Clin North Am 15:649, 1989.
41. Krause PJ, Telford SR, Spielman A, et al: Concurrent Lyme disease and babesiosis: Evidence for increased severity and duration of illness. JAMA 275:1657-1660, 1996.
42. Kujala GA, Steere AC, Davis JS IV: IgM rheumatoid factor in Lyme disease: Correlation with disease activity, total serum IgM and IgM antibody to *Borrelia burgdorferi*. J Rheumatol 14:772, 1987.
43. Lawson JP, Rahn DW: Lyme disease and radiologic findings in Lyme arthritis. AJR Am J Roentgenol 158:1065, 1992.
44. Lightfoot RW Jr, Luft BJ, Rahn DW, et al: Empiric parenteral antibiotic treatment of patients with fibromyalgia and fatigue and a positive serologic result for Lyme disease: A cost-effective analysis. Ann Intern Med 119:503, 1993.
45. Logigian EL, Kaplan RF, Steere AC: Chronic neurologic manifestations of Lyme disease. N Engl J Med 323:1438, 1990.
46. Logigian EL, Steere AC: Clinical and electrophysiologic findings in chronic neuropathy of Lyme disease. Neurology 42:303, 1992.
47. Ma B, Christen B, Leung D, Vigo-Pelfrey C: Serodiagnosis of Lyme borreliosis by western immunoblot: Reactivity of various significant antibodies against *Borrelia burgdorferi*. J Clin Microbiol 30:370, 1992.
48. Magnarelli LA: Laboratory diagnosis of Lyme disease. Rheum Dis Clin North Am 15:735, 1989.
49. Magnarelli LA, Anderson JF, Barbour AG: The etiologic agent of Lyme disease in deer flies, horse flies and mosquitoes. J Infect Dis 154:355, 1986.
50. McAlister HF, Klementowicz PT, Andrews C, et al: Lyme carditis: An important cause of reversible heart block. Ann Intern Med 110:339, 1989.
51. Muellegger RR, McHugh G, Ruthazer R, et al: Differential expression of cytokine mRNA in skin specimens from patients with erythema migrans or acrodermatitis chronica atrophicans. J Invest Dermatol 115:1115-1123, 2000.

52. Nadelman RB, Nowakowski J, Fish D, et al: Prophylaxis with single-dose doxycycline for the prevention of Lyme disease after an *Ixodes* scapularis tick bite. N Engl J Med 345:79-84, 2001.
53. Nadelman RB, Wormser GP: Erythema migrans and early Lyme disease. Am J Med 98(Suppl 4A):15S, 1995.
54. Nelson JA, Wolf MD, Yah WTC, et al: Cranial nerve involvement with Lyme borreliosis demonstrated by MRI. Neurology 42:671, 1992.
55. Oliver JH Jr, Owsley MR, Hutcheson HJ, et al: Conspecificity of the ticks *Ixodes scapularis* and *I. dammini* (Acari:Ixodidae). J Med Entomol 30:54, 1993.
56. Orloski KA, Hayes EB, Campbell GL, et al: Surveillance for Lyme disease—United States 1992-1998. MMWR Morb Mortal Wkly Rep CDC Surveill Summ 49:1-11, 2000.
57. Oschmann P, Dorndorf W, Hornig C, et al: Stages and syndromes of neuroborreliosis. J Neurol 245:262-272, 1998.
58. Pachner AR: Early disseminated Lyme disease: Lyme meningitis. Am J Med 98(Suppl 4A):30S, 1995.
59. Pachner AR, Delaney E: The polymerase chain reaction (PCR) in the diagnosis of Lyme neuroborreliosis. Ann Neurol 34:544, 1993.
60. Pachner AR, Steere AC: The triad of neurologic manifestations of Lyme disease: Meningitis, cranial neuritis, and radiculoneuritis. Neurology 35:47, 1985.
61. Rahn DW: Lyme disease: Clinical manifestations, diagnosis, and treatment. Semin Arthritis Rheum 20:201, 1991.
62. Rahn DW, Malawista SE: Lyme disease: Recommendations for diagnosis and treatment. Ann Intern Med 114:472, 1991.
63. Reik L, Steere AC, Bartenhagen NH, et al: Neurologic abnormalities of Lyme disease. Medicine 58:281, 1979.
64. Reik L Jr: Lyme Disease and The Nervous System. New York, Thieme, 1991, pp 1-130.
65. Reik L Jr: Neurologic aspects of North American Lyme disease. In Coyle PK (ed): Lyme Disease. St. Louis, Mosby–Year Book, 1993, pp 101-112.
66. Rosa PA, Schwan TG: A specific and sensitive assay for the Lyme disease spirochete *Borrelia burgdorferi* using the polymerase chain reaction. J Infect Dis 160:1018, 1989.
67. Seltzer EG, Gerber MA, Carter ML, et al: Long-term outcomes of persons with Lyme disease. JAMA 283:609-616, 2000.
68. Sigal L: Summary of the first 100 patients seen at a Lyme disease referral center. Am J Med 88:577, 1990.
69. Sigal LH: Current recommendations for the treatment of Lyme disease. Drugs 43:683, 1992.
70. Sigal LH, Zahradnik JM, Lavin P, et al: A vaccine consisting of recombinant *Borrelia burgdorferi* outer surface protein A to prevent Lyme disease. N Engl J Med 339:209-215, 1998.
71. Steere AC: Lyme disease. N Engl J Med 321:586, 1989.
72. Steere AC: Lyme disease. N Engl J Med 345:115-125, 2001.
73. Steere AC: Musculoskeletal manifestations of Lyme disease. Am J Med 98(Suppl 4A):44S, 1995.
74. Steere AC, Bartenhagen NH, Craft JE, et al: The early clinical manifestations of Lyme disease. Ann Intern Med 99:76, 1983.
75. Steere AC, Batsford WP, Weinberg M, et al: Lyme carditis: Cardiac abnormalities of Lyme disease. Ann Intern Med 93:8, 1980.
76. Steere AC, Dhar A, Hernandez J, et al: Systemic symptoms without erythema migrans as the presenting picture of early Lyme disease. 114:58-62, 2003.
77. Steere AC, Dwyer E, Winchester R: Association of chronic arthritis with increased DR4 and DR3. N Engl J Med 323:219, 1990.
78. Steere AC, Green J, Schoen RT, et al: Successful parenteral penicillin therapy for established Lyme arthritis. N Engl J Med 312:869, 1984.
79. Steere AC, Grodzicki RL, Kornblatt AN, et al: The spirochetal etiology of Lyme disease. N Engl J Med 308:733, 1983.
80. Steere AC, Schoen RT, Taylor E: The clinical evolution of Lyme arthritis. Ann Intern Med 197:725, 1987.
81. Strle F, Nadelman RB, Cimperman J, et al: Comparison of culture-confirmed erythema migrans caused by *Borrelia burgforderi* sensu stricto in New York State and by *Borrelia afzelli* in Slovenia. Ann Intern Med 130:32-36, 1999.
82. Trollmo C, Meyer AL, Steere AC, et al: Molecular mimicry in Lyme arthritis demonstrated at the single cell level: LFA-1α is a partial agonist for outer surface protein A-reactive T cells. J Immunol 166:5286-5291, 2001.
83. White DJ, Chang H, Benach JL, et al: The geographic spread and temporal increase of the Lyme disease epidemic. JAMA 266:1230, 1991.
84. Wormser GP, Bittker S, Cooper D, et al: Comparison of the yields of blood cultures using serum or plasma from patients with early Lyme disease. J Clin Microbiol 38:1648-1650, 2000.

CHAPTER 13

TUMORS AND INFILTRATIVE LESIONS OF THE SPINE

Tumors and infiltrative lesions of the spine are unusual causes of spinal pain; however, of all causes, these diseases are associated with the highest morbidity, mortality, and dysfunction. Physicians who evaluate patients with low back or neck pain must be aware of the existence of neoplastic disease of the spine and must include it in their differential diagnosis. Patients with tumors of the spine usually have low back or neck pain as their initial complaint, and not infrequently, a traumatic event is thought to be the inciting cause. Only as the pain persists and increases in intensity does it become clear that the trauma was an incidental event unassociated with the underlying disease process.

A history of pain that increases with recumbency is a hallmark for tumors of the spine. Some lesions of the spinal cord may be painless even though they are associated with abnormal neurologic signs. Lesions in the cervical spine cause more extensive spinal cord lesions that result in myelopathy (quadriparesis, difficult breathing, and spasticity) than do lesions in the lumbar spine. Physical examination demonstrates localized tenderness as well as neurologic dysfunction if the spinal cord is compressed. In many circumstances, laboratory abnormalities are nonspecific, although evaluation of cerebrospinal fluid is helpful in identifying the presence of intradural tumors or myelitis. In contrast, radiographic evaluation is very useful in identifying characteristic changes in the bony and soft tissue areas of the spine that help identify the location and type of neoplastic lesion. In general, benign tumors are located in the posterior elements of vertebrae (spinous, transverse process), whereas malignant (both primary and metastatic) tumors are located in the anterior components of vertebrae (body) (Fig. 13-1). Radiographic techniques include plain roentgenograms and computed tomography (CT) for evaluating bony architecture and myelography and magnetic resonance (MR) imaging for evaluating soft tissue structures. The definitive diagnosis of a tumor, including intraspinal lesions, must be derived from histologic examination of biopsy material obtained from the lesion (tissue diagnosis). The most effective therapy for both benign and malignant tumors is removal of the lesions that are accessible to surgical excision. When excision is not possible, partial resection, radiation therapy, corticosteroids, or chemotherapy may be indicated to control symptoms and compression of the spinal cord and nerve roots. In general, patients with malignant tumors have a poorer prognosis than those with benign neoplasms.

Benign Tumors

OSTEOID OSTEOMA

Capsule Summary

	Low Back	Neck
Frequency of spinal pain	Very common	Very common
Location of spinal pain	Lumbar spine	Cervical spine
Quality of spinal pain	Ache, boring	Dull ache
Symptoms and signs	Pain worst at night, relieved with aspirin; nonstructural scoliosis	Pain worst at night, relieved with aspirin; nonstructural scoliosis
Laboratory tests	None	None
Radiographic findings	CT, bone scan	CT, bone scan
Treatment	NSAIDs are palliative; en bloc excision is curative	NSAIDs are palliative; en bloc excision is curative

PREVALENCE AND PATHOGENESIS

In the past, osteoid osteoma has been referred to as sclerosing osteomyelitis, or an osteoblastic disease, thus highlighting the confusion surrounding its pathogenesis. Osteoid osteoma was first placed in the category of benign osteoblastic tumors by Jaffe in 1935.[23]

Epidemiology

Osteoid osteomas constitute about 2.6% of all excised primary tumors of bone and about 12.1% of all benign tumors.[32,48] Young adults between 20 and 30 years of age have the greatest risk for development of this benign tumor. The ratio of men to women is 2:1.[7] Between 7% and 18% of all osteoid osteomas are located in the spine, with the lumbar area being the most common location in the axial skeleton (lumbar, 40%; thoracic, 30%; cervical, 30%).[7,13] In another series of patients with osteoid osteoma, spine involvement occurred in 27%.[47] In general, the cervical spine is second to the lumbar spine as the most common location for osteoid osteoma in the axial skeleton. Osteoid osteoma may also be located in the sacrum and pelvis in rare circumstances.[4]

Pathogenesis

The pathogenesis of osteoid osteoma is controversial.[13,22] Some investigators believe that osteoid osteoma may be the result of a chronic infection or a reparative process instead of being a neoplasm. Factors characteristic of osteoid osteoma that are unusual for a neoplasm include its limited growth potential (less than 2 cm), a histologic appearance that is independent of the duration of the lesion, a mature osseous envelope surrounding an immature nidus, and marginal sclerosis. Others believe that osteoid osteoma is a benign bone neoplasm with limited growth potential. The absence of inflammatory debris and leukocytes and the presence of a solitary blood supply and new growth of osteoid tissue are proof of the neoplastic nature of osteoid osteomas.[22]

CLINICAL HISTORY

Pain is a characteristic feature of osteoid osteoma. The pain is intermittent and vague initially, but with time it becomes constant and aching with a boring quality. The pain is not relieved by rest or the application of heat. It is frequently exacerbated at night and consequently results in disturbed sleep. The pain of osteoid osteoma is frequently relieved with small doses of aspirin or other nonsteroidal drugs. The mechanism of analgesia in this lesion by nonsteroidals has been postulated to be inhibition of osteoma prostaglandin production. The concentration of prostaglandins is greatest at night because of decreased blood flow, thus correlating with increased symptoms.[41] An alternative explanation for production of pain is irritation of nerve fibers situated near the center (nidus) of the osteoid osteoma. These nerve fibers may be irritated by the increased pressure associated with increased blood flow to the area.[43] In any case, whether from stimulation by prostaglandin or expansile pressure from the lesion itself, the nerves found near the neoplasms are the afferent pathways that facilitate the pain associated with this lesion.[11]

It is important to remember that osteoid osteomas, even those that are typical in every other way, do not always respond to aspirin or other nonsteroidal medications.[6] Moreover, some osteoid osteomas are entirely painless.[26]

In the spine, osteoid osteomas are associated with nonstructural scoliosis,[25] and scoliosis may be the initial manifestation of a vertebral osteoid osteoma.[15] The appearance of marked paravertebral muscle spasm and the sudden onset of scoliosis in a young adult require an evaluation for the presence of this lesion. The muscles closest to the nidus of the lesion exhibit the greatest amount of spasm, and a concave curvature is created. The tumor is located on the concave side, at the center of the curvature. The clinical outcome of tumor-associated scoliosis is

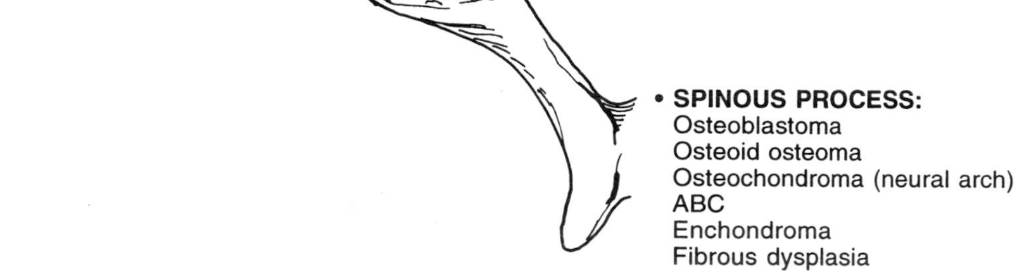

Figure 13-1 Tumors associated with the posterior components (transverse and spinous processes) and the anterior component (body) of vertebrae.

dependent on the patient's age. If an osteoma appears after skeletal maturity, excision of the lesion results in resolution of the scoliotic curve. In adolescents, postural scoliosis progresses to vertebral rotation with structural scoliosis. The lesion will result in permanent scoliosis the longer the tumor is left untreated. A search for an osteoid osteoma should be undertaken in a young patient with painful scoliosis.[18] Scoliosis may occur with osteomas in the vertebral bodies or ribs in the thoracic area.[31]

The pain associated with osteoid osteoma is slowly progressive over months. In some patients, symptoms may be present for years before the correct diagnosis is made. The symptoms of osteoid osteoma may be present for a considerable time before radiographic findings become evident.[44]

In the cervical spine, osteoid osteoma is found almost exclusively in the pedicles and the posterior elements, including the spinous processes.[19] Patients with osteoid osteoma of the cervical spine describe deep, boring pain localized to the area of the bone lesion. Associated muscle spasm may result in torticollis of the neck.[12] Occipital headache is associated with osteoid osteoma localized to the atlas.[9]

PHYSICAL EXAMINATION

The patient may have tenderness with palpation over the affected bone. Marked muscular spasm with associated scoliosis may be noted in patients with an osteoid osteoma of the spine. Approximately 63% of patients with osteoid osteoma or osteoblastoma have scoliosis secondary to asymmetric muscle spasm.[40] The spine may be curved without rotation. Early in the course of the lesion, the scoliosis is reversible. However, with prolonged spasm, muscle atrophy may occur along with structural abnormalities. Gadolinium-enhanced MR imaging of the surrounding muscles reveals derangement and destruction of muscle fibers and replacement with inflammatory cells and fat.[24] These structural changes are more likely to occur in younger individuals who are growing. Hyperemia around the neoplasm can cause localized overgrowth with subsequent vertebral deformity.[34] The hyperemia may cause swelling and erythema of the skin if the osteoid osteoma is in a superficial position in the spine. In rare circumstances, patients may complain of radicular symptoms and may exhibit sensory deficits on neurologic examination.[7]

LABORATORY DATA

Screening laboratory test results are normal in this benign neoplasm of bone.

Pathology

The nidus of an osteoid osteoma is described as a dark red or yellow-white spherical center surrounded by a margin of reactive bone (Fig. 13-2). The nidus is usually less than 1 cm in diameter and may contain more blood vessels and osteoid when red and fewer blood vessels and more woven bone when white. Histologically, the nidus contains areas of osteoid, woven bone trabeculae, and vascular fibrous tissue surrounded by dense lamellar bone (Fig. 13-3). Pathologists consider osteoid osteomas and osteoblastomas to be closely related neoplasms of osteoblastic derivation without specific histologic criteria that allow for differentiation of them. The differences between the lesions are most probably a result of the location of the tumors. Osteomas are in a cortical location and osteoblastomas in a medullary position. The slow growth potential of an osteoid osteoma versus the more actively growing osteoblastoma may be related to the intracortical position of the osteoma. The greater degree of bone sclerosis associated with osteoid osteomas is related to their compact size.[42]

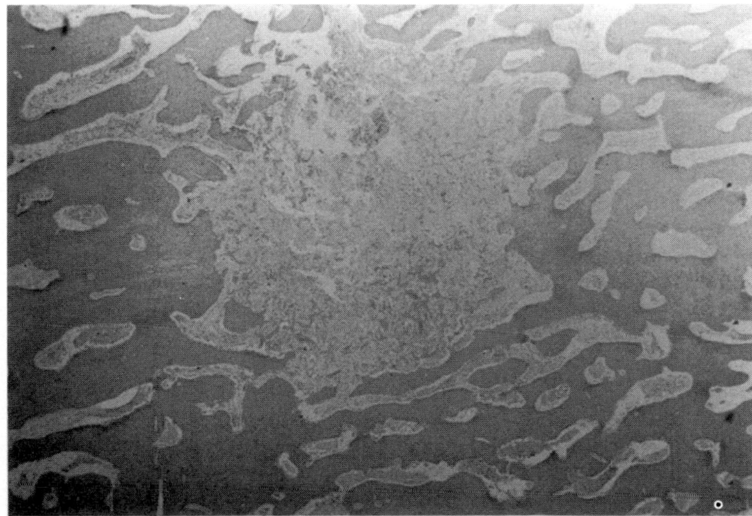

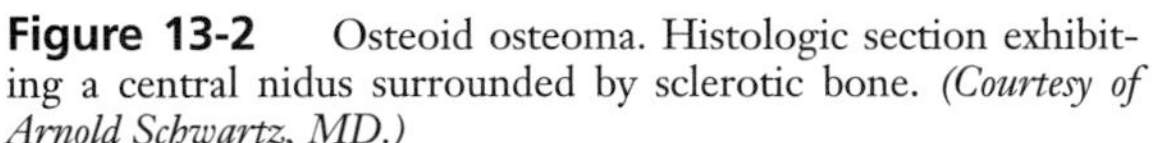

Figure 13-2 Osteoid osteoma. Histologic section exhibiting a central nidus surrounded by sclerotic bone. *(Courtesy of Arnold Schwartz, MD.)*

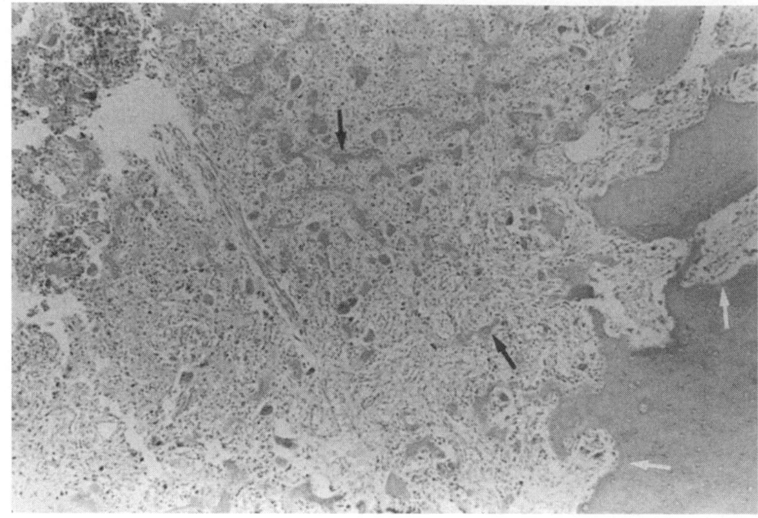

Figure 13-3 Histologic section from the central area of an osteoid osteoma demonstrating new bone formation *(black arrows)* and increased vascularity, as well as a dense sclerotic border *(white arrows)*. The presence of a sclerotic border confirms the slow growth of the tumor and helps differentiate osteoid osteoma from osteoblastoma. *(Courtesy of Arnold Schwartz, MD.)*

RADIOGRAPHIC EVALUATION

Roentgenograms

The finding of a radiolucent nidus, a lesion about 1.5 cm in diameter, and a surrounding well-defined area of dense sclerotic bone is virtually pathognomonic of osteoid osteoma. The amount of sclerosis is out of proportion to the small size of the nidus. Osteoid osteomas arise in the posterior elements of a vertebra (Fig. 13-4). The neural arch is affected in about 75% of vertebrae, the articular facets in about 18%, and the vertebral bodies in only about 7%.[3] The size and location of these lesions make them difficult to detect with plain roentgenograms (Fig. 13-5).

Scintigraphy and Computed Tomography

Bone scans are useful in localizing the lesion if plain roentgenograms are negative.[50] The nidus is demonstrated on radionuclide bone scan as an area of marked concentration of radioactivity.[14] In addition, scintigraphy may be used to monitor for local tumor recurrence.[1] CT is also helpful in localizing the nidus and in detecting encroachment of the neoplasm on the spinal canal or the neural foramen (Fig. 13-6).[49] CT is the most useful for precisely localizing the lesion and differentiating it from other bone lesions.[5] It is the best technique for demonstrating subtle osseous detail, cortical penetration by a tumor, and matrix calcification and mineralization within a tumor (Fig. 13-7).[20] CT is able to determine the specific osseous architecture associated with a bone tumor.[46] In rare circumstances, the intervertebral disc and surrounding bone may be altered if the tumor is located anteriorly in a vertebral body.[21] CT-guided percutaneous biopsy may be performed to remove accessible lesions in the skeleton, including the lumbar spine.[30,37] MR examination adds little in regard to clarifying bone architecture and is not used routinely in the evaluation of this primary bone tumor.[2]

DIFFERENTIAL DIAGNOSIS

The diagnosis of an osteoid osteoma is suggested by characteristic clinical and radiographic features and is confirmed by histologic examination of biopsy material. Despite its characteristic appearance, osteoid osteoma of

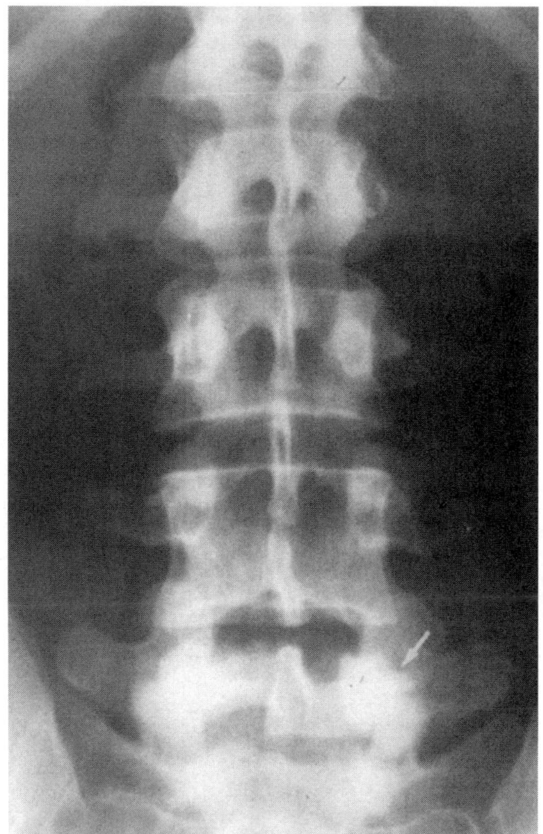

Figure 13-4 Osteoid osteoma. Anteroposterior view of the lumbar spine revealing a sclerotic pedicle of the L5 vertebra *(arrow)*. *(Courtesy of Anne Brower, MD.)*

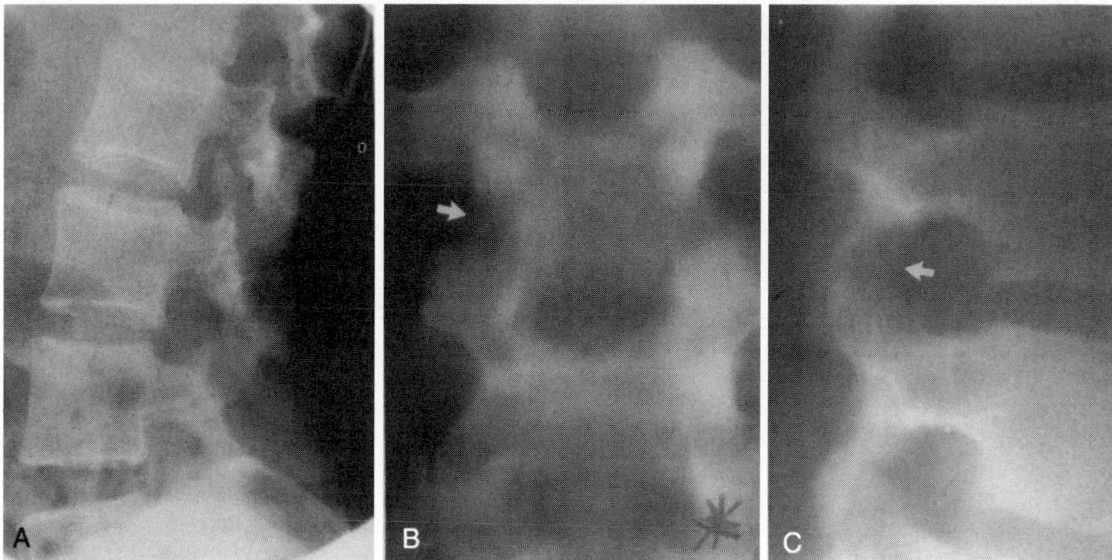

Figure 13-5 Osteoid osteoma involving the lamina of the third lumbar vertebra. *A*, A lateral plain film of the spine is normal. Tomograms in the anteroposterior *(B)* and lateral *(C)* directions reveal a radiolucent nidus *(arrows)* with a central calcific fleck. Minimal reactive bone surrounds the lucent nidus. *(Courtesy of Anne Brower, MD.)*

the spine remains an elusive diagnosis. Lumbosacral strain, psychogenic back pain, Scheuermann's disease, herniated nucleus pulposus, and nonspecific mechanical back pain are frequent previous diagnoses.[25,28] In a large series, seven patients were clinically suspected of having a herniated nucleus pulposus; three had undergone laminectomy.[48] Tomography and scintigraphy are extremely helpful in detecting lesions that are missed with screening roentgenograms. The physician's degree of suspicion should be raised when young adults with nontraumatic back pain have associated paravertebral muscle spasm and a recent onset of scoliosis. Repeat evaluation and close follow-up are necessary in individuals with negative initial evaluations. Abnormal test results may develop over a period of months in such individuals.

Other diagnoses that need to be considered include osteoblastoma, osteosarcoma, osteomyelitis, Brodie's abscess, Ewing's sarcoma, eosinophilic granuloma, metastases, fracture, aseptic necrosis, osteochondritis, and aneurysmal bone cyst. Abnormal laboratory test results (elevated white blood cell count, erythrocyte sedimentation rate, bone chemistry studies) and characteristic histologic findings help differentiate these inflammatory, infectious, or malignant lesions from osteoid osteoma.

Osteosclerosis is also associated with the presence of bone islands or endosteomas. A bone island is a homogeneous dense area of bone with distinct margins and no central radiolucent area. The absence of a nidus on pathologic section helps differentiate a bone island from an osteoid osteoma.[17] Bone islands are usually incidental roentgenographic findings and are clinically silent. Bone islands in the spine occur more commonly in the vertebral bodies. Rarely, they affect the posterior elements of the vertebrae and may expand over time.

In addition, histologic findings help differentiate the various lesions. For example, osteoblastoma is a larger lesion with less sclerosis. Ewing's sarcoma has no true nidus. Osteosarcoma may have "benign" areas that simulate osteoid osteoma, but careful examination will show areas of woven bone and osteoid of the malignant tumor infiltrating host lamellar bone. Osteoid osteoma may contain some atypical cells but does not infiltrate surrounding bone. Infiltration of any significant distance thus eliminates osteoid osteoma as a diagnostic consideration. The radiographic appearance of these lesions also helps differentiate them.

TREATMENT

Treatment of this benign lesion is simple excision of the nidus and surrounding sclerotic bone. Removal of the tumor results in relief of pain in most patients.[36] If the nidus is not entirely removed, recurrence of the lesion is possible.[16] The pathologist should carefully examine the excisional biopsy to ensure that the nidus has been fully removed.[15] Intraoperative bone scintiscans have been used to document total removal of the nidus at the time of surgery.[27] Preoperative placement of a needle into the nidus under CT guidance is another method to identify the area of bone that must be surgically ablated.[29] Ablation of osteoid osteomas has been successful in accessible lesions with the use of a percutaneously placed electrode that heats the tip to 90° C for 4 minutes.[39] When correctly performed, thermocoagulation is capable of resolving the clinical symptoms associated with the tumor.[8] Total removal of the osteoma with surgical or percutaneous techniques may be a particular problem in poorly accessible areas of the spine. If the entire lesion is not removed, unroofing a cortical lesion with removal of some surrounding sclerotic bone may relieve the symptoms.[33] However, symptoms may persist when the nidus is not entirely removed, and even total removal of an osteoma does not guarantee prevention of recurrence of the tumor. Osteoid osteomas have recurred in the same location after an asymptomatic interval of 10 years.[38] Medical therapy may alleviate the symptoms, but never to the same degree as achieved by surgical removal of the neoplasm. Some patients may use nonsteroidal anti-inflammatory drugs to control tumor pain. However, unless the lesion spontaneously recedes, these patients do not obtain complete relief of symptoms without surgical ablation. It should also be noted that occasionally, osteoid osteomas undergo spontaneous healing.[45] Removal of the tumor is able to correct preoperative spinal deformities in the vast majority of patients with osteoid osteoma.[35]

PROGNOSIS

The course of osteoid osteoma is benign once the diagnosis is made and the lesion is excised. It may be a difficult diagnostic problem, however, because clinical symptoms

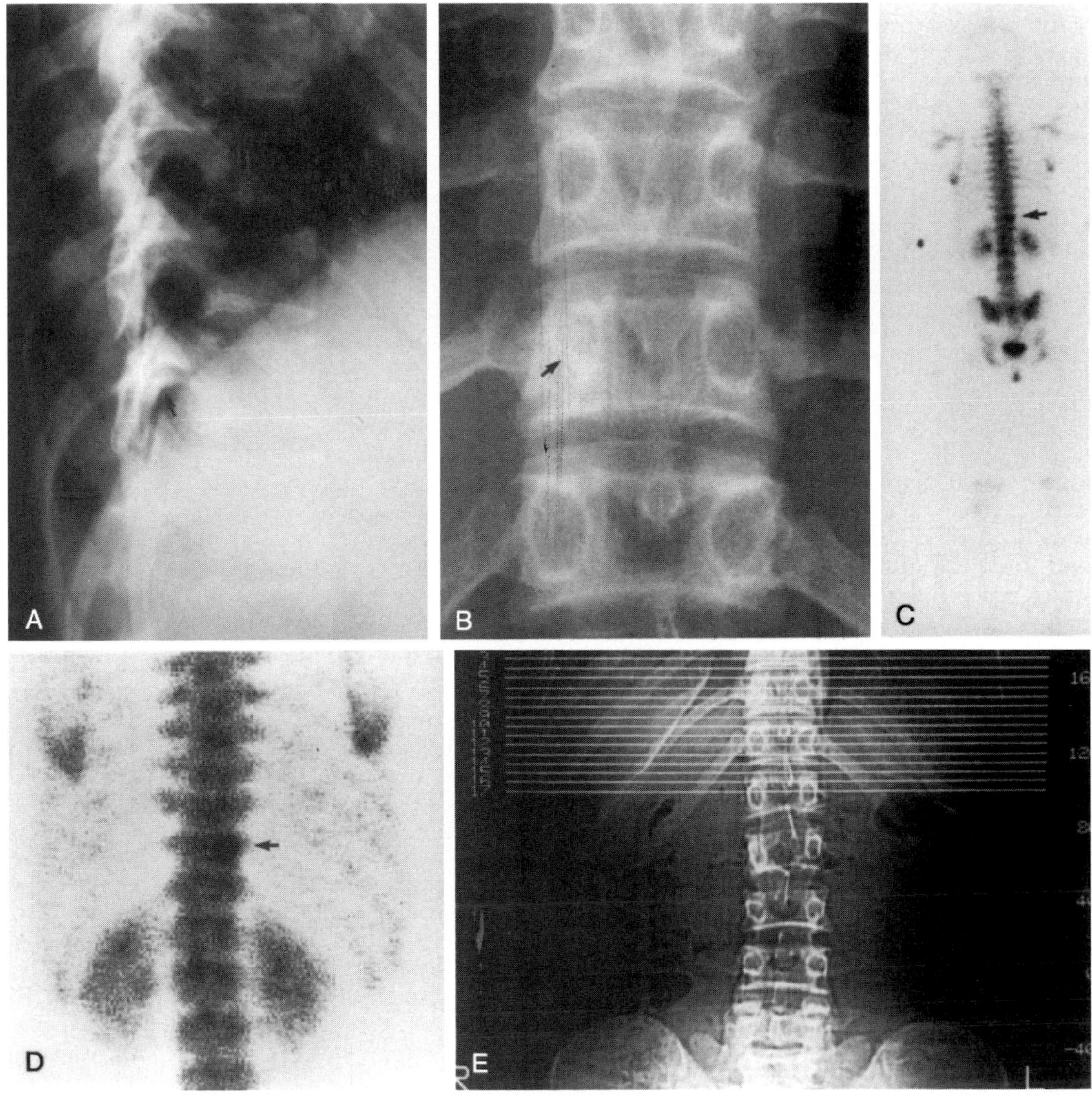

Figure 13-6 A 21-year-old woman gave a history of localized back pain of 1 year's duration over the thoracolumbar junction. The pain was increased at night and was responsive to salicylate therapy. *A,* A lateral view of the thoracolumbar junction reveals increased sclerosis in the pedicle of the T11 vertebra *(arrow). B,* Spot view of the lower thoracic vertebrae revealing an irregular border of the right pedicle *(arrow). C* and *D,* ^{99m}Tc methylene diphosphonate (MDP) bone scan. *C,* A posterior view shows increased traces of accumulation in T11 *(arrow). D,* A spot view detects increased uptake in the lateral compartment of T11 *(arrows). E* to *H,* CT scan of the thoracolumbar junction.

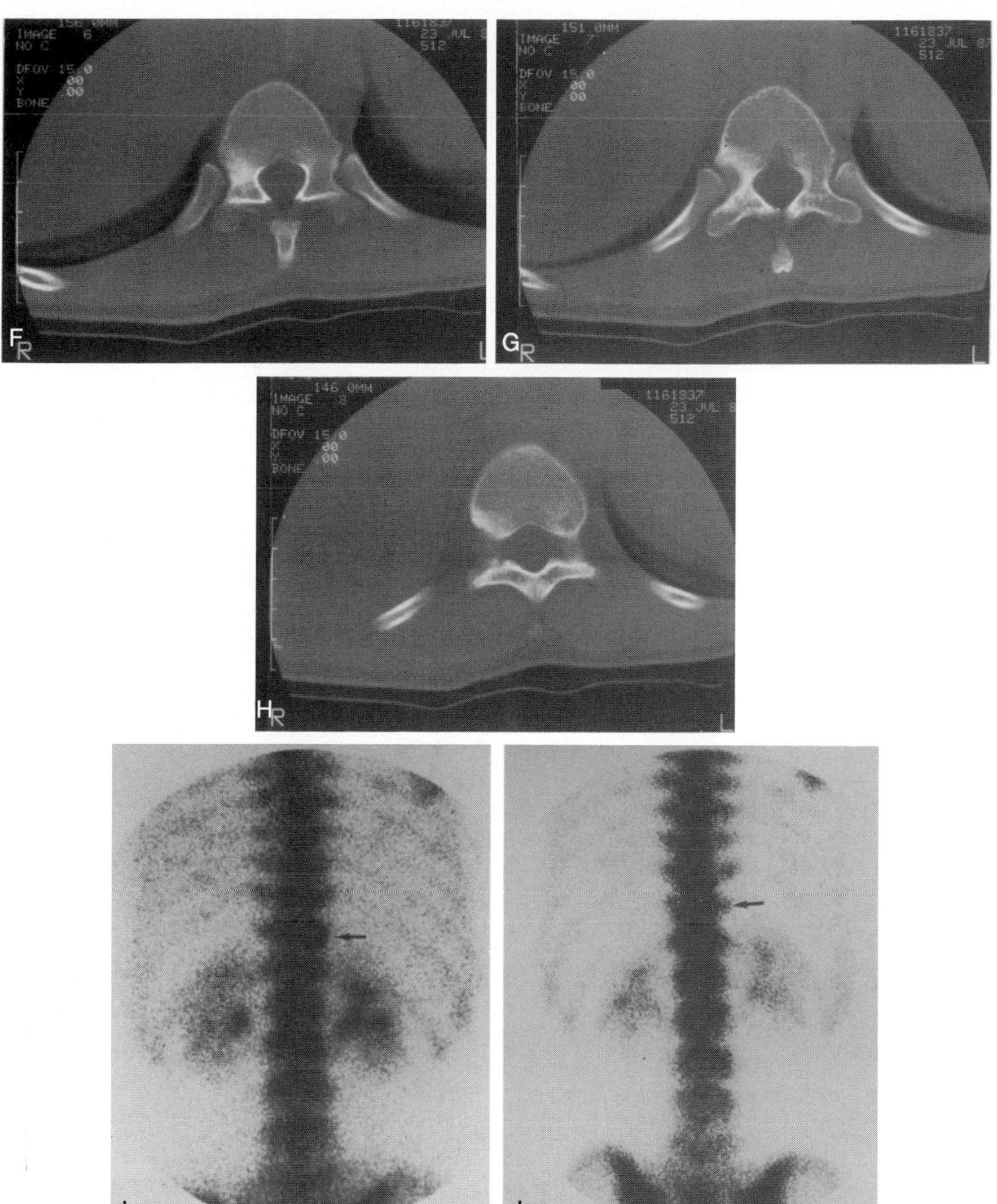

Figure 13-6, cont'd An anteroposterior view *(E)* and views of levels 6 *(F)*, 7 *(G)*, and 8 *(H)* through T11 demonstrate reactive sclerosis around an area of central clearing without soft tissue extension. The diagnosis of osteoid osteoma was made, and the patient's pain responded to diflunisal. The patient was monitored and was asymptomatic 12 months later while taking the nonsteroidal drug. She would have a biopsy of the lesion performed if it increased in size. The patient remained symptomatic when the medicines were discontinued for short periods during the following 4 years. *I*, A ^{99m}Tc MDP bone scan completed 1 year before surgery reveals persistent accumulation of tracer in T11 *(arrow)*. *J*, A repeat bone scan reveals absence of increased uptake *(arrow)* 1 day after surgical removal of the osteoid osteoma confirmed on pathologic examination.

may appear before it is radiographically evident. Low back pain and associated limitation of activities at work may be inappropriately ascribed to malingering or psychoneurosis. In a young adult with low back pain that is exacerbated at night and relieved with aspirin, a thorough evaluation for the presence of this lesion is mandatory. Osteoid osteoma is a benign lesion without reported malignant transformation. Despite its benignity, osteoid osteoma should not be considered an innocuous lesion. Osteoid osteomas have been known to recur even after removal.[10] Persistent evaluation and appropriate surgery are necessary to prevent potential physical deformities and psychic stress in patients with this elusive neoplasm.

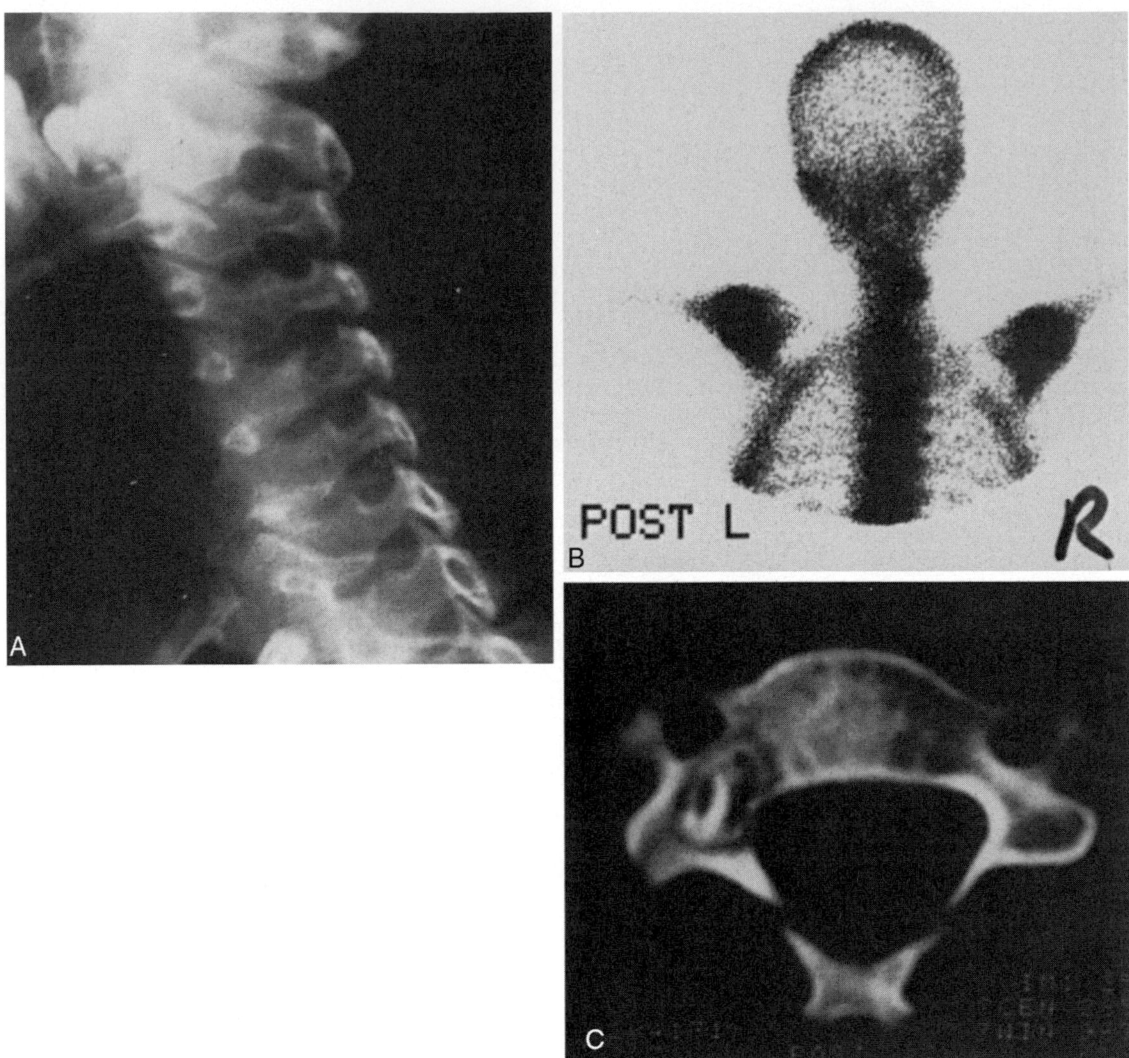

Figure 13-7 Osteoid osteoma. A 9-year-old girl had a 6-week history of progressively intractable and incapacitating right-sided neck and shoulder pain. Her general physical and neurologic examinations were normal except for neck stiffness, limitation of motion, and right paravertebral cervical tenderness. *A*, Oblique conventional radiograph. The lesion is visible as a well-developed lytic area of the pedicle of C5. *B*, Radioisotopic bone scan. *C*, A CT scan of the fifth cervical vertebra shows increased uptake at C4. Note the lytic lesion of the right pedicle with a classic central radiodensity on the CT scan. *(From Sypert GW: Osteoid osteoma and osteoblastoma of the spine. In Sundaresan N, Schmidek HH, Schiller AL, Rosenthal DI [eds]: Tumors of the Spine: Diagnosis and Clinical Management. Philadelphia, WB Saunders, 1990, p 119.)*

References

Osteoid Osteoma

1. Adams BK: Scintigraphy in benign bone tumours: A report of 4 cases. S Afr Med J 76:112, 1989.
2. Assoun J, Haldat FD, Richard G, et al: Magnetic resonance imaging in osteoid osteoma. Rev Rhum Engl Ed 60:29, 1993.
3. Banna M: Clinical Radiology of the Spine and the Spinal Cord. Rockville, MD, Aspen, 1985 pp 337-338.
4. Bettelli G, Capanna R, Van Horn Jr, et al: Osteoid osteoma and osteoblastoma of the pelvis. Clin Orthop 247:261, 1989.
5. Bilchik T, Heyman S, Siegel A, Alavi A: Osteoid osteoma: The role of radionuclide bone imaging, conventional radiography and computed tomography in its management. J Nucl Med 33:269, 1992.
6. Byers PD: Solitary benign osteoblastic lesions of bone: Osteoid osteoma and benign osteoblastoma. Cancer 22:43, 1968.
7. Cohen MD, Harrington TM, Ginsburg WW: Osteoid osteoma: 95 cases and a review of the literature. Semin Arthritis Rheum 12:265, 1983.
8. Cove JA, Taminiau AH, Obermann WR, et al: Osteoid osteoma of the spine treated with percutaneous computed tomography–guided thermocoagulation. Spine 25:1283-1286, 2000.
9. De Praeter MP, Dua GF, Seynaeve PC, et al: Occipital pain in osteoid osteoma of the atlas. A report of two cases. Spine 24:912-914, 1999.
10. Dunlop JAY, Morton KS, Elliot GB: Recurrent osteoid osteoma. Report of a case with review of the literature. J Bone Joint Surg Br 52-B:128, 1980.
11. Esquerdo J, Fernandez CF, Gomar F: Pain in osteoid osteoma. Histological facts. Acta Orthop Scand 47:520, 1976.
12. Fielding JW, Keim HA, Hawkins RJ, Kiem HA: Osteoid osteoma of the cervical spine. Clin Orthop 128:163, 1977.
13. Freiberger RH: Osteoid osteoma of the spine: A cause of backache and scoliosis in children and young adults. Radiology 75:232, 1960.
14. Ghelman B: Radiology of bone tumors. Orthop Clin North Am 20:287, 1989.
15. Gitelis S, Schajowicz F: Osteoid osteoma and osteoblastoma. Orthop Clin North Am 20:313, 1989.
16. Golding JSR: The natural history of osteoid osteoma with a report of 20 cases. J Bone Joint Surg Br 36-B:218, 1954.

17. Gower DJ, Tytle T, Brumback R: Enlarging endostoma (bone island) of the spinous process. Neurosurgery 30:608, 1992.
18. Haibach H, Farrell C, Gaines RW: Osteoid osteoma of the spine: Surgically correctable cause of painful scoliosis. Can Med Assoc J 135:895, 1986.
19. Hastings DE, Macnab I, Lawson V: Neoplasms of the atlas and axis. Can J Surg 11:290, 1968.
20. Heare TC, Enneking WF, Heare MM: Staging techniques and biopsy of bone tumors. Orthop Clin North Am 20:273, 1989.
21. Heiman ML, Cooley CJ, Bradford DS: Osteoid osteoma of a vertebral body: Report of a case with extension across the intervertebral disc. Clin Orthop 118:159, 1976.
22. Huvos AG: Bone Tumors: Diagnosis, Treatment, and Prognosis, 2nd ed. Philadelphia, WB Saunders, 1991, pp 49-66.
23. Jaffe JL: Osteoid osteoma: A benign osteoblastic tumor composed of osteoid and atypical bone. Arch Surg 31:709, 1935.
24. Kawahara C, Tanaka Y, Kato H, et al: Myolysis of the erector spinae muscles as the cause of scoliosis in osteoid osteoma of the spine. Spine 27:E313-E315, 2002.
25. Keim HA, Reina EG: Osteoid osteoma as a cause of scoliosis. J Bone Joint Surg Am 57-A:159-163, 1975.
26. Lawrie TR, Aterman K, Sinclair AM: Painless osteoid osteoma. J Bone Joint Surg Am 52-A:1357-1363, 1970.
27. Lee DH, Malawer MM: Staging and treatment of primary and persistent (recurrent) osteoid osteoma. Clin Orthop 281:231, 1992.
28. MacLellan DF, Wilson FC Jr: Osteoid osteoma of the spine. J. Bone Joint Surg 49:111, 1967.
29. Marcove RC, Heelan RT, Huvos AG, et al: Osteoid osteoma: Diagnosis, localization, and treatment. Clin Orthop 267:197, 1991.
30. Mazoyer J, Kohler R, Bossard D: Osteoid osteoma: CT-guided percutaneous treatment. Radiology 181:269, 1991.
31. Mehdian H, Summers B, Eisenstein S: Painful scoliosis secondary to an osteoid osteoma of the rib. Clin Orthop 230:273, 1988.
32. Mirra JM: Bone Tumors: Clinical, Radiologic, and Pathologic Correlations. Philadelphia, Lea & Febiger, 1989, pp 226-248.
33. Morrison GM, Hawes LE, Sacco JJ: Incomplete removal of osteoid osteoma. J Bone Joint Surg 33:166, 1951.
34. Norman A, Dorfman hd: Osteoid osteoma inducing pronounced overgrowth and deformity of bone. Clin Orthop 110:233, 1975.
35. Osaki T, Liljenqvist U, Hillmann A, et al: Osteoid osteoma and osteoblastoma of the spine: Experience with 22 patients. Clin Orthop 397:394-402, 2002.
36. Peyser AB, Makley JT, Callewart CC, et al: Osteoma of the long bones and the spine. A study of eleven patients and a review of the literature. J Bone Joint Surg Am 78-A:1172-1180, 1996
37. Poey C, Clement JL, Baunin C, et al: Percutaneous extraction of osteoid osteoma of the lumbar spine under CT guidance. J Comput Assist Tomogr 15:1056, 1991.
38. Regan MW, Galey JP, Oakeshott RD: Recurrent osteoid osteoma: Case report with a ten-year asymptomatic interval. Clin Orthop 253:221, 1990.
39. Rosenthal DI, Alexander A, Rosenberg AE, Springfield D: Ablation of osteoid osteomas with a percutaneously placed electrode: A new procedure. Radiology 183:29, 1992.
40. Saifuddin A, White J, Sherazi Z, et al: Osteoid osteoma and osteoblastoma of the spine. Factors associated with the presence of scoliosis. Spine 23:47-53, 1998.
41. Saville DP: A medical option for the treatment of osteoid osteoma. Arthritis Rheum 23:1409, 1981.
42. Schajowicz F, McGuire MH: Diagnostic difficulties in skeletal pathology. Clin Orthop 240:281, 1989.
43. Sherman MS, McFarland G: Mechanism of pain in osteoid osteomas. South Med J 58:163, 1965.
44. Silberman WW: Osteoid osteoma. J Int Coll Surgeons 38:53, 1962.
45. Sim FH, Dahlin DC, Beabout JW: Osteoid osteoma. Diagnostic problems. J Bone Joint Surg Am 57-A:154, 1975.
46. Suttner NJ, Chandy KJ, Kellerman AJ: Osteoid osteomas of the body of the cervical spine. Case report and review of the literature. Br J Neurosurg 16:69-71, 2002.
47. Sypert GW: Osteoid osteoma and osteoblastoma of the spine. In Sundaresan N, Schidek HH, Schiller AL, Roseanthal DI (eds): Tumors of the Spine: Diagnosis and Clinical Management. Philadelphia, WB Saunders, 1990, pp 117-127.
48. Unni KK: Dahlin's Bone Tumors. General Aspects and Data on 11,087 Cases, 5th ed. Philadelphia, Lippincott-Raven, 1996, pp 121-130.
49. Wedge HJ, Tchang S, MacFadyen DJ: Computed tomography in localization of spinal osteoid osteoma. Spine 6:423, 1981.
50. Winter PF, Johnson PM, Hilal SK, Feldman F: Scintigraphic detection of osteoid osteoma. Radiology, 122:177, 1977.

OSTEOBLASTOMA

CAPSULE SUMMARY

	LOW BACK	NECK
Frequency of spinal pain	Very common	Very common
Location of spinal pain	Lumbar spine	Cervical spine
Quality of spinal pain	Dull ache	Dull ache
Symptoms and signs	Localized tenderness and pain	Localized tenderness and pain
Laboratory tests	None	None
Radiographic findings	Expansive lesion of the posterior elements on plain roentgenograms	Expansive lesion of the posterior elements on plain roentgenograms
Treatment	En bloc or partial excision	En bloc or partial excision

PREVALENCE AND PATHOGENESIS

In the past, osteoblastoma has been referred to as an osteogenic fibroma, giant osteoid osteoma, spindle cell variant of giant cell tumor, and osteoblastic osteoid tissue–forming tumor. Jaffe and Mayer in 1932 described a "benign" osteoblastic tumor of bone,[18] but it was Lichtenstein in 1956 who designated the lesion a benign osteoblastoma, which is now the accepted terminology.[21]

Epidemiology

Osteoblastoma is a rare benign neoplasm of bone that accounts for about 3% of all benign bone tumors and about 0.5% of all bone tumors examined by biopsy.[27,47] A majority of the lesions appear during the second or third decade of life. Nearly 90% of patients in whom an osteoblastoma is diagnosed are 30 years or younger.[26] The tumor has a predilection for the spine, and approximately

40% of lesions are located in the axial skeleton.[24] The lumbar spine contains 50% of the lesions whereas the cervical spine is the location for 20% to 38% of the lesions.[6,30,44,47] The male-to-female ratio is 2.5 to 1.[30]

Pathogenesis

The pathogenesis of osteoblastoma is unknown.

CLINICAL HISTORY

The major clinical symptom of osteoblastoma is dull, aching, localized pain over the involved bone. The pain is insidious in onset and may have a duration of months to years before diagnosis. As opposed to osteoid osteoma, the pain of an osteoblastoma is less severe, not nocturnal, and not relieved by salicylates. In studies by Nemoto and colleagues, only 27% of patients had pain relief with aspirin therapy.[30] The pain may be aggravated by activity. Scoliosis may be an initial feature. Osteoblastomas located in the lumbar spine may be associated with pain radiating to the legs, and this pain may be accompanied by muscle spasm and limitation of motion. Pain was the initial symptom in 81% of patients, and radicular pain was present in 29% of patients with spinal involvement.[30] Torticollis may be an initial feature in a minority of patients with cervical involvement.[6,30] In general, scoliosis occurs more commonly with thoracic and lumbar lesions.[34] Radicular pain and spinal cord compression are more likely to occur with osteoblastoma than with osteoid osteoma because of its larger size, the erosion of bone cortex, and the formation of soft tissue masses.[37] Osteoblastoma may also invade the spinal canal and completely encircle nerve roots.[6] It may cause abdominal symptoms when located in the sacrum.[45] The duration of pain before diagnosis averages about 14 months.

PHYSICAL EXAMINATION

Physical examination may demonstrate local tenderness on palpation with mild swelling over the spine. Pain may be exacerbated by spine extension.[16] A positive straight leg–raising test is present in about 25% of patients.[21] Osteoblastoma associated with spinal cord compression results in abnormalities on sensory and motor examination of the upper and lower extremities that correspond to the level of the lesion. Reflexes may also be abnormal. Atrophy of surrounding muscles adjacent to the tumor may be seen.

LABORATORY DATA

This benign neoplasm does not have any associated abnormal screening blood test results. Characteristic abnormalities are present on pathologic examination, however. On gross examination, tumors are well circumscribed and composed of hemorrhagic granular tissue with variable calcification. The tumors range in size from 2 to 10 cm in length.

Pathology

Histologically, an osteoblastoma may demonstrate cellular osteoblastic tissue with a large amount of osteoid material and an absence of chondrocytes and cartilage (Fig. 13-8). Multinucleated giant cells may be present. Mitotic figures may be seen, but atypical ones are not.[16] The tumor appears loosely arranged because of the large number of capillaries between the trabeculae of bone. The vascular character of the tumor has features similar to those seen with aneurysmal bone cyst. The borders of the tumor are well demarcated and do not permeate the surrounding normal bone.

Difficulties exist in the differentiation of benign and aggressive premalignant forms of osteoblastoma.[15] Flow

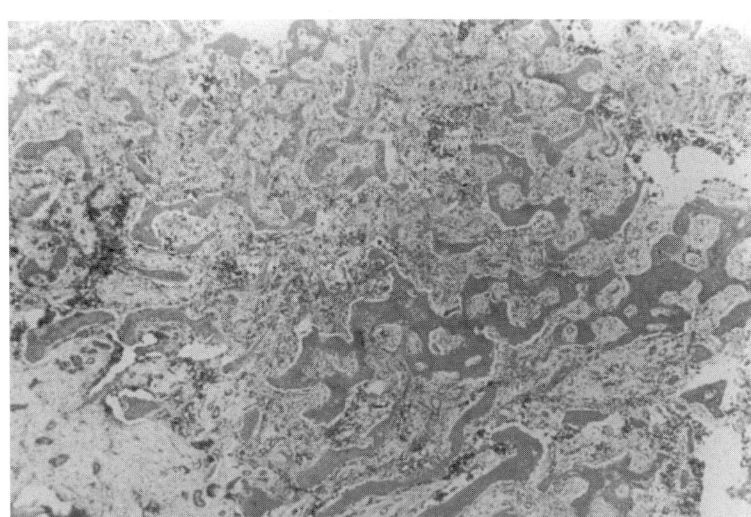

Figure 13-8 Osteoblastoma. Histologic section exhibiting a benign stroma, osteoblasts, and osteoclasts. The new osteoid matrix has a woven bone appearance. *(Courtesy of Arnold Schwartz, MD.)*

cytometry may become more useful as a means of quantifying neoplastic cells harvested from the tumor. Additional studies will be needed to correlate the aneuploidy of cells and the biologic behavior of the tumor.[36]

RADIOGRAPHIC EVALUATION

Roentgenograms

Roentgenographic findings of osteoblastoma are variable and nonspecific. In the spine, lesions are most commonly located in the posterior elements of the vertebrae, including the pedicles, laminae, and transverse and spinous processes (Fig. 13-9).[10] The vertebral body is rarely primarily involved (Fig 13-10).[1] Osteoblastoma is located in the sacrum or lumbar spine in 40% of lesions, in the cervical spine in 36%, and in the thoracic spine in 24%. In a study of 98 patients, 32 had spinal involvement.[20] The distribution of lesions was 10 (31%) in the lumbar spine, 11 (34%) in the thoracic spine, 10 (31%) in the cervical spine, and 1 (3%) in the sacrum.[20] The lumbar spine was the site of an osteoblastoma in 53% of 65 patients with this bone tumor.[20] The cervical spine was the site of osteoblastoma in 31% of 32 patients reported with this tumor in the axial skeleton.[6] Osteoblastoma has been reported to affect the atlas.[13] It also involves the axis on rare occasion.[29] Osteoblastomas are expansile and may grow rapidly as measured by serial radiographic studies. Characteristically, the lesion is well delineated and is covered by a thin layer of periosteal new bone. The extent of reactive new bone formation is much less than that associated with osteoid osteoma (Fig. 13-11).[33] The center of the lesion may be radiolucent or radiopaque. Scoliosis may be noted in association with the tumor, but the size of the tumor does not correlate with the degree of scoliosis.

Scintigraphy

Bone scintigraphy may identify the location of an osteoblastoma even in the absence of abnormalities on plain roentgenograms.[23] A bone scan is helpful in localizing the lesion, but the finding of localized high uptake is nonspecific.

Computed Tomography

CT may provide better localization of the tumor, particularly when the lesion is obscured on plain roentgenograms.[46] CT helps determine the extent of the lesion and the degree of tumor matrix mineralization.[30] The relationship of the tumor to the spinal cord is better visualized in all circumstances with CT.[20] Angiography of the lesion does not help in making a specific diagnosis, but it highlights the vascular nature of the tumor.[3]

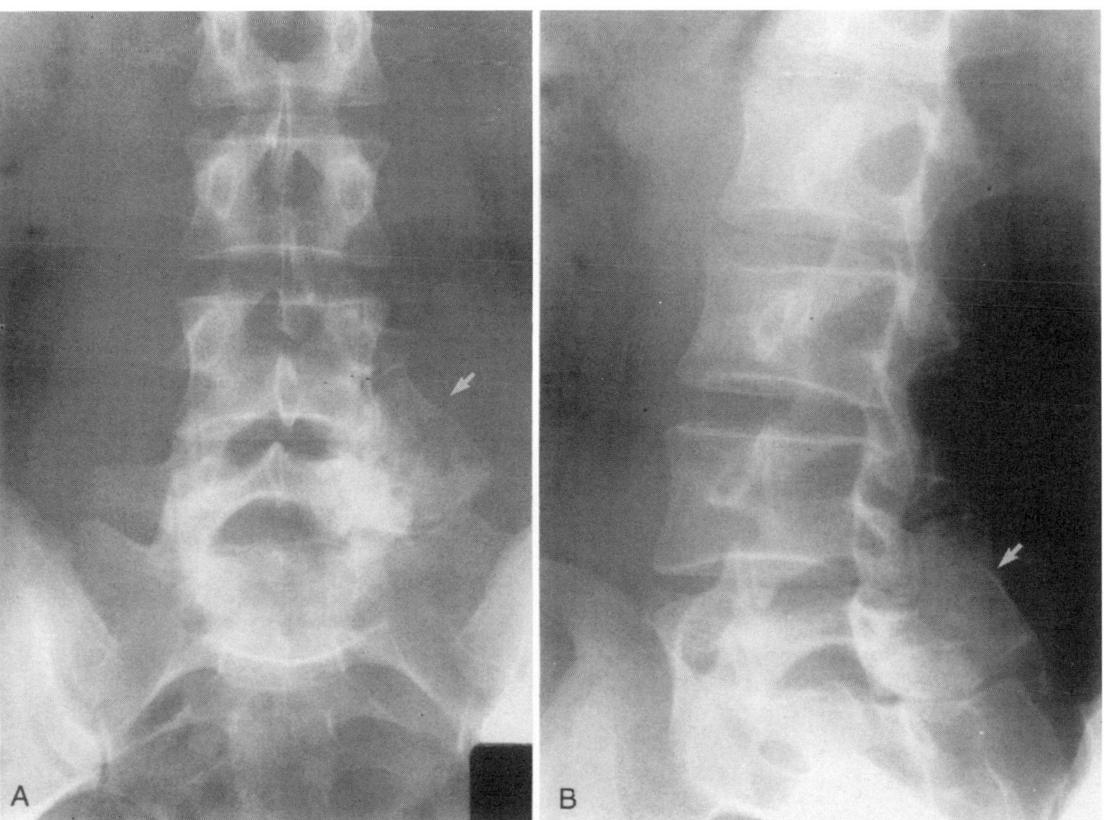

Figure 13-9 Osteoblastoma of the posterior elements of the fifth lumbar vertebra. The lesion is large and expansile, with well-circumscribed margins and homogeneous ossification *(arrows)* on anteroposterior *(A)* and oblique *(B)* views. *(Courtesy of Anne Brower, MD.)*

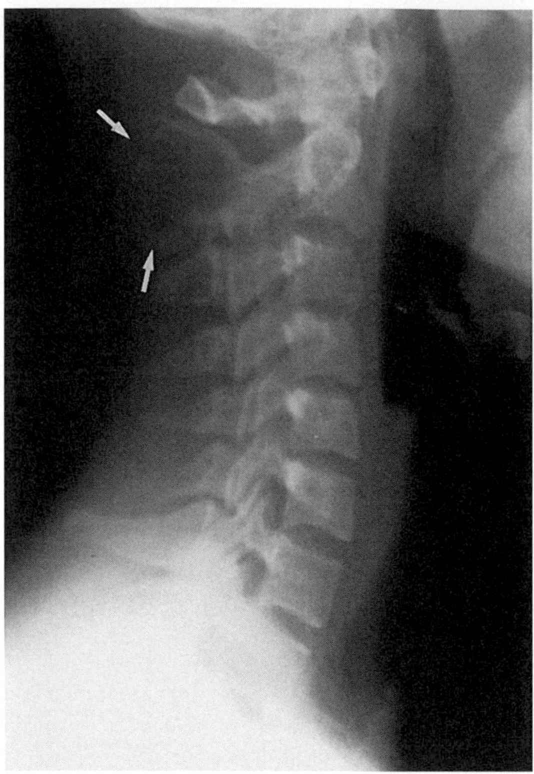

Figure 13-10 Osteoblastoma. A painless neck mass developed in a 14-year-old girl. A lateral view of the cervical spine reveals a large expansile lesion with well-circumscribed margins growing from the spinous process of C2 *(arrows)*. *(Courtesy of Anne Brower, MD.)*

Magnetic Resonance

MR is better than CT in demonstrating the extent of bone sclerosis and in differentiating the tumor from adjacent structures and marrow.[43] The increased signal intensity in soft tissues surrounding the tumor is secondary to edema.[20] On occasion, low signal intensity is noted in a wide area beyond the osteoblastoma.[31] Gadolinium contrast is occasionally needed to reveal focal enhancement not noted with other radiographic techniques.[32] This pattern may be confused with a malignant process. A marked inflammatory response to the tumor results in this MR appearance. The extent of the process may be overestimated by MR, and as a result, biopsy samples may be taken from outside the tumor. This possibility is grounds for the use of CT as the modality of choice to determine the appropriate site for biopsy of a bone tumor.[9] Biopsy of lesions in the cervical spine may be performed with CT guidance in a safe manner without the need for surgery.[2]

DIFFERENTIAL DIAGNOSIS

The diagnosis of osteoblastoma is made by thorough examination of biopsy samples. Osteogenic sarcoma, at initial evaluation, may be easily confused clinically, radiographically, and histologically with osteoblastoma. The presence of an outer rim of bone on radiographic examination and the absence of cartilage and anaplastic cells on biopsy help differentiate osteoblastoma from a malignant process.

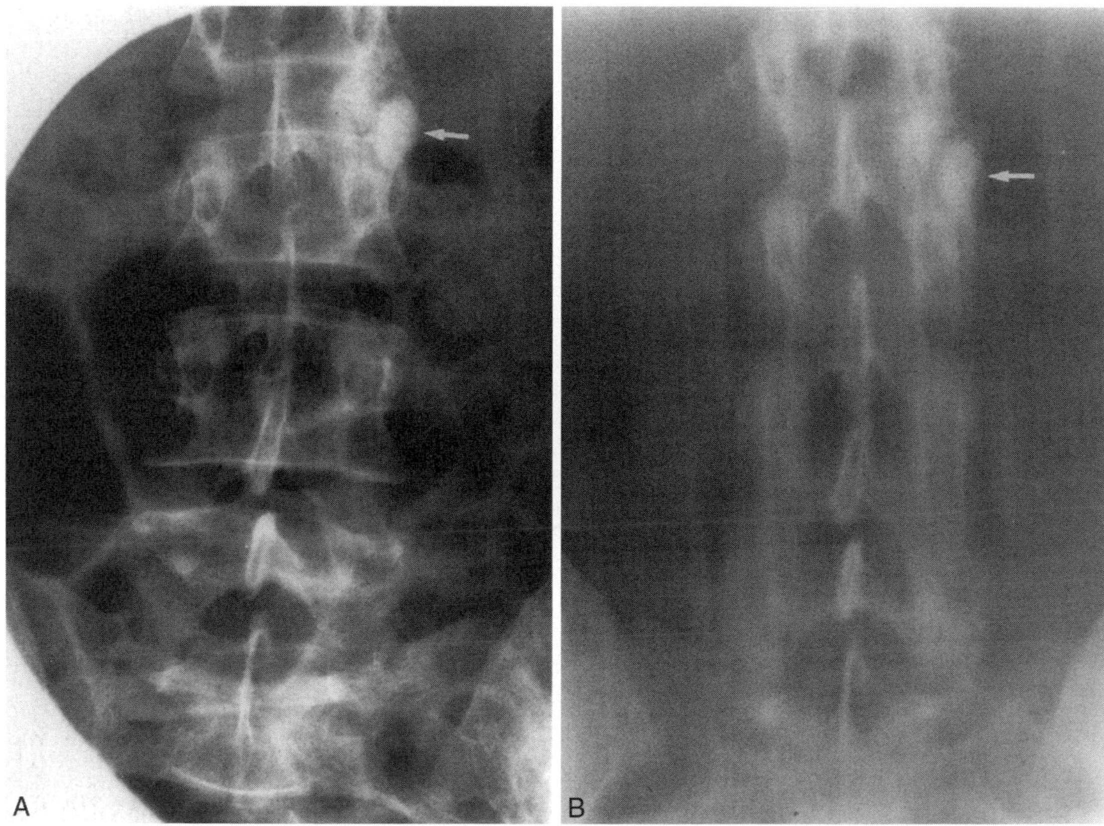

Figure 13-11 Anteroposterior *(A)* and tomographic *(B)* views of the lumbar spine reveal an oval blastic lesion of the posterior elements of L2 *(arrows)*. The size, location, and configuration are consistent with an osteoblastoma. *(Courtesy of Anne Brower, MD.)*

Osteosarcoma

Osteosarcoma is the most common primary bone tumor, and it accounts for 20% to 35% of cases.[11,42] Approximately 1500 new cases are diagnosed each year in the United States. The second decade of life is associated with the peak incidence of this tumor. The other group of individuals at risk for osteosarcoma is those older than 50 years.[14] Osteosarcoma may occur as a complication of other pathologic conditions. Common predisposing factors for secondary osteosarcoma are Paget's disease or bony infarcts secondary to radiation exposure.[7] Osteosarcoma is classified as intramedullary, juxtacortical, and extraosseous.

The spine is an unusual location for the development of osteosarcoma. The incidence of tumors arising in the spine ranges between 0.85% and 3%.[42] Approximately 50% of these tumors are secondary to other conditions, but primary osteosarcomas involving the cervical spine have been reported.[12,25,28] In the spine, 14% of patients with osteosarcoma have cervical spine involvement.[28] However, in other studies of adults with osteosarcoma, the spine is spared.[40] Localized pain and neurologic symptoms develop in most patients. The proximity of the tumor to the spinal cord and nerve roots results in an early onset of symptoms, even with small tumors. The interval between the onset of symptoms and confirmation of the diagnosis is, on average, 6 months.[39,41]

In the spine, plain roentgenograms reveal a mixed osteolytic and sclerotic bone lesion. The vertebral body is most frequently involved, with 10% or less of lesions affecting the posterior elements. CT demonstrates the extent of expansion of the tumor into soft tissues. MR has the advantage of detecting extension of tumor into the spinal canal (Fig. 13-12). Nonmineralized tumor has low signal intensity on T1-weighted images and increased signal intensity on T2-weighted images. Mineralized tumors appear dark on all sequences.

The diagnosis of osteosarcoma is confirmed by histologic evaluation of a biopsy specimen. Mirra has suggested five histologic aids that help differentiate osteoblastoma from osteosarcoma[27]:

1. Osteoblastomas do not produce cartilage.
2. Osteoblastomas produce thick trabeculae of osteoid with prominent capillaries and osteoclasts, whereas osteosarcoma produces extensive areas of poorly calcified bone with a paucity of prominent vessels.
3. The osteoid and woven bone of osteoblastoma are sharply delineated from surrounding lamellar bone. Osteosarcoma infiltrates surrounding bone, which has implications for biopsy because it is best for the surgeon to obtain an intact wedge of bone that includes a margin of normal bone to allow for examination of the lesion–host bone relationship.
4. Osteoblastomas are rimmed by osteoblasts.
5. Osteoblastomas do not have areas that contain cells with bizarre nuclei, abnormal chromatin distribution, abnormal nucleoli, or atypical mitoses.

Treatment of osteosarcoma is directed at resection of the involved vertebral body. Subsequent treatment includes chemotherapy and radiotherapy directed at the lesion.[19] The overall 5-year survival rate of 922 osteosarcoma patients, studied from 1973 to 1987, was 41%.[11] Ewing's sarcoma is a rare cause of disease in the lumbar spine. The importance of differentiating these lesions is related to the responsiveness of Ewing's sarcoma to chemotherapy.[38] In Ewing's patients without neurologic involvement, chemotherapy can be attempted without surgical resection.

Osteoid Osteoma

Osteoblastoma must also be differentiated from osteoid osteoma. Table 13-1 summarizes the features that differentiate these tumors. In brief, osteoid osteoma is associated with more intense nocturnal pain, a lesion that is less than 2 cm in size, no associated soft tissue mass, and a histologic appearance demonstrating osteoid trabeculae with continuous and regular bone formation.

Giant Cell Tumor

A giant cell tumor of bone may contain areas of woven bone. However, this lesion has areas of solidly packed giant and stromal cells without intervening osteoid. Osteoblastoma contains areas of intervening bone and osteoid between collections of giant cells.

Hyperparathyroidism

Rarely, the brown tumor of hyperparathyroidism may appear histologically similar to an osteoblastoma because of the presence of giant cells. Serum calcium and phosphorus determinations should differentiate the elevated concentrations of these factors associated with hyperparathyroidism from the normal levels associated with osteoblastoma.

TREATMENT

Local excision of the entire lesion is the treatment of choice if bone can be sacrificed without loss of function or excessive risk of neurogenic dysfunction. Osteoblastoma in the posterior elements of the spine is usually inaccessible for complete excision in up to 40% of lesions. Partial curettage of these lesions may be associated with cessation of growth and relief of symptoms for an extended period.[25] Rapidly expanding or recurrent osteoblastomas may be controlled with radiation therapy. However, radiation therapy may be ineffective and is not completely free of risk in the form of malignant transformation, spinal cord necrosis, and aggravation of spinal cord compression. Chemotherapy, including high-dose methotrexate and doxorubicin, has been reported to slow the growth of aggressive osteoblastomas that are inaccessible to surgical removal.[8]

PROGNOSIS

The course of osteoblastoma is usually benign. Bohlman and colleagues reported resolution of neck pain and

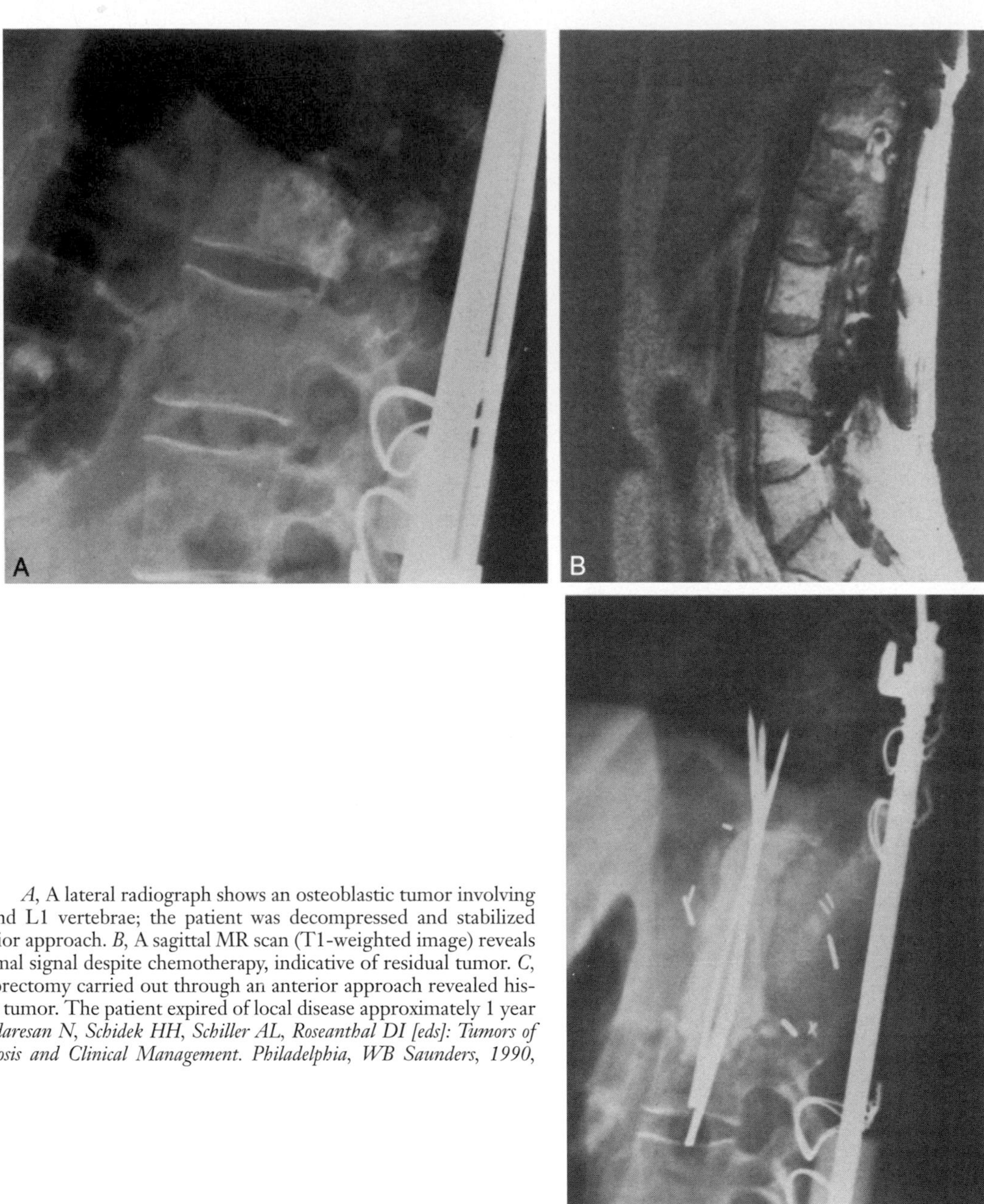

Figure 13-12 *A*, A lateral radiograph shows an osteoblastic tumor involving both the T12 and L1 vertebrae; the patient was decompressed and stabilized through a posterior approach. *B*, A sagittal MR scan (T1-weighted image) reveals persistent abnormal signal despite chemotherapy, indicative of residual tumor. *C*, A subtotal vertebrectomy carried out through an anterior approach revealed histologically viable tumor. The patient expired of local disease approximately 1 year later. *(From Sundaresan N, Schidek HH, Schiller AL, Roseanthal DI [eds]: Tumors of the Spine: Diagnosis and Clinical Management. Philadelphia, WB Saunders, 1990, p 133.)*

neurologic symptoms and signs after excision of the tumor.[5] However, tumors affecting the axial skeleton have greater morbidity and mortality.[22] The lesion is responsive to partial curettage and low-dose radiation therapy. Marsh and associates reported a series in which 1 of 13 patients with spinal osteoblastoma had a recurrence that resulted in paraplegia 7 months after surgery.[24] Laminectomy plus postoperative radiation therapy was the treatment for this complication. Less than 5% of osteoblastomas recur; however, repeated recurrences have been described.[17]

13-1 DIFFERENTIATION OF OSTEOBLASTOMA AND OSTEOID OSTEOMA

	Osteoblastoma	Osteoid Osteoma
Clinical findings	Moderate nocturnal pain	Intense nocturnal pain
	Lesion greater than 2 cm	Limited growth, less than 1.5 cm
	Rapid increase in size	Limited growth potential
Radiography	Minimal perifocal sclerosis	Marked perifocal sclerosis
	Associated soft tissue mass	No soft tissue mass
Histology	Osteoid trabeculae—discontinuous and irregular	Osteoid trabeculae—continuous and regular
	Stromal reaction—abundant	Stromal reaction—scant
	Osteoblastic giant cells—abundant	Osteoblastic giant cells—scant

Recurrences may develop after symptom-free periods of up to 17 years.[4] Malignant changes occur in a very few lesions thought to have been correctly diagnosed as benign osteoblastomas.[35]

References

Osteoblastoma

1. Alp H, Ceviker N, Baykaner K, et al: Osteoblastoma of the third lumbar vertebra. Surg Neurol 19:276, 1983.
2. Babu NV, Titus VTK, Chittaranjan S, et al: Computed tomographically guided biopsy of the spine. Spine 19:2436, 1994.
3. Banna M: Angiography of spinal osteoblastoma. J Can Assoc Radiol 30:118, 1974.
4. Beauchamp CP, Duncan CP, Dzus AK, Morton KS: Osteoblastoma: Experience with 23 patients. Can J Surg 35:199, 1992.
5. Bohlman HH, Sachs BL, Carter JR, et al: Primary neoplasms of the cervical spine: Diagnosis and treatment of twenty-three patients. J Bone Joint Surg Am 68-A:483, 1986.
6. Boriani S, Capanna R, Donati D, et al: Osteoblastoma of the spine. Clin Orthop 278:37, 1992.
7. Breton CL, Meziou M, Laredo JD, et al: Sarcoma complicating Paget's disease of the spine. Rev Rhum Engl Ed 60:17, 1993.
8. Camitta B, Wells R, Segura A, et al: Osteoblastoma response to chemotherapy. Cancer 68:999, 1991.
9. Crim JR, Mirra JM, Eckardt JJ, Seeger LL: Widespread inflammatory response to osteoblastoma: The flare phenomenon. Radiology 177:835, 1990.
10. DeSouza-Dias L, Frost HM: Osteoblastoma of the spine: A review and report of eight new cases. Clin Orthop 91:141, 1973.
11. Dorfman HD, Czerniack B: Bone cancers. Cancer 75:203, 1995.
12. Fielding JW, Fietti VG, Hughes JO, et al: Primary osteogenic sarcoma of the cervical spine. J Bone Joint Surg Am 58-A:892, 1976.
13. Gelberman RH, Olson CO: Benign osteoblastoma of the atlas: A case report. J Bone Joint Surg Am 56-A:808, 1974.
14. Ghelman B: Radiology of bone tumors. Orthop Clin North Am 20:287, 1989.
15. Gitelis S, Schajowicz F: Osteoid osteoma and osteoblastoma. Orthop Clin North Am 20:313, 1989.
16. Huvos AG: Bone Tumors: Diagnosis, Treatment, and Prognosis, 2nd ed. Philadelphia, WB Saunders, 1991, pp 67-83.
17. Jackson RP: Recurrent osteoblastoma: A review. Clin Orthop 131:229, 1978.
18. Jaffe HL, Mayer L: An osteoblastic osteoid tissue–forming tumor of a metacarpal bone. Arch Surg 24:550, 1932.
19. Jaffe N: Chemotherapy for malignant bone tumors. Orthop Clin North Am 20:487, 1989.
20. Kroon HM, Schurmans J: Osteoblastoma: Clinical and radiologic findings in 98 new cases. Radiology 175:783, 1990.
21. Lichtenstein L: Benign osteoblastoma—a category of osteoid and bone forming tumors other than classical osteoma, which may be mistaken for giant cell tumor or osteogenic sarcoma. Cancer 9:1044, 1956.
22. Lucas DR, Unni KK, McLeod RA, et al: Osteoblastoma: Clinicopathologic study of 306 cases. Hum Pathol 25:117, 1994.
23. Makhija MC, Stein IH: Bone imaging in osteoblastoma. Clin Nucl Med 8:141, 1983.
24. Marsh BW, Bonfiglio M, Brady LP, Enneking WF: Benign osteoblastoma: Range of manifestations. J Bone Joint Surg Am 57-A:1, 1975.
25. Marsh HO, Choi CB: Primary osteogenic sarcoma of the cervical spine originally mistaken for benign osteoblastoma. J Bone Joint Surg Am 52-A:1467, 1970.
26. McLeod RA, Dahlin DC, Beabout JW: The spectrum of osteoblastoma. AJR Am J Roentgenol 126:321, 1976.
27. Mirra JM: Bone Tumors: Clinical, Radiologic, and Pathologic Correlations. Philadelphia, Lea & Febiger, 1989, pp 389-430.
28. Mnaymneh W, Brown M, Tejada F, et al: Primary osteogenic sarcoma of the second cervical vertebra. J Bone Joint Surg Am 61-A:460, 1979.
29. Mori Y, Takayasu M, Saito K, et al: Benign osteoblastoma of the odontoid process of the axis: A case report. Surg Neurol 49: 274-277, 1998.
30. Nemoto O, Moser RP, Van Dam BE, et al: Osteoblastoma of the spine: A review of 75 cases. Spine 15:1272, 1990.
31. Obenberger J, Seidl Z, Plas J: Osteoblastoma in lumbar vertebral body. Neuroradiology 41:279-282, 1999.
32. Orbay T, Ataoglu O, Tali ET, et al: Vertebral osteoblastoma: Are radiologic structural changes necessary for diagnosis? Surg Neurol 51:426-429, 1999.
33. Pochaczevsky R, Yen YM, Sherman RS: The roentgen appearance of benign osteoblastoma. Radiology, 75:429, 1960.
34. Safuddin S, Sherazi Z, Shaikh MI, et al: Spinal osteoblastoma: Relationship between paravertebral muscle abnormalities and scoliosis. Skeletal Radiol 25:531-535, 1996.
35. Schajowicz F, Lemos C: Malignant osteoblastoma. J Bone Joint Surg Br 58-B:202-211, 1976.
36. Schajowicz F, McGuire MH: Diagnostic difficulties in skeletal pathology. Clin Orthop 240:281, 1989.
37. Schneider M, Sabo D, Gerner HJ, et al: Destructive osteoblastoma of the cervical spine with complete neurologic recovery. Spinal Cord 40:248-252, 2002.
38. Sharafuddin MJA, Haddad FS, Hitchon PW, et al: Treatment options in primary Ewing's sarcoma of the spine: Report of seven cases and review of the literature. Neurosurgery 30:610, 1992.
39. Shives TC, Dahlin DC, Sim FH, et al: Osteosarcoma of the spine. J Bone Joint Surg Am 66-A:660, 1986.
40. Siegel RD, Ryan LM, Antman KH: Osteosarcoma in adults: One institution's experience. Clin Orthop 240:263, 1989.
41. Sundaresan N, Rosen G, Huvos AG, Krol G: Combined modality treatment of osteosarcoma of the spine. Neurosurgery 23:714, 1988.
42. Sundaresan N, Schiller AL, Rosenthal DI: Osteosarcoma of the spine. In Sundaresan N, Schmidek HH, Schiller AL, Rosenthal DI (eds): Tumors of the Spine: Diagnosis and Clinical Management. Philadelphia, WB Saunders, 1990, pp 128-145.
43. Syklawer R, Osborn RE, Kerber CW, Glass RF: Magnetic resonance imaging of vertebral osteoblastoma: A report of two cases. Surg Neurol 34:421, 1990.
44. Sypert GW: Osteoid osteoma and osteoblastoma of the spine. In Sundaresan N, Schidek HH, Schiller AL, Roseanthal DI (eds): Tumors of the Spine: Diagnosis and Clinical Management. Philadelphia, WB Saunders, 1990, pp 117-127.
45. Tate TC, Kim SS, Ogden L: Osteoblastoma of the sacrum with intraabdominal manifestation. Am J Surg 123:735, 1972.
46. Tonai M, Campbell CT, Ahn GH, et al: Osteoblastoma: Classification and report of 16 patients. Clin Orthop 167:222, 1982.
47. Unni KK: Dahlin's Bone Tumors: General Aspects and Data on 11,087 cases, 5th ed. Philadelphia, Lippincott-Raven, 1996, pp 131-142.

OSTEOCHONDROMA

CAPSULE SUMMARY

	LOW BACK	NECK
Frequency of spinal pain	Uncommon	Uncommon
Location of spinal pain	Lumbar spine	Cervical spine
Quality of spinal pain	Mild ache	Dull ache
Symptoms and signs	Restricted motion	Restricted motion
Laboratory tests	None	None
Radiographic findings	Exostosis—single or multiple on plain roentgenograms	Exostosis—single or multiple on plain roentgenograms
Treatment	En bloc excision for lesions that cause nerve impingement	En bloc excision for lesions that cause nerve impingement

PREVALENCE AND PATHOGENESIS

The lesion was first described by Cooper in 1818.[11] Osteochondromas have been detected in skeletons dated between 3500 and 2000 BC.[9] Exostosis and osteocartilaginous exostosis are two other names associated with this benign tumor. Mirra has proposed that the term *exostosis* be reserved for marginal osteophytes associated with osteoarthritis and that *osteochondroma* be reserved for the benign bone tumor because the two lesions occur in different areas of bone, occur at different ages of the skeleton, and have different pathogenetic mechanisms.[33]

Epidemiology

Osteochondroma is a common benign tumor of bone that occurs in single or multiple locations in the skeleton. Osteochondromas represent up to 36% of all benign bone tumors and 8% to 11% of all primary tumors of bone examined by biopsy.[12,33] The lesion develops in approximately 60% of patients between the second and third decades of life. In rare instances, osteochondromas are diagnosed in middle-aged and elderly patients at a time beyond skeletal maturity.[45] In patients with multiple osteochondromas, lesions develop before 20 years of age.[33] The male-to-female ratio is 2:1.[21]

Osteochondromas occur most commonly at the ends of tubular bones. Approximately 1% to 2% of osteochondromas are located in the spine.[42] About 50% are found in the lumbosacral spine, 30% in the thoracic spine, and 20% in the cervical spine.[12] A review of 96 patients with solitary spinal osteochondromas reported the cervical spine to be the most commonly affected area with a 50% frequency; the lumbar spine was involved in 23% of individuals.[1] In the cervical spine, C2 was the most frequently affected vertebra.

Pathogenesis

The pathogenesis of osteochondroma is postulated to be related to an abnormality in cartilage growth. Keith thought that osteochondroma results from a defect in the periosteal cuff of bone that surrounds the lower end of the epiphyseal plate cartilage during embryogenesis.[25] The larger the defect, the larger the tumor will be. A single defect results in a solitary tumor, whereas multiple defects cause hereditary multiple osteochondromatoses. Nests of cartilage in a periosteal location grow out from the epiphyseal growth plate and result in a bony prominence capped by a layer of cartilage that is continuous with the cortex of the underlying bone. Osteochondromas may be thought of as slow-growing developmental anomalies that cease to enlarge once growth has stopped. This progression correlates with the clinical history of recognition of the tumor during childhood and its cessation of growth once the epiphyses close.[33]

CLINICAL HISTORY

Osteochondroma is frequently asymptomatic and is discovered only as a painless prominence of bone or as a chance finding on a radiograph. If pain is present, it is mild, deep, and usually secondary to mechanical irritation of overlying soft tissue structures. The progression of symptoms is slow and measured over years.[46] Pain may increase with activity. An osteochondroma that continues to grow may cause loss of function and decreased motion. Osteochondromas attached to the spinal column have been associated with kyphosis and spondylolisthesis.[4] The tumor may cause muscle contraction and associated scoliosis.[32] An osteochromdroma may even grow large enough to cause nerve root pain.[2] Myelopathic symptoms with spinal cord compression are also reported.[27,41] Compression of the spinal cord causes neurologic compromise, including quadriparesis. Myelopathy predominates to a greater extent in patients with multiple osteochondromas than in those with a solitary tumor in the spine. Sudden death, Brown-Séquard syndrome, and Horner's syndrome are among a variety of complications reported in patients with osteochondromas that have involved the axis and other portions of the cervical spine.*

*See references 8, 15, 22-24, 29, 31, 36, 39, 43, 48, 51.

Intermittent episodes of C2 neuralgia, tinnitus, dizziness, and blurring of vision are a result of vertebral artery occlusion by osteochondroma of the axis.[17] The onset of symptoms may be more acute when an individual has had a fall or a hyperextension injury of the neck.[22,50] Anterior spinal osteochondromas in the cervical spine may be manifested as hoarseness, dysphagia, or a slowly growing mass.[40]

In the lumbar spine, osteochondromas may be associated with radicular pain, sensory abnormalities, motor weakness, and urinary and fecal incontinence.[6,37,38,48] The lesion grows slowly over a period of months to years. The neurologic abnormality corresponds to the location of the tumor. Radiculopathy may be caused by this tumor.[49] Spinal stenosis has also been reported.[44]

PHYSICAL EXAMINATION

Physical examination may be normal, without any neurologic deficit; however, osteochondromas near facet joints of the spine may cause some restriction in motion. Osteochondromas that grow close to the body surface may cause a palpable mass that may be tender on palpation.[34] Neurologic findings, when present, will correspond to the location of the lesion and related nerve root compression.

LABORATORY DATA

Screening laboratory test results are normal with this benign tumor of bone.

Pathology

Pathologically, a gross specimen of an osteochondroma may take the form of a pedunculated stalk or a flat prominence. The tumor's cortex and its periosteal covering are continuous with those of the underlying bone. The cartilage cap may cover the entire lesion or the rounded end of a stalked exostosis. The cap's cartilage is smooth and 2 to 3 mm thick. Actively growing lesions may have cartilage 1 cm thick. As the lesion grows older, the cartilaginous cap disappears. The lesion may vary in size and is well circumscribed. Histologic examination of the tumor shows benign chondrocytes with small nuclei. The islands of cartilage and cartilage cells are embedded in the underlying cancellous bone. As the bone matures, the amount of cartilage decreases. However, residual microscopic foci of cartilage may be identified well into adult life.

RADIOGRAPHIC EVALUATION

Roentgenograms

The roentgenographic features of an osteochondroma are diagnostic. The lesion protrudes from the underlying bone on a sessile or pedunculated bony stalk that is continuous with the cortex and spongiosa of the underlying bone. The outer surface of the lesion may be smooth or irregular, but it is almost always well demarcated. If the cartilage cap is calcified, it may obscure the underlying stalk (Figs. 13-13 and 13-14). Plain roentgenogram may not identify a significant number of lesions. Among 80 tumors studied by plain roentgenograms, 21% were diagnostic, 64% had nondiagnostic anomalies, and 15% were normal.[1] In the spine, osteochondromas are located close to centers of secondary ossification, including the spinous process, pedicle, and neural arch.[22] In the cervical spine, the axis and the lateral masses of the atlas may be involved.[30,49]

Scintigraphy

Radionuclide bone scan reveals increased uptake at the site of the tumor. Malignant lesions may exhibit greater intensity of uptake, but this finding is not always a reliable distinguishing feature of malignant transformation.[13,20] The increased activity of osteochondroma is related to endochondral ossification within the cartilaginous cap.

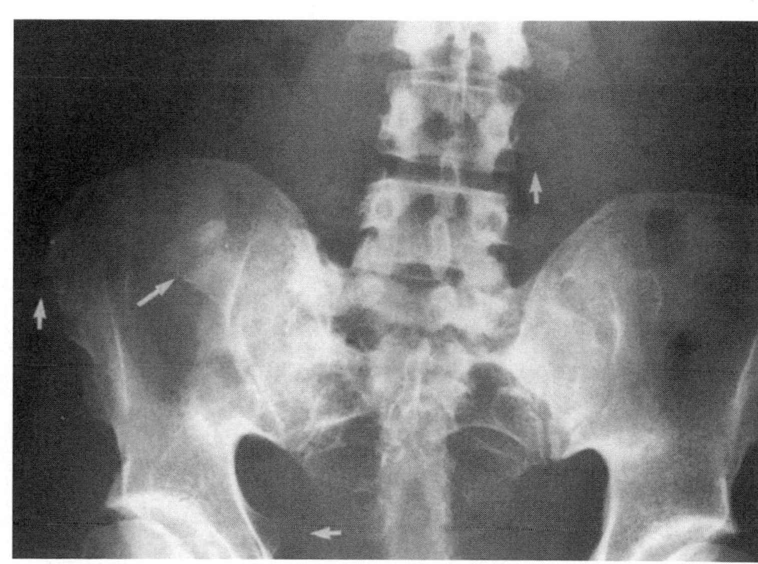

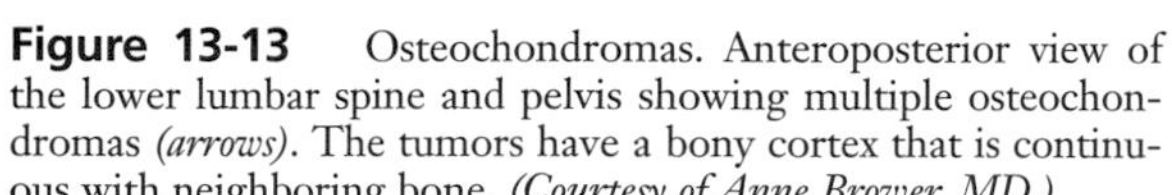

Figure 13-13 Osteochondromas. Anteroposterior view of the lower lumbar spine and pelvis showing multiple osteochondromas *(arrows)*. The tumors have a bony cortex that is continuous with neighboring bone. *(Courtesy of Anne Brower, MD.)*

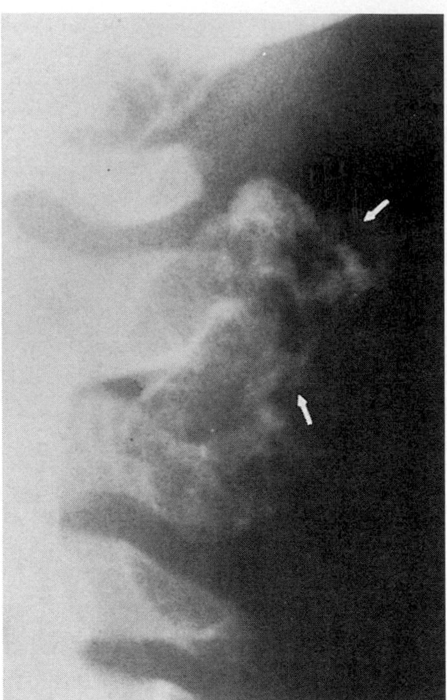

Figure 13-14 Solitary osteochondroma of the spine. This pedunculated osteochondroma *(arrows)* arises from the spinous process of the third cervical vertebra. It extends upward, behind the spinous process of the axis. *(From Resnick D, Kyriakos M, Greenway GD: Tumors and tumor-like lesions of bone: Imaging and pathology of specific lesions. In Resnick D [ed]: Diagnosis of Bone and Joint Disorders, 3rd ed. Philadelphia, WB Saunders, 1995, p 3729.)*

Computed Tomography

CT and myelography are helpful in localizing the site of the lesion in the spinal column, its size, and its relationship to the nerve roots and spinal cord, as well as in differentiating it from malignant lesions.[26,47] CT is the imaging modality of choice for identifying osteochondromas.[4] In the setting of neurologic abnormalities compatible with spinal cord compression, tumors may arise from the vertebral arch or the posterior aspect of the vertebral body.[7,19]

Magnetic Resonance

MR imaging is also a good technique for detecting spinal cord compression, but it does not image the bony architecture of the tumor as well as CT does.[35] MR imaging is able to detect the thickness of the cartilaginous cap and the continuity of the bone marrow space between the original bone and new growth. Angiography may be helpful in detecting occlusion of the vertebral artery in its location in the cervical spine by tumor.[17]

DIFFERENTIAL DIAGNOSIS

The diagnosis of an osteochondroma is based on its appearance on radiographs and the lack of clinical and laboratory findings. Chondrosarcomatous degeneration of osteochondroma occurs in less than 1% of patients. Adult patients with multiple lesions are at greater risk in this respect. However, a review of 45 secondary chondrosarcomas arising from osteochondromas reported no prognostic differences between tumors arising from solitary or multiple osteochondromas.[52] Malignant transformation is usually heralded by increasing pain, an enlarging soft tissue mass, and loss of definition of the outer border of the lesion on radiographs. However, the onset of pain in a previously asymptomatic osteochondroma is not always associated with malignant degeneration because infarction of the cartilage cap or fracture through the base of an osteochondroma may also cause pain and new bone growth.[33]

Other non-neoplastic lesions to be considered in the differential diagnosis are callus associated with fractures, chondroid metaplasia, and osteophytes associated with osteoarthritis. Other cartilage-producing tumors that must be considered include chondromas, chondroblastomas, and chondromyxoid fibromas.[16] The size and location of the benign tumor should help differentiate these non-neoplastic entities with similar histologic features. Fibrocartilaginous nodules in the ligamentum nuchae may be confused with osteochondroma or a fracture of a spinous process. These painless nodules may be noted on physical examination.[28]

TREATMENT

Osteochondromas require no therapy when they are asymptomatic.[10] Removal is indicated if the tumor is causing persistent pain or disability, has roentgenographic features suggestive of malignancy, or shows an abnormal increase in size. Patients with neurologic symptoms can be helped by removal of the lesion and decompression of the affected nerve root or spinal cord.[18] In the cervical spine, decompression, posterior stabilization, and facet fusion may be required for treatment of cord compression in patients with solitary or multiple osteochondromas (diaphyseal aclasis).[3]

Although chondrosarcoma is more common in patients with multiple osteochondromas, prophylactic removal of tumors in patients with multiple lesions is not practical. Patients must be monitored closely for a change in symptoms or size of lesions. These lesions should be removed.

PROGNOSIS

The course of a solitary osteochondroma is usually benign and asymptomatic and is not associated with any dysfunction or inability to work. In the rare patient who has a vertebral osteochondroma and neurologic dysfunction, surgical decompression of the site should result in return of function and complete cure.[14] Resolution of neck pain and neurologic dysfunction affecting the arm has been reported after surgical excision.[5] An osteochondroma may recur if the tumor, particularly its cartilaginous cap and periosteum, is not completely removed. Continuous observation of patients with osteochondromas is important, particularly those with multiple lesions, because they can occasionally become malignant. A recent review of 45 secondary chondrosarcomas arising from osteochondromas reported no prognostic differences between tumors arising from solitary or multiple osteochondromas.[52]

References

Osteochondroma

1. Albrecht S, Crutchfield S, Segall GK: On spinal osteochondromas. J Neurosurg 77:247, 1992.
2. Arasil E, Erdem A, Yuceer N: Osteochondroma of the upper cervical spine: A case report. Spine 21:516-518, 1996.
3. Bhojraj SY, Panjwani JS: A new management approach to decompression, posterior stabilization, and fusion for cervical laminar exostosis with cord compression in a case of diaphyseal aclasis: Case report and review of the literature. Spine 18:1376, 1993.
4. Blaauw G: Osteocartilaginous exostosis of the spine. In Vinken PJ, Bruyn GW (eds): Handbook of Clinical Neurology. Tumors of the Spine and Spinal Cord, Part I. New York, Elsevier, 1975, pp 313-319.
5. Bohlman HH, Sachs BL, Carter JR, et al: Primary neoplasms of the cervical spine: Diagnosis and treatment of twenty-three patients. J Bone Joint Surg Am 68-A:483, 1986.
6. Borne G, Payrot C: Right lumbo-crural sciatica due to a vertebral osteochondroma. Neurochirurgie 22:301, 1976.
7. Buckler RA, Chad DA, Smith TW, et al: Sciatica: An early manifestation of thoracic vertebral osteochondroma. Neurosurgery 21:98, 1987.
8. Calhoun JM, Chadduck WM, Smith JL: Single cervical exostosis: Report of a case and review of the literature. Surg Neurol 37:26, 1992.
9. Chamberlain AT, Rogers S, Romanowski CAJ: Osteochondroma in a British neolitic skeleton. Br J Hosp Med 47:51, 1992.
10. Chrisman OD, Goldenberg RR: Untreated solitary osteochondroma. Report of two cases. J Bone Joint Surg Am 50-A:508, 1968.
11. Cooper A: Exostosis. In Cooper A, Travers B (eds): Surgical Essays. 3rd ed. London, Cox & Son, 1818, pp 169-226.
12. Dahlin DC, Unni KK: Bone Tumors: General Aspects and Data on 8,542 cases, 4th ed. Springfield, IL, Charles C Thomas, 1986, pp 18-32.
13. Edeling CJ: Bone scintigraphy in hereditary multiple exostoses. Eur J Nucl Med 14:207, 1988.
14. Esposito PW, Crawford AH, Vogler C: Solitary osteochondroma occurring on the transverse process of the lumbar spine. Spine 10:398, 1985.
15. Fielding JW, Ratzan S: Osteochondroma of the cervical spine. J Bone Joint Surg Am 55-A:640, 1973.
16. Gaetani P, Tancioni F, Merlo P, et al: Spinal chondroma of the lumbar tract: Case report. Surg Neurol 46:534-539, 1996.
17. George B, Attallah A, Laurian C, et al: Cervical osteochondroma (C2 level) with vertebral artery occlusion and second cervical nerve root irritation. Surg Neurol 31:459, 1989.
18. Gokay H, Bucy PC: Osteochondroma of the lumbar spine: Report of a case. J Neurosurg 12:72, 1955.
19. Gottlieb A, Severi P, Ruelle A, et al: Exostosis as a cause of spinal cord compression. Surg Neurol 26:581, 1986.
20. Greenspan A: Tumors of cartilage origin. Orthop Clin North Am 20:347, 1989.
21. Huvos AG: Bone Tumors: Diagnosis, Treatment, and Prognosis, 2nd ed. Philadelphia, WB Saunders, 1991, pp 253-291.
22. Inglis AE, Rubin RM, Lewis RJ, Villacin A: Osteochondroma of the cervical spine: Case report. Clin Orthop 126:127, 1977.
23. Julien J, Riemens V, Vital C, et al: Cervical cord compression by solitary osteochondroma of the atlas. J Neurol Neurosurg Psychiatry 41:479, 1978.
24. Karian JM, DeFilipp G, Buchheit WA, et al: Vertebral osteochondroma causing spinal cord compression: Case report. Neurosurgery 14:483, 1984.
25. Keith A: Studies on the anatomical changes which accompany certain growth disorders of the human body. J Anat 54:101, 1920.
26. Kenney PJ, Gilula LA, Murphy WA: The use of computed tomography to distinguish osteochondroma and chondrosarcoma. Radiology 139:129, 1981.
27. Khosla A, Martin DS, Awwad EE: The solitary intraspinal vertebral osteochondroma: An unusual cause of compressive myelopathy: Features and literature review. Spine 24:77-81, 1999.
28. Lewinnek GE, Peterson SE: A calcified fibrocartilaginous nodule in the ligamentum nuchae: Presenting as a tumor. Clin Orthop 136:163, 1978.
29. Linkowski GD, Tsai FY, Recher L, et al: Solitary osteochondroma with spinal cord compression. Surg Neurol 23:388, 1985.
30. Lopez-Barea F, Rodriguez-Peralto JL, Hernandez-Moneo JL, et al: Tumors of the atlas: Three incidental cases of osteochondroma, benign osteoblastoma, and atypical Ewing's sarcoma. Clin Orthop 307:182, 1994.
31. MacGee EE: Osteochondroma of the cervical spine: A cause of transient quadriplegia. Neurosurgery 4:259, 1979.
32. Mexia JA, Nunez I, Garriga S, et al: Osteochondroma of the thoracic spine and scoliosis. Spine 26:1082-1085, 2001.
33. Mirra JM: Bone Tumors: Clinical, Radiologic, and Pathologic Correlations. Philadelphia, Lea & Febiger, 1989, pp 1626-1659.
34. Morard M, de Preux J: Solitary osteochondroma presenting as a neck mass with spinal cord compression syndrome. Surg Neurol 37:402, 1992.
35. Moriwaka F, Hozen H, Nakane K, et al: Myelopathy due to osteochondroma: MR and CT studies. J Comput Assist Tomogr 14:128, 1990.
36. Novick GS, Pavlov H, Bullough PG: Osteochondroma of the cervical spine: Report of two cases in preadolescent males. Skeletal Radiol 8:13, 1982.
37. O'Connon GA, Roberts TS: Spinal cord compression by an osteochondroma in a patient with multiple osteochondromatosis: Case report. J Neurosurg 60:420, 1984.
38. Palmer FJ, Blum PW: Osteochondroma with spinal cord compression. J Neurosurg 52:842, 1980.
39. Palmer FJ, Blum PW: Osteochondroma with spinal cord compression: Report of three cases. J Neurosurg 52:842, 1980.
40. Peck JH: Dysphagia due to massive exostosis of the cervical spine. In: Proceedings of the Western Orthopaedic Association. J Bone Joint Surg Am 46-A:1379, 1964.
41. Ratliff J, Voorhies R: Osteochondroma of the C5 lamina with cord compression: Case report and review of the literature. Spine 25:1293-1295, 2000.
42. Resnick D, Kyriakos M, Greenway GD: Tumors and tumor-like lesions of bone: Imaging and pathology of specific lesions. In Resnick D (ed): Diagnosis of Bone and Joint Disorders, 3rd ed. Philadelphia, WB Saunders, 1995, pp 3725-3746.
43. Rose EF, Fekete A: Odontoid osteochondroma causing sudden death: Report of a case and review of the literature. Am J Clin Pathol 42:606, 1964.
44. Royster RM, Kujawa P, Dryer RF: Multilevel osteochondroma of the lumbar spine presenting as spinal stenosis. Spine 16:992, 1991.
45. Sakai D, Mochida J, Toh E, et al: Spinal osteochondromas in middle-aged to elderly patients. Spine 27:E503-E506, 2002.
46. Sharma MC, Arora R, Deol PS, et al: Osteochondroma of the spine: An enigmatic tumor of the spinal cord. A series of 10 cases. J Neurosurg Sci 46:66-70, 2002.
47. Tigges S, Erb RE, Nance EP: Skeletal case of the day. AJR Am J Roentgenol 158:1368, 1992.
48. Twersky J, Kassner EG, Tenner MS, Camera A: Vertebral and costal osteochondromas causing spinal cord compression. AJR Am J Roentgenol 124:124, 1975.
49. van der Sluis R, Gurr K, Joseph MG: Osteochondroma of the lumbar spine: An unusual cause of sciatica. Spine 17:1519, 1992.
50. Wen DY, Bergman TA, Haines SJ: Acute cervical myelopathy from hereditary multiple exostoses: Case report. Neurosurgery 25:472, 1989.
51. Wu KK, Guise ER: Osteochondroma of the atlas: A case report. Clin Orthop 136:160, 1978.
52. Wuisman PI, Jutte PC, Ozaki T: Secondary chondrosarcoma in osteochondromas. Medullary extension in 15 of 45 cases. Acta Orthop Scand 68:396-400, 1997.

GIANT CELL TUMOR

CAPSULE SUMMARY

	LOW BACK	NECK
Frequency of spinal pain	Common	Common
Location of spinal pain	Lumbar spine, sacrum	Cervical spine
Quality of spinal pain	Intermittent ache	Intermittent ache
Symptoms and signs	Localized mass	Localized mass
Laboratory tests	None	None
Radiographic findings	Anterior vertebral body involvement on plain roentgenograms, soft tissue extension on MR	Anterior vertebral body involvement on plain roentgenograms, soft tissue extension on MR
Treatment	En bloc extension	En bloc extension

PREVALENCE AND PATHOGENESIS

The first description of the benign characteristics of this tumor was by Cooper and Travers in 1818.[8] Bloodgood in 1919 was the first to refer to this neoplasm as a benign giant cell tumor.[4] Other names that have been associated with this perplexing neoplasm include myeloid sarcoma, medullary sarcoma, and osteoclastoma.

Epidemiology

Giant cell tumor of bone is a common, locally aggressive lesion that may turn malignant. Giant cell tumors represent up to 21% of all benign tumors of bone and up to 5% of primary bone tumors examined by biopsy.[11,39] In approximately 70% of patients the diagnosis is made between the ages of 20 and 40. The average age of patients with malignant giant cell tumors is older than that of patients with benign tumors. Patients with benign tumors are predominantly women, by a ratio of 3:2, whereas those with malignant tumors are predominantly men, by a ratio of 3:1.[24]

Most giant cell tumors occur at the ends of long bones, particularly around the knee. About 8% to 12% of giant cell tumors occur in the spine,[11,26] with the sacrum being the most frequently affected area. Approximately 68% of spinal giant cell tumors occur in the sacrum, 11% in the lumbar spine, 11% in the cervical spine, and 10% in the thoracic area. Other series have found frequencies of sacral involvement in the range of 3% to 8%.[6,47] The ilium and ischium may also be involved in a small number of patients (0.05%).[32]

Pathogenesis

The pathogenesis of giant cell tumor is not known. The tumor starts after the skeleton has ceased to grow and has matured. It arises from non–bone-forming, supporting connective tissue of the bone marrow space. The factors that make this tumor inherently invasive or potentially malignant are unknown.

CLINICAL HISTORY

Giant cell tumor of bone causes intermittent, aching pain over the affected bone, which is almost always the predominant symptom. The duration of symptoms typically may vary from a few weeks to 6 months, but some patients have had pain over 2 years before diagnosis.[9] Patients with sacral or vertebral involvement may describe neurologic dysfunction, including paresthesias with radiation of pain to the lower extremities, muscle weakness, and urinary or rectal incontinence.[9,54] In one study of 26 patients with sacral giant cell tumors, 88% had neurologic symptoms, including neurogenic bladder dysfunction, sphincter weakness, and perineal hypesthesias.[58] Disc herniation and radiculopathy are misdiagnosed in some patients, and they undergo discectomy. In the cervical spine, expansion of the tumor anteriorly may be associated with the symptom of dysphagia.[42]

PHYSICAL EXAMINATION

Physical examination may demonstrate tenderness on palpation over the spine and sacrum. Localized swelling may be noted if the location of the giant cell tumor is superficial; that is, in the spinous process. Kyphosis, muscle spasm, and associated limitation of motion may also be noted in the lumbar or cervical spine. In a sacral lesion, an extracolonic mass may be found on rectal examination.[54] Neurologic examination may show sensory, motor, or reflex abnormalities, depending on the level of nerve root compression, including the sacral nerve roots.[34,60]

LABORATORY DATA

Laboratory results are normal in patients with benign giant cell tumors, but serum calcium, phosphorus, and alkaline phosphatase tests should be obtained to differentiate these tumors from hyperparathyroidism, Paget's disease, and malignant giant cell tumor. Patients with malignant giant cell tumors may show abnormalities such as anemia and an elevated sedimentation rate.

Pathology

The tumor is a soft, friable, gray to red tumor mass on gross pathologic examination. Areas of the tumor may be cystic or necrotic, or they may be filled with blood. This characteristic causes confusion with findings associated with aneurysmal bone cysts. The tumors cause expansion of host bone with cortical destruction. In most lesions the periosteum is relatively spared, with the tumor contained by a shell of new bone.

The histologic appearance of giant cell tumor of bone is not distinctively characteristic in that a number of other benign lesions may contain giant cells (Table 13-2). In general, giant cell tumors contain large numbers of osteoblast-like giant cells separated by inconspicuous mononuclear stromal cells (Fig. 13-15). The proliferating giant cells have round, oval, or spindle-shaped nuclei. Mitotic figures may be numerous. The nuclei lack the variations in size and shape that are characteristic of sarcoma. In a minority of lesions, small foci of osteoid and woven bone are seen. Thin-walled vessels with hemorrhages are also characteristic. Fine-needle aspiration of sacral lesions may produce an adequate specimen to help in the diagnosis of giant cell tumor.[45]

Great debate exists over the histologic grading of giant cell tumors. Some pathologists believe that the histologic grade is predictive of subsequent tumor behavior.[26] Others do not believe that grading, particularly at the benign end of the scale (grades I and II), is predictive of any subsequent propensity for aggressive growth.[11,39]

Cytogenic analysis of giant cell tumors reveals chromosomal abnormalities in tumor cells not detected in normal cells. Telomere-to-telomere chromosome translocations affecting the long arm of chromosomes 19 and 20 were noted in the tumors but were not predictive of the aggressiveness of the giant cell neoplasm.[48] The alteration in chromosome 19 may affect the function of transforming growth factor-beta (TGF-beta) on osteoclasts. Giant cell tumors may consist of osteoclasts that have been affected by TGF-beta activity. Researchers in another study used flow cytometric DNA analysis of giant cell tumors in an attempt to predict the biologic behavior of these neoplasms. DNA analysis was unable to predict the likelihood of the tumor metastasizing.[14]

RADIOGRAPHIC EVALUATION

Roentgenograms

The roentgenographic findings of giant cell tumors are characteristic, but not pathognomonic. The lesion is expansile, with irregular thinning of the cortical margin. It is lytic but may contain a delicate trabecular meshwork. Little bony reaction occurs in response to this lesion. Extensive sclerotic borders and periosteal reaction are not seen. In the spine, the vertebral body is frequently affected, but the spinous and transverse processes may also be involved (Figs. 13-16 and 13-17).[13] The destruction of vertebral bone, which most commonly occurs in the vertebral body as opposed to the posterior elements in other benign tumors of the spine, results in lytic lesions without surrounding reactive sclerosis or matrix mineralization.[52] The roentgenographic changes of giant cell tumor in the sacrum may be subtle, and large tumors may be missed on plain roentgenograms. The lesion may be eccentrically located in the sacrum and may spread across the sacroiliac joint to involve the ilium. When located in the superior portion of the sacrum, lesions may erode through the L5–S1 disc space.[54]

Bone Scintigraphy

If plain roentgenograms are insufficient to demonstrate abnormalities of the sacrum or spine, a bone scan may be helpful in detecting such abnormalities. However, radionuclide scintigraphy may exhibit increased tracer in bone across the adjacent joint and in other joints in the same extremity not involved with the tumor.[59]

Computed Tomography

CT is useful in localizing the extent of a lesion in the sacrum. It is superior to plain roentgenograms in detecting the extent of tumor in the extraosseous space.[7] However, clear distinction between tumor and muscle may be difficult to make with CT.

Magnetic Resonance

MR is the best imaging modality to study giant cell tumors and soft tissue extension because of superior contrast resolution. The tumor exhibits long T1 and T2 relaxation times that correspond to low intensity on T1-weighted images and high intensity on T2-weighted images. MR is better at determining the extraosseous extent of the tumor, whereas CT is better able to visualize mineralized structures, including subtle cortical breaks.[37]

DIFFERENTIAL DIAGNOSIS

A thorough review of the clinical, laboratory, pathologic, and radiologic data is necessary to make the diagnosis of a giant cell tumor of bone. Such evaluation is required because a number of benign and malignant lesions are similar in pathologic findings. Table 13-2 presents a list of benign and malignant lesions that contain giant cells that may mimic the findings of giant cell tumor of bone.[15] Not all of these neoplasms affect the lumbosacral or cervical spine. Aneurysmal bone cyst, brown tumor of hyperparathyroidism, chondroblastoma, fibrous dysplasia, osteogenic sarcoma, chondromyxoid fibroma, osteoblastoma, and enchondroma need to be included in the differential diagnosis of a giant cell–containing tumor located in the lumbosacral or cervical spine. In rare circumstances, giant cell tumor may occur in more than one location in the axial skeleton.[30]

13-2 DIFFERENTIAL DIAGNOSIS OF GIANT CELL LESIONS OF BONE

	Most Common Age Group	Location in Bone	Radiologic Appearance	Gross Features	Microscopic Features	
					Giant Cells	*Stromal Cells*
Giant cell tumor	Third and fourth decades	Epiphysis or metaphysis	Eccentric expanded radiolucent area	Fleshy soft tissue	Abundant number uniformly distributed	Plump and polyhedral cells with abundant cytoplasm
Nonossifying fibroma	First decade	Metaphysis	Eccentric oval defects	Fleshy soft tissue	Focal distribution, small and few nuclei	Slender and spindly cells with little cytoplasm; whorled pattern
Aneurysmal bone cyst	First and second decades	Vertebral column or metaphysis of long bone	Eccentric blow-out "soap bubble" appearance	Cavity filled with blood	Focal around vascular channels or hemorrhage	Large vascular channels; slender to plump cells with hemosiderin granules; metaplastic bone
Brown tumor of hyperparathyroidism	Any age	Anywhere in bone	Subperiosteal, subchondral, and subligamentous resorption of bone	Fleshy tissue or cystic spaces	Focal around hemosiderin pigment or hemorrhage	Fibrous stroma with slender spindle cells
Simple bone cyst	First and second decades	Metaphysis	Trabeculations in radiolucent area	Cyst filled with clear fluid	Focal around cholesterol clefts	Cyst wall of fibrous tissue; metaplastic bone
Chondroblastoma	Second decade	Epiphysis	Radiolucency in spotty opacities	Firm to fleshy tissue	Few and focal	Plump and round or ovoid cells with pericellular calcifications
Fibrous dysplasia	First and second decades	Metaphysis	Ground-glass appearance	Firm and gritty	Few and focal	Woven bone and whorled fibrous tissue; no osteoblasts
Giant cell reparative granuloma	Second and third decades	Maxilla and mandible	Radiolucent focus	Soft fleshy tissue	Focal around hemosiderin pigment or hemorrhage	Slender or plump spindle cells
Ossifying fibroma	Second and third decades	Maxilla and mandible	Radiopaque	Firm and gritty	Few and focal	Lamellar bony trabeculae in fibrous tissue; osteoblastic rimming
Osteosarcoma	Second and third decades	Metaphysis	Radiolucent	Soft, firm, or hard	Focal distribution	Malignant cells with direct osteoid formation
Chondromyxoid fibroma	Second and third decades	Metaphysis	Eccentric with expanded cortex	Soft to firm	Focal distribution	Chondroid, myxoid, and fibrous lobules
Osteoblastoma	Second and third decades	Vertebral column, diaphysis of long bone	Radiolucent or dense	Hemorrhagic, gritty	Focal distribution	Abundant osteoid trabeculae with osteoblasts

From Resnick D, Niwayama G: Diagnosis of Bone and Joint Disorders, 2nd ed. Philadelphia, WB Saunders, 1988. Modified from Ghandur-Mnaymneh L, Mnaymneh WA: Bone lesions with giant cells: Problems in differential diagnosis. J Med Liban 24:91, 1972.

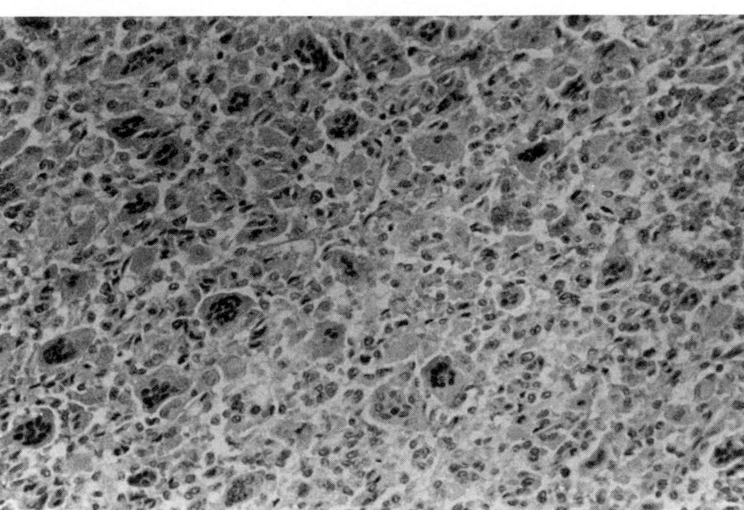

Figure 13-15 Giant cell tumor. Histologic section demonstrating an even distribution of a large number of giant cells with multiple nuclei. The tumor is very cellular but lacks fibrous or osteoid tissue. The histologic appearance of this tumor cannot be differentiated from that of a brown tumor of hyperparathyroidism. *(Courtesy of Arnold Schwartz, MD.)*

Aneurysmal Bone Cyst

An aneurysmal bone cyst is a fibrous-walled structure filled with blood that occurs in association with other neoplasms, including giant cell tumor. An aneurysmal bone cyst contains giant cells in its wall and thus may be confused with giant cell tumor.[20] A giant cell tumor with an aneurysmal bone cyst component should be treated as a giant cell tumor. Brown tumor of hyperparathyroidism contains cells that are histologically similar to those of a giant cell tumor. The elevation in serum calcium and decrease in serum phosphorus along with multiple locations of lesions help differentiate this entity. In addition, the giant cells of hyperparathyroidism are arranged in a more nodular pattern and are surrounded by areas of active bone.

Chondroblastoma

Chondroblastoma is a benign lesion that affects men younger than 30 years and is located near epiphyseal cartilage. The tumor is most commonly found in long bones and only rarely is located in the pelvis or lumbar spine.[44] On rare occasions, the tumor is situated in the cervical or thoracic spine.[5,62] Radiographically, the lesion is a solitary lytic lesion with a surrounding sclerotic border and punctate

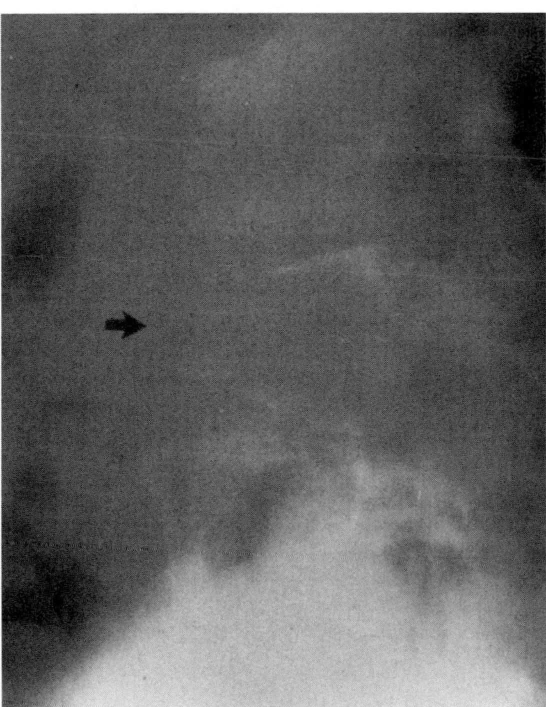

Figure 13-16 Giant cell tumor *(arrow)* showing vertebral body destruction characterized by collapse associated with loss of the anterior body margin. *(Courtesy of Anne Brower, MD.)*

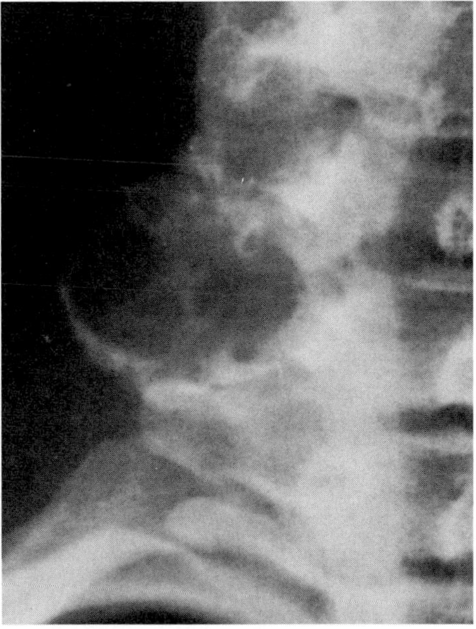

Figure 13-17 Giant cell tumor in a 21-year-old woman with a radiolucent, well-marginated expansile mass with a sclerotic rim that has been growing over a 7-year period in the lateral articular process of C7. *(From Campanacci M, Boriani S, Giunti A: Giant cell tumors of the spine. In Sundaresan N, Schmidek HH, Schiller AL, Rosenthal DI [eds]: Tumors of the Spine: Diagnosis and Clinical Management. Philadelphia, WB Saunders, 1990, p 169.)*

calcification. Histologically, the tumor contains a variable number of giant cells with multiple nuclei, polygonal to round stromal cells with distinct borders, "chicken wire" calcification, and variable amounts of chondroid.[39]

Fibrous Dysplasia

Fibrous dysplasia is a benign process affecting either one bone or multiple bones in the skeleton. The disease is more common in women than men and becomes prominent before the second decade of life. Fibrous dysplasia occasionally affects the pelvis, particularly the iliac wing and to a lesser degree the lumbar spine. Fibrous dysplasia rarely affects the cervical spine.[16,22,55] Cervical spine involvement occurs in 7% of patients with polyostotic fibrous dysplasia.[43] Radiologically, the medullary cavity of bone is replaced with fibrous tissue, which appears as a predominantly radiolucent, albeit hazy matrix (often described as "ground glass") that may contain focal calcific deposits. Lesions appear matted, loculated, or trabeculated with well-defined, sclerotic margins. The affected bone may be expanded, bowed, and deformed.[43] Histologically, the lesion contains a benign fibrous tissue matrix with variable quantities of woven bone, little to no cartilage, and only small foci of giant cells, which are associated with areas of cystification or hemorrhage. The small number of these cells helps differentiate fibrous dysplasia from giant cell tumor.

Osteosarcoma

Osteosarcoma is a very rare tumor of the axial skeleton and pelvis. Approximately 1% to 2% of osteosarcomas are located in the lumbar spine or pelvis.[1] It most commonly affects males between 10 and 30 years of age. The tumor may be osteoblastic or osteolytic. An osteoblastic lesion in a vertebral body affects one area of the body with dense sclerosis, which may extend into the neural arch. Irregular areas of calcification or ossification in the paravertebral soft tissues are usual. Osteolytic lesions are also associated with soft tissue masses and collapse of the anterior portion of a vertebra. Giant cell tumors, when untreated, are pure lytic lesions without any new bone formation. Histologic examination of osteosarcoma may demonstrate areas of osteoclast-like giant cells that superficially resemble giant cell tumor. However, close inspection of the specimen reveals frank anaplastic cells in areas away from bone-producing tissue.

Chondromyxoid Fibroma

Chondromyxoid fibroma is a very rare benign tumor that represents less than 1% of all primary bone neoplasms. The lesion occurs in men during the second and third decades of life. About 16% of these lesions occur in the ilium, ischium, or sacrum.[11] In the vertebral column, the lesion may affect the neural arch, vertebral body, or posterior elements. Radiographically, the tumor causes an area of osteolysis with bone expansion and variable calcification, which may be difficult to differentiate from other causes of bone damage.[38] On gross pathologic examination, this lesion is sharply delineated from surrounding bone. A thin sclerotic zone may be found in neighboring host bone. Histologically, the tumor contains different zones composed of myxomatous, fibrous, and chondroid tissue. The nuclei of cells may be round, oval, or spindle shaped. Giant cells, when present, are found in focal collections and are fewer in number than those associated with giant cell tumor.

Osteoblastoma

Osteoblastoma may be considered in the differential diagnosis because a giant cell tumor rich in osteoid and woven bone may be mistaken for an osteoblastoma. However, concentrating on areas in giant cell tumors with no bone production will show masses of stromal and giant cells, which are not seen in osteoblastoma.

Enchondroma

Enchondroma (EN) is a benign hyaline cartilage growth that develops within the medullary cavity of a single bone.[25] EN accounts for 1.4% of primary benign tumors. It develops most frequently in the small bones of the hands and feet, with only 0.88% of cases occurring in the axial skeleton.[31] In the axial skeleton, the distribution of EN is 31% in the cervical spine, 32% in the thoracic spine, 23% in the lumbosacral spine, and 14% in the sacrum.[25] Most patients with EN are asymptomatic, and it is identified as an incidental finding on roentgenographic examination. In the spinal column, EN may expand into the spinal canal or neural foramen and cause spinal cord or nerve root compression, respectively.[36,53,61] EN is a well-defined osteolytic lesion with sharp sclerotic margins. The lytic quality of this tumor may be confused with giant cell tumor. The lesion is radiolucent, although it may contain areas of cartilage matrix calcification. In vertebral bodies, the posterior elements are most frequently affected. The lesion may expand the surrounding bone. Pathologically, the lesion contains translucent hyaline cartilage with a varying amount of chondrocyte cellularity and little atypia. Most lesions do not require any intervention. The usual treatment of symptomatic tumors consists of curettage and filling the defect with bone chips.

Paget's Disease

Giant cell tumors may also be associated with Paget's disease.[23] The lesions of Paget's disease are more common in the skull and facial bones than in the axial skeleton. The realization that giant cell tumors may complicate extensive Paget's disease is important. Not every expansion of a pagetoid bone is sarcomatous degeneration. The presence of lytic lesions with soft tissue extension in patients with Paget's disease does not necessarily imply a grave prognosis.[3,41]

Pigmented Villonodular Synovitis

In very rare circumstances, pigmented villonodular synovitis may be confused with giant cell tumor of bone.

Villonodular synovitis may proliferate and enter the spinal canal. The occasional multinucleated giant cells of this lesion should not be confused with giant cell tumor of bone or malignant processes.[29]

TREATMENT

The lesion must be staged before therapy is instituted.[19] Staging of a giant cell tumor includes CT scanning to determine the exact extent of the tumor, along with MR imaging to determine the soft tissue distribution of the neoplasm in multiple planes. A staging system measuring the extent of intraosseous and paraspinal soft tissue extension helps determine the appropriate surgical procedure.[17] Angiography may be used to embolize the tumor before surgery.[6]

The therapy of choice for a giant cell tumor is en bloc excision if the lesion is in an accessible location. Recurrence rates of 10% to 15% are reported after excision.[40] Curettage may control growth of the tumor, but the local recurrence rate is 50% within 5 years.[27] Radiation therapy is rarely curative, is associated with frequent recurrences, and may promote malignant transformation.[24] It is reserved for lesions that are inaccessible for surgical removal or curettage.[10] Lesions treated with radiation do not necessarily undergo malignant degeneration. Patients who were monitored for up to 35 years after receiving radiation therapy had remission of their tumor without any recurrence.[2,12,28,49,50]

The ideal treatment of giant cell tumor of the spine is complete removal of accessible lesions.[46] Decompression of the spine is necessary once neurologic symptoms appear. A delay of more than 3 months after the onset of nerve root symptoms may result in irreversible nerve deficits.[34] However, complete resection is frequently impossible because of the location and size of the lesions and the potential for critical blood loss with resection. In large sacral tumors, partial excision with irradiation or irradiation alone may be the only reasonable option.[18] More sensitive radiographic techniques and advanced surgical methods have increased the success of total resection and reconstruction of sacral and vertebral lesions.[51,56] Patients who undergo these extensive procedures have a 33% mortality rate at 4 years.[63] Giant cell tumor of the cervical spine may be approached by splitting the mandible and tongue.[21] Posterior decompression and autografting to stabilize the spine have also been used for cervical lesions.[28] Chemotherapy is not effective in controlling the growth of this benign tumor.[7] Embolization of tumors in the spine may be used to treat inaccessible tumors. Long-term follow-up reports suggest that 50% of patients have a durable response to embolization of sacral tumors.[35] The procedure may be repeated for persistent control of tumor growth.[33] A potential risk associated with embolization of spinal lesions is ischemic injury to peripheral nerves and the spinal cord.[7]

PROGNOSIS

Giant cell tumors of bone are invasive, benign tumors and have a high local recurrence rate. Patients with benign giant cell tumors of the sacrum have died because of local invasion, malignant transformation, or secondary complications such as renal failure related to neurogenic bladder and obstruction.[54] Pulmonary metastases from benign giant cell tumors have been reported in patients with sacral tumors. The metastases occurred after a recurrence of the tumor and up to 10 years after diagnosis.[57] Regardless of treatment, patients must continue to be examined for signs of recurrence. In some circumstances, up to five courses of therapy were needed to eradicate the disease successfully.[24]

References

Giant Cell Tumor

1. Barwick KW, Huvos AG, Smith J: Primary osteogenic sarcoma of the column: A clinicopathologic correlation of ten patients. Cancer 46:595, 1980.
2. Bennett CJ, Marcus RB Jr, Million RR, Enneking WF: Radiation therapy for giant cell tumor of bone. Int J Radiat Oncol Biol Phys 26:299, 1993.
3. Bhambhani M, Lamberty BGH, Clements MR, et al: Giant cell tumours in mandible and spine: A rare complication of Paget's disease of bone. Ann Rheum Dis 51:1335, 1992.
4. Bloodgood JG: Bone tumors. Central (medullary) giant cell tumor (sarcoma) of lower end of ulna, with evidence that complete destruction of the bony shell or perforation of the bony shell is not a sign of increased malignancy. Ann Surg 69:345, 1919.
5. Buraczewski J, Lysakowska J, Rudowski W: Chondroblastoma (Codman's tumour) of the thoracic spine. J Bone Joint Surg Br 39-B:705, 1957.
6. Campanacci M, Boriana S, Giunti A: Giant cell tumors of the spine. In Sundaresan N, Schmidek HH, Schiller AL, Rosenthal DI (eds): Tumors of the Spine: Diagnosis and Clinical Management. Philadelphia, WB Saunders, 1990, pp 163-172.
7. Carrasco CH, Murray JA: Giant cell tumors. Orthop Clin North Am 20:395, 1989.
8. Cooper A, Travers B: Surgical Essays, 3rd ed. London, Cox & Son, 1818.
9. Dahlin DC: Giant cell tumor of vertebrae above the sacrum: A review of 31 cases. Cancer 39:1350, 1977.
10. Dahlin DC, Cupps RE, Johnson EW: Giant-cell tumor: A study of 195 cases. Cancer 25:106 1970.
11. Dahlin DC, Unni KK: Bone Tumors: General Aspects and Data on 8,542 cases, 4th ed. Springfield, IL, Charles C Thomas, 1986, pp 119-140.
12. DeGroof E, Verdonk R, Vercauteren M, et al: Giant-cell tumor involving a lumbar vertebra. Spine 15:835, 1990.
13. DiLorenzo N, Spallone A, Nolletti A, Nardi P: Giant cell tumor of the spine: A clinical study of six cases, with emphasis on the radiological features, treatment, and follow-up. Neurosurgery 6:29, 1980.
14. Fukunaga M, Nikaido T, Shimoda T, et al: A flow cytometric DNA analysis of giant cell tumors of bone including two cases with malignant transformation. Cancer 70:1886, 1992.
15. Ghandur-Mnaymneh L, Mnaymneh WA: Bone lesions with giant cells; problems in differential diagnosis. J Med Liban 24:91, 1972.
16. Harris WH, Dudley HR, Barry RJ: The natural history of fibrous dysplasia: An orthopaedic, pathological, and roentgenographic study. J Bone Joint Surg Am 44-A:207, 1962.
17. Hart RA, Boriani S, Biagini R, et al: A system for surgical staging and management of spine tumors. A clinical outcome study of giant cell tumors of the spine. Spine 22:1773-1782, 1997.
18. Harwood AR, Fornasier VL, Rider WD: Supervoltage irradiation in the management of giant cell tumor of bone. Radiology 125:223, 1977.
19. Heare TC, Enneking WF, Heare MM: Staging techniques and biopsy of bone tumors. Orthop Clin North Am 20:273, 1989.
20. Hess WE: Giant cell tumor of the cervical spine. J Bone Joint Surg Am 42-A:480, 1960.
21. Honma G, Murota K, Shiba R, Kondo H: Mandible and tongue-splitting approach to giant cell tumor of the axis. Spine 14:1204, 1989.
22. Hu SS, Healey JH, Huvos AG: Fibrous dysplasia of the second cervical vertebra: A case report. J Bone Joint Surg Am 72-A:781, 1990.
23. Hutter RVP, Foote FW, Frazell EL, Francis KC: Giant-cell tumors complicating Paget's disease of bone. Cancer 16:1044, 1963.

24. Hutter RVP, Worcester JW Jr, Francis KC, et al: Benign and malignant giant cell tumors of bone: A clinicopathological analysis of the natural history of the disease. Cancer 15:653, 1962.
25. Huvos AG: Bone Tumors: Diagnosis, Treatment, and Prognosis, 2nd ed. Philadelphia, WB Saunders, 1991, pp 268-291.
26. Huvos AG: Bone Tumors: Diagnosis, Treatment, and Prognosis, 2nd ed. Philadelphia, WB Saunders, 1991, pp 429-467.
27. Johnson EW Jr, Gee VR, Dahlin DC: Giant cell tumors of bone. J Bone Joint Surg Am 41-A:895, 1959.
28. Khan DC, Malhotra S, Stevens RE, et al: Radiotherapy for the treatment of giant cell tumor of the spine: A report of six cases and review of the literature. Cancer Invest 17:110-113, 1999.
29. Kleinman GM, Dagi TF, Poletti CE: Villonodular synovitis in the spinal canal: Case report. J Neurosurg 52:846-848, 1980.
30. Kos CB, Taconis WK, Fidler MW, et al: Multifocal giant cell tumors in the spine: A case report. Spine 22:821-822, 1997.
31. Kricun ME: Tumors of the Spine. In Kricun ME (ed): Imaging of Bone Tumors. Philadelphia, WB Saunders, 1993, p 262.
32. Kuritzky AS, Joyce ST: Giant cell tumor in the ischium: A therapeutic dilemma. JAMA 238:2392, 1977.
33. Lackman RD, Khoury LD, Esmail A, et al: The treatment of sacral giant-cell tumours by serial arterial embolization. J Bone J Surg Br 84-B:873-877, 2002.
34. Larrson SE, Lorentzon R, Boquist L: Giant cell tumors of the spine and sacrum causing neurological symptoms. Clin Orthop 111:201, 1975.
35. Lin PP, Guzel VB, Moura MF, et al: Long-term follow-up of patients with giant cell tumor of the sacrum treated with selective arterial embolization. 95:1317-1325, 2002.
36. Lozes G, Fawaz A, Perper H, et al: Chondroma of the cervical spine: Case report. J Neurosurg 66:128, 1987.
37. Masaryk TJ: Neoplastic disease of the spine. Radiol Clin North Am 29:829, 1991.
38. Mayer BS: Chondromyxoid fibroma of the lumbar spine. J Can Assoc Radiol 29:271, 1978.
39. Mirra JM: Bone Tumors: Clinical, Radiologic, and Pathologic Correlations. Philadelphia, Lea & Febiger, 1989, pp 942-1020.
40. Parrish F: Treatment of bone tumors by total excision and replacement with massive autologous and homologous grafts. J Bone Joint Surg Am 48-A:968, 1966.
41. Potter HG, Schneider R, Ghelman B, et al: Multiple giant cell tumors and Paget disease of bone: Radiographic and clinical correlations. Radiology 180:261, 1991.
42. Regen EM, Haber A: Giant cell tumor of cervical vertebra with unusual symptoms. J Bone Joint Surg Am 39-A:196, 1957.
43. Resnick CS, Lininger JR: Monostatic fibrous dysplasia of the cervical spine. Case report. Radiology 151:49, 1984.
44. Reyes CV, Kathuria S: Recurrent and aggressive chondroblastoma of the pelvis with late malignant neoplastic changes. Am J Surg Pathol 3:449, 1979.
45. Saikia B, Goel A, Gupta SK: Fine-needle aspiration cytologic diagnosis of giant-cell tumor of the sacrum presenting as a rectal mass: A case report. Diagn Cytopathol 24:39-41, 2001.
46. Savini R, Gherlinzoni F, Morandi M, et al: Surgical treatment of giant cell tumor of the spine. J Bone Joint Surg Am 65-A:1283, 1983.
47. Schajowicz F, Granato DB, McDonald DJ, Sundaram M: Clinical and radiological features of atypical giant cell tumours of bone. Br J Radiol 64:877, 1991.
48. Schwartz HS, Jenkins RB, Dahl RJ, Dewald GW: Cytogenic analysis on giant cell tumors of bone. Clin Orthop 240:250, 1989.
49. Schwartz LH, Okunieff PG, Rosenberg A, Suit hd: Radiation therapy in the treatment of difficult giant cell tumors. Int J Radiat Oncol Biol Phys 17:1085, 1989.
50. Seider MJ, Rich TA, Ayala AG, Murray JA: Giant cell tumors of bone: Treatment with radiation therapy. Radiology 161:537, 1986.
51. Shikata J, Yamamuro T, Shimizu K, et al: Surgical treatment of giant cell tumors of the spine. Clin Orthop 278:29, 1992.
52. Sim FJ, McDonald DJ, McLeod RA, Unni KK: Giant cell tumors: Mayo Clinic experience. In Sundaresan N, Schmidek HH, Schiller AL, Rosenthal DI (eds): Tumors of the Spine: Diagnosis and Clinical Management. Philadelphia, WB Saunders, 1990, pp 173-180.
53. Slowik T, Bittner-Manioka M, Grochowski W: Chondroma of the cervical spine: Case report. J Neurosurg 29:276, 1968.
54. Smith J, Wixon D, Watson RC: Giant cell tumor of the sacrum: Clinical and radiologic features in 13 patients. J Can Assoc Radiol 30:34, 1979.
55. Smith MD, Bohlman HH, Gidonse N: Fibrous dysplasia of the cervical spine: A fatal complication of treatment: A case report. J Bone Joint Surg Am 72-A:1254, 1990.
56. Tomita K, Tsuchiya H: Total sacrectomy and reconstruction for huge sacral tumors. Spine 15:12, 1990.
57. Tubbs WS, Brown LR, Beabout JW, et al: Benign giant-cell tumor of bone with pulmonary metastases: Clinical findings and radiologic appearance of metastases in 13 cases. AJR Am J Roentgenol 158:331, 1992.
58. Turcotte RE, Sim FH, Unni KK: Giant cell tumor of the sacrum. Clin Orthop 291:215, 1993.
59. Van Nostrand D, Madewell JE, McNeish LM, et al: Radionuclide bone scanning in giant cell tumor. J Nucl Med 27:329, 1986.
60. Verhagen WI, Bartels RH, Schaafsma HE, et al: A giant cell tumor of the sacrum or a soft tissue giant cell tumor? A case report. Spine 23:1609-1611, 1998.
61. Willis BK, Heilbrun MP: Enchondroma of the cervical spine. Neurosurgery 19:437, 1986.
62. Wisniewski M, Toker C, Anderson PJ, et al: Chondroblastoma of the cervical spine: Case report. J Neurosurg 38:763, 1973.
63. Wuisman P, Lieshout O, Sugihara S, et al: Total sacrectomy and reconstruction: Oncologic and functional outcome. Clin Orthop 381:192-203, 2000.

ANEURYSMAL BONE CYST

Capsule Summary

	Low Back	Neck
Frequency of spinal pain	Common	Common
Location of spinal pain	Lumbar spine	Cervical spine
Quality of spinal pain	Acute onset, increasing severity	Acute onset, increasing severity
Symptoms and signs	Localized bone tenderness, overlying skin erythema	Localized bone tenderness, overlying skin erythema
Laboratory tests	None	None
Radiographic findings	Expansile lesion of the posterior elements on plain roentgenograms	Expansile lesion of the posterior elements on plain roentgenograms
Treatment	En bloc excision	En bloc excision

PREVALENCE AND PATHOGENESIS

The first descriptions of the distinctive characteristics of this lesion are attributed to Jaffe and Lichtenstein in 1950.[22,26] Other names that have been associated with aneurysmal bone cysts (ABCs) include ossifying hematoma, plain bone cysts, and atypical giant cell tumor.

Epidemiology

An ABC is a benign, non-neoplastic, cystic vascular lesion of bone that occurs de novo or in the setting of another bone condition such as giant cell tumor, chondroblastoma, chondromyxoid fibroma, or fibrous dysplasia. ABC represents about 1% to 2% of primary bone lesions.[14,31] Other reports suggest that ABC accounts for 6% of primary bone lesions.[22] The vast majority of young adults in whom ABCs develop are younger than 30 years. Schajowicz has reported on 217 ABCs, a number approximately 50% of the frequency of giant cell tumors.[37] In contrast to the distribution of other primary bone tumors, most series report a slight female preponderance.[3,12] A review of 238 patients with ABCs found that slightly more women were affected (54%).[41] ABCs are occasionally reported in close family members.[15]

Pathogenesis

The cause of ABC remains uncertain. Trauma may play a role in its initiation because injuries may induce the formation of arteriovenous malformations (AVMs). These malformations consist of abnormal vascular channels. Several reports have suggested that the trauma that initiated an AVM may have led to the development of an ABC.[2,16]

In a third of cases, ABC is superimposed on another pathologic process, which may be either a benign or a malignant bone tumor. Primary lesions that may be complicated by an ABC include giant cell tumor, chondroblastoma, chondromyxoid fibroma, nonossifying fibroma, osteoblastoma, fibrosarcoma, fibrous histiocytoma, osteosarcoma, and fibrous dysplasia.[30] The basic abnormality in both circumstances is a local change in intraosseous blood flow. The blood pools in bone, and pooling results in increasing intraosseous pressure followed by resorption, expansion, and cyst formation.[9] The recognition of an underlying causative process is important because the clinical course of the patient may more closely follow that of the primary lesion.

A majority of ABCs occur in the long bones of the extremities; 15% to 25% occur in the spine.[11,25] The lumbosacral spine is affected in 36% of cases, the thoracic spine in 32%, and the cervical spine in 32%. In a review of 256 cases, the cervical spine was the location for 26% of ABCs affecting the axial skeleton.[23]

CLINICAL HISTORY

Patients with ABCs usually have symptoms of pain or swelling in the affected area. The pain is generally of acute onset and increases in severity over a short period. The duration of symptoms can range from months to several years. The patient may also experience limitation of motion.

The clinical manifestations of a spinal ABC vary with the location and size of the lesion. A lesion of the spinous or transverse process may be entirely asymptomatic. Neurologic symptoms and signs include a spectrum of abnormalities from sensory changes to myelopathy or paraplegia, and such manifestations may occur if expansion of the lesion results in nerve root or cauda equina compression.[13,19] Sacral lesions are associated with greater bone destruction, more pathologic fractures, and higher local recurrence rates than lesions in other locations in the spine are.[35] An ABC tends to involve the posterior elements of the vertebra, and giant cell tumor affects the vertebral body. The posterior elements and the vertebral body may be affected simultaneously in large ABCs.[40]

PHYSICAL EXAMINATION

Physical examination may demonstrate tenderness to palpation over the site of involvement. The overlying skin may be erythematous and warm if the ABC is close to the surface. Patients will demonstrate decreased range of motion with muscle spasm.[8] Slightly over 10% of patients may have associated scoliosis or kyphosis.[7] Neurologic findings correlate with the location of nerve root, spinal cord, or cauda equina compression.

LABORATORY DATA

Screening blood test results are normal in this benign, vascular lesion of bone. Patients with secondary cysts will have abnormal results that correspond to their underlying lesion (malignant tumor).

Pathology

On gross inspection, the cyst contains anastomosing cavernous spaces that compose the bulk of the lesion. The blood is unclotted. The presence of unclotted blood indicates that the lesion is a hemodynamically active lesion with pools of blood filling and draining. The pressure in the tumors is arterial.[21] Subperiosteal new bone that is eggshell thin separates the lesion from surrounding tissue.

Histologically, the cystic cavities are composed of vascular channels filled with fibrous connective tissue, osteoid, granulation tissue, and multinucleated giant cells (Fig. 13-18).[3] The solid portions of an ABC may be fibrous but may contain a lacework of osteoid trabeculae.

The "solid" variant of ABC occurs most commonly in long tubular bones but occasionally affects the axial skeleton. Histologically, the lesion is characterized by florid fibroblastic proliferation with osteoclast-like giant cell–rich areas, stromal hemorrhage, and newly formed osteoid. The histology is similar to that of an ABC except for the presence of blood-filled spaces.[33]

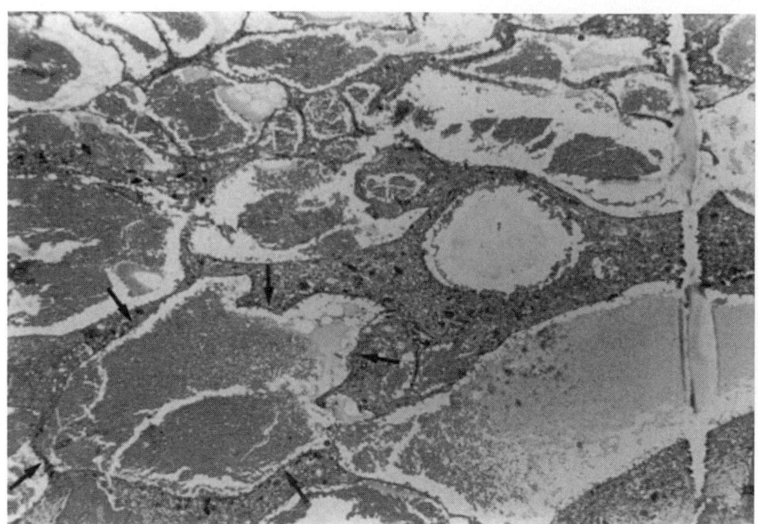

Figure 13-18 Aneurysmal bone cyst. Histologic section exhibiting large vascular channels *(arrows)*. The intravascular stroma contains giant cells that are benign. In contrast to normal vessels, the vascular spaces are not lined by endothelial cells. This lesion must be differentiated from telangiectatic osteosarcoma, which will contain vascular channels but will also show atypical cells with bizarre mitotic figures within a sarcomatous stroma. *(Courtesy of Arnold Schwartz, MD.)*

RADIOGRAPHIC FINDINGS

The roentgenographic features of an ABC consist of a solitary, eccentrically located, osteolytic expansile lesion that is sharply demarcated by a thin subperiosteal shell of bone. The cyst cavity is traversed by fine strands of bony cortex. A soft tissue mass may also be associated with the bony lesion. When in the spine, ABCs occur most commonly in the lumbar and thoracic areas and affect the posterior elements of the vertebrae, including the pedicles, laminae, and spinous and transverse processes in 60% of lesions (Fig. 13-19). About 30% to 40% occur in the vertebral bodies.[16] A lesion within the vertebral body may involve more than one vertebra by extension across the apophyseal joint or disc space.[1] Lesions may attain a considerable size. In the lumbar or sacral area, cysts may displace the kidney or ureter and may compress other pelvic organs.[17] The lesion may also expand to encroach on the neural canal.[10]

Computed Tomography

CT is useful in the diagnosis of ABCs, especially for lesions in the axial skeleton. Multiple fluid levels (layering of solid blood components) on CT are suggestive, but not diagnostic of an ABC.[20] CT may show a thin rim of bone not evident on roentgenograms, which helps exclude calcified tumor matrix (Fig. 13-20).

Magnetic Resonance

MR may be useful in identifying the extent of lesions in bone and soft tissue.[42] MR images show the expansile appearance of the lesion. The soft tissue extension of all cysts is well defined with a sharp interface. The fibrous tissue in the periphery of the tumor is highlighted by a low-intensity signal in the rim of the lesion on both T1- and T2-weighted sequences. By increasing the T2-weighting of sequences, fluid levels are also detected by MR evaluation.[32] Fluid levels may likewise accompany telangiectatic osteosarcoma, giant cell tumor, and chondroblastoma.

DIFFERENTIAL DIAGNOSIS

The characteristic radiographic appearance of an ABC helps differentiate it from other benign and malignant lesions. The posterior arch and the transverse or spinous process are the common locations of involvement in the spine. A solitary lytic lesion of the anterior body of a vertebra is more likely to be a metastasis, infection, or giant cell tumor. It is also important to remember that some primary bone tumors, including chondroblastoma and giant cell tumor, may have areas that histologically appear like

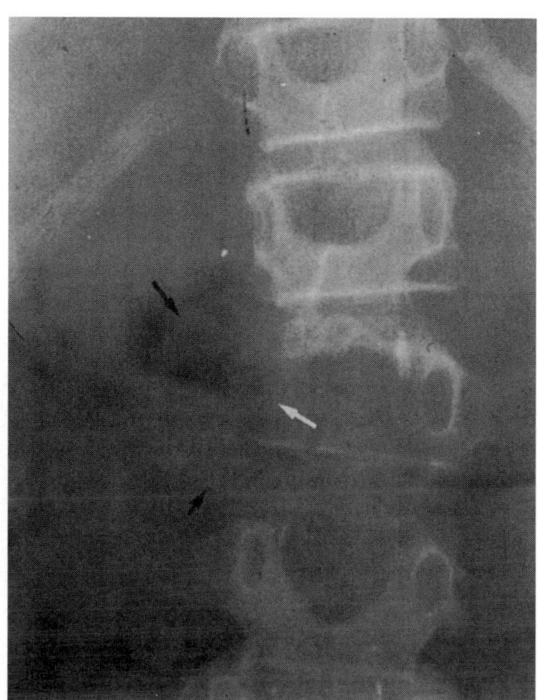

Figure 13-19 Aneurysmal bone cyst arising from the posterior elements of the second lumbar vertebra. Notice the loss of the pedicle *(white arrow)* and the faint line of calcification lateral to the vertebral body *(black arrows)*. *(Courtesy of Anne Brower, MD.)*

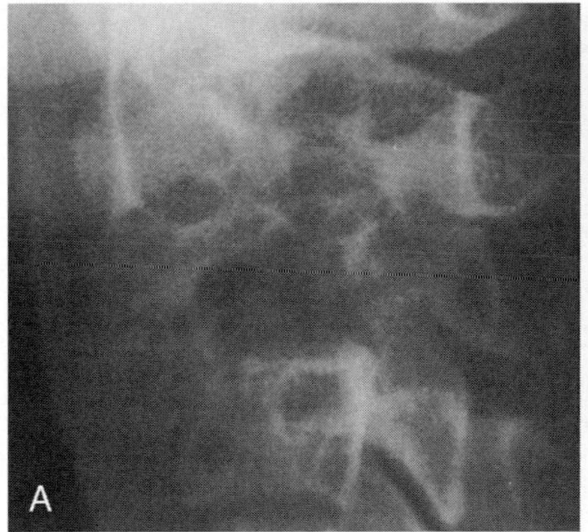

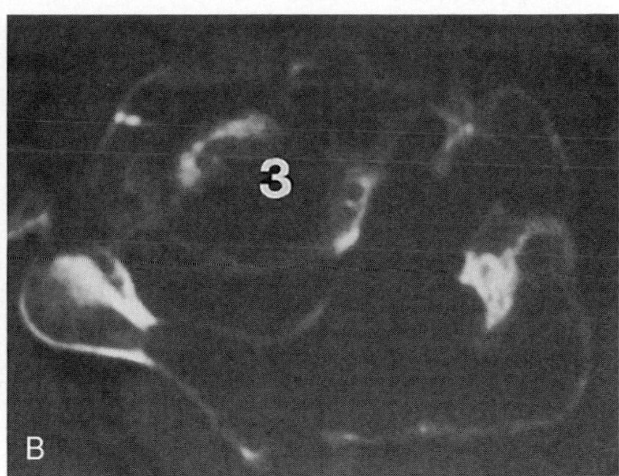

Figure 13-20 In this child, routine radiography, *A*, shows an expansile, osteolytic lesion of the body and posterior elements of the third cervical vertebra. Transaxial CT, *B*, confirms the extent of involvement and the expansile nature of the lesion. *(Courtesy of L. Pinckney, MD, San Diego, California.)*

ABCs. Careful evaluation of the entire specimen should alert the pathologist to the underlying lesion.

TREATMENT

ABCs can be treated by surgery, radiotherapy, or cryotherapy. Although they are benign lesions, they are highly prone to local recurrence after curettage. If the location of an ABC allows removal of a section of bone without loss of function, en bloc resection is the treatment of choice, and lesions in the posterior elements of the spine may be treated by resection and bone grafting.[6,36,39] Excision of the tumor is associated with postoperative resolution of pain.[4] Lesions that are too large or involve a vertebral body are treated with radiotherapy.[38] Radiation therapy controls the growth of lesions in inaccessible locations.[27] The benefit of radiotherapy must be weighed against the potential for radiation-induced sarcoma many years later. In a large series of 41 patients, the combination of curettage and radiotherapy produced the greatest frequency of late axial deformity.[5] Cryosurgery, or freezing the lesion, has also been reported to halt expansion of the cyst and prevent recurrence.[3,29]

Embolization of the tumor with polyvinyl alcohol particles may slow the growth of tumors. Lesions may then calcify over a period of months.[10] On occasion, spontaneous healing of a cyst may occur. Lesions may stabilize for extended periods. Older patients are more likely candidates for spontaneous tumor healing.[28]

PROGNOSIS

An ABC is a benign lesion but may cause severe dysfunction because of its expansile characteristics. In a study of 52 consecutive patients, 96% were tumor free after excision. Only 10% had a recurrence within 10 years.[34] If the lesion is diagnosed early and treated appropriately, dysfunction may be kept to a minimum. However, if it is located in the spine and allowed to expand unchecked, serious neurologic deficits may result. In addition, an ABC weakens the bone and increases the risk of pathologic fracture. Lesions in the cervical spine may require excision and fusion with a bone graft and wire.[18] In rare circumstances, the cyst may transform into a malignant tumor, particularly after irradiation.[24]

References

Aneurysmal Bone Cyst

1. Banna M: Clinical Radiology of the Spine and the Spinal Cord. Rockville, Md, Aspen, 1985, pp 347-348.
2. Barnes R: Aneurysmal bone cyst. J Bone Joint Surg Br 38-B:301, 1956.
3. Biesecker JL, Marcove RC, Huvos AG, and Mike V: Aneurysmal bone cyst: A clinicopathologic study of 66 cases. Cancer 26:615, 1970.
4. Bohlman HH, Sachs BL, Carter JR, et al: Primary neoplasms of the cervical spine. J Bone Joint Surg Am 68-A:483, 1986.
5. Boriani S, De Lure F, Campanacci L, et al: Aneurysmal bone cyst of the mobile skeleton. 26:27-35, 2001.
6. Buck RE, Bailey RW: Replacement of a cervical vertebral body for aneurysmal bone cyst. J Bone Joint Surg Am 51-A:1656, 1969.
7. Capanna R, Albisinni U, Picci P, et al: Aneurysmal bone cyst of the spine. J Bone Joint Surg Am 67-A:527, 1985.
8. Chakravarty K, Brett F, Merry P: Aneurysmal bone cyst: An unusual presentation of neck pain in a young adult. Br J Rheumatol 33:597, 1994.
9. Clough JR, Price CHG: Aneurysmal bone cyst: Pathogenesis and long term results of treatment. Clin Orthop 97:52, 1973.
10. Cory DA, Fritsch SA, Cohen MD, et al: Aneurysmal bone cysts: Imaging findings and embolotherapy. AJR Am J Roentgenol 153:369, 1989.
11. Dabska M, Buraczewski J: Aneurysmal bone cyst: Pathology, clinical course and radiologic appearance. Cancer 23:371, 1969.
12. Dahlin DC, Besse BE, Pugh DG, Ghormley RK: Aneurysmal bone cysts. Radiology 64:56, 1955.
13. Dahlin DC, McLeod RA: Aneurysmal bone cyst and other nonneoplastic conditions. Skeletal Radiol 8:243, 1982.
14. Dahlin DC, Unni KK: Bone Tumors. General Aspects and Data on 8,542 Cases, 4th ed. Springfield, IL, Charles C Thomas, 1986, pp 420-430.
15. DiCaprio MR, Murphy MJ, Camp RL: Aneurysmal bone cyst of the spine with familial incidence. Spine 25:1589-1592, 2000.
16. Donaldson WF: Aneurysmal bone cyst. J Bone Joint Surg Am 44-A:25, 1962.
17. Faure C, Boccon-Gibod L, Herve J, Pernin P: Case report 154. Skeletal Radiol 6:229, 1981.
18. Gupta VK, Gupta SK, Khosla VK, et al: Aneurysmal bone cysts of the spine. Surg Neurol 42:428, 1994.
19. Hay MC, Patterson D, Taylor TKF: Aneurysmal bone cysts of the spine. J Bone Joint Surg Br 60-B:406, 1978.
20. Hudson TM: Fluid levels in aneurysmal bone cysts: A CT feature. AJR Am J Roentgenol 141:1001, 1984.
21. Huvos AG: Bone Tumors: Diagnosis, Treatment, and Prognosis, 2nd ed. Philadelphia, WB Saunders, 1991, pp 727-743.
22. Jaffe HL: Aneurysmal bone cyst. Bull Hosp Jt Dis 11:3, 1950.
23. Kricun ME: Tumors of the Spine. In Kricun ME (ed): Imaging of Bone Tumors. Philadelphia, WB Saunders, 1993, pp 260-262.
24. Kyriakos M, Hardy D: Malignant transformation of aneurysmal bone cyst, with an analysis of the literature. Cancer 68:1770, 1991.
25. Lichtenstein L: Aneurysmal bone cyst: Observations on fifty cases. J Bone Joint Surg Am 39-A:873, 1957.

26. Lichtenstein L: Aneurysmal bone cyst: A pathological entity commonly mistaken for a giant cell tumor and occasionally for hemangioma and osteogenic sarcoma. Cancer 3:279, 1950.
27. Maeda M, Tateishi H, Takaiwa H, et al: High-energy, low-dose radiation therapy for aneurysmal bone cyst: Report of a case. Clin Orthop 243:200, 1989.
28. Malghem J, Maldague B, Esselinckx W, et al: Spontaneous healing of aneurysmal bone cysts: A report of three cases. J Bone Joint Surg Br 71-B:645, 1989.
29. Marcove RC, Miller TR: The treatment of primary and metastatic bone localized tumors by cryosurgery. Surg Clin North Am 49:421, 1969.
30. Martinez V, Sissons HA: Aneurysmal bone cyst: A review of 123 cases including primary lesions and those secondary to other bone pathology. Cancer 81:2291, 1988.
31. Mirra J: Bone Tumors: Clinical, Radiologic, and Pathologic Correlations. Philadelphia, Lea & Febiger, 1989, pp 1267-1312.
32. Munk PL, Helms CA, Holt RG, et al: MR imaging of aneurysmal bone cysts. AJR Am J Roentgenol 153:99, 1989.
33. Oda Y, Tsuneyoshi M, Shinohara N: Solid variant of aneurysmal bone cyst (extragnathic giant cell reparative granuloma) in the axial skeleton and long bones. Cancer 70:2642, 1992.
34. Papgelopoulos PJ, Choudhury SN, Frassica FJ, et al: Treatment of aneurysmal bone cysts of the pelvis and sacrum. J Bone Joint Surg Am 83-A:1674-1681, 2001.
35. Papagelopoulos PJ, Currier BL, Shaughnessy WJ, et al: Aneurysmal bone cyst of the spine. Management and outcome. Spine 23:621-628, 1998.
36. Parrish FF, Pevey JK: Surgical management of aneurysmal bone cyst of the vertebral column. J Bone Joint Surg Am 49-A:1597, 1967.
37. Schajowicz F: Tumors and Tumorlike Lesions of Bone: Pathology, Radiology, and Treatment, 2nd ed. Berlin, Springer-Verlag, 1994, pp 514-531.
38. Slowick FA, Campbell CJ, Kettelkamp DB: Aneurysmal bone cyst. J Bone Joint Surg Am 50-A:1142, 1968.
39. Stillwell WT, Fielding JW: Aneurysmal bone cyst of the cervicodorsal spine. Clin Orthop 187:144, 1984.
40. Tillman BP, Dahlin DC, Lipscomb PR, et al: Aneurysmal bone cyst: An analysis of ninety-five cases. Mayo Clin Proc 43:478, 1968.
41. Vergel AM, Bond JR, Shives TC, et al: Aneurysmal bone cyst: A clinicopathologic study of 238 cases. Cancer 69:2921, 1991.
42. Zimmer WD, Berquist TH, Sim FH, et al: Magnetic resonance imaging of aneurysmal bone cysts. Mayo Clin Proc 59:633, 1984.

HEMANGIOMA

Capsule Summary

	Low Back	Neck
Frequency of spinal pain	Uncommon	Rare
Location of spinal pain	Lumbar spine	Cervical spine
Quality of spinal pain	Throbbing, ache	Throbbing, ache
Symptoms and signs	Localized tenderness, decreased motion	Localized tenderness, decreased motion
Laboratory tests	None	None
Radiographic findings	Prominent vertical vertebral body striations on plain roentgenograms	Prominent vertical vertebral body striations on plain roentgenograms
Treatment	Radiation for symptomatic lesions	Radiation for symptomatic lesions

PREVALENCE AND PATHOGENESIS

Hemangioma is a benign vascular lesion composed of cavernous, capillary, or venous blood vessels that may affect soft tissues or bone. The first reference to a hemangioma was reported by Toynbee in 1845.[41] A multitude of types of this vascular lesion have been described, including capillary, cavernous, venous, hypertrophic, juvenile, arteriovenous, intramuscular, synovial, and histiocytic hemangioma.

Epidemiology

Hemangiomas account for less than 1% of clinically symptomatic primary bone tumors.[31,42] However, necropsy studies by a number of investigators have demonstrated that asymptomatic vertebral lesions are found in 12% of autopsied specimens.[29,37] The prevalence of hemangioma increases with age, with 25% of the lesions present in adults by the fifth decade of life. They are usually identified in patients between the fourth and fifth decades. Taking into account hemangiomas from all sites, women and men are equally affected.

Approximately 50% of patients with a hemangioma will have the lesion in the spine or skull. The thoracic spine is the location for 65% of spinal lesions; the cervical spine, 25%; and the lumbar spine, 10%.[42] In a review of 59 patients with vertebral hemangiomas, the distribution of lesions was the thoracic spine in 54%, the lumbar spine in 39%, and the cervical spine in 7%.[14]

Pathogenesis

The pathogenesis of hemangioma remains unknown. The lesions are thought to be congenital vascular malformations by some and benign neoplasms by others.

CLINICAL HISTORY

The initial complaints of patients with symptomatic vertebral hemangiomas are localized pain and tenderness over the involved vertebra along with associated muscle spasm.[21] The pain usually starts as a vague, nondescript ache that gradually increases in intensity and duration until it becomes constant and throbbing. Neurologic manifestations of cord compression by a vertebral hemangioma may include sensory changes, motor weakness, radiculitis, and transverse myelitis.[3,30] In a study reported by Fox and Onofrio, 22% of vertebral hemangiomas were initially manifested as neck or back pain.[14]

Multiple hemangiomas may cause spinal cord compression resembling metastatic disease to the spine.[44] Neurologic symptoms tend to occur at the time of expansion of a lesion in the vertebral body into the epidural space, pathologic fracture, or extradural hematoma.[33] Symptoms may include radicular pain, weakness or paralysis in a leg, and sensory deficits. When a lumbar vertebra is involved, patients may experience bilateral sciatica and sphincter and sexual abnormalities.[35] Neurologic symptoms may occur acutely and recurrently.[34] Many of the hemangiomas that cause neurologic symptoms are located in the thoracic spine where the spinal canal is narrow.[43] In women who are pregnant, increased venous pressure may develop and result in hemangiomas becoming symptomatic and causing nerve compression secondary to bleeding.[10,39] In the study by Fox and Onofrio, one in four cervical hemangiomas was associated with a neurologic deficit.[14]

PHYSICAL EXAMINATION

Physical examination may demonstrate tenderness with palpation over the affected vertebral body. Limitation of motion may be present if the related muscle spasm is severe.

Hemangiomas that expand bone may cause palpable swelling. Increased weakening of the vertebral body may result in fractures, which will markedly increase tenderness, and muscle spasm.[7] Increased pain and spasm may also result in kyphoscoliosis.[17] Hemangiomas may occur in the setting of systemic hemangiomatosis. Peripheral hemangiomas in the skin are associated with hemangiomas in the vertebral bodies.[1] In these circumstances, hemangiomas may be noted on the skin, mucous membranes, and other organs (multiple hemangiomatosis of bone or Osler-Weber-Rendu disease).[19,32]

LABORATORY DATA

Screening blood test results are normal in this benign lesion of bone. Occasionally, the erythrocyte sedimentation rate (ESR) is elevated.[18] Rarely, a consumptive coagulopathy with thrombocytopenia has been reported in patients with multiple vertebral hemangiomas.[27] This syndrome, Kasabach-Merritt syndrome, is characterized by multiple hemangiomas and hemangioendotheliomas.[9]

Pathology

On gross examination, the well-demarcated lesion is reddish brown and either is confined to the vertebral body or extends into the surrounding soft tissue. The vertebral body is the preferential location of primary involvement, with secondary extension into the arch or transverse process. Microscopically, a hemangioma is composed of numerous capillary and larger vascular channels contained in a fibrous stroma. The trabeculae that are not affected by the tumor are thickened in comparison to the lesional, thinned osseous trabeculae.[21]

RADIOGRAPHIC EVALUATION

Roentgenograms

Vertebral hemangiomas primarily involve the vertebral bodies.[40] In an affected vertebral body, vertical striations are prominent, but horizontal striations are absent because of absorption. This pattern gives rise to a "corduroy" appearance of the vertebral body (Fig. 13-21), most prominent on the lateral projection. The alteration in vertebral striations is diffuse, and the configuration of the vertebral body is usually unchanged (see Fig. 13-23). Occasionally, vertebral body hemangiomas may extend from the body to the laminae, pedicles, or transverse or spinous processes. Rarely, expansion or enlargement of a vertebra may occur.[30]

Symptomatic vertebral hemangiomas may have thinner and wider vertical striations. They may be associated with vertebral body collapse, hemorrhage, and soft tissue masses.[2] Hemangiomas rarely cause compression fractures because of buttressing of the weaker components by the coarse, remaining trabeculations.[30] A radiologic study of 57 solitary vertebral hemangiomas identified six factors associated with a greater likelihood of spinal cord compression. These factors

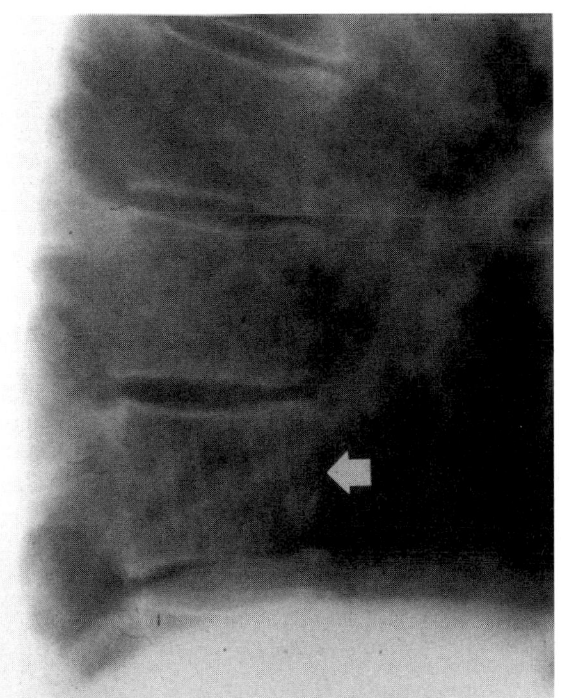

Figure 13-21 Hemangioma of a thoracic vertebra revealing radiolucency of the vertebral body and accentuation of the vertical trabeculation, which gives it a corduroy appearance *(arrow)*. *(Courtesy of Anne Brower, MD.)*

included location in the thoracic spine, involvement of the entire vertebral body, extension into the neural arch, an expanded cortex with indistinct margins, an irregular honeycomb pattern, and a soft tissue mass. Only one hemangioma at the L3 level was associated with compressive signs.[24]

Scintigraphy

Bone scintigraphy demonstrates increased uptake of tracer at the site of the vertebral hemangioma. The bone scan may demonstrate decreased uptake if the hemangioma has become thrombosed.[16]

Computed Tomography

Examination by CT demonstrates the bony changes of hemangioma, including expansion of the body and involvement of the arch (Figs. 13-22 and 13-23). Soft tissue extension is also noted on CT examination with or without contrast.[38]

Magnetic Resonance

MR examination of hemangiomas demonstrates increased signal intensity on both T1- and T2-weighted images. Increased signal intensity corresponds with fatty stroma (T1) and vascularization (T2) (Fig. 13-24). Histologic evaluation of hemangiomas confirmed the higher T1 and T2 signal intensities to be related to adipocytes and interstitial edema, respectively.[5] The aggressiveness of hemangiomas associated with expansion has been related to the absence of fat and increased degree of vascularity as measured by MR.[25]

Angiography

Angiography may help in identifying blood vessels that are feeding the tumor. Occasionally, hemorrhage may impede filling of the tumor during angiography.[38] Angiography does not distinguish hemangioma from other vascular tumors.

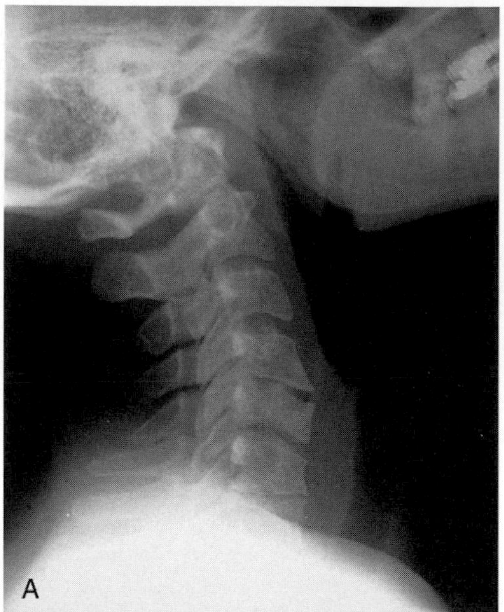

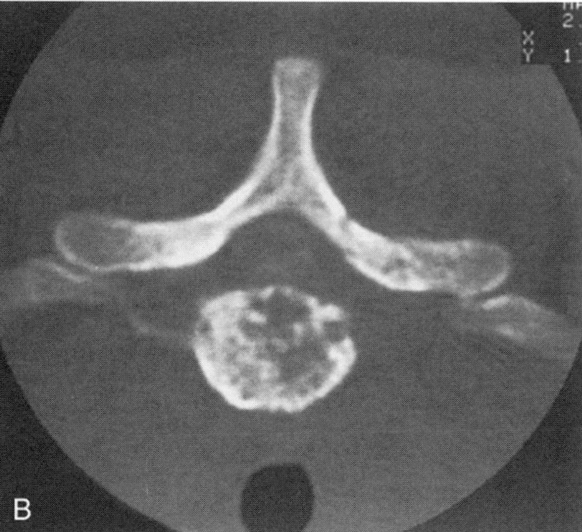

Figure 13-22 Hemangiomas in the cervical vertebral bodies (C4, C5, and C7) of an 18-year-old woman. *A*, A lateral view of the cervical spine shows prominence of the vertical striations. *B*, A CT scan of the cervical spine shows areas of osteolysis of the vertebral body and posterior lamina. *(Courtesy of Anne Brower, MD.)*

DIFFERENTIAL DIAGNOSIS

The diagnosis of a vertebral hemangioma is uncomplicated when one vertebral body demonstrates the characteristic radiographic changes. It is more difficult when portions of a vertebra other than the body are affected. Bony resorption of a pedicle may mimic the destructive changes of metastatic cancer. A vertebral body fracture may occur with a hemangioma, but it is more frequently seen in metastatic tumor.

Skeletal Lymphangiomatosis

Skeletal lymphangiomatosis may affect vertebral bodies and cause increased striation, bony lysis with bone compression, and progressive scoliosis. Lymphangiography may be required to confirm this diagnosis. Histologically, lymphoid tissue is present to an increased degree in the vascular channels of the bone.[36]

Gorham's Disease

A closely related, but very rare cause of vertebral bone loss that may resemble hemangiomatosis is Gorham's disease (massive osteolysis).[21,42] Multiple hemangiomas develop with total lysis of the affected bone and periosteum. The bone is replaced by fibrous tissue. The disease may either be self-limited or progress to a fatal outcome.[20] A fatal outcome may occur despite therapy with radiation.[8] Patients with structural instability of the cervical spine secondary to Gorham's disease have been reported.[11]

Other Vascular Tumors

Hemangiopericytoma is also a very rare vascular tumor that may mimic hemangioma.[29] Angiolipoma is another tumor affecting vertebrae that may cause spinal cord compression, and it must be differentiated from a hemangioma.[23]

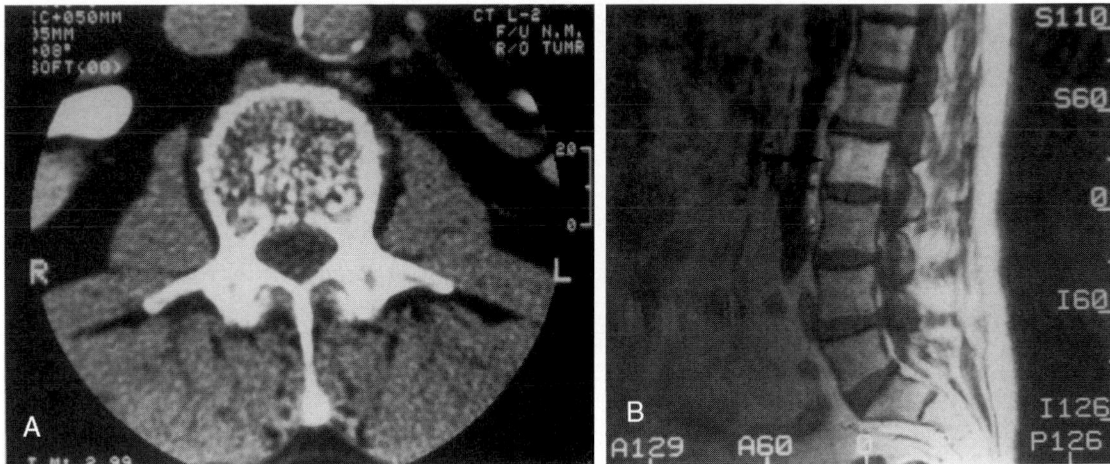

Figure 13-23 CT *(A)* and MR *(B)* scans of the lumbosacral spine in a 68-year-old man with neck pain and headaches secondary to osteoarthritis of the cervical spine. CT demonstrates loss of trabeculae in the vertebral body secondary to increased vascular channels. MR reveals increased signal in a T1-weighted image of the same vertebral body *(arrow)*. This lesion was asymptomatic.

Angiosarcoma is a very rare malignant tumor that may affect similar areas of the vertebral column as hemangiomas.[12]

Coarse trabeculation of a vertebral body may also be seen in Paget's disease. Abnormal laboratory tests (elevated ESR, serum alkaline phosphatase) should differentiate tumor and Paget's disease from a hemangioma.

TREATMENT

The treatment of choice for symptomatic vertebral hemangiomas is irradiation because the lesions are radiosensitive. Radiation therapy effectively relieves symptoms even though the appearance of the lesion remains unchanged.[28] Postoperative radiotherapy is recommended when tumor removal is subtotal.[26] Surgical intervention in the form of laminectomy is associated with excessive morbidity and mortality because of profuse hemorrhage. Therefore, laminectomy should be reserved for patients with neurologic deficits who require decompression of the spinal cord. Embolization of feeder vessels before surgery may render surgical decompression a safer procedure.[22] Embolization alone may be successful in controlling growth of the tumor, or it may be used in combination with radiation therapy or surgery to reverse neurologic symptoms.[6,13,35] A new technique is injection of methylmethacrylate into symptomatic vertebral bodies containing hemangiomas under the guidance of CT and fluoroscopy. Although the efficiency of this technique in preventing collapse cannot be evaluated, the injection is associated with resolution of pain.[15] Injection with ethanol can also relieve the pain of hemangiomas.[4]

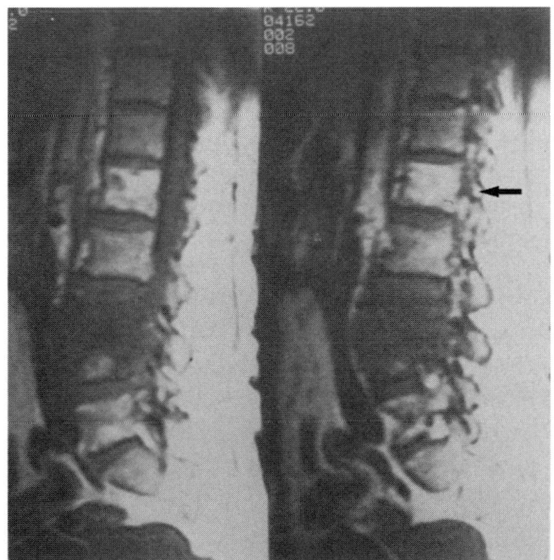

Figure 13-24 A T1-weighted MR image demonstrates an incidental finding of a hemangioma at L1 *(black arrow)* with discitis at the L3–L4 level.

PROGNOSIS

Vertebral hemangiomas are usually asymptomatic and have a benign course; however, when they become symptomatic, therapy is required to prevent expansion of the lesion. The major complication of a vertebral hemangioma is neural compression. Compression fractures may occur in vertebrae affected by a hemangioma. Hemangiomas may cause neural compression by compression fracture, expansion of an involved vertebra, direct extension of the hemangioma into the extradural space, or extradural hemorrhage. Appropriate diagnosis and treatment may help prevent such potentially disabling complications of this vascular neoplasm.

References

Hemangioma

1. Asumu TO, Williamson B, Hughes DG: Symptomatic spinal hemangiomas in association with cutaneous hemangiomas: A case report. Spine 21:1082-1084, 1996.
2. Banna M: Clinical Radiology of the Spine and the Spinal Cord. Rockville, Md, Aspen, 1985, pp 341-345.
3. Barnard L, Von Nuys RG: Primary hemangioma of the spine. Ann Surg 97:19, 1933.

4. Bas T, Aparisi F, Bas J: Efficacy of safety of ethanol injections in 18 cases of vertebral hemangioma: A mean follow-up of 2 years. Spine 26:1577-1582, 2001.
5. Baudrez V, Galant C, Vande Berg BC: Benign vertebral hemangiomas: MR-histological correlation. Skeletal Radiol 30:442-446, 2001.
6. Bednar DA, Esses SI: Double hemangioma of the spine with paraparesis: A case report. Spine 15:1377, 1990.
7. Bergstrand A, Hook O, Lidvall H: Vertebral hemangiomas compressing the spinal cord. Acta Neurol Scand 39:59, 1963.
8. Bohlman HH, Sachs BL, Carter JR, et al: Primary neoplasms of the cervical spine. J Bone Joint Surg Am 68-A:483, 1986.
9. Brower TD: Case records of the Massachusetts General Hospital. N Engl J Med 320:854, 1989.
10. Castel E, Lazennec JY, Chiras J, et al: Acute spinal cord compression due to intraspinal bleeding from a vertebral hemangiomas: Two case-reports. Eur Spine J 8:244-248, 1999.
11. Castleman B: Case records of the Massachusetts General Hospital. N Engl J Med 270:731, 1964.
12. Dagi TF, Schmidek HH: Vascular tumors of the spine. In Sundaresan N, Schmidek HH, Schiller AL, Rosenthal DI (eds): Tumors of the Spine: Diagnosis and Clinical Management. Philadelphia, WB Saunders, 1990, pp 181-191.
13. Djindijian M, Nguyen J, Gaston A, et al: Multiple vertebral hemangiomas with neurological signs: Case report. J Neurosurg 76:1025, 1992.
14. Fox MW, Onofrio BM: The natural history and management of symptomatic and asymptomatic vertebral hemangiomas. J Neurosurg 78:36, 1993.
15. Gangi A, Kastler BA, Dietmann JL: Percutaneous vertebroplasty guided by a combination of CT and fluoroscopy. AJNR Am J Neuroradiol 15:83, 1994.
16. Gerard PS, Wilck E: Spinal hemangioma: An unusual photopenic presentation on bone scan. Spine 17:607, 1992.
17. Ghormley RK, Adson AW: Hemangioma of vertebrae. J Bone Joint Surg 23:887, 1941.
18. Govender S, Charles RW, Kelman IE: Vertebral haemangiomas: A report of 2 cases. S Afr Med J 72:640, 1987.
19. Gutierrez R, Spjut J: Skeletal angiomatosis: Report of 3 cases and review of the literature. Clin Orthop 85:82, 1972.
20. Hambach R, Pujman J, Maly V: Massive osteolysis due to hemangiomatosis. Report of a case of Gorham's disease with autopsy. Radiology 71:43, 1958.
21. Huvos AG: Bone Tumors: Diagnosis, Treatment, and Prognosis, 2nd ed. Philadelphia, WB Saunders, 1991, pp 553-578.
22. Kapur P, Banna M: Spinous osseous angioma: Gelfoam embolization. J Can Assoc Radiol 31:271, 1980.
23. Kuroda S, Abe H, Akino M, et al: Infiltrating spinal angiolipoma causing myelopathy: Case report. Neurosurgery 27:315, 1990.
24. Laredo J, Reizine D, Bard M, Merland J: Vertebral hemangions: Radiologic evaluation. Radiology 161:183, 1986.
25. Laredo J, Assouline E, Gelbert F, et al: Vertebral hemangiomas: Fat content as a sign of aggressiveness. Radiology 177:467, 1990.
26. Lee S, Hadlow AT: Extraosseous extension of vertebral hemangiomas, a rare cause of spinal cord compression. Spine 24:2111-2114, 1999.
27. Lozman J, Holmblad J: Cavernous hemangiomas associated with scoliosis and a localized consumptive coagulopathy: A case report. J Bone Joint Surg Am 58-A:1021, 1976.
28. Manning JH: Symptomatic hemangioma of the spine. Radiology 56:58, 1951.
29. Marcial-Rojas RA: Primary hemangiopericytoma of bone: Review of the literature and report of the first case with metastasis. Cancer 13:308, 1960.
30. McAllister VL, Kendall BE, Bull JWD: Symptomatic vertebral hemangiomas. Brain 98:71, 1975.
31. Mirra J: Bone Tumors: Clinical, Radiologic, and Pathologic Correlations. Philadelphia, WB Saunders, 1989, pp 1338-1377.
32. Mirra JM, Arnold WD: Skeletal hemangiomatosis in association with hereditary hemorrhagic telangiectasia. J Bone Joint Surg Am 55-A:850, 1973.
33. Mohan V, Gupta SK, Tuli SM, Sanyal B: Symptomatic vertebral hemangiomas. Clin Radiol 31:575, 1980.
34. Newmark J, Jones HR Jr, Thomas CB, et al: Vertebral hemangioma causing acute recurrent spinal cord compression. J Neurol Neurosurg Psychiatry 54:471, 1991.
35. Raco A, Ciappetta P, Artico M, et al: Vertebral hemangiomas with cord compression: The rolè of embolization in five cases. Surg Neurol 34:164, 1990.
36. Reilly BJ, Davison JW, Bain H: Lymphangiectasis of the skeleton: A case report. Radiology 103:385, 1972.
37. Schmorl G, Junghanns H: The Human Spine in Health and Disease, 2nd ed. New York, Grune & Stratton, 1971, p 325.
38. Schnyder P, Frankhauser H, Mansouri B: Computed tomography in spinal hemangioma with cord compression. Report of two cases. Skeletal Radiol 15:372, 1986.
39. Schwartz DA, Nair S, Hershey B, et al: Vertebral arch hemangioma producing spinal cord compression in pregnancy: Diagnosis by magnetic resonance imaging. Spine 14:888, 1989.
40. Sherman RS, Wilner D: The roentgen diagnosis of hemangioma of bone. AJR Am J Roentgenol 86:1146, 1961.
41. Toynbee J: An account of two vascular tumors developed in the substance of bone. Lancet 2:676, 1845.
42. Unni KK: Dahlin's Bone Tumors: General Aspects and Data on 11,087 Cases, 5th ed. Philadelphia, Lippincott-Raven, 1996, pp 307-316.
43. Yung BC, Loke TK, Yuen NW, et al: Spinal cord compression caused by thoracic vertebra hemangiomas involving only the posterior elements of two contiguous vertebrae. Skeletal Radiol 27: 169-172, 1998.
44. Zito G, Kadis GW: Multiple vertebral hemangiomas resembling metastases with spinal cord compression. Arch Neurol 37:247, 1980.

EOSINOPHILIC GRANULOMA

Capsule Summary

	Low Back	Neck
Frequency of spinal pain	Common	Common
Location of spinal pain	Lumbar spine	Cervical spine
Quality of spinal pain	Localized aching	Localized aching
Symptoms and signs	Nontender swelling	Nontender swelling
Laboratory tests	Occasional peripheral eosinophilia	Occasional peripheral eosinophilia
Radiographic findings	Osteolysis without sclerosis in a vertebral body on plain roentgenogram, epidural extension of granuloma on MR	Osteolysis without sclerosis in a vertebral body on plain roentgenogram, epidural extension of granuloma on MR
Treatment	Curettage	Curettage

PREVALENCE AND PATHOGENESIS

Eosinophilic granuloma (EG) occurs in solitary and multifocal forms and is characterized by the infiltration of bone with histiocytes, mononuclear phagocytic cells, and eosinophils. EG, Hand-Schüller-Christian disease, and Letterer-Siwe disease are thought to have the same pathogenesis and are referred to collectively as histiocytosis X. EG is the mildest form and Letterer-Siwe disease the most aggressive form of histiocytosis X.

The first reference to the term *eosinophilic granuloma* was made by Jaffe and Lichtenstein in 1944.[18] In the past, this lesion has gone by many different names, including pseudotuberculous granuloma, Taratynov's disease, traumatic myeloma, and histiocytic granuloma.

Epidemiology

EG is a rare lesion that occurs in less than 1% of primary infiltrative lesions of bone examined by biopsy.[28] It occurs most commonly in children and adolescents, with approximately 10% of patients being 20 years or older.[8] It has a higher incidence in males with a 3:1 ratio in adults.[17] EG is more frequent in whites than blacks. Approximately 1200 new cases of EG are reported yearly in the United States.[25]

Pathogenesis

The pathogenesis of EG is not known. This disease belongs to the nonlipid histiocytoses, which are characterized by proliferation of histiocytes without a demonstrable disorder in lipid metabolism. These histiocytes accumulate cytoplasmic lipid, but unlike true lipid metabolic disorders (Gaucher's disease), these lipids develop as a consequence of the ingestion of necrotic debris rather than an inborn error of metabolism. The cause of this lipid accumulation is unknown. Some investigators have suggested that EG may be the result of a viral infection, but this hypothesis remains unproven.[33] Immunologic alterations have been demonstrated in patients with EG. The immunologic changes are associated with abnormal histologic findings in the thymus.[34] Autoimmune complexes have been implicated as a possible cause of this disorder, thus suggesting an immunologic origin for the disease.[30] Another suggested immunologic abnormality includes a deficiency of suppressor T lymphocytes that results in uncontrolled proliferation of monocytes and macrophages.[37]

Approximately 10% of patients with unifocal EG have lesions in the spine. They are equally dispersed through the lumbar, thoracic, and cervical spine.[28] EG involving the spine was first recognized by Compere and colleagues in 1954.[9] Macnab first described EG in the cervical spine in 1955.[26] A review of 32 cases of EG affecting the cervical spine was reported by Dickson and Farhat.[11] Unifocal (solitary) bone involvement is twice as common as multifocal osseous involvement. EG may affect multiple spinal levels.[36]

CLINICAL HISTORY

The symptoms of spinal EG vary with the location and severity of the lesion. Spinal pain that is constant is the most common complaint in up to 87% of patients.[11] The pain is not relieved with rest or aspirin. The lesion may cause restricted motion and muscle spasm. A palpable mass may be noted if a lesion is close to the skin. Symptoms of spinal cord compression are uncommon but may occur secondary to vertebral body collapse or dislocation. Patients with EG may have neurologic symptoms, including radicular pain and paresthesias.[20] In the cervical spine, the extremities (arms and legs) and visceral functions may be affected in patients with cervical cord compression.[1,2,35]

PHYSICAL EXAMINATION

A palpable mass may be present over the affected bone, but it is neither tender nor associated with redness or heat. Tenderness on palpation has been noted in patients with cervical EG.[1] Pain may be provoked by neck movement, and limited cervical range of motion may be noted. Torticollis has also been reported.[11] A low-grade fever is present in few patients.[28] Spinal cord and nerve root compression secondary to vertebral body collapse results in corresponding abnormalities on neurologic examination.

LABORATORY DATA

EG is associated with peripheral eosinophilia in 6% to 10% of patients. An occasional patient also has an elevated erythrocyte sedimentation rate. Bone marrow examination of an uninvolved area of bone will yield increased numbers of eosinophils, even with normal differential counts.[27]

Pathology

Examination of gross pathologic specimens usually reveals a soft reddish brown tissue with hemorrhage and cysts. The histologic appearance of EG is characterized by collections of eosinophils and histiocytes without the formation of local, distinct granulomas (Fig. 13-25). The characteristic cell of EG is similar to the Langerhans cell of the epidermis. On electron microscopy, Langerhans cells contain Birbeck bodies, which are granules shaped like tennis rackets. These pentalaminar cytoplasmic inclusions are thought to be formed by invagination of the cell membranes of Langerhans cells. Birbeck granules are found in cells from EG lesions. Special stains may also be used to detect S-100 nuclear–positive, dendritic system histiocytes, lysozyme, and esterase-positive and S-100–negative macrophage system histiocytes.[28] S-100 protein cells are ubiquitous and may be found in a variety of neoplastic and benign conditions. Peanut agglutinin (PNA) is a more specific histiocyte marker. The paranuclear and surface pattern of PNA binding helps define Langerhans histiocytes.[32] The histiocytes have striking

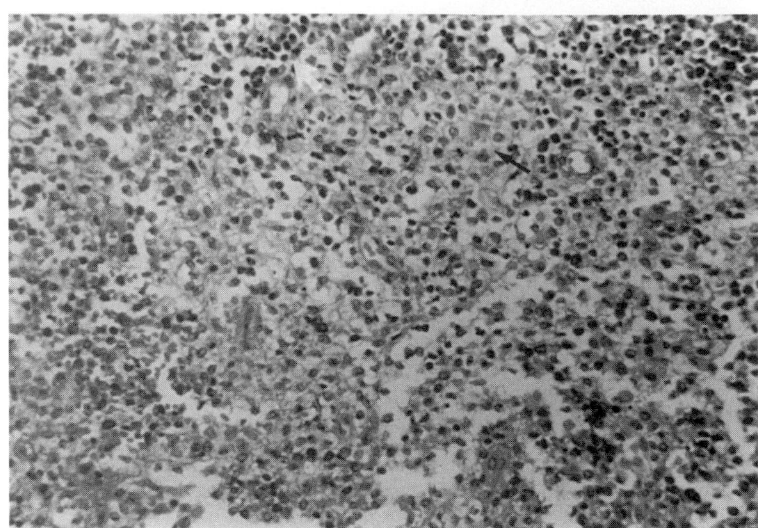

Figure 13-25 Histologic appearance of an eosinophilic granuloma with histiocytes containing large vesicular nuclei *(arrow)*. Other components of the polymorphous infiltrate include eosinophilic granulocytes and occasional lymphocytes. *(Courtesy of Arnold Schwartz, MD.)*

phagocytic activity. Some foci contain multinucleated giant cells with areas of hemorrhage and necrosis. The cytoplasm of phagocytic cells often exhibits double-refractile, neutral fat deposition. In areas where eosinophilic leukocytes are undergoing fragmentation, Charcot-Leyden crystals are noted. As an EG heals, eosinophils markedly diminish in number and are replaced by large histiocytes and fibrous tissue.[14,15]

The pleomorphic appearance of the histiocytes may superficially resemble malignant cells of Hodgkin's disease. The histiocytes of EG are benign. With time, they may form giant cells and take on the appearance of foam cells after they have ingested necrotic tissue and converted it into cytoplasmic lipids. The presence of lipid in EG is a secondary phenomenon and is not of pathogenetic importance as it is in Gaucher's disease.

RADIOGRAPHIC EVALUATION

Roentgenograms

EG in the spine is associated with a spectrum of roentgenographic abnormalities. The features of early lesions are those of a destructive, radiolucent oval area of bone lysis without peripheral sclerosis. Progressive destruction of a vertebral body results in a flattened vertebral body termed *vertebra plana* (Figs. 13-26 and 13-27), first described by Calvé.[6] In adults, C2 is the most common level of involvement.[5] The degree of compression may be symmetrical or asymmetric with preservation of the intervertebral disc. The body of the vertebra is affected, with sparing of the posterior elements.[10] The compressed vertebra may project anteriorly and, in extreme circumstances, cause spinal dislocation. The association of vertebra plana and EG has been verified by biopsy.[22] EG is the most common cause of vertebra plana in children. It may erode the posterior elements of a vertebral body and spare the vertebral body. In the cervical spine, the vertebra may be involved without signs of vertebral body collapse.[4] One pedicle, a lamina, or one of the lateral masses may be affected. These lesions are not associated with vertebral collapse.[21] Rarely, EG can produce expansile lesions with extensive destruction of multiple vertebrae and paraspinal extension.[13] Vertebral height may be restored spontaneously or after treatment, with the affected vertebra reverting to an almost normal configuration.[29] Reconstitution of body height occurs more regularly in young children with continued vertebral growth.[23]

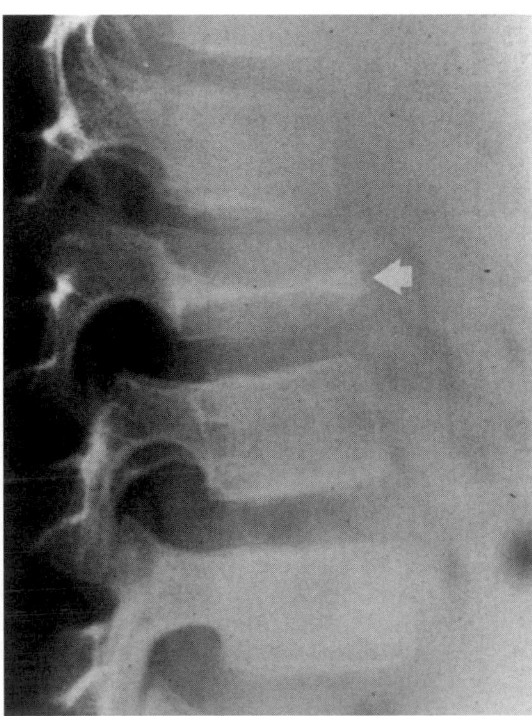

Figure 13-26 Eosinophilic granuloma involving a vertebral body *(arrow)* associated with some flattening of the vertebral body (vertebra plana) and preservation of disc spaces. *(Courtesy of Anne Brower, MD.)*

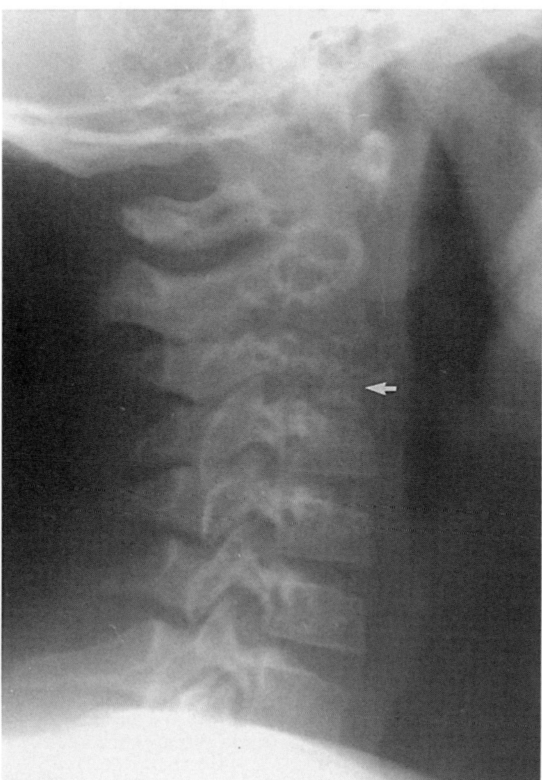

Figure 13-27 Eosinophilic granuloma. A lateral view of the cervical spine shows some flattening of the C3 vertebral body (vertebra plana) *(arrow)* with preservation of disc spaces. *(Courtesy of Anne Brower, MD.)*

Scintigraphy, Computed Tomography, Magnetic Resonance

Other radiographic techniques may be useful in the determination of bone involvement and the extent of soft tissue extension of lesions in the spinal canal. Bone scintigraphy may detect lesions in complex bones, but roentgenograms may be superior for the detection of early lesions.[24] CT is particularly helpful in confirming periosteal reaction and cortical invasion.[11] MR is very useful in determining the epidural extension of extraosseous EGs associated with neurologic compromise.[20] MR imaging is able to determine the level and extent of spinal cord compression.[1,22] It is also able to monitor resolution of the lesions over time.[19]

DIFFERENTIAL DIAGNOSIS

The diagnosis of EG is made from close inspection of biopsy material. Laboratory and radiographic features are too nonspecific to ensure an accurate diagnosis. Careful inspection of biopsy material is essential for making the correct diagnosis. There are many pitfalls that may cause misinterpretation of biopsy specimens. The characteristic cells associated with this tumor are eosinophils and monocytoid histiocytes. Improperly stained eosinophils may be mistaken for neutrophils. The large number of "neutrophils" might be mistaken for osteomyelitis caused by bacterial, tuberculous, or fungal organisms. The histiocytes associated with EG may have single or multiple nuclei that are round, oval, or lobulated in shape. This pleomorphism of histiocytes can lead to the erroneous impression of a reticulum cell sarcoma or Hodgkin's disease. Histiocytes in these malignant diseases have greater nuclear pleomorphism and more irregular nucleoli.

During the healing phase of EG, masses of multinucleated giant cells are seen in areas of the tumor that are being revascularized. The presence of these giant cells may result in an inappropriate diagnosis of giant cell tumor. The clinical, radiologic, and histologic features should prevent an erroneous diagnosis.

TREATMENT

Spontaneous healing of EG is manifested as partial restoration of vertebral body height. Restoration of vertebral height occurs most commonly in younger patients.[36] Therefore, surgical treatment or radiotherapy may not be indicated unless specific manifestations such as neurologic complications are present.[31] In patients with biopsy evidence of the neoplasm and intractable symptoms, the treatment of choice for EG is curettage, with or without packing of the lesion with bone chips. Patients with cervical lesions and neurologic impairment may require anterior or posterior exploration, vertebral body fusion, and halo traction.[15,22] Inaccessible lesions in the spine that may lead to pathologic fractures are best treated with low-dose radiation therapy of 300 to 600 rad. Lumbar braces are not usually required while affected vertebral bodies heal.[16] Healing may occur over a period of months to years. Corticosteroids have been used in pediatric patients and have been effective in reversing bone lesions.[3] Steroids have been chosen for patients with lesions in a difficult operative location.[7] Biphosphonates have been used in a small number of patients to decrease bone pain and prevent the progression of bone lesions. Clodronate given in a dose of 1.6 g/day for a 6-month period allowed healing of bone lesions in two adult patients. The remission lasted for 3 years in one patient and 5 years in the other.[12]

PROGNOSIS

EG is a benign lesion, and the prognosis is good. Patients with vertebra plana may heal in time with partial reconstitution of the affected vertebral body. The prognosis of patients with multifocal EG may not be as good if their illness progresses to the diffuse involvement associated with other components of histiocytosis X. Such progression is more of a concern for younger patients than for adults. If a patient has only a single lesion for 6 months, chances are that the lesion will remain unifocal.[28]

References

Eosinophilic Granuloma

1. Acciarri N, Paganini M, Fonda C, et al: Langerhans' cell histiocytosis of the spine causing cord compression: Case report. Neurosurgery 31:965, 1992.

2. Alley RM, Sussman MD: Rapidly progressive eosinophilic granuloma: A case report. Spine 17:1517, 1992.
3. Avioli LV, Lasersohn JT, Lopresti JM: Histiocytosis X (Schüller-Christian disease): A clinicopathological survey, review of ten patients and the results of prednisone therapy. Medicine (Baltimore) 42:119, 1963.
4. Baber WW, Numaguchi Y, Nadell JM, et al: Eosinophilic granuloma of the cervical spine without vertebrae plana. J Comput Tomogr 11:346, 1987.
5. Bertram C, Madert J, Eggers C: Eodinophilic granuloma of the cervical spine. Spine 27:1408-1413, 2002.
6. Calvé JA: Localized affection of spine suggesting osteochondritis of vertebral body, with clinical aspects of Pott's disease. J Bone Joint Surg 7:41, 1925.
7. Carmago OPD, Oliveira NRBD, Andrade JS, et al: Eosinophilic granuloma of the ischium: Long-term evaluation of a patient treated with steroids. J Bone Joint Surg Am 74-A:445, 1992.
8. Cheyne C: Histiocytosis X. J Bone Joint Surg Br 53-B:366, 1971.
9. Compere EL, Johnson WE, Coventry MD: Vertebra plana (Calve's disease) due to eosinophilic granuloma. J Bone Joint Surg Am 36-A:969, 1954.
10. David R, Oria RA, Kumar R, et al: Radiologic features of eosinophilic granuloma of bone. AJR Am J Roentgenol 153:1021, 1989.
11. Dickson LD, Farhat SM: Eosinophilic granuloma of the cervical spine: A case report and review of the literature. Surg Neurol 35:57, 1991.
12. Elomaa I, Blomqvist C, Porkka L, Holmstrom T: Experiences of clodronate treatment of multifocal eosinophilic granuloma of bone. J Intern Med 225:59, 1989.
13. Ferris RA, Pettrone FA, McKelvie AM, et al: Eosinophilic granuloma of the spine: An unusual radiographic presentation. Clin Orthop 99:57, 1974.
14. Green WT, Farber S: "Eosinophilic or solitary granuloma" of bone. J Bone Joint Surg 24:499, 1942.
15. Huvos AG: Bone Tumors: Diagnosis, Treatment, and Prognosis, 2nd ed. Philadelphia, WB Saunders, 1991, pp 695-711.
16. Ippolito E, Farsetti P, Tudisoc C: Vertebra plana. J Bone Joint Surg Am 66-A:1364, 1984.
17. Islinger RB, Kuklo TR, Owens BD, et al: Langerhan's cell histiocytosis in patients older than 21 years. Clin Orthop 379:231-235, 2000.
18. Jaffe HL, Lichtenstein L: Eosinophilic granuloma of bone: A condition affecting one, several or many bones, but apparently limited to the skeleton and representing the mildest clinical expression of the peculiar inflammatory histiocytosis also underlying Letterer-Siwe disease and Schüller-Christian disease. Arch Pathol 37:99, 1944.
19. Kamimura M, Kinoshita T, Itoh H, et al: Eosinophilic granuloma of the spine: Early spontaneous disappearance of tumor detected on magnetic resonance imaging. Case report. J Neurosurg 93(2 suppl):312-316, 2000.
20. Kantererewicz E, Condom E, Canete JD, Del Olmo JA: Spinal cord compression by a unifocal eosinophilic granuloma: A case report of an adult with unusual roentgenological features. Neurosurgery 23:666, 1988.
21. Kaye JJ, Freiberger RH: Eosinophilic granuloma of the spine without vertebra plana: A report of two unusual cases. Radiology 92:1188, 1969.
22. Kieffer SA, Nesbit ME, D'Angio GJ: Vertebra plana due to histiocytosis X: Serial studies. Acta Radiol 8:241, 1969.
23. Kricun ME: Tumors of the Spine. In Kricun ME (ed): Imaging of Bone Tumors. Philadelphia, WB Saunders, 1993, pp 266-267.
24. Kumar R, Balachandran S: Relative roles of radionuclide scanning and radiographic imaging in eosinophilic granuloma. Clin Nucl Med 5:538, 1980.
25. Lavin PT, Osband ME: Evaluating the role of therapy in histiocytosis X. Hematol Oncol Clin North Am 1:35, 1987.
26. Macnab GH: Discussion: Eosinophilic granuloma, Letterer-Siwe disease, Hand-Schüller-Christian disease. Proc R Soc Med 48:711, 1955.
27. Marcove RC: Bone marrow eosinophilia with solitary eosinophilic granuloma of bone: A report of two cases. J Bone Joint Surg Am 41-A:1521, 1959.
28. Mirra JM: Bone Tumors: Clinical, Radiologic, and Pathologic Correlations. Philadelphia, Lea & Febiger, 1989, pp 1023-1045.
29. Nesbit ME, Kieffer S, D'Angio GJ: Reconstitution of vertebral height in histiocytosis X: A long-term follow-up. J Bone Joint Surg 51:1360, 1969.
30. Osband ME: Histiocytosis X: Langerhans' cell histiocytosis. Hematol Oncol Clin North Am 1:737, 1987.
31. Raab P, Hohmann F, Kuhl J, et al: Vertebral remodeling in eosinophilic granuloma of the spine. A long-term follow-up. Spine 23:1351-1354, 1998.
32. Ree HJ, Kadin ME: Peanut agglutinin: A useful marker for histiocytosis-X and interdigitating reticulum cells. Cancer 57:282, 1986.
33. Schajowicz F, Slullitel J: Eosinophilic granuloma and its relationship to Hand-Schüller-Christian and Lettere-Siwe syndromes. J Bone Joint Surg Br 55-B:545, 1973.
34. Sessa S, Sommelet D, Lascombes P, Prevot J: Treatment of Langerhans' cell histiocytosis in children: Experience at the Children's Hospital of Nancy. J Bone Joint Surg Am 76-A:1513, 1994.
35. Sweasey TA, Dauser RC: Eosinophilic granuloma of the cervicothoracic junction: Case report. J Neurosurg 71:942, 1989.
36. Tomita T: Special considerations in surgery of pediatric spine tumors. In Sundaresan N, Schmidek HH, Schiller AL, Rosenthal DI (eds): Tumors of the Spine: Diagnosis and Management. Philadelphia, WB Saunders, 1990, pp 258-271.
37. Willman CL, Busque L, Griffith BB, et al: Langerhans' cell histiocytosis (histiocytosis X): A clonal proliferative disease. N Engl J Med 331:154, 1994.

GAUCHER'S DISEASE

Capsule Summary

	Low Back	Neck
Frequency of spinal pain	Common	Not applicable (NA)
Location of spinal pain	Lumbar spine	NA
Quality of spinal pain	Persistent ache	NA
Symptoms and signs	Generalized fatigue, abdominal distention, bleeding	NA
Laboratory tests	Pancytopenia, increased nonprostatic acid phosphatase, decreased leukocyte acid beta-glucocerebrosidase, Gaucher's cells in bone marrow	NA
Radiographic findings	Vertebra plana on plain roentgenogram	NA
Treatment	Alglucerase, gene therapy	NA

PREVALENCE AND PATHOGENESIS

Gaucher's disease (GD) is a lipid metabolism disorder associated with the accumulation of ceramide glucoside in histiocytes. Massive accumulation of this lipid in cells of the reticuloendothelial system results in an enlarged spleen, destruction of bone, and abnormalities in bone marrow. The first reference to the disease was made by Gaucher in 1882.[10]

Epidemiology

GD is an uncommon illness that can become manifested at any time of life. However, manifestations of the illness become more prominent as the affected individual ages. Ashkenazi Jews are at greatest risk for development of this illness, although whites, blacks, and Asians can also be affected.[14,22] Of the three forms of the disease, type 1 is the most common, with involvement limited to the spleen, liver, and skeletal system.[35] Type 1 is the most frequent form in Ashkenazi Jews. Types 2 and 3 are associated with neurologic involvement and differ from type 1. Most patients (94%) have type 1, with type 2 found in 1% and type 3 in 5%.[5] The age at appearance of the first symptoms is 25 years. Men and women are equally affected.

Pathogenesis

The pathogenesis of the disease is related to an inborn error of metabolism that causes the accumulation of complex lipids within histiocytes. In the past, the cause of GD was thought to be excessive production of a lipid ceramide glucoside. More recently, the abnormality has been traced to a defective enzyme, beta-glucosidase, that is unable to degrade accumulating lipid.[32] Glucose is not cleaved from the lipid portion of sphingolipids. Accumulation of this material in cells throughout the body results in the manifestations of GD. The autosomal recessive inheritance of the disease suggests that a single biochemical defect does account for the abnormalities associated with this illness. Investigators have identified a gene mutation causing a single base substitution (leucine to proline) that accounts for the loss of enzymatic activity.[29]

The gene that encodes the glucocerebrosidase enzyme is located on chromosome 1. A number of mutations have been identified in the various forms of GD. The most common alleles are *N370S* and *L444P*. In the Jewish population, a mutation that results in the substitution of serine for asparagine at amino acid 370 of the processed protein accounts for most of the abnormalities of the Ashkenazi Jewish population. In the non-Jewish population, a larger number of mutations are associated with GD,[3] which is the reason for the different clinical manifestations in non-Jewish patients with GD.

In adults, the axial skeleton is frequently involved. GD causes vertebral body osteolysis, compression fractures, and spinal deformities. Any portion of the axial skeleton may be affected.

CLINICAL HISTORY

Clinical symptoms depend on the organ involved and the degree of involvement. Adult patients have abdominal distention secondary to hepatosplenomegaly, which may result in pancytopenia in association with episodes of bleeding and infections. Constitutional symptoms of generalized fatigue and weakness are common. Patients with skeletal disease have persistent bone pain, tenderness, difficulty walking, back pain, and loss of height. Symptoms related to the skeletal system have been reported in up to 86% of patients.[12] Asplenic individuals are more likely than those with spleens to have bone pain and radiographic abnormalities.[5] Acute bone crisis, including the lumbar spine and pelvis, develops in up to 37% of patients with type 1 GD.[34] The pain is severe and resistant to narcotics. The involved bone is warm, swollen, and tender, and systemic fever is present. Later in the course of the illness, bone pain becomes the major cause of morbidity. Neurologic symptoms are usually limited to children with more severe disease. Manifestations include strabismus, seizures, tremors, clonus, mental retardation, and loss of sensation. Neurologic symptoms, including radicular pain, occur in rare circumstances in the setting of spinal cord compression. Cord compression occurs in later stages of the disease secondary to vertebral pathologic fractures.[11,16]

PHYSICAL EXAMINATION

Patients with GD have massive splenomegaly, moderate hepatomegaly, and minimal lymphadenopathy. Deposits of lipid in the dermis give exposed skin a tan color, whereas deposits in the sclera of the eye cause tan pingueculae to appear. Patient may complain of bone tenderness on palpation, and such tenderness may be particularly prominent in those in whom acute vertebral compression fractures develop. These individuals have percussion tenderness over the lumbar spine.

LABORATORY DATA

Anemia, leukopenia, and thrombocytopenia, which may be associated with occasional episodes of bleeding, result from replacement of bone marrow cells with lipid-filled histiocytes. The abnormal blood counts are related to the status of the individual's spleen. Splenectomized patients are more likely to have normalized blood counts than nonsplenectomized patients.[35] Serum acid phosphatase of nonprostatic origin is elevated.[30,31] Other findings include abnormal liver function test results, prolonged prothrombin and partial thromboplastin times, elevated serum ferritin levels, and increased angiotensin-converting enzyme activity. In one study, 15 of 23 (65%) patients with GD had elevated IgG levels, whereas a smaller percentage (43%) had diffuse hypergammaglobulinemia.[20]

Pathology

Bone marrow aspiration is usually adequate for obtaining tissue that reveals characteristic Gaucher cells. Gaucher cells have two round-to-oval eccentric nuclei with striated cytoplasm that readily stains with periodic acid–Schiff reagent (Fig. 13-28). In affected bones, the histiocytic cells form small nests that coalesce into large masses.[21] Gaucher

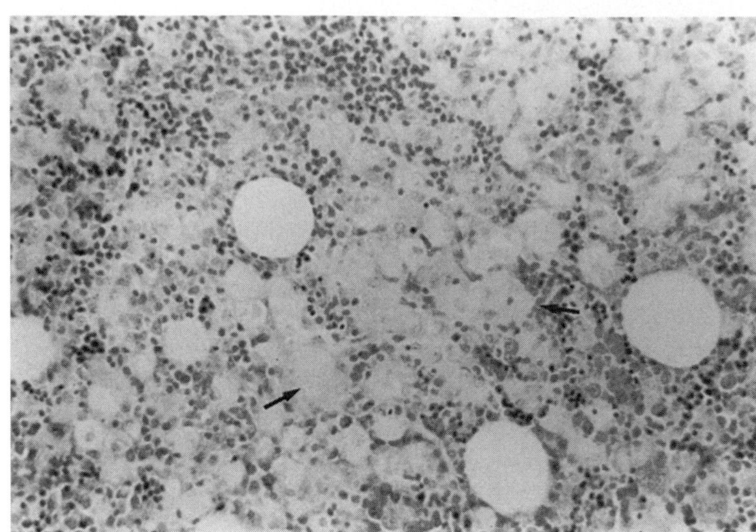

Figure 13-28 Gaucher's disease. A bone marrow specimen exhibits large, lipid-filled histiocytes (Gaucher cells) *(arrows)* that have replaced most of the other bone marrow elements. *(Courtesy of Arnold Schwartz, MD.)*

cells may be found in other body tissues, including the intervertebral discs.[26]

RADIOGRAPHIC EVALUATION

Roentgenograms

Infiltration of marrow by Gaucher cells results in characteristic roentgenographic abnormalities. In the spine, cellular infiltrates result in increased radiolucency of vertebral bodies, accentuation of vertical trabeculae, and compression fractures (Fig. 13-29).[13] Fractures may cause complete flattening of a vertebral body (vertebra plana) or the development of depressions in the superior and inferior margins of a vertebral body, referred to as an "H vertebra" (Fig. 13-30).[27] These lesions occur secondary to occlusion of vessels that are distributed to the chondro-osseous junction in the middle of the endplate. Disc spaces are usually spared. In an occasional patient, widespread disc degeneration with vertebral body overgrowth occurs.[7] GD is also associated with aseptic necrosis of bone, usually at the ends of long bones, but it has been described near the sacroiliac joint as well. This process results in apparent obliteration of the articulation, similar to changes associated with ankylosing spondylitis.[18,27]

Scintigraphy

Bone scan abnormalities include increased uptake surrounding the large joints of the extremities. On occasion, increased bone scan activity precedes roentgenographic abnormalities.[35] Bone scan abnormalities associated with GD that may be identified by scintigraphy include aseptic necrosis, bone infarction, pathologic fractures, and osteomyelitis.[17]

Computed Tomography

CT is useful in quantifying the extent of skeletal involvement, as well as delineating the degree of bone marrow

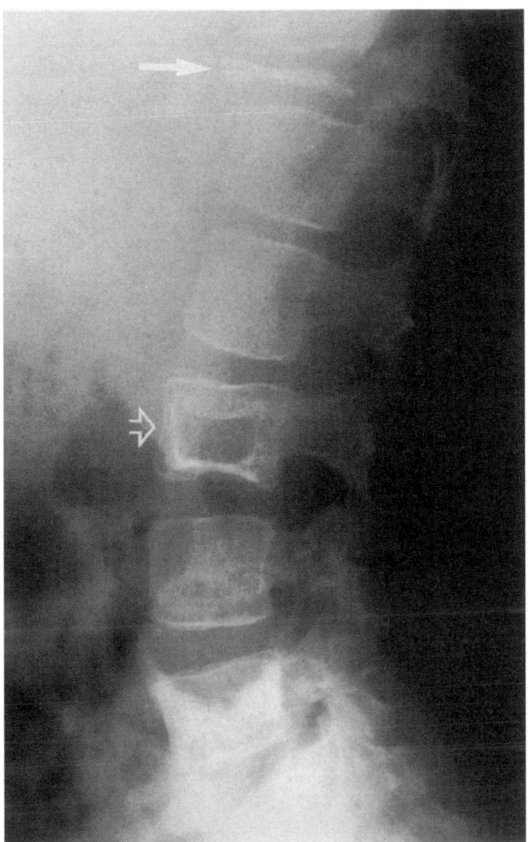

Figure 13-29 Gaucher's disease of the lumbar spine manifested by vertebra plana *(arrow)* and a rectangular lytic lesion in a vertebral body *(open arrow)*. *(Courtesy of Anne Brower, MD.)*

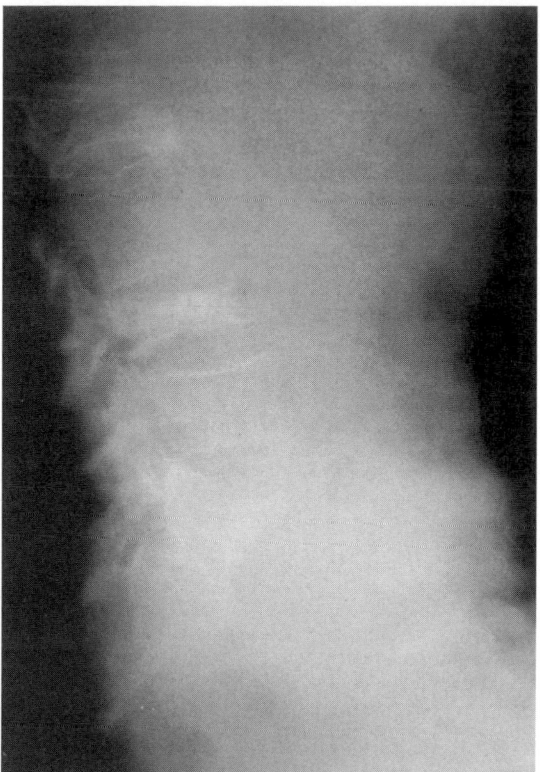

Figure 13-30 Lateral view of the lumbar spine in a 58-year-old woman with a 2-year history of intermittent low and mid back pain. The patient had marked thoracic kyphosis. Mild anemia, thrombocytopenia, and elevated acid phosphatase were noted. Bone marrow aspiration revealed Gaucher cells. The roentgenogram reveals generalized osteopenia and multiple compression fractures. *(Courtesy of Peter Levitin, MD.)*

replacement. The progression of disease reflects the infiltration of marrow with Gaucher cells moving from the axial to the appendicular skeleton. A combination of CT and technetium 99m sulfur colloid bone marrow scanning offers assessment of gradations of increasing severity of bone disease.[15] Combined use of these two tests shows that some patients with minimal to moderate roentgenographic evidence of bone disease have extensive skeletal involvement. Quantitative CT, a method for measuring bone calcium, is useful for determining the progression of disease as reflected by replacement of bone calcium.[25]

Magnetic Resonance

MR imaging of patients with GD is useful in detecting the extent of organ replacement with Gaucher cells. Replacement of normal fat with Gaucher cells results in a characteristic hyposignal of bone marrow on T1- and T2-weighted sequences. Liver and spleen enlargement is readily visible with MR. MR detects increased fluid in bone associated with episodes of acute avascular necrosis. MR is useful in the evaluation of orthopedic patients with an acute onset of skeletal pain.[8,19] It is able to document sacroiliac joint involvement, including bone infarcts, effusions, and hematomas in surrounding muscle.[4]

DIFFERENTIAL DIAGNOSIS

The diagnosis of GD is confirmed by the presence of characteristic cells obtained by biopsy of affected tissues. Because pseudo-Gaucher cells may be present in bone marrow specimens, enzymatic assay of leukocyte acid beta-glucosidase is a more specific test.[35] A group of experts who care for such patients recommend determination of beta-glucocerebrosidase activity.[6] In the future, DNA analysis for GD mutations will become the best method for diagnosis. The radiographic findings have considerable overlap with other disorders that produce osteoporosis and aseptic necrosis. Metabolic disorders associated with axial skeletal osteopenia include osteoporosis, osteomalacia, and hyperparathyroidism. Sickle cell anemia and thalassemia may cause similar radiographic findings. Tumors, including myeloma and metastatic lesions or leukemia, may cause loss of bone calcium, localized radiolucent areas, and cystic lesions, which are also seen in GD.

Osteosclerosis is not specific for GD. This radiographic finding occurs in Hodgkin's disease, myelofibrosis, mastocytosis, metastatic lesions, and tuberous sclerosis.

Patients with GD are at greater risk for infections, including osteomyelitis.[23] This diagnosis should be considered in a patient with GD who has increased bone pain with an associated fever.

TREATMENT

Splenectomy is a surgical procedure used in patients with cytopenia and abdominal discomfort from splenomegaly. The procedure is most helpful for improving the rate of growth in children and adolescents. The effect of splenectomy on progression of the disease in other organs is questionable. In a study of the relationship between splenectomy and bone disease, an equal incidence of bone disease in splenectomized and nonsplenectomized patients was noted.[35] Splenectomy has no effect on the progression of skeletal disease.[28]

New treatments have been developed for GD. Alglucerase is a mannose-terminated form of human placental glucocerebrosidase that was developed to treat patients with GD.[33] Primary therapy for GD focuses on removal of the lipid metabolite that causes organ failure. Alglucerase is taken up by Gaucher cells in the liver, spleen, and bone marrow, where accumulated lipid is broken down. The drug is given intravenously (60 U/kg) over a period of 1 to 2 hours, usually every 2 weeks. Treatment must be continued indefinitely. In one study, 12 patients treated with infusions of alglucerase for 9 to 12 months showed an increase in hemoglobin concentration and platelet count and a decrease in organ size.[1] Skeletal improvement was also noted in a quarter of patients. The cost of this enzyme is prohibitive and is estimated to be $382,200 per year. More effective methods to deliver the enzyme to macrophages are being investigated. A retroviral vector with normal human DNA for the glucocerebrosidase gene has transduced bone marrow cells in long-term culture. This method may prove useful to replace enzyme in patients. Bone marrow transplantation is curative for the disease but is associated with the higher risks of the procedure. Transplantation is usually considered only for young patients with severe disease.[3,9]

Patients with multiple bone fractures may benefit from treatment with bisphosphonates. Pamidronate (aminohydroxypropylidene bisphosphonate) has been associated with a reduction in bone resorption, increased calcium absorption, improved calcium balance, and improvement in bone density in the axial and appendicular skeleton in patients with GD. Decreased bone pain was a result of the therapy.[24]

PROGNOSIS

GD has a protracted course punctuated with periods of increased symptoms. Compression fractures of the spine, aseptic necrosis of bone, and pathologic fractures in long bones can cause severe morbidity. Adult patients usually die of infection, bleeding, anemia, or severe weight loss.

The younger the age at initial clinical involvement, the more severe the disease. Patients with type 2 disease may die at birth.[9] A factor more closely linked with disease severity is the genotype of the patient. Certain genotypes are associated with milder disease (1226G/1226G), whereas others are associated with neuropathic disease and a poor prognosis (1226G/1448C).[35]

GD is commonly regarded as a progressive disorder leading to death.[2] Recent studies have suggested that the disease is most progressive up to young adulthood with stabilization thereafter. Hematologic and biochemical involvement should be assessed with a complete blood count including platelets, acid phosphatase, and liver enzymes at 12 months in untreated patients and every 3 months in individuals who receive enzyme replacement therapy.[6] Patients with long-standing disease are at risk for progressive skeletal disease involving the hip joints and the vertebral column. Skeletal disease, including compression fractures of the spine, aseptic necrosis of bone, and pathologic fractures in long bones, has the potential to become a source of morbidity in later life. Adult patients remain at risk for bleeding, anemia, and infection.

References

Gaucher's Disease

1. Barton NW, Brady RO, Dambrosia JM, et al: Replacement therapy for inherited enzyme deficiency—macrophage-targeted glucocerebrosidase for Gaucher's disease. N Engl J Med 324:1464, 1991.
2. Beutler E: Gaucher's disease. N Engl J Med 325:1354, 1991.
3. Beutler E: Gaucher disease: New molecular approaches to diagnosis and treatment. Science 256:794, 1992.
4. Bisagni-Faure A, Dupont A, Chazerain P, et al: Magnetic resonance imaging assessment of sacroiliac joint involvement in Gaucher's disease. J Rheumatol 19:1984, 1992.
5. Charrow J, Andersson HC, Kaplan P et al: The Gaucher registry: Demographics and disease characteristics of 1698 patients with Gaucher disease. Arch Intern Med 160:2835-2843, 2000.
6. Charrow J, Esplin JA, Gribble J, et al: Gaucher disease: Recommendations on diagnosis, evaluation, and monitoring. Arch Intern Med 158:1754-1769, 1998.
7. Colhoun EN, Cassar-Pullicino V, McCall IW, David MW: Unusual discovertebral changes in Gaucher's disease. Br J Radiol 60:925, 1987.
8. Cremin BJ, Davey H, Goldblatt J: Skeletal complications of type I Gaucher disease: The magnetic resonance features. Clin Radiol 41:244, 1990.
9. Erikson A, Groth CG, Mansson JE, et al: Clinical and biochemical outcome of marrow transplantation for Gaucher disease of the Norrbottnian type. Acta Paediatr Scand 79:680, 1990.
10. Gaucher P: De l'epithelioma primitif de la rate, hypertrophie idiopathique de la rate sans l'eucemie. These de Paris, 1882.
11. Goldblatt J, Keet P, Dall D: Spinal cord decompression for Gaucher's disease. Neurosurgery 21:227, 1987.
12. Goldblatt J, Sacks S, Beighton P: The orthopedic aspects of Gaucher's disease. Clin Orthop 137:208, 1978.
13. Greenfield GB: Bone changes in chronic adult Gaucher's disease. AJR Am J Roentgenol 110:800, 1970.
14. Greenfield GB: Miscellaneous diseases related to the hematologic system. Semin Roentgenol 9:241, 1974.
15. Hermann G, Goldblatt J, Levy RN, et al: Gaucher's disease type 1: Assessment of bone involvement by CT and scintigraphy. AJR Am J Roentgenol 147:943, 1986.
16. Hermann G, Wagner LD, Gendal ES, et al: Spinal cord compression in type I Gaucher disease. Radiology 170:147, 1989.
17. Israel O, Jerushalmi J, Front D: Scintigraphic findings in Gaucher's disease. J Nucl Med 27:1557, 1986.
18. Kulowski J: Gaucher's disease in bone. AJR Am J Roentgenol 63:840, 1950.
19. Lanir A, Hadar H, Cohen I, et al: Gaucher disease: Assessment with MR imaging. Radiology 161:239, 1986.
20. Marti GE, Ryan ET, Papadopoulos NM, et al: Polyclonal B-cell lymphocytosis and hypergammaglobulinemia in patients with Gaucher disease. Am J Hematol 29:189, 1988.
21. Mirra JM: Bone Tumors: Clinical, Radiologic, and Pathologic Correlations. Philadelphia, Lea & Febiger, 1989, pp 1060-1074.
22. Novy SB, Naletson E, Stuart L, Whittock G: Gaucher's disease in a black adult. AJR Am J Roentgenol 133:947, 1979.
23. Noyes FR, Smith WS: Bone crisis and chronic osteomyelitis in Gaucher's disease. Clin Orthop 79:132, 1971.
24. Ostlere L, Warner T, Meunier PJ, et al: Treatment of type I Gaucher's disease affecting bone with aminohydroxypropylidene bisphosphonate (pamidronate). Q J Med 79:503, 1991.
25. Rosenthal DI, Mayo-Smith W, Goodsitt MM, et al: Bone and bone marrow changes in Gaucher disease: Evaluation with quantitative CT. Radiology 170:143, 1989.
26. Sack GH Jr: Clinical diversity in Gaucher's disease. Johns Hopkins Med J 146:166, 1980.
27. Schwarz AM, Homer MJ, McCauley RGK: "Step off" vertebral body. Gaucher's disease vs. sickle cell hemoglobinopathy. AJR Am J Roentgenol 132:81, 1979.
28. Stowens DW, Teitelbaum SL, Kahn AJ, Barranger JA: Skeletal complications of Gaucher disease. Medicine (Baltimore) 64:310, 1985.
29. Tsuji S, Choudary PV, Martin BM, et al: A mutation in the human glucocerebrosidase gene in neuronopathic Gaucher's disease. N Engl J Med 316:570, 1987.
30. Tuchman LR, Suna H, Carr JJ: Elevation of serum acid phosphatase in Gaucher's disease. J Mt Sinai Hosp 23:227, 1956.
31. Tuchman LR, Swick M: High acid phosphatase level indicating Gaucher's disease in patients with prostatism. JAMA 164:2034, 1957.
32. Volk BW, Adachi M, Schneck L: The pathology of the sphingolipidoses. Semin Hematol 9:317, 1972.
33. Whittington R, Goa KL: Alglucerase: A review of its therapeutic use in Gaucher's disease. Drugs 44:72, 1992.
34. Yosipovitch Z, Katz K: Bone crisis in Gaucher's disease: An update. Isr J Med Sci 26:593, 1990.
35. Zimran A, Kay A, Gelbart T, et al: Gaucher disease: Clinical, laboratory, radiologic, and genetic features of 53 patients. Medicine (Baltimore) 71:337, 1992.

SACROILIAC LIPOMA

CAPSULE SUMMARY

	LOW BACK	NECK
Frequency of spinal pain	Common	Not applicable (NA)
Location of spinal pain	Sacroiliac junction	NA
Quality of spinal pain	Intermittent ache	NA
Symptoms and signs	Pain increased with sleeping, point tenderness	NA
Laboratory tests	None	NA
Radiographic findings	None	NA
Treatment	Local injection, surgical excision	NA

PREVALENCE AND PATHOGENESIS

Sacroiliac lipomas are fatty tumors located over the sacroiliac joints. They herniate through weak areas in the overlying fascia and become painful when they are strangulated by the fascia. The pain associated with herniation of these fatty tumors may be severe, may radiate to the buttock and thigh, and may be associated with limitation of flexion of the lumbosacral spine.

Epidemiology

The prevalence of sacroiliac lipoma in the general population is unknown. Studies reporting on patients with sacroiliac lipomas suggest that the incidence is relatively high.[7,11] Approximately 10% to 26% of the population may have these nodules, but the lipomas are symptomatic in only a small fraction of individuals.[3,12] They become symptomatic most frequently when the patient is in the fifth decade. The male-to-female ratio is 1:4. Ries in 1937 was the first to describe the presence of sacroiliac lipomas and the clinical syndrome associated with them.[9]

Pathogenesis

The pathogenesis of sacroiliac lipomas is related to weaknesses in the fascia that runs from the cervical to the lumbosacral spine. The lipoma may herniate through a weakened area with deficiencies in fascia fibers or through one of the foramina where the lateral branches of the posterior primary division of the first, second, and third lumbar nerves pass.[2] The three types of herniations are pedunculated, nonpedunculated, and foraminal. With certain motions, the fascia strangulates the herniated fatty tumor and compresses its blood supply and nerves, and such compression results in local pain with possible radiation in the distribution of the cutaneous nerves. The lipomas may also develop as a manifestation of trauma. Trauma may stimulate prelipocytes to form lipomas.[10]

CLINICAL HISTORY

The typical patient is a middle-aged, obese female with unilateral low back pain radiating to the buttock or anterior of the thigh. Most symptomatic patients will have local pain or pain radiating to the thigh.[13] Patients with pain radiating to the calf or foot without other causes of radicular pain have been reported but are rare.[4] Flexion of the lumbosacral spine increases the pain, as does activity. The pain has an aching quality and occasionally may be bilateral. Compression of the area at night while sleeping may cause severe distress. No constitutional symptoms such as fatigue, weight loss, fever, or anorexia are associated with the lesion.

PHYSICAL EXAMINATION

Physical examination demonstrates a tender nodule near the dimples in the sacroiliac area. Sacroiliac lipomas are very tender to palpation. Direct pressure on the nodule may re-create pain in the referral pattern of the sclerotome of the affected nerve.[4] Forward flexion causes pain, and such motion can be limited. The nodules may occur singly or in clusters. Neurologic examination, including the straight leg–raising test, is normal.

LABORATORY DATA

Laboratory tests, including hematologic, chemical, and immunologic studies, are normal in patients with sacroiliac lipomas. The gross pathologic findings demonstrate rounded cylindric bodies that measure 1 to 5 cm in diameter. Microscopically, the lipomas consist of normal adipose tissue with little interposed connective tissue and a fibrous capsule. Nerve fibers are detected in some specimens.[6] Signs of edema and hemorrhage may be seen in some portions of the specimens.[5]

RADIOGRAPHIC EVALUATION

Sacroiliac lipomas are not associated with any radiographic abnormalities. MR may develop to a sufficient degree to identify the presence of these soft tissue tumors. At present, however, no MR studies have systematically imaged the lumbar soft tissues for the presence of these soft tissue nodules.

DIFFERENTIAL DIAGNOSIS

The diagnosis of sacroiliac lipoma is not made unless physicians are aware of the existence of this entity as a cause of low back pain. Frequently, patients undergo extensive examinations before the correct diagnosis is made. Patients who have a history of pain that is increased by rolling over in bed and can be re-created by palpation of a tender nodule may have a sacroiliac lipoma as the cause of their symptoms.

Patients may have pain over the pelvic brim. Entrapment of the medial superior cluneal nerve causes pain that radiates in a similar distribution.[8] A lipoma may cause compression that may result in low back pain.

TREATMENT

The initial treatment of sacroiliac lipoma is injection of the nodules with a local anesthetic such as lidocaine (Xylocaine). These injections frequently produce relief of pain. Patients may notice relief for extended periods even from a single injection.[11] Pain may also be relieved by dry needling of the lesion. The pathogenesis of the pain may be distention of the nodule by pressure. Multiple punctures of the nodule relieve this distention, which may be the mechanism of pain relief. Symptoms may increase for a few hours after the procedure. Surgical removal of a painful sacral lipoma is beneficial if injections do not relieve the symptoms.[1]

PROGNOSIS

Because patients with sacral lipomas may experience severe pain and limitation of motion of the lumbosacral spine, they frequently undergo extensive evaluations, including a variety of radiographic studies that are consistently normal. When no specific abnormality is discovered, these patients are thought to have psychogenic rheumatism and are referred for psychiatric evaluation. Some have had symptoms for as long as 7 years before the correct diagnosis was made.[2] The prognosis is excellent with the correct diagnosis and appropriate therapy. These patients suffer no functional impairment once they respond to therapy.

References

Sacroiliac Lipoma

1. Bonner CD, Kasdon SC: Herniation of fat through lumbosacral fascia as a cause of low-back pain. N Engl J Med 251:1102, 1954.
2. Copeman WSC: Fibro-fatty tissue and its relation to certain "rheumatic" syndromes. BMJ 2:191, 1949.
3. Copeman WSC, Ackerman WL: Edema or herniation of fat lobules as a cause of lumbar and gluteal "fibrositis." Arch Intern Med 79:22, 1947.
4. Curtis P: In search of the "back mouse." J Fam Pract 36:657, 1993.
5. Herz R: Herniation of fascial fat as a cause of low back pain. JAMA 128:921, 1945.
6. Hittner VJ: Episacroiliac lipomas. Am J Surg 78:382, 1949.
7. Hucherson DC, Gandy JR: Herniation of fascial fat: A cause of low back pain. Am J Surg 76:605, 1948.
8. Maigne J, Doursounian L: Entrapment neuropathy of the medial superior cluneal nerve: Nineteen cases surgically treated, with a minimum of 2 years' follow-up. Spine 22:1156-1159, 1997
9. Ries E: Episacroiliac lipoma. Am J Obstet Gynecol 34:490, 1937.
10. Signorini M, Campiglio GL: Postraumatic lipomas: Where do they really come from? Plast Reconstr Surg 101:699-705, 1998.
11. Singewald ML: Sacroiliac lipomata: An often unrecognized cause of low back pain. Bull Johns Hopkins Hosp 118:492, 1966.
12. Swezey RI: Non-fibrositic lumbar subcutaneous nodules: Prevalence and clinical significance. Br J Rheumatol 30:376, 1991.
13. Wollgast GF, Afeman CE: Sacroiliac (episacral) lipomas. Arch Surg 83:147, 1961.

Malignant Tumors

MULTIPLE MYELOMA

CAPSULE SUMMARY

	LOW BACK	NECK
Frequency of spinal pain	Common	Common
Location of spinal pain	Lumbar spine	Cervical spine
Quality of spinal pain	Ache of increasing intensity	Ache of increasing intensity
Symptoms and signs	Generalized fatigue, bone pain, fever	Generalized fatigue, bone pain, fever
Laboratory tests	Pancytopenia, hypergammaglobulinemia	Pancytopenia, hypergammaglobulinemia
Radiographic findings	Diffuse osteolysis without reactive sclerosis on plain roentgenograms	Diffuse osteolysis without reactive sclerosis on plain roentgenograms
Treatment	Chemotherapy for general disease, radiation therapy for cord compression	Chemotherapy for general disease, radiation therapy for cord compression

PREVALENCE AND PATHOGENESIS

Multiple myeloma is a malignant tumor of plasma cells. Plasma cells produce immunoglobulins and antibodies and are located throughout the bone marrow. Multiplication of these cells in bone marrow is associated with diffuse bone destruction characterized by bone pain, pathologic fractures, and increases in serum calcium.

The term *plasmacytoma* is used when one bone is involved by the disease. *Multiple myeloma* denotes the involvement of several bones throughout the skeleton. *Myelomatosis* refers to disseminated disease throughout the hematopoietic system, including extraosseous locations. *Extramedullary plasmacytoma* refers to lesions in soft tissues independent of bone.[6]

Three physicians, Bence-Jones, Dalrymple, and Macintyre, first identified the bone lesion and urinary protein in the 1840s.[16,30,58] Von Rustizky in 1873 was the first to call the disease multiple myeloma.[81]

Epidemiology

Multiple myeloma is the most common primary malignancy of bone in adults, and it accounts for 27% of bone tumors examined by biopsy and 45% of all malignant bone tumors.[61,79] The incidence is 3 to 4 cases per 100,000 people in the United States.[42,86] Patients are usually in an older age group ranging from 50 to 80, with a median age of 71 years.[49,86] Multiple myeloma is rare in a patient younger than 40 years but has been reported in some as young as 30.[19,41] The male-to-female ratio is slightly increased, but the ratio may be increased further for solitary plasmacytomas.[78] A majority of patients with multiple myeloma have lesions in the axial skeleton. The thoracic spine is involved in 59% of patients, the lumbosacral spine in 31%, and the cervical spine in 10%. In Unni's series of 11,087 surgical cases of multiple myeloma, axial skeletal involvement was noted in 60%, 29%, and 11% in the thoracic, lumbosacral, and cervical spine, respectively.[79] A review by Clarke of the medical literature before 1956 reported that 33 of 193 (17%) patients with multiple myeloma had cervical spine lesions.[28] The spine is affected in 30% to 50% of patients with solitary plasmacytomas.[61] Most frequently, the thoracic and lumbar spine are affected by solitary plasmacytomas rather than the cervical spine.[47] Solitary plasmacytomas involve the cervical spine in 9% to 13% of patients with spinal lesions.

Pathogenesis

The pathogenesis of this plasma cell tumor is unknown. Viral infections, chronic inflammation, exposure to toxins (including dioxin), and myeloproliferative diseases have been suggested as possible initiating factors. Interleukin-6 (IL-6) is an important cytokine for the growth and survival of myeloma cells. IL-6 may increase the resistance of myeloma cells to apoptosis.[11] Although the symptoms of a fracture associated with trauma are frequently the reason for a patient's initial evaluation by a physician, trauma is not a factor in the etiology of multiple myeloma. The lesions tend to occur in bones with the greatest hematopoietic activity, such as the spine, pelvis, ribs, skull, and proximal ends of the femora and humeri.

CLINICAL HISTORY

Skeletal Manifestations

Pain is the most common initial complaint of patients with multiple myeloma and occurs in 75% of patients.[42] Low back pain is the initial symptom in 35%. Localized neck pain is a symptom of individuals with cervical spine disease.[28] The spinal pain is mild, aching, and intermittent at the onset and is aggravated by weight bearing and relieved by bed rest. Pain when lying down is one of the symptoms that should raise the possibility of a spinal tumor, including multiple myeloma.[64] The duration of pain before diagnosis may be 6 months or longer.[10] Some patients have radicular symptoms, and a herniated intervertebral disc, sciatica, or arthritis is diagnosed.[13,53,55] Approximately 20% of patients give a history of insignificant trauma that causes pathologic fractures of vertebral bodies and results in acute, severe localized pain. Paraplegia more often develops with a solitary plasmacytoma than with multiple myeloma.[80] Spinal cord or cauda equina compression also occurs in myeloma patients.[43,76] Quadriplegia may develop after minor trauma in patients with multiple myeloma affecting the cervical spine. Fracture with extrusion of bony fragments into the spinal canal and resultant compression of the cervical spinal cord has been reported in myeloma patients.[25] Approximately 10% of patients with multiple myeloma may at initial evaluation have a solitary lesion.[66] Monoclonal antibodies will develop as a sign of progression of isolated plasmacytoma to multiple myeloma.[67] Involvement of the ribs, sternum, and thoracic spine may result in kyphosis and loss of height. In this illness, pain is not confined to the low back or neck region because bone pain may be found in any part of the skeleton and may be secondary to bone marrow expansion or microfractures.[26]

Extraosseous Manifestations

As a consequence of widespread bone destruction, abnormal immunoglobulin production, and infiltration of bone marrow, patients with multiple myeloma have a broad range of clinical symptoms. Hypercalcemia from bone destruction is associated with bone weakness, easy fatigability, anorexia, nausea, vomiting, mental status changes (including coma), and kidney stones. Increased abnormal immunoglobulin concentrations cause progressive renal insufficiency, increased susceptibility to infection, and amyloidosis. Amyloid is a protein that forms from portions of abnormal myeloma immunoglobulins. This protein infiltrates certain structures, including bone, muscle, perivascular connective tissue, kidney, and bladder.[48] Primary amyloidosis in the absence of multiple myeloma may infiltrate bone marrow and lead to radiographic changes in the vertebral column, including the cervical spine, that are similar to those of multiple myeloma.[4,69] Infiltration of bone marrow is associated with anemia, bleeding secondary to a deficiency of platelets, thrombocytopenia, and generalized weakness. Most patients have symptoms for less than 6 months before seeking medical attention. Patients in whom solitary lesions are subsequently diagnosed may have had symptoms for several years. Fever of unknown origin as an initial complaint is an unusual manifestation of myeloma when unassociated with an infection.[62]

PHYSICAL EXAMINATION

In the early stages of the illness, the results of physical examination may be unremarkable. As the duration of illness increases and bone marrow infiltration progresses, diffuse bone tenderness, fever, pallor, and purpura become prominent findings on examination. Fever is usually a manifestation of a complicating infection. Fever associated with myeloma alone is not common.[33] Rib cage and spine deformities are common in later stages of the illness. Neurologic examination may demonstrate signs of compression of the spinal cord or nerve roots if vertebral collapse has progressed to a significant extent.[31] Neurologic signs of cervical spine nerve root compression include muscle weakness, sensory changes, and reflex asymmetry. Spinal cord compression is manifested by upper motor neuron signs, including spasticity, hyperreflexia, and a positive Babinski sign.

LABORATORY DATA

Laboratory examination may reveal many abnormalities, including normochromic normocytic anemia, rouleau formation on blood smear, an elevated leukocyte count, thrombocytopenia, a positive Coombs test, and an elevated erythrocyte sedimentation rate. Abnormal serum chemistry studies include hypercalcemia, hyperuricemia, and elevated creatinine.[68] Impaired coagulation is mediated through inhibitors of clotting factors, clearance of clotting factors, and abnormalities in platelet function.[47]

Serum alkaline phosphatase is normal in most patients with multiple myeloma. Normal leukocyte alkaline phosphatase is associated with benign paraproteinemias, but an elevated level does not necessarily indicate a malignant condition.[60] Characteristic serum protein abnormalities occur in the vast majority of patients with multiple myeloma. Total serum protein concentrations are increased secondary to an increase in the globulin fraction. The increase in globulins is due to the presence of abnormal immunoglobulins of the G, A, D, E, or M classes. Immunoglobulins are composed of light and heavy chains. Multiple myeloma, instead of having a multitude of antibodies, has one single antibody composed of a light and a heavy chain, an M protein. It is produced to the exclusion of others. The balance between light and heavy chains may also be disturbed, with excess light chain production resulting in Bence-Jones protein in urine or excess heavy chain production resulting in heavy chain disease. Serum protein electrophoresis demonstrates the elevation in globulin levels, whereas quantitative immunoglobulin determination detects the class of immunoglobulin that is present in increased concentration. Serum protein electrophoresis demonstrates a spike in 76% of patients, hypogammaglobulinemia in 9%, and no abnormality in 15%.[49] Urine protein electrophoresis will detect the presence of Bence-Jones proteinuria. Other findings associated with abnormal immunoglobulins include increased serum viscosity, which results in blockage of blood vessels, and a positive test for rheumatoid factor.

Pathology

Bone marrow aspirates and biopsy show the characteristic changes of multiple myeloma. Bone marrow aspirates demonstrate increased numbers of plasma cells at levels greater than 30%. Bone marrow biopsy demonstrates diffuse infiltration of bone marrow with plasma cells (Fig. 13-31). Plasma cells may be classified into three histologic grades: well differentiated, moderately differentiated, and poorly differentiated.[12] Well-differentiated plasma cells look much like normal plasma cells. Anaplastic myeloma cells may mimic undifferentiated carcinomas or small cell sarcomas. Differentiating myeloma cells from non-neoplastic plasma cells is difficult. Subtle abnormalities in the size of the nucleus, nucleocytoplasmic disproportion, and the absence of inclusions are a few of the many factors that may help differentiate normal from malignant cells.[42]

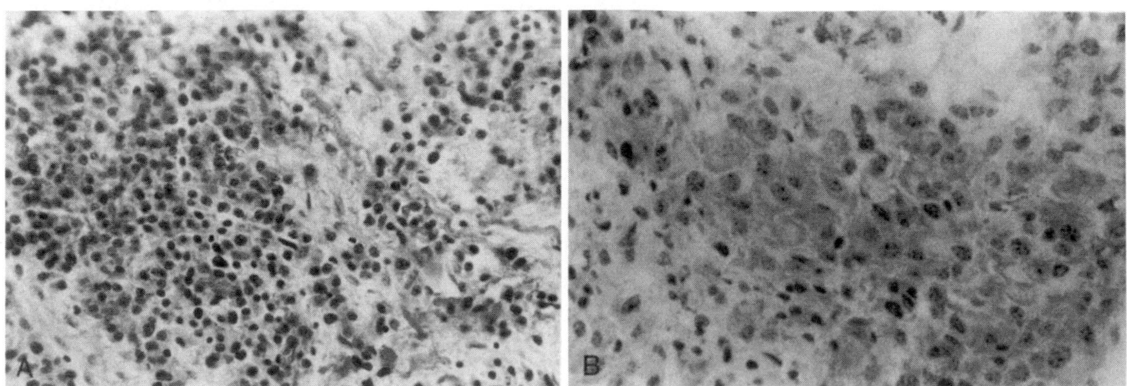

Figure 13-31 Histologic sections of multiple myeloma exhibiting numerous atypical plasma cells. *(Courtesy of Arnold Schwartz, MD.)*

Gross pathologic examination of bone shows a soft, gray, friable tumor in bone. The tumor frequently expands beyond the confines of the bone into soft tissue. In the spine, pathologic fractures are commonly identified.

Bone lesions are frequently associated with myeloma lesions. Most patients have lytic abnormalities in association with unbalanced bone remodeling leading to reduced bone mass and bone destruction.[7] Patients with sclerotic bone lesions had increased osteoblastic activity in the setting of increased bone resorption. These patients had a lambda-subtype IgG myeloma, an immunoglobulin subtype associated with sclerotic myeloma.[8] An early manifestation of myeloma is enhancement of osteoblastic recruitment with increased generation of new osteoclasts that cause increased bone resorption. The early stimulation of osteoblasts results in increased amounts of IL-6, a potent myeloma growth factor and a cytokine associated with the formation of osteoclasts in bone marrow.[9]

RADIOGRAPHIC EVALUATION

Roentgenograms

The predominant roentgenographic abnormality in multiple myeloma is osteolysis (Figs. 13-32 and 13-33). The diffuse osteolysis of the axial skeleton resembles osteoporosis.[23] A characteristic finding is the absence of reactive sclerosis surrounding lytic lesions in the spine. Preferential destruction of vertebral bodies with sparing of the posterior

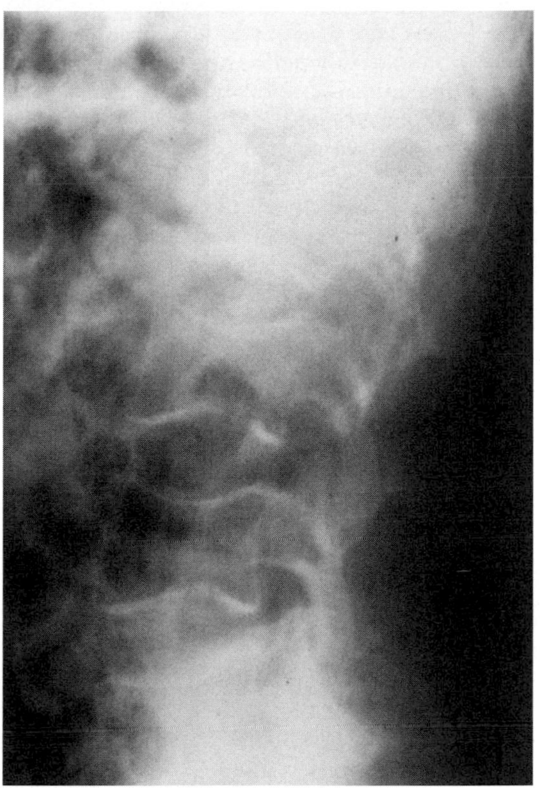

Figure 13-32 Multiple myeloma demonstrated by diffuse osteopenia. Diffuse osteopenia may be the sole radiographic abnormality in a majority of patients with this entity. *(Courtesy of Anne Brower, MD.)*

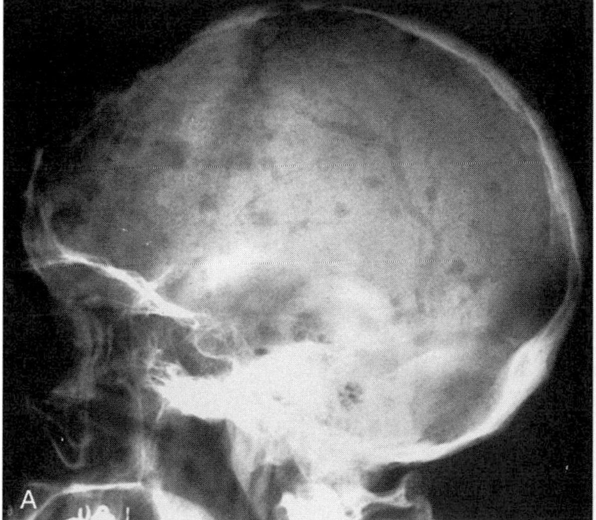

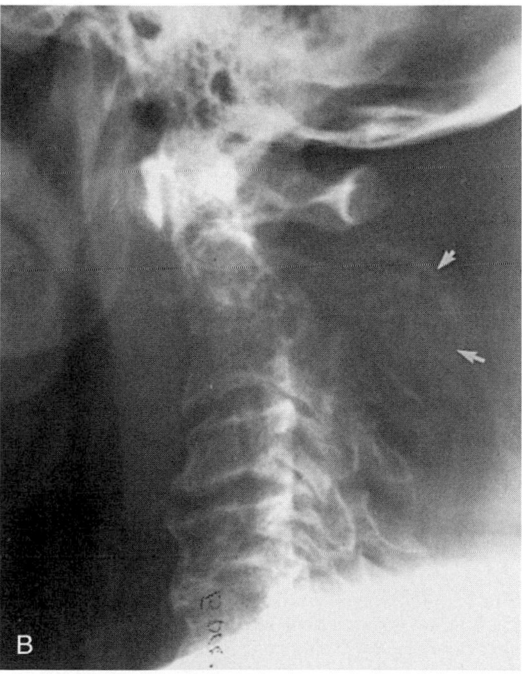

Figure 13-33 Multiple myeloma in a 62-year-old man with neck pain. *A*, A lateral view of the skull reveals multiple osteolytic "punched-out" lesions involving the entire calvarium. *B*, A lateral view of the cervical spine shows generalized osteopenia and an expansile, osteolytic lesion of the posterior elements of C2 *(arrows)*. *(Courtesy of Anne Brower, MD.)*

elements helps in differentiating multiple myeloma from osteolytic metastasis, which affects the vertebral pedicle and body (Figs. 13-34 and 13-35).[44] Paraspinous and extradural extension of tumor is seen in patients with multiple myeloma.

Benign solitary plasmacytoma may occur almost anywhere in the body, including bone and the kidney. Bone plasmacytomas are most common in the vertebral column, pelvis, and long bones, in order of decreasing frequency.[36] Solitary plasmacytomas, when located in the spine, have variable radiographic features. A purely osteolytic area without expansion or an expansile lesion with thickened trabeculae may be observed. An involved vertebral body may fracture and disappear completely, or the lesion may extend across the intervertebral disc and invade an adjacent vertebral body, similar to the appearance of an infection.[80] The lesion may have coarse trabeculae with vertical striations simulating vertebral angioma or Paget's disease.[56] Occasionally, osteoblastic lesions have been reported in patients with multiple myeloma and plasmacytoma.[20,74]

Scintigraphy

Although bone scans are used in the early detection of metastatic lesions, they are not helpful in multiple myeloma because the osteolytic lesions, which lack bone-forming (blastic) activity, will not be positive.[82,85] In the unusual patient with a positive scintiscan, regression of tumor activity may be characterized by the disappearance of scan abnormalities with treatment.[6]

Computed Tomography

CT may demonstrate vertebral body involvement before plain roentgenograms because radiographs detect

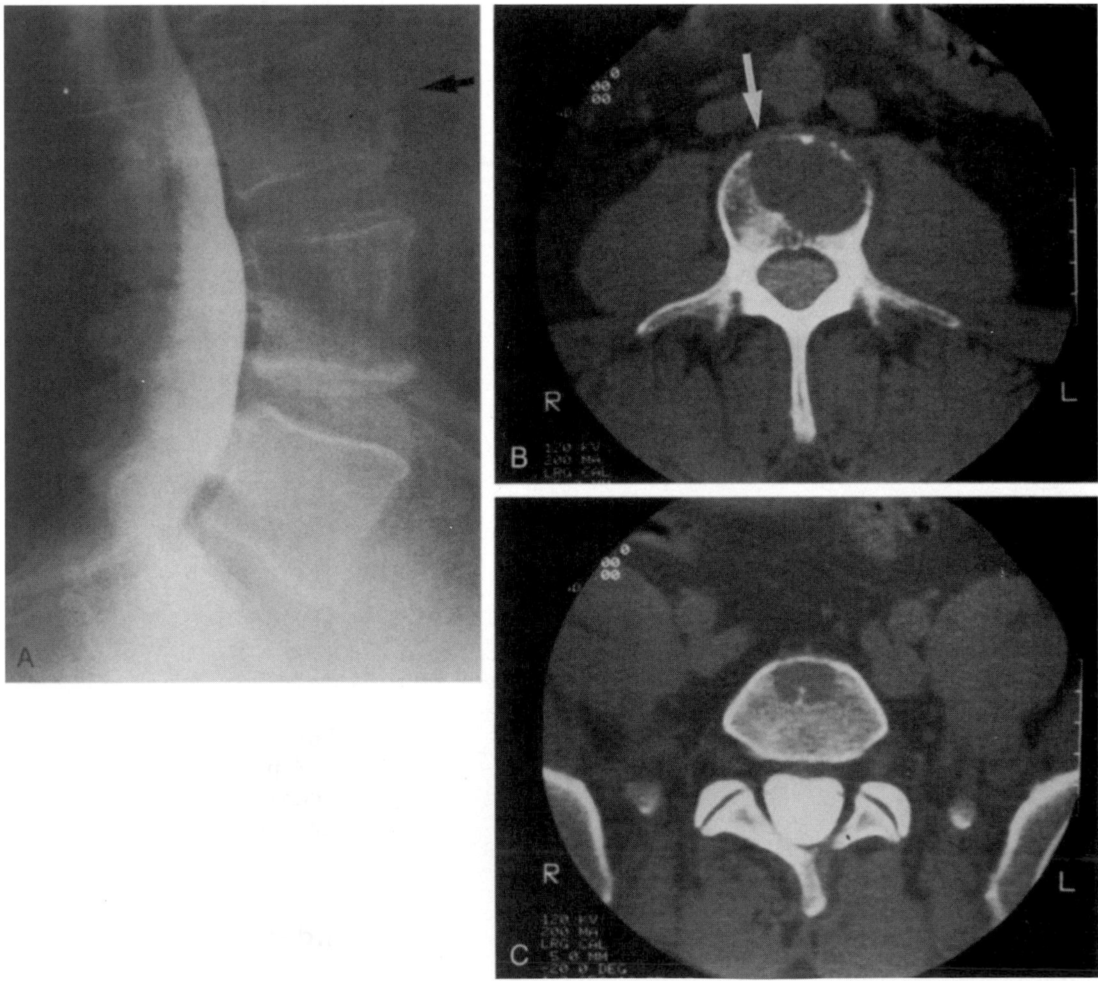

Figure 13-34 A 48-year-old man had a 6-week history of acute-onset back pain and radiation to the pelvis and right thigh associated with left leg weakness. Tenderness was demonstrated over the L3 vertebral body, and the patient had decreased sensation in a left L2 dermatome and decreased strength in the left iliopsoas muscle. *A*, Myelogram revealing an expansile lesion of L3 *(arrow)*. The spinal cord is normal. *B*, CT scan of the L3 vertebral body demonstrating a sharply marginated hypodense area occupying the greater part of L3 associated with interruption of the anterior cortex *(arrow)*. *C*, CT scan of the L5 vertebral body revealing a similar, smaller lesion. A bone biopsy of the L3 vertebral body revealed collections of plasma cells consistent with multiple myeloma. Subsequently, lesions in the thoracic spine were noted and a monoclonal IgG kappa protein was identified. The diagnosis of multiple myeloma was made, and the patient was started on a regimen of chemotherapy along with radiation therapy to the spine.

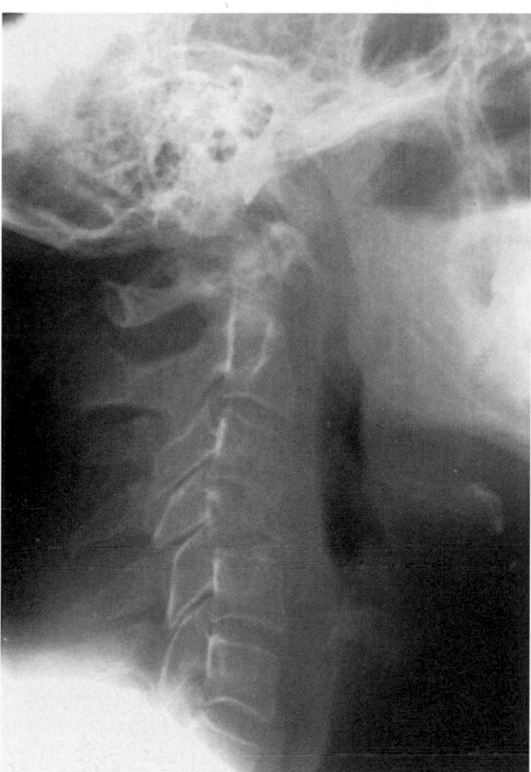

Figure 13-35 Multiple myeloma. A lateral view of the cervical spine reveals generalized osteopenia and collapse of the vertebral body of C3 without any reactive sclerosis. *(Courtesy of Anne Brower, MD.)*

abnormalities in bone calcium only after 30% of the calcium is lost.[40] CT is useful in demonstrating the extent of tumor, delineating the soft tissue component of an osseous lesion, or detecting an extramedullary plasmacytoma. CT can be used to detect early bone or extraosseous lesions in areas of the spine that are difficult to image with simple radiographic techniques.[77] Multidetector CT scans can produce re-formation projections of osseous lesions in the coronal and sagittal planes that are missed by conventional roentgenograms and MR imaging.[59]

Magnetic Resonance

MR imaging detects abnormalities in bone marrow that are not readily visualized by other techniques. On T1- and T2-weighted images, myeloma will appear as decreased or increased signal intensity, respectively. Alterations in signal may occur with fatty infiltration of marrow. Foci of tumor are better visualized with T2-weighted images (Fig. 13-36). The MR appearance does not correlate with laboratory or bone marrow findings.[54] The use of gadolinium as a contrast agent does not improve the ability of MR imaging to detect deposits of myeloma cells in the bone marrow of vertebral bodies.[3,71] Many compression fractures associated with myeloma have a benign appearance on MR imaging. In an MR study of myeloma patients, a minority (33%) of vertebral compression fractures had a malignant appearance.[52]

DIFFERENTIAL DIAGNOSIS

The diagnosis of multiple myeloma requires the inclusion of clinical, radiographic, and laboratory data along with the presence of abnormal plasma cells on histologic examination. A combination of major and minor criteria for establishing the diagnosis of myeloma has been developed by the Southwest Oncology Group.[34] Major criteria include a plasmacytoma demonstrated on biopsy, bone marrow plasmacytosis with more than a 30% content of plasma cells, and a monoclonal spike of more than 3.5 g for IgG, 2.0 g/100 mL for IgA, or 1.0 g/24 hr for urinary light chains. Minor criteria include bone marrow plasmacytosis, a monoclonal spike with small globulin concentrations, a lytic bone lesion, and serum immunoglobulin values less than 50 mg for IgM, 100 mg for IgA, and 600 mg/100 mL for IgG. The presence of characteristic abnormalities, Bence-Jones protein and M protein, on electrophoresis makes the diagnosis an easy one, but the diagnosis is more difficult in patients with diffuse osteoporosis and no detectable myeloma protein.[2] Low back or neck pain in a middle-aged to elderly patient with osteoporosis on radiographs must be evaluated thoroughly for possible myeloma.[33]

Plasmacytoma

Solitary plasmacytoma is also a difficult entity to diagnose. The diagnosis may be assumed if the character of the lesion is established by biopsy, if a bone survey is negative, if a bone marrow specimen is free of plasma cells, if hypergammaglobulinemia and Bence-Jones proteinuria are absent, and if the patient has been monitored closely for years.

Gammopathies

A differential diagnosis of monoclonal gammopathy must also be considered in patients with elevated globulin.[37] Some of the gammopathies have elevated globulin levels but do not cause bone lesions to the same degree as multiple myeloma does. Examples of these gammopathies include benign monoclonal gammopathy, Waldenström's macroglobulinemia, IgE myeloma, and alpha heavy chain disease.[47] Monoclonal gammopathy of undetermined significance (MGUS) can be differentiated from myeloma by an absence of abnormalities in the vertebral column on MR imaging.[15] The rate of progression of MGUS to myeloma is about 1% per year.[50] Liver disease, connective tissue disease, or chronic infection develops in patients with polyclonal gammopathies, but not in those with myeloma.[32]

Osteolytic Disorders

The list of other diseases that must be considered in the differential diagnosis of multiple myeloma is quite broad. Metastatic tumors and malignant lymphoma must be considered. Focal osteolysis on roentgenograms may be associated with a hemangioma. Infections, pyogenic and tuberculous, are associated with similar roentgenographic

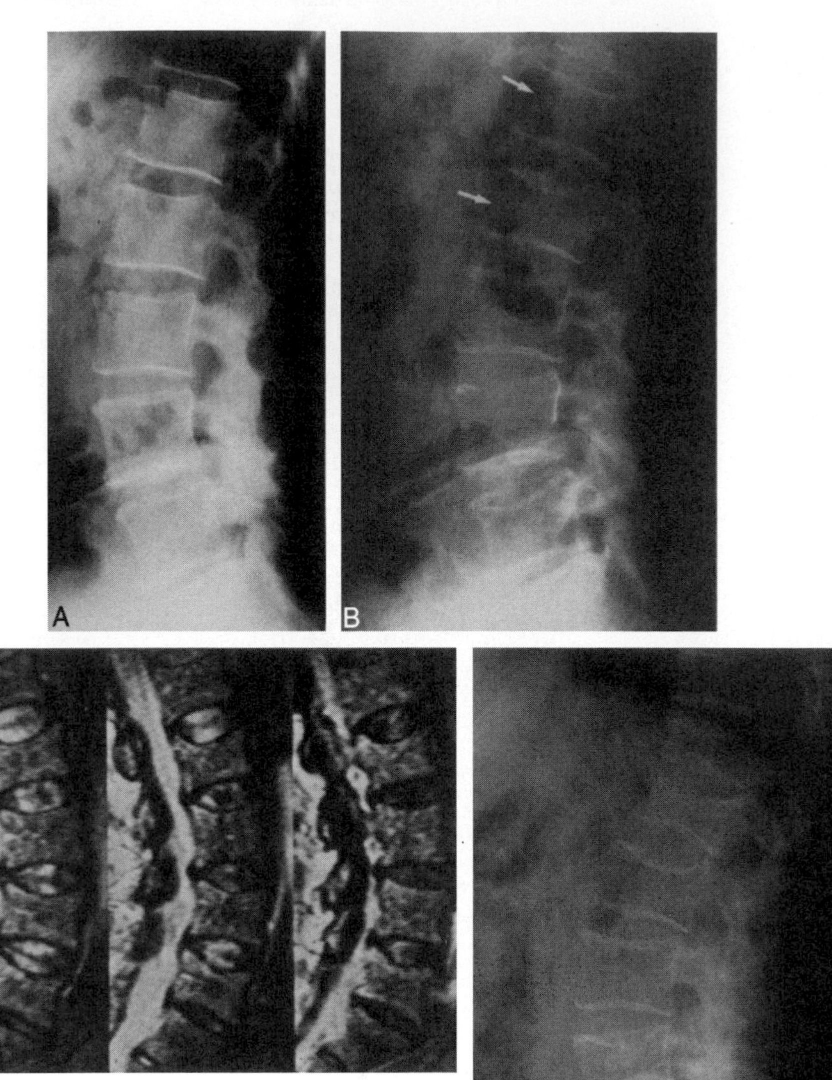

Figure 13-36 A 64-year-old man had nonspecific low back pain that increased with spine extension. *A,* A lateral plain roentgenogram on 9/30/88 revealed disc degeneration at the L5–S1 intervertebral space. *B,* The pain increased over the ensuing 8 weeks. A lateral plain roentgenogram on 12/5/88 revealed a marked increase in generalized osteopenia with evidence of vertebral fractures *(white arrows). C,* A T2-weighted MR image of the lumbar spine revealed increased signal found diffusely in the vertebral bone marrow. The diagnosis of multiple myeloma was confirmed, and the patient received prednisone and melphalan. *D,* A lateral plain roentgenogram on 12/12/90 revealed increased generalized osteopenia with additional compression fractures. The patient's myeloma was in remission, and he had little back pain. *(From Borenstein DG: Low back pain. In Klippel J, Dieppe P [eds]: Rheumatology. St Louis, CV Mosby, 1994.)*

findings.[21] Hyperparathyroidism may be associated with generalized bone lesions and hypercalcemia. Appropriate evaluation of blood tests and biopsy material should give the treating physician the information to make the appropriate diagnosis.

Multiple myeloma is usually associated with osteolytic bone activity. In rare circumstances, osteoblastic activity has been associated with this neoplasm. Patients with IgG monoclonal proteins of the lambda subtype are the ones with osteosclerotic bone lesions.[10]

TREATMENT

Treatment of multiple myeloma is an intricate combination of therapies, including chemotherapy, radiation therapy, bone marrow transplantation (autologous and allogeneic), and surgery.[86] Clinically active multiple myeloma usually requires systemic therapy with melphalan and prednisone over an extended course.[29] Approximately 70% of patients respond to this therapy and have a reduction in bone destruction and pain, a decreased concentration of abnormal proteins, and normalization of hematocrit, urea nitrogen, creatinine, and calcium. Some patients have responded well to high-dose dexamethasone alone without the toxicities associated with other therapies.[1] Patients with more aggressive disease may benefit by the M-2 drug program, a combination of vincristine, melphalan, cyclophosphamide, prednisone, and BCNU (carmustine).[24] Other treatments include high-dose melphalan, autologous bone marrow transplantation, interferon, and cytokines.[22] Thalidomide at doses up to 800 mg/day is an effective agent in resistant patients.[75] Response to therapy with changes in bone marrow cells can be seen on serial MR scans with the use of contrast media.[72] The MR changes are important for documenting a positive response to therapy in patients who may remain symptomatic from bony changes that are not related to the growth of plasma cells. In patients with cord compression secondary to multiple myeloma, decompressing laminectomy and/or local radiotherapy is indicated.[38] Radiotherapy is also indicated for a solitary plasmacytoma.

Patients with cervical spine instability caused by compression fractures secondary to multiple myeloma or plasmacytoma should be considered for surgical stabilization. Instability at the upper cervical levels may require occipitocervical fusion with a bone graft and bone cement.[57] Stability may be maintained despite progression of the neoplastic lesion in the bone. Cervical lesions may invade the adventitia of the vertebral artery. Presurgical embolization of the lesion may be required to obliterate the tumor's blood supply before surgery.[47]

Bisphosphonates inhibit calcium release from bone and prevent bone resorption through inhibition of osteoclastic activity. These drugs are most effective in patients with idiopathic osteoporosis. Pamidronate given over a 1- to 2-hour period intravenously (90 mg) every 4 weeks reduces skeletal complications and may promote tumor cell apoptosis.[18] Daily etidronate is not effective in reversing the osteopenia associated with myeloma.[14] Individuals with vertebral body fractures secondary to myeloma may benefit from percutaneous vertebroplasty.[45]

PROGNOSIS

The usual course of multiple myeloma is one of gradual progression. Myeloma patients may be asymptomatic at initial evaluation but are at risk of rapid progression, particularly if serum myeloma globulin is greater than 30 g/L.[83] Therapy may have an effect on clinical symptoms and the amount of myeloma protein, but the average survival remains about 3 to 5 years. A review of 1027 myeloma patients reported a median survival from time of diagnosis of 33 months, which had not changed from 1985 through 1998.[50a] Three patients with cervical spine disease and spinal cord compression were dead in 2 years in one study.[17] Patients with nerve compression secondary to myeloma may respond to chemotherapy with decreased paraproteinemia and tumor volume. However, the decrease in tumor size may be associated with increased instability of the spine requiring stabilization.[73] Because myeloma patients have a longer survival than other patients with malignancies do, surgical intervention does offer improvement in quality of life for up to 4 years.[35] Patients with D and G myeloma have poorer prognoses than A myeloma patients do.[39,70] Many patients may have more extensive disease than is clinically apparent. Individuals with diffuse bone marrow involvement on MR imaging have shorter survival than those with normal or focal findings.[51] Over 50% of patients may have compression fractures at autopsy.[46] In addition, the effects of myeloma may extend beyond the involvement of bone alone. Even in the absence of marrow packed with plasma cells, erythropoiesis may be depressed by an effect of the disease on progenitor cells.[65] Plasmacytosis, hypoalbuminemia, elevated alkaline phosphatase, hyperuricemia, or renal insufficiency in a male patient is a predictor of poor outcome at 2 years.[27] In a study of 130 Japanese patients, only 9 (6.9%) patients were alive at 10 years. Prognostic factors for survival included a younger age at diagnosis, low tumor mass, chemotherapy with cyclophosphamide, disappearance of myeloma protein, and a positive response to retreatment.[63]

Patients with solitary plasmacytomas have a better prognosis than do those who initially have multiple lesions.[80] However, it is important to remember that disseminated disease may eventually develop in some patients with solitary lesions, in some cases 20 or more years after their initial diagnosis.[84] Neurologic complications develop in patients with plasmacytoma. These individuals may require surgical stabilization for neurologic improvement.[5]

References

Multiple Myeloma

1. Alexanian R, Dimopoulos MA, Delasalle, Barlogie B: Primary dexamethasone treatment of multiple myeloma. Blood 80:887, 1992.
2. Arend WP, Adamson JW: Nonsecretory myeloma: Immunofluorescent demonstration of paraprotein within bone marrow plasma cells. Cancer 33:721, 1974.
3. Avrahami E, Tadmor R, Kaplinsky N: The role of T2-weighted gradient echo in MRI demonstration of spinal multiple myeloma. Spine 18:1812, 1993.
4. Axelsson U, Hallen A, Rausing A: Amyloidosis of bone: Report of two cases. J Bone Joint Surg Br 52-B:717, 1970.
5. Baba H, Maezawa Y, Furusawa N, et al: Solitary plasmacytoma of the spine associated with neurological complications. Spinal Cord 36:470-475, 1998.
6. Bataille R, Chevalier J, Rossi M, Sany J: Bone scintigraphy in plasma cell myeloma. A prospective study of 70 patients. Radiology 145:801, 1982.
7. Bataille R, Chappard D, Marcelli C, et al: Mechanisms of bone destruction in multiple myeloma: The importance of an unbalanced process in determining the severity of lytic bone disease. J Clin Oncol 7:1909, 1989.
8. Bataille R, Chappard D, Marcelli C, et al: Osteoblast stimulation in multiple myeloma lacking lytic bone lesions. Br J Haematol 76:484, 1990.
9. Bataille R, Chappard D, Marcelli C, et al: Recruitment of new osteoblasts and osteoclasts is the earliest critical event in the pathogenesis of human multiple myeloma. J Clin Invest 88:62, 1991.
10. Bataille R, Delmas PD, Chappard D, Sany J: Abnormal serum bone Gla protein levels in multiple myeloma: Crucial role of bone formation and prognostic implications. Cancer 66:167, 1990.
11. Bataille T, Horousseau JL: Multiple myeloma. N Engl J Med 336:1657-1664, 1997.
12. Bayrd ED: The bone marrow on sternal aspiration in multiple myeloma. Blood 3:987, 1948.
13. Bayrd ED, Heck FJ: Multiple myeloma: A review of 83 proven cases. JAMA 133:147, 1947.
14. Belch AR, Bergsagel DE, Wilson K, et al: Effect of daily etidronate on the osteolysis of multiple myeloma. J Clin Oncol 9:1397, 1991.
15. Bellaiche L, Laredo J, Liote F, et al: Magnetic resonance appearance of monoclonal gammopathies of unknown significance and multiple myeloma. Spine 22:2551-2557, 1997.
16. Bence-Jones H: On a new substance occurring in the urine of a patient with mollities ossium. Philos Trans R Soc Lond (Biol) 1:55, 1848.
17. Benson WJ, Scarffe JH, Todd IDH, et al: Spinal cord compression in myeloma. BMJ 1:1541, 1979.
18. Berenson JR, Lichtenstein A, Porter L, et al: Long-term pamidronate treatment of advanced multiple myeloma patients

reduces skeletal events: Myeloma Aredia Study Group. J Clin Oncol 16:593-602, 1998.
19. Blade J, Kyle RA, Greipp PR: Multiple myeloma in patients younger than 30 years: Report of 10 cases and review of the literature. Arch Intern Med 156:1463-1468, 1996.
20. Brown TS, Paterson CR: Osteosclerosis in myeloma. J Bone Joint Surg Br 55-B:621, 1973.
21. Burton CH, Fairham SA, Millet B et al: Unusual aetiology of persistent back pain in a patient with multiple myeloma: Infectious discitis. J Clin Pathol 52:633-634, 1998.
22. Camba L, Durie BGM: Multiple myeloma: New treatment options. Drugs 44:170, 1992.
23. Carson CP, Ackerman LV, Maltby JD: Plasma cell myeloma: A clinical, pathologic and roentgenologic review of 90 cases. Am J Clin Pathol 25:849, 1955.
24. Case DC Jr, Lee BJ III, Clarkson BD: Improved survival times in multiple myeloma treated with melphalan, prednisone, cyclophosphamide, vincristine and BCNUBM-2 protocol. Am J Med 63:897, 1977.
25. Chan L, Snyder HS, Verdile VP: Cervical fracture as the initial presentation of multiple myeloma. Ann Emerg Med 24:1192, 1994.
26. Charkes ND, Durant J, Barry WE: Bone pain in multiple myeloma: Studies with radioactive 87m Sr. Arch Intern Med 130:53, 1972.
27. Cherng NC, Asal NR, Kuebler JP, et al: Prognostic factors in multiple myeloma. Cancer 67:3150, 1991.
28. Clarke E: Spinal cord involvement in multiple myelomatosis. Brain 79:332, 1956.
29. Costa G, Engle RL Jr, Schilling A, et al: Melphalan and prednisone—an effective combination for the treatment of multiple myeloma. Am J Med 54:589, 1973.
30. Dalrymple J: On the microscopical character of mollities ossium. Dublin Q J Med Sci 2:85, 1846.
31. Davison C, Balser BH: Myeloma and its neural complications. Arch Surg 35:913, 1937.
32. Dispenzieri A, Gertz MA, Therneau TM, et al: Retrospective cohort study of 148 patients with polyclonal gammopathy. Mayo Clin Proc 76:476-487, 2001.
33. Duffy TP: The many pitfalls in the diagnosis of myeloma. N Engl J Med 326:394, 1992.
34. Durie BGM, Salmon SE: A clinical staging system for multiple myeloma: Correlation of measured myeloma cell mass with presenting clinical features, response to treatment and survival. Cancer 36:842, 1975.
35. Durr HR, Wegener B, Krodel A, et al: Multiple myeloma: Surgery of the spine: Retrospective analysis of 27 patients. Spine 27:320-324, 2002.
36. Eichner ER: The plasma cell dyscrasias: Diverse presentations, pathophysiology and management. Postgrad Med 67:44, 1980.
37. Gandara DR, Mackenzie MR: Differential diagnosis of monoclonal gammopathy. Med Clin North Am 72:1155, 1988.
38. Gilbert RW, Kim JH, Posner JB: Epidural spinal cord compression from metastatic tumor: Diagnosis and treatment. Ann Neurol 3:40, 1978.
39. Gompels BM, Votaw ML, Martel W: Correlation of radiological manifestations of multiple myeloma with immunoglobulin abnormalities and prognosis. Radiology 104:509, 1972.
40. Helms CA, Genant HK: Computed tomography in the early detection of skeletal involvement with multiple myeloma. JAMA 248:2886, 1982.
41. Hewell GM, Alexanian R: Multiple myeloma in young persons. Ann Intern Med 84:441, 1976.
42. Huvos AG: Bone Tumors: Diagnosis, Treatment, and Prognosis, 2nd ed. Philadelphia, WB Saunders, 1991, pp 653-676.
43. Jacobs P, King HS, Le Roux I, Handler L: Extradural spinal myeloma and emergency neurosurgery. S Afr Med J 77:316, 1990.
44. Jacobsen HG, Poppel MH, Shapiro JH, Grossberger S: The vertebral pedicle sign: A roentgen finding to differentiate metastatic carcinoma from multiple myeloma. AJR Am J Roentgenol 80:817, 1958.
45. Jensen ME, Kallmes DE: Percutaneous vertebroplasty in the treatment of malignant spine disease. Cancer J 8:194-206, 2002.
46. Kapadia SB: Multiple myeloma: A clinicopathologic study of 62 consecutively autopsied cases. Medicine (Baltimore) 59:380, 1980.
47. Kempin S, Sundaresan N: Disorders of the Spine Related to Plasma Cell Dyscrasias. In Sundaresan N, Schmidek HH, Schiller AL, Rosenthal DI (eds): Tumors of the Spine: Diagnosis and Clinical Management. Philadelphia, WB Saunders, 1990, pp 214-225.
48. Klein LA: Case Record 7B1986. N Engl J Med 314:500, 1986.
49. Kyle RA: Multiple myeloma: Review of 869 cases. Mayo Clin Proc 50:29, 1975.
50. Kyle RA, Therneau TM, Rajkumar V, et al: A long-term study of prognosis in monoclonal gammopathy of undetermined significance. N Engl J Med 346:564-569, 2002.
50a. Kyle RA, Gertz MA, Witzig TE, et al: Review of 1027 patients with newly diagnosed multiple myeloma. Mayo Clin Proc 78:21-33, 2003.
51. Lecouvet FE, Vande Berg BC, Michaux L, et al: Stage III multiple myeloma: Clinical and prognostic value of spinal bone marrow MR imaging. Radiology 209:653-656, 1998.
52. Lecouvet FE, Vande Berg BC, Maldague BE, et al: Vertebral compression fractures in multiple myeloma. Part 1. Distribution and appearance at MR imaging. Radiology 204:195-199, 1997.
53. Lehmann O: Problems of pathological fractures. Bull Hosp Jt Dis 12:90, 1951.
54. Libshitz HI, Malthouse SR, Cunningham D, et al: Multiple myeloma: Appearance at MR imaging. Radiology 182:833, 1992.
55. Lichtenstein L, Jaffee HL: Multiple myeloma: A survey based on 35 cases, 18 of which came to autopsy. Arch Pathol Lab Med 44:207, 1947.
56. Loftus CM, Micheisen CB, Rapoport F, Antunes JL: Management of plasmacytomas of the spine. Neurosurgery 13:30, 1983.
57. Lofvenberg R, Lofvenberg EB, Ahlgren O: A case of occipitocervical fusion in myeloma. Acta Orthop Scand 61:81, 1990.
58. Macintyre W: Case of mollities and fragilitas ossium accompanied with urine strongly charged with animal matter. Med Chir Soc Trans 33:211, 1850.
59. Mahnken AH, Wildberger JE, Gehbauer G, et al: Multidetector CT of the spine in multiple myeloma: Comparison with MR imaging and radiography. AJR Am J Roentgenol 178:1429-1436, 2002.
60. Majumdar G, Hunt M, Singh AK: Use of leukocyte alkaline phosphatase (LAP) score in differentiating malignant from benign paraproteinaemias. J Clin Pathol 44:606, 1991.
61. Mirra JM: Bone Tumors: Diagnosis and Treatment. Philadelphia, JB Lippincott, 1980, pp 398-406.
62. Mueller PS, Terrell CL, Gertz MA: Fever of unknown origin caused by multiple myeloma. Arch Intern Med 162:1305-1309, 2002.
63. Murakami H, Nemoto K, Miyawaki S, et al: Ten-year survivors with multiple myeloma. J Intern Med 231:129, 1992.
64. Nicholas JJ, Christy WC: Spinal pain made worse by recumbency: A clue to spinal cord tumors. Arch Phys Med Rehabil 67:598, 1986.
65. Oken MM: Multiple myeloma: Symposium on hematology and hematologic malignancies. Med Clin North Am 68:757, 1984.
66. Osserman EF: Plasma-cell myeloma. II. Clinical aspects. N Engl J Med 261:952, 1959.
67. Otto S, Vegh Z, Hindy I, Peter I: Multiple myeloma arising from solitary plasmacytoma of bone. Oncology 47:84, 1990.
68. Paredes JM, Mitchell BS: Multiple myeloma: Current concepts in diagnosis and management. Med Clin North Am 64:729, 1980.
69. Porchet F, Sonntag VK, Vrodos N: Cervical amyloidoma of C2. Case report and review of the literature. Spine 23:133-138, 1998.
70. Pruzanski W, Rother I: IgD plasma cell neoplasia: Clinical manifestations and characteristic features. Can Med Assoc J 102:1061, 1970.
71. Rahmouni A, Divine M, Mathieu D, et al: Detection of multiple myeloma involving the spine: Efficacy of fat-suppression and contrast-enhanced MR imaging. AJR Am J Roentgenol 160:1049, 1993.
72. Rahmouni A, Divine M, Mathieu D, et al: MR appearance of multiple myeloma of the spine before and after treatment. AJR Am J Roentgenol 160:1053, 1993.
73. Rapoport AP, Rowe JM: Plasma cell dyscrasia in a 15-year-old boy: Case report and review of the literature. Am J Med 89:816, 1990.
74. Roberts M, Rianudo PA, Vilinskas J, Owens G: Solitary sclerosing plasma-cell myeloma of the spine: Case report. J Neurosurg 40:125, 1974.
75. Singhal S, Mehta J, Desikan R, et al: Antitumor activity of thalidomide in refractory multiple myeloma patients. N Engl J Med 341:1565-1571, 1999.
76. Sinoff CL: Spinal cord compression due to myeloma. S Afr Med J 78:434, 1990.
77. Solomon A, Rahamani R, Seligsohn U, Ben-Artzi F: Multiple myeloma: Early vertebral involvement assessed by computerized tomography. Skeletal Radiol 11:258, 1984.

78. Todd IDH: Treatment of solitary plasmacytoma. Clin Radiol 16:395, 1965.
79. Unni KK: Dahlin's Bone Tumors: General Aspects and Data on 11,087 Cases, 5th ed. Philadelphia, Lippincott-Raven, 1996, pp 225-236.
80. Valderrama JAF, Bullough PG: Solitary myeloma of the spine. J Bone Joint Surg Br 50-B:82, 1968.
81. Von Rustizky J: Multiple myeloma. Dtsch Z Chir 3:162, 1873.
82. Wahner HW, Kyle RA, Beabout JW: Scintigraphic evaluation of the skeleton in multiple myeloma. Mayo Clin Proc 55:739, 1980.
83. Weber DM, Dimopoulos MA, Moulopoulos LA, et al: Prognostic features of asymptomatic multiple myeloma. Br J Haematol 97:810-814, 1997.
84. Woodruff RK, Malpas JS, White FE: Solitary plasmacytoma II. Solitary plasmacytoma of bone. Cancer 43:2344, 1979.
85. Wooltenden JM, Pitt MJ, Durie BGM, Moon TE: Comparison of bone scintigraphy and radiography in multiple myeloma. Radiology 134:723, 1980.
86. Zaidi AA, Vesole DH: Multiple myeloma: An old disease with new hope for the future. CA Cancer J Clin 51:273-285, 2001.

CHONDROSARCOMA

CAPSULE SUMMARY

	LOW BACK	NECK
Frequency of spinal pain	Uncommon	Uncommon
Location of spinal pain	Lumbar spine or sacrum	Cervical spine
Quality of spinal pain	Mild ache	Mild ache
Symptoms and signs	Painless mass	Painless mass
Laboratory tests	None	None
Radiographic findings	Expansile, calcified mass on plain roentgenograms	Expansile, calcified mass on plain roentgenograms
Treatment	En bloc resection	En bloc resection

PREVALENCE AND PATHOGENESIS

Chondrosarcoma is a malignant tumor that forms cartilaginous tissue. It is frequently located in the pelvis, sacrum, or lumbar spine. Chondrosarcoma is rarely located in the cervical spine, but it occurs more commonly there than osteosarcoma or Ewing's sarcoma does.[30] Because the tumor has extremely slow growth and lesions are usually painless, chondrosarcoma of the pelvis and spine may be present for a long time before it is discovered.

Chondrosarcoma has been known by many different names, including chondroblastic sarcoma, malignant chondroblastoma, myxoid chondrosarcoma, and clear cell chondrosarcoma, among others.

Epidemiology

Chondrosarcoma accounts for 11% to 22% of primary bone tumors examined by biopsy.[18,34] Among malignant tumors, chondrosarcoma is the third most common neoplasm, after multiple myeloma and osteogenic sarcoma. The usual age at onset is between 40 and 60 years, and the ratio of men to women is 3:2.[25]

Pathogenesis

The pathogenesis of chondrosarcoma is unknown. Primary chondrosarcomas arise de novo from previously normal bone, whereas secondary chondrosarcomas develop from other cartilaginous tumors such as osteochondroma or enchondroma. Chondrosarcoma may be induced by irradiation, and it accounts for 9% of radiation-induced cases of bone sarcoma.[12] It also develops in a small number of patients with Paget's disease, fibrous dysplasia, or Maffucci's syndrome (enchondromas with soft tissue hemangiomas).[11,22,33]

Approximately 9% of patients with chondrosarcoma have lesions involving the spine. A review of 553 chondrosarcoma patients documented spinal involvement in 6% of individuals.[30] The lumbosacral spine is the site of the tumor in 50% of patients, with the thoracic spine involved in 32% and the cervical spine in 18%. In another review of 151 cases of spinal chondrosarcoma, the frequency of involvement was the lumbar spine in 28.5%, the sacrum in 28.5%, the thoracic spine in 23%, the cervical spine in 12%, and unspecified location in 8%.[21]

CLINICAL HISTORY

Chondrosarcoma may be symptomless or may be characterized by only mild discomfort and palpable swelling. Tumors in the pelvis are detected when they are palpable through the abdominal wall or cause nerve compression with radicular pain, similar to the symptoms of a herniated disc.[18,24,32] Tumors in the cervical spine are associated with neck pain. Pain, when it occurs, is strongly suggestive of an actively growing tumor. This is particularly important in a patient who has had an osteochondroma for decades that suddenly becomes painful. Chondrosarcoma is a very slowly growing tumor, so a history of symptoms for several years before the patient seeks medical evaluation is usual. Patients commonly complain of nocturnal pain with exacerbation on recumbency.[7,26] Almost 50% of patients have neurologic symptoms at the time of diagnosis. Unilateral radicular pain is associated with chondrosarcoma of the cervical spine.[31] Referred arm pain may precede local neck pain, thereby delaying discovery of the tumor. With increased tumor growth, the pain becomes more severe and persistent.[31]

PHYSICAL EXAMINATION

Physical examination may demonstrate a painless tumor mass or one that is mildly painful on palpation.[5] Range of motion of the spine is decreased secondary to pain and muscle spasm. Rectal examination may be helpful in detecting a mass originating in the pelvis or sacrum. Neurologic examination may be abnormal if neural elements are compressed by the tumor. With progression of compression, increasing weakness is noted. Lesions in the lumbar spine produce lower motor neuron weakness with flaccidity of muscles and loss of reflexes. Corresponding sensory deficits are also present. Lesions in the cervical spine produce sensory deficits in the corresponding nerve root distribution. Radicular involvement produces numbness, paresthesias, and dysesthesias in a dermatomal pattern in the arm. Myelopathic abnormalities, including paresis, have been reported in patients with tumors invading the spinal canal.[30] Compression of the spinal cord produces upper motor neuron weakness with spasticity, an abnormal Babinski sign, and increased reflexes. Spinal cord lesions produce a progression of sensory deficits from impaired vibratory, joint position, and temperature sensation to pain on light touch.[31]

LABORATORY DATA

Laboratory findings may not be abnormal until late in the course of the tumor. Abnormalities may correlate with tumor size and the extent of metastasis. Useful data to obtain include blood counts, serum chemistry studies, and sedimentation rates. As many as 75% of patients with chondrosarcomas have an abnormal glucose tolerance curve and high insulin levels. Insulin and insulin growth factor are documented stimulators of cartilage metabolism.[7] However, the relationship of insulin to the development of abnormal cartilage growth is unknown.[7]

Pathology

Gross pathologic inspection of chondrosarcomas reveals a pearly, translucent tissue that is lobulated. Areas of calcification within the lesion are represented by yellow-white areas of speckling. The extent and exact boundaries of the lesion are difficult to identify.[15] More reactive new bone is seen with slow-growing tumors than with high-grade anaplastic chondrosarcomas.[14] Peripheral chondrosarcomas may grow to very large size, particularly when situated in the pelvis.[27]

The microscopic appearance of chondrosarcoma is graded by the degree of abnormality in the nuclei of the cells. Grade 1 is the most benign form of chondrosarcoma and does not have any associated cellular atypia. Some lesions have double nuclei and abundant hyaline matrix. Microscopically, a grade 1 chondrosarcoma differs only slightly from a benign enchondroma. The malignant lesion is more cellular with larger cells that are binucleate. These changes may be present in only parts of the tumor, thus necessitating review of many sections of a biopsy specimen to confirm the diagnosis (Fig. 13-37).[16] Grades 2 and 3 are increasingly malignant and are associated with higher degrees of cellularity, nuclear size, and mitoses (Fig. 13-38).[23] Grade 2 lesions have increased atypia, are more densely cellular, and have multiple nuclei and foci of necrosis. Grade 3 lesions have marked atypia, mitotic figures, multinucleate cells, little matrix, and numerous areas of necrosis. In a study of 152 pelvic chondrosarcomas, 56 were grade 1, 53 were grade 2, and 43 were grade 3.[18] Rare types of chondrosarcomas include clear cell, mesenchymal (characterized by a calcified soft tissue mass), myxoid, and

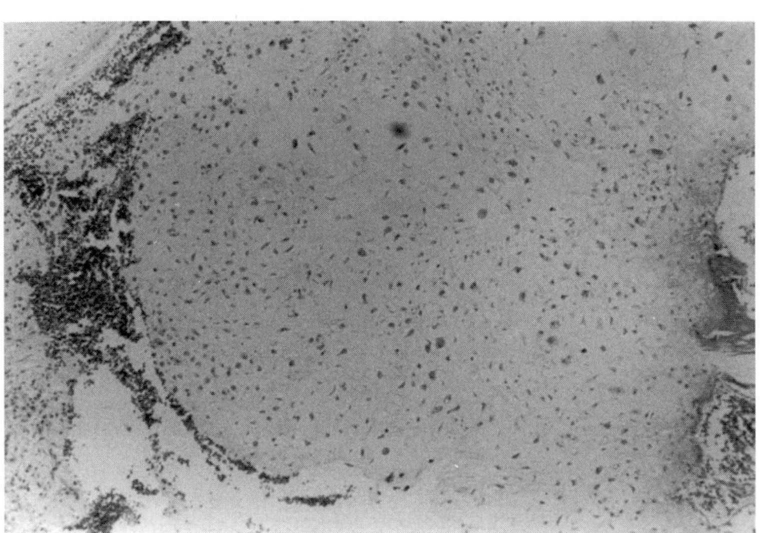

Figure 13-37 Histologic section of chondrosarcoma exhibiting increased cellularity of chondrocytes with atypical nuclei and increased mitotic activity. *(Courtesy of Arnold Schwartz, MD.)*

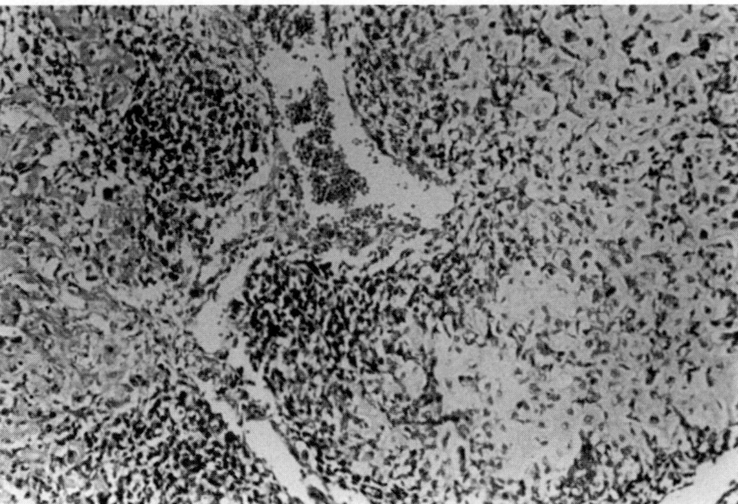

Figure 13-38 Histologic section of a high-grade chondrosarcoma with marked atypia and clumps of chondroid matrix in a disorganized pattern. *(Courtesy of Arnold Schwartz, MD.)*

periosteal. Dedifferentiation refers to the appearance of a more anaplastic connective tissue tumor in a grade 1 chondrosarcoma.[13]

RADIOGRAPHIC EVALUATION

Roentgenograms

The characteristic roentgenographic findings of chondrosarcoma include a well-defined lesion with expansile contours (Figs. 13-39 and 13-40). The interior of the lesion may demonstrate lobular or fluffy calcification with scalloping of the interior cortex of bone. Periosteal and endosteal reactive bone formation leads to a thickened cortex of bone, which is typical of a slow-growing tumor.[3] Cortical destruction and soft tissue invasion are indicative of more aggressive lesions. In the spine, the vertebral body or posterior elements may be the site of origin. The tumor may cause neural foraminal widening.[38] Plain roentgenographs are useful in detecting tumors that have calcified. However, soft tissue extension may not be appreciated on these roentgenograms. A chondrosarcoma may develop in the cartilaginous cap of an osteochondroma. Malignancy should be suspected if the cap of the benign lesion becomes thicker than 1 cm, especially after skeletal maturity, and has the appearance of irregular calcification.[13] Plain roentgenograms are the most effective means of establishing the diagnosis of a cartilaginous tumor. This technique detects calcifications, ossifications, and periosteal reaction more readily than CT or MR does.[13]

Scintigraphy/Computed Tomography/ Magnetic Resonance

For the evaluation of extraosseous extension of a tumor, CT and MR are essential. Both CT and MR can determine the presence or absence of soft tissue invasion by the tumor. CT depicts calcification in tumor matrix and cortical destruction that may be missed on MR.[16] Studies using gadolinium contrast–enhanced MR have detected scalloped margins and curvilinear septa of chondrosarcomas that correspond to fibrovascular bundles surrounding hyaline cartilage lobules.[1] Neither CT nor MR is specific enough to establish a precise diagnosis before biopsy of the lesion. Particularly with MR, benign and malignant chondrogenic lesions have similar MR characteristics that do not allow for accurate differentiation of tumors.[28] Bone scintigraphy is helpful in detecting remote skeletal lesions and local intraosseous metastases.[16]

Arteriography

Arteriography may be useful in determining the extent of extraosseous involvement associated with a chondrosarcoma and in defining the major feeding blood vessels to the tumor.[20] The evaluation is helpful in determining the most effective surgical approach to the lesion.

DIFFERENTIAL DIAGNOSIS

The diagnosis of grade 1 chondrosarcoma must be based on clinical, radiographic, and pathologic findings. For the histopathologist, chondrosarcoma is the most difficult of the malignant bone tumors to diagnose. The histologic appearance of a low-grade chondrosarcoma may be similar to that of a cellular enchondroma, a benign lesion. Malignant tumors with similar histologic appearance may have different aggressive properties. The findings of pain, rapid growth, cortical destruction, soft tissue extension, and anaplastic cells on biopsy are characteristic of higher-grade, more malignant chondrosarcoma.[25]

A wide range of benign and malignant processes may mimic the characteristics of chondrosarcoma. Processes that may cause lesions of the spine include giant cell tumor, chordoma, and osteogenic sarcoma. Careful attention to the clinical symptoms of the patient along with a

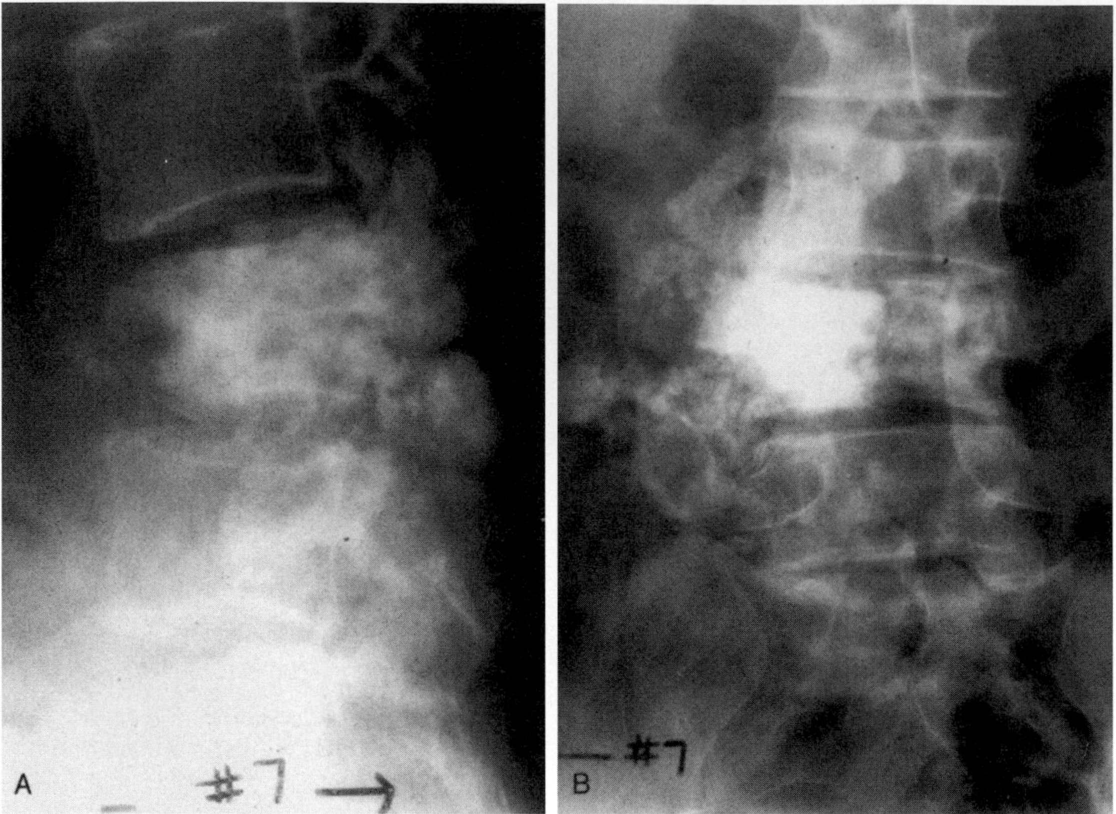

Figure 13-39 Chondrosarcoma. Lateral *(A)* and anterior *(B)* views of a vertebral body with soft tissue extension of the tumor associated with disorganized chondroid matrix calcification. The lateral view shows relative sparing of the disc spaces. *(Courtesy of Anne Brower, MD.)*

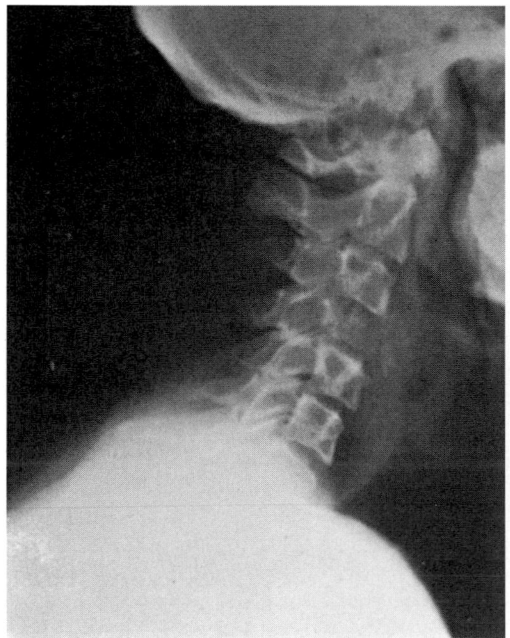

Figure 13-40 Chondrosarcoma of C4. Poorly marginated lytic destruction of the vertebral body combined with an anterior soft tissue mass indicates malignancy. *(From Sim FH, Frassica FJ, Wold LE, McLeod RA: Chondrosarcoma of the spine: Mayo Clinic experience. In Sundaresan N, Schmidek HH, Schiller AL, Rosenthal DI [eds]: Tumors of the Spine: Diagnosis and Clinical Management. Philadelphia, WB Saunders, 1990, p 157.)*

thorough review of biopsy material should give the pathologist adequate information to make the appropriate diagnosis. Pathologic differentiation of chondrosarcoma and chordoma is difficult because of histologic similarities. Immunohistochemical evaluation of cartilaginous tumors with a panel of antibodies to cytokeratin, epithelial membrane antigen, vimentin, S-100 protein, carcinoembryonic antigen, and type II collagen is helpful in differentiating these tumors.[36]

TREATMENT

Surgery is the treatment of choice for chondrosarcoma. En bloc resection of the tumor with a margin of normal tissue so that malignant cells are not implanted in the surgical wound offers the best chance of long-term survival.[4,6] Five-year survival rates for grades 1, 2, and 3 pelvic chondrosarcoma after excisional surgery were 47%, 38%, and 15%, respectively.[24] Tumors that are partially resected frequently recur with increased cytologic malignancy.[8] Recurrences develop in a majority of patients over a number of years.[37] Chondrosarcomas are radioresistant, so radiotherapy is reserved for tumors that are inaccessible to excision. Chemotherapy may play an adjunctive role in these difficult situations. A combination of surgical removal, irradiation, and chemotherapy has been associated with prolonged survival.[9]

PROGNOSIS

Patients with chondrosarcoma and frequent pain have more malignant tumors.[19] Those with low-grade, well-differentiated chondrosarcoma have a longer survival rate and longer interval between treatment and recurrence than do those with higher-grade tumors. These facts hold true for chondrosarcoma of the lumbar and cervical spine, pelvis, and sacrum. Chondrosarcoma with a low degree of malignancy grows slowly, recurs locally, and metastasizes late. High-grade tumors grow rapidly and metastasize early. Patients with the best outcome are those with low-grade tumors and successful en bloc excision. Patients without en bloc excision have progression of disease and are more likely to die of their tumor. In one study, 50% of patients with contaminated marginal excisions died after a local recurrence.[30] Patients with high-grade pelvic chondrosarcomas have a poor outcome, with a 5-year survival rate of only 20%.[17] In individuals with pelvic recurrences, successful excision of the recurrent tumor is associated with improved survival.[35]

Patients with cervical spine lesions and larger tumors that limit the opportunity to remove the entire tumor have a higher risk of recurrence.[2] Patients with a cervical lesion may survive up to 20 years after successful surgical excision.[30] In a study comparing chondrosarcoma, osteosarcoma, chordoma, and malignant fibrous histiocytoma in 2627 patients with primary malignant bone tumors, chondrosarcoma had the best 5-year survival rate (72.7%, 41.0%, 63.8%, and 42.9%, respectively), despite being the tumor in this group most commonly detected in patients older than 50 years.[10]

New immunologic techniques are being developed to categorize the potential of bone tumors to respond to different types of therapy. A Ki-67 monoclonal antibody specific for a nuclear antigen that is expressed throughout the cell cycle of an actively dividing cell has been used to determine the proliferative activity of chondrosarcoma. The level of Ki-67 expression correlates with the level of malignancy of the tumor. In the future, this information may be useful for making therapeutic decisions concerning specific grades of tumors, and it may have prognostic importance.[29]

References

Chondrosarcoma

1. Aoki J, Sone S, Fujioka F, et al: MR of enchondroma and chondrosarcoma: Rings and arcs of Gd-DTPA enhancement. J Comput Assist Tomogr 15:1011, 1991.
2. Austin JP, Urie MM, Cardenosa G, Muzenrider JE: Probable cause of recurrence in patients with chordoma and chondrosarcoma of the base of skull and cervical spine. Int J Radiat Oncol Biol Phys 25:439, 1993.
3. Barnes R, Catto M: Chondrosarcoma of bone. J Bone Joint Surg Br 48-B:729, 1966.
4. Bergh P, Gunterberg B, Meis-Kindblom JM, et al: Prognostic factors and outcome of pelvic, sacral, and spinal chondrosarcomas: A center-based study of 69 cases. Cancer 91:1202-1212, 2001.
5. Bohlman HH, Sachs BL, Carter JR, et al: Primary neoplasms of the cervical spine: Diagnosis and treatment of twenty-three patients. J Bone Joint Surg Am 68-A:483, 1986.
6. Boriani S, De Iure F, Bandiera S, et al: Chondrosarcoma of the mobile spine: Report of 22 cases. Spine 25:804-812, 2000.
7. Cammisa FP Jr, Glasser DB, Lane JM: Chondrosarcoma of the spine: Memorial Sloan-Kettering Cancer Center experience. In Sundaresan N, Schmidek, Schiller AL, Rosenthal DI (eds): Tumors of the Spine: Diagnosis and Clinical Management. Philadelphia, WB Saunders, 1990, pp 149-154.
8. Dahlin DC, Henderson ED: Chondrosarcoma: A surgical and pathological problem—review of 212 cases. J Bone Joint Surg Br 38-B:1025, 1956.
9. Di Lorenzo N, Palatinsky E, Artico M, Palma L: Dural mesenchymal chondrosarcoma of the lumbar spine: Case report. Surg Neurol 31:470, 1989.
10. Dorfman HD, Czerniak B: Bone cancers. Cancer 75:203, 1995.
11. Feintuch TA: Chondrosarcoma arising in a cartilaginous area of previously irradiated fibrous dysplasia. Cancer 31:877, 1973.
12. Fitzwater JE, Caboud HE, Farr GH: Irradiation-induced chondrosarcoma: A case report. J Bone Joint Surg Am 58-A:1037, 1976.
13. Ghelman B: Radiology of bone tumors. Orthop Clin North Am 20:287, 1989.
14. Gilmer WS Jr, Kilgore W, Smith H: Central cartilage tumors of bone. Clin Orthop 26:81, 1963.
15. Goldenbeg RR: Chondrosarcoma. Bull Hosp Jt Dis 25:30, 1964.
16. Greenspan A: Tumors of cartilage origin. Orthop Clin North Am 20:347, 1989.
17. Henderson ED, Dahlin DC: Chondrosarcoma of bone: A study of 280 cases. J Bone Joint Surg Am 45-A:1450, 1963.
18. Huvos AG: Bone Tumors: Diagnosis, Treatment, and Prognosis, 2nd ed. Philadelphia, WB Saunders, 1991, pp 343-381.
19. Kaufman JH, Douglass HO Jr, Blake W, et al: The importance of initial presentation and treatment upon the survival of patients with chondrosarcoma. Surg Gynecol Obstet 145:357, 1977.
20. Kenney PJ, Gilola LA, Murphy WA: The use of computed tomography to distinguish osteochondroma and chondrosarcoma. Radiology 139:129, 1981.
21. Kricun ME: Imaging of Bone Tumors. Philadelphia, WB Saunders, 1993, p 263.
22. Lewis RJ, Ketcham AS: Maffucci's syndrome: Functional and neoplastic significance—case report and review of the literature. J Bone Joint Surg Am 55-A:1465, 1973.
23. Lichtenstein L, Jaffe HL: Chondrosarcoma of bone. Am J Pathol 19:553, 1943.
24. Marcove RC, Mike V, Hutter RVP, et al: Chondrosarcoma of the pelvis and upper end of the femur: An analysis of factors influencing survival time in 113 cases. J Bone Joint Surg Am 54-A:561, 1972.
25. Mirra JM: Bone Tumors: Diagnosis and Treatment. Philadelphia, JB Lippincott, 1980, pp 178-218.
26. Nicholas JJ, Christy WC: Spinal pain made worse by recumbency: A clue to spinal cord tumors. Arch Phys Med Rehabil 67:598, 1986.
27. Norman A, Sissons HA: Radiographic hallmarks of peripheral chondrosarcoma. Radiology 151:589, 1984.
28. Petterson H, Sloane RM, Spanier S, et al: Primary musculoskeletal tumors: Examination with MR imaging compared with conventional modalities. Radiology 164:237, 1987.
29. Scotlandi K, Serra M, Manara C, et al: Clinical relevance of Ki-67 expression in bone tumors. Cancer 75:806, 1995.
30. Shives TC, McLeod RA, Unni KK, Schray MF: Chondrosarcoma of the spine. J Bone Joint Surg Am 71-A:1158, 1989.
31. Sim FH, Frassica FJ, Wold LE, McLeod RA: Chondrosarcoma of the spine: Mayo Clinic experience. In Sundaresan N, Schmidek HH, Schiller AL, Rosenthal DI (eds): Tumors of the Spine: Diagnosis and Clinical Management. Philadelphia, WB Saunders, 1990, pp 155-162.
32. Smith FW, Nandi SC, Mills K: Spinal chondrosarcoma demonstrated by Tc-99m-MDP bone scan. Clin Nucl Med 7:111, 1982.
33. Thomson AD, Turner-Warwick RT: Skeletal sarcomata and giant cell tumor. J Bone Joint Surg Br 37-B:266, 1955.
34. Unni KK: Dahlin's Bone Tumors: General Aspects and Data on 11,087 Cases, 5th ed. Philadelphia, Lippincott-Raven, 1996, pp 71-108.
35. Weber KL, Pring ME, Sim FH: Treatment and outcome of recurrent pelvic chondrosarcoma. Clin Orthop 397:19-28, 2002.
36. Wojno KJ, Hruban RH, Garin-Chesa P, Huvos AG: Chondroid chordomas and low-grade chondrosarcomas of the craniospinal axis: An immunohistochemical analysis of 17 cases. Am J Surg Pathol 16:1144, 1992.
37. York JE, Berk RH, Fuller GN, et al: Chondrosarcoma of the spine: 1954-1997. J Neurosurg 90 (1 suppl):73-789, 1999.
38. Yunten N, Calli C, Zileli M, et al: Chondrosarcoma causing cervical neural foramen widening. Eur Radiol 7:1028-1030, 1997.

CHORDOMA

Capsule Summary

	Low Back	Neck
Frequency of spinal pain	Common	Common
Location of spinal pain	Lumbar spine and sacrum	Cervical spine
Quality of spinal pain	Ache	Ache
Symptoms and signs	Painless mass	Dysphagia, painless mass
Laboratory tests	Anemia	Anemia
Radiographic findings	Vertebral osteolysis with calcific soft tissue mass on plain roentgenograms	Vertebral osteolysis with calcific soft tissue mass on plain roentgenograms
Treatment	En bloc resection, radiation therapy	En bloc resection, radiation therapy

PREVALENCE AND PATHOGENESIS

Chordoma is a malignant tumor that originates from the remnants of embryonic tissue, the notochord. The notochord is the structure that develops into a portion of the vertebral bodies of the spine in the embryo. Chordomas are located exclusively in the axial skeleton. These tumors are slow growing and may be present for an extended period before symptoms secondary to the compression of vital structures bring the patient to a physician.

Virchow in 1857 was the first to suggest the persistence of cells from the notochord in skeletal structures. Horwitz in 1941 proposed that chordomas arise from abnormal chordal remnants in vertebral bones.[22]

Epidemiology

Chordomas account for 3% to 4.14% of primary bone tumors.[35,53] Another study found chordomas to represent 1.3% of primary bone tumors.[42] The tumor usually becomes evident between the ages of 40 and 70, and it is rarely reported in patients 30 years or younger. The ratio of men to women with sacrococcygeal chordomas is 3:1, whereas the ratio is 1:1 for chordomas in other locations in the spine.[34] A Mayo Clinic study of 40 patients with chordomas, exclusive of the sacrum, reported the ratio of men to women to be 2:1.[6] A study of 88 chordoma patients, including those with sacral tumors, had a similar 2:1 ratio of men to women.[50] The mean age of sacral tumor patients was 56 years, whereas 47 was the mean age of those with tumors in the mobile spine.

All chordomas are located in the axial skeleton, from the spheno-occipital area in the skull to the tip of the coccyx. The most common location for chordomas is the sacrum, which is the site of 50% of the lesions. The skull is the location for 38% of the tumors. The cervical, lumbar, and thoracic spine are unusual locations for this neoplasm; these regions account for 6%, 4%, and 2% of lesions, respectively.[28] The extent of involvement of the cervical spine with chordoma has ranged from 48% to 6% in a variety of studies of this tumor in the axial skeleton.[15,50,52] Chordoma has been reported to affect the axis and the atlas.[18,31,36,61] Occasionally, chordomas may be present in other areas of the spine, such as the transverse process, and in extraosseous locations, including the epidural space.[19,44,52]

Pathogenesis

The cause of factors that initiate the regrowth of notochordal vestigial cells in the spine is unknown, although trauma has been suggested as a possible initiating factor.[39] At Memorial Hospital in New York, 15% of patients with sacrococcygeal chordoma gave a history of previous low back trauma of a degree significant enough to require medical attention. The frequency of a history of trauma to the lower back area requiring medical evaluation in patients with sacral chordoma may be as high as 50%.[28] Whether trauma is a causative factor or a chance event in pathogenesis of the lesion remains conjectural at this time.

CLINICAL HISTORY

Patients with sacrococcygeal chordoma have nondescript lower back pain. The pain may be characterized as dull or sharp and intermittent or constant and is localized in the sacrum. In the cervical spine, the pain is localized to the neck. The pain may be of long duration because the patient may not have thought it to be a significant problem.[25] Some patients initially have severe constipation, urinary frequency or hesitancy, dysuria, incontinence, or muscular weakness.[25] These symptoms are secondary to direct pressure on pelvic structures or compression of neural elements. Patients with chordomas of the lumbar spine may experience pain in the hip, knee, groin, or sacroiliac region. This pattern of referred pain to the lower extremities may be confusing and delay discovery of the true location of the spinal tumor. Pain is not relieved by lying down, and night pains are characteristic symptoms.[19]

In the cervical spine, the mean duration of symptoms in the mobile spine between the onset of symptoms and the time of diagnosis was 14 months.[6] The neurologic symptoms associated with the tumor depend on its location. Patients with cervical chordoma may complain of unilateral weakness and paresthesias.[52] Dysphagia is a symptom of patients with chordoma projecting anteriorly from the cervical spine.[44]

PHYSICAL EXAMINATION

Lumbar Spine

Rectal and neurologic examinations are helpful in detecting the presence of chordomas in the sacrum and spine. Chordomas of the sacrum extend anteriorly into the pelvis, and the presacral extension of a chordoma is detected on rectal examination. The tumor is a firm, roundish mass that is palpable through the posterior wall of the rectum. The examining finger glides easily over the tumor because the rectal mucosa and muscularis are rarely affected by the tumor. Neurologic examination may demonstrate flaccidity, whereas lesions higher in the axial skeleton are associated with muscle spasticity.

Cervical Spine

Chordoma of the cervical spine may occur in an anterior, lateral, or posterior location. Physical and neurologic examination may demonstrate a wide variety of abnormalities corresponding to the location of the tumor. Anterior lesions, which may form a soft tissue mass, may cause swelling in the retropharyngeal area. Lateral lesions may cause signs of radiculopathy. Posterior lesions may have symptoms consistent with myelopathy.

LABORATORY DATA

Laboratory findings may be unremarkable early in the course of this tumor. Abnormalities in hematologic and chemical parameters may appear late, after the tumor has grown extensively or has metastasized.

Pathology

Gross examination of the tumor reveals a soft, lobulated, grayish mass that is usually well encapsulated except in the region of bony invasion. Sacral chordomas have a presacral extension that is covered by periosteum. In the vertebral column, it originates in the vertebral body and spreads either along the posterior longitudinal ligament or through the intervertebral disc.

Histologically, chordomas are characterized by physaliphorous cells of notochordal origin (Fig. 13-41). These cells contain a large, clear area of cytoplasm with an eccentric, flattened nucleus and form columns that are interspersed in fibrous tissue.[13] The tumor is also characterized by the production of large amounts of mucin, and this histologic appearance bears a close resemblance to that of an adenocarcinoma. The nuclear size of tumor cells

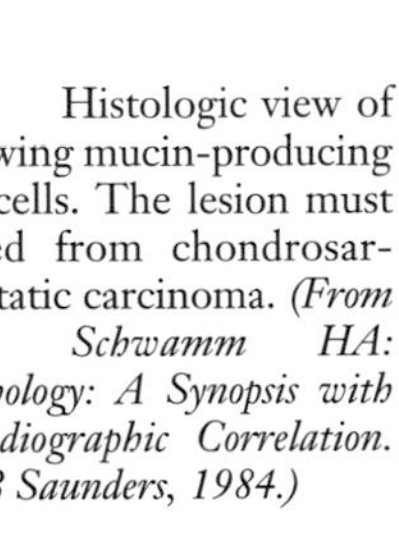

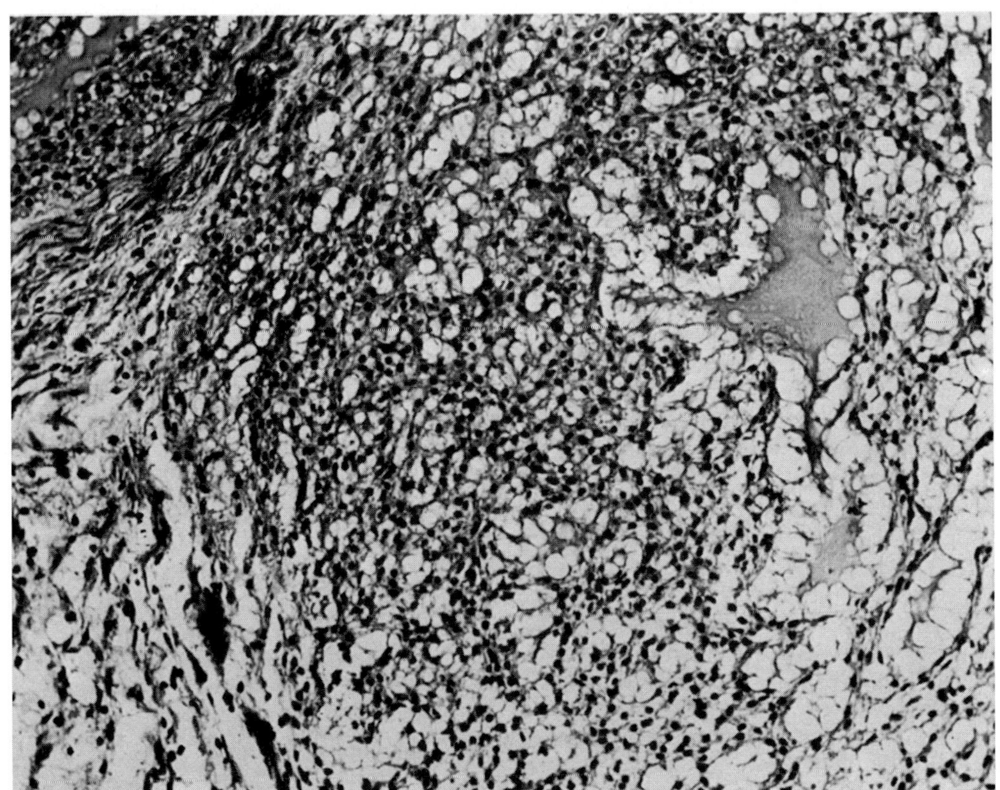

Figure 13-41 Histologic view of a chordoma showing mucin-producing physaliphorous cells. The lesion must be differentiated from chondrosarcoma and metastatic carcinoma. *(From Bogumill GP, Schwamm HA: Orthopaedic Pathology: A Synopsis with Clinical and Radiographic Correlation. Philadelphia, WB Saunders, 1984.)*

may vary greatly. Mitotic figures are rare. The tumor may show a wide range in its histologic appearance, including physaliphorous cells along with cells in arrangements that mimic spindle cell sarcomas or epithelial tumors.[55] Chordomas may be differentiated from cartilage tumors and adenocarcinomas with special stains. Chordomas are positive for keratin and S-100 protein, whereas cartilage tumors are keratin negative and adenocarcinomas are S-100 negative.[50,60]

Chondroid chordoma is a variant of chordoma with histologic features that may mimic chondrosarcoma.[29] Chordomas that contain chondroid components are usually limited to the spheno-occipital region of the spine. However, chondroid chordomas of the lumbosacral region have been reported. Distinction of conventional from chondroid chordomas is important because patients with the latter have longer survival.[23]

RADIOGRAPHIC EVALUATION

Roentgenograms

Sacrococcygeal and vertebral chordomas produce lytic bone destruction with calcific foci and a soft tissue mass (Figs. 13-42 and 13-43).[21] The tumor originates in a single vertebral body in the mobile spine. The lesion is osteosclerotic in most circumstances.[9] The soft tissue may extend superiorly to the tumor with amorphous, peripheral calcification. Sacral chordomas produce destruction of several sacral segments, along with a presacral soft tissue mass. Lesions may be difficult to identify because of the angle of the sacrum and overlying bowel gas. Soft tissue extension may be determined best by evaluation with intravenous pyelography, ultrasound, arteriography, venography, or CT (Fig. 13-44).[32,48] Vertebral chordoma initially causes destruction of a vertebral body without intervertebral disc involvement. Subsequently, the intervertebral discs become narrowed and opposing vertebral endplates are eroded.[40] Myelography is helpful in determining extradural extension of the tumor even in the absence of neurologic symptoms. However, it is important to remember that the sacral canal ends at the first or second sacral vertebra. Myelography may miss the intraspinal extension of tumor distal to the thecal sac.[2]

Scintigraphy

Bone scintigraphy may not detect sacral chordomas because of increased accumulation of tracer in the bladder. Lateral scans may be needed to evaluate the sacrum. Reduced uptake in the sacrum, or a "cold spot," should raise the possibility of a chordoma.[41] In other portions of the spinal column, bone scintigraphy may establish the solitary nature of the tumor.

Computed Tomography

CT is superior to plain roentgenograms for the evaluation of chordomas. The total extent of the tumor mass and soft tissue component can be determined by CT without any need for angiography or myelography. CT detects calcific debris not apparent on plain roentgenograms.[46] Chordoma is a solitary mass, but CT is able to detect extension of the tumor to neighboring spinal bones.[33]

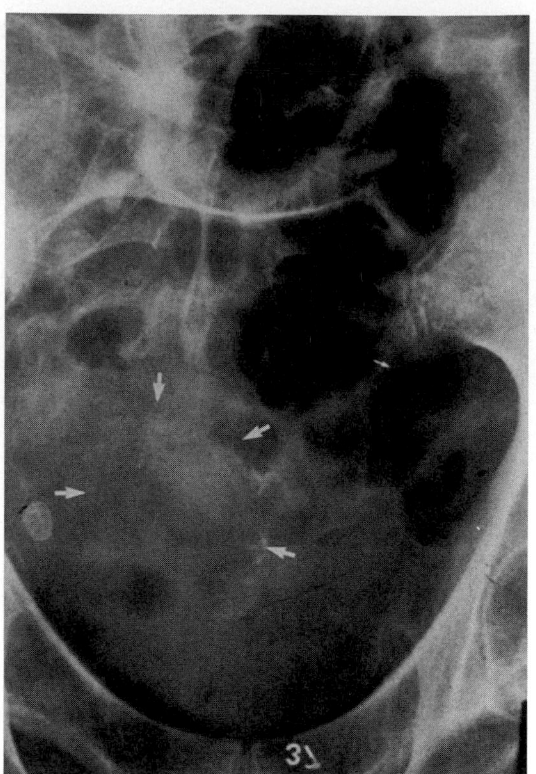

Figure 13-42 Chordoma of the sacrococcygeal spine associated with extensive bone destruction *(arrows)* and no calcification. *(Courtesy of Anne Brower, MD.)*

Magnetic Resonance

MR allows for imaging of the sacral and cervical region in three planes. MR detects the presence of bone diseases and is particularly helpful in determining the extent of the soft tissue mass accompanying the chordoma (Fig. 13-45).[58] MR characteristics of chordomas include signal intensity similar to that of muscle on T1-weighted images and increased intensity on T2-weighted images.[64,65] MR evaluation of the gluteal muscles can identify infiltration of tumor, which can be removed to help prevent local recurrences.[62] MR imaging is the best method to identify local recurrence after patients have received therapy for their tumors.[19]

DIFFERENTIAL DIAGNOSIS

The diagnosis of chordoma is suggested by its location and radiographic features, but a definitive diagnosis is dependent on examination of a biopsy specimen. Needle biopsy of a vertebral chordoma is usually adequate. Fine-needle aspiration biopsy of chordomas produces adequate specimens

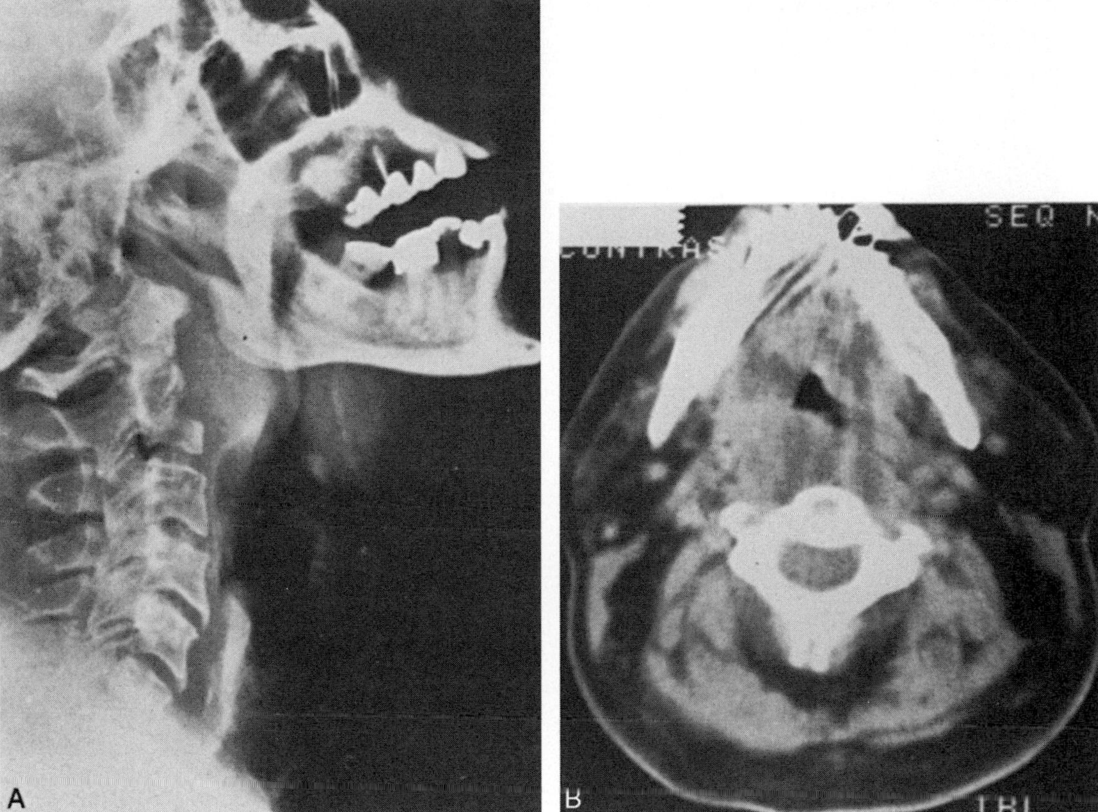

Figure 13-43 Chordoma. *A*, Lateral cervical spine. Note the retropharyngeal soft tissue mass with minimal involvement of the C2 vertebra. *B*, Axial CT scan. Note the parapharyngeal soft tissue extension of tumor. *(From Sundaresan N, Rosenthal DI, Schiller AL, Krol G: Chordomas. In Sundaresan N, Schmidek HH, Schiller AL, Rosenthal DI [eds]: Tumors of the Spine: Diagnosis and Clinical Management. Philadelphia, WB Saunders, 1990, p 200.)*

for diagnosis.[7] Specimens may be examined by microscopic, histochemical, and immunocytochemical methods, including tests for cytokeratin, epithelial membrane antigen, vimentin, carcinoembryonic antigen, and protein S-100. The use of these methods allows differentiation of chondrogenic and metastatic adenocarcinomas from chordomas.[28,31,56,60] Open biopsy is frequently required for sacral chordoma because of the tumor's location.

A number of lesions need to be considered in the differential diagnosis of a chordoma. Giant cell tumor of bone frequently involves the sacrum. Other lesions include osteochondroma, chondrosarcoma, metastases, multiple myeloma, osteosarcoma, osteoblastoma, aneurysmal bone cyst, and intrasacral cysts. Undifferentiated sarcomas may also involve the sacrum.[54] Neurofibromas cause lytic lesions of the sacrum.[59] Chordoma may cause widening of the cervical foramen, similar to neurofibroma.[45] Tumor may cause intervertebral disc narrowing that may be confused with an inflammatory disorder such as osteomyelitis.[33]

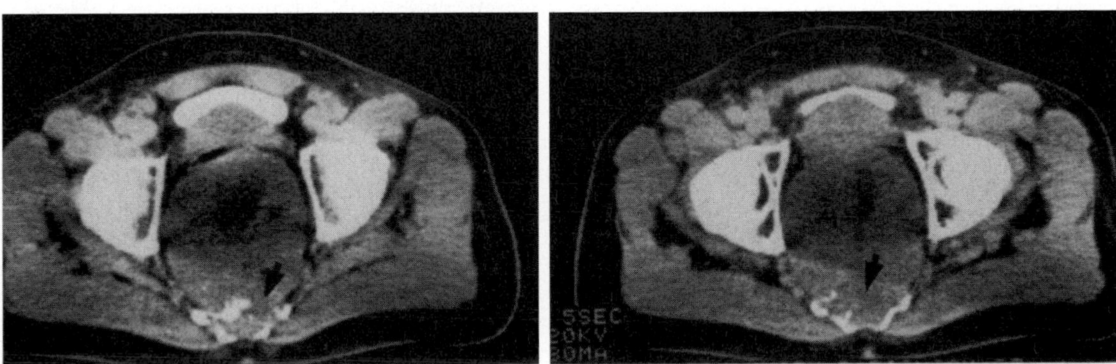

Figure 13-44 A 60-year-old man with minimal back discomfort and a mass detected on rectal examination. CT reveals a large mass anterior to the sacrum. The sacrum contains lytic lesions with destruction of the bony cortex *(arrows)*. Biopsy of this lesion revealed a chordoma.

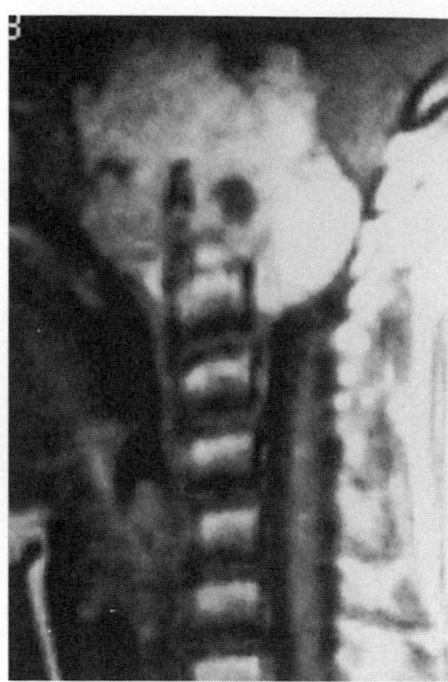

Figure 13-45 Chordoma: MR imaging abnormalities. In a 12-year-old child, a sagittal T1-weighted (TR/TE 600/20) spin echo MR image obtained after the intravenous injection of a gadolinium compound shows a large lesion in the base of the skull with inferior extension into the upper cervical vertebrae and spinal canal. The tumor is of high signal intensity, with enhancement related to the injected contrast agent. The tumor is lobulated, and there appear to be septations of low signal intensity. *(Courtesy of S. K. Brahme, MD, La Jolla, California.)*

Teratoma

Teratomas are benign or malignant tumors that occur in the sacrum and may be confused with chordoma. Most teratomas are recognized at birth. However, a number have remained undiagnosed in adults for extended periods.[27] The symptoms of these tumors, such as rectal dysfunction, may be very similar to those seen with chordoma.[17] These tumors probably arise from Hensen's node near the coccyx.

TREATMENT

Medical

Chemotherapy is usually ineffective.[30]

Radiation Therapy

In patients with inaccessible sacral chordomas, radical radiation therapy may slow tumor growth.[38] Improved long-term local control of axial skeletal chordoma has been reported with the combined use of high-dose proton and photon radiation therapy and three-dimensional planning to pinpoint the site of the radiation beam.[26]

Surgical

Lumbosacral Spine

The definitive treatment of chordoma is en bloc excision. Unfortunately, because of the size of the tumor at the time of diagnosis and approximation of the tumor to vital structures, partial resection may be the only surgical option. Staging of the tumor before surgery with radiographic techniques and percutaneous biopsy helps determine the possible surgical options for removal of the tumor.[47] Sacrococcygeal tumors are best treated by surgical excision, if the superior portion of the sacrum is not involved, followed by irradiation.[14] Postoperative radiation therapy results in reasonable local control of tumor without significant toxicity.[43] Vertebral chordomas are treated by decompression laminectomy with excision of accessible tumor located in bone, soft tissues, and the extradural space. Aggressive surgical techniques have been developed that provide the ability to remove an entire vertebra or the sacrum with little residual dysfunction.[47,51]

Cervical Spine

Lesions in the upper cervical spine may be approached through a mandibular approach; midcervical lesions may be approached from a lateral interscalene incision. Fusion with bone is preferable to methylmethacrylate for those with an unstable spine after removal of the tumor.[19]

PROGNOSIS

Chordomas are slowly growing tumors that metastasize in 10% of patients late in the course of the illness.[57] Common locations for metastatic lesions are the lung, bone, and lymph nodes.[20] Patients who undergo total resection of the tumor have a better survival rate than do those with partial resection.[5,12] Five-year survival rates for sacrococcygeal tumors and vertebral tumors are 66% and 50%, respectively. Ten-year survival rates range between 10% and 40%.[48] A few patients have survived with a chordoma for 20 years. A number of studies report that the best long-term outcome is achieved with en bloc excision of all components of the tumor.[3,8,24,37,63] Preservation of the S3 nerve roots is necessary to ensure retention of normal urinary and bowel function.[11] Cervical spine chordomas, particularly those that are larger, have a higher rate of recurrence than do those at the base of the skull.[1] Adequate removal at the time of initial cervical spine surgery is associated with a fivefold decrease in the recurrence rate in comparison to surgical removal after tumor relapse.[10] DNA analysis (diploid versus aneuploid) does not offer additional prognostic data regarding local recurrence or survival.[4] In a large study of 2627 primary malignant bone tumors in which chordoma, chondrosarcoma, osteosarcoma, and malignant fibrous histiocytoma were compared, chordoma had a 5-year survival rate of 63.8% versus 72.7%, 41.0%, and 42.9%, respectively.[16]

These data support the impression that chordoma is a tumor with a wide spectrum of behavior from slow and indolent to rapidly progressive destructive growth. The prognosis of each patient must be determined by taking into account the location, pathologic characteristics, and invasiveness of the tumor. With the advent of more sensitive radiographic techniques, smaller tumors are identified with an improved opportunity for total removal of the tumor. Such identification has resulted in a larger number of patients being disease free.[49]

References

Chordoma

1. Austin JP, Urie MM, Cardenosa G, Muzenrider JE: Probable causes of recurrence in patients with chordoma and chondrosarcoma of the base of skull and cervical spine. Int J Radiat Oncol Biol Phys 25:439, 1993.
2. Banna M: Clinical Radiology of the Spine and the Spinal Cord. Rockville, Md, Aspen, 1985, pp 353-357.
3. Bergh P, Kindblom LG, Gunterberg B, et al: Prognostic factors in chordoma of the sacrum and mobile spine: A study of 39 patients. Cancer 88:2122-2134, 2000.
4. Berven S, Zurakowski D, Mankin HJ, et al: Clinical outcome in chordoma: Utility of flow cytometry in DNA determination. Spine 27:374-379, 2002.
5. Bethke KP, Neifeld JP, Lawrence W Jr: Diagnosis and management of sacrococcygeal chordoma. J Surg Oncol 48:232, 1991.
6. Bjornsson J, Wold LE, Ebersold MJ, Laws ER: Chordoma of the mobile spine: A clinicopathologic analysis of 40 patients. Cancer 71:735, 1993.
7. Bommer KK, Ramzy I, Mody D: Fine-needle aspiration biopsy in the diagnosis and management of bone lesions: A study of 450 cases. Cancer 81:148-156, 1997.
8. Boriani S, Chevalley F, Weinstein JN, et al: Chordoma of the spine above the sacrum. Treatment and outcome in 21 cases. Spine 21:1569-1577, 1996.
9. Bruine FTD, Kroon HM: Spinal chordoma: Radiologic features in 14 cases. AJR Am J Roentgenol 150:861, 1987.
10. Carpentier A, Polivka M, Blanquet A, et al: Suboccipital and cervical chordomas: The value of aggressive treatment at first presentation of the disease. J Neurosurg 97:1070-1077, 2002.
11. Cheng EY, Ozerdemoglu RA, Transfeldt EE, et al: Lumbosacral chordoma. Prognostic factors and treatment. Spine 24:1639-1645, 1999.
12. Chetty R, Levin CV, Kalan MR: Chordoma: A 20-year clinicopathologic review of the experience of Groote Schuur Hospital, Cape Town. J Surg Oncol 46:261, 1991.
13. Congdon CC: Benign and malignant chordomas: A clinicoanatomical study of twenty-two cases. Am J Pathol 28:793, 1952.
14. Dahlin DC, MacCarthy CS: Chordoma: A study of fifty-nine cases. Cancer 5:1170, 1952.
15. deBruine FT, Kroon HM: Spinal chordoma: Radiologic features in 14 cases. AJR Am J Roentgenol 150:861, 1988.
16. Dorfman HD, Czerniack B: Bone cancers. Cancer 75:203, 1995.
17. Graham DF, McKenzie WE: Adult pre-sacral teratoma. Postgrad Med J 55:52, 1979.
18. Harwick RD, Miller AS: Craniocervical chordomas. Am J Surg 138:512, 1979.
19. Healey JH, Lane JM: Chordoma: A critical review of diagnosis and treatment. Orthop Clin North Am 20:417, 1989.
20. Hertzanu Y, Glass RBJ, Mendelsohn DC: Sacrococcygeal chordoma in young adults. Clin Radiol 34:327, 1983.
21. Higinbotham NL, Phillips RF, Farr HW, Husty HO: Chordoma: Thirty-five-year study at Memorial Hospital. Cancer 20:1841, 1967.
22. Horwitz T: Chordal ectopia and its possible relationship to chordoma. Arch Pathol 31:354, 1941.
23. Hruban RH, May M, Marcove RC, Huvos AG: Lumbosacral chordoma with high-grade malignant cartilaginous and spindle cell components. Am J Surg Pathol 14:384, 1990.
24. Hsu KY, Zucherman JF, Mortensen N, et al: Follow-up evaluation of resected lumbar vertebral chordoma over 11 years: A case report. Spine 25:2537-2540, 2000.
25. Hudson TM, Galceran M: Radiology of sacrococcygeal chordoma: Difficulties in detecting soft tissue extension. Clin Orthop 175:237, 1983.
26. Hug EB, Fitzek MM, Liebsch NJ, Munzenrider JE: Locally challenging osteo- and chondrogenic tumors of the axial skeleton: Results of combined proton and photon radiation therapy using three-dimensional treatment planning. Int J Radiat Oncol Biol Phys 31:467, 1995.
27. Hunt PT, Davidson KC, Ashcraft KW, Holder TM: Radiography of hereditary presacral teratoma. Radiology 122:187, 1977.
28. Huvos AG: Bone Tumors: Diagnosis, Treatment and Prognosis, 2nd ed. Philadelphia, WB Saunders, 1991, pp 599-624.
29. Jeffrey PB, Biava CG, Davis RL: Chondroid chordoma: A hyalinized chordoma without cartilaginous differentiation. Am J Clin Pathol 103:271, 1995.
30. Kamrin RP, Potanos JN, Pool JL: An evaluation of the diagnosis and treatment of chordoma. J Neurol Neurosurg Psychiatry, 27:157, 1964.
31. Kricun ME: Imaging of Bone Tumors. Philadelphia, WB Saunders, 1993, pp 263-265.
32. Krol G, Sundaresan N, Deck M: Computed tomography of axial chordomas. J Comput Assist Tomogr 7:286, 1983.
33. Meyer JE, Lepke RA, Lindfors KK, et al: Chordomas: Their CT appearance in the cervical, thoracic, and lumbar spine. Radiology 153:693, 1984.
34. Mindell ER: Chordoma. J Bone Joint Surg Am 63-A:501, 1981.
35. Mirra JM: Bone Tumors: Clinical, Radiologic, and Pathologic Correlation. Philadelphia, Lea & Febiger, 1989, pp 648-690.
36. Murali R, Rovit R, Benjamin MV: Chordoma of the cervical spine. Neurosurgery 9:253, 1981.
37. Ozaki T, Hillmann A, Winkelmann W: Surgical treatment of sacrococcygeal chordoma. J Surg Oncol 64:274-279, 1997.
38. Pearlman AW, Friedman M: Radical radiation therapy of chordoma. AJR Am J Roentgenol 108:333, 1970.
39. Peyron A, Mellissinos J: Chordome, tumeur tramatique. Ann Med Legale 15:478, 1935.
40. Pinto RS, Lin JP, Firooznia H, LeFleur RS: The osseous and angiographic manifestations of vertebral chordomas. Neuroradiology, 9:231, 1975.
41. Rossleigh MA, Smith J, Yeh SD: Scintigraphic features of primary sacral tumors. J Nucl Med 27:627, 1986.
42. Schajowicz F: Tumors and Tumorlike Lesions of Bone. Pathology, Radiology, and Treatment, 2nd ed. Berlin, Springer-Verlag, 1994, pp 459-468.
43. Schoenthaler R, Castro JR, Petti PL, et al: Charged particle irradiation of sacral chordomas. Int J Radiat Oncol Biol Phys 26:291, 1993.
44. Sebag G, Dubois J, Benianinovitz A, et al: Extraosseous spinal chordoma: Radiographic appearance. AJNR Am J Neuroradiol 14:205, 1993.
45. Shallat RF, Taekman MS, Nagle RC: Unusual presentation of cervical chordoma with long-term survival: Case report. J Neurosurg 57:716, 1982.
46. Smith J, Ludwig RL, Marcove RC: Sacrococcygeal chordoma. A clinicoradiological study of 60 patients. Skeletal Radiol 16:37, 1987.
47. Stener B: Complete removal of vertebrae for extirpation of tumors: A 20-year experience. Clin Orthop 245:72, 1989.
48. Sundaresan N, Galicich JH, Chu FCH, Huvos AG: Spinal chordomas. J Neurosurg 50:312, 1979.
49. Sundaresan N, Huvos AG, Krol G, et al: Surgical treatment of spinal chordomas. Arch Surg 122:1479, 1987.
50. Sundaresan N, Rosenthal DI, Schiller AL, Krol G: Chordomas. In Sundaresan N, Schmidek HH, Schiller AL, Rosenthal DI (eds): Tumors of the Spine: Diagnosis and Clinical Management. Philadelphia, WB Saunders, 1990, pp 192-213.
51. Tomita K, Tsuchiya H: Total sacrectomy and reconstruction for huge sacral tumors. Spine 15:12, 1990.
52. Tomlinson FH, Scheithauer BW, Miller GM, Onofrio BM: Extraosseous spinal chordoma. J Neurosurg 75:980, 1991.
53. Unni KK: Dahlin's Bone Tumors: General Aspects and Data on 11,087 Cases, 5th ed. Philadelphia, Lippincott-Raven, 1996, pp 291-305.
54. Uppal GS, Kollmer CE, Rhodes A, et al: Unique sacral sarcoma. Spine 16:594, 1991.
55. Volpe R, Mazabrund A: A clinicopathologic review of 25 cases of chordoma: A pleomorphic and metastatic neoplasm. Am J Surg Pathol 7:161, 1983.
56. Walaas L, Kindblom L: Fine-needle aspiration biopsy in the preoperative diagnosis of chordoma: A study of 17 cases with application of electron microscopic, histochemical, and immunocytochemical examination. Hum Pathol 22:22, 1991.
57. Wang CC, James AE Jr: Chordoma: Brief review of the literature and report of a case with widespread metastases. Cancer 22:162, 1968.

58. Wetzel LH, Levine E: MR imaging of sacral and presacral lesions. AJR Am J Roentgenol 154:771, 1990.
59. Whelan MA, Hila SK, Gold RP, et al: Computed tomography of the sacrum 2. Pathology. AJR Am J Roentgenol 139:1191, 1982.
60. Wojno KJ, Hruban RH, Garin-Chesa P, Huvos AG: Chondroid chordomas and low-grade chondrosarcomas of the craniospinal axis: An immunohistochemical analysis of 17 cases. Am J Surg Pathol 16:1144, 1992.
61. Wu KK, Mitchell DC, Guise ER: Chordoma of the atlas: A case report. J Bone Joint Surg Am 59-A:140, 1979.
62. Yonemoto T, Tatezaki S, Takenouchi T, et al: The surgical management of sacrococcygeal chordomas. Cancer 85:878-883, 1999.
63. York JE, Kaczaraj A, Abi-Said D, et al: Sacral chordoma: 40-year experience at a major cancer center. Neurosurgery 44:74-79, 1999.
64. Yuh WTC, Flickinger FW, Barloon TJ, Montgomery WJ: MR imaging of unusual chordomas. J Comput Assist Tomogr 12:30, 1988.
65. Yuh WTC, Lozano RL, Flickinger FW, et al: Lumbar epidural chordoma: MR findings. J Comput Assist Tomogr 13:508, 1989.

LYMPHOMA

Capsule Summary

	Low Back	Neck
Frequency of spinal pain	Uncommon	Uncommon
Location of spinal pain	Lumbar spine and sacrum	Cervical spine
Quality of spinal pain	Persistent ache	Persistent ache
Symptoms and signs	Pain that increases with recumbency, generalized fatigue, localized tenderness	Pain that increases with recumbency, generalized fatigue, localized tenderness
Laboratory tests	Anemia	Anemia
Radiographic findings	Osteolytic lesion with compression fracture on plain roentgenogram	Osteolytic lesion with compression fracture on plain roentgenogram
Treatment	Chemotherapy and/or radiation therapy	Chemotherapy and/or radiation therapy

PREVALENCE AND PATHOGENESIS

Lymphomas are malignant disease of lymphoreticular origin. They usually arise in lymph nodes, rarely initially in bone, and are classified into two major groups: Hodgkin's and non-Hodgkin's lymphoma. Hodgkin's lymphoma occasionally and non-Hodgkin's lymphoma rarely may be manifested as spinal pain in an adult patient.

Epidemiology

The incidence of Hodgkin's and non-Hodgkin's lymphoma is approximately 40 to 60 cases per million persons per year. Primary Hodgkin's and non-Hodgkin's lymphomas of bone unassociated with lymph node involvement are rare tumors occurring in 1% to 7% of tumors examined by biopsy.[8,28] Most bone involvement is secondary to hematogenous spread or direct extension of the tumor.[37] Approximately 30% of malignant lymphomas involve the skeletal system during the course of the illness.[6] The majority of patients in whom lymphomas develop are between the ages of 20 and 60, and the male-to-female ratio is approximately 2:1. The disease occurs with increasing frequency in each successive decade from the second to the eighth, after which the frequency declines.[1]

In a study of 25 patients with primary lymphoma of bone, 24% of the lesions occurred in the axial skeleton.[10] About the same percentage was noted in a larger retrospective study of 246 patients with primary lymphoma of bone.[30] Another study found 14% of lymphomas in the axial skeleton. The cervical spine was the location of 11% of lesions; the thoracic spine, 34%; and the lumbosacral spine, 55%.[8] A study of 422 patients found 16% (66) to have axial skeleton disease, with cervical spine lesions noted in 3% (2) of the 66.[32] A study of non-Hodgkin's lymphoma also found only 8% (1 of 13) of lesions in the axial skeleton affecting the cervical spine.[22] Other studies have found lumbar, thoracic, and sacral lesions without cervical spine involvement.[5]

Pathogenesis

The pathogenesis of lymphomas remains unknown. Although viral infections have been implicated as etiologic agents that result in lymphomas, the exact pathogenetic factors causing lymphoreticular malignancy remain to be identified.

The pathogenesis of extraosseous lesions without extensive osteolysis detected by roentgenograms of lymphoma of bone may be related to the production of cytokines with osteoclastic activity by the malignant cells. These cytokines include interleukin-1, interleukin-6, and tumor necrosis factor-alpha. Production of these factors allows for channels to form through the cortex of bone, thereby permitting spread of tumor cells into surrounding soft tissues.[17]

CLINICAL HISTORY

Patients with primary Hodgkin's or non-Hodgkin's lymphoma of bone have persistent pain over the affected bone. Bone pain may increase when the patient goes to bed. The pain often precedes the radiographic changes of lymphoma by months. A peculiar clinical finding is an increase in bone pain after the consumption of alcohol.[7] The duration of pain is usually measured in months before patients seek medical evaluation. Most patients with solitary lesions have no constitutional symptoms. Constitutional symptoms are more closely associated with multiple lesions of bone. The diagnosis of lymphoma of bone should be considered in elderly patients with fever and compression fractures.[36] Patients with spinal epidural lymphoma may complain of symptoms compatible with spinal stenosis.[39] Lesions above the lumbar spine may be associated with an acute onset of paraparesis.[29] Symptoms and signs compatible with cauda equina syndrome may develop.[14] Not only can radicular pain in the upper or lower extremity be caused by nerve compression from an expanding mass in the spinal canal, but lymphoma may also infiltrate peripheral nerves and cause multifocal polyneuropathy and radicular pain.[21]

PHYSICAL EXAMINATION

The bone affected by primary lymphoma is tender to palpation, and soft tissue swelling may be associated with the bony tenderness. Patients with axial skeletal disease may demonstrate neurologic deficits. Those with primary disease of bone may not have any peripheral signs of their tumor. Patients with generalized disease, of which bone infiltration is a part, may have lymphadenopathy and splenomegaly.

LABORATORY DATA

Patients with primary disease of bone will not have hematologic, chemical, or immunologic abnormalities associated with disseminated disease. The appearance of anemia, an elevated sedimentation rate, and increased serum proteins in a patient with bone disease suggests either that the disease has extended to other tissue or that the bone lesion was secondary to disseminated disease and occurred late in its development.

Pathology

Gross pathologic examination of affected bone reveals a main tumor mass in bone with a variable amount of soft tissue extension.[19] The architecture of the bone is destroyed to a variable extent, and areas of necrosis are noted. The margins of the tumor and the involved bone are indistinct. The histologic picture of Hodgkin's disease includes typical Reed-Sternberg cells, atypical mononuclear cells, and an inflammatory component composed of lymphocytes, plasma cells, and scattered eosinophils. The reactive histiocytes and eosinophils look superficially like eosinophilic granuloma. In an older adult, a lesion that resembles eosinophilic granuloma may be Hodgkin's disease.[20] Non-Hodgkin's lymphomas may exhibit marked histologic variation.[35] These lesions lack Reed-Sternberg cells and demonstrate different combinations of abnormal lymphocytes and supporting cells. New staining techniques may better characterize cells that cause the various kinds of lymphoma.[41] In a study of 34 Japanese patients with primary non-Hodgkin's lymphoma of bone, Ueda and colleagues identified T-cell markers in 10% of tumors.[40] The frequency of T-cell lymphomas may be related to the increased frequency of retrovirus-associated lymphoma that is common in Japan. In a series from the United States, a B-lineage large cell lymphoma was the cause of primary bone neoplasms.[34]

RADIOGRAPHIC EVALUATION

Roentgenograms

Both primary Hodgkin's and non-Hodgkin's lymphomas have a predilection for the axial skeleton.[33] The bone changes of Hodgkin's disease may include lytic (75%), sclerotic (15%), mixed (5%), or periosteal (5%) lesions.[16] In the axial skeleton, Hodgkin's disease most frequently involves a vertebral body, and involvement of the posterior elements of a vertebral body is much less common (Figs. 13-46 and 13-47). Occasionally, an osteoblastic lesion, or an "ivory" vertebra, may be seen with Hodgkin's disease.[9]

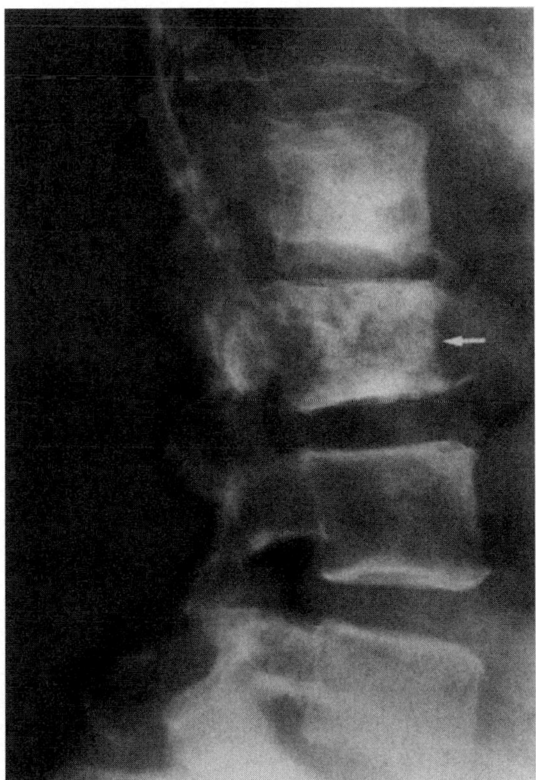

Figure 13-46 Lymphoma of the spine characterized by patchy sclerosis and radiolucency of two vertebral bodies with loss of body height. The anterior portion of one of the vertebral bodies *(arrow)* is eroded secondary to adjacent lymph node involvement. *(Courtesy of Anne Brower, MD.)*

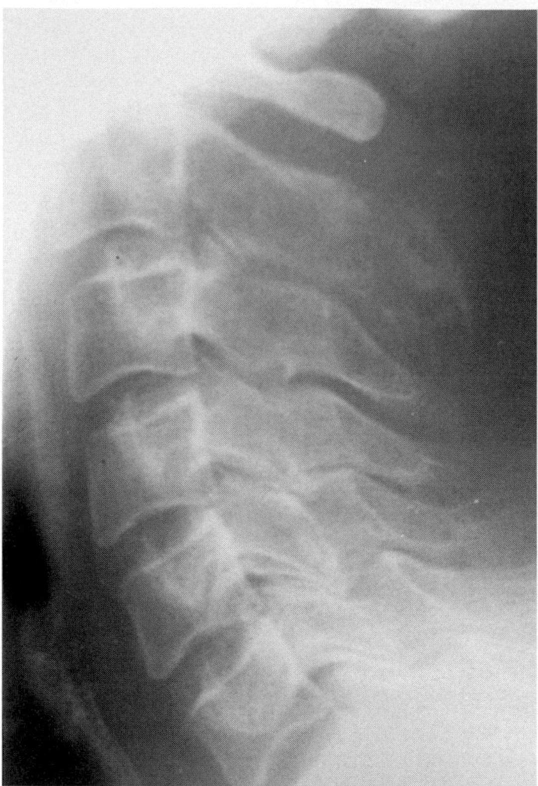

Figure 13-47 Lymphoma in a 32-year-old man with neck pain. A lateral view of the cervical spine reveals an expansile, lytic lesion of the posterior spine at C2. Lymphoma affects the vertebral body more commonly. *(Courtesy of Anne Brower, MD.)*

Hodgkin's involvement of the axial skeleton may result in compression fractures that spare the vertebral discs. Non-Hodgkin's lymphoma of bone has similar features characterized by lytic and blastic areas, cortical destruction, and little reactive new bone. The lesion may also be associated with soft tissue extension.[31]

The degree and type of bony lesions may vary with the histologic classification of the lymphoma. In a study of 179 patients with primary lymphoma of bone, 33% had two or more bones involved.[32] Skeletal lesions are more frequent and destructive in the more aggressive tumors. Sclerotic lesions are more common in less aggressive forms. Only 11% of patients with less aggressive tumors had bone lesions, in contrast to 64% of those with more malignant disease.[3]

Scintigraphy

Although CT remains the commonly used modality for staging bone lymphoma before therapy, bone scintigraphy may also be helpful in detecting multiple lesions that may not be suspected on initial evaluation of the patient. Gallium scan may detect lesions in the cervical spine, including C2, that may be overlooked on a plain roentgenogram.[13] Bone scintigraphy may also be helpful in monitoring the response of bone lesions to chemotherapy.[42]

Computed Tomography/Magnetic Resonance

CT and MR are helpful techniques for determination of any extraosseous, paravertebral extension of the neoplasm. CT reveals sequestra in 11% of patients with primary lymphoma of bone.[30] Sequestra not only are indicative of primary lymphoma but may also be associated with osteomyelitis, multiple myeloma, metastases, and bone sarcomas. CT scan is helpful in staging lymphomas, or differentiation of primary lymphoma of bone (stage I) from bone lesions associated with disease in other sites (stage IV).[26] MR evaluation demonstrates low-intensity signal on T1-weighted images and high-intensity signal on T2-weighted images. Lymph gland enlargement can be identified with MR, but it is unable to differentiate lymphadenopathy secondary to Hodgkin's disease, non-Hodgkin's disease, infection, or metastatic disease.[18] MR imaging may detect early changes in bones that may not be detected by plain bone scintigraphy or CT.[15]

DIFFERENTIAL DIAGNOSIS

The diagnosis of lymphoma is based on careful examination of adequate biopsy material. CT-guided biopsy is able to obtain adequate material from the spine without need for an open surgical procedure.[2] Even with adequate histologic material, however, the diagnosis of a specific lymphoma is difficult to make because of the pleomorphic forms of the disease. The differential diagnosis of a single osteoblastic vertebral body must include Paget's disease and carcinoma of the breast or prostate. In younger patients with vertebra plana, the possibility of eosinophilic granuloma must be investigated. Careful review of all the clinical and pathologic data should render enough information for the treating physician to make the appropriate diagnosis.

Lymphoma may also develop in the spinal epidural space without a specific osseous origin. These patients have varying degrees of spinal cord compression. Radiographic techniques identify their location. Cerebrospinal fluid analysis will reveal elevated protein levels but no specific cytopathologic findings.[24]

TREATMENT

Treatment of lymphomas is based on the extent of the illness. All patients must be staged before treatment is initiated. Staging of lymphomas continues to be modified as additional information related to prognosis is gathered. A new predictive model for aggressive non-Hodgkin's lymphoma includes extranodal sites as one of the factors determining outcome.[38] Once the stage of disease is known, the patient should receive appropriate therapy for that degree of involvement. Treatment may include radiation therapy and/or chemotherapy.[4,11,23] Monoclonal antibodies such as anti-CD20 (rituximab) are newer therapies directed at specific cellular antigens. CD20 is an attractive target because it is found on most B-cell lymphomas. One current dose regimen of rituximab includes 375 mg/m^2 once weekly for

4 weeks. Rituximab may also be used with other immune modulators such as interferon-alpha.[27]

PROGNOSIS

Therapy for lymphoma has become more effective in controlling the disease, and patients have the potential for cure if the disease is not too extensive. In many circumstances, they are able to live productive lives for an extended time. Five-year survival rates of 40% to 50% have been reported. Recent studies have continued to report 50% survival rates in patients with lymphoma of bone.[12] Patients with solitary bone lesions have a better prognosis than the 42%, 5-year survival rate for patients with multiple lesions.[1] The prognosis may also be related to the pattern of cells associated with the tumor. Favorable patterns include noncleaved and multilobated cells. Unfavorable patterns are associated with cleaved cells and immunoblasts. The 5-year survival rate is 67% for cleaved cells and 21% for uncleaved cells.[5] Young patients with neural compression should receive aggressive radiotherapy and chemotherapy. Decompression is reserved for young patients with rapidly progressive paralysis. The results of decompression in the elderly are poor.[22] Patients with disease in the pelvis have the same survival rates as patients with bone involvement in other parts of the skeleton.[8] Patients with primary epidural non-Hodgkin's lymphoma in the cervical spine may have a good response to medical and radiation therapy.[25]

References

Lymphoma

1. Aisenberg AC: Malignant Lymphoma: Biology, Natural History, and Treatment. Philadelphia, Lea & Febiger, 1991, pp 288-290.
2. Babu NV, Titus VTK, Chittaranjan S, et al: Computed tomographically guided biopsy of the spine. Spine 19:2436, 1994.
3. Braunstein EM: Hodgkin disease of bone: Radiographic correlation with the histological classification. Radiology 137:643, 1980.
4. Canellos GP, Come SE, Skarin AT: Chemotherapy in the treatment of Hodgkin's disease. Semin Hematol 20:1, 1983.
5. Clayton F, Butler JJ, Ayala AG, et al: Non-Hodgkin's lymphoma of bone: Pathologic and radiologic features with clinical correlates. Cancer 60:2492, 1987.
6. Coles WC, Schulz MD: Bone involvement in malignant lymphoma. Radiology 50:458, 1948.
7. Conn HO: Alcohol-induced pain as a manifestation of Hodgkin's disease. Arch Intern Med 100:241, 1957.
8. Dahlin DC, Unni KK: Bone Tumors: General Aspects and Data on 8,542 Cases, 4th ed. Springfield, IL, Charles C Thomas, 1986, pp 206-226.
9. Dennis JM: The solitary dense vertebral body. Radiology 77:618, 1961.
10. Desai S, Jambhekar NA, Soman CS, Advani SH: Primary lymphoma of bone: A clinicopathologic study of 25 cases reported over 10 years. J Surg Oncol 46:265, 1991.
11. Dosoretz DE, Murphy GF, Raymond AK, et al: Radiation therapy for primary lymphoma of bone. Cancer 51:44, 1983.
12. Edeiken-Monroe B, Ediken J, Kim EE: Radiologic concepts of lymphoma of bone. Radiol Clin North Am 28:841, 1990.
13. Fertakos RJ, Swayne LC, Yablonsky TM: Gallium SPECT detection of lymphomatous involvement of the cervical dens. Clin Nucl Med 20:70, 1995.
14. Freedman AS: Weekly clinicopathological exercises. Case 11-1999. N Engl J Med 340:1188-1196, 1999.
15. Gaudin P, Juvin R, Rozand Y, et al: Skeletal involvement as the initial disease manifestation in Hodgkin's disease: A review of 6 cases. J Rheumatol 19:146, 1992.
16. Granger W, Whitaker R: Hodgkin's disease in bone, with special reference to periosteal reaction. Br J Radiol 40:939, 1967.
17. Hicks DG, Gokan T, O'Keefe RJ, et al: Primary lymphoma of bone: Correlation of magnetic resonance imaging features with cytokine production by tumor cells. Cancer 75:973, 1995.
18. Holtas SL, Kido DK, Simon JH: MR imaging of spinal lymphoma. J Comput Assist Tomogr 10:111, 1986.
19. Huvos AG: Bone Tumors: Diagnosis, Treatment, and Prognosis, 2nd ed. Philadelphia, WB Saunders, 1991, pp 625-637.
20. Jaffe HL: Metabolic, Degenerative and Inflammatory Diseases of Bones and Joints. Philadelphia, Lea & Febiger, 1972, p 887.
21. Krendel DA, Stahl RL, Chan WC: Lymphomatous polyneuropathy: Biopsy of clinically involved nerve and successful treatment. Arch Neurol 48:330, 1991.
22. Laing RJ, Jakubowski J, Kunkler IH, Hancock BW: Primary spinal presentation of non-Hodgkin's lymphoma: A reappraisal of management and prognosis. Spine 17:117, 1992.
23. Leslie NT, Mauch PM, Hellman S: Stage IA to IIB supradiaphragmatic Hodgkin's disease: Long-term survival and relapse frequency. Cancer 55:2072, 1985.
24. Lyons MK, O'Neill BP, Kurtin PJ, et al: Diagnosis and management of primary spinal epidural non-Hodgkin's lymphoma. Mayo Clin Proc 71:453-457, 1996.
25. Lyons MK, O'Neill BP, Marsh WR, Kurtin PJ: Primary spinal epidural non-Hodgkin's lymphoma: Report of eight patients and review of the literature. Neurosurgery 30:675, 1992.
26. Malloy PC, Fishman EK, Magid D: Lymphoma of bone, muscle, and skin: CT findings. AJR Am J Roentgenol 159:805, 1992.
27. McCune SL, Gockerman JP, Rizzieri DA: Monoclonal antibody therapy in the treatment of non-Hodgkin lymphoma. JAMA 286:1149-1152, 2001.
28. Mirra JM: Bone Tumors: Clinical, Radiologic, and Pathologic Correlation. Philadelphia, Lea & Febiger 1989, pp 1119-1185.
29. Moridaira K, Handa H, Murakami H, et al: Primary Hodgkin's disease of the bone presenting with an extradural tumor. Acta Haematol 92:148, 1994.
30. Mulligan ME, Kransdorf MJ: Sequestra in primary lymphoma of bone: Prevalence and radiologic features. AJR Am J Roentgenol 160:1245, 1993.
31. Mulligan ME, McRae GA, Murphey MD: Imaging features of primary lymphoma of bone. AJR Am J Roentgenol 173:1691-1697, 1999.
32. Ostrowski ML, Unni KK, Banks PM, et al: Malignant lymphoma of bone. Cancer 58:2646, 1986.
33. Perttala Y, Kijanen I: Roentgenologic bone lesions in lymphogranulomatosis maligna: Analysis of 453 cases. Ann Chir Gynaecol Fenn 54:414, 1965.
34. Pettit CK, Zukerberg LR, Gray MH, et al: Primary lymphoma of bone. A B-cell neoplasm with a high frequency of multilobated cells. Am J Surg Pathol 14:329, 1990.
35. Reimer RR, Chabner BA, Young RC, et al: Lymphoma presenting in bone: Results of histopathology, staging, and therapy. Ann Intern Med 87:50, 1977.
36. Smith KY, Bradley SF, Kauffman CA: Fever of unknown origin in the elderly: Lymphoma presenting as vertebral compression fractures. J Am Geriatr Soc 42:88, 1994.
37. Steiner PE: Hodgkin's disease: The incidence, distribution, nature and possible significance of lymphogranulomatous lesions in bone marrow; review with original data. Arch Pathol 36:627, 1943.
38. The International Non-Hodgkin's Lymphoma Prognostic Factors Project: A predictive model for aggressive non-Hodgkin's lymphoma. N Engl J Med 329:987, 1993.
39. Travlos J, du Toit G: Primary spinal epidural lymphoma mimicking lumbar spinal stenosis: A case report. Spine 16:377, 1991.
40. Ueda T, Aozasa K, Ohasawa M, et al: Malignant lymphomas of bone in Japan. Cancer 64:2387, 1989.
41. Warnke RA, Gotter KC, Falini B, et al: Diagnosis of human lymphoma with monoclonal antileukocyte antibodies. N Engl Med 309:1275, 1983.
42. White LM, Gray BG, Ichise M, et al: Scintigraphic flare in skeletal lymphoma. Clin Nucl Med 19:661, 1994.

SKELETAL METASTASES

Capsule Summary

	Low Back	Neck
Frequency of spinal pain	Very common	Very common
Location of spinal pain	Lumbar spine and sacrum	Cervical spine
Quality of spinal pain	Ache of increasing intensity	Ache of increasing intensity
Symptoms and signs	Increased pain with recumbency, previous malignancy	Increased pain with recumbency, previous malignancy
Laboratory tests	Anemia; bone biopsy may or may not show characteristics of the primary tumor	Anemia; bone biopsy may or may not show characteristics of the primary tumor
Radiographic findings	Bone scintigraphy most sensitive test	Bone scintigraphy most sensitive test
Treatment	Palliative with radiation therapy, corticosteroids, decompressive laminectomy for neural compression	Palliative with radiation therapy, corticosteroids, decompressive laminectomy for neural compression

PREVALENCE AND PATHOGENESIS

A principal characteristic of malignant neoplastic lesions is the growth of tumor cells distant from the primary lesion. These distant lesions are referred to as metastases and are found commonly in the skeletal system. Skeletal lesions result either from dissemination through the bloodstream or by direct extension. The axial skeleton and pelvis are frequent sites of metastatic disease.

Epidemiology

Metastatic lesions in the skeleton are much more common than primary tumors of bone, with the overall ratio being 25:1.[35,63] In a study of 1971 patients with neoplasms, only 29 (1.5%) had primary neoplasms of the lumbar spine.[25] The 18 primary lesions that occurred in adults were malignant. The prevalence of metastases increases with increasing age. This increase with age follows from the increasing number of tumors in a population of individuals as they grow older. Patients who are 50 years or older are at greatest risk for the development of metastatic disease. The ratio of men and women in whom metastases develop varies for each type of malignancy. If all neoplasms with the potential to metastasize are considered, men and women are equally at risk for metastatic lesions.

Each tumor has a different propensity for metastasizing to bone, and the true incidence of skeletal metastases from each tumor is difficult to ascertain. Complete examination of the skeleton cannot be performed with the same degree of care as evaluation of other body organs. Therefore, great variability may be reported in the incidence of metastases from the same type of tumor. Neoplasms that are frequently associated with skeletal metastasis include tumors of the prostate, breast, lung, kidney, thyroid, and colon (Table 13-3).[39] Data from autopsy material suggest that pathologic evidence of metastasis to vertebral bodies in the thoracolumbar spine will develop in up to 70% of patients with a primary neoplasm.[34] In an autopsy study of 832 individuals with malignant neoplasms, 36% had evidence of metastases to the spine. Occult metastases visible on autopsy but not detected by plain radiographs were present in 78 of 300 cases (26%).[90]

Lumbar Spine

Metastases occur more commonly in the axial skeleton than in the appendicular skeleton. The axial skeleton is the third most common site of metastases after the lung and liver.[81] In the axial skeleton, the thoracic and lumbar spine are most frequently affected. The lumbar spine and thoracic spine are involved in approximately 46% to 49%

13-3 INCIDENCE OF SKELETAL METASTASES

Tumor Origin	Incidence (%)	
	High	*Low*
Breast	85	47
Prostate	85	33
Thyroid	60	28
Kidney	64	30
Esophagus	7	5
Intestine	11	3
Rectum	61	8
Bladder	42	
Uterine cervix	56	50
Ovary	9	
Liver	16	
Melanoma	7	

Modified from Galasko CSB: Skeletal Metastases. Boston, Butterworths, 1986.

of cases, with the cervical spine affected to a lesser degree (6%).[77]

Cervical Spine

Metastatic lesions affect the cervical spine less frequently than other portions of the axial skeleton. Many large studies of metastatic disease of the spine do not include the cervical spine, either because of the extra dissection needed for autopsy evaluation or because of the notion that the cervical spine was less frequently involved.[33,34,90] A number of studies of the entire axial skeleton have, however, identified cervical spine metastatic disease. The frequency of cervical spine involvement ranged from 6% to 19% in these studies.[5,9,20,56,67,77] A higher prevalence of 34% involvement of the cervical spine was reported with metastatic adenocarcinoma of unknown origin.[76] Metastases to the cervical spine associated with breast cancer were reported in 26% of individuals with that disease as detected by bone scintigraphy.[39] In general, the frequency of cervical spine metastases is less than that associated with the thoracic and lumbar spine.

Pathogenesis

The propensity of bone, and the axial skeleton in particular, to be the site of metastases may be explained in part by the presence of Batson's plexus around the vertebral column and the presence of bone marrow inside bone (Fig. 13-48). Batson's plexus is a network of veins located in the epidural space between the bony spinal column and the dura mater covering the spinal cord. It is connected to the major veins that return blood to the heart and the inferior and superior vena cava. This plexus of veins is unique in that there are no valves to control blood flow, and therefore any increased pressure in the vena cava system results in increased flow into Batson's plexus. Metastatic cells may enter this plexus and be deposited in the venous and sinusoidal systems of bones that are connected to Batson's plexus.[6] Supporting

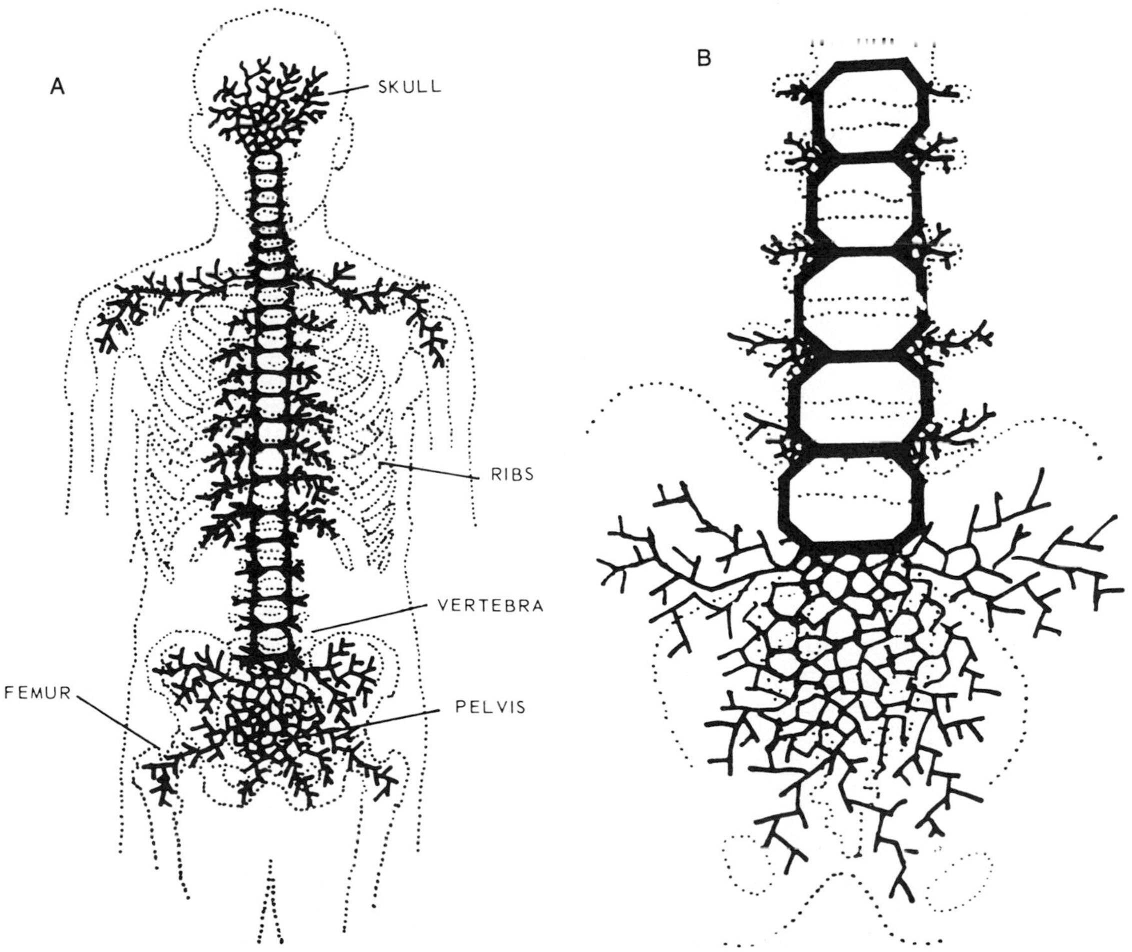

Figure 13-48 Diagrammatic representation of the vertebral vein system. This venous network is a common two-way path of metastatic spread of pelvic, abdominal, and thoracic tumors. A large proportion of bony metastases result from dissemination of neoplastic cells through the vertebral venous system. *(From del Regato JA: Pathways of metastatic spread of malignant tumors. Semin Oncol 4:33, 1977.)*

data for the importance of Batson's plexus in the distribution of skeletal metastasis are the frequency of axial skeletal metastases and the predilection of metastasis to the lumbar spine.[42,58] Breast cancer tends to occur in the thoracic spine, and prostate cancer metastasizes to the lumbar spine. The red bone marrow, located inside vertebral bodies, long bones, and flat bones, has a rich sinusoidal system. Sinusoidal vessels are usually under low hemodynamic pressure, thus allowing for pooling of blood. This pooling of blood, along with other factors such as fibrin deposits and thrombosis, may encourage tumor growth. Each vertebra has barriers to the spread of tumor, with the posterior longitudinal ligament being the weakest. The most common path for tumor spread is through the posterior longitudinal ligament into the epidural space.[38]

The incidence of skeletal metastases also may be related to the ability of tumor cell emboli to develop into secondary tumors. This ability is a property of each form of tumor. The effects of tumor cells on bone also vary for each type of neoplasm. Tumor cells may cause bone destruction or bone formation. Osteoclasts may be stimulated by products of tumor cells (in myeloma, for example), thereby resulting in osteolysis.[65] On the other hand, osteoblasts may also be directly stimulated by tumor cell factors (as in prostatic carcinoma) that stimulate bone formation or may produce bone in reaction to increased bone destruction.[37,40,41,50,74] The effects of these processes of tumor cells on bone result in osteolysis or osteosclerosis that is discernible by radiographic techniques.

A number of chemical factors related to metastases have an effect on bone mineralization. Such factors include parathyroid hormone, osteoclast-activating factor, prostaglandins (PGE_2), and transforming growth factor.[36,81] Tumors associated with osteoblastic activity (prostate cancer) release factors that stimulate osteoblasts to produce bone.[75]

CLINICAL HISTORY

A high index of suspicion for the presence of metastasis is important in the evaluation of a patient with a previous history of malignancy or an adult older than 50 years with spinal pain that is not associated with trauma.[69]

Lumbar Spine

In a study of 1975 patients with low back pain, 13 individuals (0.66%) had cancer.[27] The patients with cancer were older than 50 years, had a previous history of cancer, had pain for over 1 month, and failed to respond to conservative therapy. Pain in the lumbar or cervical spine has a gradual onset and increases in intensity over time. It tends to be localized initially but may radiate in a radicular pattern over time. Pain in the spine is commonly increased with motion, cough, or strain. Radicular pain may increase at night as the spine lengthens with recumbency. Pain with recumbency is a symptom frequently associated with spinal tumors.[66]

Not all patients with skeletal metastases will have pain. In a review of 86 patients with breast cancer and radiographic evidence of skeletal metastases, only 65% complained of pain. Similar results have been reported by other investigators.[37,77] When clinical symptoms develop, they are a consequence of one or more of the following: (1) an enlarging lesion in a vertebral body that fractures the cortex and invades surrounding soft tissues, (2) invasion or compression of adjacent nerve roots, (3) vertebral pathologic fractures, (4) destructive lesions of the posterior elements that result in spinal instability, and (5) compression of the spinal cord.[46] In patients with spinal cord or nerve root compression secondary to bony or epidural lesions, neurologic dysfunction develops and correlates with the location of the lesion. Neurologic symptoms may include numbness, tingling, unsteadiness of gait, weakness, bladder or bowel incontinence, and sexual dysfunction.[31,74]

Three patterns of progression of neurologic symptoms may be noted. In 30% of patients, symptoms occur acutely, with progression to maximal neurologic deficit in 48 hours. Subacute deterioration over a period of 7 to 10 days is noted in 60%. In the remaining 10% of individuals, symptoms develop over a 4- to 6-month period.[20]

Cervical Spine

Patients with involvement of the atlas or axis may have decreased neck rotation.[48] In a study of 51 patients with metastatic disease to the cervical spine, 14 (27%) had cervical spine disease with pain as the initial manifestation of their illness.[53]

The clinical symptoms of metastatic disease of the upper cervical spine (C1 and C2) are markedly different from those of the lower cervical spine.[70] Metastases tend to affect the anterior components of vertebrae. The anterior elements of C1 and C2 are different from those of the lower cervical vertebrae. The spinal canal is wide at the C1–C2 level, thus making neural impingement a late manifestation of metastatic disease in this location. Impingement occurs from mechanical compression of the cord as a result of gross instability, not from direct tumor growth.[79] The stability of the upper cervical spine depends on the lateral masses of C1 and C2. Destruction of the lateral masses results in rotatory instability and severe pain.[52] Pathologic fracture of the dens leads to anterior or posterior instability.[80]

In the lower cervical spine, vertebral body disease results in kyphosis and direct tumor impingement on the anterior portion of the dural sac. Flexion instability and kyphosis may be the result of metastases to the lower portion of the cervical spine.[80]

PHYSICAL EXAMINATION

Physical examination may demonstrate pain on palpation over the affected bone. Muscle spasm and limitation of motion are associated findings. Careful attention to neurologic deficits (hyperesthesia, segmental muscular weakness, asymmetric reflexes, sphincter dysfunction) may help locate the lesion in the axial skeleton.

Frankel's classification is used to grade degrees of neurologic deficit. Grade A is associated with complete motor and sensory loss, whereas grade E has normal motor and sensory function.[81]

Lumbar Spine

Lesions that affect the T12 or L1 vertebra may compress the conus medullaris, which contains the S3 through coccygeal nerve segments. Nerves originating from these segments innervate the urinary bladder, the bladder and rectal sphincter, and the sensory fibers of the perineal (saddle) region. Lesions that affect the conus may cause sphincter dysfunction and saddle anesthesia without neurologic abnormalities in the lower extremities. In contrast, lesions below L1 affect the nerve roots that are part of the cauda equina. Lesions of the cauda equina cause lower motor neuron abnormalities associated with motor and sensory loss and hyporeflexia.[30]

Cervical Spine

Invasion of the spinal canal from the vertebral body results in compression of the anterior portion of the spinal cord, and such compression affects motor function. Sensory abnormalities follow as the cord is displaced posteriorly and impacts on the lamina. The thoracic spine is most commonly associated with neurologic compromise because the spinal cord is at its largest in comparison to the diameter of the spinal canal.[46] Upper motor neuron signs, including hyperreflexia, spasticity, and abnormal Babinski's signs, are present in patients with spinal cord compression of the cervical spine. Patients with lesions in the upper cervical spine have decreased rotation as a manifestation of disease in the atlantoaxial articulation.[48]

LABORATORY DATA

Early in the course of lesions, laboratory parameters may be unremarkable. However, subsequent evaluation may demonstrate anemia, an elevated erythrocyte sedimentation rate, abnormal urinalysis, or abnormal chemistry studies, including increased serum alkaline phosphatase and increased prostatic acid phosphatase in metastatic prostate carcinoma. Therefore, initial negative laboratory data should not dissuade a physician from pursuing further diagnostic evaluation in an older patient with a recent onset of spinal pain.

Biochemical tests are not always positive in patients. Bishop and associates found false-negative alkaline (18%) and acid phosphatase (36%) levels in patients with skeletal metastases from prostatic carcinoma.[11] In another study, only 30% of patients with a positive scintiscan for metastatic disease had elevated alkaline phosphatase.[21]

Pathology

In patients without a known primary tumor, bone biopsy may provide the first evidence of a malignancy. Occasionally, the histologic features of the biopsy specimen may suggest the source of the lesion, such as colloid material with thyroid adenocarcinoma, clear cells with renal cell carcinoma, or melanin with melanoma. On many occasions, the histologic features, squamous cells or mucin cells, may be associated with primary lesions in various organs (Figs. 13-49 and 13-50). Some lesions may be so undifferentiated that the pathologic findings offer no clue to the possible source of the tumor.[63] Radiologic identification of lesions may help localize the area for biopsy.[44]

No consistent histologic abnormalities are described for compressive lesions of the spinal cord.[46] The gray matter is preserved, whereas edema and cellular degeneration affect the white matter. Venous occlusion has been suggested as the most important factor leading to neuronal degeneration, although the distribution of pathologic changes does not conform to the arterial or venous drainage of the cord.[12]

RADIOGRAPHIC EVALUATION

A number of studies have investigated the initial location for metastases in individual vertebrae. The loss of a pedicle

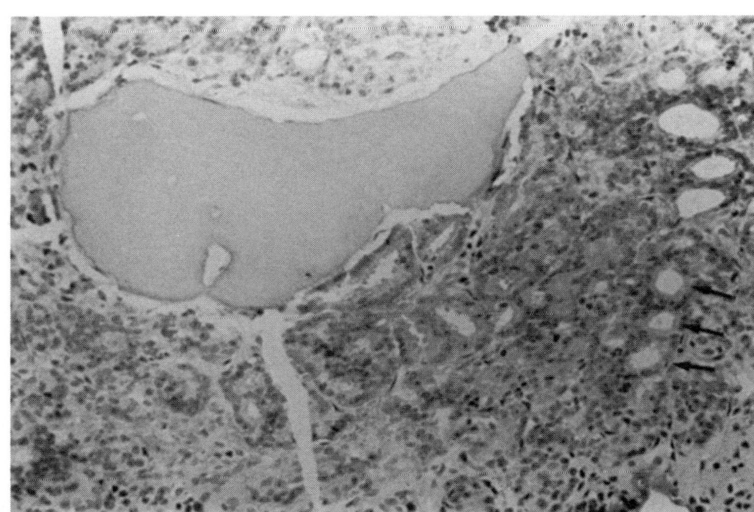

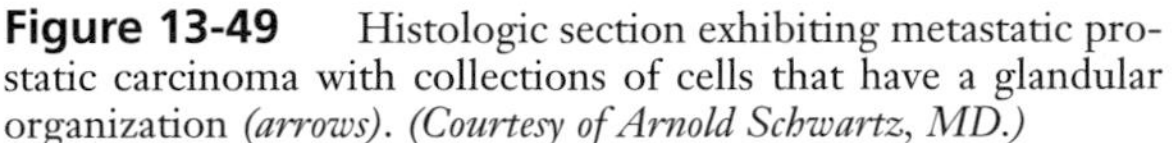

Figure 13-49 Histologic section exhibiting metastatic prostatic carcinoma with collections of cells that have a glandular organization *(arrows)*. *(Courtesy of Arnold Schwartz, MD.)*

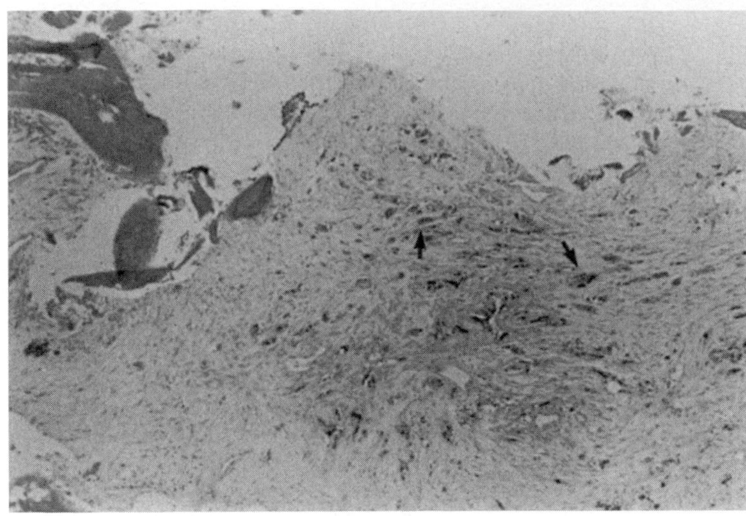

Figure 13-50 Histologic section of metastatic breast carcinoma exhibiting a lytic area of bone containing desmoplastic stroma with islands of malignant cells *(arrows)*. *(Courtesy of Arnold Schwartz, MD.)*

as the first roentgenographic finding of metastatic disease suggested that structure as the location for the initial nidus of cancerous cells. Studies by a variety of investigators have demonstrated the posterior vertebral body near the spinal venous plexus as the initial location for vertebral metastases. CT studies have demonstrated vertebral body involvement without lesions of the pedicle.[1] Pedicle involvement has been documented by MR imaging to be a direct extension from the vertebral body or the posterior elements.[2] The reason why loss of the pedicle is the first abnormality noted despite earlier vertebral body disease is related to loss of the cortical bone of the pedicle and the insensitivity of plain roentgenograms to detect loss of trabecular bone.

Roentgenograms

Lumbar Spine

Roentgenographic abnormalities associated with the axial skeleton include osteolytic, osteoblastic, or mixed lytic and blastic lesions.[91] Osteolytic lesions that affect a vertebral body or a posterior element such as a pedicle are associated with carcinoma of the lung, kidney, breast, and thyroid. Multiple osteoblastic lesions are associated with prostatic, breast, and colon carcinoma and bronchial carcinoid (Figs. 13-51 and 13-52). A single blastic vertebral body may be seen with prostatic carcinoma but is more closely associated with Hodgkin's or Paget's disease. Vertebral lesions that contain both lytic and blastic metastases are associated with carcinoma of the breast, lung, prostate, or bladder. Because of their usual slow growth, kidney and thyroid carcinoma may cause an expansile lesion from periosteal growth without destruction. Osteolytic lesions are more frequently associated with vertebral body collapse than osteoblastic lesions are (Fig. 13-53). Vertebral body destruction is not associated with changes in the intervertebral disc, so the presence of vertebral body destruction and loss of intervertebral disc space suggests infection. However, radiographic and pathologic studies suggest that intervertebral discs may degenerate more rapidly, indent weakened vertebral bone, and form a Schmorl node. Rarely, it may be invaded by tumor and result in loss of disc integrity.[49,73] Fracture of L5 is not specific enough to predict the presence of metastasis, but it should be considered in the appropriate patient.[59] Multiple lesions of varying size imply metastatic disease.[28] Some metastases of tumors in the pelvis will affect the left side of the vertebral column more than the right; this predilection for the left side is related to the proximity of lymph nodes to the axial skeleton.[32]

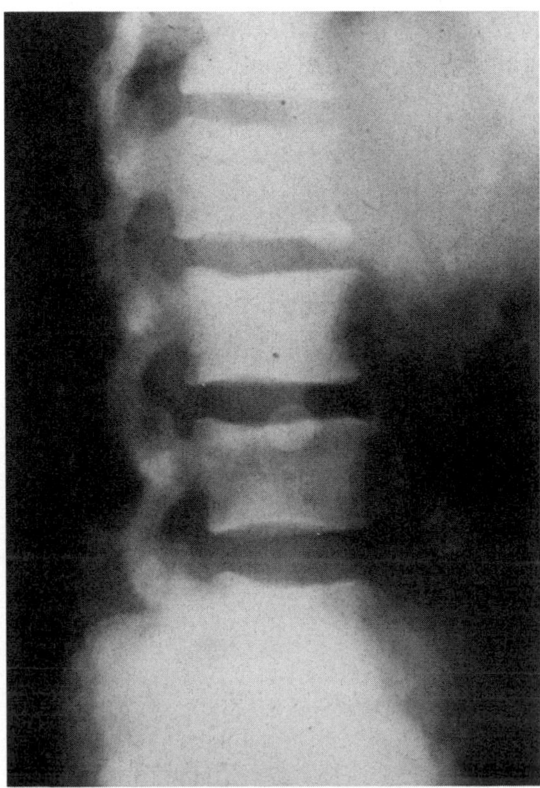

Figure 13-51 Metastatic tumor. A lateral view of the lumbar spine shows generalized osteoblastic skeletal lesions throughout the lumbar spine. Blastic lesions are most commonly associated with prostate carcinoma. *(Courtesy of Anne Brower, MD.)*

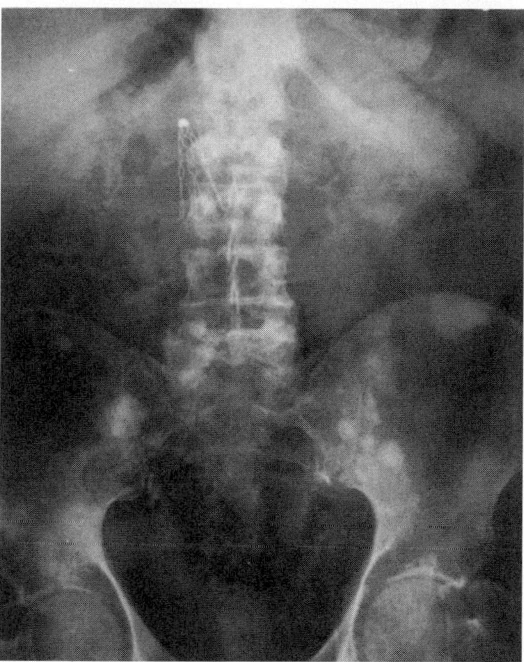

Figure 13-52 An anteroposterior view of the lumbosacral spine and pelvis in a 66-year-old man with a 3-month history of back pain reveals multiple, discrete osteoblastic lesions that proved to be metastatic prostatic carcinoma on biopsy.

Cervical Spine

Lesions of the upper cervical spine may not be identified by plain roentgenographic evaluation. Overlapping of the dens and atlantoaxial joint may obscure early alterations in bony architecture and thus delay timely diagnosis of a metastasis. In a study of 16 patients with upper cervical spine metastases, only 7 had identifiable diagnostic changes on plain roentgenogram of the cervical spine.[70] The open-mouth view may be helpful but is not routinely obtained (Fig. 13-54). In the lower cervical spine, alterations of the anterior vertebral body are easier to identify. However, the changes of degenerative disc disease seen frequently in elderly patients may draw attention away from the site of tumor involvement. Subsequently, progressive destruction may appear at a site distant from the location of degenerative disease.[70]

Involvement of the upper cervical spine as described by Phillips and Levine occurred in three patterns.[70] The most common pattern was disease in the anterior body of C2, including fracture of the dens. The second pattern was destruction of the lateral mass of C1. The third pattern was defined by involvement of the posterior portion of C2 and was the most difficult in which to make a definitive diagnosis. These patients have severe pain near the insertion of the ligamentum nuchae but do not exhibit instability.

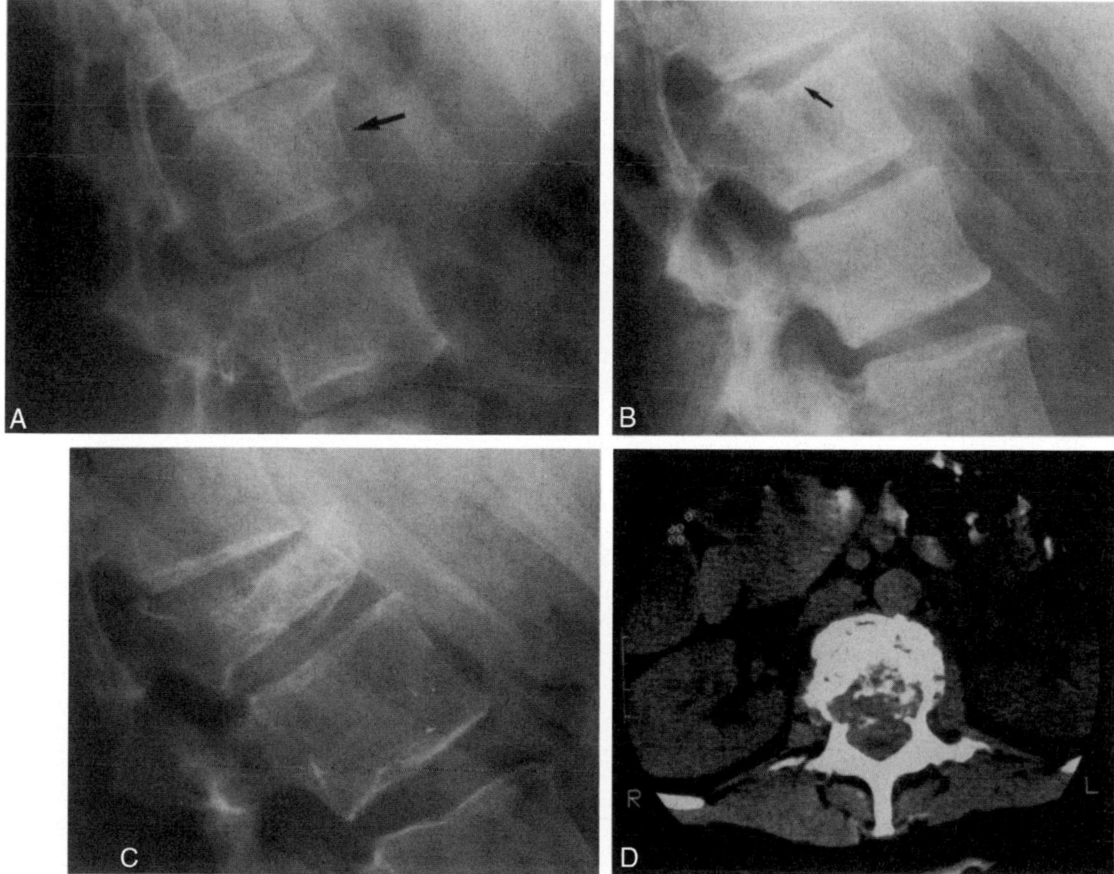

Figure 13-53 Serial view of L1 in a 43-year-old woman with metastatic breast cancer. *A*, 10/3/85. This patient had radicular symptoms associated with an acute herniated lumbar disc. Her back pain resolved with conservative management. Calcification of bone is normal in L1 *(arrow)*. *B*, 2/9/87. This patient had acute-onset, localized back pain over the L1 vertebra. The lateral view reveals sclerosis of the superior endplate of L1 associated with mild loss of vertebral body height. *C*, 4/17/87. The patient's pain persisted. A repeat roentgenogram demonstrated marked destruction of the L1 vertebral body. *D*, CT scan of L1 revealing marked destruction of the vertebral body and incipient encroachment of tumor into the spinal canal.

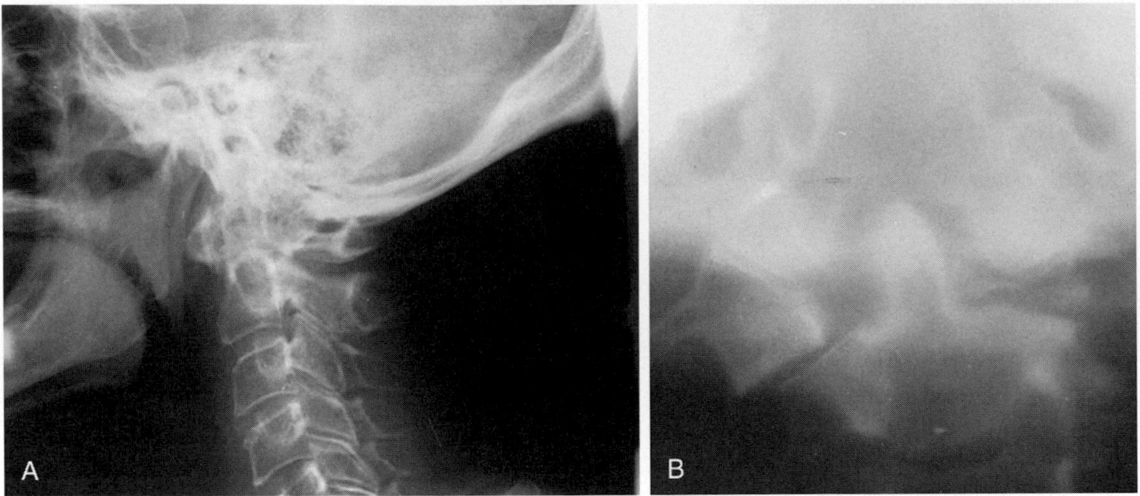

Figure 13-54 Metastatic tumor in a 64-year-old woman with a history of breast cancer and neck pain. *A*, A lateral view of the cervical spine shows no detectable abnormality. *B*, A CT open-mouth view shows loss of the left portion of the C1 ring, compatible with metastatic breast cancer. *(Courtesy of Anne Brower, MD.)*

Scintigraphy

Early in the course of a metastatic lesion, plain roentgenographic examination will be unremarkable because between 30% and 50% of bone must be destroyed before a lesion is evident on plain roentgenograms (Fig. 13-55).[29] However, scintigraphic examination with a bone scan makes it possible to detect areas of symptomatic and asymptomatic bone involvement in up to 85% of patients with metastases (Figs. 13-56 and 13-57).[22,31] A bone scan may also suggest the presence of tumor in patients with coincident degenerative disease or osteoporosis. In one study, bone scan was the single most useful diagnostic test for differentiating pain from metastatic disease from pain caused by a benign lesion.[43] It is important to remember that there are reasons for false-negative and false-positive scintiscans (Table 13-4).[39] One of the most important to remember is the "superscan." In these scans, markedly increased, symmetrical, generalized uptake by diffuse metastases may be interpreted as normal. The reduction of tracer in the kidneys and urine should alert the radiologist to this possibility (Fig. 13-58).[83] A bone scintiscan is the most sensitive and economic test for detecting bone metastases.[62] However, MR imaging is able to detect medullary abnormalities without cortical involvement that are missed by scintigraphy.[85]

Computed Tomography

CT may also be useful in localizing lesions that are difficult to identify on plain radiographs.[88] Upper cervical spine lesions missed by plain roentgenograms are detected by CT. CT is normally reserved for the assessment of patients with positive isotope scans but negative radiographs. It enables differentiation among bony metastases, benign lesions, and no abnormality.[64,72] With CT, differentiation can be made between metastases and degenerative joint disease when both coexist in apophyseal articulations.[72] CT may also be useful in detecting the presence and extent of pelvic metastases, an area inadequately evaluated by scintiscan.[24] CT scan is particularly useful in demonstrating small areas of bone destruction and bone and tumor impingement on the spinal canal.[87] CT may also prove to be more useful than MR imaging for upper cervical spine lesions at the C1–C2 level. In this location, neural impingement is a late consequence of metastasis. CT is more helpful in determining the status of bone architecture, which has implications for surgical therapeutic intervention.[22]

It should not be used as a screening technique because of the considerable exposure to radiation.

Myelography

Myelography was the definitive diagnostic procedure for any patient with a metastatic lesion and spinal cord or nerve root compression. Injection of dye in two locations, the lumbar spine and the cisterna magna (cervical spine), was necessary to locate all potential areas of neural compression because lesions in the lumbar spine were accompanied by "silent" lesions in the proximal part of the spine.[45] Myelography may be used to identify whether the lesion is extradural or intradural in location.

Magnetic Resonance

The role of MR in the evaluation of patients with metastases continues to evolve as the technique becomes more sensitive in detecting neoplasms that replace normal tissue in the spine. MR imaging is an effective method for detecting upper spinal cord compression, particularly soft tissue lesions, that may not be adequately visualized by other radiographic techniques (Fig. 13-59).[7] Some studies have demonstrated MR to be better at showing the extent of tumor inside the cord, the degree of extraosseous extension, and bone marrow invasion and CT to be better at showing cortical bone destruction and the degree of bone mineralization.[60,93] MR is able to identify compression fractures secondary to osteopenia as a result of replacement of bone marrow with malignant cells.[92] MR detects lesions that are not identified by roentgenograms or scintiscan.[55]

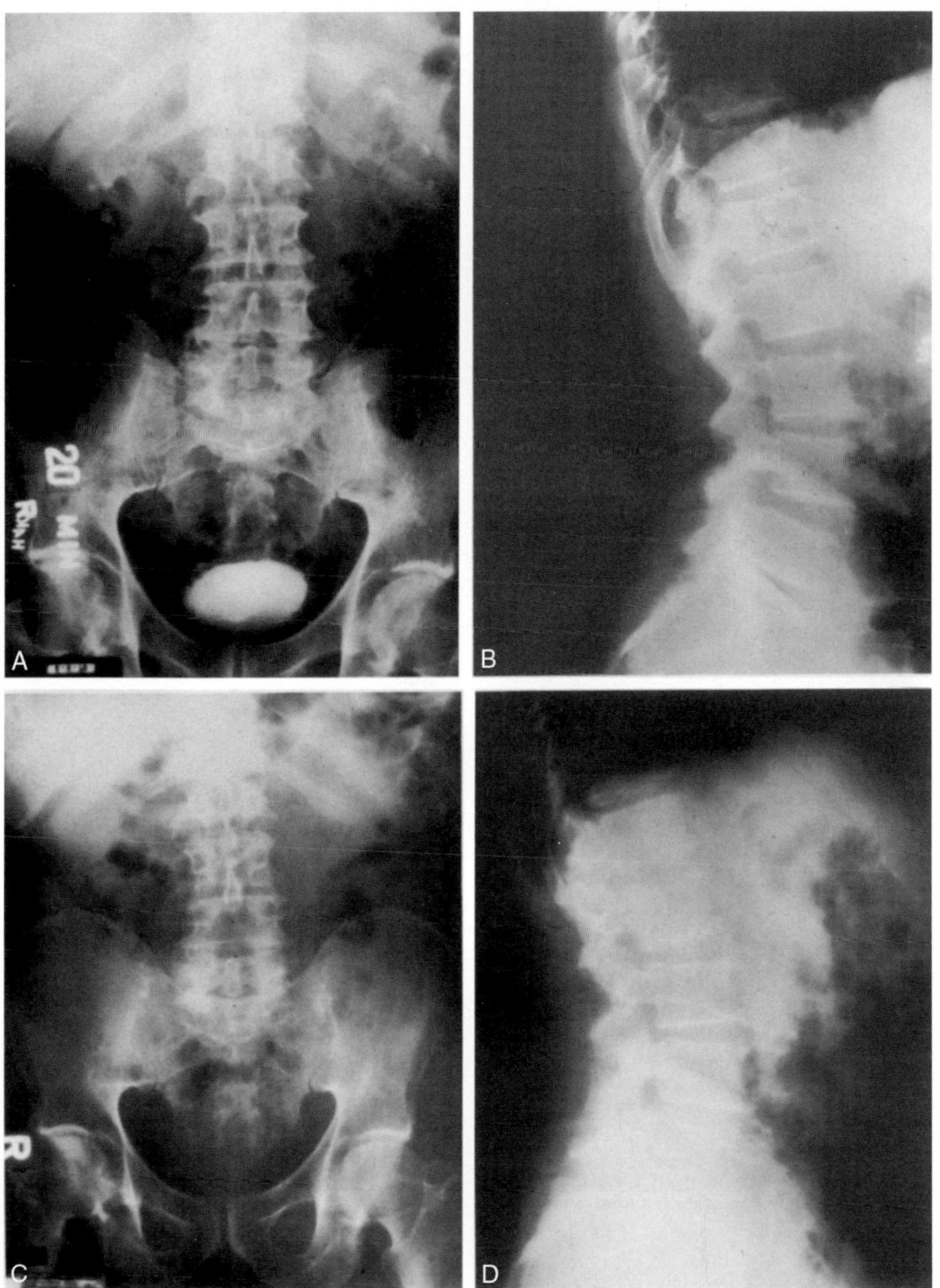

Figure 13-55 A 64-year-old man was examined for diffuse low back pain. Evaluation included an intravenous pyelogram, which showed no abnormalities. The anteroposterior (AP) *(A)* and lateral *(B)* views reveal osteoarthritic changes associated with degenerative disc disease. The patient returned 6 months later with severe pain over the L4 vertebra. The AP *(C)* and lateral *(D)* views are presented.

Continued

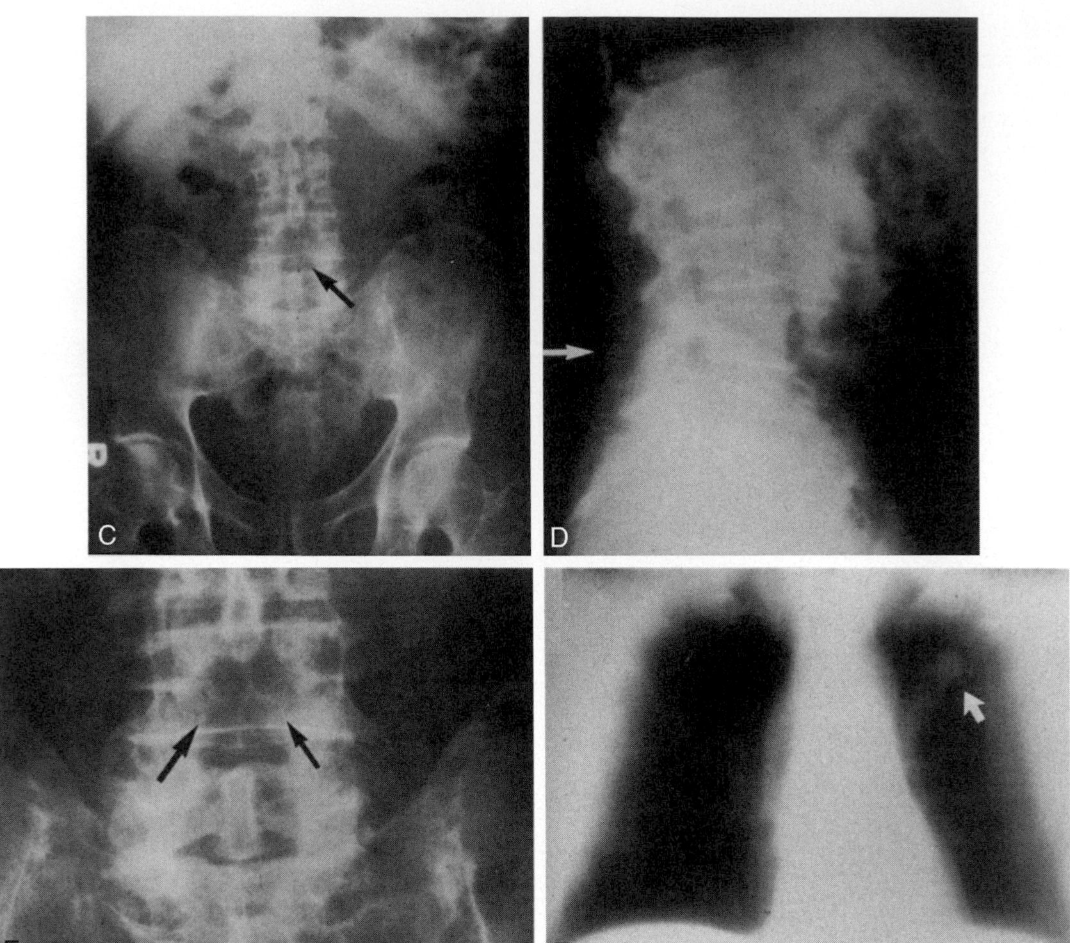

Figure 13-55, cont'd Anteroposterior *(C)* and lateral *(D)* views reveal loss of the spinous process of L4 *(arrows)*. A close-up *(E)* shows osteolysis of the process *(arrows)*. A tomogram *(F)* of the lung revealed the primary source of tumor in the upper lobe of the left lung *(arrow)*.

A study of 40 patients with metastatic disease revealed patients with breast, kidney, and prostate cancer and multiple myeloma that was abnormal on MR but normal with other radiographic techniques, including CT and scintiscan (Fig. 13-60).[3] MR is also sensitive to lesions in the pelvis that are not detected by other radiographic techniques.[7] The importance of MR as a diagnostic tool has been further advanced by the availability of gadolinium-diethylenetriaminepentaacetic acid as a paramagnetic contrast agent. MR with contrast demonstrates the size, location, configuration, and characteristics of spinal tumors.[84] MR is the first procedure to be used for patients with spinal cord compression. It is a noninvasive technique that is sensitive in detecting extradural masses.[17] MR of the entire spinal cord should be obtained if compression is suspected because 10% of patients have multiple levels of impingement.[13] CT and myelography should be reserved for patients in whom MR is not feasible or does not satisfactorily explain the neurologic findings.

DIFFERENTIAL DIAGNOSIS

In a patient with a known primary tumor and spinal pain, a destructive spinal lesion is associated with the primary neoplasm in the vast majority of cases. These patients may not require biopsy of the spinal lesion for diagnosis; however, patients with no known primary neoplasm in whom destructive lesions of the spine develop require biopsy for tissue diagnosis. CT-guided closed needle biopsy of lesions in the lumbar or cervical spine can safely yield useful information.[4,16,23] A transpedicular biopsy of lesions between T1 and L4 can be accomplished with retrieval of adequate tissue to confirm a diagnosis.[51]

Other conditions may cause bony changes on radiographs and "hot spots" on scintiscans. Elevated alkaline phosphatase may be seen with osteomalacia, Paget's disease, hyperparathyroidism, and sarcoidosis. Only by careful review of all the data can the various diagnoses be eliminated. In

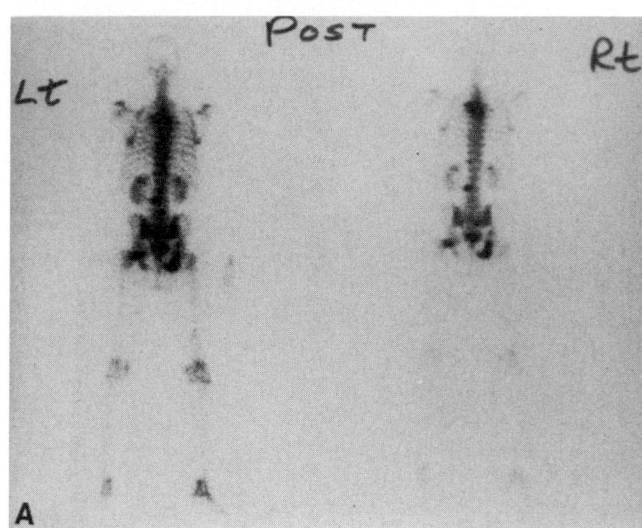

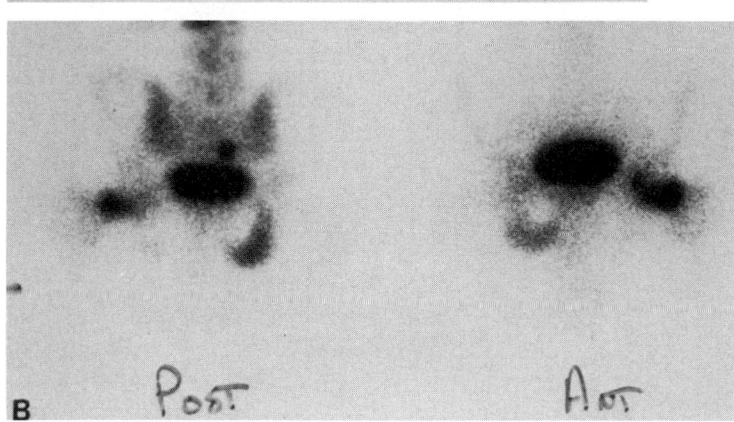

Figure 13-56 A 60-year-old man with a hard nodule in the prostate gland and bone pain. *A*, A ^{99m}Tc MDP bone scan reveals uptake in the midthoracic spine, upper lumbar spine, left femoral neck, right ischium, and sacrum. *B*, A spot view reveals focal uptake in the same areas.

some circumstances, tissue biopsy is the only sure way to obtain the data needed to make an accurate diagnosis.

Pancoast's Tumor

Lesions in the superior sulcus (Pancoast's tumors) may invade the brachial plexus and extend into the epidural

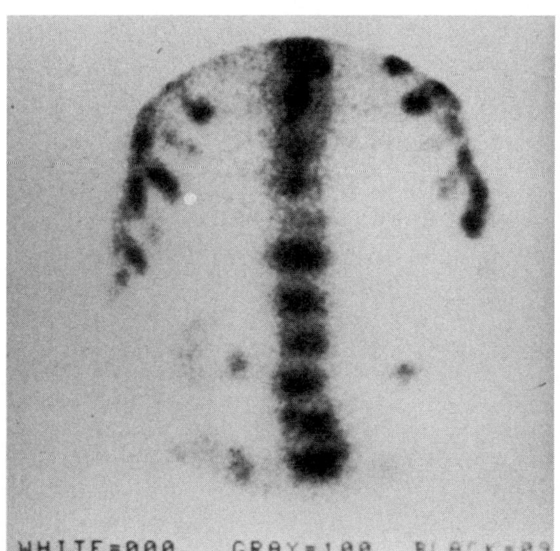

Figure 13-57 Bone scan of a 70-year-old man with metastatic prostatic carcinoma. Most of these "hot spots" on the scan were asymptomatic.

13-4 BONE SCAN

False Negative	False Positive
1. Tumor lacks an osteoblastic response (myeloma)	1. Site of injection (elbow)
2. Small deposits	2. Urinary incontinence
3. Lesions of the sacrum and ischium masked by the bladder	3. Abnormal bladder collections (diverticulum)
4. Generalized increased uptake ("superscan")	4. Incomplete isotope
	5. Superimposition of uptake

Modified from Galasko CSB: Skeletal Metastases. Boston, Butterworths, 1986.

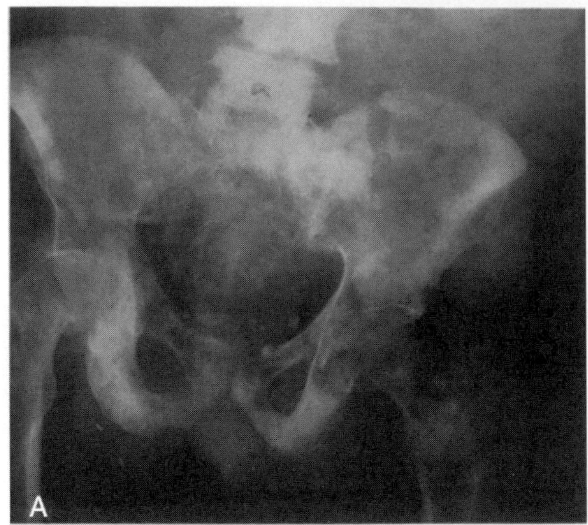

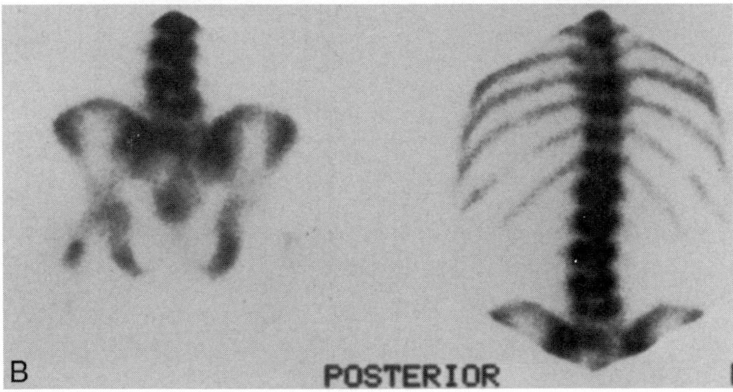

Figure 13-58 *A*, Posteroanterior view of the pelvis of a middle-aged man with metastatic prostate cancer (8/2/90). *B*, Bone scintiscan (9/26/90) with a marked increase in uptake over the axial skeleton without tracer in the kidney or bladder. *(From Borenstein DG: Low back pain. In Klippel J, Dieppe P [eds]: Rheumatology. St. Louis, CV Mosby, 1994.)*

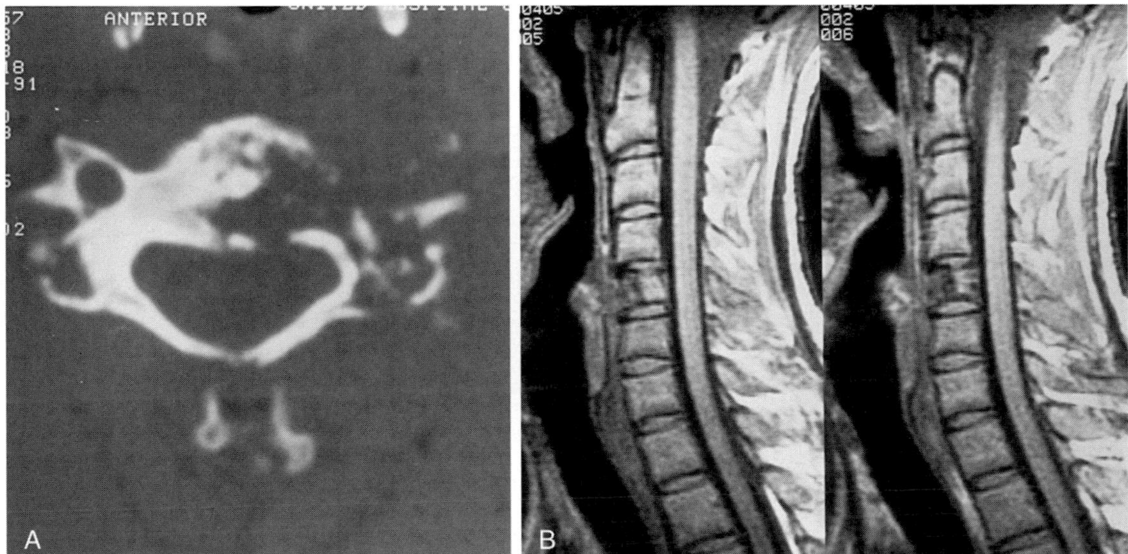

Figure 13-59 A 28-year-old man with a history of human immunodeficiency virus infection had increasing neck pain and swelling. *A*, A CT scan of the C4 vertebral body shows an osteolytic lesion of the vertebral body and transverse process. *B*, A sagittal T1-weighted MR image shows replacement of the anterior portion of C4 with anterior soft tissue extension. Biopsy of the lesion revealed metastatic follicular thyroid cancer. *(Courtesy of Thomas Dina, MD.)*

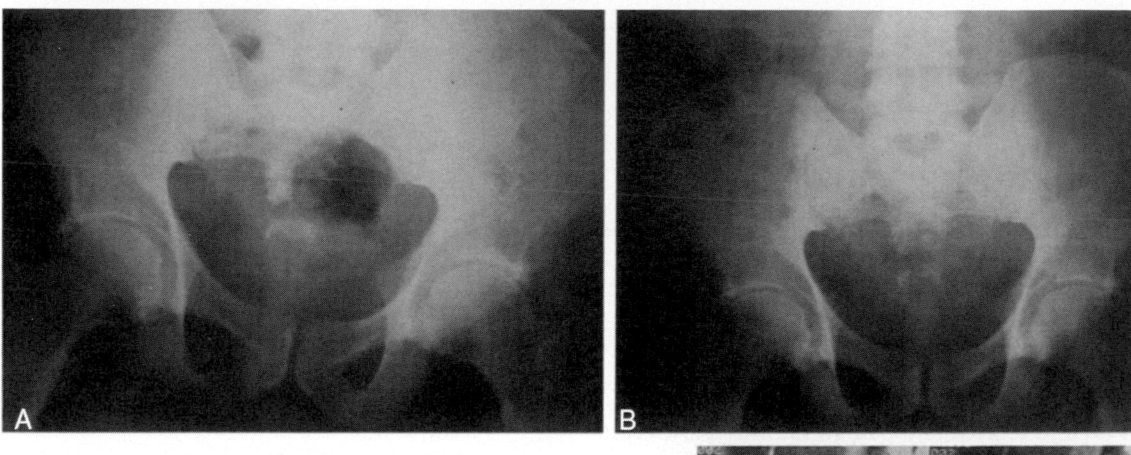

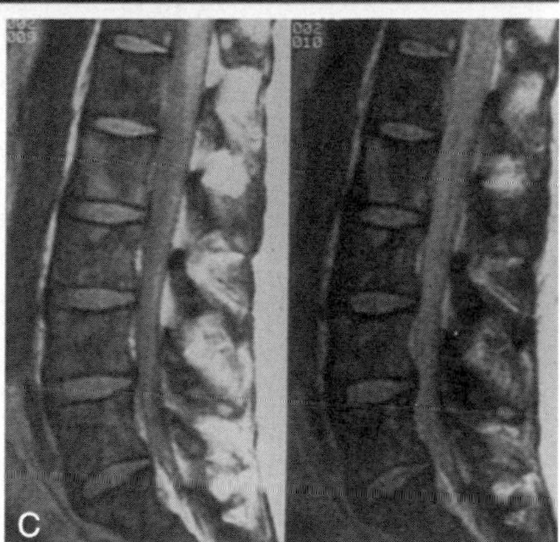

Figure 13-60 A 52-year-old man had right-sided low back and buttock pain. A plain roentgenogram *(A)* taken on 4/1/91 was unremarkable. He did not respond to conservative management and complained of increasing pain. A repeat roentgenogram *(B)* taken on 5/1/91 was suggestive of increased sclerosis in the pelvis. Serum acid phosphatase was elevated. *C*, MR of the lumbar spine (5/3/91) on proton density *(left)* and T2-weighted *(right)* sequences demonstrated decreased signal intensity in multiple vertebral bodies indicative of marrow replacement. Biopsy of the prostate revealed adenocarcinoma. The patient expired from extensive metastatic disease in 6/93.

space through an intervertebral foramen.[18,57,68] These lesions cause radicular pain in the setting of normal plain roentgenograms and bone scintigraphy. MR imaging or CT/myelographic evaluation of the spinal column detects these lesions.

TREATMENT

Treatment of metastatic disease of the spine is directed toward palliation of pain. Cure is rarely possible because most solitary metastatic lesions are accompanied by a number of "silent" deposits that become evident only over time. The pain of a metastatic spine lesion may be secondary to bone destruction or pathologic fracture.[10] Treatment directed specifically at spinal lesions may include radiation therapy, corticosteroids, and decompression. Radiotherapy may be used alone as primary treatment to decrease pain and slow growth or as adjunctive therapy after surgical decompression.[14,54] The use of bisphosphonates (pamidronate or zoledronic acid) is effective in decreasing the risk of vertebral fracture related to osteolytic metastatic disease.[8] If instability develops, patients may require the placement of rods to control their pain.[26] Metastatic lesions from breast, thyroid, and lymphomatoid tumors are most sensitive to radiotherapy. Corticosteroids may help reduce edema and alleviate symptoms in patients with spinal cord compression.[19] Surgery should be considered when the diagnosis of a spinal lesion is in doubt, in those with neurologic deterioration from metastatic epidural compression at a previously irradiated level, in those with progressive neurologic deterioration during radiotherapy despite large doses of corticosteroids, and in patients with symptomatic spinal instability or compression of neural structures by bone.[15]

Lumbar Spine

Decompression of the neural elements is usually of little help in returning function to patients with long-standing paraplegia, but it is recommended for those in whom neurologic symptoms have recently developed.[86] Laminectomy has the best chance of success if decompression is performed before the development of compressive symptoms.[78] A number of new surgical procedures have been developed for spine stabilization in patients with an unstable vertebral column.[81] Patients with breast and prostate carcinoma who undergo laminectomy improve to a greater degree than do those with lung or kidney carcinoma.[58] Individuals with solitary metastasis from a solid tumor have a median survival of 30 months if the entire lesion can be extirpated before radiation therapy.[82]

Cervical Spine

In the cervical spine, the extent and location of tumor, the spinal level, bone integrity, and patient debility play a role in regard to choosing the appropriate surgical procedure.[69] Surgery should be considered before radiotherapy if the cervical spine is unstable or has a significant neurologic deficit secondary to compression.[67] A posterior approach to cervical metastatic lesions may decompress the spinal cord or root but may result in continued pain secondary to spinal instability. Attempts have been made to decrease the risk of instability by using methylmethacrylate (bone cement) for neck stabilization.[47] Subsequently, other investigators reported the failure of bone cement for cervical spine stabilization without the additional use of bone grafts and wire stabilization.[61] Anterior decompression allows for direct resection of the tumor but requires prolonged neck bracing for stabilization. In general, combined anterior and posterior stabilization may be required for cervical spine instability secondary to neoplastic destruction.

PROGNOSIS

The course of each patient with skeletal metastasis is dependent on a number of factors, including the type of tumor, extent of involvement, sensitivity to therapy, and degree of neurologic symptoms; however, in general, the prognosis is poor. In one study, cord compression developed in 20% of patients with vertebral metastases.[30] Unless decompression is accomplished quickly, return of function is minimal and the outcome debilitating. Metastatic disease from an unknown primary is uncommon, but particularly aggressive. The survival time of these patients is extremely short—a 6-month survival rate of 6%.[76] Surgical intervention to prevent progression of structural instability can result in a mean survival time of 26 months after surgical intervention.[89] However, for patients with metastatic disease affecting the cervical spine, surgical treatment improves the quality of life.[71]

References

Skeletal Metastases

1. Algra PR, Heimans JJ, Valk J, et al: Do metastases in vertebrae begin in the body or the pedicles? Imaging in 45 patients. AJR Am J Roentgenol 158:1275, 1992.
2. Asdourian PL, Weidenbaum M, DeWald RL, et al: The pattern of vertebral involvement in metastatic vertebral breast cancer. Clin Orthop 250:164, 1990.
3. Avrahami E, Tadmor R, Dally O, Hadar H: Early MR demonstration of spinal metastases in patients with normal radiographs and CT and radionuclide bone scans. J Comput Assist Tomogr 13:598, 1989.
4. Babu NV, Titus VTK, Chittaranjan S, et al: Computed tomographically guided biopsy of the spine. Spine 19:2436, 1994.
5. Barron KD, Hirano A, Araki S, Terry RD: Experiences with metastatic neoplasms involving the spinal cord. Neurology 9:91, 1959.
6. Batson OV: The function of the vertebral veins and their role in the spread of metastasis. Ann Surg 112:138, 1940.
7. Beatrous TE, Choyke PL, Frank JA: Diagnostic evaluation of cancer patients with pelvic pain: Comparison of scintigraphy, CT, and MR imaging. AJR Am J Roentgenol 155:85, 1990.
8. Berenson JR, Rosen LS, Howell A, et al: Zoledronic acid reduces skeletal-related events in patients with osteolytic metastases. Cancer 91:1191-1200, 2001.
9. Bernat JL, Greenberg ER, Barrett J: Suspected epidural compression of the spinal cord and cauda equina by metastatic carcinoma. Cancer 51:1953, 1983.
10. Bhalla SK: Metastatic disease of the spine. Clin Orthop 73:52, 1970.
11. Bishop MC, Hardy JG, Taylor MC, et al: Bone imaging and serum phosphatase in prostatic carcinoma. Br J Urol 57:317, 1985.
12. Boland PJ, Lane JM, Sundaresan N: Metastatic disease of the spine. Clin Orthop 169:95, 1982.
13. Bonner JA, Lichter AS: A caution about the use of MRI to diagnose spinal cord compression. N Engl J Med 322:556, 1990.
14. Bruckman JE, Bloomer WD: Management of spinal cord compression. Semin Oncol 5:135, 1978.
15. Byrne TN: Spinal cord compression from epidural metastases. N Engl J Med 327:614, 1992.
16. Camins MB, Rosenblum BR: Osseous lesions of the cervical spine. Clin Neurosurg 37:722, 1991.
17. Carmody RF, Yang PJ, Seeley GW, et al: Spinal cord compression due to metastatic disease: Diagnosis with MR imaging versus myelography. Radiology 173:225, 1989.
18. Cascino TL, Kori S, Krol G, Foley KM: CT of the brachial plexus in patients with cancer. Neurology 33:1553, 1983.
19. Clark PRR, Saunders M. Steroid-induced remission in spinal canal reticulum cell sarcoma: Report of two cases. J Neurosurg 42:346-348, 1975.
20. Constans JP, De Divitiis E, Donzelli R, et al: Spinal metastases with neurological manifestations: Review of 600 cases. J Neurosurg 59:111, 1983.
21. Cowan RJ, Young KA: Evaluation of serum alkaline phosphatase determination in patients with positive bone scans. Cancer 32:887, 1973.
22. Craig FS: Metastatic and primary lesions of bone. Clin Orthop 73:33, 1970.
23. Craig FS: Vertebral body biopsy. J Bone Joint Surg Am 38-A:93, 1956.
24. Cranston PE, Patel RB, Harrison RB: Computed tomography for metastatic lesions of the osseous pelvis. South Med J 76:1503, 1983.
25. Delmarter RB, Sachs BL, Thompson GH, et al: Primary neoplasms of the thoracic and lumbar spine: An analysis of 29 consecutive cases. Clin Orthop 256:87, 1990.
26. Dewald RL, Bridwell KH, Prodromas C, Rodts MF: Reconstructive spinal surgery as palliation for metastatic malignancies of the spine. Spine 10:21, 1985.
27. Deyo RA, Diehk AK: Cancer as cause of back pain: Frequency, clinical presentation, and diagnostic strategies. J Gen Intern Med 3:230, 1988.
28. Disler DG, Miklic D: Imaging findings in tumors of the sacrum. AJR Am J Roentgenol 73:1699-1706, 1999.
29. Edelstyn GA, Gillespie PG, Grebbel FS: The radiological demonstration of skeletal metastases: Experimental observations. Clin Radiol 18:158, 1967.
30. Emsellem HA: Metastatic disease of the spine: Diagnosis and management. South Med J 76:1405, 1986.
31. Fager CA: Management of malignant intraspinal disease. Surg Clin North Am 47:743, 1967.
32. Fisher MS: Lumbar spine metastasis in cervical carcinoma: A characteristic pattern. Radiology 134:631, 1980.
33. Fornasier VL, Czitrom AA: Collapsed vertebrae: Review of 659 autopsies. Clin Orthop 131:261, 1978.

34. Fornasier VL, Horne JG: Metastases to the vertebral column. Cancer 36:590, 1975.
35. Francis KC, Hutter RVP: Neoplasms of the spine in the aged. Clin Orthop 26:54, 1963.
36. Frassica FJ, Sim FH: Pathophysiology. In Sim FH (ed): Diagnosis and Management of Metastatic Bone Disease: A Multidisciplinary Approach. New York, Raven Press, 1988, pp 7-14.
37. Front D, Schenck SO, Frankel A, Robinson E: Bone metastases and bone pain in breast cancer. Are they closely associated? JAMA 242:1747, 1979.
38. Fujita T, Ueda Y, Kawahara N, et al: Local spread of metastatic vertebral tumors. A histologic study. Spine 22:1905-1912, 1997.
39. Galasko CSB: Skeletal Metastases. Boston, Butterworths, 1986.
40. Galasko CSB: Skeletal metastases and mammary cancer. Ann R Coll Surg Engl 50:3, 1972.
41. Galasko CSB: The pathological basis for skeletal scintigraphy. J Bone Joint Surg Br 57-B:353, 1975.
42. Galasko CSB, Doyle FH: The detection of skeletal metastases from mammary cancer. A regional comparison between radiology and scintigraphy. Clin Radiol 23:295, 1972.
43. Galasko CSB, Sylvester BS: Back pain in patients treated for malignant tumors. Clin Oncol 4:273, 1978.
44. Gatenby RA, Mulhearn CB Jr, Moldofsky PJ: Computed tomography guided thin needle biopsy of small lytic bone lesions. Skeletal Radiol 11:289, 1984.
45. Gilbert RW, Kim JH, Posner JB: Epidural spinal cord compression from metastatic tumor: Diagnosis and treatment. Ann Neurol 3:340, 1978.
46. Harrington KD: Metastatic disease of the spine. J Bone Joint Surg Am 68-A:1110, 1986.
47. Harrington KD: The use of methylmethacrylate for vertebral-body replacement and anterior stabilization of pathological fracture-dislocations of the spine due to metastatic malignant disease. J Bone Joint Surg Am 63-A:36, 1981.
48. Hastings DE, Macnab I, Lawson V: Neoplasms of the atlas and axis. Can J Surg 11:290, 1968.
49. Hubbard DD, Gunn DR: Secondary carcinoma of the spine with destruction of the intervertebral disc. Clin Orthop 88:86, 1972.
50. Jacobs SC, Pikna D, Lawson RK: Prostate osteoblastic factor. Invest Urol 17:195, 1979.
51. Jelinek JS, Kransdorf MJ, Gray R, et al: Percutaneous transpedicular biopsy of vertebral body lesions. Spine 21:2035-2040, 1996.
52. Jenis LG, Dunn EJ, An HS: Metastatic disease of the cervical spine. A review. Clin Orthop 359:89-103, 1999.
53. Jonsson B, Jonsson H Jr, Karlstom G, Sjostrom L: Surgery of cervical spine metastases: A retrospective study. Eur Spine J 3:76-83, 1994.
54. Khan FR, Glickman AS, Chu FCH, Nickson JJ: Treatment by radiotherapy of spinal cord compression due to extradural metastases. Radiology 89:495, 1967.
55. Khurana JS, Rosenthal DI, Rosenberg A, Mankin HJ: Skeletal metastases in liposarcoma detectable only by magnetic resonance imaging. Clin Orthop 243:204, 1989.
56. Kleinman WB, Kiernan HA, Michelsen WJ: Metastatic cancer of the spinal column. Clin Orthop 138:166, 1978.
57. Kori SH, Foley KM, Posner JB: Brachial plexus lesions in patients with cancer: 100 cases. Neurology 31:45, 1981.
58. Lenz M, Fried JR: Metastasis to skeleton, brain, and spinal cord from cancer of the breast and effects of radiotherapy. Ann Surg 93:278, 1931.
59. Lo LD, Schweitzer ME, Juneja V, et al: Are L5 fractures an indicator of metastasis? Skeletal Radiol 29:454-458, 2000.
60. Maravilla KR, Lesh P, Weinre JC, et al: Magnetic resonance imaging of the lumbar spine with CT correlation. AJNR Am J Neuroradiol 6:237, 1985.
61. McAfee PC, Bohlman HH, Ducker T, Eismont FJ: Failure of stabilization of the spine with methylmethacrylate. J Bone Joint Surg Am 68-A:1145, 1986.
62. McNeil BJ: Value of bone scanning in neoplastic disease. Semin Nucl Med 4:277, 1984.
63. Mirra JM: Bone Tumors: Clinical, Radiologic, and Pathologic Correlation. Philadelphia, Lea & Febiger, 1989, pp 1495-1517.
64. Muindi J, Coombes RC, Golding S, et al: The role of computed tomography in the detection of bone metastases in breast cancer patients. Br J Radiol 56:233, 1983.
65. Mundy GR, Raisz LG, Cooper RA, et al: Evidence for the secretion of an osteoclast activating factor in myeloma. N Engl J Med 291:1041, 1974.
66. Nicholas JJ, Christy WC: Spinal pain made worse by recumbency: A clue to spinal cord tumors. Arch Phys Med Rehabil 67:598, 1986.
67. Onimus M, Schraub S, Bertin D, et al: Surgical treatment of vertebral metastasis. Spine 11:883, 1986.
68. Pancoast HK: Superior pulmonary sulcus tumor: Tumor characterized by pain, Horner's syndrome, destruction of bone and atrophy of hand muscles. JAMA 99:1391, 1932.
69. Perrin RG, McBroom RJ, Perrin RG: Metastatic tumors of the cervical spine. Clin Neurosurg 37:740, 1991.
70. Phillips E, Levine AM: Metastatic lesions of the upper cervical spine. Spine 14:1071, 1989.
71. Raycroft JF, Hockman RP, Southwick WO: Metastatic tumors involving the cervical vertebrae: Surgical palliation. J Bone Joint Surg Am 60-A:763, 1978.
72. Redmond J, Spring DB, Munderloh SH, et al: Spinal computed tomography scanning in the evaluation of metastatic disease. Cancer 54:253, 1984.
73. Resnick D, Niwayama G: Intervertebral disc abnormalities associated with vertebral metastasis: Observations in patients and cadavers with prostatic cancer. Invest Radiol 13:182, 1978.
74. Rodriguez M, Dinapoli RP: Spinal cord compression with special reference to metastatic epidural tumors. Mayo Clin Proc 55:442, 1980.
75. Rubens RD, Fogelman I: Bone Metastases: Diagnosis and Treatment. New York, Springer-Verlag, 1991, pp 1-247.
76. Saengnipanthkul S, Jirarattanaphochai K, Rojviroj S, et al: Metastatic adenocarcinoma of the spine. Spine 17:427, 1992.
77. Schaberg J, Gainor BJ: A profile of metastatic carcinoma of the spine. Spine 10:19, 1985.
78. Schoeggl A, Reddy M, Matula C: Neurological outcome following laminectomy in spinal metastases. Spinal Cord 40:363-366, 2002.
79. Sherk HH: Lesions of the atlas and axis. Clin Orthop 109:33, 1975.
80. Sundaresan N, Galcich JH, Lane JM, Greenberg HS: Treatment of odontoid fractures in cancer patients. J Neurosurg 54:187, 1981.
81. Sundaresan N, Krol G, Digiacinto GV, Hughes JEO: Metastatic tumors of the spine. In Sundaresan N, Schmidek HH, Schiller AL, Rosenthal DI (eds): Tumors of the Spine: Diagnosis and Clinical Management. Philadelphia, WB Saunders, 1990, pp 279-304.
82. Sundaresan N, Rothman A, Manhart K, et al: Surgery for solitary metastases of the spine: Rationale and results of treatment. Spine 27:1802-1806, 2002.
83. Sy WM, Patel D, Faunce H: Significance of absent or faint kidney sign on bone scan. J Nucl Med 16:454, 1975.
84. Sze G, Stimac GK, Bartlett C, et al: Multicenter study of gadopentetate dimeglumine as an MR contrast agent: Evaluation in patients with spinal tumors. AJNR Am J Neuroradiol 11:967, 1990.
85. Taoka T, Mayr NA, Lee HJ, et al: Factors influencing visualization of vertebral metastases on MR imaging versus bone scintigraphy. AJR Am J Roentgenol 176:1525-1530, 2001.
86. Vieth RG, Odom GL: Extradural spinal metastases and their neurosurgical treatment. J Neurosurg 23:501, 1965.
87. Weissman DE, Gilbert M, Wang H, Grossman SA: The use of computed tomography of the spine to identify patients at high risk for epidural metastases. J Clin Oncol 3:1541, 1985.
88. Wilson JS, Korobkin M, Genant HK, Bovill EG: Computed tomography of musculoskeletal disorders. AJR Am J Roentgenol 13:55, 1978.
89. Wise JJ, Fischgrund JS, Herkowitz HN, et al: Complication, survival rates, and risk factors of surgery for metastatic disease of the spine. Spine 24:1943-1951, 1999.
90. Wong DA, Fornasier VL, MacNab I: Spinal metastases: The obvious, the occult, and the impostors. Spine 15:1, 1990.
91. Young JM, Fung FJ Jr: Incidence of tumor metastasis to the lumbar spine: A comparative study or roentgenographic changes and gross lesions. J Bone Joint Surg Am 35-A:55, 1953.
92. Yuh WT, Zachar CK, Barloon TJ, et al: Vertebral compression fractures: Distinction between benign and malignant causes with MR imaging. Radiology 172:215, 1989.
93. Zimmer WD, Berquist TH, McLeod RA, et al: Bone tumors: Magnetic resonance imaging versus computed tomography. Radiology 155:709, 1985.

INTRASPINAL NEOPLASMS

Capsule Summary

	Low Back	Neck
Frequency of spinal pain		
Extradural (E):	Very common	Very common
Intradural-extramedullary (IE):	Common	Common
Intramedullary (I):	Rare	Rare
Location of spinal pain		
E:	Lumbar spine	Cervical spine
IE:	Low back and leg	Neck and arm
I:	Low back and leg	Neck and arm
Quality of spinal pain		
E:	Increasing local ache	Increasing local ache
IE:	Referred pain	Referred pain
I:	Radicular	Radicular
Symptoms and signs		
E:	Increasing spinal pain with recumbency, neurologic deficit	Increasing spinal pain with recumbency, neurologic deficit
IE:	Pain with recumbency, slow onset	Pain with recumbency, slow onset
I:	Neurologic deficit, painless	Neurologic deficit, painless
Laboratory tests		
E:	None	None
IE:	None	None
I:	None	None
Radiographic findings		
E:	MR (magnetic resonance)	MR
IE:	MR	MR
I:	MR	MR
Treatment		
E:	Radiation therapy, corticosteroids, laminectomy	Radiation therapy, corticosteroids, laminectomy
IE:	Surgical excision	Surgical excision
E:	Surgical excision	Surgical excision

PREVALENCE AND PATHOGENESIS

Although bone is the tissue in the axial skeleton most frequently affected by primary and metastatic tumors, less commonly, tissues inside the spinal column may be affected by neoplastic processes. These intraspinal neoplasms may be extradural—between bone and the covering of the spinal cord, the dura; intradural-extramedullary—between the dura and the spinal cord; and intramedullary—in the spinal cord proper (Fig. 13-61). Extradural tumors are most commonly metastatic in origin. Intradural-extramedullary tumors are predominantly meningiomas, neurofibromas, or lipomas. Intramedullary tumors are ependymomas and gliomas (Table 13-5).

Epidemiology

Tumors of the spinal cord and its coverings are uncommon and account for 10% to 15% of primary central nervous system neoplasms with an incidence of 1.3 per 100,000 per year.[124] Intraspinal tumors occur less frequently than tumors of the brain.[124] A study in Norway revealed the annual incidence of primary intraspinal neoplasms to be 5 per million for females and 3 per million for males.[93] They occur in individuals between the ages of 20 and 60 years and have equal distribution in men and women.

Extradural tumors are metastatic lesions that have invaded the intraspinal space from contiguous structures. They are the most common tumors of the spinal canal. Of the intradural lesions, extramedullary neoplasms occur more commonly than intramedullary neoplasms. Intraspinal neoplasms predominantly occur in adults between 30 and 50 years of age.[70]

Pathogenesis

The extradural, or epidural, space is the predominant site of intraspinal malignant tumors. Metastatic tumors in the spinal canal are extradural in location because the dura is resistant to invasion from lesions that extend from foci in vertebral bone. The extradural space is also the location of Batson's plexus, which is a site for hematogenous spread of tumor.[18] Major structures in the intradural-extramedullary space are the meninges and spinal nerve roots. Meningiomas and neurofibromas arise from these structures. Depending on the population of patients being studied, meningiomas

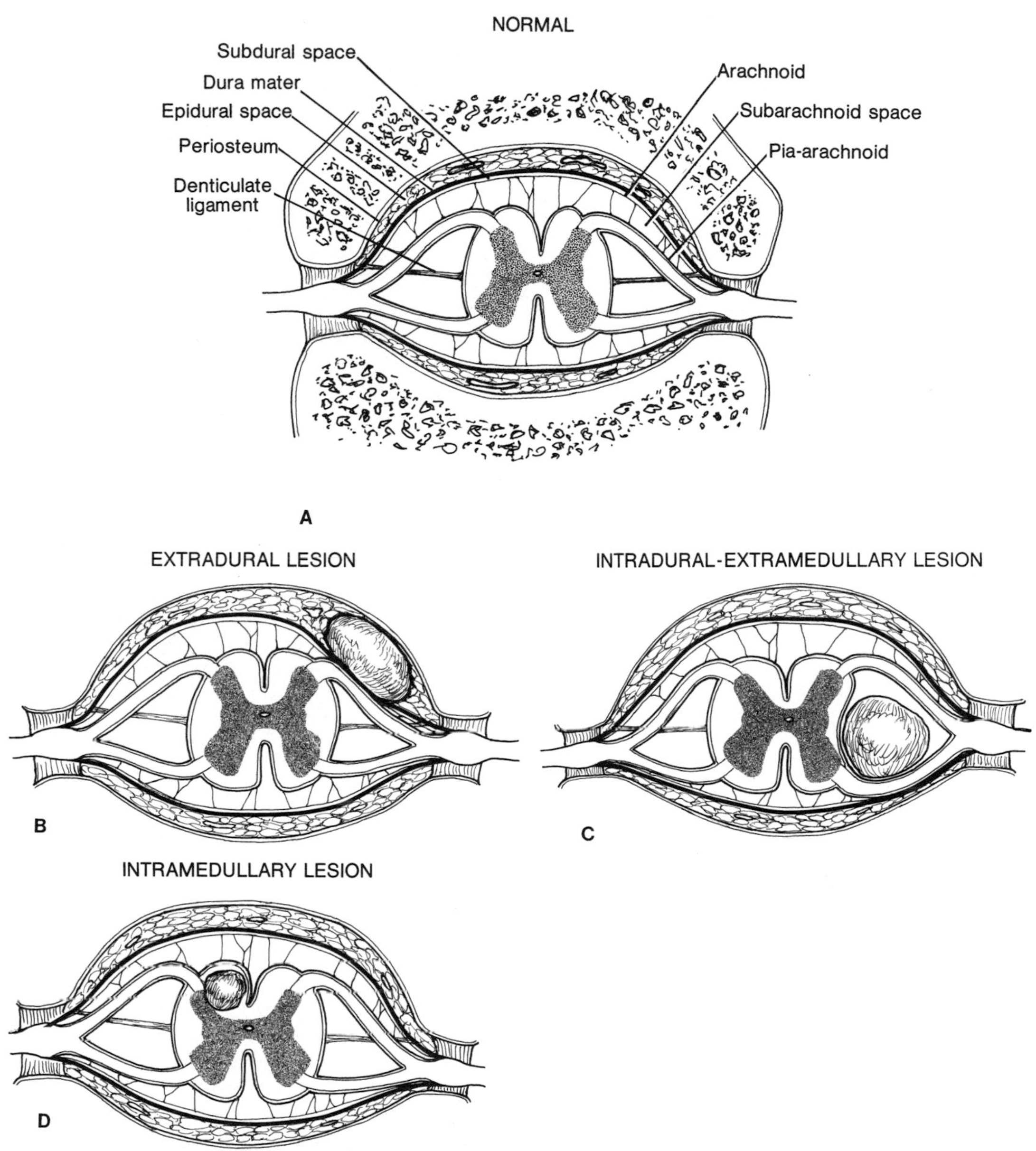

Figure 13-61 Location of intraspinal tumors. *A*, normal anatomy. *B*, Extradural lesion (metastases). *C*, Intradural-extramedullary lesion (neurofibroma). *D*, Intramedullary lesion (glioma).

may cause 25% of intraspinal neoplasms. Intramedullary tumors arise in the spinal cord itself and are composed of cells that make up the support structure of the cord, ependymal and glial cells. Metastatic lesions to the spinal cord are extremely rare.[67] Gliomas of the spinal cord occur less frequently than neurofibromas or meningiomas. Gliomas affect men more commonly than women.

CLINICAL HISTORY

Intraspinal tumors may demonstrate a wide variety of symptoms. Clinical symptoms associated with spinal cord disease may include a combination of pain, motor weakness, sensory changes, reflex alterations, and bladder incontinence.[224] Pain, which may be local, radicular, or causalgic, may develop in minutes, days, months, or years. Specific clinical disorders are associated with specific patterns of onset and location of pain. Acute local pain may be related to trauma, spinal hemorrhage, cord infarction, or disc herniation. Subacute pain may develop as a result of tumor growth or infection. Chronic pain may be related to syringomyelia or spondylosis.

Acute paralysis is a manifestation of acute trauma or cord infarction. Weakness occurring in a subacute period is frequently secondary to epidural tumor, epidural abscess, or transverse myelitis. Slowly progressive weakness is associated with multiple sclerosis, spondylosis, vitamin B_{12} deficiency, and amyotrophic lateral sclerosis. Muscle weakness may be associated with muscle atrophy and fasciculations affecting the hand muscles, whereas cervical myelopathy affects the anterior horn cells.[85]

13-5 INTRASPINAL MASSES

EXTRADURAL (50%–60%)

Metastases
- Lung
- Prostate
- Breast

Lymphoma
Chordoma
Meningioma
Fibroma
Lipoma/lipomatosis
Vascular malformation with bleeding
Abscess

INTRADURAL-EXTRAMEDULLARY (30%–35%)

Neurofibroma
Neurilemoma
Meningioma
Neurinoma
Lipoma
Arachnoid cyst
Leptomeningeal metastasis
Vascular abnormalities

INTRAMEDULLARY (10%–20%)

Glioma
- Ependymoma
- Astrocytoma

Arteriovenous malformation
Syringomyelia

Sensory symptoms may help define the spinal cord tracts affected by a disorder. Symptoms of tingling, buzzing, or a pins and needles sensation are a manifestation of dorsal column disease. Complaints of warmth, cold, or itching are more closely associated with lesions of the dorsal horn and spinothalamic tract, which mediates temperature sensation. Brown-Séquard syndrome is associated with loss of pinprick sensation on one side of the body and loss of position and vibratory sensation on the contralateral side.

Reflex changes are dependent on the time course and location of the lesions. Spinal shock secondary to severe trauma to the cord is associated with areflexia, atonia, and nonresponsiveness to plantar stimulation. More slowly progressive lesions may be associated with hyperreflexia. Hyperactivity of all lower and upper extremity reflexes with a normal jaw jerk is indicative of a high cervical spine lesion. Hyperactive lower extremity and finger reflexes with a normal biceps reflex suggest a lower cervical cord lesion.

Bladder incontinence is not an early symptom of spinal cord disease. Urinary incontinence is the hallmark of bladder involvement. Flaccid bladder paralysis is associated with overflow incontinence, whereas more slowly progressive abnormalities result in a spastic bladder with the features of frequency and urgency.

Patients with extradural metastatic disease have pain as their initial complaint. Pain may localize to the affected area in the spine or may radiate to the extremities if neural elements are compressed. The pain characteristically increases in intensity and is unrelenting. It is increased at night with recumbency because of lengthening of the spine. Pain during recumbency may occur with extradural or intradural-extramedullary lesions such as multiple myeloma, meningioma, or neurilemoma.[144] Activity may also exacerbate the discomfort. The pain is unresponsive to mild analgesics and requires narcotics for control. Not uncommonly, neurologic dysfunction rapidly follows axial pain. Neurologic symptoms include weakness, loss of sensation, and incontinence. The symptomatic course of a cervical spine extradural lesion may be precipitous if the spinal canal becomes blocked. Respiratory distress and diaphragmatic paralysis may occur with high cervical cord lesions.

Intradural-extramedullary tumors grow in proximity to nerve roots and are associated with radicular pain or axial skeletal pain. Meningiomas and neurofibromas are slow-growing tumors, and this slow growth corresponds to the slow evolution of symptoms in patients. Nocturnal symptoms are increased in these patients. Activity during the day may not be associated with symptoms. Neurologic symptoms are slower to develop than in patients with metastatic disease.

Symptoms may persist and increase to the degree of complaints associated with a herniated lumbar disc. The slow, insidious onset of pain, without intermittency, may be helpful in identifying these patients but is not of great enough specificity to distinguish patients with neurofibroma from those with disc disease.[221] It is also important to remember that these tumors affect the nerves that travel to the extremities. Patients may have dysesthesias in the buttock and lower part of the leg or in the shoulder and arm without back or neck pain, respectively. This pattern of symptoms may occur with generalized neurofibromatosis (von Recklinghausen's disease), solitary neurofibroma, or other intramedullary-extradural neoplasms (lipoma).[51,164]

Intramedullary tumors are frequently painless because of their location within the spinal cord proper, which disrupts the normal transmission of pain impulses. However, not all of these neoplasms are painless. Radicular or a girdle type of pain may develop in some patients as an early and persistent symptom. The onset may be insidious and the progression unrelenting. Not infrequently, weakness, spasticity, and sensory deficits below the level of the lesion develop. Conus medullaris tumors may cause stress incontinence as an early complaint associated with bladder dysfunction.[193] Some authors have described dysesthesias, or "electricity-like" sensations, in patients with intramedullary tumors.[11]

The pain associated with intraspinal tumors is different from that associated with mechanical disease of the spine. Patients with intraspinal tumors will often tell of sleeping sitting up in a chair because of a marked increase in the severity of pain when trying to sleep in a normal position. In contrast, in mechanical spinal disease, the sitting position increases pressure on the anatomic structures of the spine and therefore increases pain. The presence of this one aspect of the history should lead to a thorough evaluation for an intraspinal tumor.[55]

The motor and sensory features of compression are dependent on the extent and pattern of cord and nerve root distribution. Pure intramedullary tumors do not disturb nerve roots, but ependymomas may involve the lower sacral cord and involve the corresponding roots. Therefore, pain is common at the level of the lesion but is not radicular. Sensory and motor loss is routinely worse at the level of the lesion and less severe distally. This pattern is in contradistinction to that of a nerve root lesion or extramedullary tumor.[124] Corticospinal tract involvement with quadriparesis and spasticity is late in onset. Incontinence also occurs later in the course of the tumor. Blockage of cerebrospinal fluid occurs only when the tumor is extensive throughout the cord.

Extramedullary tumors between T11 and L2 compress the cord and roots. Lesions below the cord cause cauda equina symptoms. Distinguishing conus (S2–S5) lesions from tumors in the cauda equina is difficult.[90]

PHYSICAL EXAMINATION

Lumbar Spine

Examination of patients with extradural tumors may demonstrate pain on palpation with associated muscle spasm and limitation of motion. Neurologic findings correspond to the level and extent of compression of the spinal roots and cord. Patients with intradural-extramedullary tumors have slowly changing neurologic abnormalities, including gait disturbance, sensory changes, and urinary or rectal incontinence. They may also have lower extremity muscle atrophy. Patients with multiple neurofibromas may demonstrate spinal angulation, scoliosis, and/or kyphosis.[222] Those with von Recklinghausen's disease progress to paraplegia.[52] Patients with intramedullary tumors may have specific sensory changes that correlate with the location of these tumors in the center of the cord. Light touch and position sensation is normal, whereas pain and temperature sensation is lost. Hyperreflexia is a result of pressure on the pyramidal tracts. This finding helps differentiate patients with intramedullary tumors from those with a herniated disc, in whom hyperreflexia is a distinctly unusual finding.[133] Hyperreflexia may also be associated with spasticity.

Cervical Spine

Lesions at the level of the foramen magnum, upper cervical spine, and lower cervical spine are associated with different neurologic signs characteristic of compression of components of the spinal cord (Table 13-6).[52] Clinical findings may correspond to damage to the specific level of the spinal cord, or the effects may be proximal, secondary to descending fibers from cranial nerve V, or distal to that level, secondary to compromise of the vascular system supplying the cord, including the anterior spinal artery. In addition, extradural, intradural-extramedullary, and intramedullary tumors have distinct clinical signs that help the clinician determine the site of the tumor.

Examination of patients with extradural tumors may demonstrate pain on palpation of the neck with associated muscle spasm and limited motion. Neurologic findings correspond to the level and extent of compression of the cord and nerve roots. Patients with intradural-extramedullary tumors have slowly changing neurologic abnormalities, including arm weakness and sensory changes. They may also have upper extremity muscle atrophy. Patients with multiple neurofibromas may demonstrate spinal angulation, scoliosis, and kyphosis.[222] Patients with intramedullary tumors may have specific sensory changes that correlate with the location of these tumors in the center of the cord. Light touch and position sensation is normal, but pain and temperature sensation is lost. Hyperreflexia is a result of pressure on the pyramidal tracts and may also be associated with spasticity.

Other Organs

In addition to the neurologic examination, careful inspection of other organ systems may reveal abnormalities that will suggest possible diagnoses. Examination of the skin may reveal café au lait patches or axillary freckles associated with neurofibromatosis. The presence of a tuft of hair, a pigmented nevus, or a skin dimple suggests spina bifida or tumors such as lipoma, dermoid, or epidermoid cyst. Kyphosis may be related to wedge collapse of a vertebral body secondary to extension of an extradural tumor.

LABORATORY DATA

Abnormal laboratory values are most closely associated with extradural metastatic lesions. The location, degree of spread, and histologic type of the tumor will have an effect on the pattern of laboratory abnormalities. Intradural

13-6 CLINICAL SYMPTOMS AND SIGNS OF LESIONS AT DIFFERENT CERVICAL SPINAL CORD LEVELS

	Foramen Magnum	Upper Cervical Spine	Lower Cervical Spine
Pain	Occiput/neck	Neck/shoulder	Shoulder
Pain radiation	Shoulder/ipsilateral arm	Posterior scalp	Lower arm/hand
Sensory loss location	Face	Scalp	Arm/hand
Type	Decreased pin/temperature sensation Intact tactile sensation	Astereognosis	Paresthesias
Motor	Spastic weakness	Ipsilateral upper motor neuron	Ipsilateral arm/leg (extradural) Bilateral upper arm (intramedullary)
Reflex	Depressed arm/hand reflexes (decreased cord blood flow)	Increased or decreased	C5—biceps; C6—brachioradialis; C7—triceps; C8—Hoffman's syndrome
Other	Cranial nerves dysarthria, dysphonia, dysphagia	Diaphragmatic weakness	Horner's syndrome

tumors do not metastasize outside the spinal canal and are not associated with abnormal hematologic or chemical factors. Evaluation of cerebrospinal fluid obtained by lumbar puncture may demonstrate a marked elevation in spinal fluid protein in all these tumors. The fluid is usually obtained during myelographic study in a patient with suspected intraspinal tumor.

Pathology

Histologic findings depend on the cell of origin of the tumor. The most common primary tumor causing extradural metastases in women is carcinoma of the breast, whereas carcinoma of the lung is most common in men.[16,175,207]

Meningioma and neurofibroma are intradural tumors. Meningioma is an encapsulated, nodular soft tumor with a wide range of histologic patterns, including meningotheliomatous, fibroblastic, and psammomatous types.[125] The most common forms of cord meningiomas, in decreasing incidence, are psammomatous, angioblastic, fibrous, and anaplastic. The lumbosacral spine is a relatively infrequent location for these tumors when compared with the thoracic area.[55] Neurofibromas may appear as a fusiform swelling of a nerve root or as a pedunculated mass. Intraspinal neurofibromas may take on a dumbbell form with a central mass inside the vertebral canal connected by a shaft of tumor passing through the intervertebral foramen and forming a peripheral mass.[120] Histologic patterns of neurofibromas may vary but usually contain fibrous tissue in an interlacing configuration.

Intramedullary tumors are most frequently gliomas, including ependymoma and astrocytoma. Ependymomas arise from cells that line the central ventricular system of the spinal cord. Gliomas arise from glial cells, which are supporting cells for the nerve cells of the nervous system. Gliomas may be peripherally or centrally located in the spinal cord. Ependymomas and gliomas are associated with a variety of histologic forms. In adults, the forms most often encountered are ependymomas (60%), astrocytomas (20%), glioblastomas (7%), and oligodendrogliomas (4%).[55,94]

RADIOGRAPHIC EVALUATION

Radiographic evaluation of a patient with an intraspinal tumor can be very helpful in determining the exact location of tumor in the caudal-rostral orientation and its position in the extradural, intradural-extramedullary, or intramedullary space. Abnormalities noted on plain roentgenograms, CT scans, or MR images can pinpoint the location of lesions and help determine their potential source (Fig. 13-62).

Roentgenograms

Roentgenographic abnormalities on plain roentgenograms of extradural tumors are characterized by destruction of bone in proximity to the growing lesion. Malignant tumors are associated with rapid destruction of bone and loss of the posterior elements of the vertebral body or collapse of the vertebral body. On lateral roentgenograms, intraspinal lesions may be associated with posterior scalloping of the vertebral bodies, a consequence of their location and slow growth (Table 13-7).[136] Plain roentgenograms are insensitive to the presence of metastatic disease because at least 30% to 50% of bone must be destroyed before a lesion is identified.[68] In patients with identifiable lesions in the spine, cervical spine involvement occurs less frequently than involvement of other portions of the axial spine.[192] Neurofibromas may grow through intervertebral foramina, which results in uniform dilation of affected as opposed to adjacent foramina (Fig. 13-63). Intramedullary tumors rarely cause anatomic alterations that are discernible on plain roentgenogram. Changes on plain roentgenogram are seen in 10% or less of patients with spinal meningioma.[147]

Myelography

Myelographic studies are very useful in determining the exact location of an intraspinal tumor.[4,14,162] Extradural tumors frequently cause complete blockage of the myelographic dye at the point of spinal cord compression. The block has irregular edges and varying radiographic densities and displaces the spinal contents. In a study of patients with metastatic cancer of the spine, 15% of 130 patients had a complete block or a high-grade partial block on myelograms in the absence of bony abnormalities on plain roentgenograms.[81]

Myelographic features may be divided into the following four basic forms: (1) a lesion may be situated peripherally and displace the dura and cord, thereby resulting in widening of the space between the dye column and pedicle on the side with the tumor and narrowing contralaterally; (2) an anterior or posterior tumor may cause flattening of the cord—this finding may simulate that associated with intramedullary tumors; (3) a shallow filling defect without cord displacement may be seen; and (4) a lesion that encircles the cord may cause constriction of the subarachnoid space without cord displacement.

Intradural-extramedullary lesions produce a sharp, smooth, concave outline because the tumor is in direct contact with the dye. The spinal cord may be displaced to one side, and spinal nerve roots may be stretched over the lesion.

Intramedullary tumors arise in the spinal cord. The myelogram demonstrates fusiform enlargement of the spinal cord with tapering of the column of dye superiorly and inferiorly. Not all fusiform swellings of the cord are secondary to intramedullary tumors. Extradural tumors may flatten the contralateral aspect of the cord. Therefore, films must be taken at 90-degree angles so that intramedullary lesions are not confused with extradural lesions.

Computed Tomography

CT may be used after the placement of myelographic dye to better delineate the status of the spinal cord. CT/my-

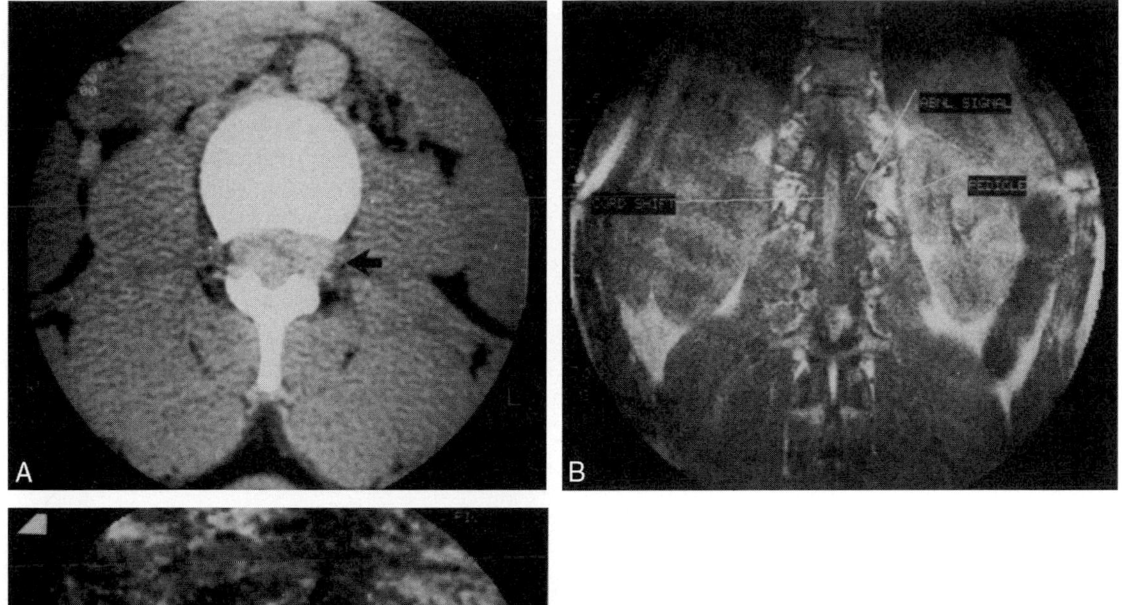

Figure 13-62 An 18-year-old man had three episodes of midback pain that radiated to the right and left sides of the groin. *A*, A CT scan suggested a mass increasing the size of the L1 neural foramen *(arrow)*. *B*, MR revealed abnormal signal from T12 to L2 on the left. *C*, An MR cross-sectional view demonstrated a mass pushing the spinal cord to the right. Hemilaminectomy of T12 to L2 revealed an intradural cyst filled with clear fluid extending from L2 to T11. Postoperatively, the patient had resolution of his pain.

elography is helpful in locating extension of tumor from the vertebrae and paravertebral structures to the epidural space.[217] For example, lesions in the superior pulmonary sulcus (Pancoast's tumors) may invade the brachial plexus and extend into the epidural space through an intervertebral foramen.[39,111,151] These lesions cause radicular pain in the setting of normal plain roentgenograms and bone scintigraphy. CT/myelographic evaluation of the spinal column detects these lesions missed by other radiographic techniques. CT techniques are useful for detecting alterations in bone architecture in individuals unable to undergo MR imaging studies (Fig. 13-64). CT technology has progressed to the development of three-dimensional imaging of the bony architecture of the spine.[231] The technique has been used in the lumbar spine for the detection of foraminal stenosis and determination of the status of postoperative fusions. In anticipation of stabilization surgery, the same technology may also be applied to the cervical spine to determine the extent of damage to structures from extradural tumors.

Magnetic Resonance

MR imaging has revolutionized the visualization of intraspinal lesions.[137] MR is the single best modality for imaging spinal tumors.[137] It is the best technique for distinguishing soft tissue densities (normal versus neoplastic) inside bony structures.[115] Extradural, intradural-extramedullary, and intramedullary tumors can be clearly depicted by MR imaging in multiple planes and can be distinguished from cerebrospinal fluid without the need for contrast media (Figs. 13-65 and 13-66).

The addition of gadolinium contrast to the technique of MR has helped increase the sensitivity of this method for the detection of intraspinal tumors. In one study of intraspinal tumors, gadolinium enhancement detected ependymomas (intense, homogeneous, sharply margined lesions), and astrocytomas (patchy, ill-defined lesions).[152] The difference in appearance of the two lesions was not adequate to allow MR to be useful in differentiating the histology of these intraspinal tumors. However, enhancement with gadolinium helps define the location, size, configuration, and character of the lesion.[197] Extramedullary-intradural tumors are also visualized better by gadolinium-enhanced MR. The mechanism of enhancement is not breakdown of the blood-brain barrier, but the highly vascular characteristics of tumors such as meningiomas and neurinomas. Gadolinium is helpful in detecting leptomeningeal spread of a metastatic tumor and in differentiating cystic lesions (syringomyelia) from intramedullary tumors that have similar radiographic

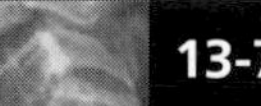

13-7 POSTERIOR VERTEBRAL SCALLOPING

INCREASED INTRASPINAL PRESSURE

Generalized: communicating hydrocephalus
Localized: syringomyelia, intraspinal cysts, intradural neoplasms

BONE RESORPTION

Acromegaly

CONGENITAL DISORDERS

Idiopathic
Neurofibromatosis
Marfan's syndrome
Ehlers-Danlos syndrome
Mucopolysaccharidosis IV (Morquio's disease)
Dysostosis multiplex (Hurler's syndrome)
Osteogenesis imperfecta

SMALL SPINAL CANAL

Achondroplasia

NORMAL VARIANT

Physiologic scalloping

Modified from Mitchell GE, Lourie H, Berne AS: The various causes of scalloped vertebrae with notes on their pathogenesis. Radiology 89:67–74, 1967.

characteristics on unenhanced MR. In patients with unexpected neurologic signs, contrast-enhanced MR may detect metastases to the pial membrane secondary to lymphoma, leukemia, adenocarcinoma of the lung, prostate carcinoma, malignant melanoma, and other tumors.[121] However, the changes in MR parameters have significant effects on the resulting images. For example, on T1-weighted images, gadolinium enhancement results in marrow metastases becoming isointense with normal bone marrow, thereby obscuring their presence. Consequently, discussion with neuroradiologists concerning the techniques used in obtaining the MR images is essential for determining the clinical significance of images.

DIFFERENTIAL DIAGNOSIS

The diagnosis of an intraspinal tumor is suggested by the presence of spinal pain that is persistent and increased by recumbency, by the presence of neurologic dysfunction, and by visualization of myelographic abnormalities. Definitive diagnosis requires histologic confirmation. A high level of suspicion is necessary to make this diagnosis. Patients with intradural tumor may have lower or upper extremity symptoms of long duration. This association must be kept in mind or the correct diagnosis may be missed.[164]

Extradural Lesions

The differential diagnosis of extradural tumors includes neoplastic and non-neoplastic lesions. Metastatic lesions from the lung, prostate, or breast are frequent causes of

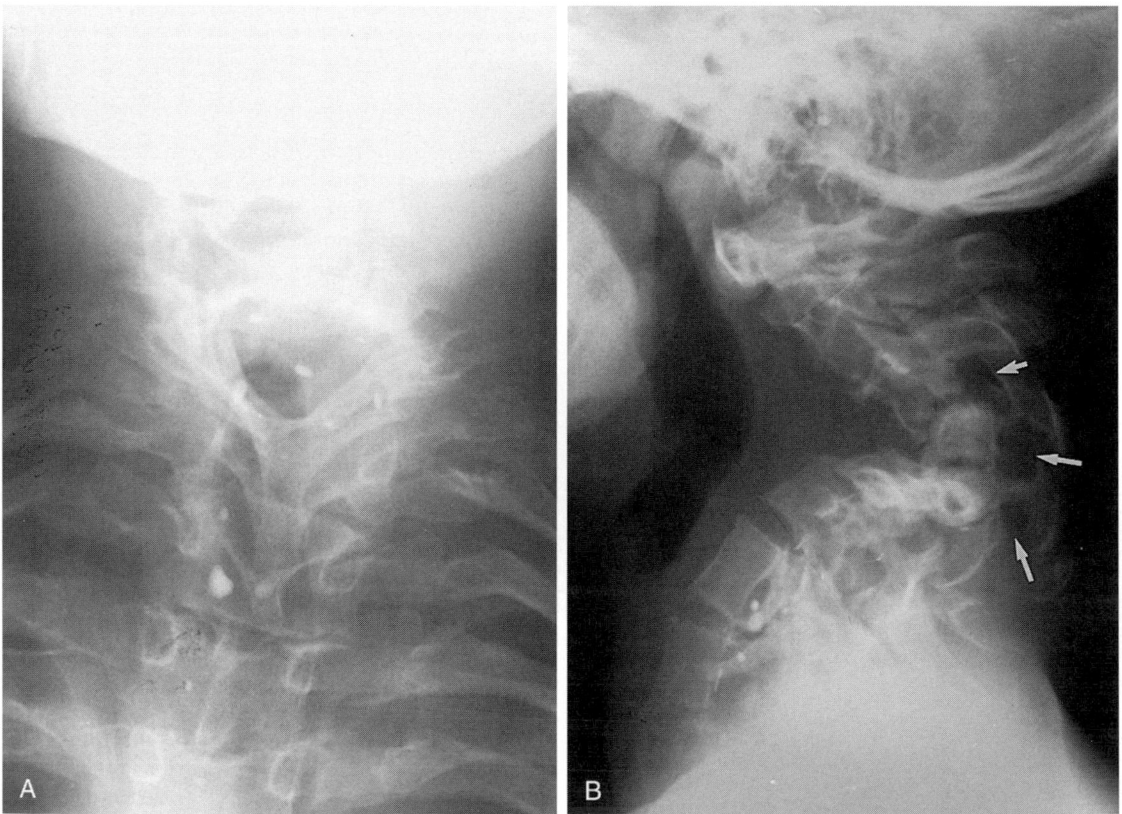

Figure 13-63 Neurofibromatosis. Anteroposterior, *A*, and lateral, *B*, views of the cervical spine revealed a marked scoliotic curve of the cervical spine with reversal of the normal lordotic curve. Expansion of the neural foramina corresponds to growth of the neurofibroma *(arrows)*. *(Courtesy of Anne Brower, MD.)*

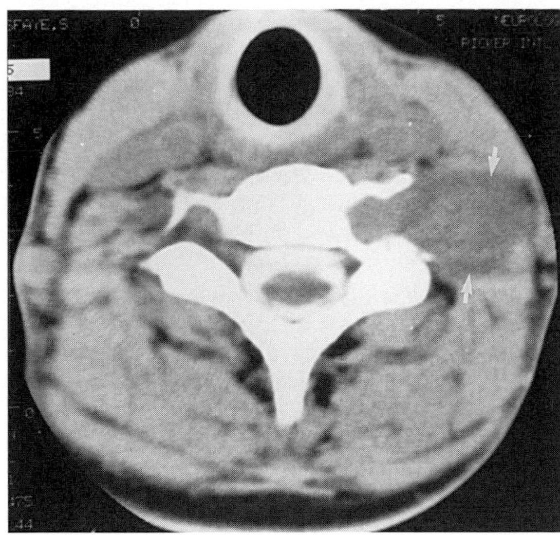

Figure 13-64 Neurofibromatosis. CT scan of the C6 vertebral body with a soft tissue mass growing from the neural foramen compatible with neurofibroma *(arrows)*. *(Courtesy of Thomas Dina, MD.)*

epidural lesions. Primary tumors—lymphoma, chordoma, meningioma, fibroma, or lipoma—may also cause epidural lesions. Fibrosarcoma is a rare extradural tumor of the cervical spine.[101,176] This tumor may need to be differentiated from benign lesions, such as giant cell tumor, and from malignant lesions, such as osteosarcoma.

Angiolipoma

Angiolipomas make up approximately 2.2% of extradural tumors of the spine.[92] They occur more commonly in the thoracic spine, with occasional lumbar involvement. Lumbar lesions cause radicular symptoms with leg weakness. MR evaluation of these lesions reveals a homogeneous mass on T1- and T2-weighted images with signal close to that of subcutaneous fat. Increased uptake of gadolinium contrast reveals the vascular nature of this benign tumor.[215] Angiolipoma is more common than lipoma and liposarcoma as a tumor of epidural fat. The tumor is amenable to surgical excision. Careful review of the CT scan and myelogram is helpful in differentiating herniated discs from metastatic tumors.[114]

Epidural Abscess

A potentially disastrous non-neoplastic epidural lesion associated with delayed diagnosis is epidural abscess. Patients with an epidural abscess in the lumbar spine may have acute-onset, severe back pain with progressive neurologic dysfunction that can evolve to complete paraplegia in 2 hours.[155] Similarly, patients with an epidural abscess in the cervical spine may have acute-onset, severe neck pain and progressive neurologic dysfunction that can evolve to quadriparesis within hours.[119] In a study of 43 spinal epidural abscesses, 7 (16%) were in the cervical spine and 14 (33%) were in the lumbar spine.[54] These patients, who are predominantly men, usually have evidence of a bacterial infection elsewhere, are acutely ill with fever and disoriented, and exhibit signs of a parameningeal infection on cerebrospinal fluid examination. On myelography, the extradural defect may extend over several vertebral levels.[13] MR has increased the opportunity to make the correct diagnosis of extradural abscess without the need for invasive procedures such as myelography (see Chapter 12).[54] MR evaluation of the cervical spine is able to determine the extent of the abscess and differentiate it from the spinal cord, vertebral bodies, intervertebral discs, and paraspinal soft tissues.[112] MR evaluation with contrast

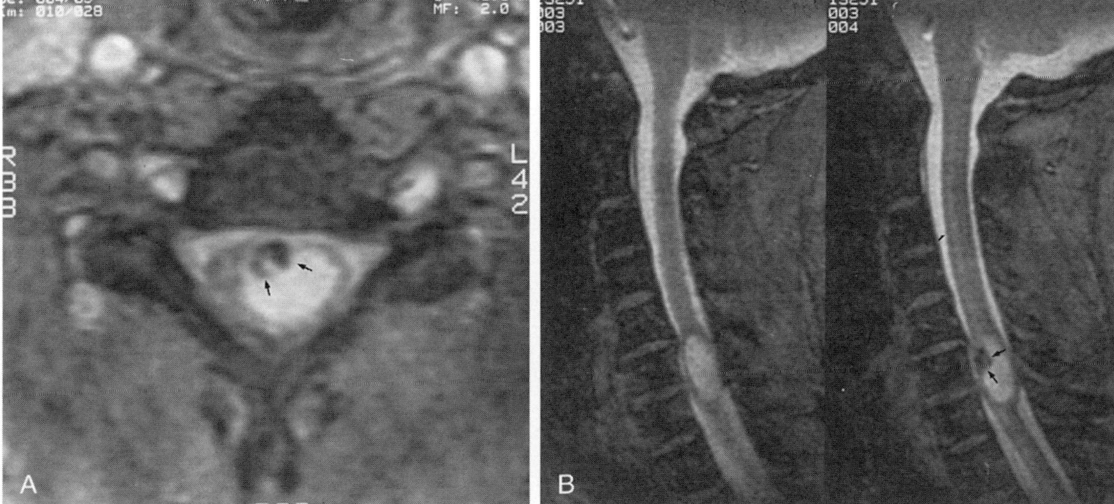

Figure 13-65 Intramedullary tumor. T1-weighted axial, *A*, and sagittal, *B*, MR images of the cervical spinal cord. A large intramedullary tumor (glioma) with a possible area of hemorrhage *(arrows)* is noted. *(Courtesy of Thomas Dina, MD.)*

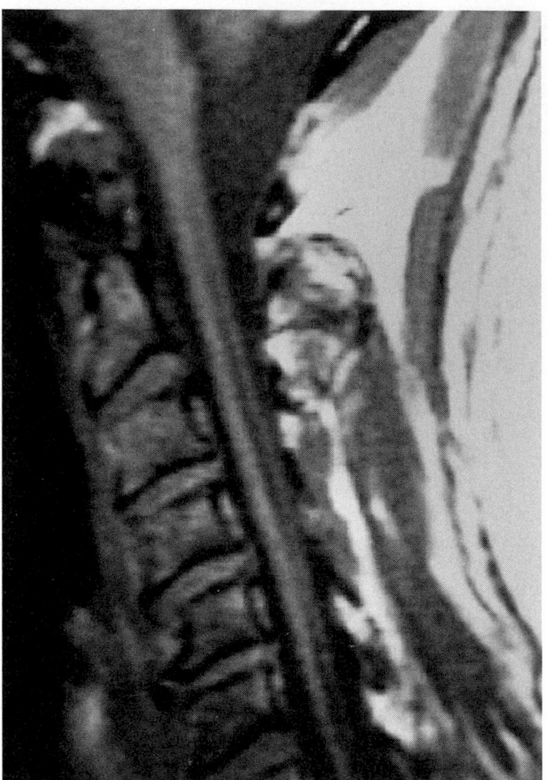

Figure 13-66 Syringomyelia. T1-weighted sagittal MR image of the cervical spine with an enlarged central cavity that is isodense with cerebrospinal fluid. *(Courtesy of Thomas Dina, MD.)*

enhancement remains the most effective test to determine the presence of epidural abscesses.[163]

Epidural Hematoma

A spontaneous epidural hematoma may mimic the time course and symptoms of an epidural abscess.[128] The bleeding may be associated with a small extradural vascular malformation or occur spontaneously without any specific anatomic abnormality. Most reported epidural hematomas are spontaneous and acute. The decreasing order of frequency of axial involvement is the cervical, thoracic, and lumbar spine.[118] Cervical epidural hematoma occurs more commonly in children and young adults.[5] Most hematomas extend two or more segments and are located in a posterolateral position.[89] Chronic epidural hematoma is rare but does occur in the cervical spine.[220]

In the lumbar spine, the spinal canal is larger than in the cervical and thoracic spine, and the cauda equina is better able to tolerate pressure than the spinal cord is. Patients with extradural cavernous hemangiomas and bleeding have had symptoms of sciatica secondary to nerve root compression in the lumbar spine,[96] as well as symptoms of neck pain and stiffness and radicular arm pain secondary to nerve root compression in the cervical spine.[1] Epidural hematomas have been associated with neurogenic claudication suggestive of lumbar spinal stenosis.[141] They have been reported as complications of invasive procedures, including surgery and myelography, and may occur in patients who are normotensive with normal blood coagulability (Fig. 13-67).[60,194] Bleeding may also occur in individuals taking anticoagulants.[209] A hematoma may be a complication of patients with a bleeding diathesis secondary to a connective tissue disease (Fig. 13-68). Hematoma may also be a complication of patients with axial arthritis, including ankylosing spondylitis.[97] Spontaneous epidural hematoma may complicate plasma cell myeloma.[199]

Most patients with spinal epidural hematoma have axial pain that may radiate in a radicular pattern.[129] The abnormalities in motor, sensory, and sphincter function correspond to the level of the spinal axis damaged. Dysfunction usually has an onset in minutes to hours. The diagnosis is corroborated by a mass with increased signal intensity on T1-weighted and decreased signal intensity on T2-weighted MR images.[50] Surgical intervention is required in the setting of neurologic dysfunction. Fresh frozen plasma and vitamin K may be given to patients to

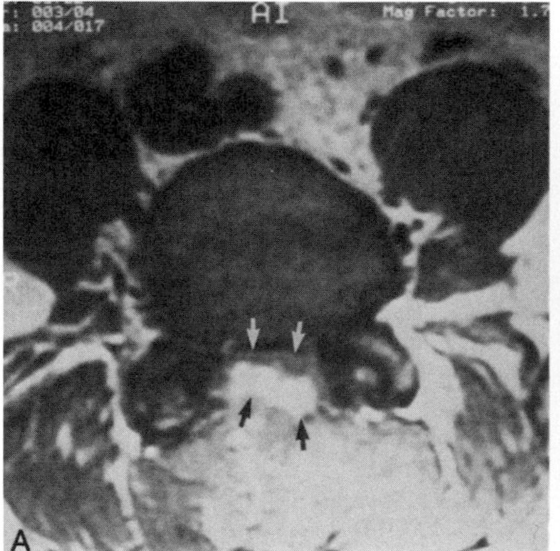

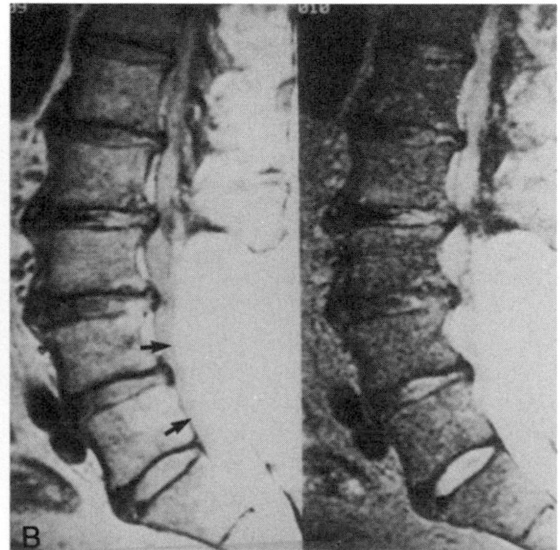

Figure 13-67 Postoperative axial *(A)* and sagittal *(B)* T1-weighted MR image demonstrating a collection of fluid *(black arrows)* with high signal intensity compressing the cauda equina *(white arrows)*. This collection was an epidural hematoma that required surgical evacuation. *(From Borenstein DG: Low back pain. In Klippel J, Dieppe P [eds]: Rheumatology. St. Louis, CV Mosby, 1994.)*

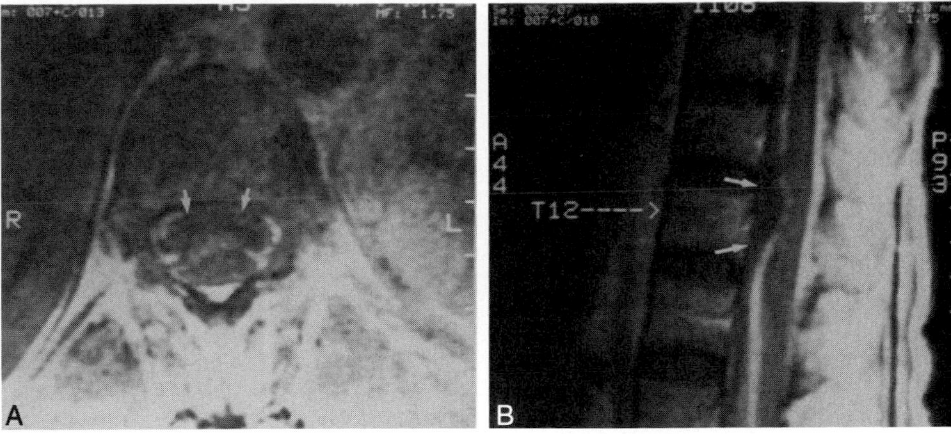

Figure 13-68 Axial *(A)* and sagittal *(B)* T1-weighted MR images of the T12 level demonstrating extradural and intradural fluid collections *(white arrows)* compressing the spinal cord. The signal in the subarachnoid space is compatible with blood. These lesions in this patient with systemic lupus erythematosus resulted in paraparesis. She subsequently expired from extension of the hematoma and overwhelming sepsis.

treat anticoagulation. Platelet transfusions may be tried in patients with thrombocytopenia. Prompt surgical decompression is required because the prognosis for neurologic recovery depends on the extent of damage and the duration of neurologic dysfunction. Patients with the best chance of recovery undergo surgical decompression rapidly and have incomplete sensorimotor deficits. Cervical and thoracic hematomas have a poorer prognosis than lumbar hematomas do.[129]

Epidural Lipomatosis

High-dose corticosteroid therapy may cause fat to accumulate in an epidural location. Epidural lipomatosis develops in patients who have renal transplants, asthma, rheumatoid arthritis, radiation pneumonitis, polyarteritis nodosa, Cushing's disease, and morbid obesity.[72] It has also been associated with protease inhibitor therapy for human immunodeficiency virus infection.[40] Corticosteroids in doses ranging from 5 to 180 mg/day have been associated with lipomatosis. Local corticosteroid epidural injection may also cause lipomatosis.[172] The onset of lipomatosis may occur in 6 months to 13 years after starting therapy. Cervical spine involvement is rare in comparison to disease located in the thoracic and lumbar areas.[171] Epidural lipomatosis can cause neurologic symptoms of lower extremity weakness and loss of sensation. Symptoms associated with epidural lipomatosis include back pain, radicular pain, loss of sensation, burning dysesthesia, and lower extremity weakness. Upper motor neuron signs (Babinski's sign, hyperreflexia) and lower motor neuron signs (hyporeflexia) have been reported, depending on the location of epidural compression of the spinal cord or cauda equina, respectively. Additional signs include weakness, decreased proprioception, decreased pain sensation, positive straight leg–raising test, and sphincter dysfunction. Transaxial CT reveals abundant soft tissue surrounding the thecal sac. T1-weighted MR reveals increased signal intensity in the lipid mass. Fat has almost a pathognomonic appearance on MR (increased T1-weighted signal and intermediate T2-weighted signal intensity). MR is an ideal technique to identify extradural fat.[160] Treatment of this condition may be surgical or medical. Surgical decompression is required for individuals with cauda equina symptoms.[122] Multilevel laminectomy may improve the symptoms and signs but is also associated with significant mortality in patients requiring high-dose steroid treatment.[72] However, with cessation of steroid therapy, the epidural fat deposits may disappear with resolution of the symptoms.[33]

Spinal Synovial Cyst

Intraspinal synovial cysts arise from the joint lining of the apophyseal joint and have been reported in the lumbar and, rarely, in the cervical spine.[42] The cysts occur most frequently at the L4–L5 level.[117] These lesions are associated with degenerative joint disease, trauma, and rheumatoid arthritis.[75,154] A cervical spine cyst may develop in individuals whose occupations entail considerable neck movement, including assembly line workers, dentists, and salespeople.[42] These extradural lesions may be asymptomatic or may cause radicular symptoms associated with sensory and motor dysfunction, including paraparesis.[158] Spinal synovial cysts may appear and cause symptoms in less than 1 year with a traumatic event or may evolve slowly throughout a number of years.[36,146,219] The CT appearance of lumbar intraspinal synovial cysts is characterized by a cystic mass with a broad base extending from the apophyseal joint. Hemorrhage into the cyst causes increased CT attenuation. Calcification of the cyst may occur in a chronic stage after hemorrhage.[146] The presence of an attachment between the apophyseal joint and the synovial cyst can be proved by injecting contrast material into the joint and noting its subsequent dispersal throughout the cyst.[24] MR evaluation of cysts is difficult because the contents of the cyst have a significant effect on varying signal intensities. Cysts with clear serous fluid show an isointense T1 and a hyperintense T2 pattern, whereas a cyst with more viscous contents shows a hyperintense signal pattern relative to cerebrospinal fluid on all pulse sequences.[226] MR imaging permits evaluation of synovial cysts at the C1–C2 level.[84] Cysts that cause nerve root compression or neurogenic claudication require surgical decompression.[42,98] Cysts may recede spontaneously and do not require surgery. Those filled with serosanguineous fluid can be aspirated by needle and may not recur.[102] Ganglion cysts arising from the ligamentum flavum in the cervical spine, independent of the neighboring apophyseal joint, have been described as causing myelopathic signs secondary to cervical spinal cord compression. These lesions also require surgical removal.[198]

Intradural-Extramedullary Lesions

Intradural-extramedullary lesions in adults are predominantly neurofibromas, neurilemomas (schwannomas), and meningiomas. Neurofibromas arise from proliferating nerve fibers, fibroblasts, and Schwann cells. A neurilemoma consists of Schwann cells and collagen fibers. Meningiomas arise from the meninges that support the spinal cord. The arachnoid may also be a source of lesions, as well as vessel abnormalities.

Neurofibroma

Neurofibromatosis type 1 (peripheral neurofibromatosis) is the most common hereditary syndrome predisposing to neoplasms; it occurs at a rate of 1 per 3000 live births in the United States.[189] Neurofibromatosis type 2 is associated with bilateral acoustic neuromas. These entities are genetically separate: type 1 is associated with a locus on chromosome 17 and type 2 with a deletion on the long arm of chromosome 22.[218] Neurofibromas, like neurilemomas, contain Schwann cells but can be differentiated by histologic examination because they have a more disorganized, plexiform appearance. Among 322 patients with nerve sheath tumors, the cervical spine was affected in 26% of cases, the thoracic spine in 41%, the lumbar spine in 31%, and the sacrum in 2%.[27,80,161] They may involve sensory or motor roots or the entire nerve. Neurofibromas may occur singly or multiply, as in Von Recklinghausen's disease. This autosomal dominant illness with variable penetrance may be easily recognized when the cutaneous manifestations (café au lait spots, axillary freckling, and cutaneous neurofibromas) are present. The disease may become evident when the patient is a child, or it may be recognized in an adult by the presence of kyphoscoliosis, vertebral scalloping, and intervertebral foramen widening.[213] Malignant deterioration of neurofibromas is noted in 3% of patients and is more likely to occur in those with multiple tumors as opposed to solitary lesions.[201]

Neurofibroma occurs in adults 30 to 60 years of age.[80] The primary symptom is pain that may be axial, radicular, or referred. Pain is exacerbated at night by recumbency, Valsalva's maneuver, or sneezing. Abnormalities, including loss of reflexes, motor function (muscle atrophy), and sensory function (loss of touch), are present at the time of diagnosis. Signs of spinal cord compression are asymmetric. Motor function is impaired on the side of the tumor, and pain and temperature loss are experienced on the opposite side. The motor loss is usually spastic, with involvement of the flexor muscles rather than the extensor muscles. The time from the onset of symptoms to diagnosis may average 1 to 4 years. The shortest period before diagnosis is associated with cervical lesions.[80]

Plain roentgenograms demonstrate widening of the intervertebral foramen, erosion of a pedicle, or widening of the interpedicular distance with tumors that extend into the extradural area. A normal roentgenogram is associated with a completely intradural tumor.[30] MR findings in patients with type 1 and type 2 neurofibromatosis include multiple masses in both extramedullary and intradural locations.[69] Skeletal abnormalities include dural ectasia and posterior scalloping. In a study of 47 neurofibromatosis patients, scoliosis occurred in 17% of cases.[61] The primary location for spinal deformation secondary to neurofibromatosis is the thoracic spine.[77] A rare abnormality is spondyloptosis with verticalization of the sacrum.[223] On occasion, tumors of the peripheral sciatic nerve must be differentiated from tumors in the central nervous system.[200] In patients with type 1 and type 2 neurofibromatosis, MR findings include multiple masses in both extramedullary and intradural locations.[69] Neurofibroma in the cervical vertebrae may be associated with abnormalities affecting the vertebral arteries.[177] Arterial disease may cause symptoms that may be attributed to neurofibroma. Angiographic evaluation identifies patients with both anomalies. Surgical removal of tumors is the preferred therapy if spinal cord or nerve root compression is present. The opportunity for tumor removal is diminished in the setting of multiple lesions. Neurofibromatosis may also be associated with malignant bone tumors, but rarely.[66] A minority of patients will have no spinal abnormalities.

Neurilemoma

Neurilemomas are common cord tumors that account for 30% to 35% of all primary intraspinal neoplasms; they occur most often in adults between 30 and 40 years of age. Neurilemoma is a solitary tumor consisting of Schwann cells and is more frequently found on sensory nerve roots than on motor roots.[90] Approximately 30% of these tumors occur in the lumbar area, 70% of which are in an intradural-extramedullary position. These tumors are considered benign and slow growing and cause symptoms by exerting pressure on adjacent structures.[55] In keeping with lesions exerting pressure on adjacent structures, neurilemoma is one of the extraosseous spinal lesions mimicking disc disease.[91] Patients with intraspinal tumors have painless neurologic deficits, pain with recumbency, pain disproportionate to that expected with disc disease, no improvement with disc surgery, and elevated spinal fluid protein. Neurilemoma is not limited to the spine but also may appear in the sacrum.[204] Lesions in the sacrum may become very large and cause minimal symptoms. MR of the lumbar spine is a noninvasive means of scanning the conus and cauda equina for the presence of these tumors. In the cervical spine, neurilemoma may also affect the cervical sympathetic plexus, brachial plexus, and spinal accessory nerve.[107] MR evaluation of the cervical spine identifies these tumors outside the spinal cord. This tumor is encapsulated and is amenable to surgical removal without loss of neurologic function.[107]

Meningioma

Meningioma is a benign, well-circumscribed tumor that represents about 25% of all primary intraspinal neoplasms.[34] This tumor affects adults older than 50 years, and approximately 80% of patients are women.[120] As opposed to neurofibroma, meningioma tends to remain intradural, with only 10% of meningiomas being extradural.[120] They are more common in the thoracic spine but occasionally occur at the lumbosacral level.[56] Only 2% occur in the lumbar spine.[90] In two studies of 705 and 97 spinal meningiomas, the cervical spine was the site of involvement in 17% of patients.[120,147] Meningioma differs from neurofibroma in that it occurs in adults 50 to 70 years of age, is commonly located in a lateral position, has a dumbbell shape only on occasion, calcifies more often, and produces sensory abnormalities more prominently than motor symptoms. Midline back pain is the most common early complaint with spinal meningiomas. The pain is axial or radicular in radiation. Sensory disturbances include paresthesias and numbness. Motor weakness in the form of hemiplegia has been reported in patients with meningiomas affecting the upper cervical spine near the craniocervical junction.[216] The average duration of symptoms before diagnosis is 2 years, but about 50% of patients come to surgery within a year of onset. Plain roentgenograms are not helpful in identifying the location of an intradural tumor, but its location may be identified if it contains calcium.[64,78] The ideal treatment is surgical excision of the tumor and its dural attachment. CT scan may be helpful if the location of the lesion has been identified by another radiographic technique. MR imaging with contrast is the most sensitive technique for identifying the location of the tumor.[196] Extensive tumors may be successfully removed with the appropriate surgical approach and technique.[174,180]

Intradural Lipoma

Intradural lipoma may occur in the presence or absence of a spinal malformation. The prevalence of spinal lipoma with spinal dysraphism is 90%. This type of lesion is found in pediatric patients with congenital abnormalities. In adults, spinal lipoma may be present without evidence of other structural abnormalities. However, about a third of intradural lesions in adults are associated with some malformation. Therefore, a distinction may not truly exist between the childhood and adult lesions. The cervicothoracic region is the most common location for adult lesions.[82] Without spina bifida, intraspinal lipoma is a rare tumor that rarely affects the conus medullaris.[14]

The duration of symptoms before diagnosis is usually measured in years. Numbness and ataxia rather than pain may be the initial symptoms.[82] In time, the symptoms of cord compression become more obvious. MR imaging is the best radiographic technique for identifying the location of an intradural lipoma.[113] Surgical excision of the lesion is the most effective therapy.[22,51]

Arachnoid Cyst

Cysts may arise from the arachnoid of the spinal cord. They are known by the terms *arachnoid cyst* or *diverticulum*.[3,44] These lesions occur in young adults, most commonly in the thoracic spine and occasionally in the lumbar or cervical area (Fig.13-69). Most cysts are asymptomatic. Patients may have fluctuating pain in the appendages made worse with activity. Pain is relieved with recumbency. Lesions may also cause sphincter malfunction, scoliosis, and paraparesis.[212] The presence of posterior scalloping of a vertebral body helps raise the possibility of this lesion in a patient with neurologic symptoms. Perineural cysts in the sacral region (Tarlov cysts) are associated with perineal pain.[139] Atypical sciatic pain radiating to the groin may be present without difficulty in voiding.[140] Neurologic examination may reveal decreased sensation in the perineal area, or it may be normal. MR of these patients is superior to CT with myelography in identifying the presence of sacral perineural cysts. In a study of 17 patients with perineal pain and no urologic, gynecologic, or anorectal abnormalities, MR detected sacral cysts in 13 (76%) patients.[206] Surgical removal of the cyst is associated with resolution of perineal pain in a majority of patients with Tarlov cysts.[44]

Arachnoiditis

Arachnoiditis is a nonspecific inflammatory process causing fibrosis of the arachnoid membrane. The pathogenesis of arachnoiditis involves the development of a mild, inflammatory cellular exudate similar to the inflammatory response necessary to repair serous membranes such as the peritoneum.[58] A fibrous exudate covers the nerve roots and causes them to adhere to one another and the thecal sac. Proliferating fibrocytes form dense collagenous adhesions around the roots. Arachnoiditis evolves from a stage of inflammation of the pia-arachnoid with hyperemia and swelling of the nerve roots, followed by arachnoiditis and fibroblast proliferation and adhesion. The final stage of arachnoiditis causes complete encapsulation of the structure with hypoxia and atrophy of the nerve root.[32]

Causes of arachnoiditis are listed in Table 13-8.[26,159,183] A frequently implicated agent in the development of arachnoiditis is the oily contrast agent iophendylate when it is not removed from the spinal canal after myelography. However, in a study of 98 patients who underwent iophendylate ventriculography, arachnoiditis did not develop in a remote location in the lumbar spine despite a follow-up period of up to 28 years.[100] Oily contrast agents have been replaced with water-soluble contrast agents not associated with the development of arachnoiditis. Other exogenous causes of arachnoiditis include infection (tuberculosis),[76] intrathecal medications, and anesthetic agents such as bupivacaine.[181,188] Arachnoiditis may be the cause of unsuccessful back surgery in more than 11% of individuals.[21,31,37] Retained swab debris may be the source of the inflammatory response.[99]

The clinical symptoms associated with arachnoiditis include diffuse constant neck or back pain, radicular pain, paresthesias, dysesthesias, causalgia, motor weakness, and sphincter dysfunction. Physical signs include spinal tenderness, muscular spasm, atrophy, scoliosis, limited straight leg–raising, hyporeflexia in the upper extremities, hyperreflexia in the lower extremities, and urinary sphincter dysfunction.

Inflammatory changes of the arachnoid space (arachnoiditis) may cause changes on myelography that should not be confused with an arachnoid cyst. Cysts cause localized lesions. Arachnoiditis causes loculations of contrast dye, partial or complete obstruction of dye flow, and obliteration of nerve root sleeves (Fig. 13-70).

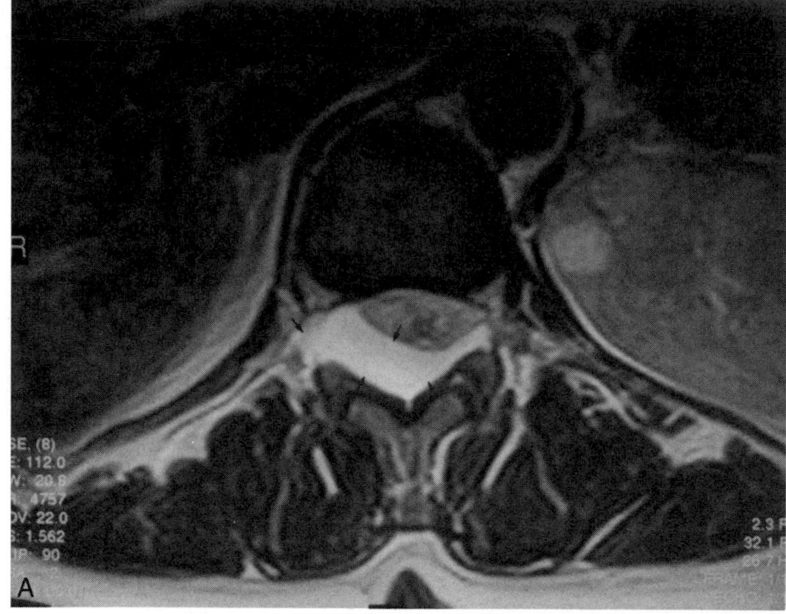
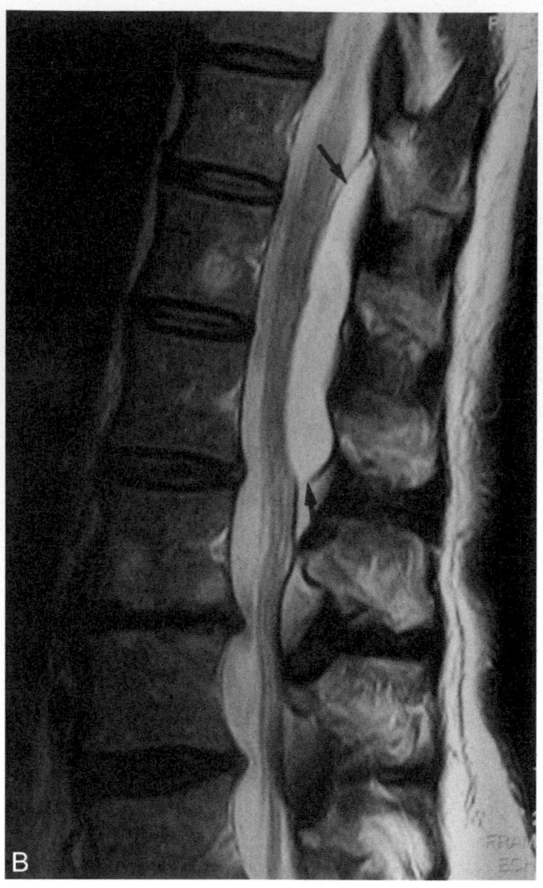

Figure 13-69 Extradural arachnoid cyst in a 60-year-old woman with chronic right hip pain. Axial *(A)* and sagittal *(B)* T2-weighted MR images of the thoracic spine demonstrated a posterior arachnoid cyst *(black arrows)* and impingement of the T12 and L1 roots in the T12/L1 and L1/L2 foramina on the right posterior canal.

MR is the best radiographic technique to evaluate arachnoiditis. The three MR patterns of arachnoiditis are conglomerations of adherent nerve roots residing centrally within the thecal sac, nerve roots adherent to the meninges, and a soft tissue mass replacing the subarachnoid space (Fig. 13-71).[106,170] In the upper spinal cord, arachnoiditis may be visualized as thickening of the leptomeninges. If the cord is involved in the inflammation, it lies eccentrically within the canal.[169] Arachnoiditis that fills the subarachnoid space may have MR characteristics that mirror those of a spinal cord tumor.[210] Gadolinium-enhanced MR does not increase the signal intensity of arachnoiditis, and the absence of enhancement helps differentiate neoplastic lesions from arachnoiditis.[106]

13-8 CAUSES OF ARACHNOIDITIS

- Surgery
  - Extradural
    - Discectomy
    - Laminectomy
    - Lumbar spine fusion
  - Intradural
    - Closure of spinal fistula
    - Nerve root severed
- Injected agents
  - Contrast media
  - Anesthetic agents
  - Intradural steroids
- Space-occupying lesion
  - Neurofibroma
- Infection
- Intrathecal hemorrhage

The disability associated with arachnoiditis is severe pain. The physical impairments change relatively little during the course of the illness. Urinary symptoms characterized by urgency, frequency, and incontinence develop late in the course of the illness. These patients have a poor prognosis because no therapy has been developed that consistently decreases inflammation or diminishes their symptoms.

Another disorder associated with thickening of the dura is pachymeningitis hypertrophica.[168] This disorder may affect the dura in the cervical spinal cord. The natural history is one of progression from local pain to radiculopathy and spinal cord compression. Surgical removal of the thickened dura is associated with resolution of neurologic symptoms. The response to surgical therapy is in clear distinction to the lack of improvement with surgery for arachnoiditis.

Arteriovenous Malformation

Arteriovenous malformations (AVMs) may be located in any part of the spinal column. Lesions may be arterial, cap-

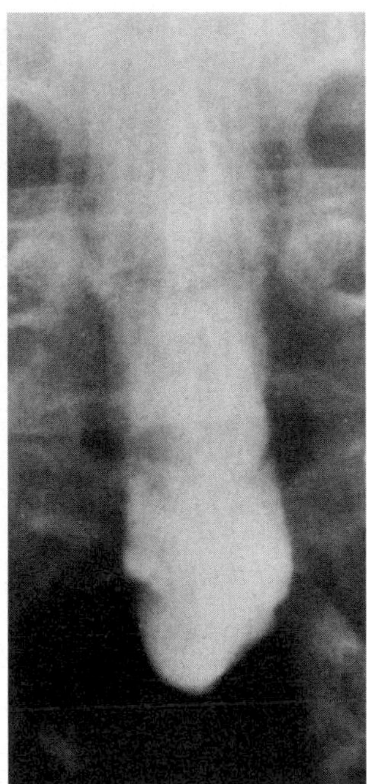

Figure 13-70 Arachnoiditis in patient who had undergone multiple back operations. Metrizamide was used, but because of scar tissue, it looks as though Pantopaque was used previously. *(From Wiesel SW, Bernini P, Rothman RH: The Aging Lumbar Spine. Philadelphia, WB Saunders, 1982.)*

illary, cavernous, or arteriovenous (Table 13-9). Vascular malformations and neoplasms account for 5% to 10% of space-occupying lesions of the spine.[34] Malformations are more common than tumors. Vascular lesions affect the thoracic spinal cord more commonly than the other portions, with about 20% of AVMs being located in the cervical segments.[5] Increased pressure in vessels causes structural alterations that result in vessel enlargement. Dysfunction of the spinal cord may occur secondary to

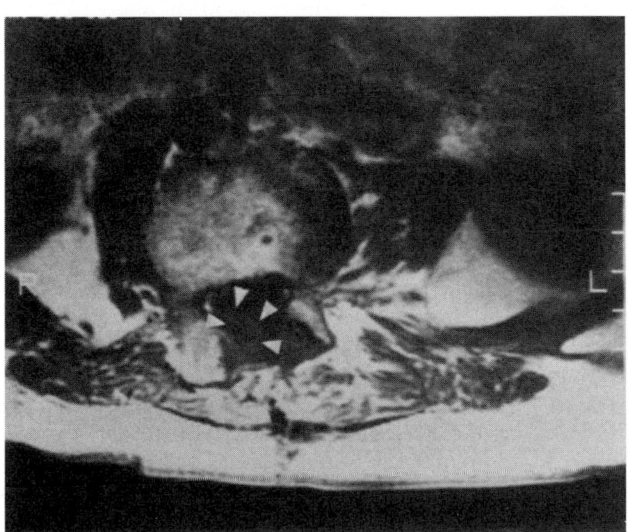

Figure 13-71 An 80-year-old woman had persistent burning leg pain after multiple surgical lumbar spine procedures. A T1-weighted axial MR view revealed a clumped mass of nerve roots *(white arrows)* in the dural sac characteristic of arachnoiditis.

13-9 SPINAL CORD VASCULAR TUMORS AND MALFORMATIONS

Vascular tumors
  Capillary hemangioblastoma
Vascular tumors of the meninges
  Hemangioblastoma
  Hemangiopericytoma
Vascular malformations
  Capillary telangiectasia
  Cavernous angioma
  Arteriovenous malformation
    Dural
    Intradural
  Venous malformation

Modified from Byrne TN, Waxman SG: Spinal Cord Compression: Diagnosis and Principles of Management. Philadelphia, FA Davis, 1990, pp 1–278.

impingement by the vessel mass, or impairment of normal venous drainage may occur as a result of abnormally high pressure in spinal cord capillaries. The majority of adults with AVMs are older than 30 years and are men.[166]

The clinical course is one of progressive symptoms of spine and radicular pain, dysesthesias, and painful claudication. Episodes of vessel thrombosis may accentuate the symptoms and signs. The course of symptoms in these patients may be hours to weeks. The symptom of exercise claudication with gradual onset of neurologic symptoms, including quadriparesis, helps distinguish vascular abnormalities from other tumors.[127] A cavernous angioma of the cauda equina may be manifested as subarachnoid hemorrhage.[205] Low back pain and sciatica may also be associated with a cavernoma of the cauda equina.[150] In addition, patients with cervical AVM and other vascular tumors are at risk for subarachnoid hemorrhage.[6] Some of these vascular lesions causing hemorrhage may be extramedullary or intramedullary.[1,23,41] Cervical subarachnoid bleeding may be difficult to differentiate from intracranial bleeding. Patients may have photophobia, change in mentation, and meningismus, as well as signs of cord compression. Physical examination of patients with bleeding should include inspection for cutaneous angioma and auscultation over the spine for bruits associated with vascular malformations.[189]

Electrophysiologic signs associated with AVM of the spinal cord include scattered, multiple bilateral thoracolumbosacral radiculopathies consistent with axonal or neuronal destruction, paraspinal fibrillations, and abnormal activation of motor unit potentials. The presence of these abnormalities depends on the caudal extension of the AVM, its arterial supply, and the duration of symptoms.[9]

Vascular lesions, including feeding vessels, draining veins, and a vascular nidus, are best localized by spinal angiography.[43,63] AVM may not always be visualized by MR.[167] However, MR is a useful technique for the study of AVMs because it is able to detect myelomalacia, edema, and reversible scalloping of the spinal cord; thrombosis and thickening of blood vessels; new bleeding versus old hematoma; and alterations associated with angiographic or surgical correction of the lesion.[20,104,135] Cerebrospinal fluid evaluation may demonstrate an elevated protein level and red blood cell count in the setting of recent bleeding.

Normal cerebrospinal fluid does not eliminate the possibility of AVM. Indications for therapy are prevention of recurrent bleeding and progressive neurologic dysfunction. Asymptomatic lesions are left undisturbed. Therapy for AVMs and vascular tumors includes the use of embolization, alone or preoperatively.[83,145] Embolization or surgery may decrease the risk of bleeding, but at the risk of increased neurologic dysfunction.

Vascular malformations may also be identified in an intramedullary location. These intramedullary vascular lesions are located in the cervical and thoracic spine. Lesions in the cervical spine are associated with arm and leg dysfunction, whereas thoracic cord lesions are associated with lower extremity motor or sensory abnormalities.[74,148] Once identified, these lesions may be left alone, embolized, or surgically treated.[123] Clinical improvement is common in patients who have had operative resection or angiographic ablation.[126,131] Patients with neurogenic claudication may undergo surgery for suspected spinal stenosis but may have an AVM as the cause of their symptoms. Relief of venous hypertension in both conditions may be one of the mechanisms by which surgical or angiographic intervention improves the symptoms of neurogenic claudication.[127]

Leptomeningeal Metastases

Leptomeningeal spread of tumor is relatively rare because the dura is a barrier to the spread of malignant tumors. In adults, this form of metastasis occurs with lymphoma, lung or oat cell carcinoma, leukemia, and breast cancer.[214] In one study, 5% of patients with breast cancer had leptomeningeal involvement.[225] Lung carcinoma is the second most common primary tumor causing leptomeningeal disease, followed by melanoma.[214] Patients may also have concomitant intraparenchymal brain metastases or epidural lesions. Leptomeningeal metastasis develops in patients with widespread metastatic disease, and it is occasionally the cause of the initial symptoms of back pain in an individual patient.

The clinical hallmark of this lesion is the multifocal nature of the neurologic deficits. The symptom of neck or back pain, as part of the list of multiple abnormalities, occurs in 25% of patients with widespread leptomeningeal disease.[214] Findings may include extremity weakness, paresthesias, back or radicular pain, causalgia, sphincter dysfunction, or all the symptoms of cauda equina compression. On physical examination, patients have focal weakness, asymmetric reflexes, and spotty sensory loss. The diagnosis is confirmed by cytologic examination of cerebrospinal fluid.[138] A variety of biochemical markers may be obtained from cerebrospinal fluid to better determine the source of cancerous cells and the response to therapy.[34] MR scan, with or without contrast enhancement, is able to identify leptomeningeal metastases in a minority of patients (Fig. 13-72).[229] Patients may be treated with irradiation or intrathecal therapy.[48] The prognosis is usually poor, and median survival of patients with leptomeningeal tumors is 4 to 6 months.[25]

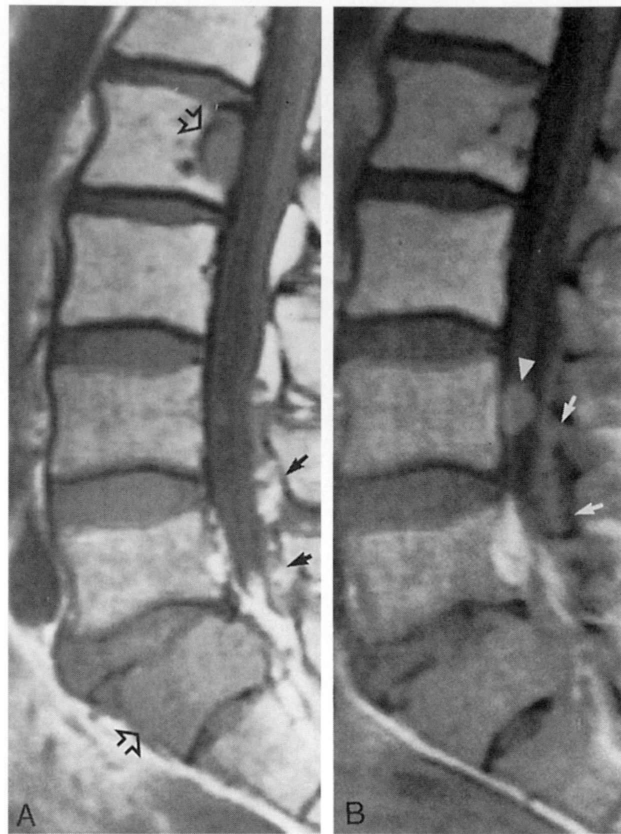

Figure 13-72 Intradural metastasis visualized by spin echo MR imaging with and without gadolinium enhancement. In this 72-year-old woman with metastatic breast carcinoma, precontrast, *A*, and postcontrast, *B*, sagittal T1-weighted (TR/TE 400/20) spin echo MR images are shown. The linear streak of enhancement agent along the dorsal surface of the spinal cord *(arrows)* represents the site of pial metastasis. *(From Lim V, Sobel DF, Zyroff J: Spinal cord pial metastases: MR imaging with gadopentetate dimeglumine. AJNR Am J Neuroradiol 11:975-982, 1990.)*

Intramedullary Lesions

Intramedullary lesions are primarily gliomas, vascular malformations, syringomyelia, lipoma, lymphoma, and melanoma. Other lesions that may cause intramedullary cord lesions include multiple sclerosis, sarcoidosis, abscess, myelitis, radiation exposure, nutritional deficiency, cord infarction, and vasculitis. These lesions may cause neurologic dysfunction without pain.

Syringomyelia

Syringomyelia is a fluid-filled cyst lined with benign glial cells that is located in the central portion of the spinal cord. Syringomyelia may be classified into communicating and noncommunicating types (Table 13-10). Communicating types are associated with obstructive lesions at the foramen magnum that result in alterations in cerebrospinal fluid flow. These cysts are attached to the central canal and lined with glial cells. Noncommunicating types are a consequence of lesions of the spinal cord. For example, arachnoiditis may cause syrinx formation by obliterating the spinal vasculature supplying the center of the cord, thereby causing ischemia. These cysts are lined with cells associated with the pathologic process that caused the lesion (tumor cells). Syringomyelia is associated with congenital abnormalities (Arnold-Chiari malformations, or cerebellar tissue extending through the foramen magnum, and downward

13-10 CLASSIFICATION OF SYRINGOMYELIA

COMMUNICATING (SYRINGOHYDROMYELIA)

Associated with developmental abnormalities of the cranial-cervical junction and posterior fossa (e.g., Arnold-Chiari malformation)
Associated with acquired obstructive lesions of the foramen magnum (basilar meningitis)

NONCOMMUNICATING

Traumatic myelopathy
Spinal arachnoiditis
Spinal cord tumors
Idiopathic

Modified from Byrne TN, Waxman SG: Spinal Cord Compression: Diagnosis and Principles of Management. Philadelphia, FA Davis, 1990, pp 1–278.

displacement of the medulla), trauma, infections (meningitis), or inflammatory abnormalities (arachnoiditis).[19,37]

This lesion is found most commonly in the cervical spine and only occasionally in the lumbar spine.[132] The cyst often extends from below the first cervical segment to the thoracic spinal cord. Cysts frequently span seven or more cord levels.[186] The cavity is located within the gray matter of the cord, posterior to the central canal. The cyst contains fluid with the composition of cerebrospinal fluid but may not always be connected to the central canal. The lesion most commonly occurs in men 25 to 40 years of age.

Syringomyelia, by its growth laterally and longitudinally through the spinal cord, first causes loss of pain sensation, then abnormalities in motor function, with weakness in the extremities and scoliosis in the axial skeleton, long tract signs (Babinski's reflex), and autonomic dysfunction of the bladder and rectum. The sensory loss is bilateral, over the shoulders secondary to the loss of decussating pain and temperature fibers, with preservation of posterior column fibers. The onset or exacerbation of symptoms may be marked by minor trauma, a sneeze, or a cough. Pain in the neck is a symptom in 24% of patients.[19] If pain is exacerbated by the Valsalva maneuver or minor strain, the cyst may be associated with a compressive lesion such as an Arnold-Chiari malformation.[230] This lesion may result in brain stem and cerebellar signs. Muscle weakness is associated with atrophy and loss of reflexes. Neuropathic joint disease, particularly in the shoulder, is a recognized complication of a cervical syringomyelia.[187] Lesions of the cervicothoracic junction affect the intermediolateral column and result in Horner's syndrome.

Plain roentgenograms of the cervical spine may demonstrate a variety of abnormalities associated with congenital lesions and syringomyelia, including canal widening, basilar impression, atlantoaxial dislocation, and occipitalization of the atlas.[191] In the past, the diagnosis was made by myelography or CT.[10] MR has become the technique of choice to localize syringomyelias.[227] MR is able to differentiate intramedullary neoplasms from cysts (Fig. 13-73).[184]

Treatment of syringomyelia is guided by progression of the symptoms and signs associated with the lesion. Approximately 22% of patients may have no progression of symptoms over a 20-year period.[34] Patients with progressive symptoms require therapy that includes surgical removal of the fluid in the cystic cavity by needle aspiration or myelotomy.[79] Surgical therapy for syringomyelia must be approached with consideration of the pathogenesis of the specific lesion. Different shunting procedures are required, depending on the location of the lesion.[134] Without effective therapeutic intervention to halt the progressive growth of the lesion, patients with syringomyelia experience marked disability consisting of spastic paraplegia, arthropathy, and infectious complications. Syringomyelia may develop years after surgical removal of lesions from the spinal cord.[53]

Spinal Cord Neoplasms

Intramedullary tumors, mostly ependymoma and astrocytoma, grow slowly and insidiously in adults with few symptoms for many years.[179] In adults, ependymomas account for the majority of intramedullary tumors, nearly 65% of the lesions.[90] More than 50% of intraspinal ependymomas arise from the filum terminale, with the lumbar spine being the next most commonly affected structure (Fig. 13-74). Astrocytomas cause 20% to 25% of primary intraspinal neoplasms but affect the lumbar spine only 20% of the time. The cervical spinal cord is involved in 33% of patients with astrocytoma,[90] and it is the location of ependymoma in 20% of patients.[73] Men are affected more frequently than women, 63% and 57%, respectively.[15] Glioblastoma and oligodendroglioma occur much less frequently.

Ependymoma is the most common primary tumor in the region of the conus and cauda equina. The tumor originates from the ependymal lining of the central canal or filum terminale and has very little capacity to invade the spinal cord. The tumor frequently grows posteriorly and separates the proprioceptive columns. Tumors around the conus and cauda equina are of the myxopapillary variety.[90] Myxopapillary ependymomas may cause slow-growing tumors in the sacrococcygeal region as well.[65] Benign astrocytomas are slow-growing tumors associated with slowly progressive clinical symptoms. Astrocytomas cause enlargement of the cord, are relatively avascular, and may not have an identifiable plane of separation from the cord.

The symptomatology of ependymoma and astrocytoma is similar. Clinical symptoms associated with ependymomas may include local, radicular, or funicular (ascending spinal tract involvement) pain. Spinal pain is a symptom in a minority of patients. Patients may or may not have spinal pain with a sensory deficit to pinprick as their initial neurologic abnormality. The symptoms are of gradual onset and progress slowly, and the average duration of symptoms before diagnosis is 3 years. Sudden bleeding into the tumor causes the onset of acute sciatic pain (Fincher's syndrome).[185] Astrocytoma occurs more frequently than ependymoma in the medullary portion of the spinal cord. Astrocytoma most commonly affects men 34 to 40 years of age. Clinical symptoms and signs are similar to those of cervical ependymoma. When the lesion is in the cervical spine, upper extremity atrophy may be associated with lower extremity spasticity. Cerebrospinal fluid evaluation of both types of tumors demonstrates an elevated protein concentration with a minimal increase in cerebrospinal leukocytes.

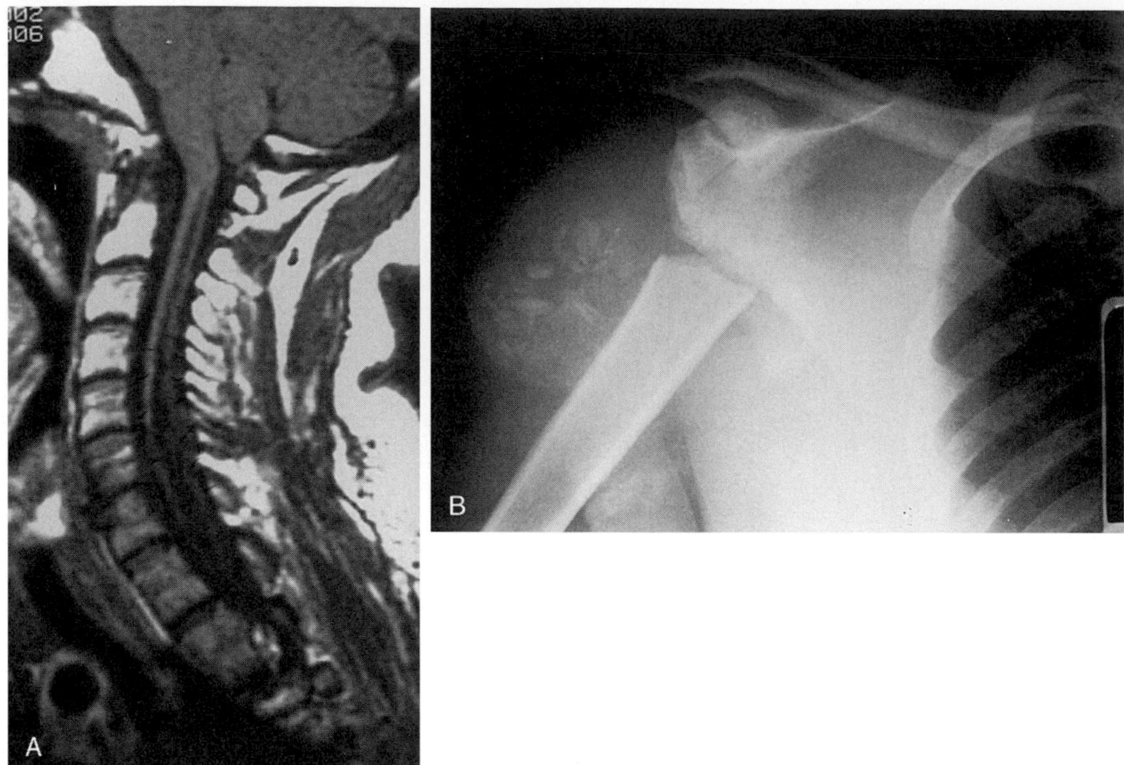

Figure 13-73 Syringomyelia. A neuropathic shoulder joint developed in a 52-year-old woman over a 6-week period. *A*, A T1-weighted sagittal MR image of the cervical spinal cord shows an isodense area in the central cord extending from the level of C1 to the thoracic spine. *B*, An anteroposterior view of the right shoulder shows disorganization, destruction, and decidua characteristic of a neuropathic joint. *(Courtesy of Anne Brower, MD.)*

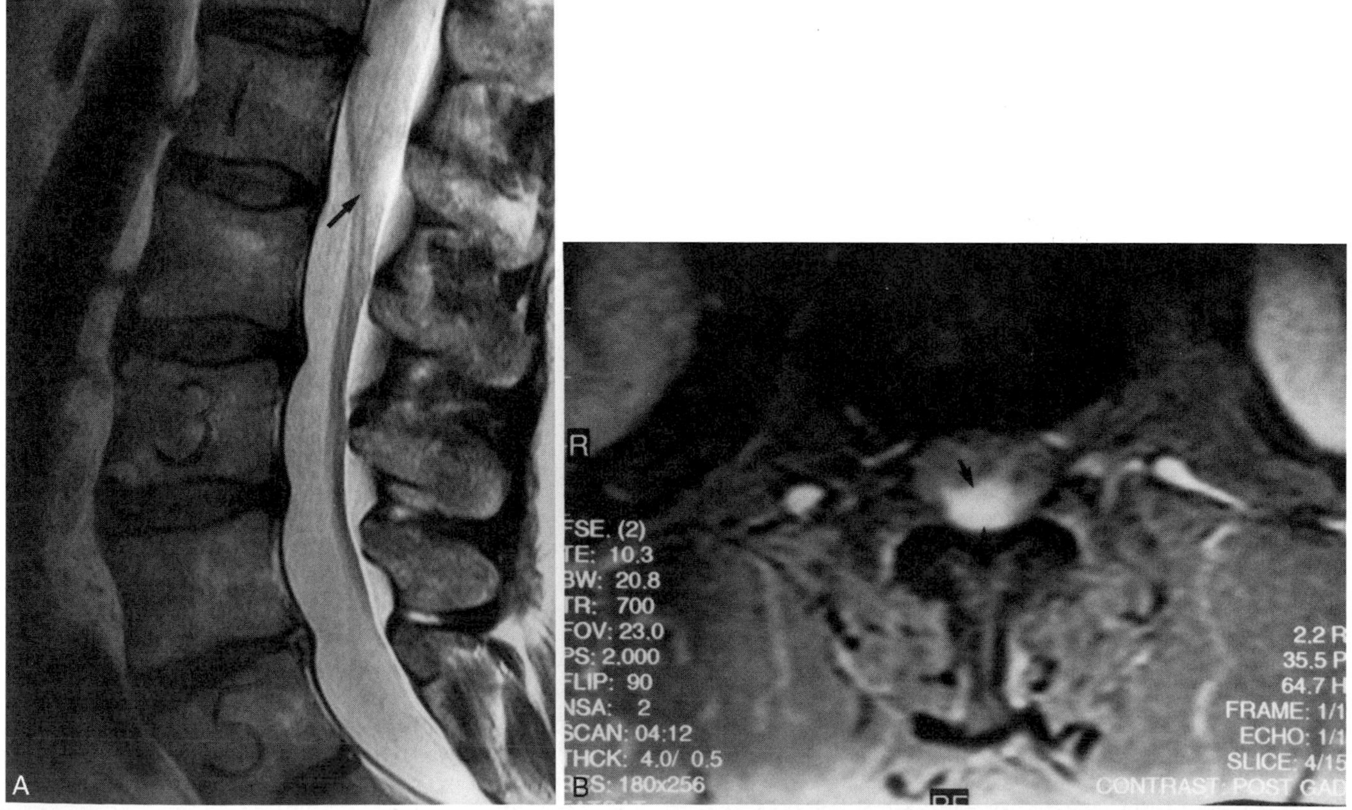

Figure 13-74 Filum terminale tumor. A 64-year-old man was evaluated for lower extremity dysesthesias. A sagittal MR image *(A)* demonstrates an intradural tumor compressing the distal tip of the conus and cauda equina compatible with an ependymoma of the filum termilae *(black arrows)*. An axial view *(B)* with gadolinium demonstrates partial enhancement of a cystic mass. Surgical removal of the ependymoma resulted in resolution of his symptoms without any recurrence as of 2/03.

Radiographic evaluation with myelography demonstrates a fusiform expansion of the spinal cord. Ependymomas of the filum may cause marked deformity of vertebral bodies without producing symptoms.[55] Some conus intramedullary ependymomas have an exophytic extramedullary component extending into the lumbosacral canal. Contrast-enhanced MR is particularly effective in identifying the presence of intramedullary tumors, including those in the cauda equina. In one study of 32 spinal tumors, 30 neoplasms were enhanced. Ependymomas and astrocytomas were located with enhanced MR.[152] Enhanced MR has advantages over other radiographic techniques in differentiating a solid tumor component from syrinx and from cysts. MR imaging is also able to detect hemorrhage within tumor masses.[142] Moreover, recurrent or residual tumor can be differentiated from scar tissue in postoperative patients. The diagnosis of lesions in the spinal cord requires biopsy of the lesion. MR imaging is unable to differentiate neoplastic from benign lesions in all cases.[28]

Treatment of these neoplasms is microsurgical removal of accessible lesions. Resection is completed to the extent consistent with preservation of neurologic function. Ependymomas are more readily removed in their entirety than astrocytomas are.[89] Postoperative irradiation is helpful in patients who have not had complete resection of the lesion, but it does not result in as good a clinical outcome.[220] The presence of urinary difficulties at the time of diagnosis is a poor prognostic sign.[178] The 10-year survival rate of patients with ependymoma is 80%.[47,71,130,220] Only a minority of these patients have experienced neurologic deterioration during the follow-up period. Crisante and Herrmann described the functional outcome of 69 patients with intramedullary tumors, including ependymoma, astrocytoma, lipoma, neurofibroma, and oligodendroglioma.[49] Surgery on lesions in the lower cervical spinal cord was associated with a greater morbidity rate than those in other locations in the cord. Patients with ependymoma had a better recovery rate than those with astrocytoma.

Primary tumors such as lipomas, lymphomas, and melanomas are very rare causes of intramedullary tumor. For example, lipomas represent 2% of intramedullary tumors.[90] In contrast to extradural metastases, intramedullary metastatic lesions are very uncommon.[67] Symptoms may develop in some patients with intramedullary metastases over a 6-month period. Common sources of metastases to the cord are lung, breast, lymphoma, colorectal, head and neck, and renal cell carcinoma, in descending order. Positron emission tomography is a diagnostic test that detects intramedullary metastases by documenting metabolically active tissue that may appear necrotic on MR imaging.[110,156] The prognosis is poor, with a 20% survival rate at 3 months in one study.[88] Angioma may also be an intramedullary lesion. The cervical spinal cord is affected less frequently than the thoracic cord. This lesion may be confused with syringomyelia.[95] Surgical removal is possible without significant neurologic deficit.[148]

Vasculitis/Infarction

In the region below T8, the spinal cord is supplied anteriorly by the anterior spinal artery, which arises from a single large vessel, the artery of Adamkiewicz. The artery of Adamkiewicz arises from a segmental vessel between T9 and L2 on the left side. This artery is the largest vessel to reach the spinal cord and supplies 25% of the cord in 50% of individuals.[190] Branches of the anterior and posterior spinal arteries form a plexus around the cord that supplies the white matter and posterior horns of the gray matter. The largest branches of the anterior spinal artery form a central artery that supplies the anterior gray matter and the innermost white matter.[5] Radicular arteries supply individual nerve roots. In the cervical spine, the anterior spinal artery receives branches from three or more segmental arteries, including one from the costocervical trunk.

In rare circumstances, connective tissue disorders that cause vasculitis may affect the blood vessels that supply blood to the spinal cord and cauda equina. Isolated granulomatous angiitis of the central nervous system is a form of vasculitis more commonly associated with cerebral vasculitis. Spinal cord symptoms, with or without cerebral involvement, may develop in patients with isolated angiitis.[35,103,211] An acute onset of neurologic symptoms may be secondary to hemorrhage from a ruptured inflammatory aneurysm.[228] Such patients describe lower extremity weakness accompanied by sensory abnormalities, including loss of pain proprioception and vibratory sense. Incontinence also develops. In a study of 40 patients with isolated angiitis, 23% had spinal cord disease.[211] The prognosis for return of function is poor, although patients may survive for a number of years after corticosteroid and radiation therapy. Polyarteritis nodosa may cause neurologic dysfunction by affecting spinal cord arteries or by compression secondary to subarachnoid hemorrhage.[149,165]

Infarction of the conus medullaris or cauda equina may occur by mechanisms other than inflammation of blood vessels, occlusion of the abdominal aorta during surgery, or formation of an atheroma. Occlusion of the artery of Adamkiewicz results in paraplegia with relative sparing of the sacral roots. Blockage of this artery usually leads to watershed ischemia in its peripheral extension. Infarction of the conus may simulate the appearance of a spinal cord tumor on MR.[7] Severe prolapse of an intervertebral disc at the T12–L1 level may compress the anterior spinal artery and result in secondary ischemia. A very rare cause of infarction is embolization of disc material to the spinal arteries.[108] Severe atherosclerosis, emboli, and sustained hypotension may be associated with cord infarction.[173] Patients with conus infarction have a poor prognosis unless definite improvement occurs within the first 48 hours after the onset of symptoms. Spinal cord infarction may also occur in the cervical spinal cord after exposure to radiation therapy.[173]

Miscellaneous Lesions

Infections

Intramedullary spinal cord abscess is a rare, but overwhelming infection.[62] This cord infection occurs in the setting of systemic infection. The onset of symptoms is rapid. Local pain with neurologic dysfunction is found in most patients with this acute infection. MR evaluation is able to identify the location and extent of the lesion, but it is not pathognomonic.[12] In a study of 93 patients with intramedullary abscesses, 32% of the abscesses occurred in the cervical spine.[17] The prognosis for these patients is poor.

Sarcoidosis

Sarcoidosis affects the central nervous system in 5% of patients.[59] Involvement of the spinal cord is rare. Granuloma affecting the spinal cord causes expansion of the cord. Granuloma may also cause vascular compression with ischemic changes in the cord. Signs of myelopathy may develop.[203] MR scan is able to determine the location of granuloma in the spinal cord.[46] Biopsy of the lesion is necessary. This lesion requires decompression and corticosteroid therapy.

Multiple Sclerosis

Multiple sclerosis (MS) is a demyelinating disease that affects the white matter of the nervous system, including the spinal cord. Although involvement of the cerebrum is more common, spinal cord disease occurs in 9% of patients.[157] Another study reported involvement in 25% of patients.[116] The signs and symptoms of the disease develop over weeks and include muscle weakness, decreased light touch and temperature sensation, and sphincter dysfunction. MR imaging demonstrates "plaque" lesions in the spinal cord.[195] MR imaging is positive in 86% of patients with clinically suspected spinal cord MS (Fig. 13-75).[86] In the cervical spine, 48% of patients, with or without myelopathic symptoms, have positive MR findings. In addition to MR imaging, visual, auditory, and somatosensory evoked potentials are helpful diagnostic tests.[2] Cerebrospinal fluid evaluation for oligoclonal bands or immunoglobulin G synthesis may be helpful when the diagnosis is in doubt. No pathognomonic tests are available for the diagnosis of MS.[153] Therapy for MS includes immunosuppressive drugs.[38]

Myelitis

Myelitis, in its various forms, may also cause lesions in the cervical spinal cord (Table 13-11). Categories of myelitis include postinfectious (postvaccinal), primary infectious (viral, bacterial, and spirochetal), primary intraspinal infectious (meningitis), toxic (drugs), physical agent (radiation), metabolic (vitamin B_{12} deficiency), blood vessel (connective tissue disease and systemic lupus erythematosus), and paraneoplastic.[209] Parainfectious myelitis may be differentiated from MS by the presence of spinal shock, MR evidence of cord swelling, and absence of oligoclonal bands.[105] Connective tissue disease may also cause transverse myelitis that may mimic MS. For example, in a study of 31 patients with central nervous system systemic lupus erythematosus, 16% had symptoms and signs of transverse myelitis.[143] Patients with Behçet's syndrome may have neurologic involvement that may also include myelitis.[182] MR evaluation of the cerebral cortex may be a useful additional test for myelitis if the diagnosis is not evident with spinal cord tests. Plaques compatible with MS may be noted in the cortex.[8] Myelitis usually occurs in a single episode; however, repeated episodes may occur, but they are not associated with any specific diagnostic group.[202] The diagnosis of myelitis should be considered when other causes of spinal cord dysfunction have been eliminated as possibilities.[57]

TREATMENT

Therapy directed at extradural metastatic lesions may include radiation therapy, corticosteroids, or spinal decom-

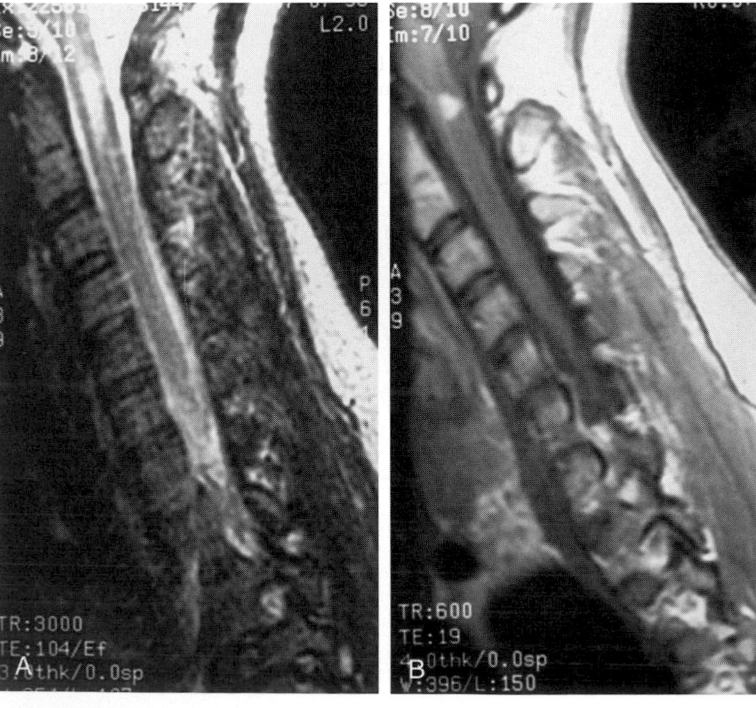

Figure 13-75 Multiple sclerosis in a 26-year-old woman with a history of facial and right arm numbness. Pain and paresthesias developed in her legs when she bent her neck. She had a positive Lhermitte sign and a positive Babinski sign. A T2-weighted sagittal MR image of the cervical spinal cord, *A*, revealed an area of increased signal approximately one vertebral body in length. Abnormal gadolinium enhancement is visible on the T1-weighted sagittal image, *B*. This appearance is compatible with demyelinating plaque in the cord substance.

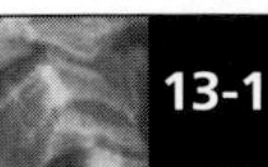

13-11 CAUSES OF MYELITIS AND NONCOMPRESSIVE MYELOPATHY

POSTINFECTIOUS/PARAINFECTIOUS
Vaccination for smallpox
Viral infection
Spontaneous

DEMYELINATING
Multiple sclerosis
Neuromyelitis optica
Acute necrotizing myelitis

PRIMARY INFECTIOUS

Viral
Poliomyelitis/postsyndrome
Acute encephalomyelitis
Herpes zoster
Rabies
Subacute myoclonic spinal neuritis
Human T-cell lymphotropic virus type 1
Acquired immunodeficiency syndrome

Bacterial/Spirochetal
Spinal abscess
Tuberculoma
Syphilis
Lyme disease
Rickettsial/fungal/parasitic

INTRASPINAL INFECTIONS
Bacterial meningitis
Tuberculous meningitis

PHYSICAL AGENTS
Irradiation
Electrical injury

METABOLIC/NUTRITIONAL
Diabetes mellitus
Cyanocobalamin deficiency
Pellagra
Chronic liver disease

BLOOD VESSELS
Arteriosclerosis
Dissecting aortic aneurysm
Coarctation of the aorta
Vascular malformations

CONNECTIVE TISSUE DISEASE
Polyarteritis nodosa
Systemic lupus erythematosus
Sjögren's syndrome
Behçet's syndrome

TOXIC
Organic iodide contrast media
Penicillin
Spinal anesthetics
Arsenic
Lathyrism
Orthocresyl phosphate

PARANEOPLASTIC

Modified from Byrne TN, Waxman SG: Spinal Cord Compression: Diagnosis and Principles of Management. Philadelphia, FA Davis, 1990.

pression.[29,45,109] Treatment of intradural-extramedullary tumors is complete surgical removal. Intramedullary tumors accessible to surgical excision should be removed.[87,208] Some physicians suggest postsurgical radiation therapy for the spinal cord.

PROGNOSIS

In general, extradural and intramedullary tumors are malignant, and intradural-extramedullary tumors are benign. The course and prognosis of these tumors correspond to their invasiveness, rapidity of growth, and location. Extradural and intramedullary tumors have poor prognoses, whereas intradural-extramedullary tumors may be cured with surgical removal.

References

Intraspinal Neoplasms

1. Acciarri N, Padovani R, Pozzati E, et al: Spinal cavernous angioma: A rare cause of subarachnoid hemorrhage. Surg Neurol 37:453, 1992.
2. Adams RD, Salam-Adams M: Chronic nontraumatic disease of the spinal cord. Neurol Clin 9:605, 1991.
3. Adams RD, Wegner W: Congenital cyst of the spinal meninges as cause of intermittent compression of the spinal cord. Arch Neurol Psychiatry 58:57, 1947.
4. Alazraki N: Radionuclide techniques. In Resnick D, Niwayama G (eds): Diagnosis of Bone and Joint Disorders. Philadelphia, WB Saunders, 1981, pp 432-445.
5. Aminoff MJ: Spinal vascular disease. In Critchley E, Eisen A (eds): Diseases of the Spinal Cord. London, Springer-Verlag, 1992, pp 281-299.
6. Aminoff MJ, Logue V: Clinical features of spinal vascular malformation. Brain 97:197, 1974.
7. Andrews BT, Kwei U, Greco C, Miller RG: Infarct of the conus medullaris simulating a spinal cord tumor: Case report. Surg Neurol 35:139, 1991.
8. Arlien-Soborg P, Kjaer L, Praestholm J: Myelography, CT and MRI of the spinal canal in patients with myelopathy: A prospective study. Acta Neurol Scand 87:95, 1993.
9. Armon C, Daube JR: Electrophysiological signs of arteriovenous malformations of the spinal cord. J Neurol Neurosurg Psychiatry 52:1176, 1989.
10. Aubin ML, Vignaud J, Jardin C, Bar D: Computed tomography in 75 clinical cases of syringomyelia. AJNR Am J Neuroradiol 2:199, 1981.
11. Austin GM: The significance and nature of pain in tumors of the spinal cord. Surg Forum 10:782, 1959.
12. Babu R, Jafar JJ, Huang PP, et al: Intramedullary abscess associated with a spinal cord ependymoma: Case report. Neurosurgery 30:121, 1992.
13. Baker AS, Ojemann RG, Swartz MN, Richardson EP Jr: Spinal epidural abscess. N Engl J Med 293:463, 1975.
14. Banna M: Clinical Radiology of the Spine and the Spinal Cord. Rockville, Md, Aspen, 1985.
15. Barone BM, Elvidge AR: Ependymomas: A clinical survey. J Neurosurg 33:428, 1970.
16. Barron KD, Hirano A, Araki S, Terry RD: Experiences with metastatic neoplasms involving the spinal cord. Neurology 9:91, 1959.
17. Bartels RH, Gonera EG, van der Spek JAN, et al: Intramedullary spinal cord abscess: A case report. Spine 20:1199, 1995.
18. Batson OV: The function of vertebral veins and their role in the spread of metastases. Ann Surg 112:138, 1940.
19. Batzdorf U (ed): Syringomyelia: Current Concepts in Diagnosis and Treatment. Baltimore, Williams & Wilkins, 1991.
20. Bemporad JA, Sze G: Magnetic resonance imaging of spinal cord vascular malformations with an emphasis on the cervical spine. Neuroimaging Clin N Am 11:111-129, 2001.
21. Benoist M, Ficat C, Baraf P, Cauchoix J: Postoperative lumbar epiduro-arachnoiditis: Diagnosis and therapeutic aspects. Spine 5:432, 1980.
22. Bertalanffy H, Mitani S, Otani M, et al: Usefulness of hemilaminectomy for microsurgical management of intraspinal lesions. Keio J Med 41:76, 1992.
23. Biondi A, Merland JJ, Hodes JE, et al: Aneurysms of spinal arteries associated with intramedullary arteriovenous malformations I: Angiographic and clinical aspects. AJNR Am J Neuroradiol 13:913, 1992.
24. Bjokengren AG, Kurz LT, Resnick D, et al: Symptomatic intraspinal synovial cysts: Opacification and treatment by percutaneous injection. AJR Am J Roentgenol 149:105, 1987.
25. Bleyer WA, Byrne TN: Leptomeningeal cancer in leukemia and solid tumors. Curr Probl Cancer 12:185, 1988.
26. Bourne IHJ: Lumbo-sacral adhesive arachnoiditis: A review. J R Soc Med 83:262, 1990.
27. Broager B: Spinal neurinoma. Acta Psychiatr Scand Suppl 85:1, 1953.
28. Brotchi J, DeWitte O, Levivier M, et al: A survey of 65 tumors within the spinal cord: Surgical results and the importance of preoperative magnetic resonance imaging. Neurosurgery 29:651, 1991.
29. Bruckmas JE, Bloomer WD: Management of spinal cord compression. Semin Oncol 5:135, 1978.
30. Bull JWD: Spinal meningiomas and neurofibromas. Acta Radiol 40:283, 1953.
31. Burton CV: Causes of failure of surgery on the lumbar spine: Ten-year follow-up. Mt Sinai J Med 58:183, 1991.
32. Burton CV: Lumbosacral arachnoiditis. Spine 3:24, 1978.
33. Butcher DL, Sahn SA: Epidural lipomatosis: A complication of corticosteroid therapy. Ann Intern Med 90:60, 1979.
34. Byrne TN, Waxman SG: Spinal Cord Compression: Diagnosis and Principles of Management. Philadelphia, FA Davis, 1990, pp 1-278.

35. Caccamo DV, Garcia JH, Ho K: Isolated granulomatous angiitis of the spinal cord. Ann Neurol 32:580, 1992.
36. Cameron SE, Hanscom DA: Rapid development of a spinal synovial cyst. A case report. Spine 17:1528, 1992.
37. Caplan LR, Norohna AB, Amico LL: Syringomyelia and arachnoiditis. J Neurol Neurosurg Psychiatry 53:106, 1990.
38. Carter JL, Hafler DA, Dawson DM, et al: Immunosuppressive with high-dose IV cyclophosphamide and ACTH in progressive multiple sclerosis: Cumulative 6-year experience in 164 patients. Neurology 38(suppl 2):9, 1988.
39. Cascino TL, Kori S, Krol G, Foley KM: CT of the brachial plexus in patients with cancer. Neurology 33:1553, 1983.
40. Cersosimo MG, Lasala B, Folgar S, et al: Epidural lipomatosis secondary to indinavir in an HIV positive patient. Clin Neuropharmacol 25:51-54, 2002.
41. Chalif DJ, Black K, Rosenstein D: Intradural spinal cord tumor presenting as a subarachnoid hemorrhage: Magnetic resonance imaging diagnosis. Neurosurgery 27:631, 1990.
42. Choe W, Walot I, Schlesinger C, et al: Synovial cyst of dens causing spinal cord compression: Case report. Paraplegia 31:803, 1993.
43. Choi IS, Berenstein A: Surgical neuroangiography of the spine and spinal cord. Radiol Clin North Am 26:1131, 1988.
44. Cillufo JM, Gomez MR, Reese DF, et al: Idiopathic ("congenital") spinal arachnoid diverticula: Clinical diagnosis and surgical results. Mayo Clin Proc 56:93, 1981.
45. Clark PRR, Saunders M: Steroid-induced remission in spinal canal reticulum cell sarcoma. Report of two cases. J Neurosurg 42:346, 1975.
46. Clifton AG, Stevens JM, Kapoor R, Rudge P: Spinal cord sarcoidosis with intramedullary cyst formation. Br J Radiol 63:805, 1990.
47. Clover LL, Hazuke MB, Kinzie JJ: Spinal cord ependymomas treated with surgery and radiation therapy. A review of 11 cases. Am J Clin Oncol 16:350, 1993.
48. Collins BT, Reddy AA, Akyiirekli D, et al: Radiation therapy for metastatic disease of the spine. Semin Spine Surg 12:17-20, 2000.
49. Crisante L, Herrmann H: Surgical management of intramedullary spinal cord tumors: Functional outcome and sources of morbidity. Neurosurgery 35:69, 1994.
50. Crisi G, Sorgato P, Colombo A, et al: Gadolinium-DTPA–enhanced MR imaging in the diagnosis of spinal epidural haematoma: Report of a case. Neuroradiology 32:64, 1990.
51. Crols R, Appel B, Klaes R: Extensive cervical intradural and intramedullary lipoma and spina bifida occulta of C1: A case report. Clin Neurol Neurosurg 95:39, 1993.
52. Curtis BH, Fisher RL, Butterfield WL, Sauders FP: Neurofibromatosis in paraplegia. J Bone Joint Surg Am 51-A:843, 1969.
53. Cusick JF, Bernardi R: Syringomyelia after the removal of benign spinal extramedullary neoplasms. Spine 20:1289, 1995.
54. Darouiche RO, Hamill RJ, Greenberg SB, et al: Bacterial spinal epidural abscess: Review of 43 cases and literature survey. Medicine (Baltimore) 71:369, 1992.
55. Davidoff RA: Handbook of the Spinal Cord, Vol 4 and 5. Congenital Disorders, Trauma, Infections, and Cancer. New York, Marcel Dekker, 1987.
56. Davis RA, Washburn PL: Spinal cord meningiomas. Surg Gynecol Obstet 131:15, 1970.
57. Dawson DM, Potts F: Acute nontraumatic myelopathies. Neurol Clin 9:585, 1991.
58. Delamarter RB, Ross JS, Masaryk TJ, et al: Diagnosis of lumbar arachnoiditis by magnetic resonance imaging. Spine 15:304, 1990.
59. Delaney P: Neurologic manifestations in sarcoidosis: Review of the literature with a report of 23 cases. Ann Intern Med 87:336, 1977.
60. DiLauro L, Poli R, Bortoluzzi M: Paresthesia after lumbar disc removal and their relationship to epidural haematoma. J Neurosurg 57:135, 1982.
61. Disimone RE, Berman AT, Schwentker EP: The orthopedic manifestation of neurofibromatosis: A clinical experience and review of the literature. Clin Orthop 230:277, 1988.
62. Ditulio MV: Intramedullary spinal abscess: A case report with a review of 53 previously described cases. Surg Neurol 7:351, 1977.
63. Djindjian R: Arteriography of the spinal cord. AJR Am J Roentgenol 107:461, 1969.
64. Doita M, Harada T, Nishida K, et al: Recurrent calcified spinal meningioma detected by plain radiograph. Spine 26:E249-E252, 2001.
65. Domingues RC, Mikulis D, Swearingen B, et al: Subcutaneous sacrococcygeal myxopapillary ependymoma: CT and MR. AJNR Am J Neuroradiol 12:171, 1991.
66. Ducatman BS, Scheithauer BW, Dahlin DC: Malignant bone tumors associated with neurofibromatosis. Mayo Clin Proc 58:578, 1983.
67. Edelson RN, Deck MDF, Posner JB: Intramedullary spinal cord metastases: Clinical and radiographic findings in nine cases. Neurology 22:1222, 1972.
68. Edelstyn GA, Gillespie PJ, Grebbell FS: The radiological demonstration of skeletal metastases. Clin Radiol 18:158, 1967.
69. Egelhoff JC, Bates DJ, Ross JS, et al: Spinal MR findings in neurofibromatosis types 1 and 2. AJNR Am J Neuroradiol 13:1071, 1992.
70. Elsberg CA: Diagnosis and Treatment of Surgical Diseases of the Spinal Cord and Its Membranes, 2nd ed. Philadelphia, WB Saunders, 1941.
71. Ferrante L, Mastronardi L, Celli P, et al: Intramedullary spinal cord ependymomas: A study of 45 cases with long-term follow-up. Acta Neurohr (Wien) 119:74, 1992.
72. Fessler RG, Johnson DL, Brown FD, et al: Epidural lipomatosis in steroid-treated patients. Spine 17:183, 1992.
73. Fischer G, Tommasi M: Spinal ependymomas. In Vinken PJ, Bruyn GW (eds): Handbook of Clinical Neurology, vol 20. Amsterdam, North Holland Publishing, 1976, pp 759-780.
74. Fontaine S, Melanson D, Cosgrove R, Bertrand G: Cavernous hemangiomas of the spinal cord: MR imaging. Radiology 166:839, 1988.
75. Franck JI, King RB, Petro GR, Kanzer MD: A post-traumatic lumbar spinal synovial cyst. Case report. J Neurosurg 68:293, 1987.
76. Freilick D, Swash M: Diagnosis and management of tuberculosis paraplegia with special reference to tuberculosis radiculomyelitis. J Neurol Neurosurg Psychiatry 42:12, 1979.
77. Funasaki H, Winter RB, Lonstein JB, Denis F: Pathophysiology of spinal deformities in neurofibromatosis: An analysis of seventy-one patients who had curves associated with dystrophic changes. J Bone Joint Surg Am 76-A:692, 1994.
78. Gamache FW Jr, Wang JC, Deck M, et al: Unusual appearance of an en plaque meningioma of cervical spinal canal. A case report and literature review. Spine 26:E87-E89, 2001.
79. Gardner WJ, Bell HS, Poolos PN, et al: Terminal ventriculostomy for syringomyelia. J Neurosurg 46:609, 1977.
80. Gautier-Smith PC: Clinical aspects of spinal neurofibromas. Brain 90:359, 1970.
81. Gilbert RW, Kim JH, Posner JB: Epidural spinal cord compression from metastatic tumor: Diagnosis and treatment. Ann Neurol 3:40, 1978.
82. Giuffre R: Spinal lipomas. In Vinken PJ, Bruyn GW (eds): Handbook of Clinical Neurology, vol 20. Amsterdam, North Holland Publishing, 1976, pp 389-414.
83. Glasser R, Masson R, Mickle P, Peters KR: Embolization of a dural arteriovenous fistula of the ventral cervical spinal canal in a nine-year-old boy. Neurosurgery 33:1089, 1993.
84. Goffin J, Wilms G, Plets C, et al: Synovial cyst at the C1–C2 junction. Neurosurgery 30:914, 1992.
85. Goodridge AE, Feasby TE, Ebers GC, et al: Hand wasting due to mid-cervical spinal cord compression. Can J Neurol Sci 14:309, 1987.
86. Greenberg JO: Neuroimaging of the spinal cord. Neurol Clin 9:679, 1991.
87. Greenwood J: Surgical removal of intramedullary tumors. J Neurosurg 26:275, 1967.
88. Grem JL, Burgess J, Trump DL: Clinical features and natural history of intramedullary spinal cord metastasis. Cancer 56:2305, 1985.
89. Guidetti B, Mercuri S, Vagnozzi R: Long-term results of the surgical treatment of 129 intramedullary spinal gliomas. J Neurosurg 54:323, 1981.
90. Gurusinghe NT: Spinal cord compression and spinal cord tumours. In Critchley E, Eisen A (eds): Diseases of the Spinal Cord. London, Springer-Verlag, 1992, pp 351-408.
91. Guyer RD, Collier RR, Ohnmeiss DD, et al: Extraosseous spinal lesions mimicking disc disease. Spine 13:328, 1988.
92. Haddad FS, Abla A, Allam CK: Extradural spinal angiolipoma. Surg Neurol 26:473, 1986.
93. Helseth A, Mork SJ: Primary intraspinal neoplasms in Norway 1955 to 1986: A population based survey of 467 patients. J Neurosurg 71:842, 1989.

94. Heshmat MY, Kovi J, Simpson C, et al: Neoplasms of the central nervous system. Cancer 38:2135, 1976.
95. Hida K, Tada M, Iwasaki Y, Abe H: Intramedullary disseminated capillary hemangioma with localized spinal cord swelling: Case report. Neurosurgery 33:1099, 1993.
96. Hillman J, Bynke O: Solitary extradural cavernous hemangiomas in the spinal canal: Report of five cases. Surg Neurol 36:19, 1991.
97. Hissa E, Boumphrey F, Bay J: Spinal epidural hematoma and ankylosing spondylitis. Clin Orthop 208:225, 1986.
98. Howington JU, Connolly ES, Voorhies RM: Intraspinal synovial cysts: 10-year experience at the Ochsner Clinic. J Neurosurg 91 (2 suppl):193-199, 1999.
99. Hoyland JA, Freemont AJ, Denton J, et al: Retained surgical swab debris in post-laminectomy arachnoiditis and peridural fibrosis. J Bone Joint Surg Br 70-B:659, 1988.
100. Hughes DG, Isherwood I: How frequent is chronic lumbar arachnoiditis following intrathecal Myodil? Br J Radiol 65:758, 1992.
101. Huvos AG: Bone Tumors: Diagnosis, Treatment, and Prognosis, 2nd ed. Philadelphia, WB Saunders, 1991, pp 413-427.
102. Imai K, Nakamura K, Inokuchi K, et al: Aspiration of intraspinal synovial cyst: Recurrence after temporal improvement. Arch Orthop Trauma Surg 118:103-105, 1998.
103. Inwards DJ, Piepgras DG, Lie JT, et al: Granulomatous angiitis of the spinal cord associated with Hodgkin's disease. Cancer 68:1318, 1991.
104. Isu T, Iwasaki Y, Akino M, et al: Magnetic resonance imaging in cases of spinal dural arteriovenous malformation. Neurosurgery 24:919, 1989.
105. Jeffrey DR, Mandler RN, David LE: Transverse myelitis: Retrospective analysis of 33 cases, with differentiation of cases associated with multiple sclerosis and Parainfectious events. Arch Neurol 50:532, 1993.
106. Johnson CE, Sze G: Benign lumbar arachnoiditis: MR imaging with gadopentetate dimeglumine. AJR Am J Roentgenol 155:873, 1990.
107. Katz AD, McAlpin C: Face and neck neurogenic neoplasms. Am J Surg 166:421, 1993.
108. Kestle JRW, Resch L, Tator CH, Kucharczyk W: Intervertebral disc embolization resulting in spinal cord infarction: Case report. J Neurosurg 71:938, 1989.
109. Khan FR, Glickman AS, Chu FCH, Nickson JJ: Treatment by radiotherapy of spinal cord compression due to extradural metastases. Radiology 89:495, 1967.
110. Komori T, Delbeke D: Leptomeningeal carcinomatosis and intramedullary spinal cord metastases from lung cancer: Detection with FDG positron emission tomography. Clin Nucl Med 26:905-907, 2001.
111. Kori SH, Foley KM, Posner JB: Brachial plexus lesions in patients with cancer: 100 cases. Neurology 31:45, 1981.
112. Kricun R, Shoemaker EI, Chovanes GI, Stephens HW: Epidural abscess of the cervical spine: MR findings in five cases. AJR Am J Roentgenol 158:1145, 1992.
113. Lantos G, Epstein F, Kory L: Magnetic resonance imaging of intradural spinal lipoma. Neurosurgery 20:469, 1987.
114. Le May M, Jackson DM: Intervertebral disc protrusion masquerading as an intramedullary tumor. Br J Radiol 37:463, 1964.
115. Lee RR: Spinal tumors. Spine 9:261, 1995.
116. Leibowitz U, Halpern L, Alter M: Clinical studies of multiple sclerosis in Israel: Progressive spinal syndromes and multiple sclerosis. Neurology 17:988, 1967.
117. Lemish W, Apsimon T, Chakera T: Lumbar intraspinal synovial cysts: Recognition and CT diagnosis. Spine 14:1378, 1989.
118. Levitan LH, Wiens CW: Chronic lumbar extradural haematoma: CT findings. Radiology 148:707, 1983.
119. Levy ML, Wieder BH, Schneider J, et al: Subdural empyema of the cervical spine: Clinicopathological correlates and magnetic resonance imaging. J Neurosurg 79:929, 1993.
120. Levy WJ, Bay J, Dohn D: Spinal cord meningioma. J Neurosurg 57:804, 1982.
121. Lim V, Sobel DF, Zyroff J: Spinal cord pial metastases: MR imaging with gadopentetate dimeglumine. AJNR Am J Neuroradiol 11:975, 1990.
122. Lisai P, Doria C, Crissantu L, et al: Cauda equina syndrome secondary to idiopathic spinal epidural lipomatosis. Spine 26:307-309, 2001.
123. Logue V: Angiomas of the spinal cord: Review of the pathogenesis, clinical features, and results of surgery. J Neurol Neurosurg Psychiatry 42:1, 1979.
124. Long DM: Cervical cord tumors. In Sherk HH, Dunn EJ, Eismont FJ, et al (eds): The Cervical Spine, 2nd ed. Philadelphia, JB Lippincott, 1989, pp 526-543.
125. Love JG, Dodge HW: Dumbbell (hourglass) neurofibromas affecting the spinal cord. Surg Obstet Gynecol 94:161, 1952.
126. Lundqvist C, Berthelsen B, Sullivan M, et al: Spinal arteriovenous malformations: Neurological aspects and results of embolization. Acta Neurol Scand 82:51, 1990.
127. Madsen JR, Heros RC: Spinal arteriovenous malformations and neurogenic claudication: Report of two cases. J Neurosurg 68:793, 1988.
128. Markham JW, Lynge HN, Stahlman GEB: The syndrome of spontaneous spinal epidural hematoma: Report of three cases. J Neurosurg 26:334, 1967.
129. Mattle H, Sieb JP, Rohner M, Mumenthaler M: Nontraumatic spinal epidural and subdural hematomas. Neurology 37:1351, 1987.
130. McCormack PC, Torres R, Post K, Stein BM: Intramedullary ependymoma of the spinal cord. J Neurosurg 72:523, 1990.
131. McCormick PC, Michelsen WJ, Post KD, et al: Cavernous malformations of the spinal cord. Neurosurgery 23:459, 1988.
132. McIlory WJ, Richardson JC: Syringomyelia: A clinical review of 75 cases. Can Med Assoc J 93:731, 1965.
133. McKraig W, Svien HJ, Dodge HW Jr, Camp JD: Intraspinal lesions masquerading as protruded lumbar intervertebral discs. JAMA 149:250, 1952.
134. Milhorat TH, Johnson WD, Miller JI, et al: Surgical treatment of syringomyelia based on magnetic resonance imaging criteria. Neurosurgery 31:231, 1992.
135. Minami S, Sagoh T, Nishimura K, et al: Spinal arteriovenous malformations: MR imaging. Radiology 169:109, 1988.
136. Mitchell GE, Lourie H, Berne AS: The various causes of scalloped vertebrae with notes on their pathogenesis. Radiology 89:67, 1967.
137. Modic MT, Masaryk T, Paushter D: Magnetic resonance imaging of the spine. Radiol Clin North Am 24:229, 1986.
138. Murray JJ, Greco FA, Wolff SN, Hainsworth JD: Neoplastic meningitis: Marked variations of cerebrospinal fluid composition in the absence of extradural block. Am J Med 75:289, 1983.
139. Nabors MW, Pait TG, Byrd E, et al: Updated assessment and current classification of spinal meningeal cysts. J Neurosurg 68:366, 1988.
140. Nadler SF, Bartoli LM, Stitik TP, et al: Tarlov cyst as a rare cause of S1 radiculopathy. Arch Phys Med Rehabil 82:689-690, 2001.
141. Nakagami W, Yokota S, Ohishi Y, et al: Chronic spontaneous lumbar spinal epidural hematoma. Spine 17:1509, 1992.
142. Nemoto Y, Inoue Y, Tahiro T, et al: Intramedullary spinal cord tumors: Significance of associated hemorrhage at MR imaging. Radiology 182:793, 1992.
143. Neuwelt CM, Lacks S, Kaye BR, et al: Role of intravenous cyclophosphamide (IV-CYC) in the treatment of severe neuropsychiatric lupus erythematosus (NOSLE). Am J Med 98:32, 1995.
144. Nicholas JJ, Christy WC: Spinal pain made worse by recumbency: A clue to spinal cord tumors. Arch Phys Med Rehabil 67:598, 1986.
145. Nichols DA, Rufenacht DA, Jack CR Jr, Forbes GS: Embolization of spinal dural arteriovenous fistula with polyvinyl alcohol particles: Experience with 14 patients. AJNR Am J Neuroradiol 13:933, 1992.
146. Nijensohn E, Russell EJ, Milan M, Brown T: Calcified synovial cyst of the cervical spine: CT and MR evaluation. J Comput Assist Tomogr 14:473, 1990.
147. Nittner K: Spinal meningiomas, neurinomas, and neurofibromas and hourglass tumors. In Vinken PJ, Bruyn GW (eds): Handbook of Clinical Neurology, vol 20. Amsterdam, North Holland Publishing, 1976, pp 177-322.
148. Oglivy CS, Louis DN, Ojemann RG: Intramedullary cavernous angiomas of the spinal cord: Clinical presentation, pathological features, and surgical management. Neurosurgery 31:219, 1992.
149. Ojeda VJ: Polyarteritis affecting the spinal cord arteries. Aust N Z J Med 13:287, 1983.
150. Pagni CA, Canavero S, Forni M: Report of a cavernoma of the cauda equina and review of the literature. Surg Neurol 33:124, 1990.
151. Pancoast HK: Superior pulmonary sulcus tumor: Tumor characterized by pain, Horner's syndrome, destruction of bone and atrophy of hand muscles. JAMA 99:1391, 1932.

152. Parizel PM, Baleriaux D, Rodesch G, et al: Gd-DTPA enhanced MR imaging of spinal tumors. AJNR Am J Neuroradiol 10:249, 1989.
153. Paty DW, McFarlin DE, McDonald WI: Magnetic resonance imaging and laboratory aids in the diagnosis of multiple sclerosis. Ann Neurol 29:3, 1991.
154. Pendleton B, Carl B, Pollay M: Spinal extradural benign synovial or ganglion cyst: Case report and review of the literature. Neurosurgery 13:322, 1983.
155. Phillips GE, Jefferson A: Acute spinal epidural abscess: Observations from fourteen cases. Postgrad Med J 55:712, 1979.
156. Poggi MM, Patronas N, Buttman JA, et al: Intramedullary spinal cord metastasis from renal cell carcinoma: Detection by positron emission tomography. Clin Nucl Med 26:837-839, 2001.
157. Poser S, Hermann-Gremmeis I, Wikstrom J, Poser W: Clinical features of the spinal form of multiple sclerosis. Acta Neurol Scand 57:151, 1978.
158. Quaghebeur G, Jeffree M: Synovial cyst of the high cervical spine causing myelopathy. AJNR Am J Neuroradiol 13:981, 1992.
159. Quiles M, Marchisello PJ, Tsairis P: Lumbar adhesive arachnoiditis: Etiologic and pathologic aspects. Spine 3:45, 1978.
160. Quint DJ, Boulos RS, Sanders WP, et al: Epidural lipomatosis. Radiology 169:485, 1988.
161. Rasmussen TB, Kernohan JW, Adson AW: Pathologic classification with surgical consideration of intraspinal tumors. Ann Surg 111:513, 1940.
162. Resnick D, Niwayama G: Diagnosis of Bone and Joint Disorders. Philadelphia, WB Saunders, 1981, pp 432-445.
163. Rigamonti D, Liem L, Sampath P, et al: Spinal epidural abscess: Contemporary trends in etiology, evaluation, and management. Surg Neurol 52:189-196, 1999.
164. Robinson SC, Sweeney JP: Cauda equina lipoma presenting as acute neuropathic arthropathy of the knee. A case report. Clin Orthop 178:210, 1983.
165. Rodgers H, Veale D, Smith P, Corris P: Spinal cord compression in polyarteritis nodosa. Ann Neurol 32:580, 1992.
166. Rosenblum B, Oldfield EH, Doppman JL, DiChiro G: Spinal arteriovenous malformations: A comparison of dural arteriovenous fistulas and intradural AVM's in 81 patients. J Neurosurg 67:795, 1987.
167. Rosenblum DS, Myers SJ: Dural spinal cord arteriovenous malformation. Arch Phys Med Rehabil 72:233, 1991.
168. Rosenfeld JV, Kaye AH, David S, Gonzales M: Pachymeningitis cervicalis hypertrophica: Case report. J Neurosurg 66:137, 1987.
169. Ross JS: Inflammatory disease. In Modic MT, Masaryk TJ, Ross JS (eds): Magnetic Resonance Imaging of the Spine. Chicago, Year Book, 1989, pp 167-182.
170. Ross JS, Masaryk TJ, Modic MT, et al: MR imaging of lumbar arachnoiditis. AJR Am J Roentgenol 149:1025, 1987.
171. Roy-Camille R, Mazel C, Husson JL, Saillant G: Symptomatic spinal epidural lipomatosis induced by a long-term steroid treatment: Review of the literature and report of two additional cases. Spine 16:1365, 1991.
172. Sandberg DI, Lavyne MH: Symptomatic spinal epidural lipomatosis after local epidural corticosteroid injections: Case report. Neurosurgery 45:162-165, 1999.
173. Sandson TA, Friedman JH: Spinal cord infarction: Report of 8 cases and review of the literature. Medicine (Baltimore) 68:282, 1989.
174. Sawa H, Tamaki N, Kurata H, Nagashima T: Complete resection of a spinal meningioma extending from the foramen magnum to the second thoracic vertebral body via the anterior approach: Case report. Neurosurgery 33:1095, 1993.
175. Schaberg J, Gainor BJ: A profile of metastatic carcinoma of the spine. Spine 10:19, 1985.
176. Schierholz U: Fibrosarcoma of the cervical spine. Arch Orthop Trauma Surg 93:145, 1979.
177. Schievink WI, Piepgras DG: Cervical vertebral artery aneurysms and arteriovenous fistulae in neurofibromatosis type 1: Case reports. Neurosurgery 29:760, 1991.
178. Schweitzer JS, Batzdorf U: Ependymoma of the cauda equina region: Diagnosis, treatment, and outcome in 15 patients. Neurosurgery 30:202, 1992.
179. Sekula RF, Sandhu FA, Oliverio PJ, et al: Intramedullary tumors of the cord. Semin Spine Surg 12:21-29, 2000.
180. Sen CN, Sekhar LN: An extreme lateral approach to intradural lesions of the cervical spine and foramen magnum. Neurosurgery 27:197, 1990.
181. Sghirlanzoni A, Marazzi R, Pareyson D, et al: Epidural anaethesia and spinal arachnoiditis. Anaesthesia 44:317, 1989.
182. Shakir RA, Sulaiman K, Rudman M: Neurological presentation of Behçet's syndrome: Clinical categories. Eur Neurol 30:249, 1990.
183. Shaw MDM, Russel JA, Grossart KW: The changing pattern of spinal arachnoiditis. J Neurol Neurosurg Psychiatry 41:97, 1978.
184. Shen W, Lee S: MRI of concurrent spinal meningioma, ependymoma, and syringomyelia. J Comput Assist Tomogr 16:665, 1992.
185. Shen WC, Ho YJ, Lee SK, Lee KR: Ependymoma of the cauda equina presenting with subarachnoid hemorrhage. AJNR Am J Neuroradiol 14:399, 1993.
186. Sherman JL, Barkovich AJ, Citrin CM: The MR appearance of syringomyelia: New observations. AJR Am J Roentgenol 148:381, 1987.
187. Singer GL, Brust JCM, Challenor YB: Syringomyelia presenting as shoulder dysfunction. Arch Phys Med Rehabil 73:285, 1992.
188. Sklar EML, Quencer RM, Green BA, et al: Complications of epidural anesthesia: MR appearance of abnormalities. Radiology 181:549, 1991.
189. Skuse GR, Kosciolek BA, Rowley PT: The neurofibroma in von Recklinghausen neurofibromatosis has a unicellular origin. Am J Hum Genet 49:600, 1991.
190. Sliwa JA, Maclean IC: Ischemic myelopathy: A review of spinal vasculature and related clinical syndromes. Arch Phys Med Rehabil 73:365, 1992.
191. Spillane JD, Pallis C, Jones AM: Developmental abnormalities in the region of the foramen magnum. Brain 80:11, 1957.
192. Stark RJ, Henson RA, Evans SJW: Spinal metastases: A retrospective survey from a general hospital. Brain 105:189, 1982.
193. Stein BM: Intramedullary spinal cord tumors. Clin Neurosurg 30:717, 1983.
194. Stevens JM, Kendall BE, Gedroyc W: Acute epidural haematoma complicating myelography in a normotensive patient with normal blood coagulability. Br J Radiol 64:860, 1991.
195. Sze G: Gadolinium-DTPA in spinal disease. Radiol Clin North Am 26:1009, 1988.
196. Sze G, Abramson A, Krol G, et al: Gadolinium-DTPA in the evaluation of intradural extramedullary spinal disease. AJNR Am J Neuroradiol 9:153, 1988.
197. Sze G, Stimac GK, Bartlett C, et al: Multicenter study of gadopentetate dimeglumine as a MR contrast agent: Evaluation in patients with spinal tumors. AJNR Am J Neuroradiol 11:967, 1990.
198. Takano Y, Homma T, Okumura H, Takahashi HE: Ganglion cyst occurring in the ligamentum flavum of the cervical spine: A case report. Spine 17:1531, 1992.
199. Tang HJ, Lin HJ, Liu YC, et al: Spinal epidural abscess—experiences with 46 patients and evaluation of prognostic factors. J Infect 45:76-81, 2002.
200. Thomas JE, Piepgras DG, Scheithauer B, et al: Neurogenic tumors of the sciatic nerve. A clinicopathologic study of 35 cases. Mayo Clin Proc 58:640, 1983.
201. Thomeer RT, Bots GTAM, Van Dulken H, et al: Neurofibrosarcoma of the cauda equina. Case report. J Neurosurg 54:409, 1981.
202. Tippett DS, Fishman PS, Panitch HS: Relapsing transverse myelitis. Neurology 41:703, 1991.
203. Tuel SM, Meythaler JM, Cross LL: Rehabilitation of quadriparesis secondary to spinal cord sarcoidosis. Am J Phys Med Rehabil 70:63, 1991.
204. Turk PS, Peters N, Libbey P, Wanebo HJ: Diagnosis and management of giant intrasacral schwannoma. Cancer 70:2650, 1992.
205. Ueda S, Saito A, Inomori S, Kim I: Cavernous angioma of the cauda equina producing subarachnoid hemorrhage: Case report. J Neurosurg 66:134, 1987.
206. Van de Kelft E, Van Vyve M: Chronic perineal pain related to sacral meningeal cysts. Neurosurgery 29:223, 1991.
207. Vieth RG, Odom GL: Extradural spinal metastases and their neurosurgical treatment. J Neurosurg 23:501, 1965.
208. Vijayakumar S, Estes M, Hardy RW Jr, et al: Ependymoma of the spinal cord and cauda equina: A review. Cleve Clin J Med 55:163, 1988.

209. Vinters HV, Barnett HJM, Kaufmann JCE: Subdural hematoma of the spinal cord and widespread subarachnoid hemorrhage complicating anticoagulant therapy. Stroke 11:459, 1980.
210. Vloeberghs M, Herregodts P, Stadnik T, et al: Spinal arachnoiditis mimicking a spinal cord tumor: A case report and review of the literature. Surg Neurol 37:211, 1992.
211. Vollmer TL, Guarnaccia J, Harrington W, et al: Idiopathic granulomatous angiitis of the central nervous system. Arch Neurol 50:925, 1993.
212. Voyadzis JM, Bhargava P, Henderson FC: Tarlov cysts: A study of 10 cases with review of the literature. J Neurosurg 95(1 suppl): 25-32, 2001.
213. Wander JV, Das Gupta TK: Neurofibromatosis. Curr Probl Surg 14:1, 1977.
214. Wasserstrom WR, Glass JP, Posner JB: Diagnosis and treatment of leptomeningeal metastases from solid tumors: Experience with 90 patients. Cancer 49:759, 1982.
215. Weill A, del Carpio-O'Donovan R, Tampieri D, et al: Spinal angiolipomas: CT and MR aspects. J Comput Assist Tomogr 15:83, 1991.
216. Weil SM, Gewirtz RJ, Tew JM Jr: Concurrent intradural and extradural meningiomas of the cervical spine. Neurosurgery 27:629, 1990.
217. Weissman DE, Gilberg M, Wang H, et al: The use of computed tomography of the spine to identify patients at high risk for epidural metastases. J Clin Oncol 3:1541, 1985.
218. Wertelecki W, Rouleau G, Superneau D, et al: Neurofibromatosis: Clinical and DNA linkage studies at a large kindred. N Engl J Med 319:278, 1988.
219. Weymann CA, Capone P, Kinkel PR, Kinkel WR: Synovial cyst of the upper cervical spine: MRI with gadolinium. Neurology 43:2151, 1993.
220. Whitaker SJ, Bessell EM, Ashley SE, et al: Postoperative radiotherapy in the management of spinal ependymoma. J Neurosurg 74:720, 1991.
221. Wiesel SW, Ignatius P, Marvel JP, Rothman RH: Intradural neurofibroma simulating lumbar disc disease. J Bone Joint Surg Am 58-A:1040, 1976.
222. Winter RB, Moe JH, Bradford DS, et al: Spine deformity in neurofibromatosis: A review of 102 patients. J Bone Joint Surg Am 61-A:677, 1979.
223. Wong-Chung J, Gillespie R: Lumbosacral spondyloptosis with neurofibromatosis: Case report. Spine 16:986, 1991.
224. Woolsey RM, Young RR: The clinical diagnosis of disorders of the spinal cord. Neurol Clin 9:573, 1991.
225. Yap HY, Yap BS, Tashima CK, et al: Meningeal carcinomatosis in breast cancer. Cancer 42:283, 1978.
226. Yarde WL, Arnold PM, Kepes JJ, et al: Synovial cysts of the lumbar spine: Diagnosis, surgical management, and pathogenesis. Report of eight cases. Surg Neurol 43:459-465, 1995.
227. Yeates A, Brant-Zawadzki M, Norman D, et al: Nuclear magnetic resonance of syringomyelia. AJNR Am J Neuroradiol 4:234, 1983.
228. Yoong MF, Blumberg PC, North JB: Primary (granulomatous) angiitis of the central nervous system with multiple aneurysms of spinal arteries: Case report. J Neurosurg 79:603, 1993.
229. Yousem DM, Patrone PM, Grossman RI: Leptomeningeal metastases: MR evaluation. J Comput Assist Tomogr 14:255, 1990.
230. Zager EL, Ojemann RG, Poletti CE: Acute presentations of syringomyelia: Report of three cases. J Neurosurg 72:133, 1990.
231. Zinreich SJ: Three-dimensional computed tomography of the spine: Evaluation of failed back surgery syndrome and spinal stenosis. Spine 9:287, 1995.

CHAPTER 14

ENDOCRINOLOGIC AND METABOLIC DISORDERS OF THE SPINE

Endocrinologic and metabolic disorders are systemic illnesses that can affect components of the musculoskeletal system throughout the body. Those endocrinologic and metabolic illnesses that produce symptoms of low back and neck pain and characteristic laboratory and radiologic abnormalities include osteoporosis, osteomalacia, parathyroid disease, ochronosis, acromegaly, and microcrystalline disorders. Patients with these systemic diseases may present to a physician with low back or neck pain as their initial or primary complaint, and a minor traumatic event is frequently thought to be the cause of the spinal discomfort. Evaluation by the physician, however, demonstrates compression fractures of the vertebral bodies secondary to inadequate bone stock, extensive degenerative disease of the spine, or accumulation of crystals, amino acids, or mucopolysaccharides in bone. A characteristic finding of endocrinologic and metabolic disorders is that, although symptoms may be limited to the axial skeleton, these illnesses cause bone changes in many locations. The bone abnormalities may be subtle but can be discovered if looked for carefully.

The history of back or neck pain in patients with endocrinologic and metabolic diseases is usually nonspecific. Back pain is located predominantly in the lumbosacral spine, with occasional radiation into the lower extremities. Neck pain is located over the osseous components of the cervical spine. Pain may be insidious in onset or acute, associated with a vertebral body compression fracture or acute gouty arthritis of the sacroiliac joint. Patients frequently have symptoms of bone or joint pain in other locations. In addition, the systemic manifestations of the endocrinologic or metabolic bone disorder may include symptoms of muscle weakness, renal stones, gastrointestinal malabsorption, or change in facial configuration. Patients with abnormalities associated with the deposition of mucopolysaccharide in soft tissues or laxity of ligamentous structures are at risk for development of myelopathic symptoms. Physical examination may demonstrate the systemic quality of the underlying disorder. Not only will patients have vertebral pain with percussion over the spine, loss of height, and dorsal kyphosis, but they may also demonstrate muscle weakness, peripheral joint inflammation, tetany, pigmentation of cartilage, enlargement of the hands and jaw, or tophaceous deposits. Neurologic examination may demonstrate spasticity, hyperreflexia, and positive Babinski's sign, indicative of spinal cord compression. Laboratory evaluation may be very helpful in making a specific diagnosis of the underlying disorder.

Abnormalities of calcium and phosphorus may raise the suspicion of osteomalacia or hyperparathyroidism. Bone biopsy confirms the diagnosis of osteoporosis or osteomalacia. Measurement of parathyroid hormone confirms the diagnosis of hyperparathyroidism or hypoparathyroidism. Nonsuppressibility of growth hormone during a glucose tolerance test is characteristic of acromegaly. Detection of homogentisic acid in urine is diagnostic of ochronosis. Detection of urate or calcium pyrophosphate dihydrate crystals is essential for the diagnosis of gout or pseudogout, respectively. Prominent radiographic findings may indicate decreased bone stock, periosteal resorption, disc calcification, widened joint space, or bone erosions, but they are nonspecific. Although radiologic evaluation is not diagnostic, it is important in documenting the global involvement of the skeletal system with these diseases.

Therapy is tailored for each endocrinologic or metabolic illness. Calcium and vitamin D supplements are useful in patients with osteoporosis or osteomalacia. Surgical ablation of parathyroid or pituitary tumors is the therapy of choice for hyperparathyroidism or acromegaly, respectively. Patients with episodes of acute microcrystalline arthritis are benefitted by courses of nonsteroidal anti-inflammatory drugs (NSAIDs). Patients with myelopathy benefit from spinal decompression and stabilization.

OSTEOPOROSIS

See page 570 for Capsule Summary.

PREVALENCE AND PATHOGENESIS

Osteoporosis, a metabolic bone disease related to several different disorders, is associated with loss of bone mass per unit volume even though the ratio of bone mineral content and bone matrix remains normal. The reduction of bone

CAPSULE SUMMARY

	LOW BACK	NECK
Frequency of spinal pain	Uncommon	Not applicable (NA)
Location of spinal pain	Lumbar spine	NA
Quality of spinal pain	Chronic, dull ache; acute, sharp with fracture	NA
Symptoms and signs	Back pain increases with motion, marked percussion tenderness over spine	NA
Laboratory tests	Anemia, elevated sedimentation rate (ESR) with secondary forms	NA
Radiographic findings	Diffuse vertebral involvement, compression fractures on plain roentgenograms; bone densitometry: DEXA or QCT	NA
Treatment	Calcium, vitamin D, estrogens, calcitonin, bisphosphonates, parathyroid hormone	NA

mass occurs predominantly in the axial skeleton, femoral neck, and pelvis. Loss of bone mass in the axial skeleton predisposes vertebral bodies to fracture, which results in back pain and deformity. Patients with osteoporosis may sustain multiple vertebral fractures over the years, with persistent mechanical pain and limitation of work potential. The diagnosis of osteoporosis is usually made on clinical grounds in a patient with a history of back pain and radiographic findings consistent with the disease. Other significant causes of osteoporosis, including tumors, hematologic disease, endocrinologic disorders, and drugs, must be considered in patients whose history, physical examination, or laboratory findings are not consistent with idiopathic osteoporosis.

Epidemiology

The absolute prevalence of osteoporosis is unknown. The frequency of the disorder depends on the definition of the illness. In the United States, 10 million persons have osteoporosis, whereas another 18 million have low bone mass.[83] Patients who are symptomatic or who have radiographic changes of osteoporosis are easily recognized; however, many osteoporotic individuals are asymptomatic and have not come to medical attention. By radiographic criteria, 29% of women and 18% of men between 45 and 79 years of age have osteoporosis.[7] By a more sensitive method for determining vertebral bone mineral density (BMD), however, 50% of women past age 65 may be found to have asymptomatic osteoporosis.[110] By age 80, 70% of women have osteoporosis.[112] Bone resorption increases with age, with bone loss normally beginning after age 40. In general, males have more bone mass than females, and blacks have more than whites. These facts correlate with the clinical finding of osteoporosis being more common in white women, particularly those of Northern European extraction. In at least 3% of patients with osteoporosis the disease is progressive, disabling, and an impediment to the activities of daily living.[126] During the course of their lifetime, women lose 50% of cancellous bone and 30% of cortical bone, whereas men lose 30% and 20%, respectively. The number of fractures related to osteoporosis in the United States is estimated to be 1.5 million per year.[108] In 1995, the estimated health care costs in the United States were $13.8 billion.[97]

Pathogenesis

The cause of increased bone resorption on the endosteal (inner) surfaces of bone with inadequate compensatory bone formation, osteoporosis, is not well understood. Bone is living tissue that is constantly undergoing remodeling. Before adulthood, during growth, bone formation is greater than bone resorption. In the adult skeleton, up to the age of 30, the deposition and resorption of bone are equal and bone mass in both men and women is maximum at this age. Soon after, men start losing 0.3% of their skeletal bone calcium per year. In women, the rate is initially the same as in men but at menopause it increases to 3% per year.[18,49] Patients with osteoporosis are individuals who either mature with a decreased skeletal mass or have an accelerated rate of bone loss after achieving peak bone density.

Primary Causes

The causes of osteoporosis are listed in Table 14-1.[67] Primary osteoporosis includes postmenopausal or senile osteoporosis and idiopathic, adult or juvenile, osteoporosis. Senile osteoporosis is found in aging men and women, whereas postmenopausal osteoporosis occurs in women after menopause (Table 14-2).[107] Postmenopausal osteoporosis is the most common form of this illness. Juvenile idiopathic osteoporosis occurs in early adolescence and is manifested by fragility in the axial skeleton. The disease may be severe and may cause vertebral fractures, kyphosis, and loss of height. Remissions can occur spontaneously, but the patients seldom achieve normal adult bone mass.

Idiopathic adult osteoporosis is found in men younger than 50 years of age.[51] This illness is often associated with

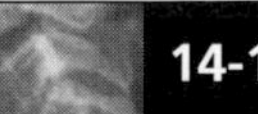

14-1 CAUSES OF OSTEOPOROSIS

PRIMARY

Involutional (postmenopausal or senile)
Idiopathic (juvenile or adult)

SECONDARY

Endocrine

Hypogonadism
Adrenocortical hormone excess (primary or iatrogenic)
Hyperthyroidism
Hyperparathyroidism
Diabetes mellitus
Growth hormone deficiency

Nutritional

Calcium deficiency
Phosphate deficiency
Phosphate excess
Vitamin D deficiency
Protein deficiency
Vitamin C deficiency
Intestinal malabsorption

Drug

Heparin
Anticonvulsants
Ethanol
Methotrexate

Genetic

Osteogenesis imperfecta
Homocystinuria

Miscellaneous

Rheumatoid arthritis
Chronic liver disease
Chronic renal disease
Immobilization
Malignancy (multiple myeloma)
Metabolic acidosis
Cigarette smoking

14-2 TYPES OF INVOLUTIONAL OSTEOPOROSIS

Factor	Type 1 (Postmenopausal)	Type 2 (Senile)
Age (yr)	50-75	Over 70
Sex ratio (M/F)	1:6	1:2
Type of bone loss	Trabecular	Trabecular and cortical
Fracture site	Vertebrae (crush), distal radius	Vertebrae (multiple wedge), hip
Main causes	Menopause	Aging
Calcium absorption	Decreased	Decreased
1,25-$(OH)_2$-vitamin D synthesis from 25-(OH) vitamin D	Secondary decrease	Primary
Parathyroid function	Decreased	Increased

Modified from Riggs BL, Melton LJ III: Involutional osteoporosis. N Engl J Med 314:1676, 1986.

idiopathic hypercalcemia, and the axial skeleton is the area most severely affected.

In men, osteoporosis was thought to be related to hypogonadism related to a depletion of testosterone. A prospective study of 405 men revealed a correlation of low estradiol, not testosterone, as the important hormone in men for maintenance of BMD. Aromatase is an enzyme that converts testosterone to estradiol at the level of the osteoblasts. In elderly men, the effect of testosterone treatment on BMD may be due to conversion of testosterone to estradiol.[4]

Secondary Causes

Hormonal. Secondary forms of osteoporosis may be caused by specific abnormalities, such as a hormonal imbalance that affects bone metabolism. Endocrine abnormalities that can cause osteoporosis should be investigated in any young or middle-aged person with decreased skeletal mass. Hypogonadism with decreased sex hormones can cause bone loss in both men and women, and this also plays a role in postmenopausal osteoporosis, particularly in women who undergo oophorectomy at an early age.[13] Amenorrhea may also play a role in women who exercise excessively.[55] Men undergoing hormonal modifications for prostate cancer with leuprolide develop rapid bone loss.[120] Adrenocortical hormone excess leads to decreased bone mass.[25] Glucocorticoids reduce bone calcium by decreasing intestinal absorption of calcium, by stimulating parathyroid hormone so as to increase bone resorption, and by exerting a direct inhibitory effect on bone metabolism and bone formation. Corticosteroids may also decrease the response of luteinizing hormone to gonadotropin-releasing hormone, thereby decreasing gonadal hormone production.[27] This dual effect may explain the rapid bone loss associated with corticosteroid therapy. The glucocorticoids from endogenous (Cushing's syndrome) or exogenous (cortisone) sources can cause osteoporosis.[1] The effects of corticosteroids are rapid, with significant bone loss occurring during the first 6 months of therapy. The effects are greater on the hip and spine than on the forearm.[127] Patients receiving inhaled corticosteroids for asthma may experience a decrease in BMD.[50] Hyperthyroidism, by increasing general metabolic levels, increases bone turnover and remodeling. Continuous parathyroid hormone excess exerts a direct effect on bone that causes an increase in resorption. Osteoporosis in hyperparathyroidism may develop because of parathyroid tumors or from illnesses that result in parathyroid gland hypertrophy. Whether or not diabetes contributes to the loss of bone mass is controversial, but studies suggest that bone density is decreased in patients with this illness.[78] Growth hormone is important for skeletal growth and maturation, and deficiencies are associated with decreased bone formation and mass.

Nutritional. The mineralization of bone is a complicated process involving a balance between calcium, phosphate, pH levels, hormones, and other factors. A nutritional deficiency of bone minerals or excess of any one of them may have a profound effect on bone mineralization. Low calcium consumption and decreased bone density are typical in women older than 45 years of age.[2] The ratio of calcium to phosphorus or phosphate is altered by fluctuations in phosphorus concentration in nutritional sources, which may lead to bone resorption.[70] Vitamin D in its activated form, 1,25-dihydroxyvitamin D_3, helps maintain serum calcium and phosphate levels by increasing both absorption of these substances from the intestine and their resorption from bone. Sources of vitamin D include fortified milk and fish, along with the endogenous sources created by exposure of skin to the ultraviolet rays in sunlight. Osteoporosis may also be caused by deficiencies of protein and ascorbic acid (vitamin C) as well as by disorders such as celiac disease that result in intestinal malabsorption. Increased intake of vitamin A (>3000 μg/day of retinal equivalents) is associated with a 1.48 relative risk of hip fracture.[37]

Drug. With extended use, certain drugs can lead to osteoporosis but the mechanisms are unknown. They include the anticoagulant heparin, anticonvulsants (e.g., phenytoin), and methotrexate, an antimetabolite used in cancer chemotherapy. Chronic alcoholism is a common cause of bone loss in young men. Osteoporosis in alcoholics is probably related to poor dietary habits and decreased intestinal absorption. In addition, alcohol impairs vitamin D metabolism, has toxic effects on bone tissue, and decreases body mass, resulting in decreased forces on skeletal structures.[114]

Genetic. Genetic causes of osteoporosis are rare. Osteogenesis imperfecta is a severely deforming congenital disease occurring in children and, to a lesser extent, in adults and characterized by skeletal fragility, fractures, blue sclerae, and deafness. Specific disorders of collagen metabolism also result in weakened bones. Homocystinuria, a very rare heritable disorder related to a deficiency in the enzyme cystathionine beta-synthetase, causes mental retardation, tall stature, scoliosis, dislocated lens, and skeletal fragility.

Miscellaneous. A number of unrelated disorders may also cause osteoporosis. Increased blood flow related to synovial inflammation in rheumatoid arthritis causes osteoporosis that is periarticular. Immobilization results in osteoporosis. Mechanical stress increases bone mass and is necessary for maintenance of normal bone architecture.[70] Prolonged immobilization causes a proportionate loss of bone matrix and mineral. Focal loss occurs in bones that have been fractured and have been placed in casts. Generalized bone loss occurs in elderly patients who are chronically ill and are placed in bed.[119] Malignancies, particularly multiple myeloma and other hematologic neoplasms, cause local or general osteoporosis. Acidosis causes increased calcium resorption and, if present on a chronic basis, results in osteoporosis. Women who smoke cigarettes may also be at risk of developing osteoporosis.[23]

Bone Remodeling

Bone loss results from a disturbance of bone remodeling. Bone remodeling replaces old bone matrix with new matrix with an annual turnover rate of 25% in cancellous bone and 3% in cortical bone.[31] In adults, remodeling is the only important mechanism by which new bone is formed. Remodeling occurs in units of bone. A bone remodeling unit is composed of a group of cells removing and replacing bone. These cells include osteoclasts, reversal cells, and osteoblasts.

The process of remodeling is initiated by denuding the bone surface of lining cells derived from osteoblasts. The retraction of these cells allows mononucleated osteoclasts to coalesce into multinucleated, mature osteoclasts in the area vacated by the surface lining cells. The two molecules that are essential and sufficient to promote the differentiation of macrophages to osteoclasts are macrophage colony-stimulating factor (M-CSF) and receptor for activation of nuclear factor kappa B (NF-κB) (RANK) ligand (RANKL).[122] RANKL is expressed by activated T lymphocytes. This may explain the increased osteoclastogenesis associated with inflammatory arthropathies, such as rheumatoid arthritis. An inhibitor of RANKL is osteoprotegrin (OPG). The balance between RANKL and OPG dictates the quantity of bone resorbed. RANKL and RANK are associated with tumor necrosis factor (TNF). RANK and TNF induce similar intracellular signals that result in activation of NF-κB and c-Jun NH_2-terminal kinase. The activated osteoclasts resorb a predetermined volume of bone over 1 to 2 weeks. Once attached to the bone, the osteoclasts generate a local microenvironment on the bone surface. The inorganic mineral phase of hydroxyapatite resorption occurs before type 1 collagen removal. An acidic pH of 4.5 is generated within the microenvironment that mobilizes bone mineral. Subsequently, the collagen is degraded by a lysosomal protease, cathepsin K. Osteoclasts then disappear from the surface and are replaced by mononucleated cells that prepare the surface for new bone formation by osteoblasts. During the reversal phase, a factor is released that signals the change from resorption to formation. Likely candidates for this factor are insulin-like growth factor (IGF)-II or transforming growth factor (TGF)-beta, examples of osteoblast mitogens.[81]

Osteoblasts are of mesenchymal origin and are sophisticated fibroblasts. Mouse models have allowed for a greater understanding of the transcription factors that promote osteoblast function.[33] Cbfa1 is a osteoblast-specific transcription factor and is an activator of transcription that induces osteoblast-specific gene expression in fibroblasts. Once osteoblasts are generated, IGF and TGF-beta control the steady-state level of osteoblasts differentiation. Cbfa1 also regulates the expression of osteocalcin, a gene product expressed only in terminally differentiated osteoblasts. Osteocalcin inhibits osteoblast function. Another important component of bone formation may be under central nervous system control through the effects of leptin on the hypothalamus. Leptin, a product of adipocytes, inhibits bone formation through effects on osteoblasts. The signals to the osteoblasts are mediated through the hypothalamus. This may explain, in part, the effect of obesity on bone density. Once osteoblasts are differentiated and stimulated, bone formation occurs. The recruitment of osteoblasts results in the filling in of the cavity made by the osteoclasts. The filling-in process progresses and is concluded by mineralization of the osteoid manufactured by these cells after a 25- to 35-day delay. Disruption of the process results in an imbalance of resorption and formation, causing a loss of bone mineral. Increased activity of osteoclasts results in larger lacunae. Lack of the reversing factor may stall formation. Osteoblasts may have inadequate amounts of factors, such as calcium, phosphate, and vitamin D, to mineralize bone fully (osteomalacia).

As mentioned previously, parathyroid hormone (PTH), 1,25-dihydroxyvitamin D, and calcitonin are important in the maintenance of serum calcium levels. With increasing age, calcium intestinal absorption declines and renal function falls, limiting the amount of activated vitamin D manufactured. The increase in PTH levels is a secondary response to the lower calcium levels. Increased PTH causes activation of more remodeling units and greater loss of bone.

In postmenopausal women, the loss of estrogens results in the activation of increased numbers of remodeling units. The increased calcium levels inhibit the release of PTH and decrease the intestinal absorption of calcium. Estrogens may also have effects on a number of factors that affect bone metabolism, including calcitonin, interleukin (IL)-1 and IL-6, TGF-beta, prostaglandin E_2, tumor necrosis factor, and IGF.[52,93] Increased levels of IL-1 and IL-6 recruit osteoclasts, resulting in increased bone resorption. IL-1 stimulates M-CSF expression by marrow stromal cells. M-CSF stimulates osteoclast differentiation. Estrogen treatment reverses the increased production of IL-1 in menopausal women.[86]

Local factors that have effects on bone metabolism may also play a role in the development of osteoporosis. Prostaglandins, osteoclast-activating factors, and bone-derived growth factors are a few of the substances that are the targets of studies researching the overall pathogenesis of osteoporosis.[92]

CLINICAL HISTORY

Certain risk factors predispose particular patients to osteoporosis, especially of the involutional (senile or postmenopausal) variety. Risk factors for osteoporosis include (1) female gender, (2) age 20 years post menopausal, (3) white or Asian race, (4) positive family history, (5) premature menopause, (6) inactivity, (7) associated diseases (bowel resection, thyrotoxicosis, hyperparathyroidism), and (8) drugs (corticosteroids, anticonvulsants, ethanol, smoking). Low body weight is also considered a risk factor for osteoporosis.[72] For example, anorexia nervosa is associated with an increased risk for decreased BMD.[66]

Patients with vertebral osteoporosis may be asymptomatic, with the diagnosis being made on radiographs taken for other purposes. Symptomatic osteoporosis presents as midline back pain localized over the thoracic or lumbar spine, the most common location for fractures. Most vertebral body fractures occur after some mechanical stress such as slipping on a stair, lifting, or jumping. The patient with an acute fracture has severe pain localized over the affected vertebral body.

Occasionally the pain radiates into the flanks, upper portion of the posterior thighs, or abdomen. Spasm of the paraspinous muscles contributes to the back pain. Back motion aggravates the discomfort, and many patients attempt to reduce the pain by remaining motionless in bed, frequently lying on their side. Prolonged sitting, standing, and the Valsalva maneuver intensify the pain. Severe pain usually lasts 3 to 4 months and then resolves. However, some patients are left with persistent, nagging, dull spinal pain after vertebral body fracture secondary to osteoporosis, and this pain may persist even in the absence of new fractures on radiographs. The source of this pain may be microfractures too small to be detected by radiographs or biomechanical effects of the deformity on the lumbar spine below. Recurrent pain, increased deformity, and loss of height suggest new fractures. Most patients do not have constant, sharp pain in the interval between fractures. Vertebral fractures of the dorsal spine result in anterior compression of the vertebral body. This kyphotic deformity (dowager's or widow's hump) can cause a compensatory flattening of the lumbar lordosis and low back pain. Multiple compression fractures may also cause persistent pain due to mechanical stress on ligaments, muscles, and apophyseal joints. They also result in a loss in height, and this is one of the parameters used to follow the progression of the disease. Because the disease affects only the anterior components of the vertebral bodies, neural compression is not associated with vertebral osteoporosis. Neurologic or radicular symptoms distant from an area of fracture are unusual; and if they are present, other pathologic conditions must be considered.

PHYSICAL EXAMINATION

Physical findings commonly include pain over the spinous process of the fractured vertebral body on percussion and associated spasm of surrounding paraspinous muscles. Patients with multiple fractures may demonstrate a loss of height and kyphoscoliosis. Neurologic examination is normal. On abdominal examination, patients with severe pain secondary to acute fracture may demonstrate a loss of bowel sounds, ileus, or bladder distention secondary to acute urinary retention.

LABORATORY DATA

Laboratory parameters in primary osteoporosis, such as serum calcium, phosphate, and alkaline phosphatase, are normal. Although urinary concentrations of calcium are normal, the amount of urinary calcium is high in relation to oral intake. Urinary hydroxyproline, an indicator of collagen breakdown, is normal. The presence of anemia, elevated ESR, rheumatoid factor, elevated serum proteins, or increased serum calcium suggests a secondary form of osteoporosis and requires further investigation. If there is a concern that osteomalacia may be playing a role in osteopenia, vitamin D levels should be measured. Thyroid hormone determinations along with any additional tests to eliminate renal, liver, parathyroid, and gastrointestinal disorders may be indicated in the setting of the appropriate history.

Bone Turnover Measures

New methods have been developed to detect bone resorption based on the measurement of the breakdown products of collagen. Pyridinoline (Pyr) and deoxypyridinoline (D-Pyr) are nonreducible crosslinks that stabilize the collagen chains in extracellular matrix. Pyr and D-Pyr are released from bone matrix during its degradation by osteoclasts.[29] These nonreducible crosslinks are excreted in the urine in free form and can be measured by fluorimetry after high-pressure liquid chromatography (HPLC) extraction of hydrolized urine. Cross-linked N-telopeptides (NTX) of type 1 collagen are also a marker of bone resorption.[115] Increased levels of NTX are associated with decreased BMD levels. There is a correlation between markers of bone turnover and subsequent rates of bone loss.[14,113] Elevated levels of D-Pyr are associated with patients with vertebral osteoporosis.[30] Currently, the test has assay variability with no synthetic standard. The amount excreted also varies with time of day and menstrual cycle. A consensus does not exist in regard to the need for bone turnover markers in the treatment and monitoring of osteoporosis. Controversy also exists regarding the best markers to monitor. One approach using bone turnover markers suggests that measuring BMD and markers at baseline, followed by a repeat measurement of markers after 3 months of antiresorptive therapy, is useful. Patients who have a fall of urinary NTX excretion of 50% will have a maintenance of BMD with bisphosphonate therapy.[95] The use of bone turnover markers may be most appropriate for women with alterations in the lumbar spine that make serial BMD measurements problematic.[34]

Pathology

Biopsy of osteoporotic bone reveals a reduction of thickness of cortical bone. In trabecular bone, the trabeculae within the medullary cavity are markedly thin and reduced in number. The biopsy contains no osteoid (Fig. 14-1).

RADIOGRAPHIC EVALUATION

Roentgenograms

Roentgenographic evaluation of osteopenia is best made from the lateral projection of the spine. Roentgenographic abnormalities of vertebral osteoporosis include changes in radiolucency, trabecular pattern, and shape of vertebral bone (Fig. 14-2).[89] Early osteoporosis may not be demonstrated on roentgenograms until 30% of bone mass has been lost.[6] An early finding is the accentuation of the mineral density of the vertebral endplates because osteoporosis causes increasing lucency of the central portion of the vertebral body; however, the outer dimensions of the body remain the same, with sharply defined margins.[123] Horizontal trabeculae are thinned, accentuating the vertical trabeculae that remain. This pattern is similar to that seen with hemangiomas. Prominent vertical trabeculae are limited to one vertebral body with a hemangioma, whereas multiple vertebrae are affected with osteoporosis. Osteoporosis may progress to the point where vertebral body contours may be affected, and "fish" or "codfish" vertebrae occur when intervertebral discs expand into weakened vertebral bone, causing an exaggerated biconcavity. "Fish" vertebrae are particularly common in the lower thoracic and upper lumbar spine. This deformity is more likely to be seen in young adults with osteopenia.

An anterior wedge compression fracture is manifested by a decrease in anterior height, usually 4 mm or greater, compared with the vertical height of the posterior body. A transverse compression fracture results in equal loss of both anterior and posterior heights. Many patients will demonstrate roentgenographic changes of "fish," anterior wedging, and compression vertebrae in the thoracic and lumbar spine. The changes in osteoporotic vertebrae are unevenly distributed along the spine,[8] with no two affected exactly alike (Fig. 14-3). "Fish" vertebrae may occur asymptomatically. Anterior wedging and compression in osteoporosis indicate a fracture of the vertebral body and are associated with sudden, severe episodes of incapacitating back pain in most circumstances (Fig. 14-4).

Scintigraphy

For the most part, bone scintigraphy is not useful in differentiating the various forms of metabolic bone disease.[129]

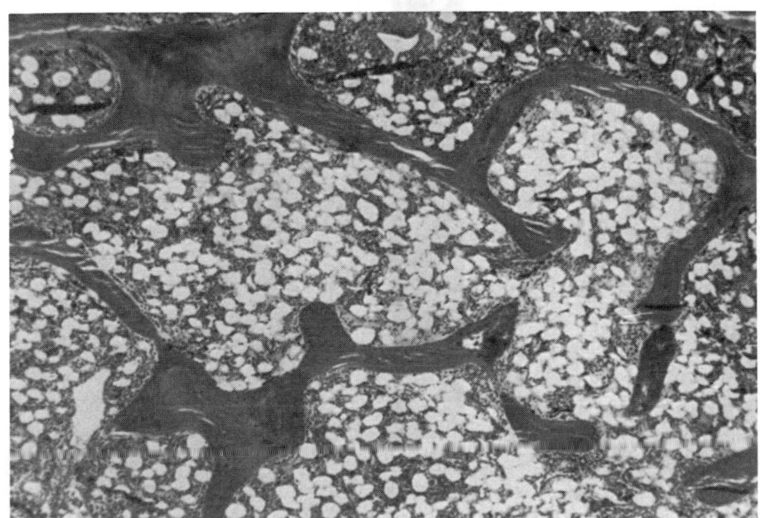

Figure 14-1 Osteoporosis. Histologic section demonstrating decreased bone and no osteoid. *(Courtesy of Arnold Schwartz, MD.)*

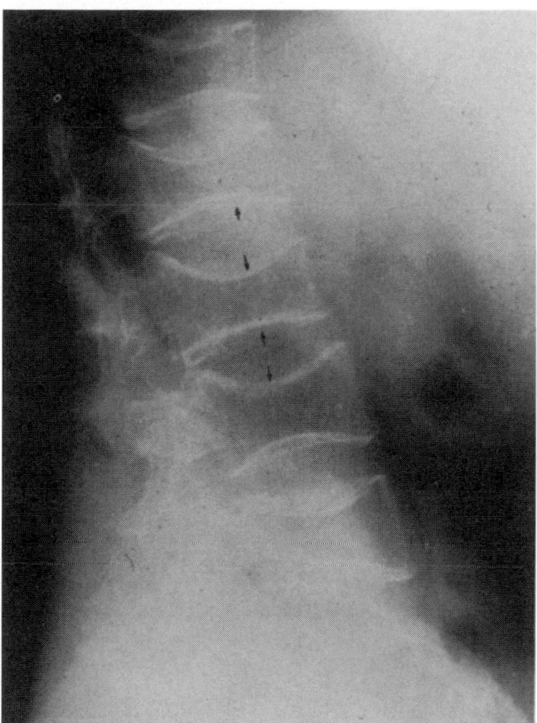

Figure 14-2 Osteoporosis. Roentgenogram shows generalized loss of bone mineral in multiple vertebral bodies along with thin cortical endplates in a 60-year-old woman with diffuse midline back pain. Disc expansion into vertebral bodies is associated with weakened bone structures *(arrows)*. *(Courtesy of Anne Brower, MD.)*

Bone scan is more helpful in detecting increased focal bone formation associated with acute spinal compression fractures. However, old fractures may remain "hot" on bone scan for months and may make identifying the most recent fracture site difficult.

Bone Mineral Density Measurements

A number of radiographic techniques exist to measure bone calcium. They include radiographic photodensitometry, photon absorptiometry (single and dual), neutron activation, and CT.[41,89] Controversy surrounds the utility of these radiographic techniques in predicting those individuals at risk for vertebral fractures. Two editorials in respected journals suggest that these techniques are not indicated in the common office setting.[45,85] Since these editorials were written, greater sophistication has developed in the measurement of bone mineral calcium.[60] The major questions that concern bone densitometry are the accuracy and reproducibility of calcium measurement and associated risk of fracture. Characteristics of the more commonly utilized densitometry methods are listed in Table 14-3.[133] Plain roentgenograms may be helpful at estimating bone loss but are relatively inaccurate.[79] Physicians have been divided into two major camps in regard to the utility of vertebral bone densitometry. Some physicians believe that clinical risk factors should be used to identify women needing preventive therapy and that

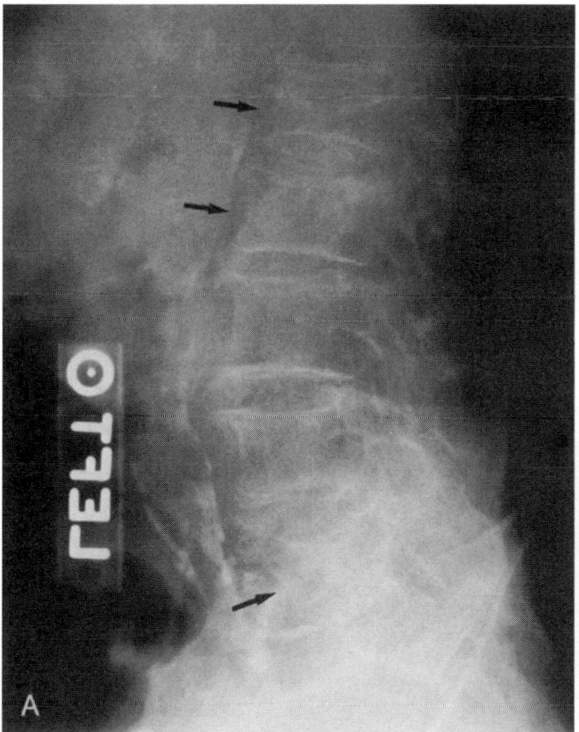

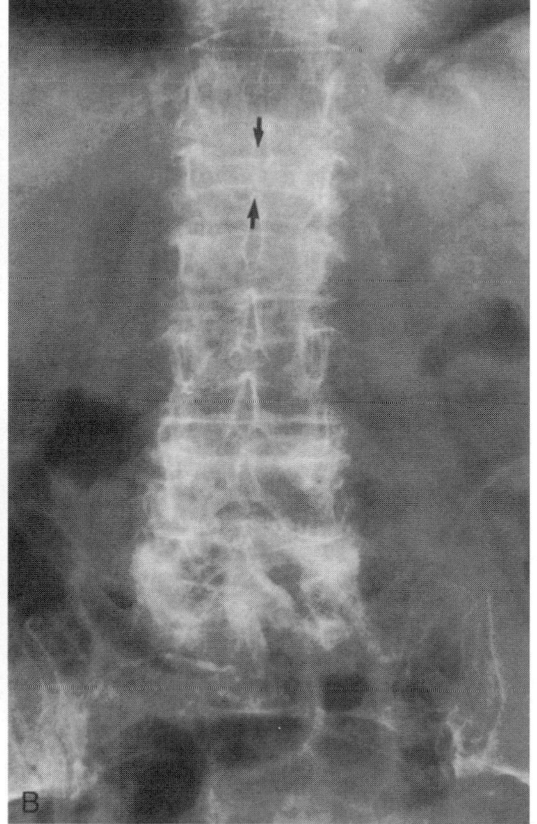

Figure 14-3 An 83-year-old woman presented with a history of acute low back pain localized to the thoracolumbar junction. *A*, Lateral view reveals generalized osteoporosis with diminished height of L1, L2, and L5 *(arrows)*. *B*, Anteroposterior view reveals marked loss of height of the L1 vertebral body *(arrows)*.

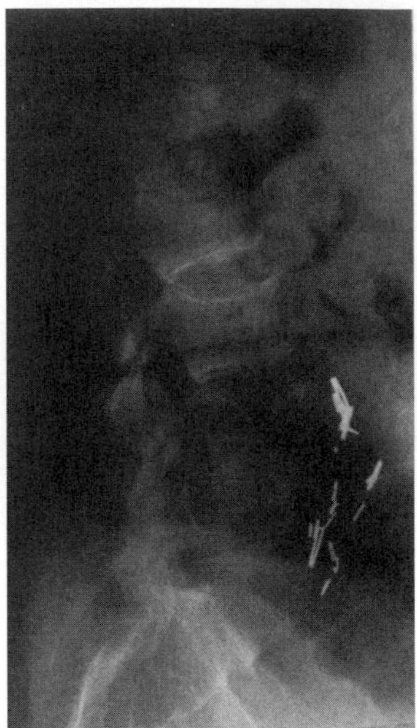

Figure 14-4 Osteoporosis. Lateral roentgenogram demonstrates vertebral compression fractures in vertebral bodies L1, L2, L3, and L4. Disc degeneration is noted at L4-L5 with complete obliteration of the disc space with degenerative spondylolisthesis. *(From Borenstein DG: Low back pain. In Kippel J, Duppe P [eds]: Rheumatology. St Louis, CV Mosby, 1994, Sec 5, p 4.18.)*

vertebral fractures are a better way to measure outcome than densitometry. Others believe that not all women with clinical risk factors should receive treatment because of toxicities of therapy, and treatment should be restricted to those whose bone mass is 1 to 2 standard deviations (SDs) below age-matched controls.[75]

Quantitative Computed Tomography

The two techniques most commonly thought to be accurate for the determination of vertebral bone density are dual energy x-ray absorptiometry (DEXA) and quantitated computed tomography (QCT).[44,87] Both methods have their advantages and disadvantages. QCT is better able to separate the contribution of cortical and cancellous bone to bone density. QCT allows for three-dimensional BMD calculation. It has somewhat better predictive value for spine fractures than DEXA. The test has a high cost compared with other techniques.

Dual Energy X-ray Absorptiometry

Central DEXA (spine, hip, and wrist examination) is the "gold standard" for BMD evaluation. DEXA has better approximation of bone mineral with the use of lateral images that remove osteophytes and calcified ligaments from the measurement. This change in method has improved its accuracy. DEXA has 1/100 the x-ray exposure of QCT in the measurement of bone mineral, about one tenth of a chest roentgenogram. The test can be completed rapidly in minutes. This difference in exposure is important when screening postmenopausal healthy women.[57]

Other Measurements

Other forms of measurement of BMD include evaluation of the calcaneus with DEXA (peripheral) and ultrasonometry. Although these forms of measurement are convenient, they are not as accurate as a central DEXA of the spine and hip. Peripheral DEXA provides less precise T scores that do not correlate well with data generated by central DEXA. Ultrasonometry uses sound wave attenuation and speed of sound to measure BMD of the heel. The technique has also been used to measure tibia, wrist, and phalanges. The test is limited by reproducibility and variations in heel shapes. The test is available, quick, and inexpensive. However, full-body DEXA remains the measurement of choice.

The important measurement determined by DEXA is the T score. The T score measures BMD as matched to normal, healthy young control subjects at peak bone

14-3 BONE DENSITOMETRY METHODS FOR THE SPINE

Technique	Radiation	Precision/ Accuracy (%)*	Scan Time (min)	Comments
Plain x-ray	400-1000 mrem			Available; insensitive
Dual photon absorptiometry (DPA)	5 mrem	2-4/4-6	20-30	Density correlates with risk for fracture; repositioning problem for sequential studies
Dual energy x-ray absorptiometry (DEXA)	5 mrem	1-2/2-6	7	Sequential studies are reliable; spurs increase bone density
Quantitative computed tomography (QCT)	400-1000 mrem	3-5/2-10	20	Density correlates with risk for spine fracture; expensive; low reading for extra marrow fat

*Precision: reproducibility of test; accuracy: correct amount measured against standards.
Modified from White PH: Osteopenic disorders of the spine. Semin Spine Surg 2:121, 1990.

mass.[116] A T score of −1.0 signifies a 10% to 12% loss of bone mass compared with mean values for young normal adults. The Z score represents an individual's BMD compared with a healthy age-matched and sex-matched person and may detect the presence of secondary causes of osteoporosis. An individual within 1 SD of normal is considered normal; between 1 and 2.5 SD below normal is osteopenia, more than 2.5 SD is osteoporotic; and more than 2.5 SD and one or more fractures is considered severe osteoporosis. For each one SD fall in BMD below the mean, the hip is associated with an increased relative risk of 2.6 for a hip fracture. The same decrease of BMD at the lumbar spine causes an increased relative risk of 2.4 for vertebral fractures.[73] Therefore, for each 1-SD decrease in BMD, there is a doubling of fracture risk.

The role of bone densitometry continues to evolve. The use of bone densitometry in general clinical practice will be decided on scientific and financial (reimbursement) concerns. The U.S. Preventive Services Task Force has recommended DEXA screening of the femur for osteoporosis for women who are older than 65 years. Women between 60 and 65 years of age should be screened if they have an additional risk factor.[125]

Concerns also exist in regard to monitoring of osteoporosis therapy with repeat bone densitometry measurements. The measurements that are used to monitor the effects of treatment are imperfect. The measurement values vary from time to time because of inherent variations in the patient. This variability may produce changes in values that could be mistaken as therapeutic benefit or failure. Patients who lose BMD in the first year of therapy with alendronate or raloxifene will gain BMD when the same therapy is continued. Changes in therapy should not be considered only on the basis of DEXA data.[24]

DIFFERENTIAL DIAGNOSIS

In most patients with diffuse osteoporosis of the axial skeleton, vertebral compression fractures, and no abnormalities on laboratory evaluation, the diagnosis of osteoporosis is made on clinical grounds alone. Suspicion for the diagnosis is also heightened if the patient has any risk factors that are associated with osteoporosis, such as sedentary lifestyle; low calcium intake; early menopause or oophorectomy; cigarette smoking; excessive consumption of alcohol, protein, or caffeine; slender build; or a family history of osteoporosis.[48] Low levels of estrogen in the bloodstream of menstruating women may also be a risk factor for decreased bone mass.[54]

Secondary causes of osteoporosis as listed in Table 14-1 should be considered in patients with abnormal laboratory findings such as anemia, elevated ESR, abnormal serum proteins, or hypovitaminosis D. Osteoporosis may be complicated by osteomalacia in 8% of postmenopausal women. Osteomalacia is a metabolic bone disease characterized by decreased bone mineralization with normal bone matrix, usually secondary to inadequate vitamin D. Osteomalacia is usually associated with normal or low concentrations of serum calcium, decreased concentration of phosphorus, and increased levels of alkaline phosphatase. Osteoporosis and osteomalacia may be indistinguishable by clinical and radiologic criteria. Bone biopsy is useful in detecting the presence of osteomalacia complicating osteoporosis and is indicated when the diagnoses are in doubt, because specific therapy is available for osteomalacia. Other methods for measuring bone calcium include dual-photon absorptiometry (DPA), neutron activation analysis, and QCT; however, the significance of the measurement results remains to be determined. Therefore, these methods should not be utilized to predict patients at risk for osteoporosis in the usual clinical setting.

The differential diagnosis of abnormalities in vertebral body shape depends on the configuration of the alteration and its focal or generalized distribution. Biconcave ("fish") vertebrae occur with osteomalacia, Paget's disease, and hyperparathyroidism. Schmorl's nodes occur with Scheuermann's disease, trauma, and hyperparathyroidism. Flattened vertebrae occur with eosinophilic granuloma.

Sacral Insufficiency Fractures

Trauma to the spine can cause vertebral fractures. Patients with such injuries experience acute pain over the area traumatized. Not only are the bones of the vertebral column affected, but the bony pelvis may also be traumatized and cause back pain (Fig. 14-5). Insufficiency fractures of the sacrum may occur independent of trauma to the pelvis. Patients with metabolic bone disease, pelvic irradiation, or corticosteroid therapy may be at increased risk of fracture.[21,22] The typical patient is a woman who is 55 years of age or older with dull buttock pain and with risk factors. Patients experience acute onset of back pain with radiation into the buttock or leg with no antecedent history of trauma. Subtle alterations in bone architecture seen on plain roentgenograms are frequently missed on initial readings (Fig. 14-6). Bone scintiscan or CT scans are useful to detect the presence of fractures. Most patients improve with resolution of pain and healing of fractures with an extended period of controlled mobilization. Nonsurgical therapy also consists of analgesics, including calcitonin.

Vertebral Osteonecrosis

One other entity associated with vertebral collapse is Kümmell's disease or osteonecrosis of a vertebral body.[11] Not infrequently these patients are receiving long-term corticosteroid therapy and develop pain localized over a vertebral body (Fig. 14-7).[42] Plain roentgenograms demonstrate vertebral collapse with intravertebral body gas (Fig. 14-8). CT scan demonstrates the gas in the cortical margins of the vertebral body. The presence of gas in the body is distinctive. Metastatic lesions and fractures do not exhibit an intravertebral vacuum sign. Although it has not been reported in the spine, intraosseous gas accumulation does occur in osteomyelitis.[94] This possibility must be considered in the patient taking corticosteroids who develops intraosseous gas and collapse of a vertebral body. In these patients, MR examination may be useful in identifying spinal cord or nerve root compression associated with vertebral body collapse.[15] With MR, a distinction can be

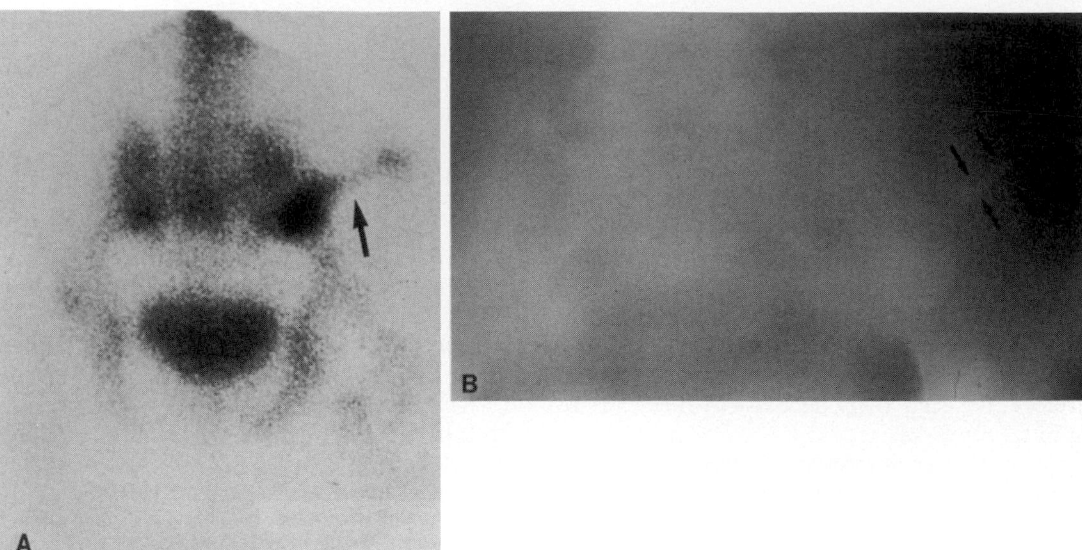

Figure 14-5 A 69-year-old woman was receiving nonsteroidal drugs and prednisone for an asymmetrical polyarthritis. After a number of months on therapy, she developed excruciating low back pain without antecedent trauma. *A*, Bone scan reveals linear uptake in the left ilium *(arrow)*. *B*, Tomogram of left ilium reveals healing fracture that resulted from osteoporosis *(arrows)*. *(Courtesy of David Caldwell, MD.)*

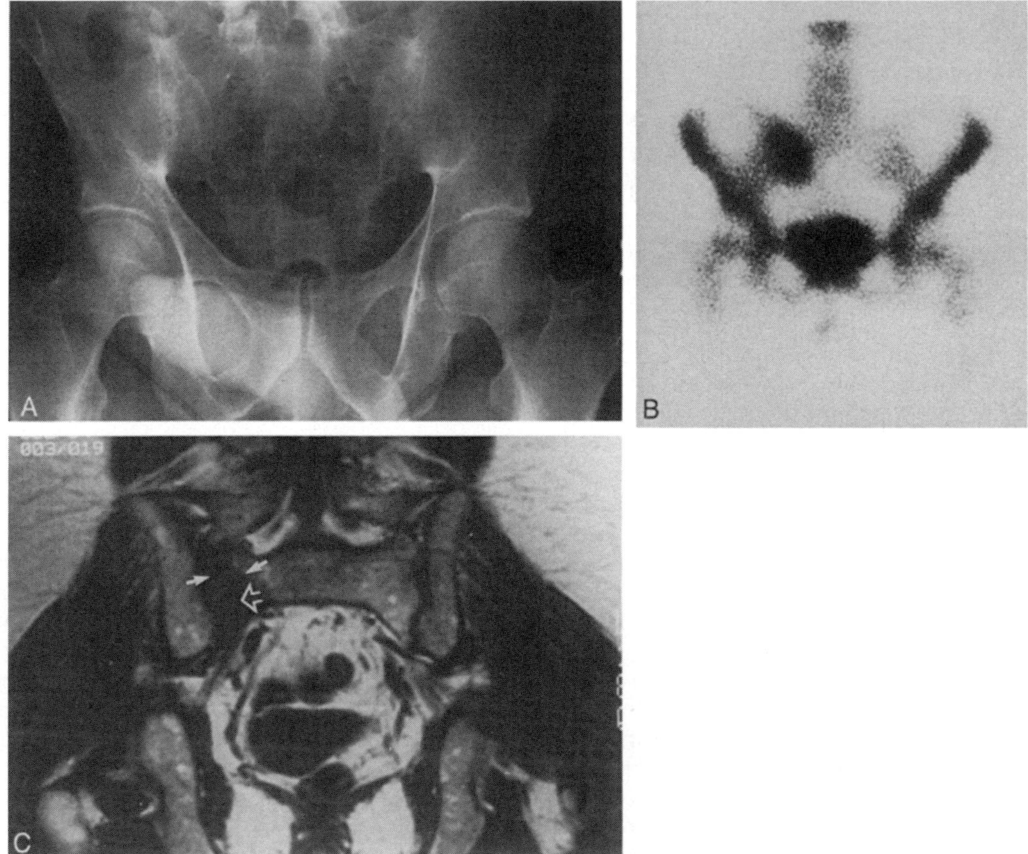

Figure 14-6 Sacral insufficiency fracture. A 57-year-old woman with severe asthma requiring high-dose corticosteroids for many years developed spontaneous right-sided low back pain with radiation into the right buttock. *A*, Plain roentgenogram of the pelvis. No specific abnormality was noted. Persistent pain continued despite maximum medical therapy. *B*, Bone ^{99m}Tc MDP scintiscan. Marked increase in tracer uptake was noted over the right sacrum. *C*, MR of the pelvis. The coronal section of this T1-weighted image reveals abnormal signal in the right sacrum. The changes are compatible with inflammation surrounding a fracture *(white arrows)*. The fracture is noted in the lateral aspect of the sacrum *(open arrow)*. This MR image was originally misread as being normal. The patient improved with 6 weeks of controlled physical activity and crutch walking.

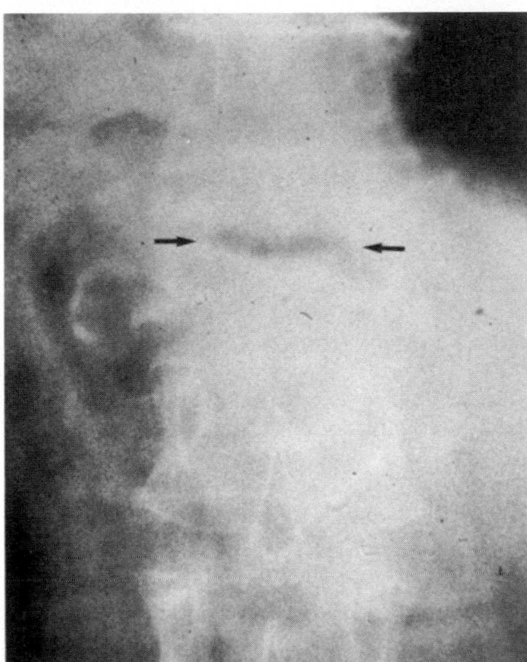

Figure 14-7 Osteonecrosis. Anteroposterior view of the lumbar spine of a patient on long-term corticosteroid therapy who developed acute-onset low back pain. Osteonecrosis has resulted in an intravertebral vacuum sign *(arrows)*. *(Courtesy of David Caldwell, MD.)*

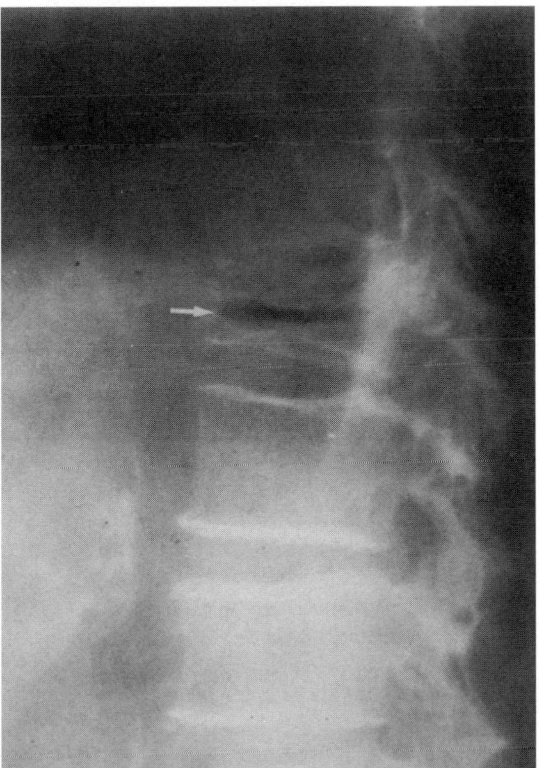

Figure 14-8 Osteonecrosis of a vertebral body in a patient with systemic lupus erythematosus receiving corticosteroids, demonstrated by linear lucency of the vertebral body *(arrow)*, vertebral body collapse, and relative preservation of intervertebral disc spaces. *(Courtesy of Anne Brower, MD.)*

made between malignant compression fractures and those caused by benign processes.[136]

TREATMENT

Prevention

The treatment of osteoporosis should be primarily directed at young adult women at risk to help prevent the disease. Preventive factors include a high calcium intake, at least 1000 mg/day, regular exercise, and avoidance of excessive protein, alcohol, smoking, and caffeine.[3] In postmenopausal women, preventive measures may also be helpful in slowing bone calcium loss. These measures include increased calcium intake and regular exercise against gravity, which must be performed at least 3 hours per week.[16,19] Exercise improves BMD and decreases all-cause mortality.[59] Tai chi is a form of exercise that improves balance and decreases risk of falling, which is another factor associated with fractures.[134]

Combinations of these various therapies have been associated with varying degrees of slowing or preventing bone loss. Combined calcium and exercise is effective at slowing bone loss.[91] Calcium alone may be more helpful at slowing bone loss at the radius and hip than at the spine, and calcium citrate malate is more effective than supplementation with calcium carbonate according to one study.[28] Alendronate, a bisphosphonate, at a dose of 5 mg/day, prevents loss of BMD at the spine and hip in early postmenopausal women.[76]

Acute Therapy

Patients who sustain an acute compression fracture experience severe pain and require bed rest for relief of the discomfort associated with physical activity. The period of bed rest, however, should be kept to a minimum, because immobilization speeds bone resorption. Bed rest is usually kept to about a week. Analgesics in the form of salicylates or other NSAIDs are useful in controlling pain. Pain from paravertebral muscle spasm is responsive to muscle relaxants. Lumbosacral corsets increase intra-abdominal pressure and provide comfort but are usually poorly tolerated and tend to weaken abdominal muscles. The back pain usually resolves spontaneously over 3 to 4 months, and patients are encouraged to participate in non–weight-bearing exercises (such as swimming initially) and resume normal weight-bearing activity (e.g., walking) as soon as possible.

Chronic Therapy

The long-term goal in patients with osteoporotic fractures is to slow the rate of bone resorption, thereby reducing the possibility of additional fractures and progressive deformity. Medical therapies are directed at increasing calcium absorption and improving bone mineralization. No one regimen has been shown to be effective for all patients with osteoporosis (Table 14-4). Calcium supplements

14-4 THERAPY FOR OSTEOPOROSIS

1. Encourage gravity exercises, including back extension exercises and balance exercises, strengthening abdominal muscles; acute fracture—analgesics, nasal calcitonin, braces
2. Recommended therapy:

Drug	Positive Effects	Negative Effects	Recommended Doses and Duration
Calcium	Prevents further bone loss Overcomes malabsorption	Rare Constipation	1000-1500 mg minimal daily requirement Milk: three to four 8-oz glasses Calcium citrate most easily absorbed
Vitamin D: 1-alpha-OH D_3 25-OH D_3 1,25-$(OH)_2$ D_3	Overcomes calcium malabsorption of advancing age	Hypercalciuria Hypercalcemia	50,000 units two times weekly or 25-OH D_3 50 mg MWF in patients with 24-hr urine calcium < 150 mg Do not allow urine calcium to exceed 300 mg/24 hr
Estrogens	Reduce bone resorption	Bone formation rates will decrease over several months Cancer of uterus Breast cancer Vascular clotting	No longer recommended
SERM	Reduces bone resorption	Poorly tolerated in women with hot flashes No significant effect on nonvertebral fractures	Raloxifene, 60 mg/day FDA approved
Calcitonin	Reduces bone resorption Best effect in high turnover osteoporosis, fracture pain reduction	Allergic reactions Hypocalcemia	25-100 MRC units SQ daily or every other day Need rest period off drug every 12-18 mo 100 MRC units intranasally per day FDA approved
Thiazides	Decrease urinary excretion of calcium	Hypokalemia Efficacy unproven	≥25 mg daily?
Bisphosphonates	Reduce bone resorption	Continuous use can result in osteomalacia Occasional gastrointestinal upset	Alendronate, 10 mg/day or 70 mg/wk Risedronate, 5 mg/day or 35 mg/wk FDA approved Intravenous preparations: Pamidronate and zoledronic acid for hypercalcemia of malignancy FDA approved; FDA approval pending for osteoporosis therapy Poor absorption with calcium or food (taken with large glass of water 30 minutes before food) MUST REMAIN UPRIGHT
Sodium fluoride	Stimulates osteoid formation Reduces bone resorption Replaces calcium in hydroxyapatite: crystal is denser	Osteomalacia may occur Bone crystal may be brittle and cortical fractures increased Gastrointestinal discomfort Acne Arthralgias/arthritis Periostosis	No longer recommended

FDA, Food and Drug Administration; SERM, selective estrogen receptor modulator.

alone have been shown to decrease the vertebral fracture rate in osteoporosis in some studies.[109] Other studies have demonstrated the inability of calcium alone in increasing BMD.[38] The daily requirement of calcium in perimenopausal women is 1.3 to 1.5 g/day.[98] In a double-blind, controlled study, it was shown that calcium supplements alone are not as effective as estrogen for the prevention of trabecular bone loss associated with postmenopausal osteoporosis.[111] It is important to remember that urinary calcium increases by about 6% of any increase in dietary intake of calcium. Therefore, an increase of 1000 mg of calcium will increase urinary calcium about 60 mg in 24 hours.

Calcium

A study has tested the absorption of calcium from calcium salt preparations (e.g., calcium gluconate or calcium carbonate) and milk. Approximately a third of the available calcium was absorbed from the calcium salts and milk. The applicability of the findings of the study to the absorption of calcium from over-the-counter calcium preparations is not clear, because the study used analytic grade preparations of the salts in capsules. In addition, the subjects used for the study were normal men. The application of the study findings to women and older individuals remains to be determined.[117] The management of symptomatic individuals with osteoporosis in whom urinary calcium is less than 100 mg/24 hr should include calcium, 1000 to 1500 mg/day, and vitamin D, 50,000 units twice a week. Urinary calcium should be kept under 300 mg for 24 hours and should be monitored every 4 months. The bioavailablity of the calcium preparation is also important (Fig. 14-9). The calcium tablet can be tested by observing the dissolution of the tablet in a small volume of acetic acid in less than 30 minutes. Studies using calcium alone as a study group have demonstrated that this supplement is inadequate by itself to treat osteoporosis.[38]

Vitamin D

Vitamin D helps increase calcium absorption from the gut. The improvement in bone mineralization after the institution of vitamin D therapy may be related to the presence of osteomalacia in some elderly patients with osteoporosis.[69] The principal effect of calcium supplements and vitamin D therapy may be to decrease bone turnover and increase intestinal absorption. Vitamin D does not increase bone mass or decrease fracture rates.[106] Doses of 50,000 units of vitamin D once a week are usually well tolerated; however, complications of vitamin D therapy given in more frequent doses include hypercalcemia, nephrocalcinosis, and/or nephrolithiases (renal stones). Measurement of 24-hour urinary calcium excretion every 4 to 6 months is indicated to detect the presence of hypercalciuria, a condition associated with the formation of calcium-containing renal stones.

Hormone Replacement

Estrogens, female sex hormones, tend to decrease bone resorption and enhance bone mass by slowing the rate at which bone loss occurs.[17] A beneficial effect of estrogens in combination with calcium in preventing the progression of osteoporosis has been reported.[36] Estrogens are effective at decreasing the risk of fractures.[62] The effects of estrogens seem to be maximal when treatment is initiated early in the postmenopausal period. Patients are usually treated for a minimum of 5 to 10 years. Estrogens also are helpful in patients with well-established osteoporosis.[64] These

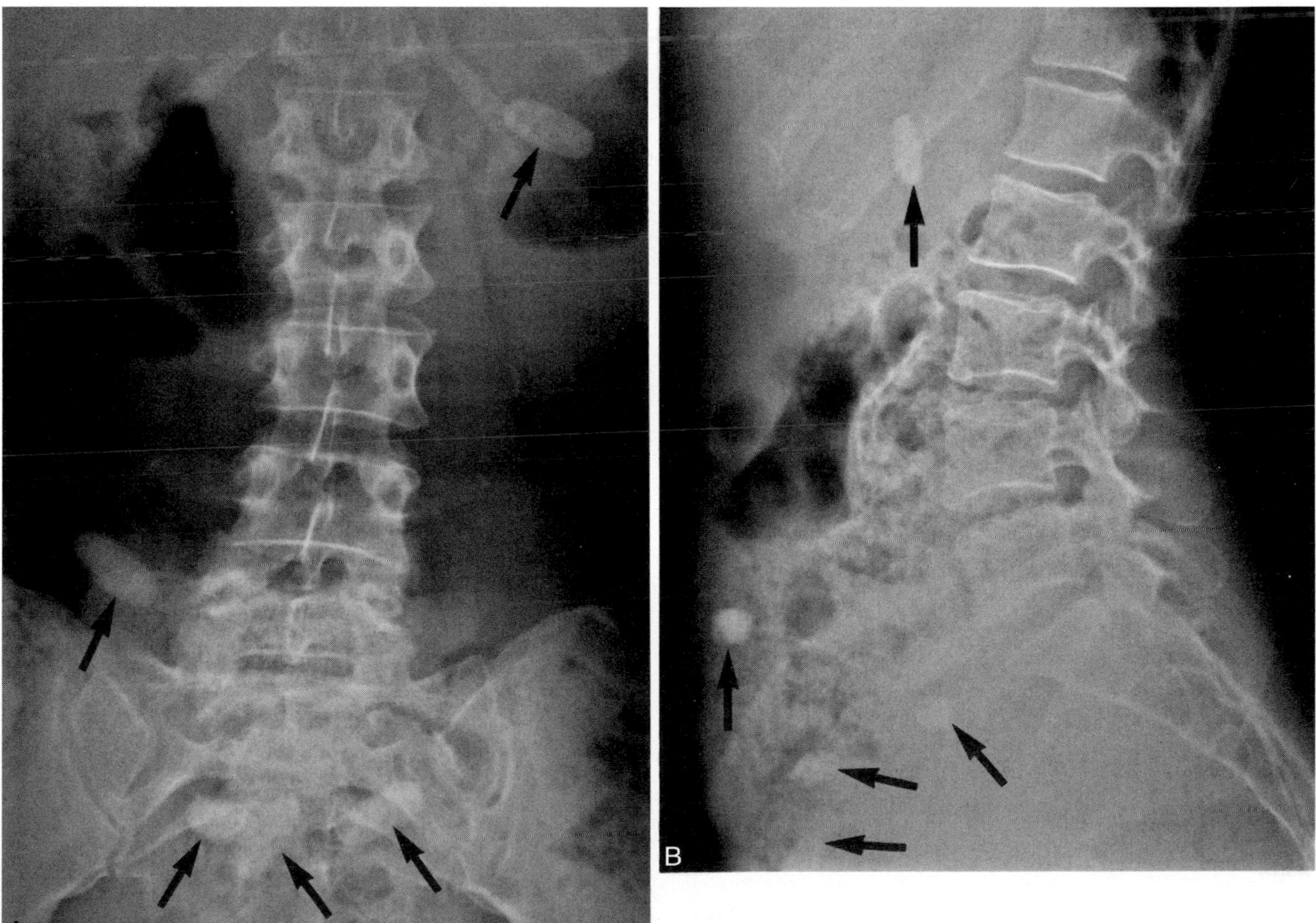

Figure 14-9 Calcium tablets. A 48-year-old woman was taking calcium tablets for osteoporosis. Anteroposterior *(A)* view and lateral *(B)* view demonstrate five *(black arrows)* undissolved calcium tablets.

hormones are given daily for 3 weeks and then withheld for 5 to 7 days to allow withdrawal bleeding and endometrial shedding. Estrogens also may be given by transdermal patches. This form of estrogen therapy is associated with decreased bone loss.[103] The use of low-dose progesterone may limit side effects of estrogen in postmenopausal women. Estrogens are not used routinely in patients with osteoporosis because of side effects, which include vaginal bleeding and breast engorgement. Another significant potential complication of estrogen therapy is the increase in risk of endometrial cancer.[5] The use of progesterone decreases this risk. The effects of estrogen last only as long as the patient takes the hormone replacement. Rapid bone loss occurs once the estrogen is stopped.[63] Estrogens may also be a cause of low back pain. In a postal questionnaire of 1324 women between 55 and 56 years of age, 48.2% of hormone recipients had back pain compared with 42% without replacement. The risk factor associated with hormonal back pain was low back pain with pregnancy.[12] Patients taking these replacement female hormones need to be followed closely by a gynecologist.

The Women's Health Initiative randomized controlled trial reported data that have had a significant impact on the use of estrogen replacement therapy. Overall health risks exceeded benefits from the use of combined estrogen plus progestin. Increased risks were documented for breast cancer, myocardial infarction, stroke, pulmonary emboli, and deep venous thrombosis. This large study sponsored by the National Institutes of Health of 16,608 postmenopausal women was stopped prematurely because of these data. The recommendations of the study included the discontinuation of combination hormonal therapy for any indication.[135]

SERM

Raloxifene is a nonsteroidal selective estrogen receptor modulator (SERM) that suppresses bone turnover, improves BMD, and decreases total and low-density lipoprotein cholesterol levels, without any effect on the uterus or breast. Raloxifene is approved by the U.S. Food and Drug Administration (FDA) for the prevention and treatment of osteoporosis in postmenopausal women only. It reduces vertebral fractures by 50%, a rate that mirrors bisphosphonates.[35,53] Another drug that may decrease bone loss is tamoxifen.[65] Tamoxifen is a synthetic antiestrogen that is effective as an adjuvant therapy for invasive breast cancer. Tamoxifen is not a pure antiestrogen. It has agonist estrogen effects, decreases levels of cholesterol, and increases sex hormone binding globulin. It might have either an agonist or antagonist effect on bone loss. Recent studies of BMD in postmenopausal women with breast cancer demonstrated preservation of bone mineral. The effect on risk for fracture remains to be determined.

Bisphosphonates

Bisphosphonates are analogues of pyrophosphate that inhibit bone resorption. Etidronate, a bisphosphonate, is effective at decreasing bone fractures associated with osteoporosis.[131] The effect of this drug is similar to the effect of estrogen and calcitonin on bone.[131] The recommended dosage for etidronate is 400 mg daily for 2 weeks followed by 12 weeks off the drug. This cycle is continued for a 2-year period. Etidronate must be given on an empty stomach. Food should not be consumed 4 hours before and after taking the tablet. The time frame free of the drug is important to decrease the risk of osteomalacia, allowing bone to remineralize. The beneficial effect of therapy continues for 7 years when the drug is used for this duration. Bone mass is maintained, but not increased, for 2 years after the drug is stopped.[80] The drug has never received approval for treatment in osteoporosis. The availability of newer, more convenient bisphosphonates has limited its use in current clinical practice.

Alendronate, 10 mg/day or 70 mg/wk, increases BMD by 5% to 10% over 2 to 4 years and reduces fracture risk by 30% to 50%.[10,61] The duration of bisphosphonate therapy is not known. Alendronate is effective in increasing spine, hip, and total-body BMD and helps prevent vertebral fractures and decreases in height in men.[84] Conflicting data exist concerning the effect of discontinuation of alendronate on BMD. Some studies demonstrate a maintenance of BMD whereas others report a loss of BMD.[96,124] Benefits from continued alendronate therapy are evident at 7 years of continuous use.[124]

Risedronate, 5 mg/day or 35 mg/wk, is another bisphosphonate with clinical trials demonstrating improved BMD and reduced risk of fracture.[39] At 3 years, risedronate is associated with a 65% reduction of vertebral fractures compared with placebo.[46] Risedronate is also effective in decreasing hip fractures in women who are 70 years or older with confirmed osteoporosis.[77]

Other forms of bisphosphonate therapy exist in the form of pamidronate and zoledronic acid. These therapies require intravenous administration and have not been approved for therapy for osteoporosis. These bisphosphonates are utilized for the control of hypercalcemia in the setting of malignancy.[9] Pamidronate is given for osteoporosis in a dose of 30 mg over a 4-hour infusion. These infusions are repeated every 3 to 4 months. Zoledronic acid is given in a dose of 2 to 4 mg over a 5-minute infusion. This infusion is required only once a year. Zoledronic acid has demonstrated BMD effects similar to other oral bisphosphonates for the treatment of osteoporosis.[102]

Fluoride

Sodium fluoride increases skeletal mass by boosting osteoblastic activity. Calcium supplements must be given with fluoride to ensure adequate bone mineralization. Sodium fluoride is given in daily doses of 40 to 65 mg in conjunction with calcium (1.5 g daily) and vitamin D (50,000 units once or twice weekly). Fluoride dose may need to be increased to 75 mg daily. Lower doses of fluoride (50 mg/day) in a slow-release form are associated with prevention of new vertebral fractures whereas higher doses increase the risk of nonvertebral fractures.[88,105] Fluoride therapy is associated with a number of potential toxicities. Although fluoridic bone may appear more dense on radiographic examination, it may be less elastic and more prone to fracture. Preliminary data suggest, however, that patients treated with fluoride for osteoporosis may have a decreased incidence of fracture.[104,109] Other adverse side effects of fluorides include synovitis, gastric irritation, plantar fasciitis of the feet, and anemia. Sodium monofluorophosphate (MFP) is readily absorbed and has fewer gastrointestinal toxicities than sodium fluoride. Patients taking MFP, 20 mg/day, plus calcium had fewer vertebral fractures than women receiving calcium alone.[100] Most patients with vertebral osteoporotic fractures will heal spontaneously and will not require therapy other than the usual calcium and vitamin D. In patients with progressive bone loss, recurrent fractures, and deformity, sodium fluoride may be a useful drug to prevent progressive osteoporosis. Additional prospective studies investigating the fracture rate of postmenopausal women with osteoporosis using fluoride have been completed. Fluoride therapy increases cancellous bone but decreases cortical BMD and increases skeletal fragility.[105] Fluoride is not effective at decreasing osteoporotic fractures. With all the concerns regarding the efficacy of fluoride and its toxicities, this therapy is not recommended except for those who are unable to tolerate any other form of therapy.

Calcitonin

Calcitonin, a hormone produced by C cells in the thyroid gland that suppresses bone resorption, is increased when postmenopausal women receive exogenous estrogen therapy. Intramuscular calcitonin injections along with calcium supplements may retard the rate of bone loss in osteoporotic women.[43] A recent study has reported the prevention of early postmenopausal bone loss in 30 women who used intranasal calcitonin (50 IU/day) and calcium 500 mg/day in comparison to 30 women who received calcium 500 mg/day alone.[99] Further studies are required to determine the efficacy of calcitonin to decrease fractures. Intranasal calcitonin is easier to administer than the intramuscular form and is effective at decreasing bone loss.[99] Calcitonin also may prove beneficial by controlling pain of fractures in osteoporotic patients through the release of endogenous analgesics such as beta-endorphin.

Parathyroid (PTH) Therapy

PTH is usually associated with osteoporosis. This occurs with tonic presence of the hormone. Intermittent exposure of PTH given as a subcutaneous injection results in enhanced bone formation. A study of 1000 women with vertebral fractures demonstrated increased BMD in the spine of 10% with 20 μg/day and 14% with 40 μ/day over a 2-year period.[82] The frequency of vertebral fractures was also reduced by 53% compared with placebo. Fewer adverse events occurred with the 20-μg injection. Teriparatide (PTH) is given at a dose of 20 μg/day SQ for up to 24 months. Teriparatide is indicated for osteoporosis patients at high risk for fragility fractures. High-risk patients are those with previous fractures who are unresponsive or intolerant of other osteoporosis therapies. The therapy should not be used in patients with metabolic bone disease other than osteoporosis or those with radiation therapy exposure. Rats treated with teriparatide at a dose 3- to 60-fold the therapeutic dose had an increased incidence of osteosarcoma. The therapy is also expensive.

Thiazides

Thiazide diuretics block renal excretion of calcium. Studies have shown that bone mineral is increased in patients taking thiazides as compared with age-matched controls. The therapeutic effect of thiazides on osteopenia remains to be determined.[130] Hydrochlorothiazide (HCTZ) at a dose of 50 mg/day slows cortical bone loss in normal postmenopausal women. No effect occurs on the lumbar spine or femoral neck. HCTZ may be useful in preventing osteoporosis but is not appropriate monotherapy for treating osteoporosis.[101]

If the patient's urine contains greater than 100 mg of urinary calcium, then calcium, vitamin D, and estrogen 0.625 mg every day to be cycled monthly should be considered. If new fractures occur within 6 to 12 months, the addition of calcitonin or fluoride should be considered.

Patients who receive corticosteroids are at risk of developing symptomatic osteoporosis, including vertebral fractures. Patients who take corticosteroids should be considered for treatment with drugs that prevent osteoporosis, including calcium, vitamin D, and thiazide diuretics. In patients with fractures, calcitonin and bisphosphonates may be helpful in decreasing symptoms.[68]

Vertebroplasty/Kyphoplasty

A percutaneous technique of treating metastatic lesions with polymethylmethacrylate (PMMA) was the idea behind the instillation of PMMA in osteoporotic vertebral fractures. Vertebroplasty is utilized in individuals with fractures older than 6 weeks in duration that remain painful. The technique starts with the placement of a large-bore needle through a pedicle into a vertebral body. PMMA is injected under pressure. The use of curved needles allows the use of one entry to obtain uniform placement of cement. The posterior vertebral cortex must be intact during vertebroplasty to avoid leakage into the spinal canal.[90] A majority of patients may experience decreased pain within 24 hours after the injection.[26] Vertebroplasty is also successful for individuals with corticosteroid-induced osteoporotic compression fractures.[74]

Kyphoplasty is a procedure that reexpands the collapsed vertebral bodies.[40] This procedure is possible within 6 weeks after an acute fracture. A tract is drilled into the vertebral body through the pedicle followed by an inflatable balloon (bone tamp). The expanded balloon creates a cavity. The balloon is removed before the injection of the PMMA cement. Kyphoplasty is done bilaterally for each vertebral body fracture. No more than six levels should be completed at one time, with one or two levels the usual number (Fig.14-10). The larger-gauge needle allows for a more viscous PMMA mixture to be injected under a lower pressure. This reduces the risk for cement leakage. The onset of pain relief is rapid. A component of the pain relief may be due to heat that affects nociceptors in vertebral bodies.[132]

PROGNOSIS

Vertebral compression fractures occur episodically and are usually self-limited. Patients will usually have more than one fracture, and a recurrence usually occurs within a few

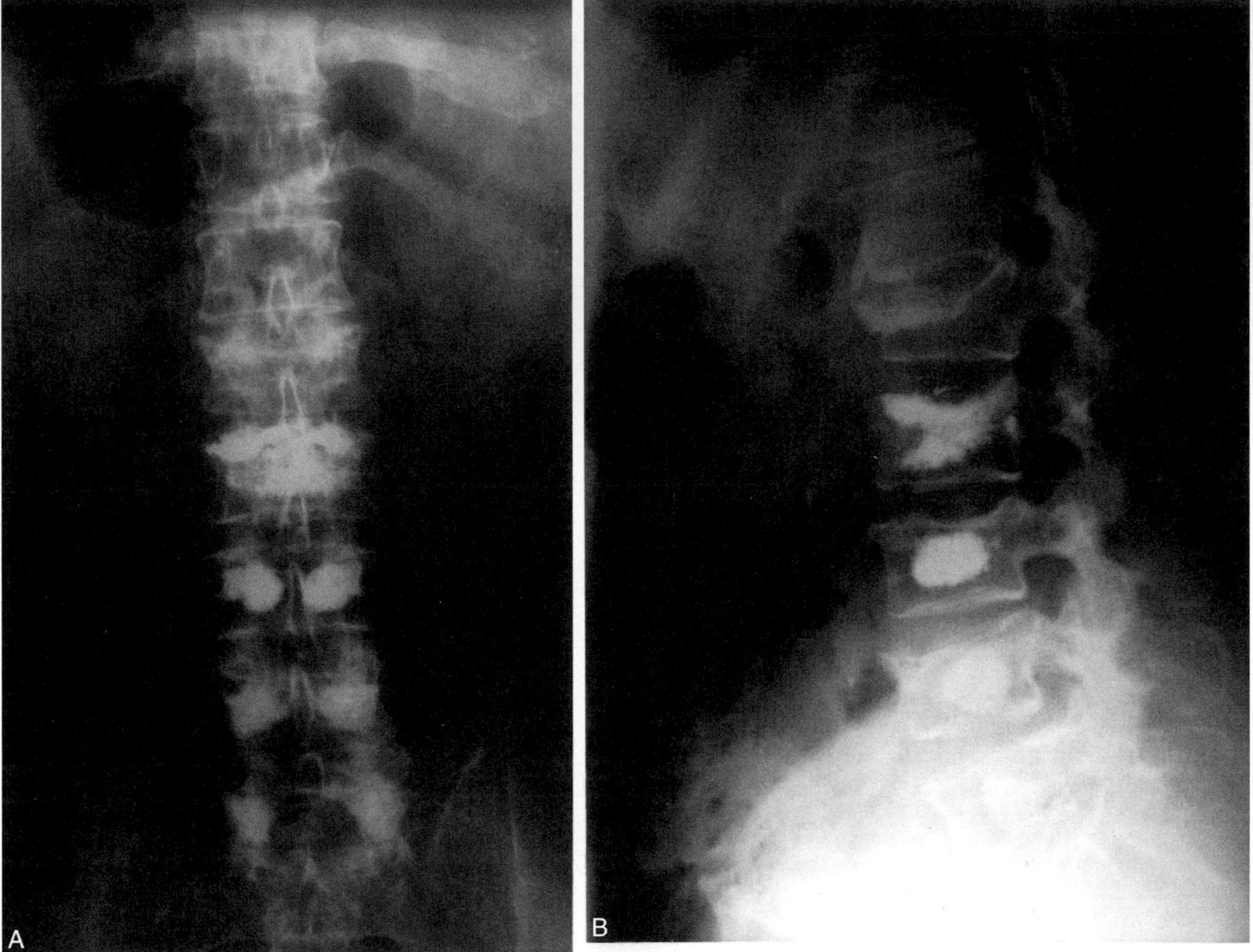

Figure 14-10 Kyphoplasty. A 64-year-old-woman presented with severe osteoporosis with multiple vertebral compression fractures. Anteroposterior *(A)* and lateral *(B)* views show the lumbar spine after kyphoplasty at four vertebral levels. *(Courtesy of Norman Koval, MD.)*

years of the first incident. Back pain may resolve within months of a fracture or may persist if increasing deformity causes a mechanical strain in the lumbar spine. The course of osteoporosis is variable, and it is impossible to predict the severity and frequency of fractures. Patients with osteoarthritis in conjunction with osteoporosis may be at less risk of bone fracture. Patients with both disorders are older, with a longer period of menopause, and are physically smaller in stature and body weight than those with the individual disorders.[128]

Patients with osteoporosis who continue to work are at risk of repeated fractures, and they should not be required to lift or carry heavy objects. They should refrain from work activities that jar the spine. Measures such as structured exercise and drug therapy may be helpful at slowing the progression of the disease. Individuals with strong back extensor muscles may have greater BMD than individuals with weaker muscles.[118] Maintenance of muscle strength is worthwhile in a treatment program.

Osteoporosis and associated vertebral fractures cause significant morbidity in patients. Patients with fractures have decreased spinal motion and have difficulty walking. Psychologic perceptions of illness are also increased in the group with fractures. Osteoporosis is a significant medical disorder with physical and psychiatric impairments.[71] Long-term benefits may be found with the prolonged use of etidronate. A 4-year study demonstrated a decreased number of vertebral fractures in patients treated with cyclic etidronate therapy.[47]

The mortality of osteoporosis is associated with hip fracture. Men and women are two to five times more likely to die during the 12 months after a hip fracture than age- and sex-matched individuals in the general population without fracture. Mortality associated with hip, vertebral, or other major fractures is higher in men than women.[32] Men are less likely than women to receive antiresorptive therapy after hip fracture.[58] Much of the increased mortality occurs in the first 6 to 12 months after the fracture.[20]

Vertebral fractures also have an associated increased mortality. Women with vertebral fractures had a 1.23-fold greater age-adjusted mortality rate compared with women without a fracture. Increased mortality was associated with cancer and pulmonary disease.[56]

References

Osteoporosis

1. Adinoff AD, Hollister JR: Steroid induced fractures and bone loss in patients with asthma. N Engl J Med 309:265, 1983.
2. Albanese AA, Edelson AH, Lorenze EJ Jr, et al: Problems of bone health in elderly. NY State J Med 75:326, 1975.
3. Aloia JF, Vaswani AN, Yeh JK, Cohn SH: Premenopausal bone mass is related to physical activity. Arch Intern Med 148:121, 1988.
4. Amin S, Zhang Y, Swain CT: Association of hypogonadism and estradiol levels with bone mineral density in elderly men from the Framingham study. Ann Intern Med 133:951-963, 2000.
5. Antunes CMF, Stolley PD, Rosenshein NB, et al: Endometrial cancer and estrogen use: Report of a large case-controlled study. N Engl J Med 300:9, 1979.
6. Ardan GM: Bone destruction not demonstrable by radiography. Br J Radiol 24:107, 1951.
7. Avioli LV: The osteoporosis problem. Curr Concepts Nutr 5:99, 1977.
8. Barnett E, Nordin BEC: The radiologic diagnosis of osteoporosis: A new approach. Clin Radiol 11:166, 1960.
9. Berenson JR, Lichtenstein A, Porter L, et al: Efficacy of pamidronate in reducing skeletal events in patients with advanced multiple myeloma. Myeloma Aredia study group. N Engl J Med 334:488-493, 1996.
10. Black DM, Cummings SR, Karpf DB, et al: Randomized trial of effect of alendronate on risk of fracture in women with existing vertebral fractures: Fracture intervention trial research group. Lancet 348:1535-1541, 1996.
11. Brower AC, Downey EF: Kümmell disease: Report of a case with serial radiographs. Radiology 141:363, 1981.
12. Brynhildsen JO, Bjors E, Skarsgard C, et al: Is hormone replacement therapy a risk factor for low back pain among postmenopausal women? Spine 23:809-813, 1998.
13. Cann CE, Genant HK, Ettinger B, Gordon GS: Spinal mineral loss in oophorectomized women: Determination by quantitative computed tomography. JAMA 244:2056, 1980.
14. Chestnut CH III, Bell NH, Clark GS, et al: Hormone replacement therapy in postmenopausal women: Urinary N-telopeptide of type 1 collagen monitors therapeutic effect and predicts response of bone mineral density. Am J Med 102:29-37, 1997.
15. Chevalier X, Wrona N, Avouac B, et al: Thigh pain and multiple vertebral osteonecroses: Value of magnetic resonance imaging. J Rheumatol 18:1627, 1991.
16. Chow R, Harrison JE, Notarius C: Effect of two randomised exercise programmes on bone mass of healthy postmenopausal women. BMJ 295:1441, 1987.
17. Christiansen C, Christensen MS, Tansbol I: Bone mass in postmenopausal women after withdrawal of oestrogen/gestagen replacement therapy. Lancet 1:459, 1981.
18. Cohn SH, Vaswani A, Zanzi I, Ellis KJ: Effect of aging on bone mass in adult women. Am J Physiol 230:140, 1976.
19. Consensus Conference: Osteoporosis. JAMA 252:799, 1984.
20. Cooper C, Atkinson EJ, Jacobsen SJ, et al: Population-based study of survival after osteoporotic fractures. Am J Epidemiol 137: 1001-1005, 1993.
21. Crayton HE, Bell CL, De Smet AA: Insufficiency fractures of the sacrum: Twenty cases and review of the literature. Spine 18: 2507-2512, 1993.
22. Crayton HE, Bell CL, De Smet AA: Sacral insufficiency fractures. Semin Arthritis Rheum 20:378, 1991.
23. Cummings SR, Kelsey JL, Hevitt MC, O'Dowd KJ: Epidemiology of osteoporosis and osteoporotic fractures. Epidemiol Rev 7:178, 1985.
24. Cummings SR, Palermo L, Browner W, et al: Monitoring osteoporosis therapy with bone densitometry: Misleading changes and regression to the mean. JAMA 283:1318-1321, 2000.
25. Cushing H: The basophil adenomas of the pituitary body and their clinical manifestations. Bull Johns Hopkins Hosp 50:137, 1932.
26. Cyteval C, Sarrabere MPB, Roux JO, et al: Acute osteoporotic vertebral collapse: Open study on percutaneous injection of acrylic surgical cement in 20 patients. AJR 173:1685-1690, 1999.
27. Dawson-Hughes B: Bone loss accompanying medical therapies. N Engl J Med 345:989-991, 2001.
28. Dawson-Hughes B, Dallal GE, Krall EA, et al: A controlled trial of the effect of calcium supplementation on bone density in postmenopausal women. N Engl J Med 323:878, 1990.
29. Delmas PD: Markers of bone formation and resorption. In Favus MJ (ed): Primer on the Metabolic Bone Disease and Disorders of Mineral Metabolism, 2nd ed. New York, Raven, 1993, pp 108-112.
30. Delmas PD, Schlemmer A, Gineyts E, et al: Urinary excretion of pyridinoline crosslinks correlates with bone turnover measured on iliac crest biopsy in patients with vertebral osteoporosis. J Bone Miner Res 6:639, 1991.
31. Dempster DW, Lindsay R: Pathogenesis of osteoporosis. Lancet 341:797, 1993.
32. Diamond TH, Thornley SW, Sekel R, et al: Hip fracture in elderly men: Prognostic factors and outcomes. Med J Aust 167:412-415, 1997.
33. Ducy P, Schinke T, Karsenty G: The osteoblasts: A sophisticated fibroblast under central surveillance. Science 289:1501-1504, 2000.
34. Eastell R: Treatment of postmenopausal osteoporosis. N Engl J Med 338:736-746, 1998.
35. Ettinger B, Black DM, Mitlak BH, et al: Reduction of vertebral fracture risk in postmenopausal women with osteoporosis treated with raloxifene: Results from a 3-year randomized clinical trial. Multiple outcomes of raloxifene evaluation investigators. JAMA 282:637-645, 1999.
36. Ettinger B, Genant HK, Cann CE: Postmenopausal bone loss is prevented by treatment with low-dosage estrogen with calcium. Ann Intern Med 106:40, 1987.
37. Feskanich D, Singh V, Willett WC, et al: Vitamin A intake and hip fractures among postmenopausal women. JAMA 287:47-54, 2002.
38. Fogelman I, Ribot C, Smith R, et al: Risedronate reverses bone loss in postmenopausal women with low bone mass: Results from a multinational, double-blind, placebo-controlled trial. BMD-MN study group. J Clin Endocrinol Metab 85:1895-1900, 2000.
39. Fogelman I, Ribot C, Smith R, et al: Risedronate reverses bone loss in postmenopausal women with low bone mass: Results from a multinational, double-blind, placebo-controlled trial. BMD-MN study group. J Clin Endocrinol Metab 85:1895-1890, 2000.
40. Garfin SR, Yuan HA, Reiley MA: New technologies in spine: Kyphoplasty and vertebroplasty for the treatment of painful osteoporotic compression fractures. Spine 26:1511-1515, 2001.
41. Genant HK, Cann CE, Ettinger B, Gordon GS: Quantitative computed tomography of vertebral spongiosa: A sensitive method for detecting early bone loss after oophorectomy. Ann Intern Med 97:699, 1982.
42. Golimbu C, Firooznia H, Rafi M: The intravertebral vacuum sign. Spine 11:1040, 1986.
43. Gruber HE, Ivey JL, Baylink DJ, et al: Long-term calcitonin therapy in postmenopausal osteoporosis. Metabolism 33:295, 1984.
44. Haddaway MJ, Davie MWJ, McCall IW: Bone mineral density in healthy normal women and reproducibility of measurements in spine and hip using dual-energy x-ray absorptiometry. Br J Radiol 65:213, 1991.
45. Hall FM, Davis MA, Baran DT: Bone mineral screening for osteoporosis (Editorial). N Engl J Med 316:212, 1987.
46. Harris ST, Watts NB, Genant HK, et al: Effects of risedronate treatment on vertebral and nonvertebral fractures in women with postmenopausal osteoporosis—a randomized controlled trial. JAMA 282:1344-1352, 1999.
47. Harris ST, Watts NB, Jackson RD, et al: Four-year study of intermittent cyclic etidronate treatment of postmenopausal osteoporosis: Three years of blinded therapy followed by one year of open therapy. Am J Med 95:557, 1993.
48. Heaney RP: Prevention of age-related osteoporosis in women. In Avioli LV (ed): The Osteoporotic Syndrome. New York, Grune & Stratton, 1983, pp 123-144.
49. Heaney RP, Recker RR, Saville PD: Calcium balance and calcium requirements in middle-aged women. Am J Clin Nutr 30:1603, 1977.

50. Israel E, Banerjee TR, Fitzmaurice GM, et al: Effects of inhaled glucocorticoids on bone density in premenopausal women. N Engl J Med 345:941-947, 2001.
51. Jackson WPU: Osteoporosis of unknown cause in younger people. J Bone Joint Surg Br 40B:420, 1958.
52. Jilja R, Hangoc G, Girasole G, et al: Increased osteoclast development after estrogen loss: Mediation by interleukin-6. Science 257:88, 1992.
53. Johnston CC Jr, Bjarnason NH, Cohen FJ, et al: Long-term effects of raloxifene on bone mineral density, bone turnover, and serum lipid levels in early postmenopausal women: Three-year data from 2 double-blind, randomized, placebo-controlled trials. Arch Intern Med 160:3444-3450, 2000.
54. Johnston CC Jr, Hui SL, Witt RM, et al: Early menopausal changes in bone mass and sex steroids. J Clin Endocrinol Metab 61:905, 1985.
55. Jones KP, Raunikar VA, Tulchinsky D, Schiff I: Comparison of bone density in amenorrheic women due to athletics, weight loss, and premature menopause. Obstet Gynecol 66:5, 1985.
56. Kado DM, Browner WS, Palmero L, et al: Vertebral fractures and mortality in older women: A prospective study. Arch Intern Med 159:1215-1220, 1999.
57. Kellie SE: DEXA (letter). JAMA 268:475, 1992.
58. Kiebzak GM, Beinart GA, Perser K, et al: Undertreatment of osteoporosis in men with hip fracture. Arch Intern Med 162: 2217-2222, 2002.
59. Kushi LH, Fee RM, Folsom AR, et al: Physical activity and mortality in postmenopausal women. JAMA 277:1287-1292, 1997.
60. Lang P, Steiger P, Faulkner K, et al: Osteoporosis: Current techniques and recent developments in quantitative bone densitometry. Radiol Clin North Am 29:49, 1991.
61. Liberman UA, Weiss SR, Broll J, et al: Effect of oral alendronate on bone mineral density and the incidence of fractures in postmenopausal osteoporosis: The alendronate phase III osteoporosis treatment study group. N Engl J Med 333:1437-1443, 1995.
62. Lindsay R: Prevention and treatment of osteoporosis. Lancet 341:801, 1993.
63. Lindsay R, Hart DM, MacLean A, et al: Bone response to termination of estrogen treatment. Lancet 1:1325, 1978.
64. Lindsay R, Tohme J: Estrogen treatment of patients with established postmenopausal osteoporosis. Obstet Gynecol 76:1, 1990.
65. Love RR, Mazess RB, Barden HS, et al: Effects of tamoxifen on bone mineral density in postmenopausal women with breast cancer. N Engl J Med 326:852, 1992.
66. Lucas AR, Melton LJ, Crowson CS, et al: Long-term fracture risk among women with anorexia nervosa: A population-based cohort study. Mayo Clin Proc 74:972-977, 1999.
67. Lukert BP: Osteoporosis: A review and update. Arch Phys Med Rehab 63:480, 1982.
68. Lukert BP, Raisz LG: Glucocorticoid-induced osteoporosis: Pathogenesis and management. Ann Intern Med 112:352, 1990.
69. Lund B, Kjaer I, Friis T, et al: Treatment of osteoporosis of aging with 1-hydroxycholecalciferol. Lancet 2:1168, 1975.
70. Lutwak L, Singer FR, Urist MR: Current concepts of bone metabolism. Ann Intern Med 80:630, 1974.
71. Lyles KW, Gold DT, Shipp KM, et al: Association of osteoporotic vertebral compression fractures with impaired functional status. Am J Med 94:595, 1993.
72. Margolis KL, Ensrud KE, Schreiner PJ, et al: Body size and risk for clinical fractures in older women. Ann Intern Med 133:123-127, 2000.
73. Marshall D, Johnell O, Wedel H: Meta-analysis of how well measures of bone mineral density predict occurrence of osteoporotic fractures. BMJ 312:1254-1259, 1996.
74. Mathis JM, Petri M, Naff N: Percutaneous vertebroplasty treatment of steroid-induced osteoporotic compression fractures. Arthritis Rheum 41:171-175, 1998.
75. Mazess RB, Barden HS, Ettinger M: Radial and spinal bone mineral density in a patient population. Arthritis Rheum 31:891, 1988.
76. McClung M, Clemmesen B, Daifotis A, et al: Alendronate prevents postmenopausal bone loss in women without osteoporosis: A double-blind, randomized, controlled trial. Ann Intern Med 128: 253-261, 1998.
77. McClung MR, Geusens P, Miller PD, et al: Effect of risedronate on the risk of hip fracture in elderly women. N Engl J Med 344: 333-340, 2001.
78. McNair P, Madsbad S, Christiansen C, et al: Osteopenia in insulin treated diabetes mellitus: Its relation to age at onset, sex, and duration of disease. Diabetologia 15:87, 1978.
79. Michel BA, Lane NE, Jones HH, et al: Plain radiographs can be useful in estimating lumbar bone density. J Rheumatol 17:528, 1990.
80. Miller PD, Watts NB, Licata AA, et al: Cyclical etidronate in the treatment of postmenopausal osteoporosis: Efficacy and safety after seven years of treatment. Am J Med 103:468-476, 1997.
81. Mohan S, Baylink D: Bone growth factors. Clin Orthop 263:30, 1992.
82. Neer RM, Arnaud CD, Zanchetta JR, et al: Effect of parathyroid hormone (1-34) on fractures and bone mineral density in postmenopausal women with osteoporosis. N Engl J Med 344: 1434-1441, 2001.
83. NIH Consensus development panel on osteoporosis presentation, diagnosis and therapy: Osteoporosis prevention, diagnosis, and therapy. JAMA 285:785-795, 2001.
84. Orwoll E, Ettinger M, Weiss S, et al: Alendronate for the treatment of osteoporosis in men. N Engl J Med 343:604-610, 2000.
85. Ott S: Should women get screening bone mass measurements? (Editorial.) Ann Intern Med 104:874, 1986.
86. Pacific R, Brown C, Puscheck E, et al: The effect of surgical menopause and estrogen replacement on cytokine release from human blood monocytes. Proc Natl Acad Sci U S A 88:5134, 1991.
87. Pacifici R, Rupich R, Griffin M, et al: Dual energy radiography versus quantitative computer tomography for the diagnosis of osteoporosis. J Clin Endocrinol Metab 70:705, 1990.
88. Pak CY, Sakhaee K, Adams-Huet B, et al: Treatment of postmenopausal osteoporosis with slow-release sodium fluoride: Final report of a randomized controlled trial. Ann Intern Med 123: 401-408, 1995.
89. Parfitt AM, Duncan H: Metabolic bone disease affecting the spine. In Rothman RH, Simeone FA (eds): The Spine, 2nd ed. Philadelphia, WB Saunders, 1982, pp 775-905.
90. Phillips FM, Wetzel FT, Lieberman I, et al: An in vivo comparison of the potential for extravertebral cement leak after vertebroplasty and kyphoplasty. Spine 27:2173-2178, 2002.
91. Prince RL, Smith M, Dick IM, et al: Prevention of postmenopausal osteoporosis: A comparative study of exercise, calcium supplementation, and hormone-replacement therapy. N Engl J Med 325:1189, 1991.
92. Raisz LG: Local and systemic factors in the pathogenesis of osteoporosis. N Engl J Med 318:818, 1988.
93. Ralston SH, Rusell RGG, Gowen M: Estrogen inhibits release of tumor necrosis factor from peripheral blood mononuclear cells in postmenopausal women. J Bone Miner Res 5:983, 1990.
94. Ram PC, Martinez S, Korobkin M, et al: CT detection of intraosseous gas: A new sign of osteomyelitis. AJR Am J Roentgenol 137:721, 1981.
95. Ravn P, Hoking D, Thompson D, et al: Monitoring of alendronate treatment and prediction of effect on bone mass by biochemical markers in the early postmenopausal intervention cohort study. J Clin Endocrinol Metab 84:2363-2368, 1999.
96. Ravn P, Weiss SR, Rodriguez-Portales JA, et al: Alendronate in early postmenopausal women: Effects on bone mass during long-term treatment and after withdrawal. Alendronate osteoporosis prevention study group. J Clin Endocrinol Metab 85:1492-1497, 2000.
97. Ray NF, Chan JK, Thamer M, et al: Medical expenditures for the treatment of osteoporotic fractures in the United States in 1995: Report from the National Osteoporosis Foundation. J Bone Miner Res 12:24-35, 1997.
98. Recker RR, Saville PD, Heaney RP: Effect of estrogens and calcium carbonate on bone loss in postmenopausal women. Ann Intern Med 87:649, 1977.
99. Reginster JY, Denis D, Albert A, et al: One-year controlled randomised trial of prevention of early postmenopausal bone loss by intranasal calcitonin. Lancet 2:1481, 1987.
100. Reginstar JY, Meurmans L, Zegels B, et al: The effect of sodium nonfluorophosphate plus calcium on vertebral fracture rate in postmenopausal women with moderate osteoporosis: A randomized, controlled trial. Ann Intern Med 129:1-8, 1998.
101. Reid IR, Ames RW, Orr-Walker BJ, et al: Hydrochlorothiazide reduces loss of cortical bone in normal postmenopausal women: A randomized controlled trial. Am J Med 109:362-370, 2000.

102. Reid IR, Burckhardt P, Horowitz Z, et al: Intravenous zoledronic acid in postmenopausal women with low bone mineral density. N Engl J Med 346:653-661, 2002.
103. Ribot C, Tremollieres F, Pouilles JM, et al: Preventive effects of transdermal administration of 17β-estradiol on postmenopausal bone loss: A 2-year prospective study. Obstet Gynecol 75(Suppl 4):43S, 1990.
104. Riggs BL, Hodgson SF, Hoffman DL, et al: Treatment of primary osteoporosis with fluoride and calcium: Clinical tolerance and fracture occurrence. JAMA 243:446, 1980.
105. Riggs BL, Hodgson SF, O'Fallon WM, et al: Effect of fluoride treatment on the fracture rate in postmenopausal women with osteoporosis. N Engl J Med 322:802, 1990.
106. Riggs BL, Jowsey J, Kelley PJ, et al: Effects of oral therapy with calcium and vitamin D in primary osteoporosis. J Clin Endocrinol Metab 42:1139, 1976.
107. Riggs BL, Melton LJ III: Involutional osteoporosis. N Engl J Med 314:1676, 1986.
108. Riggs BL, Melton LJ III: The prevention and treatment of osteoporosis. N Engl J Med 327:620, 1992.
109. Riggs BL, Seeman E, Hodgson SF, et al: Effect of the fluoride/calcium regimen on vertebral fracture occurrence in postmenopausal osteoporosis: Comparison with conventional therapy. N Engl J Med 306:446, 1982.
110. Riggs BL, Wahner HW, Dunn WL, et al: Differential changes in bone mineral density of appendicular and axial skeleton with aging. J Clin Invest 67:328, 1981.
111. Riis B, Thomsen K, Christiansen C: Does calcium supplementation prevent postmenopausal bone loss? N Engl J Med 316:173, 1987.
112. Ross PD: Osteoporosis: Frequency, consequences, and risk factors. Arch Intern Med 156:1399-1411, 1996.
113. Ross PD, Knowlton W: Rapid bone loss is associated with increased levels of biochemical markers. J Bone Miner Res 13: 297-302, 1998.
114. Schapira D: Alcohol abuse and osteoporosis. Semin Arthritis Rheum 19:371, 1990.
115. Schneider DL, Barrett Connor EL: Urinary N-telopeptide levels discriminate normal, osteopenic, and osteoporotic bone mineral density. Arch Intern Med 157:1241-1245, 1997.
116. Seeger LL: Bone density determination. Spine 22:49S-57S, 1997.
117. Sheikh MS, Santa Ana CA, Nicar MJ, et al: Gastrointestinal absorption of calcium from milk and calcium salts. N Engl J Med 317:532, 1987.
118. Sinaki M, McPhee MC, Hodgson SF, et al: Relationship between bone mineral density of spine and nutritional strength of back extensors in healthy postmenopausal women. Mayo Clin Proc 61:116, 1986.
119. Smith EL, Reddon W: Physical activity: A modality for bone accretion in the aged. AJR Am J Roentgenol 126:1297, 1976.
120. Smith MR, McGovern FJ, Zeitman AL, et al: Pamidronate to prevent bone loss during androgen-deprivation therapy for prostate cancer. N Engl J Med 345:948-955, 2001.
121. Storm T, Thamsborg G, Steiniche T, et al: Effect of intermittent cyclical etidronate therapy on bone mass and fracture rate in women with postmenopausal osteoporosis. N Engl J Med 322:1265, 1990.
122. Teitelbaum SL: Bone resorption by osteoclasts. Science 289: 1504-1508, 2000.
123. Thomson DL, Frame B: Involutional osteopenia: Current concepts. Ann Intern Med 85:789, 1976.
124. Tonino RP, Meunier PJ, Emkey R, et al: Skeletal benefits of alendronate: 7-year treatment of postmenopausal osteoporotic women. Phase III osteoporosis treatment study group. J Clin Endocrinol Metab 85:3109-3115, 2000.
125. U.S. Preventive Services Task Force: Screening osteoporosis in postmenopausal women: Recommendations and rationale. Ann Intern Med 137:526-528, 2002.
126. Urist MP, Gurvey MS, Fareed DO: Long-term observations on aged women with pathologic osteoporosis. In Barzel US (ed): Osteoporosis. New York, Grune & Stratton, 1970, pp 3-37.
127. Van Staa TP, Leufkens HGM, Abenhaim L, et al: Use of oral corticosteroids and risk of fractures. J Bone Miner Res 15:993-1000, 2000.
128. Verstraeten A, Van Ermen H, Haghebaert G, et al: Osteoarthrosis retards the development of osteoporosis. Clin Orthop 264:169, 1991.
129. Wahner HW: Assessment of metabolic bone disease: Review of new nuclear medicine procedures. Mayo Clin Proc 60:827, 1985.
130. Wasnich RD, Benfante RJ, Yano K, et al: Thiazide effect on the mineral content of bone. N Engl J Med 309:344, 1983.
131. Watts NB, Harris ST, Genant HK, et al: Intermittent cyclical etidronate treatment of postmenopausal osteoporosis. N Engl J Med 323:73, 1990.
132. Watts NB, Harris ST, Genant HK: Treatment of painful osteoporotic vertebral fractures with percutaneous vertebroplasty or kyphoplasty. Osteoporos Int 12:429-437, 2001.
133. White PH: Osteopenic disorders of the spine. Semin Spine Surg 2:121, 1990.
134. Wolfson L, Whipple R, Derby C, et al: Balance and strength training in older adults: Intervention gains and Tai Chi maintenance. J Am Geriatr Soc 44:498-506, 1996.
135. Writing group for the Women's Health Initiative Investigators: Risks and benefits of estrogen plus progestin in healthy postmenopausal women: Principal results from the Women's Health Initiative randomized controlled trial. JAMA 288:321-333, 2002.
136. Yuh WT, Zachar CK, Barloon TJ, et al: Vertebral compression fractures: Distinction between benign and malignant causes with MR imaging. Radiology 172:215, 1989.

OSTEOMALACIA

Capsule Summary

	Low Back	Neck
Frequency of spinal pain	Very common	Not applicable (NA)
Location of spinal pain	Lumbar spine	NA
Quality of spinal pain	Chronic, dull ache; acute, sharp with fracture	NA
Symptoms and signs	Pain increases with activity and standing	NA
Laboratory tests	Decreased serum calcium, phosphate, vitamin D; increased alkaline phosphatase; decreased urinary calcium; increased parathyroid hormone	NA
Radiographic findings	"Codfish" vertebrae on plain roentgenograms; multiple Looser's zones on bone scan	NA
Treatment	Vitamin D, calcium, phosphate	NA

PREVALENCE AND PATHOGENESIS

Osteomalacia is a metabolic bone disease associated with loss of bone mass per unit volume and a decrease in the ratio of bone mineral content to bone matrix. In essence, it is an abnormality in the mineralization of bone. Any disorder that affects calcium or phosphorus concentrations or alters the physiologic conditions needed for the formation of hydroxyapatite crystals may result in osteomalacia. It may occur in any of the long bones, pelvis, scapula, ribs, or axial skeleton. Loss of bone mineralization weakens the bone, which makes it vulnerable to fracture. Osteomalacia in the axial skeleton is associated with back pain, vertebral body weakening, fracture, and progressive kyphoscoliosis. It should be suspected in a patient with bone pain, radiographic evidence of decreased bone mass (osteopenia), and depressed levels of serum calcium and inorganic phosphate. The definitive diagnosis of osteomalacia is made based on the presence of a widened osteoid seam and decreased mineralization found in an undemineralized bone section. Osteomalacia may be caused by vitamin D deficiency, intestinal disorders, drugs, metabolic acidosis (usually associated with renal disorders, including tubular defects), phosphate deficiencies, and mineralization defects, both primary and secondary.

Evaluation of a patient with osteomalacia is directed at identifying the underlying disease process that results in the decreased bone mineralization. Treatment is directed toward the specific illness causing the osteomalacia and may include vitamin D supplements, pancreatic enzyme supplements, dietary modifications to increase intake of calcium and phosphorus, reduction of metabolic acidosis, and the discontinuation of drugs associated with osteomalacia.

Epidemiology

The prevalence of osteomalacia is unknown. The number of illnesses associated with osteomalacia prohibits the computation of prevalence from all sources (Table 14-5).[22] Osteomalacia in children, rickets, is common outside the United States in areas of the world with malnutrition.[73] Up to 9% of young children may demonstrate radiographic findings of rickets in impoverished urban areas.[61] Osteomalacia has been reported in 3% to 5% of acutely ill elderly patients.[14] Before the 1930s, vitamin D–sensitive osteomalacia was the most common form of osteomalacia. With the addition of vitamin D to the diet, the frequency of nutritional vitamin D osteomalacia has decreased. In the 1990s, some variant of vitamin D–resistant osteomalacia is a more commonly recognized form of disease.[56]

Pathogenesis

Osteomalacia includes a group of disorders with similar clinical symptoms and signs but with diverse causes. The most frequent abnormality associated with osteomalacia is vitamin D deficiency. Vitamin D in its activated form increases intestinal calcium absorption, renal tubular resorption of calcium and phosphate, and promotion of bone mineralization.[37] The sources of vitamin D are exogenous (fortified dairy products) and endogenous (exposure of skin to ultraviolet rays in sunlight). Dairy products are fortified with vitamin D_2 (ergocalciferol, irradiation product of plant sterols) or vitamin D_3 (cholecalciferol). Adequate gastrointestinal absorption of dietary vitamin D requires an intact and functioning mucosal surface of the small intestine as well as an intact biliary system with adequate concentrations of bile salts. A more important source of vitamin D_3 is endogenous production generated by the exposure of 7-dehydrocholesterol in the skin to ultraviolet light.

Vitamin D

Metabolism. Vitamin D (either D_2 or D_3) is transported to the liver by a carrier protein. Hepatic enzymes hydroxylate the precursor vitamin at the 25 position to form 25-hydroxyvitamin D. The 25-hydroxyvitamin D is then transported to the kidney, where hydroxylation at the 24 position will form 24,25-dihydroxyvitamin D, an active form of vitamin D. This form of vitamin D may contribute to mineralization of bone and modulation of parathyroid function, but it is less potent than the 1,25-dihydroxy form of vitamin D. Increased activity of 1-hydroxylase, the enzyme that controls hydroxylation at the 1 position, is mediated by decreased dietary intake of calcium, increased parathyroid hormone secretion, and hypophosphatemia.[37] Both inadequate intake of vitamin D–supplemented nutrition and an avoidance of the sun must occur to cause deficiency severe enough to result in osteomalacia.

Absorption. Normal vitamin D absorption in the gut requires an intact intestinal mucosa, normal hepatobiliary circulation of bile salts, and, to a lesser degree, exocrine pancreatic function. Osteomalacia may occur despite adequate production of vitamin D_3 in the skin since the hepatic product 25-hydroxyvitamin D undergoes enterohepatic circulation like bile salts.[3] Most vitamin D is absorbed in the mid-jejunum, whereas a smaller component is absorbed in the terminal ileum.[64] Diseases associated with small bowel malabsorption, such as sprue, celiac disease, Crohn's disease, scleroderma, and jejunal diverticula and bowel bypass surgery, may all be complicated by osteomalacia.[67] Postgastrectomy patients are also prone to develop osteomalacia. Patients with hepatocellular disorders (cirrhosis, alcoholic hepatitis, or chronic active hepatitis) and those with biliary system disease (primary biliary cirrhosis) are unable to absorb vitamin D and develop osteomalacia.[16,46] Malabsorption associated with pancreatic insufficiency may cause osteomalacia not only by decreasing levels of 25-hydroxyvitamin D but also by decreasing calcium absorption.[35] Osteomalacia may be the only symptom in some patients with gluten-sensitive enteropathy.[17]

Mode of Action. 1,25-Dihydroxyvitamin D_3 is responsible for calcium and phosphorus homeostasis and maintenance of bone mineralization.[48] In the intestine, vitamin D increases the absorption of calcium and phosphorus. Parathyroid hormone binds to receptors on intestinal cells, activating adenyl cyclase and cyclic adenosine monophosphate to allow calcium to enter the cell. Activated 1,25-$(OH)_2$ vitamin D acts

14-5 DISEASES ASSOCIATED WITH OSTEOMALACIA

Disorder	Metabolic Defect
VITAMIN D	
Deficiency	Decreased generation of vitamin D_3
Dietary	
Ultraviolet light exposure	
Malabsorption	Decreased absorption of vitamins D_2 and D_3
Small intestine	
Inadequate bile salts	
Pancreatic insufficiency	
Abnormal metabolism	
Hereditary enzyme deficiency	Decreased 1-alpha-hydroxylation of 25-(OH)-vitamin D
Vitamin D–dependent rickets type I	
Chronic renal failure	Decreased 25-hydroxylation of vitamin D
Mesenchymal tumors	?P450 enzyme alteration of 25-hydroxyvitamin D conversion vs. decreased sunlight exposure
Systemic acidosis	
Hepatic failure	
Anticonvulsant drugs	
Peripheral resistance	
Vitamin D–dependent rickets type II	Absent or abnormal 1.25-$(OH)_2$-vitamin D receptors
PHOSPHATE DEPLETION	
Dietary	
Malnutrition (rare)?	Inadequate bone mineralization secondary to low serum concentrations
Aluminum hydroxide ingestion	
Renal tubular wasting	
Hereditary	Decreased serum phosphate concentrations
X-linked hypophosphatemic osteomalacia	
Acquired	
Hypophosphatemic osteomalacia	
Renal disorders	
Fanconi's syndrome	
Mesenchymal tumors	
Fibrous dysplasia	
MINERALIZATION DEFECTS	
Hereditary	
Hypophosphatasia	Abnormal alkaline phosphatase activity
Acquired	
Sodium fluoride	Inhibition of bone mineralization
Disodium etidronate	
MISCELLANEOUS	
Osteopetrosis	Abnormal osteoclast activity
Fibrogenesis imperfecta	Unknown
Axial osteomalacia	Unknown
Calcium deficiency	Inadequate bone mineralization secondary to low serum calcium concentration

to enhance the message to synthesize cholecalcin or calbindin, binding proteins, that transport calcium across the cell membrane into the extracellular space.[11] The vitamin also affects skeletal tissues by mobilizing calcium and phosphorus from old bone and promotes mineralization in newly formed organic bone matrix.[56] 1,25-Dihydroxyvitamin D also has effects on osteocalcin production, osteoclastic resorption, monocytic maturation, myelocytic resorption, skin growth, and insulin secretion.[18,59]

The regulation of 1,25-dihydroxyvitamin D is determined by the interaction of serum calcium, serum phosphorus, and parathyroid hormone. Decreased serum calcium levels cause secretion of parathyroid hormone that stimulates 1,25-dihydroxyvitamin D production. The result is an increase in absorption and mobilization of bone calcium and phosphorus. The increased phosphorus is excreted by the kidney, resulting in increased serum calcium. In the setting of decreased vitamin D, gastrointestinal absorption of calcium is decreased, resulting in decreased serum calcium concentration. This change in calcium results in secondary hyperparathyroidism, causing a mobilization of bone calcium along with a phosphate diuresis. The chemical results of these changes are low serum calcium, diminished serum phosphate, decreased urinary calcium, reduced tubular resorption of phosphate, and increased alkaline phosphatase. The levels of vitamin D are decreased, and those of parathyroid hormone are increased. The metabolic effects on bone are secondary to reduced mineral and secondary hyperparathyroidism.

Abnormalities. Abnormalities, hereditary or acquired, in the metabolism necessary for the formation of 1,25-dihydroxyvitamin D result in rickets or osteomalacia. Patients with an autosomal recessive genetic condition or an absence of the renal 25-hydroxyl-1-hydroxylase are incapable of manufacturing adequate concentrations of

1,25-dihydroxyvitamin D. These patients develop vitamin D–dependent rickets.[30] Patients with chronic parenchymal liver disease are unable to form 25-hydroxyvitamin D.[38] Renal osteodystrophy is the bone disease associated with chronic renal failure. Osteomalacia, osteoporosis, osteosclerosis (particularly in the axial skeleton), and secondary hyperparathyroidism are all potential complications of renal disease. Osteomalacia in renal osteodystrophy occurs secondary to the impaired conversion of 25-hydroxyvitamin D to 1,25-dihydroxyvitamin D due to a decrease in kidney cell mass.[5] Hyperphosphatemia and systemic acidosis, complications of chronic renal failure, also may contribute to the deficiency of the renal metabolite.[45] Anticonvulsant drugs, phenytoin (Dilantin) and phenobarbital, induce hepatic hydroxylase enzymes that alter 25-hydroxyvitamin D, producing inactive metabolites.[34] Phenytoin also may decrease calcium absorption from the gut.[75] A rare cause of abnormal vitamin D metabolism is mesenchymal soft tissue tumors associated with low levels of 1,25-hydroxyvitamin D.[25] A study of 72 patients with tumor-associated osteomalacia and low levels of 1,25-dihydroxyvitamin D included about a third of tumors of vascular origin, such as hemangiopericytomas. Other common tumors included nonossifying fibromas, mesenchymal tumors, and giant cell tumors. Only 10 of the 72 tumors were malignant.[53] Patients with hypophosphatemia and mesenchymal tumors may have clinical and radiologic findings in the sacroiliac joints that may resemble those of ankylosing spondylitis.[50] Patients may develop osteomalacia in the presence of normal concentrations of 1,25-dihydroxyvitamin D when impaired end organ (gut and bone) responsiveness to the renal metabolite exists. This may occur with chronic renal failure or use of anticonvulsant drugs.[10] When no other cause is evident, peripheral resistance to vitamin D associated with hypocalcemia, osteomalacia, and secondary hyperparathyroidism is referred to as vitamin D–dependent rickets type II.[12]

Phosphate Abnormalities

Phosphate, as well as calcium, in the appropriate concentration is essential for normal bone mineralization and muscle function. Any disorder that causes phosphate deficiency will result in osteomalacia. Phosphorus is present in most foodstuffs. Therefore, phosphate deficiency on the basis of malnutrition is rare. Patients who ingest large quantities of phosphate-binding aluminum antacids for ulcer or renal disease are at risk of developing osteomalacia.[24] Aluminum may cause phosphate malabsorption by precipitation of aluminum phosphates in the gut. The result is decreased serum levels of phosphate, normal serum levels of calcium, and elevated levels of alkaline phosphatase.[42] The most common cause of hypophosphatemia is related to hereditary or acquired renal tubular wasting of phosphate. A hereditary form of phosphate depletion is X-linked (male) hypophosphatemic osteomalacia. Phosphate reabsorption in the kidney is modulated predominantly by parathyroid hormone and, to a lesser degree, by serum calcium concentration.[32] Patients with X-linked hypophosphatemic osteomalacia (or familial vitamin D–resistant rickets) have complete absence of the parathyroid hormone–sensitive component of phosphate reabsorption. The disease is transmitted as a dominant trait in men, has onset in childhood, and results in short stature and bowing of legs in adults.[47] The disease may have an onset in adulthood (hypophosphatemic osteomalacia) in patients with no evidence of rachitic deformities.[31] Patients with familial vitamin D–resistant rickets develop increases in bone density in the axial skeleton along with ectopic calcification, which resembles ankylosing spondylitis.[69] Enthesopathy is a universal finding in adults with hypophosphatemic osteomalacia.[60] Many of these individuals are disabled secondary to degenerative joint disease in the lower extremities. A new form of hypophosphatemic osteomalacia is associated with hypercalciuria and increased levels of 1,25-dihydroxyvitamin D. The differentiation of these patients from those with other forms of hypophosphatemic osteomalacia is that the use of phosphate reverses osteomalacia and the use of vitamin D exacerbates the condition.[74]

Fanconi's Syndrome

Fanconi's syndrome comprises a heterogeneous group of disorders that cause dysfunction in the renal tubules.[20] The syndromes have been classified by Mankin into proximal, distal, or combination of proximal and distal tubular diseases.[47] Tubular disorders may result in phosphate wasting, glycosuria, aminoaciduria, renal tubular acidosis, hypokalemia, or polyurias. A number of disorders, including cystinosis, Lowe's syndrome (oculocerebrorenal syndrome), Wilson's disease, tyrosinemia, nephrotic syndrome, and multiple myeloma may cause tubular dysfunction resulting in osteomalacia. Tumors, both benign and malignant, that inhibit renal phosphate absorption may cause osteomalacia.[36] Tumors associated with osteomalacia include giant cell tumor, nonossifying fibroma, osteoblastoma, and angiosarcoma.[33] Osteosarcoma may also be associated with the development of osteomalacia.[72] These tumors may be producing a factor that is an antagonist to vitamin D.[66] Phosphatonins are hormones produced by mesenchymal tumors that cause renal phosphate wasting resulting in osteomalacia.[26] Fibroblast growth factor type 23 in tumor cells acts as a phosphatonin and causes osteomalacia.[65] Evidence for this proposal is the report of two patients who did not respond to increasing doses of vitamin D but became responsive to normal doses of vitamin D with removal of the tumors.[68] Neurofibromatosis also is associated with hypophosphatemia and osteomalacia.[43] The mechanism of phosphate wasting is of renal origin. These patients may improve with increased doses of vitamin D. Fibrous dysplasia, a disorder of unknown cause that causes bone lesions with a ground-glass appearance in combination with precocious puberty and skin pigmentation, has been associated with osteomalacia.[21]

Hypophosphatasia

Alkaline phosphatase is an enzyme required for the normal mineralization of bone. Patients with hypophosphatasia have a deficiency in this enzyme resulting in elevated levels of plasma and urinary inorganic pyrophosphate, phosphorylethanolamine, and osteomalacia.[39] Adults with the disease have osteomalacia with axial skeletal ligamentous and tendinous calcification and develop marked limitation of motion in the lumbosacral spine.[2] Fluoride in increased concentrations causes inhibition of bone mineralization. Patients in areas where fluorosis is endemic or those who received sodium fluoride for osteoporosis are at risk of developing osteomalacia.[71] Bisphosphonates, synthetic analogues of pyrophosphate, are inhibitors of bone formation and are used in the therapy for patients with Paget's disease. Patients receiving bisphosphonates at increased doses for extended periods may develop inadequate mineralization of bone and pathologic fractures.[41] Aluminum causes osteomalacia by interfering with bone mineralization at the mineralization front in bone.[9]

Miscellaneous Disorders

A number of miscellaneous disorders may be associated with osteomalacia. Axial osteomalacia is a disease occurring in adult men who develop typical osteomalacic changes in bone limited to the axial skeleton, including the cervical and lumbar spine.[27] Some of these patients have features on radiographs that are similar to those of ankylosing spondylitis.[51] Fibrogenesis imperfecta ossium is a rare lesion in men older than 50 who develop increased bone density, pseudofractures, and bone pain.[28] Osteopetrosis, also called marble bone or Albers-Schönberg disease, is a rare inherited disorder associated with increased osteosclerosis.[40] The benign form, autosomal dominant in inheritance, is associated with bone pain, fracture, osteomyelitis, and cranial nerve palsies due to bone overgrowth. The pathogenesis of the illness is related to the absence of osteoclastic activity in resorbing bone.

CLINICAL HISTORY

Patients with osteomalacia may present with a wide variety of symptoms depending on the underlying cause of their bone disease. The major complaint relating to their bone disease is bone pain. In nutritional osteomalacia, backache along with spine tenderness is present in over 90% of cases.[54] It is maximal in the lower extremities and axial skeleton and is worsened by activity. Lumbar pain increases with standing as opposed to the sudden and severe pain associated with osteoporosis. Back pain starts in the lumbar area and hips and then spreads to the upper portion of the spine and extremities.[29] Fractures of the spine causing sudden changes in height do not occur with osteomalacia unless the patient has concomitant osteoporosis.[23] The pain of osteomalacia tends to be more diffuse and less intense, but of longer duration. Muscle weakness and tenderness, along with episodes of muscle spasm, particularly in the proximal muscles in the lower extremities, may occur with hypocalcemia or hypophosphatemia. Movement of the spine is not necessarily painful. Patients with osteomalacia with long-standing disease may also have a history of fractures in appendicular bones. In rare circumstances, patients with X-linked hypophosphatemic osteomalacia may develop symptoms of spinal stenosis associated with lower leg weakness. The level of stenosis is frequently the lower thoracic spine and is secondary to ossification of the ligamentum flavum.[1]

PHYSICAL EXAMINATION

Physical findings are sparse in osteomalacia. The affected bones are tender on palpation, and proximal muscles may be tender as well. Muscle weakness, exemplified by inability to climb stairs or to rise from a seated position, also may be present. The patient has a waddling gait similar to that associated with inflammatory proximal myopathies. Kyphoscoliosis of the thoracic and lumbar spine is prominent if osteomalacia of the axial skeleton is of long standing. Adult patients with a history of rickets may have short stature, bowing of the lower extremities, and enlargement of the costochondral junctions (rachitic rosary).

LABORATORY DATA

Laboratory abnormalities are frequent in patients with osteomalacia, which is in marked distinction to the normal values found in patients with osteoporosis.[22] Patients with abnormalities in vitamin D concentration or metabolism have low serum calcium and phosphate concentration, elevated serum alkaline phosphatase concentration, a reduced renal phosphate threshold, generalized aminoaciduria, reduced urinary calcium excretion, increased parathyroid hormone levels (hyperparathyroidism secondary to hypocalcemia), and decreased serum concentrations of vitamin D (Table 14-6). The forms of vitamin D that are assayed are 25-hydroxyvitamin D and 1,25-dihydroxyvitamin D. These tests have assay variation and cross react with materials that may not be vitamin constituents. Therefore, vitamin D assay results must be viewed critically and in light of other independent data (calcium, phosphate, and parathyroid hormone levels).[4] Urinary calcium excretion is less than 75 mg/day in 95% of patients with osteomalacia, and this measurement is a useful screening test.[52] Laboratory abnormalities associated with phosphate wasting include low serum phosphate concentration, normal serum calcium levels, elevated serum alkaline phosphatase concentration, a reduced renal phosphate threshold, normal amino acid excretion, reduced urinary calcium excretion, increased parathyroid hormone concentration with therapy, and normal vitamin D concentrations. Additional laboratory abnormalities may be present depending on the underlying disease causing osteomalacia. Examples of these abnormalities might include decreased serum carotene, increased fecal fat in gastrointestinal malabsorption, increased urea nitrogen and creatinine in renal failure, and anemia and elevated erythrocyte sedimentation rate (ESR) with a tumor. Patients with osteomalacia secondary to gastrectomy may not demonstrate typical laboratory abnormalities. These patients may have normal serum calcium and alkaline phosphatase concentrations. In some patients, 25-hydroxyvitamin D was normal but bone biopsy revealed osteomalacia.[8] Osteocalcin is a marker of osteoblast function. In patients with osteomalacia, levels of osteocalcin are elevated along with those of serum alkaline phosphatase. The increase in osteocalcin is related to increased osteoid synthesis but not the mineralization defect.[19]

14-6 LABORATORY FINDINGS IN SELECTED OSTEOMALACIC DISORDERS

	Serum Calcium	Serum Phosphorus	Serum Alkaline Phosphatase	Serum Bicarbonate	Urinary Calcium Excretion	Serum 25-(OH)-Vitamin D	Serum 1,25 $(OH)_2$ Vitamin D	Serum Parathormone	Other
Vitamin D deficiency	N, L	L	H	N, L	L	L	L, N	H	
Intestinal malabsorption	N, L	L	H	N, L	L	L	L, N	H	Malabsorption tests positive
Chronic renal failure	L, N	H	H	L	L	N	L	H	Abnormal kidney function
Phosphate depletion (antacids)	N	L	N, L	N	N, H	N	N, H	N	Urinary phosphate low
Phosphate depletion (renal wasting)	N, L	L	H	L	N, H	N	N	N	Urinary phosphate high
Phosphate depletion (tumor-related)	N	L	H	N	N	L	N	N	Tumor interference with renal tubular phosphate reabsorption
Axial osteomalacia	N	N	N	N	N	N	N	N	

N, normal; H, high; L, low.

Pathology

The definitive diagnosis of osteomalacia must be made by biopsy of undemineralized sections of a bone (Fig. 14-11). Tetracycline, which will fix to newly forming mineralized bone, is given to patients before the biopsy sample is taken. The extent of tetracycline fluorescence in bone is used to measure the decrease in the mineralization front. There is also an increase in osteoid thickness (more than 20 μ) and an increase in osteoid seams covering cortical and trabecular bone associated with osteomalacia.

RADIOGRAPHIC EVALUATION

Roentgenograms

The radiographic findings of osteomalacia are osteopenia and loss of bone mass, and they mimic the changes of osteoporosis. The generalized loss of bone density in osteomalacia is indistinguishable from bone loss in osteoporosis. In osteomalacia, the remaining trabeculae are thickened between radiolucent areas blurring the trabecular pattern. One of the major radiologic findings in osteomalacia is pseudofractures (Looser's zones, milkman's fractures).[70] They occur in long or flat bones, are usually oriented at right angles to the cortex, and incompletely span the diameter of the bone. Pseudofractures, which usually occur symmetrically, may or may not be associated with pain. Radiographic findings in the spine may include expansion of the intervertebral discs with "codfish" vertebrae and scoliosis if osteomalacia occurs during periods of growth. In contrast to osteoporosis, most vertebral bodies are involved to a similar degree (Figs. 14-12 and 14-13). Pseudofractures may occur in the ribs, pelvis, femoral neck, ulna, radius, scapula, clavicles, and phalanges. With long-standing disease and minimal trauma, patients with weakened areas of bone secondary to pseudofractures develop true fractures.

Patients with hypophosphatemic osteomalacia may develop roentgenographic enthesopathic changes in the axial skeleton that may mimic ankylosing spondylitis. The changes in the sacroiliac joints included mild widening, symmetric intra-articular and anterior para-articular bony bridging, and enthesopathic calcification. These changes may occur without marked changes of osteomalacia in other areas of the skeleton.[13]

Patients with renal osteodystrophy will have changes of osteomalacia but also will have findings associated with secondary hyperparathyroidism, which are predominant. These patients have areas of osteosclerosis in the spine (49% in one study), bone cysts, and erosion of bone that may be noted around the sacroiliac joints.[15,63]

Scintigraphy

Some investigators have suggested that bone scintigraphy is useful in the evaluation of metabolic bone decrease. Increased uptake of tracer is noted in areas of active bone metabolism. Although helpful, quantitative results from a number of conditions overlap, making the differentiation of these disorders by bone scintigraphy difficult.[76]

DIFFERENTIAL DIAGNOSIS

The diagnosis of osteomalacia can be suspected in a patient with bone pain and deformity, muscle weakness and tenderness, abnormal laboratory data consistent with disordered bone metabolism, and radiographic evidence of inadequate bone mineralization; and it can be confirmed, if necessary, by bone biopsy. A recent study reviewed the significance of clinical, radiographic, and biochemical abnormalities in the diagnosis of osteomalacia.[7] Patients with osteomalacia had at least two of the following abnormalities: low serum calcium, low serum phosphate, elevated serum alkaline phosphatase, or radiographic evidence of pseudofractures. Tests that were not helpful included parathyroid hormone levels, 1,25-dihydroxyvitamin D, and decreased urinary calcium excretion. Histologic examination of a bone biopsy specimen is a useful test for patients in whom the diagnosis of osteomalacia remains in question after noninvasive screening tests are performed. Osteomalacia, like acute pain, is a sign of an underlying disease process that requires additional evalua-

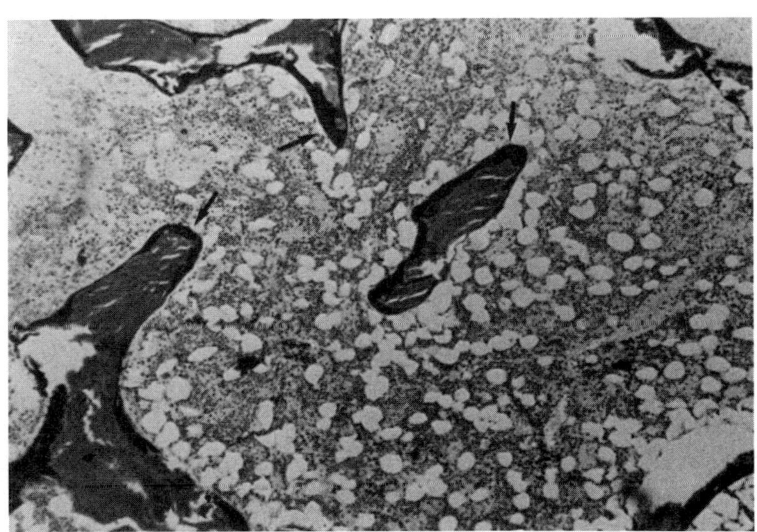

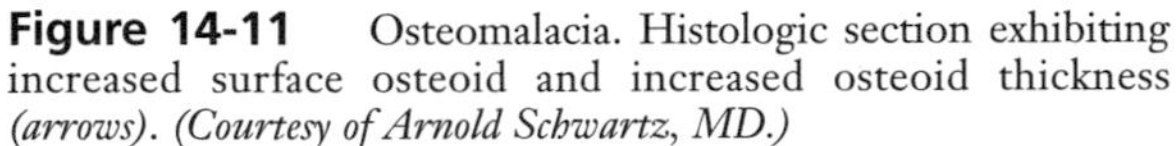

Figure 14-11 Osteomalacia. Histologic section exhibiting increased surface osteoid and increased osteoid thickness *(arrows)*. *(Courtesy of Arnold Schwartz, MD.)*

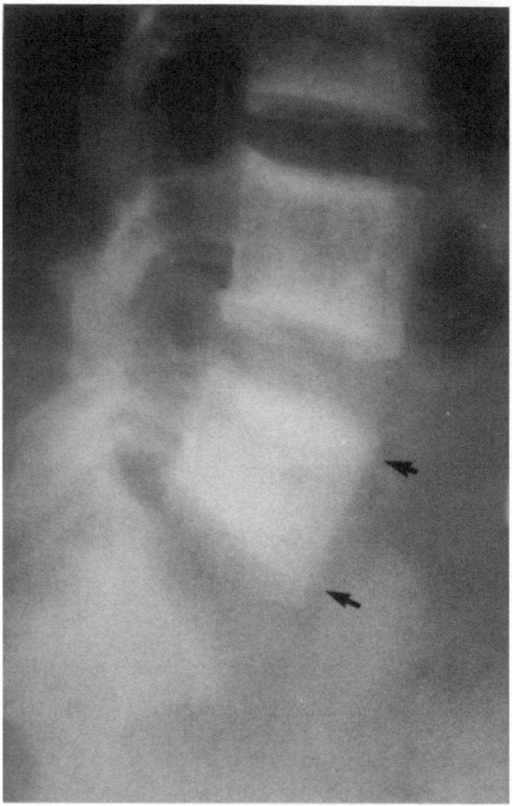

Figure 14-12 Osteomalacia. "Rugger jersey" spine of osteomalacia characterized by smudgy increased density of vertebral endplates *(arrows)* and osteopenia of the midportion of vertebral bodies with indistinct trabeculae. *(Courtesy of Anne Brower, MD.)*

tion. The possibility that a patient has one of the diseases associated with osteomalacia listed in Table 14-5 would need to be investigated. In addition to osteoporosis, diffuse carcinomatosis of bone, polymyositis, or rhabdomyolysis would also have to be considered in a patient with bone pain or muscle weakness. The acute onset of pain, with pain-free intervals, and normal calcium and phosphate concentrations help differentiate patients with osteoporosis from those with osteomalacia. It should be remembered that vitamin D deficiency is not uncommon in the elderly, many of whom are not exposed to the sun and do not drink milk. These individuals may have a combination of metabolic bone diseases, osteomalacia, and osteoporosis.[6] Anemia and abnormal serum proteins are associated with diffuse carcinomatosis (multiple myeloma). Elevated muscle enzyme levels identify patients with primary muscle diseases.

Osteomalacia may occur in the setting of another illness that causes abnormalities of the skeleton. A notable prevalence of unrecognized osteomalacia was present in hospitalized patients with rheumatoid arthritis.[57] In these patients, 12.9% had unrecognized osteomalacia. They were elderly, had a poor diet, and were housebound. Osteomalacia should be considered in patients with other reasons for musculoskeletal pain who are at risk for vitamin D deficiency.

TREATMENT

The treatment of osteomalacia must be directed at the underlying abnormality that results in abnormal bone

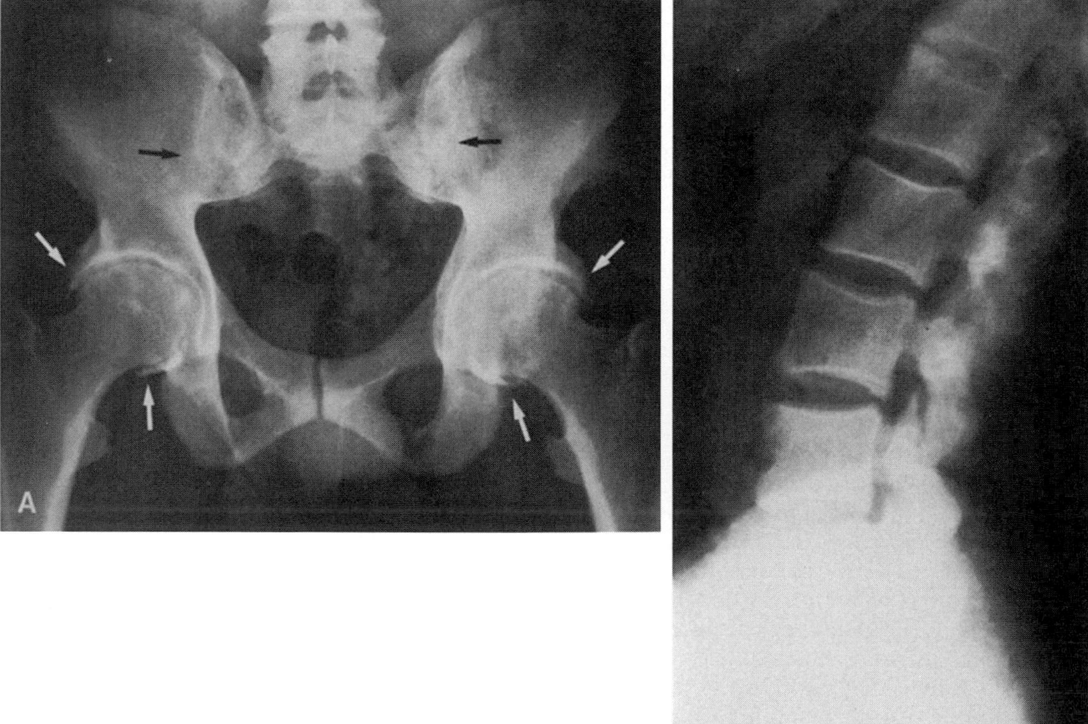

Figure 14-13 Hypophosphatasia. A 37-year-old man presented with marked stiffness of the spine. Laboratory evaluation revealed low serum alkaline phosphatase concentrations. *A*, Pelvic view reveals sclerosis of the sacroiliac joints *(black arrows)* and marked bony overgrowth of both acetabula *(white arrows)*. *B*, Lateral view of spine reveals generalized coarsening of vertebral trabeculae.

mineralization. The recommended daily intake of vitamin D is 400 IU for children and 100 IU for adults. This amount of vitamin D is adequate to heal bone lesions secondary to vitamin D nutritional deficiency, although higher doses can be given to speed healing.[29] Vitamin D comes in many different forms. These include vitamin D_2 (calciferol), dihydrotachysterol, 25-hydroxyvitamin D_3 (calcifediol, Calderol), and 1,25-dihydroxyvitamin D_3 (calcitriol, Rocaltrol).[44] Adequate calcium and phosphate intake are also required to ensure normal mineralization of bone. Therapy for patients with osteomalacia secondary to gastrointestinal disorders should be directed at the underlying gut disease. For instance, a gluten-free diet may in itself correct osteomalacia in a patient with celiac disease. Patients with refractory gastrointestinal disease may benefit from pharmacologic doses of vitamin D (1 to 10 mg/day). Oral pancreatic enzymes may improve vitamin D absorption in pancreatic insufficiency. Increased oral intake of vitamin D (1 to 2 mg/day), along with correction of acidosis or removal of a tumor, will improve bone mineralization in patients with abnormal vitamin D metabolism. Patients with chronic renal failure may benefit from replacement with physiologic doses of 1,25-dihydroxyvitamin D_3. Discontinuing antiepileptic drugs may be helpful in improving calcium absorption, decreasing osteomalacia, and improving musculoskeletal pain.[62]

Patients with phosphate-wasting forms of osteomalacia require phosphate supplementation and vitamin D to reduce the possibility of decreased serum ionized calcium concentrations and secondary hyperparathyroidism. Some patients may also require alkali therapy to control renal tubular acidosis. Patients with osteomalacia secondary to hypophosphatemia associated with mesenchymal tumors improve with removal of the neoplasm.[49]

Mineralization defects caused by fluoride may be prevented if calcium supplements are administered. The pathologic fractures associated with disodium etidronate used in therapy for Paget's disease may be prevented by using doses of 5 mg/kg along with an alternating monthly schedule of giving and not giving the drug. Medical therapy for adult hypophosphatasia is ineffective. Treatment of aluminum-associated osteomalacia has a number of options. Discontinuing aluminum-containing medications is helpful. Desferrioxamine has been utilized to allow mineralization of bone despite the presence of aluminum. The proposed mechanism of action is relief of the inhibitory action of aluminum on parathyroid cells and osteoblasts.[58] Others have suggested that iron in patients with chronic renal failure may be the cause of osteomalacia.[55] Desferrioxamine may be helpful by removing iron from these patients, allowing for improved bone metabolism.

The degree that sun exposure is needed for adequate levels of vitamin D is mitigated by the concern of the development of melanoma. Relatively little sun exposure is adequate to produce vitamin D levels that prevent osteomalacia. However, dermatologists prefer oral supplements instead of sun exposure. In 1997, the Institute of Medicine's Food and Nutrition Board established the recommended daily allowance for vitamin D to be 200 IU/day (5 μg) for persons up to 50 years of age, 400 IU/d (10 μg) for persons 51 to 70 years of age, and 600 IU/d (15 μg) for persons older than 70 years of age.

PROGNOSIS

The prognosis of osteomalacia is based not only on the time of onset of the illness (rickets) and the extent of the bone disease but also on the underlying disease and its reversibility with therapy. Many forms of osteomalacia are reversible with adequate vitamin D, calcium, and phosphorus supplementation. Pseudofractures heal and bone can be restored to normal mineralization and strength. Deformities secondary to bone weakening, lower extremity bowing, and kyphoscoliosis remain but do not progress. Patients with these reversible forms of osteomalacia are able to resume normal work activities without increased risk of fracture. Patients with hereditary abnormalities tend to be less responsive to therapy, and areas of bone may continue to be osteomalacic in these patients despite therapy. Patients with chronic renal failure and those on chronic dialysis may continue to have osteomalacia despite efforts at maintaining calcium and phosphorus concentrations close to normal and correcting acidosis. Secondary hyperparathyroidism, which complicates renal osteodystrophy, may necessitate the removal of hypertrophied parathyroid tissue to prevent additional bone destruction. Patients with tumors and osteomalacia will have a prognosis that corresponds to the characteristics of the neoplasms. With so many diseases associated with osteomalacia, the prognosis for that disease must be evaluated on an individual basis, taking into account all factors that deal with the underlying disease process, extent of bone disease, and potential response to therapy.

References

Osteomalacia

1. Adams JE, Davies M: Intraspinal new bone formation and spinal cord compression in familial hypophosphataemic vitamin D–resistant osteomalacia. Q J Med 236:1117, 1986.
2. Anderton JM: Orthopedic problems in adult hypophosphatasia. J Bone Joint Surg Br 61B:82, 1979.
3. Arnaud SB, Goldsmith RS, Lambert PN, Go VLW: 25-Hydroxyvitamin D_3: Evidence of an enterohepatic circulation in man. Proc Exp Biol Med 149:570, 1975.
4. Audran M, Kumar R: The physiology and pathophysiology of vitamin D. Mayo Clin Proc 60:851, 1985.
5. Avioli LV: Controversies regarding uremia and acquired defects in vitamin D_3 metabolism. Kidney Int 13(Suppl 8):36, 1978.
6. Barzel US: Vitamin deficiency: A risk factor for osteomalacia in the aged. J Am Geriatr Soc 31:598, 1983.
7. Bingham CT, Fitzpatrick LA: Noninvasive testing in the diagnosis of osteomalacia. Am J Med 95:519, 1993.
8. Bisballe S, Eriksen EF, Melsen F, et al: Osteopenia and osteomalacia after gastrectomy: Interrelations between biochemical markers of bone remodelling, vitamin D metabolites, and bone histomorphometry. Gut 32:1303, 1991.
9. Boyce BF, Byars J, McWilliams S, et al: Histological and electron microprobe studies of mineralization in aluminum-related osteomalacia. J Clin Pathol 45:502, 1992.
10. Brickman AS, Coburn JW, Massey SG: 1,25-Dihydroxyvitamin D_3 in normal man and patients with renal failure. Ann Intern Med 80:161, 1974.
11. Bronner F: Intestinal calcium absorption: Mechanisms and applications. J Nutr 117:1347, 1987.
12. Brooks MD, Bell NH, Love L, et al: Vitamin D–dependent rickets type II: Resistance of target organs to 1,25-dihydroxyvitamin D. N Engl J Med 298:996, 1978.

13. Burnstein MI, Lawson JP, Kottamasu SR, et al: The enthesopathic changes of hypophosphatemic osteomalacia in adults: Radiologic findings. AJR Am J Roentgenol 153:785, 1989.
14. Campbell GA: Osteomalacia: Diagnosis and management. Br J Hosp Med 44:332, 1990.
15. Chan Y, Furlong TJ, Cornish CJ, Posen S: Dialysis osteodystrophy: A study involving 94 patients. Medicine 64:296, 1985.
16. Compston JE, Thompson RPH: Intestinal absorption of 25-hydroxyvitamin D and osteomalacia in primary biliary cirrhosis. Lancet 1:721, 1977.
17. De Boer WA, Tytgat GN: A patient with osteomalacia as single presenting symptom of gluten-sensitive enteropathy. J Intern Med 232:81, 1992.
18. DeLuca HF: The vitamin D story: A collaborative effort of basic science and clinical medicine. FASEB J 2:224, 1988.
19. Demiaux B, Arlot ME, Chapuy MC, et al: Serum osteocalcin is increased in patients with osteomalacia: correlations with biochemical and histomorphometric findings. J Clin Endocrinol Metab 74:1146, 1992.
20. Dent CE: Rickets (and osteomalacia), nutritional and metabolic (1919-1969). Proc R Soc Med 63:401, 1970.
21. Dent CE, Gertner JM: Hypophosphatemic osteomalacia in fibrous dysplasia. Q J Med 45:411, 1976.
22. Dent CE, Stamp TCB: Vitamin D, rickets, and osteomalacia. In Avioli LV, Krane SM (eds): Metabolic Bone Disease. New York, Academic Press, 1977, pp 237-305.
23. Dent CE, Watson L: Osteoporosis. Postgrad Med J (Suppl) 42:582, 1966.
24. Dent CE, Winter CS: Osteomalacia due to phosphate depletion from excessive aluminum hydroxide ingestion. BMJ 1:551, 1974.
25. Drezner MK, Feinglos MN: Osteomalacia due to 1,25-dihydroxycholecalciferol deficiency: Association with a giant cell tumor of bone. J Clin Invest 60:1046, 1977.
26. Econs MJ, Drezner MK: Tumor-induced osteomalacia—unveiling a new hormone. N Engl J Med 330:1679-1681, 1994.
27. Frame B, Frost HM, Ormond RS, Hunter RB: Atypical osteomalacia involving the axial skeleton. Ann Intern Med 55:632, 1961.
28. Frame B, Frost HM, Pac CYC, et al: Fibrogenesis imperfecta ossium: A collagen defect causing osteomalacia. N Engl J Med 285:769, 1971.
29. Frame B, Parfitt AM: Osteomalacia: Current concepts. Ann Intern Med 89:966, 1978.
30. Fraser D, Kooh SW, Kind HP, et al: Pathogenesis of hereditary vitamin D–dependent rickets: an inborn error of vitamin D metabolism involving defective conversion of 25-hydroxyvitamin D to 1,25-dihydroxyvitamin D. N Engl J Med 289:817, 1973.
31. Frymoyer JW, Hodgkin W: Adult-onset vitamin D–resistant hypophosphatemic osteomalacia: A possible variant of vitamin D–resistant rickets. J Bone Joint Surg Am 59A:101, 1977.
32. Glorieux FH, Scriver CR: Loss of a parathyroid hormone-sensitive component of phosphate transport in X-linked hypophosphatemia. Science 175:997, 1972.
33. Goldring SR, Krane SM: Disorders of calcification: Osteomalacia and rickets. In De Groot L (ed): Endocrinology, vol. 2. New York, Grune & Stratton, 1979, pp 853-871.
34. Hahn TJ, Birge SJ, Scharp CR, Avioli LV: Phenobarbital-induced alterations in vitamin D metabolism. J Clin Invest 51:741, 1972.
35. Hahn TJ, Squires AE, Halstead LR, Strominger DB: Reduced serum 25-hydroxyvitamin D concentration and disordered mineral metabolism in patients with cystic fibrosis. J Pediatr 94:38, 1979.
36. Harrison HE: Oncogenous rickets: Possible elaboration by a tumor of a humeral substance inhibiting tubular reabsorption of phosphate. Pediatrics 52:432, 1973.
37. Haussler MR, McCain TA: Basic and clinical concepts related to vitamin D metabolism and action. N Engl J Med 297:974, 1977.
38. Imawari M, Akanuma Y, Itakura H, et al: The effects of diseases of the liver on serum 25-hydroxyvitamin D and on the serum binding protein for vitamin D and its metabolites. J Lab Clin Med 93:171, 1979.
39. Jardon OM, Burney DW, Fink RL: Hypophosphatasia in an adult. J Bone Joint Surg Am 52A:1477, 1970.
40. Johnston CC Jr, Lavy N, Lord T, et al: Osteopetrosis: A clinical genetic, metabolic, and morphologic study of the dominantly inherited, benign form. Medicine 47:149, 1968.
41. Kantrowitz FG, Byrne MH, Krane SM: Clinical and metabolic effects of the diphosphonate in Paget's disease of bone. Clin Res 23:445A, 1975.
42. Kassem M, Eriksen EF, Melsen F, Mosekilde L: Antacid-induced osteomalacia: A case report with a histomorphometric analysis. J Intern Med 229:275, 1991.
43. Konishi K, Nakamura M, Yamakawa H, et al: Hypophosphatemic osteomalacia in von Recklinghausen neurofibromatosis. Am J Med Sci 301:322, 1991.
44. Kumar R, Riggs BL: Vitamin D in the therapy of disorders of calcium and phosphorus metabolism. Mayo Clin Proc 56:327, 1981.
45. Lee SW, Russell J, Avioli LV: 25-Dihydroxycholecalciferol to 1,25-dihydroxycholecalciferol: Conversion impaired by systemic metabolic acidosis. Science 195:994, 1977.
46. Long RG, Skinner RK, Willes MR, Sherlock S: Serum 25-hydroxyvitamin D in untreated parenchymal and cholestatic liver disease. Lancet 2:650, 1976.
47. Mankin HJ: Rickets, osteomalacia and renal osteodystrophy: II. J Bone Joint Surg Am 56A:352, 1974.
48. Mankin HJ: Rickets, osteomalacia, and renal osteodystrophy: An update. Orthop Clin North Am 21:81, 1990.
49. McGuire MH, Merenda JT, Etzkorn JR, Sundaram M: Oncogenic osteomalacia: A case report. Clin Orthop 244:305, 1989.
50. Moser CR, Fessel WJ: Rheumatic manifestations of hypophosphatemia. Arch Intern Med 134:674, 1974.
51. Nelson AM, Riggs BL, Jowsey JO: Atypical axial osteomalacia: Report of four cases with two having features of ankylosing spondylitis. Arthritis Rheum 21:715, 1978.
52. Nordin BEC, Hodgkinson A, Peacock M: The measurement and the meaning of urinary calcium. Clin Orthop 52:293, 1967.
53. Nuovo MA, Dorfman HD, Sun CC, Chalew SA: Tumor-induced osteomalacia and rickets. Am J Surg Pathol 13:588, 1989.
54. Parfitt AM, Duncan H: Metabolic bone disease affecting the spine. In Rothman RH, Simeone FA (eds): The Spine, 2nd ed. Philadelphia, WB Saunders, 1982, pp 775-905.
55. Phelps KR, Vigorita VJ, Bansal M, Einhorn TA: Histochemical demonstration of iron but not aluminum in a case of dialysis-associated osteomalacia. Am J Med 84:775, 1988.
56. Pitt MJ: Rickets and osteomalacia are still around. Radiol Clin North Am 29:97, 1991.
57. Ralson SH, Willocks L, Pitkeathly DA, et al: High prevalence of unrecognized osteomalacia in hospital patients with rheumatoid arthritis. Br J Rheumatol 27:202, 1988.
58. Rapoport J, Chaimovitz C, Abulfil A, et al: Aluminum-related osteomalacia: Clinical and histological improvement following treatment with desferrioxamine. Isr J Med Sci 23:1242, 1987.
59. Reichel H, Koeffler P, Norman AW: The role of vitamin D endocrine system in health and disease. N Engl J Med 320:980, 1989.
60. Reid IR, Hardy DC, Murphy WA, et al: X-linked hypophosphatemia: A clinical, biochemical, and histopathologic assessment of morbidity in adults. Medicine 68:336, 1989.
61. Richards IDG, Sweet EM, Arneil GC: Infantile rickets persists in Glasgow. Lancet 1:803, 1968.
62. Ronin DI, Wu YC, Sahgal V, MacLean IC: Intractable muscle pain syndrome, osteomalacia, and axonopathy in long-term use of phenytoin. Arch Phys Med Rehabil 72:755, 1991.
63. Rubin LA, Fam AG, Rubenstein J, et al: Erosive azotemic osteoarthropathy. Arthritis Rheum 27:1086, 1984.
64. Schachter D, Finkelstein JD, Kowarski S: Metabolism of vitamin D: I. Preparation of radioactive vitamin D and its intestinal absorption in the rat. J Clin Invest 43:787, 1964.
65. Shimada T, Mizutani S, Muto T, et al: Cloning and characterization of FGF23 as a causative factor of tumor-induced osteomalacia. Proc Natl Acad Sci U S A 98:6500-6505, 2001.
66. Siris ES, Clemens TL, Dempster DW, et al: Tumor-induced osteomalacia: Kinetics of calcium, phosphorus, and vitamin D metabolism and characteristics of bone histomorphometry. Am J Med 82:307, 1987.
67. Sitrin M, Meredith S, Rosenberg IH: Vitamin D deficiency and bone disease in gastrointestinal disorders. Arch Intern Med 138:886, 1978.
68. Sparagana M: Tumor-induced osteomalacia: Long-term follow-up of two patients cured by removal of their tumors. J Surg Oncol 36:198, 1987.

69. Steinbach HL, Kolb FO, Crane JT: Unusual roentgen manifestations of osteomalacia. AJR Am J Roentgenol 82:875, 1959.
70. Steinbach HL, Noetzli M: Roentgen appearance of the skeleton in osteomalacia and rickets. AJR Am J Roentgenol 92:955, 1964.
71. Teotia SPS, Teotia M: Secondary hyperparathyroidism in patients with endemic skeletal fluorosis. BMJ 1:637, 1973.
72. Terek RM: Case 29-2001: N Engl J Med 345:903-908, 2001.
73. Thacher TD, Fischer PR, Pettifor JM, et al: A comparison of calcium, vitamin D, or both for nutritional rickets in Nigerian children. N Engl J Med 341:563-568, 1999.
74. Tieder M, Arie R, Bab I, et al: A new kindred with hereditary hypophosphatemic rickets with hypercalciuria: Implications for correct diagnosis and treatment. Nephron 62:176, 1992.
75. Villareale ME, Chiroff RT, Bergstron WH, et al: Bone changes induced by diphenylhydantoin in chicks on a controlled vitamin D intake. J Bone Joint Surg Am 60A:911, 1978.
76. Wahner HW: Assessment of metabolic bone disease: Review of new nuclear medicine procedures. Mayo Clin Proc 60:827, 1985.

PARATHYROID DISEASE

CAPSULE SUMMARY

	LOW BACK	NECK
Frequency of spinal pain	Rare	Not applicable (NA)
Location of spinal pain	Lumbar spine	NA
Quality of spinal pain	Diffuse ache, severe localized (hyperparathyroidism); stiffness (hypoparathyroidism)	NA
Symptoms and signs	Ulcers, renal stones, bone pain with percussion (hyperparathyroidism); muscle spasm, tetany, decreased motion (hypoparathyroidism)	NA
Laboratory tests	Hypercalcemia, hypophosphatemia, increased serum parathyroid hormone (hyperparathyroidism); hypocalcemia, hyperphosphatemia, decreased serum parathyroid hormone (hypoparathyroidism)	NA
Radiographic findings	"Rugger-jersey" spine (hyperparathyroidism); calcified spinal ligaments (hypoparathyroidism)	NA
Treatment	Surgical (hyperparathyroidism); vitamin D, calcium (hypoparathyroidism)	NA

PREVALENCE AND PATHOGENESIS

Parathyroid hormone (PTH) is the dominant factor in the maintenance of serum calcium in a normal range. Hyperparathyroidism results in excess concentrations of parathyroid hormone in the bloodstream and elevated serum calcium levels. Primary hyperparathyroidism is caused by abnormal growth of the parathyroid glands. Secondary hyperparathyroidism results from the secretion of PTH in response to persistently low serum concentrations of calcium. Hyperparathyroidism, regardless of type, leads to bone disease and abnormal physiology in a number of organ systems that are dependent on calcium for normal function (nervous, genitourinary, and gastrointestinal). The loss of calcium from bone results in pain, weakening, and fracture. Untreated disease causes marked osteopenia of the vertebral column with progressive vertebral body fractures and spinal deformity.

Hypoparathyroidism, an illness associated with deficient activity of parathyroid hormone, causes hypocalcemia with associated soft tissue calcification and bony overgrowth. Paravertebral calcification of ligamentous structures in the lumbar spine leads to progressive stiffness and limitation of motion.

Epidemiology

The absolute prevalence of parathyroid disease is unknown, although an incidence of 1 per 1000 patients was reported from data obtained at a diagnostic clinic.[5] The ratio of men to women affected is 1:3. After age 50, the incidence is 1 per 1000 males and 2 to 3 per 1000 females.[38] Rarely, hyperparathyroidism occurs in two familial syndromes associated with multiple endocrine neoplasms, type I (anterior pituitary, enteropancreatic, parathyroid tumors), and type IIa (medullary thyroid carcinoma, pheochromocytoma).[32,57]

Pathogenesis

PTH maintains serum calcium levels by stimulating intestinal calcium absorption, activating osteoclasts for bone resorption, and stimulating renal tubular calcium reabsorption, phosphate excretion, and enzyme synthesis of the active form of vitamin D.[43] The concentration of serum calcium perfusing the four parathyroid glands located posterior to the thyroid gland is the dominant factor in the control of secretion of PTH. PTH is secreted in response to low serum calcium concentrations initiated by means of a calcium-sensing receptor on the surface of parathyroid cells.[9]

PTH increases the rate of bone turnover. Persistent increases result in catabolic effects on bone. Intermittent elevations cause anabolic effects. The catabolic effects cause demineralization distributed variably between trabecular (vertebral body) and cortical (femur) bones. Osteopenia is a risk of this illness in 25% of patients.[50] The risk for fractures in individuals with mild hyperparathyroidism is similar to age-matched controls (one new fracture per decade). However, individuals with more severe involvement have an increased number of vertebral fractures when measured in large population studies.[27]

The hormone is released in an inactive form and is broken into at least two fragments (amino-terminal, short half-life, active component; and carboxyl-terminal, long half-life, inactive component) by the liver and kidney.[45] PTH is stored and secreted as an 84-amino-acid peptide. The active component is 34 amino acids in length. The effects of PTH on mineral metabolism are mediated by binding of PTH on the type 1 PTH receptor in target tissues.[30] PTH exerts its effects through activation of membrane-bound adenylate cyclase generating cyclic adenosine monophosphate.

PTH-related peptide is synthesized by cartilage cells and is not regulated by serum calcium levels. Its local release activates the type 1 PTH receptor. This peptide has similar affinity for this receptor as PTH.[52]

Hyperparathyroidism

Primary hyperparathyroidism is a disease process within the parathyroid glands. In approximately 90% of cases, the abnormality is a neoplasm, usually the overgrowth of one gland forming an adenoma. Less often, the abnormality consists of multiple adenomas (2%), diffuse hyperplasia (6%), or a carcinoma of the parathyroids (2%).[42] Secondary hyperparathyroidism is the increased secretion of PTH in response to low serum calcium levels caused by abnormalities in other organ systems, such as the kidney, or when there is inadequate vitamin D metabolism. Alterations in calcium metabolism and relevant hormones occur with aging. The mean serum PTH level is 20% to 40% higher in persons older than 70 years.[17] Calcitriol, the active form of vitamin D, is lower in older individuals.[14] Calcitonin levels are lower in older women. Tertiary hyperparathyroidism occurs when PTH is irrepressible in patients with normal or low serum calcium levels.[55]

A few patients have an inherited disorder. These inherited disorders include multiple endocrine neoplasia type 1, multiple endocrine neoplasia type 2a, hyperparathyroidism-jaw tumor syndrome (cemento-ossifying fibromas of the jaw, Wilms' tumor, renal cysts), and familial hypocalciuric hypercalcemia.[8,30,31]

Hypoparathyroidism

Hypoparathyroidism also occurs in primary and secondary forms. Primary or idiopathic hypoparathyroidism associated with cessation of function of the four parathyroid glands is uncommon and occurs more frequently in female children. These abnormalities include DiGeorge syndrome and autoimmune polyendocrinopathy/candidiasis/ectodermal dystrophy syndrome.[1] The usual form of hypoparathyroidism is secondary and is caused by damage to or accidental removal of the parathyroid glands during thyroid gland surgery.[35]

CLINICAL HISTORY

The vast array of symptoms associated with hyperparathyroidism is related to direct effects of PTH and hypercalcemia. The patient with the florid syndrome of hyperparathyroidism is unusual, because many patients are discovered with hypercalcemia by multiphasic blood screening at an early stage of disease. Many individuals are asymptomatic when mild hypercalcemia is first discovered.[39] They complain of bone pain and may present with a history of back pain from vertebral compression fractures.[15] Dull back pain also may be related to renal colic secondary to nephrolithiasis. Approximately 20% of patients with hyperparathyroidism develop nephrolithiasis.[51] Other renal manifestations include polyuria and polydipsia. Gastrointestinal symptoms associated with hypercalcemia include anorexia, nausea, vomiting, constipation, and abdominal pain secondary to peptic ulcer disease or pancreatitis.[29] Subtle changes in neurologic function, manifested as fatigue and weakness, occur in 50% of patients at modest elevations of calcium.[10] Markedly elevated serum levels of calcium may affect mental status and cause muscle weakness, hypotonia, and coma. Band keratopathy occurs in the eye. Musculoskeletal abnormalities may include generalized arthralgias and microcrystalline diseases.[23] The frequency of clinical symptoms is 40% for fatigue, 20% for musculoskeletal complaints, 20% for gastrointestinal complaints, 15% for renal failure, 10% for renal stones, and 10% for hypertension.[38]

The most prominent symptom of hypoparathyroidism is tetany. Tetany is tonic muscle spasm that occurs secondary to abnormally low concentrations of calcium. Persistent hypocalcemia may cause irritability, depression, and decrease in mental activity.

PHYSICAL EXAMINATION

Patients with hyperparathyroidism show muscle weakness on examination. Examination of the back may demonstrate percussion tenderness over a recently fractured vertebral body. Kyphosis occurs with wedging of vertebral bodies. Musculoskeletal examination may show joint inflammation (swelling, heat, redness, pain, loss of motion) in patients with acute gout or pseudogout. Both illnesses are commonly found in patients with hyperparathyroidism.[11,48] Acute pseudogout occurs in about 3.8% of patients with hyperparathyroidism.[18]

Patients with hypoparathyroidism may show signs of tetany when stressed with percussion over the facial nerve (Chvostek's sign) or carpal spasm with reduced blood flow from a blood pressure cuff (Trousseau's sign). They also may have limitation of motion of the lumbosacral spine secondary to soft tissue calcification.[25] These patients do not have spinal or pelvic tenderness on palpation but complain of pain with motion.

LABORATORY DATA

The laboratory parameter of greatest importance in the evaluation of a patient with suspected hyperparathyroidism is the serum calcium concentration. The serum calcium level is elevated in over 96% of patients with primary hyperparathyroidism.[24] Mild disease can be associated with intermittent elevations, so repeated determinations are indicated if suspicion is great and the initial calcium value is normal. Other chemical tests are useful but not diagnostic. Findings associated with hyperparathyroidism include low serum phosphorus, elevated serum chloride, elevated serum alkaline phosphatase, and elevated urinary calcium excretion.[36] Measurement of PTH by radioimmunoassay includes the detection of both amino-terminal and carboxyl-terminal epitopes of the peptide. The better assays do not cross react with PTH-related peptide.[26] The antibody tests for intact PTH have improved to a significant degree. In a study of 101 patients with a variety of disorders of calcium homeostasis including hyperparathyroidism, hypoparathyroidism, hypercalcemia of malignancy, or chronic renal failure, intact PTH assay was superior to midregion/carboxyl-terminal PTH assay in reflecting parathyroid function.[46] PTH molecules that are reactive in the two-site immunoassays are intact but may have no bioactivity. A slight modification of the PTH molecule will result in inactivity of the molecule.[33]

Hypoparathyroidism is associated with low serum calcium, elevated serum phosphorus, and normal alkaline phosphatase levels. Secondary hyperparathyroidism, usually associated with chronic renal failure, seldom produces hypercalcemia but is associated with elevated phosphorus concentrations. The electrocardiogram may demonstrate a shortened QT interval with hyperparathyroidism and a prolonged interval with hypoparathyroidism.

Patients with hyperparathyroidism have little evidence of clinical bone disease at presentation, and bone biopsy is rarely performed. When it is, it usually demonstrates the effects of PTH on bone. Characteristic findings include an increased number of osteoclasts resorbing bone, osteoblasts repairing bone that is being resorbed, and numerous fibroblasts producing dense fibrous tissue. Bone resorption may result in bone cyst formation, and bleeding into the cysts results in brown discoloration of the fibrous tissue and is referred to as a brown tumor. *Osteitis fibrosa cystica* is the term used in reference to the bone disease of hyperparathyroidism (Fig. 14-14).

RADIOGRAPHIC EVALUATION

Hyperparathyroidism

Roentgenograms

A variety of roentgenographic lesions are associated with hyperparathyroidism, including subperiosteal bone resorption, particularly on the radial aspects of the middle phalanges, resorption of the terminal tufts of the phalanges, "salt and pepper" appearance of the skull, and cystic lesions of the long bones.[19]

The axial skeleton is also involved in hyperparathyroidism. Most severely affected are the sacroiliac joints. Subchondral resorption affects the iliac side of the joint more than the sacrum, mimicking the "pseudowidening," sclerotic articular margins and bilateral symmetric distribution associated with ankylosing spondylitis. Resorption may also occur in the symphysis pubis (Fig. 14-15). Axial skeletal changes include osteopenia with wedging of vertebral bodies. Marked kyphosis may also be present. Sclerosis may develop at the superior and inferior margins of vertebral bodies, resulting in a "rugger-jersey" spine. This form of vertebral bony sclerosis may be associated with vertebrae of normal configuration or those that have undergone fracture and collapse. In one study, 20% of patients who underwent parathyroidectomy for primary hyperparathyroidism had evidence of vertebral body fractures, compared with 13% in an age-matched control group. The difference in fracture rates was statistically significant.[28] Subchondral resorption at the discovertebral junction results in bone weakening and Schmorl's nodes. Other axial skeleton and joint manifestations of hyperparathyroidism include instability of the sacroiliac joints, calcium pyrophosphate dihydrate deposition disease, and gout.[40,44] Hyperparathyroidism secondary to renal failure causes renal osteodystrophy and has radiologic similarities to primary hyperparathyroidism. Osteosclerosis with soft tissue and arterial calcification occurs more commonly with secondary hyperparathyroidism than with the primary disease.[22] Osteomalacia is also more frequently associated with renal osteodystrophy.

Brown tumors of bone are large cystic areas containing fibrous tissue. Brown tumors are most commonly found in the appendicular skeleton in hyperparathyroidism. Occasionally, brown tumors may involve the vertebral column and may be associated with vertebral collapse and spinal cord compression presenting as paraplegia.[49,54] Brown tumors will appear as large cystic areas in bone.

Scintigraphy/Computed Tomography

The methods for identifying the location of hyperfunctioning parathyroid tissue utilize thallium 201/technetium-99m parathyroid scan. The accuracy of these scans to identify parathyroid tissue is 87%.[55] The test was associated with false-positive results, particularly in patients with concomitant thyroid disease, resulting in the sestamibi scan not being used routinely.[37,56] Single-photon emission CT scan may be better able to detect the presence of parathyroid adenomas.[34] Ultrasound and CT also may be helpful to localize enlarged glands. In patients with an enlarged adenoma, CT scan may be the most effective test for localizing the malfunctioning parathyroid gland.[12]

Hypoparathyroidism

Roentgenograms

Hypoparathyroidism is most commonly associated with osteosclerosis. Subcutaneous calcification and calcification of the longitudinal ligaments of the spine are the most

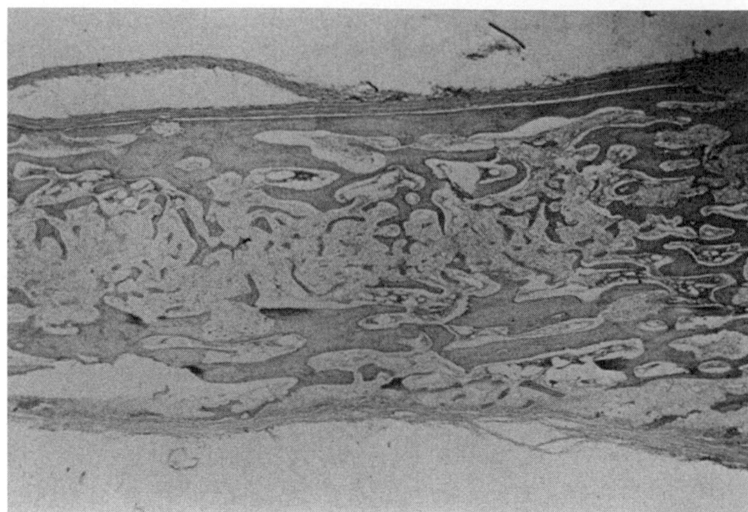

Figure 14-14 Secondary hyperparathyroidism associated with renal osteodystrophy. Histologic section exhibiting a combination of osteoporosis and osteomalacia. Bone matrix is decreased. Cortical osteoclastic activity is increased in association with bone resorption. *(Courtesy of Arnold Schwartz, MD.)*

common axial skeletal abnormalities.[25] The calcifications may become prominent to the same degree as those associated with ankylosing spondylitis.[13] In contrast to spondylitis, the sacroiliac joints are generally spared in hypoparathyroidism.

DIFFERENTIAL DIAGNOSIS

The diagnosis of hyperparathyroidism can be suspected in a patient who presents with hypercalcemia. The symptoms and signs of the more severe, classic disease are seldom observed. Evaluation of corroborating chemical and radiographic parameters help firm up the diagnosis, which can be definitively made by the surgical removal of abnormal parathyroid tissue.

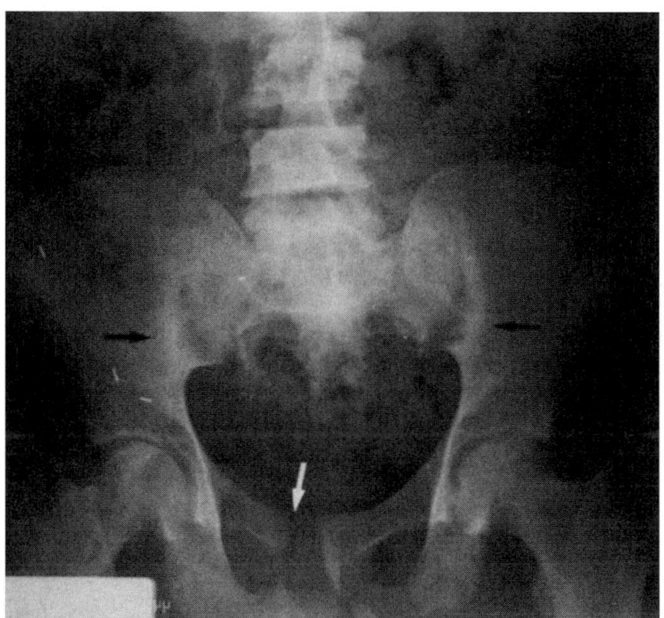

Figure 14-15 A 42-year-old man on hemodialysis after a failed kidney transplant with secondary hyperparathyroidism. Anteroposterior view of pelvis reveals "pseudowidening" of both sacroiliac joints with sclerosis most prominent in the ilium *(black arrows)*. Bone resorption of the symphysis pubis is noted *(white arrow)*.

Hypercalcemia

A number of illnesses cause hypercalcemia and must be considered in the differential diagnosis of hyperparathyroidism.[20] The major categories to consider in the patient with back pain, vertebral fracture, and hypercalcemia include malignancies, secondary hyperparathyroidism, and granulomatous disorders such as sarcoidosis. Careful examination for the presence of a malignancy, urinalysis, chemical testing for renal function, and chest radiographs should help differentiate these illnesses from primary hyperparathyroidism.

Hypophosphatemia

Hypophosphatemia is a complication of hyperparathyroidism. Phosphorus is the most abundant intracellular ion with only 1% of the 700-g total body concentration in the plasma. Most phosphate is present in creatine phosphate and adenosine monophosphate and triphosphate. The normal plasma concentration is 2.7 to 4.5 mg/dL. Severe hypophosphatemia occurs at concentrations less than 1.5 mg/dL. Causes of hypophosphatemia include hyperparathyroidism, chronic antacid ingestion, increased renal excretion, and malabsorption, among others. Adding phosphate to patients with hyperparathyroidism after correction of hypercalcemia can have a beneficial effect, particularly on muscular function.[53]

Hypocalcemia

The diagnosis of hypoparathyroidism is made based on the presence of decreased serum calcium in a patient who has undergone parathyroid surgery. Other diseases that cause generalized osteosclerosis (osteoblastic metastases, myelofibrosis, Paget's disease, fluorosis, and mastocytosis) rarely cause hypocalcemia.

TREATMENT

Hyperparathyroidism

The treatment of hyperparathyroidism is the surgical removal of the malfunctioning parathyroid tissue in symptomatic patients. There is no effective medical therapy to control the effects of excessive parathyroid hormone. MR evaluation of the parathyroid glands identifies the size of the glands, and by the signal intensity of the lesions, the histologic characteristics of the adenomas.[3] Most patients have a single parathyroid adenoma, and its removal brings the hyperparathyroidism under control without recurrence.[2] In a smaller group of patients with diffuse hyperplasia of all the glands, total removal of all but a small portion of a single parathyroid gland is required.[4] Occasionally, reoperation is needed for patients who have recurrence of the tumor or hyperplasia.[47] Patients with hypercalcemia who have clinically severe bone disease may require postoperative therapy with supplemental calcium, phosphorus, vitamin D, and magnesium. This is necessary to mineralize bone that has been chronically resorbed.[21] Most patients do not require this therapy unless tetany ensues after surgery. Bisphosphonates such as alendronate inhibit bone resorption but may be less effective in patients with hyperparathyroidism than in those with hypercalcemia from other causes.[7] Therapy for patients with secondary hyperparathyroidism is directed toward control of the underlying disease process. For example, renal transplantation may slow down the bone regression of secondary hyperparathyroidism.[16]

Patients with back pain from hyperparathyroidism are treated for their underlying disease. Patients with compression fractures receive symptomatic therapy, analgesics, anti-inflammatory drugs, intranasal calcitonin, and braces while their skeletal lesions heal but there may be residual deformity of the spine despite bone healing.

Hypoparathyroidism

The logical replacement therapy for hypoparathyroidism would be PTH, but hormone replacement is not practical for clinical use. Vitamin D provides a satisfactory alternative because it has actions similar to those of PTH. Acute hypocalcemia requires intravenous calcium gluconate. Vitamin D, 25,000 to 50,000 units/day, is needed to maintain serum calcium concentrations at 8.5 mg/dL. Urine calcium needs to be checked for concentrations greater than 250 mg/day, which require increased fluid intake to prevent renal stone formation.

PROGNOSIS

Patients who have mildly elevated calcium concentrations and are asymptomatic may be followed closely without surgical intervention. In one 4-year study, 20% of 141 patients with hypercalcemia required surgical intervention.[41] Many patients may be followed by testing serum calcium, alkaline phosphatase, and renal function twice a year. Patients who become symptomatic require surgical intervention. Surgery is effective at controlling the disease, although an occasional patient may require reoperation. Postoperative hypercalcemia may be persistent or recurrent. Persistent postoperative hypercalcemia is a level that is unresolved by surgery or returns shortly thereafter. The causes of persistent hypercalcemia include a second adenoma, unrecognized hyperplasia, or parathyroid carcinoma. Recurrent (after 6 months) postoperative hypercalcemia occurs secondary to continuous hyperplasia or indolent parathyroid carcinoma.[6] Bone lesions heal after the source of excess PTH is removed. Brown tumors usually heal, but large cysts may not heal and carry a risk of pathologic fractures through areas of weakened bone. Lesions in the spine may heal, but areas of fracture and angular deformity are not reversible. Hypoparathyroidism is treated with calcium and vitamin D supplements.

References

Parathyroid Disease

1. Ahonen P, Myllarniemi S, Sipila I, et al: Clinical variation of autoimmune polyendocrinopathy-candidiasis-ectodermal dystrophy (APECED) in a series of 68 patients. N Engl J Med 322:1829-1836, 1990.
2. Attie JN, Wise L, Mir R, Ackerman LV: The rationale against routine subtotal parathyroidectomy for primary hyperparathyroidism. Am J Surg 136:437, 1978.
3. Auffermann W, Guis M, Tavares NJ, et al: MR signal intensity of parathyroid adenomas: Correlation with histopathology. AJR Am J Roentgenol 153:873, 1989.
4. Block MA, Frame B, Jackson CE, Horn RC Jr: The extent of operation for primary hyperparathyroidism. Arch Surg 109:798, 1974.
5. Boonstra CE, Jackson CE: Serum calcium survey for hyperparathyroidism: Results in 50,000 clinic patients. Am J Clin Pathol 55:523, 1971.
6. Broadus A: Case 7-2002. N Engl J Med 346:694-700, 2002.
7. Brown DL, Robbins R: Developments in the therapeutic applications of bisphosphonates. J Clin Pharmacol 39:651-660, 1999.
8. Brown EM, Pollak M, Hebert SC: The extracellular calcium-sensing receptor: Its role in health and disease. Annu Rev Med 49: 15-29, 1998.
9. Brown EM, Vassilev PM, Quinn S, et al: G-protein–coupled, extracellular Ca^{2+}-sensing receptor: A versatile regulator of diverse cellular functions. Vitam Horm 55:1-71, 1999.
10. Burney RE, Jones KR, Christy B, et al: Health status improvement after surgical correction of primary hyperparathyroidism in patients with high and low preoperative calcium levels. Surgery 125:608-614, 1999.
11. Bywaters EGL: Discussion of simulations of rheumatic disorders by metabolic bone disease. Ann Rheum Dis 18:64, 1959.
12. Carmalt HL, Gillett DJ, Chan J, et al: Perspective comparison of radionuclide, ultrasound and computed tomography and the preoperative localization of parathyroid glands. World J Surg 12:830, 1988.
13. Chaykin LB, Frame B, Sigler JW: Spondylitis: A clue to hypoparathyroidism. Ann Intern Med 70:955, 1970.
14. Clemens TL, Zhou XY, Myles M, et al: Serum vitamin D_2 and vitamin D_3 metabolite concentrations and absorption of vitamin D_2 in elderly subjects. J Clin Endocrinol Metab 63:656, 1986.
15. Dauphine RT, Riggs BL, Scholz DA: Back pain and vertebral crush fractures: An unemphasized mode of presentation for primary hyperparathyroidism. Ann Intern Med 83:365, 1975.
16. David DS, Sakai S, Brennan L, et al: Hypercalcemia after renal transplantation: Long-term follow-up data. N Engl J Med 289:298, 1973.

17. Endres DB, Morgan CH, Garry PJ, et al: Age-related changes in serum immunoreactive parathyroid hormone and its biological action in healthy men and women. J Clin Endocrinol Metab 65:724, 1987.
18. Geelhoed GW, Kelly TR: Pseudogout as a clue and complication in primary hyperparathyroidism. Surgery 106:1036, 1989.
19. Genant HK, Heck LL, Lanzi LH, et al: Primary hyperparathyroidism: A comprehensive study of clinical, biochemical, and radiographic manifestations. Radiology 109:513, 1973.
20. Goldsmith RS: Differential diagnosis of hypercalcemia. N Engl J Med 274:674, 1966.
21. Gonzales-Villapando C, Porath A, Berelowitz M, et al: Vitamin D metabolism during recovery from severe osteitis fibrosa cystica of primary hyperparathyroidism. J Clin Endocrinol Metab 51:1180, 1980.
22. Greenfield GB: Roentgen appearance of bone and soft tissue changes in chronic renal diseases. AJR Am J Roentgenol 116:749, 1972.
23. Hamilton EBD: The arthritis of hyperparathyroidism, haemochromatosis, and Wilson's disease. Clin Rheum Dis 1:109, 1975.
24. Hect A, Gershberg H, St Paul H: Primary hyperparathyroidism: Laboratory and clinical data in 73 cases. JAMA 233:519, 1975.
25. Jimenea CV, Frame B, Chaykin LB, Sigler JW: Spondylitis of hypoparathyroidism. Clin Orthop 74:84, 1971.
26. Kao PC, van Heerden JA, Grant CS, et al: Clinical performance of parathyroid hormone immunometric assays. Mayo Clin Proc 67:637-645, 1992.
27. Khosla S, Melton LJ III, Wermers RA, et al: Primary hyperparathyroidism and the risk of fracture: A population-based study. J Bone Miner Res 14:1700-1707, 1999.
28. Kochersberger G, Buckley NJ, Leight GS, et al: What is the clinical significance of bone loss in primary hyperparathyroidism? Arch Intern Med 147:1951, 1987.
29. Lockwood K, Bruun E, Tansbol I: Disease of the parathyroid glands. Adv Surg 9:177, 1975.
30. Marx SJ: Hyperparathyroidism and hypoparathyroid disorders. N Engl J Med 343:1863-1875, 2000.
31. Marx SJ, Spiegel AM, Skarulis MC, et al: Multiple endocrine neoplasia type 1: Clinical and genetic topics. Ann Intern Med 129: 484-494, 1998.
32. Melvin KEW, Miller HH, Tashjian AH Jr: Early diagnosis of medullary carcinoma of the thyroid gland by means of calcitonin assay. N Engl J Med 285:115, 1971.
33. Michelangeli VP, Heyma P, Colman PG, et al: Evaluation of a new, rapid and automated immunochemiluminometric assay for the measurement of serum intact parathyroid hormone. Ann Clin Biochem 34:97-103, 1997.
34. Moka D, Voth E, Dietlein M, et al: Technetium 99m-MIBI-SPECT: A highly sensitive diagnostic tool for localization of parathyroid adenomas. Surgery 128:29-35, 2000.
35. Nusynowitz ML, Frame B, Kolb FO: The spectrum of the hypoparathyroid states: A classification based on physiologic principles. Medicine 55:105, 1976.
36. O'Riordan JLH, Adami S: Pathophysiology of hyperparathyroidism. Horm Res 20:38, 1984.
37. Pattou F, Torres G, Mondragon-Sanchez, et al: Correlation of parathyroid scanning and anatomy in 261 unselected patients with sporadic primary hyperparathyroidism. Surgery 126:1123-1131, 1999.
38. Petti GH Jr: Hyperparathyroidism. Otolaryngol Clin North Am 23:339, 1990.
39. Potts JT Jr: Management of asymptomatic hyperparathyroidism. J Clin Endocrinol Metab 70:1489, 1990.
40. Pritchard MH, Jessop JD: Chondrocalcinosis in primary hyperparathyroidism: Influence of age, metabolic bone disease, and parathyroidectomy. Ann Rheum Dis 36:146, 1977.
41. Purnell DC, Scholz DA, Smith LH, et al: Treatment of primary hyperparathyroidism. Am J Med 56:800, 1974.
42. Pyrah LN, Hodgkinson A, Anderson CK: Primary hyperparathyroidism. Br J Surg 53:234, 316, 1966.
43. Raisz LG, Kream BE: Regulation of bone formation. N Engl J Med 309:29, 83, 1983.
44. Resnick D, Niwayama G: Subchondral resorption of bone in renal osteodystrophy. Radiology 118:315, 1976.
45. Rosenblatt M: Pre-proparathyroid hormone: Intracellular transport and processing. Miner Electrolyte Metab 8:118, 1982.
46. Rudnicki M, McNair P, Tansbol I, Lindgren P: Diagnostic applicability of intact and midregion/C-terminal parathyroid hormone assays in calcium metabolic disorders. J Intern Med 228:465, 1990.
47. Sayle AW, Brennan MF: Strategy and technique of reoperative parathyroid surgery. Surgery 89:417, 1981.
48. Scott JT, Dixon ASJ, Bywaters EGL: Association of hyperuricemia and gout with hyperparathyroidism. BMJ 1:1070, 1964.
49. Shaw MT, Davies M: Primary hyperparathyroidism presenting as a spinal cord compression. BMJ 4:230, 1968.
50. Silverberg SJ, Locker FG, Bilezikian JP: Vertebral osteopenia: A new indication for surgery in primary hyperparathyroidism. J Clin Endocrinol Metab 81:4007-4012, 1996.
51. Silverberg SJ, Shane E, Jacobs TP, et al: A 10-year prospective study of primary hyperparathyroidism with or without surgery. N Engl J Med 341:1249-1255, 1999.
52. Strewler GJ: The physiology of parathyroid hormone–related protein. N Engl J Med 342:177-185, 2000.
53. Subramanian R, Khardori R: Severe hypophosphatemia: Pathophysiologic implications, clinical presentations, and treatment. Medicine 70:1-8, 2000.
54. Sundarim M, Scholz C: Primary hyperparathyroidism presenting with acute paraplegia. AJR Am J Roentgenol 128:674, 1977.
55. Voorman GS, Petti GH Jr, Schulz E, et al: The pitfalls of technetium Tc 99 mm/thallium 201 parathyroid scanning. Arch Otolaryngol Head Neck Surg 114:993, 1988.
56. Wei JP, Burke GJ: Cost utility of routine imaging with Tc-99m-sestamibi in primary hyperparathyroidism before initial surgery. 63:1097-1100, 1997.
57. Yamaguchi K, Kameya T, Abe K: Multiple endocrine neoplasm type I. Clin Endocrinol Metab 9:261, 1980.

PITUITARY DISEASE

Capsule Summary

	Low Back	Neck
Frequency of spinal pain	Common	Not applicable (NA)
Location of spinal pain	Lumbar spine	NA
Quality of spinal pain	Ache	NA
Symptoms and signs	Headache, visual disturbance, muscle weakness, normal range of spine motion, coarsened facial features	NA
Laboratory tests	Increased growth hormone and somatomedin C	NA
Radiographic findings	Posterior scalloping vertebral bodies, increased disc space on plain roentgenograms	NA
Treatment	Surgical ablation of pituitary tumor	NA

PREVALENCE AND PATHOGENESIS

Excessive growth hormone (GH) secretion from tumors in the anterior pituitary gland causes gigantism in growing children and acromegaly in adults. A number of morphologic and physiologic abnormalities occur secondary to hypersecretion of GH, including increased growth of bone, cartilage, and visceral organs; hypermetabolism resulting in impaired glucose tolerance; and osteoporosis. Low back pain is a prominent symptom of patients with acromegaly, although the range of motion of the lumbosacral spine remains normal.

Epidemiology

The prevalence and incidence of pituitary tumors are unknown. In one study, 13% of patients had small pituitary tumors that were asymptomatic and were only discovered at autopsy.[18] In symptomatic disease, recent epidemiologic studies have indicated an incidence rate of 3.3/million/year and a prevalence rate of 66/million.[2] The disease usually begins insidiously at 30 to 50 years of age and affects men and women equally.

Pathogenesis

GH has multiple actions, including maintenance of serum glucose levels, protein synthesis, calcium absorption from the gut, renal tubular absorption of phosphate, epiphyseal periosteal bone growth, production of connective tissue, and collagen synthesis. GH stimulates the hepatic secretion of insulin-like growth factor-I (IGF-I). IGF-I is the factor that results in the clinical appearance of acromegaly. GH secretion is stimulated primarily by hypoglycemia and, to a lesser degree, by exercise, sleep, and stress. Overproduction of GH while the growth plates are still open causes a marked overgrowth of bone, resulting in extreme height, which is referred to as hyperpituitary gigantism. In the adult with closed growth plates, new bone formation is endochondral, with periosteal growth resulting in widening bones and excess cartilage formation. The newly formed cartilage is friable and is easily damaged, causing fissuring and ulceration of the articular surface. Degeneration of the cartilage initiates increased cartilage and bone repair, and secondary osteoarthritis. Acromegaly is the disease associated with excessive GH production in the adult.[27] The source of GH is usually an acidophilic or chromophobic adenoma of the anterior lobe of the pituitary gland, which is located in the center of the skull in the sella turcica. This tumor accounts for about one third of all hormone-secreting pituitary adenomas. GH may also be produced by nonendocrine tumors that produce GH-releasing hormone (i.e., small cell lung cancers) or ectopic GH (i.e., non-Hodgkin's lymphoma).[3]

CLINICAL FINDINGS

The symptoms associated with acromegaly are related to the growth of the tumor intracranially as well as to the effect of GH and IGF-I on the musculoskeletal system and other viscera. Headaches and visual disturbances are directly related to the growth of a tumor in the sella turcica. Rheumatic disease symptoms of carpal tunnel syndrome, backache, limb pain, muscle weakness, and Raynaud's phenomenon are common.[6] Carpal tunnel syndrome is a result of edema of the median nerve rather than the increased volume of extraneural structures in the canal.[16] Arthropathy is the mode of presentation of acromegaly in a small minority of patients.[26] Spinal stenosis and disc herniation are unusual complications of acromegaly but have been more frequently recognized as a complication of this illness.[8,28] Back pain is a symptom in 50% of patients. The pain is localized to the lumbosacral spine in most circumstances but may radiate into the lower extremities when there is secondary cauda equina compression from spinal stenosis.[14] Pain in the lumbar area is insidious in onset and slowly progressive. In general, acromegalic patients with longer duration disease have more severe musculoskeletal symptoms and signs.[20,22] In the axial skeleton, the lumbosacral region is most often affected; the next most often is the cervical spine and, rarely, the thoracic spine.[27,29] Pain may be related to bony overgrowth and osteophyte formation. The effect of acromegaly on bone mineral density is variable. In women with estrogens, bone mineral density may increase in the spine and hip.[30] In others, osteoporosis of vertebral bodies may occur, whereas bone mineral density of the femoral neck may not be diminished.[23] The bone mineral status of the acromegalic patient is related to the gonadal status.[21] In addition to musculoskeletal abnormalities, a patient may also notice a gradual enlargement of facial features, deepening of the voice, thickening of the tongue, enlargement of the extremities, particularly the fingers, and diminished libido.

PHYSICAL EXAMINATION

Facial characteristics of the patient with acromegaly usually are prominent and alert the physician to the potential diagnosis. The jaw is large, and the skin over the face is thickened and coarse. A broad-based nose is usual, and the forehead is bossed. The musculoskeletal examination is characterized by joint swelling owing to periarticular thickening and noninflammatory synovial hypertrophy. Coarse crepitation with motion is common. The hands become "spade-like" and broad, with blunted fingers. Compression of the median nerve in the carpal tunnel elicits paresthesias in the sensory distribution of the nerve, and there is a positive Phalen test (wrist flexion test).

Lumbar spine examination may be unremarkable even in the 50% of acromegalic patients with back pain. Examination of the back may demonstrate percussion tenderness over the spine. The range of motion of the lumbar spine remains normal. This preservation of motion may be related to thickened intervertebral discs that retain their turgor. However, with progressive disease, painful kyphosis of the axial skeleton may occur. Acromegalic adults are not taller. Long tract signs indicative of spinal cord compression also may be found in some patients.[15] Secondary osteoarthritic changes may appear in the knees, hips, and shoulders. Rarely, an acute episode of joint inflammation may be seen secondary to crystal-induced synovitis from calcium pyrophosphate dihydrate deposition.[31]

LABORATORY DATA

Abnormal laboratory parameters include elevated GH levels, excessive insulin-like growth factor I, elevated serum glucose levels indicative of glucose intolerance, and elevated levels of serum phosphorus and alkaline phosphatase in proportion to skeletal growth.[7] Basal GH levels are elevated and are nonsuppressible during a standard glucose tolerance test. Glucose tolerance is impaired and is relatively resistant to insulin therapy. GH levels may be measured 2 hours after a patient ingests 75 to 100 g of glucose. A value greater than 5 ng/mL should initiate definitive testing for acromegaly.[36]

The activity of acromegaly and the pathologic effects of the disease on cartilage may be more closely correlated with IGF-I than with GH itself.[9] Unlike those of GH, the IGF-I concentrations are not modified acutely by food intake, sleep, or exercise. IGF-I production is a reflection of GH excretion over a day or more.[33] Increased IGF-I concentrations may be an indication of acromegaly in those individuals with the disease and equivocally elevated GH levels.[35]

RADIOGRAPHIC EVALUATION

Roentgenographic findings in the axial skeleton are prominent in patients with acromegaly. Anterior and lateral osteophytes of the lumbar and thoracic vertebral bodies are very prominent and may resemble diffuse idiopathic skeletal hyperostosis (DISH). Posterior osteophytes are less prominent. Posteriorly, the vertebral bodies are scalloped as a result of bone resorption.[19,34] Disc spaces are well maintained and may be increased in size (Figs. 14-16 and 14-17). Anterior intervertebral disc calcification, thought to be secondary to calcium pyrophosphate deposition, also may be seen. Other characteristic roentgenographic findings of acromegaly include increased heel pad thickness and widening of joint spaces secondary to growth of cartilage.[32]

Bone mineral density varies in the skeleton depending on the effects of excess GH and the hypogonadism resulting from the inhibition of gonadotropin production by the pituitary tumor. Peripheral bone densities are increased in the forearm secondary to increased GH, whereas vertebral values are decreased secondary to hypogonadism.[11]

MR evaluation is necessary for visualization of the sella turcica. Pituitary tumors as small as 2 mm in diameter may be identified. If the sella is normal, a CT of the chest and abdomen is indicated to identify an ectopic source of GH or GH-releasing factor.

DIFFERENTIAL DIAGNOSIS

The diagnosis of acromegaly can be suspected in a patient with the clinical symptoms and signs previously described and confirmed by measurement of GH in basal and suppressible states. Once abnormalities of GH are determined, evaluation of the sella turcica by CT scan or MR is essential.[10]

The differential diagnosis of a patient with symptoms and signs of headaches, head and extremity enlargement, and glucose intolerance is essentially limited to acromegaly. The radiographic changes of acromegaly with increased articular space and increased bone surface are easily differentiated from those of other disease processes. The later stages of joint disease of acromegaly are similar to those of primary osteoarthritis and are difficult to differentiate from this disorder. Unusual locations for osteophytes (metacarpophalangeal joints) and the lack of subchondral erosions have been suggested as factors differentiating acromegaly from secondary osteoarthritis.[37] Scalloped vertebral bodies, although associated with acromegaly, also may be seen as other disease processes associated with increased intraspinal pressure, weakness of the dural sac, or genetic abnormalities with tissue accumulation of mucopolysaccharides.[25] Lesions associated with increased intraspinal pressure include intraspinal tumors and cysts, syringomyelia, and communicating hydrocephalus. Disorders of connective tissue that result in weakness in the covering of the spinal cord dura predispose vertebral bodies to scalloping. These disorders, which occasionally cause low back pain, include Marfan and Ehlers-Danlos syndromes. Tumors of spinal nerves, neurofibromas, also may cause vertebral body indentation. The mucopolysaccharidoses, a heterogeneous group of genetic abnormalities that result in the excessive accumulation of mucopolysaccharides in various organs, may cause skeletal abnormalities. Hurler's and Morquio's syndromes are most closely associated with posterior skeletal abnormalities.[24] The physical appearance of these patients helps differentiate them from patients with acromegaly.

TREATMENT

The goals of therapy to cure acromegaly include the total elimination of the pituitary tumor and its mass effects, along with complete restoration of normal GH physiology.[13] Surgery is the preferred means to obtain the goals of therapy.[35] A transsphenoidal approach is adequate to remove the pituitary tumor unless massive suprasellar extension requires a craniotomy. The mortality rate is 1%. GH levels are reduced to 10 ng/mL or less in 70% of patients.[13] The life expectancy of acromegalic patients is the same as the general population if postsurgical IGF-I levels are in the normal reference range.[1] Surgical removal is successful in controlling growth hormone levels in a majority of patients with follow-up as long as 16 years.[5] Surgical hypopituitarism occurs in 10% to 18% of patients. Patients who suffer from spinal stenosis may benefit from surgical decompression to relieve nerve compression.[17]

Radiation therapy may normalize GH levels but may require 2 to 4 years to achieve this goal. Between 10% and 15% of patients may continue with elevated levels of GH despite 10 years of radiation therapy. The toxicity of radi-

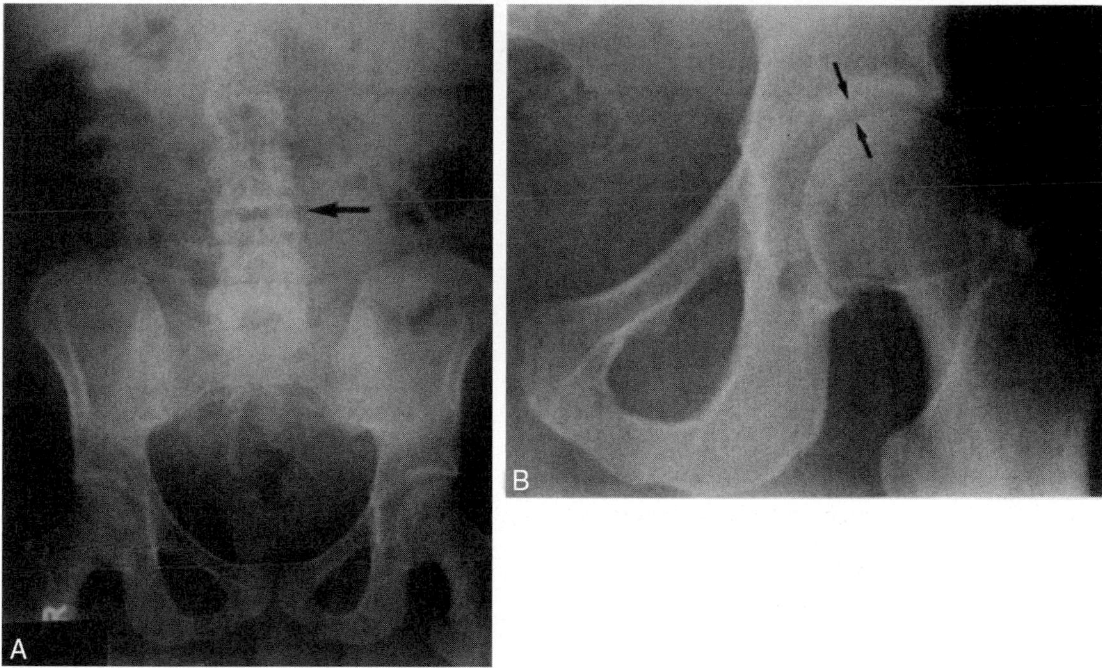

Figure 14-16 Acromegaly in a 34-year-old man. *A*, Anteroposterior view of the lumbosacral spine demonstrating well-maintained disc spaces *(arrow)*. *B*, Left hip joint with increased joint space *(arrows)*.

ation therapy is the risk of multihormonal pituitary insufficiency in between 15% and 50% of irradiated patients.

The somatostatin analogues are the medical therapy of choice for the treatment of acromegaly. These analogues inhibit GH secretion more potently and selectively than does somatostatin. Octreotide acetate inhibits the secretion of GH. Octreotide is indicated in individuals with macroadenoma that will not be cured by surgery or if surgery is refused or contraindicated.[12] Octreotide treatment results in a significant reduction in GH levels in up to 94% of patients.[39] The drug is injected subcutaneously two to three times a day. Sandostatin, a long-acting octreotide, is an intramuscular form of this therapy. This injection given once a month has been associated with a volume reduction of adenomas and normalization of growth hormone and IGF-I levels.[4] The most common toxicities include loose acholic stools, abdominal discomfort, and gallstones.

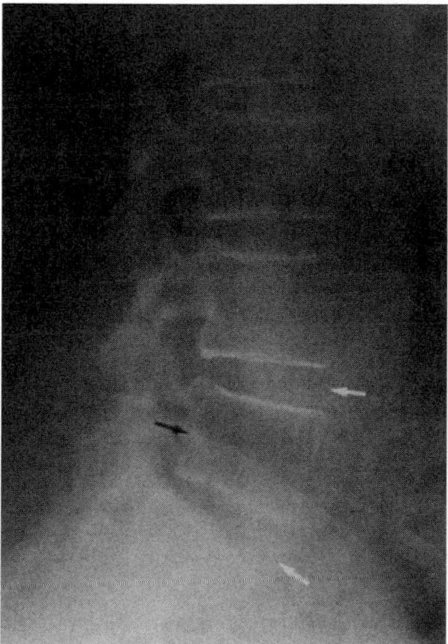

Figure 14-17 Acromegaly in a 46-year-old woman with a 5-year history of clinical symptoms of the disease. Lateral view of the lumbosacral spine reveals large intervertebral disc spaces *(white arrows)* and early scalloping of the L5 vertebral body *(black arrow)*.

Medical therapy may include bromocriptine, pergolide, or cabergoline, which are dopamine agonists. The doses of bromocriptine needed to reduce GH are higher than the doses needed to reduce prolactin secretion. Although 70% of acromegaly patients experience clinical improvement when treated with bromocriptine, GH levels are only reduced to 5 ng/mL in 20% of patients. Bromocriptine is taken orally every 8 to 12 hours. The side effects include malaise, nausea, vomiting, postural hypotension, nasal congestion, and depression.

A new form of therapy is a GH receptor antagonist. Pegvisomant, a genetically engineered analogue of GH, blocks the binding of the hormone to its receptor. A daily dose of 15 or 20 mg SQ of pegvisomant resulted in a normalization of IGF-I levels in 81% and 89% of patients, respectively.[38]

Unfortunately, therapeutic measures that are effective in controlling the pituitary lesion have little effect on the progression of acromegalic arthropathy in the axial skeleton or peripheral joints once the joint disease has developed. These patients develop progressive degenerative joint disease and are treated in a similar fashion with nonsteroidal anti-inflammatory drugs, physical therapy, and orthopedic surgery.

PROGNOSIS

Articular symptoms of acromegaly may range from mild joint pain to severe disabling arthritis of the peripheral joints and axial skeleton. Degenerative changes may be progressive, causing marked joint destruction that requires joint replacement of the hip or knee. Bony or disc enlargement in the spine may cause compressive symptoms requiring decompression procedures. The usual course of the illness, in general, is one of benign chronicity; however, some patients have a premature demise from congestive heart failure, complications of diabetes, or unrecognized hypopituitarism.

References

Pituitary Disease

1. Abosch A, Tyrrell JB, Lamborn KR, et al: Transsphenoidal microsurgery for growth hormone-secreting pituitary adenomas: Initial outcome and long-term results. J Clin Endocrinol Metab 83:3411, 1998.
2. Bengtsson BA, Eden S, Ernest I, et al: Epidemiology and long-term survival in acromegaly: A study of 166 cases diagnosed between 1955 and 1984. Acta Med Scand 223:327, 1988.
3. Beuschlein F, Strasburger CJ, Siegerstetter V, et al: Acromegaly caused by secretion of growth hormone by a non-Hodgkin's lymphoma. N Engl J Med 342:1871, 2000.
4. Bevan JS, Atkin SL, Atkinson AB, et al: Primary medical therapy for acromegaly: An open, prospective, multicenter study of the effects of subcutaneous and intramuscular slow-release octreotide on growth hormone, insulin-like growth factor-I, and tumor size. J Clin Endocrinol Metab 87:4554-4563, 2002.
5. Biermasz NR, van Dulken H, Roelfsema F: Ten-year follow-up results of transsphenoidal microsurgery in acromegaly. J Clin Endocrinol Metab 85:4596, 2000.
6. Bluestone R, Bywaters EGL, Hartog M, et al: Acromegalic arthropathy. Ann Rheum Dis 30:243, 1971.
7. Chang-DeMoranville BM, Jackson IMD: Diagnosis and endocrine testing in acromegaly. Endocrinol Metab Clin North Am 21:649, 1992.
8. Cheng CL, Chow SP: Lumbar disc protrusion in an acromegalic patient. Spine 15:50, 1990.
9. Clemmons DR, Van Wyk JJ, Ridgway EC, et al: Evaluation of acromegaly by radioimmunoassay of somatomedin-C. N Engl J Med 301:1138, 1979.
10. Daughaday WH: New criteria for evaluation of acromegaly. (Editorial.) N Engl J Med 301:1175, 1979.
11. Diamond T, Nery L, Posen S: Spinal and peripheral bone mineral densities in acromegaly: The effects of excess growth hormone and hypogonadism. Ann Intern Med 111:567, 1989.
12. Freda PU: Somatostatin analogs in acromegaly. J Clin Endocrinol Metab 87:3013-3018, 2002.
13. Frohman LA: Therapeutic options in acromegaly. J Clin Endocrinol Metab 72:1175, 1991.
14. Gelman MI: Cauda equina compression in acromegaly. Radiology 112:357, 1974.
15. Hornstein S, Hambrook G, Eyerman E: Spinal cord compression by vertebral acromegaly. Trans Am Neurol Assoc 96:254, 1971.
16. Jenkins PJ, Sohaib A, Akker S, et al: The pathology of median neuropathy in acromegaly. Ann Intern Med 133:197-201, 2000.
17. Kaufman HH, Ommaya AK, Dopman JL, Roth JA: Hypertrophy of the ligamentum flavum: Secondary cord syndrome in an acromegalic. Arch Neurol 25:256, 1971.
18. Kovacs K, Bryan N, Horvath E, et al: Pituitary adenomas in old age. J Gerontol 35:16, 1980.
19. Lang EK, Bessler WT: The roentgenologic features of acromegaly. AJR Am J Roentgenol 86:321, 1961.
20. Layton MW, Fudman EJ, Barkan A, et al: Acromegalic arthropathy: Characteristics and response to therapy. Arthritis Rheum 31:1022, 1988.
21. Lesse GP, Fraser WD, Farquharson R, et al: Gonadal status is an important determinant of bone density in acromegaly. Clin Endocrinol 48:59-65, 1998.
22. Lieberman SA, Bjorkengren AG, Hoffman AR: Rheumatologic and skeletal changes in acromegaly. Endocrinol Metab Clin North Am 21:615, 1992.
23. Longobardi S, Di Somma C, Di Rella F, et al: Bone mineral density and circulating cytokines in patients with acromegaly. J Endocrinol Invest 21:688-693, 1998.
24. McKusick VA, Kaplan D, Wise D, et al: The genetic mucopolysaccharidoses. Medicine 44:445, 1965.
25. Mitchell GE, Lourie H, Berne AS: The various causes of scalloped vertebrae with notes on their pathogenesis. Radiology 89:67, 1967.
26. Molitch ME: Clinical manifestations of acromegaly. Endocrinol Metab Clin North Am 21:597, 1992.
27. Ney RL: The anterior pituitary gland. In Bondy PK, Rosenberg LE (eds): Duncan's Diseases of Metabolism, 7th ed, Vol II, Endocrinology. Philadelphia, WB Saunders, 1974, p 966.
28. Parikh M, Iyer K, Elias AN, Gwinup G: Spinal stenosis in acromegaly. Spine 12:627, 1987.
29. Podgorski M, Robinson B, Weissberger A, et al: Articular manifestations of acromegaly. Aust N Z J Med 1828, 1988.
30. Scillitani A, Chiodini I, Carnevale V, et al: Skeletal involvement in female acromegalic subjects: The effects of growth hormone excess in amenorrheal and menstruating patients. J Bone Miner Res 12:1729, 1997.
31. Silcox DC, McCarty DJ: Measurement of inorganic pyrophosphate in biologic fluids: Elevated levels in some patients with osteoarthritis, pseudogout, acromegaly, and uremia. J Clin Invest 52:1836, 1973.
32. Steinbach HL, Russell W: Measurement of the heel pad as an aid to diagnosis of acromegaly. Radiology 82:418, 1964.
33. Stoffel-Wagner B, Springer W, Bidlingmaier F, et al: A comparison of different methods for diagnosing acromegaly. Clin Endocrinol 46:531, 1997.
34. Stuber JL, Palacios E: Vertebral scalloping in acromegaly. AJR Am J Roentgenol 112:397, 1971.
35. Thomas JP: Treatment of acromegaly. BMJ 286:330, 1983.
36. Thorner MO, Vance ML, Horvath E, Kovacs K: The anterior pituitary. In Wilson JD, Foster DW (eds): Textbook of Endocrinology, 8th ed. Philadelphia, WB Saunders, 1992, pp 221-310.
37. Tornero J, Castaneda S, Vidal J, Herrero-Beaumont G: Differences between radiographic abnormalities of acromegalic arthropathy and those of osteoarthritis. Arthritis Rheum 33:455, 1988.
38. Trainer PJ, Drake WM, Katznelson L, et al: Treatment of acromegaly with the growth hormone-receptor antagonist pegvisomant. N Engl J Med 342:1171-1177, 2000.
39. Vance ML, Harris AG: Long-term treatment of 189 acromegalic patients with the somatostatin analog octreotide: Results of the International Multicenter Acromegaly Study Group. Arch Intern Med 151:1573, 1991.

MICROCRYSTALLINE DISEASE

CAPSULE SUMMARY

	LOW BACK	NECK
Frequency of spinal pain	Rare	Rare
Location of spinal pain	Sacroiliac joints (gout), lumbar spine (CPPD)	Cervical spine
Quality of spinal pain	Acute and sharp, chronic ache	Acute and sharp, chronic ache
Symptoms and signs	Generalized microcrystalline disease, straightened lumbar spine	Generalized microcrystalline disease, straightened cervical spine
Laboratory tests	Monosodium urate or calcium pyrophosphate dihydrate crystals	Monosodium urate or calcium pyrophosphate dihydrate crystals
Radiographic findings	Joint erosions, disc calcification on plain roentgenograms	Joint erosions, disc calcification on plain roentgenograms
Treatment	NSAIDs, colchicine, corticosteroids	NSAIDs, colchicine, corticosteroids

PREVALENCE AND PATHOGENESIS

Microcrystalline disease, gout, and calcium pyrophosphate dihydrate disease (CPPD) are commonly associated with peripheral joint arthritis. Occasionally, patients with gouty axial skeletal disease may develop episodes of acute low back pain secondary to spinal or sacroiliac joint involvement. CPPD is associated with radiographic findings of disc calcification and degenerative changes of the discs and vertebral bodies. Symptoms of spinal pain may develop secondary to these degenerative changes. Calcification of the ligamentum flavum or atlantoaxial ligaments within the cervical canal may cause compression of the spinal cord, resulting in symptoms and signs of myelopathy.

Epidemiology

Gout

The actual prevalence of gout is not known. In one report, approximately 5% of a large adult population had hyperuricemia[21]: men develop gout during the fourth or fifth decade; women develop it after menopause. In a study of 37 women with gout, 86% developed gout after menopause.[50] The premenopausal women developed gout secondary to renal insufficiency or increased activity of phosphoribosylpyrophosphate synthetase. Prevalence increases with age in both sexes and is higher among males at all ages.[63] In North America, gout develops at rates of 1.7 and 0.2 cases/1000 person-years among men and women, respectively, aged 30 and older.[1] A similar rate was found in a cohort of male physicians who were enrolled in a study at Johns Hopkins.[60] The majority of people with primary gout are men, with a 20:1 ratio to women. In secondary gout, approximately 30% of patients are women.[14]

CPPD

CPPD causes symptomatic disease in about half the number of patients affected by gouty arthritis.[48] CPPD occurs in 5% to 10% of all adults. In one report 6% of an elderly population had CPPD in a joint.[44] CPPD shows a marked increase with age, with a prevalence as high as 30% in those older than 75.[20] Like gout, CPPD affects men more than women. The disease becomes symptomatic in patients in the sixth or seventh decade.

Pathogenesis

Gout

The cause of gout is related to the inability of the body to eliminate uric acid. This may occur secondary to underexcretion of uric acid through the kidney or to overproduction during protein metabolism. Uric acid accumulates in tissues throughout the body. The abnormality may relate to an inability of cells to transport uric acid out of the cytoplasm. A human transporter protein has been identified.[36] The transporter is present in not only renal tubular cells but also all nucleated cells. The inability to transport uric acid outside of cells may play a role in the pathogenesis of hypertension, cardiovascular, and renal disorders.[27] The presence of crystals in joints, soft tissues, and other areas may initiate the inflammatory response that results in acute symptoms. Uric acid may accumulate into large collections, tophi, which may be located in superficial structures such as the olecranon bursae, as well as in deep areas such as the kidney, heart, and sacroiliac joints.[35] Risk factors for the development of acute gout include hyperuricemia primarily, obesity, hypertension, alcohol consumption, lead exposure, and renal insufficiency.[12]

High concentrations of uric acid alone are not adequate for the formation of crystals in synovial fluid. Gouty synovial fluids promote urate crystal formation significantly better than fluids from rheumatoid arthritis and osteoarthritis. A heat-sensitive macromolecule in gout fluid may promote the formation of crystals.[45] Crystals may act as antigens that induce IgG antibodies. These antibodies may act as a nucleating matrix for new uric acid crystallization.[29] The ability of crystals to trigger attacks of acute inflammation is linked to their capacity to induce the release of a plethora of inflammatory mediators from phagocytes, serum proteins, and synovial lining cells into the synovial space.[64-66] The ingress of polymorphonuclear leukocytes supplies the soluble inflammatory mediators that initiate and perpetuate the acute attack.

CPPD

Calcium pyrophosphate dihydrate is the crystal in CPPD that initiates the inflammatory response, but the factors that facilitate the deposition of these crystals in cartilage and surrounding articular structures are poorly understood. Inorganic pyrophosphate (PP) is a byproduct in the formation of cyclic adenosine monophosphate. PP is normally hydrolyzed by an inorganic pyrophosphatase, resulting in very low tissue concentrations of PP. Elevated levels of PP are noted in individuals who develop CPPD.[26] PP levels are increased 5- to 8-fold in individuals with CPPD compared with those with other arthropathies. Pyrophosphatase is inhibited by the presence of divalent cations including iron, calcium, and copper. This may be reflected in the illnesses that are associated with CPPD. The disease may be associated with a number of metabolic conditions, including hyperparathyroidism, hemochromatosis, hypothyroidism, Wilson's disease, and ochronosis. The disorders that are currently believed to be associated with chondrocalcinosis and pseudogout include hypophosphatasia, hypomagnesemia, hyperparathyroidism, and hypothyroidism. Chronic arthropathy of CPPD is associated with hemochromatosis, acromegaly, and ochronosis.[28]

CLINICAL FINDINGS

Gout

Spinal pain secondary to gout is a rare occurrence. Those patients who present with spinal pain secondary to gout have a long history of peripheral gouty arthritis, are mostly men older than 50 years of age, and have nonradiating spinal pain due to chronic gouty arthritis.[39] Occasionally they may have a sudden onset of spinal pain associated with an acute gouty attack in the sacroiliac joints. These patients may experience pain-limiting back motion to a severe degree.[34] Tophaceous deposits may affect the spine and spinal cord to the point of the development of radicular symptoms, paraparesis, or quadriparesis.[56,62,67] Patients with spinal cord compression from tophi frequently have chronic polyarthritis.[35,38,52]

CPPD

Patients with CPPD of the spine may also have symptoms of axial skeleton pain associated with straightening and stiffening of the spine.[52] Rarely do they have neurologic symptoms. Back pain associated with CPPD is an uncommon symptom. In one study, only 7% of patients had back pain as part of their symptom complex.[54] In rare circumstances, patients with CPPD may develop symptoms of spinal stenosis secondary to calcification in the spinal canal.[17] Neurologic symptoms compatible with myelopathy occur in the occasional patient with CPPD involvement of the ligamentum flavum in the foramen magnum and cervical spine.[13] Involvement of the cervical spine may occur independent of CPPD in other areas of the skeleton.[8] CPPD deposits may be found throughout the cervical, thoracic, and lumbar spine.[55] Pseudogout may cause an acute attack that causes spasm of the cervical spine that mimics the symptoms and signs associated with meningitis.[24]

PHYSICAL EXAMINATION

Gout

Physical findings in the spine of a patient with gout may demonstrate spinal stiffness, loss of motion, and muscle spasm with pain on motion. Patients with acute gout of the axial skeleton may be febrile on initial presentation.[34] Examination of extensor surfaces (elbows, Achilles tendons) and ears may demonstrate tophaceous deposits. Peripheral joints may be affected at the same time as the spine. However, even in patients with polyarticular gout, involvement of the spine is unusual.[33]

CPPD

Patients with CPPD disease may have restricted motion as a result of associated degenerative disease of the spine. Neurologic signs with CPPD are rare.[19] Patients with CPPD may also develop prolonged fever and elevated erythrocyte sedimentation rate (ESR).[6]

LABORATORY DATA

Gout

Hyperuricemia is a prerequisite for the diagnosis of gout and many patients will have an elevated level of uric acid during an acute attack. However, a normal level does not eliminate the possibility of gout since uric acid concentrations fluctuate, particularly with anti-inflammatory medications. The presence of arthritis and elevated uric acid concentration does not equate with a diagnosis of gout. Hyperuricemia may occur without acute gout. The diagnosis of gout is established definitively by the demonstration of characteristic crystals of monosodium urate monohydrate in synovial fluid or from aspirates of tophaceous deposits. These crystals are negatively birefringent. Other synovial fluid characteristics of gout include a fair mucin clot test, elevated white blood cell count, and increased protein concentration. In a patient with gouty nephropathy, renal function as measured by blood urea nitrogen and creatinine may be impaired, and red blood cells may be present in the urine of the patient with uric acid renal stones. Components of the acute phase response, including serum leukocytes, platelet count, ESR, and C-reactive protein, are elevated in patients with acute gout.[59]

CPPD

Blood studies in CPPD are of no use except to detect associated diseases such as hemochromatosis or hyperparathyroidism. Synovial fluid aspiration of acute effusions will demonstrate calcium pyrophosphate dihydrate crystals in the vast majority of patients. A careful examination for these crystals is necessary because they are less numerous than uric acid crystals in an inflamed joint and they polarize light weakly in contrast to urate crystals. White blood cell count and protein concentration in synovial fluid will be elevated, at levels similar to those occurring in gout.

RADIOGRAPHIC EVALUATION

Roentgenograms

Gout

Roentgenographic abnormalities in the sacroiliac joint and axial skeleton are unusual in gout, but gout may cause joint margin sclerosis with cystic areas of erosion in the ilium, sacrum, and vertebral bodies.[2] Gout also may cause erosions of endplates of vertebral bodies, disc space narrowing, and vertebral subluxation (Figs. 14-18 and 14-19).[22] The changes associated with gout in the intervertebral disc may be confused with infectious discitis. Biopsy material from suspected areas should be placed in absolute alcohol and not formalin so that crystals will not be leached out from the specimen.[16] Occasionally, extradural deposits of urate may cause nerve compression and can be detected by myelographic examination.[37] Pathologic fractures in posterior elements of vertebral bodies are also found in patients with extensive gouty involvement.[10]

CPPD

Roentgenographic manifestations of CPPD in the spine include intervertebral disc calcifications, primarily in the annulus fibrosus. The nucleus pulposus is not involved.[9,43] Calcification also may be present in the symphysis pubis, sacroiliac joint, and throughout the cervical spine, most commonly at the C5-C6 interspace.[5] The ligamentum flavum may be calcified.[19]

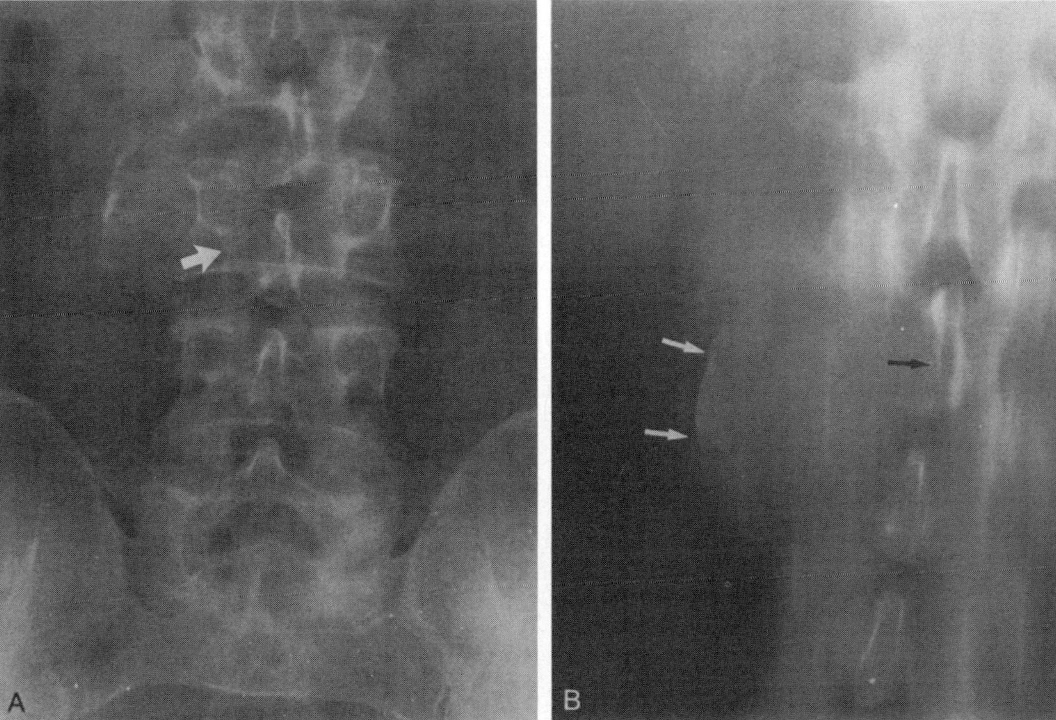

Figure 14-18 Gout. *A*, Huge tophus of gout eroding the R lamina *(arrow)* of L2. *B*, Tomogram shows erosion of the posterior spinous process *(black arrow)*. There is a rim of expanding cortex present *(white arrows)*. *(Courtesy of Anne Brower, MD.)*

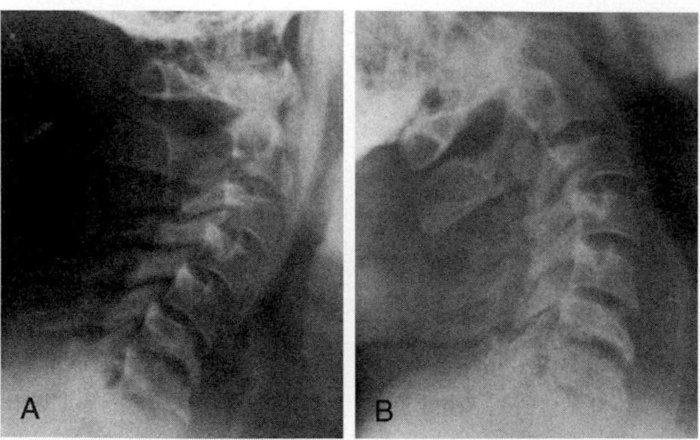

Figure 14-19 Gout. Flexion *(A)* and extension *(B)* cervical spine roentgenograms demonstrate endplate erosive changes in C6-C7. *(From Alarçon G, Reveille J: Gouty arthritis of the axial skeleton including the sacroiliac joints. Arch Intern Med 147:2018-2019, 1987. Copyright 1987, American Medical Association.)*

Scintigraphy

Gout

Indium-111–labeled leukocyte scintigraphy will identify accumulation of tracer in involved joints during an acute attack. This type of scan has been utilized in patients with appendicular arthritis. The utility of this type of scan with axial involvement with gout is not known.[49] Repeat scan will demonstrate decreased uptake after therapy corresponding to the patient's course.

Computed Tomography/Magnetic Resonance

Gout/CPPD

Calcifications of the ligamentum flavum may be better visualized by computed tomography (CT) or magnetic resonance (MR) imaging (Fig 14-20). MR is able to detect tophaceous deposits that mimic discovertebral infection or an epidural abscess.[7,18] Patients with spinal stenosis secondary to ligamentum flavum calcification frequently have evidence of CPPD in peripheral joints.[8] Disc space narrowing associated with vertebral osteophyte formation may occur and is a common finding in the spine.[68] Vertebral body destruction may become severe enough to cause degenerative spondylolisthesis.[54,57] On CT, the calcifications are contiguous to the laminae but not continuous with the spinal cord. Subluxation of the atlantoaxial joint has been reported with CPPD.[53] Ninety to 100 patients with CPPD of the spine have been reported in the medical literature.[5]

DIFFERENTIAL DIAGNOSIS

The diagnosis of microcrystalline disease is confirmed by the detection of the specific crystal in a clinical specimen. Patients with spinal pain secondary to microcrystalline disease usually have extensive disease in other locations, so that aspiration of the facet or sacroiliac joints is not necessary. Careful monitoring of response to therapy will show rapid improvement if the diagnosis is correct.

Infection must always be considered if the patient has extreme pain, fever, and an elevated peripheral white blood cell count. Patients with septic sacroiliac joints or osteomyelitis will not improve with anti-gout therapy, and they will require further evaluation with blood cultures and joint aspiration to rule out infection.

Cervical spine subluxation in the upper cervical spine in CPPD disease resembles the findings of rheumatoid arthritis. The absence of diffuse osteopenia, apophyseal erosions, and rheumatoid factor helps distinguish the diseases.

Hemochromatosis

Hemochromatosis, a disease associated with increased body stores of iron, is an important illness to consider in the differential diagnosis of CPPD.[23] The pathologic processes associated with iron deposition do occur in the spine in patients with hemochromatosis. Roentgenographic changes

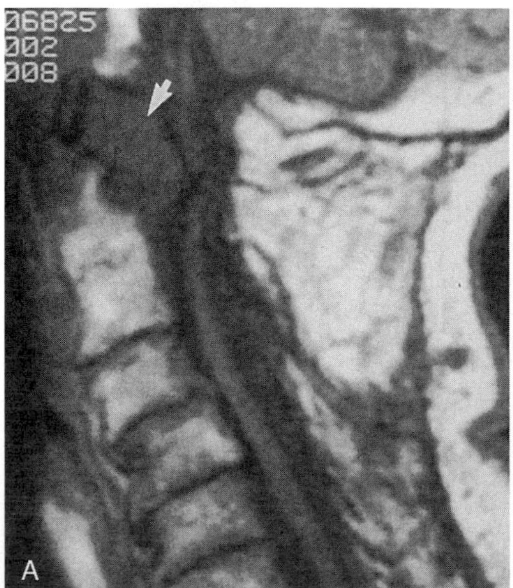

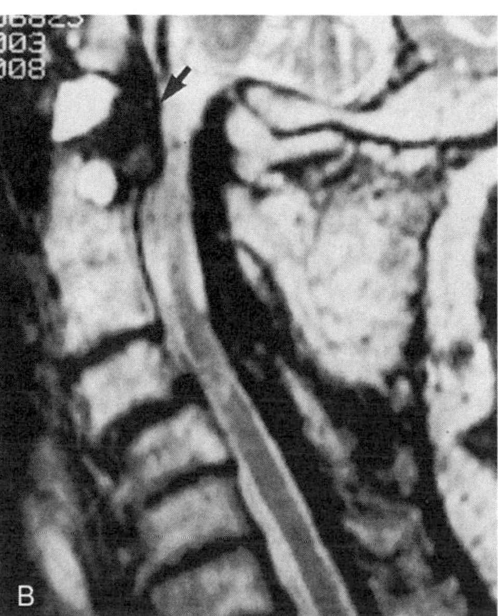

Figure 14-20 Calcium pyrophosphate dihydrate disease (CPPD). In this 70-year-old man, sagittal T1-weighted (TR/TE 500/12) *(A)* and T2-weighted (TR/TE 3400/96) *(B)* spin-echo MR images show a mass *(arrows)* about the eroded odontoid process. Note adjacent areas of high-signal intensity in *B*. The spinal cord is displaced. On CT scans, the mass was found to be calcified. CPPD crystal deposition was documented when the mass was surgically removed. *(From Resnick D, Niwayama G: Calcium pyrophosphate dihydrate (CPPD) crystal deposition disease. In Resnick D [ed]: Diagnosis of Bone and Joint Disorders, 3rd ed. Philadelphia, WB Saunders, 1995, p 1598.)*

are seen in the lumbosacral spine in 15% of patients, but patients rarely have symptoms in the axial skeleton associated with these changes.[11] Most patients with symptomatic hemochromatosis are men between the ages of 40 and 60 years. Arthritis occurs in 20% to 50% of patients and is a late manifestation of the disease. The arthritis may have characteristics of chronic disease similar to that of osteoarthritis or symptoms of acute disease similar to those of CPPD. Roentgenographic features associated with hemochromatosis include axial skeleton osteoporosis associated with "fish vertebrae"; chondrocalcinosis affecting the symphysis pubis, intervertebral discs, and sacroiliac joints; joint space narrowing; and osteophytosis (Fig. 14-21).[19] These spinal abnormalities may lead to fracture and vertebral collapse, back pain, and deformity.[25] The diagnosis of hemochromatosis is suspected because of the presence of bronze skin, diabetes, cirrhosis, and elevated levels of iron and the iron-binding complex, ferritin. The diagnosis is confirmed by the presence of excessive amounts of iron on liver biopsy. MR is a noninvasive method of confirming excess iron deposition in the liver. MR is able to detect excess iron of 400 μg/g of tissue. Liver biopsy is not always required. The therapy for hemochromatosis is the removal of iron through phlebotomy. Unfortunately, the changes of arthritis are progressive despite control of iron concentrations.

Calcific Retropharyngeal Tendinitis

Acute calcific retropharyngeal tendinitis is a rare form of calcific periarthritis and is associated with acute upper neck pain and transient calcification of the tendon of the longus colli muscle, the principal flexor of the neck.[61] Middle-aged persons of both sexes are affected. These patients develop painful restriction of motion and pain on swallowing. Tenderness may occur over the C2 and C3 spinous processes. A lateral roentgenogram of the cervical spine reveals a calcific deposit anterior to the atlantoaxial junction and below the anterior arch of C1 (Fig. 14-22). Resorption of the deposit may occur throughout a 14-day period. Therapy is a cervical collar and nonsteroidal anti-inflammatory drugs. This form of calcific tendinitis is one of the forms of hydroxyapatite calcification that may cause calcification in and around structures of the cervical spine and spinal canal. These calcifications look similar to those of CPPD and may be associated with radiculopathy and myelopathy.[47]

Destructive Spondyloarthropathy Associated with Hemodialysis

Patients who have chronic renal failure on dialysis and those with chronic renal failure alone may develop a destructive lesion of the cervical spine.[32] The prevalence of destructive lesions in the cervical spine in patients with chronic hemodialysis is 15%.[30] The mean period on dialysis before the development of spondyloarthropathy is 34 months.[15] Symptoms associated with this disorder include neck pain and radiculopathy.[70] The mechanism by which destructive spondyloarthropathy occurs is not clear. Some investigators have suggested that the destructive lesions are related to hyperparathyroidism.[41] This fact correlates with the presence of the syndrome in patients who have chronic renal failure who have not received dialysis. Other investigators have reported beta$_2$-microglobulin amyloid deposits in the destructive lesions in the spine.[46,69] Amyloid deposits in the ligaments of the spine cause laxity, resulting in excess motion and eventual bony destruction. Although CPPD crystals are not frequently detected in these lesions, calcium hydroxyapatite crystals have been recovered from involved joints. Amyloid deposits may reach adequate size in the cervical spine to cause spinal cord impingement and signs of myelopathy.[3] Radiographic abnormalities of disc space narrowing may simulate changes of osteomyelitis. The use of MR and CT to exclude the presence of soft tissue alterations helps exclude the possibility of infection

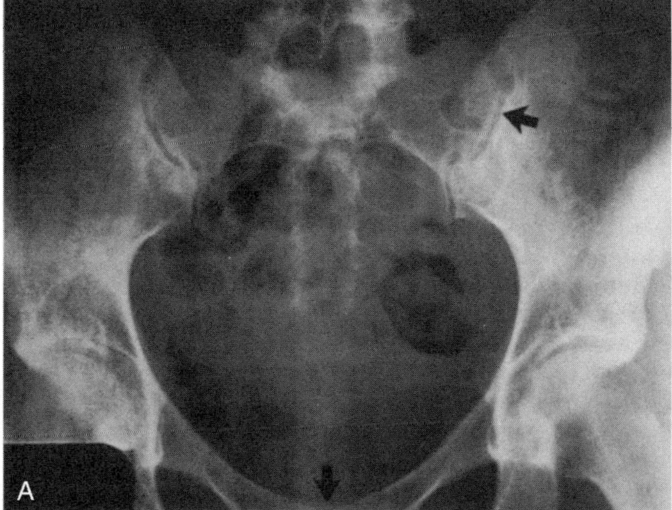

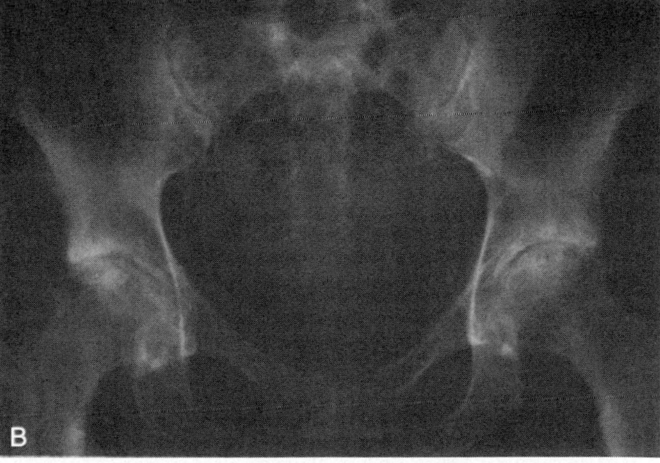

Figure 14-21 Hemochromatosis. *A*, A 53-year-old woman presented with occasional low back pain with an elevated level of serum ferritin. Anteroposterior view of pelvis reveals chondrocalcinosis of the left sacroiliac joint and symphysis pubis *(arrows)*. Degenerative disease of the right hip is noted. *B*, A roentgenogram of the same patient at age 63 demonstrated progressive degenerative disease of both hips. The patient's primary clinical complaint was hip pain. The chondrocalcinosis in the symphysis pubis and sacroiliac joint was no longer visible. The patient was treated with phlebotomy with normalization of serum ferritin levels.

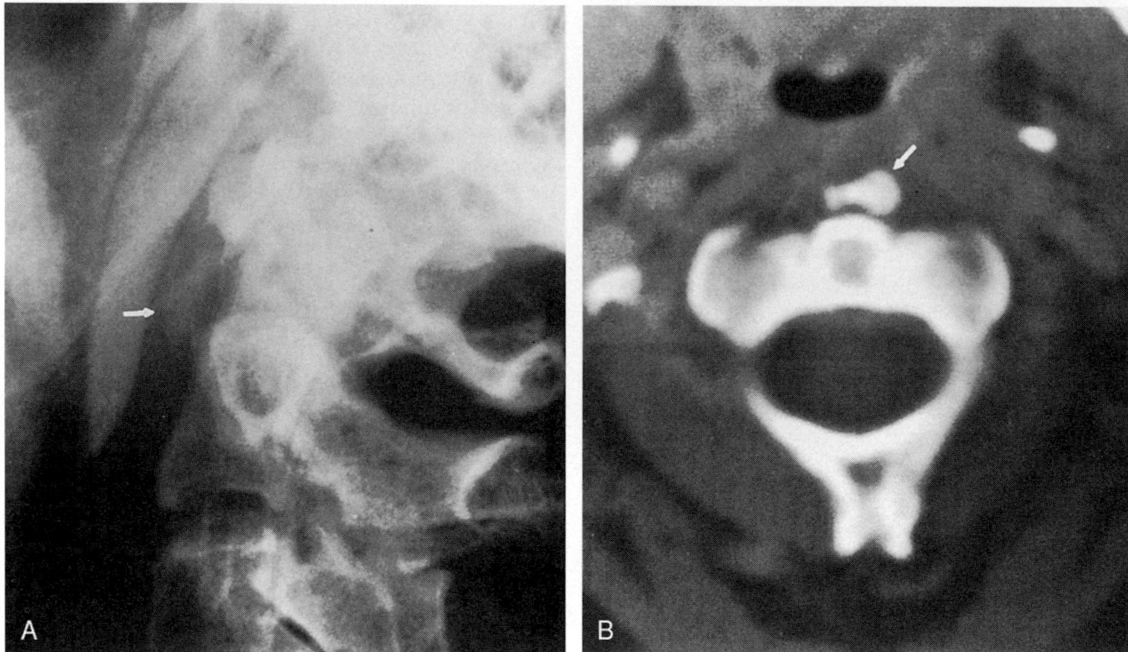

Figure 14-22 Longus colli calcification. A 46-year-old woman developed neck pain, fever, and decreased range of motion over a 2-week period. A lateral roentgenogram *(A)* and transaxial CT scan *(B)* at the level of the base of the odontoid process document calcification *(arrows)* within the longus colli muscle. The symptoms and imaging abnormalities disappeared over a period of weeks.*(Courtesy of G. Greenway, MD, Dallas, Texas.)*

(Fig. 14-23).[51] Patients may require surgical stabilization if subluxation occurs. Most patients with destructive spondyloarthropathy improve with stabilization.[15]

TREATMENT

Gout

Therapy for gout requires the immediate control of inflammation during the acute attack and the chronic control of hyperuricemia to prevent tophaceous deposits.[71] An acute gouty attack may be controlled with intravenous colchicine or nonsteroidal anti-inflammatory drugs, particularly indomethacin. The nonsteroidal drug (indomethacin, 150 mg/day) is continued for 7 to 10 days or until the attack is alleviated. In patients in whom nonsteroidal drugs or colchicine is contraindicated, corticotropin in the form of an intramuscular injection of 40 to 80 IU is used. Corticosteroids given by either oral or intravenous route may also be effective. The corticosteroids are gradually tapered over a 2- to 3-week period as the attack subsides. A maximum dose of intravenous colchicine for the treatment of an acute attack of gout should not exceed 2 mg. The use of a maximum dose less than 4 mg per attack may prevent potential toxicities of cytopenias and renal failure.[58] The dose of colchicines should be reduced in the setting of renal or hepatic failure. Once the acute inflammation has subsided, uric acid concentrations may be controlled by increasing uric acid excretion with probenecid or sulfinpyrazone or by inhibiting uric acid production with the xanthine oxidase inhibitor allopurinol, along with colchicine prophylaxis.[31,42] New concerns regarding the pathogenesis of uric acid in the development and perpetuation of cardiovascular disease, as well as gouty attacks, require uric acid concentrations to be maintained at levels of 5.5 mg/dL. These levels may require allopurinol at doses greater than 300 mg/day.[40]

CPPD

Therapy for CPPD is primarily directed toward control of inflammation with nonsteroidal anti-inflammatory drugs. Occasionally, aspiration of a joint to remove crystals is helpful in controlling joint symptoms, but this is not practical for axial skeletal involvement. Oral colchicine is not as effective in preventing attacks in CPPD as it is in gout. Controlling diseases associated with CPPD may help to arrest its progression, but the calcium pyrophosphate deposits are not resorbed.[42] In the rare circumstance of spinal cord compression in the foramen magnum, surgical removal by a transoral route of CPPD deposits may be required to restore neurologic function.[4]

PROGNOSIS

Acute attacks of gout and CPPD do not occur with any specific intervals between episodes. Some patients have only one attack, whereas others have frequent, painful bouts of inflammatory arthritis. Both the acute and chronic manifestations of gout can be well controlled with available therapy; if diagnosed early enough, patients should have limited dysfunction from the disease. Those with CPPD also have a variable period between attacks, but anti-inflammatory therapy is usually effective at controlling the associated inflammation. There is, however,

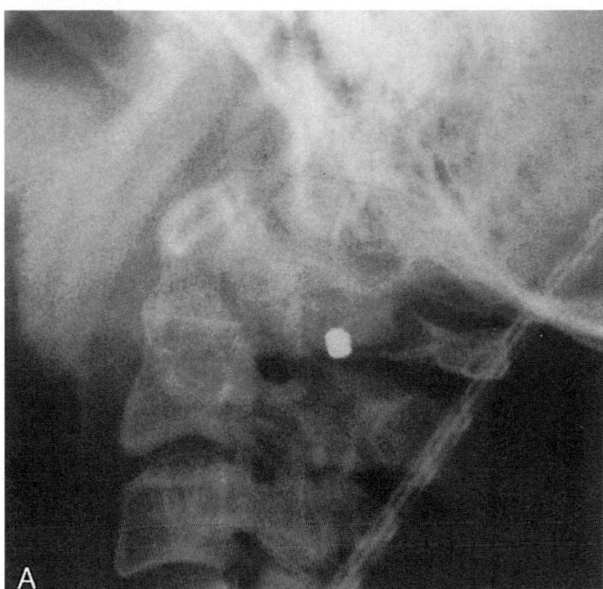

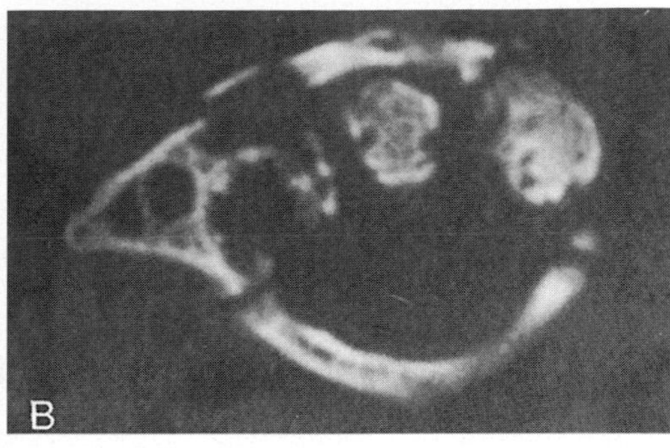

Figure 14-23 *A* and *B*, Spondyloarthropathy during hemodialysis. In this patient on long-term hemodialysis, findings included bone destruction of the atlas, odontoid erosions, a pathologic fracture at the base of the dens, fractures of the ring of the atlas, and posterior atlantoaxial subluxation. *(Courtesy of S. Moreland, MD, San Diego, California.)*

no effective therapy to either control or reverse the calcification of tissues or the secondary degenerative changes associated with crystal deposition. Patients with severe disease may develop progressive axial skeletal involvement with limited function. However, these circumstances are rare.

References

Microcrystalline Disease

1. Abbott RD, Brand FN, Kannel WB, Castelli WP: Gout and coronary heart disease: The Framingham study. J Clin Epidemiol 41:237, 1988.
2. Alarcon-Segovia D, Cetina JA, Diza-Jouanen E: Sacroiliac joints in primary gout: Clinical and roentgenographic study of 143 patients. AJR Am J Roentgenol 118:438, 1973.
3. Allain TJ, Stevens PE, Bridges LR, et al: Dialysis myelopathy: Quadriparesis due to extradural amyloid of beta$_2$-microglobulin origin. BMJ 296:752, 1988.
4. Assaker R, Louis E, Boutry N, et al: Foramen magnum syndrome secondary to calcium pyrophosphate crystal deposition in the transverse ligament of the atlas. Spine 26:1396-1400, 2001.
5. Baba H, Maezawa Y, Kawahara N, et al: Calcium crystal deposition in the ligamentum flavum of the cervical spine. Spine 18:2174, 1993.
6. Berger RG, Levitin PM: Febrile presentation of calcium pyrophosphate dihydrate deposition disease. J Rheumatol 15:642, 1988.
7. Bonaldi VM, Duong H, Starr MR, et al: Tophaceous gout of the lumbar spine mimicking an epidural abscess: MR features. AJNR Am J Neuroradiol 17:1949-1952, 1996.
8. Brown TR, Quinn SF, D'Agostino AN: Deposition of calcium pyrophosphate dihydrate crystals in the ligamentum flavum: Evaluation with MR imaging and CT: Radiology 178:871, 1991.
9. Bundens WD Jr, Brighton CT, Weitzman G: Primary articular cartilage calcification with arthritis (pseudogout syndrome). J Bone Joint Surg Am 47A:111, 1965.
10. Burnham J, Fraker J, Steinbach H: Pathologic fracture in an unusual case of gout. AJR Am J Roentgenol 129:116, 1977.
11. Bywaters EGH, Hamilton CBP, Williams R: The spine in idiopathic haemochromatosis. Ann Rheum Dis 30:453, 1971.
12. Campion EW, Glynn RJ, DeLabry LO: Asymptomatic hyperuricemia: Risks and consequences in the Normative Aging Study. Am J Med 82:421, 1987.
13. Circillo SF, Weinstein PR: Foramen magnum syndrome from pseudogout of the atlanto-occipital ligament: Case report. J Neurosurg 71:141, 1989.
14. Cornelius R, Schneider HJ: Gouty arthritis in the adult. Radiol Clin North Am 26:1267, 1988.
15. Cuffe MJ, Hadley MN, Herrera GA, Morawetz RA: Dialysis-associated spondyloarthropathy: Report of 10 cases. J Neurosurg 80:694, 1994.
16. De AD: Intervertebral disc involvement in gout: brief report. J Bone Joint Surg Br 70B:671, 1988.
17. Delamarter RB, Sherman JE, Carr J: Lumbar spinal stenosis secondary to calcium pyrophosphate crystal deposition (pseudogout). Clin Orthop 289:127, 1993.
18. Duprez TP, Malghem J, Vande Berg BC, et al: Gout in the cervical spine: MR pattern mimicking diskovertebral infection. Am J Neuroradiol 17:151-153, 1996.
19. Ellman MH, Vazquez T, Ferguson L, Mandel N: Calcium pyrophosphate deposition in ligamentum flavum. Arthritis Rheum 21:611, 1978.
20. Felson DT, Anderson JJ, Naimark A, et al: The prevalence of chondrocalcinosis in the elderly and its association with knee osteoarthritis: The Framingham study. J Rheumatol 16:1241, 1989.
21. Hall AP, Barry PE, Dawber TR, McNamara PM: Epidemiology of gout and hyperuricemia: A long-term population study. Am J Med 42:27, 1967.
22. Hall MC, Selin G: Spinal involvement in gout. J Bone Joint Surg Am 42A:341, 1960.
23. Hamilton E, Williams R, Barlow KA, Smith PM: The arthropathy of idiopathic haemochromatosis. Q J Med 37:171, 1968.
24. Hammoudeh M, Siam AR: Pseudogout mimicking meningitis. Br J Rheumatol 32:351, 1993.
25. Hirsch JH, Killien C, Troupin RH: The arthropathy of hemochromatosis. Radiology 118:591, 1976.
26. Jensen PS: Chondrocalcinosis and other calcifications. Radiol Clin North Am 26:1315, 1988.
27. Johnson RJ, Kivlighn SD, Kim YG, et al: Reappraisal of the pathogenesis and consequences of hyperuricemia in hypertension, cardiovascular disease, and renal disease. Am J Kidney Dis 33:225-234, 1999.
28. Jones AC, Chuck AJ, Arie EA, et al: Diseases associated with calcium pyrophosphate deposition disease. Semin Arthritis Rheum 22:188, 1992.
29. Kam M, Perl-Treves D, Caspi D, Addadi L: Antibodies against crystals. FASEB J 6:2608, 1992.
30. Kerr R, Bjorkengren A, Bielecki DK, et al: Destructive spondyloarthropathy in hemodialysis patients. Skeletal Radiol 17:176, 1988.

31. Klinenberg JR, Goldfinger S, Seegmiller JE: The effectiveness of the xanthine oxidase inhibitor allopurinol in the treatment of gout. Ann Intern Med 62:639, 1965.
32. Kuntz D, Bertrand N, Bardin T, et al: Destructive spondyloarthropathy in the hemodialyzed patients: A new syndrome. Arthritis Rheum 27:369, 1984.
33. Lawry GV, Fan PT, Bluestone R: Polyarticular versus monoarticular gout: A prospective, comparative analysis of clinical features. Medicine 67:335, 1988.
34. Leventhal LJ, Levin RW, Bomalaski JS: Peripheral arthrocentesis in the work-up of acute low back pain. Arch Phys Med Rehabil 71:253, 1990.
35. Lichtenstein L, Scott HW, Levin MH: Pathologic changes in gout: Survey of eleven necropsied cases. Am J Pathol 32:871, 1956.
36. Lipkowitz MS, Leal-Pinto E, Rappoport JZ, et al: Functional reconstitution, membrane targeting genomic structure, and chromosomal localization of a human urate transporter. J Clin Invest 107:1103-1115, 2001.
37. Litvak J, Briney W: Extradural spinal depositions of urates producing paraplegia: Case report. J Neurosurg 39:656, 1973.
38. Magid SK, Gray GE, Arand A: Spinal cord compression by tophi in a patient with chronic polyarthritis: Case report and literature review. Arthritis Rheum 24:1431, 1984.
39. Malawista SE, Seegmiller JE, Hathaway BE, Sokoloff L: Sacroiliac gout. JAMA 194:954, 1965.
40. Mandell BF: Hyperuricemia and gout: A reign of complacency. Cleve Clin J 69:589-593, 2002.
41. McCarthy JT, Dahlberg PJ, Kriegshauser JS, et al: Erosive spondyloarthropathy in long-term dialysis patients: Relationship to severe hyperparathyroidism. Mayo Clin Proc 63:446, 1988.
42. McCarty DJ: Calcium pyrophosphate dihydrate crystal deposition disease (pseudogout syndrome)—clinical aspects. Clin Rheum Dis 3:61, 1977.
43. McCarty DJ Jr, Haskin ME: The roentgenographic aspects of pseudogout (articular chondrocalcinosis): An analysis of 20 cases. AJR Am J Roentgenol 90:1248, 1963.
44. McCarty DJ, Hogan JM, Gatter RA, Grossman M: Studies on pathological calcifications in human cartilage: I. Prevalence and types of crystal deposits in the menisci of 215 cadavers. J Bone Joint Surg Am 48A:309, 1966.
45. McGill NW, Dieppe PA: Evidence for a promoter of urate crystal formation in gouty synovial fluid. Ann Rheum Dis 50:558, 1991.
46. Moriniere P, Marie A, el Esper N, et al: Destructive spondyloarthropathy with beta$_2$-microglobulin amyloid deposits in a uremic patient before chronic hemodialysis. Nephron 59:654, 1991.
47. Nakajima K, Miyaoka M, Sumie H, et al: Cervical radiculomyelopathy due to calcification of the ligamenta flava. Surg Neurol 21:479, 1984.
48. O'Duffy JD: Clinical studies of acute pseudogout attacks: Comments on prevalence, predispositions and treatment. Arthritis Rheum 19:349, 1976.
49. Palestro CJ, Vega A, Kim CK, et al: Appearance of acute gouty arthritis on indium-111–labeled leukocyte scintigraphy. J Nucl Med 31:682, 1990.
50. Puig JG, Michan AD, Jimenez ML, et al: Female gout: Clinical spectrum and uric acid metabolism. Arch Intern Med 151:726, 1991.
51. Rafto SE, Dalinka MK, Schiebler ML, et al: Spondyloarthropathy of the cervical spine in long-term hemodialysis. Radiology 166:201, 1988.
52. Reginato A, Valenzuela F, Martinez V, et al: Polyarticular and familial chondrocalcinosis. Arthritis Rheum 13:197, 1970.
53. Resnick D, Niwayama G: Calcium pyrophosphate dihydrate (CPPD) crystal deposition disease. In Resnick D (ed): Diagnosis of Bone and Joint Disorders, 3rd ed. Philadelphia, WB Saunders, 1995, pp 1556-1614.
54. Resnick D, Niwayama G, Goergen TG, et al: Clinical, radiographic, and pathologic abnormalities in calcium pyrophosphate dihydrate deposition disease (CPPD): Pseudogout. Radiology 122:1, 1977.
55. Resnick D, Pineda C: Vertebral involvement in calcium pyrophosphate dihydrate crystal deposition disease. Radiology 153:55, 1984.
56. Reynolds AF, Wyler AR, Norris HT: Paraparesis secondary to sodium urate deposits in the ligamentous flavum. Arch Neurol 33:795, 1976.
57. Richards AJ, Hamilton EBD: Spinal changes in idiopathic chondrocalcinosis articularis. Rheumatol Rehabil 15:138, 1976.
58. Roberts WN, Liang MH, Stern SH: Colchicine in acute gout: Reassessment of risks and benefits. JAMA 257:1920, 1987.
59. Roseff R, Wohlgethan JR, Sipe JD, et al: The acute phase response in gout. J Rheumatol 14:794, 1987.
60. Roubenoff R, Klag MJ, Mead LA, et al: Incidence and risk factors for gout in white men. JAMA 266:3004, 1991.
61. Saskozi J, Fam AG: Acute calcific retropharyngeal tendinitis: An unusual cause of neck pain. Arthritis Rheum 27:708, 1984.
62. Sequeria W, Bouffard A, Salgia K, et al: Quadriparesis in tophaceous gout. Arthritis Rheum 24:1428, 1981.
63. Star VL, Hochberg MC: Prevention and management of gout. Drugs 45:212, 1993.
64. Terkeltaub R: Pathogenesis and treatment of crystal-induced inflammation. In McCarty DJ, Koopman WJ (eds): Arthritis and Allied Conditions, 12th ed. Philadelphia, Lea & Febiger, 1993, pp 1819-1833.
65. Terkeltaub RA: What stops a gouty attack? J Rheumatol 19:8, 1992.
66. Terkeltaub RA, Zachariae C, Santoro D, et al: Monocyte-derived neutrophil chemotactic factor/IL-8 is a potential mediator of crystal-induced inflammation. Arthritis Rheum 34:894, 1991.
67. Varga J, Giampaolo C, Goldenberg DL: Tophaceous gout of the spine in a patient with no peripheral tophi: Case report and review of the literature. Arthritis Rheum 28:1312, 1985.
68. Webb J, Deodhar S, Lee P: Chronic destructive polyarthritis due to pyrophosphate crystal arthritis ("pseudogout" syndrome). Med J Aust 2:206, 1974.
69. Welk LA, Quint DJ: Amyloidosis of the spine in a patient on long-term hemodialysis. Neuroradiology 32:334, 1990.
70. Westmark KD, Weissman BN: Complications of axial arthropathies. Orthop Clin North Am 21:423, 1990.
71. Yu TF, Gutman AB: Principles of current management of primary gout. Am J Med Sci 254:893, 1967.

OCHRONOSIS

Capsule Summary

	Low Back	Neck
Frequency of spinal pain	Very common	Not applicable (NA)
Location of spinal pain	Lumbar spine	NA
Quality of spinal pain	Ache	NA
Symptoms and signs	Decreased back motion; pigmentation of sclerae, ears, nose	NA
Laboratory tests	Homogentisic acid in urine	NA
Radiographic findings	Extensive disc calcifications on plain roentgenograms	NA
Treatment	Anti-inflammatory drugs	NA

PREVALENCE AND PATHOGENESIS

Ochronosis is a rare metabolic disorder associated with the deposition of homogentisic acid in connective tissue throughout the body. The accumulation of homogentisic acid results in darkened pigmentation and progressive degeneration of connective tissue. Ochronotic arthropathy develops in the fourth decade of life and is associated with progressive low back pain, stiffness, and obliteration of the normal lumbar lordosis. Peripheral joint disease also may occur in the hips, knees, and shoulders.

Epidemiology

The prevalence of ochronosis is approximately 1 in 10 million.[22] The illness has a wide geographic distribution, although most large series have been reported from Central European countries.[24] Men are slightly more often affected than women.

Pathogenesis

The cause of this illness is the congenital absence of the enzyme homogentisic acid oxidase.[11] The complete human gene for homogentisate 1,2-dioxygenase has been sequenced and contains 54,363 base pairs.[8] A number of mutations within this gene sequence results in the phenotypic appearance of ochronosis.[2] Without the enzyme there is an accumulation of homogentisic acid. Alkaptonuria is the disease associated with the excretion of homogentisic acid in the urine. Ochronosis, which is caused by the same enzyme deficiency, is the discoloration of connective tissue from the deposition of a black pigment that is thought to be a polymer of homogentisic acid.[14] The pigment affects the integrity of cartilage matrix and chondrocytes and results in cartilage damage and degeneration.[21] The inheritance of the disorder is autosomal recessive.[24]

CLINICAL HISTORY

Alkaptonuria is usually unrecognized during childhood, although occasionally discoloration of urine is detected before adulthood. Symptoms of ochronosis first appear in the fourth decade of life. Low back pain and stiffness are frequently the initial symptoms of the illness.[13] Herniation of an intervertebral disc, particularly in men, can be the initial symptom of disease in some patients.[4,16] This is associated with severe sharp pain.[1,5,17] Peripheral joint involvement may cause loss of motion and pain in the hips, knees, and shoulders. Pain in some patients is most intense in the morning. Some also describe episodes of acutely swollen, inflamed joints, particularly the knees. This symptom is related to the association of calcium pyrophosphate dihydrate deposition disease (CPPD) and ochronosis.[20] Ochronotic deposition in other organs may cause prostatic enlargement with calculi, renal calculi with renal failure, and myocardial infarction.

PHYSICAL EXAMINATION

Physical examination demonstrates limited motion of the lumbar spine and localized tenderness with percussion. Muscle spasm is usually absent. With advanced disease, there is rigidity of the axial skeleton. Chest wall expansion is also limited. Kyphosis may be prominent and is associated with a loss in height. Dark pigmentation may be discovered in the nose, ears, sclerae, and fingernails.

LABORATORY DATA

The characteristic laboratory finding is the presence of homogentisic acid in urine. Alkalinization of a urine specimen will cause darkening, which is indicative of the presence of homogentisic acid.[21] Synovial fluid analysis may demonstrate a "ground-pepper" appearance of the fluid or pyrophosphate crystals.[9,20] Ochronotic patients are HLA-B27 negative.[10]

Pathology

Pathologic examination demonstrates pigment deposition in connective tissue, including articular cartilage, tendons, and ligaments. Pathologic changes in the axial skeleton first occur in the lumbar spine. Pigment is located in the nucleus pulposus and annulus fibrosus. The discs become brittle.[3,12] The ligaments may also become calcified. Transmission electron microscopy has demonstrated the binding of ochronotic pigment to collagen fibrils in the presence of mucopolysaccharide ground substance.[6] The presence of mucopolysaccharide ground substance may be the factor located in tissues that attracts deposition of ochronotic pigment.

RADIOGRAPHIC FINDINGS

Roentgenograms

Roentgenographic examination of the lumbar spine in ochronosis demonstrates marked disc space narrowing, osteophyte formation, and disc calcification (Fig. 14-24). "Vacuum" phenomena may be seen in an intervertebral disc and are suggestive of the diagnosis of ochronosis when it occurs at multiple levels. Disease of long duration may be associated with total obliteration of disc spaces, bony fusion, and loss of lumbar lordosis, and may be confused with the axial skeletal changes of ankylosing spondylitis (Fig. 14-25).[23] Osteoporosis of the vertebral bodies is common and accentuates the prominence of disc calcification.

Scintigraphy

Bone scintigraphy may demonstrate a "whisker sign" in the axial skeleton in patients with ochronosis.[18] The increased uptake near the axial skeleton is a result of intervertebral discs

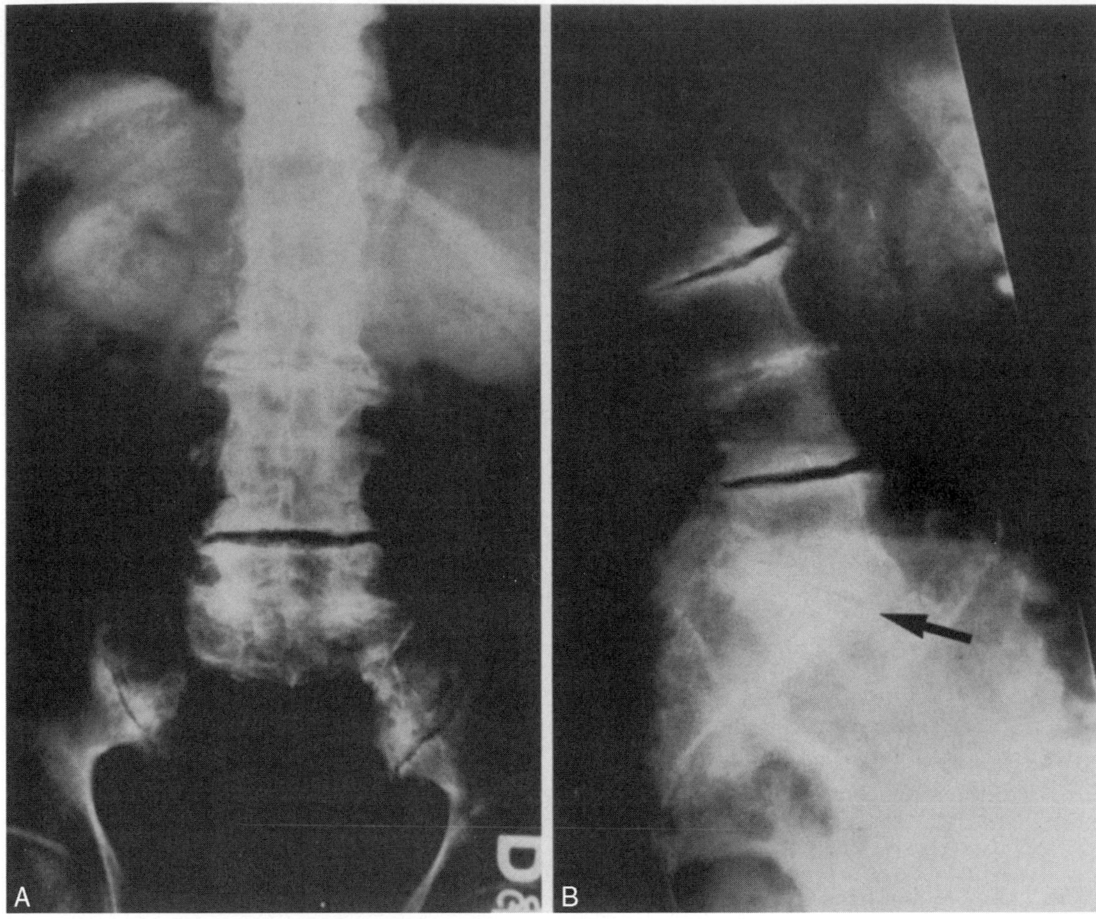

Figure 14-24 Ochronosis. *A*, Anteroposterior view reveals disc space narrowing and marked osteophyte formation of the vertebral bodies and sacroiliac joints. *B*, Lateral view shows disc space calcification *(arrow)*. *(Courtesy of Randall Lewis, MD.)*

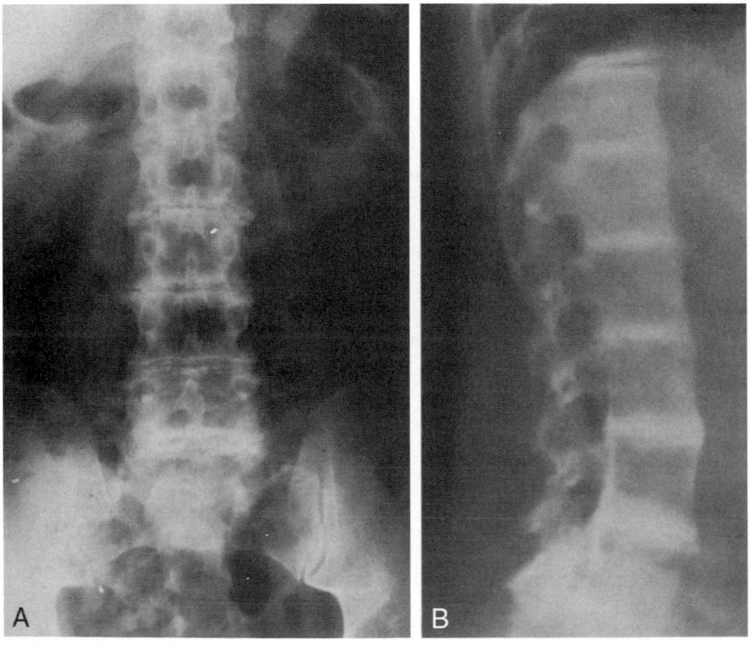

Figure 14-25 Ochronosis. *A*, Anteroposterior view demonstrating generalized disc space narrowing and diffuse disc calcification. *B*, Lateral view of lumbar spine simulating ankylosing spondylitis. Notice multiple disc calcifications, which are not characteristic of ankylosing spondylitis. *(Courtesy of Anne Brower, MD.)*

14-7 DISC CALCIFICATION

Disease	Character of Disc	Diagnosis
Ochronosis	Diffuse distribution, "wafer-like" configuration Broad outer band-like osteophytes	Homogentisic acid in urine
Ankylosing spondylitis	Preservation of disc space Central calcification Vertically oriented thin syndesmophytes	Radiographic distribution Clinical history (iritis)
Calcium pyrophosphate dihydrate disease (hemochromatosis, hyperparathyroidism)	Outer portion of the annulus fibrosus Disc narrowing	Presence of crystals
Acromegaly	Anterior portion of disc Increased disc height	Increased growth hormone

accumulating radioactivity allowing spread of the uptake bilaterally beyond the confines of the vertebral column.

DIFFERENTIAL DIAGNOSIS

A diagnosis of ochronosis is based on the characteristic clinical symptoms and radiographic findings along with the presence of homogentisic acid in urine. Other diseases, such as CPPD, hemochromatosis, hyperparathyroidism, and acromegaly, may involve intervertebral disc calcification and must be considered in the differential diagnosis (Table 14-7).[25] Patients with ankylosing spondylitis may have symptoms and signs similar to those of ochronosis but will not have skin pigmentation or disc calcification. The coexistence of ochronosis and ankylosing spondylitis in patients has been reported.[7,26,27] These patients have characteristic evidence of ochronosis, including increased urinary homogentisic acid, along with bilateral sacroiliac joint fusion. Interestingly, HLA-B27 is positive in only 1 of 3 patients with both illnesses.

Patients with generalized degenerative disc disease (intervertebral osteochondrosis) will have loss of disc space, vacuum phenomena, traction osteophytes, and marginal sclerosis. The absence of widespread disc calcification should help differentiate these diseases.[19]

TREATMENT

Specific treatment for this disease, replacement of homogentisic acid oxidase, is not available. Treatment is symptomatic and includes rest, exercise, analgesics, and anti-inflammatory drugs. Low tyrosine/low phenylalanine diets lower homogentisic acid levels but do not seem to produce major benefits in regard to the course of the illness.[21]

PROGNOSIS

The course of ochronosis is progressive and disabling. Ochronosis is a generalized disease that affects the appendicular and axial skeleton with destructive disease. The disease may progress to the degree that patients have severely limited function because of musculoskeletal disease. The osteoporotic spine of the ochronotic patient is at risk for fracture from minimal injury.[15]

References

Ochronosis

1. Acosta C, Watts CC, Simpson CW: Ochronosis and degenerative lumbar disc disease: A case report. J Neurosurg 28:488, 1968.
2. Beltran-Valero de Bernabe D, Granadino B, Chiarelli I, et al: Mutation and polymorphism analysis of the human homogentisate 1,2-dioxygenase gene in alkaptonuria patients. Am J Hum Genet 62:776-784, 1998.
3. Bywaters EGL, Dorling J, Sutor J: Ochronotic densification. Ann Rheum Dis 29:563, 1970.
4. Emel E, Karagoz F, Aydin IH, et al: Alkaptonuria with lumbar disc herniation: A report of two cases. Spine 25:2141-2144, 2000.
5. Feild JR, Higley GB, Disaussare RL Jr: Case report: Ochronosis with ruptured lumbar disc. J Neurosurg 20:348, 1963.
6. Gaines JJ: The pathology of alkaptonuric ochronosis. Hum Pathol 20:40, 1989.
7. Gemignani G, Olivieri I, Semeria R, et al: Coexistence of ochronosis and ankylosing spondylitis. J Rheumatol 17:1707, 1990.
8. Granadino B, Beltran-Valero de Bernabe D, Fernandez-Canon JM, et al: The human homogentisate 1,2 dioxygenase (HGO) gene. Genomics 43:115-122, 1997.
9. Hunter T, Gordon DA, Ogryzlo MA: The ground pepper sign of synovial fluid: A new diagnostic feature of ochronosis. J Rheumatol 1:45, 1974.
10. Kocyigit H, Gutgan A, Terzioglu R, et al: Clinical, radiographic and echocardiographic findings in a patient with ochronosis. Clin Rheumatol 17:403-406, 1998.
11. LaDu BN, Zannoni VG, Laster L, Seegmiller JE: The nature of the defect in tyrosine metabolism in alkaptonuria. J Biol Chem 230:251, 1985.
12. Lagier R, Sitaj S: Vertebral changes in ochronosis: Anatomical and radiological study of one case. Ann Rheum Dis 33:86, 1974.
13. McCollum DE, Odom GL: Alkaptonuria, ochronosis, and low back pain: A case report. J Bone Joint Surg Am 47A:1389, 1965.
14. Milch RA: Biochemical studies on the pathogenesis of collagen tissue changes in alkaptonuria. Clin Orthop 24:213, 1962.
15. Millea TP, Segal LS, Liss RG, Stauffer ES: Spine fracture in ochronosis: Report of a case. Clin Orthop 281:208, 1992.
16. O'Brien WM, LaDu BN, Bunim JJ: Biochemical, pathologic, and clinical aspects of alkaptonuria, ochronosis, and ochronotic arthropathy. Am J Med 34:813, 1963.
17. Ortiz AC, Neal EG: Alkaptonuria and ochronotic arthritis: A general review and report of two cases. Clin Orthop 25:147, 1962.
18. Paul R, Ylinen S: The "whisker sign" as an indicator of ochronosis in skeletal scintigraphy. Eur J Nucl Med 18:222, 1991.
19. Resnick D, Niwayama G: Radiographic and pathologic features of spinal involvement in diffuse idiopathic skeletal hyperostosis (DISH). Radiology 119:559, 1976.
20. Rynes RI, Sosman JL, Holdsworth DE: Pseudogout in ochronosis: Report of a case. Arthritis Rheum 18:21, 1975.

21. Schumacher HR, Holdsworth DE: Ochronotic arthropathy: I. Clinicopathologic studies. Semin Arthritis Rheum 6:207, 1977.
22. Seradge H, Anderson MG: Alkaptonuria and ochronosis: Historical review and update. Orthop Rev 7:41, 1978.
23. Simon G, Zorab PA: The radiological changes in alkaptonuric arthritis: A report of 3 cases (one an Egyptian mummy). Br J Radiol 34:384, 1961.
24. Srsen S: Alkaptonuria. Johns Hopkins Med J 145:217, 1979.
25. Weinberger A, Myers AR: Intervertebral disc calcification in adults: A review. Semin Arthritis Rheum 8:69, 1978.
26. Weinberger KA: The coexistence of ochronosis and ankylosing spondylitis. J Rheumatol 18:1948, 1991.
27. Zanetakis E, Khan MA, Yagan R, Kushner I: Ochronotic arthropathy, post-traumatic spinal pseudoarthrosis and HLA-B27. J Orthop Rheumatol 2:48, 1989.

FLUOROSIS

CAPSULE SUMMARY

	LOW BACK	NECK
Frequency of spinal pain	Rare	Rare
Location of spinal pain	Lumbar spine	Cervical spine
Quality of spinal pain	Ache	Ache
Symptoms and signs	Bone pain, decreased spine motion, spasticity, discolored teeth	Bone pain, decreased spine motion, spasticity, hyperreflexia, discolored teeth
Laboratory tests	Increased urinary fluoride, increased alkaline phosphatase	Increased urinary fluoride, increased alkaline phosphatase
Radiographic findings	Osteosclerosis and osteophytes on plain roentgenograms	Osteosclerosis and osteophytes on plain roentgenograms
Treatment	Limit exposure to fluoride	Limit exposure to fluoride

PREVALENCE AND PATHOGENESIS

Fluorine is an element that is found extensively throughout the environment because, like silicon and phosphorus, it is a common constituent of the earth's crust. Fluorine serves as a trace element in the human body. At optimal concentrations, fluoride compounds stabilize the crystalline structure of teeth and bone. At high concentrations, fluoride is a cell poison. Between optimum (1 mg/day) and toxic (100 mg/day) intake levels, fluoride ingestion causes alterations primarily of bone.

Fluoride poisoning occurs in three circumstances:

1. Endemic fluorosis occurs in regions of the world where drinking water contains fluoride in concentrations greater than 4 parts/million (ppm).[19] Endemic fluorosis occurs in parts of India, Africa, and South America where water supplies are contaminated with fluorine compounds. Fluoride is added to water in developed countries to help reduce the incidence of dental caries. The concentration of fluoride in water in developed countries is 1 ppm and causes no harm to people.
2. Industrial fluorosis occurs in industrial workers exposed to fluoride compounds (aluminum mining, phosphate fertilizer industries), in laboratory workers who inhale fluorine fumes, or with exposure to insecticides. This form of fluorosis occurs with exposure over many years.[2]
3. Iatrogenic fluorosis occurs in patients treated with sodium fluoride for osteoporosis or with other medications or liquids that contain increased concentrations of fluoride.[10,12,15]

Epidemiology

The prevalence of fluorosis in the United States is unknown. For the most part, it is a very rare illness outside of endemic areas. In endemic areas, fluoride intoxication of bone is the most common form of bone disease.

Pathogenesis

The effects of fluoride on the skeleton are related to the interaction of fluoride ions with bone and the parathyroid glands. Fluoride ions enter the surface of bone from the extracellular fluid. Fluoride ions, because of their similarity to hydroxyl ions, substitute for hydroxyl groups in the hydroxyapatite lattice structure of bone. The new crystals, hydroxyfluoroapatite, are harder and more resistant to dissolution and growth and to the actions of parathyroid hormone.[4,21] Fluoride causes simultaneous increases in bone formation and bone resorption.[1] These findings are reflected in the osteoblastic appearance of bone and the increased plasma levels of alkaline phosphatase.[21] The new bone that is formed is osteomalacic secondary to inadequate mineralization.

CLINICAL HISTORY

In the initial stages of exposure, the patients have no specific complaints. As the skeletal disease advances, patients complain of vague pains in the small joints of hands and feet. As the spine becomes involved, patients complain of back stiffness and loss of motion. With severe disease, patients complain of inability to flex the fingers, rigidity of the spine, flexion deformities of the appendicular skeleton, and shortness of breath secondary to decreased chest expansion. With increasing sclerosis in the spinal canal, symptoms of spinal cord compression may appear. In the cervical spine, myelopathy may occur.[9,13] Paraplegia has been reported in the lumbar spine.[6]

PHYSICAL EXAMINATION

Physical examination may demonstrate abnormalities of the teeth. Tooth enamel is weakened by high concentrations of fluoride. The enamel becomes mottled, with discoloration and pitting. Examination of the musculoskeletal system reveals decreased range of motion of the spine along with percussion tenderness. Appendicular joints also have decreased motion. In advanced disease, kyphosis and spinal angulation occur, which may result in neurologic signs, including sensory disturbance, muscle weakness, and atrophy proceeding to paralysis.[18] Cervical cord compression results in signs of myelopathy including sensory deficits, leg weakness, spasticity, and positive Babinski's signs.

LABORATORY DATA

Laboratory evaluation of patients with fluorosis reflects the increased bone and parathyroid hormone activity. Plasma levels of alkaline phosphatase are extremely high. In the urine, increased phosphate clearance in association with decreased tubular reabsorption of phosphate is noted along with decreased concentrations of calcium. Urinary fluoride concentrations are elevated.[21] Bone biopsy specimens may be measured for fluoride content.[6]

RADIOGRAPHIC EVALUATION

Involvement of the axial skeleton, including the spine and pelvis, is commonplace in patients with fluorosis.[11,20] Roentgenographic abnormalities include osteosclerosis and osteopenia, associated with overall decreased bone density or osteomalacia. Osteosclerosis is the predominant finding in adults who have ingested fluoride for many years. In a study of 127 patients with endemic fluorosis, 89% of the adults had evidence of calcification or ossification of ligaments, tendons, muscles, or interosseous membranes.[22] Osteosclerosis was present in 43% of patients and osteopenia in 40%. Osteomalacia occurred in 18% of individuals.

Osteoblastic activity occurs along trabecular surfaces, leading to thickening of trabeculae and loss of detail in bony architecture. Osteophytes are numerous and large and may encroach on the spinal canal. Encroachment on the spinal canal may result in compromise of nerve function, resulting in myelopathy or neuropathy.[6] Calcification of supporting ligaments also is common. In severe cases, osteophytosis may resemble a "bamboo spine" and corresponds to the symptom of spinal rigidity.

DIFFERENTIAL DIAGNOSIS

In the United States the diagnosis of fluorosis should be considered in an individual with an industrial exposure to the chemical or someone who is ingesting sodium fluoride as part of a therapeutic regimen for osteoporosis.[16] Workers in the manufacture of aluminum, nickel, copper, gold, glass-works, and pesticides are at risk. Fluorosis also has occurred in communities neighboring fluoride-polluting industries.[14] Fluorosis should also be considered in individuals whose primary source of drinking water is ground wells.[5] Acute fluoride poisoning has also been reported from excess fluoridation of water from a public water system in Alaska.[8] The diagnosis is confirmed by the presence of increased fluoride concentration in the urine. The combination of generalized axial skeletal sclerosis, osteophytosis, and ligamentous calcification is almost diagnostic of the illness.

Osteosclerosis alone may be noted in patients with bone metastases, hematologic disorders (myelofibrosis), renal osteodystrophy, and Paget's disease. Vertebral osteophytosis is found in patients with diffuse idiopathic skeletal hyperostosis (DISH), spondyloarthropathy, neuroarthropathy, and ochronosis. Ligamentous calcifications are also associated with DISH. It is the combination of all three findings in a single patient that helps differentiate fluorosis from these other more common illnesses.

TREATMENT

The most important aspect of therapy for patients with fluorosis is to limit any additional exposure to the chemical. Excess body stores of fluoride trapped in bone crystals are released only when bone resorption occurs and some of the liberated fluoride is redeposited at sites of new bone formation. If intake is minimized, urinary excretion of the chemical will gradually decrease.

PROGNOSIS

Questions remain concerning the strength of fluorotic bone and whether it is at greater risk for fracture than normal bone. Evans and Woods have suggested that fluorotic bone is weaker and prone to fracture.[3] In contrast, Franke and colleagues observed increased strength of fluorotic bone.[7] Clinically, fluoride in combination with calcium may improve bone strength and decrease bone fracture.[17] Additional studies are needed to determine the effect of fluorine on bone.

References

Fluorosis

1. Aggarwal ND: Structure of human fluorotic bone. J Bone Joint Surg Am 55A:331, 1973.
2. Boillat MA, Garcia J, Velebit L: Radiological criteria of industrial fluorosis. Skel Radiol 5:161, 1980.
3. Evans FG, Wood JL: Mechanical properties and density of bone in a case of severe endemic fluorosis. Acta Orthop Scand 47:489, 1976.
4. Faccini JM, Teotia SPS: Histopathological assessment of endemic skeletal fluorosis. Calcif Tissue Res 16:45, 1974.
5. Felsenfeld AJ, Roberts MA: A report of fluorosis in the United States secondary to drinking well water. JAMA 265:486, 1991.
6. Fisher RL, Medcalf TW, Henerson MC: Endemic fluorosis with spinal cord compression: A case report and review. Arch Intern Med 149:697-700, 1989.
7. Franke J, Runge H, Grau P, et al: Physical properties of fluorosis bone. Acta Orthop Scand 47:20, 1976.
8. Gessner BD, Beller M, Middaugh JP, et al: Acute fluoride poisoning from a public water system. N Engl J Med 330:95, 1994.
9. Gupta RK, Agarwal P, Kumar S, et al: Compressive myelopathy in fluorosis: MRI. Neuroradiology 38:338-342, 1996
10. Johnson FF, Fischer LL: Report on fluorine in urine. Am J Pharm 107:512, 1939.
11. Largent EJ, Bovard PG, Heyroth FF: Roentgenographic changes and urinary fluoride excretion among workmen engaged in the manufacture of inorganic fluorides. AJR Am J Roentgenol 65:42, 1951.
12. Meunier PJ, Courpron P, Smoller JS, Briancon D: Niflumic acid–induced skeletal fluorosis: Iatrogenic disease or therapeutic perspective for osteoporosis? Clin Orthop 148:304, 1980.
13. Mrabet A, Fredj M, Ben Ammou S, et al: Spinal cord compression in bone fluorosis: Apropos of 4 cases. Rev Med Interne 16:533-535, 1995.
14. Nemeth L, Zsogon E: Occupational skeletal fluorosis. Clin Rheumatol 3:81, 1989.
15. O'Duffy JD, Wahner HW, O'Fallon WM, et al: Mechanism of acute lower extremity pain syndrome in fluoride-treated osteoporotic patients. Am J Med 80:561, 1986.
16. Riggs BL, Hodgson SF, Hoffman DL, et al: Treatment of primary osteoporosis with fluoride and calcium. JAMA 243:446, 1980.
17. Riggs BL, Seeman E, Hodgson SF, et al: Effect of the fluoride/calcium regimen on vertebral fracture occurrence in postmenopausal osteoporosis. N Engl J Med 306:446, 1982.
18. Singh A, Jolly SS, Bansal BC: Skeletal fluorosis and its neurological complications. Lancet 1:197, 1961.
19. Singh A, Jolly SS, Bansal BC, Mathur CC: Endemic fluorosis: Epidemiological, clinical, and biochemical study of chronic fluorine intoxication in the Punjab (India). Medicine 42:229, 1963.
20. Stevenson CA, Watson AR: Fluoride osteosclerosis. AJR Am J Roentgenol 78:13, 1957.
21. Teotia SPS, Teotia M: Secondary hyperparathyroidism in patients with endemic skeletal fluorosis. BMJ 1:637, 1973.
22. Wang Y, Yin Y, Gilula LA, et al: Endemic fluorosis of the skeleton: Radiographic features in 127 patients. AJR Am J Roentgenol 162:93-98, 1994.

HERITABLE GENETIC DISORDERS

Capsule Summary

	Low Back	Neck
Frequency of spinal pain	Common	Common
Location of spinal pain	Lumbar spine	Cervical spine
Quality of spinal pain	Chronic ache	Chronic ache
Symptoms and signs	Structural abnormalities noticeable early in life; alterations—kyphoscoliosis, short stature	Structural abnormalities noticeable early in life; alterations—kyphoscoliosis, short stature
Laboratory tests	Specific for each illness	Specific for each illness
Radiographic findings	Specific for each illness	Specific for each illness
Treatment	Symptomatic bracing	Surgical decompression of stenosis

This section will review a number of heritable disorders of connective tissue that are associated with spinal pain. Some disorders are more commonly associated with lumbar spine pain (Table 14-8). Heritable disorders may also be associated with neck pain and cervical spinal cord compression. For the most part, these diseases are rare. Many of the patients with these disorders are not evaluated by internists, because many of these patients do not live to adulthood.

Within the major categories of heritable disorders of connective tissue, impairment of the spine is common. However, not all of the entities included in a single disorder (e.g., Ehlers-Danlos syndrome) have associated back pain. Those subclasses of these disorders associated with back or neck pain will be identified and the clinical characteristics of each group listed. The disorders of connective tissue may involve fibrous connective tissue elements (collagen or elastin), ground substance (mucopolysaccharide), cartilage, or bone.[8,82]

MARFAN SYNDROME

Marfan syndrome is a connective tissue disorder associated with arachnodactyly, myopia, and aortic disease.[84] The musculoskeletal abnormalities associated with this syndrome include loose-jointedness, scoliosis, and prominent ribs. Marfan syndrome is a familial disorder that is inherited as an autosomal dominant trait. Both sexes are equally affected. The incidence is 1 in 10,000 to 20,000 individuals. The cause of this disease is related to an abnormality in the fibrillin gene *(FBN1)*. *FBN1* is a gene with 65 exons

14-8 HERITABLE DISORDERS ASSOCIATED WITH BACK PAIN

Disorder	Spinal Manifestations
Marfan syndrome	Kyphoscoliosis Vertebral body—posterior scalloping, increased height
Homocystinuria	Kyphoscoliosis Vertebral body—posterior scalloping, compression fractures
Ehlers-Danlos syndrome	Kyphoscoliosis Vertebral body—posterior scalloping, anterior wedging Spondylolysis Spondylolisthesis
Achondroplasia	Kyphoscoliosis Lumbar lordosis, small spinal canal Vertebral body—decreased height, posterior scalloping Pedicles short and thick
Osteogenesis imperfecta	Kyphoscoliosis Fractures Osteoporosis Vertebral body—flattening, "fish" vertebrae, anterior wedging
Mucopolysaccharidoses	
Hunter's syndrome	Vertebral bodies—ovoid, hypoplastic Kyphoscoliosis Osteoporosis
Morquio's syndrome	Vertebral bodies—flattening, central beaking Kyphoscoliosis
Maroteaux-Lamy	Vertebral bodies—central beaking, hypoplasia
Tuberous sclerosis	Osteosclerosis of sacroiliac joints and vertebrae
Spondyloepiphyseal dysplasia	Vertebral bodies—flattened irregular endplates Intervertebral disc space narrowing

located at chromosome 15q-21.1.[121] A variety of mutations on chromosome 15 result in alterations in fibrillin polypeptides that result in the phenotypic expression of Marfan syndrome.[53]

Over 90 different mutations involving this protein have been described in Marfan patients.[34] Different forms of gene mutations (shortened mutant transcripts with milder disease and exon deletion with more severe disease) have been described.[81] Fibrillin is a large glycoprotein that is one of the structural components of microfibrils. Microfibrils are components of a number of 666 tissues in the body that are abnormal in Marfan syndrome, including the suspensory ligament of the lens, periosteum of bone, and the media of the aorta.[70] These connective tissue microfibrils are essential to normal elastic fibrillogenesis.

Clinically, these patients are tall and thin with disproportionately long arms in comparison to the trunk (dolichostenomelia). The thoracic kyphosis is lost (straight back) with scoliosis at multiple levels. Joint laxity is prominent (Fig. 14-26). Abnormal curvature of the vertebral column is a consequence of generalized ligamentous laxity. Radiographic evaluation reveals a high proportion of patients with scoliosis of the thoracolumbar spine, which is similar in configuration to that seen with idiopathic scoliosis. However, scoliosis associated with Marfan syndrome

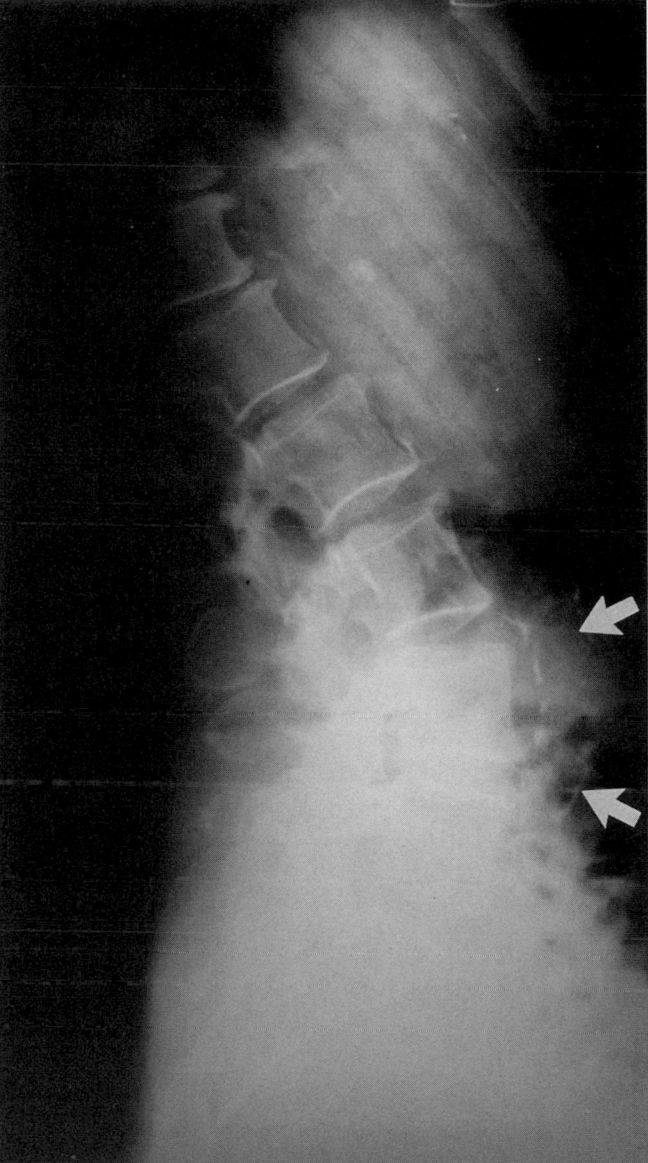

Figure 14-26 Marfan syndrome. A 46-year-old-woman presented with chronic low back pain with history of aortic root dilatation with aortic valve replacement and abdominal aneurysm. A lateral view of the lumbar spine reveals marked hyperlordosis as a manifestation of hypermobility and evidence of atherosclerosis in the abdominal aorta *(white arrows)*.

starts at an earlier age and does not have a female predominance. In a study of 113 people with Marfan syndrome, 52% had evidence of scoliosis.[109] Other roentgenographic findings include posterior scalloping of the vertebral bodies and increased vertebral height. Measurement of osseous lumbar spinal anatomy has detected reduced pedicle width and laminar thickness in Marfan syndrome patients.[107] Dural ectasia, a result of hydraulic forces of pulsatile cerebrospinal fluid on weakened connective tissue, may be noted in 63% of Marfan patients by roentgenographic techniques in areas of osseous weakness.[71] Osseous weakness may also result in fractures of pedicles as a cause of back pain.[24] MR evaluation of the spine is able to detect dural ectasias in 92% of Marfan patients.[27] Dural ectasia results in Tarlov, or perineural, cysts, arachnoid cysts, or pelvic meningoceles that are associated with neurologic signs including sensory deficits.[112] The spinal deformity is progressive and potentially painful.[52] Dural ectasias may be present in the absence of pain.[1] Sinclair reported that 7 of 40 patients with Marfan syndrome had associated back pain.[105] Cervical spine involvement is manifested by increased atlantoaxial subluxations (54%) and basilar impression (36%). Atlantoaxial rotatory subluxations is another rare form of spinal instability.[38] Cervical spinal stenosis occurs in 3% of patients.[39]

The diagnosis of Marfan syndrome is a clinical one, because most patients have only some of the characteristic manifestations of disease.[83] In one study, arachnodactyly occurred in 89%, aortic murmurs in 62%, and ectopia lentis in 57%.[91] Schlesinger has suggested the possibility of Marfan syndrome in patients with refractory low back syndrome, dural ectasia, and protracted pain after lumbar puncture with a marfanoid habitus.[96] New diagnostic criteria for Marfan syndrome were proposed in 1996.[22] These criteria include major criteria (4 of 8 skeletal manifestations, ectopia lentis, aortic root dilatation, and lumbosacral dural ectasias) and minor criteria (joint hypermobility, mitral valve prolapse, myopia, and recurrent hernias). Criteria for establishing the diagnosis include major manifestations in two organ systems and involvement of a third organ system with a major or minor criterion.

The treatment of Marfan syndrome starts early in life with bracing to decrease abnormal spinal curvature. A retrospective study of brace treatment is effective in only a small proportion of delaying curvature progression in Marfan patients.[108] Surgical stabilization is needed if scoliosis progresses to too great a degree (usually 40 degrees). Surgical intervention also may be required to control the growth of arachnoid cysts.[86] Surgical correction of spinal deformity is associated with surgical complications in a significant proportion of patients. Instrumentation fixation failure was reported in 21% of 39 Marfan patients who underwent surgical correction. Pseudoarthrosis, perioperative infections, and dural tears occurred in about 10% of individuals. One patient died of valvular insufficiency.[49]

Homocystinuria

Homocystinuria is the disease that must be differentiated from Marfan syndrome. Homocystinuric patients are long limbed and tall but have restricted movements as opposed to lax ones. In addition, homocystinuria is associated with nervous system disorders including mental retardation and seizures. Between 25% and 60% of homocystinuric patients have skeletal abnormalities, including scoliosis, posterior scalloping, and osteoporosis with compression fractures.[14,15] Unlike in Marfan syndrome, a specific biochemical abnormality is detectable in homocystinuria. Levels of homocysteine, homocystine, and methionine are elevated. Cystathionine B-synthetase deficiency is the most common cause of homocystinuria.[106]

Stickler's Syndrome

Stickler's syndrome is a hereditary, progressive arthro-ophthalmopathy with an autosomal dominant inheritance pattern. The incidence is 1 in 10,000 individuals, which is similar to that of Marfan syndrome. Stickler's syndrome patients develop kyphoscoliosis, wedging or flattening of vertebrae, or platyspondylia. Other manifestations of the disorder include mitral valve prolapse, retinal detachment, hearing loss, and mandibular hypoplasia.[66] In adulthood, arthropathy may progress to limit joint movement. The abnormality associated with Stickler's syndrome may be associated with mutation in the *COL2A1* gene of type II collagen.[58]

EHLERS-DANLOS SYNDROME

Ehlers-Danlos syndrome (EDS) comprises a group of disorders characterized by skin hyperelasticity and fragility, loose-jointedness, and decreased tensile strength of elastic tissues. Eleven different forms of EDS have been reclassified into nine entities that have been separated on the basis of clinical or biochemical differences.[9,74] In 1998, a revised nosology was proposed for the forms of EDS (Table 14-9). Classic type includes types I (gravis) and II (mitis). The new hypermobility type is the former type III (hypermobile).[10] Classic and hypermobility types account for 80% of all cases of EDS. The phenotypic heterogeneity within the EDS syndrome results from mutations in collagen genes that affect type I procollagen, type III procollagen, or enzymes that modify collagens.[17] Mutations in the type V collagen genes *(COL5A1)* account for up to 50% of cases of classic EDS.[98] Tenascin-X deficiency is an example of an autosomal recessive trait that codes an abnormality in extracellular-matrix proteins that results in EDS.[95]

In general, EDS patients have hyperelastic skin that tears with minimal trauma. Patients experience easy bruisability. Loose-jointedness ("India rubber man") is characteristic of the disorder. Hypermobility results in back pain in 6% of patients, with radiographic evidence of spinal deformity appearing in 23%.[11] Spinal deformity is noted in patients with classic type, kyphoscoliosis type, and, most commonly, arthrochalasis type. Radiographically, EDS patients present with kyphoscoliosis at the thoracolumbar junction in association with anterior wedging and posterior scalloping of the vertebral bodies.[31] Patients may also develop spondylolysis and spondylolisthesis secondary to tissue laxity. EDS is associated with vascular fragility, bleeding, compartment syndromes, and sciatic neuropathy.[97] The treatment of EDS is nonsurgical. Bracing and muscle strengthening exercises are used to prevent deformities. Swimming may strengthen muscles to help stabilize loose joints. Bracing of the spine may be worthwhile early in the course of the illness before scoliosis appears.

ACHONDROPLASIA

Achondroplasia is a skeletal defect associated with a quantitative decrease in endochondral bone growth and is the

14-9 CLASSIFICATION OF EHLERS-DANLOS SYNDROMES (1998)

New	Former	Inheritance
Classical type	Gravis (EDS type I)	AD
	Mitis (EDS type II)	AD
Hypermobility type	Hypermobile (EDS type III)	AD
Vascular type	Arterial-ecchymotic (EDS type IV)	AD
Kyphoscoliosis type	Ocular-scoliotic (EDS type VI)	AR
Arthrochalasis type	Arthrochalasis multiplex congenita (EDS types VIIA and VIIB)	AD
Dermatosparaxis type	Human dermatosparaxis (EDS type VIIC)	AR
Other forms	X-linked EDS (EDS type V)	XL
	Periodontitis type (EDS type VIII)	AD
	Fibronectin-deficient EDS (EDS type X)	?
	Familial hypermobility syndrome (EDS type XI)	AD
	Progeroid EDS	?
	Unspecified forms	?

AD, autosomal dominant; AR, autosomal recessive; XL, X-linked.

most frequent cause of dwarfism. The cause of the disease in more than 98% of individuals is related to a single base-pair missense mutation at a specific site of the *FGFR3* (fibroblast growth factor receptor) gene.[100] The disease is transmitted as an autosomal dominant trait, but only 20% have an affected parent. Spontaneous mutations occur in 90%.[40]

The diagnosis of achondroplasia is made at birth. Patients have short limbs, prominent forehead with frontal bossing, low nasal bridge, hypotonia, kyphoscoliosis, and prominent buttocks associated with accentuated lumbar lordosis. Patients have normal intelligence and no visceral lesions.

Achondroplasts have abnormalities affecting the entire axial skeleton.[59] The vertebral bodies of the spine have normal width, are slightly elongated, but have diminished diameter in the spinal canal. The space for the spinal cord is narrowed throughout the length of the spine.[69] Patients may also have critical narrowing at the level of the foramen magnum. Cerebrospinal fluid may accumulate in the brain secondary to narrowing of all the foramina and venous channels exiting the skull.[35] Infants may have respiratory difficulties secondary to both central (cervical medullary compression) and peripheral (small chest) causes.[89] Sudden death may occur when the child stands upright, with the increased weight of the head increasing cord compression.[8] Quadriplegia may occur at any age.[130] Syringomyelia may also be a complication along with cord thinning.[62] Achondroplasts also have severe and persistent sciatica secondary to disc disease and stenosis in the lower lumbar canal.[5] These patients also develop cord or cauda equina compression at the thoracic or upper lumbar level.[25]

Achondroplasts have increasing back pain as they become adults, which is associated with their hyperlordosis and small spinal canal.[85] Patients develop facet joint hypertrophy, which further narrows the canal. Achondroplasts have severe and persistent sciatica secondary to disc disease in the lower lumbar canal, which often requires surgery.[5]

Roentgenographically, the height of vertebral bodies is reduced with flaring of the upper and lower endplates resulting in posterior scalloping. The pedicles are short and thick. The interpediculate distances become progressively smaller from L1 to L5.[3] Increased disc spaces are also noted. Hyperlordosis is marked, with the sacrum directed sharply posterior.[65] The spinal canal is very narrow (Fig. 14-27).[19] Dynamic lumbar myelography may be one method to determine the most significant level caus-

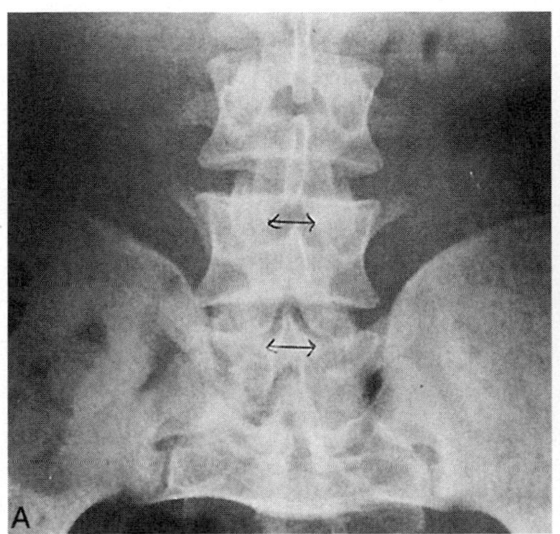

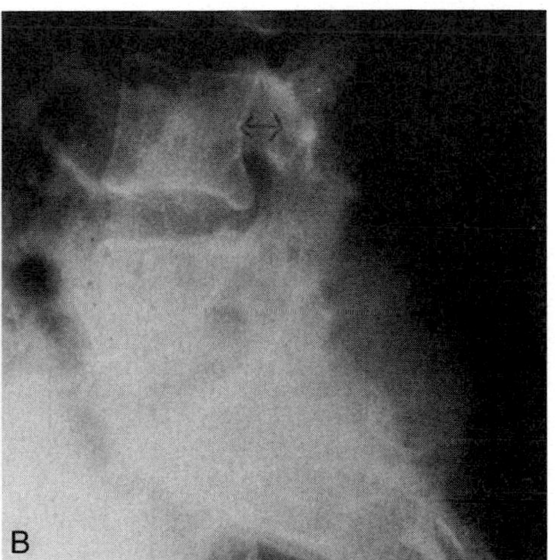

Figure 14-27 Anteroposterior *(A)* and lateral *(B)* views of an achondroplast showing decreased spinal canal size and posterior scalloping of the vertebral bodies. *(From Wiesel SW, Bernini P, Rothman RH [eds]: The Aging Lumbar Spine. Philadelphia, WB Saunders, 1982, p 12.)*

ing symptoms.[118] Reconstructed sagittal CT may be the most sensitive radiographic technique for detecting craniocervical stenosis with medullary compression.[89] Somatosensory evoked potential (SEP) is a specific but not a sensitive test for documenting cervical cord compression. SEP may be a confirmatory test of compression in patients with signs of compression on CT evaluation.[89]

Treatment of neurologic complications is surgical, including extensive laminectomy.[101] As the achondroplastic dwarf ages, stenosis is increased with hypertrophy of the ligamentum flavum and degenerative spondylosis.[32] Leg lengthening also has been proposed as a means to decrease lumbar hyperlordosis in achondroplastic dwarfs.[124] Physiotherapy, nonsteroidal anti-inflammatory drugs, and injections are useful for back pain. Some patients may benefit from bracing.[52,103]

Repetitive compression injuries to the cord and spinal nerves lead to irreversible atrophy. Patients with signs of myelopathy require surgical decompression. Reoperation is required for those individuals who develop increasing motor weakness because of restenosis. The interval between surgeries is 8 years. Restenosis is secondary to disc degeneration and facet hypertrophy.[2] Patients with severe stenosis of the spinal canal may require surgical decompression from the foramen magnum to the sacrum (Fig. 14-28).[122]

OSTEOGENESIS IMPERFECTA

Osteogenesis imperfecta (OI) is an inherited disorder of connective tissue affecting bones, ligaments, skin, sclerae, and teeth. In all its forms, OI affects between 1/5000 to 1/10,000 individuals of all racial and ethnic backgrounds.[18] The primary abnormality of OI is abnormal maturation of collagen. Significant progress has been made in determining the exact mutations resulting in alterations of collagen production. The principal collagen genes, *COL1A1* for the alpha-1 chain on chromosome 17 and *COL1A2* for the alpha-2 chain on chromosome 7, code for the formation of procollagen.[30] Collagen is a heterotrimer consisting of two alpha-1 and one alpha-2 chains. A number of defects, including decreased rate of collagen synthesis, abnormal aldehyde cross-linkages, and alterations in the usual proportions of type I and type II collagen, have been reported.[29,78,113,123] OI has several phenotypically distinct entities with different inheritance patterns.[67] Type I OI, the most common variety, has an autosomal dominant pattern of inheritance with variable penetrance and is associated with short stature, blue sclerae, hearing loss, and variable bone fragility.[104] Type II OI has autosomal dominant inheritance and is the lethal form with in utero fractures associated with rearrangements of the *COL1A1* and *COL1A2* genes and substitution of

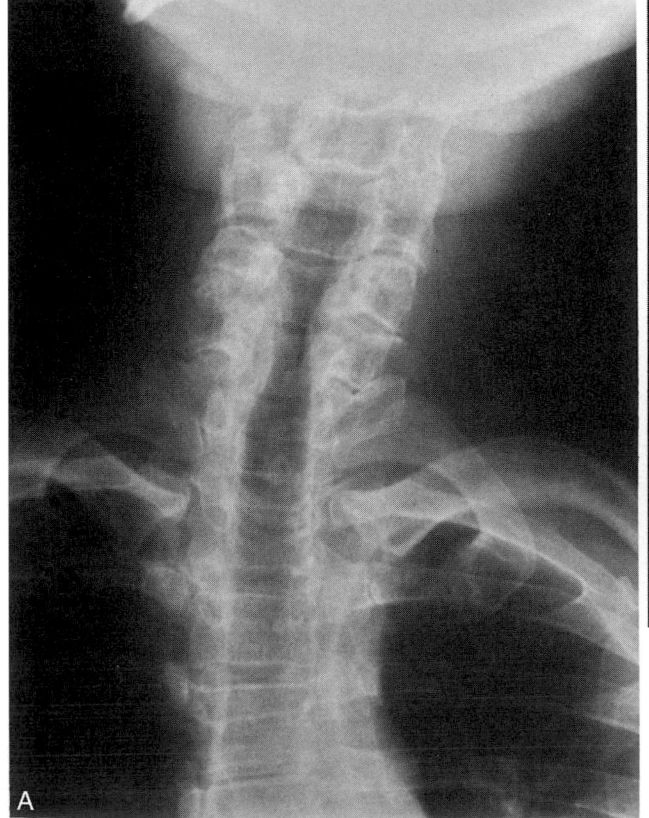

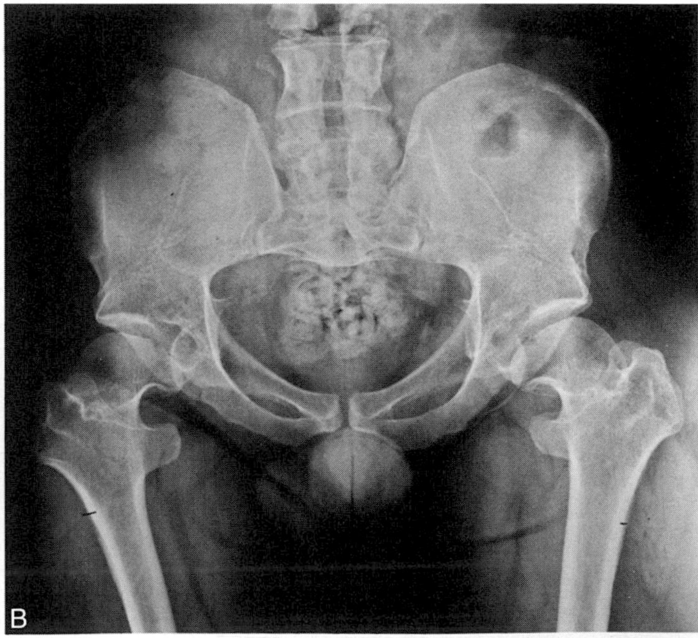

Figure 14-28 Achondroplasia. A 36-year-old achondroplastic dwarf developed severe spinal stenosis in the cervical and lumbar spine. He underwent total decompression surgery of the cervical and lumbar spine. Anteroposterior views of the cervical spine *(A)* and lumbar spine *(B)* reveal the wide decompression with absence of all the spinous processes in these areas of the spine.

bulkier amino acids for glycine in the alpha-1 chain.[30] Type III OI has autosomal recessive inheritance and a variable phenotypic appearance with marked deformity, scoliosis, joint laxity, and variable scleral color associated with a deletion in alpha-2 chains. Type IV has autosomal dominant inheritance with point mutations in the alpha-2 chain and is like type I with normal sclerae. The diagnosis of OI is confirmed by the presence of two of three criteria: (1) abnormal fragility of the skeleton, (2) blue sclerae, and (3) dentinogenesis imperfecta. Other features of OI include premature otosclerosis, ligamentous laxity, episodic diaphoresis, easy bruisability, constipation, and premature vascular calcification.[26]

Skeletal manifestations of OI include short stature secondary to multiple fractures, kyphoscoliosis, and bowing of the long bones. Fractures are very numerous before puberty. Back pain may be present secondary to vertebral body fractures or chronic muscle strain resulting from scoliosis.[72] Scoliosis may affect up to 80% of patients. The presence of six or more biconcave vertebrae before puberty is associated with the development of a scoliosis greater than 50 degrees.[45] Pulmonary compromise is the leading cause of death secondary to thoracic scoliosis of 60 degrees or greater in adult OI patients.[128] Facial features, including temporal bulging, micrognathia, and blue sclerae, are common. The teeth are frequently discolored. Hearing loss secondary to otosclerosis is common.

Roentgenographic features of OI include diffuse osteopenia of the axial and appendicular skeleton. Spine studies reveal flattening of vertebral bodies, "fish" vertebrae, and anterior wedge deformity. Severe kyphoscoliosis results from ligamentous laxity, fractures, and osteopenia (Fig. 14-29).[55]

Therapy for OI is essentially symptomatic, but new therapies are being tested. Growth hormone therapy may result in improved linear growth rate in type IV OI.[72] Fractures are casted. Sofield procedures (intramedullary rodding) may be needed to add support to bones that are chronically fractured. Intravenous pamidronate can have beneficial results on bone density and pain.[4] Acute vertebral fractures may respond to percutaneous vertebroplasty.[87] Hanscom and co-workers have reported the natural history of radiographic changes in six defined groups of patients with OI.[33] Patients with mild disease (type A) that maintained the contours of vertebral bodies had a halt to progression of spinal curvature with spinal fusion. More severely affected patients with OI (type BBF) had a less successful response to bracing and surgery. For scoliosis greater than 50 degrees, surgical fusion is required to maintain maximum pulmonary function.

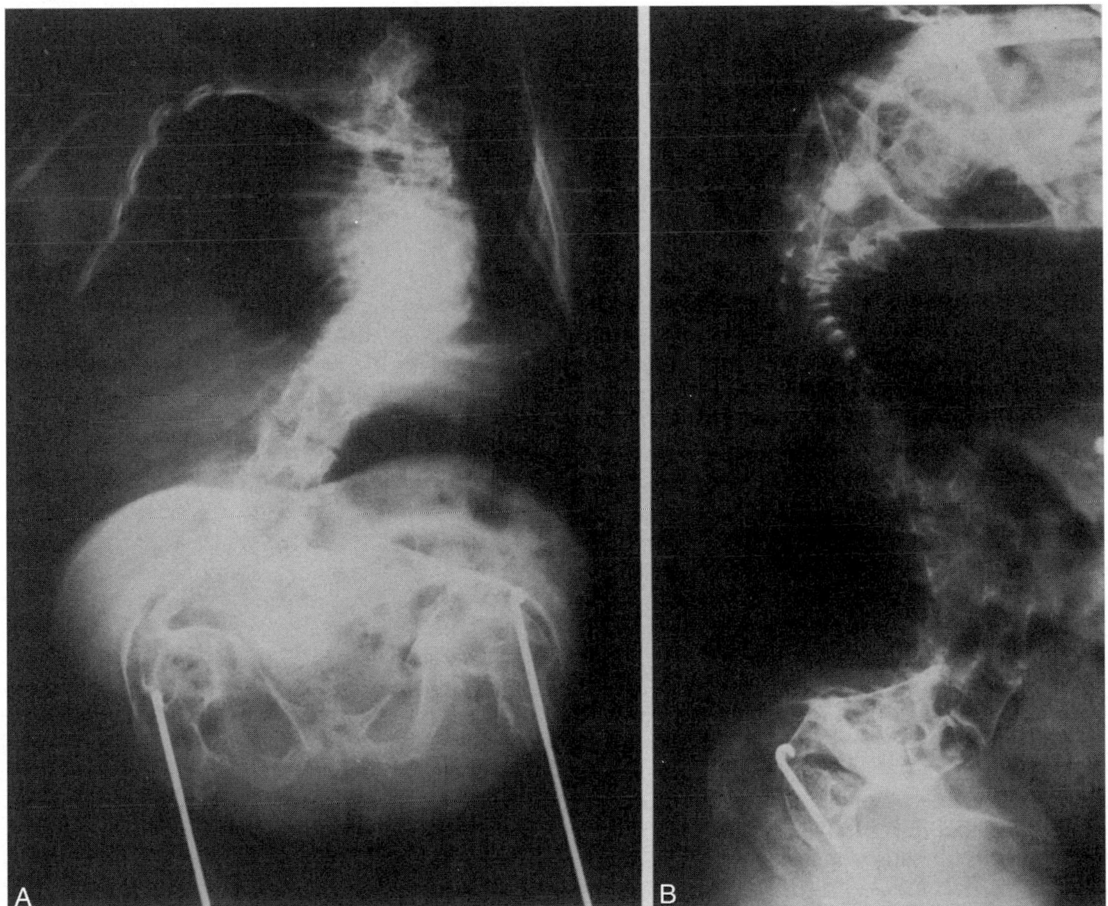

Figure 14-29 Osteogenesis imperfecta. Anteroposterior *(A)* and lateral *(B)* views of a 24-year-old woman with type III osteogenesis imperfecta who has sustained over 100 fractures. Severe kyphoscoliosis is noted associated with generalized osteoporosis and flattening of the vertebral bodies. Sofield procedures have been performed in the femoral bones for added support to decrease fractures.

Nonsteroidal anti-inflammatory and analgesic drugs are necessary to diminish pain associated with skeletal fractures. The use of sodium fluoride and anabolic steroids has not decreased fracture rates and is not recommended.[102]

MUCOPOLYSACCHARIDOSES

The diseases in the mucopolysaccharidosis class of inborn errors of metabolism result in deposition of mucopolysaccharides in various tissues. The distinct types of mucopolysaccharidosis are distinguished on the basis of combined clinical, genetic, biochemical, and allelic subtypes.[126] Many of the patients with mucopolysaccharidoses do not live into adulthood. For example, type I, Hurler's syndrome, causes abnormalities of the odontoid, severe kyphoscoliosis resulting in spinal claudication in children.[115] The forms of mucopolysaccharidoses that may be seen by an internist include type II, Hunter's syndrome; type IV, Morquio's syndrome; and type VI, Maroteaux-Lamy syndrome.

Hunter's syndrome (type II) is an X-linked syndrome with a deficiency of iduronate sulfatase resulting in accumulation of dermatan sulfate and heparan sulfate. The patients are men with mild mental retardation and mild hearing loss. The roentgenographic abnormalities include ovoid vertebral bodies with hypoplasia of vertebrae near the thoracolumbar junction resulting in kyphosis and osteoporosis (Fig.14-30).[43] Hunter's syndrome is considered a milder form of Hurler's syndrome (type I), a disorder associated with severe deficiency of iduronate sulfatase and death before the age of 10 years. In Hurler's syndrome, cervical spine laxity with subluxation occurs in patients with hypoplasia of the odontoid process.[117] In Hunter's syndrome, compressive myelopathy is a complication of the illness. A combination of progressive thickening of the dura with glycosaminoglycan deposition (pachymeningitis cervicalis) and stenosis of the cervical canal results in myelopathy.[50]

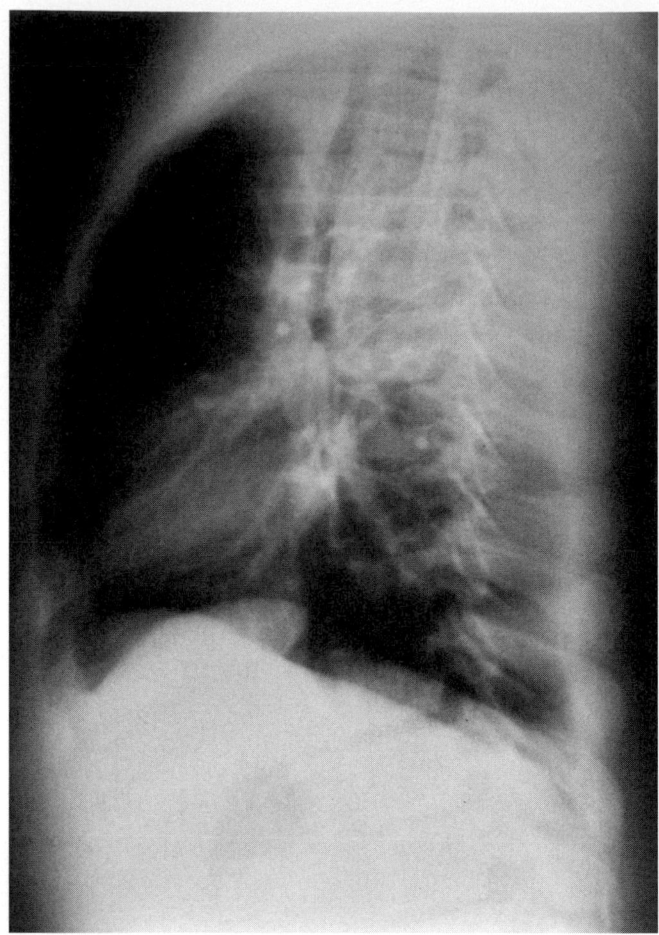

Figure 14-30 Hunter syndrome. A 26-year-man presented with Hunter syndrome with polyarthritis including back pain and mild mental retardation. Lateral view of the thoracic spine reveals ovoid vertebral bodies, widened chest cavity, and broad ribs.

Morquio's syndrome (type IV) is an autosomal recessive disorder with abnormalities in galactosamine-6-sulfate sulfatase (type A) or beta-galactosidase (type B), resulting in ineffective keratan sulfate catabolism and keratan sulfaturia. The incidence of this disorder is 1 per 300,000 live births.[59] The chromosomal defect is on chromosome 16, at band q24.3.[6] Clinical manifestations of Morquio's syndrome include dwarfism, facial deformity, corneal opacification, deafness, pectus carinatum, ligamentous laxity, hepatomegaly, and normal intelligence.[129] The spinal roentgenograms of Morquio's syndrome patients reveal platyspondyly with central beaking of vertebral bodies, atlantoaxial subluxation, and kyphoscoliosis.[73] High spinal cord compression related to ligamentous laxity and hypoplasia of the odontoid is a frequent complication of Morquio's syndrome (Fig. 14-31). MR scan is able to detect abnormal odontoid process anatomy and varying degrees of cord compression associated with anterior soft tissue masses.[41] These individuals have myelopathic signs, spastic paraplegia, and decreased physical endurance secondary to repeated trauma and atrophy of the cervical spinal cord.[13,68,120] Compression of the spinal cord is a major cause of death in these individuals. Surgical fusion of the cervical spine is indicated in the majority of these patients.[126] Fusion may result in reossification of odontoid once fusion is performed and instability is eliminated.[88] Patients who have symptomatic back pain may benefit from analgesics and anti-inflammatory drugs.[52] The use of a Milwaukee corset can prevent the appearance of medullary compressions of the spinal cord.[13]

Maroteaux-Lamy syndrome (type VI) is an autosomal recessive syndrome with arylsulfatase B deficiency that results in accumulation of dermatan sulfate. Clinical manifestations of the syndrome include kyphoscoliosis, pectus carinatum, genu valgum, hepatosplenomegaly, and joint contractures.[67] Variations in the severity of clinical manifestations of the illness may be related to the heterogeneity of genetic mutations that result in corresponding alterations in the activity or amounts of the arylsulfatase B enzyme.[47] Roentgenograms of the spine may demonstrate beaked vertebral bodies, hypoplasia of vertebral bodies, abnormal ossification of ring epiphyses, and atlantoaxial subluxations with hypoplasia of the odontoid process. Compressive myelopathy may be the result of chronic spinal cord compression secondary to cervical spine instability.[7,114,125] Patients with this syndrome require surgical decompression of the cervical spinal cord. Bone marrow transplant may be used early in the course of the disorder

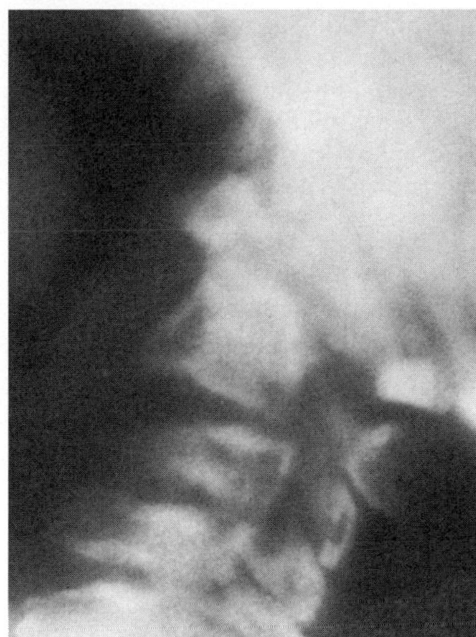

Figure 14-31 Mucopolysaccharidoses IV (Morquio's syndrome). A lateral computerized tomogram of the cervical spine shows odontoid hypoplasia and narrowing of the spinal canal. *(From McAlister WH, Herman TE: Osteochondrodysplasias, dysostoses, chromosomal aberrations, mucopolysaccharidoses, and mucolipidoses. In Resnick D [ed]: Diagnosis of Bone and Joint Disorders, 3rd ed. Philadelphia, WB Saunders, 1995, p 4233.)*

to prevent harmful deposition of mucopolysaccharide systemically.[61]

Tuberous Sclerosis

Tuberous sclerosis is a phakomatosis, a disorder of neuroectodermal tissues. The illness is also termed *Bourneville's disease*. Tuberous sclerosis is a rare disorder with a variable pattern of inheritance and an estimated incidence of 1 to 2/100,000 population.[20] Abnormalities have been localized to chromosome 9 associated with the protein hamartin and chromosome 16 associated with the protein tuberin.[54] A more recent study suggests the point prevalence of tuberous sclerosis in Olmstead County, Minnesota, to be 6.9/100,000 persons. The higher rate of diagnosis is related to the use of CT and MR to detect cerebral lesions.[99] The classic diagnostic triad consists of facial adenoma sebaceum, mental retardation, and epilepsy. Depigmented nevi, café-au-lait spots, and shagreen patches are other associated cutaneous manifestations. The cause of these abnormalities is considered to be hamartomas of the skin, brain, and other body organs. Although some of the manifestations of tuberous sclerosis are present at birth, some do not appear until adulthood.[75,92] Therefore, it is possible for the diagnosis to be overlooked.

Skull films will demonstrate calcification in up to 80% of patients. The calcifications are usually multiple and are located in the basal ganglia and paraventricular areas.[28,63]

In the axial skeleton, osteoblastic lesions are common and have multiple discrete shapes (round and ovoid). Patchy areas of increased density are also noted. The sacroiliac joints, vertebral bodies, and posterior elements are also involved (Fig. 14-32). Bone scintiscans can identify areas of uptake that correspond to bone sclerosis on roentgenograms.[48] These areas may have a mottled appearance. The lesions do not expand the bone.[56] These lesions are usually asymptomatic. Other areas of the skeleton that frequently have abnormalities include the hands and feet. Skeletal involvement is present in approximately 50% of patients with tuberous sclerosis.[12]

Tuberous sclerosis is a generalized disease and affects other organ systems in addition to the musculoskeletal and neurologic systems. Hamartomas affect the kidneys, heart, liver, lungs, and gastrointestinal tract. There is no specific therapy for the disorder. Therapy is directed at symptomatic relief of clinical complaints.

Spondyloepiphyseal Dysplasia

The epiphyseal dysplasias have been defined by Spranger as a group of heterogeneous disorders characterized by defective or excessive bone formation in the secondary ossification centers of tubular bones and vertebrae.[110] Because there is no known biochemical abnormality to differentiate these disorders, they have been divided into two large categories based on skeletal disease: (1) spondyloepiphyseal dysplasias (SD) with vertebral beaking and (2) multiple epiphyseal dysplasia without spinal involvement.[93] Abnormalities in type II collagen have been identified in some of the forms of SD.[90] One abnormality is associated with a higher ratio of hydroxylysine to lysine than in normal collagen.[76] The spectrum of clinical severity of SD may be related to the extent of

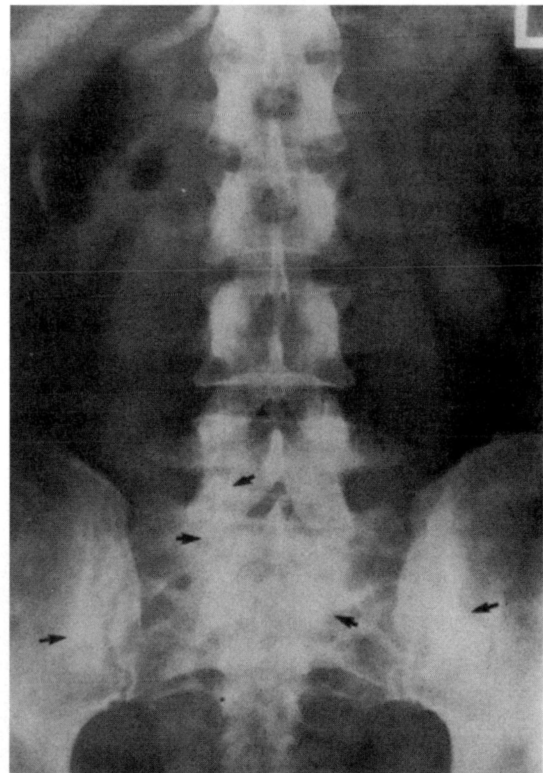

Figure 14-32 Tuberous sclerosis. Anteroposterior view of a 50-year-old woman with adenoma sebaceum and episodes of middle back pain. Pain was worse with bending or rotation. Irregular areas of osteosclerosis are noted in the ilium, sacrum, and vertebral bodies *(arrows)*. *(Courtesy of Eric Gall, MD.)*

alteration and proximity of defects to the carboxyl terminus of the collagen molecule.

The disorder has an autosomal dominant inheritance. X-linked recessive inheritance is associated with spondyloepimetaphyseal dysplasia, which is associated with spinal abnormalities.[127] Most cases are the result of spontaneous mutations. The prevalence of this disorder is estimated at 3.4 per 1 million.[59] Spinal involvement in multiple epiphyseal dysplasia, if it occurs, is mild compared with the marked alterations that occur in the appendicular skeleton. Most forms of the illness affect the phalanges, shoulders, hips, or elbow and knee joints. The vertebral changes mimic those of Scheuermann's disease. The vertebral bodies are wedge shaped, with mild platyspondyly and scoliosis. The spine is also osteoporotic.[42] This disorder is occasionally confused with Morquio's syndrome. Patients with SD of Maroteaux also mimic Morquio's syndrome but have no abnormality at birth and have no biochemical abnormality.[23] Morquio's syndrome is not manifest at birth and results in increased mucopolysaccharide in the urine.[94]

SD is recognized to have two primary forms: congenita and tarda. The spine and some appendicular bones are involved in the congenita form. The vertebrae are flattened with an irregular aspect to the superior and inferior endplates along with a bulging configuration to the posterior portion of the vertebral body (Fig. 14-33).[111] People with this disorder have a short neck and odontoid hypoplasia and are at risk for C1-C2 subluxation and myelopathy.[90] Up to 40% of children with this form of SD have atlantoaxial subluxations.[37] They may require cervical stabilization with fusion.[57]

The tarda form of SD is a male sex-linked recessive disorder that becomes manifest in late childhood as short stature with spinal abnormalities, pectus carinatum, and a broad thorax.[64] Roentgenograms of patients with this form of dysplasia reveal generalized flattening of vertebral bodies with irregular endplates, intervertebral disc space narrowing, and small iliac bones. The appendicular skeleton is minimally affected (Fig. 14-34).

A review of 30 patients with epiphyseal dysplasia reported by Kahn determined that 13% had lumbar stiffness and pain suggestive of ankylosing spondylitis.[51] Six patients with the tarda form of disease had disc narrowing to a severe degree. Fusion of the disc space occurred in these patients and has been reported previously.

One other rare form of dysplasia is spondylometaphyseal dysplasia, reported by Kozlowski and Beighton.[60] These patients are dwarfs with a waddling gait, kyphoscoliosis, and decreased joint motion. As opposed to the abnormalities in the dysplasias described earlier, the epiphyses are normal in this disorder, and the metaphyseal areas of bone are the primary locations of the bony abnormalities.[116]

Engelmann Disease

Diaphyseal dysplasia is characterized by expansion and sclerosis of the diaphyses of the long bones associated with cranial hyperostosis. This is a rare, autosomal dominant disorder with abnormalities localized to chromosome 19.[46] The main clinical features are severe pain in the legs, mus-

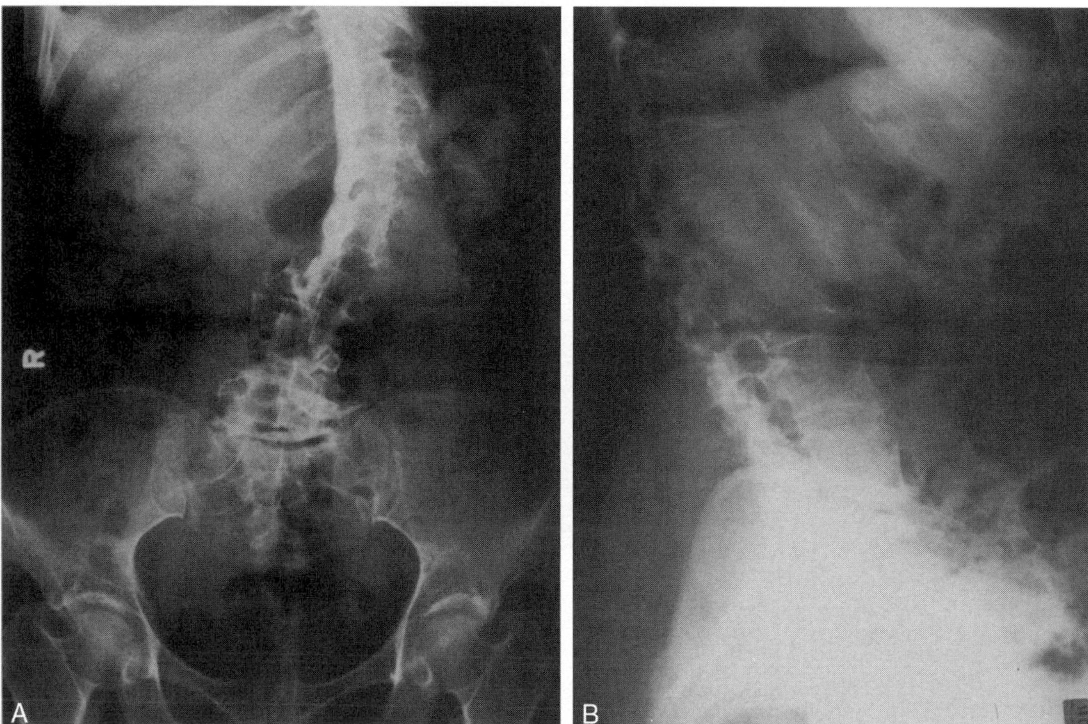

Figure 14-33 Spondyloepiphyseal dysplasia. *A*, Anteroposterior view of the lumbar spine and pelvis demonstrating marked scoliosis and hypoplastic ilia. *B*, Lateral view reveals generalized osteopenia associated with flattening of the vertebrae (platyspondyly) and irregularity of the contour of the vertebral bodies.

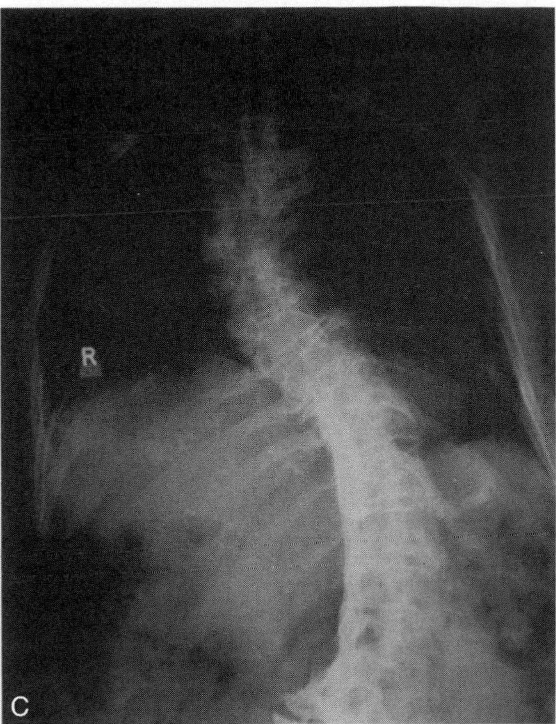

Figure 14-33, cont'd *C,* Anteroposterior view of the thoracolumbar spine shows postsurgical fusion from T9 to L2. This 64-year-old woman had progressive kyphoscoliosis as a young adult and had surgery to prevent additional deformity. She experienced diffuse low back pain with occasional episodes of L5 radiculopathy manifested by weakness in her foot. Electromyography documented radiculopathy. Her symptoms responded to a 6-day course of oral corticosteroid therapy. In 1991, progressive leg pain and motor weakness in the left foot associated with calf atrophy was noted. Laminectomy was undertaken to decompress the L5 and S1 nerve roots. Surgery was successful in decreasing pain. In 1993, the patient's weakness was slowly progressive. An ankle brace was being considered to improve ambulation. In 1999, the patient developed increasing pulmonary dysfunction and died.

cular weakness, and a waddling gait. These patients may complain of lower back and buttock pain (Fig 14-35). These patients have a favorable response to corticosteroids as compared with bisphosphonates in decreasing bone pain.[44]

DOWN SYNDROME

Patients with Down syndrome have a trisomy of chromosome 21. Down syndrome occurs in 1 of 700 live births.[37] These people are recognized at birth with certain phenotypic characteristics, including epicanthal folds, hypotonia, brachycephaly, and large tongue. At any age, they are at risk of developing atlantoaxial subluxation (Fig. 14-36). A prevalence of 15% has been reported in these patients.[16,80] Although the transverse ligaments are attenuated, the alar ligaments remain intact and protect the spinal cord from compression. Therefore, although excess motion may be measured, few individuals are symptomatic from this abnormality.[21] The incidence of occipitocervical instability is reported to be as high as 61%.[119] Patients with Down syndrome may also develop lower cervical spondylosis and myelopathy below C1-C2.[77] No single assessment technique is available to determine those patients with increased risk for neurologic compromise.[79] Progressive cervical instability and neurologic deficits are

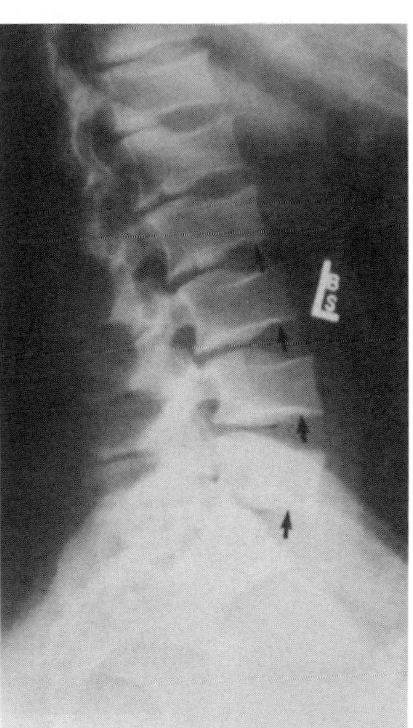

Figure 14-34 Spondyloepiphyseal dysplasia. A 26-year-old man presented with progressive scoliosis and broadening of the thorax. Lateral view of the lumbar spine demonstrates elongation of vertebral bodies at all levels *(black arrows). (From Borenstein DG: Low back pain. In Klippel JH, Dieppe P (eds): Rheumatology. St Louis, CV Mosby, 1994, Sec 5, p 4.8.)*

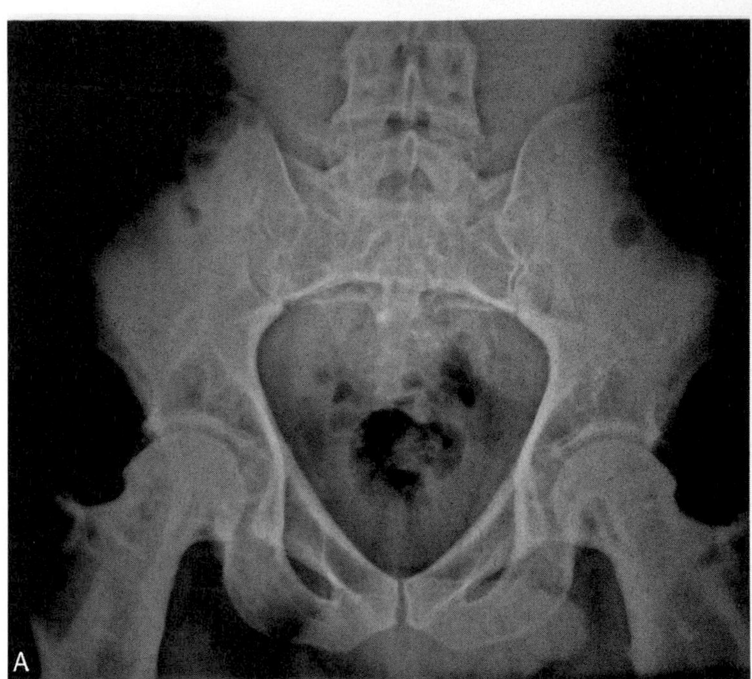

Figure 14-35 Engelmann disease. A 38-year-old man presented with appendicular and low back pain associated with diaphyseal dysplasia. Anteroposterior pelvis *(A)* and lateral spine *(B)* views demonstrate cortical thickening of the periosteal and endosteal surfaces of the femur with extension into the pelvis and vertical striations of the vertebral bodies.

more common in boys than girls with Down syndrome. In general, routine clinical and radiographic evaluation is indicated for Down syndrome patients, particularly those involved in athletics, including the Special Olympics. Patients with atlantoaxial subluxation should not engage in contact sports or those activities associated with flexion of the neck.[36]

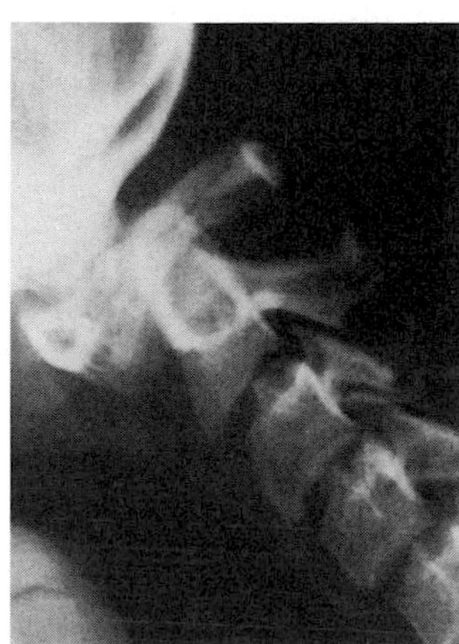

Figure 14-36 Down syndrome. Note the considerable atlantoaxial subluxation. *(From McAlister WH, Herman TE: Osteochondrodysplasias, dysostoses, chromosomal aberrations, mucopolysaccharidoses, and mucolipidoses. In Resnick D [ed]: Diagnosis of Bone and Joint Disorders, 3rd ed. Philadelphia, WB Saunders, 1995, p 4227.)*

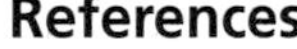

References

Heritable Genetic Disorders

1. Ahn NU, Sponseller PD, Ahn UM, et al: Dural ectasia is associated with back pain in Marfan syndrome. Spine 25:1562-1568, 2000.
2. Ain MC, Elmaci I, Hurko O, et al: Reoperation for spinal restenosis in achondroplasia. J Spinal Disord 13:168-173, 2000.
3. Alexander E Jr: Significance of the small lumbar spinal canal: Cauda equina compression syndromes due to spondylosis: V. Achondroplasia. J Neurosurg 31:513, 1969.
4. Astrom E, Soderhall S: Beneficial effect of long term intravenous bisphosphonate treatment of osteogenesis imperfecta. Arch Dis Child 86:356-364, 2002.
5. Bailey JA: Orthopaedic aspects of achondroplasia. J Bone Joint Surg Am 52A:1285, 1970.
6. Baker E, Gua XH, Orsborn AM, et al: The Morquio A syndrome (mucopolysaccharidosis IVA) gene maps to 16q24.3. Am J Hum Genet 52:96-98, 1993.
7. Banna M, Hollenberg R: Compressive meningeal hypertrophy in mucopolysaccharidosis. AJNR Am J Neuroradiol 8:385, 1987.
8. Beighton P (ed): McKusick's Heritable Disorders of Connective Tissue, 5th ed. St. Louis, CV Mosby, 1993, p 748.
9. Beighton P: The Ehlers-Danlos syndromes. In Beighton P (ed): McKusick's Heritable Disorders of Connective Tissue, 5th ed. St. Louis, CV Mosby, 1993, pp 189-251.

10. Beighton P, De Paepe A, Steinmann B, et al: Ehlers-Danlos syndromes: Revised nosology, Villefranche, 1997. Am J Med Genet 77:31-37, 1998.
11. Beighton P, Horan F: Orthopaedic aspects of the Ehlers-Danlos syndrome. J Bone Joint Surg Br 51B:444, 1969.
12. Bell DG, King BF, Hattery RR, et al: Imaging characteristics of tuberous sclerosis. AJR Am J Roentgenol 156:1081, 1991.
13. Blaw ME, Langer LO: Spinal cord compression in Morquio-Brailsford disease. J Pediatr 74:593, 1969.
14. Brenton DP, Dow CJ, James JIP, et al: Homocystinuria and Marfan's syndrome: A comparison. J Bone Joint Surg Br 54B:277, 1972.
15. Brill PW, Mitty HA, Gaull GE: Homocystinuria due to cystathionine synthetase deficiency: Clinical roentgenologic correlation. AJR Am J Roentgenol 121:45, 1974.
16. Burke SW, French HG, Roberts JM, et al: Chronic atlanto-axial instability in Down's syndrome. J Bone Joint Surg Am 67A:1356, 1985.
17. Byers PH: Inherited disorders of collagen gene structure and expression. Am J Med Genet 34:72, 1989.
18. Byers PH, Steiner RD: Osteogenesis imperfecta. Ann Rev Med 43:269, 1992.
19. Caffey J: Achondroplasia of pelvis and lumbosacral spine: Some roentgenographic features. AJR Am J Roentgenol 80:449, 1958.
20. Critchley M, Earl CJC: Tuberose sclerosis and allied conditions. Brain 55:311, 1932.
21. Davidson RG: Atlantoaxial instability in individuals with Down's syndrome: A fresh look at the evidence. Pediatrics 81:857, 1988.
22. DePaepe A, Devereux RB, Dietz HC, et al: Revised diagnostic criteria for the Marfan syndrome. Am J Med Genet 62:417-426, 1996.
23. Doman AN, Maroteaux P, Lyne ED: Spondyloepiphyseal dysplasia of Maroteaux. J Bone Joint Surg Am 72A:1364, 1990.
24. Duncan R, Esses S: Marfan syndrome with back pain secondary to pedicular attenuation. Spine 20:1197-1198, 1995.
25. Epstein JA, Malis LI: Compression of spinal cord and cauda equina in achondroplastic dwarfs. Neurology 5:875, 1955.
26. Falvo KA, Root L, Bullought PG: Osteogenesis imperfecta: Clinical evaluation and management. J Bone Joint Surg Am 56A:783, 1974.
27. Fattori R, Nienaber CA, Descovich B, et al: Importance of dural ectasia in phenotypic assessment of Marfan's syndrome. Lancet 354:910-913, 1999.
28. Fitz CR, Harwood-Nash DCF, Thompson JR: Neurobiology of tuberous sclerosis in children. Radiology 110:635, 1974.
29. Fugi K, Tanzer ML: Osteogenesis imperfecta: Biochemical studies of bone collagen. Clin Orthop 124:271, 1977.
30. Gertner JM, Root L: Osteogenesis imperfecta. Orthop Clin North Am 21:151, 1990.
31. Goldman AB: Collagen diseases, epiphyseal dysplasias, and related conditions. In Resnick D, Niwayama G (eds): Diagnosis of Bone and Joint Disorders, 2nd ed. Philadelphia, WB Saunders, 1988, pp 3374-3441.
32. Hancock DO, Phillips DG: Spinal compression in achondroplasia. Paraplegia 3:23, 1965.
33. Hanscom DA, Winter RB, Luther L, et al.: Osteogenesis imperfecta: Radiographic classification, natural history, and treatment of spinal deformities. J Bone Joint Surg 74:598, 1992.
34. Hayward C, Porteous ME, Brock DJH: Mutation screening of all 65 exons of the fibrillin-1 gene in 60 patients with Marfan syndrome: Report of 12 novel mutations. Hum Mutat 10:280-289, 1997.
35. Hecht JT, Butler IJ: Neurologic morbidity associated with achondroplasia. J Child Neurol 5:84, 1990.
36. Hensinger RN: Congenital anomalies of the cervical spine. Clin Orthop 264:16, 1991.
37. Herman MJ, Pizzutillo PD: Cervical spine disorders in children. Orthop Clin North Am 30:457-466, 1999.
38. Herzka A, Sponseller PD, Pyeritz RE: Atlantoaxial rotatory subluxations in patients with Marfan syndrome: A report of three cases. Spine 25:524-526, 2000.
39. Hobbs WR, Sponseller PD, Weiss AC, et al: The cervical spine in Marfan syndrome. Spine 22:983-989, 1997.
40. Horton WA, Hecht JT: The chondrodysplasias. In Royce PM, Steinmann B (eds): Connective Tissue and Its Heritable Disorders: Molecular, Genetic, and Medical Aspects. New York, Wiley-Liss, 1993, pp 641-675.
41. Hughes DG, Chadderton RD, Cowle RA, et al: MRI of the brain and craniocervical junction in Morquio's disease. Neuroradiology 39:381-385, 1997.
42. Hulvey JT, Keats T: Multiple epiphyseal dysplasia: A contribution to the problem of spinal involvement. AJR Am J Roentgenol 106:170, 1969.
43. Hunter C: A rare disease in two brothers. Proc R Soc Med 10:104, 1971.
44. Inaoka T, Shuke N, Sato J, et al: Scintigraphic evaluation of pamidronate and corticosteroid therapy in a patient with progressive diaphyseal dysplasia (Camurati-Engelmann disease). Clin Nucl Med 26:680-682, 2001.
45. Ishikawa S, Kumar SJ, Takahashi HE, et al: Vertebral body shape as a predictor of spinal deformity in osteogenesis imperfecta. J Bone Joint Surg Am 78A:212-219, 1996.
46. Janssens K, Gershoni-Baruch R, van Hul E, et al: Localization of the gene causing diaphyseal dysplasia Camurati-Engelmann to chromosome 19q13. J Med Genet 37:245-249, 2000
47. Jin W, Jackson CE, Desnick RJ, Schuchman EH: Mucopolysaccharidosis type IV: Identification of three mutations in the arylsulfatase B gene of patients with the severe and mild phenotypes provides molecular evidence for genetic heterogeneity. Am J Hum Genet 50:795, 1992.
48. Jonard P, Lonneux M, Boland B, et al: Tc-99m HDP bone scan showing bone changes in a case of tuberous sclerosis or Bourneville's disease. Clin Nucl Med 26:50-52, 2001.
49. Jones KB, Erkula G, Sponseller PD, et al: Spine deformity correction in Marfan syndrome. Spine 27:2003-2012, 2002.
50. Kaendler S, Bockenheimer S, Grafin VIH, et al: Cervical myelopathy in mucopolysaccharidosis type II (Hunter's syndrome): Neuroradiologic, clinical and histopathologic findings. Dtsch Med Wochenschr 115:1348, 1990.
51. Kahn MF, Corvol MT, Jarmand SH, et al: Le rhumatisme chondrodysplastique. Rev Rheum 37:825, 1970.
52. Kahn MF, De Sese S: Rheumatic manifestations of heritable disorders of connective tissue. Clin Rheum Dis 1:3, 1975.
53. Kainulainen K, Sakai LY, Child A, et al: Two mutations in Marfan syndrome resulting in truncated fibrillin polypeptides. Proc Natl Acad Sci 89:5917, 1992.
54. Kimmelman A, Liang BC: Familial neurogenic tumor syndromes. Hematol Oncol Clin North Am 15:1073-1084, 2001.
55. King JD, Bobechko WP: Osteogenesis imperfecta: An orthopaedic description and surgical review. J Bone Joint Surg Br 53B:72, 1971.
56. Komar NN, Gabrielsen TO, Holt JF: Roentgenographic appearance of lumbosacral spine and pelvis in tuberous sclerosis. Radiology 89:701, 1967.
57. Kopits S: Orthopedic complications of dwarfism. Clin Orthop 114:153, 1976.
58. Korkko J, Ritvaniemi P, Haataja L, et al: Mutation in type II procollagen (COL2A1) that substitutes aspartate for glycine α1-67 and that causes cataracts and retinal detachment: Evidence for molecular heterogeneity in the Wagner syndrome and the Stickler syndrome (arthro-ophthalmopathy). Am J Hum Genet 53:55-61, 1993.
59. Kornblum M, Stanitski DF: Spinal manifestations of skeletal dysplasias. Orthop Clin North Am 30:501-520, 1999.
60. Kozlowski K, Beighton P: Radiographic features of spondyloepimetaphyseal dysplasia with joint laxity and progressive kyphoscoliosis. Fortschr Roentgenstr 141:337, 1984.
61. Krivit W, Pierpont ME, Ayaz KL, et al: Bone-marrow transplant in Maroteaux-Lamy syndrome (mucopolysaccharidoses type VI biochemical and clinical status 24 months after transplantation). N Engl J Med 311:1606, 1984.
62. Lachman RS: Neurologic abnormalities in the skeletal dysplasia: A clinical and radiological perspective. Am J Med Gen 69:33-43, 1997.
63. Lagos JC, Holman CB, Gomez MR: Tuberous sclerosis. Neuroroentgenologic observations. AJR Am J Roentgenol 104:171, 1968.
64. Langer LO Jr: Spondyloepiphyseal dysplasia tarda: Hereditary chondrodysplasia with characteristic vertebral configuration in the adult. Radiology 82:833, 1964.
65. Langer LO Jr, Baumann PA, Gorlin RJ: Achondroplasia. AJR Am J Roentgenol 100:12, 1967.
66. Letts M, Kabir A, Davidson D: The spinal manifestations of Stickler's syndrome. Spine 24:1260, 1999.
67. Levin LS, Salinas CF, Jogenson RJ: Classification of osteogenesis imperfecta by dental characteristics. Lancet 1:332, 1978.
68. Lipson SJ: Dysplasia of the odontoid process in Morquio's syndrome causing quadriparesis. J Bone Joint Surg Am 59A:340, 1977.

69. Lutter LD, Langer LO: Neurological symptoms in achondroplastic dwarfs: Surgical treatment. J Bone Joint Surg Am 59A:87, 1977.
70. Maddox BK, Sakai LY, Keene DR, Glanville RW: Connective tissue microfibrils. J Biol Chem 264:21381, 1989.
71. Magid D, Pyeritz RE, Fishman EK: Musculoskeletal manifestations of the Marfan syndrome: Radiologic features. AJR Am J Roentgenol 155:99, 1990.
72. Marini JC, Gerber NL: Osteogenesis imperfecta: Rehabilitation and prospects for gene therapy. JAMA 277:746-750, 1997.
73. McAlister WH: Osteochondrodysplasias, dysostoses, chromosomal aberrations, mucopolysaccharidoses, and mucolipidoses. In Resnick D, Niwayama G (eds): Diagnosis of Bone and Joint Disorders, 2nd ed. Philadelphia, WB Saunders, 1988, pp 3442-3515.
74. McKusick VA, Scott CI: A nomenclature for constitutional disorders of bone. J Bone Joint Surg 53A:978, 1971.
75. Medley BE, McLeod RA, Houser OW: Tuberous sclerosis. Semin Roentgenol 11:35, 1976.
76. Murray LW, Baustista J, James PL, Rimoin DL: Type II collagen defects in the chondrodysplasias: I. Spondyloepiphyseal dysplasias. Am J Hum Genet 45:5, 1989.
77. Olive PM, Whitecloud TS III, Bennett JT: Lower cervical spondylosis and myelopathy in adults with Down's syndrome. Spine 13:781, 1988.
78. Prockop DJ, Constantinou CD, Dombrowski KE, et al: Type I procollagen: The gene-protein system that harbors most of the mutations causing osteogenesis imperfecta and probably more common heritable disorders of connective tissue. Am J Med Gen 34:60, 1989.
79. Pueschel SM, Findley TW, Furia J, et al: Atlantoaxial instability in Down syndrome: Roentgenographic, neurologic, and somatosensory evoked potential studies. J Pediatr 110:515, 1987.
80. Pueschel SM, Scola FH: Atlantoaxial instability in individuals with Down's syndrome: Epidemiologic, radiographic, and clinical studies. Pediatrics 80:555, 1987.
81. Putnam EA, Cho M, Zinn AB, et al: Delineation of the Marfan phenotype associated with mutations in exons 23-32 of the *FBN1* gene. Am J Med Genet 62:233-242, 1996.
82. Pyeritz RE: Heritable and development disorders of connective tissue and bone. In McCarty DJ, Koopman WJ (eds): Arthritis and Allied Conditions, 12th ed. Philadelphia, Lea & Febiger, 1993, pp 1483-1509.
83. Pyeritz RE: The Marfan syndrome. In Royce PM, Steinmann B (eds): Connective Tissue and Its Heritable Disorders: Molecular, Genetic, and Medical Aspects. New York, Wiley-Liss, 1993, pp 437-468.
84. Pyeritz RE, McKusick VA: The Marfan syndrome: Diagnosis and management. N Engl J Med 300:772, 1979.
85. Pyeritz RE, Sack GH Jr, Udvarhelyi GB: Cervical and lumbar laminectomy for spinal stenosis in achondroplasia. Johns Hopkins Med J 146:203, 1980.
86. Raftopoulos C, Pierard GE, Retif C, et al: Endoscopic cure of a giant sacral meningocele associated with Marfan's syndrome: Case report. Neurosurgery 130:765, 1992.
87. Rami PM, McGraw JK, Heatwole EV, et al: Percutaneous vertebroplasty in the treatment of vertebral bony compression fracture secondary to osteogenesis imperfecta. Skel Radiol 31:162-165, 2002.
88. Ransford AO, Crockard HA, Stevens JM, et al: Occipito-atlantofusion in Morquio-Brailsford syndrome. J Bone Joint Surg Br 78B:307-313, 1996.
89. Reid CS, Pyeritz RE, Kopits SE, et al: Cervicomedullary compression in young patients with achondroplasia: Value of comprehensive neurologic and respiratory evaluation. J Pediatr 110:522, 1987.
90. Rimoin DL, Lachman RS: Genetic disorders of the osseous skeleton. In Beighton P (ed): McKusick's Heritable Disorders of Connective Tissue. St Louis, CV Mosby, 1993, pp 557-689.
91. Robins PR, Moe JH, Winter RB: Scoliosis in Marfan syndrome: Its characteristics and results of treatment in thirty-five patients. J Bone Joint Surg Am 57A:358, 1975.
92. Rosenberg S, Mendez MF: Tuberous sclerosis in the elderly. J Am Geriatr Soc 37:1058, 1989.
93. Rubin P: Dynamic Classification of Bone Dysplasias. Chicago, Year Book Medical, 1964, p 120.
94. Saldino RM: Radiographic diagnosis of neonatal short-linked dwarfism. Med Radiogr Photogr 48:61, 1973.
95. Schalkwijk J, Zweers MC, Steijlen PM, et al: A recessive form of the Ehlers-Danlos syndrome caused by tenascin-X deficiency. N Engl J Med 345:1167-1175, 2001.
96. Schlesinger EB: The significance of genetic contributions and markers in disorders of spinal structure. Neurosurgery 26:944, 1990.
97. Schmalzried TP, Eckardt JJ: Spontaneous gluteal artery rupture resulting in compartment syndrome and sciatic neuropathy: Report of a case in Ehlers-Danlos syndrome. Clin Orthop 275:253, 1992.
98. Schwarze U, Atkinson M, Hoffman GG, et al: Null alleles of the *COL5A1* gene of type V collagen are a cause of the classical forms of Ehlers-Danlos syndrome (types I and II). Am J Hum Genet 66:1757-1765, 2000.
99. Shepherd CW, Beard CM, Gomez MR, et al: Tuberous sclerosis complex in Olmstead County, Minnesota, 1950-1989. Arch Neurol 48:400, 1991.
100. Shiang R, Thompason L, Zhu Y, et al: Mutations in the transmembrane domain of *FGFR3* cause the most common genetic form of dwarfism, achondroplasia. Cell 78:335-342, 1994.
101. Shikata J, Yamamuro T, Iida H, et al: Surgical treatment of achondroplastic dwarfs with paraplegia. Surg Neurol 29:125, 1988.
102. Shoenfeld Y, Fried A, Ehrenfeld NE: Osteogenesis imperfecta: Review of the literature with presentation of 29 cases. Am J Dis Child 129:679, 1975.
103. Siebens AA, Hungerford DS, Kirby NA: Achondroplasia: Effectiveness of an orthosis in reducing deformity of the spine. Arch Phys Med Rehabil 68:384, 1987.
104. Sillence DO, Senn A, Danks DM: Genetic heterogeneity in osteogenesis imperfecta. J Med Genet 16:101, 1979.
105. Sinclair RJG: The Marfan syndrome. Bull Rheum Dis 8:153, 1958.
106. Skovby F: The homocystinurias. In Royce PM, Steinmann B (eds): Connective Tissue and Its Heritable Disorders: Molecular, Genetic, and Medical Aspects. New York, Wiley-Liss, 1993, pp 469-486.
107. Sponseller PD, Ahn NU, Ahn UM, et al: Osseous anatomy of the lumbosacral spine in Marfan syndrome. Spine 25:2797-2802, 2000.
108. Sponseller PD, Bhimani M, Solacoff D, et al: Results of brace treatment of scoliosis in Marfan syndrome. Spine 25:2350-2354, 2000.
109. Sponseller P, Hobbs W, Riley L, et al: The thoracolumbar spine in Marfan syndrome. J Bone Joint Surg Am 77A:867-876, 1995.
110. Spranger J: The epiphyseal dysplasias. Clin Orthop 114:46, 1976.
111. Spranger JW, Langer LO Jr: Spondyloepiphyseal dysplasia congenita. Radiology 94:313, 1970.
112. Stern WE: Dural ectasia and the Marfan syndrome. J Neurosurg 69:221, 1988.
113. Sykes B, Francis MJO, Smith R: Altered relation of two collagen types in osteogenesis imperfecta. N Engl J Med 296:1200, 1977.
114. Tamaki N, Kojima N, Tanimoto M, et al: Myelopathy due to diffuse thickening of the cervical dura mater in Maroteaux-Lamy syndrome. Neurosurgery 21:416, 1987.
115. Tandon V, Williamson JB, Cowie RA, et al: Spinal problems in mucopolysaccharidosis I. (Hurler syndrome). J Bone Joint Surg Br 78B:938-948, 1996.
116. Thomas PS, Nevin NC: Spondylometaphyseal dysplasia. AJR Am J Roentgenol 128:89, 1977.
117. Thomas SL, Childress MH, Quinton B: Hypoplasia of the odontoid with atlanto-axial subluxation in Hurler's syndrome. Pediatr Radiol 15:353, 1985.
118. Thomeer RTWM, van Dijk JMC: Surgical treatment of lumbar spinal stenosis in achondroplasia. J Neurosurg 96:292-297, 2002.
119. Tredwell SJ, Newman DE, Lockith G: Instability of the upper cervical spine in Down syndrome. J Pediat Orthop 10:602-606, 1990.
120. Trojak JE, Ho C, Roesel RA, et al: Morquio-like syndrome (MPS IV B) associated with deficiency of a beta-galactosidase. Johns Hopkins Med J 146:75, 1980.
121. Tsipouras P, Del Mastro R, Sarfarazi M, et al: Genetic linkage of the Marfan syndrome, ectopia lentis, and congenital contractural arachnodactyly to the fibrillin genes on chromosomes 15 and 5. N Engl J Med 326:905, 1992.
122. Uematsu S, Wang H, Kopits SE, et al: Total craniospinal decompression in achrondroplastic stenosis. Neurosurgery 35:250, 1994.

123. Uitto J, Murray LW, Blumberg B, Shamban A: Biochemistry of collagen in diseases. Ann Intern Med 105:740, 1976.
124. Vilarrubias JM, Ginebreda I, Jimeno E: Lengthening of the lower limbs and correction of lumbar hyperlordosis in achondroplasia. Clin Orthop 250:143, 1990.
125. Wald SL, Schmidek HH: Compressive myelopathy associated with type IV mucopolysaccharidosis (Maroteaux-Lamy syndrome). Neurosurgery 14:83, 1984.
126. Whitley CB: The mucopolysaccharidoses. In Beighton P (ed): McKusick's Heritable Disorders of Connective Tissue. St. Louis, CV Mosby, 1993, pp 367-499.
127. Whyte MP, Gottesman GS, Eddy MC, et al: X-linked recessive spondyloepiphyseal dysplasia tarda: Clinical and radiographic evolution in a 6-generation kindred and review of the literature. Medicine 78:9-25, 1999.
128. Widmann RF, Bitan FD, Laplaza J, et al: Spinal deformity, pulmonary compromise, and quality of life in osteogenesis imperfecta. Spine 24:1673, 1999.
129. Wraith J: The mucopolysaccharidoses: A clinical review and guide to management. Arch Dis Child 72:263-267, 1995.
130. Yang SS, Corbett DP, Bough AJ, et al: Upper cervical myelopathy in achondroplasia. Am J Clin Pathol 68:68, 1977.

CHAPTER 15

HEMATOLOGIC DISORDERS OF THE SPINE

Disorders of the hematologic system may involve any area of the body where bone marrow is located. Since the axial skeleton contains a significant proportion of an adult's bone marrow, disorders that cause hyperplasia of bone marrow or the replacement of normal bone marrow cells with abnormal ones may be associated with spinal pain. A characteristic of hematopoietic disorders is that although symptoms may be localized to various areas of the skeleton, these illnesses are systemic in origin and cause significant abnormalities in a number of other organ systems. In the axial skeleton, the lumbar and thoracic spine are affected to a much greater degree than the cervical spine. This follows the relative proportion of bone marrow cells in these osseous structures. The hematologic disorders that produce symptoms of spinal pain include the hemoglobinopathies, myelofibrosis, and mastocytosis.

The symptom of spinal pain in a patient with a hemoglobinopathy (sickle cell anemia) occurs at the height of a vaso-occlusive crisis. These crises occur secondary to the blockage of small vessels and the infarction of tissue by sickled cells. Back pain is acute in onset and has a duration of 4 to 5 days. Patients frequently have bone pain in the extremities as well. Patients with myelofibrosis have an insidious onset of spinal pain secondary to the fibrosis and osteosclerosis that occurs as the bone marrow is replaced with fibrous tissue. Patients with mastocytosis may also have insidious onset of back pain in the setting of a systemic illness characterized by skin eruptions, flushing, weight loss, and diarrhea.

Physical examination of a patient with a hemoglobinopathy demonstrates a chronically ill individual in acute distress during a crisis. Abnormal findings may include fever, tachycardia, and tenderness to palpation over the spine and extremities with associated muscle spasm. The patient with myelofibrosis has pallor, splenomegaly, and bone tenderness on palpation. The patient with mastocytosis has skin rash, hepatosplenomegaly, and bone tenderness.

Laboratory evaluation of these patients is helpful in making a specific diagnosis of the underlying disorder. Patients with hemoglobinopathies have characteristic abnormalities on blood smear, including sickle and target cells. The specific hemoglobin abnormality is identified by hemoglobin electrophoresis. The blood smear in myelofibrosis contains abnormal red blood cell forms, mature and immature white blood cell forms, and variable numbers of platelets. The diagnosis of myelofibrosis is confirmed by bone marrow biopsy, which characteristically reveals marrow fibrosis, an increased number of megakaryocytes, and osteosclerosis. Findings in mastocytosis include increased urinary histamine, increased fibrosis, and mast cells, which may be confused with granulomatous cells on bone marrow biopsy.

Radiographic findings associated with hemoglobinopathies include evidence of marrow expansion secondary to hyperplasia, characterized by loss of trabeculae and cortical thinning, distinctive cuplike depression in vertebral bodies ("H" vertebrae), sclerosis, and fractures compatible with aseptic necrosis of bone. Radiographic findings of myelofibrosis include diffuse osteosclerosis in the axial skeleton and proximal long bones. Mastocytosis may cause osteosclerosis, osteoporosis, or a mixed picture on plain roentgenograms. Bone scintiscan may show diffusely increased uptake.

Therapy for these hematopoietic disorders is essentially symptomatic. Patients with sickle cell anemia are educated to avoid circumstances that may precipitate a painful crisis. They are treated with hydration and analgesics during vaso-occlusive crises. Transfusions are reserved for life-threatening complications such as a cerebrovascular accident. There is no effective therapy that alters the course of myelofibrosis, although bone marrow stem cell transplants offer a temporary remission of the disorder. Antihistamines are the cornerstone of therapy for mastocytosis. These drugs counteract the effects of the chemical mediators released by mast cells. The prognosis of patients with hematologic disorders is related to the severity of the illness in sickle cell disease and the possibility of malignant degeneration in myelofibrosis and mastocytosis. Hemoglobinopathies are systemic illnesses that affect the musculoskeletal, pulmonary, cardiovascular, renal, and nervous systems. Patients with severe sickle cell anemia die prematurely from cardiac failure or infection.

Patients with myelofibrosis are at risk of developing acute leukemia. Many patients die from leukemia within 5 years of the diagnosis of their illness.

Mastocytosis is associated with a broad spectrum of diseases, including urticaria pigmentosa with or without systemic disease. The patients with the worst prognosis are those with marked systemic involvement who develop mast cell leukemia.

HEMOGLOBINOPATHIES

Capsule Summary

	Low Back	Neck
Frequency of spinal pain	Common	Not applicable (NA)
Location of spinal pain	Lumbar spine	NA
Quality of spinal pain	Aching, boring	NA
Symptoms and signs	Intermittent episodes of pain with crises, bone tenderness	NA
Laboratory findings	Anemia, abnormal blood smear	NA
Radiographic findings	Coarsened trabeculae with "fish" vertebrae on plain roentgenograms	NA
Treatment	Hydration, analgesics, hydroxyurea	NA

PREVALENCE AND PATHOGENESIS

Hemoglobinopathies are a clinical group of disorders associated with defects in the physical properties or manufacture of the polypeptide chains that are the protein parts of hemoglobin. The presence of abnormal hemoglobin in red blood cells causes continuous premature destruction of these cells and chronic hemolytic anemia. Abnormal hemoglobins also change the shape of red blood cells, causing sickling and obstruction of the vascular microcirculation. Vascular obstruction leads to deoxygenation, tissue necrosis, and pain, and this condition is referred to as a *vaso-occlusive* or *thrombotic crisis*. In adults with hemoglobinopathies, particularly sickle cell anemia, acute back pain and extremity pain are the most common symptoms of vascular crises. Persistent bone destruction secondary to vaso-occlusion and hyperplasia of bone marrow in the axial skeleton results in compression fractures, accentuated dorsal kyphosis, and lumbar lordosis.

Herrick in 1910 was the first to describe the sickle-shaped erythrocytes of sickle cell anemia.[25] Cooley and Lee in 1925 used the Greek word for "the sea" to propose thalassemia as the name for the severe anemia associated with splenomegaly in patients of Mediterranean origin.[15]

The most common clinically significant hemoglobinopathies include sickle cell anemia (hemoglobin SS), sickle cell–hemoglobin C disease (hemoglobin SC), and sickle cell–β-thalassemia. Human adult hemoglobin consists of two pairs of coiled polypeptide chains, alpha and beta, and is referred to as *hemoglobin A*. Substitution of gamma or delta chains for beta chains results in hemoglobin F (fetal) or hemoglobin A_2. Patients with hemoglobin S have normal alpha chains but have glutamic acid replaced with valine at the sixth amino acid position in the beta chain. Chromosome 16 is the location for the gene that produces the alpha chain and chromosome 11 is the location for the gene that produces the beta chain.[10] Hemoglobin C has lysine substituted in the sixth position of the beta chain.

Epidemiology

Sickle cell anemia, or hemoglobin SS, is a relatively common disorder, present in 1 in 625 black Americans.[32] Hemoglobin SC affects 1 in 833 black Americans. Hemoglobin S–β-thalassemia occurs in 1 in 1667. Sickle cell trait (hemoglobin having only one abnormal beta chain with valine) occurs in 8% of black Americans. Sickle cell trait may also be seen infrequently in persons from the eastern Mediterranean, India, or Saudi Arabia. The overlap of geographic areas of sickle trait hemoglobin and endemic falciparum malaria suggests a protective advantage of this hemoglobin against malaria.[34]

Pathogenesis

The function of hemoglobin is to carry oxygen in red blood cells to cells throughout the body. When hemoglobin S is oxygenated, it has normal solubility. However, on deoxygenation, hemoglobin S has decreased solubility and polymerizes into rigid, elongated rods that alter the biconcave shape of red blood cells into a sickle form.[16] The polymerization of sickle hemoglobin is dependent on the cell's degree of deoxygenation, the intracellular hemoglobin concentration, and the presence or absence of hemoglobin F.[9] Sickled erythrocytes retain the K^+/Cl^- cotransport function that stabilizes cell hydration. The Gardos efflux channel regulates calcium ion concentration. Increased levels of calcium result in activation of the Gardos channel, modifying K^+ concentrations and resulting in cell dehydration. Increased hemoglobin S concentration promotes polymerization and sickling. Hemoglobin F inhibits polymerization because the glutamine residue at position 87 blocks lateral contact of the sickle fiber.[9] When hypoxemia and the hemoglobin S concentration reach a critical level, polymerization occurs after a variable delay during which a nidus of deoxyhemoglobin S tetramers associate to form a nucleus. When the nucleus reaches a critical size, gelation occurs, resulting in the formation of long, tubelike fibers forming the sickled cell. Sickling occurs if the time to polymerization is less than 1 second or if cells become trapped in the microcirculation. Sickle cells have greater adherence to vascular endothelium, increasing the risk for stasis and sickling.[28] For example, sickle cells have on their surface the integrin complex alpha$_4$-beta$_1$, which binds to fibronectin and vascular cell adhesion molecule-1. Disruption of the membrane phospholipid bilayer, with exposure of phosphatidylserine, increases the risk of thrombo-occlusion.

The change in morphology results in two major clinical features of sickle cell disease: chronic hemolysis with anemia and acute vaso-occlusive crises associated with pain, organ necrosis, and significant morbidity and mortality. Red blood cells that are sickled are irreversibly deformed. They are removed by the reticuloendothelial system at an earlier stage in their life span than are normal red blood cells. Marrow hyperplasia is unable to produce an adequate supply to replace those prematurely removed from the bloodstream. Chronic anemia is the result.

Sickle cell crises occur when acute sickling of red blood cells causes a rise in blood viscosity, decreased blood flow, and vessel obstruction. Vessel blockage leads to ischemia, increased concentrations of deoxygenated hemoglobin, and a progression to sickle crises. Some of the initiating factors that may result in sickle crises include infections, acidosis, fever, and dehydration.[18] These factors play a role as manifestations of systemic infection. The most important factor is the degree of deoxygenation. Sickle cell trait cells sickle at oxygen tensions of about 15 mm Hg, whereas sickle anemia cells sickle at about 40 mm Hg. Low temperatures causing vasoconstriction also may predispose to crises. Acidosis shifts the oxygen dissociation curve to the right, favoring the deoxy conformation of hemoglobin and resulting in polymerization of hemoglobin S. Increases of mean corpuscular hemoglobin concentration secondary to dehydration promote sickling. The vascular endothelium of patients with severe disease has increased propensity to cause red blood cell adherence.[53] The severity of crises varies from patient to patient and may be related to the concentration of hemoglobin S and other hemoglobins in red blood cells. The frequency of painful crises cannot be predicted.

Sickle cell crises occur most commonly in patients with hemoglobin SS. Patients with sickle trait usually do not have sufficient hemoglobin S in their red blood cells to cause sickling. Patients with hemoglobin SC have equal amounts of hemoglobin S and C and very small quantities of hemoglobin F and A_2 in each red blood cell. Hemoglobin SC causes milder diseases and relatively infrequent crises.[35] The degree of anemia is less in hemoglobin SC disease partly because of the red blood cell survival for 29 days versus 17 days for erythrocytes from patients with sickle cell disease.[33] Crises may occur when patients are stressed during surgery or medical emergencies.[5] In addition, patients with hemoglobin SC have a higher frequency of aseptic necrosis of bone.[46]

Thalassemia is a defect in the production of an entire polypeptide chain of hemoglobin. Patients with β-thalassemia produce normal alpha chains but no beta chains in the homozygous state. Patients with thalassemia minor are usually heterozygous for a beta-globin mutation and have either mild or no anemia. Patients with β-thalassemia have abnormalities in the production of the alpha chains and accumulate beta chains. The imbalance in chain production causes an accumulation of unpaired chains in developing erythroblasts, which eventually causes the death of the cell, giving rise to changes in the bone marrow that result in ineffective erythropoiesis.[12] In sickle cell–B-thalassemia, the β-thalassemia defect is combined with sickle trait to produce a disease similar to sickle cell anemia.

The severity of sickle cell–β-thalassemia is related to the amount of normal hemoglobin that is produced.[44] Patients with sickle cell–β^0-thalassemia produce no normal beta chains and have a disease quite similar to sickle cell anemia. Patients with β^+-thalassemia produce hemoglobin A but in reduced amounts. These patients have milder disease. β-Thalassemia is associated with four clinical syndromes corresponding to the concentrations of hemoglobin produced. These syndromes include thalassemia major, thalassemia intermedia, thalassemia trait, and silent carrier. Bone and joint pathology is noted most frequently in patients with thalassemia major and thalassemia intermedia who have not received sufficient blood transfusions. Normalizing hemoglobin levels suppresses ineffective erythropoiesis that results in bone pathology.[26] α-Thalassemia also may be found in patients with hemoglobin SS. The decreased levels of alpha chains results in decreased amounts of sickle hemoglobin per cell and prolonged red blood cell survival. However, the persistence of cells with sickle hemoglobin promotes vaso-occlusive events by blocking microvasculature that might otherwise be able to accommodate more rigid cells at a lower hematocrit. The end result is that patients with α-thalassemia and sickle hemoglobin are less anemic but experience frequent vaso-occlusive episodes, including an increased incidence and severity of aseptic necrosis of bone.[50]

CLINICAL HISTORY

Patients with sickle cell anemia usually present with a painful vaso-occlusive crisis during childhood. The hand-foot syndrome may be the first manifestation of their disease. Diffuse swelling of the hands and feet occurs along with associated warmth and pain. Infarction of bone marrow, which is present in bones of the hands and feet in children, is the cause of this syndrome.[38]

In adults, the most common manifestation of vaso-occlusive crises is back and extremity pain. Back pain may be most severe over the axial skeleton but frequently radiates to the flanks. Muscle spasm may also contribute to the severity of pain in the lumbosacral area. In the extremities, pain is usually asymmetrical and unassociated with soft tissue swelling. The duration of symptoms is 4 to 5 days. The patient may be left with no residual pain and resolution of the crisis. Sickle cell crises may also present as severe abdominal pain, which may mimic an acute surgical abdomen. The presence of bowel sounds and the absence of peritoneal signs in sickle cell crisis help differentiate it from the acute abdomen. The use of pain drawings has been helpful in detecting an amplification of pain symptoms during crises. Patients with pain amplifications have pain drawings with sites inconsistent with expected sickle cell disease pain patterns. These patients may benefit from specific psychological evaluation for improved pain control.[22] Other forms of acute crises include the splenic sequestration, aplastic, and hyperhemolytic.[27] Patients with hemoglobin SC and sickle cell–β^+-thalassemia have milder disease and as adults may present with occasional bone pain along with a history of abdominal or bone pain in childhood.

Tissue infarction secondary to chronic vaso-occlusion is associated with abnormalities in a number of organ systems in patients with sickle cell anemia. In the musculoskeletal system, sickle cell anemia causes bone infarctions, joint effusions, hemarthroses, septic arthritis, and osteomyelitis.[46] In a study of 15 sickle cell patients, Epps described two individuals who had osteomyelitis in the ilium and lumbar vertebrae.[19] These patients were infected with *Salmonella* and *Proteus mirabilis*. Although *Salmonella* has been more frequently associated with bone infection in sickle cell patients, *Staphylococcus aureus* was a more frequent cause of osteomyelitis in the individuals in this study.[10,19] In one study of 57 sickle cell patients, 35 (61%) had osteomyelitis.[7] Five (aged 9 to 27 years) had osteomyelitis of the spine. Of the 35 individuals with osteomyelitis, *Salmonella* caused infection in 25 (71%) and *S. aureus* caused infection in 10 (29%). Propensity to *Salmonella* infections is related to a number of abnormalities, including reduced function of the reticuloendothelial system suppressing clearance of the organisms, abnormal opsonizing and complement functions, and sluggish blood flow allowing pooling.[3]

Cholelithiasis from chronic hemolysis and hepatitis from congestive, viral, or intrahepatic cholestasia are complications in the gastrointestinal system.[11] Pneumonia and pulmonary infarction are frequently the cause of hospitalization of sickle cell patients.[6] Renal function may be impaired by glomerular sclerosis, papillary necrosis, and a renal concentrating defect.[8] Stroke and subarachnoid hemorrhage are potentially life-threatening complications of the central nervous system in sickle cell anemia.[40]

Patients with thalassemia major become symptomatic by the first 2 years of life. The anemia is severe and requires transfusion. Hyperplasia of the bone marrow causes organomegaly, including splenomegaly, and skeletal abnormalities, including osteopenia, which is associated with fractures.[20] Patients with thalassemia may rarely develop neurologic symptoms secondary to spinal cord compression resulting from extramedullary hematopoiesis.[1]

PHYSICAL FINDINGS

Physical findings demonstrate obvious distress when the patient is in sickle crisis. The affected areas (back, extremities) are tender to palpation. The patient is febrile, often with tachycardia, systolic hypertension, and tachypnea. Other physical signs found in painful crises include a tender, rigid abdomen and normal bowel sounds. Abnormal breath sounds and signs of pleural disease are present in the patient with pneumonia or pulmonary infarction.

Patients with thalassemia have hyperpigmented skin. Abdominal examination reveals hepatosplenomegaly. Marrow hyperplasia may cause bone expansion manifested by frontal bossing and maxillary prominence. Patients with vertebral compression fractures have percussion tenderness over the affected vertebrae.

LABORATORY DATA

Laboratory test results demonstrating abnormalities in the hematologic system are universal in patients with sickle cell anemia. Hematocrit values are in a range of 16% to 36%, with hemoglobin of 5 to 12 g/100 mL.[27] Leukocyte counts are usually elevated in the 20,000/mm range, with increased reticulocytosis to levels of 33%. In general, hemoglobin, hematocrit, and reticulocyte counts remain unchanged during a crisis. A leukocytosis and mild thrombocytopenia may occur.[53]

Blood smear shows the presence of sickled cells and erythrocytes with Howell-Jolly bodies. Howell-Jolly bodies are cytoplasmic remnants of nuclear chromatin that are normally removed by the spleen.

The inability to concentrate urine is manifested by a low urine specific gravity. Evidence of persistent hemolysis is reflected in increased serum bilirubin and lactic dehydrogenase concentrations.

Thalassemia also causes anemia. The anemia is hypochromic and microcytic on smear. Nucleated red blood cells, reticulocytes, and "target" cells are seen in increased numbers.

RADIOGRAPHIC EVALUATION

Roentgenograms

The radiographic abnormalities of sickle cell anemia are not unique but are distinctive and are diagnostic when detected in multiple sites.[43] In the spine, marrow hyperplasia causes loss of bone trabeculae and cortical thinning. This results in osteoporosis and coarsening of the remaining trabeculae in the axial skeleton. Vertebral bodies develop a distinctive cuplike depression on the superior and inferior endplates ("fish vertebrae") (Figs. 15-1 and 15-2).[42] Central depression of the vertebral endplate with "squared off" edges may be caused by a growth abnormality of the subchondral bone, and the resulting deformity is referred to as an *H vertebra* (Fig. 15-3).[45] H vertebrae may be seen in other conditions as well (Table 15-1). Irregular sclerosis of the sacroiliac joints secondary to bone infarctions may mimic the radiologic abnormalities of ankylosing spondylitis.[47] Infarction or osteomyelitis may result in bony ridging in the axial skeleton and hip.[17]

β-Thalassemia causes osteopenia of the vertebrae, which is most evident in the vertebral bodies. Reduction of trabeculae, thinning of vertebral endplates, and biconcave deformities are common. H vertebrae occur more rarely in thalassemia major than they do in sickle cell anemia.[13]

Scintigraphy

Bone scintigraphic abnormalities are common in sickle cell patients who experience osseous and bone marrow infarctions. Abnormal uptake also may be noted in patients with osteomyelitis. Expansion of the bone marrow space, in the absence of infarction, may be associated with increased uptake on scintigraphic scan. The differentiation of these abnormalities by scintigraphy may be difficult.[23] The use of gallium-67 and indium-111 leukocyte scans is helpful in differentiating infection from infarction.[2,41]

Magnetic Resonance

Magnetic resonance (MR) may be extremely helpful in differentiating the disease processes that complicate the

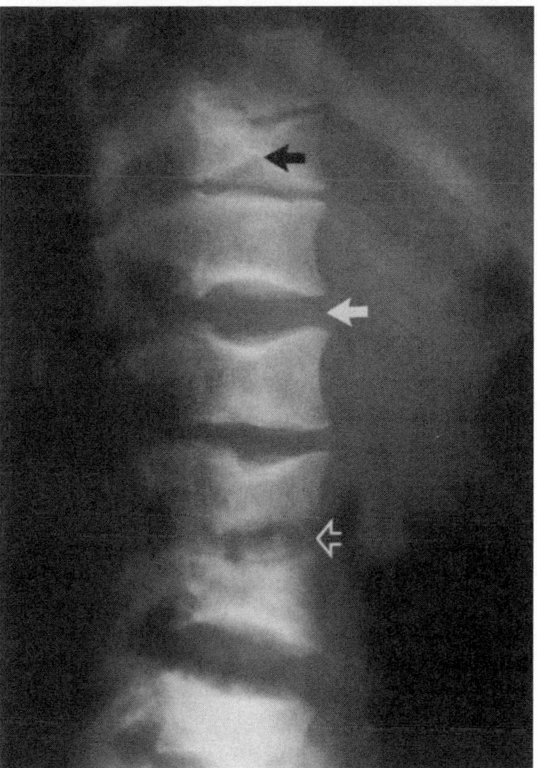

Figure 15-1 Sickle cell anemia. "Fish vertebrae" with widening of the intervertebral disc space *(white arrow)* are associated with sickle cell anemia. Also demonstrated is an H-shaped vertebral body *(black arrow)* and a chronic disc space infection *(open arrow)*. *(Courtesy of Anne Brower, MD.)*

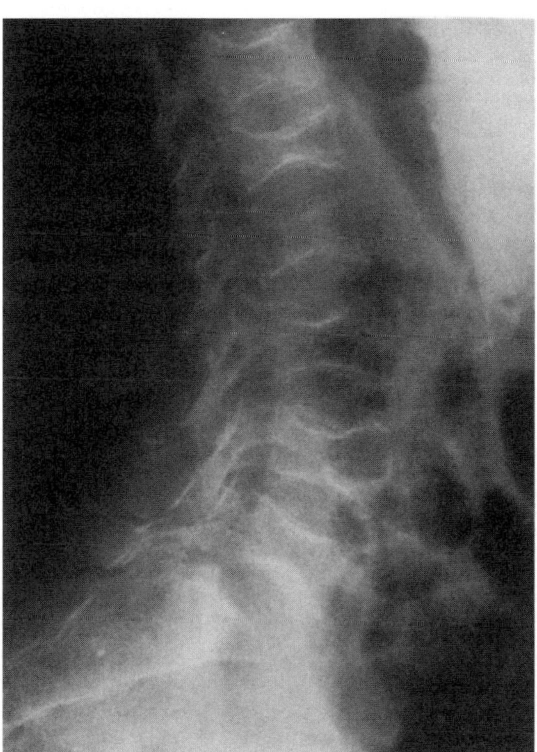

Figure 15-2 Lateral view of the lumbosacral spine in a 30-year-old woman with severe sickle cell anemia manifested by frequent, painful crises. The roentgenogram reveals diffuse osteopenia and multiple "fish vertebrae."

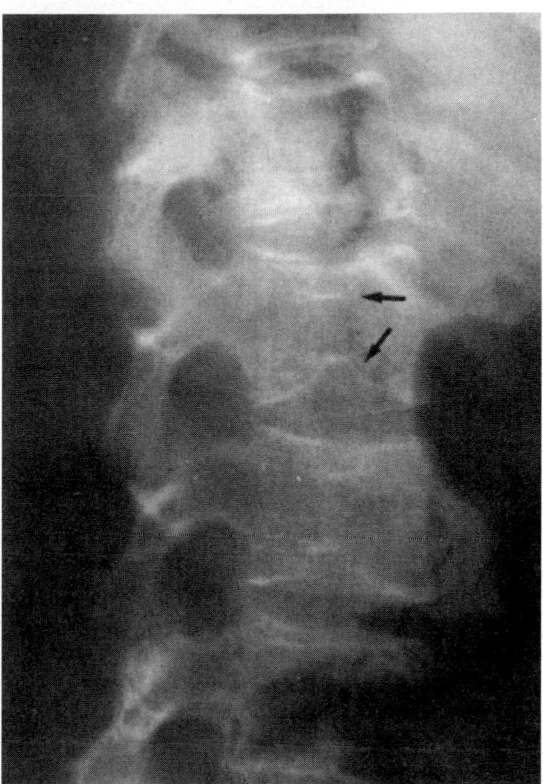

Figure 15-3 Sickle cell anemia resulting in H-shaped vertebral bodies. There is a square indentation of the endplates *(arrows)*. The indented area corresponds to areas of ischemia beneath the cartilaginous endplates, which result in abnormalities of bone growth. *(Courtesy of Anne Brower, MD.)*

course of patients with sickle cell disorders.[52] The expansion of bone marrow is noted by the replacement of fat signal. Osteonecrosis is readily identified in the femoral heads and other bony locations by MR. Acute infarction, characterized by areas of low signal intensity on T1-weighted pulse sequences and high signal intensity on T2-weighted pulse sequences, may be determined in the spine by MR evaluation. Old infarction is associated with low signal with T1 and T2 images. Although the signal intensities of osteomyelitis and acute infarction are similar, the presence of defined cortical involvement, marrow edema beyond the infarcted zone, sinus tracts, and a soft tissue mass suggests the presence of osteomyelitis.[30] MR is also an excellent method to determine the extent of extramedullary hematopoiesis near the vertebral column. Thalassemia patients with neurologic dysfunction can be studied with MR to determine the location and extent of spinal cord or nerve root impingement.[24]

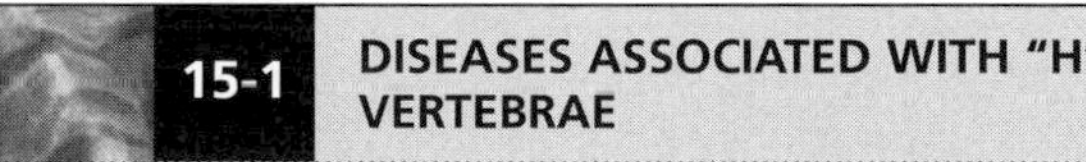

15-1 DISEASES ASSOCIATED WITH "H" VERTEBRAE

Sickle cell anemia
Sickle cell–hemoglobin C disease
Sickle cell–thalassemia disease
Thalassemia
Gaucher's disease
Congenital hereditary spherocytosis
Osteoporosis

DIFFERENTIAL DIAGNOSIS

The diagnosis of sickle cell anemia is suspected in a child or young adult black patient with diffuse back, bone, or abdominal pain with anemia. A blood smear shows sickled cells and red blood cells with Howell-Jolly bodies, which are usually removed by a normally functioning spleen. A "sickle prep" helps confirm the diagnosis. Red blood cells are circulated with 2% sodium metabisulfite for 1 hour, which causes sickling. The exact proportion of normal and abnormal hemoglobins is determined by the separation of the individual hemoglobins on hemoglobin electrophoresis.

The diagnosis of sickle cell anemia is not in doubt when a patient demonstrates the symptoms and signs of crisis and has abnormal hemoglobin on electrophoresis. However, patients with sickle cell anemia are susceptible to infection and must be evaluated for that possibility when they present with a crisis. The spine may be infected occasionally with *Salmonella*, or more commonly with *S. aureus*.[49]

The diagnosis of thalassemia major is usually made when the affected child has severe anemia. Hemoglobin electrophoresis measures increased concentrations of hemoglobin F and A_2, which occur secondary to the inadequate amounts of hemoglobin A.

TREATMENT

Medical management of sickle cell crises includes hydration, analgesics for pain, and antibiotic therapy in crises when there is an ongoing infection. Narcotic therapy for sickle cell patients can be a difficult problem for the treating physician. The patient complains of pain but may have no objective physical signs of an ongoing crisis. Ballas has reviewed some of the behavioral patterns used by patients during a vaso-occlusive crisis.[4] A better understanding of the patient's fears, a knowledge of the pharmacokinetics of the narcotic analgesics, and trust between the patient and physician are important in optimizing medical care for these individuals. Nonsteroidal anti-inflammatory drugs may be useful adjuncts to the narcotics for individuals with musculoskeletal pain. The use of alkali to reverse acidosis does not seem to be effective during acute crises. Oxygen is not needed if the patient has no ventilatory hypoxia. Oxygen therapy may be detrimental owing to a re-emergence of irreversible sickled cells appearing with oxygen cessation.[10] Standard red blood cell transfusions and exchange transfusions are reserved for patients with severe complications of sickle cell anemia such as strokes. Transfusions also may be useful preoperatively for patients who are undergoing surgery.

Hydroxyurea increases fetal hemoglobin synthesis. Hydroxyurea, at a starting dose of 15 mg/kg/day, decreases the number of painful crises, hospital admissions, and the need for transfusions.[14] This therapy has the potential to reduce mortality by 40% over an 8-year period.[51] Hydroxyurea is also a cost-effective method of reducing the frequency of crises with a saving of $5210 on an annualized basis.[31] Nitric oxide inhalation at 80 parts per million in air for 45 minutes shifts the hemoglobin dissociation curve, resulting in a decreased affinity of normal and sickle hemoglobin for oxygen. This reduction in oxygen partial pressure releases nitric oxide at a vascular level causing vasodilation, resulting in decreased pooling in the microcirculation. The effect remains for 1 hour after inhalation.[21] Nitric oxide may also decrease vascular adhesion by downregulating vascular adhesion molecule-1.[48] Another factor that may decrease endothelial adhesion is poloxamer 188. This material works as a surfactant, reducing cell adhesion to endothelium. In a study of 225 patients, infusion of purified poloxamer 188, 100 mg/kg for 1 hour, followed by 30 mg/kg per hour for 47 hours, resulted in a modest reduction of the duration of painful crises.[36] Allogeneic bone marrow transplantation can result in a cure or substitution of sickle trait for sickle cell anemia. In a study of 22 patients, 15 patients had a cure, although 2 died and 5 had graft failure.[54]

Animal models exist using viral vectors that have reversed the point mutation in hemoglobin synthesis resulting in correction of the production of red blood cells.[37] This is a prime example of how gene therapy can reverse a life-threatening human disease.

Thalassemia is treated with transfusions maintaining a hemoglobin level of 12 g/100 mL. Iron overload is limited as much as possible with deferoxamine. Occasionally, splenectomy is required to control hypersplenism. In patients with greater risk for infection, including pneumonia and osteomyelitis, pneumococcal vaccine is indicated. Bone marrow transplantation using HLA-matched sibling donors has a potential cure rate of 54% to 90%.[29]

PROGNOSIS

The course of sickle cell anemia is difficult to predict. Some patients with the disease have occasional crises, once every year or two, and have little in the way of organ dysfunction from their disease. On the other end of the spectrum are patients who are in almost continuous crises and are frequently hospitalized. These patients commonly show evidence of generalized disease affecting many organ systems. Patients must avoid situations that predispose to sickle crisis (dehydration) and receive comprehensive medical care. Immunization with pneumococcal vaccine, good nutrition, vitamins, and psychological support have improved their long-term outlook. However, until the time comes when the genetic defect of sickle hemoglobin is corrected, patients with sickle cell anemia will be at risk for the complications of their disease and can expect a decreased work potential as well as a shortened life span.

A study of 4000 patients with sickle cell anemia has provided updated information on the longevity of individuals with this illness. The median age of death is 42 years for men and 48 years for women. This life expectancy is 25 years less than that of the general black American population. Poor outcome was associated with a white blood cell count higher than 15,000/mm^3, a low hemoglobin F level, and organ involvement manifested by neurologic and renal diseases and acute chest syndrome.[39]

Thalassemia major is also a cause of shortened life span. Either the results of the chronic anemia or the complications of chronic transfusion therapy are detrimental. As with sickle cell anemia, correction of the underlying genetic defect is the most appropriate therapy for this illness.

References

Hemoglobinopathies

1. Abbassioun K, Amir-Jamshidi A: Curable paraplegia due to extradural hematopoietic tissue in thalassemia. Neurosurgery 11:804, 1982.
2. Amundsen TR, Siegel MF, Siegel BA: Osteomyelitis and infarction in sickle cell hemoglobinopathies: Differentiation by combined technetium and gallium scintigraphy. Radiology 153:807, 1984.
3. Anand A, Glatt AE: *Salmonella* osteomyelitis and arthritis in sickle cell disease. Semin Arthritis Rheum 24:211-221, 1994.
4. Ballas SK: Treatment of pain in adults with sickle cell disease. Am J Hematol 34:49, 1990.
5. Bannerman RM, Serjeant B, Seakins M, et al: Determinants of hemoglobin level in sickle cell–hemoglobin C disease. Br J Haematol 43:39, 1979.
6. Barret-Connor E: Pneumonia and pulmonary infarction in sickle cell anemia. JAMA 224:997, 1973.
7. Bennett OM, Namnyak SS: Bone and joint manifestations of sickle cell anaemia. J Bone Joint Surg Br 72-B:494-499, 1990.
8. Buckalew VM Jr, Someren A: Renal manifestations of sickle cell disease. Arch Intern Med 133:660, 1974.
9. Bunn HF: Pathogenesis and treatment of sickle cell disease. N Engl J Med 337:762-769, 1997.
10. Bunn HF, Forget BG (eds): Hemoglobin: Molecular, Genetic, and Clinical Aspects. Philadelphia, WB Saunders, 1986.
11. Cameron JL, Maddrey WC, Zuidema GD: Biliary tract disease in sickle cell anemia: Surgical considerations. Ann Surg 174:702, 1971.
12. Canale V: Beta-thalassemia: A clinical review. Pediatr Annu 3:6, 1974.
13. Cassady JR, Berdon WE, Baker DH: The "typical" spine changes of sickle cell anemia in a patient with thalassemia major (Cooley's anemia). Radiology 89:1065, 1967.
14. Charache S, Terrin ML, Moore RD, et al: Effect of hydroxyurea on the frequency of painful crises in sickle cell anemia. N Engl J Med 332:1317, 1995.
15. Cooley TB, Lee P: A series of cases of splenomegaly in children with anemia and peculiar bone changes. Trans Am Pediatr Soc 37:29, 1925.
16. Dean J, Schechter AN: Sickle cell anemia: Molecular and cellular bases of therapeutic approaches. I, II, III. N Engl J Med 299:752, 804, 863, 1978.
17. Diggs LW: Bone and joint lesions in sickle cell disease. Clin Orthop 52:119, 1967.
18. Diggs LW: Sickle cell crises. Am J Clin Pathol 44:1, 1965.
19. Epps Ch, Bryant DD III, Coles MJM, Castro O: Osteomyelitis in patients who have sickle cell disease. J Bone Joint Surg Am 73-A:1281, 1991.
20. Finsterbush A, Farber I, Mogle P, Goldfarb A: Fracture patterns in thalassemia. Clin Orthop 192:132, 1985.
21. Gladwin MT, Schecthter AN, Shelhamer JH, et al: The acute chest syndrome in sickle cell disease: Possible role of nitric oxide in its pathophysiology and treatment. Am J Respir Crit Care Med 159:1368-1376, 1999.
22. Gil KM, Phillips G, Abrams MR, Williams DA: Pain drawings and sickle cell disease pain. Clin J Pain 6:105, 1990.
23. Glaser AM, Chen DCP, Siegel ME, et al: An unusual scintigraphic pattern in sickle cell patients. Eur J Nucl Med 15:357, 1989.
24. Hassoun H, Lawn-Tsao L, Langevin R Jr, et al: Spinal cord compression secondary to extramedullary hematopoiesis: A noninvasive management based on MRI. Am J Hematol 37:201, 1991.
25. Herrick JB: Peculiar elongated and sickle-shaped red blood corpuscles in a case of severe anemia. Arch Intern Med 6:517, 1910.
26. Johanson NA: Musculoskeletal problems in hemoglobinopathy. Orthop Clin North Am 21:191, 1990.
27. Karayalcin G, Rosner F, Kim KY, et al: Sickle cell anemia: Clinical manifestations in 100 patients and review of the literature. Am J Med Sci 269:51, 1975.
28. Kasschau MR, Barabino GA, Bridges KR, et al: Adhesion of sickle neutrophils and erythrocytes to fibronectin. Blood 87:771-780, 1996.
29. Lucarelli G, Galimberti M, Giardini C, et al: Bone marrow transplantation in thalassemia. Ann N Y Acad Sci 850:270, 1998.
30. Modic MT, Pflanze W, Fieglin DH, Belhobek G: Magnetic resonance imaging of musculoskeletal infections. Radiol Clin North Am 24:247, 1986.
31. Moore RD, Charache S, Terrin ML, et al: Cost-effectiveness of hydroxyurea in sickle cell disease. Am J Hematol 64:26-31, 2000.
32. Motulsky AG: Frequency of sickling disorders in U. S. blacks. N Engl J Med 288:31, 1973.
33. Nagel RL, Lawrence C: The distinct pathobiology of sickle cell–hemoglobin C disease: Therapeutic implications. Hematol Oncol Clin North Am 5:433, 1991.
34. Nagel RL, Ranney HM: Genetic epidemiology of structural mutations of the beta-globin gene. Semin Hematol 27:342, 1990.
35. Neel JV, Kaplan E, Zuelzer WW: Further studies on hemoglobin C. I. A description of three additional families segregating for hemoglobin C and sickle cell hemoglobin. Blood 8:724, 1953.
36. Orringer EP, Casella JF, Ataga KI, et al: Purified poloxamer 188 for treatment of acute vaso-occlusive crisis of sickle cell disease. JAMA 286:2099-2106, 2001.
37. Pawliuk R, Westerman KA, Fabry ME: Correction of sickle cell disease in transgenic mouse models by gene therapy. Science 294:2368-2371, 2001.
38. Pearson HA, Diamond LK: The critically ill child: Sickle cell disease crises and their management. Pediatrics 48:629, 1971.
39. Platt OS, Brambilla DJ, Rosse WF, et al: Mortality in sickle cell disease: Life expectancy and risk factors for early death. N Engl J Med 330:1639, 1994.
40. Powars D, Wilson B, Imbus C, et al: The natural history of stroke in sickle cell disease. Am J Med 65:461, 1978.
41. Rao VM, Sebes JI, Steiner RM, Ballas SK: Noninvasive diagnostic imaging in hemoglobinopathies. Hematol Oncol Clin North Am 5:517, 1991.
42. Reynolds J: A re-evaluation of the "fish vertebra" sign in sickle cell hemoglobinopathy. AJR Am J Roentgenol 97:693, 1966.
43. Reynolds J: Radiologic manifestations of sickle cell hemoglobinopathy. JAMA 238:247, 1977.
44. Reynolds J, Pritchard JA, Ludders D, Mason RA: Roentgenographic and clinical appraisal of sickle cell beta-thalassemia. AJR Am J Roentgenol 118:378, 1973.
45. Rohifing BM: Vertebral end-plate depression: Report of two patients with hemoglobinopathy. AJR Am J Roentgenol 128:599, 1973.
46. Schumacher HR: Rheumatological manifestations of sickle cell disease and other hereditary haemoglobinopathies. Clin Rheum Dis 1:37, 1975.
47. Schumacher HR, Andrews R, McLaughlin G: Arthropathy in sickle cell disease. Ann Intern Med 78:203, 1978.
48. Space SL, Lane PA, Pickell CK, et al: Nitric oxide attenuates normal and sickle red blood cell adherence to pulmonary endothelium. Am J Hematol 63:200, 2000.
49. Specht CE: Hemoglobinopathic *Salmonella* osteomyelitis: Orthopedic aspects. Clin Orthop 79:110, 1971.
50. Steinberg MH: The interactions of alpha-thalassemia with hemoglobinopathies. Hematol Oncol Clin North Am 5:453, 1991.
51. Steinberg MH, Barton F, Castro O, et al: Hydroxyurea is associated with reduced mortality in adults with sickle cell anemia [Abstract]. J Am Soc Hematol 96:485a, 2000.
52. Steiner RM, Mitchell DG, Rao VM, et al: Magnetic resonance imaging of bone marrow: Diagnostic value in diffuse hematologic disorders. Magn Reson Q 6:17, 1990.
53. Steingart R: Management of patients with sickle cell disease. Med Clin North Am 76:669, 1992.
54. Walters MC, Patience M, Leisenring W, et al: Bone marrow transplantation for sickle cell disease. N Engl J Med 335:369, 1996.

MYELOFIBROSIS

Capsule Summary

	Low Back	Neck
Frequency of spinal pain	Uncommon	Not applicable (NA)
Location of spinal pain	Lumbar spine	NA
Quality of spinal pain	Aching, or sharp	NA
Symptoms and signs	Weakness, weight loss, bone pain	NA
Laboratory findings	Anemia, leukoerythroblastic smear	NA
Radiographic findings	Osteosclerosis on plain roentgenograms	NA
Treatment	Transfusions, chemotherapy, bone marrow transplant	NA

PREVALENCE AND PATHOGENESIS

Myelofibrosis is a disease of the hematopoietic system characterized by fibrosis of bone marrow and myeloid metaplasia, or the production of blood cells in non–marrow-containing organs such as the liver and spleen. The primary pathogenetic mechanism is a clonal stem cell disorder that leads to ineffective erythropoiesis, dysplastic megakaryocyte hyperplasia, and an increase in the ratio of immature granulocytes to total granulocytes.[41] The disease is characterized by anemia, organomegaly, osteosclerosis, and extramedullary hematopoiesis. Bone and joint pain in the axial and peripheral skeleton is associated with myeloid metaplasia. Patients may develop localized masses of hematopoietic tissue near the spinal cord that can cause neurologic symptoms of weakness, hyperreflexia, and sensory deficit.

Epidemiology

Myelofibrosis is a relatively uncommon disorder that appears in patients during the sixth decade of life.[34] Approximately 22% of patients are 56 years of age or younger, whereas 11% are younger than 46 years.[4] Population-based epidemiologic studies estimate the incidence of agnogenic myeloid metaplasia at between 0.5 and 1.5 per 100,000 population.[24,25] Both sexes are equally afflicted.

Pathogenesis

The pathogenesis of this disorder is unknown. Although initially thought to be a compensatory mechanism for bone marrow failure, myelofibrosis is part of the spectrum of primary myeloproliferative disorders that affect blood stem cells, including erythrocytes, granulocytes, and platelets.[1] The marrow fibrosis that is characteristic of the illness is a secondary phenomenon. Marrow fibroblasts are functionally normal, marrow-derived fibroblasts and are polyclonal in origin. The disease increases the number of stromal cells, extracellular matrix proteins, increased angiogenesis, and osteosclerosis. Cytokines (platelet-derived growth factor, basic fibroblast growth factor, transforming growth factor-beta, vascular endothelial growth factor, tumor necrosis factor-alpha) produced by the cellular components of the clonal proliferation result in the manifestations of the disorder.[8,22,27] In the past the disease has been considered a primary bone disease, a reactive response to marrow necrosis, a leukemic variant, or a myeloproliferative disorder. The term *myeloproliferative disorder* was proposed by Dameshek, who noticed a spectrum of illnesses (polycythemia rubra vera, chronic myelocytic leukemia, essential thrombocythemia, and agnogenic myeloid metaplasia [myelofibrosis]) that were associated with marked marrow proliferation that evolved into an illness progressing to a blast crisis similar to acute myeloblastic leukemia.[9] The unity of these disorders under the concept of myeloproliferation has been challenged.[46] In the light of these proposed etiologies of myelofibrosis, it should not be surprising to find a number of terms used in the description of this illness. Starting in the 1870s, the disease has been known as *leukocythemia*, *agnogenic myeloid metaplasia*, *aleukemic myelosis*, *leukoerythroblastic anemia*, *osteosclerosis*, *myelosclerosis*, and *myelofibrosis*.[21,47]

Myelofibrosis is probably mediated through a number of different pathologic processes.[37] It has been associated with toxin exposure to benzol, paint thinners, and thorium dioxide. Radiation exposure has been associated with myelofibrosis in survivors of the Hiroshima atomic bomb explosion. A number of karyotypic abnormalities (in ~ 60% of patients), including loss of the Y chromosome, trisomy 8, and trisomy 1q, deletion of the long arm of chromosome 13 or 20, along with familial predisposition, have been reported.[41] The primary abnormality of myelofibrosis seems to reside in the bone marrow stem cells and not the bone marrow fibroblasts.[26] All the bone marrow stem cells contain the same glucose-6-phosphate dehydrogenase isoenzymes that are separate from the isoenzyme in the fibroblasts. This suggests that the bone marrow fibrosis is mediated by nonmalignant bone marrow fibroblasts in response to a malignant process.

CLINICAL HISTORY

Patients with myelofibrosis present with symptoms secondary to anemia (weakness, fatigue, weight loss) and abdominal pain associated with fullness or heaviness. The onset of symptoms is insidious, with a usual delay of 1 to 2 years before the diagnosis is made.[2] Patients may also experience a gradual progressive weight loss, acute gouty arthritis, nephrolithiasis, jaundice, peripheral edema, and lymphadenopathy. As many as 13% of patients may have an episode of acute gout before the diagnosis of myelofibrosis is recognized.[14] Systemic lupus erythematosus has been associated with rare patients with steroid-responsive autoimmune myelofibrosis.[28] Bone pain in the extremities and axial skeleton may be mild to severe.[11] Neurologic symptoms of lower extremity weakness and sensory loss may be present with spinal cord compression secondary to extramedullary erythropoiesis.[7]

PHYSICAL EXAMINATION

Physical examination reveals a patient who appears chronically ill with pallor. Abdominal examination is remarkable with a markedly enlarged spleen. Hepatomegaly and ascites occur less frequently. Portal hypertension with variceal bleeding occurs in 7% of patients.[36] Bones affected in the lumbar spine by myelofibrosis may be tender to palpation. Examination of the extremities demonstrates edema and purpura. Hyperreflexia and Babinski's sign are seen in the patients with spinal cord compression.

LABORATORY DATA

Myelofibrosis is associated with a number of hematologic abnormalities. Anemia is found in the vast majority of patients and is initially normochromic but becomes hypochromic with progression of the illness. Blood smears reveal an abnormal configuration of cells, polychromatic cells (reticulocytes), and increased numbers of white blood cells with both mature and immature forms. This blood smear is characteristic of leukoerythroblastic anemia.[43] Platelets may be present in high, normal, or low numbers. The bleeding time may be prolonged even with normal numbers of platelets, indicating a platelet functional disorder. The neutrophil alkaline phosphatase score is high.

Bone marrow in myelofibrosis is unobtainable by needle aspiration because of the fibrosis and hypocellularity. Bone marrow biopsy, which protects the positional integrity of bone and marrow elements, shows fibrosis, increased numbers of megakaryocytes, and osteosclerosis.[31] Cytogenic studies of bone marrow are helpful in excluding chronic myeloid leukemia. Some of the chromosome abnormalities include the deletion of the long arm of chromosome 13, trisomy 8, and a deletion of the long arm of chromosome 20.[41]

Other laboratory features include an elevated serum or urinary uric acid concentration in most patients with myelofibrosis.[10] Secondary gout, with tophi and uric acid stones, occurs in an occasional patient.[49] An elevation in lactate dehydrogenase, a decrease in albumin, or prolongation in prothrombin time is noted in most patients.[14] A number of autoimmune factors are abnormal in patients with myelofibrosis, including complement components indicative of activation, presence of excess immune complexes, elevated antinuclear antibodies, rheumatoid factor, positive direct Coombs' test, lupus anticoagulant, polyclonal increases in serum immunoglobulins, and platelet-associated IgG and IgM.[14,37]

The fibroblasts in the bone marrow produce a number of collagens, including I, III, IV, and V with a predominance of III. The procollagen III molecule is cleaved and the amino-terminal fragments are released into the serum. The serum level of fragments has been associated with the degree of marrow fibrosis associated with primary and secondary myelofibrosis.[17] Marrow fibrosis has also been associated with type IV collagen metabolites.[16] Hyaluronan is a polysaccharide that is a component of ground substance of connective tissues. This material is detected by a radioimmunoassay and has been found elevated in a variety of fibrosing conditions.[15] Although a differentiation between normal subjects and individuals with myelofibrosis is not possible, serial samples of hyaluronan follow the response of patients to therapy for myelofibrosis.

RADIOGRAPHIC FINDINGS

Roentgenograms

The radiologic findings of myelofibrosis are those of osteosclerosis in the axial skeleton and proximal long bones.[29] Osteosclerosis is observed in 40% to 50% of patients.[18] In vertebral bodies, the sclerosis is increased at the superior and inferior endplates. The sclerosis may be uniformly dense or disrupted by small areas of radiolucency (Fig. 15-4). In the spine, increased radiodensity or

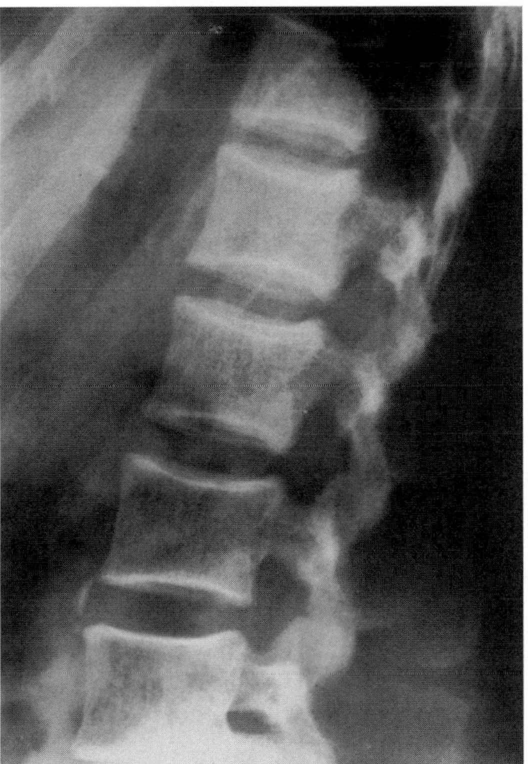

Figure 15-4 Myelofibrosis. Lateral view of the lumbar spine showing diffuse increased density of bone associated with a thickened trabecular pattern. *(Courtesy of Anne Brower, MD.)*

condensation of bone at the superior and inferior margins of the vertebral body may result in a "sandwich vertebrae."[30] Other bones that may show sclerosis include the pelvis, skull, ribs, proximal femur, and humerus. Long bones may demonstrate alterations associated with hypertrophic osteoarthropathy and periostitis.[23]

Magnetic Resonance

MR of patients with myelofibrosis can identify the extent of bone marrow replacement.[18] Through the use of spin-echo images, the degree of replacement of normal marrow with fat, fibrosis, and hemosiderosis secondary to transfusions is possible.[39] MR is able to differentiate myelofibrosis from essential thrombocythemia. In essential thrombocythemia, the marrow fat is preserved and MR signals in the vertebrae and femur are normal. In myelofibrosis, the fat is replaced with hematopoietic cells, reducing the fat signal seen on MR scans.[33] Reduced MR signal is associated with the location and extent of extramedullary hematopoiesis that causes spinal cord compression.[20] Paravertebral soft tissue masses may be identified in patients with spinal cord compression and neurologic abnormalities.[6,7] Transcortical leakage of bone marrow associated with vertebral fractures may be a source of bone marrow stem cells resulting in extramedullary hematopoiesis.[13]

DIFFERENTIAL DIAGNOSIS

The diagnosis of myelofibrosis may be suspected in the patient with anemia, splenomegaly, and osteosclerosis and can be confirmed by identifying the characteristic abnormalities on bone marrow biopsy. However, splenomegaly and osteosclerosis are not found exclusively in myelofibrosis.

Disseminated carcinoma that involves the bone marrow may produce a leukoerythroblastic smear. It may also cause sclerosis of bone, particularly if the primary lesion is in the prostate.

Patients with chronic myelogenous leukemia (CML) have splenomegaly and abnormal blood smears. These patients also may present with back pain.[19] Leukocyte counts are higher with CML, and there is an increased proportion of immature cells. CML rarely produces a leukoerythroblastic smear. The Philadelphia chromosome is positive in 90% of patients with CML. CML is associated with a low neutrophil alkaline phosphatase score. Radiographic abnormalities are uncommon.[5] Other neoplastic disorders associated with myelophthisis with or without bone marrow fibrosis include lymphoma, Hodgkin's disease, and plasma cell dyscrasias.[41]

The differential diagnosis of osteosclerosis is quite broad. These entities include osteoblastic metastases, mastocytosis, lymphomas, Paget's disease, fluorosis, renal osteodystrophy, and axial osteomalacia. Careful review of blood tests and bone biopsy material should differentiate these entities from myelofibrosis (Table 15-2).[30]

A variety of disorders may cause spinal cord compression associated with extramedullary hematopoiesis. These disorders are listed in Table 15-3.[13]

TREATMENT

The treatment of myelofibrosis is mostly supportive. Anemia is helped by transfusions and, occasionally, by androgen therapy (oral oxymetholone, 150 mg/day). The anemia is unresponsive to epoetin therapy.[32] Patients with bone pain or spinal cord compression may benefit from local radiation therapy.[20] Hydroxyurea is the drug of choice for control of organomegaly, thrombocytosis, and leukocytosis.[26] The dose of hydroxyurea ranges from 10 to 30 mg/kg/day with a goal of a white blood cell level of 2500 cells/mm^3 or greater. Individuals with advanced disease and lower cell counts may be controlled with every-other-day hydroxyurea. Hydroxyurea has been implicated as a leukemogenic agent. Therefore, anagrelide is useful to decrease elevated platelet counts in individuals with thrombocythemia. Anagrelide is given 1 mg twice daily. The maximum daily dose is 10 mg divided over a day.[48] Chemotherapy with low doses of busulfan (2 to 4 mg/day) may decrease spleen size but may cause pancytopenia. Alkylating agents may cause a leukemic transformation and are not a first-choice therapy. Splenectomy is not always helpful in improving blood counts, and it may be associated with excessive bleeding postoperatively. This may be increased by a history of splenic irradiation. Surgical mortality may be as high as 31%.[42]

Debate remains concerning the potential risk of splenectomy initiating a leukemic transformation.[41] Hyperuricemia may be controlled with allopurinol. Patients who develop aggressive disease with increasing organomegaly, peripheral blast cells, anemia, and thrombocytopenia are generally resistant to therapeutic intervention.[45] Bone marrow transplantation has been used with patients with acute or secondary myelofibrosis. Young individuals with two or more of the following—(1) decreased hemoglobin (<10 g/dL), (2) constitutional symptoms, (3) isolated cytogenetic abnormality, or (4) blasts higher than 1%—are candidates for bone marrow transplant early in the course of the illness.[3] The degree of marrow fibrosis does not appear to limit the efficiency of engraftment.[37,38] Allogeneic hematopoietic stem cell transplantation engraftment may be successful in 90% of patients.[12] Complete hematologic remission may occur in 70% of patients, with a regression of fibrosis in 40%.

PROGNOSIS

Occasionally, the course of myelofibrosis is benign, with a survival greater than 5 years after diagnosis.[34] Individuals younger than 56 years of age, with no anemia or constitutional symptoms, may survive as long as 15 years.[3] Bone marrow fibrosis may be reversed through the use of alkylating agents, ^{32}P therapy, or splenectomy.[40] In the usual circumstance, the disease is progressive, with a survival of only 2 to 3 years after diagnosis.[2] Many patients die from infections or thromboembolic events.[14] Bad prognostic factors include advanced age, a short period between the first symptoms and diagnosis, anemia, significant leukocytosis (10,000 to 30,000 mm^3), and the presence of immature granulocyte precursors in the peripheral blood.[44]

15-2 DIFFERENTIAL DIAGNOSIS OF OSTEOSCLEROSIS*

	Skeletal Metastasis	**Mastocytosis**	**Myelofibrosis**	**Lymphomas**	**Paget's disease**	**Fluorosis**	**Renal Osteodystrophy**	**Axial Osteomalacia**
Distribution	Axial > appendicular	Axial > appendicular	Axial > appendicular	Axial > appendicular	Axial > appendicular	Axial > appendicular	Axial > appendicular	Axial
Diffuse sclerosis	+	+	+	+	+	+	+	+
Focal sclerosis	+	+	–	+	+	–	–	–
Osteopenia or bone lysis	+	+	+	+	+	–	+	–
Bony enlargement	–	–	–	–	+	–	–	–
Osteophytosis, ligament ossification	–	–	–	–	–	+	–	–
Splenomegaly	–	+	+	+	–	–	–	–

* +, Common; –, uncommon or rare.

From Resnick D, Niwayama G (eds): Diagnosis of Bone and Joint Disorders, 2nd ed. Philadelphia, WB Saunders, 1988, p 2486.

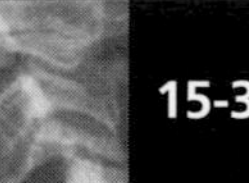

15-3 SPINAL CORD COMPRESSION ASSOCIATED WITH EXTRAMEDULLARY HEMATOPOIESIS

Myelofibrosis
Polycythemia rubra vera
Thalassemia
Hemoglobin S
Hemoglobin E
Pyruvate kinase deficiency
Sideroblastic anemia
Transposition of the great vessels
Paget's disease

Rarely, patients may have an acute myelofibrosis that is highly aggressive, with death occurring within a year. This is heralded by fever, weight loss, and increased anemia and thrombocytopenia in the absence of organomegaly and a hypercellular marrow with bone marrow biopsy. Approximately 20% of patients with myelofibrosis develop acute myelogenous leukemia and usually are resistant to therapeutic intervention.[35]

References

Myelofibrosis

1. Adamson JW, Fialkow PJ: The pathogenesis of myeloproliferative syndromes. Br J Haematol 38:229, 1978.
2. Bouruncle BA, Doan CA: Myelofibrosis: Clinical, hematologic, and pathologic study of 110 patients. Am J Med Sci 243:697, 1962.
3. Cervantes F, Barosi G, Demory JL, et al: Myelofibrosis with myeloid metaplasia in young individuals: Disease characteristics, prognostic factors, and identification of risk groups. Br J Haematol 102:684-690, 1998.
4. Cervantes F, Pereira A, Esteve J, et al: Identification of "short-lived" and long-lived" patients at presentation of idiopathic myelofibrosis. Br J Haematol 97:635-640, 1997.
5. Chabner BA, Haskell CM, Canellos GP: Destructive bone lesions in chronic granulocytic leukemia. Medicine 48:401, 1969.
6. Close AS, Taira Y, Cleveland DA: Spinal cord compression due to extramedullary hematopoiesis. Ann Intern Med 48:421, 1958.
7. Cromwell LD, Kerber C: Spinal cord compression by extramedullary hematopoiesis in agnogenic myeloid metaplasia. Radiology 128:118, 1978.
8. Dalley A, Smith JM, Reilly JT, et al: Investigation of calmodulin and basic fibroblast factor (bFGF) in idiopathic myelofibrosis: Evidence for a role of extracellular calmodulin in fibroblast proliferation. Br J Haematol 93:856-862, 1996.
9. Dameshek W: Some speculations on myeloproliferative syndromes. Blood 6:372, 1951.
10. Gilbert HS: The spectrum of myeloproliferative disorders. Med Clin North Am 57:355, 1973.
11. Glew RH, Haese WH, McIntyre PA: Myeloid metaplasia with myelofibrosis: The clinical spectrum of extramedullary hematopoiesis and tumor formation. Johns Hopkins Med J 132:253, 1973.
12. Guardiola P, Anderson JE, Bandini G, et al: Allogeneic stem cell transplantation for agnogenic myeloid metaplasia: A European Group for Blood and Marrow Transplantation, Societe Francaise de Greffe de Moelle, Gruppo Italiano per il Trapianto Midollo Osseo, and Fred Hutchinson Cancer Research Center collaborative study. Blood 93:2381-2388, 1999.
13. Haran M, Ni S: Recurrent reversible paraplegia. Lancet 357:1092, 2001.
14. Hasselbalch H: Idiopathic myelofibrosis: A clinical study of 80 patients. Am J Hematol 34:291, 1990.
15. Hasselbalch H, Junker P, Lisse I, et al: Circulating hyaluronan in the myelofibrosis/osteomyelosclerosis syndrome and other myeloproliferative disorders. Am J Hematol 36:1, 1991.
16. Hasselbalch H, Junker P, Lisse I, et al: Serum markers for type IV collagen and type III procollagen in the myelofibrosis-osteomyelosclerosis syndrome and other chronic myeloproliferative disorders. Am J Hematol 23:101, 1986.
17. Hochweiss S, Fruchtman S, Hahn EG, et al: Increased serum procollagen III amino-terminal peptide in myelofibrosis. Am J Hematol 15:343, 1983.
18. Kaplan KR, Mitchell DG, Steiner RM, et al: Polycythemia vera and myelofibrosis: Correlation of MR imaging, clinical, and laboratory findings. Radiology 183:331, 1992.
19. Klier I, Santo M: Low back pain as a presenting symptom of chronic granulocytic leukemia. Orthop Rev 11:111, 1982.
20. Klippel ND, Dehou MF, Bourgain C, et al: Progressive paraparesis due to thoracic extramedullary hematopoiesis in myelofibrosis. J Neurosurg 79:125, 1993.
21. Leigh TF, Corley CC Jr, Huguley CM Jr, Rogers JV Jr: Myelofibrosis: The general and radiologic findings in 25 proven cases. AJR Am J Roentgenol 82:183, 1959.
22. Martyre MC, Le Bousse-Kerdiles MC, Romquin N, et al: Elevated levels of basic fibroblast growth factor in megakaryocytes and platelets from patients with idiopathic myelofibrosis. Br J Haematol 97:441-448, 1997.
23. Mason BA, Kressel BR, Cashdollar MR, et al: Periostitis associated with myelofibrosis. Cancer 43:1568-1571, 1979.
24. McNally RJ, Rowland D, Roman E, et al: Age and sex distributions of hematological malignancies in the UK. Hematol Oncol 15:173-189, 1997.
25. Mesa RA, Silverstein MN, Jacobsen SJ, et al: Population-based incidence and survival figures in essential thrombocythemia and agnogenic myeloid metaplasia: An Olmstead County study, 1976-1995. Am J Hematol 61:10-15, 1999.
26. Mintzer D, Bagg A: Clinical syndromes of transformation in clonal hematologic disorders. Am J Med 111:480-488, 2001.
27. Mohle R, Green D, Moore MA, et al: Constitutive production and thrombin-induced release of vascular endothelial growth factor by human megakaryocytes and platelets. Proc Natl Acad Sci U S A 94:663-668, 1997.
28. Paquette R, Meshkinpour A, Rosen PJ: Autoimmune myelofibrosis: A steroid-responsive cause of bone marrow fibrosis associated with systemic lupus erythematosus. Medicine 73:145-152, 1994.
29. Pettigrew JD, Ward HP: Correlation of radiologic, histologic, and clinical findings in agnogenic myeloid metaplasia. Radiology 93:541, 1969.
30. Resnick D, Niwayama G (eds): Diagnosis of Bone and Joint Disorders. Philadelphia, WB Saunders, 1981, p 2011.
31. Roberts BE, Miles DW, Woods CG: Polycythaemia vera and myelosclerosis: A bone marrow study. Br J Haematol 16:75, 1969.
32. Rodriguez JN, Martino ML, Dieguez JC, et al: rHuEpo for the treatment of anemia in myelofibrosis with myeloid metaplasia: Experience in six patients and meta-analytical approach. Haematologica 83:616-621, 1998.
33. Rozman C, Cervantes F, Rozman M, et al: Magnetic resonance imaging in myelofibrosis and essential thrombocythaemia: Contribution to differential diagnosis. Br J Haemotol 104:574-580, 1999.
34. Silverstein MN, Gomes MR, ReMine WH, Elveback LR: Agnogenic myeloid metaplasia. Arch Intern Med 120:546, 1967.
35. Silverstein MN, Linman JW: Causes of death in agnogenic myeloid metaplasia. Mayo Clin Proc 44:36, 1969.
36. Silverstein MN, Wollaeger EE, Baggenstoss JK: Gastrointestinal and abdominal manifestations of agnogenic myeloid metaplasia. Arch Intern Med 131:532-537, 1973.
37. Smith RE, Chelmowski MK, Szabo EJ: Myelofibrosis: A concise review of clinical and pathologic features and treatment. Am J Hematol 29:174, 1988.
38. Soll E, Massumoto C, Clift RA, et al: Relevance of marrow fibrosis in bone marrow transplantation: A retrospective analysis of engraftment. Blood 86:4667-4673, 1995.
39. Steiner RM, Mitchell DG, Rao VM, et al: Magnetic resonance imaging of bone marrow: Diagnostic value in diffuse hematologic disorders. Magn Reson Q 6:17, 1990.
40. Talarico L, Wolf BC, Kumar A, Weintraub LR: Reversal of bone marrow fibrosis and subsequent development of polycythemia in patients with myeloproliferative disorders. Am J Hematol 30:248, 1989.

41. Tefferi A: Myelofibrosis with myeloid metaplasia. N Engl J Med 342:1255-1265, 2000.
42. Tefferi A, Mesa R, Nagorney D, et al: Splenectomy in myelofibrosis with myeloid metaplasia: A single-institution experience with 223 patients. Blood 95:2226-2233, 2000.
43. Vaugh JM: Leuco-erythroblastic anaemia. J Pathol 42:541, 1936.
44. Visani G, Finelli C, Castelli U, et al: Myelofibrosis with myeloid metaplasia: Clinical and haematological parameters predicting survival in a series of 133 patients. Br J Haematol 75:4, 1990.
45. Ward HP, Block MH: The natural history of agnogenic myeloid metaplasia (AMM) and a critical evaluation of its relationship with the myeloproliferative syndrome. Medicine 50:357, 1971.
46. Ward HP, Vautrin E, Kurnick J: Presence of a myeloproliferative factor in patients with polycythemia vera and agnogenic myeloid metaplasia. I. Expansion of the erythropoietin responsive stem cell compartment. Proc Soc Exp Biol Med 147:305, 1974.
47. Wood HC: On relations of leukocythemia and pseudoleukemia. Am J Med Sci 62:373, 1871.
48. Yoon SY, Li CY, Mesa RA, et al: Bone marrow effects of anagrelide therapy in patients with myelofibrosis with myeloid metaplasia. Br J Haematol 106:682-688, 1999.
49. Yu TF: Secondary gout associated with myeloproliferative disorders. Arthritis Rheum 8:765, 1965.

MASTOCYTOSIS

CAPSULE SUMMARY

	LOW BACK	NECK
Frequency of spinal pain	Uncommon	Not applicable (NA)
Location of spinal pain	Lumbar spine	NA
Quality of spinal pain	Ache	NA
Symptoms and signs	Urticaria, diarrhea, flushing, bone tenderness, hepatosplenomegaly	NA
Laboratory findings	Anemia, increased mast cells on bone marrow biopsy associated with increased fibrosis	NA
Radiographic findings	Lytic and/or sclerotic vertebral body lesions on plain roentgenograms	NA
Treatment	H1- and H2-receptor blockers, oral cromolyn	NA

PREVALENCE AND PATHOGENESIS

Systemic mastocytosis is a rare disorder associated with the proliferation of mast cells in skin, bone, liver, spleen, and lymph nodes.[32] Mast cells contain vasoactive compounds, such as histamine, that cause some of the clinical symptoms of the illness, including hives, flushing, diarrhea, and brownish skin lesions. Mast cells play an important role in protection of portals of entry (blood vessels, mucosal membranes).[9] Patients with mast cell proliferation in the axial skeleton may have back pain.

Epidemiology

The prevalence of disease associated with mast cells is unknown. Approximately 1 in 1000 to 8000 patients in dermatology clinics have mastocytosis.[12] However, an unknown number of patients may have disease without skin involvement.[55] The disease may start at any age. The disease usually becomes manifest after the age of 20. The age range is 25 to 80 years, with a median of 60 years. Men and women are equally affected.[24] A study of 58 cases revealed a male-to-female ratio of 1.33:1.[52]

Pathogenesis

The pathogenesis of mastocytosis is unknown. Mast cells originate from pluripotent bone marrow cells that are disseminated as precursors and then undergo proliferation and maturation in specific tissues.[3] Mast cells originate from a CD34-positive, Fc epsilon RI-negative cell population.[42] Mast cells in the skin or in other organs start to proliferate. Mast cells in the skin, gastrointestinal tract, liver, spleen, lymph nodes, and bone produce chemical mediators that have effects on a number of these organ systems. The mediators include histamine, arachidonic acid metabolites (possibly including leukotrienes C_4 and B_4), and platelet-activating factor.[28] Mast cells contain secretory granules and membrane-derived factors that are from three biologically active categories. These categories include (1) histamine, a proteoglycan, and neutral proteinases; (2) cysteinyl and dihydroxyleukotrienes, prostaglandin D_2, and platelet-activating factor; and (3) interleukin-1 (IL-1), IL-3, IL-4, IL-5, IL-6, tumor necrosis factor-alpha, granulocyte-macrophage colony-stimulating factor, and interferon-gamma.[3] Mast cells may also promote the synthesis of IgE.[30] These factors have potent effects on immune function, inflammation, blood vessels, and fibroblasts. The clinical manifestations of the disease can be directly correlated with the products released by mast cells.[34] The number of tissue mast cells is regulated by the kit ligand, stem cell factor.[23] Kit is part of the tyrosine kinase receptor group. Activation of kit by its ligand causes phosphorylation in a wide array of signal transduction cascades. This results in the production of a variety of cytokines.[51] Mast cells undergo apoptosis on withdrawal of stem cell factor.

Nettleship in 1869 was the first to describe the cutaneous manifestations of the disease,[33] whereas Sangster in 1878 coined the term *urticaria pigmentosa*.[45] In 1958, Ende and Cherniss were the first to report the occurrence of systemic mastocytosis in the absence of skin involvement.[10]

CLINICAL HISTORY

Systemic mastocytosis may manifest itself in a number of ways. The clinical manifestations may be divided into five distinct syndromes: (1) urticaria pigmentosa (95% to 99% of all mastocytoses); (2) cutaneous involvement with bone disease; (3) systemic mastocytoses with cutaneous and other internal organ involvement, including bone; (4) systemic mastocytosis without urticaria pigmentosa; and (5) mast cell leukemia.[5,17,53,56] A consensus conference held in 1991 classified mastocytosis into the following four forms (Table 15-4)[31]:

Type 1: indolent mastocytosis (limited to skin or extracutaneous)
Type 2: mastocytosis with hematologic disorders (*V816D* mutation)
Type 3: aggressive mastocytosis
Type 4: mast cell leukemia

The symptoms of patients with the illness depend on the extent and degree of mast cell organ involvement and physiologic response to histamine. Approximately 10% to 20% of patients with a systemic disease have bone pain, including back pain. Fractures may be present in 16%.[52] Patients have attacks that begin with a sensation of flushing, followed by palpitations and lightheadedness due to vasodilation with associated hypotension.[25] Skin lesions may precede systemic disease by 10 to 20 years.[56] Other common symptoms include generalized fatigue, night sweats, weakness, vomiting, diarrhea, and weight loss. Gastrointestinal abnormalities in systemic mastocytosis include esophagitis, acid hypersecretion, dysmotility, small bowel dilation, and malabsorption.[21] Patients may also complain of cutaneous flushing, pruritus, dizziness, syncope, and various neuropsychiatric disorders, including irritability and inability to concentrate.[12]

15-4 MASTOCYTOSIS CLASSIFICATION

1. Indolent mastocytosis
   A. Cutaneous disease*
      Urticaria pigmentosa
      Diffuse cutaneous mastocytosis
   B. Systemic disease†
      Bone marrow
         Mast cell aggregates
      Gastrointestinal
         Ulcer disease
         Malabsorption
         Hepatosplenomegaly
      Skeletal disease
      Lymphadenopathy
2. Mastocytosis with a hematologic disorder
   A. Myeloproliferative‡
      Nonlymphatic leukemia
      Malignant lymphoma
   B. Myelodysplastic
      Chronic neutropenia
3. Aggressive
   A. Lymphadenopathic mastocytosis with eosinophilia§
4. Mast cell leukemia¶

*Major form.
†Unaltered life expectancy.
‡Prognostic of hematologic disorder.
§Prognostic of extent of organ infiltration.
¶Invariably fatal.
Modified from Metcalfe DD: Classification and diagnosis of mastocytosis: Current status. J Invest Dermatol 96:2S-4S, 1991; conclusions, 65S.

PHYSICAL EXAMINATION

The most frequent site of organ involvement with any form of mastocytosis is the skin. Skin lesions include urticaria pigmentosa, mastocytoma, diffuse and erythrodermic cutaneous mastocytosis, and telangiectasia macularis eruptive perstans.[49] Skin or mucous membrane lesions include confluent macules, papules, or nodules, which may become pigmented. Progressive disease affects the oral, nasal, and rectal mucosa. Dermatographism is also a common finding. Cutaneous manifestations are the most prevalent abnormality on physical examination.[4] Other prominent findings in systemic disease include hepatosplenomegaly, generalized lymphadenopathy, and tenderness on palpation of affected bones in the vertebral column.

LABORATORY DATA

The infiltration of mast cells into the bone marrow, the release of mast cell products, and the associated fibrosis have marked effects on laboratory parameters. Anemia is seen in about 50% of patients in association with normal leukocyte counts.[36] A minority of patients have leukopenia, whereas leukocytosis with eosinophilia occurs in 10% to 20% of patients.[28,58] A minority of patients may be thrombocytopenic.[52] Patients with systemic mastocytosis with urticaria pigmentosa may have normal blood parameters. Patients with malignant mastocytosis have blood abnormalities involving the red blood cells, white blood cells, or platelets, invariably.[19] The erythrocyte sedimentation rate is elevated. The biochemical diagnosis of mastocytosis may be suspected even in the absence of histologic proof of the illness. In patients with episodes of systemic mastocytic activation, mast cell mediators are elevated during these episodes and are normal at quiescent times. In contrast, patients with proliferative mast cell disease, such as leukemia, usually exhibit chronic overproduction of mast cell mediators.[39] Mast cell secretory products include heparin, histamine, prostaglandin D_2, and tryptase. Episodes of mast cell activation are short-lived, usually lasting up to 60 minutes. Blood samples should be obtained while a patient is experiencing an episode of mast cell activation.

Heparin from mast cells may cause a prolongation of the partial thromboplastin time (PTT). An abnormal PTT is encountered only during severe episodes of activation. The specificity of the abnormal PTT secondary to heparin may be increased by the presence of a normal prothrombin time that is less sensitive to heparin and the reversal of the abnormal PTT by the addition of protamine, a heparin antagonist. Measurement of urinary histamine and its metabolites documents increased concentrations along with increased prostaglandin D_2 metabolites.[22,40] Many difficulties are associated with the quantification of histamine in plasma and urine. Mass spectrometric analysis is the most accurate but least available means to measure histamine.[39] Plasma histamine may be increased by basophils activated during phlebotomy. Bacteria add to the levels of urinary histamine. Elevated levels of histamine during a period of mast cell activation with a return to normal may be more indicative of overproduction of histamine secondary to systemic mastocytosis. Prostaglandin D_2 metabolites are elevated but are difficult to quantify since mass spectrometric analysis is necessary. Tryptase is a neutral protease found in mast cell granules and not in basophil granules. Tryptase is more specific than histamine as a measure of mast cell activation.[47] Tryptase is measured by an enzyme-linked immunosorbent assay. Samples may be obtained up to 2 or more hours after an attack of mast cell activation.[48] Total tryptase levels of 20 ng/mL in a baseline sample suggest underlying systemic mastocytosis.[46] Elevated alkaline phosphatase may be seen in a minority of patients with significant bone involvement. Patients have also been described with abnormal lipoproteins, particularly pre-beta-lipoprotein. These patients had accelerated coronary atherosclerosis.[14]

Pathology

Bone marrow biopsy is the definitive diagnostic procedure for systemic mastocytosis. Bone marrow is hypercellular with increased reticulin and increased myeloid elements.[43] Superficially, the lesions have a granulomatous appearance, but there are no giant cells. The mast cells are present but may be difficult to recognize, since the mast cells of systemic mastocytosis are immature and contain fewer granules than mature mast cells.[27] Mast cells are paratrabecular and perivascular in location. The bone cells, osteoblasts and osteoclasts, are prominent in this disease. Both types of cells are enlarged. In certain areas, osteoclasts predominate and there is associated bone lysis. In other areas, bone density is increased corresponding to increased osteoblastic activity. A study of nine patients with mastocytosis investigated the pathologic changes associated with osteopenia and osteosclerosis.[16] Patients with osteopenia had active bone-forming surfaces that were outpaced by bone resorption by osteoclasts. In these patients, bone marrow infiltration by mast cells and fibrosis was not as extensive as that with osteosclerosis. Patients with osteosclerosis had extensive skin and visceral organ involvement. Bone marrow mast cells and fibrosis was significantly increased. Skin biopsy may also demonstrate increased numbers of mast cells.[34]

RADIOGRAPHIC EVALUATION

Roentgenograms

Although bone pain may be a symptom in a minority of patients, skeletal changes on radiographic evaluation occur in up to 70% of patients with mastocytosis. The abnormalities include either diffuse or localized osteoblastic or osteolytic lesions (Fig. 15-5). In the axial skeleton, diffuse lesions predominate. In a number of reviews, generalized osteosclerosis was the most common pattern (16% to 45%) (Fig. 15-6). Mixed osteosclerosis with focal osteolytic areas and generalized osteoporosis occur less commonly (Fig 15-7).[5,37,38,44,56] Patients with mastocytosis may present with compression fractures as a manifestation of osteopenia. This may occur in the thoracic or lumbar spine.[13] Osteopenia may be the sole manifestation of mastocytosis independent of skin disease (see Fig 15-7).[7] In the axial skeleton, the loss of delineation of the bony trabeculae results in a homogeneous, radiodense appearance of bone. Osteolytic areas are discrete (≤5 cm in diameter), with a thin rim of sclerotic bone.

Scintigraphy

Bone scan may also have a variable pattern. In one study, patients had a variety of scans ranging from normal to unifocal, multifocal, or diffuse increased uptake.[41] The finding of osteolytic and osteosclerotic bone abnormalities on plain roentgenograms and a diffuse increased uptake on bone scan should suggest the possibility of mast cell disease.[15] Mast cells absorb gallium. Gallium scans may identify the location of increased numbers of mast cells.[11] Dual-photon absorptiometry has been used to document the increased amount of bone mineral calcium in patients with systemic mastocytosis.[2]

DIFFERENTIAL DIAGNOSIS

The diagnosis of mastocytosis is not difficult in the patient with urticaria pigmentosa, positive Darier's sign (urticaria formation with gentle stroking of the skin), cutaneous flushing, hepatosplenomegaly, histaminuria, and osteosclerosis on plain films associated with back pain. A problem exists in making the diagnosis because mastocytosis has a broad spectrum of disease. Patients may present with systemic involvement without cutaneous lesions.[8] In these patients, biopsy of an involved area (bone marrow, liver, skin) should yield tissue with mast cells. The histologic demonstration of increased numbers of mast cells in the appropriate clinical setting is diagnostic.

Flushing or diarrhea may occur in a variety of disorders including angioedema, carcinoid syndrome, pheochromocytoma, vasoactive intestinal peptide (VIP)-secreting tumors, and Zollinger-Ellison syndrome. Angioedema patients have C1 esterase deficiency. Carcinoid syndrome has elevations of serum serotonin but not tryptase. Pheochromocytoma is associated with urinary free catecholamines. VIP tumors produce increased serum levels of VIPs. Zollinger-Ellison syndrome is associated with elevated levels of gastrin.

The radiographic picture of mastocytosis may be confused with that of other diseases that cause osteosclerosis. These include myelofibrosis, fluorosis, sickle cell anemia, Paget's disease, and metastatic lesions, particularly prostatic carcinoma (see Table 15-2).[54] Each disease has laboratory or clinical parameters that differentiate it from mastocytosis.

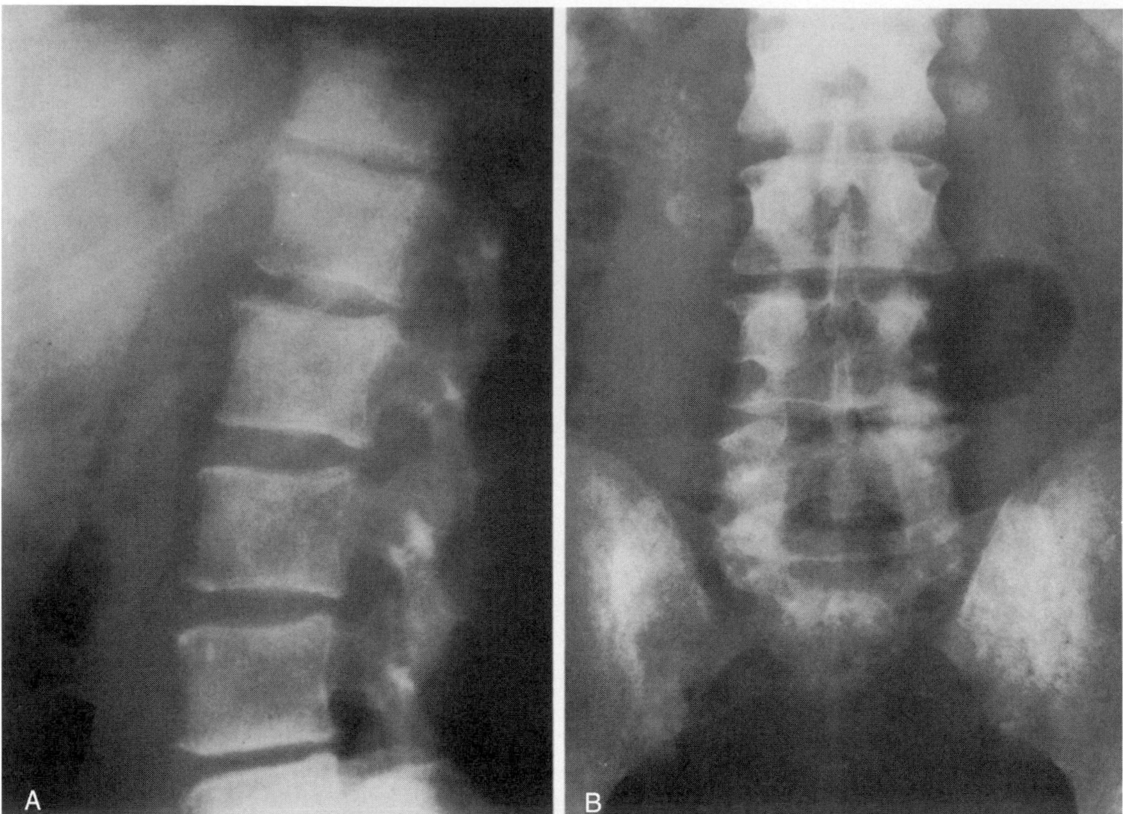

Figure 15-5 *A* and *B*, Mastocytosis demonstrated by diffuse osteosclerosis involving ilium, sacrum, and vertebral bodies. *(Courtesy of Anne Brower, MD.)*

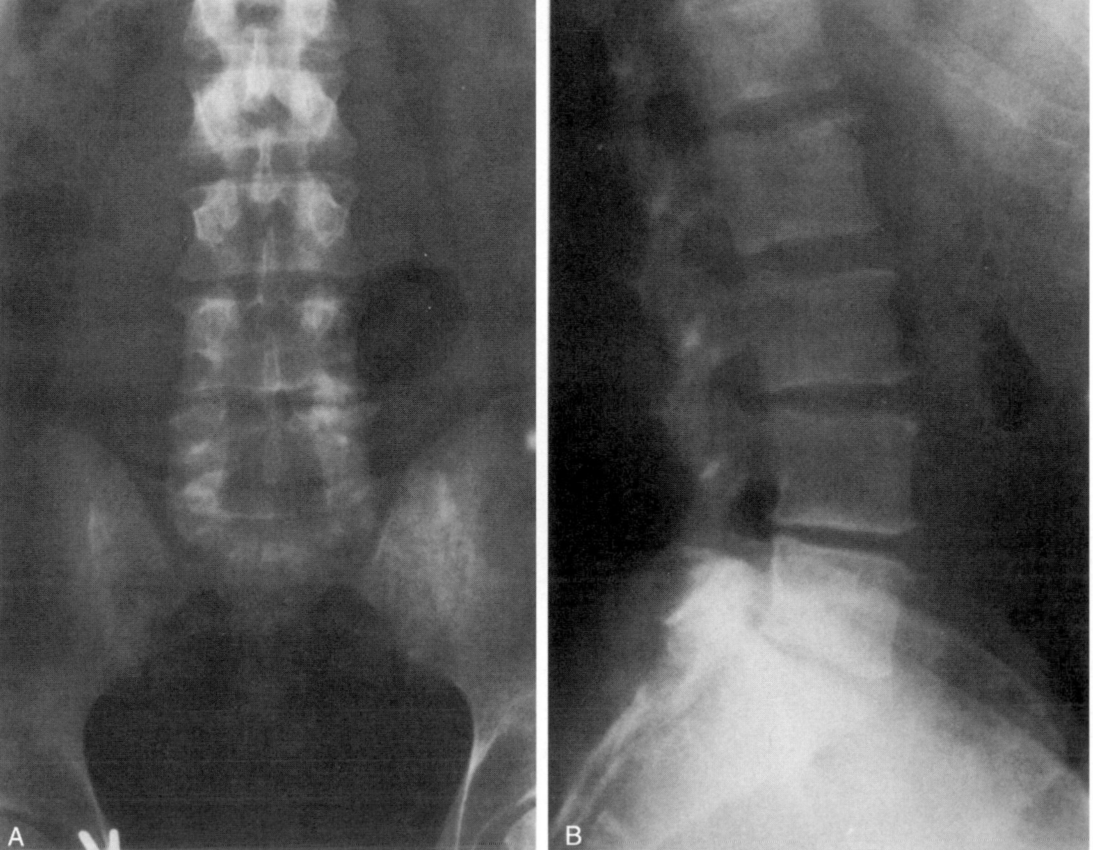

Figure 15-6 Anteroposterior *(A)* and lateral *(B)* views of the lumbosacral spine of a 55-year-old man with systemic mastocytosis. The patient had urticaria pigmentosa. The patient had chronic low back pain since a fall as a child. In the past year, the pain had increased. The roentgenograms reveal advanced lower lumbar spondylosis. The bones reveal a granular quality consistent with early osteosclerosis, most evident in the pelvis.

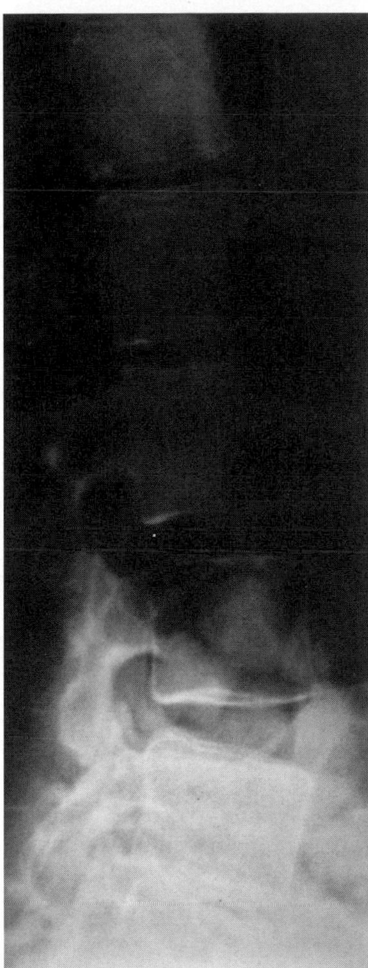

Figure 15-7 Lateral view of the lumbosacral spine of a 43-year-old woman with urticaria pigmentosa. The roentgenograms reveal generalized osteoporosis with thinning of the vertebral endplates, with some vertebral bodies containing areas of sclerosis.

TREATMENT

Treatment of mastocytosis is directed at counteracting the effects of mast cell products. A major part of therapy is antihistamines. Treatment may include histamine-1 (H_1)-receptor antagonists, such as chlorpheniramine 12 to 24 mg/day, oral cetirizine 10 mg/day, and hydroxyzine 25 mg four times a day.[57] H_2-receptor antagonists, such as cimetidine 800 to 1200 mg/day, famotidine 10 mg twice daily, or ranitidine 300 to 600 mg/day, are also effective.[1] The H_1 antagonists inhibit flushing and pruritus, whereas the H_2 antagonists limit gastrointestinal manifestations.

Oral cromolyn sodium (100 to 400 mg/day) may ameliorate pruritus, abdominal pain, and neuropsychiatric dysfunction.[50] The mechanism of action of this agent may be to block absorption of factors from the gut that stimulate mast cell discharge of active products. At 800 mg/day, oral cromolyn is significantly better than placebo for the gastrointestinal manifestations of mastocytosis.[18]

The use of nonsteroidal anti-inflammatory drugs (NSAIDs) is controversial. Some patients with mastocytosis are sensitive to aspirin and develop bronchospasm with aspirin ingestion. Other patients have used NSAIDs to block the production of prostaglandin D_2 by mast cells, thereby decreasing symptoms.[40] In patients with severe disease who have not responded to antihistamines, a trial of aspirin is warranted. Small doses of aspirin (60 to 120 mg) along with antihistamines should be given as tolerated.

Radiation therapy has been used in patients with severe spinal involvement. Mast cell degranulation with increased histamine levels does not occur with radiation therapy.[20]

In patients who develop shock, emergency procedures are needed. These patients require intravenous fluids and dopamine or epinephrine. Transfusions may be indicated for patients who develop profound anemia.

Type 3 disease are treated with interferon alfa-2b and hydroxyurea.[26] Interferon alfa-2b is administered at 4 million units three times per week to start and may be increased to a maximum of 3 million units per day. This therapy may relieve pain and improve bone lesions in those patients with multiple fractures.[6]

Targeting specific mast cells with mutated c-*kit* receptors holds promise as a potential therapy to control the number of diseased mast cells. The limitation of this therapy is the presence of c-*kit* ligand on stem cells and melanocytes. These cells may also be damaged by treatments directed at this receptor, affecting the repopulation of other hematopoietic lineages in the bone marrow.[29]

PROGNOSIS

The prognosis in mastocytosis varies with two factors: age at onset and absence of systemic disease. Patients who are older at time of onset or have systemic manifestations have a worse prognosis. About 15% to 30% of adult patients with skin disease may progress to systemic mastocytosis. The patients at greatest risk of developing mast cell leukemia are those with no skin disease, marked splenomegaly, and severe myeloid hyperplasia.[43] In one study, 40% of 43 patients with mastocytosis developed leukemia. The leukemias included myelogenous, monocytic, and mast cell malignancies. This suggests that systemic mastocytosis may be part of a spectrum of myeloproliferative disorders that includes polycythemia, chronic myelogenous leukemia, and essential thrombocythemia. Patients with systemic mast cell disease without associated hematologic disorders have a poor prognosis with shortened survival, with elevated serum alkaline phosphatase, increased bone marrow mast cell numbers, and bone marrow eosinophilia.[35]

The prognosis of 58 patients with mast cell disease was evaluated by univariate and multivariate analysis.[52] Most of the deaths from mastocytosis occurred during the first 3 years after diagnosis. Older men with constitutional symptoms, anemia, thrombocytopenia, abnormal liver function tests, lobulated mast cell nuclei, and few cells in bone marrow biopsy were at greatest risk.

References

Mastocytosis

1. Achord JL, Langford H: The effect of cimetidine and propantheline on the symptoms of a patient with systemic mastocytosis. Am J Med 69:610, 1980.
2. Arrington ER, Eisenberg B, Hartshorne MF, et al: Nuclear medicine imaging of systemic mastocytosis. J Nucl Med 30:2046, 1989.
3. Austen KF: Systemic mastocytosis [Editorial]. N Engl J Med 326:639, 1992.
4. Austen KF, Horan RF: Systemic mastocytosis: Retrospective review of a decade's clinical experience at the Brigham and Women's Hospital. J Invest Dermatol 96:5S, 1991.
5. Brunning RD, McKenna RW, Rosai J: Systemic mastocytosis: Extracutaneous manifestations. Am J Surg Pathol 7:425, 1983.
6. Butterfield JH: Response of severe systemic mastocytosis to interferon-alpha. Br J Dermatol 138:489-495, 1998.
7. Chines A, Pacifici R, Avioli LV, et al: Systemic mastocytosis presenting as osteoporosis: A clinical and histomorphometric study. J Clin Endocrinol Metab 72:140, 1991.
8. Duffy TP: Clinical problem solving. N Engl J Med 328:1333, 1993.
9. Echtenacher B, Mannel DN, Hultner L: Critical protective role of mast cells in a model of acute septic peritonitis. Nature 381:75-77, 1996.
10. Ende W, Cherniss EL: Splenic mastocytosis. Blood 13:631, 1958.
11. Ensslen RD, Jackson FI, Reid AM: Bone gallium scans in mastocytosis: Correlation with count rates, radiography, and microscopy. J Nucl Med 24:568, 1983.
12. Fine J: Mastocytosis. Int J Dermatol 19:117, 1980.
13. Floman Y, Amir G: Systemic mastocytosis presenting with severe osteopenia and multiple compression fractures. J Spinal Disord 4:369-373, 1991.
14. Frieri M, Papadopoulos NM, Kaliner MA, Metcalfe DD: An abnormal pre-beta-lipoprotein in patients with systemic mastocytosis. Ann Intern Med 97:227, 1982.
15. Gagnon JH, Kalz F, Kadri AM, Von Graefe I: Mastocytosis: Unusual manifestations; clinical and radiologic changes. Can Med Assoc J 112:1329, 1975.
16. Gennes CD, Kuntz D, Vernejoul CD: Bone mastocytosis: A report of nine cases with a bone histomorphometric study. Clin Orthop 279:281, 1992.
17. Hills E, Dunstan CR, Evans RA: Bone metabolism in systemic mastocytosis. J Bone Joint Surg Am 63-A:665, 1981.
18. Horan RF, Sheffer AL, Austen KF: Cromolyn sodium in the management of systemic mastocytosis. J Allergy Clin Immunol 85:852, 1990.
19. Horny HP, Ruck M, Wehrmann M, Kaiserling E: Blood findings in generalized mastocytosis: Evidence of frequent simultaneous occurrence of myeloproliferative disorders. Br J Haematol 76:186, 1990.
20. Janjan NA, Conway P, Lundberg J, Derfus G: Radiation therapy in a case of systemic mastocytosis: Evaluation of histamine levels and mucosal effects. Am J Clin Oncol 15:337, 1992.
21. Jensen RT: Gastrointestinal abnormalities and involvement in systemic mastocytosis Hematol Oncol Clin North Am 14:579-623, 2000.
22. Keyzer JJ, de Monchy JGR, Van Doormaal JJ, van Voorst Vader PC: Improved diagnosis of mastocytosis by measurement of urinary histamine metabolites. N Engl J Med 309:1603, 1983.
23. Kirshenbaum A: Regulation of mast cell number and function. Hematol Oncol Clin North Am 14:497-516, 2000.
24. Korenblat PE, Wedner HJ, Whyte MP: Systemic mastocytosis. Arch Intern Med 144:2249, 1984.
25. Kuter I: Case records of the Massachusetts General Hospital. N Engl J Med 326:472, 1992.
26. Lehmann T, Beyeler C, Lammle B, et al: Severe osteoporosis due to systemic mast cell disease: Successful treatment with interferon alpha-2B. Br J Rheumatol 35:898-900, 1996.
27. Lennert K, Parwaresch MR: Mast cells and mast cell neoplasia: A review. Histopathology 3:349, 1979.
28. Lewis RA: Mastocytosis. J Allergy Clin Immunol 74:755, 1984.
29. Longley BJ, Ma Y, Carter E, et al: New approaches to therapy for mastocytosis: A case for treatment with *kit* kinase inhibitors. Hematol Oncol Clin North Am 14:689-695, 2000.
30. Mekori YA: Lymphoid tissues and the immune system in mastocytosis. Hematol Oncol Clin North Am 14:569-577, 2000.
31. Metcalfe DD: Classification and diagnosis of mastocytosis: Current status. J Invest Dermatol 96:2S, 1991.
32. Mutter RD, Tannenbaum M, Ultmann JE: Systemic mast cell disease. Ann Intern Med 59:887, 1963.
33. Nettleship E: Rare forms of urticaria. BMJ 2:323, 1869.
34. Olafsson JH: Cutaneous and systemic mastocytosis in adults: A clinical, histopathological, and immunological evaluation in relation to histamine metabolism. Acta Derm Venereol Suppl 115:1, 1985.
35. Pardanani A, Baek J, Li C, et al: Systemic mast cell disease without associated hematologic disorder: A combined retrospective and prospective study. Mayo Clin Proc 77:1169-1175, 2002.
36. Parker RI: Hematologic aspects of systemic mastocytosis. Hematol Oncol Clin North Am 14:557-568, 2000.
37. Poppel MH, Gruber WF, Silber R, et al: The roentgen manifestations of urticaria pigmentosa (mastocytosis). AJR Am J Roentgenol 82:239, 1959.
38. Rafii M, Firooznia H, Golimbu C, Bathazar E: Pathologic fracture in systemic mastocytosis. Clin Orthop 180:260, 1983.
39. Roberts LJ, Oates JA: Biochemical diagnosis of systemic mast cell disorders. J Invest Dermatol 96:19S, 1991.
40. Roberts LJ II, Sweetman BJ, Lewis RA, et al: Increased production of prostaglandin D_2 in patients with systemic mastocytoses. N Engl J Med 303:1400, 1980.
41. Rosenbaum RC, Frieri M, Metcalfe D: Patterns of skeletal scintigraphy and their relationship to plasma and urinary histamine levels in systemic mastocytosis. J Nucl Med 25:859, 1984.
42. Rottem M, Okada T, Goff JP, et al: Mast cells cultured from the peripheral blood of normal donors and patients with mastocytosis originate from a CD34+/Fc epsilon RI– cell population. Blood 84:2489, 1994.
43. Rudders RA: Case records of the Massachusetts General Hospital: Weekly clinicopathological exercises. Case 38-1986: A 73-year-old man with diffuse osteosclerotic lesions. N Engl J Med 315:816, 1986.
44. Sagher F, Cohen C, Schorr S: Concomitant bone changes in urticaria pigmentosa. J Invest Dermatol 18:425, 1952.
45. Sangster A: An anomalous mottled rash, accompanied by pruritus, factitious urticaria, and pigmentation: Urticaria pigmentosa? Trans Clin Soc Lond 11:161, 1878.
46. Schwartz LB, Irani AA: Serum tryptase and the laboratory diagnosis of systemic mastocytosis. Hematol Oncol Clin North Am 14:641-657, 2000.
47. Schwartz LB, Metcalfe DD, Miller JS, et al: Tryptase levels as an indicator of mast cell activation in systemic anaphylaxis and mastocytosis. N Engl J Med 316:1622, 1987.
48. Schwartz LB, Yunginger JW, Miller J, et al: Time course of appearance and disappearance of human mast cell tryptase in the circulation after anaphylaxis. J Clin Invest 83:1551, 1989.
49. Soter NA: Mastocytosis and the skin. Hematol Oncol Clin North Am 14:537-555, 2000.
50. Soter NA, Austen KF, Wasserman SI: Oral disodium cromoglycate in the treatment of systemic mastocytosis. N Engl J Med 301:465, 1979.
51. Taylor ML, Metcalfe DD: Kit signal transduction. Hematol Oncol Clin North Am 14:517-535, 2000.
52. Travis WD, Li C, Bergstralh EJ, et al: Systemic mast cell disease: Analysis of 58 cases and literature review. Medicine 67:345, 1988.
53. Travis WD, Li C, Hoagland HC, et al: Mast cell leukemia: Report of a case and review of the literature. Mayo Clin Proc 61:957, 1986.
54. Tubiana JM, Dana A, Petit-Perrin D, Duperray B: Lymphographic patterns in systemic mastocytosis with diffuse bone involvement and hematological signs. Radiology 131:651, 1979.
55. Turk J, Oates JA, Roberts LJ II: Intervention with epinephrine in hypotension associated with mastocytosis. J Allergy Clin Immunol 71:189, 1983.
56. Webb TA, Li CY, Yam LT: Systemic mast cell disease: A clinical and hematopathologic study of 26 cases. Cancer 49:927, 1982.
57. Worobec A: Treatment of systemic mast cell disorders. Hematol Oncol Clin North Am 14:659-687, 2000.
58. Yam LT, Yam CF, Li CY: Eosinophilia in systemic mastocytosis. Am J Clin Pathol 73:48, 1980.

CHAPTER 16

NEUROLOGIC AND PSYCHIATRIC DISORDERS OF THE SPINE

Disorders of the neurologic system may be associated with systemic illnesses that alter nerve function or with local compression that causes isolated neurologic abnormalities. Charcot joint disease, which affects the spine, occurs in the setting of decreased sensation in the skeletal system and results in marked destruction of bony structures. Syphilis and diabetes remain the most common causes of this arthropathy of the spine.

In addition to systemic disorders, peripheral neuropathy may affect nerves that course through the lumbosacral or the cervical spine to the leg and arm, respectively. Abnormalities of these nerves may superficially resemble impingement of a nerve root by a herniated nucleus pulposus or spinal stenosis. However, careful history and physical examination should localize the lesion outside the central nervous system and should raise the possibility of a wide range of disorders that affect the structures embedded in the retroperitoneum (retroperitoneal bleeding) or neck (tumor), for example.

The diagnosis of neurologic disorders is made by the careful review of the findings discovered during the physical examination and data obtained from a limited number of electrophysiologic and radiographic tests.

The therapy for neurologic disorders associated with spinal pain must be directed at the underlying disorder causing nerve dysfunction. Most commonly, strict control of glucose metabolism in diabetes is necessary. When compression of a peripheral nerve is relieved, total return of function is possible.

Psychiatric disorders are also associated with spinal pain. A small minority of patients with psychiatric illness actually complain of spinal pain. The hallucinations and other psychotic thoughts of these patients do not usually involve pain.

In contrast, those patients with chronic spinal pain very frequently develop neurotic behavior. Neurosis increases with the duration of pain. Patients with chronic pain lose control over their lives and become depressed. The initial injury that caused the pain may have healed entirely, but the patient continues to exhibit pain behavior. The diagnosis of chronic pain syndrome is made in a patient who has no new organic disease, has had pain for 6 months or longer, and has experienced progressive physical and emotional deterioration. In patients with chronic pain, therapy must take a multidisciplinary form including drugs, physical therapy, psychiatric therapy, and vocational rehabilitation.

Malingerers are individuals who feign their symptoms and signs willfully to gain some advantage. The number of patients with spinal pain who are malingering is very small. A careful history and physical examination frequently reveal the inconsistencies between malingerers' symptoms and signs and those of patients with organic disease. If the patient is thought to be malingering, that fact should be corroborated by another physician. Extensive evaluations and prolonged courses of treatment are counterproductive in the patient with feigned illness.

NEUROPATHIES

Lumbar Spine

Neurologic disorders most commonly associated with the lumbosacral spine are radiculopathies associated with alterations of the lumbar disc (herniation) and the spinal canal (spinal stenosis). These entities are discussed in Chapter 10. Patients with herniated disc and spinal stenosis may have back pain as part of their symptom-complex but more prominently have symptoms that affect the lower extremities. The involvement of the lower extremities follows a specific pattern that correlates with motor and sensory abnormalities associated with dysfunction of a specific nerve root.

Distal to the neural foramen, nerve roots from multiple levels form trunks that are incorporated into the lumbar and sacral plexuses. Because the structures are continuous, the lumbar and sacral plexuses can be considered as one unit, the lumbosacral plexus (see Fig. 5-16). A nerve distal to the spinal cord will have a distribution not as a single root but as a peripheral nerve with abnormalities in cutaneous or muscular structures innervated by multiple nerve root segments.

The lumbosacral plexus forms from the spinal roots of L1 through S5 and lies just lateral to both sides of the vertebral column in a retroperitoneal and posterior pelvic position. Any pathologic disease process that alters the anatomy of retroperitoneal or posterior pelvic areas may affect the plexus (tumor, fibrosis). Systemic disorders that affect the vasa nervorum may also have marked effects on plexus function (vasculitis).

NEUROLOGIC DISORDERS

Capsule Summary

	Low Back	Neck
Frequency of spinal pain	Rare	Rare
Location of spinal pain	Radicular distribution: thigh, lower leg	Radicular distribution: shoulder, arm
Quality of spinal pain	Neuropathic: burning, stinging, radiating	Neuropathic: burning, stinging, radiating
Symptoms and signs	Burning pain or painless, diabetes most common illness, loss of sensation, local muscle wasting	Tingling pain or numbness, loss of sensation, local muscle wasting
Laboratory tests	Glucose intolerance	Electromyogram nerve compression
Radiographic findings	Neuroarthropathy—marked destruction and disorganization of vertebral bodies	Chest radiograph—Pancoast's tumor
Treatment	Glucose control, antidepressants, anticonvulsants	Nonsteroidal anti-inflammatory drugs (NSAIDs), surgical decompression

Lumbosacral Plexus

Tumors. Tumors of the pelvic organs spread by direct or lymphatic extension to involve the lumbosacral plexus.[175] Tumors in the pelvis (cervix, prostate, bladder, and rectum) spread to pelvic lymph nodes that neighbor the sacral plexus. The nerves supplying the gluteal muscles, the posterior cutaneous nerve of the thigh, and the sciatic nerve are affected. Tumors that spread to abdominal lymph glands in the lower aortic chain (testicular, ovarian) involve the lumbar plexus and are more likely to affect obturator, femoral, and genitofemoral nerves along with the psoas muscle. Lymphoma involving the retroperitoneal nodes may invade the lumbar plexus. Lymph nodes near the pelvic brim may affect the femoral and obturator nerves. Primary retroperitoneal sarcomas may have a similar effect.[272] Nonmalignant processes that cause fibrosis of the retroperitoneum (retroperitoneal fibrosis) may also cause a similar clinical picture.[156]

The clinical symptom commonly associated with tumors affecting the lumbosacral plexus is constant, deep boring pain. The pain is predominantly in the hip and posterolateral thigh. With involvement of the motor neurons, atrophy of the gluteal and thigh muscles results in increasing hip instability and gait abnormalities. Radiographic evaluation of the retroperitoneum may demonstrate mass lesions or increased osteoblastic activity on scintigraphy. Radiation treatment of the affected area is used to decrease pain and halt progressive paralysis.[151]

Vasculitis. Systemic vasculitis can affect the blood vessels supplying nerves.[123] When blood flow to a nerve is compromised, neurologic dysfunction in the form of motor and/or sensory loss occurs. Most often, mononeuritis multiplex is associated with this pathologic process.[108] Mononeuritis multiplex is associated with a variety of connective tissue disorders including polyarteritis nodosa, systemic lupus erythematosus, and rheumatoid arthritis. However, in a review of 35 patients with mononeuritis, 15 had no identifiable rheumatic disease. Of the 14 patients with mononeuritis multiplex and a connective tissue disease, 5 had systemic lupus erythematosus.[108] A significant number of individuals may develop mononeuritis without an identifiable, associated connective tissue disorder.

Ischemic nerve lesions may be distributed along the entire length of the affected nerves, although the majority of lesions are located in the proximal nerve trunks.[56] These lesions occur only with extensive disease, because the peripheral nerves receive extensive collateral circulation. Multiple small vessels of the aorta must be occluded before limb nerve ischemia occurs. Chronic, severe peripheral arterial insufficiency is associated with neurologic deficits in the lower extremities. Up to 88% of individuals with chronic arterial disease may demonstrate sensory abnormalities in the lower extremities.[241] The vasculitides associated with these lesions are listed in Table 16-1. Connective tissue disorders include polyarteritis nodosa, allergic granulomatosis, Wegener's granulomatosis, vasculitis associated with cryoglobulinemia, and rheumatoid arthritis.[66] Other vasculitides associated with peripheral neuropathy include systemic lupus erythematosus, Sjögren's syndrome, and temporal arteritis.[241] Peripheral nerve lesions in inflammatory vascular disorders occur less frequently than with atherosclerotic vascular disease. A variety of peripheral neuropathic syndromes occur in 14% of patients with temporal arteritis.[36] Approximately 10% of patients with systemic lupus erythematosus have a peripheral neuropathy.[173] The frequency of peripheral neuropathy associated with Sjögren's syndrome has been quantified at 30% of individuals with primary disease.[135]

The clinical symptoms associated with vasculitis of a plexus or major nerve branch is the sudden onset of profound weakness or paralysis of a group of muscles supplied

16-1 RHEUMATIC DISORDERS ASSOCIATED WITH NEUROPATHY

Disorder	Percent with Neuropathies	Reference
Polyarteritis nodosa	67%	95
Wegener's granulomatosis	20%	67
Rheumatoid vasculitis	42%	244
Systemic lupus erythematosus	10%	68
Sjögren's syndrome	30%	177
Temporal arteritis	14%	36
Scleroderma	1%	15,16,155,199
Cryoglobulinemia/myeloma	13%	81,270,282,289
Lyme disease	5%	206

by a major nerve and radiating, burning, aching, or shooting pain associated with dysesthesias or numbness in a matching cutaneous distribution. Footdrop is a manifestation of mononeuritis multiplex.[262] The onset may take hours to days but is maximal at the beginning of the insult to the nerve. The damage to the nerve can be profound, so that function does not return. If the damage is not complete, return of function may occur over months to a year or longer. Laboratory evaluation will reveal systemic factors associated with the specific form of vasculitis (rheumatoid factor—rheumatoid vasculitis; eosinophils—allergic granulomatosis) and nonspecific signs of generalized vessel inflammation (elevated erythrocyte sedimentation rate [ESR], thrombocytosis). Antibodies to neutrophil cytoplasmic antigens (ANCAs) are associated with Wegener's granulomatosus and microscopic polyangiitis.[111] c-ANCA (cytoplasmic pattern of staining) is highly specific for Wegener's granulomatosus. p-ANCA (perinuclear pattern of staining) is associated with microscopic polyangiitis and a variety of inflammatory disorders, including ulcerative colitis, rheumatoid arthritis, and systemic lupus erythematosus.[180] The cerebrospinal fluid (CSF) level remains normal in most cases because the nerve lesions are extraspinal. Electromyography (EMG) reveals denervation in the affected muscle along with slowed conduction in the corresponding nerve on nerve conduction studies. Biopsy of nerve (sural) and muscle has the best opportunity to obtain pathologic specimens to satisfy a diagnosis.[92] The appearance of neurologic abnormalities in the setting of vasculitis is indicative of more aggressive, potentially life-threatening disease. These patients usually require large doses of corticosteroids and immunosuppressive drugs such as cyclophosphamide.[95,185] Cyclophosphamide (2 mg/kg orally each day, or 0.6 g/m^2 intravenously every month) is the usual dose required.[97] Individuals who may benefit from cyclophosphamide therapy at the time of diagnosis of polyarteritis nodosa include those with gastrointestinal bleeding, perforation, infarction, or pancreatitis; renal insufficiency (serum creatinine level >1.58 mg/dL; proteinuria higher than 1 g/day; central nervous system involvement; and cardiomyopathy.[96] Other manifestations of connective tissue diseases may also cause neurologic dysfunction similar to a radiculopathy or plexopathy. On rare occasions, rheumatoid arthritis causes a pachymeningitis of the cauda equina and lumbosacral meninges. These patients develop abnormal CSF leukocytosis and elevated CSF protein levels. Cauda equina symptoms are associated with this meningeal inflammation and resolve after treatment with high doses of corticosteroids.[167]

Bradley and associates reported an inflammatory lesion of the lumbosacral plexus associated with perivascular inflammation in epineural arterioles associated with markedly ESRs in six patients.[24] All patients presented with buttock or thigh pain or with mononeuritis multiplex symptoms of the lower extremities. Involvement was characterized by asymmetrical radicular involvement initially associated with weakness and pain in a sciatic nerve distribution. Subsequently the process became bilateral and was associated with progressive motor and sensory dysfunction. Sural nerve biopsies demonstrated axonal degeneration and epineural arteriolar inflammation. Patients who were treated with immunosuppressive drugs had resolution of their symptoms.[24]

Radiation Therapy. Radiation therapy to the pelvis has been reported to cause damage to the lumbosacral plexus.[9] Radiation is given for gynecologic cancers in women, testicular cancer in men, and lymphoma in both sexes.[179] Patients receiving 5900 to 6760 rads to the pelvis developed signs of neurologic injury 6 to 48 months after exposure. Other reports have symptoms appearing three decades after exposure. Asymmetrical patchy involvement of the entire plexus was manifested by spotty sensory, motor, and reflex abnormalities in both lower extremities. Painless weakness is an initial manifestation followed by limb paresthesias in 50% of patients. Bowel and bladder disturbances are rare findings. The major difficulty for the clinician in this circumstance is to distinguish plexus abnormalities from recurrent tumor. EMG evaluation may demonstrate myokymic potentials that are associated with radiation damage.[179] Patients with radiation damage develop neurologic dysfunction secondary to fibrosis.[283] Fibrosis may also be a manifestation of recurrent tumor. Surgical exploration may be needed to differentiate the possible diagnoses. No specific therapy is effective for this form of nerve damage.

Other causes of lumbosacral plexopathy include bleeding disorders, including iatrogenic events associated with anticoagulants, pregnancy, psoas abscesses, hip surgery, and therapeutic injections. Nondiabetic lumbosacral plexopathy has similar natural history and outcome to the diabetic variant.[57]

These forms of immune-mediated plexopathy should be separated from chronic inflammatory demyelinating polyneuropathy and from systemic necrotizing vasculitis.[58]

Peripheral Nerve Syndromes

Peripheral nerves are the extension of the spinal nerve roots that comprise the lumbosacral plexus. These nerves supply sensory function alone or a combination of sensory and motor function. Pathologic processes that compress (tunnel syndromes) or decrease blood flow (diabetes) to peripheral nerves are associated with neurologic symptoms of dysesthesias and muscular weakness in the distribution of the corresponding nerve. Many of the rheumatic diseases that cause mononeuritis multiplex may also be associated with a peripheral polyneuropathy or a multifocal mononeuropathy.[201] A number of nerves are affected in different locations in the lower extremity. Careful physical examination allows for the differentiation of spinal root from peripheral nerve lesions. Specific areas of sensory loss are characteristic of individual peripheral nerve lesions such as meralgia paresthetica and ilioinguinal syndrome. A complete listing of lower extremity tunnel syndromes is presented in Table 16-2.

Femoral Neuropathy. The femoral nerve, the largest branch of the lumbar plexus, arises from the posterior divisions of the L2, L3, and L4 nerve roots (Fig. 16-1). The nerve emerges through the lower lateral border of the psoas muscle and descends along the line of junction of the psoas and iliacus muscles. The nerve supplies innervation to these muscles, runs with them under the inguinal ligament, and enters the femoral triangle, at which point it divides into superficial and deep branches. The superficial branch supplies cutaneous innervation to the anterior thigh and medial aspect of the lower leg. The deep branches innervate the rectus femoris, pectineus, vastus lateralis, vastus medialis, and vastus internus and the knee joint and its medial ligament. In its course from the spine to the leg, the nerve is at greatest risk for compression in the iliac fossa, where it is included in a fascial compartment.

Patients with femoral neuropathy have deep pain that radiates into the flank, low back, and groin. Burning dysesthesias may also be felt in the cutaneous distribution of the nerve in the thigh and lower leg. Muscle weakness is manifested by weakness in hip flexion and loss of the patellar reflex. In pure femoral neuropathy, the patellar reflex is abolished while the adductor reflex is preserved. There are many causes for femoral neuropathy secondary to compression, traction, or direct injury to the nerve (Table 16-3). The most common cause of femoral neuropathy is diabetes.[43]

Femoral neuropathy may also be caused by bleeding disorders. In hemophilia, 75% to 80% of episodes of nerve compression are caused by bleeding into muscles.[61,117]

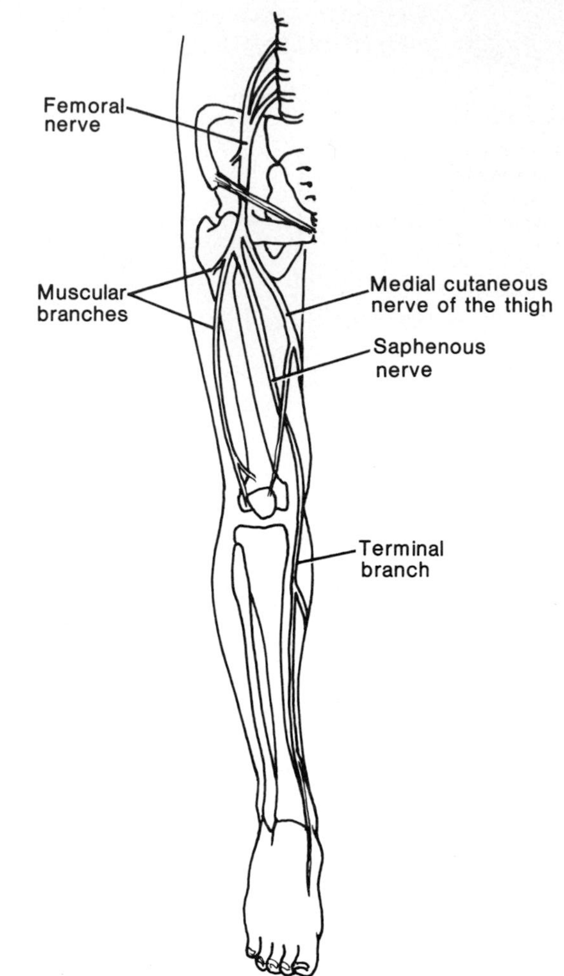

Figure 16-1 Femoral nerve. The nerve supplies hip flexors proximally and the cutaneous structures of the medial aspect of the lower leg distally.

16-2 COMPRESSION NEUROPATHIES OF THE LOWER EXTREMITY

Syndrome	Nerve	Location of Compression	Clinical Manifestations
Lumbosacral tunnel	L5 nerve root	Iliolumbar ligament	L5 dysesthesias
Iliacus/femoral	Femoral nerve (L2, L3, L4)	Iliopectineal arch	Iliopsoas weakness (hip flexion); patellar reflex; dysesthesias: medial lower leg
Obturator	Obturator (L2, L3, L4)	Obturator tunnel	Dysesthesias: medial thigh, posterior knee; leg adductor weakness (partial)
Piriformis	Sciatic (L4-S3)	Sciatic notch	Sciatica; Freiberg's sign +; gluteal muscle atrophy, distal leg muscles
Meralgia paresthetica	L2, L3 nerve roots (lateral femoral cutaneous nerve)	Inguinal ligament, fascia lata	Dysesthesias: anterolateral thigh
Ilioinguinal	L1 nerve root	Transversus abdominis muscle	Dysesthesias: scrotum, labia, inguinal ligament
Saphenous	Femoral (cutaneous)	Adductor canal mid thigh	Dysesthesias: medial lower leg
Common peroneal	Peroneal (L4-S2)	Fibular head	Dysesthesias: lateral lower leg, dorsal foot; foot weakness dorsiflexion
Superficial peroneal	Peroneal (L4-S1)	Crural fascia mid lower leg	Dysesthesias: dorsal foot; foot weakness eversion
Deep peroneal	Peroneal (L5-S1)	Dorsal pedis fascia; anterior tarsal tunnel	Dysesthesias: dorsum great and second toes; weakness great toe extension
Tarsal tunnel	Tibial (L5-S1)	Medial malleolus	Dysesthesias: medial plantar foot; weakness intrinsic foot flexors

16-3 ETIOLOGY OF FEMORAL NEUROPATHY

Diabetes mellitus
Bleeding disorders
  Inherited
    Hemophilia
  Iatrogenic
    Anticoagulants
  Acquired
    Ruptured aneurysm
Retroperitoneal tumors
  Benign
  Malignant
Surgical
  Leg traction
  Thermal injury
Femoral hernia
Postanesthetic
Idiopathic

About 35% of hemophilic neuropathies involve the femoral nerve or lumbar plexus secondary to a psoas hematoma. Iatrogenic forms of bleeding secondary to anticoagulant therapy may also cause femoral neuropathy or lumbar plexus compression. Bleeding occurs in the iliopsoas.[33,63] If bleeding occurs in the buttock, sciatica from sciatic nerve compression can occur.[212] A differentiation of the location of bleeding can be made in that bleeding into the psoas muscle causes hip muscle paralysis as well as quadriceps weakness. Sensory loss involves the anterior thigh, medial leg, medial upper thigh, and anterolateral thigh, corresponding to the femoral, saphenous, obturator, and lateral femoral cutaneous nerves, respectively.[63] Hemorrhage into the iliacus muscle, which affects the femoral nerve alone, results in quadriceps weakness. Hemorrhage may occur spontaneously in rare circumstances.[168] Iliacus hematoma may occur as a complication of hip arthroplasty.[98] The development of femoral nerve palsy is more likely related to the complexity of the hip replacement surgery (e.g., previous surgery, defect in acetabulum) as opposed to the degree of limb lengthening.[60] Femoral neuropathy has also been a rare complication at 8 weeks after a posterior spinal decompression surgery.[230] Although some have suggested fasciotomy to relieve nerve compression, most allow healing to occur without surgical intervention.[61,193,212,300] It is also important to remember that femoral neuropathy and psoas weakness may be a sign of a ruptured abdominal aneurysm (Fig. 16-2).[204]

Other causes of femoral neuropathy include retroperitoneal masses. These may be benign, such as appendiceal or renal abscesses, or malignant, such as retroperitoneal lymphoma or metastatic lesions.[20,192] Femoral nerve palsies also occur secondary to leg traction during orthopedic procedures, to thermal injuries during hip replacement, or to bleeding from a bone biopsy site.[290,291]

Hernias may also be associated with femoral neuropathy. This occurs more commonly with femoral hernias. The repair of hernias and other pelvic operations have been associated with postoperative femoral nerve palsies.[139,174,248]

Patients with femoral neuropathy must be evaluated for the possibility of an L3–L4 disc herniation. This lesion is uncommon compared with lesions at the L4–L5, and L5–S1 intervertebral disc interspaces. However, it is a lesion that is easily overlooked unless the possibility is kept in the differential diagnosis. Careful physical examination (hip and knee weakness or knee weakness alone) helps localize the area of compression. When there is doubt, CT

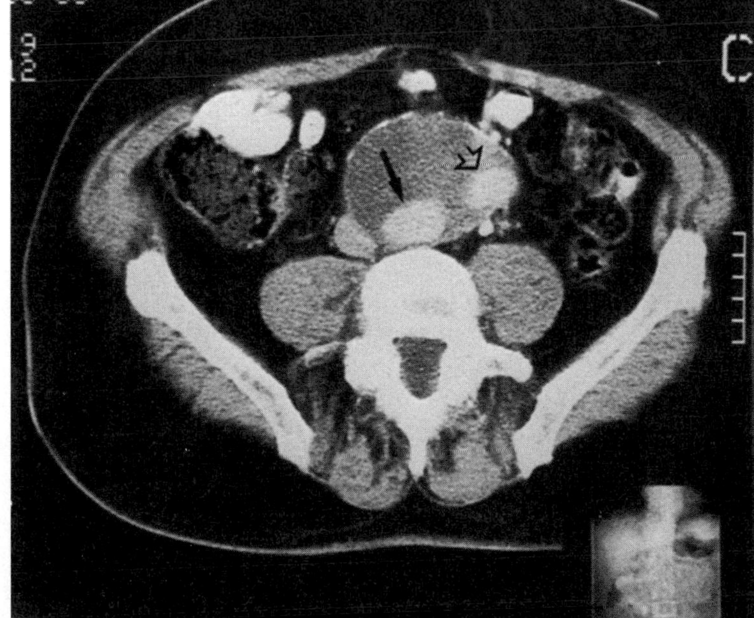

Figure 16-2 Abdominal aneurysm. CT scan with contrast dye reveals the aorta *(black arrow)* and left iliac artery *(open arrow)* involved with an expanding aneurysm. This is a patient at risk of developing rupture, retroperitoneal bleeding, and femoral neuropathy.

scan of the retroperitoneum is very helpful in identifying anatomic abnormalities.

Femoral neuropathy resolves spontaneously in most circumstances. The degree of axonal loss in the nerve is most closely associated with the eventual course of the neuropathy.[145] Axonal loss of less than 50% was associated with improvement within 1 year in 65% of patients. Fewer than 50% had improvement if femoral axonal loss was more than 50%.

Piriformis Syndrome. The piriformis muscle arises from the pelvic surface of the second, third, and fourth sacral vertebrae. The muscle is directed toward the greater sciatic foramen and inserts into the upper border and medial side of the greater trochanter of the femur. The sciatic nerve, which arises from L4-S3 nerve roots, passes over the lower edge of the sciatic notch and lies just beneath the piriformis muscle and just above the obturator internus muscle (Fig. 16-3). Branches of the sciatic nerve that supply the gluteus medius and minimus and tensor fasciae latae separate from the nerve before the main branch travels beneath the piriformis muscle. The sciatic nerve continues down the leg to supply innervation to the hamstring and muscles of the lower leg along with sensory innervation of the leg and foot. Any disease process that irritates the piriformis muscle will cause it to contract, compressing the sciatic nerve against the obturator internus and the sharp edge of the greater sciatic notch. Trauma to the buttock may result in scar formation that involves the sciatic nerve and piriformis muscle.[18] Patients with piriformis syndrome have sciatic pain that radiates down the leg to the foot, following the course of the sciatic nerve but in no specific dermatome. Females may experience dyspareunia. Both sexes may develop a limp with dragging of the lower leg on the affected side.[205,299] The pain associated with the piriformis syndrome is referred to as "pseudosciatica." The straight leg–raising test is usually negative. The patient may have sciatic notch tenderness. The characteristic test that is positive in the patient with piriformis syndrome is re-creation of pain with internal rotation of the hip (Freiburg's sign).[79] (The piriformis is a lateral rotator of the hip.) Internal rotation puts stretch on the muscle and causes reflex pain and spasm. A more consistent positive finding is pain and weakness on resisted abduction and external rotation of the thigh. Rectal examination also may identify the increased tone in the affected muscles.

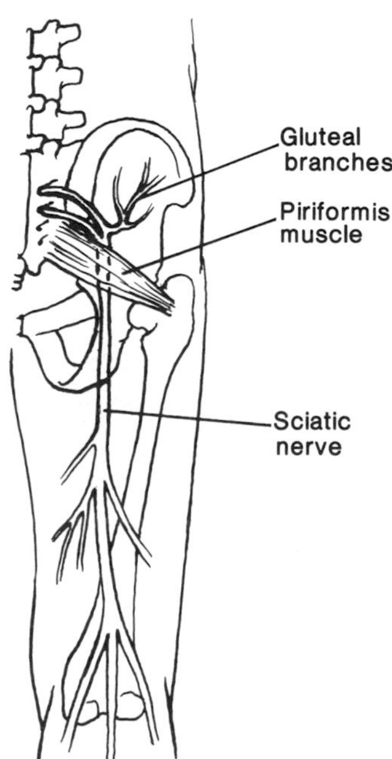

Figure 16-3 Piriformis syndrome. The piriformis muscle originates from the sacrum and inserts on the medial side of the greater trochanter of the femur. Spasm of the piriformis muscle will affect motor and sensory supply to the lower extremity but will spare the proximal gluteal muscles.

EMG of the upper sciatic muscles (gluteal, tensor fasciae latae) and paraspinous lumbosacral muscles will be normal, whereas EMG of those below the piriformis muscle may show mild denervation potentials. These findings are consistent with an entrapment neuropathy of the upper sciatic nerve. Abnormal H-reflex may be noted when forcible pressure is placed on the sciatic nerve with internal rotation of an affected limb in an adducted, flexed position.[75] The abnormal H-reflex in the hip flexed, adducted, and internally rotated position is sensitive and specific for the piriformis syndrome.[74] CT or MR may identify soft tissue enlargement of the piriformis muscle on the lateral wall of the pelvis.[122,234]

Therapy for the piriformis syndrome is bed rest, analgesic medications, and anti-inflammatory drugs. Injection of the piriformis muscle is difficult to do and is rarely done. Caudal injection of an anesthetic and corticosteroids may be of value because the medication diffuses along the nerve root sleeves to the proximal portion of the sciatic nerve.[187] Preliminary studies have reported the benefit of botulinum toxin A injections compared with corticosteroid and placebo injections for piriformis syndrome.[73] A dose of 100 units of botulinum toxin type A intramuscularly improves pain to a greater degree than a saline injection.[41] Section of the piriformis by surgical means is rarely indicated. In a study of 918 patients with piriformis syndrome, only 6.47% had surgical intervention.[74] Anatomic variations in the location of the sciatic nerve in the piriformis may make surgical intervention less effective.[253] However, sectioning of the piriformis muscle at its tendinous origin causes little functional loss and may relieve sciatic symptoms.[284]

Piriformis syndrome may complicate the symptoms of patients with other disease processes. Abnormalities of the inferior gluteal artery are associated with piriformis syndrome.[207] Disorders that cause inflammation of the sacroiliac joints may irritate the origin of the muscle and cause "pseudosciatica." Patients with spondyloarthropathy may be prone to the development of this disorder. The following case report illustrates the difficulty of diagnosing piriformis syndrome:

Case Study 16-1

A 26-year-old man with ankylosing spondylitis (AS) was referred for evaluation of persistent right leg pain. The diagnosis of AS was made on the basis of a history of sacroiliac (SI) joint pain, morning stiffness, and bilateral sacroiliitis on plain roentgenograms of the pelvis. The patient required indomethacin therapy at a dose of 75 mg/day on an intermittent basis. The patient stopped his medicine and within a few months developed bilateral low back pain, more severe on the right, with radiation of pain down the leg to the foot. His physical examination by his family physician revealed bilateral SI joint pain, a negative straight leg–raising test, and no sensory or motor abnormalities. The patient underwent an evaluation for a herniated disc, including CT scan and myelogram, which was unrevealing for disc pathology. Evaluation by the rheumatologist at the time of his referral for continued back and leg pain revealed bilateral SI joint percussion tenderness, positive Faber tests, increased pain with internal rotation of the right hip, and increased pain with palpation of the right lateral wall of the rectum on rectal examination. A diagnosis of AS with piriformis syndrome was made and the patient started on indomethacin 75-mg slow-release capsules twice a day. Within 4 weeks, the leg pain resolved and the SI joint symptoms were remarkably improved.

Other Lower Extremity Peripheral Neuropathies

Obturator Neuropathy. *Obturator neuropathy* occurs secondary to an obturator hernia or osteitis pubis. Patients develop groin pain that radiates to the medial thigh. Physical examination reveals weakness of the thigh adductors. Atrophy of the muscles is not seen, since the adductor magnus and longus may receive innervation from the sciatic and femoral nerves, respectively. Patients with adductor weakness will have an increased lateral swing to their gait associated with the unopposed action of the thigh abductors. If oral medications are ineffective, obturator nerve block may be performed. Surgical neurolysis is effective treatment for those who fail medical therapy.[25]

Meralgia Paresthetica. *Meralgia paresthetica* is compression of the lateral femoral cutaneous nerve. A number of disorders are associated with the development of meralgia paresthetica (Table 16-4).[214] Meralgia paresthetica can be a complication of hip surgery, abdominal aneurysm, and abdominal surgery.[137a] Middle-aged, obese men are more commonly affected.[263] The nerve may be compressed near the inguinal ligament, the aponeurotic expansion of the sartorius muscle, or at its emergence from the iliac fascia. Patients have symptoms of numbness manifest as paresthesias in the anterolateral thigh.[94] Physical examination reveals numbness in the distribution of the nerve (see Fig 16-4). Individuals who have a herniated disc at L2-L3 may have symptoms that mimic meralgia paresthetica. An MR evaluation is indicated if individuals do not improve with medical therapy.[278] Treatment in the form of weight reduction can be helpful. Most patients have resolution of the syndrome without the need for injection or decompression of the nerve. Surgical decompression is indicated if medical therapies (NSAIDs, local analgesic injections, removal of constrictions) are ineffective.[119] Surgical intervention is less successful if compression has been present longer than 18 months.[163]

16-4 ETIOLOGY OF MERALGIA PARESTHETICA

Retroperitoneal hematoma, tumor, metastasis
Iliopsoas muscle abscess
Abdominal aortic aneurysm
Abdominal/inguinal surgery
Direct injury, stretching, scar formation
Iliac graft harvest
Seat belt trauma
Tight clothing
Obesity
Abnormal path through muscles
Weight loss

Modified from Pecina MM, Krmpotic-Nemanic J, Markiewitz AD: Tunnel Syndromes: Peripheral Nerve Compression Syndromes, 3rd ed. Boca Raton, FL, CRC Press, 2001, p 313.

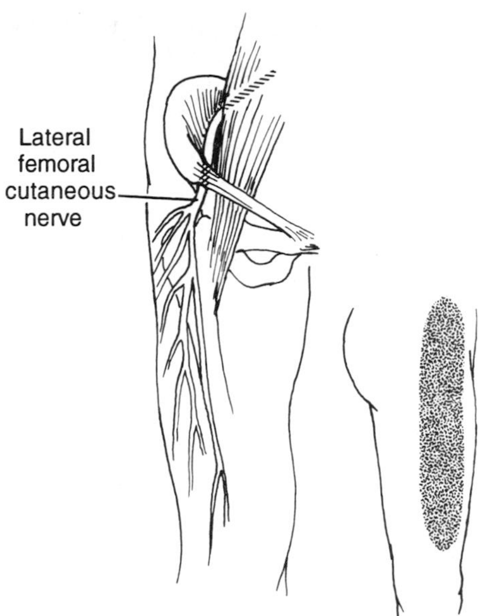

Figure 16-4 Meralgia paresthetica. The lateral femoral cutaneous nerve supplies the cutaneous structures of the lateral thigh. An area from the inguinal ligament to the knee may be affected.

Ilioinguinal Syndrome. *Ilioinguinal syndrome* is associated with pain in the inguinal region above the inguinal ligament (Fig 16-5). The nerve is compressed in the transversus

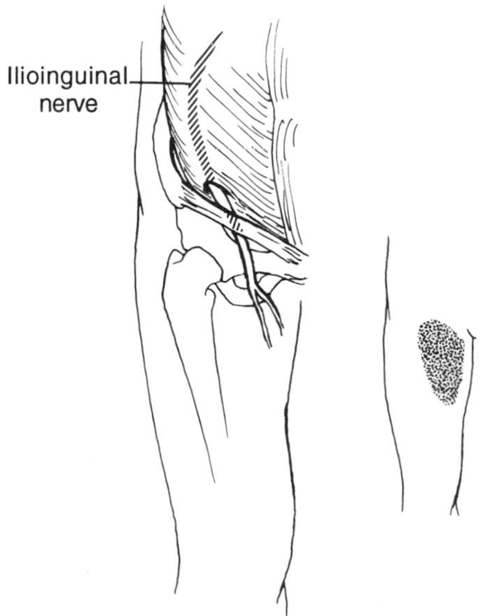

Figure 16-5 Ilioinguinal syndrome. The ilioinguinal nerve lies within the transversus abdominis and emerges below the inguinal ligament. An area near the medial thigh near the genitalia is affected.

abdominis muscle. Patients may develop this syndrome after repair of an inguinal hernia or blunt abdominal trauma.[257] Laparoscopic hernia repair is commonly associated with ilioinguinal compression if care is not given to placement of mesh and surgical clips.[256] Injection of a trigger point medial and below the anterior-superior iliac spine is diagnostic and therapeutic for this syndrome.[141]

Iliohypogastic Syndrome. The iliohypogastic nerve originates from L1 and supplies the skin over the gluteus medius, tensor fascia latae, rectus abdominis, and inguinal ligament and symphysis. Abdominal wall weakness may be exacerbated in the standing position. Athletes may develop groin pain related to iliohypogastric entrapment in the external oblique aponeurosis. Local injection and posture modification are helpful in resolving symptoms. Surgical repair of the aponeurosis may result in improvement in groin pain in those who fail medical mangement.[302]

Genitofemoral Syndrome. The genitofemoral nerve passes through the psoas muscle and branches into the femoral branch and genital branch supplying the skin over the medial thigh, scrotum/labia, and abdominal wall below the inguinal ligament. Surgical removal of the nerve is associated with a poorer prognosis than resection of the ilioinguinal or iliohypogastric nerves.[153]

Cutaneous Femoris Posterior Nerve Syndrome. The cutaneous femoris posterior nerve is a cutaneous nerve innervating the distal part of the gluteal region, perineum, labia majora, scrotum, and the posterior part of the thigh to the knee.[214] The nerve originates from the posterior surface of the sacral plexus and travels through the piriformis muscle in the infrapiriformis foramen, between the biceps femoris and semitendinosus muscles, supplying the posterior thigh. Compression of the nerve causes burning similar to meralgia paresthetica. Sensory loss may occur after intragluteal injections.[276] Treatment consists of avoiding sitting for a long time, physical therapy, and injections.

Saphenous Nerve. The saphenous nerve is a purely sensory nerve and is the longest cutaneous branch of the femoral nerve. *Entrapment of the saphenous nerve* causes pain along the medial aspect of the knee and lower leg. The nerve is frequently compressed in the adductor canal. Electrodiagnostic testing can distinguish between femoral, obturator, and saphenous nerve compression.[32a] Injection into the adductor canal provides improvement in 80% of patients with saphenous nerve compression.[231]

Common Peroneal Nerve. Lesions of the lower leg include involvement of the common peroneal nerve. *Compression of the common peroneal nerve* is associated with footdrop with weakness of ankle dorsiflexion or eversion. Involvement of the common peroneal nerve occurs more frequently than selective disease of the deep or superficial peroneal nerve. Paresthesias may be noted over the dorsum of the foot if the common nerve is compressed in the fibular tunnel.[52] The similarities in clinical symptoms between L5 radiculopathy and common peroneal compression may be differentiated by EMG studies.[128]

Tarsal Tunnel Syndrome. The extensions of the tibial nerve and medial and lateral plantar nerve pass around the medial malleolus at the ankle, through a fibro-osseous tunnel, the tarsal tunnel. The nerves supply sensation to the heel and plantar surface of the foot. Compression of the nerves in the tarsal tunnel results in burning pain, numbness, and dysesthesias. The pain is worse at night and with prolonged standing. Tinel's sign over the tunnel is a more constant objective finding of the compression. Maximal eversion and dorsiflexion of the ankle while passively dorsiflexing the toes exacerbates symptoms in those with surgically proven tarsal tunnel syndrome.[137] Compression may occur with inflammatory (rheumatoid arthritis) and noninflammatory (ganglion) lesions.[188]

Conservative management with splinting oral medications and local injections are helpful. Surgical decompression is indicated and successful in patients who fail conservative management.[12,280]

Diabetic Neuropathy. *Diabetic neuropathy* describes a heterogeneous and often overlapping group of neuropathic syndromes associated with diabetes mellitus. The absolute prevalence of neuropathy in diabetes is not known, but at time of diagnosis 8% of patients have signs of neurologic dysfunction and electrophysiologic abnormalities are encountered in 100% of patients.[78] The prevalence of physical signs of neurologic disease increases with longer duration of the disease.[35] The pathogenesis of diabetic mononeuropathies is ischemia of the nerve. Multiple infarctions of the femoral nerve and other peripheral nerves were demonstrated by Raff and Asbury.[221] Pathologic evaluation of the nerves demonstrated thickening and hyalinization of the arteriolar capillary walls, leading to luminal narrowing of nutrient vessels, with resultant discrete ischemic lesions. The pathogenesis of symmetric diabetic neuropathy is related to a deficiency of myoinositol, a sugar alcohol that has a myriad of biochemical effects on peripheral nerves resulting in decreased oxygen uptake, decreased high-energy phosphates, decreased glutathione, and increased oxygen-derived free radicals and membrane peroxidation. The end result of these biochemical abnormalities is slowed conduction.[91] Depletion of peripheral nerve myoinositol results in alterations of phosphoinositide metabolism that reduces protein kinase C–mediated Na^+/K^+-ATPase activity. The decrease in Na^+/K^+-ATPase activity results in impairment of nerve conduction velocity.[90] Therefore, myoinositol abnormalities in peripheral nerves seem to play a role in the pathogenesis of diabetic mononeuropathies. The nerves most commonly affected by mononeuropathy are those anatomically exposed to external mechanical compression. In patients with peripheral mononeuropathy, the nerve may be sensitized to the noxious effects of compression by the abnormality in carbohydrate metabolism. Most diabetic mononeuropathies are reversible over time with strict control of glucose metabolism, diminished compression of the nerve (removal of tight garments), and analgesics for pain.

Diabetic Radiculopathy. Other forms of diabetic neuropathy that might be confused with femoral neuropathy include diabetic radiculopathy and diabetic amyotrophy. *Diabetic radiculopathy* is associated with the acute onset of radicular pain in an older patient, whose pain is worse at night. The trunk and areas supplied by the upper lumbar nerve roots are affected. The upper extremities are involved less frequently. In a study of 60 patients with diabetic lumbosacral radiculoplexopathy, 9 had upper extremity involvement.[132] The pain may be confused with pain of pulmonary, cardiac, or gastrointestinal origin. The relationship of pain with physical activities, such as Valsalva maneuver, is variable. Patients may have a history of weight loss of 15 to 40 pounds. The pain does not cross the midline. Physical examination reveals dysesthesia and a loss of muscle tone. Involvement may include the intercostal and abdominal muscles. The diagnosis is confirmed by nerve conduction and EMG studies. This form of neuropathy, like the mononeuropathy, resolves spontaneously. The period of time of resolution may be as long as 2 years.[8]

Diabetic Amyotrophy. *Diabetic amyotrophy*, or proximal motor neuropathy, is a rare form of proximal muscle weakness that affects men between 50 and 60 years of age with new-onset or mild diabetes.[266] Neurologic symptoms begin after a period of weight loss followed by severe thigh pain.[42] The pain is also experienced in the low back and hip. It is unilateral and radiates down the leg. The pain may be confused with that associated with a lumbar disc or hip disease. The pain has a burning, causalgic component with dysesthesias of the overlying skin. Simultaneously, the patient develops increasing weakness and wasting of the proximal muscles of one leg, then the other. In a study of 17 patients, 14 (82%) had unilateral involvement that became bilateral over a 3-day to 8-month period.[13] Involvement of the quadriceps, iliopsoas, and adductors of the thigh is common.[8,53] Walking becomes increasingly difficult. Physical examination reveals wasting and weakness of the proximal thigh muscle that does not conform to any one nerve root or peripheral nerve. Scapulohumeral and lumbar spinal muscles are affected rarely and to a lesser degree. The straight leg–raising test is normal, and hip motion is unrestricted. Reflexes are reduced if the corresponding muscle is weak from the disease. Laboratory abnormalities include increased CSF protein and abnormal EMG findings consistent with denervation. Biopsy studies have identified inflammatory vascular infiltrates.[133,161] The usual course of the illness is progressive over the first 6 months, followed by a partial and variable recovery over the subsequent 2- to 3-year period. Strict glucose control is recommended, although proof of improvement of amyotrophy with glucose control is lacking.[62] The weakness and pain remit during the same time frame.[8] The pain associated with diabetic neuropathy and amyotrophy may improve with carbamazepine, 300 mg three times a day.[235] Other drugs, which may be helpful but have not been tested in double-blind studies, include trazodone and doxepin.[146] Amitriptyline and fluphenazine were helpful in controlling pain associated with diabetic neuropathy in one study.[48] However, a more recent small double-blind study of the same drugs demonstrated no greater improvement from these drugs than from placebo.[178]

Aldose reductase inhibitors, drugs that limit the conversion of glucose to sorbitol in nerves, are a new class of agents that may improve nerve conduction velocities and diminish pain associated with diabetic neuropathy. The accumulation of sorbitol and its conversion to fructose is thought to play a role in the pathogenesis of diabetic neuropathy. Aldose reductase inhibitors (e.g., sorbinil) have been reported to decrease neuropathic pain in diabetic patients.[65] However, the inefficacy and toxicity of aldose reductase inhibitors including sorbinil, ponalrestat, and tolrestat have limited the utility of these agents for diabetics with neuropathy.[87] A new aldose reductase inhibitor, fidarestat, has demonstrated some initial improvement in patients with diabetic neuropathy.[118] The full risk-benefit comparison for this agent remains to be determined.

In patients with diabetic or other peripheral neuropathies (traumatic, compressive, post-herpetic), the oral administration of mexiletine, a class IB antiarrhythmic agent, is helpful in decreasing neuropathic pain that is resistant to conventional therapies of glucose control, antidepressants, anticonvulsants, and NSAIDs. Mexiletine at doses between 150 to 900 mg in two or three divided doses per day is required. Patients with congestive heart failure may have difficulty with this agent secondary to worsening of their cardiac condition.[50]

Cervical Spine

Neurologic disorders most commonly involved with the cervical spine are also radiculopathies associated with alterations of cervical intervertebral discs (herniation) and the spinal canal (spinal stenosis with myelopathy). These entities are discussed in Chapter 10. Patients with a herniated disc or myelopathy may have neck pain as part of their symptom-complex, but more prominently they have symptoms that affect the upper extremities. The involvement of the arms follows a specific pattern that correlates with motor and sensory abnormalities associated with dysfunction of a specific nerve root.

Distal to the neural foramen, spinal nerve roots from multiple levels form trunks that are incorporated into the cervical and brachial plexi (see Fig. 5-5). Pathologic processes that affect nerves distal to the spinal cord have a distribution not as a single root but as a peripheral nerve with abnormalities in cutaneous or muscular structures innervated by multiple nerve root segments.

Spinal Nerves

Spinal nerve roots become spinal nerves as they leave the spinal canal and lose their dural covering. Spinal nerves may continue as individual nerves or coalesce to form plexi. Different clinical syndromes are produced by problems affecting different segments of the spinal nerves. In the cervical area, paravertebral tumors may damage spinal nerves before they form the brachial plexus.

Pancoast's Syndrome. Pancoast's syndrome (superior sulcus tumor) arises near the pleural surface at the apex of the lung. The source of tissue for Pancoast's tumor is bronchopulmonary in origin. This tumor may grow outward and posteriorly into the paravertebral space and posterior chest wall.[209] Pancoast's syndrome occurs as the tumor extends posteriorly toward the costovertebral joints, invading the sympathetic nerve chain (stellate ganglion) and the spinal roots proximal to the brachial plexus from C8 to T3.[151] Because Pancoast's tumor involves extraspinal nerve roots in the paravertebral gutter proximal to the brachial plexus, clinical syndromes associated with individual cervical nerve root dysfunction are compatible with Pancoast's tumor.[286] Other structures that may be involved less frequently include the lower trunk of the brachial plexus, subclavian artery and vein, internal jugular vein, phrenic nerve, vagus nerve, common carotid artery, and recurrent laryngeal nerve. Tumors may also invade the first three ribs, the transverse processes of C7 through T3. Further invasion results in compromise of the bone surrounding the spinal canal and eventual compression of the spinal cord.[15] Pancoast's tumor comprises 3% of all lung cancers.[301] This tumor is the most common malignancy to invade the brachial plexus.[286] The condition occurs most commonly in smokers. In one study, 49 of 51 patients with Pancoast's tumor were smokers.[251]

The clinical syndrome associated with this tumor includes aching pain in the shoulder of 90% of patients, followed by upper anterior chest wall pain and medial scapular pain posteriorly.[286] Subsequently, pain and numbness develop down the medial aspect of the lower arm and hand (C8 and T1). The arm may become discolored or edematous.[181] Motor weakness and wasting of intrinsic hand muscles occur with further compression. Invasion of the sympathetic ganglia results in decreased autonomic function, with increased warmth of the appendage (without perspiration) and Horner's syndrome. The presence of Horner's syndrome associated with dysfunction of the entire plexus and a primary lung tumor suggests epidural involvement.[264] Movement of the arm may cause muscle spasm and radiating arm pain with lower arm paresthesias. Reflex sympathetic dystrophy of the upper extremity has been associated with Pancoast's tumor.[51]

Radiographic evaluation of the apex of the lung with plain roentgenogram, apical lordotic view, or computed tomography (CT) is able to detect the presence of a lung lesion once the diagnosis is suspected. Plain roentgenograms in 40% of instances may show only apical thickening. Findings on plain roentgenograms include unilateral apical cap of more than 5 mm, asymmetry of both apical caps of more than 5 mm, an apical mass, or bone destruction. The tumor may grow from areas of old subpleural scarring.[151] Magnetic resonance (MR) imaging is useful for assessing the local extent of the tumor and predicting the possibility of resection of the tumor.[16]

The causes of a superior sulcus lesion include non-small cell bronchogenic carcinoma (squamous, adenocarcinoma), other primary thoracic neoplasms, metastatic lesions, infectious diseases, neurogenic thoracic outlet syndromes, and pulmonary amyloid nodules.[7] The diagnosis requires pathologic evaluation of tissue. Expectorated sputum cytologic analysis yields a diagnosis in 20% of cases. Bronchoscopy is not helpful because the lesion is peripheral in the lung. Percutaneous transthoracic needle biopsy can be accomplished with ultrasonographic or CT guidance. EMG is able to determine the presence of a radiculopathy and the location of the lesion proximal to the brachial plexus.[286] The diagnosis of Pancoast's syndrome is frequently delayed. The onset of symptoms and the determination of the correct diagnosis may take more than 7 months.[110] Other disorders confused with Pancoast's tumor include shoulder bursitis, cervical osteoarthritis, and thoracic outlet syndrome. Treatment of presumed cervical osteoarthritis or bursitis of the shoulder is not uncommon and is associated with a delay of 5 to 10 months before a correct diagnosis is made.[7]

The treatment of Pancoast's syndrome requires appropriate staging. Superior sulcus tumors are either stage IIb or stage III (a or b) in the absence of distal metastasis.[186] Therapy includes a combination of preoperative irradiation, pulmonary wedge resection of the lung, and excision of the involved chest wall and rib.[164] Mediastinoscopy should be accomplished before surgery to determine the extent of involvement of mediastinal lymph nodes.[225] The best outcome is found in those patients with complete resection of the tumor. Different median survival rates are associated with involvement of various chest structures. Factors associated with a poor prognosis include extension of the tumor to the neck; involvement of mediastinal lymph nodes, vertebral bodies, or great vessels; Horner's syndrome; and prolonged presence of symptoms. A survival of 4 months is associated with brachial plexus disease, and 7 months is associated with vertebral body invasion. Five-year survival rates for combined preoperative radiotherapy and surgical resection is 35% with a median survival of 7 to 31 months.[86] Early diagnosis is essential for the best outcome. Patients with bilateral Pancoast's tumors may survive 6 years or longer with complete resection and irradiation.[224]

Cervical Plexus

The cervical plexus is composed of the anterior primary rami of the upper four cervical nerves, the superior cervical sympathetic ganglia, the spinal accessory nerve, and the hypoglossal nerve. The plexus supplies cutaneous nerves to the lateral occipital portion of the scalp, the pinna, the angle of the jaw, the neck, the supraclavicular area, and the upper thorax. The motor branches supply the scalene, levator, sternocleidomastoid, trapezius, infrahyoid, diaphragm, and posterior vertebral muscles. The plexus forms the greater and lesser occipital, greater auricular, and supraclavicular nerves. The plexus is located behind the sternocleidomastoid and anterior to the levator muscle.

Brachial Plexus

The brachial plexus is composed of the anterior primary rami of the lower four cervical nerves and the first thoracic nerve. The upper portion supplies the supraclavicular nerve, innervating the supraspinatus and infraspinatus muscles. The lateral cord forms the anterior thoracic nerve supplying the pectoralis muscle. The medial cord supplies the medial brachiocutaneous nerves. The posterior cord forms the subscapular nerve supplying the subscapular muscle, teres major, and the latissimus dorsi. The brachial plexus also receives sympathetic nerves from the lower cervical ganglia.

Tumors. Metastatic lesions of the axillary or cervical lymph nodes, causing compression or direct invasion of nerves in the neck, axilla, or upper arm, are the most common cause of neoplasms affecting the brachial plexus.[151] The pattern of involvement corresponds to the location of the nodes or the primary source of the tumor. Breast cancer causes compression of the medial cord and medial cutaneous nerves of the arm and forearm (median and ulnar) secondary to involvement of axillary nodes that compress the anteromedial aspect of the plexus. Metastatic cancer of the deep cervical nodes at the base of the neck involves the upper portion of the brachial plexus and the cervical sympathetic chain.

The clinical symptom commonly associated with tumors affecting the brachial plexus is constant, deep, boring pain with dysesthesias. The pain is predominantly in the medial aspect of the arm, forearm, and hand. Weakness in the hand, in a distribution similar to that of Pancoast's lesions, occurs with motor involvement. These lesions may be differentiated from Pancoast's tumors by the absence of paravertebral and subscapular pain and ocular sympathetic nerve abnormalities.

In a study of 100 patients with brachial plexus cancer lesions, Kori and colleagues reported 78 with metastatic disease and 22 with radiation therapy lesions.[142] Lung and breast cancer were the most frequent, causing diseases in 32 and 38 individuals, respectively. Other tumors included lymphoma, melanoma, and sarcoma. Pain was the most constant symptom in individuals with metastatic disease. Physical examination demonstrates dysesthesias in the arm and intrinsic hand muscle atrophy with lower brachial plexus lesions. MR imaging is a useful radiographic technique for identifying mass lesions adjacent to the brachial plexus.[274] MR imaging detects tumor infiltration, which helps to distinguish lesions from damage associated with exposure to radiation. MR imaging also identifies the presence of anatomic abnormalities that may cause brachial plexus dysfunction (cervical rib).[44] A latent period of 16 years has been reported in individuals who have developed brachial plexus metastatic lesions after treatment for primary breast cancer.[271] Radiation treatment is used in the area to decrease pain, but there may not be improvement in arm or hand weakness.[142]

Vasculitis. Systemic vasculitis can affect the blood vessels supplying nerves. When blood flow to a nerve is compromised, neurologic dysfunction in the form of motor or sensory loss, or both, occurs. Most often, mononeuritis multiplex is associated with this pathologic process.[108] Medium-sized arteries are most frequently associated with mononeuritis. Mononeuritis multiplex is associated with a variety of connective tissue disorders, including polyarteritis nodosa, systemic lupus erythematosus, and rheumatoid arthritis (see Table 16-1).[244] In Wegener's granulomatosis, mononeuritis multiplex affects 12% of patients.[55] The most frequently involved nerves include the median, ulnar, peroneal, and tibial.[194] Mononeuritis multiplex may affect as many as 75% of individuals with Churg-Strauss allergic granulomatosis.[157] In general, mononeuritis multiplex occurs less commonly in systemic lupus erythematosus than isolated sensory neuropathy.[11] A significant number of individuals may develop mononeuritis without an identifiable, associated connective tissue disorder. Dyck and colleagues reported that ischemic nerve lesions are located in the proximal nerve trunks of the upper arms in patients with necrotizing arteritis associated with rheumatoid arthritis.[56] The extent of lesions is throughout the length of the nerve. The areas of nerve ischemic degeneration are watershed zones of poor perfusion. Because peripheral nerves have extensive collateral circulations, vasculitis must be extensive to cause dysfunction.

Upper extremities are less frequently affected than lower extremities. Sensory abnormalities affected 5 of 35 mononeuritis patients with upper extremity symptoms versus 15 of 35 patients with lower extremity symptoms.[108] Eleven patients had both upper and lower extremity symptoms. In the upper extremities, the median (9 of 35 patients) and ulnar (9 of 35 patients) nerves were affected. Weakness in a nerve distribution occurred in the setting of a corresponding sensory loss. Motor loss affected the same number of patients with median and ulnar nerve weakness.

The clinical symptoms associated with vasculitis of a plexus or major nerve branch is sudden onset of profound weakness or paralysis of a group of muscles supplied by a major nerve and radiating, burning, aching, or shooting pain associated with dysesthesias or numbness in a matching cutaneous distribution.[201] The onset may take hours to days, but the condition is maximal at the beginning of the insult to the nerve. The damage to the nerve can be profound so that function does not return. If the damage is not complete, return of function may occur from months to a year or later. Laboratory evaluation reveals systemic factors associated with the specific form of vasculitis (rheumatoid factor—rheumatoid vasculitis; eosinophils—allergic granulomatosis) and nonspecific signs of generalized vessel inflammation (elevated erythrocyte sedimentation rate, thrombocytosis). ANCA is useful in the diagnosis of some forms of vasculitis. Antibodies directed against proteinase 3, a granular cytoplasmic pattern (c-ANCA), are most closely associated with Wegener's granulomatosis.[111] Antibodies directed against myeloperoxidase, a perinuclear pattern (p-ANCA), are associated with microscopic polyangiitis.[93,180] The CSF remains normal in most cases because the nerve lesions are extraspinal. EMG reveals denervation in the affected muscle along with slowed conduction in the corresponding nerve on nerve conduction studies. Nerve biopsies are most commonly limited to the lower extremities, primarily the sural nerve. Upper extremity biopsies result in neurologic deficits and are not done. Muscle biopsy is a reasonable alternative. A diagnosis may be established in 38% of patients with a muscle biopsy alone.[237] The appearance of neurologic abnormalities in the setting of vasculitis is indicative of more aggressive, potentially life-threatening disease. Patients with this condition usually require large doses of corticosteroids and immunosuppressive drugs such as cyclophosphamide.[95,185]

Radiation Therapy. Radiation therapy to the apex of the lung or neck has been reported to cause damage to the brachial plexus.[142] Patients receiving greater than 6000 rads to the brachial plexus developed signs of neurologic injury about a year after exposure. The major difficulty for the clinician in this circumstance is to distinguish plexus abnormalities from recurrent tumor. Patients with radiation damage develop neurologic dysfunction primarily in the upper portion of the brachial plexus, involving the C5, C6, or C7 roots. Radiation damage is usually painless, is associated with lymphedema of the treated arm, and is not associated with Horner's syndrome. Patients with neoplastic invasion of the brachial plexus have lower branch involvement, with arm pain, and Horner's syndrome. MR imaging is helpful in differentiating radiation injury from other forms of plexopathy. High signal intensity on T2-weighted images is indicative of fibrosis and may enhance with gadolinium 21 years after exposure.[297]

Brachial Neuritis. Neuralgic amyotrophy, or Parsonage-Turner syndrome, is a viral infection of motor nerves solely with acute onset of pain and weakness of the shoulder and arm.[279] Multiple nerve roots are affected without any sensory deficit, and it occurs most commonly in middle-aged men. The relative absence of sensory abnormalities helps differentiate this disorder from root or plexus abnormalities. The phrenic nerve with diaphragmatic paralysis is a rare finding associated with acute dyspnea.[147] Chest roentgenograms reveal an elevated diaphragm.[189] Pain is exacerbated by arm movement but is relatively unaffected by neck motion or maneuvers that increase intervertebral disc pressure. Pain of sudden onset is the initial manifestation followed by weakness in the proximal muscles of the shoulder.[46] The absence of exacerbation of symptoms with mechanical stresses helps differentiate this disorder from radiculopathy secondary to an osteophyte or herniated disc. Other examples of disorders causing plexopathy include a hereditary autosomal dominant neuropathy manifested by a long nasal bridge and upslanting palpebral fissures in association with a gene located on the distal long arm of chromosome 17(17q24-qter).[37] Immunologic-mediated mechanisms of nerve injury may play a role in postpartum neuralgic amotrophy.[152] In other patients, immune mediating mononuclear cell infiltrates have been documented in brachial plexus biopsy specimens.[265] In rare instances, acute diabetic ketoacidosis can cause severe, bilateral, asymmetrical brachial plexopathy.[239] Infective endocarditis may also be a cause.[64] No specific therapy is effective for this disorder. Treatment is chiefly supportive, with analgesics initially followed by range of motion exercises.[172] Mild weakness may persist for years.[183]

Erb's Palsy. Injury to the upper and middle trunk of the brachial plexus, affecting C5 and C6 cervical roots, causes paralysis to the deltoid, biceps, brachial, and brachioradial muscles and less often to the supraspinatus, infraspinatus, and rhomboid muscles. The arm hangs down and cannot be abducted or externally rotated; the forearm cannot be flexed or supinated. The sensory changes are more variable because of overlapping distribution. This disorder occurs secondary to excessive traction on the arm.

Dejerine-Klumpke Palsy. Injury to the lower trunk of the brachial plexus affecting the C8 and T1 roots causes paralysis to the flexors of the wrist, fingers, adductor thumb muscles, interossei, and hypothenar muscles, and, to a lesser extent, to the thumb flexors. Sensory abnormalities correspond to the distribution of the ulnar and median nerves. Causes of this syndrome are apical tumors, aneurysm of the aortic arch, fracture of the clavicle or humerus, and sudden upward traction on the arm.

Peripheral Nerve Syndromes

Peripheral nerves are the extension of the spinal nerve roots that comprise the brachial plexus. These nerves supply sensory function alone or a combination of sensory and motor function. Pathologic processes that compress (tunnel syndromes) or decrease blood flow (diabetes) to peripheral nerves are associated with neurologic symptoms of dysesthesias and muscular weakness in the distribution of the corresponding nerve. In diabetes, mononeuropathies of acute onset are located almost exclusively in the lower extremities.[221] Diabetes may increase the sensitivity of peripheral nerves to compression syndromes. Many of the rheumatic diseases that cause mononeuritis multiplex may also be associated with a peripheral polyneuropathy or a multifocal mononeuropathy. A number of nerves are affected in different locations in the upper extremity. Careful physical examination allows for the differentiation of spinal root from peripheral nerve lesions. Specific areas of sensory loss are characteristic of individual peripheral nerve lesions, such as carpal tunnel syndrome (CTS). A complete listing of upper extremity tunnel syndromes is shown in Table 16-5.

Upper Extremity Compression Neuropathies

Thoracic Outlet Syndrome. This syndrome is caused by compression of the brachial plexus and subclavian vessels as they course from the neck into the arm. The area before the division of the plexus into its component parts is called the thoracic outlet. Compression of structures in this area is called thoracic outlet syndrome and was named by Peet and colleagues in 1956.[215] The upper portion, the cervical outlet (nerve roots C5, C6, C7), and the lower portion, the thoracic outlet (subclavian vessels, C8, T1), fill this anatomic structure.[223] Depending on the location of compression, thoracic outlet syndrome patients may have symptoms associated with anterior scalene syndrome, costoclavicular syndrome, or hyperabduction syndrome (Fig. 16-6).[213]

Anterior Scalene Syndrome. The brachial plexus and subclavian artery may be compressed between the anterior and medial scalene muscles and the first rib, causing the anterior scalene syndrome. A cervical rib was thought to be the most common cause of this syndrome.[26] However, only 10% of patients who underwent surgery for thoracic outlet syndrome had a cervical rib.[3] Hypertrophy of the scalene muscles, fibrous bands, and vibration injuries are a few of the alternative reasons for this syndrome.[76,160,294]

The symptoms of this syndrome are related to compression of the lower roots of the brachial plexus on the first rib. Symptoms include pain in the shoulder, arm, forearm, hand, and fingers in a C8 and T1 distribution. The neck and shoulders are in a forward flexed position. Overhead activity stretches the plexus and causes compression by the scalene muscles. Tightness of the scalene muscles may produce occipital headaches.[162] Distal structures are more consistently affected with numbness in the fingers. The degree of arterial compression corresponds to the extent of ischemic changes in the hand, including mottled skin color, swelling, and ulcerations. Motor abnormalities include weakness and atrophy of the hypothenar eminence and interossei. The diagnosis is best determined by reproduction of symptoms with compression and positional provocative testing. Examples of provocative tests include Adson's test and Phalen's maneuver.[196] Adson's test stretches the scalene muscles to create neurovascular compression in the region of the first rib. Loss of pulse volume is not pathognomonic of the syndrome because 15% of normal individuals have similar findings.[49] Electrodiagnostic testing is usually normal

16-5 COMPRESSION NEUROPATHIES OF THE UPPER EXTREMITY

Syndrome	Nerve	Location	Clinical Manifestations
Thoracic outlet	C8-T1 nerve roots	Anterior scalene muscle, first rib	Hand dysesthesias
Suprascapular	Suprascapular (C5, C6)	Scapular notch	Abduction, external humeral rotation, shoulder joint capsule
Quadrilateral tunnel	Axillary (C5, C6)	Lateral axillary hiatus	Dysesthesias: shoulder joint, upper arm; deltoid weakness
Supracondylar process	Median (C6, C7, C8)	Supracondylar process (elbow)	Dysesthesias: palmar, dorsal hand; wrist, finger flexor weakness
Pronator teres tunnel	Median (C6, C7)	Pronator teres (anterior lower arm near elbow)	Dysesthesias: palmar, dorsal hand; wrist, finger flexor weakness
Radial tunnel	Radial (C5, C6, C7) (motor branch) (posterior interosseus)	Supinator (lateral elbow)	Weakness of extensors, wrist, fingers
Anterior interosseus	Median (C7, C8)	Medial forearm	Weakness of thumb, index finger flexors (motor only)
Ulnar (ulnar sulcus)	Ulnar (C7, C8)	Medial epicondyle (elbow)	Dysesthesias: ring, little fingers; weakness of finger flexors
Cubital	Ulnar (C7, C8)	Distal to epicondyle (between heads of flexor carpi ulnaris)	Dysesthesias: ring, little fingers; weakness of finger flexors
Carpal	Median (C8, T1)	Wrist	Dysesthesias: palmar surface fingers; weakness of thumb
Guyon's	Ulnar (C8, T1)	Lateral wrist, hypothenar	Dysesthesias: ring, little fingers; weakness of hypothenar eminence
Cheiralgia paresthetica	Radial (C7, C8) (superficial)	Medial thumb, forearm	Dysesthesias: dorsal wrist, thumb, web space
Collateral digital nerve	Median, ulnar (C8, T1)	Fingers	Dysesthesias: neighboring fingers

because compression changes are reversible with alteration of position. Arteriography may be considered for those patients with signs of vascular compression. Poststenotic dilatation may be found in these patients.[213] No individual test is adequate to determine the presence of this syndrome.

Primary treatment of anterior scalene syndrome is physical therapy with exercises to increase the range of motion of the neck and shoulders, strengthen the trapezius and rhomboid muscles, and improve posture. Increased tone in the shoulder muscles has the potential to reduce tension in the cervical muscles. Conservative therapy, including exercises, can be successful in the majority of patients.[136] Chemodenervation of the scalene muscles has been achieved through fluoroscopically guided selective muscle injection with botulinum toxin. In a study of 22 patients, 64% had a 50% reduction in symptoms at 1 month.[126] Transient dysphagia was a complication in 2 patients. If conservative therapy is ineffective, surgical intervention in the form of scalenotomy or rib resection may be considered. The success rate for these operations is 50% or less and is associated with risk of damage to the brachial plexus.[40,213] In a study of 45 patients with thoracic outlet syndrome treated with

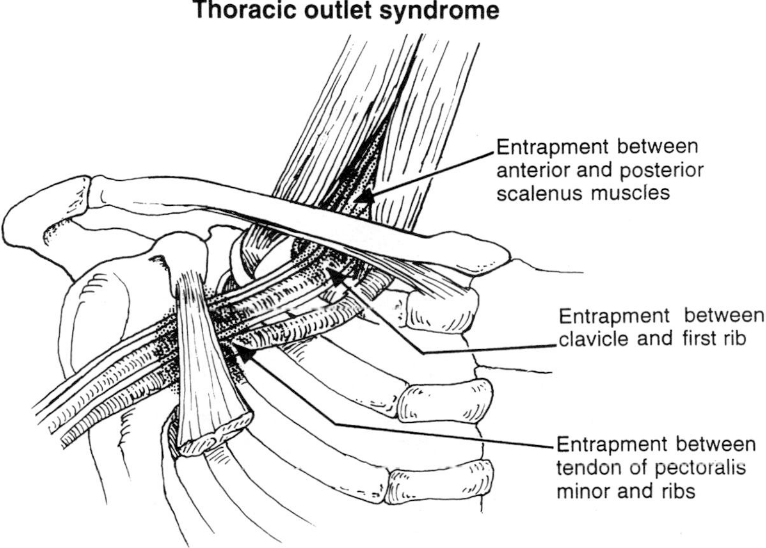

Figure 16-6 Compression of the brachial plexus and subclavian artery may occur near the anterior scalenus muscle or the costoclavicular area or under the pectoralis minor muscle.

surgery and followed for a mean of 8 years, successful outcome was reported in 43%.[158]

Costoclavicular Syndrome. Compression of the subclavian artery and vein and brachial plexus between the clavicle and the first rib causes symptoms of vascular insufficiency. The costoclavicular space is bordered by the medial third of the clavicle, the anterior third of the first rib, and insertions of the scalene muscles. The brachial plexus and subclavian artery run through this triangle, with the subclavian vein medial to the insertion of the anterior scalene muscle. Arm raising, posterior movement of the shoulder, or deep inhalation move the clavicle posteriorly in the first two instances or raise the first rib to narrow the costoclavicular space.[295]

Vascular symptoms, as opposed to neurogenic symptoms with the anterior scalene syndrome, tend to predominate and are characterized by claudication or edema. Symptoms may be exacerbated by carrying weight on the back, as in backpacking. The costoclavicular maneuver, rotating shoulders backward and downward, increases symptoms and causes a decrease in pulse volume. Control individuals may also have diminution in pulse volume.[83] Arteriography with movement of the affected shoulder may be required to determine the location of the vascular compression.[236] Helical CT shows significant narrowing of the costoclavicular space in patients with arterial stenosis as the cause of symptoms.[227] Functional imaging in an open MR scanner with the arm in abduction can document the compression of the brachial plexus.[249]

Conservative therapy with isometric shoulder girdle exercises, improved posture, and avoidance of movements of the arm above the head are useful means of decreasing symptoms. Conservative therapy should be tried for a minimum of 6 months before surgical intervention is considered. Patients with evidence of vascular insufficiency with digital ischemia may require more immediate surgical intervention.[275]

Hyperabduction Syndrome. The neurovascular bundle continues to the axilla, passing under the attachment of the pectoralis minor muscle tendon to the coracoid process. With abduction of the arm to 180 degrees, the neurovascular bundle is stretched around the tendon and humeral head.[72]

Symptoms of pain, paresthesias, and numbness develop in the fingers and then the hand. Vascular changes may resemble Raynaud's phenomenon, which has been reported in 38% of individuals with the syndrome.[19] Neurologic symptoms tend to be temporary because returning the arm to normal position resolves the pain. Hyperabduction of the arm during physical examination initiates symptoms in most patients. The Adson test and hyperabduction test, along with Doppler ultrasonography, in combination help with determining a more specific diagnosis of thoracic outlet syndrome versus alternative diagnoses.[85]

Treatment consists of avoiding hyperabduction of the arm. This may be difficult for individuals who work overhead, such as painters, bricklayers, or electricians. Operative intervention consists of dividing the pectoralis minor tendon.

The benefit of surgery for the treatment of thoracic outlet syndrome remains unclear. Reports from surgical departments using various techniques (supraclavicular approach, removal of cervical and first rib) reported benefits in a majority of patients.[171, 238] However, others reported equal success in individuals treated with nonsurgical interventions.[148] In addition, the presence of depression, marital status, and lower educational level had a detrimental effect on surgical outcome and increased disability.[10]

Carpal Tunnel Syndrome. Compression of the wrist-to-palm segment of the median nerve under the flexor retinaculum causes the clinical condition known as CTS.[233] Patients with CTS have numbness in the palmar side of the thumb and the three medial fingers, excluding the lateral half of the ring finger and the little finger (Fig. 16-7). Pain may spread proximally from the hand to the level of the shoulder. The symptoms increase at night and with movement during the day. Motor weakness occurs in the thenar eminence with more severe compression. The usual pressure in the tunnel is 7 or 8 mm Hg. In CTS, the resting pressure is 30 mm Hg, a pressure associated with nerve dysfunction.[267] Pressure may increase to 90 mm Hg with extremes of wrist motion.[49] Two-point discrimination and thenar atrophy are late findings with low sensitivity and high specificity.[131] Tinel's sign has a greater specificity than Phalen's maneuver for the diagnosis (87% vs. 60%, respectively). History and physical findings have poor predictive value particularly in workplace screening programs.

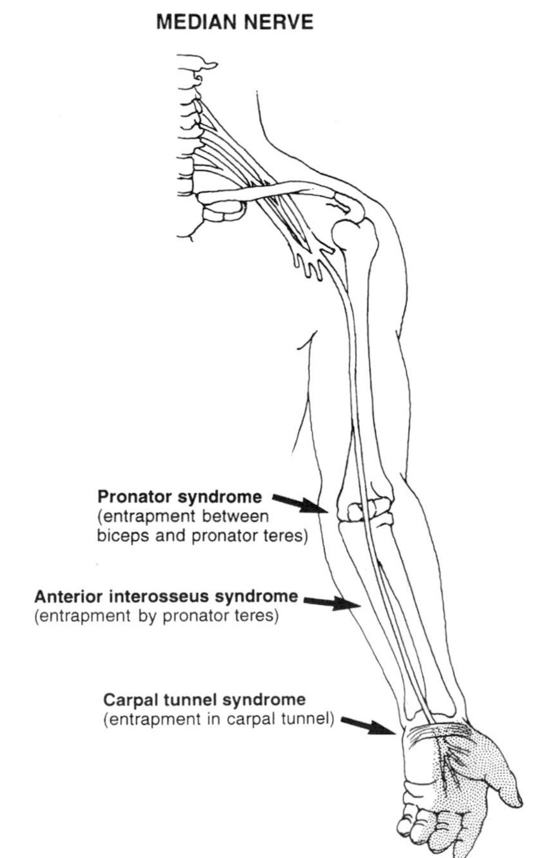

Figure 16-7 Median nerve distribution in the upper extremity. Shaded area in the hand corresponds to the area of numbness with carpal tunnel syndrome.

CTS is the most common entrapment neuropathy.[14] In a national health survey in 1988, 2.65 million of 170 million adults (1.55%) reported CTS.[268] White women were most frequently affected. In another study, an incidence of 125 per 100,000 general population was reported.[260] The incidence of CTS in workers covered by workers' compensation is 15 times that in the general population, with a greater proportion of men (60% vs. 25%) and a younger peak age at onset (37.4 years vs. 51 years).[77] Occupations with awkward wrist positions, increased force across the wrist, and repetitive hand motions have been proposed as causes of this compression syndrome. Musician, assembly line worker, and dental hygienist are a few of the occupations associated with CTS.[114,170] Overuse or repetitive motion syndromes, including CTS, account for 50% of occupational illnesses in the United States.[226] However, continued debate exists concerning the specific criteria for diagnosis of CTS and the importance of nonergonomic factors (age and obesity) on the development of symptoms.[130,191] CTS is also associated with a wide variety of medical conditions that cause swelling of the contents of the carpal tunnel, resulting in nerve compression. The idiopathic group remains the most common cause of CTS (Table 16-6).[259]

Electrodiagnostic studies in the form of median sensory and motor nerve conduction studies provide the greatest diagnostic accuracy for CTS.[120] These tests are able to differentiate upper-limb numbness caused by cervical radiculopathy, peripheral neuropathy, and entrapment syndromes. Of the electrodiagnostic tests, the predictive value of sensory conduction is greatest with the maximum latency difference.[190] Uncini and colleagues reported the difference between median and ulnar sensory latencies at digit-four stimulation being the most sensitive test for mild CTS.[281] Distal motor latency determinations are the most helpful tests for detecting severe CTS.[246] Nerve conduction and EMGs are required to determine the extent of nerve compression.[293] The sensitivity of these tests is not total. Normal studies may be found in up to 8% of patients with CTS.[21] Electrophysiologic studies are most abnormal when large myelinated fibers are damaged. Symptoms of CTS may be related to damage of smaller-diameter myelinated and nonmyelinated fibers or to a small number of large fibers to be detected by conduction tests.

Double-crush syndrome refers to the coexistence of CTS and cervical spondylosis causing a C6 radiculopathy.[203] Patients with cervical radiculopathy have pain in the neck, shoulder, arm, and hand, whereas the pain of CTS is primarily in the hand, with radiation to the shoulder but not to the neck. Pain radiating to the chest wall or the scapula suggests radiculopathy. When both lesions are present, the neurologic examination may demonstrate findings beyond those expected with pure median nerve compression, such as decrease of biceps (C6) or triceps (C7) reflexes.

Radiographic evaluation of the carpal tunnel is not necessary for diagnosis of CTS. MR imaging is able to determine a causative lesion in a minority of CTS patients.[247] MR imaging detects tenosynovitis, cysts, and aberrant muscles. Edema or enlargement of the nerve may also be detected, which may be unrecognized at time of surgery. However, MR imaging does not have greater diagnostic accuracy than electrodiagnostic tests and should be reserved for the patient who does not respond to usual treatment.

Conservative treatment with wrist splints, patient education, NSAIDs, and occasional carpal tunnel corticosteroid injection is effective therapy for the majority of patients with CTS. In a study of 265 patients, 188 (71%) improved without the need for carpal tunnel release surgery.[104] Follow-up electrodiagnostic studies obtained normal results in 72 (27%) and improvement in 106 (40%).[104] Potential indicators of poor response to conservative therapy include age greater than 50 years, duration of disease of more than 10 months, and constant paresthesias.[127] Clinical trials have demonstrated the short-term benefits of oral corticosteroids, splinting, and yoga for CTS.[198] Doses of prednisolone, 10 mg to 20 mg daily for 2 to 4 weeks, have resulted in improvement.[39] Local corticosteroid injection has greater efficacy than oral corticosteroids at 3 months after treatment.[169] Patients who have a poor response to conservative therapy and demonstrate motor weakness confirmed with electrodiagnostic tests are candidates for sectioning of the volar carpal tunnel ligament. This outpatient procedure has good to excellent improvement of symptoms in 80% to 86% of patients, with 40% regaining normal function.[47,106] In a study of 176 patients with CTS, open surgical decompression resulted in better outcomes at 18 months compared with splinting alone.[84] No particular benefit is found between the use of the usual open surgical procedure versus alternative methods, including endoscopic techniques.[242] Patients with a poor result from surgery may have had only partial sectioning of the retinaculum or they develop neural fibrosis as a complication of surgery.[27] Re-exploration of the tunnel, with internal neurolysis of the median nerve, may be required to relieve symptoms in these patients.[38,202] A thorough evaluation for concurrent conditions is required for these patients with recurrent symptoms.[261] Patients with occupations that do not require excessive use of the hands may return to work in 7 to 14 days. Patients whose

16-6 CAUSES OF CARPAL TUNNEL SYNDROME

Condition	Patients (n = 1,016) No.	%
Idiopathic	439	43.2
Associated Conditions	577	56.8
Trauma	136	13.4
Collagen vascular (rheumatoid arthritis, subacute lupus erythematosus)	66	6.5
Hormone replacement	65	6.4
Diabetes mellitus	62	6.1
Excessive hand use	60	5.9
Wrist osteoarthritis	54	5.3
Pregnancy	47	4.6
Tenosynovitis	31	3.1
Miscellaneous (tumors, amyloidosis)	25	2.5
Myxedema	14	1.4
Other (acromegaly, tuberculosis)	17	1.7

Modified from Stevens JC, Beard CM, O'Fallon WM, et al: Conditions associated with carpal tunnel syndrome. Mayo Clin Proc 67:531, 1992. By permission.

occupations involve exposure of the hands to repeated trauma (such as carpenters) may not return for months. Some people may need to change jobs because of stress to the hands.[49] Women who have CTS early in the course of pregnancy may be at risk of experiencing persistent symptoms 1 year after delivery.[208]

Other Median Nerve Syndromes. Other conditions associated with compression of the median nerve in the upper extremity include supracondylar process syndrome, pronator syndrome, and anterior interosseous syndrome.[23] The supracondylar process is an atavistic bone connected to the anteromedial surface of the distal humerus. A fibrous band (ligament of Struthers) attaches this bone to the median epicondyle. The median nerve can be compressed under this band, causing pain and paresthesias in the median nerve distribution in the hand, motor signs of decreased thumb opposition, and flexion of the first three fingers. Nerve conduction tests document slowing across the supracondylar tunnel. Pronator syndrome occurs as the median nerve leaves the cubital fossa at the elbow, passing between the heads of the pronator teres and the tendinous arch of the flexor digitorum superficialis. The test on physical examination that helps differentiate this syndrome from CTS is the absence of Phalen's sign at the wrist, Tinel's sign in the forearm, pain on resistance to pronation, and pain in the forearm on resistance to isolated flexion of the proximal joints of the long and ring fingers.[23] Anterior interosseous syndrome affects the anterior interosseous nerve, which is a pure motor branch of the median nerve that supplies the flexor pollicis longus (thumb) and flexor digitorum profundus (index finger). The nerve appears from the posterior portion of the median nerve distal to the medial humeral epicondyle and travels to the deep fascial layer to run with the interosseous membrane, ending under the pronator quadratus. Individuals are unable to pinch the thumb and index finger and are usually unable to write.[258]

Ulnar Nerve Entrapments

The ulnar nerve entrapment syndromes occur less commonly than median nerve syndromes. Ulnar nerve syndromes include ulnar nerve sulcus syndrome, cubital tunnel syndrome, and ulnar tunnel (Guyon's canal) syndrome (Fig. 16-8).

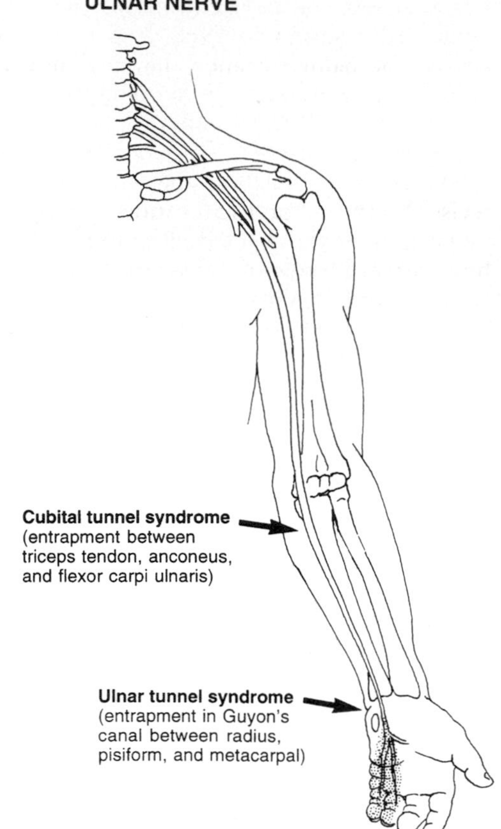

Figure 16-8 Ulnar nerve distribution in the upper extremity. Shaded area in the hand corresponds to the area of numbness with ulnar tunnel syndrome.

Ulnar Nerve Sulcus Syndrome. The ulnar nerve is compressed in the sulcus at the medial side of the distal humerus. The sulcus is covered by the epicondylo-olecranon ligament to prevent subluxation with forearm movement. Swelling of or trauma to the sulcus may result in ulnar nerve dysfunction. Pain and dysesthesias appear in the lateral aspect of the hand. Pain may also radiate to the shoulder. Further compression results in atrophy of intrinsic hand muscles, including hypothenar wasting.

Cubital Tunnel Syndrome. Cubital tunnel syndrome occurs as the ulnar nerve passes under the aponeurosis of the flexor carpi ulnaris 1.5 to 3.5 cm distal to the humeral sulcus. When the elbow is flexed, the aponeurosis becomes taut, compressing the ulnar nerve, increasing symptoms. External compression results from resting the elbow on a flat surface and may occur in anesthetized patients.[182] Patients develop pain, paresthesias, and weakness in the hand in an ulnar nerve distribution. The location of Tinel's sign helps differentiate this syndrome from the sulcus syndrome. Nerve conduction tests detect pathologic conditions near the elbow. Intrinsic hand muscles are used to determine motor velocity and the little finger for sensory abnormalities. Despite careful examination, the exact location of the lesion may not be found in up to 50% of patients.[49] The differential diagnosis for cubital tunnel syndrome includes C8–T1 radiculopathy, compression of the medial cord of the brachial plexus with Pancoast's tumor, or thoracic outlet syndrome. Conservative therapy with decreased elbow flexion and NSAIDs is only partially effective. Surgical therapy is not necessarily a preferred option because the exact location of impingement may not be identified. Splinting with or without a corticosteroid injection is associated with improved function at 6 months.[112] Surgical decompression should be reserved for individuals with disability associated with muscle weakness. Surgical intervention may include transposition of the nerve with protective muscle flap or removal of the epicondyle.[2,107] Transposition of the nerve is an effective option for those who do not have accompanying thoracic outlet syndrome.[149]

Ulnar Tunnel Syndrome. Ulnar tunnel syndrome occurs on compression of the nerve in Guyon's canal in the hand. The tunnel's floor is formed by the transverse carpal ligament and its roof by the insertion of the flexor carpi ulnaris muscle. Only the superficial and deep palmar branches of the nerve run in the ulnar tunnel. The superficial portion of the palmar branch supplies the palmaris brevis muscle, the palmar skin of the little finger, and the ulnar skin of the ring finger. The deep branch supplies the hypothenar muscles, the two lateral lumbrical muscles, the interossei muscles, the adductor pollicis, and the flexor pollicis brevis. Depending on the location of nerve injury, ulnar nerve symptoms may be mixed or purely motor in origin. The differential diagnosis between compression at the wrist or elbow of the ulnar nerve may be made by involvement of the flexor to the little finger, because this muscle is only affected by ulnar nerve compression at the elbow. Conservative therapy may be used for a 6-month trial. If symptoms persist, surgical decompression of the canal with release of sensory and motor branches is indicated.[213]

Radial Nerve Entrapments

The radial nerve may be involved in radial tunnel syndrome, posterior interosseous syndrome, and compression of the superficial branch of the radial nerve (cheiralgia paresthetica) (Fig. 16-9). The terminal motor branch of the radial nerve passes under the tendinous arch (Frohse's arcade, present in only 30% of adults) of the supinator muscle at the elbow, with the superficial sensory nerve branching proximal to the muscle.[252] The component of the radial nerve supplying the extensors of the elbow and wrist also branches before the supinator muscle so motion of these joints remains unaffected by radial tunnel syndrome.

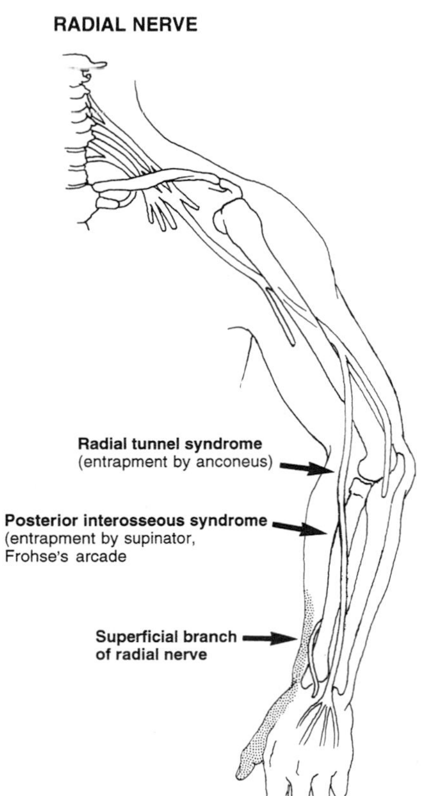

Figure 16-9 Radial nerve distribution in the upper extremity. Shaded area in the hand corresponds to the area of numbness with cheiralgia paresthetica.

Radial Tunnel Syndrome. The radial nerve may be compressed by fibrous bands in the region of the radiocapitellar joint, the radial recurrent vessels, the tendinous origin of the extensor carpi radialis brevis, the tendon of the supinator, and the distal edge of the supinator muscle. Workers who require full extension of the elbow associated with a twisted posture of the forearm to complete their work are at greater risk of developing radial tunnel syndrome.[232] Finger weakness in association with pain over the lateral epicondyle is a finding associated with this nerve entrapment. Pain may be elicited with forced resistance to middle finger extension with the wrist and elbow extended.[159] Approximately 10% of patients with radial tunnel syndrome may also have lateral epicondylitis.[292] Treatment of the entrapment includes avoidance of repetitive trauma to the nerve in the tunnel. Physical therapy, splinting, and local injections may be helpful in a majority of patients.[240] Surgical decompression of the radial tunnel along with decompression of the epicondyle is frequently done because these areas of inflammation coexist.

Posterior Interosseous Syndrome. Posterior interosseous syndrome occurs with compression of the deep branch of the radial nerve at the distal end of the supinator muscle. Patients with this entrapment have transient pain and weakness of thumb extension. Electrodiagnostic tests are able to differentiate this nerve compression from those affecting the brachial plexus or more proximal lesions of the radial nerve. This syndrome is treated in a fashion similar to that for radial tunnel syndrome. Improvement of paralysis may occur with conservative or surgical treatment.[105]

Cheiralgia Paresthetica. Cheiralgia paresthetica is caused by damage to the superficial cutaneous portion of the radial nerve supplying the dorsal skin over the wrist and the thumb and index and middle fingers to the base of the second phalanx. The superficial branch of the radial nerve passes over the supinator muscle, dips under the brachioradialis muscle, and emerges in the skin near the radial styloid. Any trauma to the radial side of the hand results in a burning sensation in the wrist, thumb, and first two fingers. A variety of traumas, including those resulting from plaster casts, watchbands, handcuffs, and intravenous infusions, may irritate the nerve. Patients present with paresthesias without motor signs. Trophic changes in the skin appendages occur if the damage is chronic and extensive. The symptoms may respond to conservative therapy, including topical agents. If scar tissue develops, reduction of tissue with neurolysis is indicated.

Other Peripheral Neuropathies

Greater Occipital Nerve (C2). The greater occipital nerve ascends through the semispinalis capitis and trapezius muscles close to their attachments to the occipital bone and travels with the occipital artery over the medial portion of the scalp to the vertex of the skull. Entrapment of this nerve causes pain over the occiput without lower neck or shoulder pain. Increased pain with flexion or extension may suggest C1–C2 joint disease as a cause of nerve irritation. Palpation over the occipital prominence frequently increases scalp pain. Conservative management in the form of exercises and oral anti-inflammatory medications may be helpful. Injection over the maximum point of tenderness near the occiput with a local anesthetic may offer temporary relief of pain.

Dorsal Scapular Nerve (C5). The dorsal scapular nerve arises from the upper trunk of the brachial plexus, primarily from C5. The nerve passes through the body of the scalenus medius muscle. The nerve approaches the levator at its anterior border, passing under the muscle and the rhomboids adjacent to the medial border of the scapula. The nerve is the sole nerve supply to the rhomboids, and it supplies the lower portion of the levator scapulae. Pain is located over the rhomboid muscle and may be associated with muscular spasm. Subjective weakness may also be noted by the patient. On examination, pain is aggravated by turning the head toward the affected extremity and by lateral flexion to the opposite side. Physical therapy for strengthening the shoulder girdle muscles is helpful in decreasing compression of the nerve. Surgical decompression is limited to those with EMG evidence of denervation of the appropriate muscles.

Long Thoracic Nerve (Bell's Nerve). The long thoracic nerve arises from roots from C5, C6, and C7 and supplies the serratus anterior muscle. The nerve passes through the scalenus medius muscle. Loss of function results in winging of the scapula. The nerve may be injured by continuous heavy effort with the arm above the shoulder or by heavy objects being carried on the shoulder.

Suprascapular Nerve. The suprascapular nerve is derived from the upper trunk of the brachial plexus (C5, C6). The nerve passes behind the brachial plexus to enter the suprascapular notch under the transverse ligament. This pure motor nerve supplies the supraspinous and infraspinous muscles. Stretching of the arm causes a deep pain that is poorly localized. The pain results in decreased motion of the shoulder. In a patient with adhesive capsulitis with decreased motion of the humerus, forward flexion of the arm causes increased stretch of the nerve under the transverse ligament, resulting in pain. Persistent injury results in weakness in abduction and external rotation of the arm, tenderness on palpation, and atrophy of the muscles. Injection in the suprascapular notch may decrease pain. Division of the transverse ligament is indicated if conservative therapy is ineffective and muscle weakness is persistent. Individuals with spinoglenoid notch cysts as the cause of suprascapular nerve compression have better outcome with surgical decompression.[6]

MISCELLANEOUS DISORDERS

Lumbar Spine

Neuropathic Arthropathy (Charcot Joints)

Neuropathic arthropathy is a joint disease that occurs secondary to a wide range of neurologic disorders with a common characteristic—diminished sensory function. Although Charcot described the relationship between joint disease and neurologic dysfunction with tabes dorsalis (syphilis), Charcot joint disease has become synonymous with any articular disorder associated with neurologic deficits.[89]

John Kearsley Mitchell, in 1831, was the first to describe vertebral column abnormalities with spinal cord disease.[184] Vertebral neuroarthropathy (Charcot spine) was first reported with syphilitic tabes dorsalis by Kronig in 1884.[34] In modern times, Charcot spine is more likely secondary to diabetes mellitus or syringomyelia.[303] Lumbar spine involvement is most commonly associated with tabes dorsalis and occasionally occurs in patients with diabetes and syringomyelia.[28,102,222] Individuals with trauma to the spinal cord that results in quadriparesis or paraplegia may also develop neuropathic changes in the spine.[254]

Epidemiology

Vertebral neuroarthropathy accounts for up to 12% of all neuropathic joints.[176] In tabetic patients, the proportion may rise to 21%.[70] The patients are between 50 and 60 years of age and the male:female ratio is 3 to 1. In the axial skeleton, the thoracolumbar and lumbar spine are most frequently affected.[176] Up to 20% of patients with neuropathic joints may have no sign of neurologic dysfunction at the time of presentation.[129]

Pathogenesis

The pathogenesis of neuropathic joint disease, regardless of the anatomic site, is the result of a combination of factors, including an absence of normal pain sensation, preservation of motor strength, repeated trauma to the anesthetic part, and damage to afferent proprioceptive neurons, that lead to joint instability and destruction.[69] The deprivation of normal protective reactions results in repeated trauma to articular constituents (neurotropic mechanism). Severe cumulative injury damages the articular cartilage, fractures subchondral bone, and disorganizes the joint. Some patients undergo rapid destruction of a joint without bone repair. The rapid resorption of bone without accompanying bone repair has been proposed as evidence for a neurovascular mechanism in the pathogenesis of Charcot joint disease.[29] In this hypothesis, neurally initiated vascular reflex mediated through the sympathetic nerves leads to increased blood flow, resulting in dissolution of bone and cartilage.[4] Proof supporting this theory is the development of Charcot joints in patients who have been immobilized with limited exposure to trauma.[195] Local microfractures lead to hyperemia and hyperactive resorption of bone. Hyperactive resorption of bone results in osteopenia. These weakened bones are then at greater risk from local fracture secondary to minor trauma. Fracturing and repair are a secondary phenomenon.

Other factors that predispose to joint destruction include chondrocalcinosis (CPPD neuropathic joints in absence of neurologic disturbance) and increased stress on subchondral bone that has stiffened as a result of healing of trabecular fractures.[71] Increased bone stiffness may hasten articular cartilage dissolution and accelerate the breakdown of Charcot joints.[109,121,220]

The pathologic findings associated with Charcot joint disease include fibrillation and erosion of articular cartilage, formation of loose bodies, and marginal osteophytes.[217] The marginal osteophytes are markedly larger than those ordinarily associated with osteoarthritis. Dense subchondral sclerosis is common. Subluxation in association with juxta-articular fractures, which may involve articular facet joints, results in formation of additional callus. Parts of osteophytes may fracture and become incorporated into the joint capsule and synovium.[116,124] These pathologic abnormalities have also been reported in the axial skeleton.[176]

The pathology of acute neuropathic joint disease reveals an intact articular surface.[4] Most of the bone directly beneath the articular cartilage is replaced by a vascular connective tissue reticulum. Remaining bone trabeculae are surrounded by numerous dilated vascular channels and are being resorbed by numerous osteoclasts. The increase in vascular channels correlates with increased vascularity noted with neuropathic lesions of the lower extremity.[59]

Neurologic disorders that cause Charcot joints may be of central (upper motor neuron) or peripheral (lower motor neuron) origin (Table 16-7). In general, central lesions and those that spare the sympathetic nervous system result in hypertrophic joint changes whereas peripheral lesions and those that affect the postganglionic sympathetic nerve fibers are more closely associated with destructive joint alterations.[228,296]

CLINICAL HISTORY

In contrast to peripheral Charcot joints, axial involvement is frequently symptomatic. The patients have pain in the low back that may radiate to the lower extremities. The source of pain is posterior nerve root compression resulting from malalignment of vertebral bodies, disc protrusion, and facet joint hypertrophy.[69] Some patients are asymptomatic or are only slightly uncomfortable, and the diagnosis of these patients is made as an incidental finding on roentgenographic evaluation of the lumbosacral spine.[222]

16-7 CHARCOT ARTHROPATHY[242]

CENTRAL (UPPER MOTOR NEURON)

Trauma
Syringomyelia
Meningomyelocele
Syphilis (tabetic)
Multiple sclerosis
Congenital vascular anomalies
Charcot-Marie-Tooth syndrome[30]
Cervical myelopathy (compression)
Arachnoiditis
Diabetes
Tuberculosis
Pernicious anemia

PERIPHERAL (LOWER MOTOR NEURON)

Diabetes[303]
Alcoholism
Infections (leprosy)
Trauma
Pernicious anemia[99]
Corticosteroids

UNKNOWN

Congenital insensitivity to pain[273]
Familial dysautonomia[32]

PHYSICAL EXAMINATION

Physical examination reveals kyphosis, scoliosis, sensory disturbances, and lack of local tenderness. Neurologic dysfunction is discovered in those patients with nerve impingement secondary to extradural compression of the spinal cord associated with marked destruction of the vertebral column.

RADIOGRAPHIC EVALUATION

Roentgenographic abnormalities may occur solely in the spine or in combination with peripheral lesions. Axial neuropathy is limited to one to three contiguous vertebral bodies and is characterized by either marked sclerosis or destruction (lysis). Associated with this appearance of the vertebrae is fragmentation of bone with compression of vertebral bodies and discs, bony debris in the paravertebral soft tissues, and subluxation. Kyphoscoliosis is associated with facet joint involvement. The atrophic, or resorbed, lesions of the spine are a diagnostic problem. These lesions may be mistaken for a rampant infection or an aggressive bone tumor. There is extensive bone resorption with no evidence of accompanying bone repair. There is a sharp zone of transition between the area of resorption and the remaining bone.

Roentgenograms. The more common roentgenographic abnormality is vertebral sclerosis. Sclerosis involves the vertebral bodies, facet joints, spinous processes, and laminae. Large osteophytes, out of proportion to disc space narrowing, are usual. Sclerosis is a result of bone reaction to fracture. Sclerosis occurs early in the course of the disease. Osteolysis is less common and is associated with rapidly progressive disease. The disc spaces and facet joints may narrow or dissolve (Fig. 16-10).[69] A mixed pattern containing areas of lysis and bone production may also be noted. The progression of disease is vertebral fracture, followed by bone sclerosis, large osteophytes, and loss of disc space, which may be associated with a large paraspinal mass, a result of improper fracture healing. A final development may be the formation of a pseudoarthrosis.[211]

Scintigraphy. Nuclear imaging is often used to differentiate Charcot arthropathy from infection and tumor. The three-phase bone scan (blood flow, blood pool [1-minute image]) and delayed uptake (2- to 4-hour images) of ^{99m}Tc methylene diphosphonate in the bone and joint uniformly demonstrates abnormality of high turnover and increased uptake in the neuropathic lesion. This corresponds to the increased blood flow to the lesion.[4] A differentiation between Charcot joint and septic arthritis may be made by the initial increased blood flow in the area of interest versus the increase in the third phase of the scan in septic arthritis.[80] Gallium-67 citrate scan has been utilized for detection of infectious lesions but has been capable of detecting lesions in only 80% of patients with chronic osteomyelitis.[4] Indium-111 white blood cell scan has differentiated infectious from noninfectious lesions in patients with diabetic neuroarthropathy.[140] However, subsequent evaluation of indium-111 scans reported a significant number of false-positive and false-negative results. The use of MR in this same study also resulted in a number of false-positive tests for infection. The conclusion of these studies suggests that a

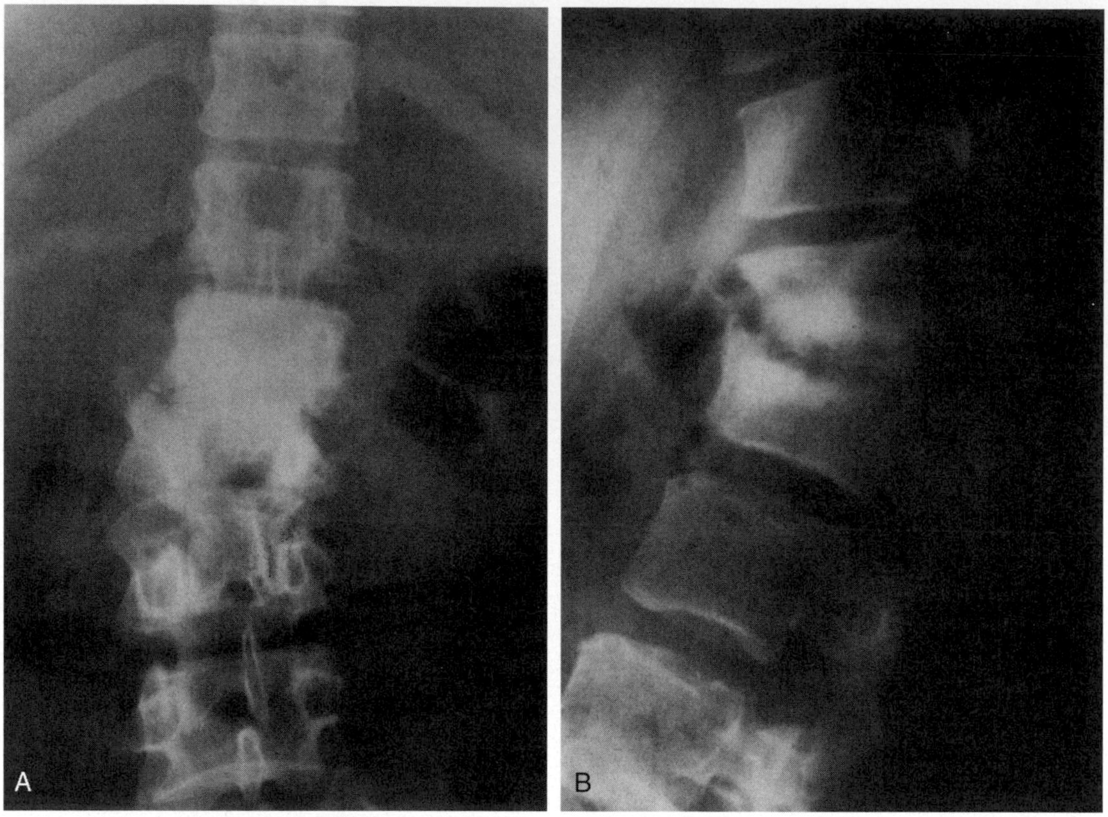

A

B

Figure 16-10 Neuropathic spine. Anteroposterior *(A)* and lateral *(B)* views of the lumbar spine demonstrate total disintegration of the L1-L2 intervertebral disc space with associated extensive osteosclerosis. L1 appears to be "tumbling" into L2. This patient had congenital insensitivity to pain. *(Courtesy of Anne Brower, MD.)*

negative result with indium scan and MR makes a diagnosis of osteomyelitis unlikely.[245]

Magnetic Resonance. MR imaging is able to differentiate neuropathic spinal alterations from disc space infection. Facet joint involvement, disc vacuum phenomenon, debris, and disorganization are found more commonly on radiographs with Charcot joint disease. Gadolinium enhancement of the periphery of a disk (rim enhancement) and diffusely in the vertebral body was more commonly seen in spinal neuropathic arthropathy than in disc infection. As opposed to prior reports, T2-weighted images were not helpful in differentiating the entities. Endplate sclerosis and erosions, osteophytes, paraspinal soft tissue mass, and decreased disc height were not helpful.[288]

Differential Diagnosis

The discovery of vertebral neuroarthropathy requires the identification of the underlying neurologic disorder. An evaluation for patients with lumbar disease should include, at a minimum, a work-up for syphilis and diabetes. The differential diagnosis of sclerotic axial neuropathy includes spondylosis, vertebral osteomyelitis, and osteoblastic metastasis. Unlike degenerative spondylosis, neuropathic joint disease is rapidly progressive and is associated with florid osteophyte formation. In contrast to osteomyelitis, sclerosis of axial neuropathy parallels the vertebral endplates, involves the posterior arch, and is associated with paraspinal debris but not a soft tissue mass. Unlike blastic metastases, Charcot spine involves the disc spaces and preferentially affects the facet joints and vertebral bodies. Similar explanations could be given for the differential diagnosis of the lytic form of spinal neuroarthropathy. Bacterial infection must be considered in the patients with a progressive destructive lesion.[218] Tuberculosis and osteolytic metastases need to be considered in this form of the disease.[89]

Treatment

Therapy for Charcot spine disease is directed at immobilization of the vertebral column by the use of a corset or brace.[113] Arthrodesis of Charcot joints is frequently unsuccessful. Infection and nonunion are frequent complications of the surgical procedure. Failures of surgery in the past were likely due to early mobilization and inadequate instrumentation. Staged procedures with anterior and posterior fusion, instrumentation, and prolonged immobilization have been associated with successful fusion of the unstable Charcot segment that is frequently located at the thoracolumbar junction.[103,216] However, the same forces that led to spinal destruction and instability remain present. These patients are at risk of developing accelerated degenerative abnormalities at vertebral levels contiguous to the fusion.

Other Conditions

Other conditions that may on occasion be associated with back pain or cause symptoms that may be confused with sciatica include *coccydynia* (pain in the coccyx, usually secondary to fracture); *hip arthritis*, which usually radiates pain to the groin but on occasion radiates up to the buttock and lumbar region; and *iliopsoas bursitis* (pain in the inguinal area).

Coccydynia. The coccyx is usually protected by the buttocks and is not usually traumatized by a fall. However, a fall on a projecting object or a fall by a thin individual may damage the bone. Lumbosacral disc prolapse is not an associated factor.[298] The primary symptom is pain that is produced by sitting and relieved with standing or walking. Rectal examination re-creates pain with palpation and movement of the coccyx. Instability of the coccyx may be documented with radiographs of the coccyx in a seated position.[165] Therapy will include a circular cushion for sitting, NSAIDs, injection of anesthetics, and transcutaneous nerve stimulation. Surgery is successful in patients with coccygeal instability.[166] Although surgery may be contemplated, it is not helpful in all patients because the patient may still have pain secondary to the surgical scar.

Hip Arthritis. Hip arthritis may cause back pain on a referred basis (hip joint capsule is supplied by branches of nerves that innervate muscle and skin of the back) or by a change in gait that puts strain on the lumbar spine on a mechanical basis. The diagnosis is apparent after the patient is observed walking and examination of hip motion re-creates hip pain. Most patients will have roentgenographic evidence of hip disease.

Iliopsoas Bursitis. Iliopsoas bursitis occurs in individuals with inflammation of the bursa that complicates the course of degenerative or inflammatory arthropathy of the hip joint. The bursa is located between the iliopsoas muscle and the anterior capsule of the hip joint. Awareness of the syndrome as a cause of pain in the inguinal area has increased with the availability of radiographic methods that image the pelvis. MR evaluation may reveal a fluid-filled distended bursa.[144] The diagnosis should be suspected in patients presenting with anterior hip pain or an inguinal mass. Oral medications are usually effective in controlling the pain associated with bursitis. A home exercise program including internal and external hip rotator muscle strengthening exercises, along with stretching of the hip flexors, quadriceps, and hamstring muscles.[125] Injection therapy is limited to refractory cases.[277]

Cervical Spine

Other conditions that may, on occasion, be associated with neck pain or cause symptoms that may be confused with radicular arm pain include complex regional pain syndrome (reflex sympathetic dystrophy) and shoulder arthritis. These disorders cause radiating pain into the arm, to the trapezius and, on occasion, pain up to the base of the neck.

Complex Regional Pain Syndrome

Complex regional pain syndrome (CRPS), also known as reflex sympathetic dystrophy (RSD), is a syndrome associated with causalgia, extremity swelling, and vascular instability. The International Association for the Study of Pain has defined CRPS as "continuous pain in a portion of an extremity after trauma which may include fracture but does not involve a major nerve, associated with sympathetic hyperactivity."[210] The pain is associated with findings of abnormal skin color, temperature change, abnormal sudomotor activity, or edema. CRPS is separated into two forms. CRPS type I corresponds to RSD without a definable nerve lesion. Type II, associated with causalgia, is the form associated with a definable nerve lesion.[255] Kozin has suggested that a patient may experience pain as the sole manifestation of CRPS and other patients may have only vasomotor or sudomotor changes without pain or tenderness.[143] The American Association for Hand Surgery considered CRPS to be a pain syndrome in which pain is accompanied by loss of function and evidence of autonomic dysfunction.[5] Not only is there debate about the components of CRPS, but also the syndrome has had a number of different names, including Sudeck's atrophy, algodystrophy, and shoulder-hand syndrome.

PATHOGENESIS

The pathogenesis of the syndrome is a matter of debate in the medical literature. Some reports have suggested that peripheral sensory nerve increases afferent input to the internuncial nerve in the spinal cord, which results in continuous stimulation of the sympathetic system. Others have suggested vasomotor reflex spasm resulting in loss of vascular tone. Abnormalities in blood flow control result in atrophy of affected tissues.[210] Recent experiments suggest that alterations in blood flow are related to supersensitivity to sympathetic neurotransmitters rather than overactivity of the sympathetic system because levels of epinephrine and norepinephrine are lower in affected limbs compared with the unaffected limb. This finding suggests that the manifestations of CRPS are a result of disruption of efferent sympathetic modulation of pain.[54] Hannington-Kiff suggested that failure of natural opioid modulation of pain mediated by regional sympathetic ganglia after injury results in dystrophic alterations of a limb.[101] Others believe that CRPS is a disorder of the psyche associated with personality traits of rigidity and somatization.[285] Others promote the idea that the sympathetic system plays little role in CRPS and consider neuropsychiatric mechanisms the cause of the syndrome.[197]

CRPS is usually incited after a trauma (fracture), central or peripheral nerve injuries (stroke and shingles), cardiovascular events (myocardial infarction), drugs (barbiturates), pulmonary disease (tuberculosis), and immobilization. The clinical symptoms and signs of CRPS include severe, burning pain; vasomotor instability; diffuse swelling of the appendage; and dystrophic skin changes. Most patients do not demonstrate all the manifestations of the syndrome. Many patients do not recall a traumatic event. Bonica defined three stages of CRPS, starting with dysesthesias, swelling, increased blood flow, and increased skin temperature; followed by burning pain, decreased blood flow, decreased skin temperature, and decreased limb motion; and concluding with subcutaneous tissue atrophy and contractures.[22] Another study of 829 patients did not find a chronologic progression in this syndrome.[287] Patients could be divided according to warm and cold appendages. Individuals with a longer duration of CRPS were in the cold group. Another study of 113 patients also did not discover a sequential pattern to the development of CRPS signs.[31] CRPS may spread to affect other limbs without additional trauma,[269] or it may affect only part of a limb, such as a single digit.[150]

Laboratory/Radiographic Evaluation

Routine laboratory test results are normal or reflect abnormalities with associated conditions. Plain roentgenograms of the affected limb may demonstrate diffuse osteopenia, which is greater than what would be expected from disuse alone.[82] Three-phase ^{99m}Tc-methylene diphosphonate bone scintiscans are useful in identifying individuals with CRPS. Scintiscans taken immediately after injection show decreased perfusion of the affected limb soon after the onset of the disorder. After 6 weeks, delayed scintigraphy may reveal increased uptake in the peripheral joint of the affected limb.[154] The delayed images are better than blood flow or pool phase images to determine the presence of CRPS.[200] The utility of scintiscans diminishes after 6 months. Roentgenograms will reveal patchy osteoporosis that occurs secondary to sustained increased blood flow to the limb. MR imaging is useful in CRPS in the initial stages by identifying skin thickening, tissue enhancement with a contrast agent, and soft tissue edema.[243]

Treatment

Treatment of CRPS should be initiated as soon as the diagnosis is suspected. Physiotherapy for mobilization of the limb is essential to avoid progression of the syndrome. Physiotherapy is the cornerstone of therapy for CRPS.[229] Patients should receive analgesics, NSAIDs, temperature modalities, and exercises to increase range of motion. Systemic corticosteroids in the range of 20 to 40 mg should be added if symptoms persist. Persistent low-dose therapy with corticosteroids may be required for severe cases. Bisphosphonate therapy in the form of pamidronate or alendronate has been associated with decreased pain in patients with CRPS.[1,45] Intramuscular calcitonin therapy (100 IU) for 4 weeks has also been used for analgesia.[100] Sympathetic blocks may be used to decrease pain to increase movement of the affected limb.[115] Surgical sympathectomy may be considered for those patients who have responded to injections. Some individuals have a sustained response to surgical sympathectomy.[138] Others have suggested that sympathectomy is not helpful and that symptoms return after operation.[197] Other therapies that have been used include guanethidine and nifedipine.[210,219] Intrathecal morphine has been used for CRPS patients whose intractable pain is resistant to all other therapies.[17] This technique has been used for only a few patients and requires additional study with prolonged follow-up to determine its efficacy. Dorsal column stimulation may be helpful for individuals with disease limited to one extremity. In a randomized study of 36 individuals, electrical stimulation reduced pain and improved quality of life but did not change functional outcome measures.[134]

Shoulder Arthritis

Shoulder abnormalities cause pain primarily over the joint itself.[250] Instability, trauma, arthritis, bursitis, rotator cuff lesions, and bicipital tendinitis are a partial list of the lesions that affect the shoulder.[88] Referred pain from the shoulder may radiate proximally toward the base and lateral aspect of the neck. This radiation of pain may be mediated through tension in the trapezius muscle. Patients complain of pain in both locations. Acromioclavicular joint disease may also refer pain toward the base of the neck. C5 radiculopathy is associated with pain over the deltoid area that coincides with the location of pain associated with shoulder problems. Careful examination of the shoulder joint and cervical spine, including careful palpation of the structures, can help differentiate the primary focus of pain. Cervical spine disorders frequently refer pain to both shoulders. The absence of any tenderness in the neck or exacerbation of symptoms on manipulation of the cervical spine is important evidence that another musculoskeletal structure is the source of pain. The shoulder is usually more sensitive to mechanical enhancement of symptoms. Pain is more acute with movement and may remain more persistent. Shoulder disorders are also accompanied with stiffness or instability that would not be expected with primary cervical spine disease.

References

Neurologic Disorders

1. Adami S, Fossaluzza V, Gatti D, et al: Bisphosphonate therapy of reflex sympathetic dystrophy syndrome. Ann Rheum Dis 56:201-204, 1997.
2. Adelaar RS, Foster WC, McDowell C: The treatment of the cubital tunnel syndrome. J Hand Surg 9A:90, 1984.
3. Adson AW: Surgical treatment for symptoms produced by cervical ribs and scalenus anticus muscle. Clin Orthop 207:3, 1986.
4. Allman RM, Brower AC, Kotlyarov EB: Neuropathic bone and joint disease. Radiol Clin North Am 26:1373, 1988.
5. Amadio PC, Mackinnon SE, Merritt WH, et al: RSDS: Consensus report of an ad hoc committee of the American Association for Hand Surgery on the definition of RSDS. Plast Reconstr Surg 87:371, 1991.
6. Antoniou J, Tae SK, Williams GR, et al: Suprascapular neuropathy: Variability in the diagnosis, treatment, and outcome. Clin Orthop 386:131-138, 2001.
7. Arcasoy SM, Jett JR: Superior pulmonary sulcus tumors and Pancoast's syndrome. N Engl J Med 337:1370-1376, 1997.
8. Asbury AK: Focal and multifocal neuropathies of diabetes. In Dyck PJ, Thomas PK, Asbury AK, et al (eds): Diabetic Neuropathy. Philadelphia, WB Saunders, 1987, pp 45-55.
9. Ashenhurst EM, Quartey GRC, Starreveld A: Lumbosacral radiculopathy induced by radiation. Can J Neurol Sci 4:259, 1977.
10. Axelrod DA, Proctor MC, Geisser ME, et al: Outcomes after surgery for thoracic outlet syndrome. J Vasc Surg 33:1220-1225, 2001.
11. Bacon PA, Carruthers DM: Vasculitis associated with connective tissue disorders. Rheum Dis Clin North Am 21:1077, 1995.
12. Bailie DS, Kelikian AS: Tarsal tunnel syndrome: Diagnosis, surgical technique, and functional outcome. Foot Ankle Int 19:65-72, 1998.
13. Barohn RJ, Sahenk Z, Warmolts JR, et al: The Bruns-Garland syndrome (diabetic amyotrophy): Revisited 100 years later. Arch Neurol 48:1130-1135, 1991.
14. Barrett DS, Donnell ST: Entrapment neuropathies: I. Upper limb. Br J Hosp Med 46:94, 1991.
15. Batzdorf U, Brechner V: Management of pain associated with the Pancoast syndrome. Am J Surg 137:638, 1979.
16. Beale R, Siater R, Hennington M, et al: Pancoast tumor: Use of MRI for tumor staging. South Med J 85:1260, 1992.
17. Becker WJ, Ablett DP, Harris CJ, et al: Long-term treatment of intractable reflex sympathetic dystrophy with intrathecal morphine. Can J Neurol Sci 22:153, 1995.
18. Benson ER, Schutzer SF: Posttraumatic piriformis: Diagnosis and results of operative treatment. J Bone Joint Surg 81A:941-949, 1999.

19. Beyer JA, Wright IS: The hyperabduction syndrome: With special reference to its relationship to Raynaud's syndrome. Circulation 4:161, 1951.
20. Biedmond A: Femoral neuropathy. In Vinlen PJ, Bruyn BW (eds): Handbook of Clinical Neurology, Vol 1, Part II, Diseases of Nerves. Amsterdam, North Holland Publishing, 1970, pp 303-310.
21. Biundo JJ Jr, Mipro RC Jr, Djuric V: Peripheral nerve entrapment, occupation-related syndromes, sports injuries, bursitis, and soft tissue problems of the shoulder. Curr Opin Rheumatol 7:151, 1995.
22. Bonica JJ: Causalgia and other reflex sympathetic dystrophies. Adv Pain Res Ther 3:141, 1979.
23. Bracker MD, Ralph LP: The numb arm and hand. Am Fam Physician 51:103, 1995.
24. Bradley WG, Chad D, Verghese JP, et al: Painful lumbosacral plexopathy with elevated erythrocyte sedimentation rate: A treatable inflammatory syndrome. Ann Neurol 15:457, 1984.
25. Bradshaw C, McCrory P, Bell S, et al: Obturator nerve entrapment: A cause of groin pain in athletes. Am J Sports Med 25:402-408, 1997.
26. Brannon EW: Cervical rib syndrome: An analysis of nineteen cases and twenty-four operations. J Bone Joint Surg 45A:977, 1963.
27. Braunn RM, Rechnic M, Fowler E: Complications related to carpal tunnel release. Hand Clin 18:347-357, 2002.
28. Briggs JR, Freehafer AA: Fusion of the Charcot spine: Report of 3 cases. Clin Orthop 53:83, 1967.
29. Brower AC, Allman RM: Pathogenesis of the neurotropic joint: Neurotraumatic vs neurovascular. Radiology 139:349, 1981.
30. Bruckner FE, Kendal BE: Neuroarthropathy in Charcot-Marie-Tooth disease. Ann Rheum Dis 28:577, 1969.
31. Bruehl S, Harden RN, Galer BS, et al: Complex regional pain syndrome: Are there distinct subtypes and sequential stages of the syndrome? Pain 95:119-124, 2002.
32. Brunt PW: Unusual cause of Charcot joints in early adolescence (Riley-Day syndrome). BMJ 4:277, 1967.
32a. Busis NA: Femoral and obturator neuropathies. Neurol Clin 17:633-653, 1999.
33. Butterfield WC, Neiraser RJ, Robert MP: Femoral neuropathy and anticoagulants. Ann Surg 176:56, 1972.
34. Campbell DJ, Doyle JO: Tabetic Charcot's spine. BMJ 1:1018, 1954.
35. Campbell IW, Fraser DM, Ewing DJ, et al: Peripheral and autonomic nerve function in diabetic ketoacidosis. Lancet 2:167, 1976.
36. Casseli RJ, Daube JR, Hunder GC, Whisnant JP: Peripheral neuropathic syndromes in giant cell (temporal) arteritis. Neurology 38:685, 1988.
37. Chance PF, Windebank AJ: Hereditary neuralgic amyotrophy. Curr Opin Neurol 9:343-347, 1996.
38. Chang B, Dellon AL: Surgical management of recurrent carpal tunnel syndrome. J Hand Surg [Br] 18B:467, 1993.
39. Chang MH, Ger LP, Hsieh PF, et al: A randomized clinical trial of oral steroids in the treatment of carpal tunnel syndrome: A long term follow-up. J Neurol Neurosurg Psychiatry 73:710-714, 2002.
40. Cherington M, Happer I, Machanic B, et al: Surgery for thoracic outlet syndrome may be hazardous to your health. Muscle Nerve 9:632, 1986.
41. Childers MK, Wilson DJ, Gantz SM, et al: Botulinum toxin type A use in piriformis muscle syndrome: A pilot study. Am J Phys Med Rehabil 81:751-759, 2002.
42. Chokroverty S, Reyes MG, Rubino FA: The Bruns-Garland syndrome of diabetic amyotrophy. Trans Am Neurol Assoc 102:173, 1977.
43. Chopra JS, Hurwitz LJ: Femoral nerve conduction in diabetes and chronic occlusive disease. J Neurol Neurosurg Psychiatry 31:28, 1968.
44. Collins JD, Shaver ML, Disher AC, et al: Compromising abnormalities of the brachial plexus as displayed by magnetic resonance imaging. Clin Anat 8:1, 1995.
45. Cortet B, Flipo RM, Coquerelle P, et al: Treatment of severe, recalcitrant reflex sympathetic dystrophy: Assessment of efficacy and safety of the second generation bisphosphonate pamidronate. Clin Rheumatol 16:51-56, 1997.
46. Cruz-Martinez A, Barrio M, Arpa J: Neuralgic amyotrophy: Variable expression in 40 patients. J Peripher Nerv Syst 7:198-204, 2002.
47. Cseuz KA, Thomas JE, Lambert EH, et al: Long-term results of operation for carpal tunnel syndrome. Mayo Clin Proc 41:232, 1966.
48. David JL, Lewis SB, Gerich JE, et al: Peripheral diabetic neuropathy treated with amitriptyline and fluphenazine. JAMA 238:2291, 1977.
49. Dawson DM: Entrapment neuropathies of the upper extremities. N Engl J Med 329:2013, 1993.
50. Dejgard A, Peterson P, Kastrup J: Mexiletine for treatment of chronic painful diabetic neuropathy. Lancet 1:9, 1988.
51. Derbekyan V, Novales-Diaz J, Lisbona R: Pancoast tumor as a cause of reflex sympathetic dystrophy. J Nucl Med 34:1992, 1993.
52. Donnell ST, Barrett DS: Entrapment neuropathies: II. Lower limb. Br J Hosp Med 46:99, 1991.
53. Donovan WH, Sumi SM: Diabetic amyotrophy: A more diffuse process than clinically suspected. Arch Phys Med Rehabil 57:397, 1976.
54. Drummond PD, Finch PM, Smythe GA: Reflex sympathetic dystrophy: The significance of differing plasma catecholamine concentrations in affected and unaffected limbs. Brain 114:2025, 1991.
55. Duna GF, Galperin C, Hoffman GS: Wegener's granulomatosis. Rheum Dis Clin North Am 21:949, 1995.
56. Dyck PJ, Conn DL, Okazaki H: Necrotizing angiopathic neuropathy: Three-dimensional morphology of fiber degeneration related to sites of occluded vessels. Mayo Clin Proc 47:461, 1972.
57. Dyck PJ, Norell JE, Dyck PJ: Non-diabetic lumbosacral radiculoplexus neuropathy: Natural history, outcome and comparison with the diabetic variety. Brain 124:1197-1207, 2001.
58. Dyck PJ, Windebank AJ: Diabetic and nondiabetic lumbosacral radiculoplexus neuropathies: New insights into pathophysiology and treatment. Muscle Nerve 25:477-491, 2002.
59. Edelman SV, Kosofsky EM, Paul RA, Kozak GP: Neuro-osteoarthropathy (Charcot's joint) in diabetes mellitus following revascularization surgery: Three case reports and a review of the literature. Arch Intern Med 147:1504, 1987.
60. Eggli S, Hankemayer S, Muller ME: Nerve palsy after leg lengthening in total replacement arthroplasty for developmental dysplasia of the hip. J Bone Joint Surg Br 81B:843-845, 1999.
61. Ehrmann L, Lechner K, Mamoli B, et al: Peripheral nerve lesions in haemophilia. J Neurol 225:175, 1981.
62. Ellenberg M: Diabetic neuropathic cachexia. Diabetes 23:418, 1974.
63. Emery S, Ochoa J: Lumbar plexus neuropathy resulting from retroperitoneal hemorrhage. Muscle Nerve 1:330, 1978.
64. English P, Maciver D: Neuralgic amyotrophy as a presenting feature of infective endocarditis. Postgrad Med J 76:710-711, 2000.
65. Fagius J, Brattberg A, Jameson S, Berne C: Limited benefit of treatment of diabetic polyneuropathy with an aldose reductase inhibitor: A 24-week controlled trial. Diabetologia 28:323, 1985.
66. Fauci AS, Haynes BG, Katz P: The spectrum of vasculitis: Clinical, pathologic, immunologic and therapeutic consideration. Ann Intern Med 89:660, 1978.
67. Fauci AS, Haynes BF, Katz P, Wolff SM: Wegener's granulomatosis: Prospective and therapeutic experience with 85 patients for 21 years. Ann Intern Med 98:76, 1983.
68. Feinglass EJ, Arnett FC, Dorsch CA, et al: Neuropsychiatric manifestations of systemic lupus erythematosus: Diagnosis, clinical spectrum, and relationship to other features of the disease. Medicine 55:323, 1976.
69. Feldman F, Johnson AM, Walter JF: Acute axial neuropathy. Radiology 111:1, 1974.
70. Feldman MJ, Becher KL, Reefe WE, Longo A: Multiple neuropathic joints including the wrist in a patient with diabetes mellitus. JAMA 209:1690, 1969.
71. Fidler WK, Dewar CL, Fenton PV: Cervical spine pseudogout with myelopathy and Charcot joints. J Rheumatol 23:1445-1448, 1996.
72. Fields WS, Lemak NA, Ben-Menachem Y: Thoracic outlet syndrome: Review and reference to stroke in a major league pitcher. AJR Am J Roentgenol 146:809, 1986.
73. Fishman LM, Anderson C, Rosner B: BOTOX and physical therapy in the treatment of piriformis syndrome. Am J Phys Med Rehabil 81:936-942, 2002.
74. Fishman LM, Dombi GW, Michaelsen C, et al: Piriformis syndrome: Diagnosis, treatment, and outcome: A 10-year study. Arch Phys Med Rehabil 83:295-301, 2002.
75. Fishman LM, Zybert PA: Electrophysiologic evidence of piriformis syndrome. Arch Phys Med Rehabil 73:359, 1992.
76. Frankel SA, Hirata I Jr: The scalenus anticus syndrome and competitive swimming: Report of two cases. JAMA 215:1796, 1971.

77. Franklin GM, Haug J, Heyer N, et al: Occupational carpal tunnel syndrome in Washington State, 1984-1988. Am J Public Health 81:741, 1991.
78. Fraser DM, Campbell IW, Ewing DJ, et al: Peripheral and autonomic nerve function in newly diagnosed diabetes mellitus. Diabetes 26:546, 1977.
79. Freiburg AA, Vinke TA: Sciatica pain and its relief by operation on muscle and fascia. J Bone Joint Surg 16:126, 1934.
80. Gandsman EJ, Deutsch SD, Kahn CB, Deutsch AM: Dynamic bone scanning in diabetic osteoarthropathy. J Nucl Med 24:664, 1987.
81. Gemignani F, Pavesi G, Fiocchi A, et al: Peripheral neuropathy in essential mixed cryoglobulinaemia. J Neurol Neurosurg Psychiatry 55:116, 1992.
82. Genant HK, Kozin F, Bekerman C, et al: The reflex sympathetic dystrophy syndrome: A comprehensive analysis using fine-detail radiography, photon absorptiometry and bone and joint scintigraphy. Radiology 117:21, 1975.
83. Gergouldis R, Barnes RW: Thoracic outlet arterial compression: Prevalence in normal persons. Angiology 31:538, 1980.
84. Gerritsen AA, de Vet HC, Scholten RJ, et al: Splinting vs surgery in treatment of carpal tunnel syndrome: A randomized controlled trial. JAMA 288:1245-1251, 2002.
85. Gillard J, Perez-Cousin M, Hachulla E, et al: Diagnosing thoracic outlet syndrome: Contribution of provocative tests, ultrasonography, electrophysiology, and helical computed tomography in 48 patients. Joint Bone Spine 68:416-424, 2001.
86. Ginsberg RJ, Martini N, Zaman M, et al: Influence of surgical resection and brachytherapy in the management of superior sulcus tumor. Ann Thorac Surg 57:1440-1445, 1994.
87. Giugliano D, Marfella R, Quatraro A, et al: Tolrestat for mild diabetic neuropathy: A 52-week, randomized, placebo-controlled trial. Ann Intern Med 118:7-11, 1993.
88. Glockner SM: Shoulder pain: A diagnostic dilemma. Am Fam Physician 51:1677, 1995.
89. Goldman AB, Freiberger RH: Localized infections and neuropathic diseases. Semin Roentgenol 14:19, 1979.
90. Green DA, Lattimer SA: Altered myoinositol metabolism in diabetic nerve. In Dyck PJ, Thomas PK, Asbury AK, et al (eds): Diabetic Neuropathy. Philadelphia, WB Saunders, 1987, pp 289-298.
91. Green DA, Lattimer SA, Ulbrecht J, Carroll P: Glucose-induced alterations in nerve metabolism: Current perspective on the pathogenesis of diabetic neuropathy and future directions for research and therapy. Diabetes Care 8:290, 1985.
92. Griffin JW: Vasculitis neuropathies. Rheum Clin North Am 27:751-760, 2001.
93. Gross WL: Antineutrophil cytoplasmic autoantibody testing in vasculitides. Rheum Dis Clin North Am 21:987, 1995.
94. Grossman MG, Ducey SA, Nadler SS, et al: Meralgia paresthetica: Diagnosis and treatment. J Am Acad Orthop Surg 9:336-344, 2001.
95. Guillevin L, Du LTH, Godeau P, et al: Clinical findings and prognosis of polyarteritis nodosa and Churg-Strauss angiitis: A study in 165 patients. Br J Rheumatol 27:258, 1988.
96. Guillevin L, Lhote F: Treatment of polyarteritis nodosa and microscopic polyangiitis. Arthritis Rheum 41:2100-2105, 1998.
97. Guillevin L, Lhote F, Gayraud M, et al: Prognostic factors in polyarteritis nodosa and Churg-Strauss syndrome: A prospective study in 342 patients. Medicine 75:17-28, 1996.
98. Ha YC, Ahn IO, Jeong ST, et al: Iliacus hematoma and femoral nerve palsy after revision hip arthroplasty: A case report. Clin Orthop 385:100-103, 2001.
99. Halonen PI, Jarvinen KAJ: On the occurrence of neuropathic arthropathies in pernicious anaemia. Ann Rheum Dis 7:152, 1948.
100. Hamamci N, Dursun E, Ural C, et al: Calcitonin treatment in reflex sympathetic dystrophy: a preliminary study. Br J Clin Pract 50:373-375, 1996.
101. Hannington-Kiff JG: Does failed natural opioid modulation in regional sympathetic ganglia cause reflex sympathetic dystrophy? Lancet 338:1125, 1991.
102. Harrision BR: Charcot joint: Two new observations. AJR Am J Roentgenol 128:807, 1977.
103. Harrison MJ, Sacher M, Rosenblum BR, Rothman AS: Spinal Charcot arthropathy. Neurosurgery 29:273, 1991.
104. Harter BT Jr, McKiernan JE Jr, Kirzinger SS, et al: Carpal tunnel syndrome: Surgical and nonsurgical treatment. J Hand Surg 18A:471, 1993.
105. Hashizume H, Nishida K, Nanba Y, et al: Non-traumatic paralysis of the posterior interosseous nerve. J Bone Joint Surg 78B:771-776, 1996.
106. Haupt WF, Wintzer G, Schop A, et al: Tunnel decompression. J Hand Surg 18B:471, 1993.
107. Heithoff SJ, Millender LH, Nalebuff EA, et al: Medial epicondylectomy for the treatment of ulnar nerve compression at the elbow. J Hand Surg 15A:22, 1990.
108. Hellmann DB, Laing TJ, Petri M, et al: Mononeuritis multiplex: The yield of evaluations for occult rheumatic diseases. Medicine 67:145, 1988.
109. Helms CA, Chapman GS, Wild JH: Charcot-like joints in calcium pyrophosphate dihydrate deposition disease. Skeletal Radiol 7:55, 1981.
110. Hepper NGG, Herskovic T, Witten DM, et al: Thoracic inlet tumors. Ann Intern Med 64:979, 1966.
111. Hoffman G, Specks U: Antineutrophil cytoplasmic antibodies. Arthritis Rheum 41:1521-1537, 1998.
112. Hong CZ, Long HA, Kanakamedala RV, et al: Splinting and local steroid injection for the treatment of ulnar neuropathy at the elbow: Clinical and electrophysiological evaluation. Arch Phys Med Rehabil 77:573-577, 1996.
113. Hoppenfeld S, Gross M, Giangarra C: Nonoperative treatment of neuropathic spinal arthropathy. Spine 15:54, 1990.
114. Hoppmann RA, Patrone NA: A review of musculoskeletal problems in instrumental musicians. Semin Arthritis Rheum 19:117, 1989.
115. Hord AH, Rooks MD, Stephens BO, et al: Intravenous regional bretylium and lidocaine for treatment of reflex sympathetic dystrophy: Randomized, double-blind study. Anesth Analg 74:818, 1992.
116. Horwitz T: Bone and cartilage debris in the synovial membrane: Its significance in the early diagnosis in neuroarthropathy. J Bone Joint Surg Am 30A:579, 1948.
117. Hoskinson J, Duthie RB: Management of musculoskeletal problems in hemophilias. Orthop Clin North Am 9:455, 1978.
118. Hotta N, Toyota T, Matsuoka K, et al: Clinical efficacy of fiderestat, a novel aldose reductase inhibitor for diabetic peripheral neuropathy: A 52-week multicenter placebo-controlled double-blind parallel group study. Diabetes Care 24:1776-1782, 2001.
119. Ivins GK: Meralgia paresthetica, the elusive diagnosis: Clinical experience with 14 adult patients. Ann Surg 232:281-286, 2000.
120. Jablecki CK, Andary MT, So YT, et al: Usefulness of nerve conduction studies and electromyography for the evaluation of patients with carpal tunnel syndrome. Muscle Nerve 16:1392, 1993.
121. Jacobelli S, McCarty DJ, Silcox DS, Mall JC: Calcium pyrophosphate dihydrate crystal deposition in neuropathic joints: Four cases of polyarticular involvement. Ann Intern Med 79:340, 1973.
122. Jankiewicz JJ, Henrikus WL, Houkom JA: The appearance of the piriformis muscle syndrome in computed tomography and magnetic resonance imaging. Clin Orthop 262:205, 1991.
123. Jennette J, Falk R, Andrassy K, et al: Nomenclature of systemic vasculitides: Proposal of an international consensus conference. Arthritis Rheum 37:187-192, 1994.
124. Johnson JTH: Neuropathic fractures and joint injuries: Pathogenesis and rationale of prevention and treatment. J Bone Joint Surg Am 49A:1, 1967.
125. Johnston CAM, Kindsay DM, Wiley JP: Treatment of iliopsoas syndrome with a hip rotation strengthening program: A retrospective case series. J Orthop Sports Phys Ther 29:218-224, 1999.
126. Jordan SE, Ahn SS, Freischlag, et al: Selective botulinum chemodenervation of the scalene muscles for treatment of neurogenic thoracic outlet syndrome. Ann Vasc Surg 14:365-369, 2000.
127. Kaplan SJ, Glickel SZ, Eaton RG: Predictive factors in the nonsurgical treatment of carpal tunnel syndrome. J Hand Surg [Br] 15B:106, 1990.
128. Katirji B: Peroneal neuropathy. Neurol Clin 17:567-591, 1999.
129. Katz I, Rabinowitz JG, Dziadiw R: Early changes in Charcot's joints. AJR Am J Roentgenol 86:965, 1961.

130. Katz JN, Larson MG, Fossel AH, et al: Validation of a surveillance case definition of carpal tunnel syndrome. Am J Public Health 81:189, 1991.
131. Katz JN, Simmons BP: Carpal tunnel syndrome. N Engl J Med 346:1807-1812, 2002.
132. Katz JS, Saperstein DS, Wolfe G, et al: Cervicobrachial involvement in diabetic radiculoplexopathy. Muscle Nerve 24:794-798, 2001.
133. Kelkar P, Masood M, Parry GJ: Distinctive pathologic findings in proximal diabetic neuropathy (diabetic amyotrophy). Neurology 55:83-88, 2000.
134. Kemler MA, Barendse GA, van Kleef M, et al: Spinal cord stimulation in patients with chronic reflex sympathetic dystrophy. N Engl J Med 31:618-624, 2000.
135. Kennett R, Harding AE: Peripheral neuropathy associated with sicca syndrome. J Neurol Neurosurg Psychiatry 49:90, 1986.
136. Kenny RA, Traynor GB, Withington D, et al: Thoracic outlet syndrome: A useful exercise treatment option. Am J Surg 165:282, 1993.
137. Kinoshita M, Okuda R, Morikawa J, et al: The dorsiflexion-eversion test for diagnosis of tarsal tunnel syndrome. J Bone Joint Surg Am 83A:1835-1839, 2001.
137a. Kitson J, Ashworth MJ: Meralgia paresthetica. A complication of a patient-positioning device in total hip replacement. J Bone Joint Surg Br 84:589-590, 2002.
138. Kleinert HE, Cole NM, Wayne L, et al: Post-traumatic sympathetic dystrophy. Orthop Clin North Am 4:917, 1983.
139. Kline DG: Operative management of major nerve lesions of the lower extremity. Surg Clin North Am 52:1247, 1972.
140. Knight D, Gray HW, McKillop JH, Bessent RG: Imaging for infection: Caution required with the Charcot joint. Eur J Nucl Med 13:523, 1988.
141. Knockaert DC, O'Heygere FG, Bobbaers HJ: Ilioinguinal nerve entrapment: A little known cause of iliac fossa pain. Postgrad Med J 65:632, 1989.
142. Kori SH, Foley KM, Posner JB: Brachial plexus lesions in patients with cancer: 100 cases. Neurology 31:45, 1981.
143. Kozin F: Reflex sympathetic dystrophy syndrome: A review. Clin Exp Rheumatol 10:401, 1992.
144. Kozlov DB, Sonin AH: Iliopsoas bursitis: Diagnosis by MRI. J Comput Assist Tomogr 22:625-628, 1998.
145. Kuntzer T, van Melle G, Regli F: Clinical and prognostic features in unilateral femoral neuropathies. Muscle Nerve 20:205-211, 1997.
146. Kurana RC: Treatment of painful diabetic neuropathy with trazodone. JAMA 250:1392, 1983.
147. Lahrmann H, Grisold W, Authier FJ, et al: Neuralgic amyotrophy with phrenic nerve involvement. Muscle Nerve 22:437-442, 1999.
148. Landry GJ, Moneta GL, Taylor LM Jr, et al: Long-term functional outcome of neurogenic thoracic outlet syndrome in surgically and conservatively treated patients. J Vasc Surg 33:312-317, 2001.
149. Laskar T, Laulan J: Cubital tunnel syndrome: A retrospective review of 53 anterior subcutaneous transpositions. J Hand Surg 25:453-456, 2000.
150. Laukaitis JP, Varma VM, Borenstein DG: Reflex sympathetic dystrophy localized to a single digit. J Rheumatol 16:402, 1989.
151. Layzer RB: Neuromuscular Manifestations of Systemic Disease. Philadelphia, FA Davis, 1985.
152. Lederman RJ, Wilbourn AJ: Postpartum neuralgic amyotrophy. Neurology 47:1213-1219, 1996.
153. Lee CH, Dellon AL: Surgical management of groin pain of neural origin. J Am Coll Surg 191:137-142, 2000.
154. Lee GW, Weeks PM: The role of bone scintigraphy in diagnosing reflex sympathetic dystrophy. J Hand Surg 20:458-463, 1995.
155. Lee P. Bruni J, Sukenik S: Neurological manifestations in systemic sclerosis (scleroderma). J Rheumatol 11:480, 1984.
156. Lepor H, Walsh P: Idiopathic retroperitoneal fibrosis. J Urol 122:1, 1979.
157. Lhote F, Guillevin L: Polyarteritis nodosa, microscopic polyangiitis, and Churg-Strauss syndrome: Clinical aspects and treatment. Rheum Dis Clin North Am 21:911, 1995.
158. Lindgren K, Oksala I: Long-term outcome of surgery for thoracic outlet syndrome. Am J Surg 169:358, 1995.
159. Lister GD, Belsole RB, Kleinert HE: The radial tunnel syndrome. J Hand Surg [Am] 4A:52, 1979.
160. Liu JE, Tahmoush AJ, Roos DB, et al: Shoulder-arm pain from cervical bands and scalene muscle anomalies. J Neurol Sci 128: 175, 1995.
161. Llewelyn JG, Thomas PK, King RH: Epineural microvasculitis in proximal diabetic neuropathy. J Neurol 245:159-165, 1998.
162. Mackinnon SE, Novak CB: Clinical commentary: Pathogenesis of cumulative trauma disorder. J Hand Surg [Am] 19A:873, 1994.
163. Macnicol MF, Thompson WJ: Idiopathic meralgia paresthetica. Clin Orthop 254:270, 1990.
164. Maggi G, Casadio C, Pischedda F, et al: Combined radiosurgical treatment of Pancoast tumor. Ann Thorac Surg 57:198, 1994.
165. Maigne JY, Doursounian L, Chatellier G: Causes and mechanisms of common coccydynia: Role of body mass index and coccygeal trauma. Spine 25:3072-3079, 2000.
166. Maigne JY, Lagouche D, Doursounian L: Instability of the coccyx in coccydynia. J Bone Joint Surg Br 82B:1038-1041, 2000.
167. Markenson JA, McDougal JS, Tsairis P, et al: Rheumatoid meningitis: A localized immune process. Ann Intern Med 90:786, 1979.
168. Marquardt G, Barduzal Angles S, Leheta F, et al: Spontaneous haematoma of the iliac psoas muscle: A report and review of the literature. Arch Orthop Trauma Surg 122:109-111, 2002.
169. Marshall S, Tardiff G, Ashworth N: Local corticosteroid injection for carpal tunnel syndrome. Cochrane Database Syst Rev 4:CD001554, 2002.
170. Masear VR, Hayes JM, Hyde AG: An industrial cause of carpal tunnel syndrome. J Hand Surg 11A:222, 1986.
171. Maxwell-Armstrong CA, Noorpuri BS, Haque SA, et al: Long-term results of surgical decompression of thoracic outlet compression syndrome. J R Coll Surg Edinb 46:35-38, 2001.
172. McCarty EC, Tsairis P, Warren RF: Brachial neuritis. Clin Orthop 368:37-43, 1999.
173. McCombe PA, McLeod JG, Pollard JD, et al: Peripheral sensorimotor and autonomic neuropathy associated with systemic lupus erythematosus. Brain 110:533, 1987.
174. McDaniel GC, Kukliy WH, Gilbert SC: Femoral nerve injury associated with the Pfannenstiel incision and abdominal retractors. Am J Obstet Gynecol 87:381, 1967.
175. McKinney AS: Neurologic findings in retroperitoneal mass lesions. South Med J 66:862, 1973.
176. McNeel DP, Ehni G: Charcot joint of the lumbar spine. J Neurosurg 30:55, 1969.
177. Mellgren SI, Conn DL, Stevens JC, Dyck PJ: Peripheral neuropathy in primary Sjögren's syndrome. Neurology 39:390, 1989.
178. Mendel CM, Klein RF, Chappell DA, et al: A trial of amitriptyline and fluphenazine in the treatment of painful diabetic neuropathy. JAMA 255:637, 1986.
179. Mendell JR, Kissel JT, Cornblath DR: Diagnosis and Management of Peripheral Nerve Disorders. Oxford, Oxford University Press, 2001, p 669.
180. Merkel PA, Polisson RP, Chang Y, et al: Prevalence of antineutrophil cytoplasmic antibodies in a large inception cohort of patients with connective tissue disease. Ann Intern Med 126:866-873, 1997.
181. Miller JI, Mansour KA, Hatcher CR: Carcinoma of the superior pulmonary sulcus. Ann Thorac Surg 28:44, 1975.
182. Miller RG, Camp PE: Postoperative ulnar neuropathy. JAMA 242:1636, 1979.
183. Misamore GW, Lehman DE: Parsonage-Turner syndrome (acute brachial neuritis). J Bone Joint Surg Am 78A:1405-1408, 1996.
184. Mitchell JK: On a new practice in acute and chronic rheumatism. Am J Med Sci 8:55, 1831.
185. Moore PM, Fauci AS: Neurologic manifestations of systemic vasculitis: A retrospective and prospective study of the clinicopathologic features and response to therapy in 25 patients. Am J Med 71:517, 1981.
186. Mountain CF: Revision in the International System for Staging lung cancer. Chest 111:1710-1717, 1997.
187. Mullin V, de Rosayro M: Caudal steroid injection for treatment of piriformis syndrome. Anesth Analg 71:705, 1990.
188. Nagaoka M, Satou K: Tarsal tunnel syndrome caused by ganglia. J Bone Joint Surg 81B:607-610, 1999.

189. Nardone R, Bernhart H, Pozzera A, et al: Respiratory weakness in neuralgic amyotrophy: Report of two cases with phrenic nerve involvement. Neurol Sci 21:177-181, 2000.
190. Nathan PA, Keniston RC, Meadows KD, et al: Predictive value of nerve conduction measurements at the carpal tunnel. Muscle Nerve 16:1377, 1993.
191. Nathan PA, Meadows KD, Doyle LS: Relationship of age and sex to sensory conduction of the median nerve at the carpal tunnel and association of slowed conduction with symptoms. Muscle Nerve 11:1149, 1988.
192. Nelson LM, Hewett WJ, Chu Ang JT: Neural manifestations of para-aortic node metastasis in carcinoma of the cervix. Obstet Gynecol 40:45, 1972.
193. Niakan E, Carbone JE, Adams M, Schroeder FM: Anticoagulants, iliopsoas, hematoma and femoral nerve compression. Am Fam Physician 44:2100, 1991.
194. Nishino H, Rubino FA, DeRemee RA, et al: Neurological involvement in Wegener's granulomatosis: An analysis of 324 consecutive patients at the Mayo Clinic. Ann Neurol 33:4, 1993.
195. Norman A, Robbins H, Milgram JE: The acute neuropathic arthropathy: A rapid, severely disorganizing form of arthritis. Radiology 90:1159, 1968.
196. Novak CB, MacKinnon SE, Patterson GA: Evaluation of patients with thoracic outlet syndrome. J Hand Surg [Am] 18A:292, 1993.
197. Ochoa JL, Verdugo RJ: Reflex sympathetic dystrophy: A common clinical avenue for somatoform expression. Neurol Clin 13:351, 1995.
198. O'Connor D, Marshall S, Massy-Westropp N: Non-surgical treatment (other than steroid injection) carpal tunnel syndrome. Cochrane Database Syst Rev 1:CD003219, 2003.
199. Oddis CV, Eisenbeis CH Jr, Reidbord HE, et al: Vasculitis in systemic sclerosis: Association with Sjögren's syndrome and CREST syndrome variant. J Rheumatol 14:942, 1987.
200. O'Donoghue JP, Powe JE, Mattar AG, et al: Three-phase bone scintigraphy: Asymmetric patterns in the upper extremities of asymptomatic normals and reflex sympathetic dystrophy patients. Clin Nucl Med 18:829, 1993.
201. Olney RK: AAEM minimonograph #38: Neuropathies in connective tissue disease. Muscle Nerve 15:531, 1992.
202. O'Malley MJ, Evanoff M, Terrono AL, et al: Factors that determine reexploration treatment of carpal tunnel syndrome. J Hand Surg 17A:638, 1992.
203. Osterman AL: The double crush syndrome. Orthop Clin North Am 19:147, 1988.
204. Owens ML: Psoas weakness and femoral neuropathy: Neglected signs of retroperitoneal hemorrhage from ruptured aneurysm. Surgery 91:363, 1982.
205. Pace JB, Nagle D: Piriformis syndrome. West J Med 124:435, 1976.
206. Pachner AR, Steere AC: The triad of neurologic manifestations of Lyme disease: Meningitis, cranial neuritis, and radiculoneuritis. Neurology 35:47, 1985.
207. Padopoulos SM, McGillicuddy JE, Albers JW: Unusual cause of "piriformis muscle syndrome." Arch Neurol 47:1144, 1990.
208. Padua L, Aprile I, Caliandro P, et al: Carpal tunnel syndrome in pregnancy: Multiperspective follow-up of untreated cases. Neurology 59:1643-1646, 2002.
209. Pancoast HK: Superior pulmonary sulcus tumor: Tumor characterized by pain, Horner's syndrome, destruction of bone and atrophy of hand muscles. JAMA 99:1391, 1932.
210. Paice E: Reflex sympathetic dystrophy. BMJ 310:1645, 1995.
211. Park YH, Taylor JA, Szollar SM, et al: Imaging findings in spinal neuroarthropathy. Spine 19:1499-1504, 1994.
212. Parkes JD, Kidner PH: Peripheral nerve and root lesions developing as a result of hematoma formation during anticoagulation treatment. Postgrad Med J 46:146, 1970.
213. Pecina MM, Krmpotic-Nemanic J, Markiewitz AD: Tunnel Syndromes. Boca Raton, FL, CRC Press, 1991, pp 1-84.
214. Pecina MM, Krmpotic-Nemanic J, Markiewitz AD: Tunnel Syndromes: Peripheral Nerve Compression Syndromes, 3rd ed. Boca Raton, FL, CRC Press, 2001, p 313.
215. Peet RM, Hendricksen JD, Gunderson TP, et al: Thoracic outlet syndrome: Evaluation of a therapeutic exercise program. Mayo Clin Proc 31:281, 1956.
216. Piazza MR, Bassett GS, Bunnell WP: Neuropathic spinal arthropathy in congenital insensitivity to pain. Clin Orthop 236:175, 1988.
217. Potts WJ: The pathology of Charcot joints. Ann Surg 86:596, 1927.
218. Pritchard JC, Desoia MF: Infection of a Charcot spine: A case report. Spine 18:7674, 1993.
219. Prough DS, McLeshey CH, Poehling GG, et al: Efficacy of oral nifedipine in the treatment of reflex sympathetic dystrophy. Anesthesiology 62:796, 1985.
220. Radin EL: Mechanical aspects of osteoarthrosis. Bull Rheum Dis 26:862, 1976.
221. Raff MC, Asbury AK: Ischemic mononeuropathy and mononeuropathy multiplex in diabetes mellitus. N Engl J Med 279:17, 1968.
222. Ramani PS, Sengupta RP: Cauda equina compression due to tabetic arthropathy of the spine. J Neurol Neurosurg Psychiatry 32:260, 1973.
223. Ranney D: Thoracic outlet: An anatomical redefinition that makes clinical sense. Clin Ant 9:50-52, 1996.
224. Rea F, Mazzucco C, Breda C, et al: Bilateral Pancoast syndrome in a patient with metachronous primary lung cancer. Ann Thorac Surg 58:550, 1994.
225. Remmen HJ, Lacquet LK, Van Son JA, et al: Surgical treatment of Pancoast tumor. J Cardiovasc Surg 34:157, 1993.
226. Rempel DM, Harrison RJ, Barnhart S: Work-related cumulative trauma disorders of the upper extremity. JAMA 267:838, 1992.
227. Remy-Jardin M, Remy J, Masson P, et al: Helical CT angiography of thoracic outlet syndrome functional anatomy. AJR Am J Roentgenol 174:1667-1674, 2000.
228. Resnick D: Neuroarthropathy. In Resnick D, Niwayama G (eds): Diagnosis of Bone and Joint Disorders, 2nd ed. Philadelphia, WB Saunders, 1988, pp 3162-3185.
229. Rho RH, Brewer RP, Lamer TJ, et al: Complex regional pain syndrome. Mayo Clin Proc 77:174-180, 2002.
230. Robinson DE, Ball KE, Webb PJ: Iliopsoas hematoma with femoral neuropathy presenting as a diagnostic dilemma after spinal decompression. Spine 26:E135-138, 2001.
231. Romanoff ME, Cory PC, Kalenak A, et al: Saphenous nerve entrapment at the adductor canal. Am J Sports Med 17:478, 1989.
232. Roquelaure Y, Raimbeau G, Dano C, et al: Occupational risk factors for radial tunnel syndrome in industrial workers. Scand J Work Environ Health 26:507-513, 2000.
233. Ross MA, Kimura J: AAEM case report #2: The carpal tunnel syndrome. Muscle Nerve 18:567, 1995.
234. Rossi P, Cardinali P, Serrao M, et al: Magnetic resonance imaging findings in piriformis syndrome: A case report. Arch Phys Med Rehabil 82:519-521, 2001.
235. Rull JA, Quibrera R, Gonzales-Millan H, Castaneda OL: Symptomatic treatment of peripheral diabetic neuropathy with carbamazepine: Double-blind crossover study. Diabetologia 5:215, 1969.
236. Sadler TR Jr, Rainer WG, Twombley G: Thoracic outlet compression: Application of positional arteriographic and nerve conduction studies. Am J Surg 130:704, 1975.
237. Said G, Lacroix-Ciaudo C, Fujimura H, et al: The peripheral neuropathy of necrotizing arteritis: A clinicopathological study. Ann Neurol 23:461-465, 1994.
238. Sanders RJ, Hammond SL: Management of cervical ribs and anomalous first ribs causing neurogenic thoracic outlet syndrome. J Vasc Surg 36:52-56, 2002.
239. Santillan CE, Katirji B: Brachial plexopathy in diabetic ketoacidosis. Muscle Nerve 23:271-273, 2000.
240. Sarhadi NS, Korday SN, Bainbridge LC: Radial tunnel syndrome: Diagnosis and management. J Hand Surg 23:617-619, 1998.
241. Schaumburg HH, Berger AR, Thomas PK: Disorders of Peripheral Nerves, 2nd ed. Philadelphia, FA Davis, 1992, pp 130-135.
242. Scholten RJ, Gerritsen AA, Uitdehaag BM, et al: Surgical treatment options for carpal tunnel syndrome. Cochrane Database Syst Rev 4:CD003905, 2002.
243. Schweiter ME, Mandel S, Schwartzman RJ, et al: Reflex sympathetic dystrophy revisited: MR imaging findings before and after infusion of contrast material. Radiology 195:211-214, 1995.
244. Scott DGI, Bacon PA, Tribe CR: Systemic rheumatoid vasculitis: A clinical and laboratory study of 50 cases. Medicine 60:288, 1981.

245. Seabold JE, Flickinger FW, Kao SCS, et al: Indium-111-leukocyte/technetium-99m-MDP bone and magnetic resonance imaging: Difficulty of diagnosing osteomyelitis in patients with neuropathic osteoarthropathy. J Nucl Med 31:549, 1990.
246. Seror P: Sensitivity of various electrophysiologic studies for the diagnosis of carpal tunnel syndrome. Muscle Nerve 16:1418, 1993.
247. Seyfert S, Boegner F, Hamm B, et al: The value of magnetic resonance imaging in carpal tunnel syndrome. J Neurol 242:41, 1994.
248. Sinclair RH, Pratt JH: Femoral neuropathy after pelvic operation. Am J Obstet Gynecol 112:404, 1972.
249. Smedby O, Rostad H, Klaastad O, et al: Functional imaging of the thoracic outlet syndrome in an open MR scanner. Eur Radiol 10:597-600, 2000.
250. Smith DL, Campbell SM: Painful shoulder syndromes: Diagnosis and management. J Gen Intern Med 7:328, 1992.
251. Spengler DM, Kirsh MM, Kaufer H: Orthopaedic aspects and early diagnosis of superior sulcus tumor of the lung (Pancoast). J Bone Joint Surg Am 55A:1645, 1973.
252. Spinner MJ: The arcade of Frohse and its relationship to posterior interosseous nerve paralysis. J Bone Joint Surg Br 50B:809, 1968.
253. Spinner RJ, Thomas NM, Kline DG: Failure of surgical decompression for a presumed case of piriformis syndrome: Case report. J Neurosurg 94:652-654, 2001.
254. Standaert C, Cardenas DD, Anderson P: Charcot spine as a late complication of traumatic spinal cord injury. Arch Phys Med Rehabil 78:221-225, 1997.
255. Stanton-Hicks M, Janig W, Hassenbusch S, et al: Reflex sympathetic dystrophy: Changing concepts and taxonomy. Pain 63:127-133, 1995.
256. Stark E, Oestreich K, Wendl K, et al: Nerve irritation after laparoscopic hernia repair. Surg Endosc 13:878-881, 1999.
257. Starling JR, Harms BA, Schroeder ME, Eichman PL: Diagnosis and treatment of genitofemoral and ilioinguinal entrapment neuralgia. Surgery 102:581, 1987.
258. Stern MB: The anterior interosseous nerve syndrome (The Kiloh-Nevin syndrome): Report and followup study of three cases. Clin Orthop 187:223, 1984.
259. Stevens JC, Beard CM, O'Fallon WM, et al: Conditions associated with carpal tunnel syndrome. Mayo Clin Proc 67:541, 1992.
260. Stevens JC, Sun S, Beard CM, et al: Carpal tunnel syndrome in Rochester, Minnesota, 1961 to 1980. Neurology 38:134, 1988.
261. Steyers CM: Recurrent carpal tunnel syndrome. Hand Clin 18:339-345, 2002.
262. Stone JH: Polyarteritis nodosa. JAMA 288:1632-1639, 2002.
263. Stuart JD, Morgan RF, Persing JA: Nerve compression syndromes of the lower extremity. Am Fam Physician 40:101, 1989.
264. Stubgen J: Neuromuscular disorders in systemic malignancy and its treatment. Muscle Nerve 18:636, 1995.
265. Suarez GA, Giannini C, Bosch EP, et al: Immune brachial plexus neuropathy: Suggestive evidence for an inflammatory-immune pathogenesis. Neurology 46:559-561, 1996.
266. Subramony SH, Wilbourn AJ: Diabetic proximal neuropathy: Clinical and electromyographic studies. J Neurol Sci 53:293, 1981.
267. Szabo RM, Chidgey LK: Stress carpal tunnel pressures in patients with carpal tunnel syndrome and normal patients. J Hand Surg [Am] 14A:624, 1989.
268. Tanaka S, Wild DK, Seligman PJ, et al: The US prevalence of self-reported carpal tunnel syndrome: 1988 national health interview survey data. Am J Public Health 84:1846, 1994.
269. Teasell RW, Potter P, Moulin D: Reflex sympathetic dystrophy involving three limbs: A case study. Arch Phys Med Rehabil 75:1008, 1994.
270. Thomas FP, Lovelace RE, Ding XS, et al: Vasculitic neuropathy in a patient with cryoglobulinemia and anti-MAG IgM monoclonal gammopathy. Muscle Nerve 15:891, 1992.
271. Thomas JE, Colby MY Jr: Radiation-induced or metastatic brachial plexopathy: A diagnostic dilemma. JAMA 222:1392, 1972.
272. Thomas MH, Chisholm GD: Retroperitoneal fibrosis associated with malignant disease. Br J Cancer 28:453, 1973.
273. Thrush DG: Congenital insensitivity to pain: A clinical genetic, and neurophysiological study of four children from the same family. Brain 96:369, 1973.
274. Thyagarajan D, Cascino T, Harms G: Magnetic resonance imaging in brachial plexopathy of cancer. Neurology 45:421, 1995.
275. Toby EB, Koman LA: Thoracic outlet compression syndrome. In Szabo RM: Nerve Compression Syndromes: Diagnosis and Treatment. Thorofare, NJ, Slack, 1989, pp 209-226.
276. Tong HC, Haig A: Posterior femoral cutaneous nerve mononeuropathy: Case report. Arch Phys Med Rehabil 81:1117-1118, 2000.
277. Toohey AK, LaSalle TL, Martinez S, Polisson RP: Iliopsoas bursitis: Clinical features, radiographic findings, and disease associations. Semin Arthritis Rheum 20:41, 1990.
278. Trummer M, Flaschka G, Unger F, et al: Lumbar disc herniation mimicking meralgia paresthetica: Case report. Surg Neurol 54: 80-81, 2000.
279. Tsairis P, Dyck PJ, Mulder DW: Natural history of brachial plexus neuropathy. Arch Neurol 27:109, 1972.
280. Turan I, Rivero-Melian C, Guntner P, et al: Tarsal tunnel syndrome: Outcome of surgery in longstanding cases. Clin Orthop 343:151-156, 1997.
281. Uncini A, DiMuzio A, Awad J, et al: Sensitivity of three median-to-ulnar comparative tests in the diagnosis of mild carpal tunnel syndrome. Muscle Nerve 16:1366, 1993.
282. Vallat JM, Desproges-Gotteron R, Leboutet MJ, et al: Cryoglobulinemic neuropathy: A pathological study. Ann Neurol 8:179, 1980.
283. Van der Kogel AJ, Barendsen GW: Late effects of spinal cord irradiation with 300 KV x-rays and 15 MeV neutrons. Br J Radiol 47:393, 1974.
284. Vandertop WP, Bosma NJ: The piriformis syndrome: A case report. J Bone Joint Surg 73A:1095, 1991.
285. Van Houdenhove B, Vasquez G, Onghena P, et al: Etiopathogenesis of RSD: A review and biopsychosocial hypothesis. Clin J Pain 8:300, 1992.
286. Vargo MM, Flood KM: Pancoast tumor presenting as cervical radiculopathy. Arch Phys Med Rehabil 71:606, 1990.
287. Veldman PHJM, Reynen HM, Arntz IE, et al: Signs and symptoms of reflex sympathetic dystrophy: Prospective study of 829 patients. Lancet 342:1012, 1993.
288. Wagner SC, Schweitzer ME, Morrison WB, et al: Can imaging findings help differentiate spinal neuropathic arthropathy from disk space infection? Initial experience. Radiology 214:693-699, 2000.
289. Walsh JC: The neuropathy of multiple myeloma: An electrophysiological and histological study. Arch Neurol 25:404, 1971.
290. Walton RJ: Femoral palsy complicating iliac bone biopsy. Lancet 2:497, 1975.
291. Weber ER, Daube JR, Coventry MB: Peripheral neuropathies associated with total hip arthroplasty. J Bone Joint Surg Am 58A:66, 1976.
292. Werner CO: Lateral elbow pain and posterior interosseous nerve entrapment. Acta Orthop Scand 174(Suppl):1, 1979.
293. Werner RA, Albers JW: Relation between needle electromyography and nerve conduction studies in patients with carpal tunnel syndrome. Arch Phys Med Rehabil 76:246, 1995.
294. Wilbourn AJ: Thoracic outlet syndrome surgery causing severe brachial plexopathy. Muscle Nerve 11:66, 1988.
295. Winsor T, Brow R: Costoclavicular syndrome: Its diagnosis and treatment. JAMA 196:109, 1966.
296. Wirth CR, Jacobs RL, Rolander SD: Neuropathic spinal arthropathy: A review of Charcot spine. Spine 5:558, 1980.
297. Wouter van Es H, Engelen AM, Witkamp TD, et al: Radiation-induced brachial plexopathy: MR imaging. Skeletal Radiol 26:284-288, 1997.
298. Wray CC, Easom S, Hoskinson J: Coccydynia: Aetiology and treatment. J Bone Joint Surg 73B:335-338, 1991.
299. Yoemans WE: The relation of arthritis of the sacroiliac joint to sciatica. Lancet 2:1119, 1928.
300. Young MR, Norris JW: Femoral neuropathy during anticoagulant therapy. Neurology 26:1173, 1976.
301. Ziporyn T: Upper body pain: Possible tipoff to Pancoast tumor. JAMA 246:1759, 1981.
302. Ziprin P, Williams P, Foster ME: External oblique aponeurosis nerve entrapment as a cause of groin pain in the athlete. Br J Surg 86:566-568, 1999.
303. Zucker G, Marder MJ: Charcot spine due to diabetic neuropathy. Am J Med 12:118, 1952.

PSYCHIATRIC DISORDERS, CHRONIC PAIN, AND MALINGERING

Capsule Summary

	Low Back	Neck
Frequency of spinal pain		
P	Rare	Rare
CP	Very common	Common
M	Very common	Common
Location of spinal pain		
P	Low back	Neck
CP	Low back	Neck
M	Low back	Neck
Quality of spinal pain		
P	Unremitting, persistent, descriptive language ("burning through my back")	Unremitting, persistent, descriptive language (knife-like neck pain)
CP	Continuous with irregular fluctuations	Continuous with irregular fluctuations
M	Unremitting, unresponsive to all therapies, disabling	Unremitting, unresponsive to all therapies, disabling
Symptoms and signs		
P	Neurotic	Neurotic
CP	Traumatic injury, loss of control over life	Traumatic injury, loss of control over life
M	Incapacitating pain, attempt to impress with severity of lesion, pain not consistent with anatomic findings; entire back, entire limb affected	Incapacitating pain, attempt to impress with severity of lesion, pain not consistent with anatomic findings; entire back, entire limb affected
Laboratory tests		
P	Normal	Normal
CP	Normal	Normal
M	Normal	Normal
Radiographic findings		
P	Normal	Normal
CP	Normal	Normal
M	Normal	Normal
Treatment		
P	Antipsychotic drugs	Antipsychotic drugs
CP	Antidepressant, pain clinic	Antidepressant, pain clinic
M	None	None

P, psychiatric disorders; CP, chronic pain; M, malingering.

PSYCHIATRIC DISORDERS

Patients with psychiatric disorders may develop pain as part of the symptoms associated with their illness. The prevalence of pain as a symptom in psychiatric patients ranges from 22% to 66%, depending on the population studied (inpatient vs. outpatient, Veterans Administration system vs. private clinic).[11,26,51] In many of these patients, pain is recognized as a result of their mental illness but is not a major complaint. However, in at least 25% of psychiatric patients, pain is severe.[11]

Patients with psychiatric disorders use medical services frequently. Katon and colleagues reported on frequent medical care users at a clinic.[24] About 33% of all services were used by 10% of patients. Of this 10%, about 50% were psychologically distressed. In this group, psychiatric diagnoses were prevalent, including major depression, panic disorder, and somatization disorder. Somatoform disorders are defined as those in which the presentation of psychological conflicts and issues has taken the form of physical illness.[1]

Somatization accompanies genuine physical disease as excessive worry, elaboration of symptoms, or disproportionate disability.[33] Components of the somatoform disorders include hypochondriasis, conversion disorder, somatization disorder, pain disorder, and body dysmorphic disorder.[16]

Pain

Definition

The pain that these patients experience is as "real" to the individuals with psychiatric illness as to those with a fractured femur. *Pain* is defined by the International Association for the Study of Pain as "an unpleasant sensory and emotional experience which we primarily associate with tissue damage or describe in terms of such damage, or both."[23] The definition of pain has two parts. One part deals with tissue damage or the threat of damage. It is necessary to experience an emotional response to that injury to experience pain. Therefore, those psychiatric patients who experience an emotional response to an event that they believe to be damaging have felt pain.

Frequency

Walters was one of the first to report on pain in psychiatric patients.[57] In a study of 430 patients referred for evaluation of pain, 112 patients (26%) had low back pain. Other locations for pain included the head, neck, chest, trunk, pelvis, and whole body. Pain was usually described dramatically. The most common diagnoses in these 430 patients was "other neuroses and situational states" in 336, conversion hysteria in 26, and psychoses in 68. Psychiatric patients with minor physical trauma had greater levels of pain than would have been expected given the extent of tissue damage.

Merskey reported his experience with 76 patients with mental illness and pain. Pain associated with neurosis was more common than pain associated with schizophrenia or endogenous depression.[38] Merskey discovered a relatively high association of neurosis, hysteria, and conversion symptoms with pain. Spear also found an increased number of neurotic patients with pain.[51] He found, as in the Mersky study, that the proportion of neurotic patients with pain to psychotic individuals with pain was similar.

Psychologic test studies yield comparable results. A number of researchers reported that the Minnesota Multiphasic Personality Inventory (MMPI) scores for hypochondrosis and conversion reaction were elevated compared with those for depression in psychiatric patients who complained of back pain.[21,42] Sternbach has demonstrated that the conversion pattern on the MMPI was found in patients who had pain that was chronic in duration. An unexpected finding was the relative absence of depression as a psychiatric diagnosis.[54] In a comparison between patients in chronic pain clinics and psychiatric patients with pain, depression was identified more commonly in the psychiatric population but only 10% of the psychiatric patients.[41,43]

Psychiatric Pain Generation

Anxiety

Merskey has suggested four reasons why psychologic illness causes the appearance or exacerbation of pain.[37] The first relates to a state of anxiety. Increased anxiety or worry about a lesion or experience heightens the intensity of pain. The mechanism of anxiety-associated pain remains speculative, but from a clinical standpoint alleviation of anxiety has a beneficial effect in the reduction of pain.

Hallucination

A second mechanism is associated with psychiatric hallucination. This mechanism is a rare cause of pain and is most closely associated with schizophrenic patients. Schizophrenic patients may experience hallucinatory damage to their person but infrequently associate that with pain.[58]

Muscle Tension

The third proposed mechanism concerns increased tension in muscles, which is associated with inadequate circulation and the accumulation of metabolic byproducts (lactic acid).[31] Individuals who use muscles in a new way may develop aching and discomfort in a body part. It is proposed that generalized muscle tension in those with chronic anxiety and stress similarly causes pain. In actuality, this hypothesis is not proven in fact. In a number of studies of pain, particularly headache, increased muscle tension accounted for only a small percentage of pain in patients with chronic pain. The pain was more closely related to a patient's personality disorder than to the level of muscle contraction.[22,47]

Hysteria

The fourth mechanism of pain production in psychiatric patients is hysteria with conversion reactions. Conversion reaction or hysterical conversion is a mechanism for transforming anxiety or other emotions into a dysfunction of bodily structures or organs supplied by the voluntary portion of the nervous system. The symptoms lessen anxiety and symbolize the underlying mental conflict. The patient may gain benefits from his situation and may not be overly concerned about the dysfunction. The mental anguish associated with the patient's condition is not easily recognized by the people who surround him, but a somatic complaint, like spinal pain, is one that is readily accepted and understood. Some traditional associated phenomena such as symbolism, la belle indifférence, and histrionic personality do not occur with adequate frequency to be useful in differentiating conversion from physical disease.[13]

Psychogenic Rheumatism

Psychogenic rheumatism is a term that may be used in patients who have musculoskeletal symptoms, such as spinal pain, associated with a psychiatric disorder.[46] The criteria for this diagnosis include the absence of an organic disease or the insufficiency of disease that is present to account for the complaints, "functional" character of the complaints, and a positive diagnosis for a psychiatric illness. In one large population of rheumatology patients, approximately 7% had a diagnosis of psychogenic rheumatism. However, the separation of psychogenic rheumatism and organic disease was seldom distinct.

Camptocormia

One specific form of psychiatric disorder associated with back pain is camptocormia.[44] Camptocormia is derived from the Greek words *kamptein*, "to bend," and *kormos*, "trunk." It is a special form of conversion hysteria occurring mainly in soldiers and industrial workers. The disease consists of assumption of a position in which the back is flexed acutely, the arms hang loosely, and the eyes are directed downward after a trivial trauma. The position disappears when the patient assumes a recumbent position. Many of these individuals are men whose parents have had back disorders. Therapy for the condition is separation of the individuals from the source of stress. Patients have had quick recoveries within days of receiving the news of discharge from the Armed Forces.[44]

Case Study 16-2

A 23-year-old hotel maintenance man developed acute low back pain while lifting heavy sofa cushions at work. He had no response to conservative therapy and developed a severe headache and increased back pain after a myelogram. He described his pain as constant with radiation up his back to his neck and down to his feet. His pain was so severe that he was limited to walking 15 minutes per day. He was unable to shave or dress himself and relied on his wife for activities of daily living. His physical examination revealed an individual "stuck" in a forward flexed posture at 20 degrees. The motion of the lumbar spine was severely limited. The patient was unable to raise his arms secondary to low back pain. He also reported back pain with movement of his wrists and hands. He had cogwheeling movements of his lower extremities and "no feeling" in his entire left leg. He had back pain with vertical loading over his skull. He also had facial grimacing, muscle tremors, cramps of his hands, sweating, and gagging during his examination. Although in the standing position he was unable to straighten his spine, he was able to lie flat on the examining table when assuming a supine position. During a functional capacity examination and work hardening program, he was unable to complete minimal tasks (lifting a 1-pound weight from waist to shoulder level) secondary to pain. This individual has a form of camptocormia in which his physical condition maintains his role as a patient for all the individuals with whom he interacts including his family and his employer. The possibility of return to work for these types of individuals is poor.

Other Conversion Reactions

Conversion reactions can be dramatic to the degree of paralysis.[30] Young adult women who are disadvantaged economically, have limited education, or who have difficulty expressing distress are at risk for this disorder.[2] Individuals with hysteria may present with complete loss of extremity function. Careful examination of these individuals is required to discover the inconsistencies of their presentation. These individuals are not malingerers. Informing these individuals of normal findings may result in rapid improvement. A total of 60% will improve within 2 weeks, with 98% improved within 1 year.[3,52] These individuals require evaluation and therapy with a psychiatrist. Sometimes identifying the stress that precipitated the reaction helps resolve the symptoms.[45] If the underlying cause of the hysteria is not addressed, these individuals are at risk of repeated episodes of "physical" impairments. Recurrence rates are as high as 25% within the first year of diagnosis.[49]

Rotes-Querol has suggested a list of symptoms and signs found in patients with psychogenic rheumatism.[46] These symptoms do not have diagnostic importance until the possibility of organic disease has been ruled out. The symptoms and signs include the following:

1. Dramatic urgency for an appointment not justified by the severity of disease.
2. A written list of complaints so that no fact is left out.
3. Multiple test results including electrocardiography, EMG, electroencephalography, barium enema, upper gastrointestinal studies, CT scans, myelograms, and MR imaging.
4. The necessity to review the laboratory data first to determine the cause of the patient's symptoms. Any minor abnormalities are highlighted by the patient.
5. Preoccupation with future disability from minor physical changes.
6. Those who accompany the patient may be separated from the patient's condition or intensively supportive, highlighting every abnormality and frequently using the pronoun "we" during the description of tests or medications taken.
7. Inability to relax during the examination.
8. Marked theatrical responses to questions concerning pain.
9. Patient frequently holds on to the physician during the course of the examination as a gesture of seeking support.

Specific psychogenic syndromes involving the cervical spine and areas of referred pain are listed in Table 16-8. Benign dorsalgia is associated with pain in the interscapular area. The pain is variable in quality, consisting of com-

16-8 PSYCHOGENIC RHEUMATISM SYNDROMES OF THE CERVICAL SPINE

Benign dorsalgia
Cervicocranial syndromes
- Pain in the cervical and nuchal areas
- Fronto-occipital headaches
- Paresthesias over the vertex
- Sensations of giddiness and instability on walking; agoraphobia
- Feelings of weight and pain in the eyes or in the periorbital region
- Functional disturbances of eyesight including transitory blindness and central scotomata
- Dryness and irritation of the mouth and larynx and intermittent loss of voice
- Feelings of unreality

Nocturnal acroparesthesias
- Sensory abnormalities similar to carpal tunnel syndrome
- Occur always at night
- Relieved by moving arms in morning
- Absence of motor abnormalities
- Frequent proximal radiation of pain to the shoulder
- Symptoms increased with anxiety and tension, not position
- Difficult to differentiate from median nerve compression

Modified from Rotes-Querol J: The syndrome of psychogenic rheumatism. Clin Rheum Dis 5:797, 1979.

ponents of fatigue, aching, and burning. Diffuse pain over the corresponding spinous processes is common. In contrast, pain in a bandlike pattern may be of nerve root origin. Plain roentgenograms are unremarkable for alterations that are commensurate with the level of pain expressed by the patient. The syndrome is seen most frequently in light-duty workers who require a slight flexion of the spine, such as typists and computer operators. Cervicocranial psychogenic rheumatism affects older patients and involves the nuchal area, with radiation of pain to the vertex of the skull. These individuals experience persistent headaches and an unsteady gait. These episodes may be differentiated from vertebrobasilar insufficiency by the lack of reproducibility of symptoms and signs with specific rotatory and extension movements of the neck.[46]

The evaluation of the psychiatric patient must be complete. A thorough history is essential to remove the possibility of an organic cause of a patient's pain. This type of evaluation also gains the patient's confidence that the physician has been thorough and concerned about the problem. At a second session, the possibility of stress as a cause of the patient's pain is raised. Additional portions of the patient's history concerning job or family stresses or conflicts are asked. The patient may be willing to talk about the faults of others in the workplace but will remain reticent about sexual conflicts with spouses or conflicts with parents or children unless specifically asked about these interpersonal difficulties.

The patient must be told that the pain is of psychogenic origin. Statements by the physician denying the presence of an illness ("It is all in your own imagination") are inappropriate. The explanation of the fact that patients who are anxious, threatened, or stressed experience real pain is reassuring to the patient. These patients are referred to a mental health professional for care of their psychiatric disorders. While the patient is undergoing psychiatric therapy, the referring physician should encourage the patient to be as physically active as possible. Interaction with other people in an exercise class may be very useful.

Patients with low back pain frequently ask the question concerning the association of stress or anxiety with the onset or exacerbation of pain. Feuerstein studied the mood fluctuations of patients with recurrent low back pain with matched healthy controls. Patients with pain had higher levels of anxiety, tension, and fatigue and lower levels of vigor. No mood state was predictive of pain onset, but fatigue was more common after the onset of pain. No mood set predicted the severity of pain, but greater levels of pain were correlated with levels of fatigue. Although this study does not clearly demonstrate the correlation of anxiety and the initiation of pain, the control of established pain requires the reduction of anxiety and the improvement of functional endurance to counteract the fatigue factor associated with low back pain. A regular exercise program has the potential to decrease fatigue, relieve stress, and reduce pain.[13]

Despite careful evaluation and the institution of appropriate therapy, patients with psychogenic rheumatism may not improve. The following case study demonstrates the difficulties in the treatment of these patients:

CASE STUDY 16-3

A 26-year-old woman was referred for evaluation of back pain. The patient had worked as a bookkeeper for her husband's company but was now unemployed. She had been divorced once and had two children by her first marriage. She had remarried but had become disenchanted with her marriage because of physical threats by her spouse. Eight months before her evaluation, she was pushed down by her husband, hitting her lower back on the ground. Subsequent to that event, the patient experienced severe back pain radiating down both legs, anterior and posterior aspects. The patient felt most comfortable standing, because sitting and lying increased her pain. An extensive work-up including a CT scan, myelogram, and MR revealed a minimal protrusion of a disc without nerve impingement. A multitude of therapeutic modalities, including nonsteroidal anti-inflammatory drugs (NSAIDs), physical therapy, and nerve blocks, were ineffective.

On examination, the patient had exquisite pain of the lumbar area with slight pressure on the skin over the low back. With palpation of the back, the patient would grimace and jump. She had low back pain with lateral bending of the neck and downward pressure on her head. Her muscle tests revealed cogwheeling and resisting movements.

The possibility of a psychiatric problem as a cause of the patient's pain was offered as one explanation of her symptoms. The patient's thought that an operation to remove a disc would "cure" her problem was discounted.

Attempts at involving the patient in psychiatric therapy were not successful. The patient remained at home with her husband. On subsequent visits, she offered the history that she was fearful and anxious and could not decide whether to leave her spouse or stay at home. Her back pain continued to be severe.

Despite the best of efforts, some patients with spinal pain will not improve. Some patients with psychiatric disorders fit into this group. All the clinician can do is rule out the possibility of an organic cause of pain and discuss, in a frank but supportive fashion, the psychologic sources of the patient's symptoms. The care of these patients is time consuming. Often a busy practitioner will not have the time to treat these patients. If that is the case, these patients should be referred to a psychiatrist, psychologist, or other mental health care professional for continued evaluation and therapy.

Psychiatric disorders may be the source of physical ailments. A prime example is the effect of eating disorders and depression on the level of bone mineral density (BMD) and the risk of osteoporotic fractures. Women who have experienced a major depression during their lives had significant decreases in BMD in the spine and hip, as well as lower serum osteocalcin levels than nondepressed age-matched controls.[36] Men with depression also have decreased BMD, which may be even greater than the loss experienced by women.[48] Anorexia nervosa and bulimia are associated with osteoporosis.[60] Treatment of the eating disorder can result in improvement in BMD abnormalities if the anorexic patients are treated early.[7]

PSYCHIATRIC ILLNESS WITH CHRONIC PAIN

Patients with acute injuries recognize the linkage between pain (nociception) and tissue injury. The pain serves a purpose to warn the host that injury has occurred and removal of the body part from the injurious stimulus is warranted. The pain that remains after the immediate injury results in decreased use of that body part during the healing process. That portion of the body is protected. Once the injury heals, the pain disappears.

From a psychological perspective, neck pain is particularly disturbing to the host because the location of discomfort is close to the spinal cord and central nervous system. Referred pain from neck injury may radiate up to become a headache or down the spine to cause low back pain. Pain may also radiate into the arms, hands, or thighs. Although the pain may be severe, gradual resolution of the pain is the rule. In the usual circumstance, the process resolves with increasing improvement over 8 weeks.

The patient with chronic pain does not follow this scenario. *Chronic pain* is defined as pain that has been present for 6 months or longer.[53] The most significant factor differentiating chronic from acute pain is that the pain is no longer serving a useful biologic or survival function and has become a disease itself. The emotional state of patients, involving affective, vegetative, cognitive, and behavioral components of personality, is affected. This was noted during the Civil War by Mitchell, who described the development of dejection and anger in soldiers who developed chronic causalgia.[39] The patient undergoes a progressive physical and emotional deterioration caused by loss of appetite, insomnia, depression, anxiety, decreased physical activity, demoralization, and depressive symptoms of worthlessness, helplessness, and hopelessness. These patients have the clinical signs and symptoms of the chronic pain syndrome.[4]

The effects of the chronic pain syndrome will vary depending on the patient's ethnic background, coping skills, and self-image and the support system contributed by the patient's family and fellow workers. Understanding the patient's psychosocial dynamics has a profound effect on the prognosis and the choice of therapy. A psychosocial assessment of the patient with chronic pain can identify the strengths and weaknesses in the patient's personality structure that will influence the manifestations of the pain syndrome and identify those factors that may hinder compliance with the treatment regimen.

Pain Assessment

MMPI

The psychologic assessment of the patient with chronic pain may include evaluation of the patient's personality and conceptualization of the pain, along with a rating scale for the severity of pain. The MMPI is the most widely used personality test.[10] The purpose of the test is to categorize psychiatric patients and to discriminate between psychiatric patients and normal patients through the answers to 566 true/false questions. The questions are divided into the following 10 clinical scales: hypochondriasis, depression, hysteria, psychopathic deviance, masculinity/femininity, paranoia, psychasthenia, schizophrenia, hypomania, and social introversion.

Patients with chronic pain indicate an elevation in neuroticism manifested by increases on the hypochondriasis, depression, and hysteria scales. The basic interpretation of this profile is that it reflects a preoccupation with physical symptoms, bodily functions, depression, negativism, hostility, and use of denial to cope with psychologic conflicts. The data record for patients who have less depression forms a V shape on the MMPI, which is referred to as a "conversion V" pattern. These patients somatosize their problems when under stress. Physical symptoms are easier for these patients to understand than psychologic conflicts.

The results of the MMPI taken by chronic pain patients have been reported by a number of investigators. Sternbach reported neurotic scale elevation in patients with chronic back pain as compared with those who have acute low back pain.[56] Neurosis was not a permanent part of the patient's personality as shown by a reduction in neurotic scales in patients who had pain relief after back surgery.[55] Fordyce has noted that the degree of neuroticism in MMPI studies is related more to the chronicity of the pain than to the physical lesion.[17]

Bradley and associates have identified three homogeneous subgroups of low back pain patients based on MMPI profiles.[5] The first group is normal patients who are functioning well in their job and family life with a minimum of disruption despite back pain. The second, most common, group is composed of patients who are neurotic. The third group manifests a psychopathologic profile that shows elevations in all scales except the masculinity/femininity scale. These patient have significant psychiatric dysfunction diagnosed as schizophrenia, psychotic depression, or inadequate personality. Heaton and colleagues also have used the MMPI to characterize chronic pain patients into seven groupings.[20] A report by Love and Peck suggests that the psychologic etiology of chronic low back pain and the response of individuals to specific therapy cannot be differentiated by the MMPI.[32]

MMPI has been used in the evaluation of industrial workers who report injury associated with chronic pain. In a prospective study of industrial workers, MMPI was used to predict the likelihood of reporting back injury.[18] MMPI scale 3 (lassitude/malaise) had the greatest predictive power of those who report back pain from an injury. However, job dissatisfaction is also a contributing factor because 75% of workers in this study had back pain but only 5% reported a painful injury.

The results of all the studies of MMPI suggest that the test is helpful in characterizing the psychologic profile of some patients with chronic low back pain. However, the test is cumbersome, does not predict all individuals who will develop pain, and does not define the appropriate and effective therapy for patients with chronic pain.

McGill Pain Questionnaire

The McGill pain questionnaire assesses how patients conceptualize their pain by using words to qualify and quantify it. There are a total of 78 pain descriptors in the questionnaire. In one study, psychiatric disturbance was associated with a greater total number of pain descriptors.[27] Patients may also use visual pain analogue scales to quantify their pain. A daily log of the patient's pain level, along with degree of physical activity, and medication usage can be used to assess the patient's functional status and monitor progress. Whether estimations of pain intensity are correlated with the clinical status and health care utilization of a patient has been challenged by Fordyce.[19] Patient self-reports of pain may not accurately describe their level of functioning. However, the ratings of pain by the patient do help in monitoring progress in treatment.

In addition to those tests already mentioned, a mental status examination and a social and work history are essential. These evaluations focus on the patient's thought processes and self-image. The work history is important to list the patient's work experiences and test those job skills the patient retains that may be used in vocational rehabilitation.

Psychiatric Diagnostic Classification

The classification of psychiatric diagnoses of pain patients is difficult. *The Diagnostic and Statistical Manual of Mental Disorders*, 4th edition (DSM-IV) is the standard for the nomenclature of psychiatric diagnoses. In a study of 1801 patients seen by a psychiatric consultation service, 167 pain patients were compared with the remainder in regard to their DSM-III diagnosis. The pain patients had more serious medical problems, lack of improvement in medical condition, and decreased mobility. Patients without pain had more serious psychiatric disorders. The psychiatric diagnoses of the patients with pain were nonspecific for the problem of pain, including dysthymic disorder and depressed mood. The DSM-IV does not provide specificity of the clinical state of pain including the separation of chronic and acute syndromes.[25]

A variety of DSM diagnoses, including depression, somatosensory conversion disorder, anxiety, and personality disorders, were used for the characterization of 283 chronic pain patients at a pain center. Diagnosis of schizophrenia and psychogenic disorders was rare. The authors of this study also agree that difficulties exist in characterizing patients with chronic pain with the current DSM classification.[15]

Patients with chronic spinal pain received medical therapy consisting of NSAIDs, muscle relaxants, and physical therapy, including temperature modalities and exercises, but have not had a satisfactory response. Many of these patients seek multiple medical consultations and undergo a variety of unconventional therapies, including acupuncture and spinal manipulation. Other chronic pain patients may have undergone multiple surgical procedures or suffered substance abuse in the form of alcohol or narcotics.

Treatment of patients with chronic pain must be directed at physical-structural abnormalities if they persist and, equally important, at pain behavior of the patient. The four most important factors determining successful outcome in rehabilitation of chronic pain patients are the following in order of importance: (1) motivation, (2) social support system, (3) chronicity, and (4) degree of tissue pathology.[40] Correction of tissue pathology is important but may not be adequate to alter pain behavior. If the condition has been chronic, patients may have altered their behavior because of the pain to the point where they have lost control over their lives.[59] These individuals, in response to the loss of control, develop reduced motivation to initiate responses to the environment, inability to learn new responses, depression, and anxiety disorders. Depression was noted in over 50% of patients with chronic low back pain resistant to medical and surgical therapy.[35] The reality of being in pain and out of work can also contribute to psychologic dysfunction. Dependency becomes all-encompassing in a patient who is unemployed, is financially insecure, and is experiencing deteriorating interpersonal relationships with family members and social isolation. Therapy for these individuals must be directed at returning some control of their lives back to them.

Patients with chronic, resistant spinal pain benefit from an evaluation by a pain center. Pain centers have the resources to deal with a patient's situation in a multidisciplinary fashion. Psychiatrists, psychologists, neurosurgeons, anesthesiologists, physical therapists, vocational rehabilitation counselors, and social workers are part of the treatment team. Through the concerted effort of all these health professionals and the motivation of the patient, improvement in the patient's condition can occur. A study of 38 patients with disabling chronic pain at an inpatient/outpatient pain center demonstrated an improvement in patient function at 3 weeks. Patients at the pain center had significant reduction in addictive medications, subjective pain ratings, the number of functional activities that caused pain, and the number of health professional visits.[50]

MALINGERING

Malingering, which may be defined as conscious misrepresentation of thoughts, feelings, and facts, is a condition in which symptoms and signs associated with pain are entirely feigned for secondary gain.[14] Most commonly, malingering occurs in the setting of the workplace and workers' compensation. However, the secondary gain associated with malingering may not be financial alone. Individuals may feign spinal symptoms to continue in a less strenuous job at work. They may receive a parking space closer to their place of employment. These individuals may feign symptoms to gain control over family members or fellow workers. The injured party may allow others to do work the patient would do ordinarily.

The actual percentage of chronic spinal pain patients who are malingering is undetermined. Obviously, the ascertainment of the inaccuracy of the patient's report of pain and disability is a difficult process. Each health care provider has an internalized standard of symptoms and signs by which those with chronic spinal pain are judged. However, most physicians who see a large population of spinal pain patients believe that the number of individuals who are true malingerers—those who totally feign injury and pain in a willful manner to collect workers' compensation or disability payments—is a very small percentage of the individuals with spinal pain. A survey of a total of 300 orthopedists and neurosurgeons quantified the percentage of malingerers among back pain patients to be 5% or less.[29]

The possibility of malingering should be raised in the mind of the treating physician when major discrepancies or inconsistencies appear in the patient's medical situation. Seventeen patients with chronic low back pain with inconsistencies in their statements or behaviors were compared with subjects assessed without inconsistencies. Inconsistent subjects were more likely to have pending litigation and were more focused on pain with more dramatized complaints, lower levels of medical findings, and less interest in treatment.[8]

These inconsistencies may involve the patient's history or physical examination. The following two case studies are examples of how patients who are malingering can be identified by history or physical examination.

CASE STUDY 16-4

A 24-year-old woman slipped and fell while working at a restaurant. She experienced acute low back pain. Over the next year, the patient complained of continued pain that was unrelenting. The pain was so severe that the patient had decreased range of motion of the lumbar spine. The patient stated that the pain with motion was so severe that she was unable to bend her back. She had received courses of NSAIDs, muscle relaxants, physical therapy, and transcutaneous nerve stimulation. All these therapies had no effect on her pain. She could not go back to work because she could not bend or carry objects. Formal testing of the motion of her lumbar spine was markedly limited. No palpable muscle spasm was noted. During the physical examination, nail polish was noted on her fingers and toes. She was asked who applied the polish to her nails. She said she did her own nails. Her lack of motion was feigned. In the privacy of her home, she had full range of motion of her spine. Other distraction tests completed during the physical examination corroborated the fact that the patient was malingering.

The second case illustrates the suggestibility of the malingering patient. They are willing to agree with any of the statements of the examining physician. The patient believes that whatever the physician suggests as symptoms or signs of the disease must be correct.

CASE STUDY 16-5

A 36-year-old man was working on a construction site when he developed back pain while lifting some lumber. The patient developed localized, right-sided lumbar pain. The patient was placed on bed rest and NSAIDs. He had no response to therapy. He was referred to our office and was evaluated. A suspicion of malingering was raised, but the patient was given another course of NSAIDs to monitor his response. When he returned he reported no response to therapy. It was suggested to him that palpation of areas other than the lumbar spine may cause low back pain. The patient's nose was pressed and patient complained that the maneuver re-created his low back pain. We referred to this as "Rudolph, the Red-Nosed Reindeer" sign.

The assessment of malingering by the treating physician is very difficult. It is difficult to positively prove conscious misrepresentation of thoughts, feelings, and facts by the patient. However, the inconsistencies in history and physical examination are useful in documenting one's suspicions.

Two separate sets of criteria have been developed to document the likelihood of malingering.[6,12] Although the Emory Pain Control Center "inconsistency profile" and Ellard's profile of inconsistency were developed independently, they are remarkably similar. The Emory profile is an amalgamation of those factors that would lead the examining physician to suspect malingering. The profile includes the following:

1. Discrepancy between a person's complaint of "terrible pain" and an attitude of calmness and well-being.
2. Complete negative work-up for organic disease by two or more physicians.
3. "Dramatized" complaints that are vague or have global implications ("It just hurts" or "I hurt bad").
4. Exaggeration of trivial pathology, embellished with medical terms learned from previous contacts with physicians ("My back spasms paralyze my legs").
5. Overemphasized gait or posture abnormalities that develop suddenly, persist, and cannot be substantiated objectively (the presence of a limp that is not confirmed by a specific pattern of wear of old shoes, the use of a cane, or a back brace that is said to be used on a daily basis but shows little wear).
6. Resistance to evaluation or rehabilitation when the stated goal of therapy is return to gainful employment.
7. Lack of motivation to learn new coping skills, despite verbal reports of compliance with treatment (no increase in back motion despite claims of completing range of motion exercise on a daily basis).
8. Missed appointments for studies that measure function, motion, or vocational capabilities.
9. Unconventional response to treatment (no discrimination between saline and analgesic injection into affected areas; reports of increased symptoms with therapy that follow no anatomic or physiologic pattern—response to tranquilizers as stimulants and vice versa).
10. Resistance to treatment procedures, especially in presence of intense complaints of pain.
11. Absence of psychologic or emotional disturbances.
12. Inconsistent psychologic test profile with clinical presentations. For example, the MMPI profile is indicative of a psychotic disorder with no clinical signs of psychosis.
13. Discrepancies between reports of patient and spouse or other close relatives.
14. Unstable personal and occupational history.
15. A personal history that reflects a character disorder that might include drug and/or alcohol abuse, criminal behavior, erratic personal relationships, and violence.

As suggested by the inconsistency profile, physical examination of the malingerer is often helpful and revealing. The patient may refuse to cooperate with components of the examination.[9] Patients with low back pain may be better able to exaggerate symptoms than those individuals who are pain free when using pain questionnaires.[28] Gait abnormalities may not be present when the patient initially enters the office but are during the formal examination. A normal lumbar lordosis without paraspinous muscle spasm is unusual in the patient with persistent low back pain, in whom a decreased lordosis would be expected. A normal cervical curvature without paraspinous muscle spasm is also unusual in the patient with persistent neck pain in whom straightening would be expected. Gently touching the skin over the back or neck results in intense pain with reflex spasm. The area of tenderness may vary during the examination. It is worthwhile to retest the area of tenderness during the course of the physical examination. Not infrequently, the patient does not remember the exact location of the tenderness and an inconsistency is noted. Patients will be unable to bend the back or neck forward more than 5 degrees despite the absence of muscle spasm. (Patients without spasm should be able to rotate around the hips, resulting in flexion of the upper body despite lumbar spine disease.) Simultaneous hand strength should be checked after each hand is tested independently. The strong arm becomes weak in the simultaneous test. Patients may have a limited straight leg–raising test in the supine position but normal motion without pain with the modified straight leg–raising test in the seated position or the bilateral straight leg–raising test (see Waddell's tests, Fig. 5-20). The Hoover test will document the patient's effort to complete the requested physical test. The absence of muscle atrophy belies a history of chronic leg weakness. Sensory abnormalities may include extreme pain with pin prick, a midline loss of sensation, stocking-glove anesthesia, whole arm or leg numbness, differences in loss in supination and pronation, and inconsistent response to vibratory stimuli with a tuning fork. Deep tendon reflexes are hyperactive and out of proportion to the stimulus. Cogwheel rigidity is noted in the affected arm with sudden giving way. Patients should also complete a pain drawing documenting all areas of involvement. Many malingerers believe that more is better. Patients tend to fill out areas of involvement far from the axial skeleton including areas outside the body.

Caveats regarding the interpretation of Waddell's tests in the setting of spinal pain have been presented. The developer of the tests has cautioned about the overinterpretation of a few positive findings as a clear indication of malingering. These tests are also not a substitute for a complete psychological assessment.[34]

Once all the data have been collected, the physician should make a determination of malingering by the patient. This is a difficult process that requires the diagnostic and detective skill of the physician. Very few things in medicine are black and white. The same can be said about malingering. Very few malingerers are totally without pain or the fear of being placed back in a job situation that may be perceived as harmful.

Some physicians prefer to remove themselves from the determination of malingering and leave it to others, including lawyers, to make the determinations of impairment and disability. If the process is allowed to function without medical input, those who do not really deserve compensation or consideration will diminish the resources that rightfully belong to those who have organic difficulties and are attempting to function at their maximum capacity. If the physician believes the patient is a malingerer, he or she should terminate further treatment of the patient. The patient should be told that there is no anatomic abnormality that can explain the pain. If the patient has been evaluated only once, he or she should be referred to another physician for an additional opinion. If the first physician was in error, the second physician can initiate appropriate therapy. If the first physician was correct, no additional investigations are ordered and therapy is discontinued.

References

Psychiatric Disorders, Chronic Pain, and Malingering

1. American Psychiatric Association: Diagnostic and Statistical Manual of Mental Disorders, 3rd ed. Washington, DC, American Psychiatric Press, 1987.
2. Binzer M, Andersen PM, Kullgren G: Clinical characteristics of patients with motor disability due to conversion disorder: A prospective control group study. J Neurol Neurosurg Psychiatry 63:83-88, 1997.
3. Binzer M, Kullgren G: Motor conversion disorder: A prospective 2- to 5-year follow-up study. Psychosomatics 39:519-527, 1998.
4. Black RG: The chronic pain syndrome. Surg Clin North Am 4:999, 1975.
5. Bradley LA, Prokop CK, Margolis R, Gentry DD: Multivariate analysis of the MMPI profiles of low back pain patients. J Behav Med 1:253, 1978.
6. Brena SF, Chapman SL: Pain and litigation. In Wall PD, Melzack R (ed): Textbook of Pain. Edinburgh, Churchill Livingstone, 1984, pp 832-839.
7. Castro J, Lazaro L, Pons F, et al: Adolescent anorexia nervosa: The catch-up effect in bone mineral density after recovery. J Am Acad Child Adolesc Psychiatry 40:1215-1221, 2001.
8. Chapman SL, Brena SF: Patterns of conscious failure to provide accurate self-report data in patients with low back pain. Clin J Pain 6:178, 1990.
9. Cunnien AJ: Psychiatric and medical syndromes associated with deception. In Rogers R (ed): Clinical Assessment of Malingering and Deception. New York, Guilford Press, 1988, pp 13-33.
10. Dahlstrom WG, Welsh GS, Dahlstrom LE: An MMPI Handbook, Vols I and II. Minneapolis, University of Minnesota Press, 1972.
11. Delaplaine R, Ifabumuyi OI, Mersky H, Zarfas J: Significance of pain in psychiatric hospital patients. Pain 4:361, 1978.
12. Ellard J: Psychological reactions to compensable injury. Med J Aust 8:349, 1970.
13. Feuerstein M, Carter RL, Papciak AS: A prospective analysis of stress and fatigue in recurrent low back pain. Pain 31:333, 1987.
14. Finneson BE: Low Back Pain, 2nd ed. Philadelphia, JB Lippincott, 1981, pp 179-197.
15. Fishbain DA, Goldberg M, Meagher BR, et al: Male and female chronic pain patients categorized by DSM-III psychiatric diagnostic criteria. Pain 26:181, 1986.
16. Ford CV: Dimensions of somatization and hypochondriasis. Neurol Clin 13:241, 1955.
17. Fordyce WE: Behavioral Methods in Chronic Pain and Illness. St Louis, CV Mosby, 1976.
18. Fordyce WE, Bigos SJ, Battie MC, Fisher LD: MMPI scale 3 as a predictor of back injury report: What does it tell us? Clin J Pain 8:222, 1992.
19. Fordyce WE, Lansky D, Calsyn DA, et al: Pain measurement and pain behavior. Pain 18:53, 1984.
20. Heaton RK, Getto CJ, Lehman RAW, et al: A standardized evaluation of psychosocial factors in chronic pain. Pain 12:165, 1982.
21. Hanvik LH: MMPI profiles in patients with low-back pain. J Consult Clin Psychol 15:350, 1956.
22. Harper RC, Steger JC: Psychological correlates of frontalis EMG and pain in tension headache. Headache 18:215, 1978.
23. International Association for the Study of Pain (Subcommittee on Taxonomy): Pain terms: a list with definitions and notes on usage. Pain 6:249, 1979.
24. Katon W, Von Korff M, Lin E, et al: Distressed high utilizers of medical care. DSM-III-R diagnoses and treatment needs. Gen Hosp Psychiatry 12:355, 1990.

25. King SA, Strain JJ: The problem of psychiatric diagnosis for the pain patient in the general hospital. Clin J Pain 5:329, 1989.
26. Klee GD, Ozelis S, Greenberg I, Gallant LJ: Pain and other somatic complaints in a psychiatric clinic. MD St Med J 8:188, 1959.
27. Kremer EF, Atkinson JH, Kremer AM: The language of pain: Affective descriptors of pain are a better predictor of psychological disturbance than sensory and effective descriptors. Pain 16:185, 1983.
28. Leavitt F: Detection of simulation among persons instructed to exaggerate symptoms of low back pain. J Occup Med 29:229, 1987.
29. Leavitt F, Sweet JJ: Characteristics and frequency of malingering among patients with low back pain. Pain 25:357, 1986.
30. Letonoff EF, Williams TR, Sidhu KS: Hysterical paralysis: A report of three cases and a review of the literature. Spine 27:E441-E445, 2002.
31. Lewis T, Pickering GW, Rothschild P: Observations upon muscular pain in intermittent claudication. Heart 15:359, 1931.
32. Love AW, Peck CL: The MMPI and psychological factors in chronic low back pain: A review. Pain 28:1, 1987.
33. Mabe PA, Hobson DP, Jones LR, et al: Hypochondriacal traits in medical inpatients. Gen Hosp Psychiatry 10:236, 1988.
34. Main CJ, Waddell G: Behavioral responses to examination: A reappraisal of the interpretation of "nonorganic signs." Spine 23:2367-2371, 1998.
35. Maruta T, Swanson DW, Swenson WM: Low back pain in a psychiatric population. Mayo Clin Proc 51:57, 1976.
36. Michelson D, Stratakis C, Hill L, et al: Bone mineral density in women with depression. N Engl J Med 335:1176-1181, 1996.
37. Merskey H: Pain and Psychological Medicine. In Wall PD, Melzack R (eds): Textbook of Pain. Edinburgh, Churchill Livingstone, 1984, pp 496-502.
38. Merskey H: The characteristics of persistent pain in psychological illness. J Psychosom Res 9:291, 1965.
39. Mitchell SW, Moorehouse GR, Keen WW: Gunshot Wounds and Other Injuries of Nerves. Philadelphia, JB Lippincott, 1864.
40. Ng LKY (ed): New Approaches to Treatment of Chronic Pain: A Review of Multidisciplinary Pain Clinics and Pain Centers. US Dept HEW, NIDA, Monograph Series 36, 1981.
41. Pelz M, Merskey H: A description of the psychological effects of chronic painful lesions. Pain 14:293, 1982.
42. Pilling LF, Brannick TL, Swenson WM: Psychological characteristics of patients having pain as a presenting symptom. Can Med Assoc J 97:387, 1967.
43. Pilowsky I, Chapman CR, Bonica JJ: Pain, depression, and illness behavior in a pain clinic population. Pain 4:183, 1977.
44. Rockwood CA Jr, Eilbert RE: Camptocormia. J Bone Joint Surg Am 51A: 553, 1969.
45. Rosen JC, Frymoyer JW: A review of camptocormia and an unusual case in the female. Spine 10:325-327, 1985.
46. Rotes-Querol J: The syndrome of psychogenic rheumatism. Clin Rheum Dis 5:797, 1979.
47. Sainsbury P, Gibson JG: Symptoms of anxiety and tension and the accompanying physiological changes in the muscular system. Psychosom Med 17:216, 1954.
48. Schweiger U, Weber B, Deuchle M, et al: Lumbar bone mineral density in patients with major depression: Evidence of increased bone loss at follow-up. Am J Psychiatry 157:118-120, 2000.
49. Silver FW: Management of conversion disorder. Am J Phys Med Rehabil 75:134-140, 1995.
50. Smith GT, Hughes LB, Duvall RD, Rothman S: Treatment outcome of a multidisciplinary center for management of chronic pain: A long-term follow-up. Clin J Pain 4:47, 1988.
51. Spear FG: Pain in psychiatric patients. J Psychosom Res 11:187, 1967.
52. Speed J: Behavioral management of conversion disorder: Retrospective study. Arch Phys Med Rehabil 77:147-153, 1996.
53. Sternbach RA: Pain: A Psychophysiological Analysis. New York, Academic Press, 1968.
54. Sternbach RA: Pain Patients: Traits and Treatment. New York, Academic Press, 1974.
55. Sternbach RA, Timmermans G: Personality changes associated with reduction of pain. Pain 1:177, 1975.
56. Sternbach RA, Wolf SR, Murphy RW, Akeson WH: Traits of pain patients: The low-back "loser." Psychosomatics 14:226, 1973.
57. Walters A: Psychogenic regional pain alias hysterical pain. Brain 84:1, 1961.
58. Watson GD, Chandarana PC, Merskey H: Relationships between pain and schizophrenia. Br J Psychiatry 138:33, 1981.
59. Woodforde JM, Merskey H: Personality traits of patients with chronic pain. J Psychosom Res 16:167, 1972.
60. Zipfel S, Seibel MJ, Lowe B, et al: Osteoporosis in eating disorders: A follow-up study of patients with anorexia and bulimia nervosa. J Clin Endocrinol Metab 86:5227-5233, 2001.

CHAPTER 17

REFERRED PAIN

Low back or neck pain occurs not only with diseases that affect the bones, joints, ligaments, tendons, and other components of the spine, but also as a significant symptom of disorders of the cardiovascular, genitourinary, and gastrointestinal systems. Some of the visceral organs of the neck and chest and the abdomen and pelvis lie in proximity to the cervical and lumbosacral spine, respectively. Inflammation, infection, or hemorrhage that originates in the aorta, pancreas, or kidney may spread beyond the confines of these organs and stimulate sensory nerves within the lumbosacral spine. Such direct stimulation of sensory nerves results in pain that not only is localized to the damaged area but may also be experienced in a location other than the one being stimulated. The pain occurs in superficial tissues supplied by the same segment of the spinal cord that sends afferent sensory fibers to the diseased area. This pain is called "referred pain."

Referred pain occurs as a result of the organization of the nervous system and the embryologic location of the visceral organs. Sensory impulses of somatic origin (skin and parietal peritoneum, for example) travel by somatic afferent neurons to the dorsal root ganglia and then into the posterior horn of the spinal cord. They synapse either with a second neuron that crosses to the opposite side of the cord and ascends to the cerebral cortex through the lateral spinothalamic tract or with motor neurons in the anterior horn of the spinal cord at the same level. Sensory impulses from visceral structures, such as the duodenum or pancreas, travel in visceral afferent nerve fibers that accompany fibers of the sympathetic nervous system through the rami communicantes and the posterior horn to join somatic sensory neurons in the posterior horn of the spinal cord. The visceral afferent fibers may travel cranially or caudally in the gray matter of the dorsal horn before synapsing with neurons of the spinothalamic tract.

Sensory impulses of visceral origin travel the same path to the brain as somatic afferent nerves do. Radiation of visceral afferents to a number of spinal cord segments may explain the diffuse, poorly localized character of visceral pain. The organization of the spinal segment is further complicated by projections of neurons from higher centers in the brain that may intensify or diminish either visceral or somatic pain. Sensory stimulation of visceral origin may spill over in the dorsal horn to affect somatic sensory nerves and result in pain that is felt only in the corresponding segmental somatic distribution (a dermatome of skin). Sensory input may also stimulate motor fibers in the anterior horn, and such stimulation results in muscle contraction and spasm.

The segment of the spinal cord that supplies a visceral structure is dependent not on its anatomic location in the fully developed adult but also on its original location in the developing human embryo. Visceral organs migrate to their final location and take along their nerve and vascular supply, and referred pain from these organs will be sensed in the somatic distribution of their embryologic origin. For example, because the 12th thoracic and 1st lumbar nerves supply the visceral sensory input of the uterus, referred somatic pain originating from the uterus is felt in the groin area, which receives its somatic sensory input from the same L1 segment. In the cervical spine, because the third, fourth, and fifth cervical nerves supply the visceral sensory input of the central part of the diaphragm, referred somatic pain originating in the diaphragm is felt in the neck and shoulder, which receive their somatic sensory input from the same cervical segments.

Patients with visceral disease in the abdomen or thorax may experience three types of pain. True visceral pain is felt at the site of primary stimulation and is dull and aching in character. It has a diffuse and deep location. This type of pain is particularly true of visceral structures that originate in the midline (small intestine) and have visceral sensory input from both sides of the spinal cord. Visceral pain from the kidney is more easily localized because the sensory innervation to it is unilateral.

A second type of deep somatic pain in the abdomen is related to stimulation of the parietal peritoneum. These impulses are transmitted by somatic pathways. The pain is localized, sharp, and intense in character. Such pain is frequently associated with reflex abdominal wall muscle spasm.

A third category is referred pain to the spine from lesions in the aorta or the genitourinary or gastrointestinal tract. This pain is characteristically sharp and relatively well localized to the skin. Hyperalgesia may be noted in the area of referred pain, and reflex muscle contraction may also be present. Although referred pain usually occurs in combination with visceral and somatic pain, occasionally it may exist in the absence of visceral pain or symptoms of an underlying disease.

In the setting of spinal pain and no associated visceral symptoms, a complete history, physical examination, and laboratory evaluation are essential to discover the source of the visceral referred pain. Characteristically, spinal pain that is referred from visceral structures is not aggravated by activity or relieved by recumbency. Cardiac examination may uncover abnormal heart sounds or cardiomegaly indicative of silent myocardial infarction. Laboratory evaluation with an electrocardiogram or abdominal roentgenogram may show evidence of myocardial infarction or cholecystitis. Abdominal examination may uncover an asymptomatic pulsatile mass indicative of an abdominal aortic aneurysm, or rectal examination may reveal blood in the stool suggesting a hidden malignancy. Laboratory evaluation may show pyuria, indicative of urinary tract infection, or increased amylase, reflective of pancreatitis. Referred pain from a visceral structure must be considered as the cause of spinal pain when mechanical, rheumatologic, infectious, metabolic, and neoplastic origins of the pain have been eliminated as possibilities.

CARDIOVASCULAR DISEASES

Capsule Summary

	Low Back	Neck
Frequency of spinal pain	Rare to uncommon	Rare
Location of spinal pain	Left lumbar paraspinous area	Anterior, left arm, C8 distribution
Quality of spinal pain	Dull ache to sharp tearing	Crushing
Symptoms and signs	Epigastric pain—not affected by position; hypertension, smoking history, pulsatile mass; hypotension with rupture	Chest pain—not affected by position; increased with activity, hypertension, smoking history
Laboratory tests	Decreased hematocrit with rupture	Electrocardiogram with ischemic changes
Radiographic findings	Curvilinear calcification on plain roentgenogram, aortic enlargement on sonogram or CT scan	Angiographic evidence of coronary artery stenosis
Treatment	Surgical excision with enlargement >5 cm	Medical therapy, angioplasty, bypass procedure

LUMBOSACRAL SPINE

Abdominal Aortic Disease

Low back pain associated with disease of the abdominal aorta may occur secondary to aneurysmal dilation, rupture, or obstruction of the vessel. The abdominal aorta is located in the retroperitoneum, just to the left of the midline. The abdominal aorta splits at the L4 vertebra to form the common iliac arteries, which supply the lower extremities. An arterial aneurysm is a localized or diffuse enlargement of an artery. One or all three layers (intima, media, and adventitia) of the aorta make up the wall of the aneurysm. A dissecting aneurysm is caused by the formation of a false channel in the wall of the aorta that splits the layers of the vessel apart. Saccular aneurysms are bulbous protrusions of all three layers on one side of the vessel. A fusiform aneurysm is a diffuse, circumferential expansion of a segment of the vessel.

Epidemiology

Abdominal aneurysms occur most commonly in white men between the ages of 60 and 70[30]; however, they have been reported in patients as early as in the fourth decade of life and are quite common in people older than 50 years.[17] Aneurysms occur twice as often in whites as blacks[42] and four times more frequently in men than women. The incidence of abdominal aneurysm is increasing as the number of elderly people increases.[55] Between 10 and 40 per 1000 people older than 50 years may have this abnormality. Abdominal aortic aneurysms were responsible for 14,982 deaths in the United States in 1988 among people 55 years or older.[22] In a Swedish study, the incidence in men increased rapidly after the age of 55, with a peak of 5.9% at age 80; in women, the increase occurred after the age of 70 with a peak of 4.5% at age 90.[4] The estimated financial loss for hospitals who have patients with ruptured aneurysms is $24,655 per individual.[8]

Aneurysms are fusiform in configuration and extend from an area just inferior to the renal arteries to the common iliac artery bifurcation. Only 5% are characterized by dilation of the suprarenal aorta.[17] The inferior mesenteric artery frequently arises out of the aneurysm. The iliac arteries and common and superficial femoral arteries are occasionally affected. Patients with abdominal aneurysms may have aneurysms of other types (saccular) and location (thoracic, popliteal) in association with generalized arterial disease.

Pathogenesis

The pathogenesis of the aneurysm is related to atherosclerotic degeneration with structural weakening of the connective tissue (collagen) of the vessel wall. Patients with abdominal aneurysms are usually hypertensive and may demonstrate manifestations of generalized atherosclerosis, including angina, previous myocardial infarction, stroke, or peripheral vascular disease.[62] Smoking is the risk factor most strongly associated with abdominal aortic aneurysms.[42]

Trauma, in itself, is not an etiologic factor, although it may cause rupture of a preexistent aneurysm.[9] A number of studies have also described a familial tendency (possible genetic predisposition) for the development of abdominal aneurysms.[33,64] First-degree relatives are at significantly increased risk for the development of aneurysmal degeneration. In a study of 238 first-degree relatives of patients with aneurysm, a family history increased the risk by 4.33-fold.[58] At a minimum, review of the family history for aortic disease is warranted in patients with back pain. Noninvasive screening tests to detect early aortic disease may be indicated in those with a strong family history of aneurysm. Family studies have demonstrated an increased prevalence of aneurysm in the brothers and sons of patients who died secondary to ruptured aneurysms.[5] The highest risk for development of an aneurysm is in brothers older than 60 years, within whom the prevalence is 18%.

Two theories have been proposed for the cause of aneurysmal enlargement. The first theory is that a genetically linked deficit in the quantity and quality of collagen and elastin in the arterial wall causes generalized arteriomegaly. The decrease in elastin and collagen may be the result of degradation by proteases, including elastase, matrix metalloproteinases, and cathepsin S and K.[10] This theory would explain the fact that a number of vessels may be affected in a patient. A second theory is that plaque from atherosclerosis interferes with the blood supply of the arterial wall and thereby results in weakening of the wall.[28] Inflammatory mediators such as interleukin-8 and monocyte chemoattractant protein-1 have been identified in aortic aneurysms. These factors are chemoattractant to leukocytes and recruit inflammatory cells to the arterial wall, which leads to weakening of the wall.[37] Interleukin-6 is present in large or inflammatory aneurysms at a higher concentration than in brachial arteries.[34] Atherosclerosis may represent a secondary, nonspecific response to vessel wall injury.

Factors other than atherosclerosis may also increase the risk for aneurysm formation. Vascular infection with *Salmonella* or syphilis may cause an aneurysm.[54] Individuals with the connective tissue diseases of Marfan's syndrome and Ehlers-Danlos syndrome are at risk for aneurysms.

The risk of rupture has been associated with the size and expansion rate of the aneurysm. The average increase in size is 0.4 cm/yr. Approximately 80% of small aneurysms increase in diameter, with 20% increasing more than 0.5 cm/yr.[22] Aneurysms larger than 5 to 6 cm expand more rapidly. The rate of expansion is an important determinant of the risk of rupture. However, the rate of expansion in each patient is unpredictable. Some aneurysms remain stable for years and then expand rapidly. The risk for rupture is 2% in aortic aneurysms less than 4.0 cm in diameter.[51] The 5-year risk for rupture of aneurysms 5.0 cm or larger is up to 41%.[44,49] For aneurysms 8.0 cm in diameter, the risk of rupture is 25.7% within the next 6 months.[40]

Clinical History

The pain associated with an abdominal aortic aneurysm occurs secondary to compression of surrounding structures by expansion or rupture of the aneurysm. Evidence from the Framingham study suggests that back pain may be related, in part, to loss of blood flow to the lumbar spine causing advanced intervertebral disc degeneration.[36] Patients with stable or slowly enlarging aneurysms are asymptomatic, and such may be the case in a majority of those with an abdominal aneurysm.[30] The aneurysm may be noted as an incidental finding on a radiograph of the abdomen or as a pulsatile abdominal mass at the level of the umbilicus, which is minimally tender if found on physical examination.

Extension of the aneurysm is associated with increased pain and clinical symptoms. Most frequently, patients experience abdominal pain that is dull, steady, and unrelated to activity or eating. Some patients notice or complain of a "pounding" sensation or palpitations in their abdomen. Back pain, when it occurs, is usually associated with epigastric discomfort and may radiate to the hips or thighs. Pressure of the aneurysm on lumbar nerves may give rise to this symptom. With increasing expansion, stretching of the mesenteric root or obstruction of the duodenum is associated with acute episodes of pain and gastrointestinal symptoms of nausea and vomiting. Such symptoms may simulate gastrointestinal diseases such as pancreatitis or peptic ulcer disease.

Rupture of an abdominal aneurysm is associated with excruciating pain, circulatory shock from blood loss, and an expanding mass. The pain of rupture may be the first clinical sign in a previously asymptomatic patient with an aneurysm. An exacerbation of previously milder pain in a patient with an aneurysm is a harbinger of extension or impending rupture. Ruptures of the abdominal aorta are frequently located at the junction of the aortic attachment to the vertebral bodies and the portion that is unattached in the retroperitoneum. Blood from the ruptured aneurysm may be contained in the retroperitoneum or pass into the peritoneal cavity or a hollow viscus. Rupture into the retroperitoneum is associated with the sudden onset of severe tearing or piercing pain that is continuous and increasing in intensity. The pain is present deep in the abdomen and is referred to the back, legs, and groin.[2] Extension to the lower extremities may be confused with radiculopathy. Patients with a ruptured aorta may have a history of chronic back pain lasting a month or more.[28] The hematoma is confined to the retroperitoneal space.

Physical Examination

The common physical finding in patients with uncomplicated abdominal aortic disease is the presence of an expansile, pulsatile mass that is located near the level of the umbilicus and frequently extends into the lower part of the abdomen. Palpation of a normal aorta may cause discomfort. A normal aorta is pulsatile, expands in an anterior and lateral direction, and measures approximately 2.5 cm in diameter. As an individual ages, the aorta loses its elasticity and becomes tortuous. The aorta bulges anteriorly to the left or, less commonly, to the right. A tortuous aorta should be rolled under the examining hand to establish a true measure of its size. The ability to palpate an aneurysm in both planes separates true aneurysms from transmitted pulsations, which are palpable only in the anteroposterior direction. The size of the aneurysm, the thickness of the abdominal wall, and the state of relaxation of the abdominal wall will have a significant effect on the chance of palpating an aneurysm. The examination is best performed with the patient in the supine position, knees flexed. Pressure should be applied to the abdomen between respirations as the abdominal musculature relaxes. Examination of the aorta does not cause rupture of an aneurysm.[41] In a study of 200 subjects (99 with and 101 without aneurysms documented by ultrasonography), physical examination had a sensitivity of 68% and a specificity of 75%. The larger the aneurysm was in an individual with an abdominal girth of less than 100 cm, the greater the sensitivity of the examination was. Physical examination has adequate sensitivity to identify individuals with a large enough aneurysm to warrant elective intervention.[24]

A patient with an asymptomatic aneurysm may complain of pain with palpation of the abdomen. Tenderness may be more pronounced with impending rupture. Palpation should be gentle to avoid causing the patient discomfort or perturbing the aneurysm.

Physical examination of a patient with abdominal aortic rupture demonstrates hypotension, profuse sweating, and rarely (because of surrounding hematoma, which camouflages vessel movement), a pulsatile abdominal mass that is tender. The classic triad of hypotension, back pain, and a pulsatile mass may be present in only 50% of patients with ruptured aneurysms.[56] Palpation of the aneurysm may elicit low back pain that radiates to the thigh or lower part of the abdomen.[18] The abdominal wall is not usually rigid. Less frequently, patients have hemorrhagic discoloration of the skin in the back and flanks secondary to a retroperitoneal hematoma, or they have loss of sensation in the distribution of the femoral nerve along with weakness in the quadriceps musculature as a manifestation of rupture in the psoas region.[3,52] The status of distal pulses in both lower extremities does not correlate with the presence or absence of an aneurysmal rupture. Neurologic signs such as leg weakness may be detected if expansion of the aneurysm compromises blood flow to the spinal cord. In rare circumstances, infarction of the spinal cord may occur.[59]

Laboratory Data

Laboratory test results may be normal in patients with asymptomatic aneurysms. Patients with ruptured aneurysms may have mild to profound anemia at the time of evaluation, depending on the degree of extravascular blood loss. Thrombocytopenia may result from active thrombus deposition.

Radiographic Evaluation

Ultrasonography and computed tomography (CT) of the abdomen are noninvasive diagnostic methods used to identify the presence and extent of an aneurysm (Figs. 17-1 and 17-2). These investigations are very reliable in identifying the location of an aneurysm in the abdomen.[7,29] A normal ultrasound examination in a 65-year-old man has great significance. In a cohort of 233 65-year-old men monitored for 12 years, none of the deaths were attributed to a ruptured abdominal aneurysm. A normal ultrasound at age 65 rules out the risk of a clinically significant aneurysm for life in men.[14]

Abdominal ultrasonography detects aneurysms with a sensitivity that approaches 100%.[39] The longitudinal and transverse diameters can be determined without radiation or contrast medium. The effectiveness of ultrasound is diminished by excessive bowel gas, which obscures the infrarenal abdominal aorta, and the pancreas, which hides the suprarenal aorta. Therefore, ultrasound is a good screening tool but is not adequate for planning surgery.

CT is highly sensitive and specific for the identification of aneurysms. CT visualizes the suprarenal and infrarenal aorta and accurately determines the size and shape of the aneurysm to a greater degree than ultrasound does. Unlike ultrasonography, CT visualizes aortic anomalies, horseshoe kidneys, inferior vena cava anomalies, and involvement of the iliac and hypogastric arteries. CT identifies rupture or leakage into the retroperitoneal space. CT may be inaccurate in the evaluation of a tortuous aorta. The use of contrast media and exposure to ionizing radiation are the disadvantages of this radiographic method.

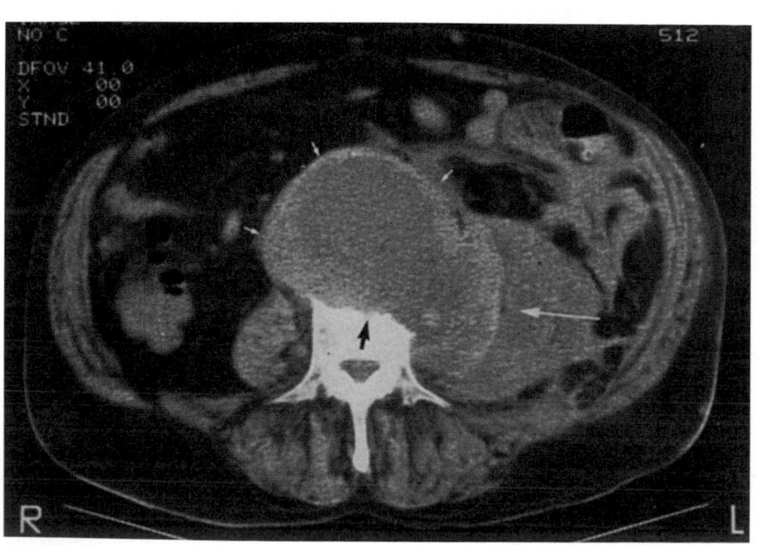

Figure 17-1 CT scan of a ruptured abdominal aneurysm in a 72-year-old man who had abdominal pain and left-sided back pain of acute onset that radiated to the left leg. The abdomen was distended with minimal pulsations of the aorta. Abdominal CT demonstrates an old aneurysm *(small white arrows)* and new retroperitoneal bleeding *(large white arrow)*. An unusual finding is remodeling of the vertebral body by the aneurysm *(black arrow)*. *(Courtesy of Joseph Giordano, MD.)*

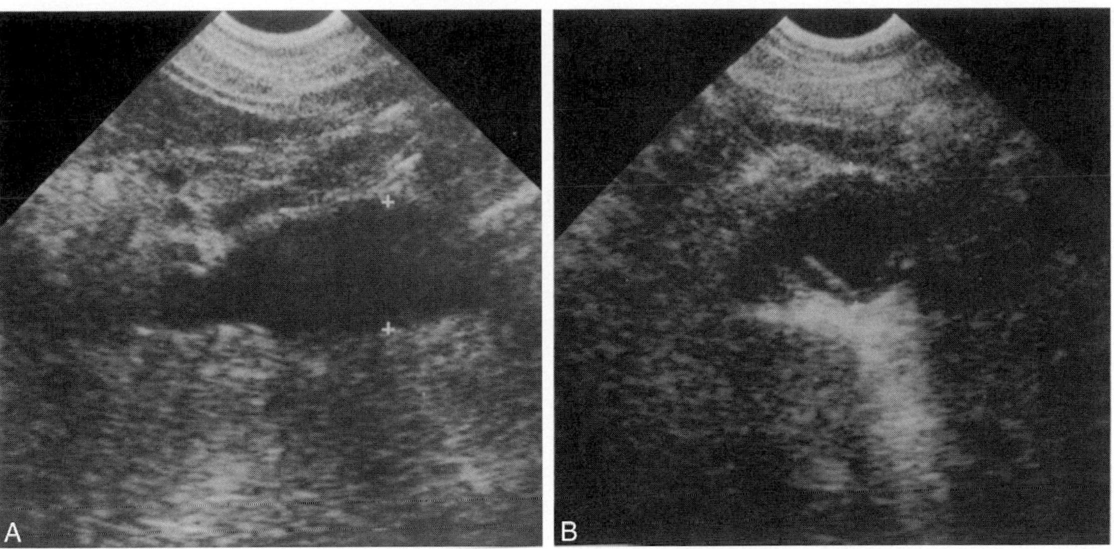

Figure 17-2 Abdominal ultrasound. Sagittal *(A)* and cross-sectional *(B)* views of an abdominal aneurysm show increased signal in the vessel wall compatible with vascular calcification. *(Courtesy of Michael Hill, MD.)*

Therefore, CT should not be used as a screening method for abdominal aneurysms. CT is most effective when the aneurysm has been identified and resection is planned. CT may be the most useful test in the emergency department setting if surgery is being contemplated because it reveals the extent of the aneurysm and extravasation of blood, which are important for preoperative evaluation of the patient by the vascular surgeon.

Magnetic resonance (MR) is another very useful imaging technique and can be used to depict involvement of the renal and iliac arteries.[1] MR imaging combined with angiography (MRA) can identify vascular anatomy in three planes without the need for contrast dye or radiation. MRA is able to determine the extent of an aneurysm, the proximal and distal extent of the lesion, and the origins of the renal arteries.[21] MR is more expensive and less available than other radiographic techniques.

Aortography is performed in patients with abdominal aneurysms to delineate the vascular anatomy. The lack of time to complete the test in a compromised patient with an acute rupture occasionally results in surgery being performed without an angiogram.[48,66] Aortography may not determine the true size of an aneurysm. Aneurysms commonly have thrombus lining the inner wall. Because the aortogram visualizes only the lumen, the thrombus obscures the true diameter of the aorta. Aortography may be useful in a patient with an aneurysm associated with occlusive disease and ischemic symptoms involving the lower extremities. It depicts the status of the iliac, femoral, and popliteal vessels of the lower extremity before surgery in these patients (Fig. 17-3). Aortography is used selectively by vascular surgeons for the preoperative planning of aneurysmal endovascular stent placement.

Review of plain films of the abdomen is helpful in detecting abdominal aneurysms. Anteroposterior and lateral projections of the abdomen may demonstrate a curvilinear thin layer of calcification in the wall of the aorta in 70% of patients.[32] Vertebral body erosion is generally not found with an abdominal aneurysm.[67]

Differential Diagnosis

The spectrum of abdominal aortic disease is quite broad with regard to both the severity of arterial disease and the extent of organs affected by the expanding aneurysm (Table 17-1). The diagnosis should be considered in an elderly patient with nondescript back pain that does not

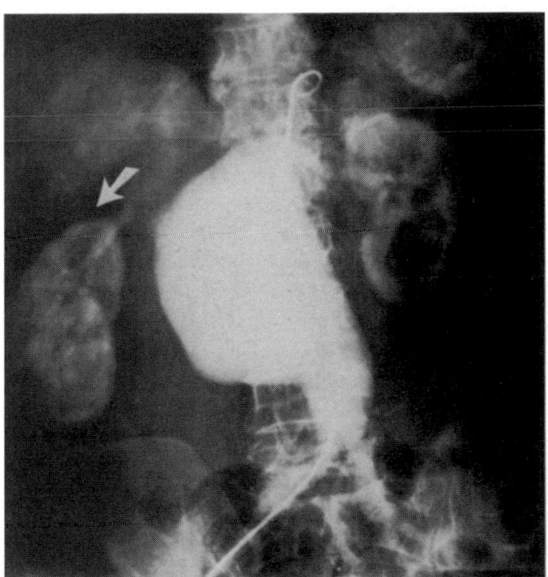

Figure 17-3 Aortogram of an abdominal aneurysm. A 70-year-old woman was evaluated for acute low back pain and had a history of a pulsatile aorta. The aortogram reveals an 8-cm aneurysm arising below the renal arteries. A right retroperitoneal mass (hematoma) has caused marked inferior displacement of the right kidney *(arrow)*. *(Courtesy of Edward Druy, MD.)*

17-1 SPECTRUM OF AORTIC DISEASE

Asymptomatic aneurysm
Symptomatic aneurysm
  Abdominal fullness or pulsation
  Pain—abdominal or lumbar
    Dull, gnawing
    Initially intermittent, then continuous
  Obstruction—ureter, duodenum, vena cava, lower aorta
    Peptic ulcer, renal colic, lower limb claudication
Dissection and/or rupture
  Sudden onset
    Severe pain radiating from the abdomen or back into the groin, buttocks, thighs
  Hypovolemic shock
  Gastrointestinal or retroperitoneal bleeding

improve with rest and is exacerbated with activity. Patients with impending rupture have more severe symptoms that may simulate a wide range of illnesses. Disorders causing back pain that may be mimicked by an aneurysm include peptic ulcer disease, pancreatitis, biliary or renal colic, acute appendicitis, and a herniated intervertebral disc. Misdiagnosis may occur in 30% of patients, with the most common incorrect diagnoses being renal colic, diverticulitis, and gastrointestinal hemorrhage.[46] Careful evaluation of the abdomen with noninvasive methods should identify the presence of an aneurysm (Fig. 17-4). *Salmonella* infection may localize in an abdominal aortic aneurysm and cause progressive symptoms that may call for surgical intervention to repair the aneurysm.[47] Inflammation of the three layers of the aorta may result in narrowing and decreased blood flow. Takayasu's arteritis occurs most commonly in young women. Back pain is a symptom in up to 10% of patients with this disease.[31]

Treatment

Therapy for an abdominal aneurysm is surgical. The presence of an aneurysm 6 cm or larger in external diameter is associated with increased mortality, and in those with no major contraindication, elective resection and bypass of the aneurysm should be considered.[25] Improved survival has been documented in patients who have undergone surgery for intact aneurysms.[13] The mortality from an elective procedure is 2% to 5%. If the aneurysm is smaller than 5.5 cm in diameter, elective repair has a 30-day operative mortality of 5.4%. At 3 years, surgery has no better advantage than surveillance does with regard to survival.[43] However, if patients with small aneurysms are monitored over an 8-year period, individuals who undergo surgery have lower mortality than do those monitored by ultrasound every 6 months.[63]

Patients with evidence of a ruptured aneurysm require immediate surgical intervention because up to 80% of patients with ruptured aneurysms live at least 6 hours after the onset of symptoms. Early surgery is the most important factor influencing survival. Recent surgical data suggest that more than 70% of patients with ruptured abdominal aneurysms can survive surgery.[19] Complications associated with surgery include shock, myocardial infarction, necrosis of viscera, and renal failure. Infection of the aneurysm may be a complicating factor both preoperatively and postoperatively.[6,19,57]

Patients for whom extensive surgery would present a high risk may be treated by alternative means. Beta-blocker therapy is indicated to prevent expansion of aneurysms. In a study of 121 patients with an aneurysm, 38 treated with beta-blockers had slower progression of expansion than did those without medical therapy.[27] Induced thrombosis by ligature of both iliac arteries or ligature of the aorta above and below the aneurysm with an axillofemoral artery bypass graft has been performed. These techniques should be considered only in patients who would not survive extensive surgery.[11,38] Another therapeutic option is percutaneous placement of implantable endovascular stents, similar to those used for renal artery, coronary artery, and peripheral artery stenosis. Endovascular repair is an option for individuals with co-morbid conditions that preclude open surgical repair.[65] Correct patient and device selection is essential for a satis-

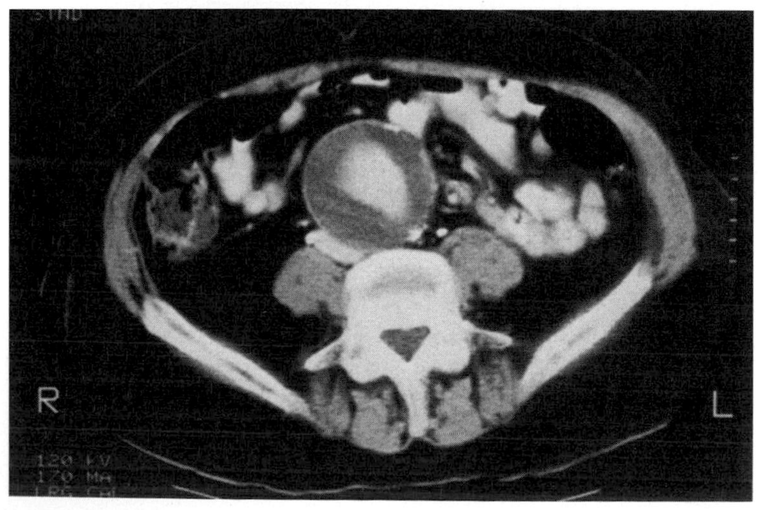

Figure 17-4 Abdominal CT scan with contrast dye in a 73-year-old man with very mild, diffuse back pain. The CT scan demonstrates an abdominal aneurysm. Contrast dye (white) accentuates the surrounding intraluminal thrombus. *(Courtesy of Joseph Giordano, MD.)*

factory outcome. Endoluminal grafting can result in decreased pressure in the aneurysm.[61]

Prognosis

The prognosis for individuals identified before aortic rupture is good. Even in patients 80 years or older, the operative mortality rate is 3%.[53] In contrast, operative mortality in individuals 80 years or older with a ruptured aneurysm is 91%.[16] In a review of data from many studies, operative mortality in all age groups of individuals is 4% with nonruptured aneurysms and 49% with ruptured aneurysms.[22] Quality of life is also different for individuals who undergo elective versus emergency surgery. Patients with ruptured aneurysms have a deterioration in quality of life even with a successful operation.[45] Young patients with small aneurysms should consider resection even with a small risk of expansion.[35] Contraindications for elective reconstruction include myocardial infarction within 6 months, intractable congestive heart failure, severe pulmonary insufficiency, intractable angina pectoris, chronic renal insufficiency, stroke, or a life expectancy of less than 2 years.[4] Individuals with aortic aneurysms are at greater risk for mortality from cardiovascular disease than are age-matched individuals with similar degrees of atherosclerosis. These individuals should decrease their exposure to risk factors (smoking) to lower the risk of aneurysmal expansion and progression of generalized vascular disease.[50] With regard to screening, an abdominal examination is inexpensive but relatively insensitive in men 60 to 80 years old.[26] A single abdominal ultrasound screening is of greater benefit, but at added cost.[46]

Aortic Occlusion

Acute Occlusion

Obstruction of the abdominal aorta is associated with pain in the muscles of the low back and gluteal areas. The pain may be of either acute or gradual onset. Patients with acute embolic obstruction of the terminal aorta experience acute claudication of the lower extremities and acute, severe low back pain.[23,60] The source of the embolus is most frequently a mural thrombus from the left side of the heart, which may be generated by a myocardial infarction, cardiomyopathy, valvular disease, atrial fibrillation, or atrial myxoma.[23] The embolus lodges at the bifurcation of the aorta and blocks blood flow to the lower half of the body.[15] Patients experience pain in the thigh, low back, buttock, and lower abdominal areas. Neurologic function is impaired, as evidenced by weakness, numbness, and paresthesias. Pulses are lost in the lower extremities, and the skin turns pale. Aortography is the diagnostic procedure of choice for acute aortic occlusion. Removal of the clot is required for the patient to survive. Embolectomy may be accomplished with the use of an intra-arterial balloon catheter. Surgical intervention is usually necessary to restore blood flow. Patients who have undergone a successful revascularization operation have a 20% mortality rate because of underlying cardiac disease.

Gradual Occlusion

Low back pain may also be a symptom in patients with gradual obstruction of the abdominal aorta.[12] Occasionally, they will have low back pain as their initial symptom, and this pain may occur without associated symptoms of claudication, neurologic dysfunction, or pallor. Back pain from arterial obstruction may be limited to repeated activity, with the pain subsiding with rest. Patients with aortic obstruction may be predisposed to the development of Leriche's syndrome, which is associated with buttock or thigh claudication and impotence. Claudication occurs in the muscles of the lower extremity, most commonly in the calf and less commonly in the thigh and buttocks. Cramping occurs with exercise and is relieved by rest in 3 to 5 minutes. Rest pain is a symptom of more severe peripheral vascular disease. Rest pain occurs in the toes or forefoot and at night while the individual is recumbent. The supine position lessens the beneficial effect of gravity, increasing blood flow to the most distal part of the lower extremity. The sleeping state also decreases cardiac output and blood pressure, thereby further reducing flow. If individuals do not have pain in their feet while recumbent, they do not have rest pain.

Claudication occurs secondary to narrowing or occlusion of major arteries in the lower extremities. With exercise, the peripheral vascular bed dilates to increase blood flow. Arterial pressure does not change despite marked increases in blood flow. In the situation of a patient with claudication, the arterial pressure in arteries distal to the obstruction is reduced to levels below the pressure generated by contracting muscles. The arteries are closed off and symptoms of claudication occur.

Examination of patients with claudication reveals absent pulses and bruits over the iliac or femoral arteries. On occasion, distal pulses may remain palpable. Measurement of ankle arterial pressure is a means to differentiate neurogenic from vascular claudication. The presence of normal ankle pressure after exercise definitively rules out vascular disease as the cause of lower extremity pain.[28] The use of a treadmill and a stationary bicycle has been suggested as a means of differentiating patients with neurogenic and vascular claudication. Patients with neurogenic pain may cycle for long distances without pain, whereas pain develops in patients with vascular disease. However, the treadmill test will not differentiate patients with neurogenic pain if they flex while walking.[20] The results of these exercise tests must be examined carefully to determine the cause of claudication. Vascular pressure measurements or Doppler tests may be required to establish vascular disease.

Bypass grafting is successful in controlling symptoms in 80% of patients undergoing such surgery. Mortality from the operation is greatest in those who have cardiac disease.[12]

References

Cardiovascular Diseases—Lumbosacral Spine

1. Amparo EG, Hoddick WK, Hricak H, et al: Comparison of magnetic resonance imaging and ultrasonography in the evaluation of abdominal aortic aneurysms. Radiology 154:451, 1985.
2. Barratt-Boye BG: Symptomatology and prognosis of abdominal aortic aneurysm. Lancet 2:716, 1957.

3. Beebe RT, Powers SR Jr, Ginouves E: Early diagnosis of ruptured abdominal aneurysm. Ann Intern Med 48:834, 1958.
4. Bengtsson H, Bergqvist D, Sternby NH: Increasing prevalence of abdominal aortic aneurysms: A necropsy study. Eur J Surg 158:19, 1992.
5. Bengtsson H, Sonesson B, Lanne T, et al: Prevalence of abdominal aortic aneurysm in the offspring of patients dying from aneurysm rupture. Br J Surg 79:1142, 1992.
6. Bennett DE, Cherry JK: Bacterial infection of aortic aneurysms: A clinicopathologic study. Am J Surg 113:321, 1967.
7. Bluth EL: Ultrasound of the abdominal aorta. Arch Intern Med 144:377, 1984.
8. Breckwoldt WL, Mackey WC, O'Donnell TF Jr: The economic implications of high-risk abdominal aortic aneurysm. J Vasc Surg 13:798, 1991.
9. Cannon JA, Van De Water J, Barker WF: Experience with surgical management of 100 consecutive cases of abdominal aneurysm. Am J Surg 106:128, 1963.
10. Carrell TW, Burnand KG, Wells GM, et al: Stromelysin-1 (matrix metalloproteinase-3) and tissue inhibitor of metalloproteinase-3 are overexpressed in the wall of abdominal aortic aneurysms. Circulation 105:477-482, 2002.
11. Compion ML, Kreel L, Rothman MT, Pardy BJ: Induced thrombosis of abdominal aortic aneurysm. J R Soc Med 78:72, 1985.
12. Crawford ES, Bomberger RA, Galeser DH, et al: Aortoiliac occlusive disease: Factors influencing survival and function following reconstruction operation over a twenty-five-year period. Surgery 90:1055, 1981.
13. Crawford ES, Saleh SA, Babb JW III, et al: Infrarenal abdominal aortic aneurysm. Ann Surg 193:699, 1981.
14. Crow P, Shaw E, Earnshaw JJ, et al: A single normal ultrasonographic scan at age 65 years rules out significant aneurysm disease for life in men. Br J Surg 88:941-944, 2001.
15. Danto LA, Fry WJ, Kraft RO: Acute aortic thrombosis. Arch Surg 104:569, 1972.
16. Dean RH, Woody JD, Enarson CE, et al: Operative treatment of abdominal aortic aneurysms in octogenarians. When is it too much too late? Ann Surg 217:721, 1993.
17. DeBakey ME, Crawford ES, Cooley DA, et al: Aneurysm of abdominal aorta. Ann Surg 160:622, 1964.
18. DeHoff JB, Finney GG: Sign of ruptured aneurysm of abdominal aorta. N Engl J Med 281:47, 1969.
19. Diehl JT, Cali RF, Hertzer NR, Beven EG: Complications of abdominal aortic reconstruction: An analysis of perioperative risk factors in 557 patients. Ann Surg 197:49, 1983.
20. Dong G, Porter RW: Walking and cycling tests in neurogenic and intermittent claudication. Spine 14:965, 1989.
21. Durham JR, Hackworth CA, Tober JC, et al: Magnetic resonance angiography in the preoperative evaluation of abdominal aortic aneurysms. Am J Surg 166:173, 1993.
22. Ernst CB: Abdominal aortic aneurysm. N Engl J Med 328:1167, 1993.
23. Filtzer DL, Bahnson HT: Low back pain due to arterial obstruction. J Bone Joint Surg Br 41:244, 1959.
24. Fink HA, Lederle FA, Roth CS, et al: The accuracy of physical examination to detect abdominal aortic aneurysm. Arch Intern Med 160:833-836, 2000.
25. Foster JH, Bolasny BL, Gobbel WG, Scott HW Jr: Comparative study of elective resection and expectant treatment of abdominal aortic aneurysm. Surg Gynecol Obstet 129:1, 1969.
26. Frame PS, Fryback DG, Patterson C: Screening for abdominal aortic aneurysm in men ages 60 to 80 years. A cost-effectiveness analysis. Ann Intern Med 119:411, 1993.
27. Gadowski GR, Pilcher DB, Ricci MA: Abdominal aortic aneurysm expansion rate: Effect of size and beta-adrenergic blockade. J Vasc Surg 19:727, 1994.
28. Giordano JM: Vascular versus spinal disease as a cause of back and lower extremity pain. Semin Spine Surg 2:136, 1990.
29. Gomes MN, Schellinger D: Abdominal aortic aneurysms: Diagnostic review and new technique. Ann Thorac Surg 27:479, 1979.
30. Gore I, Hirst AE Jr: Arteriosclerotic aneurysms of the abdominal aorta: A review. Prog Cardiovasc Dis 16:113, 1973.
31. Ishikawa K: Patterns of symptoms and prognosis in occlusive thromboaortopathy (Takayasu's disease). J Am Coll Cardiol 8:1041, 1986.
32. Janower ML: Ruptured arteriosclerotic aneurysms of the abdominal aorta. N Engl J Med 265:12, 1961.
33. Johansen K, Koepsell T: Familial tendency for abdominal aortic aneurysms. JAMA 256:1934, 1986.
34. Jones KG, Brull DJ, Brown LC, et al: Interleukin-6 (IL-6) and the prognosis of abdominal aortic aneurysms. Circulation 103:2260-2265, 2001.
35. Katz DA, Littenberg B, Cronenwett JL: Management of small abdominal aneurysms. Early surgery vs watchful waiting. JAMA 268:2678, 1992.
36. Kauppila LI, McAlindon T, Evans S, et al: Disc degeneration/back pain and calcification of the abdominal aorta: A 25-year follow-up study in Framingham. Spine 22:1642-1649, 1997.
37. Koch AE, Kunkel SL, Pearce WH, et al: Enhanced production of the chemotactic cytokines interleukin-8 and monocyte chemoattractant protein-1 in human abdominal aortic aneurysms. Am J Pathol 142:1423, 1993.
38. Kwaan JHM, Khan RJ, Connally JE: Total exclusion technique for the management of abdominal aortic aneurysms. Am J Surg 146:93, 1983.
39. LaRoy LL, Cormier PJ, Matalon TAS, et al: Imaging of abdominal aortic aneurysms. AJR Am J Roentgenol 152:785, 1989.
40. Lederle FA, Johnson GR, Wilson SE, et al: Rupture rate of large abdominal aortic aneurysms in patients refusing or unfit for elective repair. JAMA 287:2968-2972, 2002.
41. Lederle FA, Simel DL: Does this patient have abdominal aortic aneurysm? JAMA 281:77-82, 1999.
42. Lederle FA, Johnson GR, Wilson SE, et al: Prevalence and associations of abdominal aortic aneurysm detected through screening. Aneurysm detection and management (ADAM) Veterans Affairs cooperative study group. Ann Intern Med 126:441-449, 1997.
43. Lederle FA, Wilson SE, Johnson GR, et al: Immediate repair compared with surveillance of small abdominal aortic aneurysms. N Engl J Med 346:1437-1444, 2002.
44. Limet R, Sakalihassan N, Albert A: Determination of the expansion rate and incidence of rupture of abdominal aortic aneurysms. J Vasc Surg 14:540, 1991.
45. Magee TR, Scott DJ, Dunkley A, et al: Quality of life following surgery for abdominal aortic aneurysm. Br J Surg 79:1014, 1992.
46. Marston WA, Ahlquist R, Johnson G Jr, Meyer AA: Misdiagnosis of ruptured abdominal aneurysms. J Vasc Surg 16:17, 1992.
47. Mendelowitz DS, Ramstedt R, Yao JST, Bergan JJ: Abdominal aortic salmonellosis. Surgery 85:514, 1979.
48. Nano IN, Collins GM, Bardin JA, Bernstein EF: Should aortography be used routinely in the elective management of abdominal aortic aneurysm? Am J Surg 144:53, 1982.
49. Nevitt MP, Ballard DJ, Hallett JW Jr: Prognosis of abdominal aortic aneurysms: A population-based study. N Engl J Med 321:1009, 1989.
50. Newman AB, Arnold AM, Burke GL, et al: Cardiovascular disease and mortality in older adults with small abdominal aortic aneurysms detected by ultrasonography: The cardiovascular health study. Ann Intern Med 134:182-190, 2001.
51. Ouriel K, Green RM, Donayre C, et al: An evaluation of new methods of expressing aortic aneurysm size: Relationship to rupture. J Vasc Surg 15:12, 1992.
52. Owens ML: Psoas weakness and femoral neuropathy: Neglected signs of retroperitoneal hemorrhage from ruptured aneurysm. Surgery 91:363, 1982.
53. Paty PS, Lloyd WE, Chang BB, et al: Aortic replacement for abdominal aortic aneurysm in elderly patients. Am J Surg 166:191, 1993.
54. Pyne D, Mootoo R, Bhanji A, et al: Salmonella arteritis: An unusual cause of low back pain. Ann Rheum Dis 60:1086-1087, 2001.
55. Rob C: Surgical diseases of the iliac and mesenteric arteries. Arch Surg 93:21, 1966.
56. Rohrer MJ, Cutler BS, Wheeler HB: Long-term survival and quality of life following ruptured abdominal aortic aneurysm. Arch Surg 123:1213, 1988.
57. Russinovich NAE, Karem GG, Luna RF: Radiology rounds: Persistent lumbar pain and low-grade fever in a 62-year-old man. Ala J Med Sci 19:67, 1982.
58. Salo JA, Soisalon-Soininen S, Bondestam S et al: Familial occurrence of abdominal aortic aneurysm. Ann Intern Med 130:637-642, 1999.
59. Sandson TA, Friedman JH: Spinal cord infarction: Report of 8 cases and review of the literature. Medicine (Baltimore) 68:282, 1989.
60. Schalz IJ, Stanley JC: Saddle embolus of the aorta. JAMA 235:1262, 1976.

61. Seelig MH, Oldenburg A, Hakaim AG, et al: Endovascular repair of abdominal aortic aneurysms: Where do we stand? Mayo Clin Proc 74:999-1010, 1999.
62. Spittell JA: Hypertension and arterial aneurysm. J Am Coll Cardiol 1:533, 1983.
63. The United Kingdom Small Aneurysm Trial Participants: Long-term outcomes of immediate repair compared with surveillance of small abdominal aortic aneurysms. N Engl J Med 346:1445-1452, 2002.
64. Tilson MD, Seashore MR: Fifty families with abdominal aortic aneurysms in two or more first order relatives. Am J Surg 147:551, 1984.
65. Treiman GS, Lawrence PF, Edwards WH Jr, et al: An assessment of the current applicability of the EVT endovascular graft for treatment of patients with an infrarenal abdominal aortic aneurysm. J Vasc Surg 30:68-75, 1999.
66. Wheeler WE, Beachley MC, Ranniger K: Angiography and ultrasonography: A comparative study of abdominal aortic aneurysms. AJR Am J Roentgenol 126:95, 1976.
67. Wheelock F, Shaw RS: Aneurysm of abdominal aorta and iliac arteries. N Engl J Med 255:72, 1956.

CERVICAL SPINE

Angina and Myocardial Infarction

The sensory fibers of the heart, parietal pleura, and diaphragmatic surface of the parietal pericardium are supplied by nerves in the thoracic and cervical spinal cord levels. The sensory fibers of the heart are supplied by the superior, middle, and inferior cardiac nerves, which conduct impulses through the cervical and upper thoracic sympathetic ganglia to the posterior sensory roots at levels T1 to T5, with expansion to C8. Cardiac pain may radiate to the left arm in a C8 (ulnar nerve) distribution. Both sympathetic and vagal cardiac afferent fibers contribute to anginal pain. The vagal nerves synapse in the medulla and descend to the upper cervical spinothalamic tract cells. This innervation contributes to the angina pain experienced in the neck and jaw.[14]

The central diaphragmatic pleura has innervation from the phrenic nerve, with contribution from nerve roots C3, C4, and C5. Disorders that affect the central portion of the diaphragm may refer pain to the superior ridge of the trapezius muscle.[4] Inflammation of the diaphragm may occur as a result of bacterial pneumonia, pulmonary infarction, or pleurisy secondary to systemic lupus erythematosus. Right shoulder pain may occur as a result of diaphragmatic inflammation secondary to cholecystitis. Left shoulder pain may be secondary to splenic inflammation. In instances of inflammation of the diaphragm, respirations tend to exacerbate the symptoms.

Epidemiology/Pathophysiology

The epidemiology and pathophysiology of coronary artery disease are beyond the scope of this book. A wide range of articles are available that review individuals at risk for this disorder and factors that predispose to coronary artery disease.[40-43,46,54]

Clinical History

Angina occurs with increased activity or stress caused, for example, by cold weather, a large meal, and emotional upset. Resting or relieving the stress results in a decrease in the pain or pressure. The pressure or pain may be perceived as a pressure sensation or chest pain. With increasing severity, the pain may remain localized to the chest or may radiate to the anterolateral aspect of the neck, left shoulder, left arm to the hand, or lower jaw. Anginal pain may last up to 30 minutes. Relief is obtained within 3 minutes with sublingual nitroglycerin. Myocardial infarction causes pain in a similar distribution, but of greater severity and duration. In addition, sympathetic stimulation characterized by marked sweating, nausea, and vomiting is frequent.

Physical Examination

Physical examination demonstrates degrees of cardiac dysfunction in proportion to the location and severity of cardiac muscle damage. Angina may result in a transient S_4 gallop that occurs with episodes of pain. Myocardial infarction may cause alterations in blood pressure, faint heart sounds, an S_3 gallop indicative of ventricular dysfunction, and arrhythmias.

Laboratory Data

The diagnosis of acute myocardial infarction has increasingly been dependent on evaluation of serum markers. Determination of creatine kinase with its isoforms, along with troponins, is useful in the detection of myocardial muscle damage. Electrocardiography is the most readily available diagnostic method for detecting cardiac ischemia associated with angina or myocardial infarction. The electrocardiogram should show ischemic changes (ST segment elevation or depression) or pathologic Q waves.[37]

Radiographic Evaluation

A number of other diagnostic tests—exercise electrocardiography, radioisotope imaging, and angiography—are available to document the extent of coronary artery stenosis with associated increased risks.[17,58]

Differential Diagnosis

The differential diagnosis of arm pain is the clinical symptom shared by patients with coronary artery insufficiency and those with cervical radiculopathy. Determination of the cause of chest and arm pain may be quite difficult. Mechanical factors that are unassociated with significant physical exertion (such as rolling over in bed and coughing) may identify patients with arm pain secondary to nerve impingement.[1,10] Patients who have a herniated cervical disc with radiculopathy may have all the symptoms associated with myocardial ischemia (diaphoresis, nausea, vomiting, and dyspnea).[34] Patients with cervical disease may complain of radiation to the posterolateral aspect of the neck and scapula. The diagnosis of herniated cervical disc may be considered only after the possibility of myocardial ischemia has been eliminated as a diagnosis. Cardiac pain may occur in individuals in whom cord infarction develops at the C6–C7 level.[8]

Cervical Angina

Brodsky reported on a group of 438 patients with chest pain unassociated with myocardial ischemia.[6] Of this group, 88 patients underwent cervical spine surgery to improve chest and arm pain. These patients had arm pain with or without numbness, a tender chest wall, and absence of neurologic signs. Neck pain and interscapular pain were uncommon symptoms. The results of coronary angiography performed before spine surgery were normal. Cervical laminectomy was associated with an excellent or fair outcome, with arm pain being decreased in 84% of patients with cervical angina. On occasion, movement of the neck of an individual with cervical angina can result in chest pain and acute, nonspecific ST-T wave changes that are reversible with return of the neck to a neutral position.[18]

Pericarditis

Acute pericarditis may develop secondary to myocardial infarction or a wide variety of disorders that inflame serosal surfaces, including viruses, uremia, systemic lupus erythematosus, rheumatoid arthritis, tuberculosis, and drugs. Patients have chest pain that may radiate to the shoulder or lateral part of the neck that is exacerbated by the supine position and relieved by sitting forward. Physical examination may reveal a triphasic pericardial rub. Electrocardiography demonstrates characteristic diffuse ST segment elevation. Therapy is usually symptomatic.[39]

Treatment

A variety of therapies are available for preventing and limiting myocardial damage. These therapies range from the use of a daily 81-mg aspirin tablet to placement of vascular stents, thrombolytic therapy, and coronary bypass surgery to name a few.[13,16,27,28]

Carotid Artery Dissection

Dissection of the internal carotid artery is an unusual cause of anterolateral neck pain. The annual incidence of spontaneous carotid artery dissection is 3 per 100,000.[45] The carotid and vertebral arteries have a greater frequency of dissection than other arteries (renal and coronary) of similar size do. The increased frequency may relate to the greater mobility of the carotid and vertebral arteries over bony structures. In a study of 147 patients with this entity, 9% (13) had neck pain as an associated symptom.[2] In another study of 36 patients with carotid dissection, neck pain was noted in 19% (7).[36] The disorder occurs in hypertensive individuals who have no evidence of atherosclerotic vessel disease. Other risk factors include smoking and fibromuscular dysplasia. Dissection may occur with hyperextension and lateral flexion of the neck as the artery is stretched over the transverse processes of the upper cervical vertebrae.[53] Dissection may also occur with trauma induced by chiropractic manipulation.[47] In young patients, connective tissue diseases such as Takayasu's arteritis or systemic lupus erythematosus may cause carotid artery dissection.[7] Focal unilateral headache is the most common symptom in association with dissection. The headache is steady, nonthrobbing, of variable intensity, and located in the frontal, auricular, or periorbital area. Neurologic manifestations may include stroke (resulting in contralateral hemiparesis, paresthesias, aphasia, ipsilateral blindness, or abducens paralysis) or oculosympathetic palsy with ptosis and miosis but not anhidrosis. Oculosympathetic palsy is found in less than 50% of patients.[48] Focal neurologic deficits may follow the onset of headache or neck pain within minutes or hours. In rare circumstances, major strokes may be associated with severe deficits or death.[21] Bruits may be heard over the carotid. The diagnosis may be made by arteriography or MR imaging.[2,55] Heparinization is the most commonly used form of therapy for symptomatic dissection.[33] Surgery may be required for recurrent or progressive dissections resistant to medical therapy. Traumatic dissections require surgical therapy more often than spontaneous internal carotid dissections do.[35] Most spontaneous carotid dissections have a benign course and do not require surgical or catheter revascularization.[25] Recurrence of dissection in an artery that had a dissection previously is a very rare event.[3]

Vertebral Artery Dissection

Vertebral artery dissection occurs most commonly in middle-aged women.[31] People with hypertension or fibromuscular dysplasia are at greater risk for dissection. Cervical manipulation has also been reported as a cause of vertebral artery damage.[32] Signs of a stroke develop in these individuals because of brain stem dysfunction.[20,52] Individuals who sustain significant trauma to the cervical spine may have associated vertebral artery dissection. Early Doppler ultrasound and duplex sonography can identify dissection in the setting of cervical spine trauma.[44] Pain in the occiput or posterior of the neck is the initial symptom in 80% of patients, and it precedes ischemic symptoms by minutes to 30 days. Pain rarely radiates to the frontal region. Most patients are initially seen with a completed stroke, but a minority have transient ischemic attacks. The lateral medullary syndrome (pain, numbness in the ipsilateral face [trigeminal], ataxia, vertigo, nystagmus, Horner's syndrome [descending sympathetic tract], dysphagia, numbness of the ipsilateral appendages) is the most common neurologic manifestation. Severe cases may have basilar artery involvement with associated quadriparesis, dysphagia, diplopia, and preserved sensation. Unilateral pharyngeal pain that may be confused with glossopharyngeal neuralgia is associated with vertebral artery dissection.[50] In rare circumstances, young individuals with unilateral neck pain have vertebral artery dissection.[26] Some of these younger patients may have experienced a whiplash injury before the onset of neurologic symptoms.[9] The diagnosis is documented by angiography. MR imaging may demonstrate spinal cord infarction, with axial T2-weighted images documenting hyperintensities in the upper cervical cord.[56] MRA has resolution similar to that of conventional angiography and can show intramural hematomas.[29] Treatment with heparin followed by warfarin has been helpful in decreasing the risk of thrombosis. The majority of patients improve without any need for surgical intervention. The death rate in patients with dissection of the carotid or vertebral arteries is less than 5%.[5]

Thoracic Aortic Dissection

Neck pain associated with disease of the thoracic aorta occurs secondary to aneurysmal dilation or dissection of the vessel. An arterial aneurysm is a localized or diffuse enlargement of an artery. One or all three layers (intima, media, and adventitia) of the aorta make up the wall of the aneurysm. An aneurysm is caused by the formation of a false channel in the wall of the aorta that splits the layers of the vessel apart. Saccular aneurysms are bulbous protrusions of all three layers on one side of the vessel. A fusiform aneurysm is a diffuse, circumferential expansion of a segment of the vessel. A type A dissection involves the ascending aorta. Type B dissections occur distal to the left subclavian artery.

Epidemiology

Thoracic aneurysms and dissections occur most commonly in elderly patients with hypertension and atherosclerosis. Hypertension is noted in up to 90% of aneurysm patients, particularly those with distal dissections.[30] Dissections in the ascending aorta occur in middle-aged patients without hypertension who have cystic medionecrosis of the aorta.[22] Aneurysms in the ascending aorta are relatively uncommon. Dissections predominate in males in a ratio of 3:1.[19] Pregnant women younger than 40 years who are in the third trimester have half the dissections in that age group.[12]

Pathogenesis

The pathogenesis of the aneurysm is related to atherosclerotic degeneration with structural weakening of the connective tissue (collagen) of the vessel wall. Patients with aneurysms are usually hypertensive and may have manifestations of generalized atherosclerosis, including angina, previous myocardial infarction, stroke, or peripheral vascular disease.[51]

Two theories have been proposed regarding the cause of aneurysmal enlargement. The first theory is that a genetically linked deficit in the quantity and quality of collagen and elastin in the arterial wall causes generalized arteriomegaly. This theory explains the fact that a number of vessels may be affected in an individual patient. The second theory is that plaque from atherosclerosis interferes with the blood supply of the arterial wall, thereby resulting in weakening of the wall.[15] Inflammatory mediators such as interleukin-8 and monocyte chemoattractant protein-1 have been identified in aortic aneurysms. These factors are chemoattractant to leukocytes and recruit inflammatory cells to the arterial wall, which leads to weakening of the wall.[24] Atherosclerosis may represent a secondary, nonspecific response to vessel wall injury. Aortic arch calcification may be related to an increase risk for coronary artery disease risk, but not to artery dissection.[23]

Clinical History

Pain associated with thoracic aortic dissection occurs secondary to expansion of the aneurysm. Extension of the aneurysm is associated with severe chest pain, with maximal intensity at initiation of the dissection. A distinguishing feature of the pain associated with aortic dissection is its tendency to migrate from its initial site to other areas as the dissection advances through the aorta. Patients complain of a tearing pain in the chest that radiates to the lateral and posterior aspect of the neck and to the interscapular, low back, and abdominal regions. Syncope, in the absence of a stroke, is frequently associated with proximal dissection and the development of cardiac tamponade.[49] Neurologic complications include stroke, ischemic peripheral neuropathy, and paralysis related to impaired flow to the spinal cord.

Physical Examination

The physical findings in patients with thoracic aortic dissection consist of diaphoresis, vasoconstriction, and normal blood pressure in a majority with distal lesions.[12] Hypotension is common in proximal dissections. Loss of one or more peripheral pulses may be found with proximal or distal lesions.

Laboratory Data

Laboratory test results may be normal. Patients with ruptured aneurysms may have mild to profound anemia at the time of evaluation, depending on the amount of extravascular blood loss, and moderate leukocytosis.

Radiographic Findings

The most appropriate noninvasive method for detecting the presence of thoracic aneurysms and dissections is a controversial issue. Recent studies have reported the superior sensitivity of MR for detecting aneurysms in patients who are hemodynamically stable.[38] In patients who are unable to be moved, transesophageal echocardiography has sufficient sensitivity to identify the presence of aortic defects.[57]

Aortography is performed in patients with thoracic dissection to delineate the vascular anatomy. Aortography determines the site of the intimal tear and the extent of the dissection and assesses aortic insufficiency and the involvement of branch arteries.[12]

Treatment

Therapy for thoracic dissection in the early phase is lowering of blood pressure while protecting cerebral, cardiac, and renal blood flow. Therapy for acute proximal dissection is surgical. Therapy for distal dissections may be medical or surgical, depending on the extent of the aneurysm. The overall 10-year survival rate of patients with dissection is 40%.[11]

References

Cardiovascular Diseases: Cervical Spine

1. Allison DR: Pain in the chest wall simulating heart disease. BMJ 1:332, 1950.
2. Anson J, Crowell RM: Cervicocranial arterial dissection. Neurosurgery 29:89, 1991.
3. Atkinson JL, Piepgras DG, Huston J 3rd, et al: Cervical artery dissections: Evidence for redissection in previously dissected arteries: Report of three cases. Neurosurgery 51:797-801, 2002.

4. Bauwens DB, Paine R: Thoracic pain. In Blacklow RS (ed): MacBryde's Signs and Symptoms: Applied Pathologic Physiology and Clinical Interpretation, 6th ed. Philadelphia, JB Lippincott, 1983, pp 139-164.
5. Biousse V, Touboul PJ, D'Anglejan-Chatillon J, et al: Time course of symptoms in extracranial carotid artery dissections: A series of 80 patients. Stroke 26:235-239, 1995.
6. Brodsky AE: Cervical angina: A correlative study with emphasis on the use of coronary arteriography. Spine 10:699, 1985.
7. Caso V, Paciaroni M, Parnetti L, et al: Stroke related to carotid artery dissection in a young patient with Takayasu arteritis, systemic lupus erythematosus and antiphospholipid antibody syndrome. Cerebrovasc Dis 13:67-69, 2002.
8. Cheshire WP Jr: Spinal cord infarction mimicking angina pectoris. Mayo Clin Proc 75:1197-1199, 2000.
9. Chung YS, Han DH: Vertebrobasilar dissection: A possible role of whiplash injury in its pathogenesis. Neurol Res 24:129-138, 2002.
10. Davis D, Rivito M: Osteoarthritis of the cervicodorsal spine (radiculitis) simulating coronary artery disease. N Engl J Med 238:857, 1948.
11. DeBakey ME, McCollum CH, Crawford ES, et al: Dissection and dissecting aneurysms of the aorta: Twenty-year follow-up of five hundred twenty-seven patients treated surgically. Surgery 92:1118, 1982.
12. DeSanctis RW, Doroghazi RM, Austen WG, et al: Aortic dissection. N Engl J Med 317:1060, 1987.
13. Fischman DL, Leon MB, Baim DS, et al: A randomized comparison of coronary-stent placement and balloon angioplasty in the treatment of coronary artery disease. Stent restenosis study investigators. N Engl J Med 331:496-501, 1994.
14. Foreman RD: Mechanisms of cardiac pain. Annu Rev Physiol 61:143-167, 1999.
15. Giordano JM: Vascular versus spinal disease as a cause of back and lower extremity pain. Semin Spine Surg 2:136, 1990.
16. Gottlieb SS, McCarter RJ, Vogel RA: Effect of beta-blockade on mortality among high-risk and low-risk patients after myocardial infarction. N Engl J Med 339:489-497, 1998.
17. Guidelines for coronary angiography: A report of the American College of Cardiology/American Heart Association Task Force on Assessment of Diagnostic and Therapeutic Cardiovascular Procedures (Subcommittee on Coronary Angiography). J Am Coll Cardiol 10:935, 1987.
18. Guler N, Bilge M, Eryonucu B, et al: Acute ECG changes and chest pain induced by neck motion in patients with cervical hernia—a case report. Angiology 51:861-865, 2000.
19. Hagan PG, Nienaber CA, Isselbacher EM, et al: The International Registry of Acute Aortic Dissection (IRAD): New insights into an old disease. JAMA 283:897-903, 2000.
20. Haldeman S, Kohlbeck FJ, McGregor M: Stroke, cerebral artery dissection, and cervical spine manipulation therapy. J Neurol 249:1098-1104, 2002.
21. Hart RG, Easton JD: Dissections of cervical and cerebral arteries. Neurol Clin North Am 1:255, 1983.
22. Hirst AE, Gore I: Is cystic medionecrosis the cause of dissecting aortic aneurysm? Circulation 53:915, 1976.
23. Iribarren C, Sidney S, Sternfeld B, et al: Calcification of the aortic arch: Risk factors and association with coronary heart disease, stroke, and peripheral vascular disease. JAMA 283:2810-2815, 2000.
24. Koch AE, Kunkel SL, Pearce WH, et al: Enhanced production of the chemotactic cytokines interleukin-8 and monocyte chemoattractant protein-1 in human abdominal aortic aneurysms. J Pathol 142:1423, 1993.
25. Kremer C, Mosso M, Georgiadis D, et al: Carotid dissection with permanent and transient occlusion or severe stenosis: Long-term outcome. Neurology 60:271-275, 2003.
26. Krespi Y, Gurol ME, Coban O, et al: Vertebral artery dissection presenting with isolated neck pain. J Neuroimaging 12:179-182, 2002.
27. Langer A, Krucoff MW, Klootwijk P, et al: Prognostic significance of ST segment shift early after resolution of ST elevation in patients with myocardial infarction treated with thrombolytic therapy: the GUSTO-1st segment monitoring substudy. J Am Coll Cardiol 31:783-789, 1998.
28. Lauer MS: Aspirin for primary prevention of coronary events. N Engl J Med 346:1468-1474, 2002.
29. Leclerc X, Lucas C, Godefroy O, et al: Preliminary experience using contrast-enhanced MR angiography to assess vertebral artery structure for the follow-up of suspected dissection. AJNR Am J Neuroradiol 20:1482-1490, 1999.
30. Leonard JC, Hasleton PS: Dissecting aortic aneurysms: A clinicopathological study. Q J Med 48:55, 1979.
31. Mas J, Bousser M, Hasboun D, et al: Extracranial vertebral artery dissections: A review of 13 cases. Stroke 18:1037, 1987.
32. Mas JL, Henin D, Bousser MG, et al: Dissecting aneurysm of the vertebral artery and cervical manipulation: A case report with autopsy. Neurology 39:512, 1989.
33. McNeil DH, Dreisbach J, Marsden RJ: Spontaneous dissecting aneurysm of the internal carotid artery: Its conservative management with heparin sodium. Arch Neurol 37:54, 1980.
34. Mitchell LC, Schafermeyer RW: Herniated cervical disc presenting as ischemic chest pain. Am J Emerg Med 9:343, 1991.
35. Mokri B, Piepgras DG, Houser OW: Traumatic dissections of the extracranial internal carotid artery. J Neurosurg 68:189, 1988.
36. Mokri B, Sundt TM Jr, Houser OW, et al: Spontaneous dissection of the cervical internal carotid artery. Ann Neurol 19:126, 1986.
37. Myocardial infarction redefined—a consensus document of the Joint European Society of Cardiology/American College of Cardiology. J Am Coll Cardiol 36:959-969, 2000.
38. Nienaber CA, von Kodolitisch Y, Nicolas V, et al: The diagnosis of thoracic aortic dissection by noninvasive imaging procedures. N Engl J Med 328:1, 1993.
39. Permanyer-Miralda G, Sagrista-Sauleda J, Soler-Soler J: Primary acute pericardial disease: A prospective series of 231 consecutive patients. Am J Cardiol 56:623, 1985.
40. Ridker PM, Rifai N, Rose L, et al: Comparison of C-reactive protein and low-density lipoprotein cholesterol levels in the prediction of first cardiovascular events. N Engl J Med 347:1157-1565, 2002.
41. Roger VL, Weston SA, Killian JM, et al: Time trends in the prevalence of atherosclerosis: A population-based autopsy study. Am J Med 110:267-273, 2001.
42. Rogers WJ, Canto JG, Lambrew CT, et al: Temporal trends in the treatment of over 1.5 million patients with myocardial infarction in the US from 1990 through 1999: The National Registry of Myocardial Infarction 1, 2, and 3. J Am Coll Cardiol 36:2056-2063, 2000.
43. Ross R: The pathogenesis of atherosclerosis: A perspective for the 1990s. Nature 362:801, 1993.
44. Schellinger PD, Schwab S, Krieger D, et al: Masking of vertebral artery dissection by severe trauma to the cervical spine. Spine 26:314-319, 2001.
45. Schievink WI: Spontaneous dissection of the carotid and vertebral arteries. N Engl J Med 344:898-906, 2001.
46. Sempose C, Cooper R, Kovar MG, et al: Divergence of the recent trends in coronary mortality for the four major race-sex groups in the United States. Am J Public Health 78:1422, 1988.
47. Sherman DG, Hart RG, Easton JD: Abrupt change in head position and cerebral infarction. Stroke 12:2, 1981.
48. Silbert PL, Mokri B, Schievink WI: Headache and neck pain in spontaneous internal carotid and vertebral artery dissections. Neurology 45:1517-1522, 1995.
49. Slater EE, DeSanctis RW: The clinical recognition of dissecting aortic aneurysm. Am J Med 60:625, 1976.
50. Soga Y, Ito Y: Sudden onset pharyngeal pain associated with dissecting vertebral artery aneurysm. Acta Neurochir 144:835-838, 2002.
51. Spittell JA: Hypertension and arterial aneurysm. J Am Coll Cardiol 1:533, 1983.
52. Stevinson C, Honan W, Cooke B, et al: Neurological complications of cervical manipulation. J R Soc Med 94:107-110, 2001.
53. Stringer WL, Kelly DL: Traumatic dissection of the extracranial internal carotid artery. Neurosurgery 6:123, 1980.
54. Sytkowski PA, Kannel WB, D'Agostino RB: Changes in risk factors and the decline in mortality from cardiovascular disease: The Framingham study. N Engl J Med 322:1635, 1990.
55. Waespe W, Niesper J, Imhof H, et al: Lower cranial nerve palsies due to internal carotid dissection. Stroke 19:1561, 1988.
56. Weidauer S, Nichtweiss M, Lanfermann H, et al: Spinal cord infarction: MR imaging and clinical features in 16 cases. Neuroradiology 44:851-857, 2002.
57. Wiet SP, Pearce WH, McCarthy WJ, et al: Utility of transesophageal echocardiography in the diagnosis of disease of the thoracic aorta. J Vasc Surg 20:613, 1994.
58. Zaret BL, Wackers FJ: Nuclear cardiology. N Engl J Med 329:775, 1993.

GENITOURINARY DISEASES

CAPSULE SUMMARY

	LOW BACK	NECK
Frequency of spinal pain	Common	Not applicable (NA)
Location of spinal pain	Flanks, sacrum	NA
Quality of spinal pain	Colicky or dull ache	NA
Symptoms and signs	Colicky flank and referred pain, tender costovertebral angle	NA
Laboratory tests	Abnormal urinalysis, positive cultures	NA
Radiographic findings	Filling defects or masses with contrast studies or sonography, calcifications on plain roentgenograms	NA
Treatment	Surgical removal of mass, lysis or removal of stone, antibiotics	NA

The organs that compose the genitourinary tract are located in the retroperitoneum and pelvis and lie close to the lumbosacral spine. Diseases that affect the genitourinary organs may be associated with both local pain and referred pain that radiates to the lumbosacral area. Primary renal disease causes flank pain. The flank is the region of the back bounded superiorly by the ribs, inferiorly by the iliac crests, medially by the spine, and laterally by the sides of the body. Stretching of the renal capsule causes pain in the distribution of T10–T12, the source of sensory innervation. Renal pain is not exacerbated by movement or increased by palpation or percussion, except in the setting of pyelonephritis or renal infarcts.[66]

Processes that obstruct the outflow of urine will cause symptoms. Obstruction may be secondary to congenital narrowing, stones, or tumor. Tumors may also cause pain, but of a slow and insidious variety as opposed to the sharp pain associated with acute obstruction of the urinary tract. The blockage of blood flow and associated tissue necrosis (renal infarction) will also cause acute pain.

Acute inflammatory involvement of glomeruli may result in flank pain. Hereditary disorders associated with structural abnormalities of the kidney cause back pain. Blockage of vessel outflow in the form of renal vein thrombosis is associated with renal capsular swelling and low back pain.

KIDNEY

The kidneys are located at the level of the 10th through 12th thoracic and 1st lumbar vertebrae. Pain from diseases that affect the kidneys is felt at the costovertebral angle just lateral to the paraspinous muscles at T12–L1. It often radiates around the flank toward the umbilicus and is usually dull and constant. The source of the pain is thought to be sudden distention of the capsule of the kidney. Diseases that cause or are associated with acute kidney obstruction (stone, hemorrhage, hydronephrosis, or acute pyelonephritis) are painful. Disease processes that cause only gradual capsular distention are not associated with kidney pain (stone with partial obstruction, tumor, congenital obstruction).

Kidney Stones

Epidemiology

Nephrolithiasis, or urinary stones, may also be associated with back pain. Stones located in the pelvis of the kidney will cause dull flank pain in patients with capsular distention and colic in those with obstruction or spasm at the ureteropelvic junction. Approximately 2% to 3% of people in the United States and Western Europe have an attack of renal colic during their lifetime. Individuals with a positive family history have a relative risk of 2.57 of experiencing a stone in comparison to those who do not have such a history.[42] The risk for recurrent attacks ranges from 20% to 50% over the subsequent 10 years.[85,153]

Pathogenesis

The major types of stones include calcium oxalate, struvite (magnesium ammonium phosphate, or stones of infection), calcium phosphate, uric acid, and cystine. Many of the factors that predispose to renal lithiasis are unknown. However, factors that either increase urinary concentration or decrease urinary solubility do promote stone formation in general. Different types of liquids can promote or inhibit stone formation. For example, grapefruit and tomato juice increase the risk of stone formation.[43] Other factors may predispose to the formation of specific stones, including hypercalcemia, hyperoxaluria, and hyperuricosuria for calcium oxalate stones; urinary infection causing alkaline urine (urea-splitting organisms) for struvite stones; persistent alkaline urine from oral antacids, renal tubular acidosis, or primary hyperparathyroidism for calcium phosphate stones; acidic urine for uric acid stones; and cystinuria for cystine stones.[20] Stone formation is increased twofold in hypertensive individuals.[112] Vasectomy in men may also predispose to stone formation.[95]

Clinical History

The clinical symptoms associated with a kidney stone are correlated with stone size and the duration, location, and degree of obstruction. Although kidney stones frequently produce symptoms of renal colic or acute urinary tract infection (UTI), some stones are discovered incidentally during an x-ray examination for another condition. Pain, when it occurs, is secondary to stretching of the collecting system or renal capsule and is not necessarily caused by increased peristalsis. The severity of pain correlates with the rate of distention rather than the degree of dilation. Acute obstruction from a renal calculus causing sudden hydronephrosis of a mild degree may be very painful, whereas chronic obstruction of insidious onset may be painless. Patients with stones in the kidney or caliceal system may experience sharp, cramping pain or pain that is dull and persistent. Acute obstruction may be characterized by a steady crescendo of pain in the flank, which may radiate downward toward the groin and into the genitalia if the area near the ureter is affected.[157] The pain is steady and continuous in its onset and may have a duration as short as 30 minutes or as long as 24 hours. The patient may find that walking or other movement is preferred over lying still in bed. In general, the character of the pain is not changed with movement or position. The pain is associated with nausea and vomiting and may mimic an acute surgical abdomen. A history of chills and fever suggests a complicating infection.

Physical Examination

Physical examination may demonstrate costovertebral angle tenderness on percussion. Some paraspinous muscle spasm may accompany the tenderness. Acute nonstructural scoliosis may occur in severe cases. Abdominal examination may elicit tenderness in the appropriate upper quadrant, particularly with an associated infection. Abdominal distention and paralytic ileus may accompany acute renal colic.

Laboratory Data

Examination of urine is the most important part of the laboratory evaluation of a patient with a suspected stone. Hematuria may range from a few erythrocytes on microscopic evaluation to gross blood. Proteinuria is also present. The presence of hematuria with unilateral flank pain and a positive flat plate of the abdomen is found in 90% of emergency department patients. However, the absence of hematuria does not eliminate thc presence of a stone.[57] If the pH of the urine is alkaline, the stone may be struvite in origin. A pH constantly in the 6.0 to 6.5 range may be associated with renal tubular acidosis. A low pH is associated with uric acid stones. Microscopic evaluation of urine for crystals is worthwhile because the different crystals that cause stones have different shapes. Calcium oxalate and calcium phosphate are rectangular, uric acid is rhomboidal, cystine is hexagonal, and struvite is a rectangle within a rectangle. A 24-hour urine collection along with samples collected individually over a 24-hour period aids in diagnosis. Hypercalciuria favors the formation of calcium oxalate stones. Hyperuricosuria favors calcium oxalate or uric acid stones.[56]

Blood tests may also be useful in detecting the potential source of stones. Hypercalcemia is associated with oxalate stones, whereas hyperuricemia is associated with oxalate and uric acid stones. Hyperchloremia suggests renal tubular acidosis, which is associated with phosphate stones.[76] Tests of serum creatinine and urea nitrogen are obtained to assess renal function and document the extent of any renal disease that may be associated with nephrolithiasis.

Radiographic Findings

Plain roentgenograms of the abdomen may be adequate to detect the presence of stones. Radiopaque stones contain calcium and are oxalate or phosphate (Fig. 17-5). Moderate-size stones or staghorn calculi are frequently composed of struvite. Cystine stones are moderately radiopaque. Uric acid stones are radiolucent. Intravenous pyelography (IVP) is useful to localize a calcific shadow as long as the kidneys are functioning and are not acutely obstructed. However, the use of contrast increases the risk of reactions and renal dysfunction. Radiolucent stones may appear as holes in the column of dye.[89] Ultrasonography is the method of choice for individuals who cannot be exposed to radiation.[19] Non–contrast-enhanced helical CT is the method of choice for identifying the presence of stones.[28] CT is able to detect radiolucent stones missed on a plain film of the abdomen.[207] MR imaging visualizes the organs of the genitourinary system well, but it does not identify stones. The usefulness of this technique is limited in these patients.[172]

Differential Diagnosis

The diagnosis of nephrolithiasis is suggested by the patient's history, physical examination, and urinalysis and

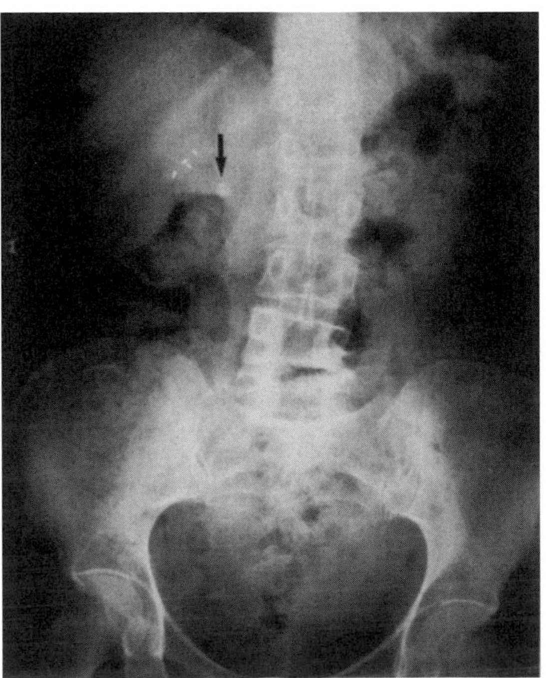

Figure 17-5 Colicky right-sided back pain, most noticeable in the flank, developed in a 55-year-old woman with rheumatoid arthritis. A plain roentgenogram of the abdomen revealed a radiopaque stone in the right kidney *(arrow)*. *(Courtesy of Arnold Kwart, MD.)*

is confirmed by the presence of the stone on radiographic studies (helical CT). Chemical analysis of passed stones specifies the type of stone that is at fault. Patients with other kidney conditions may have flank pain. Pyelonephritis may complicate nephrolithiasis, as well as occur independently. Renal tumor with an obstructive blood clot may cause pain. Papillary necrosis with obstruction of the pelvis will cause pain. Infarction of the kidney will result in flank pain. Renal tubular acidosis, independent of nephrolithiasis, may be a cause of back pain. In one study, 16% of patients with renal tubular acidosis had low back pain in the absence of a mechanical cause of pain.[76]

Treatment

A patient with acute pain associated with nephrolithiasis is treated with increased fluid intake and analgesia. The patient may pass the stone without any other therapy. Between 80% and 90% of stones will pass spontaneously, especially if the stones are 1 to 5 mm in diameter.[20] The average time for passage of a stone is 8 days for those with a diameter of 2 mm or less, 12 days for 2- to 4-mm stones, and 22 days for stones larger than 4 mm.[123] If a kidney is totally blocked for a few days, removal of the stone needs to be considered. In the past, open surgery may have been considered. The treatment of choice for upper tract stones (above the upper third of the ureter) is extracorporeal shock wave lithotripsy.[18,203] The stones are fragmented by shock waves and subsequently passed through the ureter into the bladder to be voided out. Stones as large as 2 cm can be treated with extracorporeal shock wave lithotripsy.[14] Even large stones may be fragmented by this method. Treatment has been reported to be successful in 70% of patients.[32] Two forms of percutaneous disintegration include ultrasonic lithotripsy and electrohydraulic disintegration. These procedures require endoscopic surgery.[18,34] The ability of these procedures to remove renal stones continues to improve.[163]

If the other procedures are contraindicated or ineffective, open surgery is advised. Such treatment may be particularly necessary for staghorn calculi.[111]

Prognosis

The prognosis for patients with an episode of nephrolithiasis is that they will have a recurrence. Patients with stones should undergo a careful metabolic evaluation to identify the source of their stones. After appropriate evaluation, specific therapy in the form of phosphates, thiazides, allopurinol, penicillamine, or antibiotics may be given to reverse the underlying metabolic abnormality predisposing to stone formation.[41,139,166]

Pyelonephritis

Acute pyelonephritis is a bacterial infection of the parenchyma of the kidney.[161] Bacteria are able to travel retrogradely from the bladder to the kidney when obstruction of the vesicoureteral reflux in the genitourinary system allows access to the kidney parenchyma.

Epidemiology

UTI is the most common of all bacterial infections. Between the ages of 1 and 50, when prostate infection increases the prevalence of UTI in men, the ratio of men to women with UTI is 1:50. The yearly incidence in females older than 10 years is approximately 5%.[173] Most of the infections involve the bladder (cystitis). In individuals older than 65 years, the male-to-female ratio is 1:10.

Pathogenesis

More than 95% of UTIs occur via the ascending route from the urethra, bladder, and ureter to the kidney. Only 3% to 5% are of hematogenous origin.[20] Vesicoureteral reflux allows infected urine to reach the pelvicaliceal system. Urine gains access to the kidney parenchyma at the papillary tips and then spreads along the collecting tubules. The medullary portion of the kidney is predisposed to infection because of a chemical environment characterized by high urea and ammonia concentrations and high osmolarity, which inhibits granulocyte function as well as complement activation.[88] The infection is focal and causes localized swelling with an inflammatory infiltrate composed of polymorphonuclear leukocytes initially and lymphocytes subsequently. Persistent or repeated infections will result in scarring of the kidneys.

Clinical History

Patients with pyelonephritis complain of severe, constant, aching pain over one or both costovertebral angles that is not affected by position or movement. The pain may radiate to the lower abdominal quadrants. Patients have frequency, urgency, and burning on urination. Nausea and vomiting may be part of the symptom complex.

Physical Examination

Patients with acute pyelonephritis are systemically ill with high fever, tachycardia, and chills. Fever above 37.8° C is correlated with pyelonephritis.[150] The fever is mediated through an increased concentration of interleukin-6 (IL-6) generated in the urinary tract independent of bacteremia.[138] Patients exhibit exquisite tenderness to percussion over the costovertebral angle along with associated back muscle spasm. Abdominal signs may include muscle guarding of the abdominal wall and hypoactive bowel sounds.

Laboratory Data

Laboratory tests confirm the presence of pyuria and bacteria, and cultures of urine and blood will grow the offending organism. *Escherichia coli*, staphylococcal species, and *Streptococcus faecalis* are the most common pathogens. Urine will show many white blood cells (WBCs) on an unspun specimen. The presence of bacteria on a Gram stain of an unspun urine specimen is also suggestive of a significant infection.[101] Use of the antibody-coated bacteria assay has proved to be too nonspecific to separate upper tract from lower tract infection.[159] The response to single-dose antibiotic therapy is a more sensitive means of separating lower tract from upper tract disease. Other laboratory findings include elevated WBC counts to the level of 40,000 cells/mL. The erythrocyte sedimentation rate (ESR) and C-reactive protein are also increased.

Radiographic Evaluation

Radiographic evaluation, including IVP and ultrasonography, is not routinely required for a patient with pyelonephritis. Radiographic evaluation is most appropriate for individuals with persistent or early recurrent infections. A plain film of the abdomen may show some obliteration of the renal shadow secondary to edema of the kidney. IVP or ultrasound is useful to survey the urinary tract for the presence of obstruction or vesicoureteral reflux. If the infection is severe, the involved kidney is enlarged and its nephrographic image is diminished in intensity. These investigations are most useful in patients who do not respond to antibiotic therapy. Gallium 67 can be used to localize the site of infection in the kidney. Although 86% accuracy has been claimed, both false-positive and false-negative findings can occur.[81] This technique cannot differentiate acute pyelonephritis from renal abscess.

Differential Diagnosis

The differential diagnosis of patients with acute back pain not relieved by rest and associated with systemic signs includes pancreatitis, pneumonia, acute cholecystitis, acute appendicitis, and acute diverticulitis. Gastrointestinal problems are associated with normal urinalysis and changes in bowel habits. Pleuritic pain is associated with pneumonia. Herpes zoster, before vesicles appear, can simulate the pain of pyelonephritis if the T12 or L1 dermatomes are affected.

Treatment

Treatment with appropriate antibiotics results in control of the infection and resolution of the pain.[20] Debate exists regarding the need for parenteral versus oral antibiotics for uncomplicated pyelonephritis.[125,198] The choice of antibiotic will be determined by local environmental factors affecting microbial antibiotic resistance. When the infection is resistant to cure because of structural abnormalities such as polycystic kidneys or vesicoureteral reflux, chronic pyelonephritis may develop. This disorder may be clinically silent except in acute exacerbations of the chronic infection, when localized renal pain will be present.[170] The ideal duration of antibiotic therapy depends on the location of the infection in the upper or lower portion of the genitourinary tract. For upper tract infection, intravenous therapy is given until the patient is afebrile. Oral antibiotics such as trimethoprim-sulfamethoxazole or quinolones may be used to complete a 2-week course of therapy.[175,189]

Perinephric Abscess

Infections that escape the confines of the renal capsule will lodge in the perinephric tissues and form a perinephric abscess. Frequently, patients with these abscesses have a history of chronic renal disease from UTIs, urinary calculus with hydronephrosis, trauma, or hematogenous spread from a distant infected area. The site of pain associated with perinephric abscess is the costovertebral angle, and the pain is insidious in onset. Patients may be symptomatic for weeks before seeking medical attention. Patients may have symptoms of dysuria, hematuria, or urinary retention along with anorexia, fever, and weight loss. They may have mild to severe tenderness on palpation, as well as muscle spasm with a scoliotic posture. Inflammation of the skin over the flank may be observed. A mass may be palpated over the flank in 50% of patients. Laboratory evaluation reveals anemia, leukocytosis, an elevated ESR, and abnormal urinalysis with positive urine culture for the infecting organism. Renal function is usually normal because the infection is unilateral. Urinalysis may be normal in 30% and urine culture sterile in 40% of cases. Blood cultures are positive in 40% of individuals. Radiologic findings in the abdomen include ptosis of a kidney and obliteration of the psoas shadow. Chest roentgenograms may demonstrate an elevated or fixed hemidiaphragm, pleural effusion, empyema, lung abscess, and lower lobe atelectasis. Excretory urography demonstrates poor visualization of the kidney, displacement of the kidney, and obstruction. Gallium scanning, sonography, or CT may reveal an inflammatory mass. Of these techniques, CT demonstrates the full extent of the infection to the best degree.[148] In a series of 25 patients with perinephric abscess, CT detected the abscess in 92% of individuals.[122] MR imaging may identify edema but may not be able to distinguish cysts from other inflammatory processes. Treatment includes appropriate antibiotics and percutaneous or open surgical drainage.[187] Early diagnosis and percutaneous drainage can reduce mortality from more than 40% to 12%.[42]

Ureteropelvic Junction Obstruction

Abnormalities of the ureteropelvic junction are most commonly congenital malformations that cause stenosis or obstruction. The stricture elicits symptoms associated with urinary obstruction. Rarely, stenosis of the junction may occur in adults as one of the sequelae of renal injury. Extravasation of urine or blood results in fibrosis of the junction. A historical fact that helps localize the site of the lesion to the junction is the scenario of increased water intake exacerbating back pain.[37] The pain is intermittent, but in acute circumstances the pain may be sharp and colicky. Over time, the pain becomes dull and persistent. Tenderness at the costovertebral angle or flank is common. The diagnosis is confirmed by demonstration of hydronephrosis and enlargement of the renal pelvis as seen on IVP, sonography, or renal scanning (Fig. 17-6). Surgical repair of the stenosis is indicated. The goal of surgery is to relieve obstruction at the junction.[147] If the process of obstruction continues on a chronic basis and causes hydronephrosis and atrophy of the kidney with loss of renal function, nephrectomy may be required.

Renal Infarction

Infarcts of the kidney are caused by arterial occlusion. The major causes of occlusion include thrombi in the atria or ventricles secondary to myocardial infarction, myocarditis, or infective endocarditis and embolization to the kidney

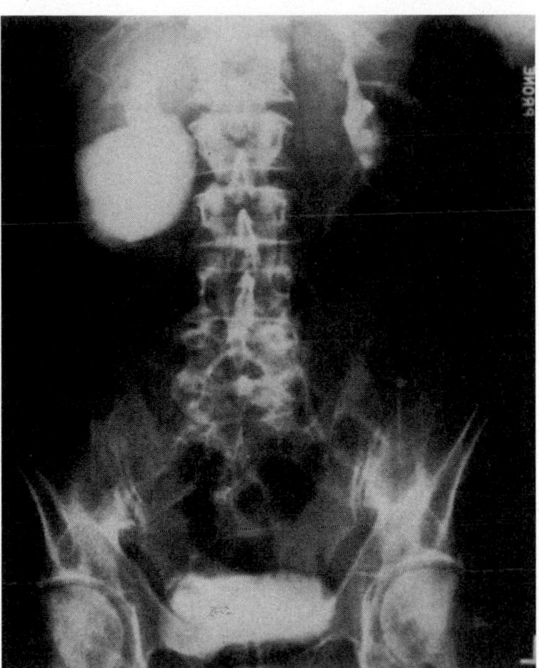

Figure 17-6 Intravenous pyelography reveals bilateral hydronephrosis and enlargement of both renal pelves in a patient with ureteropelvic junction obstruction. *(Courtesy of Arnold Kwart, MD.)*

(Fig. 17-7). Plaques associated with arteriosclerosis may also be a source of emboli. Primary vascular inflammation (e.g., polyarteritis nodosa, Churg-Strauss vasculitis) will cause vascular occlusion.[70] Trauma to the blood vessels to the kidney will also interrupt blood flow. In addition, aneurysms of the renal artery may be a source of emboli (Fig. 17-8). In a study of 17 patients with renal infarction, 14 had a risk factor: atrial fibrillation (11), previous embolism (6), mitral stenosis (6), hypertension (9), or ischemic heart disease (7).[49]

If the main renal artery is occluded, the entire kidney may become infarcted and be functionless and atrophic. This process is associated with a sudden onset of severe, sharp costovertebral angle pain. Smaller areas of infarction may cause no symptoms. Pain usually affects the flank, abdomen, or low back region.[49] The development of symptoms is due in part to the acuteness of onset and the amount of kidney tissue affected.

Physical examination elicits pain over the paraspinal muscles on the affected side. The kidney is not enlarged on abdominal examination. Bowel sounds may be hypoactive. Urinalysis will usually reveal erythrocytes. Repeated urinalysis is indicated if the first specimen is normal because blood flow to the kidney is impaired and urine containing erythrocytes may take hours to appear. IVP

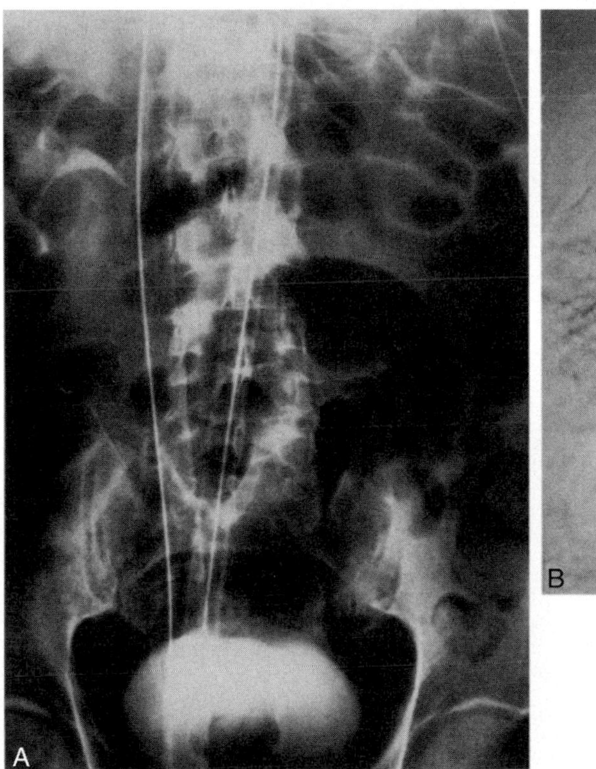

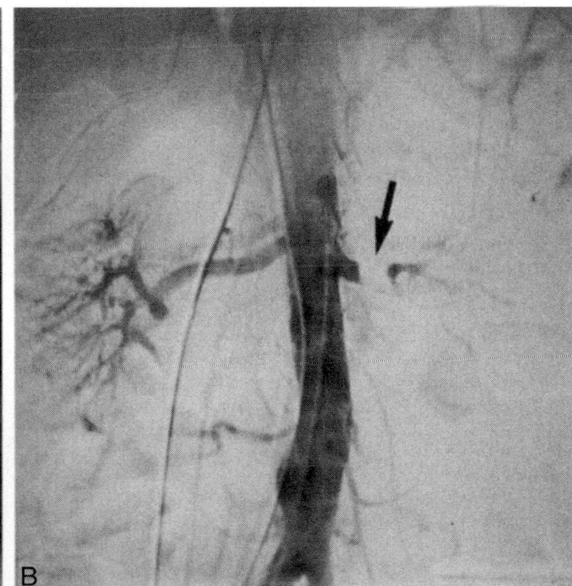

Figure 17-7 Intravenous pyelography *(A)* demonstrates no flow to the left kidney. A subtraction view *(B)* of the renal arteriogram reveals an embolus in the left renal artery *(arrow)*. The patient experienced severe left-sided back pain while recovering from a coronary artery bypass graft operation. *(Courtesy of Edward Druy, MD.)*

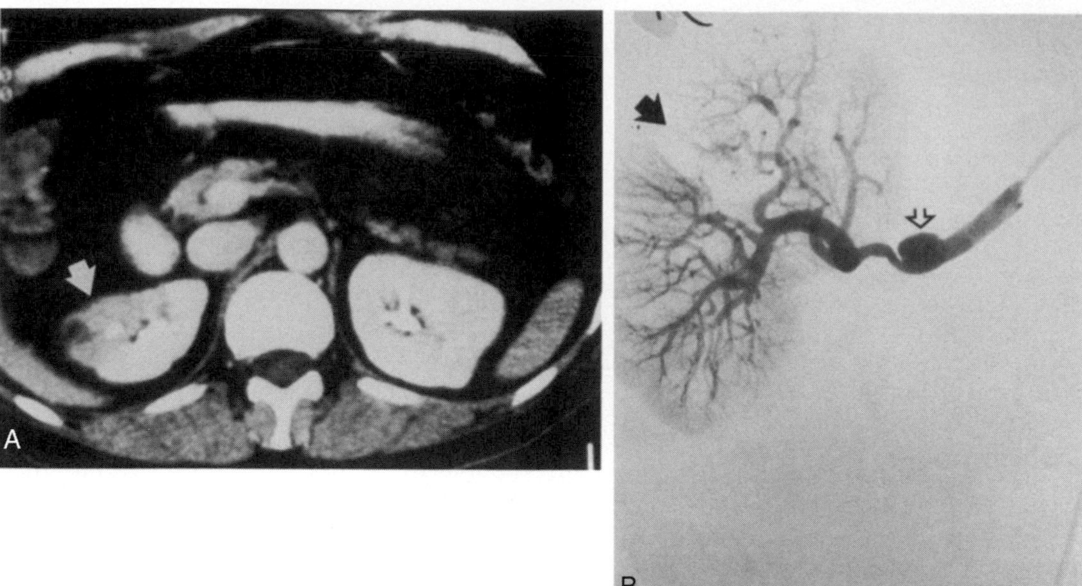

Figure 17-8 A 40-year-old man sought medical care for acute-onset, right-sided costovertebral angle pain. Urinalysis was initially normal. The pain continued and the patient became febrile. Microscopic hematuria appeared on the third day of hospitalization. *A*, A CT scan of the abdomen showed an infarct of the upper outer aspect of the right kidney *(arrow)*. *B*, A renal angiogram (subtraction view) revealed a large renal artery aneurysm *(open arrow)* with an area of decreased blood vessels corresponding to the area of infarction *(black arrow)*. Surgery was performed to correct the aneurysm. *(Courtesy of Edward Druy, MD.)*

may fail to visualize a portion of the kidney with a partial infarction. Total occlusion results in an absence of any radiographic image of the kidney.

A definitive diagnosis is made through the use of a renal scan or arteriogram. A renal scan is able to demonstrate a segmental or generalized decrease in renal perfusion. This procedure is less invasive than an arteriogram or contrast-enhanced CT scan. An arteriogram will identify the location and extent of vessel involvement. Possible sources of emboli should be investigated by the appropriate methods (echocardiogram, for example) if renal infarction is documented. Therapy for infarction, if the diagnosis is made promptly, is embolectomy by either medical or surgical means. Although surgical intervention can restore renal blood flow, the procedure has a higher associated mortality rate and no better return of renal function than seen with medical therapy. Medical therapy must be given within 3 hours to have a beneficial effect on preservation of renal function.[15] Anticoagulants are useful to prevent progressive thrombosis and may improve renal function. If hypertension ensues from partial occlusion of the renal artery that is not responsive to medical therapy, renal endarterectomy or nephrectomy may be required.[193] A study has reported the successful use of intra-arterial streptokinase to dissolve clots causing renal infarcts.[160] The mortality of patients with renal infarcts remains high because of the risk of stroke or gastrointestinal crisis from recurrent emboli.

Renal Cancer

Epidemiology

Tumors of the kidney include renal cell carcinoma (85%), renal pelvis tumor (8%), Wilms' tumor (5%), and sarcoma (2%).[20] Of all the renal tumors, renal cell carcinoma is the most prevalent and, because of the diverse and nonrenal symptoms associated with the tumor, the most difficult to diagnose. In the United States, the incidence is 35,000 new cases per year.[82] The ratio of men to women with renal cell tumor has been 2:1, but this ratio has been narrowing. The incidence has increased over time because the widespread use of noninvasive abdominal imaging allows for the recognition of smaller lesions.[140] The peak age of incidence is 60 years. The most common site of origin of renal tumors is the proximal convoluted tubular epithelium. In light of this fact, the designation of kidney tumors as renal cell carcinoma as suggested by Mostofi is a more appropriate name than hypernephroma.[126]

Clinical History

Patients with renal cell carcinoma may have a range of symptoms. They may be symptomless or have renal symptoms, or systemic complaints may develop. The classic triad of hematuria, flank pain, and a palpable renal mass occurs in 10% of patients. The most common finding is hematuria (63%), with flank or back pain occurring in 41%.[65,167] The pain is usually a constant, dull ache in the back or abdomen. The dull ache occurs as the tumor extends beyond its capsule into retroperitoneal structures. Acute low back pain that is sharp or colicky will occur with clot formation that obstructs a portion of the caliceal system. As part of the systemic or paraneoplastic manifestations of renal cell carcinoma, patients will complain of fever, anorexia, weight loss, or neurologic symptoms.[33] A polymyalgia rheumatica–like disorder is a rare manifestation of renal cell carcinoma and is alleviated by nephrectomy.[165]

Physical Examination

Physical examination will reveal fever in 20% of patients and a palpable mass in a similar number.[13] The appearance of a left-sided varicocele is noted in up to 11% of male patients. This finding is secondary to blockage of the left gonadal vein at its point of entry into the left renal vein by a tumor thrombus.[149] Edema of the lower extremities may also occur in 11% of patients.

Laboratory Data

Laboratory tests may be very helpful in documenting the systemic nature of the patient's disease. The ESR is elevated in a majority of patients. Anemia with normal WBC and platelet counts is seen in 40%. Thrombocytosis is rare but is associated with a poor prognosis.[134] Hypercalcemia secondary to a hormone effect of a material released by the tumor is noted in 15%. Urinalysis is positive for erythrocytes and protein. Pathologic evaluation of the tumor reveals adenocarcinoma in most circumstances. Tumors with more mitotic figures or anaplasia are more invasive.

Radiographic Findings

IVP will demonstrate a space-occupying lesion (Fig. 17-9). Renal ultrasonography shows a solid mass as opposed to a cyst, which lacks internal echoes and has a smooth, sharp border (Fig. 17-10). If any doubt remains in regard to whether the mass is solid or cystic, a CT scan will demonstrate the status of the lesion along with extension of the tumor within the vena cava.[156,201] The presence of a multilocular mass, thickened or enhanced septa within the mass, enhancement with contrast, or thickened irregular walls is indicative of a neoplastic lesion.[44,110] Arteriography may be necessary to document the vascular supply of the tumor to plan for operative intervention.[200] Arteriography is rarely required with newer radiographic techniques. MR imaging is able to identify the presence of a mass and is most helpful in staging the neoplasm. It determines the origin of the mass, vascular patency (renal vein or vena cava), the presence of lymph node metastases, and direct tumor invasion to adjacent organs.[80]

Treatment

Therapy for renal cell carcinoma is radical nephrectomy. This procedure includes the removal of regional lymph nodes.[156] The need for chemotherapy or radiotherapy, or both, is determined by the extension of the tumor locally and the number of metastases distally.[158] In general, chemotherapy and radiotherapy are ineffective in controlling tumor growth. No chemotherapeutic agent is adequate as a single agent. The use of interferon and IL-2 has achieved response rates of 10% to 20%.[127] Nephrectomy followed by interferon therapy is associated with longer survival than noted with interferon therapy alone.[63] The prognosis is best for patients with stage I disease (tumor confined to the kidney capsule), in whom the survival rate is 75% at 5 years. The number of tumors confined to the kidney at the time of diagnosis has increased from 47% to 78% from 1989 to 1998.[104] Patients with stage IV disease (distant metastases) have a 5-year survival rate of 25%.[199]

Miscellaneous Kidney Disorders

Glomerulonephritis

Glomerulonephritis is an inflammatory disorder of the kidney characterized by the abrupt onset of hematuria, proteinuria, decreased filtration rate, hypertension, and oliguria. Inflammation of the glomerulus may be caused by a variety of disorders, including multisystemic diseases such as systemic lupus erythematosus.[20] Patients may have malaise and a dull persistent aching in the flanks bilaterally. Interstitial edema within the renal parenchyma and stretching of the renal capsule are the cause of flank pain. Physical examination reveals hypertension and evidence of fluid overload (rales, edema, dyspnea). Laboratory evaluation reveals red cell casts and proteinuria on urinalysis. Renal function tests may demonstrate a variable degree of dysfunction. Treatment is based on the underlying disease and may include corticosteroids or cytotoxic therapy.[17]

Hereditary Disorders/Polycystic Kidneys

Hereditary disorders causing structural damage to the kidney may be associated with back pain. Autosomal dominant polycystic kidney disease may be manifested as back pain in 20% of all patients.[66] Between the ages of 20 and 24, up to 50% of affected women will have back pain as the initial symptom. The flank pain is dull in quality and

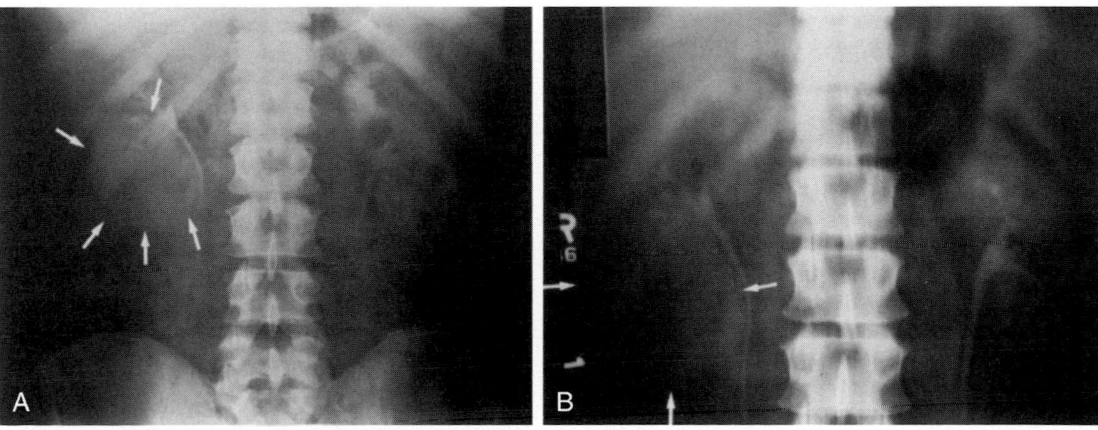

Figure 17-9 *A* and *B*, Intravenous pyelographic views of a renal mass in the lower pole of the right kidney *(arrows)*. Pathologic examination revealed renal cell carcinoma. *(Courtesy of Arnold Kwart, MD.)*

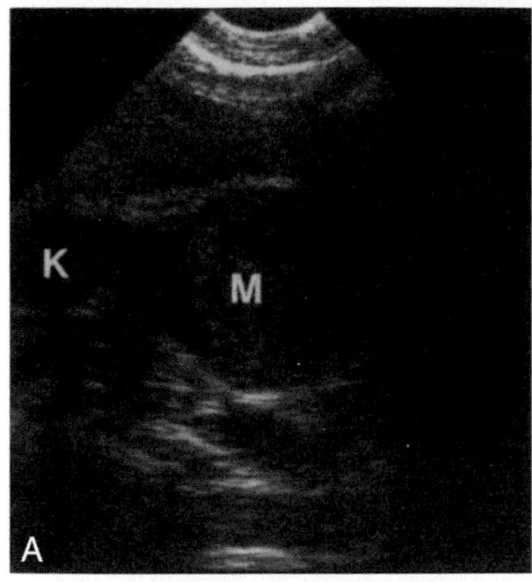

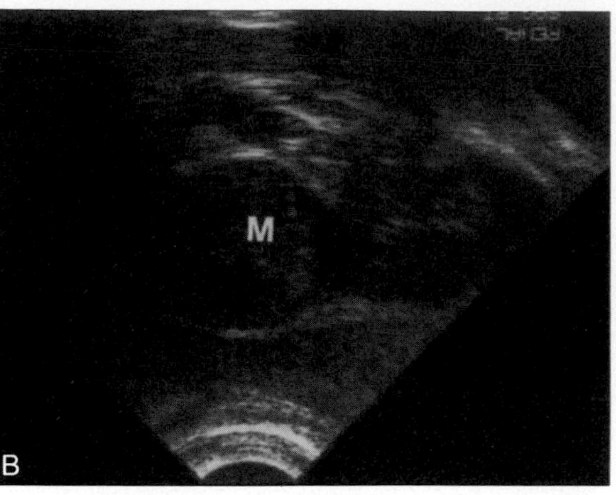

Figure 17-10 Ultrasound. *A*, Sagittal scan of the kidney (K) demonstrating a solid intrarenal mass (M) compatible with a renal cell carcinoma. *B*, Cross-sectional scan revealing a solid intrarenal mass. *(Courtesy of Michael Hill, MD.)*

associated with flank masses and gross hematuria. Patients may have renal insufficiency at initial evaluation. Ultrasound of the kidney demonstrates multiple cysts. The disease inevitably progresses to renal failure.[141]

Other disorders associated with flank pain include renal vein thrombosis and nephrotic syndrome. Renal vein thrombosis may be treated with local infusion of thrombolytic therapy if heparin is inadequate to resolve the clot.[97] When venous outflow from the kidney is obstructed, the associated swelling results in flank pain. Nephrotic syndrome is caused by excessive excretion of albumin and is the result of a wide range of kidney disorders, including glomerulosclerosis and IgA nephropathy.[72] The resulting hypoalbuminemia causes interstitial edema of the kidney. Interstitial edema within the renal parenchyma results in stretching of the renal capsule. Patients with nephrotic syndrome often complain of dull bilateral fullness in the area of the costovertebral angles. Therapy is directed at the specific disorder associated with the proteinuria.[137]

URETER

The ureter is a thin tube composed of smooth muscle that connects the renal pelvis with the bladder. The ureter is anatomically narrowed at three locations: the ureteropelvic junction, a point crossing over the iliac vessels, and the ureterovesical junction. These three locations are the ones most frequently obstructed by urinary stones. Other inflammatory (retroperitoneal fibrosis) or neoplastic (transitional cell) processes may affect the ureter along its path from the kidney to the bladder.[7,8] These processes may cause obstruction that occurs on a chronic basis (Fig. 17-11).

Ureteral Stone

Renal stones are initially formed in the proximal part of the urinary tract and pass progressively into the calices, renal pelvis, and ureter. In the ureter, specific locations that become obstructed are associated with specific symptoms.

Clinical History

In the upper or proximal part of the ureter, stones cause acute, sharp, spasmodic pain that is localized to the flank. If acute renal capsular distention occurs, pain may radiate along the course of the ureter to the ipsilateral testicle because the nerve supply to the kidney and testis is the same. As the stone passes along the ureter, it may lodge at the level where the ureter passes over the iliac vessels. The pain remains sharp and intermittent, corresponding to peristalsis of the ureter. The pain radiates to the lateral flank and lower quadrant of the abdomen.

As the stone passes into the distal part of the ureter, the pain remains intermittent and sharp and corresponds to the waves of ureteral peristalsis. In women, the pain will radiate to the genitalia, particularly the labia. In men, the pain radiates along the inguinal canal to the groin and

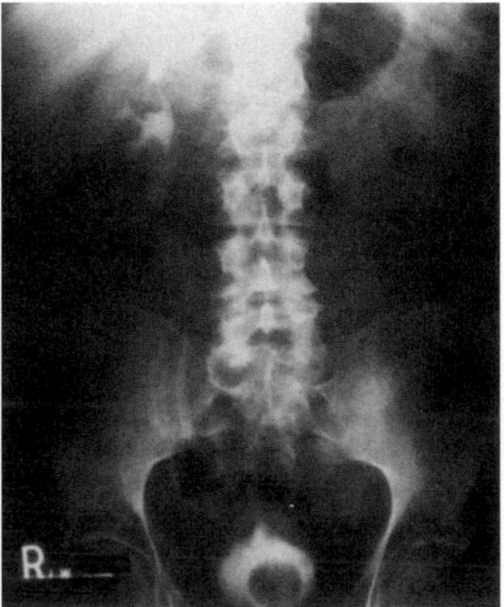

Figure 17-11 Intravenous pyelogram demonstrating an obstructive pattern involving the right kidney. An entire column of dye is visualized while the left kidney has emptied. This 56-year-old man had vague, right-sided flank pain. The cause of the obstruction was a ureteral transitional cell cancer.

scrotal wall. A stone in this location may give rise to excruciating pain and cause the patient to writhe about trying to find a comfortable position. In contrast, with abdominal disease such as peritonitis, patients lie quietly because motion increases the discomfort.[186] When the stone approaches the bladder, urgency and frequency with burning on urination develop as a result of inflammation of the bladder wall around the ureteral orifice.

The sensory innervation of the kidneys and abdominal organs is similar. Ureteral disease may cause autonomic reflex symptoms in the gastrointestinal tract manifested as nausea, vomiting, and paralytic ileus. The differential diagnosis of a ureteral stone includes abdominal or pelvic processes (appendicitis, colitis, salpingitis, or cholecystitis).

Physical Examination

Physical examination reveals a patient in significant distress who is in constant motion, unable to find a comfortable position. Fever is present if the patient has an associated infection. The costovertebral angle is tender to percussion. Bowel sounds may be hypoactive on abdominal examination.

Laboratory Data

Urinalysis is an essential part of the evaluation. Hematuria, either gross or microscopic, is frequently present.

Radiographic Findings

Plain film of the abdomen may reveal the presence of a stone inasmuch as more than 90% are radiopaque (Fig. 17-12). Oblique films will separate renal stones from other calcified structures such as gallstones, mesenteric lymph nodes, and pelvic phleboliths. IVP findings may include a delay in visualization of the collecting system on the affected side, followed by an intense nephrographic effect. The column of dye will end at the level of stone obstruction. Ultrasonography can identify hydronephrosis in patients who are allergic to intravenous dye or are anuric.

Treatment

A majority of ureteral stones will pass through the urinary tract spontaneously.[4] Hydration and analgesics are generally useful in treating the symptoms of stone obstruction. Stones in the lower tract pass spontaneously more often than those in the upper system. If fever develops or if severe nausea and vomiting or complete obstruction occurs, manipulative or surgical therapy is needed. Manipulative therapy includes lithotripsy or stone removal by endo-urologic procedures.[53] Open surgical measures are infrequently used.

Vesicoureteral Reflux

The ureterovesical junction is a specialized structure that allows urine to enter the bladder but prevents urine from reentering the ureter, particularly during voiding.[3] Because the kidney is protected from the high pressures developed in the bladder during excretion, infection is limited to the bladder. If the valve becomes incompetent on either a congenital (short intravesical ureter) or an environmental (infectious) basis, refluxed urine will reach the kidney and play a key role in the pathogenesis of infection. Hydronephrosis may also occur. About 8% of adults with bacteriuria have reflux.[169] Patients with reflux are usually

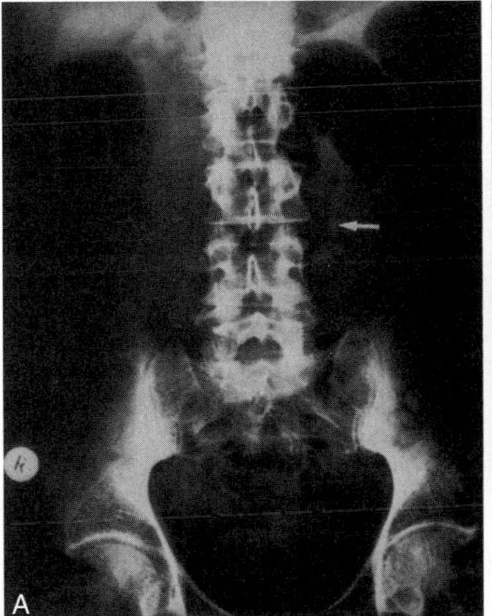

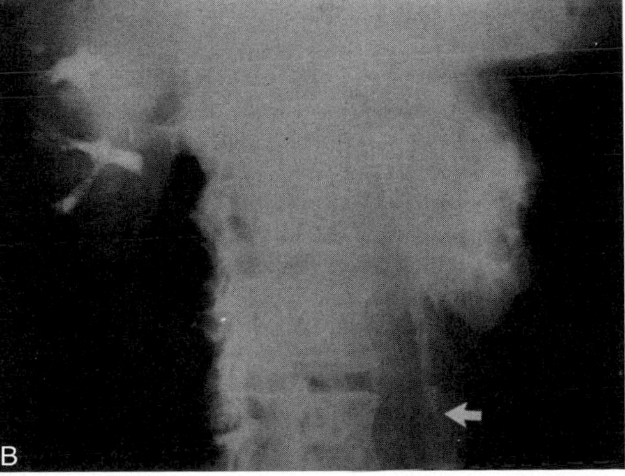

Figure 17-12 *A*, A plain roentgenogram reveals a radiopaque structure lateral to the L3–L4 intervertebral disc space *(arrow)* in a patient with left-sided back pain. *B*, An intravenous pyelogram, oblique view, confirms the object as a ureteral stone that has obstructed the left ureter *(arrow)*. *(Courtesy of Arnold Kwart, MD.)*

asymptomatic, but occasionally, dull unilateral or bilateral flank pain develops. On rare occasion, such pain may be associated with voiding. Patients may have episodes of acute pyelonephritis (particularly females) or may have pyuria without symptoms. Physical examination may be unremarkable. Laboratory evaluation may show bacteriuria without pyuria. Renal function test (creatinine, blood urea nitrogen) results are abnormal in a minority. Radiographic evaluation with IVP may be normal, but a dilated lower ureter, visualization of the entire length of the ureter, and healed pyelonephritis are clues to the presence of reflux. Cystography may directly visualize reflux. Therapy for vesicoureteral reflux in adult women is to control infection, if present in the urinary tract, with antibiotics and, if necessary, to administer chronic suppressive treatment for 6 months or longer. Surgical therapy is necessary if acute pyelonephritis recurs and is not preventable with antibiotics. Reimplantation of the ureter into the bladder may be necessary in these circumstances.[2] If reflux is not treated, the end result may be markedly diminished renal function.[9]

BLADDER

Bladder pain is visceral in origin and is usually felt in a suprapubic or lower abdominal location. It is occasionally located in the sacral area.

Bladder Retention

Urinary retention develops in patients with obstruction at the bladder neck. In acute circumstances, the bladder fills rapidly, becomes distended, and causes suprapubic pain. Slowly developing obstruction, frequently from prostatic hypertrophy, causes pain of a dull variety that may be suprapubic or sacral in location. Patients are men older than 60 years who have difficulty maintaining a normal urinary stream. Examination of these patients demonstrates a lower abdominal midline mass frequently associated with prostatic hypertrophy discovered during rectal examination. Laboratory data are consistent with renal dysfunction in a minority. IVP demonstrates a postvoid residual in the bladder with associated hydronephrosis. Sonography can be used to document bladder size if the patient is allergic to contrast media. Therapy for bladder retention is relief of the obstruction. Acute obstruction is relieved by catheterization. Special consideration must be made for individuals with a massively distended bladder that becomes unobstructed acutely.[114] Rapid decompression is ill advised. Slow removal of fluid (100 to 300 mL/hr) will decrease the likelihood of gross hematuria. Prostatectomy is required for men with outflow obstruction secondary to prostatic hypertrophy.

Bladder Infection

Pathogenesis

Bladder infections (cystitis) are very common, particularly in women. The greater frequency of this infection in women can be directly related to the length of the urethra in each sex. Bacteria on the introitus can gain entry into the bladder with greater ease in women than in men.[38] Prostatic secretions contain bacteriostatic factors that may also inhibit the entry of bacterial organisms into the bladder in men. The bladder is able to clear infections spontaneously by voiding the organism in urine. Urine also contains bacteriostatic substances, and the mucosa of the bladder has properties that inhibit bacterial invasion.[20] However, if these defense mechanisms are inadequate to clear the organisms, cystitis will occur. Patients with severe cystitis (local infection or inflammation of the bladder) may experience mild, diffuse low back pain that resolves with resolution of the inflammation.

Clinical History

Patients with acute cystitis describe a burning pain with urination, but little fever and no chills. Those with chronic cystitis in whom signs of obstruction develop, including cystoceles, may have persistent, low-grade sacral back pain. Some patients with symptoms of cystitis (nocturia, dysuria, frequency, and hematuria) may have urethral irritation without bacteriuria.[18] Patients with cystitis are frequently sexually active women.

Physical Examination

On physical examination, the patient complains of pain with palpation over the lower part of the abdomen and tenderness of the bladder on palpation during pelvic examination.

Laboratory Data

Positive laboratory tests are usually limited to urinalysis, which shows hematuria and pyuria with positive urine cultures.

Treatment

Therapy for uncomplicated cystitis is a single large dose of an effective antimicrobial agent—3 g of oral amoxicillin, two double-strength trimethoprim-sulfamethoxazole tablets, or 2 g of oral sulfisoxazole. Patients who have infections limited to the bladder will respond to single-dose therapy with eradication of bacteria and relief of symptoms.[60] However, a 3-day regimen is more effective than single-day therapy for all antibiotics tested.[78] If infection recurs subsequent to a several-week delay after the completion of therapy, the reappearance of symptoms is secondary to reinfection. If the same organism reappears in the first few days after completion of therapy, the infection is a relapse of the original infection and a hidden focus (pyelonephritis, bladder diverticulum) must be sought.[174] Cystoscopy, which allows direct visualization of the bladder wall, documents the extent of bladder inflammation and obstruction in a patient with persistent symptoms.

MALE GENITAL ORGANS

Prostate

The prostate gland is located in the pelvis at the base of the bladder in males. Diseases of the prostate are not usually associated with visceral pain from the gland itself. Instead, pain is localized to the perineal or rectal area and the sacral portion of the lumbosacral spine.

Prostatitis

Prostatitis may be defined as a disease state characterized by inflammation of the prostatic acini, which is frequently caused by bacterial infection.

EPIDEMIOLOGY

From 1990 to 1994 in an analysis of 58,955 visits by men, 5% of all ambulatory visits by men 18 years or older included genitourinary symptoms as the reason for the visit. In almost 2 million visits annually, prostatitis was listed as a diagnosis. Prostatitis was the diagnosis in 8% of urology and 1% of primary care visits.[35] In an older study among male patients, prostatitis accounted for 25% of office visits for genitourinary tract complaints.[107]

PATHOGENESIS

Bacteria gain entry into the bladder from the urethra. In a retrograde manner, bacteria travel past the urethra to the bladder and gain entry to the prostate. Antegrade infection occurs less frequently from a source in the kidney.[121] However, not all cases of prostatitis have an infectious etiology. A National Institutes of Health classification system includes four categories: (1) acute prostatitis, (2) chronic bacterial prostatitis, (3) chronic abacterial prostatitis/pelvic pain syndrome with or without inflammation, and (4) asymptomatic inflammatory prostatitis.[93] Category 1 is a bacterial infection. Category 2 is related to recurrent bacterial infections. These individuals may have urethral strictures. Category 3 contains a number of possible etiologies, including urinary reflux, psychological stress, and pelvic floor abnormalities. Category 4 includes individuals with prostate biopsy evidence of inflammation. Some of these individuals have asymptomatic infections, and some have elevated prostatic-specific antigen (PSA) levels.[151]

CLINICAL HISTORY

Acute prostatitis is characterized by severe urinary frequency, urgency, dysuria, and nocturia. Pain in the lower part of the back, perineum, or external genitalia may be noted. Symptoms of systemic infection are usual and include fever, diffuse myalgias, nausea, vomiting, and anorexia. Individuals with category 3 prostatitis may complain of severe pelvic pain with voiding.

PHYSICAL EXAMINATION

Rectal examination reveals a very tender, enlarged, warm prostate that is firm to the examining finger. Abnormalities may also be palpated in the obturator, levator ani, and sphincter muscles.

LABORATORY DATA

Laboratory evaluation reveals positive cultures of urine or prostatic fluids. The Meares-Stamey urine evaluation with three vessels is the technique that identifies the origin of bacteria in urine.[119] An increased PSA value is consistent with a diagnosis of acute prostatitis. However, PSA should not be ordered as a screening test for prostatic carcinoma until the infection is resolved.

DIFFERENTIAL DIAGNOSIS

The differential diagnosis of prostatitis includes other forms of prostatitis and infections of other parts of the urinary system (Table 17-2). The pain of acute pyelonephritis with bladder irritability is primarily lumbar in location, whereas prostatitis is sacral.

TREATMENT

The choice of therapy is limited because of the inability of most antibiotics to gain entry into the prostate. A wide variety of antibiotics are effective for the treatment of prostatitis. The choice of a specific antibiotic is dependent on the organism cultured from prostatic fluid. Trimethoprim-sulfamethoxazole enters the prostate gland and is one of the antibiotics of choice. Therapy for 6 to 12 weeks has been associated with a significantly better cure rate than has a conventional 2-week course of therapy.[68] After completion of successful therapy, the patient should undergo serial examinations with prostatic fluid culture for a minimum of 4 months to ensure resolution of the infection.

CHRONIC PROSTATITIS

Chronic prostatitis has the same pathogenesis as acute disease, but the symptoms and signs are milder. Chronic prostatitis may develop without any previous history of acute prostatitis. Patients may have symptoms of recurrent UTI. They may note an aching or "fullness" in the bladder area and a dull, aching pain in the low back region. Pain with ejaculation may be a symptom. Rectal examination reveals a boggy, indurated prostate gland with areas of fibrosis. Massage of the gland is productive of an inflammatory fluid that contains numerous leukocytes and few organisms. Reports of an increased incidence of sacroiliitis with chronic prostatitis on plain roentgenograms have not been substantiated.[124] Therapy includes long-term antibiotic therapy, particularly with trimethoprim-sulfamethoxazole.[52] Other antibiotics recommended for prolonged periods of 2 to 6 weeks include carbenicillin, erythromycin, minocycline, doxycycline, cephalexin, or fluoroquinolones (norfloxacin, ciprofloxacin, ofloxacin).[120] Sitz baths twice daily are prescribed for pain in the perineum, back, and rectum. Prostatic massage is useful to relieve the symptoms of fullness and reduce pain.

17-2 DIFFERENTIAL DIAGNOSIS OF PROSTATITIS

Acute bacterial prostatitis
Chronic bacterial prostatitis
Acute nonspecific granulomatous prostatitis—eosinophilia/vasculitis (Wegener's)
Nonbacterial prostatitis—?autoimmune
Prostatodynia—voiding dysfunction
Acute diverticulitis
Pyelonephritis with bladder irritability
Prostatic carcinoma

Prostatic Neoplasms

Neoplasms of the prostate are among the most common malignancies found in men. Benign prostatic hypertrophy, or hyperplastic growth of the glandular tissue of the prostate, develops slowly and is not associated with low back pain. Flank pain may occur with benign prostatic hypertrophy if obstruction of the outflow tract causes hydronephrosis.

Prostatic Carcinoma

Epidemiology. Each year prostate cancer will be diagnosed in approximately 190,000 men in the United States. In a year, about 30,000 die of complications of the neoplasm.[82]

Clinical History. Adenocarcinoma of the prostate does not cause back pain when the tumor is confined to the limits of the gland capsule; however, the cancer may spread through the pelvic lymph channels and through vertebral veins to bones in the pelvis and lumbosacral spine.[202] Many tumors are asymptomatic when first diagnosed by detection of a nodule or diffuse induration of the prostate on rectal examination. In other instances, symptoms of obstruction may be the initial feature. Symptoms of low back pain with radiation down one or both legs associated with symptoms of bladder obstruction in men, especially those older than 50 years, suggest metastases to the axial skeleton by prostatic cancer.

Physical Examination. Rectal examination documents a hard, fixed, nodular prostate. Symmetrical enlargement and firmness of the prostate are more indicative of benign hyperplasia. Rectal examination will not detect 25% to 35% of tumors not located in the posterior or lateral portion of the gland.

Laboratory Data. Anemia, hematuria, decreased renal function, and elevated serum acid phosphatase may be present on initial laboratory examination. Serum PSA is a serine protease produced only by prostatic epithelial cells. Malignant prostate tissue generates more PSA than normal or hyperplastic tissue does. When the PSA level is higher than 10 ng/mL, the test is 92% specific for prostate cancer.[29] However, when used as a screening test, PSA may identify individuals who do not have cancer and who then receive therapy with an unfavorable effect.[92] Some patients with prostate cancer will have a PSA level of 4.0 ng/mL. Rectal examination does not increase PSA values to any significant degree, thus allowing for testing at any time.[39] The test is most useful in detecting recurrence after radical prostatectomy.[98]

Radiographic Findings. Transrectal ultrasonography is an efficient radiographic technique for staging the local extent of disease. Malignant nodules appear hypoechoic when viewed sonographically.[105] However, the technique has a high false-positive rate with benign hypertrophy and does not identify hypertrophy of pelvic lymph nodes. MR and CT scans detect soft tissue involvement with lymph nodes but do not differentiate benign from malignant lesions limited to the prostate itself.[79] Endorectal coil MR is able to detect extracapsular spread into the seminal vesicles, which negates surgical intervention.[46] Osteoblastic lesions from metastases to bone are demonstrated on plain radiographs of the pelvis. Bone scintiscan may demonstrate multiple lesions throughout the axial skeleton (see Chapter 13). Quantitative bone scintigraphy may be used after therapy to document the response of skeletal lesions to treatment.[181]

Differential Diagnosis. The diagnosis is confirmed by biopsy of the gland.[87] Most prostatic neoplasms are adenocarcinomas.[91] The lesions are evaluated by the Gleason grading system, which identifies well, moderately, and poorly differentiated tumors.[67] Poorly differentiated tumors are the ones that have more malignant characteristics and metastasize to a greater degree.[116] The anaplastic characteristics of the tumors also may be noted by the DNA status of the cells. Patients with diploidy have a better prognosis than those with aneuploidy do.[118] Once the diagnosis is established, staging of the tumor is necessary before appropriate therapy can be instituted.[117]

Treatment. Great controversy exists regarding the optimal therapy for prostatic carcinoma.[130] The side effects of the therapies must be weighed against the opportunity for cure of the disease. Prostate cancer has a progression that may be slow, so men have mortality from other disorders (cardiovascular disease). Staging the disease is essential in making an informed decision. Involvement of pelvic lymph nodes limits therapy in that radical prostatectomy or radiotherapy will not be curative. Radical prostatectomy is associated with decreased urinary and sexual function.[176] In about 80% of patients with lymph node involvement, metastatic disease develops in 5 years.[11] Therapy for prostatic cancer includes surgical, endocrine, and radiation modalities.[55] The basic premise of therapy for metastatic disease is to deprive the tumor of androgen. Such deprivation may be achieved through surgical castration or the administration of estrogen (diethylstilbestrol), analogues of luteinizing hormone–releasing hormone (LHRH), or antiandrogens such as flutamide or cyproterone acetate. Aminoglutethimide and ketoconazole block steroid biosynthesis and may be useful in patients with advanced disease. Combination chemotherapy with cyclophosphamide, cisplatin, fluorouracil, and/or doxorubicin is reasonably effective in palliating pain from widespread bone metastases. Radiotherapy is used to decrease pain in isolated areas of metastatic disease.[96,191,192] Brachytherapy, or radioactive seed implantation, involves the placement of rice-sized pellets in the prostate gland that emit radiation for a predicted period. This therapy may be most effective with low-grade disease.[47]

Treatment of prostatic carcinoma depends on the stage of the tumor. Stages A (limited to the gland with well-differentiated cells) and B (tumor confined to the gland in one or more lobes) may be treated with transurethral prostatectomy, radical prostatectomy, or radiation therapy.[36] Stages C (extension beyond the capsule) and D (distant metastases) require radiotherapy and hormonal manipulation. A variety of treatment protocols are under study to determine the most effective means of controlling the growth of metastatic prostatic carcinoma.[40,144]

Prognosis. The prognosis is good when prostate cancer is diagnosed early (stage A or B), with a 77% to 80% 5-year survival rate.[5] In stage C disease the survival rate is 58% and in stage D, 27%.[181] Rectal examination is a simple procedure but is relatively insensitive. Transrectal ultrasound and serum markers are more expensive and are not recommended for asymptomatic men. A positive PSA test is correlated with a tumor 30% of the time. A negative test does not eliminate prostatic cancer as a possibility. Therapy for prostatic cancer does not improve survival and has significant toxicities. The best screening mechanism to detect early cancer remains to be determined.[50] Insufficient evidence is available to determine whether the benefits of screening outweigh the harm in a population screened for prostatic cancer.[194]

Testis

The testicles are rarely affected by disease processes that are associated with back pain. However, malignancies of the testicles may metastasize locally to structures that will be associated with back pain. Testicular examination is frequently omitted from the evaluation of men with back pain. Failure to perform a testicular examination in a young man may cause a scrotal mass that is indicative of testicular disease to be missed.

Testicular Carcinoma

Approximately 5000 cases of testicular cancer are diagnosed yearly in the United States. Testicular cancer accounts for 1% of all cancers in men.[82] The peak age of incidence is 20 to 35 years, with white men more commonly affected than blacks. Men with maldescended testicles are at greater risk for development of the tumor. Types of testicular tumor include seminoma (most benign), embryonal cell cancer, teratoma, and choriocarcinoma (most malignant).

Back pain may be an initial symptom in 10% to 21% of patients. Patients have back pain in the absence of any testicular symptoms.[27,143] The pain may be dull and insidious or persistent and sharp. The pain is localized over the bones of the lumbosacral spine and the para-aortic area. The source of the pain is metastatic disease to the para-aortic or caval nodes. A history of back pain that prevents sleep in a young man should raise the possibility of testicular cancer.[168] Physical examination will usually reveal a testicular mass. Seminoma tends to expand within the testicle as a rubbery enlargement. Nonseminomatous germ cell tumors have an irregular border. Diffuse induration without nodularity may be the initial finding. In rare circumstances, the testis may feel normal despite the presence of a tumor. Gynecomastia may be a rare finding. Abdominal examination is worthwhile to detect lymphadenopathy. Laboratory tests are performed to identify tumor markers. Two useful markers are alpha-fetoprotein and human chorionic gonadotropin (HCG). These markers can also be used to monitor the response to therapy.[99] Radiographic evaluation may include scrotal ultrasound. Ultrasound is able to differentiate hydrocele and epididymitis from mass lesions. Scrotal ultrasound is about 70% accurate.[113] CT scan of the abdomen is a preferred test for determining the extent of lymph gland involvement to help stage the tumor.

Once the diagnosis is established, staging of the lesion is necessary. Patients with back pain will have stage II or more advanced disease. Therapy for patients with back pain usually consists of orchiectomy along with chemotherapy that includes cisplatin and etoposide.[64,205] The use of chemotherapy helps decrease the risk of recurrence.[128] The outcome is better if the disease is recognized at stage I. The chance of diagnosis is improved if a testicular examination is added to the routine examination of young adult men. Back pain may be the initial symptom of recurrence of tumor before radiologic abnormalities are identified.[206]

FEMALE GENITAL ORGANS

Females with disease in the pelvic organs may experience visceral, somatic, or referred pain.[197] Visceral pain from the uterus, fallopian tubes, or ovary is transmitted through nerves that travel with the sympathetic nervous system to spinal segments T11–T12 and with the parasympathetic system to segments S2–S4. The pain is deep, diffuse, and not well localized. Somatic nerves supply supporting tissues of the pelvis, including the muscles, ligaments (e.g., uterosacral), peritoneum, and periosteum of bone. Irritation, traction, or pressure on these structures results in a more localized, sharp pain that is felt in the suprapubic area or sacrum. Referred pain to the low back area develops when the sympathetic or parasympathetic nerves are stimulated by a disease process in the pelvic organs and cause sensory fibers in the dorsal horn of the corresponding spinal segment (T12, S2) to be activated. Back pain secondary to a gynecologic disorder is almost invariably associated with symptoms and signs of disease in the pelvic organs. A number of pathologic processes that affect the uterus, tubes, or ovaries may be associated with low back pain.

Uterus

The uterus is an organ composed chiefly of smooth muscle lined by endometrium. New growths in the form of leiomyomas may be associated with back pain. Abnormal position of the uterus may put traction on ligamentous structures, which may cause pain. The lining of the uterus may escape the confines of that organ and become implanted on structures in the pelvis, which will result in cyclic pain. Pregnancy may cause pain on the basis of either the size of the uterus or the effects of hormones on musculoskeletal structures.

Leiomyomas

Leiomyomas are the most common form of uterine tumor.[177] One of every four or five women older than 35 years has uterine myomas. They are benign tumors composed of smooth muscle and arise in the wall of the uterus. A variety of factors, including genetic predisposition, steroid hormones, and growth factors, increase the risk for development of these benign tumors.[178] For example, the growth factors transforming growth factor-beta and granulocyte-macrophage colony-stimulating factor, which mediate fibrosis, may contribute to the development of myomas.[51] Small myomas do not usually produce symptoms; however, these tumors may become quite large. Tumors occur and grow most commonly during the reproductive years and regress after menopause. Large tumors produce symptoms of heaviness in the pelvis and may cause back or lower extremity pain if they place pressure on nerves in the sacral portion of the bony pelvis. A dull aching soreness is usual. Myomas are palpable on physical examination of the pelvis. They are firm, irregular nodules arising from the pelvis and extending into the lower part of the abdomen. The masses may be movable if they are pedunculated. The differential diagnosis may prove to be a problem. Symmetrical enlargement of the uterus may be confused with pregnancy. A soft pregnant uterus and a positive HCG test should help make the diagnosis of an intrauterine pregnancy. A pedunculated tumor may be confused with an ovarian tumor. Endometriosis can cause uterine scarring, which may be difficult to distinguish from subserous myomas. Rapid growth is rarely related to uterine sarcoma. Women who have taken tamoxifen are at a greater risk for sarcoma.[208] Ultrasonography may help differentiate among these possibilities (Fig. 17-13). MR imaging is capable of visualizing the size and location of all uterine myomas and can distinguish between myomas and adenomyomas. Surgical removal is indicated for persistent symptoms of pain, uterine bleeding, infertility, size or position of the uterus preventing proper pelvic examination, or impingement on adjacent organs (such as the ureter). Control of hormone antagonists may offer a nonsurgical method to control leiomyoma growth in the future.[178]

Malposition

The uterus is normally directed forward in the pelvis.[48] In about a third of patients the uterus is retroverted or inclined posteriorly toward the sacrum and gently retroflexed. The most common simple displacement of the uterus is retroversion. Retroversion is congenital, acquired after a pregnancy, or a result of cul-de-sac pathology. The position of the uterus in itself is not usually associated with back pain. However, a retroverted uterus may be associated with chronic congestion of the pelvic veins. Back pain may also occur as a result of permanent uterine retroversion. The pain is associated with the underlying condition (endometriosis, salpingitis). Pelvic pain, low back pain, abnormal menstrual bleeding, and infertility have been associated with retroversion of the uterus. Pelvic examination allows determination of the position of the uterus. Bimanual replacement of the uterus is inadequate to achieve appropriate positioning of the uterus. Use of a pessary is more successful in relieving symptoms.

Women who have had multiple births may experience weakening of the uterosacral and cardinal ligaments, as well as the ligaments of the pelvic musculature that supports the uterus.[184] In addition, uterine prolapse may develop in patients who have a pelvic or presacral tumor or a sacral nerve disorder. Uterine prolapse is migration of the uterus down into the vagina. Patients with moderate prolapse will complain of a sensation of heaviness in the pelvis, lower abdominal pulling discomfort, and low back pain. Pelvic examination reveals descent of the cervix into the vagina. Therapy includes the use of a pessary or surgical removal of the uterus.

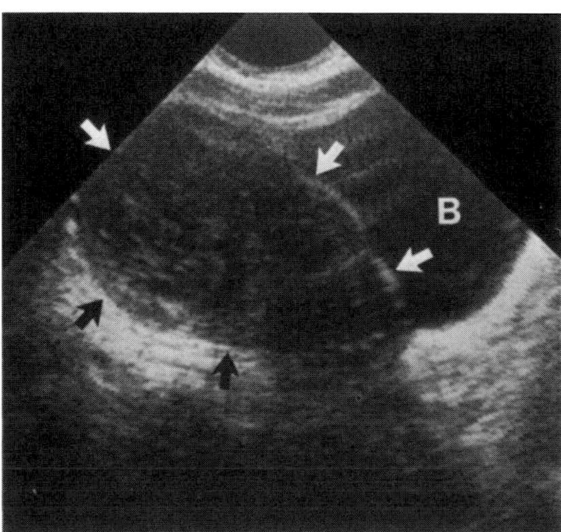

Figure 17-13 Ultrasound. A longitudinal scan through the pelvis demonstrates a large uterus *(arrows)* with multiple fibroid masses. B, Urinary bladder. *(Courtesy of Michael Hill, MD.)*

Endometriosis

Epidemiology

Endometriosis is a disease in which functioning tissue from the lining of the uterus (endometrium) is situated outside the uterine cavity. The estimated prevalence of endometriosis in women aged 15 to 50 is 2.5% to 3.3%.[71] The overall prevalence of symptomatic and asymptomatic women is 5% to 10%.[108] A total of 1% of all gynecologic surgeries are undertaken for endometriosis.[162]

Pathogenesis

Adenomyosis is the presence of endometrial tissue within the uterine musculature. Endometrial tissue may be located most commonly on the ovaries or the dependent portion of the pelvic peritoneum. However, peritoneal surfaces as well as extraperitoneal sites have been remote locations for this tissue. Three theories proposed as the cause of endometriosis include metaplastic transformation of cells lining the pelvic peritoneum, transplantation of endometrium to ectopic locations, or induction of endometrial tissue from mesenchymal tissues by factors released by shed endometrium.[136] Endometrial tissue outside the uterus undergoes the same monthly cycle of growth, shedding, and bleeding as the endometrial lining in the uterus, and symptoms of endometriosis are correlated with the site of the abnormal tissue. Cytokines, including IL-1, IL-6, IL-8, and tumor necrosis factors, are released from ectopic endometrium. These factors may facilitate cell proliferation.[75] Abnormalities in immune function may result in delayed apoptosis with the persistence of ectopic cells.[103] The disease may occur at any age after the onset of menses. Endometriosis is a familial disease, with the mothers, daughters, and sisters of patients more frequently affected than appropriate controls.[133] Recurrent disease may develop in older women who had endometriosis during their menses if they receive estrogen replacement therapy.

CLINICAL HISTORY

Implants in the rectovaginal septum, colon, and ureter are associated with low back pain that may radiate to the rectum or to the medial or posterior portions of the thighs. Radiation of pain correlates with innervation of the pelvic peritoneum by nerves from the lumbar and sacral spinal segments. The pain may be intermittent or persistent, but it characteristically increases at the time of menstruation and persists throughout the entire period of bleeding. Other symptoms associated with endometriosis include dysmenorrhea, dyspareunia, infertility, and menorrhagia. About 20% of patients may be asymptomatic. Endometriosis causes sciatica with invasion of the sciatic nerve. Laparoscopy reveals a "pocket sign" in these patients, or evagination of the pelvic peritoneum with endometriosis at its base on the sciatic nerve.[190] The stage of endometriosis is not correlated with the presence or severity of symptoms.[196] Pain starts just before the onset of bleeding and lasts 1 to 2 days after the bleeding has stopped. Secondary dysmenorrhea may be associated with pelvic inflammatory disease (PID) and pelvic neoplasms. Other symptoms of endometriosis may mimic gastrointestinal, urologic, or neurologic disorders.

Patients with endometriosis frequently experience dysmenorrhea. Painful menstruation and dysmenorrhea of all etiologies are the most common of all gynecologic complaints and are the leading causes of absenteeism of women from work. Dysmenorrhea may be primary or secondary. When primary, it is unassociated with any identifiable gynecologic disease. Secondary dysmenorrhea is caused by pelvic disease such as uterine malposition, cervical stenosis, salpingitis, or endometriosis. Painful menses occur in ovulatory cycles and are associated with nausea, vomiting, and diarrhea. Dysmenorrheic pain occurs in the pelvis, is crampy and correlated with uterine contractions, and is frequently referred to the low back region. In women with uterine retroversion, pain may be increased during menses; however, even those with normal uterine position may experience abdominal and back pain associated with their menses.

PHYSICAL EXAMINATION

Physical findings in patients with endometriosis are variable and depend on the location and size of the implants. Physical examination reveals uterine tenderness and enlargement. Ovarian tenderness and enlargement may also be discovered. The uterus may be fixed in a retroverted position. Endometriosis may lodge within surgical scars. Inguinal endometriosis may mimic the signs of an incarcerated hernia.[136]

DIFFERENTIAL DIAGNOSIS

The diagnosis of endometriosis is frequently made at the time of a pelvic operative procedure. Laparoscopy or laparotomy is essential to make an appropriate diagnosis because noninvasive tests are unreliable for making an accurate diagnosis of endometriosis. The diagnosis and extent of the disease in the pelvis can be adequately determined during laparoscopy or laparotomy.[133] MR imaging is useful in the identification of endometriosis in women with adnexal masses.[84] The sensitivity and specificity for identification by MR was 90% and 98%, respectively.[188] Endometriosis is frequently discovered in the pouch of Douglas, ureterosacral ligaments, ovaries, uterine surface, rectovaginal septum, fallopian tubes, bowel, or appendix. The urinary tract may be involved, as indicated by symptoms of obstruction. The intestinal tract also may be obstructed. Biopsy demonstrates endometrial glandular tissue. The most recently proposed classification system, from the work of the Brisbane series, is based on the severity and extent of disease (Table 17-3).[133] The American Society for Reproductive Medicine has a classification system for endometriosis that consists of four stages, with higher-numbered stages representing more extensive disease of reproductive structures. However, the classification scheme is limited in that it is designed to predict only the likelihood of future fertility.[154] The more advanced the stage of disease, the greater the chance for the patient to experience symptoms of pain and infertility. Cytologic examination of peritoneal washings and ultrasonography are inadequate to make an accurate diagnosis of endometriosis.[69,152]

TREATMENT

Therapy for endometriosis may consist of medications, including LHRH agonists (medical oophorectomy), oral contraceptives, danazol, and nonsteroidal anti-inflammatory drugs, pregnancy, and surgery to remove foci of abnormal implants and lyse adhesions.[133] Medications directed at endometriosis itself include danazol, which attenuates the midcycle surge of luteinizing hormone; progestational agents, which cause decidualization of endometrial tissue; and gonadotropin-releasing hormone (GnRH) agonists, which cause hypogonadotropic hypogonadism.[135] Many patients with primary dysmenorrhea obtain relief with the use of nonsteroidal anti-inflammatory drugs or oral contraceptives.[210] Therapies with GnRH activity and progestational agents have pain-relieving activity in endometriosis. The downside of medical therapy is the high recurrence rate after discontinuation and the risk of infertility. The need for oophorectomy in young women with endometriosis remains to be determined.[135] Prolonged LHRH treatment with low-dose estrogens may offer pain relief with little effect on bone mineral

17-3 BRISBANE SERIES CLASSIFICATION OF ENDOMETRIOSIS

Stage	Extent of Disease
0	Minimal disease, no hemorrhage
1	Minimal disease, hemorrhage, no adhesions
2	Progression with hemorrhage, adhesions
3	Progression to organ destruction, dense adhesions
4	Total loss of reproductive function, extensive organ destruction, dense adhesions, progression to "frozen pelvis"

density.[182] Danazol has been demonstrated to decrease pain even for an extended period after discontinuing the drug.[185] Infertility associated with endometriosis is treated exclusively by surgical elimination of disease and restoration of the anatomic integrity of the pelvis.

Pregnancy

Pregnant women complain of low back pain with increasing size of the gravid uterus. Low back pain may be secondary to increasing tension in the uterosacral ligaments or a marked increase in lumbar lordosis with concomitant muscle strain. Pain is experienced in the sacroiliac joints and the pubis and may radiate to the thighs. Low back pain in pregnancy may also be related to pelvic girdle relaxation. In the nonpregnant state, there is practically no motion in the joints of the pelvis, symphysis, and sacroiliac joints. During pregnancy, women produce a hormone, relaxin, that allows increased motion in the pelvic joints, and such motion causes tension in the relaxed capsule and ligaments. Pain develops about the sacroiliac joints, the symphysis pubis, and the medial part of the thighs. It is increased by active movement such as climbing stairs. Most patients have resolution of their symptoms postpartum. Rarely, they continue with symptoms of pelvic relaxation and require bracing or operative stabilization of joints to resolve their complaints.[73]

The frequency of back pain in pregnancy has been reported by Fast and associates. Whites had a statistically higher incidence of back pain than other groups did. Overall, 56% of mothers had pain. Pain radiated from the low back region to the lower extremities in 45% of patients. The pain usually started during the fifth to seventh month of pregnancy.[61] In another study, Svensson and associates reported back pain in 24% of the 1514 women who had been pregnant.[183]

Kristiansson and co-workers monitored 200 consecutive pregnant women for the development of low back pain.[94] Seventy-six percent reported back pain during the pregnancy, with 61% having the onset of pain during the current pregnancy. The prevalence rate increased to 48% until the 24th week. Postpartum pain occurred in 9.4%. The most common locations of pain were the sacrum (47%) and lumbar spine (35%). Thirty percent of pregnant women with back pain reported significant disability with activities of daily living, as well as time lost from work.[94]

Pain associated with hormone replacement therapy may develop in women who have been pregnant. In a study of 1324 postmenopausal women between 55 and 56 years of age, Bryhildsen and colleagues determined the prevalence of low back pain.[22] Low back pain occurred in 48.2% of hormone recipients versus 42% without replacement. The risk factor associated with the presence of low back pain was pregnancy.

Fallopian Tubes

The fallopian tubes are appendages of the uterus that convey ova from the ovary to the uterus. Problems that affect the fallopian tubes and cause back pain are PID and ectopic pregnancy.

Pelvic Inflammatory Disease

Epidemiology

The most common disorder that affects the fallopian tubes and is associated with low back pain is PID.[59] It is the most frequent gynecologic cause of emergency department visits, numbered at 350,000 per year.[45] PID will develop in about 1 million American women (1% of sexually active females). This group will experience ectopic pregnancy (5%), infertility (10%), pelvic pain (15%), and recurrent infection (25%).[58]

Pathophysiology

PID is a term for acute or chronic infection of the tubes and ovary. Bacteria, particularly *Neisseria gonorrhoeae*, gain access to the tube by direct spread from the endometrial lining or lymphatic dissemination. Other organisms causing infection include *Chlamydia trachomatis* (most common pathogen), *E. coli*, *Streptococcus viridans*, anaerobic cocci, and *Clostridium perfringens*. The infection may localize to the tube or spread to involve the ovary (tubo-ovarian abscess) or the pelvic peritoneum.

Clinical History

The chief clinical symptom of a patient with acute salpingitis is lower abdominal and pelvic pain, which may be unilateral or bilateral. Patients have a feeling of pelvic pressure and may have radiation of low back pain to the thighs. Nausea may also be present.

Physical Examination

Physical examination finds an acutely ill patient with or without fever, hypoactive bowel sounds, lower quadrant abdominal tenderness, purulent cervical discharge, and exquisite tenderness on movement of the pelvic organs during pelvic examination.

Laboratory Data

Laboratory examination of pelvic discharge may show pathogenic organisms on Gram stain and culture.

Differential Diagnosis

The diagnosis of PID should be considered in sexually active young women with the combination of lower abdominal, adnexal, and cervical motion pain.[31] No single laboratory test is specific for the diagnosis of PID. Tests with a negative predictive value include a normal peripheral WBC count, few WBCs in vaginal fluid, and a normal ESR.[145] A number of conditions must be considered during the evaluation of a patient with pelvic pain, including ectopic pregnancy, acute appendicitis, acute pyelonephritis, adnexal torsion, endometriosis, ovarian cysts, renal stones, myomas, and psychogenic pain syndromes.

Treatment

Therapy for acutely ill patients is hospitalization for intravenous antibiotics and bed rest in the semi-Fowler position.[6] In patients with mild to moderate PID, outpatient and inpatient antibiotic therapy has similar outcomes in regard to future pregnancy, recurrence rate, and ectopic pregnancy.[131]

PROGNOSIS

Repeated infections or inadequate treatment of acute salpingitis can result in recurrent episodes of pelvic infection or tubo-ovarian or pelvic abscess. Complications of these very serious infections include infertility, peritonitis, intra-abdominal abscesses, bowel obstruction, or septic emboli.

Ectopic Pregnancy

Ectopic pregnancy is a pregnancy that is implanted outside the uterine cavity. The most common site for ectopic pregnancy is the fallopian tube, which occurs in about 98% of cases.

EPIDEMIOLOGY

The number of hospitalizations for ectopic pregnancies in the United States in 1989 was 88,400.[54] The frequency is estimated to be 19 per 1000 pregnancies.[30] The frequency has increased as a consequence of the increasing frequency of PID.[31] The death rate is 1 in 1000 cases.[21] The major sources of disease and death with ectopic pregnancy are delay by patients in reporting early symptoms and delay by physicians in initiating appropriate treatment. One study showed delay in diagnosis in 50% or more of patients with ectopic pregnancy.[21] The problem for the examining physician is the fact that the symptoms of ectopic pregnancy mimic those of other abdominal and pelvic problems. Ectopic pregnancy should remain on the list of possible diagnoses in all women between menarche and menopause.

PATHOGENESIS

Patients with structural abnormalities of the fallopian tubes are at risk for an ectopic pregnancy. Chronic PID is a common cause of both problems. Ectopic pregnancies develop in approximately 5% of patients with PID. The chances for ectopic implantation are greater with increasing severity of salpingitis.[83] Distorted tubal anatomy may be associated with a ruptured appendix or endometriosis. Previous ectopic pregnancy or tubal surgery can increase the risk.[209] Patients who use an intrauterine device as contraception are also at greater risk for ectopic pregnancy because PID is a frequent result of its use.[24]

CLINICAL HISTORY

The first symptoms of ectopic pregnancy are a missed period, nausea, and breast tenderness. The classic triad of pain, irregular uterine bleeding, and an adnexal mass on physical examination is found in a minority of patients when seen in an emergency department setting.[179] Pain develops in the lower quadrant as rupture is imminent. As rupture occurs, blood collects in the inferior portion of the pelvis and abdomen. Pain in the sacral area may radiate to the thighs as the pelvic peritoneum is irritated. Nausea and vomiting may occur with rupture. A significant proportion of women may be asymptomatic before rupture.

PHYSICAL EXAMINATION

Physical examination reveals fever in less than 2% of patients.[21] The pulse rate is increased in patients hemorrhaging from a ruptured tubal pregnancy. Abdominal signs vary. Lower abdominal tenderness is common, with rebound tenderness and guarding occurring less often. Pelvic examination may be normal in a minority of patients. Usually, tenderness is present along with an adnexal mass in about half. A mass in the cul-de-sac, when present, is due to collection of blood in the area. A woman with a small, unruptured ectopic pregnancy may have no physical findings.

LABORATORY DATA

Anemia is found in a minority along with leukocytosis. The pregnancy test is positive in 82% of patients with the radioimmunoassay for beta-HCG.[10] A pregnancy may be detected by HCG assay or maternal serum by day 7.[72] Serum progesterone levels are higher in intrauterine than in ectopic pregnancies. A concentration less than 5 ng/mL is associated with a nonviable pregnancy.[115] However, the level of progesterone may vary among different populations, thus making the determination less reliable than beta-HCG to establish viability.[146] Culdocentesis is a valuable test for diagnosing rupture of an ectopic pregnancy. In a study of 300 surgically treated patients, culdocentesis revealed nonclotting blood in 95% of patients.[21]

RADIOGRAPHIC EVALUATION

Ultrasonography may help identify the location of the pregnancy.[100] The use of transvaginal ultrasonography is able to detect the presence of an adnexal mass that may be missed by transabdominal ultrasound (Fig. 17-14).[164] Ultrasound is most helpful in identifying normal intrauterine pregnancies. Ectopic pregnancies are imaged about 33% of the time.[25]

DIFFERENTIAL DIAGNOSIS

The differential diagnosis of ectopic pregnancy includes a wide range of disorders, including normal intrauterine pregnancy, ruptured corpus luteum cyst, acute appendicitis,

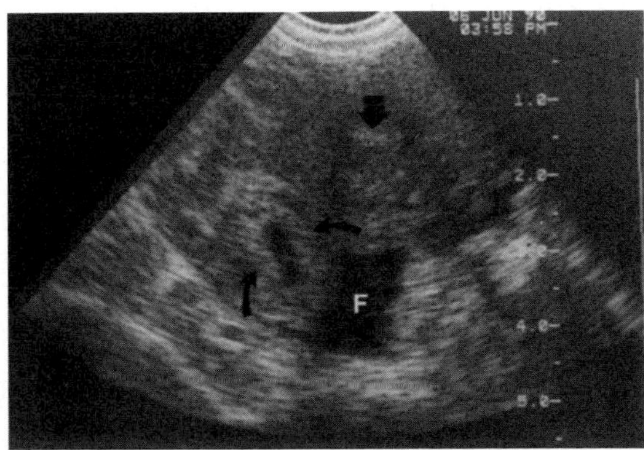

Figure 17-14 Transvaginal sonogram of a right tubal ectopic pregnancy. The uterine cavity *(large arrow)* is empty. An echogenic ringlike structure present in the right adnexa *(curved arrows)* represents the ectopic gestational sac. A small amount of fluid (F) is present in the cul-de-sac. *(Courtesy of Michael Hill, MD.)*

salpingitis, acute pyelonephritis, degenerating fibroid, and incomplete abortion. A careful history, along with pregnancy tests, may help differentiate the nonpregnant from the pregnant state. Women who have undergone in vitro fertilization are at increased risk for ectopic pregnancies.

TREATMENT

Treatment of ectopic pregnancy has evolved over the past 7 years to include medical and surgical therapies.[77] Early ectopic pregnancies may resolve spontaneously at a rate of 75% to 83%.[102] These patients are asymptomatic and have falling HCG levels. Methotrexate, 1 mg/kg intramuscularly, with leukovorin rescue, 0.1 mg/kg, has had a 96% success rate in resolving pregnancies with minimal toxicity. This therapy works best when HCG levels are less than 10,000 mU/mL.[180] In a study of 350 women treated with a single dose of methotrexate, the mean concentration of HCG was significantly lower in women with successful therapy than in those who failed (4019 versus 13,420 mIU/mL).[106] Methotrexate may also be given intravenously and locally by laparoscopic placement.[62] Surgical intervention in the form of laparoscopy has been associated with preservation of fertility. This procedure is less costly than laparotomy and has equally good results.[211] Surgery is indicated for a ruptured ectopic pregnancy with hemodynamic instability or an inability to institute medical therapy. Also to be considered are an HCG level greater than 5000 mIU/mL and tubal size greater than 3 cm. At the time of laparoscopy, the diagnosis can be made and the appropriate fallopian tube can be preserved if at all feasible. The ovary is spared unless it is involved by an extensive hematoma arising from the tube. Medical therapy may offer a more cost-effective approach but requires a longer post-treatment monitoring period.[74]

Ovary

The ovaries have great potential for producing an unusual number of neoplasms of both epithelial and connective tissue origin. Although ovarian neoplasms may occur at any age, they are most common during the reproductive years. Benign tumors occur most frequently during the years of ovulation (30 to 40 years of age), whereas malignant tumors occur after ovulation has ceased (50 years and older).

Benign Tumors

Benign tumors of the ovary encompass a wide range of lesions that may include functional cysts (corpus luteum cysts) and new growths (serous cystadenoma, granulosa cell tumor, or dermal cyst). Functional cysts occur at times of pregnancy or ineffective ovulation. These growths are associated with symptoms if they grow to a large size or are complicated by torsion, rupture, or hemorrhage. Of the benign tumors, serous cystadenoma and mucinous cystadenoma are the most common, and they constitute 25% of all benign tumors.[48]

CLINICAL HISTORY

Back pain associated with benign ovarian tumors is rare. When back pain occurs, it is localized to the sacrum. The pain has a quality of pressure and aching. Most benign tumors are asymptomatic until they reach a large size. The symptoms that these tumors cause are frequently related to pressure on neighboring structures (ureters, colon, veins, or lymphatics). Pain from benign lesions may be referred to the iliac or inguinal areas, the inner aspect of the upper part of the thigh, or the vulva. A sudden change in symptoms may occur with hemorrhage, torsion, or rupture of a cyst. These complications of benign tumors result in abdominal symptoms.

PHYSICAL EXAMINATION

Physical examination reveals a unilateral, freely movable, smooth mass. Ascites may be present. The uterus may be displaced if the tumor is large. Careful pelvic examination should be able to identify the location of the mass in relation to the ovary. Lesions of the colon, bladder, uterus, and fallopian tube must be differentiated. Ultrasonography does not replace the pelvic examination for determining the site of a lesion, but it may discriminate between uterine and adnexal masses and distinguish cystic from solid tumors (Fig. 17-15).[132]

TREATMENT

Management of ovarian neoplasms may be medical for functional growths and surgical for benign tumors. For functional cysts, a course of oral contraceptives can accelerate involution of non-neoplastic ovarian enlargement. In one study, 72% of patients had resolution of ovarian enlargement after a 6-week trial of therapy.[171] Benign tumors larger than 5 cm and those that do not respond to hormonal therapy require an exploratory operation. The extent of surgery depends on the findings at surgery, including the type of tumor and extent of the lesion. Benign tumors are usually removed. Removal of the opposite ovary and uterus depends on the age of the patient and the potential for development of the same lesion in the remaining tissue.

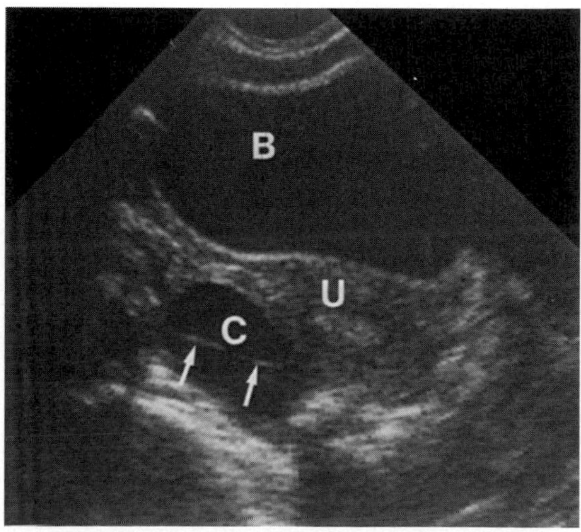

Figure 17-15 Ultrasound. Transverse section through the pelvis revealing a right ovarian cyst (C) that is septated *(arrows)*. B, Bladder; U, uterus. *(Courtesy of Michael Hill, MD.)*

Malignant Tumors

EPIDEMIOLOGY

Carcinoma of the ovary causes 6% of all cancer deaths in women in the United States. The annual incidence of cases is 22,000.[16] It is the most common cause of death among gynecologic cancers.[155] An estimated 14,000 women will die yearly of ovarian cancer.[82] Women who are nulliparous and have a family history of ovarian cancer have an increased risk. The most important risk factor is heredity, having two first-degree relatives with the tumor.[109]

CLINICAL HISTORY

Like benign tumors, malignant tumors may be asymptomatic until the tumor reaches a large size. Abdominal distention and pain are very common complaints. Back pain occurs rarely. The pain may have an aching quality, with radiation from the paraspinous area and sacrum to the thighs. The pain may occur when the blood supply to the ovary is compromised. Back pain may also develop by direct extension of the tumor or spread through the lymphatics.[86]

PHYSICAL EXAMINATION

Physical examination, including pelvic examination, is very revealing, particularly in a postmenopausal patient. The ovaries are not usually palpable in postmenopausal women. Palpable ovaries in this group of women require additional evaluation. Cul-de-sac nodularity may be secondary to metastatic disease. Examination of the inguinal and supraclavicular nodes may detect the spread of an unsuspected malignant ovarian tumor.

RADIOGRAPHIC EVALUATION

Transvaginal ultrasonography is more sensitive than CT for imaging the ovary and is predictive in detecting the presence of cancer.[195] This technique is able to differentiate simple cysts from complex cysts associated with malignancies. Doppler evaluation of blood flow in addition to ultrasonography can detect malignant tumor blood flow.[90]

DIFFERENTIAL DIAGNOSIS

Once an ovarian tumor is suspected, surgical staging is necessary for diagnosis and determination of the extent of disease. Areas of lymph drainage (iliac and para-aortic nodes) must be sampled along with the cul-de-sac, the abdominal gutters, and the diaphragm.[23] Determination of glycoprotein markers for ovarian cancer, CA 125 and DF 3, is useful for monitoring the response to treatment and detecting early disease.[12] The CA 125 test is more useful for monitoring patients in whom an ovarian tumor has been diagnosed than for detecting the presence of an ovarian neoplasm. Elevated levels may be detected with other neoplasms and with other gynecologic conditions such as endometriosis and pregnancy.[26]

TREATMENT

Therapy for early-stage disease (I and II—limited to the ovary or true pelvis, respectively) is surgical. Disease with extension beyond the pelvis (III) and distant metastases (IV) requires chemotherapy. The benefit of therapy with a single drug versus combination therapy remains to be determined.[142,204] Current chemotherapy that includes platinum has improved response rates and prolonged median survival. Therapy for advanced disease includes cyclophosphamide, doxorubicin, and cisplatin.[1] Paclitaxel (Taxol), a diterpene plant product isolated from the bark of the Pacific yew tree, has been effective as an adjunct to platinum in patients resistant to platinum and cyclophosphamide chemotherapy.[26] This therapy has efficacy for ovarian cancer patients with stage III and IV disease.[129]

References

Genitourinary Diseases

1. Aabo K, Adams M, Adnitt P, et al: Chemotherapy in advanced ovarian cancer: Four systematic meta-analyses of individual patient data from 37 randomized trials. Advanced Ovarian Cancer Trialist' Group. Br J Cancer 78:1479-1487, 1998.
2. Ahmed S, Smith AJ: Results of ureteral reimplantation in patients with intrarenal reflux. J Urol 120:332, 1978.
3. Amar AD: Vesiculoureteral reflux in adults: A 12 year study of 122 patients. Urology 3:184, 1974.
4. Anderson EE: The management of ureteral calculi. Urol Clin North Am 1:357, 1974.
5. Andriole GL, Catalona WJ: Early diagnosis of prostate cancer. Urol Clin North Am 14:657, 1987.
6. Ansbacher R: Recognition and treatment of pelvic inflammatory disease. Mod Med 55:79, 1987.
7. Babian RJ, Johnson DE: Primary carcinoma of the ureter. J Urol 123:357, 1980.
8. Baker LR, Mallinson WJ, Gregory MC, et al: Idiopathic retroperitoneal fibrosis: A retrospective analysis of 60 cases. Br J Urol 60:497, 1987.
9. Bakshandeh K, Lynne C, Carrion H: Vesicoureteral reflux and end stage renal disease. J Urol 116:557, 1976.
10. Barnes RB, Roy S, Yee B, et al: Reliability of urinary pregnancy tests in the diagnosis of ectopic pregnancy. J Reprod Med 30:827, 1985.
11. Barzel W, Bean MA, Hilaris BS, Whitmore WF Jr: Prostatic adenocarcinoma: Relationship of grade and local extent to the pattern of metastases. J Urol 118:278, 1977.
12. Bast RC Jr, Knapp RC: Immunologic approaches to the management of ovarian carcinoma. Semin Oncol 11:264, 1984.
13. Berger L, Sinkoff MW: Systemic manifestations of hypernephroma: A review of 273 cases. Am J Med 22:791, 1957.
14. Bihl G, Meyers A: Recurrent renal stone disease—advances in pathogenesis and clinical mangement. Lancet 358:651-656, 2001.
15. Blum U, Billman P, Krause T, et al: Effect of local low-dose thrombolysis on clinical outcome in patients with acute embolic renal artery occlusion. Radiology 189:549-554, 1993.
16. Boring CC, Squires TS, Tong T: Cancer statistics, 1993. CA Cancer J Clin 43:7, 1993.
17. Boumpas DT, Austin HA 3rd, Vaughn EM, et al: Controlled trial of pulse methylprednisolone versus two regimens of pulse cyclophosphamide in severe lupus nephritis. Lancet 340:741-745, 1992.
18. Brannen GF, Bush WH, Correa RJ, et al: Kidney stone removal, percutaneous versus surgical lithotomy. J Urol 133:6, 1985.
19. Brennan RE, Curtis JA, Kurtz AB, Dalton JR: Use of tomography and ultrasound in the diagnosis of non-opaque renal calculi. JAMA 244:594, 1980.
20. Brenner BM, Rector FC Jr (eds): The Kidney, 3rd ed. Philadelphia, WB Saunders, 1986.
21. Brenner PF, Roy S, Mishell DR Jr: Ectopic pregnancy. A study of 300 consecutive surgically treated cases. JAMA 243:673, 1980.
22. Brynhildsen JO, Bjors E, Skarsgard C, et al: Is hormone replacement therapy a risk factor for low back pain among postmenopausal women? Spine 23:809-813, 1998.
23. Buchsbaum HJ, Lifshitz S: Staging and surgical evaluation of ovarian cancer. Semin Oncol 11:227, 1984.
24. Burkman RT: Association between intrauterine device and pelvic inflammatory disease. The Women's Health Study. Obstet Gynecol 57:269, 1981.
25. Cacciatore B: Can the status of tubal pregnancy be predicted with transvaginal sonography? A prospective comparison of sonographic, surgical, and serum hCG findings. Radiology 177:481-484, 1990.

26. Cannistra SA: Cancer of the ovary. N Engl J Med 329:1550, 1993.
27. Cantwell BMJ, Mann KA, Harris AL: Back pain—a presentation of metastatic testicular germ cell tumors. Lancet 1:262, 1987.
28. Catalano O, Nunziata A, Altei F, et al: Suspected ureteral colic: Primary helical CT versus selective helical CT after unenhanced radiography and sonography. AJR Am J Roentgenol 178:379-387, 2002.
29. Catalona WJ, Smith DS, Ratliff TL, et al: Measurement of prostate-specific antigen in serum as a screening test for prostate cancer. N Engl J Med 324:1156, 1991.
30. Centers for Disease Control and Prevention: Ectopic pregnancy—United States, 1990-1992. MMWR Morb Mortal Wkly Rep 44:46, 1995.
31. Centers for Disease Control and Prevention: Sexually transmitted diseases treatment guidelines 2002. MMWR Recomm Rep 51(RR-6):1, 2002.
32. Chaussy C, Schuller J, Schmiedt E, et al: Extracorporeal shock-wave lithotripsy (ESWL) for treatment of urolithiasis. Urology 23:59, 1984.
33. Chisholm GD, Roy RR: The systemic effects of malignant renal tumor. Br J Urol 43:687, 1971.
34. Clayman R: Techniques in percutaneous removal of renal calculi: Mechanical extraction and electrohydraulic lithotripsy. Urology 25:11, 1984.
35. Collins MM, Stafford RS, O'Leary MP, et al: How common is prostatitis? A national survey of physician visits. J Urol 159:1224-1228, 1998.
36. Consensus Conference: The management of clinically localized prostate cancer. JAMA 258:2727, 1987.
37. Covington T Jr, Reeser W: Hydronephrosis associated with overhydration. J Urol 63:438, 1950.
38. Cox CE, Lacy SS, Hinman F Jr: The urethra and its relationships to urinary tract infections. II. The urethral flora of the female with recurrent urinary infection. J Urol 99:632, 1968.
39. Crawford ED, Schutz MJ, Clejan S, et al: The effect of digital rectal examination on prostate-specific antigen levels. JAMA 267:2227-2228, 1992.
40. Crawford ED, Eisenberger MA, McLeod DG, et al: A controlled trial of leuprolide with and without flutamide in prostatic carcinoma. N Engl J Med 321:419, 1989.
41. Crawhall JC, Scowen EF, Watts RWE: Effect of penicillamine on cystinuria. BMJ 1:588, 1963.
42. Curhan GC, Willett WC, Rimm EB, et al: Family history and risk of kidney stones. J Am Soc Nephrol 8:1568-1573, 1997.
43. Curhan GC, Willett WC, Rimm EB, et al: Beverage use and risk for kidney stones in women. Ann Intern Med 128:535-540, 1998.
44. Curry NS: Small renal masses (lesions smaller than 3 cm): Imaging evaluation and management. AJR Am J Roentgenol 164:355-362, 1995.
45. Curtis KM, Hillis SD, Kieke BA, et al: Visits to emergency departments for gynecologic disorders in the United States, 1992-1994. Obstet Gynecol 91:1007-1012, 1998.
46. D'Amico AV, Schnall M, Whittington R, et al: Endorectal coil magnetic resonance imaging identifies locally advanced prostate cancer in select patients with clinically localized disease. Urology 51:449-454, 1998.
47. D'Amico AV, Whittington R, Malkowicz SB, et al: Biochemical outcome after radical prostatectomy, external beam radiation therapy, or interstitial radiation therapy for clinically localized prostate cancer. JAMA 280:969-974, 1998.
48. Danforth DN, Scot JR, DiSaia PJ, et al (eds): Obstetrics and Gynecology. Philadelphia, JB Lippincott, 1986.
49. Domanovits H, Paulis M, Nikfardjam M, et al: Acute renal infarction. Clinical characteristics of 17 patients. Medicine (Baltimore) 78:386-394, 1999.
50. Dorr VJ, Williamson SK, Stephens RL: An evaluation of prostate-specific antigen as a screening test for prostate cancer. Arch Intern Med 153:2529, 1993.
51. Dou Q, Zhao Y, Tarnuzzer RW, et al: Suppression of transforming growth factor-β (TGF-β) and TGF-β receptor messenger ribonucleic acid and protein expression in leiomyomata in women receiving gonadotropin-releasing hormone agonist therapy. J Clin Endocrinol Metab 81:3222-3230, 1996.
52. Drach GW: Prostatitis and prostatodynia: Their relationship to benign prostatic hypertrophy. Urol Clin North Am 7:79, 1980.
53. Drach GW: Stone manipulation. Urology 12:286, 1978.
54. Ectopic pregnancy—United States. MMWR Morb Mortal Wkly Rep 41:591, 1992.
55. Elder JS, Catalona WJ: Management of newly diagnosed metastatic carcinoma of the prostate. Urol Clin North Am 11:283, 1984.
56. Elliot JS: Urinary calculus disease. Surg Clin North Am 45:1393, 1965.
57. Elton TJ, Roth CS, Berquist TH, et al: A clinical prediction rule for the diagnosis of ureteral calculi in emergency departments. J Gen Intern Med 8:57-62, 1993.
58. Eschenbach DA: Acute pelvic inflammatory disease. Urol Clin North Am 11:65, 1984.
59. Eschenbach DA, Holmes KK: Acute pelvic inflammatory disease: Current concepts of pathogenesis, etiology, and management. Clin Obstet Gynecol 18:35, 1975.
60. Fang LST, Tolkoff-Rubin NE, Rubin RH: Efficacy of single-dose and conventional amoxicillin therapy in urinary tract infection localized by the antibody-coated bacteria technic. N Engl J Med 298:413, 1978.
61. Fast A, Shapiro D, Docommun EJ, et al: Low-back pain in pregnancy. Spine 12:368, 1987.
62. Fernandez H, Yves Vincent SC, Pauthier S, et al: Randomized trial of conservative laparoscopic treatment and methotrexate administration in ectopic pregnancy and subsequent fertility. Hum Reprod 13:3239-3243, 1998.
63. Flanigan RC, Salmon SE, Blumenstein BA, et al: Nephrectomy followed by interferon alfa-2b compared with interferon alfa-2b alone for metastatic renal-cell cancer. N Engl J Med 345:1655-159, 2001.
64. Garnick MB, Canellos GP, Richie JP: Treatment and surgical staging of testicular and primary extragonadal germ cell cancer. JAMA 250:1733, 1983.
65. Gibbons RP, Montie JE, Correa RJ Jr, Mason JT: Manifestations of renal cell carcinoma. Urology 8:201, 1976.
66. Gibson SM, Kimmel PL: Genitourinary disease affecting the spine. Semin Spine Surg 2:145, 1990.
67. Gleason DF: The Veterans Administration Cooperative Urological Research Group: Histologic grading and clinical staging of prostatic carcinoma. In Tannenbaum M (ed): Urologic Pathology. The Prostate. Philadelphia, Lea & Febiger, 1977, p 171.
68. Gleckman R, Crowley M, Natsios GA: Therapy of recurrent invasive urinary-tract infection of men. N Engl J Med 301:878, 1979.
69. Goldman SM, Minkin SI: Diagnosing endometriosis with ultrasound: Accuracy and specificity. J Reprod Med 25:178, 1980.
70. Guillevin L, Cohen P, Gayraud M, et al: Churg-Strauss syndrome. Medicine (Baltimore) 78:26-37, 1999.
71. Guzick DS: Clinical epidemiology of endometriosis and infertility. Obstet Gynecol Clin North Am 16:43, 1989.
72. Haas M, Meehan SM, Karrison TG, et al: Changing etiologies of unexplained adult nephritic syndrome: A comparison of renal biopsy findings from 1976-1979 and 1995-1997. Am J Kidney Dis 30:621-631, 1997.
73. Hagen R: Pelvic girdle relaxation from an orthopaedic point of view. Acta Orthop Scand 45:550, 1974.
74. Hajenius PJ, Engelsbel S, Mol BW, et al: Randomized trial of systemic methotrexate versus laparoscopic salpingostomy in tubal pregnancy. Lancet 350:774-779, 1997.
75. Harada T, Iwabe T, Terakawa N: Role of cytokines in endometriosis. Fertil Steril 76:1-10, 2001.
76. Harrington TM, Bunch TW, Van Den Berg CJ: Renal tubular acidosis: A new look at treatment of musculoskeletal and renal disease. Mayo Clin Proc 58:354, 1983.
77. Helsa JS, Rock JA: Emergent management of ectopic pregnancy. Infertil Reprod Med Clin North Am 3:775, 1992.
78. Hooton TM, Stamm WE: Diagnosis and treatment of uncomplicated urinary tract infection. Infect Dis Clin North Am 11:551-581, 1997.
79. Hricak H, Dooms GC, Jeffrey RB, et al: Prostatic carcinoma: Staging by clinical assessment, CT, and MR imaging. Radiology 162:331, 1987.
80. Hricak H, Thoeni RF, Carroll PR, et al: Detection and staging of renal neoplasms: A reassessment of MR imaging. Radiology 166:643, 1988.
81. Hurwitz SR, Kessler WO, Alazraki NP, Ashburn WL: Gallium-67 imaging to localize urinary-tract infections. Br J Radiol 49:156, 1976.

82. Jemal A, Thomas A, Murray T, et al: Cancer statistics, 2002. CA Cancer J Clin 52:23-47, 2002.
83. Joesoef MR, Westrom L, Reynolds G, et al: Recurrence of ectopic pregnancy: The role of salpingitis. Am J Obstet Gynecol 165:46, 1991.
84. Johnson IR, Symonds EM, Worthington BS, et al: Imaging ovarian tumors by nuclear magnetic resonance. Br J Obstet Gynecol 91:260, 1984.
85. Johnson CM, Wilson DM, O'Fallan WM, et al: Renal stone epidemiology: A 24-year study in Rochester, Minnesota. Kidney Int 16:624, 1979.
86. Julian CG, Goss J, Blanchard K, Woodruff JD: Biologic behavior of primary ovarian malignancy. Obstet Gynecol 44:873, 1974.
87. Kass LG, Woyke S, Schreiber K, et al: Thin-needle aspiration biopsy of the prostate. Urol Clin North Am 11:237, 1984.
88. Kaye D, Santoro J: Urinary tract infection. In Mandell GL, Douglas RG Jr, Bennett JE (eds): Principles and Practice of Infectious Disease. New York, John Wiley & Sons, 1979, p 537.
89. Kaye AD, Pollack HM: Diagnostic imaging approach to the patient with obstructive uropathy. Semin Nephrol 2:55, 1982.
90. Kinkel K, Hricak H, Lu Y, et al: US characterization of ovarian masses: A meta-analysis. Radiology 217:803-811, 2000.
91. Klein LA: Prostatic carcinoma. N Engl J Med 300:824, 1979.
92. Kramer BS, Brown ML, Prorok PC, et al: Prostate cancer screening: What we know and what we need to know. Ann Intern Med 119:914, 1993.
93. Krieger JN, Nyberg L Jr, Nickel JC: NIH consensus definition and classification of prostatitis. JAMA 282:236-237, 1999.
94. Kristiansson P, Svardsudd K, von Schoultz B: Back pain during pregnancy: A prospective study. Spine 21:702-709, 1996.
95. Kronmal RA, Krieger JN, Coxon V, et al: Vasectomy is associated with an increased risk of urolithiasis. Am J Kidney Dis 29:207-213, 1997.
96. Labrie F, Dupont A, Belanger A: Complete androgen blockade for the treatment of prostate cancer. In Devita VT Jr, Hellman S, Rosenberg SA (eds): Important Advances in Oncology, 1985. Philadelphia, JB Lippincott, 1984, p 193.
97. Lam KK, Lui CC: Successful treatment of acute inferior vena cava and unilateral renal vein thrombosis by local infusion of recombinant tissue plasminogen activator. Am J Kidney Dis 32:1075-1079, 1998.
98. Lange PH, Ercole CJ, Lightner DJ, et al: The value of serum prostate-specific antigen determinations before and after radical prostatectomy. J Urol 141:873, 1989.
99. Lange PH, McIntire KR, Waldmann TA, et al: Serum alpha fetoprotein and human chorionic gonadotropin in the diagnosis and management of nonseminomatous germ-cell testicular cancer. N Engl J Med 295:1237, 1976.
100. Lawson TL: Ectopic pregnancy: Criteria and accuracy of ultrasonic diagnosis. AJR Am J Roentgenol 131:153, 1978.
101. Latham RH, Wong ES, Larson A, et al: Laboratory diagnosis of urinary tract infection in ambulatory women. JAMA 254:3333, 1985.
102. Leach RE, Ory SJ: Modern management of ectopic pregnancy. J Reprod Med 34:324, 1989.
103. Lebovic DI, Mueller MD, Taylor RN: Immunobiology of endometriosis. Fertil Steril 75:1-10, 2001.
104. Lee CT, Katz J, Shi W, et al: Surgical management of renal tumors 4 cm. Or less in a contemporary cohort. J Urol 163:730-736, 2000.
105. Lee F, Torp-Pedersen ST, Siders DB, et al: Transrectal ultrasound in the diagnosis and staging of prostatic carcinoma. Radiology 170:609, 1989.
106. Lipscomb GH, McCord ML, Stovall TG, et al: Predictors of success of methotrexate treatment in women with tubal ectopic pregnancies. N Engl J Med 341:1974-1978, 1999.
107. Lipsky BA: Urinary tract infections in men: Epidemiology, pathophysiology, diagnosis, and treatment. Ann Intern Med 110:138, 1989.
108. Lu PY, Ory SJ: Endometriosis: Current management. Mayo Clin Proc 70:453-463, 1995.
109. Lynch HT, Lynch JF: Hereditary ovarian carcinoma. Hematol Oncol Clin North Am 6:783, 1992.
110. Macari M, Bosniak MA: Delayed CT to evaluate renal masses incidentally discovered at contrast-enhanced CT: Demonstration of vascularity with deenhancement. Radiology 213:674-680, 1999.
111. Maddern JP: Surgery of the staghorn calculus. Br J Urol 39:237, 1967.
112. Madore F, Stampfer MJ, Willett WC, et al: Nephrolithiasis and risk of hypertension in women. Am J Kidney Dis 32:802-807, 1998.
113. Marth D, Scheidegger J, Studer UE: Ultrasonography of testicular tumors. Urol Int 45:237-40, 1990.
114. Martinez-Maldonado M, Kumjian DA: Acute renal failure due to urinary tract obstruction. Med Clin North Am 74:919, 1990.
115. McCord ML, Muram D, Buster JE, et al: Single serum progesterone as screen for ectopic pregnancy: Exchanging specificity and sensitivity to obtain optimal test performance. Fertil Steril 66:513-516, 1996.
116. McCullough DL, Prout GR Jr, Daly JJ: Carcinoma of the prostate and lymphatic metastases. J Urol 111:65, 1974.
117. McCullough DL: Diagnosis and staging of prostatic cancer. In Skinner DG, de Kemion JB (eds): Genitourinary Cancer. Philadelphia, WB Saunders, 1978, p 295.
118. McIntire TL, Murphy WM, Coon JS, et al: The prognostic value of DNA ploidy combined with histologic substaging for incidental carcinoma of the prostate gland. Am J Clin Pathol 89:139, 1988.
119. Meares EM, Stamey TA: Bacteriologic localization patterns in bacterial prostatitis and urethritis. Invest Urol 5:492-518, 1968.
120. Meares EM Jr: Acute and chronic prostatitis: Diagnosis and treatment. Infect Dis Clin North Am 1:855, 1987.
121. Meares EM Jr: Prostatitis syndromes: New perspectives about old woes. J Urol 123:141, 1980.
122. Meng MV, Mario LA, McAninch JW: Current treatment and outcomes of perinephric abscesses. J Urol 168:1337-1340, 2002.
123. Miller OF, Kane CJ: Time to stone passage for observed ureteral calculi: A guide for patient education. J Urol 162:688-690, 1999.
124. Moller P, Vinje O, Fryjordet A: HLA antigens and sacroiliitis in chronic prostatitis. Scand J Rheumatol 9:138, 1980.
125. Mombelli G, Pezzoli R, Pinoja-Lutz G, et al: Oral vs intravenous ciprofloxacin in the initial empirical management of severe pyelonephritis or complicated urinary tract infections: A prospective randomized clinical trial. Arch Intern Med 159:53-58, 1999.
126. Mostofi FK: Pathology and spread of renal cell carcinoma. In King JS Jr (ed): Renal Neoplasia. Boston, Little, Brown, 1967, p 41.
127. Motzer RJ, Russo P: Systemic therapy for renal cell carcinoma. J Urol 163:408-417, 2000.
128. Motzer RJ, Sheinfeld J, Mazumdar M, et al: Etoposide and cisplatin adjuvant therapy for patients with pathologic stage II germ cell tumors. J Clin Oncol 13:2700-2704, 1995.
129. Muggia FM, Braly PS, Brady MF, et al: Phase III randomized study of cisplatin versus paclitaxel versus cisplatin and paclitaxel in patients with suboptimal stage III or IV ovarian cancer: A gynecologic oncology groups study. J Clin Oncol 18:106-115, 2000.
130. Narayan P, Lange PH: Current controversies in the management of carcinoma of the prostate. Semin Oncol 7:460, 1960.
131. Ness RB, Soper DE, Holley RL, et al: Effectiveness of inpatient and outpatient treatment strategies for women with pelvic inflammatory disease: Results from the Pelvic Inflammatory Disease Evaluation and Clinical Health (PEACH) Randomized Trial. Am J Obstet Gynecol 186:929-937, 2002.
132. O'Brien WS, Buck DR, Nash JD: Evaluation of sonography in the initial assessment of the gynecological patient. Am J Obstet Gynecol 149:598, 1984.
133. O'Connor DT: Endometriosis. New York, Churchill Livingstone, 1987.
134. O'Keefe SC, Marshall FF, Issa MM, et al: Thrombocytosis is associated with a significant increase in the cancer specific death rate after radical nephrectomy. J Urol 168:1378-1380, 2002.
135. Olive DL, Pritts EA: Treatment of endometriosis. N Engl J Med 345:266-275, 2001.
136. Olive DL, Schwartz LB: Endometriosis. N Engl J Med 328:1759, 1993.
137. Orth SR, Ritz E: The nephritic syndrome. N Engl J Med 338:1202-1211, 1998.
138. Otto G, Braconier J, Andreasson A, et al: Interleukin-6 and disease severity in patients with bacteremic and nonbacteremic febrile urinary tract infection. J Infect Dis 179:172-179, 1999.
139. Pak CYC, Peters P, Hurt G, et al: Is selective therapy of recurrent nephrolithiasis possible? Am J Med 71:615, 1981.
140. Pantuck AJ, Zisman A, Belldegrun AS: The changing natural history of renal cell carcinoma. J Urol 166:1611-1623, 2001.

141. Parfrey PS, Bear JC, Morgan J, et al: The diagnosis and prognosis of autosomal dominant polycystic kidney disease. N Engl J Med 323:1085-1090, 1990.
142. Parker LM, Griffiths CT, Yankee RA, et al: Combination chemotherapy with Adriamycin-cyclophosphamide for advanced ovarian carcinoma. Cancer 46:669, 1980.
143. Paulson DF, Einhorn L, Peckham M, Williams SD: Cancer of the testis. In De Vita VT, Hellman S, Rosenberg SA (eds): Cancer: Principles and Practice of Oncology. Philadelphia, JB Lippincott, 1982, pp 786-822.
144. Peeling WB: Phase III studies to compare goserelin (Zoladex) with orchiectomy and with diethylstilbestrol in treatment of prostatic carcinoma. Urology 33(5 suppl):45, 1989.
145. Peipert JF, Boardman L, Hogan J, et al: Laboratory evaluation of acute upper genital tract infection. Obstet Gynecol 87:730-736, 1996.
146. Perkins SL, Al-Ramahi M, Claman P: Comparison of serum progesterone as an indicator of pregnancy nonviability in spontaneously pregnant emergency room and infertility clinic patient populations. Fertil Steril 73:499-504, 2000.
147. Perlberg S, Pfau A: Management of ureteropelvic junction obstruction associated with lower polar vessels. Urology 23:13, 1984.
148. Piccirillo M, Rigsby C, Rosenfield AT: Contemporary imaging of renal inflammatory disease. Infect Dis Clin North Am 1:927, 1987.
149. Pinals RS, Krane SK: Medical aspects of renal carcinoma. Postgrad Med J 38:507, 1982.
150. Pinson AG, Philbrick JT, Lindbeck GH, et al: Fever in the clinical diagnosis of acute pyelonephritis. Am J Emerg Med 15:148-151, 1997.
151. Potts JM: Prospective identification of National Institutes of Health category IV prostatitis in men with elevated prostate-specific antigen. J Urol 164:1550-1553, 2000.
152. Protuondo JA, Herran C, Echanojaurgei AD, Riego AG: Peritoneal flushing and biopsy in laparoscopically diagnosed endometriosis. Fertil Steril 38:538, 1982.
153. Recurrent renal calculi [Editorial]. BMJ 282:5, 1981.
154. Revised American Society for Reproductive Medicine classification of endometriosis: 1996. Fertil Steril 67:817-821, 1997.
155. Richardson GS, Scully RE, Nikrui N, Nelson JH Jr: Common epithelial cancer of the ovary. N Engl J Med 312:415, 474, 1985.
156. Richie JP, Garnick MB, Seltzer S, Bettmann MA: Computerized tomography scan for diagnosis and staging of renal cell carcinoma. J Urol 129:114, 1983.
157. Risholm L: Studies on renal colic and its treatment by posterior splanchnic block. Acta Chir Scand Suppl 184:1, 1954.
158. Robson CJ, Churchill BM, Anderson W: The results of radical nephrectomy for renal cell carcinoma. Trans Am Assoc Genitourin Surg 60:122, 1968.
159. Rubin RH, Fang LST, Jones SR, et al: Multicenter trial of single dose amoxicillin therapy of acute, uncomplicated urinary tract infection localized by the antibody-coated technique. JAMA 244:561, 1980.
160. Rudy DC, Seigel RS, Parker TW, Woodside JR: Segmental renal artery emboli treated with low-dose intra-arterial streptokinase. Urology 19:410, 1982.
161. Sanford JP: Urinary tract symptoms and infections. Annu Rev Med 26:485, 1975.
162. Sangi-Haaghpeykar H, Poindexter AN 3rd: Epidemiology of endometriosis among parous women. Obstet Gynecol 85:983-992, 1995.
163. Segura JW: The role of percutaneous surgery in renal and ureteral stone removal. J Urol 141:780, 1989.
164. Shapiro BS, Cullen M, Taylor KJ, DeCherney AH: Transvaginal ultrasound for the diagnosis of ectopic pregnancy. Fertil Steril 50:425, 1988.
165. Sidhom OA, Basalaev M, Sigal LH: Renal cell carcinoma presenting as polymyalgia rheumatica. Resolution after nephrectomy. Arch Intern Med 153:2043-2045, 1993.
166. Silverman DE, Stamey TA: Management of infection stones: The Stanford experience. Medicine (Baltimore) 62:44, 1983.
167. Skinner DG, Colvin RB, Vermillion CD, et al: Diagnosis and management of renal cell carcinoma. A clinical and pathologic study of 309 cases. Cancer 28:1165, 1971.
168. Smith DB, Newlands ES, Rustin GJ, et al: Lumbar pain in stage 1 testicular germ cell tumors: A symptom preceding radiological abnormality. Br J Urol 64:302, 1989.
169. Smith DR: Vesiculoureteral reflux and other abnormalities of the ureterovesical junction. In Campbell MF, Harrison JH (eds): Urology, 4th ed. Philadelphia, WB Saunders, 1978.
170. Smith JW, Jones SR, Reed WP, et al: Recurrent urinary tract infections in men—characteristics and response to therapy. Ann Intern Med 92:544, 1979.
171. Spanos WJ: Preoperative hormonal therapy of cystic adrenal masses. Am J Obstet Gynecol 116:551, 1973.
172. Spirnak JP, Resnick MI: Urinary stones. In Tanagho EA, McAninch JW (eds): General Urology, 13th ed. Norwalk, CT, Appleton & Lange, 1992, pp 271-298.
173. Stamey TA: Pathogenesis and Treatment of Urinary Tract Infections. Baltimore, Williams & Wilkins, 1972.
174. Stamey TA: Urinary tract infections in the female: A perspective. In Remington JS, Swartz MW (eds): Current Clinical Topics in Infectious Diseases, Vol 2. New York, McGraw-Hill, 1981, p 31.
175. Stamm WE, McKevitt M, Counts GW: Acute renal infection in women: Treatment with trimethoprim-sulfamethoxazole or ampicillin for two or six weeks. A randomized trial. Ann Intern Med 106:341, 1987.
176. Stanford JL, Feng Z, Hamilton AS, et al: Urinary and sexual function after radical prostatectomy for clinically localized prostate cancer. The Prostate Cancer Outcomes Study. JAMA 283:354-360, 2000.
177. Stearns HC: Uterine myomas: Clinical and pathologic aspects. Postgrad Med 51:165, 1972.
178. Stewart EA: Uterine fibroids. Lancet 357:293-298, 2001.
179. Stovall TG, Kellerman AL, Ling FW, Buster JE: Emergency department diagnosis of ectopic pregnancy. Ann Emerg Med 19:1098, 1990.
180. Stoval TG, Ling FW, Gray LA, et al: Methotrexate treatment of unruptured ectopic pregnancy: A report of 100 cases. Obstet Gynecol 77:749, 1991.
181. Sundkvist GMG, Ahlgren L, Mattsson S, et al: Repeated quantitative bone scintigraphy in patients with prostatic carcinoma treated with orchiectomy. Eur J Nucl Med 14:203, 1966.
182. Surrey ES, Hornstein MD: Prolonged GnRH agonist and add-back therapy for symptomatic endometriosis: Long-term follow-up. Obstet Gynecol 99:709-719, 2002.
183. Svensson H, Andersson GBJ, Hagstad A, Jansson P: The relationship of low-back pain to pregnancy and gynecologic factors. Spine 15:371, 1990.
184. Te Linde RW: Prolapse of the uterus and allied conditions. Am J Obstet Gynecol 94:444, 1966.
185. Teloimaa S, Puolakka J, Ronnberg L, Kaupilla A: Placebo-controlled comparison of danazol and high-dose medroxyprogesterone acetate in the treatment of endometriosis. Gynecol Endocrinol 1:13, 1987.
186. Thomas WC Jr: Clinical concepts of renal calculus disease. J Urol 113:423, 1975.
187. Thorley JD, Jones SR, Sanford JP: Perinephric abscess. Medicine (Baltimore) 53:441, 1974.
188. Togashi K, Nishimura K, Kimura I, et al: Endometrial cysts: Diagnosis with MR imaging. Radiology 180:73, 1991.
189. Tolkoff-Rubin NE, Rubin RH: Ciprofloxacin in management of urinary tract infection. Urology 31:359, 1988.
190. Torkelson SJ, Lee RA, Hidahl DB: Endometriosis of the sciatic nerve: A report of two cases and a review of the literature. Obstet Gynecol 71:473, 1988.
191. Torti FM, Carter SK: The chemotherapy of prostatic adenocarcinoma. Ann Intern Med 92:681, 1980.
192. Trachtenberg J: Ketoconazole therapy in advanced prostatic cancer. J Urol 132:61, 1984.
193. Tse RL, Leberman PR: Acute renal artery occlusion—etiology, diagnosis, and treatment. Report of a case with subsequent revascularization. J Urol 108:32, 1972.
194. U.S. Preventive Services Task Force: Screening for prostate cancer: Recommendation and rationale. Ann Intern Med 137:915-916, 2002.
195. van Nagell JR Jr, Higgins RV, Donaldson ES, et al: Transvaginal sonography as a screening method for ovarian cancer: A report on the first 1000 cases screened. Cancer 65:573, 1990.

196. Vercellini P, Trespidi L, DeGiorgi O, et al: Endometriosis and pelvic pain: Relation to disease stage and localization. Fertil Steril 65:299-304, 1996.
197. Walde J: Obstetrical and gynecological back and pelvic pains, especially those contracted during pregnancy. Acta Obstet Gynecol Scand 41:11, 1962.
198. Warren JW, Abrutyn E, Hebel JR, et al: Guidelines for antimicrobial treatment of uncomplicated acute bacterial cystitis and acute pyelonephritis in women. Clin Infect Dis 29:745-758, 1999.
199. Waters WB, Richie JP: Aggressive surgical approach to renal cell carcinoma: Review of 130 cases. J Urol 122:306, 1979.
200. Watson RC, Fleming RJ, Evans JA: Arteriography in the diagnosis of renal carcinoma. Radiology 91:188, 1968.
201. Weyman PJ, McCleannan BL, Stanley RJ, et al: Comparison of computed tomography and angiography in the evaluation of renal cell carcinoma. Radiology 137:417, 1980.
202. Whitmore WF Jr: Natural history and staging of prostate cancer. Urol Clin North Am 11:205, 1984.
203. Wickham JEA, Webb DR, Payne SR, et al: Extracorporeal shock wave lithotripsy: The first 50 patients treated in Britain. BMJ 290:1188, 1985.
204. Williams CJ, Mead GM, Macbeth FR, et al: Cisplatin combination chemotherapy versus chlorambucil in advanced ovarian carcinoma: Mature results of a randomized trial. J Clin Oncol 3:1455, 1985.
205. Williams SD, Einhorn LH, Greco AF, et al: VP-16-213 salvage therapy for refractory germinal neoplasms. Cancer 46:2154, 1980.
206. Woll PJ, Rankin EM: Persistent back pain due to malignant lymphadenopathy. Ann Rheum Dis 46:681, 1987.
207. Worster A, Preya I, Weaver B, et al: The accuracy of noncontrast helical computed tomography versus intravenous pyelography in the diagnosis of suspected acute urolithiasis: A meta-analysis. Ann Emerg Med 40:280-286, 2002.
208. Wysowski DK, Honig SF, Beitz J: Uterine sarcoma associated with tamoxifen use. N Engl J Med 346:1832-1833, 2002.
209. Yao M, Tulandi T: Current status of surgical and non-surgical treatment of ectopic pregnancy. Fertil Steril 67:421-433, 1997.
210. Ylikorkala O, Dawood MY: New concepts in dysmenorrhea. Am J Obstet Gynecol 130:833, 1978.
211. Zouves C, Urman B, Gomel V: Laparoscopic surgical treatment of tubal pregnancy: A safe, effective alternative to laparotomy. J Reprod Med 37:205, 1992.

GASTROINTESTINAL DISEASES

CAPSULE SUMMARY

	LOW BACK	NECK
Frequency of spinal pain	Common	Rare
Location of spinal pain	Lumbar spine	Lateral neck, shoulder, interscapular
Quality of spinal pain	Dull ache, colicky	Dull ache, colicky
Symptoms and signs	Alteration in bowel habits, abdominal tenderness	Dysphagia, fatty food intolerance, neck mass
Laboratory tests	Abnormal serum enzymes, bilirubin level, abnormal white blood cell count	Abnormal alkaline phosphatase, bilirubin, abnormal white blood cell count
Radiographic findings	Abnormal filling defects on contrast radiographs	Abnormal filling defects on contrast radiographs
Treatment	Surgical removal of mass or stones, antibiotics	Surgical removal of mass or stones, antibiotics

LUMBOSACRAL SPINE

The organs of the gastrointestinal tract associated with back pain are those in direct contact with the retroperitoneum or those with referred pain to the low back region. Diseases of the pancreas, duodenum, gallbladder, and colon may be associated with low back pain of visceral, somatic, or referred origin. A common finding in the history of patients with back pain secondary to a gastrointestinal disorder is the relationship between pain and eating or bowel function such as defecation.[58]

Pancreas

The pancreas is located at the level of the first and second lumbar vertebrae in the retroperitoneum. Pain from diseases that affect the pancreas is felt deep in the midepigastrium secondary to somatic irritation and is referred to the back in the region of L1. Acute inflammatory diseases of the pancreas cause severe, persistent pain that may be out of proportion to the physical findings. Infiltrative diseases of the pancreas, such as pancreatic carcinoma, may not cause pain until the lesion has invaded the peripancreatic nerves. Disease processes that affect the head of the pancreas cause pain to the right of the spine, whereas lesions of the body and tail are felt to the left of the spine.

Acute Pancreatitis

Acute pancreatitis is an inflammatory disease of the pancreas in which the digestive enzymes produced by that organ act on pancreatic tissue.[26] Conditions that may precipitate episodes of pancreatitis include gallstones, ethanolism, drugs (azathioprine, oral contraceptives, tetracycline, furosemide), hyperlipidemia, trauma, infections, vasculitis, hypercalcemia, and obstruction to the outflow of pancreatic enzymes. As a cause of pancreatitis, gallstones occur more frequently in women whereas ethanol is more common in men.

Epidemiology

The incidence of acute pancreatitis is 28 per 100,000 population per year.[78] The median age is 53, and men and women are affected equally.[51]

CLINICAL HISTORY

Most often the initial and most significant symptoms include steady, boring, severe epigastric pain that radiates to the upper lumbar spine and is increased in the supine position. The pain reaches peak intensity within an hour. Approximately 50% of patients have pain that radiates to the vertebral area in a bandlike distribution. Pain gradually resolves over a period of 3 to 7 days.[62]

Patients with pancreatitis are systemically ill with fever, tachycardia, hypotension (with severe disease), and abdominal tenderness without abdominal muscle guarding. They frequently assume a characteristic position in which they sit with the trunk flexed, the knees drawn up, and the arms folded across the abdomen to get relief. Bowel sounds are diminished. Nausea and vomiting occur in a majority of patients.

PHYSICAL EXAMINATION

Fever, tachycardia, and hypotension may be present. Two rare, but dramatic signs of severe pancreatitis are Cullen's sign, or faint blue discoloration about the umbilicus, and Turner's sign, or discoloration of the flanks reflecting hemorrhage into the retroperitoneum. Jaundice is present in those with obstruction of the common bile duct.

LABORATORY DATA

Laboratory tests reveal an elevated white cell count, between 10,000 and 30,000 cells/mm^3, and an elevated sedimentation rate. Elevated amylase and lipase concentrations on laboratory evaluation reflect pancreatic inflammation. Serum amylase is usually more than three times the upper limit of normal. However, increased amylase concentrations may arise from tissue other than the pancreas (salivary gland, intestine) or from disease states (renal insufficiency, pancreatic carcinoma, ruptured ectopic pregnancy). Separating pancreatic from salivary isoforms of amylase is a sensitive (90%) and specific (92%) test for the presence of acute pancreatitis.[73] Elevated lipase does not offer additional specificity to the diagnosis beyond that of amylase.[35] Trypsin levels should differentiate pancreatic disease from disorders of the salivary gland. Serum immunoreactive trypsinogen/trypsin is a specific and sensitive test for the diagnosis of acute pancreatitis.[83] If the increased amylase is more than three times normal in the presence of normal renal function, the diagnosis of pancreatitis is likely. If amylase remains elevated, a nonpancreatic source of amylase should be sought. An increase in serum alanine aminotransferase above 150 IU/L is suggestive of gallstones as the cause of pancreatitis.[77]

RADIOGRAPHIC FINDINGS

Radiographic findings in the abdomen may include the presence of a single dilated loop of small bowel with edematous walls in the left upper quadrant (a "sentinel loop") or generalized ileus. A plain roentgenogram of the abdomen is also helpful to exclude other disorders that may complicate pancreatitis. Left-sided pleural effusions may be seen on chest films.

Ultrasonography and CT are accurate methods of delineating the extent of pancreatic inflammation, but they do not have a place in the initial diagnosis of acute pancreatitis. Bowel gas may obscure the image of an abdominal sonogram, and a CT scan may not detect inflammatory changes in a significant number of patients with mild pancreatitis. The techniques are better used to detect complications that predispose to pancreatitis (gallstones—ultrasonography) or exacerbate symptoms (pseudocyst—CT scan).[43] Ultrasonography has 93% sensitivity and 96% specificity for the diagnosis of cholelithiasis and acute cholecystitis.[13] CT scans are useful in patients with severe disease because the technique detects the presence of a phlegmon or retroperitoneal necrosis. MR is no better and is more expensive than CT for the evaluation of acute pancreatitis.[67]

DIFFERENTIAL DIAGNOSIS

Once the diagnosis of acute pancreatitis has been established, differentiation of alcoholic and gallstone pancreatitis is essential. Recurrent attacks suggest ethanol as an etiology, but unrecognized gallstones can also cause frequent attacks. Among patients with acute biliary pancreatitis discharged from the hospital without a cholecystectomy, 30% to 50% will have a recurrence of pancreatitis in about 100 days.[54] In about 30% of patients, no specific cause of pancreatitis can be determined. These individuals rarely have another episode over an extended period. Evaluation for unusual causes of pancreatitis is not required after the first attack.

TREATMENT

Treatment of acute pancreatitis includes general supportive measures consisting of fluids, nasogastric suction, respiratory support if respiratory failure intervenes, surgical intervention for local complications (pseudocyst), and removal of precipitating factors that may provoke additional attacks (gallstones). In one study, 63% of patients who required surgery for acute pancreatitis had the disease as a result of biliary tract abnormalities.[42] Removal of stones by endoscopic retrograde cholangiopancreatography (ERCP) is indicated in the treatment of acute pancreatitis.[21] If patients worsen over a day, abdominal CT is indicated to determine whether necrosis of the pancreas has occurred. Those who have necrosis benefit from prophylactic antibiotics.[28,61] The use of antifungal agents is a consideration to prevent fungal infections.[31] These patients also require nutritional support.

Chronic Pancreatitis

Inflammation of the pancreas may lead to chronic, irreversible damage to the organ; such damage results in chronic abdominal pain and pancreatic insufficiency. About 75% of adult patients with chronic pancreatitis have the disease on the basis of alcohol abuse. Men are more frequently affected than women, and the average age of onset is 38 years. Other cases of chronic pancreatitis are classified as idiopathic, traumatic, familial, hypercalcemic, and nutritional.

CLINICAL HISTORY

Chronic pancreatitis is associated with a variety of pain. It may cause intermittent, aching pain or boring, constant pain that radiates from the epigastrium to the back in about 66% of patients.[30] The pain may last for up to

2 weeks and gradually diminishes. If chronic pancreatitis is associated with severe exocrine insufficiency, patients may have pain along with anorexia, weight loss, malabsorption in the form of steatorrhea, and new-onset diabetes.[68] More than 90% of pancreatic function must be lost before fat and protein deficiencies appear.[44]

PHYSICAL EXAMINATION

Patients are usually thin, and physical examination occasionally reveals a palpable right quadrant mass (pseudocyst).

LABORATORY DATA

Serum analysis of patients with quiescent chronic pancreatitis may be normal. Serum enzymes may be normal even with acute exacerbations of pain. Decreased serum trypsinogen levels determined by radioimmunoassay strongly suggest pancreatic exocrine insufficiency. Trypsinogen levels are helpful in differentiating patients with chronic pancreatic insufficiency from those with other pancreatic disorders such as acute pancreatitis, which is associated with an elevated concentration.[69] Low trypsinogen concentrations are found in both chronic pancreatitis and carcinoma of the pancreas. In these circumstances, the presence of CA 19-9 antigen with pancreatic tumors will help differentiate patients with carcinoma from those with chronic pancreatitis.

Another useful test in the evaluation of chronic pancreatitis is the bentiromide test. Bentiromide is a molecule with a terminal para-aminobenzoic acid (PABA) group. The enzymatic function of the pancreas is necessary for PABA to be separated from the molecule. The orally ingested bentiromide is absorbed through the gut and PABA is excreted by the kidney, where it is collected over a 6-hour period. A collection of less than 50% of the ingested PABA associated with bentiromide is compatible with abnormal function.[79]

RADIOGRAPHIC EVALUATION

Plain films of the abdomen may demonstrate diffuse calcification in 30% of patients with chronic pancreatitis. This calcification is pathognomonic of the illness (Fig. 17-16). Other noninvasive tests that may prove useful in detecting calcifications and pseudocysts are ultrasonography and CT. CT is a better test than ultrasound for detecting cysts, but the lower cost and lack of radiation exposure make ultrasound a worthwhile initial test.[25]

ERCP is an invasive test performed by cannulating the pancreatic duct at its junction with the duodenum (papilla of Vater) and visualizing the system for ductal architecture. The demonstration of widespread duct abnormalities during ERCP is characteristic of chronic pancreatitis.[23]

DIFFERENTIAL DIAGNOSIS

An evaluation for chronic pancreatitis would include serum amylase; Sudan stain for stool fat; a flat plate of abdomen for calcification; sonography for dilated pancreatic ducts or pseudocysts; CT scans for calcifications not detected by plain film; ERCP for stricture and dilation of ducts; and pancreatic secretory tests associated with decreased bicarbonate output after secretin stimulation and decreased trypsin with cholecystokinin stimulation, which is the most sensitive way to diagnose chronic pancreatitis.

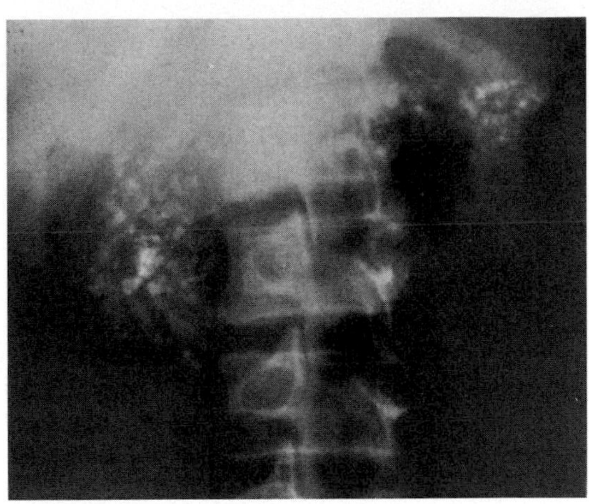

Figure 17-16 A plain roentgenogram of the abdomen reveals diffuse calcification in a patient with chronic pancreatitis. *(Courtesy of William Steinberg, MD.)*

TREATMENT

Abstinence from alcohol once chronic pancreatitis has been established has no effect on the course of recurrent attacks. Patients with pancreatic insufficiency and malabsorption benefit by replacement of pancreatic enzymes.[6] Complications associated with diabetes mellitus are treated with insulin. Surgical intervention is needed to bypass biliary tract obstruction and drain pseudocysts if they become large.[55,63] Endoscopic ductal decompression can result in pain relief in a majority of patients with obstruction.[59] It should be noted that once calcification and insufficiency appear, pain symptoms may decrease. After 5 years, many patients will have resolution of their back pain.

Pancreatic Tumor

EPIDEMIOLOGY

Carcinoma of the pancreas occurs in 10 per 100,000 persons in the general population and 100 per 100,000 in the population older than 75 years.[46] Approximately 30,300 new cases occur each year in the United States.[33] Pancreatic carcinoma is the fourth most common cause of cancer deaths in men. The sex ratio, men to women, is 2:1. Blacks are more commonly affected than whites. The disease occurs most commonly in the elderly.

PATHOGENESIS

The etiology of this neoplasm is unknown, although cigarette smoking, ingestion of animal fats, juvenile-onset diabetes, and chronic pancreatitis have been implicated.

CLINICAL HISTORY

Pancreatic tumors are frequently asymptomatic until they have metastasized to surrounding abdominal viscera. Patients may have a nondescript, dull, midepigastric pain that radiates to the back.[46] Pain that radiates to the back in patients with carcinoma implies direct invasion of adjacent retroperitoneal organs or splanchnic nerves.[32] Pain is heightened with eating. Patients also may have symptoms of anorexia, weight loss, nausea, vomiting, and jaundice.[82]

Physical Examination

Physical findings include a hard abdominal mass, which may be associated with a distended, nontender gallbladder (Courvoisier's sign). Ascites may be present in a minority of patients. Left supraclavicular lymphadenopathy (Virchow's node) is present in individuals with widespread disease.

Laboratory Data

Commonly, abnormal laboratory tests include a decreased hematocrit, elevated sedimentation rate, elevated serum alkaline phosphatase, and hyperbilirubinemia. Unfortunately, these test results are nonspecific and do not allow for early diagnosis of the tumor. Tumor antigens, particularly carcinoembryonic antigen (CEA), have been reported to be elevated in more than 70% of patients with pancreatic malignancy. Unfortunately, most patients had unresectable tumors at the time of diagnosis of their malignancy.[40] CEA has low sensitivity and is associated with benign and malignant disorders.[19] A new antigen, CA 19-9, has been shown to have greater sensitivity and specificity than CEA does. CA 19-9 was detectable in 79% of patients with resectable tumors.[70] A serum concentration of 37 U/mL or more discriminates the presence of pancreatic cancer from benign pancreatic disease.[47] However, CA 19-9 may also be present in the setting of other gastrointestinal tumors (bile duct and colon).[71] Moreover, the antigen may be negative in the early stages of pancreatic cancer and is thus not suitable for screening. CA 19-9 may be a better test for measuring response to chemotherapy in patients with pancreatic cancer.

Radiographic Evaluation

A number of radiographic techniques, including an upper gastrointestinal series, sonography, angiography, ERCP, and CT of the abdomen, may be useful in identifying the presence of a pancreatic tumor.[64] Ultrasonography and CT can detect pancreatic masses as small as 2 cm.[81] The sensitivity of abdominal ultrasound for the detection of pancreatic cancer is 90% in the hands of an experienced technician.[34] CT provides better definition of the tumor and surrounding structures.[4] Helical CT is able to detect periportal collaterals and dilated small peripancreatic veins indicative of portal vein occlusion, which increases the risk of unresectability.[80] MR imaging is not significantly better than CT in differentiating pancreatic tumors from normal pancreatic tissue.[72] However, MR cholangiopancreatography has a specificity of 97% in detecting pancreatic carcinoma,[1] similar to that of ERCP.

Differential Diagnosis

The diagnosis of pancreatic tumor is confirmed by intraoperative biopsy or fine-needle aspiration biopsy of the pancreas.[86] Single-phase CT is the initial test to diagnose pancreatic cancer.[15] Pancreatic tumors must be differentiated from other retroperitoneal tumors, which may also cause back pain. Some of the lesions associated with retroperitoneal tumors include malignant fibrous histiocytoma, liposarcoma, leiomyosarcoma, fibrosarcoma, paraganglioma, and neurofibroma.[38]

Treatment

Therapy for pancreatic carcinoma includes surgical removal of the pancreas and duodenum, as well as the surrounding lymph nodes (Whipple procedure). In most circumstances, only up to 22% have resectable tumors.[14] In experienced hands, this procedure may result in a 5-year survival rate of 20%.[75]

Chemotherapy and radiation therapy are adjunctive methods of treatment for patients with nonresectable disease. Gemcitabine is a chemotherapeutic agent that has greater effect than 5-fluorouracil in reducing symptoms of advanced pancreatic cancer.[11] Unfortunately, cures of this neoplasm are very rare.[17] The prognosis of patients with pancreatic cancer was related to the presence of back pain in one study. Patients with back pain had shorter survival than did those who did not have back pain with their tumor. This outcome correlated with the extent of disseminated disease in those with back pain.[41] Pancreatic cancer has a very poor prognosis, with a 20% survival rate at 1 year and a 3% rate at 5 years.[81]

Hollow Viscus

Stomach

The term *hollow viscus* refers to the stomach, duodenum, and small and large bowel. Most gastric ulcers tend to occur in the antrum of the stomach and are most commonly associated with epigastric pain. In very rare circumstances, gastric pain may be referred to the back at the L1 level. Gastric lesions cause back pain less often than duodenal lesions do. When gastric pain is referred to the back, it may occur in the lumbar area but is almost never felt exclusively in the back.

Duodenum

The duodenum is located retroperitoneally at the level of the first lumbar vertebra. The primary disease of the duodenum that is associated with low back pain is peptic ulceration of its posterior wall.[60] Patients taking nonsteroidal anti-inflammatory drugs have decreased protection of the mucosa by altered production of the bicarbonate and prostaglandins that maintain blood flow.[66] Patients taking these drugs on a regular basis are at risk for gastric and duodenal ulcerations. Bleeding and perforation occur less frequently than simple ulceration. Patients with *Helicobacter pylori* infection of the intestinal tract have an increased risk for the development of ulcers.[29]

Patients with duodenal peptic ulcer generally have burning, epigastric pain that occurs 1 to 3 hours after meals, awakens the patient from sleep, and is relieved with food.[16] A minority have pain that radiates to the back.[27] The pain is localized to the L1–L2 vertebral body level and to the right of the midspinal line for up to 3 cm. The pain is episodic and has no relationship to physical activity. The pain follows the same association with eating as anterior ulcer pain does. Duodenal ulcers may cause pain that occurs only in the back. Physical examination may reveal little more than epigastric tenderness. When pain is present in the back, the involved area may be tender on palpation. Laboratory evaluation is of little benefit unless a decreased hematocrit is present to suggest hemorrhage or an elevated serum amylase concentration indicates posterior penetration into the pancreas. Serologic tests for the detection of antibodies to *H. pylori* are adequate for diagnosis of the infection.[84] Follow-up tests demonstrating undetectable levels of antibody can confirm eradication of the infection.[22] Upper gastrointestinal radiography may outline the ulcer with barium, whereas endoscopy allows for direct visualization of the ulcer crater (Figs. 17-17 and 17-18).[39] Medical treatment of peptic ulcers, which includes antacids, histamine H_2 receptor antagonists, proton pump inhibitors, and sucralfate, is successful in greater than 85% of patients. Eradication of *H. pylori* infection may also be helpful in healing ulcerations.[57] Treatment of *H. pylori* in patients with positive serology is an appropriate first intervention.[50] However, persistence or a change in symptoms suggests a complication of the disease. Endoscopy offers a more specific diagnosis but is reserved for individuals who fail initial medical therapy.[24] An increase in pain, loss of relief with food, and onset of radiation to the back suggest posterior penetration through the wall of the duodenum into the underlying pancreas and acute pancreatitis, which is an unusual complication of this disease.[49] Back pain may occur in the absence of anterior abdominal pain and may become persistent.[82a] Complications of an untreated posterior penetrating ulcer include pancreatitis, obstruction, and giant duodenal ulcers.[45] In most circumstances, as the ulcer responds to therapy, the back pain begins to resolve. Back pain should be absent once the ulcer has healed.

Colon

Of the segments of the colon—ascending, transverse, descending, sigmoid, and rectum—only the transverse colon and sigmoid colon are located outside the retroperitoneum. Pain of colonic origin that is related to distention is usually felt locally in the abdomen; however, disease processes that affect the rectum may be associated with midsacral back pain. The sigmoid colon and rectum are located just anterior to the sacrum and coccyx.

DIVERTICULITIS

Diverticulitis of the colon may be associated with low back pain. Diverticula are outpouchings of the wall of a portion of the gut and are found most commonly in the colon. The cleft made by the nutrient artery passing into the wall of the gut is their most frequent location. Autopsy studies show diverticula in 50% of all individuals older than 60 years.[53] Diverticula in the gut are usually asymptomatic. However, diverticulitis, a disease associated with infection and inflammation of diverticula, causes constitutional symptoms such as fever.[3] Of those with diverticulosis, symptoms and signs of diverticulitis will develop in a small percentage. Patients suffer from acute, persistent pain that localizes to the left lower quadrant and then radiates to the low back area. The pain is often severe and gripping and lasts from hours to days. Relief of pain may occur with a bowel movement, whereas pain is increased with eating. The mechanism of pain is inflammation in the colonic wall. Patients frequently have fever and a change in bowel

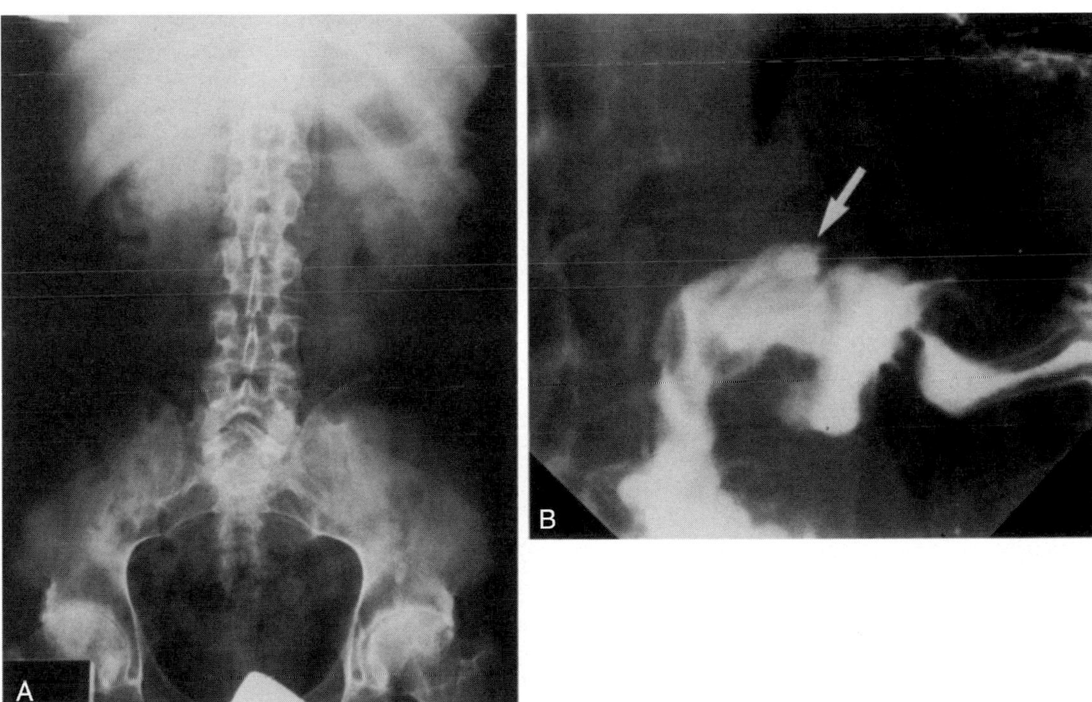

Figure 17-17 A 33-year-old man with reactive arthritis had three different types of back pain during a 1-month period. *A*, A plain roentgenogram of the abdomen reveals bilateral sacroiliitis and severe joint narrowing of both hips. The patient had continuous low back pain localized over the sacroiliac joints. Acute colicky flank pain developed along with hematuria, and the patient later passed a stone. *B*, Within 1 month of passing the stone, epigastric pain developed and radiated to the middle part of the patient's spine. An upper gastrointestinal roentgenogram revealed an ulcer crater in the duodenum *(arrow)*. The patient's symptoms resolved with anti-ulcer therapy.

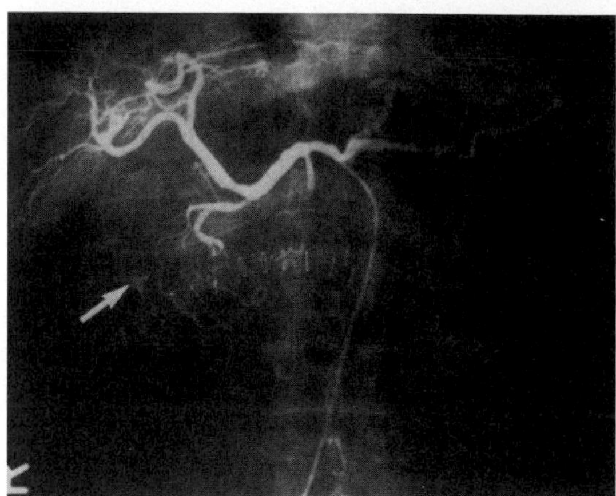

Figure 17-18 Arteriogram of a patient with an actively bleeding duodenal ulcer with dye extravasation *(arrow)*. *(Courtesy of Edward Druy, MD.)*

habits with diverticular disease. Dysuria will also be present if the bladder is involved. Physical examination demonstrates tenderness, which is more pronounced with palpation, a mass in the colon, and depressed bowel sounds.

Laboratory examination will show an elevation in white blood cells. Plain radiographs of the abdomen may reveal evidence of an ileus or intestinal obstruction. CT is a useful technique for the diagnosis of acute diverticulitis[48] because it identifies changes in the wall of the colon and pericolic fat that are induced by inflammation of the diverticulum. It also identifies colonic abscesses without any need for contrast. The noninvasive character of the test makes it a technique of choice in these patients. However, CT is limited in that marked thickening of the colonic wall cannot be differentiated from a neoplasm. Some patients may require a contrast enema to exclude carcinoma and confirm the diagnosis of acute diverticulitis.[5] The presence of fluid at the base of the sigmoid mesentery is useful for distinguishing diverticulitis from colon cancer.[52] Helical CT with water-soluble colonic contrast material is a preferred and accurate test for the diagnosis of diverticulitis.[56] Ultrasonography may also play a useful role as a technique for identifying diverticulitis that is noninvasive, and it does not involve the use of ionizing radiation. Sonography was able to identify diverticulitis confirmed by other more invasive means, such as surgery or colonoscopy, in 46 of 54 (85%) patients with clinical signs of colonic disease.[85] Treatment of acute diverticulitis includes antibiotic therapy to control infection and prevent perforation. This therapy is successful in 70% of patients with uncomplicated disease.[74] Surgical drainage of an abscess is necessary if the diverticular disease has perforated into the peritoneum. The damaged segment of bowel is removed and a colostomy may be needed. Back pain will resolve as the swelling and inflammation of diverticular disease resolve.

Colorectal Carcinoma

Epidemiology. Rectal adenocarcinoma is another colonic cause of low back pain.[20] In 1982, the incidence of colorectal cancer was reported to be 140,000 new cases per year.[2] Data from 1991 revealed 157,000 new cases in the United States with 61,000 related deaths, second only to lung cancer.[9] In 2002, the estimated deaths were 57,000.[33]

Clinical History. Patients are asymptomatic in the early stages of the illness except for a change in bowel habits. Subsequently, they may complain of fatigue, which is secondary to occult bleeding. Those in whom systemic symptoms of anorexia, weight loss, and weakness develop may have a tumor that has invaded through the wall and metastasized. Patients with infiltration of the rectum by tumor experience deep pelvic and midsacral back pain that may radiate to the lower extremities if local invasion irritates the sacral nerves. Patients with rectal carcinoma may have tenesmus and a reduction in stool diameter. Rectal examination may show a hard mass that is fixed and nontender. Carcinoma of the colon may be manifested as a localized, walled-off perforation that simulates a local diverticular abscess. Patients may also have palpable masses anywhere along the length of the colon. Metastatic disease is associated with ascites, hepatomegaly, or lymphadenopathy and occurs in 20% of patients at initial evaluation.

Differential Diagnosis. The diagnosis of rectal carcinoma may be made through the use of colonoscopy or barium enema. The role of virtual CT colonography for the diagnosis of colon and rectal cancer is under investigation.[37] Biopsy and brush cytology specimens can be obtained from lesions at the time of endoscopy. Repeat rectal examination will provide information about the fixation of the rectum and the potential for removal of the tumor. A thorough search for metastatic lesions is essential to plan for appropriate therapy. Determination of increased CEA and lactate dehydrogenase levels may be useful in detecting metastatic disease. In one study, median survival was 8 months when both tests were elevated. CEA has low predictive value in asymptomatic individuals and is not useful as a screening test.[8] This is the current recommendation of the American Society of Clinical Oncology.[7]

Treatment. Curative resection for rectal cancer involves removal of the rectal lymph nodes and surrounding perineal structures.[36] Palliative surgery is offered to patients with metastatic disease who are at risk of obstruction.[18] Stent placement may offer an alternative to excision in those with extensive disease.[12] However, complications of this therapy include perforation and infection. Radiation therapy may be helpful, but chemotherapy for rectal carcinoma has been disappointing. The median improvement in survival for patients who received 5-fluorouracil was 3.7 months.[65] A number of treatment regimens have been developed, with some improvement in survival. Surgical removal of the lesion remains the best chance for cure.[10] The chance for cure by surgery in patients with back pain associated with colon cancer is very low because the presence of back symptoms usually indicates locally invasive disease.

Miscellaneous

Other lesions of the abdominal viscera or thorax on very rare occasion may produce back pain. Subphrenic abscess, acute retrocecal appendicitis, and lower lobe pneumonia may all have a component of back pain.[76] An important consideration in differentiating these lesions from mechanical abnormalities of the lumbosacral spine is that the former also produce either anterior pain or additional symptoms in the organ system involved. Rarely is back pain the exclusive sensory symptom of visceral disease. Other examples might include femoral inguinal or obturator hernias, which may cause chronic aching pelvic and sacral pain associated with radiation to the anteromedial or inner aspect of the thigh. Retroperitoneal bleeding from anticoagulant therapy may also cause back pain that is not associated with mechanical factors.

References

Gastrointestinal Diseases: Lumbosacral Spine

1. Adamek HE, Albert J, Breer H, et al: Pancreatic cancer detection with magnetic resonance cholangiopancreatography and endoscopic retrograde cholangiopancreatography: A prospective study. Lancet 356:190-193, 2000.
2. American Cancer Society: Cancer Facts and Figures. New York, American Cancer Society, 1982.
3. Asch MJ, Markowitz AM: Diverticulosis coli: A surgical appraisal. Surgery 62:239, 1967.
4. Balthazar EJ, Chako AC: Computed tomography of pancreatic masses. Am J Gastroenterol 85:343, 1990.
5. Balthazar EJ, Megibow A, Schinella RA, Gordon R: Limitations in the CT diagnosis of acute diverticulitis: Comparison of CT, contrast enema, and pathologic findings in 16 patients. AJR Am J Roentgenol 154:281, 1990.
6. Bank S: Chronic pancreatitis: Clinical features and medical management. Am J Gastroenterol 81:153, 1986.
7. Bast RC Jr, Ravdin P, Hayes DF, et al: 2000 update on recommendations for the use of tumor markers in breast and colorectal cancer: Clinical practice guidelines of the American Society of Clinical Oncology. J Clin Oncol 19:1865-1878, 2001.
8. Bates SE: Clinical applications of serum tumor markers. Ann Intern Med 115:623, 1991.
9. Boring CC, Squires TS, Tong T: Cancer statistics, 1991. CA Cancer J Clin 41:19, 1991.
10. Bresalier RS, Kim YS: Malignant neoplasms of the large intestine. In Sleisenger MH, Fordtran JS (eds): Gastrointestinal Disease: Pathophysiology, Diagnosis, Management, 5th ed, Vol 2. Philadelphia, WB Saunders, 1993, pp 1449-1493.
11. Burris HA 3rd, Moore MJ, Andersen J, et al: Improvements in survival and clinical benefit with gemcitabine as first-line therapy for patients with advanced pancreas cancer: A randomized trial. J Clin Oncol 15:2403-2413, 1997.
12. Camunez F, Echenagusia A, Simo G, et al: Malignant colorectal obstruction treated by means of self-expanding metallic stenets: Effectiveness before surgery and in palliation. Radiology 21:492-497, 2000.
13. Carroll BA: Preferred imaging techniques for the diagnosis of cholecystitis and cholelithiasis. Ann Surg 21:1, 1989.
14. Connolly MM, Dawsin PJ, Michelassi F, et al: Survival in 1001 patients with carcinoma of the pancreas. Ann Surg 206:366, 1987.
15. DiMagno EP, Reber HA, Tempero MA: AGA technical review on the epidemiology, diagnosis, and treatment of pancreatic ductal adenocarcinoma. Gastroenterology 117:1464-1484, 1999.
16. Earlam R: A computerized questionnaire analysis of duodenal ulcer symptoms. Gastroenterology 71:314, 1976.
17. Edis AJ, Kiernan PD, Taylor WF: Attempted curative resection of ductal carcinoma of the pancreas: Review of Mayo Clinic experience, 1951-1975. Mayo Clin Proc 55:531, 1980.
18. Enker WE, Laffer UT, Block GE: Enhanced survival of patients with colon and rectal cancer is based upon wide anatomic resection. Ann Surg 190:350, 1979.
19. Fabris C, Del Favero G, Basso D, et al: Serum markers and clinical data in diagnosing pancreatic cancer: A contrastive approach. Am J Gastroenterol 83:549, 1988.
20. Falterman KW, Hill CB, Markey JC, et al: Cancer of the colon, rectum and anus: A review of 2,313 cases. Cancer 34:951, 1974.
21. Fan ST, Lai EC, Mok FP, et al: Early treatment of acute biliary pancreatitis by endoscopic papillotomy. N Engl J Med 329:1228, 1993.
22. Feldman M, Cryer B, Lee E, et al: Role of seroconversion in confirming cure of *Helicobacter pylori* infection. JAMA 280:363-365, 1998.
23. Feller ER: Endoscopic retrograde cholangiopancreatography in the diagnosis of unexplained pancreatitis. Arch Intern Med 144:1797, 1984.
24. Fendrick AM, Chernew ME, Hirth RA, et al: Alternative management strategies for patients with suspected peptic ulcer disease. Ann Intern Med 123:260-268, 1995.
25. Foley WD, Stewart ET, Lawson TL, et al: Computed tomography, ultrasonography, and endoscopic retrograde cholangiopancreatography in the diagnosis of pancreatic disease: A comparative study. Gastrointest Radiol 5:29, 1980.
26. Geokas MC, Van Lancker JL, Kadell BM, Machleder HI: Acute pancreatitis. Ann Intern Med 76:105, 1972.
27. Gibson SB: Back pain in peptic ulcer. N Y State J Med 61:625, 1961.
28. Golub R, Siddiqi F, Pohl D: Role of antibiotics in acute pancreatitis: A meta-analysis. J Gastrointest Surg 2:496-503, 1998.
29. Graham DY: *Campylobacter pylori* and peptic ulcer disease. Gastroenterology 96:615, 1989.
30. Grendell JH, Cello JP: Chronic pancreatitis. In Sleisenger MH, Fordtran JS (eds): Gastrointestinal Disease: Pathophysiology, Diagnosis, and Management. Philadelphia, WB Saunders, 1983, pp 1485-1514.
31. Grewe M, Tsiotos GG, Luque de-Leon E, et al: Fungal infection in acute necrotizing pancreatitis. J Am Coll Surg 188:408-414, 1999.
32. Hermann RE, Cooperman AM: Current concepts in cancer: Cancer of the pancreas. N Engl J Med 301:482, 1979.
33. Jemal A, Thomas A, Murray T, et al: Cancer statistics, 2002. CA Cancer J Clin 52:23-47, 2002.
34. Karlson BM, Ekborn A, Lindgren PG, et al: Abdominal US for diagnosis of pancreatic tumor: Prospective cohort analysis. Radiology 213:107-111, 1999.
35. Keim V, Teich N, Fiedler F, et al: A comparison of lipase and amylase in the diagnosis of acute pancreatitis in patients with abdominal pain. Pancreas 16:45-49, 1998.
36. Kemeny N, Braun DE: Prognostic factors in advanced colorectal carcinoma: The importance of lactic dehydrogenase, performance status and white blood cell count. Am J Med 74:786, 1983.
37. Kim HJ, Kim MH, Myung SJ, et al: A new strategy for the application of CA 19-9 in the differentiation of pancreatobiliary cancer: Analysis using a receiver operating characteristic curve. Am J Gastroenterol 94:1941-1946, 1999.
38. Lane RH, Stephens DH, Reiman HM: Primary retroperitoneal neoplasms: CT findings in 90 cases with clinical and pathologic correlation. AJR Am J Roentgenol 152:83, 1989.
39. Laufer I, Mullens JE, Hamilton J: The diagnostic accuracy of barium studies of the stomach and duodenum: Correlation with endoscopy. Radiology 115:569, 1975.
40. Mackie CR, Moosa AR, Go VLW, et al: Prospective evaluation of some candidate tumor markers in the diagnosis of pancreatic cancer. Dig Dis Sci 25:161, 1980.
41. Mannell A, van Heerden JA, Weiland LH, Istrup DM: Factors influencing survival after resection for ductal adenocarcinoma of the pancreas. Ann Surg 203:403, 1986.
42. Martin JK Jr, van Heerden JA, Bess MA: Surgical management of acute pancreatitis. Mayo Clin Proc 59:259, 1984.
43. Mendez G Jr: CT of acute pancreatitis: Interim assessment. AJR Am J Roentgenol 135:463, 1980.
44. Mergener K, Baillie J: Chronic pancreatitis. Lancet 350:1379-1385, 1997.
45. Mistilis SP, Wiot JF, Nedelman SH: Giant duodenal ulcer. Ann Intern Med 59:155, 1963.
46. Morgan RGH, Wormsley KG: Progress report—cancer of the pancreas. Gut 18:580, 1977.
47. Morrin MM, Farrell RJ, Raptopoulos V, et al: Role of virtual computed tomographic colonography in patients with colorectal cancers and obstructing colorectal lesions. Dis Colon Rectum 43:303-311, 2000.
48. Morris J, Stellato TA, Haaga JR, Lieberman J: The utility of computed tomography in colonic diverticulitis. Ann Surg 204:128, 1986.

49. Norris JR, Haubrich WS: The incidence and clinical features of penetration in peptic ulceration. JAMA 178:386, 1961.
50. Ofman JJ, Etchason J, Fullerton S, et al: Management strategies for *Helicobacter pylori*–seropositive patients with dyspepsia: Clinical and economic consequences. Ann Intern Med 126:280-291, 1997.
51. O'Sullivan JW, Nobrega FT, Morlock CG, et al: Acute and chronic pancreatitis in Rochester, Minnesota, 1940-1969. Gastroenterology 62:373, 1972.
52. Padidar AM, Jeffrey RB Jr, Mindelzun RE, et al: Differentiating sigmoid diverticulitis from carcinoma on CT scans: Mesenteric inflammation suggests diverticulitis. AJR Am J Roentgenol 163:81-83, 1994.
53. Painter NS, Buckett DP: Diverticular disease of the colon, a 20th century problem. Clin Gastroenterol 4:3, 1975.
54. Paloyan D, Simonowitz D, Skinner DB: The timing of biliary tract operations in patients with pancreatitis associated with gallstones. Surg Gynecol Obstet 141:737-739, 1975.
55. Prinz RA, Greelee HB: Pancreatic duct drainage in 100 patients with chronic pancreatitis. Ann Surg 194:313, 1981.
56. Rao PM, Rhea JT, Novelline RA, et al: Helical CT with only colonic contrast material for diagnosing diverticulitis: Prospective evaluation of 150 patients. AJR Am J Roentgenol 170:1445-1449, 1998.
57. Rauws EAJ, Tytgat GNJ: Cure of duodenal ulcer associated with eradication of *Helicobacter pylori.* Lancet 335:1233, 1990.
58. Roberts I: Gastrointestinal disorders presenting with back pain. Semin Spine Surg 2:141, 1990.
59. Rosch T, Daniel S, Scholz M, et al: Endoscopic treatment of chronic pancreatitis: A multicenter study of 1000 patients with long-term follow-up. Endoscopy 34:765-761, 2002.
60. Ross JR, Reave LE III: Syndrome of posterior penetrating peptic ulcer. Med Clin North Am 50:461, 1966.
61. Sainio V, Kemppainen E, Puolakkainen P et al: Early antibiotic treatment in acute necrotizing pancreatitis. Lancet 346:663-667, 1995.
62. Scholhamer CF Jr, Spiro HM: The first attack of acute pancreatitis: A clinical study. J Clin Gastroenterol 1:325, 1979.
63. Shatney CH, Lillehei RC: Surgical treatment of pancreatic pseudocysts: Analysis of 119 cases. Ann Surg 189:386, 1979.
64. Simeone JF, Wittenberg H, Ferruci JT: Modern concepts of imaging of the pancreas. Invest Radiol 15:620, 1980.
65. Simmonds PC: Palliative chemotherapy for advanced colorectal cancer: Systematic review and meta-analysis. Colorectal Cancer Collaborative Group. BMJ 321:531-535, 2000.
66. Soll AH (moderator): Nonsteroidal anti-inflammatory drugs and peptic ulcer disease. Ann Intern Med 114:307, 1991.
67. Stark DD, Moss AA, Goldberg HI, et al: Magnetic resonance and CT of the normal and diseased pancreas. A comparative study. Radiology 250:153, 1984.
68. Steer ML, Waxman I, Freedman SD: Chronic pancreatitis. N Engl J Med 332:1482-1490, 1995.
69. Steinberg WM, Goldstein SS, Davis ND, et al: Predictive value of low serum trypsinogen. Dig Dis Sci 30:547, 1985.
70. Steinberg WM, Gelfand R, Anderson KK, et al: Comparison of the sensitivity and specificity of the CA 19-9 and carcinoembryonic antigen assays in detecting cancer of the pancreas. Gastroenterology 90:343, 1986.
71. Steinberg W: The clinical utility of the CA 19-9 tumor-associated antigen. Am J Gastroenterol 85:350, 1990.
72. Steiner E, Stark DD, Hahn PF, et al: Imaging of pancreatic neoplasms: Comparison of MR and CT. AJR Am J Roentgenol 152:487, 1989.
73. Sternby B, O'Brien JF, Zinmeister AR, et al: What is the best biochemical test to diagnose acute pancreatitis? A prospective clinical study. Mayo Clin Proc 71:1138-1144, 1996.
74. Stollman NH, Raskin JB: Diagnosis and management of diverticular disease of the colon in adults. Ad Hoc Practice Parameters Committee of the American College of Gastroenterology. Am J Gastroenterol 94:3110-3121, 1999.
75. Strasberg SM, Drebin JA, Soper NJ: Evolution and current status of the Whipple procedure: An update for gastroenterologists. Gastroenterology 113:983-994, 1997.
76. Sullivan JE: Backache due to visceral lesions of the chest and abdomen. Clin Orthop 26:67, 1963.
77. Tenner S, Dubner H, Steinberg W: Predicting gallstone pancreatitis with laboratory parameters. A meta-analysis. Am J Gastroenterol 89:1863-1899, 1994.
78. The Copenhagen Pancreatitis Study Group: An interim report from a prospective epidemiological multicenter study. Scand J Gastroenterol 26:305, 1981.
79. Toskes PP: Bentiromide as a test of exocrine pancreatic function in adult patients with pancreatic exocrine insufficiency. Determination of appropriate dose and urinary collection interval. Gastroenterology 85:565, 1983.
80. Vedantham S, Lu DS, Reber HA, et al: Small peripancreatic veins: Improved assessment in pancreatic cancer patients using thin-section pancreatic phase helical CT. AJR Am J Roentgenol 170: 377-383, 1998.
81. Warshaw AL, Fernandez-del Castillo C: Pancreatic carcinoma. N Engl J Med 326:455, 1992.
82. Weingarten L, Gelb AM, Fischer MG: Dilemma of pancreatic ductal carcinoma. Am J Gastroenterol 71:473, 1979.
82a. Weiss DJ, Conliffe T, Tata N: Low back pain caused by a duodenal ulcer. Arch Phys Med Rehabil 79:1137-1139, 1998.
83. Werner M, Steinberg WM, Pauley C: Strategic use of individual and combined enzyme indicators for acute pancreatitis analyzed by receiver-operator characteristics. Clin Chem 35:967, 1989.
84. Wilcox MH, Dent TH, Hunter JO, et al: Accuracy of serology for the diagnosis of *Helicobacter pylori* infection—a comparison of eight kits. J Clin Pathol 49:373-376, 1996.
85. Wilson SR, Toi A: The value of sonography in the diagnosis of acute diverticulitis of the colon. AJR Am J Roentgenol 154:1199, 1990.
86. Yamanaka T, Kimura K: Differential diagnosis of pancreatic mass lesion with percutaneous fine-needle aspiration biopsy under ultrasonic guidance. Dig Dis Sci 24:694, 1979.

LUMBOSACRAL/CERVICAL SPINE

Gallbladder

The gallbladder receives its innervation from both greater splanchnic nerves (T5–T9). The brain interprets biliary pain to be in the midline in relation to the bilateral innervation of the gallbladder. When biliary pain is severe, the discomfort may radiate to the back in a T5–T9 distribution, which corresponds to an interscapular location. Occasionally, patients may experience pain lower in the thoracic area that they consider to be low back pain or that radiates to the right shoulder.

Acute Cholecystitis

Epidemiology

In certain patients, the bile that is stored in the gallbladder crystallizes to form gallstones (cholelithiasis).[12] The presence of these stones may cause inflammation of the gallbladder, which results in chronic cholecystitis. Gallstones are a common medical problem, with 5 million men and 15 million women affected in the United States.[6]

Clinical History

Women younger than 30 years who have had more than three pregnancies are at greatest risk for gallstones.[9] A majority of gallstones are asymptomatic. When the cystic duct is obstructed by a gallstone, acute cholecystitis occurs. Cholelithiasis is present in 95% of patients with acute cholecystitis. Acalculous cholecystitis is usually associated with previous surgery, trauma, or sepsis.[4] This entity is the cause of cholecystitis in about 10% of individuals but is associated with significant morbidity and mortality.[13] Bacterial infection and ischemia may play a role in the pathogenesis of acute cholecystitis. Lodging of a gallstone in the cystic duct or common bile duct causes severe, steady pain lasting 15 minutes to 1 hour. The pain typically occurs in the midepigastrium and moves to the right upper quadrant. Pain may radiate around the sides to the back or directly through to an area below the tip of the right scapula, the dorsolumbar spine, or occasionally the right shoulder.[5] The pain is intense, begins abruptly, and subsides gradually. The quality of the pain varies from excruciating or lancinating to aching or cramping. Nausea, vomiting, and dyspepsia may develop.

PHYSICAL EXAMINATION

Physical examination demonstrates an abnormal Murphy sign (inspiratory arrest on palpation in the right subcostal area), abdominal guarding, rebound tenderness, fever, and jaundice. The gallbladder is palpable in 30% of patients. Generalized rebound tenderness suggests the possibility of rupture. In a study of patients referred for gallstones, the most characteristic signs and symptoms were pain in the upper part of the abdomen, radiation to the back, a steady quality of the pain, duration for 1 to 24 hours, and onset more than an hour after meals. These clinical findings required confirmation by radiographic imaging.[2]

LABORATORY DATA

Laboratory tests demonstrate an elevated white blood cell count to 15,000 cells/mm^3. An increased alkaline phosphatase level suggests a common bile duct stone. An elevated amylase level also suggests pancreatic inflammation and a common bile duct stone.

RADIOGRAPHIC EVALUATION

The primary imaging modality for the diagnosis of cholelithiasis is ultrasonography. Ultrasonography has 93% sensitivity and 96% specificity for the diagnosis of cholelithiasis and acute cholecystitis[10] (Fig. 17-19). Ultrasonography is able to detect biliary duct obstruction, as well as the presence of an abscess or tumor. However, the technique is unable to determine the extent of inflammation in the gallbladder.[3,7,14] Cholescintigraphy is a reasonably specific test to confirm the diagnosis of acute cholecystitis.[1] Under normal circumstances, technetium-labeled iminodiacetic acid is preferentially concentrated in the biliary tree and enters the gallbladder. In acute cholecystitis, radiolabeled material enters the common bile duct but does not enter the gallbladder. The scan may not be helpful in patients with severe hyperbilirubinemia. These tests have taken the place of the oral cholecystogram.

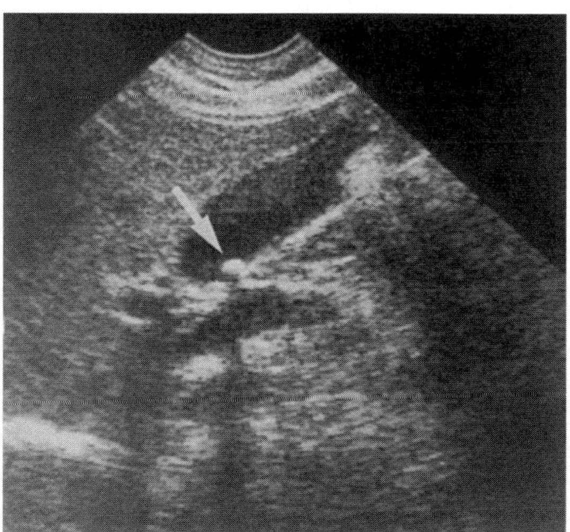

Figure 17-19 Ultrasound of the gallbladder demonstrates a large gallstone *(arrow)*. *(Courtesy of Michael Hill, MD.)*

DIFFERENTIAL DIAGNOSIS

The presence of cholelithiasis in the correct clinical setting, including fever and sustained abdominal pain, is diagnostic of cholecystitis. Biliary colic is pain associated with cystic duct blockage but no inflammation of the gallbladder wall. Biliary colic pain is intense but resolves over a period of hours. Other disorders that must be differentiated from biliary colic include esophageal spasm, esophageal reflux, irritable bowel syndrome, renal colic, and coronary artery disease.

TREATMENT

Frequently, treatment of acute cholecystitis is surgical removal of the gallbladder once the patient's condition has been optimized with the use of antibiotics, fluid replacement, and nasogastric suction. Patients who do not elect to undergo cholecystectomy may be at risk for perforation. Laparoscopic cholecystectomy has become the surgical method of choice for removal of the gallbladder.[12] When compared with laparotomy, postoperative pain is reduced, hospitalization is shortened, and a quicker return to normal function is common.[11] Laparoscopic cholecystectomy can be used in patients who have a delay in diagnosis.[8]

For those who choose to forego surgery, symptoms may resolve in as little time as 48 hours or continue for weeks despite antibiotics. The interscapular pain or upper back pain associated with cholecystitis follows a similar course. Those who have had one attack of cholecystitis are at risk for another. Patients with recurrent attacks should consider surgical removal of the gallbladder.

References

Gastrointestinal Tract: Lumbosacral/Cervical Spine

1. Boucher IAD: Imaging procedures to diagnose gallbladder disease. BMJ 288:1632, 1984.
2. Dieh AK, Sugarek NJ, Todd KH: Clinical evaluation for gallstone disease: Usefulness of symptoms and signs in diagnosis. Am J Med 69:29, 1990.
3. Fink-Bennett D, Freitas JE, Ripley SD, et al: The sensitivity of hepatobiliary imaging and real time ultrasonography in the detection of acute cholecystitis. Arch Surg 120:904, 1985.
4. Frazee RC, Nagorney DM, Mucha P Jr: Acute acalculous cholecystitis. Mayo Clin Proc 64:163, 1989.
5. French EG, Robb WAT: Biliary and renal colic. BMJ 2:135, 1963.
6. Friedman GD, Kannel WB, Dawber TR: The epidemiology of gallbladder disease: observations in the Framingham study. J Chronic Dis 19:273, 1966.
7. Laing FC, Federle MP, Jeffrey RB, et al: Ultrasonic evaluation of patients with acute right upper quadrant pain. Radiology 140:449, 1981.
8. Lo CM, Liu CL, Fan ST, et al: Prospective randomized study of early versus delayed laparoscopic cholecystectomy for acute cholecystitis. Ann Surg 227:461-467, 1998.

9. Maringhini A, Ciambra M, Baccelliere P, et al: Sludge, stones, and pregnancy. Gastroenterology 95:1160, 1988.
10. Marton KI, Doubilet P: How to image the gallbladder in suspected cholecystitis. Ann Intern Med 109:722, 1988.
11. McMahon AJ, Russell IT, Baxter JN, et al: Laparoscopic versus minilaparotomy cholecystectomy: A randomized trial. Lancet 343:135, 1994.
12. Roberts I: Gastrointestinal disorders presenting with back pain. Semin Spine Surg 2:141, 1990.
13. Shapiro MJ, Luchtefeld EB, Kurzwell S, et al: Acute acalculous cholecystitis in the critically ill. Am Surg 60:335-339, 1994.
14. The Southern Surgeons Club: A prospective analysis of 1518 laparoscopic cholecystectomies. N Engl J Med 324:1073, 1991.

CERVICAL SPINE

The organs of the gastrointestinal tract associated with neck pain are those with referred pain distribution to the neck and shoulder. Diseases of the esophagus and gallbladder may be associated with neck pain of visceral, somatic, or referred origin. A common finding in the history of patients with neck pain secondary to a gastrointestinal disorder is the relationship between pain and eating or bowel function.[15]

Esophagus

The esophagus is a midline structure that is innervated with a distribution from C7 to T12. Most esophageal pain is substernal in location. Acid reflux disorders are associated with substernal, burning pain that may radiate to the anterior of the neck and between the shoulder blades.[13] Other esophageal disorders that may cause chest, posterior thoracic, and anterior neck pain include esophageal spasm, dysmotility disorders, and carcinoma.[4] Hiatal hernia caused by slippage of the lower esophageal sphincter through the diaphragm may also be associated with left arm, anterior neck, and posterior thorax pain. In general, esophageal pain is altered by eating and the recumbent position. Esophageal pain is relieved by antacid therapy or by nitroglycerin therapy in the setting of esophageal spasm. Diagnostic techniques include barium swallow, esophagoscopy, and manometry to evaluate the cause of esophageal dysfunction. Therapy is directed at both decreasing the damage caused by acid secretion and normalizing peristalsis.

Esophageal Diverticulum

Zenker's diverticulum (ZD) occurs in the upper portion of the esophagus at the level of the cricopharyngeal muscle. ZD is caused by motor abnormalities of the esophagus. This area of the esophagus has a weakness in the wall. Most patients are initially seen at 50 years of age or older. Symptoms are insidious in onset, with dysphagia and regurgitation being most common. As the diverticulum expands, food lodges in the sac and is regurgitated hours after eating. Increasing size may result in a neck mass and local neck pain. Patients are at risk for aspiration pneumonia. A barium esophagogram is useful for identifying the location and size of the diverticulum. Esophagoscopy is not recommended because of the risk of perforation, unless a malignancy is suspected.[4] Surgical removal of the diverticulum in a one-step procedure is indicated if the size of the lesion is large enough to cause obstruction.[12] A variety of intraluminal techniques are available to close the ZD. A stapling procedure can offer benefit with less risk than surgical removal.[17]

Esophageal Cancer

Esophageal cancer is one of the more common malignant tumors, but it affects the upper part of the esophagus in a minority of patients.[14] The middle and lower portions of the esophagus are involved more frequently. The tumors arise from the squamous epithelium of the lumen and cause squamous cell carcinomas. Adenocarcinomas occur in the columnar epithelium near the end of the esophagus (Barrett's esophagus) and account for the remainder of the tumors.[3] Dysphagia and weight loss are frequent early symptoms. The esophagus does not have a serosal layer, which allows neoplasms to grow to significant size and extent before evaluation is undertaken. The rich lymphatic supply to the esophagus permits early metastatic spread before the diagnosis is considered. Upper esophageal cancer may be manifested as upper neck discomfort along with dysphagia and weight loss. Difficulty with solids progresses to dysphagia with liquids. Advanced tumors may cause local mass lesions, infections, and fistulas. Bronchoscopy may be needed to determine bronchial invasion from the esophagus. The diagnosis of esophageal cancer is confirmed by biopsy at time of endoscopy.[8] The prognosis is poor for most individuals with esophageal cancer whose manifestation is neck pain.[4]

Therapy that includes chemotherapy with 5-fluorouracil and cisplatin, radiation therapy, and surgical removal of the tumor offers a better survival advantage than surgery alone does for resectable tumors.[22]

Miscellaneous

Anterior Neck Lesions

Lesions of the oropharynx, thyroid, cervical lymph glands, salivary glands (parotid and submandibular), and vascular structures (carotid) may cause anterior and lateral neck pain. These lesions may refer pain to the throat, anterior chest wall, and occasionally the posterior aspect of the neck. Many of these disorders are mass lesions. In patients 60 years or older, a mass in the lateral part of the neck has an 80% chance of being malignant. Lesions found in the upper portion of the anterior neck region have sources in lesions of the tongue, larynx, mouth floor, or salivary glands. Lesions in the lower portion of the neck have an origin in the thyroid gland. Enlarged lymph glands are the most frequent cause of masses in the anterior cervical triangle.

The history and physical examination are essential for determining the potential etiologies of neck lesions. The duration and amount of smoking are an essential part of the history. A change in voice quality, dysphagia, and the onset of cough, fever, chills, and night sweats have the implication that tumor or infection is the cause of the anterior neck pain. A history of migraine headaches may be associated with vascular pain. Physical examination, including bimanual palpation of the oropharynx, may identify small masses in the parotid and submandibular regions and in the base of the tongue and tonsillar areas. Careful examination of the thyroid identifies any nodules and free movement of the gland anterior to the trachea.

Technologic advances, including fiberoptic laryngoscopy, CT and MR imaging, and fine-needle biopsies, have improved the opportunity to identify the location and pathologic condition of lesions with less invasive procedures. Laryngoscopy allows for direct visualization of lesions in the nasal cavity, base of the tongue, epiglottis, larynx, and vocal cords. CT and MR scans visualize the extent of soft tissue lesions and the number of masses present. Fine-needle aspiration is able to obtain specimen samples for cytopathology, Gram stain, and culture.

Benign masses in the neck are most frequently lymph glands (cervical lymphadenitis). Primary infections in the mouth, pharynx, tonsils, dental structures, and skin over the face or head cause lymph gland enlargement.[2] Midline masses are of thyroid origin or are caused by thyroglossal cysts. The thyroid gland may be involved with acute infection (suppurative thyroiditis), subacute thyroiditis (de Quervain's thyroiditis), Hashimoto's thyroiditis, Riedel's struma, or thyroid malignancy.[7,18-20] Branchial cleft cysts are lateral masses with a fistulous opening found near the anterior border of the sternocleidomastoid muscle. These congenital cysts may be asymptomatic masses or acutely inflamed masses associated with suppurative infections.[10] Infections not associated with congenital cysts or lymph glands may occur from superficial structures (skin) or deep structures such as the parotid gland, mastoid process, mandible, or muscles in the fascial compartments. Superficial infections cause a tender mass at the anterior border of the sternocleidomastoid muscle. Deep fascial infections require radiographic evaluation to identify the location of the abscess in the lateral pharyngeal, pretracheal, submandibular, or deep fascial planes (retropharyngeal and prevertebral).[1,6] Deep fascial infections are rare, but potentially catastrophic if swelling in soft tissue planes results in airway compromise. *Ludwig's angina* is the term associated with submandibular space infection. Most of these infections are associated with dental abscesses or postextraction infections.[11] Carotidynia may be caused by vascular and soft tissue structures near the carotid sheath. Carotid body tumors are found close to the bifurcation of the carotid artery. Migraine headaches may cause carotid tenderness. Calcification or inflammation of tendons (stylohyoid), bone (hyoid), and muscles (digastric and stylohyoid) may cause pain in the lateral aspect of the neck.[9,16]

Lymphomas may be manifested as cervical lymphadenopathy or as mass lesions involving the tonsils in Waldeyer's ring. Metastatic lesions may also cause lymph gland swelling. The presence of metastatic lesions in the upper portion of the neck suggests that the primary lesion (squamous cell carcinoma, melanoma, or adenocarcinoma) is localized to the head or neck. Unknown primary neck metastases are the most common cause of node swelling in the lower third of the neck. Surgical intervention in the form of neck dissection depends on the location of the mass and the probably primary source of the tumor.[21]

The advances in salvage of tissue by current surgical techniques have led to improved function after removal of tumors.[5]

References

Gastrointestinal Diseases: Cervical Spine

1. Blomquist IK, Bayer AS: Life-threatening deep fascial space infections of the head and neck. Infect Dis Clin North Am 2:237, 1988.
2. Brook I: The swollen neck: Cervical lymphadenitis, parotitis, thyroiditis, and infected cysts. Infect Dis Clin North Am 21:221, 1988.
3. Cameron AJ, Ott BJ, Payne WS: The incidence of adenocarcinoma in columnar-lined (Barrett's) esophagus. N Engl J Med 313:857, 1985.
4. Castell DO: The Esophagus, 2nd ed. Boston, Little, Brown, 1995, p 795.
5. Forastiere A, Koch W, Trotti A, et al: Head and neck cancers. N Engl J Med 345:1890-1900, 2001.
6. Hall MB, Arteaga DM, Mancuso A: Use of computerized tomography in the localization of head-and-neck-space infections. J Oral Maxillofac Surg 43:978, 1985.
7. Hamburger JI: The various presentations of thyroiditis: Diagnostic considerations. Ann Intern Med 104:219, 1986.
8. Lightdale CJ: Esophageal cancer: American College of Gastroenterology. Am J Gastroenterol 94:20-29, 1999.
9. Lim RY: Carotodynia exposed: Hyoid bone syndrome. South Med J 80:444, 1987.
10. McManus K, Holt R, Aufdemorte TM, et al: Bronchogenic cyst presenting as deep neck abscess. Otolaryngol Head Neck Surg 92:109, 1984.
11. Moreland LW, Corey J, McKenzie R: Ludwig's angina: Report of a case and review of the literature. Arch Intern Med 148:461, 1988.
12. Payne WS, King RM: Pharyngoesophageal (Zenker's) diverticulum. Surg Clin North Am 63:815, 1983.
13. Pope CE: Acid-reflux disorders. N Engl J Med 331:656, 1994.
14. Puhakka HJ, Aitsalo K: Oesophageal carcinoma: Endoscopic and clinical findings in 258 patients. J Laryngol Otol 102:1137, 1988.
15. Roberts I: Gastrointestinal disorders presenting with back pain. Semin Spine Surg 2:141, 1990.
16. Sarkozi J, Fam AG: Acute calcific retropharyngeal tendinitis: An unusual cause of neck pain. Arthritis Rheum 27:708, 1984.
17. Scher RL, Richtsmeier WJ: Long-term experience with endoscopic staple-assisted esophagodiverticulostomy for Zenker's diverticulum. Laryngoscope 108:200-205, 1998.
18. Shervo J, Gal R, Avidor I, et al: Anaplastic thyroid carcinoma: A clinical, histologic, and immunohistochemical study. Cancer 62:319, 1988.
19. Szabo S, Allen DB: Thyroiditis: Differentiation of acute suppurative and subacute—case report and review of the literature. Clin Pediatr (Phila) 28:171, 1989.
20. Tupchong L, Phil D, Hughes F, et al: Primary lymphoma of the thyroid: Clinical features, prognostic factors, and results of treatment. Int J Radiat Oncol Biol Phys 12:1813, 1986.
21. Vokes EE, Weichselbaum RR, Lippman SM, et al: Head and neck cancer. N Engl J Med 328:184, 1993.
22. Walsh TN, Noonan N, Hollywood D, et al: A comparison of multimodal therapy and surgery for esophageal adenocarcinoma. N Engl J Med 335:462-467, 1996.

CHAPTER 18

MISCELLANEOUS DISEASES

PAGET'S DISEASE OF BONE

CAPSULE SUMMARY

	LOW BACK	NECK
Frequency of spinal pain	Uncommon	Rare
Location of spinal pain	Lumbar spine	Cervical spine
Quality of spinal pain	Deep, boring ache	Deep, boring ache
Symptoms and signs	Pain with walking	Decreased spine motion
Laboratory tests	Increased alkaline phosphatase	Increased alkaline phosphatase
Radiographic findings	Lytic and sclerotic Enlarged vertebrae on plain roentgenograms	Lytic and sclerotic Enlarged vertebrae on plain roentgenograms
Treatment	Bisphosphonates, calcitonin, nonsteroidal anti-inflammatory drugs	Bisphosphonates, calcitonin, nonsteroidal anti-inflammatory drugs

PREVALENCE AND PATHOGENESIS

Paget's disease of bone (PD) is a localized disorder of bone characterized by a remarkable degree of bone resorption and subsequent formation of disorganized and irregular new bone. The disease was first described by Sir James Paget in 1877.[73]

Epidemiology

PD is a common disorder in certain areas of the world. It is more common in Western Europe, Australia, and New Zealand than in the United States. Most Americans with PD are of Western European or Mediterranean descent. PD is rare in blacks in Africa but is reported in blacks in the United States.[104] The risk for the disease is also rare in Asians. It affects up to 3% of people older than 40 years of age,[96] and this number increases to 10% in individuals 80 years or older.[9] The prevalence increases to 10% to 20% with a positive family history.[91] Men are slightly more commonly affected than women by a ratio of 1.3:1.[5] In New York State between 1980 to 1983, the rate for PD for hospitalized patients was 26 per 100,000 for the age group 65 to 74 years and 34 for the group 75 years and older. The average length of hospitalization for these groups was 9 and 11 days, respectively.[75]

Pathogenesis

Osteoclasts

The pathogenesis of PD is unknown. There is little evidence to support abnormalities in hormone secretion, vascular supply, or connective tissue metabolism as a cause of this illness. The primary abnormality resides in osteoclasts, cells that resorb bone. Histologic examination of pagetic bone reveals increased numbers of osteoclasts, with marked increases in size and number of nuclei in these cells. Pagetic osteoclasts in long-term marrow cultures have a 10-fold to 20-fold increase in number compared to normal marrow cultures, are larger in size, have more nuclei per cell, have increased levels of tartrate-resistant acid phosphatase activity, and are hyper-responsive to 1,25$(OH)_2$ vitamin D.[57] The hyper-responsiveness is mediated through the vitamin D receptor but is not associated with increased number or affinity of the receptor.[79] Levels of interleukin-6 (IL-6) are increased in long-term marrow cultures of PD bone cells. IL-6 is an important regulator of bone function, acting as a stimulator of osteoclast cell formation.[87] This change in the number of osteoclasts results in increased bone resorption and inadequate new bone formation. New pagetic bone is less compact, more vascular, and weaker than normal bone.[22]

Osteoblasts

Other investigators have suggested that the osteoblast is the source of the primary abnormality of PD.[11,53] The evidence for this hypothesis is the focal nature of PD and the presence of viral genome in cells other than osteoclasts in bone, including the osteoblast. Osteoblasts are not distributed via the bloodstream. The osteoclasts are derived from progenitor cells in bone marrow and distributed through the peripheral circulation. If osteoclasts were the putative cause of PD, the illness should be systemic following the body-wide distribution of the osteoclasts. In addition, osteoblasts produce large amounts of IL-6. Additional evidence has been reported suggesting that deregulation of c-*fos* protooncogene expression in bone cells by the insertion of a paramyxovirus may be the primary lesion of PD. Animal models with overexpression of the c-*fos* gene develop increased number of osteoclasts with phenotypic changes characteristic of PD.[12]

Viral Etiology

Ultrastructural studies of pagetic bone have demonstrated the presence of nuclear and cytoplasmic inclusions that resemble portions of paramyxoviruses.[100] Immunohistologic data have suggested a role for measles, respiratory syncytial virus, and canine distemper virus in PD.[23] The characteristics of a slow virus infection—long latent period, single organ disease, and lack of inflammatory response—match closely those of PD. However, the infectious agent has not been isolated from cultured pagetic cells and the specific virus has not been identified. Infection with paramyxovirus promotes the fusion of infected cells, with subsequent formation of multinucleated giant cells.[69] Polymerase chain reaction techniques have been used to screen for paramyxovirus sequences in RNA extracted from bone from patients with PD. No evidence of viral products was identified in RNA extracts from 10 patients.[77] Therefore, any conclusion concerning the role of viruses as the etiologic agent of PD cannot be made at this time.

Genetic Factors

Family studies suggest that a genetic component plays a role in the expression of the illness. Between 14% and 25% of family members of patients with PD contract the illness.[102] First-degree relatives have a sevenfold increased risk of developing PD.[105] Four susceptibility loci on three different chromosomes (5, 6, 18) have been identified. These loci include 18q21-22, 5q35-qter, 5q31, and 6q.[34,44,59] Questions remain regarding the effect of these genes on age of onset and/or the severity of disease. Family studies suggest a variable onset and expression of disease with individuals with the same haplotype.[60]

CLINICAL HISTORY

Most patients with PD are asymptomatic.[19] Frequently the possibility that a patient may have the disease is raised by the presence of an elevated serum alkaline phosphatase level on screening chemistry tests or by the discovery of an area of bony change on radiographs. When patients become symptomatic, however, they frequently develop rheumatologic complaints. Back pain is common, affecting 34% of 290 patients in one study and 43% in another.[5,90] However, other investigators have reported prevalences as low as 11% and have suggested that PD has been inappropriately diagnosed as the cause of back pain in a large proportion of patients.[10,32] A study has documented spine involvement in 35% of 248 patients with PD.[39] The problem arises that these patients may have osteoarthritis of the spine, which may be the actual cause of back pain. A study investigating this specific point reported only 3 (12%) of 25 patients with PD having back pain directly related to their underlying illness. The remaining patients had back pain that could be related to PD and/or coexistent osteoarthritis.[6] A similar frequency (13%) of back pain related to PD alone was reported in the study.[39]

Axial skeleton disease occurs in the sacrum, lumbar spine, thoracic spine, and cervical spine in descending order. Cervical spine disease occurs in only 3% to 8% of patients with axial skeleton disease.[33,39]

Pain of PD is of a deep boring quality and is not increased at night. Pain secondary to PD uncomplicated by mechanical disorders is unrelated to activity, is not relieved by rest, and is not significantly relieved with nonsteroidal anti-inflammatory drugs (NSAIDs).[39] The pain may radiate with a radicular pattern in the gluteal region, thighs, legs, or feet. Cauda equina symptoms with saddle anesthesia, progressive weakness, and bladder or bowel incontinence are present in a small percentage of patients.[5,111] Spinal stenosis occurs in 10% to 20% of patients, with half experiencing neurologic deficits.[76] The lumbosacral spine is the area of the axial skeleton most commonly symptomatic. The pelvis and sacrum are the most common primary sites of bone involvement with the polyostotic form of PD.[38]

In the cervical spine, radicular pain may involve the shoulders, arms, or hands. PD may affect the upper portion of the cervical spine, resulting in symptoms of radiculopathy, myelopathy, or quadraparesis.[15,29,50,61,67,78,89,112]

The pain of PD involving the axial skeleton may be of bone, joint, or nerve origin.[3] Vertebral bodies may fracture, facet joints may develop secondary osteoarthritis due to deformity, and neural elements may become compressed by new bone growth including extradural structures such as ligamentum flavum.[25,32,40,46,72] Monostotic PD affecting a vertebral body may be associated with pain not related to fracture or compression of neural elements.[18] Pain also may be generated by compression of neural elements by intraspinal soft tissue, neural ischemia produced by arterial steal phenomenon, interference with blood supply to the cord by compression of expanding bone, or platybasia with compression of the medulla.[39] The increased vascularity associated with PD has been implicated as the cause of spontaneous spinal epidural hematomas associated with neurologic dysfunction, including cauda equina syndrome.[41,85] Neurologic complications are relatively uncommon but may cause significant disability such as myelopathy, radiculopathy, and cranial nerve signs, including optic atrophy, deafness, and cerebellar dysfunction.[17] Spinal cord compression occurs most commonly in the thoracic spine where vertebral width is narrowed.[95] Cervical spinal stenosis secondary to PD may occur with or without neck pain.[89] Occasionally, cord compression develops suddenly as a result of a collapse of a vertebra.[97]

Other frequently affected sites are the skull, pelvis, femurs, and tibias. Patients may experience pain in weight-bearing bones with walking. PD may also cause deformities in bones and results in increased size of the skull, hip joint disease (osteoarthritis), and bowing of the legs. Bone softening may give rise to invagination of the base of the skull, which may result in obstructive hydrocephalus.[104]

Other complications of PD include hyperuricemia with gout,[63] hypercalcemia in the immobilized patient, and high-output cardiac failure due to the increased blood flow to bones. Malignant degeneration develops in patients with polyostotic PD but is a rare occurrence. Less than 1% of PD patients develop osteosarcoma or fibrosarcoma.[113] Metastases also may involve pagetic bone and may only be differentiated from sarcomas by tissue biopsy.[94]

PHYSICAL EXAMINATION

Physical examination may be entirely normal in the patient with asymptomatic PD. Increasing disease activity, manifested by rapid bone growth, may correspond to physical findings consistent with rapid bone metabolism, and the temperature over bones may be elevated from increased blood flow. Bone growth of the skull is manifested by increased skull circumference and dilated scalp veins. Angioid streaks are an occasional finding on funduscopic examination. Resting tachycardia is seen in patients with high cardiac output.

Lumbar Spine

Musculoskeletal abnormalities may include a pagetic stature (dorsal kyphosis) and abnormal gait. In the weight-bearing bones, new bone formation leads to lateral bowing in the femur and anterior bowing in the tibia. Decreased motion may be demonstrated in the lumbar spine, and point tenderness may be elicited over vertebral bodies that have sustained fractures. The lumbar spine may be straightened, fixed, or reversed on examination. Scoliosis may be present. Straight-leg raising may be reduced.

Cervical Spine

The cervical spine may be straightened, fixed, or reversed on examination. Patients with upper cervical involvement have decreased rotation.[89] Neurologic examination may be remarkable for cranial nerve, sensory, motor, or cerebellar dysfunction if bone growth has resulted in nerve compression in the cervical area.

LABORATORY DATA

The most characteristic laboratory abnormality is an elevation of the serum alkaline phosphatase level, since this mirrors the extent of new bone, osteoblastic activity. A measure of bone resorption is 24-hour total urinary hydroxyproline. This amino acid is formed from collagen matrix during bone breakdown. Another bone marker of increased bone resorption is increased urinary excretion of the pyridinium cross-link pyridinoline. Pyridinoline and *N*- and *C*-telopeptides of collagen are more specific components of bone matrix than is hydroxyproline.[23] Together the tests can provide an indication of bone disease, its progression, and its response to therapy. From a practical standpoint, measurement of serum alkaline phosphatase is used routinely, since 24-hour urine collections are difficult to obtain on a regular basis.

Serum levels of calcium and phosphorus are normal, since bone resorption and formation are closely linked. Elevations of calcium concentration occur in pagetic patients who are immobilized, who have coexistent primary hyperparathyroidism, or who have metastatic disease to bone. In rare circumstances, hypercalcemia has been reported in monostotic PD unassociated with immobilization.[8] Serum uric acid concentrations may be increased in men with extensive disease. Serum osteocalcin is a vitamin K–dependent protein that has a high affinity for hydroxyapatite, binds calcium, and is produced by osteoblasts. Osteocalcin levels have lower sensitivity and specificity than other biochemical markers for activity of PD.[20] Histocompatibility testing of a small group of patients has demonstrated a greater frequency of HLA-DR2 compared to controls.[31] This test has no diagnostic significance at this time.

Pathology

Pathologic abnormalities of early disease are characterized by an increased number of osteoclasts. Subsequently new bone is produced in a chaotic, mosaic pattern, and woven bone, as opposed to normal lamellar bone, is produced. The amount of minerals in pagetic new bone appears normal. Histologically, the bone contains irregular, broad trabeculae, with numerous osteoclasts and fibrous vascular tissue replacement of the bone marrow space (Fig. 18-1). Malignant tumors may arise in pagetoid lesions. The most common is osteosarcoma. Other neoplasms include fibrosarcoma and malignant giant cell tumor.[107]

RADIOGRAPHIC EVALUATION

Roentgenograms

Roentgenographic abnormalities vary with the stage of disease. The osteolytic phase corresponds to localized lytic lesions of bone. There is a well-demarcated area of lucency without associated bony reaction. These lesions are most commonly discovered in the skull and are referred to as *osteoporosis circumscripta*. Lytic lesions may be seen in long

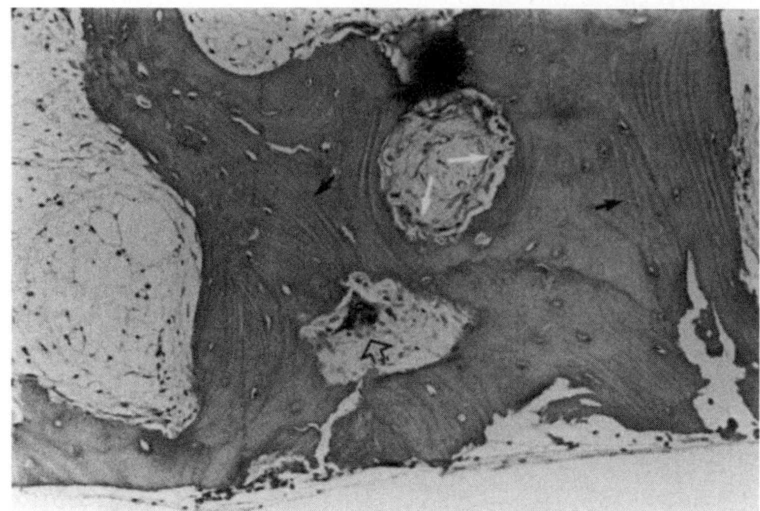

Figure 18-1 Paget's disease. Histologic section of late stage of Paget's disease exhibiting thickened trabeculae with a prominent mosaic bone pattern *(black arrows)*. Osteoblastic *(white arrows)* and osteoclastic *(open black arrow)* activity is present. *(Courtesy of Arnold Schwartz, MD.)*

bones but are rarely seen in the spine.[88] PD is monostotic in 35% of cases (Fig. 18-2).[82] Monostotic disease may also be found in the cervical spine (Fig. 18-3).

The mixed phase consists of bone sclerosis combined with osseous demineralization. The bone increases in size with greatly thickened and widely spaced trabeculae, cortical thickening, and irregularly distributed zones of increased and reduced density. A "cotton wool" appearance is a term used to describe the patchy involvement.

The sclerotic phase of disease appears as areas of homogeneous increase in bone density. This form of disease may be too difficult to distinguish clearly from the mixed form of disease.

In the spine, mixed or sclerotic radiographic changes are usually demonstrated.[106] Vertebral bodies may develop coarse, parallel, vertical striations that may simulate the appearance of a hemangioma. Increased cortical thickening at the inferior and superior vertebral borders may result in a "picture frame" appearance (Fig. 18-4). Marked osteoblastic changes may result in a homogeneously sclerotic "ivory" vertebra (Fig. 18-5). The "ivory" vertebra is usually enlarged in PD, and this helps differentiate it from metastatic disease (Fig. 18-6).[61] Compression fractures and large osteophytes may also be seen. PD may invade soft tissue and cartilage structures such as intervertebral discs. This process, causing disc space narrowing, may be entirely asymptomatic.[58]

Scintigraphy

Bone scintiscans are sensitive in detecting increased bone activity even in locations where plain radiographs are normal. In a patient with localized disease and normal biochemical parameters, a bone scan may give the only objective indication of the presence and activity of disease.[110] In a patient with PD, a positive scan in a "normal" area of skeleton suggests involvement at that location.[55] Multiple areas of increased activity also may be associated with diffuse skeletal metastases. Roentgenographic evaluation of areas of increased scintiscan activity may be able to differentiate areas with PD from those with a malignancy.[99] A characteristic appearance of a "mouse face" (increased uptake on the vertebral body, posterior elements, and the spinous processes) is most indicative of PD.[56] Response to treatment is characterized by radiographic changes in an area of normal activity on scan. PD may be noted on indium 111 white blood cell scintigraphy as "cold" areas. The cold bone defects are related to the loss of the bone marrow component in pagetic bone.[26]

Computed Tomography

Computed tomography (CT) generally is not required for the evaluation of uncomplicated PD.[84] CT demonstrates

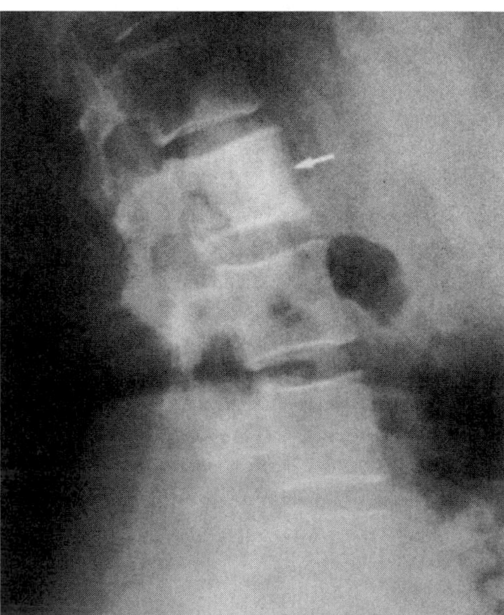

Figure 18-2 Paget's disease appearing as a monostotic lesion in the second lumbar vertebra *(arrow)*. This early lesion has vertical striations simulating a hemangioma (see Fig. 13-14). This 51-year-old woman was asymptomatic and had a normal serum alkaline phosphatase level. *(From Borenstein DG: Low back pain. In Klippel JH, Dieppe P [eds]: Rheumatology. St Louis, Mosby, 1994, p 4.18.)*

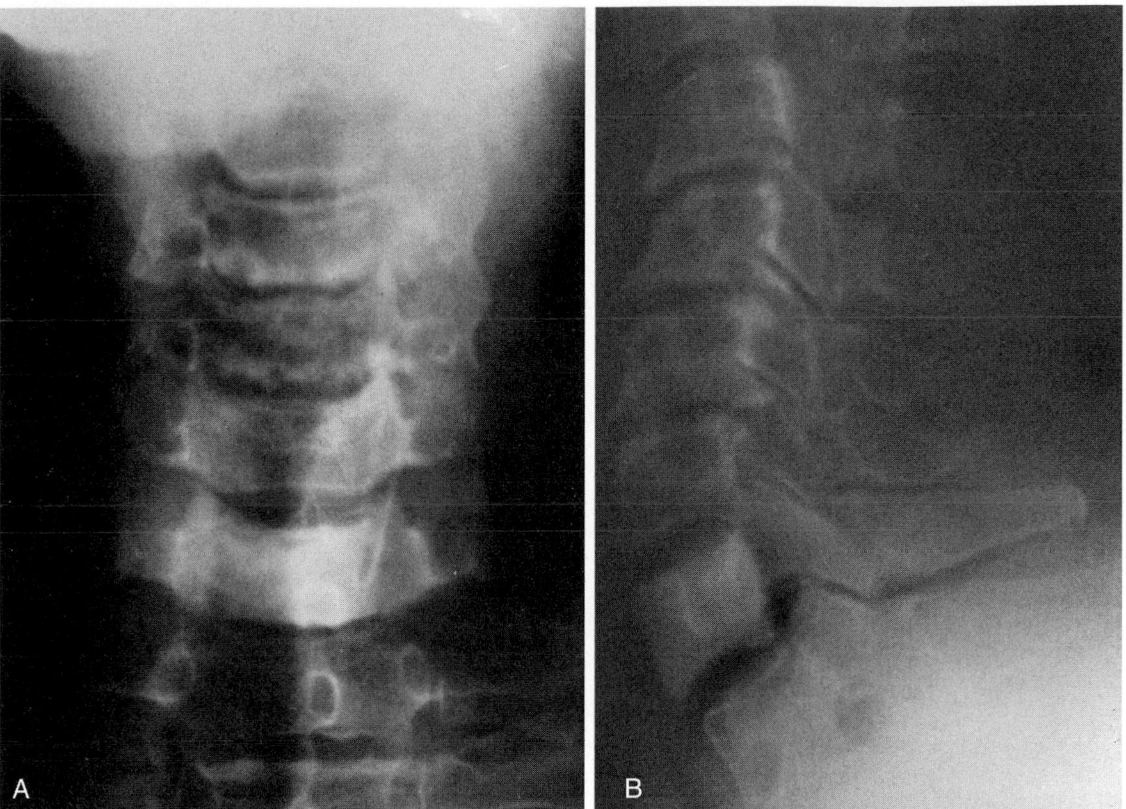

Figure 18-3 Paget's disease—"ivory" vertebra in the cervical spine. Posteroanterior *(A)* and lateral *(B)* views of the cervical spine demonstrating ivory vertebra at the C7 level. *(Courtesy of Anne Brower, MD.)*

the coarsened trabeculae of PD (Fig. 18-7). It is most useful at identifying complications of PD, including articular disease, neoplastic degeneration, and neurologic impingement secondary to vertebral involvement.[114]

Magnetic Resonance

Magnetic resonance (MR) also is not required for the diagnosis of PD. However, the frequent use of MR in a variety of skeletal conditions results in the identification of PD serendipitously. Complications of spinal stenosis secondary to PD are readily identified by MR.[86]

DIFFERENTIAL DIAGNOSIS

In most patients, the history, physical examination, and chemical, plain roentgenographic, and bone scan abnormalities are adequate to confirm the diagnosis of PD. In an occasional patient with unusual clinical or radiologic presentation, bone biopsy may be necessary to confirm the diagnosis.

The problem for the clinician may not be discovering the presence of PD in the spine but rather the association of the patient's back or neck symptoms with spinal pagetoid lesions. PD causes alterations of the lumbar spine, many of which can cause back pain (Table 18-1). Altman and associates have suggested that for a patient's symptoms to be directly related to PD and not another disorder (osteoarthritis), they should fulfill the following characteristics: (1) nonspecific low back pain without radiculopathy; (2) normal or minimal findings on examination; (3) radiographically demonstrated vertebral sclerosis (ivory vertebra) with facet sclerosis and normal disc space and facet joint; (4) bone scan revealing isolated vertebral PD; and (5) CT demonstrating an enlarged vertebra and neural arch but no facet joint arthritis or bony impingement.[6]

The differential diagnosis of PD is broad, since all lesions that may cause sclerosis of bone must be included. Diseases associated with sclerotic vertebral bodies, including metastatic tumor, lymphoma, myelofibrosis, fluorosis, mastocytosis, renal osteodystrophy, tuberous sclerosis, axial osteomalacia, and fibrogenesis imperfecta ossium, may be confused with PD. Abnormalities on physical and radiologic examination, such as hepatosplenomegaly (myelofibrosis) or anemia (metastatic tumor), help differentiate these disorders from PD. A history of renal disease along with laboratory evidence of renal failure helps with the diagnosis of renal osteodystrophy. A history of urticaria pigmentosa is common in patients with mastocytosis. Fibrous dysplasia may also cause sclerosis of vertebral bodies. A careful history, physical examination, and review of laboratory data should help the clinician in making the appropriate diagnosis.

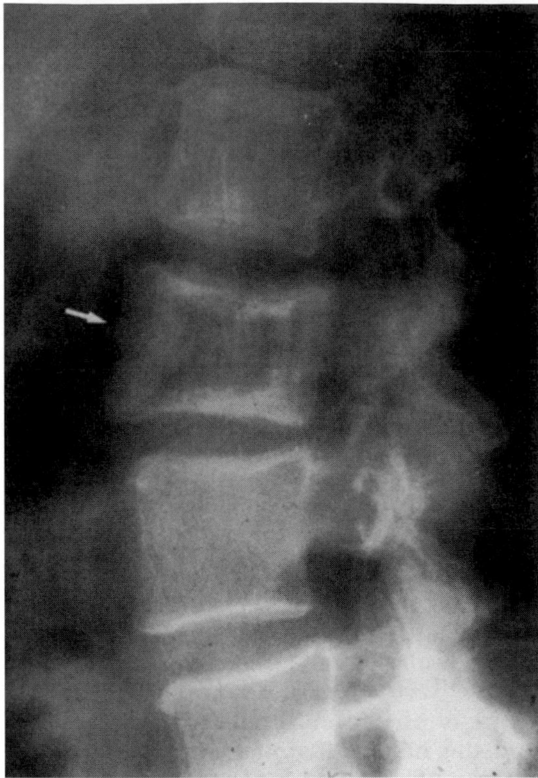

Figure 18-4 Paget's disease seen as a "picture frame" vertebral body. Lateral view demonstrates generalized enlargement of the vertebral body associated with thickening of the vertebral endplates and the cortex. Also visible are the straightening of the convexity of the anterior surface of the body *(arrow)* and thickening of the trabecular pattern. *(Courtesy of Anne Brower, MD.)*

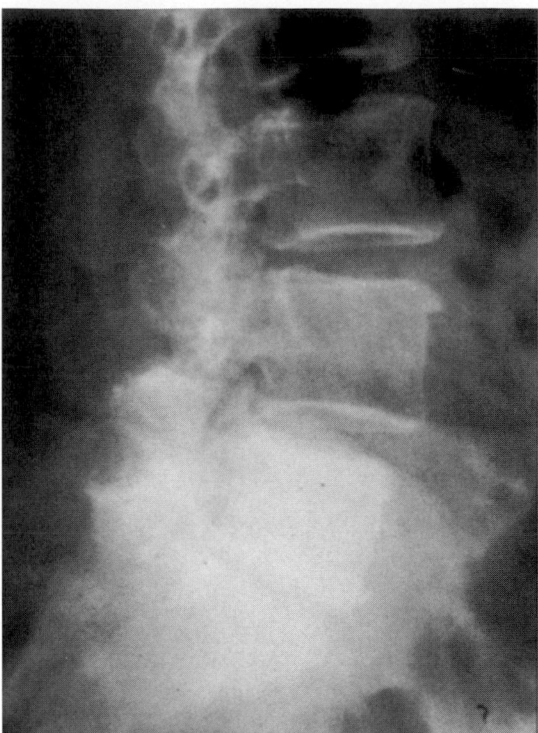

Figure 18-5 Paget's disease—"ivory" vertebra in the lumbar spine. Lateral view of the lumbar spine of a 72-year-old black woman with a 3-year history of low back and right leg pain. Abnormal findings include narrowing of the L5–S1 disc space and dense sclerosis of the L5 vertebral body. Craig needle biopsy revealed Paget's disease. *(Courtesy of Randall Lewis, MD.)*

Fibrous Dysplasia

Fibrous dysplasia is a developmental anomaly of the bone-forming mesenchymal tissue of bone that may occur in a monostotic or polyostotic form. It was first described by Lichtenstein in 1938.[62] It also may be associated with endocrine abnormalities (precocious female development) and café au lait spots, which is associated with Albright's syndrome and neurofibromatosis.[2] The diverse metabolic abnormalities arise from cells that respond to extracellular signals through the activation of the hormone-sensitive adenylyl cyclase system.[65] McCune-Albright syndrome may occur secondary to a mutation of the gene encoding a subunit of the stimulatory G protein of adenylyl cyclase.[98] Being a developmental abnormality, this illness is usually diagnosed in adolescents, particularly if they suffer from polyostotic lesions. Occasionally, patients with monostotic lesions are not discovered to have fibrous dysplasia until adulthood. In the skeleton, the pelvis is involved in 80% of patients and the axial skeleton in 8% of patients with polyostotic disease.[70] Bone involvement may be associated with localized pain if the lesion is large or if a pathologic fracture occurs. Neurologic deficits, including paralysis, have been described in association with vertebral compression, osseous expansion, or fibrous tissue extending into the spinal canal.[28] Fibrous dysplasia causes the replacement of normal bone with a slow-growing mass of fibrous tissue and woven bone, which leads to expansion of bone that is structurally weak

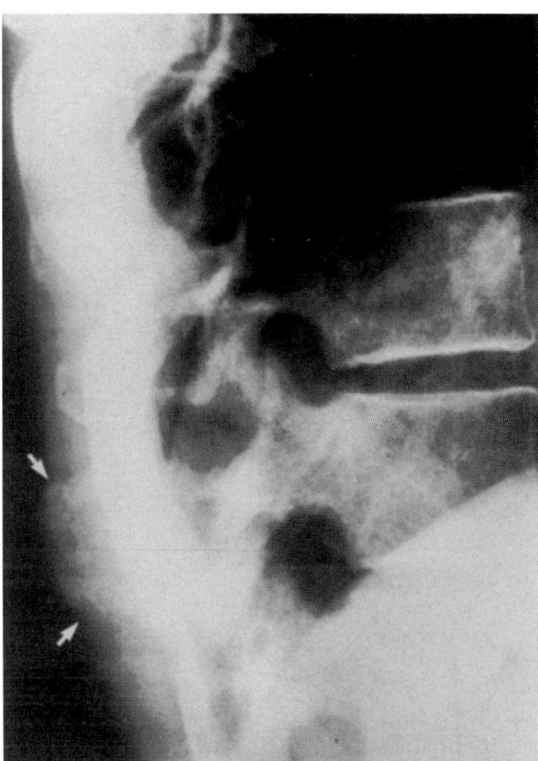

Figure 18-6 Paget's disease—expanded bone. Lateral view of the lumbar spine in a 60-year-old white man with an expanded spinous process of T12 *(white arrows)*. This isolated lesion was asymptomatic. *(Courtesy of Randall Lewis, MD.)*

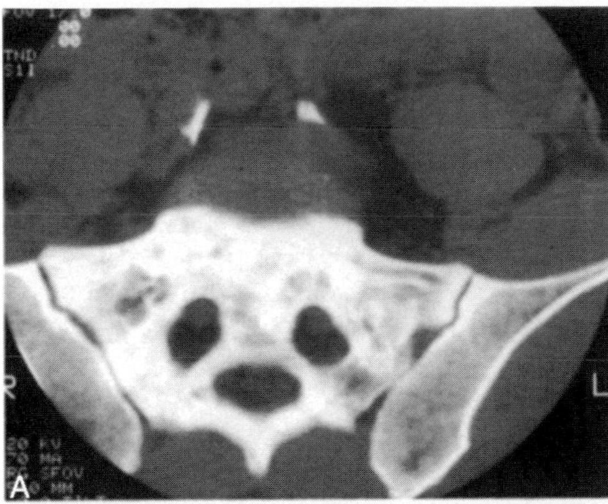

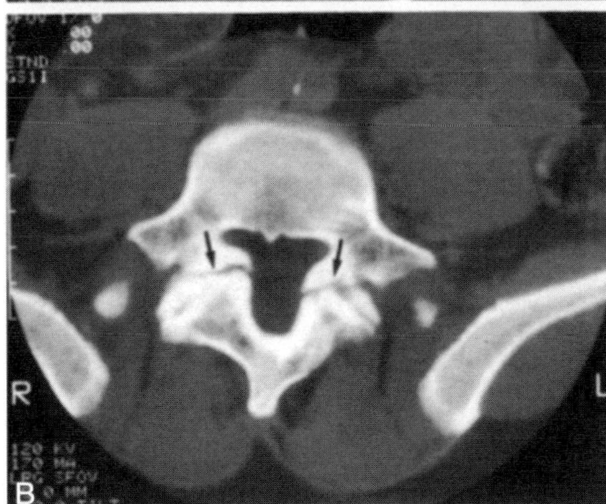

Figure 18-7 Paget's disease. CT scan of the sacrum *(A)* and fifth lumbar vertebral body *(B)* of a 61-year-old white man with a history of parathyroid adenoma with hyperparathyroidism, prostatic hypertrophy, and right sacral and anterior thigh pain. Pelvic radiographs and bone scan were suggestive of Paget's disease. The axial view of the sacrum *(A)* demonstrated replacement of normal trabecular pattern with hyperdense bony pattern compatible with Paget's disease. At level L5 *(B)*, a spondylolysis *(black arrows)* is surrounded by reactive sclerosis that is not Paget's disease. His back and leg pain were responsive to nonsteroidal anti-inflammatory therapy, suggesting a mechanical source of his pain.

and results in marked deformity. A helpful test in differentiating fibrous dysplasia from PD is measurement of the alkaline phosphatase levels, which is minimally elevated in a minority of patients with fibrous dysplasia in contrast with the markedly elevated levels in PD. The radiographic features of fibrous dysplasia include a radiolucent, "ground-glass" appearance of the bone. These areas are bordered by a sclerotic rim (Fig. 18-8). The interior of the bone contains variable amounts of calcification and bony septa. Vertebral changes may show deformed vertebral bodies or posterior elements with variable areas of lucency and cysts (Fig. 18-9).[83] Monostotic fibrous dysplasia of the spine has been reported.[52,66] The bone scan is not helpful in differentiating fibrous dysplasia from PD.[27] MR reveals an expanded bone contour, a decreased signal on T1-weighted image, and variable signal on T2-weighted images. MR is most helpful in determining the extent of fibrous dysplasia within an affected bone.[108] The age of the patient (<30 years in fibrous dysplasia vs. >30 years in PD) and the radiographic and alkaline phosphatase differences should allow the differentiation of these diseases.

TREATMENT

Most patients with PD are asymptomatic and do not require therapy. Indications for treatment include disabling bone pain that is not relieved with NSAIDs, progressive skeletal deformity with frequent fractures, vertebral compression, acetabular protrusion, neurologic complications, deafness, high-output congestive heart failure, or immobilization. A variety of oral, injectable, and intravenous therapies are available for the treatment of PD (Table 18-2).

Calcitonin

None of the three classes of agents used for PD to produce symptomatic improvement and better control of bone

18-1 MANIFESTATIONS OF LUMBAR SPINE PAGET'S DISEASE

Anatomic Part	Mechanism	Clinical Correlate
Vertebra	Total enlargement	Altered lordosis/scoliosis
	Posterior element enlargement	Spinal stenosis/paraplegia
	Uneven subchondral enlargement (disc fracture)	Degenerative disc
	Enlargement stressing ligamentous attachment	Osteophytes
	Spinal osteoporosis, fibrous replacement, bone weakening	Compression fractures (kyphosis)
	Hypervascularity	Paraplegia (spinal artery steal syndrome)
Neural arch	Medial facet enlargement	Lateral recess syndrome, stenosis, loss or reversal of lordosis
	Facet joint enlargement	Facet osteoarthritis
	Altered joint congruity	
Spinal ligaments	Ligamentous calcifications	
	Ankylosing hyperostosis form	Back pain?
	Ankylosing spondylitis form	Back pain?
Any bone	Sarcomatous degeneration	Severe pain
	Metastatic disease to hypervascular bone	Severe pain
Pelvis	Protrusion acetabulae with hip flexion contractures	Forward bend to trunk
Lower extremity	Tibial bowing	Forward or altered pelvic tilt, abnormal gait, muscle spasm

Modified from Altman R: Low back pain in Paget's disease of bone. Clin Orthop 217:152, 1987.

metabolism cures the illness.[47] Calcitonin, a polypeptide hormone from the parafollicular cells of the thyroid gland, slows osteoclastic bone resorption. Injection of 50 to 100 IU of calcitonin three or more times per week results in a gradual decrease in serum alkaline phosphatase to about half of the initial elevated concentrations and resolution of bone pain; however, patients may develop antibodies to calcitonin, which abrogates its beneficial effects.[24] Salmon calcitonin is the most commonly used form of calcitonin and the type most commonly associated with antibody production. Human calcitonin differs from salmon calcitonin at 16 of the 32 amino acid sites.[49] Anti–salmon calcitonin antibodies do not bind human calcitonin. Patients resistant to salmon calcitonin have responded to human calcitonin.[7] Intranasal salmon calcitonin is available for the treatment of PD.[21] Intranasal calcitonin is more convenient than parenteral calcitonin, but the efficacy relative to parenteral calcitonin remains to be determined. The absence of side effects is probably related to the 60% reduction in plasma levels obtained from intranasal installation compared to the same dose given by subcutaneous injection. Intranasal doses of 200 to 400 IU daily are

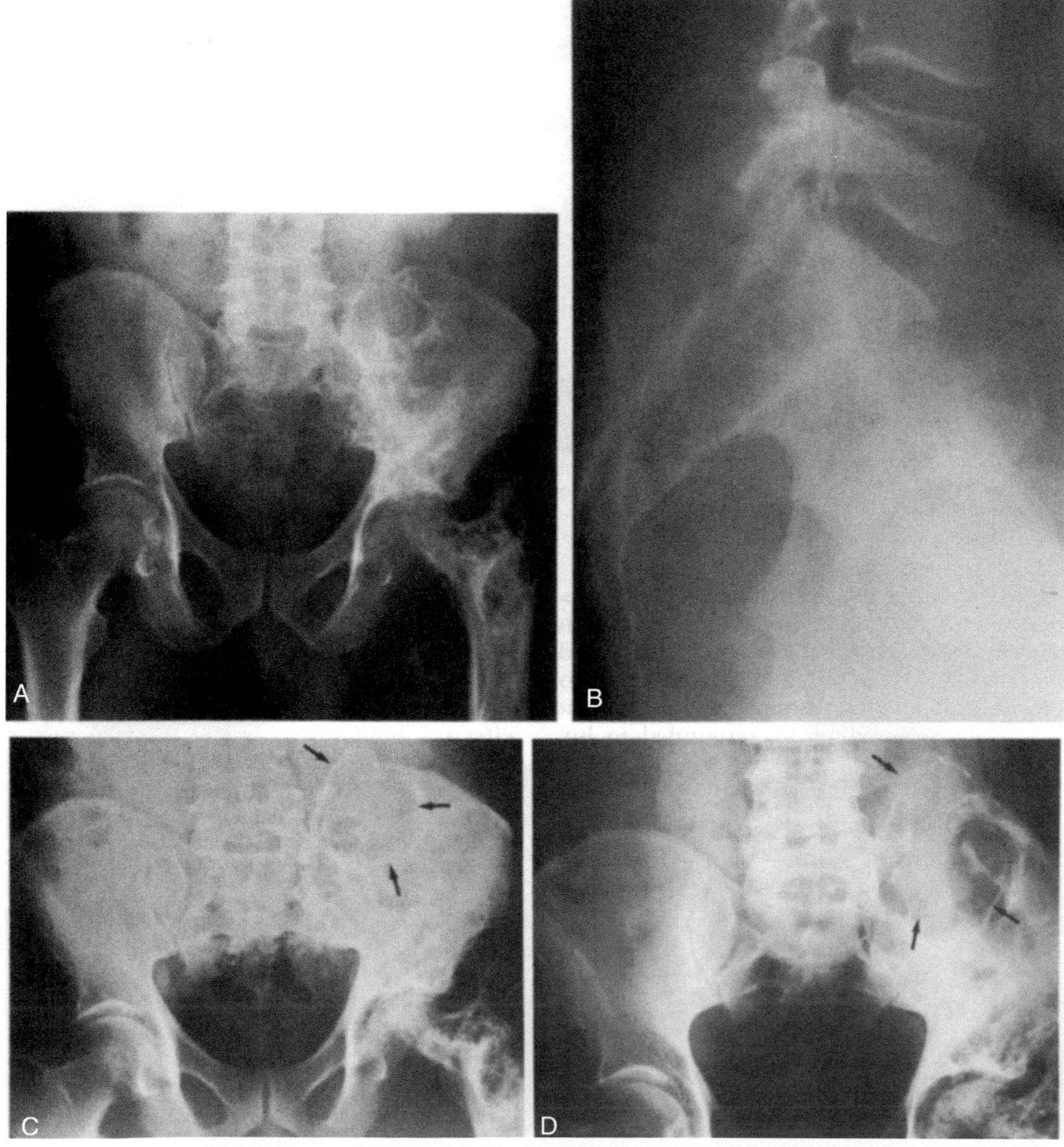

Figure 18-8 Fibrous dysplasia. Anteroposterior (AP) *(A)* and lateral *(B)* views of the pelvis of a 56-year-old black man with left-sided back and leg pain. An expansile lesion with areas of sclerosis is present involving the left hemipelvis and left femur. The alkaline phosphatase level of this patient was normal. The patient's symptoms improved with a heel lift for a leg-length discrepancy and indomethacin 75 mg every evening. These radiographs were obtained in 1983. *C* is an AP view of the pelvis taken in 1988. The left hemipelvis has increased in size. The superior rim of the left pelvis *(black arrows)* has expanded the cortex, which is compatible with an aneurysmal bone cyst. The patient complained of left buttock pain. *D* is an AP view of the pelvis taken in 1991. The area of the aneurysmal bone cyst has expanded. The patient complained of an enlarging mass that was warm to the touch that expanded intermittently.

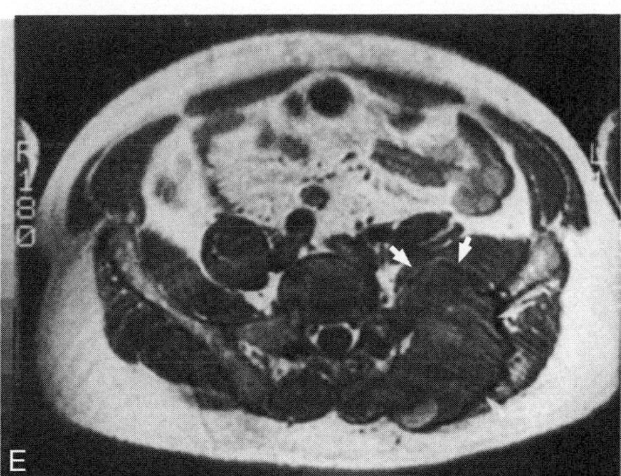

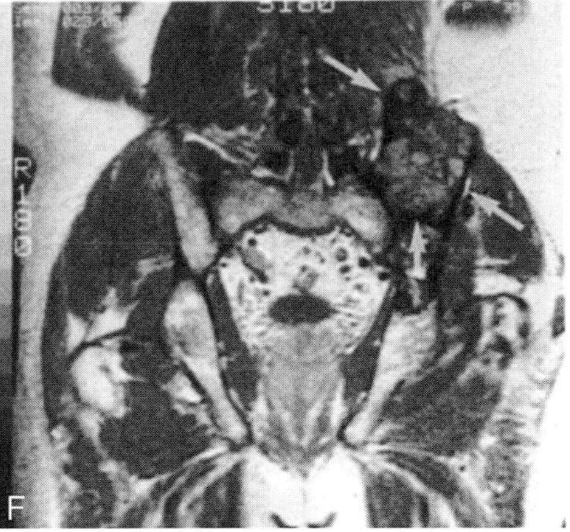

Figure 18-8, cont'd *E,* MR exam of the pelvis, axial T1-weighted image, demonstrates a huge expansile lesion in the left ilium *(white arrows). F,* MR coronal view of pelvis demonstrates extensive involvement of the left ilium with a mixed signal abnormality compatible with fibrous dysplasia *(white arrows).* As of 1993, the lesion is cool to touch on physical examination and had not expanded further. The patient's symptoms are controlled with indomethacin 75 mg twice a day.

needed to decrease bone turnover.[16] Intranasal calcitonin produces a maximum reduction in bone turnover of 30% to 40% after 6 months of therapy. Calcitonin in either form is effective in reducing bone-related pain. Pain relief onset occurs within 2 weeks and may be sustained for months.

Toxicities of calcitonin occur in 20% to 30% of patients, manifested by nausea and flushing. These effects may be minimized by injecting calcitonin after dinner.

Figure 18-9 Fibrous dysplasia of the vertebral bodies and posterior elements. The bones have multiple lytic lesions caused by the fibrous replacement. *(Courtesy of Anne Brower, MD.)*

Other symptoms include vomiting, diarrhea, and abdominal pain.

Bisphosphonates

Bisphosphonates are structural analogues of pyrophosphate that, when ingested by osteoclasts, decrease the osteoclast's ability to resorb bone. In addition, to a variable extent, they interfere with the mineralization of normal bone, and this limits the dose and duration of a course of bisphosphonate therapy. Bisphosphonates are given at a dose of 5 mg/kg/day for 6 months of the year. Some physicians give a course for a 6-month period and discontinue therapy for 6 months, while others give therapy every other month for 6 months and then re-evaluate the response. Bisphosphonates may increase the tendency of PD to develop pathologic fractures.[16] Etidronate was a commonly used bisphosphonate before more easily administered bisphosphonates became available.

Pamidronate, an aminohydroxypropilidene bisphosphonate, has been used in the United States for intravenous treatment of hypercalcemia associated with malignancy.[74] In Europe, pamidronate is used regularly for the control of PD. The drug may be used orally or intravenously. As opposed to other bisphosphonates, pamidronate inhibits bone resorption without any significant detrimental effect on bone growth and mineralization.[30] Pamidronate decreases serum alkaline phosphatase to near-normal values, almost completely relieves bone pain, and maintains the response for 6 months or longer after the cessation of therapy.[64] A single intravenous infusion of 60 mg administered over 4 hours may be adequate for those with mild disease. Repeated doses of 60 mg are infused over 4 hours administered consecutively for 3 days, weekly, or monthly for those with more severe disease. The infusions may be repeated every 3 to 18 months, depending on response. The dose range of pamidronate has been between 300 and 1200 mg/day. An oral dose of 600 mg/day has been associated with low back pain relief in 56% of 156 patients with PD but is not

18-2 RECOMMENDED THERAPY FOR PAGET'S DISEASE

Drug	Dose	Duration	Effect
INITIAL			
Pamidronate	30–60 mg IV/day	3 days	80% decrease in alkaline phosphatase level
Alendronate	40 mg/day	6 months	80% decrease in alkaline phosphatase level
Risedronate	30 mg/day	3 months	80% decrease in alkaline phosphatase level
SECONDARY			
Calcitonin (salmon)	50 U SC daily first week, then 100 U SC daily 6 months, then 100 U SC three times a week	Indefinite	50% decrease in alkaline phosphatase level; escape of efficacy related to neutralizing antibodies
Calcitonin (human)	50 U SC daily first week, then 100 U SC daily 6 months, then 100 U SC three times a week	Indefinite	50% decrease in alkaline phosphatase level Nausea, flushing more common than for salmon calcitonin

IV, intravenous; SC, subcutaneous.
Modified from Siris ES: Paget's disease of bone. J Clin Endocrinol Metab 80:335-338, 1995. ©The Endocrine Society; and Delmas PD, Meunier PJ: The management of Paget's disease of bone. N Engl J Med 336:558-566, 1997.

available in the United States.[42] Hypocalcemia, with tetany, may occur with high-dose pamidronate therapy. Ingestion of 1000 mg calcium daily for 1 to 2 weeks after the infusion diminishes the risk of this toxicity. Doses of pamidronate higher than 180 mg may result in bone mineralization defects.[1]

Alendronate and risedronate are other bisphosphonates with efficacy against PD. Alendronate is administered at 40 mg/day for 6 months, whereas risedronate is taken at a dose of 30 mg/day for 2 months.[35] In studies compared to placebo or etidronate, alendronate has a greater reduction and a greater frequency of normalization of alkaline phosphatase.[81,101] Radiologic improvement in osteolysis was 48% in the alendronate group and 4% in the placebo group.[81] Risedronate also has efficacy in decreasing serum alkaline phosphatase compared to editronate.[68] In a study of 179 PD patients, the relapse rates were 3% for the risedronate group and 15% for the etidronate group. Reduction in pain was also greater in the risedronate group.

A number of bisphosphonates are currently available (clodronate, tiludronate, zoledronate) or are being studied (ibandronate) for the treatment of PD.[35,47,80] An inadequate response to a bisphosphonate does not preclude an excellent response to another.[37] The availability of additional bisphosphonates will allow for more specific therapy for individuals who may not tolerate oral medicines or who are resistant to intravenous drugs.

Bisphosphonate therapy has been shown to cause improvement of symptoms in 60% or more of patients even in the presence of secondary osteoarthritis.[4] Bisphosphonates may be helpful in patients with low back pain secondary to PD alone or to PD and associated osteoarthritis.[6]

Mithramycin

Mithramycin is an antibiotic that binds to DNA and inhibits RNA synthesis. It has a cytotoxic effect on osteoclasts and is used as a treatment for hypercalcemia related to cancer. The drug is potent and rapidly effective, but, since it is associated with toxicity, it cannot be used as a first-line agent.[93] It is administered intravenously to patients with progressive neurologic compression syndromes secondary to PD. Pamidronate may control hypercalcemia with less toxicity than mithramycin.

Other therapies used for PD include gallium nitrate. Gallium nitrate inhibits bone resorption by inhibiting the adenosine triphosphate–dependent proton pump of osteoclasts. One study of 49 patients with advanced disease suggested that a cyclical regimen (doses of 0.25 to 0.5 mg/kg/day) may be effective in patients who had previously received moderate to extensive treatment with other drugs.[14] This agent is associated with a beneficial effect on the clinical symptoms and biochemical parameters of PD.[109]

Goals for Treatment

The current therapy for PD is more potent than etidronate and calcitonin. The current therapy is able to reduce activity indices of bone turnover by 80%. A majority of patients achieve biochemical remission, and the duration of remission may exceed 1 year or more with a single course of therapy. The new bone formed is lamellar in appearance but with no mineralization abnormality.[103]

Physicians usually use one agent at a time, following the patient's symptoms, serum alkaline phosphatase, and bone activity on bone scan. A single agent should normalize biochemical indices, primarily alkaline phosphatase since hydroxyproline, pyridinolines, and telopeptides do not adequately follow response to therapy.[13] Many have remission of their disease after a course of therapy and may not need to resume the drug for an extended period. More complete biochemical suppression is associated with more prolonged clinical remission not requiring a resumption of therapy.[36] The alkaline phosphatase level should be measured every 4 to 6 months after a course of therapy. Retreatment is indicated if indices rise above the upper limit of normal or by 25% above the previous nadir. Patients with persistent neurologic syndromes may require a combination of agents for adequate control.[48]

Surgical intervention is not required as frequently with the advent of more effective medical therapy. Surgical therapy is useful for weight-bearing joint replacement and decompressive laminectomy for spinal stenosis. Complications of surgery on pagetic bone include hemorrhage, infection, pathologic fracture, delayed union, nonunion, and aseptic loosening of joint replacements.[54] In rare circumstances, surgical amputation or limb salvage reconstruction of a limb is necessary because of the very aggressive nature of osteosarcoma associated with PD.[43]

PROGNOSIS

Most patients with PD have an asymptomatic illness. In others, more active disease can usually be controlled with NSAIDs and agents that modify bone metabolism. Patients with PD uncomplicated by osteoarthritis may respond to a combination of calcitonin and bisphosphonates or bisphosphonates alone.[18,51] Improvement may be manifested by a decrease in bone scintiscan activity. However, complete resolution of increased activity is unusual.[92] The complications of PD that cause disability and mortality are rare. Occasionally patients develop neurologic symptoms from spinal cord compression. Increased drug therapy or laminectomy can be effective in controlling these complications. Malignant transformation of PD is associated with a very poor prognosis but is fortunately a rare occurrence. The most common site of tumor is the femur, with the proximal humerus second most frequent. In a series of 22 cases of sarcoma complicating PD, one patient had involvement of the sacrum and another, the thoracic spine.[71] Sarcoma occurred in areas of advanced disease and presented as a destructive lesion without periosteal reaction. The 5-year survival is 15% of patients.[45]

References

Paget's Disease of Bone

1. Adamson BB, Gallacher SJ, Byars J, et al: Mineralisation defects with pamidronate therapy for Paget's disease. Lancet 342:1459-1460, 1993.
2. Albright F, Butler AM, Hampton AO, Smith P: Syndrome characterized by osteitis fibrosa disseminata, areas of pigmentation, and endocrine dysfunction with precocious puberty in females. N Engl J Med 216:727, 1937.
3. Altman R: Arthritis in Paget's disease of bone. J Bone Miner Res 14(suppl 2):85-87, 1999.
4. Altman RD: Long-term follow-up of therapy with intermittent etidronate disodium in Paget's disease of bone. Am J Med 79:583, 1985.
5. Altman RD: Musculoskeletal manifestations of Paget's disease of bone. Arthritis Rheum 23:1121, 1980.
6. Altman RD, Brown M, Gargano GA: Low back pain in Paget's disease of bone. Clin Orthop 217:152, 1987.
7. Altman RD, Collins-Yudiskas B: Synthetic human calcitonin in refractory Paget's disease of bone. Arch Intern Med 147:1305, 1987.
8. Bannister P, Roberts M, Sheridan P: Recurrent hypercalcemia in a young man with mono-ostotic Paget's disease. Postgrad Med J 62:481, 1986.
9. Barker DJ: The epidemiology of Paget's disease of bone. Metab Bone Dis 3:231, 1981.
10. Barry HC: Paget's Disease of Bone. Edinburgh, E & S Livingstone, 1969.
11. Bataille R: Etiology of Paget's disease of bone: A new perspective [Letter]. Calcif Tissue Int 50:293, 1992.
12. Beedles KE, Sharpe PT, Wagner EF, et al: A putative rule for c-*fos* in pathophysiology of Paget's disease. J Bone Miner Res 14(suppl 2):21-28, 1999.
13. Blumsohn A, Naylor KE, Assiri AMA, et al: Different responses of biochemical markers of bone resorption to bisphosphonate therapy in Paget's disease. Clin Chem 41:1592-1598, 1995.
14. Bockman RS, Wilhelm F, Siris E, et al: A multicenter trial of low-dose gallium nitrate in patients with advanced Paget's disease of bone. J Clin Endocrinol Metab 80:595, 1995.
15. Brown HP, LaRocca H, Wickstrom JK: Paget's disease of the atlas and axis. J Bone Joint Surg Am 53:1441, 1971.
16. Canfield R, Rosner W, Skinner J, et al: Diphosphonate therapy of Paget's disease of bone. J Clin Endocrinol Metab 44:96, 1977.
17. Chen J, Rhee RSC, Wallach S, et al: Neurologic disturbances in Paget diseases of bone: Response to calcitonin. Neurology 29:448, 1979.
18. Chines A, Villareal D, Pacifici R: Paget's disease of bone affecting a single vertebra: Clinical, radiologic, and histopathologic correlations. Calcif Tissue Int 50:115, 1992.
19. Collins DH: Paget's disease of bone: Incidence and subclinical forms. Lancet 2:51, 1956.
20. Coulton LA, Preston CJ, Couch M, Kanis JA: An evaluation of serum osteocalcin in Paget's disease of bone and its response to diphosphonate treatment. Arthritis Rheum 31:1142, 1988.
21. D'Agostino HR, Barnett CA, Zielinski XJ, Gordan GS: Intranasal salmon calcitonin treatment of Paget's disease of bone: Results in nine patients. Clin Orthop 230:223, 1988.
22. de Deuxchaisnes CN, Krane SM: Paget's disease of bone: Clinical and metabolic observations. Medicine 43:233, 1964.
23. Delmas PD, Meunier PJ: The management of Paget's disease of bone. N Engl J Med 336:558-566, 1997.
24. De Rose NJ, Singer FR, Avramides A, et al: Response of Paget's disease to porcine and salmon calcitonins: Effects of long-term treatment. Am J Med 56:858, 1974.
25. Dinneen SF, Buckley TF: Spinal nerve root compression due to monostotic Paget's disease of a lumber vertebra. Spine 12:948, 1987.
26. Dunn EK, Vaquer RA, Strashun AM: Paget's disease: A cause of photopenic skeletal defect in indium 111 WBC scintigraphy. J Nucl Med 29:561, 1988.
27. Ehara S, Kattapuram SV, Rosenberg AE: Fibrous dysplasia of the spine. Spine 17:977, 1992.
28. Feldman F: Tuberous sclerosis, neurofibromatosis, and fibrous dysplasia. In Resnick D, Niwayama G (eds): Diagnosis of Bone and Joint Disorders, 2nd ed. Philadelphia, WB Saunders, 1988, pp 4057-4072.
29. Feldman F, Seaman WB: The neurologic complications of Paget's disease in the cervical spine. AJR Am J Roentgenol 105:375, 1969.
30. Fitton A, McTavish D: Pamidronate: A review of its pharmacological properties and therapeutic efficacy in resorptive bone disease. Drugs 41:289, 1991.
31. Foldes J, Shamir S, Brautbar C, et al: HLA-D antigens and Paget's disease of bone. Clin Orthop 266:301, 1991.
32. Frank WA, Bress NM, Singer FR, Krane SM: Rheumatic manifestations of Paget's disease of bone. Am J Med 56:592, 1974.
33. Freeman DA: Southwestern Internal Medicine Conference: Paget's disease of bone. Am J Med Sci 295:144, 1988.
34. Good D, Busfield F, Duffy D, et al: Familial Paget's disease of bone: Nonlinkage to the PDB1 and PDB2 loci on chromosomes 6p and 18q in a large pedigree. J Bone Miner Res 16:33, 2001.
35. Grauer A, Bone H, McCloskey E, et al: Newer bisphosphonates in the treatment of Paget's disease of bone: Where we are and where we want to go. J Bone Miner Res 14(Suppl 2):74-78, 1999.
36. Gray RE, Yates AJ, Preston CJ, et al: Duration of effect of oral diphosphonate therapy in Paget's disease of bone. Q J Med 64:755, 1987.
37. Gutteridge DH, Ward LC, Stewart GO, et al: Paget's disease: Acquired resistance to one aminobisphosphonate with retained response to another. J Bone Miner Res 14(Suppl 2):79, 1999.
38. Guyer PB: Paget's disease of bone: The anatomical distribution. Metab Bone Dis 4:239, 1981.
39. Hadjipavlou A, Lander P: Paget disease of the spine. J Bone Joint Surg Am 73:1376, 1991.

40. Hadjipavlou A, Shaffer N, Lander P, Srolovitz H: Pagetic spinal stenosis with extradural pagetoid ossification: A case report. Spine 13:128, 1988.
41. Hanna JW, Ball MR, Lee KS, McWhorter JM: Spontaneous spinal epidural hematoma complicating Paget's disease of the spine. Spine 14:900, 1989.
42. Harinck HI, Bijvoet OL, Blanksma HJ, Dahlinghaus-Nienhuys PJ: Efficacious management with aminobisphosphonate (APD) in Paget's disease of bone. Clin Orthop 217:79, 1987.
43. Harrington KD: Surgical management of neoplastic complications of Paget's disease. J Bone Miner Res 14(Suppl 2):45-48, 1999.
44. Haslam SI, Hul WV, Morales-Piga A, et al: Paget's disease of bone: Evidence for a susceptibility locus on chromosome 18q and for genetic heterogeneity. J Bone Miner Res 13:911-917, 1998.
45. Healey JH, Buss D: Radiation and pagetic osteogenic sarcomas. Clin Orthop 270:128, 1991.
46. Hepgul K, Nicoll JA, Coakham HB: Spinal cord compression due to pagetic spinal stenosis with involvement of extradural soft tissues: A case report. Surg Neurol 35:143, 1991.
47. Hosking DJ: Advances in the management of Paget's disease of bone. Drugs 40:829, 1990.
48. Hosking DJ, Bijovoet OL, van Aken J, Will EJ: Paget's bone disease treated with diphosphonate and calcitonin. Lancet 1:615, 1976.
49. Human calcitonin for Paget's disease. Med Lett Drugs Ther 29:47, 1987.
50. Janetos GP: Paget's disease in the cervical spine. AJR Am J Roentgenol 97:655, 1966.
51. Jawad ASM, Berry H: Spinal cord compression in Paget's disease of bone treated medically. J R Soc Med 80:319, 1987.
52. Kahn A, Rosenberg PS: Monostotic fibrous dysplasia of the lumbar spine. Spine 13:592, 1988.
53. Kahn AJ: The viral etiology of Paget's disease of bone: A new perspective [Editorial]. Calcif Tissue Int 47:127, 1990.
54. Kaplan FS: Surgical management of Paget's disease. J Bone Miner Res 14(Suppl 2):34-83, 1999.
55. Khairi MR, Wellman HN, Robb JA, Johnston CC Jr: Paget's disease of bone (osteitis deformans): Symptomatic lesions and bone scan. Ann Intern Med 79:348, 1973.
56. Kim CK, Estrada WN, Lorberboym M, et al: The "mouseface" appearance of the vertebrae in Paget's disease. Clin Nucl Med 22:104-108, 1997.
57. Kukita A, Chenu C, McManus LM, et al: Atypical multinucleated cells form in long-term marrow cultures from patients with Paget's disease. J Clin Invest 85:1280, 1990.
58. Lander P, Hadjipavlou A: Intradiscal invasion of Paget's disease of the spine. Spine 16:26, 1991.
59. Laurin N, Brown JP, Lemainque A, et al: Paget's disease of bone: Mapping of two loci at 5q35-qter and 5q31. Am J Hum Genet 69:528-543, 2001.
60. Leach RJ, Singer FR, Cody JD, et al: Variable disease severity associated with a Paget's disease predisposition gene. J Bone Miner Res 14(Suppl 2):17-20, 1999.
61. Lewis RJ, Jacobs B, Marchisello PJ, Bullough PG: Monostatic Paget's disease of the spine. Clin Orthop 127:208, 1977.
62. Lichtenstein L: Polyostotic fibrous dysplasia. Arch Surg 36:874, 1938.
63. Lluberas-Acosta G, Hansell JR, Schumacher HR Jr: Paget's disease of bone in patients with gout. Arch Intern Med 146:2389, 1986.
64. Mallette LE: Successful treatment of resistant Paget's disease of bone with pamidronate. Arch Intern Med 149:2765, 1989.
65. Mansfield FL: Case records of the Massachusetts General Hospital. N Engl J Med 328:1836, 1993.
66. Marks KE, Bauer TW: Fibrous tumors of bone. Orthop Clin North Am 20:377, 1989.
67. Mawhinney R, Jones R, Worthington BS: Spinal cord compression secondary to Paget's disease of the axis. Br J Radiol 58:1203, 1985.
68. Miller PD, Brown JP, Siris ES, et al: A randomized, double-blind comparison of risedronate and etidronate in the treatment of Paget's disease of bone. Am J Med 106:513-520, 1999.
69. Mills BG, Fausto A, Singer FR, et al: Multinucleated cells formed in vitro from Paget's bone marrow express viral antigens. Bone 15:443-448, 1994.
70. Mirra JM: Bone Tumors: Clinical, Radiologic, and Pathologic Correlations. Philadelphia, Lea & Febiger, 1989, pp 191-226.
71. Moore TE, King AR, Kathol MH, et al: Sarcoma in Paget disease of bone: Clinical, radiologic, and pathologic features in 22 cases. AJR Am J Roentgenol 156:1199, 1991.
72. Nichjolson DA, Roberts T, Sanville PR: Spinal cord compression in Paget's disease due to extradural pagetic ossification. Br J Radiol 64:864, 1991.
73. Paget J: On a form of chronic inflammation of bones (osteitis deformans). Trans R Chir Soc London 60:37, 1877.
74. Pamidronate. Med Lett Drugs Ther 34:1, 1992.
75. Polednak AP: Rates of Paget's disease of bone among hospital discharges, by age and sex. J Am Geriatr Soc 35:550, 1987.
76. Poncelet A: The neurologic complications of Paget's disease. J Bone Miner Res 14(Suppl 2):88-91, 1999.
77. Ralston SH, Digiovine FS, Gallacher SJ, et al: Failure to detect paramyxovirus sequences in Paget's disease of bone using the polymerase chain reaction. J Bone Miner Res 6:1243, 1991.
78. Ramamurthi B, Visvanathan GS: Paget's disease of the axis causing quadriplegia. J Neurosurg 14:580, 1957.
79. Reddy SV, Menaa C, Singer FR, et al: Cell biology of Paget's disease. J Bone Miner Res 14(Suppl 2):3-8, 1999.
80. Reginster JY, Colson F, Morlock G, et al: Evaluation of the efficacy and safety of oral tiludronate in Paget's disease of bone: A double-blind, multiple-dosage, placebo-controlled study. Arthritis Rheum 35:967, 1992.
81. Reid IR, Nicholson GC, Weinstein RS, et al: Biochemical and radiologic improvement in Paget's disease of bone treated with alendronate: A randomized, placebo-controlled trial. Am J Med 171:341-348, 1996.
82. Resnick D: Paget disease of bone: Current status and a look back to 1943 and earlier. AJR Am J Roentgenol 150:249, 1988.
83. Resnick D, Niwayama G: Tuberous sclerosis, neurofibromatosis and fibrous dysplasia. In Feldman F: Diagnosis of Bone and Joint Disorders. Philadelphia, WB Saunders, 1981, pp 2949-2961.
84. Resnick D, Niwayama G: Paget's disease. In Resnick D, Niwayama G (eds): Diagnosis of Bone and Joint Disorders, 2nd ed. Philadelphia, WB Saunders, 1988, pp 2127-2170.
85. Richter RL, Semble EL, Turner RA, Challa VR: An unusual manifestation of Paget's disease of bone: Spinal epidural hematoma presenting as acute cauda equina syndrome. J Rheumatol 17:975, 1990.
86. Roberts MC, Kressel HY, Fallon MD, et al: Paget disease: MR imaging findings. Radiology 173:341, 1989.
87. Roodman GD, Kukihara N, Ohsaki Y, et al: Interleukin 6: A potential autocrine/paracrine factor in Paget's disease of bone. J Clin Invest 89:46, 1992.
88. Rosen MA, Matasar KW, Irwin RB, et al: Osteolytic monostotic Paget's disease of the fifth lumbar vertebra: A case report. Clin Orthop 262:119, 1991.
89. Rosen MA, Wesolowski DP, Herkowitz HN: Osteolytic monostotic Paget's disease of the axis: A case report. Spine 13:125, 1988.
90. Rosenkrantz JA, Wolfe J, Karcher JJ: Paget's disease (osteitis deformans). Arch Intern Med 90:610, 1952.
91. Rosenthal MJ, Hartnell JM, Kaiser FE, et al: Paget's disease of bone in older patients. Am J Geriatr Soc 37:639, 1989.
92. Ryan PJ, Gibson T, Fogelman I: Bone scintigraphy following intravenous pamidronate for Paget's disease of bone. J Nucl Med 33:1589, 1992.
93. Ryan W, Schwartz TB, Perlia CP: Effects of mithramycin on Paget's disease of bone. Ann Intern Med 70:549, 1969.
94. Schajowicz F, Velan O, Araujo ES, et al: Metastases of carcinoma in the pagetic bone. Clin Orthop 228:290, 1988.
95. Schmidek HH: Neurologic and neurosurgical sequelae of Paget's disease of bone. Clin Orthop 127:70, 1977.
96. Schmorl G: Ueber Osteitis deformans Paget. Virchows Arch Pathol Anat Physiol 283:694, 1932.
97. Schreiber MH, Richardson GA: Paget's disease confined to one lumbar vertebra. AJR Am J Roentgenol 90:1271, 1963.
98. Schwindinger WF, Francomano CA, Levine MA: Identification of a mutation in the gene encoding the alpha subunit of the stimulatory G protein of adenylyl cyclase in McCune-Albright syndrome. Proc Natl Acad Sci U S A 89:5152, 1992.
99. Shih W, Riley C, Maggoun S, Ryo Y: Paget's disease mimicking skeletal metastases in a patient with coexistent prostatic carcinoma. Eur J Nucl Med 14:422, 1988.

100. Singer FR, Mills BG: Evidence for a viral etiology of Paget's disease of bone. Clin Orthop 178:245, 1983.
101. Siris E, Weinstein RS, Altman R, et al: Comparative study of alendronate versus etidronate for the treatment of Paget's disease of bone. J Clin Endorincol Metal 81:961-967, 1996.
102. Siris ES: Epidemiologic aspects of Paget's disease: Family history and relationship to other medical conditions. Semin Arthritis Rheum 23:222, 1994.
103. Siris ES: Goals of treatment for Paget's disease of bone. J Bone Miner Res 14(Suppl 2):49-52, 1999.
104. Siris ES, Jacobs TP, Canfield RE: Paget's disease of bone. Bull NY Acad Med 56:285, 1980.
105. Siris ES, Ottoman R, Flaster E, et al: Familial aggregation of Paget's disease of bone. J Bone Miner Res 6:495, 1991.
106. Steinbach HL: Some roentgen features of Paget's disease. AJR Am J Roentgenol 86:950, 1961.
107. Unni KK: Dahlin's Bone Tumors: General Aspects and Data on 11,087 Cases, 5th ed. Philadelphia, Lippincott-Raven, 1996, pp 416-417.
108. Utz JA, Kranedorf MJ, Jelinek JS, et al: MR appearance of fibrous dysplasia. J Comput Assist Tomogr 13:845, 1989.
109. Warrell RP Jr, Bosco B, Weinerman S, et al: Gallium nitrate for advanced Paget disease of bone: Effectiveness and dose-response analysis. Ann Intern Med 113:847, 1990.
110. Waxman AD, Ducker S, McKee D, et al: Evaluation of 99m Tc diphosphonate kinetics and bone scans in patients with Paget's disease before and after calcitonin treatment. Radiology 125:761, 1977.
111. Weisz GM: Lumbar canal stenosis in Paget's diseases: The staging of the clinical syndrome, its diagnosis, and treatment. Clin Orthop 206:223, 1986.
112. Whalley N: Paget's disease of atlas and axis. J Neurol Neurosurg Psychiatry 9:84, 1946.
113. Wick MR, Siegal GP, Unni KK, et al: Sarcomas of bone complicating osteitis deformans (Paget's disease): Fifty years' experience. Am J Surg Pathol 5:47, 1981.
114. Zlatkin MB, Lander PH, Hadjipavlou AG, Levine JS: Paget's disease of the spine: CT with clinical correlation. Radiology 160:155, 1986.

INFECTIVE ENDOCARDITIS

CAPSULE SUMMARY

	LOW BACK	NECK
Frequency of spinal pain	Rare	Not applicable (NA)
Location of spinal pain	Lumbar spine	NA
Quality of spinal pain	Diffuse ache	NA
Symptoms and signs	Back pain an initial symptom in a minority, fever, weight loss	NA
Laboratory tests	Anemia, leukocytosis, hematuria, rheumatoid factor, blood cultures	NA
Radiographic findings	Echocardiogram—vegetations	NA
Treatment	Antibiotics	NA

PREVALENCE AND PATHOGENESIS

Infective endocarditis (IE) is a microbial infection of a heart valve or the mural endocardium. A similar disease occurs with intravascular infection of the endothelial surface of large arteries. Infections of these anatomic areas are not limited to bacteria alone but can be caused by fungi, rickettsiae, and chlamydiae as well.

A variety of classification systems have been proposed for the definition of endocarditis.[30] Initial classification systems were based on the duration of illness before the demise of the patient. Acute bacterial endocarditis caused fatal disease in less than 6 weeks and was associated with infection of normal valves with virulent organisms, such as *Staphylococcus aureus* and *Streptococcus pneumoniae*. Subacute and chronic endocarditis affected structurally abnormal valves with less virulent organisms, such as *Streptococcus viridans*, and would cause death between 3 months and 2 years of the onset of infection. This arbitrary system based on duration of illness has been supplanted in current medical literature for classification systems for IE based on the type of valve (native, prosthetic), host infected (intravenous drug abuser), and infecting organism *(Streptococcus pyogenes)*. Other systems have defined the infection as definite, probable, or possible depending on clinical and pathologic features.[30] Definite endocarditis is defined by histologic or bacteriologic evidence of infection of a valvular vegetation or peripheral embolus. Probable endocarditis is defined as persistently positive blood cultures in the setting of clinical evidence of infection including new heart murmur, fever, and embolic phenomena. Possible endocarditis has positive cultures and only one of the three clinical features.

Epidemiology

The clinical manifestations of IE include fever, cardiac murmurs, splenomegaly, and embolic events. When patients present with these signs, the diagnosis is an easy one to make. The difficulty arises when a patient presents with low back pain as the initial manifestation of the infection. The diagnosis of this potentially life-threatening infection is more difficult in those circumstances. The actual prevalence and incidence of this infection are not known. A number of studies from the 1960s and 1970s reported on large groups of patients with IE, but the relative numbers of patients with this infection compared with groups of patients with other infectious diseases was not known.[8,32,44] The incidence of IE in the United States in the 1980s was 1.7 to 4 cases per 100,000 person-years.[18,22,31] The epidemiologic features of IE in developed countries are changing as a result of increasing longevity, new predisposing factors, and nosocomial cases.[40] In the 1990s, the incidence of community-acquired native-valve endocarditis is 1.7 to 6.2 cases per 100,000 person-years.[4,25] A 1-year survey of hospitals in six regions of France in 1999 reported 3.1 cases per 100,000 person-years.[23] Individuals with IE associated with drug abuse are younger persons. The incidence of IE in this group is 150 to 2000 per 100,000 person-years.[12] The overall proportion of men to women with IE is 3:1.[55] The ratio may be as high as 8:1 in individuals older than 60 years of age.[14] The proportion of individuals who are 60 years of age or older with endocarditis has increased over recent decades. In Olmstead County, Minnesota, the comparison of individuals older than 65 years of age to those younger with endocarditis is 8.8:1.[18] The increased risk of the elderly to endocarditis is related to increased exposure to intravascular invasive procedures, genitourinary infections, and bowel lesions.[51] Other risk factors include poor dental hygiene, long-term hemodialysis, diabetes mellitus, and human immunodeficiency virus infection.[35,36,50] Mitral valve prolapse is the most common cardiovascular disorder with increased risk for IE. The incidence of IE in these patients is 100 per 100,000 patient-years.[60] Prosthetic valve IE accounts for 7% to 25% of IE. The risk is 1% at 12 months and 2% to 3% at 5 years, postoperatively.[54]

Although the disease had been recognized at an earlier time, the disease complex that is associated with IE was formulated by Sir William Osler. Osler, in the Gulstonian lecture in 1885, described the myriad of manifestations of malignant endocarditis, many of which are recognized during the present era.[43]

Pathogenesis

The pathogenesis of IE seems to follow a regular sequence of events. Microbial proliferation occurs within a vegetation located within the circulatory system. These vegetations may occur in areas of endothelial damage (valvular heart diseases, prosthetic heart valves, indwelling catheters), hypercoagulable states, and cancer (marantic endocarditis). Once the organisms gain entry into the vegetation, they multiply within the interstices of the vegetation. Constant bloodstream dissemination of microorganisms is a hallmark of this disease. Constant bacteremia occurs despite normal systemic host defense mechanisms, including antibodies and polymorphonuclear leukocytes. The process becomes a vicious circle as constant bacteremia reinfects the vascular vegetation. Over time, the host defense mechanism mounts an increasingly intensive antibody response, which leads to the formation of antigen-antibody immune complexes. As the vegetation increases in size, small pieces may loosen and embolize to any part of the body. In addition, if located on a heart valve, the increasing size of the vegetation may cause hemodynamic alterations in cardiac function. In its final stages, endocarditis can cause damage through local invasion of cardiac tissue, resulting in cardiac collapse. The problem in diagnosing this process is that the clinical symptoms associated with this disease are nonspecific and the possibility of the infection as a diagnosis is raised late in the course of the infection.[11,30] The clinical manifestations of these pathogenic mechanisms are the damage to heart valves and the associated hemodynamic cardiac complications, septic or bland embolization to distant organs causing necrosis of tissues, metastatic infections, and circulating immune complexes causing disease similar to that associated with serum sickness.

The classic case of indolent, subacute endocarditis with multiple systemic complications in the young patient has decreased in frequency. The disease has evolved, in part, since the discovery and use of increasing numbers of antibiotics. Subacute presentation with presence of microvascular phenomenon, including Osler nodes, splinter hemorrhages, and Roth's spots is an uncommon event.[48] The number of young individuals with heart lesions from rheumatic fever has diminished. Older individuals are the persons with degenerative valvular heart disease predisposed to infection. Other factors that have changed the spectrum of the illness include the increased prevalence of prosthetic heart valves and vascular shunts, intravenous drug abuse, and hospital-acquired infections and antibiotic resistance.[34]

Back pain occurs in patients with IE. Although musculoskeletal symptoms of any sort have been reported in 40% of endocarditis patients, between 9% and 12% of patients have had back pain as an initial symptom or during the course of their disease.[9,19,37,52] The frequency of back pain as a symptom during the course of native-valve or drug abuse–associated IE ranges from 15.4% to 19% of individuals.[5,16,48] The pathogenesis of back pain in endocarditis remains obscure. Proposed mechanisms have included septic foci in muscles, reactive arthritis, renal disease with kidney infarction, or circulating immune complexes. Of all these mechanisms, the presence of increased amounts of immune complexes is the most likely mechanism of pain production in the musculoskeletal system. Immune complexes are normally present in musculoskeletal structures.[2,39] As a result of chronic antigenic stimulation and overriding of normal T-lymphocyte suppression mechanisms, a hypergammaglobulinemic state is created. The bypassing of normal controls results in a polyclonal B-lymphocyte proliferation and immunoglobulin secretion. Increased levels of antibodies activate the complement cascade, which helps kill bacteria but also contributes to the pathologic destruction of host tissues. The variable manifestations of the disease may correlate to the physicochemical nature of the immune complexes, their deposition in tissues, and their clearance by the reticuloendothelial system.[46] Musculoskeletal complaints develop later in the course of the illness. Also probably related is the fact that back pain resolves within 2 weeks of the initiation of antibiotic therapy. Arterial embolization also has been proposed as a possible mechanism.[28] Although an occasional patient has evidence of emboli, many individuals with endocarditis have symptoms of the disease without any evidence of embolization of vegetations.

CLINICAL HISTORY

The bacterial organisms that are the cause of the infection determine the clinical picture presented to the physician.

A listing of these organisms and the relative frequency of each as a cause of endocarditis is presented in Table 18-3. Acute IE develops over days or weeks and is associated with *S. aureus*, *S. pneumoniae*, *S. pyogenes*, or *Neisseria gonorrhoeae*. Patients with acute disease develop musculoskeletal symptoms about half as often as patients with subacute IE. Subacute endocarditis develops over weeks to months and is associated with low-virulence organisms such as the viridans streptococci, including *Streptococcus mutans*, *Streptococcus sanguis*, *Streptococcus mitior*, and *Streptococcus salivarius*. The HACEK group *(Haemophilus parainfluenzae, Haemophilus aphrophilus, Haemophilus paraphrophilus, Actinobacillus actinomycetemcomitans, Cardiobacterium hominis, Eikenella corrodens, and Kingella kingae)* cause 3% of community-acquired cases of IE.[3]

Patients with subacute IE may present with generalized malaise, fever, fatigue, and weight loss. Fever may be minimal or absent in patients with congestive heart failure, chronic renal or liver failure, prior use of antibiotics, or less virulent organisms.[40] The onset of these symptoms is insidious. Back pain may be a presenting symptom in a minority. Other musculoskeletal complaints may include arthralgias, arthritis, or diffuse myalgias. The arthralgias and arthritis tend to involve proximal and lower extremity joints. Up to 44% of patients may have a musculoskeletal complaint during the course of their illness. Occasionally, a patient may develop vertebral osteomyelitis or septic arthritis as a result of endocarditis.[17,29] Although the usual organisms causing vertebral osteomyelitis are more closely associated with acute endocarditis, more indolent microorganisms associated with subacute endocarditis have also caused vertebral osteomyelitis.[1,53] Spondylodiscitis may occur in 10% of patients with IE.[38] Patients with endocarditis may complain of radicular pain without muscle weakness on rare occasions.[26] A mechanical cause may be suspected in these patients because they complain of increased pain with cough. However, no specific area of disc degeneration can be found in these patients. The source of their pain is undetermined.[52] Subacute bacterial endocarditis also has been reported to affect a patient with ankylosing spondylitis and aortic valvular disease.[27]

18-3 MICROBIOLOGIC ETIOLOGY IN 2345 EPISODES OF INFECTIVE ENDOCARDITIS*

Organism	Total Episodes	Percent of Total
Streptococci†	1322	56.4
Enterococci‡	142	6.1
Pneumococci	71	3.0
Staphylococci	583	24.9
Coagulase-positive	447	19.1
Coagulase-negative	136	5.8
Gram-negative bacteria	135	5.7
Fungi	24	1.0
Other§	63	2.7
Culture negative	218	9.3

*Representing cases from 1933–1987.
†Total includes viridans streptococci, enterococci, pneumococci, and other streptococcal species (e.g., *Streptococcus bovis*).
‡Now considered a separate genus.
§Includes *Erysipelothrix, Pharyngis sicca, Micrococcus, Spirillium, Bacillus, Corynebacterium, Clostridium perfringens, Lactobacillus, Listeria, Coxiella burnetti, Chlamydia*, and nonstreptococcal anaerobes.
Modified from Kaye D (ed): Infective Endocarditis, 2nd ed. New York, Raven Press, 1992, p 86.

Other manifestations of subacute bacterial endocarditis include mental status changes, transient ischemic attacks, progressive heart failure, and skin rash. Neurologic disorders may occur in 25% of IE patients.[20]

PHYSICAL EXAMINATION

The duration of the infection before diagnosis plays a major role in determining the manifestations that will be apparent on physical examination. Since the diagnosis is considered earlier in the course of the disease than in the preantibiotic era, those manifestations that take a considerable time to develop (clubbing, splenomegaly, Osler and Janeway lesions, and glomerulonephritis) are less evident when the diagnosis is established.

Physical findings usually include fever and a heart murmur in 90% and 80% of patients, respectively. Splenomegaly occurs in a smaller proportion of patients. Skin rash is found in 20% to 40% of patients at the time of hospital admission.[13,44]

Back examination may demonstrate spinal tenderness and decreased motion. Scoliosis and a list may be noted in patients with unilateral paraspinous muscle spasm. Muscle spasm may be the sole presenting symptom on occasion. Percussion tenderness without sacroiliitis on radiographs has been reported.[55]

Examination of the eyes may demonstrate a wide variety of lesions including petechiae, hemorrhages, cotton-wool exudates, Roth's spots, or endophthalmitis. Neurologic manifestations may include hemiparesis, seizures, or transient ischemic attacks.

Patients with acute endocarditis develop high spiking fever, rigors, and chills. Petechiae may be very prominent if *S. aureus* is the cause of the infection. Meningitis along with signs of intravascular coagulation may be present. Septic emboli, which cause localized infections in various areas of the body, are characteristic. These manifestations may occur even in the absence of a heart murmur. Isolated right-sided IE is not associated with peripheral emboli. Pulmonary signs predominate.

LABORATORY DATA

Screening blood tests are frequently positive but the findings are nondiagnostic. Anemia occurs in 90% and thrombocytopenia in 15%. The erythrocyte sedimentation rate (ESR) is universally elevated. However, ESR does not decrease rapidly in response to antibiotic therapy. C-reactive protein is also increased in all IE patients. Serial C-reactive protein does follow response to therapy. Persistence of C-reactive protein suggests a complicated course without full eradication of the infection.[42] Gamma globulins, particularly rheumatoid factor, are present in patients with longer duration disease. Rheumatoid factor is detectable in patients with disease over 6 weeks in duration. Urinalysis may reveal proteinuria and microscopic hematuria. Elevated creatinine levels suggest renal failure secondary to immune complex glomerulonephritis. Hypocomplementemia is frequently present when endocarditis is complicated by glomerulonephritis.

The blood culture is the most important laboratory test in IE. In patients with fulminant disease, three venous samples over a 1-hour period should be obtained. In patients with subacute disease, three or four venous samples drawn over a 24-hour period are adequate. Two more cultures should be drawn if the initial sets are negative for growth of an organism. Cultures should be incubated for 4 weeks to detect fastidious pathogens. The bacteremia of endocarditis is continuous, so blood cultures may be obtained at any time and not exclusively at times of temperature spikes. Only 5% to 7% of patients who have been given a diagnosis of IE by strict criteria and who have not recently received antibiotics have sterile blood cultures.[40] For example, 88 (14%) of 620 cases were culture negative in a 1-year study of IE in France. In 42 of 88 cases, antibiotics were administered prior to venesection for blood cultures.[24]

Polymerase chain reaction (PCR) analysis is useful for the detection of fastidious organisms that may be missed by standard culture techniques. PCR may be particularly useful for the detection of organisms in excised surgical specimens or vegetations.[15,41]

IE is usually caused by gram-positive cocci, with streptococci and staphylococci accounting for 80% to 90% of cases (see Table 18-3). *S. viridans* is the leading cause of streptococcal infection. Viridans streptococci normally inhabit the oral cavity. After dental manipulation, the organisms may enter the bloodstream to infect abnormal heart valves. *Streptococcus bovis* is a group D streptococcus that inhabits the gastrointestinal tract. *S. bovis* bacteremia has occurred in patients with carcinoma of the colon and other lesions of the gastrointestinal tract. Gastrointestinal evaluation is appropriate in patients with *S. bovis* endocarditis.[49,56]

Staphylococci cause 30% of cases, with *S. aureus* the most common organism of that group.[45] *S. aureus* affects the elderly and drug abusers most often. *Staphylococcus epidermidis* has become an increasingly important cause of endocarditis, particularly in individuals with prosthetic heart valves.

Enterococci are normal inhabitants of the gastrointestinal tract, genital tract, and occasionally, the anterior urethra and mouth. They cause infections in older men after prostatectomy and young women after obstetric procedures.

Gram-negative organisms are infrequent causes of endocarditis except in intravenous drug abusers, recipients of prosthetic valves, persons with cirrhosis, and immunocompromised hosts. Among gram-negative organisms, *Pseudomonas aeruginosa* is the most common cause of endocarditis.

Fungal endocarditis is a problem for drug abusers and those who have been receiving prolonged parenteral antibiotic therapy. *Candida albicans* is the prime culprit in this group.

Approximately 5% of endocarditis is culture negative. Reasons for the absence of growth may include use of antibiotics by patients and the presence of slow-growing fastidious organisms, anaerobic organisms, and obligate intracellular parasites as the infecting organisms.

Other laboratory measurements that may be obtained are complement, which is decreased, and immune complexes or cryoglobulins, which are increased. These tests help document the immune nature of the disease but are too nonspecific to help in the diagnosis. However, like the C-reactive protein and rheumatoid factor, these test results may normalize as the patient responds to therapy.

RADIOGRAPHIC EVALUATION

Radiographic evaluation of the back in patients with endocarditis is unrevealing. Any changes that may be present are more likely to be related to the patient's age than to the infection. Rarely, a hematogenous infection may involve the spine. These patients have the radiographic changes associated with vertebral osteomyelitis or discitis.[53]

Great advances have occurred in the radiographic evaluation of endocarditis. Echocardiography is able to detect vegetations and intracardiac complications of endocarditis noninvasively. Transesophageal imaging has increased the sensitivity of detecting lesions compared to two-dimensional echocardiography. Transthoracic echocardiography may be inadequate in as many as 20% of adult patients because of obesity, chest wall deformities, or pulmonary disease.[57] Transesophageal echocardiography is particularly useful for prosthetic valve IE and for evaluation of myocardial abscesses. Doppler with color-flow mapping has been a sensitive method for depicting the abnormal flow of blood in the heart.[30]

DIFFERENTIAL DIAGNOSIS

The diagnosis of IE is considered in the patient with back pain who has associated constitutional symptoms. It may also be considered in the patient who is older and has "mechanical" back pain if there is no history of injury or previous episode of pain and roentgenograms are normal or show minimal degenerative arthritis. The diagnosis may not be apparent initially, but persistent surveillance of patients should alert the clinician that the problem is not a mechanical one but is associated with a systemic illness. These are the patients who may be identified in the low back pain algorithm as the cohort of individuals with fever. They also might be identified as one of the group with persistent muscle pain. Laboratory evaluation of these patients would identify anemia, leukocytosis, elevated ESR, or C-reactive protein, which would alert the physician to the likelihood of a systemic illness.

Criteria for the diagnosis of IE are listed in Table 18-4. These criteria have been modified from those proposed by physicians at Duke University in 1994. Modifications were proposed because of misclassification of culture-negative cases and the overly broad categorization of cases as "possible."[40]

TREATMENT

Once the cultures have been obtained and the diagnosis is established, antibiotic therapy is begun. The basic compo-

18-4 CRITERIA FOR THE DIAGNOSIS OF INFECTIVE ENDOCARDITIS*

MAJOR CRITERIA

Microbiologic

Typical microorganism isolated from two separate blood cultures: *Streptococcus viridans*, *Streptococcus bovis*, HACEK group, *Staphylococcus aureus*, or community-acquired enterococcal bacteremia without a primary focus

or

Microorganism consistent with infective endocarditis isolated from persistently positive blood cultures

or

Single positive blood culture for *Coxiella burnetii* or phase I IgG antibody titer to *C. burnetii* > 1:800

Endocardial Involvement

New valvular regurgitation (change in preexistent murmur not sufficient)

or

Positive echocardiogram (transesophageal test recommended for patients with prosthetic heart valves, rated as possible endocarditis by clinical criteria, or who have complicated infective endocarditis)

MINOR CRITERIA

Predisposition—cardiac conditions or injection drug use

High risk—previous IE, aortic valve disease, rheumatic heart disease, prosthetic valve, coarctation of the aorta, congenital heart disease

Moderate risk—mitral valve prolapse with regurgitation or leaflet thickening, mitral stenosis, tricuspid valve disease, pulmonary stenosis, hypertrophic cardiomyopathy

Low risk—secundum atrial septal defect, ischemic heart disease, previous coronary artery bypass graft surgery, mitral valve prolapse without regurgitation or thickening

Fever: temperature > 38°C (100.4°F)

Vascular phenomena: major arterial emboli, septic pulmonary infarctions, mycotic aneurysm, intracranial hemorrhage, conjunctival hemorrhages, Janeway lesions

Immunologic phenomena: rheumatoid factor, glomerulonephritis, Osler's nodes, Roth's spots

Microbiologic findings: positive blood cultures that do not meet major criterion, or serologic evidence of active infection with organisms consistent with infective endocarditis

*Definite—2 major criteria, 1 major criterion + 3 minor criteria, or 5 minor criteria; Possible—1 major + 1 minor criterion, or 3 minor criteria.

Modified from Li JS, Sexton DJ, Mick N, et al: Proposed modifications to the Duke criteria for the diagnosis of infective endocarditis. Clin Infect Dis 30:633-638, 2000; and Heiro M, Nikoskelainen J, Hartiala J, et al: Diagnosis of infective endocarditis: Sensitivity of the Duke versus von Reyn criteria. Arch Intern Med 158:18-24, 1998.

nent of therapy is bactericidal drugs, administered parenterally, for a long enough period to eradicate the infection. The reasons for prolonged therapy are that host defense mechanisms do not work well in vegetations and that older bacteria in vegetations are in a static state, less susceptible to the effects of antibiotics.

Antibiotic Therapy

In subacute endocarditis, the usual therapy is penicillin G, 24 million units/day, along with an aminoglycoside (gentamicin) for penicillin-resistant organisms. Bactericidal levels are measured routinely and antibiotic doses are given to maintain bactericidal levels. The course of therapy is 4 to 6 weeks, depending on the organism and its antibiotic sensitivity.[10,58,59]

Patients with acute endocarditis, which is usually secondary to staphylococci or gram-negative organisms, require parenteral oxacillin or nafcillin, 12 g/day, for a 4- to 6-week period and gentamicin or tobramycin, 3 to 5 mg/kg/day, for the first 3 to 5 days. Alterations in dose, duration of therapy, or choice of antibiotic are determined by local environmental factors such as bacterial sensitivity to antibiotics.

The therapy for each form of endocarditis must be individualized. Antibiotic regimens change for specific organisms (streptococcal vs. enterococcal vs. staphylococcal disease) versus HACEK organisms (ceftriaxone—4 weeks), the sensitivity of the organism to antibiotics in that hospital at the time of the infection (i.e., hospital acquired), and the medical condition of the host (human immunodeficiency virus infection). For example, the same species of bacteria in two different hospitals may have different antibiotic sensitivities. Current information from the hospital's bacteriology laboratory concerning antibiotic sensitivity should be reviewed to formulate the best therapeutic regimen.[54]

Surgical Therapy

Surgical replacement of an infected valve may be required for eradication of infection by certain organisms. Optimal therapy for *Bartonella* and Q fever infections usually requires valve replacement. Congestive heart failure, myocardial abscesses or persistent infection despite maximum antibiotic therapy are indications for surgical intervention.[40]

Prophylaxis

Another important component of therapy is antibiotic prophylaxis before invasive medical procedures.[47] This includes amoxicillin 2 g orally 1 hour before a dental, respiratory, or esophageal procedure, or azithromycin or clarithromycin 500 mg 1 hour before a similar procedure if the patient is penicillin sensitive. Genitourinary or gastrointestinal procedures in high-risk patients require ampicillin 2 g orally and gentamicin 1.5 mg/kg intramuscularly followed 6 hours later by ampicillin 1 g orally. Penicillin-sensitive patients should receive vancomycin 1 g intravenously over 1 to 2 hours plus gentamicin 1.5 mg/kg intramuscularly. The application of the recommendations has not been consistent. In one study of 108 patients undergoing transesophageal echocardiography, 45.9% received instructions concerning prophylaxis. Of this group, 13.2% elected not to follow medical recommendations.[6]

PROGNOSIS

The prognosis of patients with IE is good if the diagnosis is recognized and prompt therapy is given. Back pain resolves within 2 weeks of the start of antibiotic treatment if the pain is related to the infection.[9]

The overall survival rate for IE is about 75%. The rate depends in large measure on the timeliness of initiation of therapy and the nature of the infecting organism. Survival is 90% with *S. viridans* and 50% with *S. aureus*. With *S. aureus*, mortality is associated with late congestive heart failure, older age, and central nervous system involvement.[45] *S. aureus* infection is associated with greater mortality within the first 30 days of the infection (16.4% in one study).[7] Endocarditis in the elderly is associated with a significantly higher mortality rate than in middle-aged and young patients (45.3%, 32.6%, and 9.1%, respectively, in one study).[6] Cardiac failure is a grave prognostic sign and is the most common cause of death. Valve replacement may be required not only in patients with acute endocarditis but also in patients with native-valve endocarditis with indolent organisms (coagulase-negative staphylococci), if recognition of the infection is delayed.[7] Patients with cardiac failure may require valve replacement, but they may not receive any benefit if their cardiac function has been too severely compromised.[46]

References

Infective Endocarditis

1. Allen SL, Salmon JE, Roberts RB: *Streptococcus bovis* endocarditis presenting as acute vertebral osteomyelitis. Arthritis Rheum 24:1211, 1981.
2. Bayer AS, Theofilopoulous AN, Eisenberg R, et al: Circulating immune complexes in infective endocarditis. N Engl J Med 295:1500, 1976.
3. Berbari EF, Cockerill FR, Steckelberg JM: Infective endocarditis due to unusual or fastidious microorganisms. Mayo Clin Proc 72:532-542, 1997.
4. Berlin JA, Abrutyn E, Strom BL, et al: Incidence of infective endocarditis in the Delaware Valley, 1988–1990. Am J Cardiol 76:933-936, 1995.
5. Bouza E, Menasalvas A, Munoz P, et al: Infective endocarditis—a prospective study at the end of the twentieth century: New predisposing conditions, new etiologic agents, and still a high mortality. Medicine 80:298-307, 2001.
6. Cabal CH, Jollis JG, Peterson GE, et al: Changing patient characteristics and the effect on mortality in endocarditis. Arch Intern Med 162:90-94, 2002.
7. Caputo GM, Archer GL, Calderwood SB, et al: Native valve endocarditis due to coagulase-negative staphylococci: Clinical and microbiologic features. Am J Med 83:619, 1987.
8. Cherubin CE, Neu HC: Infective endocarditis at the Presbyterian Hospital in New York City from 1938–1967. Am J Med 51:83, 1971.
9. Churchill MA Jr, Geraci J, Hunder GG: Musculoskeletal manifestations of bacterial endocarditis. Ann Intern Med 87:754, 1972.
10. Dajani AS, Taubert KA, Wilson W, et al: Prevention of bacterial endocarditis: Recommendations by the American Heart Association. JAMA 339:135-139, 1997.
11. Freedman LR: Infective Endocarditis and Other Intravascular Infections. New York, Plenum, 1982.
12. Frontera JA, Gradon JD: Right-side endocarditis in injection drug users: Review of proposed mechanisms of pathogenesis. Clin Infect Dis 30:374-379, 2000.
13. Garvey GJ, Neu HC: Infective endocarditis—an evolving disease. Medicine 57:105, 1978.
14. Gladstone JL, Recco R: Host factors and infectious disease in the elderly. Med Clin North Am 60:1225, 1976.
15. Goldenberger D, Kunzli A, Vogt P, et al: Molecular diagnosis of bacterial endocarditis by broad-range PCR amplification and direct sequencing. J Clin Microbiol 35:2733-2739, 1997.
16. Gonzalez-Juanatey C, Gonzalez-Gay MA, Llorca J, et al: Rheumatic manifestations of infective endocarditis in non-addicts: A 12-year study. Medicine 80:9-19, 2001.
17. Good AE, Hague JM, Kauffmann CA: Streptococcal endocarditis initially seen as septic arthritis. Arch Intern Med 138:805, 1978.
18. Griffen MR, Wilson WR, Edward WD, et al: Infective endocarditis: Olmstead County, Minnesota, 1950 through 1981. JAMA 254:1199, 1985.
19. Harkonen M, Olin PE, Wenstrom J: Severe backache as a presenting sign of bacterial endocarditis. Acta Med Scand 210:329, 1981.
20. Heiro M, Nikoskelainen J, Engblom E, et al: Neurologic manifestations of infective endocarditis: A 17-year experience in a teaching hospital in Finland. Arch Intern Med 160:2781-2787, 2000.
21. Heiro M, Nikoskelainen J, Hartiala J, et al: Diagnosis of infective endocarditis: Sensitivity of the Duke versus von Reyn criteria. Arch Intern Med 158:18-24, 1998.
22. Hickey AJ, MacMahon SW, Wilcken DE: Mitral valve prolapse and bacterial endocarditis: When is antibiotic prophylaxis necessary? Am Heart J 109:431, 1985.
23. Hoen B, Alla F, Selton-Suty C, et al: Changing profile of infective endocarditis: Results of a 1-year survey in France. JAMA 288:75-81, 2002.
24. Hoen B, Selton-Suty C, Lacassin F, et al: Infective endocarditis in patients with negative blood cultures: Analysis of 88 cases from a one-year nationwide survey in France. Clin Infect Dis 20:501-506, 1995.
25. Hogevik H, Olaison L, Andersson R, et al: Epidemiologic aspects of infective endocarditis in an urban population: A 5-year prospective study. Medicine 74:324-339, 1995.
26. Holler JW, Pecora JS: Backache in bacterial endocarditis. NY State J Med 70:1903, 1970.
27. Hoppmann RA, Wise CM, Challa VR, Peacock JE: Subacute bacterial endocarditis in a patient with ankylosing spondylitis. Ann Rheum Dis 47:423, 1988.
28. Irvin RG, Sade RM: Endocarditis and musculoskeletal manifestations. Ann Intern Med 88:578, 1978.
29. Kahn MF: Vertebral osteomyelitis and bacterial endocarditis. Arthritis Rheum 25:600, 1982.
30. Kaye D (ed): Infective Endocarditis, 2nd ed. New York, Raven Press, 1992.
31. King JW, Nguyen VQ, Conrad SA: Results of a prospective statewide reporting system for infective endocarditis. Am J Med Sci 295:517, 1988.
32. Lerner PI, Weinstein L: Infective endocarditis in the antibiotic era. N Engl J Med 274:199, 259, 353, 388, 1966.
33. Li JS, Sexton DJ, Mick N, et al: Proposed modifications to the Duke criteria for the diagnosis of infective endocarditis. Clin Infect Dis 30:633-638, 2000.
34. Littler WA, Shanson DC: Infective endocarditis. In Shanson DC (ed): Septicemia and Endocarditis: Clinical and Microbiological Aspects. Oxford, Oxford University Press, 1989, pp 143-171.
35. Manoff SB, Vlahov D, Herkowitz A, et al: Human immunodeficiency virus infection and infective endocarditis among injecting drug users. Epidemiology 7:566-570, 1996.
36. McCarthy JT, Steckelberg JM: Infective endocarditis in patients receiving long-term hemodialysis. Mayo Clin Proc 75:1008-1014, 2000.
37. Meyers OL, Commerford PJ: Musculoskeletal manifestations of bacterial endocarditis. Ann Rheum Dis 36:527, 1977.

38. Morelli S, Carmenini E, Caporossi AP, et al: Spondylodiscitis and infective endocarditis: Case studies and review of the literature. Spine 26:499-500, 2001.
39. Myers AR, Schumacher HR Jr: Arthritis of subacute bacterial endocarditis (SBE). Arthritis Rheum 19:813, 1976.
40. Mylonakis E, Calderwood SB: Infective endocarditis in adults. N Engl J Med 345:1318-1330, 2001.
41. Nikkari S, Gotoff R, Bourbeau PP, et al: Identification of *Cardiobacterium hominis* by broad-range bacterial polymerase chain reaction analysis in a case of culture-negative endocarditis. Arch Intern Med 162:477-479, 2002.
42. Olaison L, Hogevik H, Alestig K: Fever, C-reactive protein, and other acute-phase reactants during treatment of infective endocarditis. Arch Intern Med 157:885-892, 1997.
43. Osler W: The Gulstonian Lectures on malignant endocarditis. BMJ 1:467, 522, 577, 1885.
44. Pelletier LL, Petersdorf RG: Infective endocarditis: A review of 125 cases from the University of Washington Hospitals, 1963–1972. Medicine 56:287, 1977.
45. Roder BL, Wandall DA, Frimodt-Moller N, et al: Clinical features of *Staphylococcus aureus* endocarditis: A 10-year experience in Denmark. Arch Intern Med 159:462-469, 1999.
46. Sande MA, Kaye D, Root RK (eds): Endocarditis. Edinburgh, Churchill Livingstone, 1984.
47. Seto TB, Kwiat D, Taira DA, et al: Physicians' recommendations to patients for use of antibiotic prophylaxis to prevent endocarditis. JAMA 284:68-71, 2000.
48. Siddiq S, Missri J, Silverman DI: Endocarditis in an urban hospital in the 1990s. Arch Intern Med 156:2454-2458, 1996.
49. Steinberg D, Naggar CZ: *Streptococcus bovis* endocarditis with carcinoma of the colon. N Engl J Med 297:1354, 1977.
50. Strom BL, Abrutyn E, Berlin JA, et al: Risk factors for infective endocarditis: Oral hygiene and nondental exposures. Circulation 102:2842-2848, 2000.
51. Terpenning MS, Buggy BP, Kauffman CA: Infective endocarditis: Clinical features in young and elderly. Am J Med 83:626, 1987.
52. Thomas P, Allal J, Bontoux D, et al: Rheumatological manifestations of infective endocarditis. Ann Rheum Dis 43:716, 1984.
53. Ullman RF, Strampfer MJ, Cunha BA: *Streptococcus mutans* vertebral osteomyelitis. Heart Lung 17:319, 1988.
54. Vlessis AA, Hovaguimian H, Jaggers J, et al: Infective endocarditis: Ten-year review of medical and surgical therapy. Ann Thorac Surg 61:1217-1222, 1996.
55. Watanakunakorn C: Changing epidemiology and newer aspects of infective endocarditis. Adv Intern Med 22:21, 1977.
56. Watanakunakorn C: *Streptococcus bovis* endocarditis associated with villous adenoma following colonoscopy. Am Heart J 116:1115, 1988.
57. Werner GS, Schulz R, Fuchs JB, et al: Infective endocarditis in the elderly in the era of transesophageal echocardiography: Clinical features and prognosis compared to younger patients. Am J Med 100:90-97, 1996.
58. Wilson WR, Karchmer AW, Dijani AS, et al: Antibiotic treatment of adults with infective endocarditis due to streptococci, enterococci, staphylococci, and HACEK organisms. JAMA 274:1706-1713, 1995.
59. Working Party of the British Society for Antimicrobial Chemotherapy: Antibiotic treatment of streptococcal, enterococcal, staphylococcal endocarditis. Heart 79:207-210, 1998.
60. Zuppiroli A, Rinaldi M, Kramer-Fox R, et al: Natural history of mitral valve prolapse. Am J Cardiol 75:1028-1032, 1995.

VERTEBRAL SARCOIDOSIS

CAPSULE SUMMARY

	LOW BACK	NECK
Frequency of spinal pain	Rare	Rare
Location of spinal pain	Lumbar spine	Cervical spine
Quality of spinal pain	Intermittent, dull or stabbing pain	Intermittent, dull or stabbing pain
Symptoms and signs	Cough, dyspnea, vertebral percussion tenderness	Cough, dyspnea, vertebral percussion tenderness
Laboratory tests	Increased calcium, gamma globulin levels	Increased calcium, gamma globulin levels
Radiographic findings	Mixed lytic-sclerotic lesions on plain roentgenograms	Mixed lytic-sclerotic lesions on plain roentgenograms
Treatment	Corticosteroids, surgical decompression	Corticosteroids, surgical decompression

PREVALENCE AND PATHOGENESIS

Sarcoidosis is a disease of unknown cause that causes the formation of granulomas, a form of inflammation consisting of epithelioid cells surrounded by a border of mononuclear cells, in any organ in the body. It is most closely associated with granuloma formation in the lung and thoracic lymph nodes. Fibrosis is a result of granuloma formation. Fibrosis disrupts organ architecture and may result in dysfunction and ultimate failure.[27] Less commonly, a smaller proportion of patients develop bony involvement, including vertebral bodies. The disease was first described by Hutchinson in 1877.[26]

Epidemiology

The exact prevalence of sarcoidosis is unknown but may be as high as 1 case per 10,000 population. Autopsy studies suggest that the prevalence of sarcoidosis may be as high as 641 cases per 100,000 population in Scandinavian countries.[48] In the United States sarcoidosis is 14 times more common in blacks than in whites.[30] The incidence rate of sarcoidosis in the United States is 10.9 per 100,000 for whites and 35.5 per 100,000 for blacks. The lifetime risk of sarcoidosis for U.S. blacks is 2.4% and for U.S. whites is 0.85%.[45] The age of onset is between 20 and 40 years. The male-to-female ratio is 1:1. Vertebral sarcoidosis is a rare entity.[42] Most patients with vertebral sarcoidosis are black men, with a mean age of 26 years.

Pathogenesis

The pathogenesis of sarcoidosis is unknown. However, environmental and genetic factors play a role in this disease's development. Community outbreaks, occupational exposures, and case contacts suggest person-to-person transmission or shared exposure to an environmental agent.[40] Cell wall–deficient mycobacteria have been grown from the blood of a group of sarcoid patients. However, other sarcoid patients do not show evidence of a mycobacterial infection, ranging from 0% to 50% positivity.[31] Human herpesvirus 8 has also been implicated as a possible environmental initiator of sarcoidosis.[4] Both organic (endotoxin) and inorganic (metallic dust) agents may initiate this disorder. No single gene seems solely responsible for the illness. Genetically predisposed hosts would have altered immune dysregulation that would affect antigen recognition, T-cell function, and granuloma formation. A genetic predisposition is associated with HLA-A1 and B8 and class II HLA-DR3.[3]

The presence of granulomas in the lung and other tissues suggests an abnormality in immune function. Sarcoidosis has a dichotomy of depressed systemic cellular immunity in the setting of increased T-lymphocytic activity in affected organs.[31] The immune dysfunction is characterized by depression of delayed hypersensitivity, imbalance of CD4/CD8 T-cell subsets, an influx of Th1 helper cells to sites of activity, hyperactivity of B cells , and circulation of immune complexes.[2] On a focal level, Th1 activity predominates, whereas on a systemic level Th2 activity is stimulated manifested by hypergammaglobulinemia. Bronchoalveolar lavage has been used to sample immune cells from the lungs of sarcoid patients. Lavage fluid has a high proportion and absolute number of lymphocytes.[54] Normally, macrophages comprise 90% and lymphocytes 10% of lavage fluid. In sarcoidosis, the number of cells is increased several times the number from normal individuals, and the number of lymphocytes may be increased to 60% of total recovered cells.[50] T lymphocytes from patients with active sarcoidosis release substances that promote the formation of granulomas. T-helper cells, as opposed to T-suppressor cells, are found in increased numbers in the lung, whereas the ratio of helper to suppressor cells in the peripheral blood is decreased. In addition to increased numbers, T lymphocytes are in an activated state manifested by active proliferation, release of migration-inhibiting factor, interleukin-2 (IL-2), and gamma interferon.[54] Th1 cytokines, such as IL-2 and IL-15, act as local growth factors for sarcoid T lymphocytes. Macrophages are also activated to produce IL-1 and IL-15. Growth stimulatory factors for macrophage proliferation (monocyte colony-stimulating factor, granulocyte-macrophage colony-stimulating factor) are released locally to facilitate the proliferation and aggregation of macrophages. IL-12 expression is enhanced in the lung of sarcoid patients and is another important cytokine in Th1-mediated immune response.[34] In addition, T lymphocytes from patients with sarcoidosis cause B lymphocytes to produce immunoglobulin. These abnormalities in the number and function of immune cells correlate with the clinical findings of granuloma formation, anergy to delayed hypersensitivity reaction, and hypergammaglobulinemia.[15,24,25] The granuloma in an organ causes disorganization of normal tissue, and the process of healing results in the production of fibrosis in areas of granulomatous inflammation. A cytokine associated with remission is transforming growth factor-beta (TGF-β). TGF-β inhibits IL-12 and interferon-gamma production. TBF-β may play an important role in down-regulating granulomatous inflammation in sarcoidosis. Granuloma-associated fibrosis in the lungs, heart, kidney, eyes, and musculoskeletal system may be associated with dysfunction in all these organ systems and correlates with the wide range of clinical findings associated with this illness.

Osseous involvement in sarcoidosis has been estimated to be 15% to 20%. A proportion of sarcoid patients as high as 34% has been reported when consistent radiologic evaluation of patients is performed.[48] This proportion of patients with osseous involvement may be an underestimate because granulomas may be present in bone and not detected by radiographic techniques. Bone lesions are more common in patients with more persistent disease with chronic skin involvement.[39] The areas of involvement include the bones of the hands and feet, skull, pelvis, femurs, humeri, and ribs. The spine is rarely involved.[44] The hips and sacroiliac joints are also rare locations for sarcoid arthropathy.[23]

CLINICAL HISTORY

Osseous sarcoidosis almost invariably occurs when there is clinical or radiographic pulmonary involvement. Pulmonary symptoms include cough and shortness of breath. Osseous lesions may be asymptomatic or discovered by chance on radiographs, but this is rarely the case in vertebral sarcoidosis since it is usually painful. Patients complain of a dull or stabbing pain localized at the involved vertebrae. It may radiate from the back to the thighs or neck to the shoulders and is relieved by rest and increased with activity. Vertebral movements may be severely limited. Patients with spinal cord compression complain of neurologic symptoms, including lower extremity weakness, loss of sensation, and abnormalities of bladder and bowel function.[16,38] Symptoms related to a single nerve root infiltrated with sarcoid also have been reported.[6]

In 20% to 50% of acute-onset sarcoid, patients present with Lofgren's syndrome. Lofgren's syndrome is characterized by erythema nodosum, bilateral hilar adenopathy, and polyarthralgias, primarily affecting the ankles. Patients with generalized sarcoidosis may also give a history of anorexia, weight loss, and fever. A significant proportion present with chronic respiratory symptoms and few constitutional complaints.[40]

PHYSICAL EXAMINATION

Physical examination of patients with vertebral sarcoidosis demonstrates percussion tenderness over the involved area of the axial skeleton. Limitation of motion of the spine may be an accompanying finding. Those with neurologic involvement may demonstrate impaired sensation, weakness, and depressed or absent lower extremity reflexes. Dactylitis ("sausage digits") like those associated with spondyloarthropathies may occur secondary to periostitis and soft tissue inflammation. General physical examination may demonstrate other organ system involvement with sarcoidosis, including skin rash (erythema nodosum, macules or papules containing granulomas), abnormal breath sounds, splenomegaly, generalized lymphadenopathy, and eye inflammation (iridocyclitis, choroidoretinitis, conjunctivitis, enlarged lacrimal glands).

LABORATORY DATA

Several biochemical abnormalities have been described in sarcoidosis. These include hypercalcemia, increased serum alkaline phosphatase level, and hypergammaglobulinemia. Hypercalcemia is a byproduct of increased production of 1,25-dihydroxyvitamin D_3 (calcitriol) by activated macrophages in sarcoid granulomas. Serum angiotensin-converting enzyme (ACE) level is elevated in patients with sarcoidosis.[36] ACE is most active in lung lining cells. Granulomatous inflammation of the lung and lymph nodes may be the source of increased concentrations of ACE. ACE is elevated in 43% to 88% of patients with sarcoidosis.[17] This variability is in part due to differences in sensitivity of the test in different laboratories. The test also lacks specificity, since miliary tuberculosis, histoplasmosis, Gaucher's disease, and biliary cirrhosis are associated with increased ACE levels. Therefore, an elevated ACE level is supportive but not diagnostic of sarcoidosis. Cutaneous anergy (loss of delayed hypersensitivity), when tested with exposure to three antigens (PPD, *Candida*, and *Trichophyton*), occurs in a minority of patients.[53] Bronchoalveolar lavage has been used for determination of elevated proportions of helper T lymphocytes in sarcoid patients.[56] The results of bronchoalveolar lavage are not specific for sarcoidosis, and difficulty in obtaining fluid has limited its utility as a diagnostic test. Most individuals with musculoskeletal disease have an elevated erythrocyte sedimentation rate and C-reactive protein level. Circulating immune complexes may also be present.

Pathology

Pathologic specimens from patients with sarcoidosis demonstrate multiple noncaseating granulomas consisting of multinucleated giant cells. They are present in any organ involved with sarcoid, including the lung, skin, bone, and muscle. Nonsarcoid causes of granulomas (tuberculosis, berylliosis) must be considered before a diagnosis of sarcoidosis is entertained. Most sarcoid granulomas gradually resolve and leave few or no residual manifestations of previous inflammation.[51]

RADIOGRAPHIC EVALUATION

Roentgenograms

Roentgenographic abnormalities associated with vertebral sarcoidosis include bone lysis with marginal sclerosis that involves the vertebral body.[10,47] Occasionally the posterior elements of vertebra also may be affected (Fig. 18-10).[8] Any portion of the axial skeleton may be affected, with the lower thoracic and the upper lumbar the most common areas of involvement.[14,19,21,35] Contiguous vertebrae may be involved, some with narrowing of the intervertebral disc.[5] Other patients have noncontiguous vertebral body disease (Fig. 18-11).[58] The inflammatory process may progress to cause vertebral body collapse.[22] Paravertebral ossification with anterior bony bridges simulating ankylosing spondylitis has been reported (Fig. 18-12).[42] It has been suggested that patients with sarcoidosis may develop sacroiliitis in addition to nonmarginal syndesmophytes and paravertebral ossification.[13,46] The sacroiliac joints may fuse. Occasionally, sarcoidosis may produce sclerotic lesions of bone that may be confused with metastatic disease to bone.[1] Sarcoidosis may cause severe disc destruction that may mimic radiographic changes of discitis.[33] Cervical spine involvement has included pathologic fracture of the odontoid process.

Myelography, Computed Tomography, Magnetic Resonance Imaging

Myelography may demonstrate defects compatible with soft tissue compression of spinal cord elements.[10] Rarely, the spinal cord and cauda equina may be affected directly. Myelography may reveal intramedullary or intradural masses, arachnoiditis, or meningeal thickening.[9] CT and MR scans are particularly well suited to the evaluation of

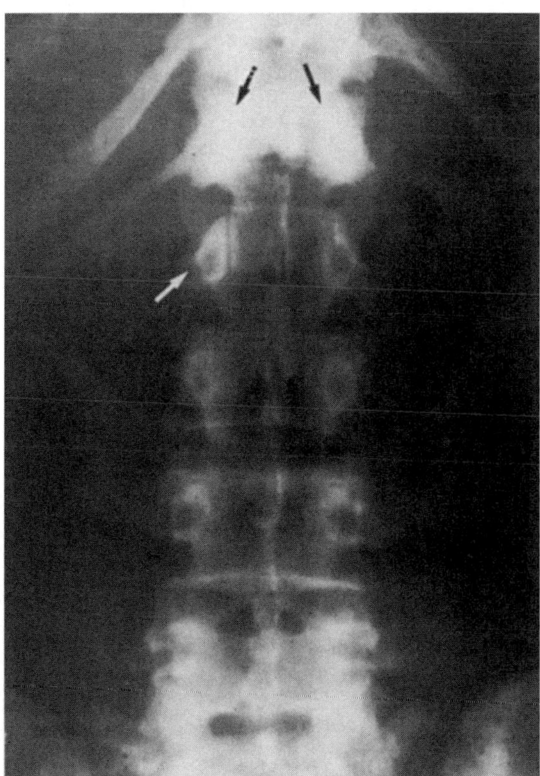

Figure 18-10 Sarcoidosis. Anteroposterior view of the lumbar spine demonstrating sclerosis of the pedicles of T12 *(black arrows)* and the right pedicle of L1 *(white arrow)* and diffuse sclerosis of L5. *(Courtesy of Anne Brower, MD.)*

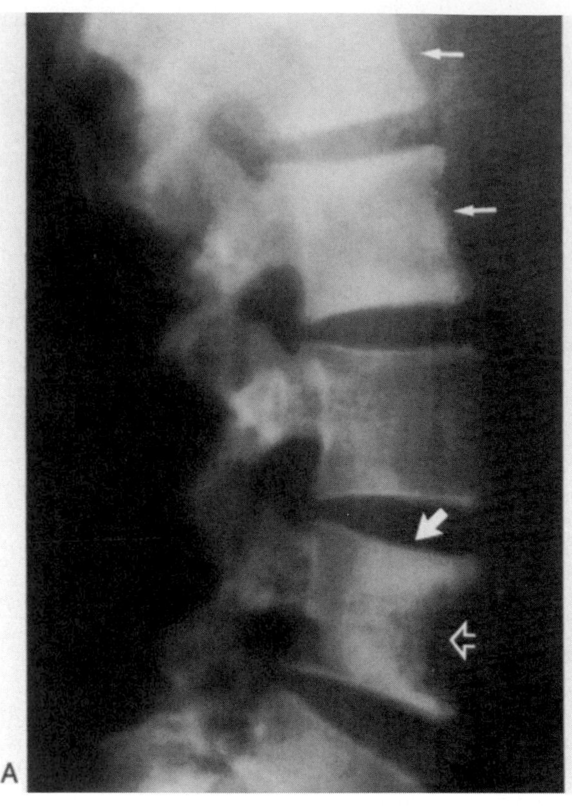

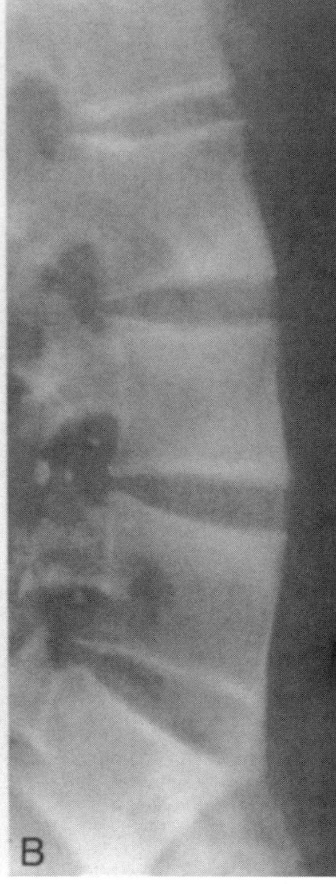

Figure 18-11 A 27-year-old black man with low back pain and sarcoidosis. *A*, Lateral view of the lumbar spine reveals sclerosis of L1 and L2 vertebral bodies *(small white arrows)* and mixed sclerosis *(white arrow)* and lysis *(open arrow)* of the L4 vertebral body. The radiograph was obtained in 1975. *B*, Lateral view of the lumbar spine taken in 1980 demonstrates continued sclerosis with paravertebral calcification. The patient developed hemoptysis secondary to an aspergilloma and died in 1989. *(Courtesy of Werner Barth, MD.)*

neurosarcoidosis.[18] They are sensitive to detecting space-occupying lesions in the spinal cord and other parts of the central nervous system.[11,49]

Scintigraphy

Bone scintigraphy is a sensitive indicator of the extent of osseous sarcoidosis.[7] Both gallium citrate Ga 67 and technetium Tc 99m methylene diphosphonate may show alterations in bone activity not evident on plain roentgenograms. The bone scan may identify more accessible sites for biopsy. Bone scintigraphic activity may decrease with response to therapy.[12]

DIFFERENTIAL DIAGNOSIS

The definitive diagnosis of vertebral sarcoidosis requires a biopsy of the lesion in patients with posterior element involvement or disc space narrowing. Diseases that may mimic sarcoid involvement of the spine include tuberculosis, pyogenic osteomyelitis, Hodgkin's disease, and metastatic carcinoma. These diseases also may cause posterior element destruction and/or disc space narrowing. Biopsy of the bone lesion may not be necessary in the patient in whom previous biopsy has proved pulmonary and skin disease secondary to sarcoid. However, if an anterior lytic lesion of a vertebral body does not respond to therapy, further diagnostic tests, including biopsy, are indicated.

A number of tests are needed as a minimum to diagnose sarcoidosis (Table 18-5).[40] A suspected case of sarcoidosis should undergo biopsy of appropriate tissues to exclude infection or malignancy, particularly if therapy will be instituted.

TREATMENT

Most patients with vertebral sarcoidosis require corticosteroids in the range of 15 to 80 mg/day to control the symptoms and the granulomatous inflammation.[16,23,30] A tapering course of therapy is continued for 6 to 12 months. Although sustained therapy for the lung may not alter long-term progression, corticosteroids for osseous lesions may offer a sustained effect.[20,41] Bone lysis and sclerosis may remain the same or lessen with therapy. Methotrexate at doses from 7.5 to 15 mg/week are effective for those individuals resistant or intolerant to corticosteroid therapy.[32,37] Methotrexate may take up to 6 months to become fully effective. Compressive neurologic symptoms secondary to vertebral sarcoidosis are uncommon and may respond to corticosteroids.[44] Antitumor necrosis factor therapy has been used for sarcoid myopathy. However, a hypercoagulable state developed that limited the usefulness of the biological therapy.[57] In patients with persistent spinal pain or neurologic symptoms of cord compression who do not respond to medical management, surgical decompression of the involved vertebrae is required.[42,43] Surgical decompression may also be necessary to relieve radicular pain for nerve roots infiltrated with sarcoid granulomas.[50] Spinal instability caused by bone destruction or progressive neurologic symptoms may require spinal fusion.[28,52]

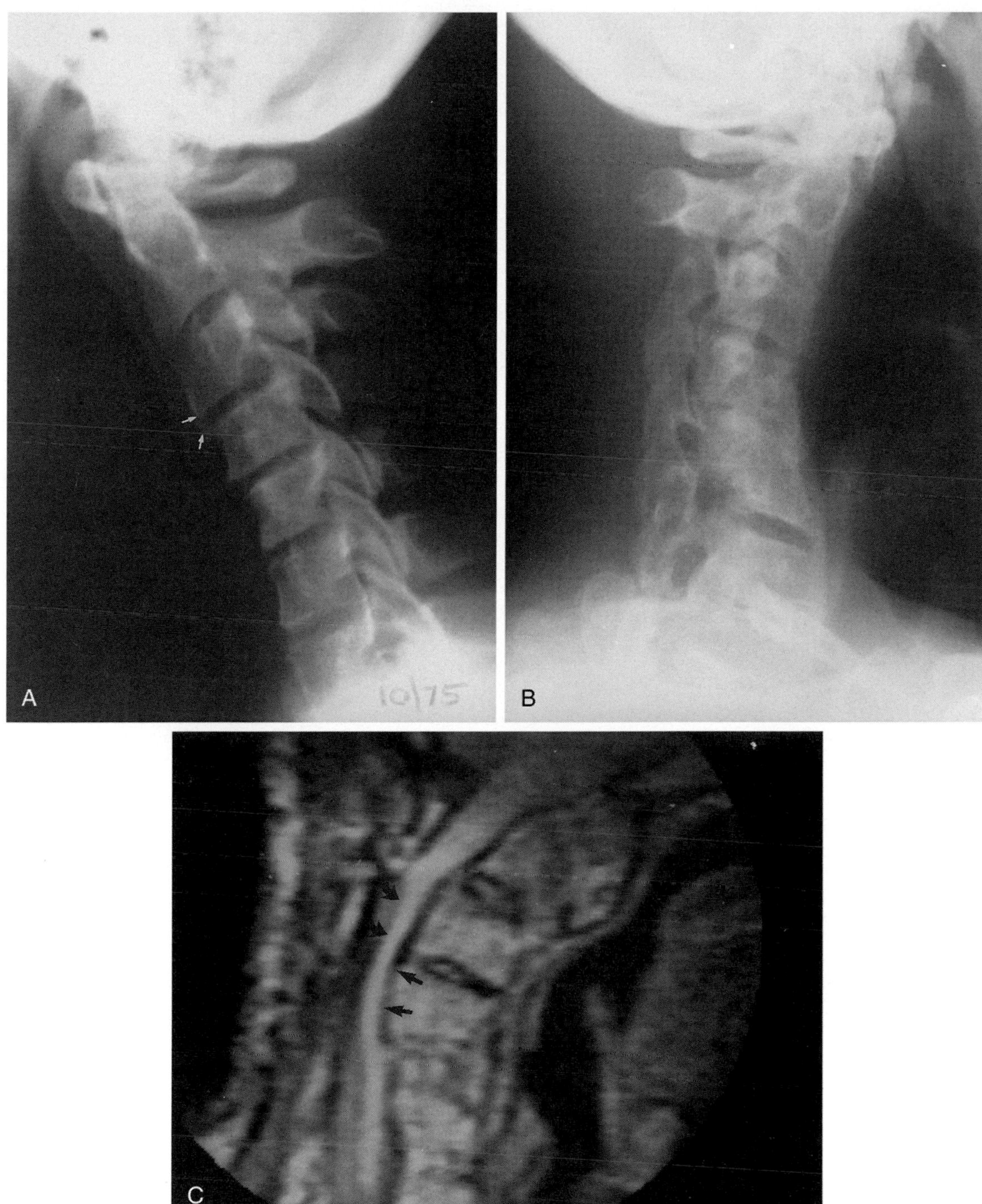

Figure 18-12 Vertebral sarcoidosis. A black man 27 years of age (same patient as in Fig. 18-11) with neck and low back pain and sarcoidosis. *A*, Lateral view of the cervical spine (October 1975) reveals early bridging of the C3–C4 interspace *(arrows)*. In November 1976 he developed an abrupt onset of quadriparesis secondary to a fall. A lateral roentgenogram and myelogram (not shown) revealed collapse of C5 as well as C3–C7 extradural blockage. An anterior C4–C6 spinal fusion was completed. *B*, Lateral view of the cervical spine in 1980 demonstrates continued paravertebral calcification. In 1986 he developed increasing neck pain and angulation. *C*, MR scan reveals reversal of normal spinal curvature, with most marked angulation at C3–C5, close adherence of the spinal cord to the posterior margin of the vertebral bodies *(straight arrows)*, and atrophy of the spinal cord *(curved arrows)*. *(Courtesy of Werner Barth, MD.)*

PROGNOSIS

The prognosis of patients with vertebral sarcoidosis has been generally good.[55] Surgical intervention for biopsies of lesions is important in eliminating other causes of vertebral lysis and sclerosis and confirming the presence of noncaseating granuloma. Decompression and/or fusion of severely affected areas of the axial skeleton has helped prevent the progression of potentially life-threatening neurologic complications. In most circumstances, corticosteroids for sarcoidosis in general, and vertebral sarcoidosis in particular, have been effective in controlling the systemic inflammatory component of this illness. However, patients with vertebral sarcoidosis have extrathoracic disease, and patients with extensive systemic

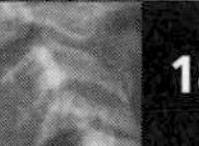

18-5 CLINICAL EVALUATION FOR SARCOIDOSIS

INITIAL

Thorough history, including occupational and environmental exposures
Physical examination—including lung, skin, eye, liver, heart
Histologic confirmation of noncaseating granuloma with special stains and cultures
Chest radiograph
Electrocardiography
Slit-lamp ophthalmologic examination
Chemistry blood tests to evaluate hepatic and renal function and serum calcium level
Tests to determine extent of organ involvement

SUBSEQUENT EVALUATION

Monitoring for resolution or progression of disease with new organ involvement
Subspecialty referral for specific organ system involvement

Modified from Newman LS, Rose CS, Maier LA: Sarcoidosis. N Engl J Med 336:1224-1234, 1997.

manifestations of sarcoidosis have a less favorable prognosis than those patients with exclusively intrathoracic disease.[27,29]

References

Vertebral Sarcoidosis

1. Abdelwahab IF, Norman A: Osteosclerotic sarcoidosis. AJR Am J Roentgenol 150:161, 1988.
2. Agostini C, Adamif, Semenzato G: New pathogenetic insights into sarcoid granuloma. Curr Opin Rheum 12:71-77, 2000.
3. Agostini C, Costabel U, Semenzato G: Sarcoidosis news: Immunologic frontiers for new immunosuppressive strategies. Clin Immunol Immunopathol 88:199-204, 1998.
4. Alberti LD, Piatelli A, Aartese L, et al: Human herpesvirus 8 variants in sarcoid tissues. Lancet 350:1655-1661, 1997.
5. Baldwin DM, Roberts JG, Croff HE: Vertebral sarcoidosis: A case report. J Bone Joint Surg Am 56:629, 1974.
6. Baron B, Goldberg AL, Rothfus WE, Sherman RL: CT features of sarcoid infiltration of a lumbosacral nerve root. J Comput Assist Tomogr 13:364, 1989.
7. Benelhadj S, Patrois F, Duet M, et al: Radioisotope bone scanning in a case of sarcoidosis. Clin Nucl Med 21:371-374, 1996.
8. Berk RN, Brower TD: Vertebral sarcoidosis. Radiology 82:660, 1964.
9. Bernstein J, Rival J: Sarcoidosis of the spinal cord as the presenting manifestation of the disease. South Med J 71:1571, 1978.
10. Brodey PA, Pripstein S, Strange G, Kohout ND: Vertebral sarcoidosis: A case report and review of the literature. AJR Am J Roentgenol 126:900, 1976.
11. Chapelon C, Ziza JM, Piette JC, et al: Neurosarcoidosis: Signs, course, and treatment in 35 confirmed cases. Medicine 69:261, 1990.
12. Cinti DC, Hawkins HB, Slavin JD: Radioisotope bone scanning in a case of sarcoidosis. Clin Nucl Med 10:192-195, 1985.
13. Curran JJ, Dennis GJ, Boling EP: Sarcoidosis and spondyloarthropathy. Arthritis Rheum 30:S42, 1986.
14. Cutler SS, Sankaranarayan G: Vertebral sarcoidosis. JAMA 240:557-558, 1978.
15. Daniele RP, Dauber JH, Rossman MD: Immunologic abnormalities in sarcoidosis. Ann Intern Med 92:406, 1980.
16. Delaney P: Neurologic manifestations in sarcoidosis: Review of literature and report of 23 cases. Ann Intern Med 87:336, 1977.
17. Fanburg BL: Angiotensin-1-converting enzyme. Infanburg BL (ed): Sarcoidosis and Other Granulomatous Diseases of the Lung. New York, Marcel Dekker, 1983, pp 263-272.
18. Fisher AJ, Giklula LA, Kyriakos M, et al: MR imagining changes of lumbar vertebral sarcoidosis. AJR Am J Roentgenol 173:354-356, 1999.
19. Franco M, Passeron C, Tieulie N, et al: Long-term radiographic follow-up in a patient with osteosclerotic sarcoidosis of the spine and pelvis. Rev Rheum Engl Ed 65:586-590, 1998.
20. Gibson GJ, Prescott RJ, Muers MF, et al: British Thoracic Society Sarcoidosis study: Effects of long-term corticosteroid treatment. Thorax 51:238-247, 1996.
21. Ginsberg LE, Williams DW III, Stanton C: MRI of vertebral sarcoidosis. J Comput Assist Tomogr 17:158-159, 1993.
22. Goobar JE, Gilmer S Jr, Carrol DS, Clark GM: Vertebral sarcoidosis. JAMA 178:162, 1961.
23. Gran JT, Bohmer E: Acute sarcoid arthritis: A favorable outcome? Scand J Rheumatol 23:874-877, 1996.
24. Hunninghake GW, Crystal RG: Mechanisms of hypergammaglobulinemia in pulmonary sarcoidosis: Site of increased antibody production and role of T lymphocytes. J Clin Invest 67:86, 1981.
25. Hunninghake GW, Crystal RG: Pulmonary sarcoidosis: A disorder mediated by excess helper T-lymphocyte activity at sites of disease activity. N Engl J Med 305:429, 1981.
26. Hutchinson J: Illustrations of Clinical Surgery, Vol 1. London, Churchill, 1877, p 42.
27. Inoue Y, King TE Jr., Tinkle SS, et al: Human mast cell basic fibroblast growth factor in pulmonary fibrotic disorders. Am J Pathol 149:2037-2054, 1996.
28. James DG, Neville E, Carstairs LS: Bone and joint sarcoidosis. Semin Arthritis Rheum 6:53, 1976.
29. James DG, Williams WJ: Sarcoidosis and Other Granulomatous Disorders. Philadelphia, WB Saunders, 1985.
30. Johns CJ, Scott PP, Schonfeld SA: Sarcoidosis. Annu Rev Med 40:353, 1989.
31. Jones RE, Chatham WW: Update on sarcoidosis. Curr Opin Rheumatol 11:83-87, 1999.
32. Kaye O, Palazzo E, Grossin M, et al: Low-dose methotrexate: An effective corticosteroid-sparing agent in the musculoskeletal manifestations of sarcoidosis. Br J Rheumatol 34:642-644, 1995.
33. Kenney CM III, Goldstein SJ: MRI of sarcoid spondylodiskitis. J Comput Assist Tomogr 16:660, 1992.
34. Kim DS, Jeon YG, Shim TS, et al: The value of interleukin-12 as an activity marker of pulmonary sarcoidosis. Sarcoidosis Vasc Diffuse Lung Dis 17:271-276, 2000.
35. Kremer P, Gallinet E, Benmansour A, et al: Sarcoidosis and spondyloarthropathy: Three cases. Rev Rheum Engl Ed 63:405-411, 1996.
36. Lieberman S: The specificity and nature of serum angiotensin-converting enzyme in sarcoidosis. Ann N Y Acad Sci 278:488, 1976.
37. Mana J, Gomez-Vaquerro C, Dorca J, et al: Vertebral and rib sarcoidosis: Long-term clinical remission with methotrexate. Clin Rheumatol 18:492-494, 1999.
38. Moldover A: Sarcoidosis of the spinal cord: Report of a case with remission associated with cortisone therapy. Arch Intern Med 102:414, 1958.
39. Neville E, Carstairs LS, James DG: Sarcoidosis of bone. Q J Med 46:215, 1977.
40. Newman LS, Rose CS, Maier LA: Sarcoidosis. N Engl J Med 336:1224-1234, 1997.
41. Paramothayan S, Jones PW: Corticosteroid therapy in pulmonary sarcoidosis: A systematic review. JAMA 287:1301-1307, 2002.
42. Perlman SG, Damergis J, Witorsch P, et al: Vertebral sarcoidosis with paravertebral ossification. Arthritis Rheum 21:271, 1978.
43. Rodman R, Funderburk EE Jr, Myerson RM: Sarcoidosis with vertebral involvement. Ann Intern Med 50:213, 1959.
44. Rua-Figueroa I, Gantes MA, Erausquin C, et al: Vertebral sarcoidosis: Clinical and imaging findings. Semin Arthritis Rheum 31:346-352, 2002.
45. Rybicki BA, Major M, Popovich J Jr, et al: Racial differences in sarcoidosis incidence: A 5-year study in a health maintenance organization. Am J Epidemiol 145:234-241, 1997.
46. Sartoris DJ, Resnick D, Resnick C, et al: Musculoskeletal manifestations of sarcoidosis. Semin Roentgenol 20:376-386, 1985.
47. Shaikh S, Soubani AO, Rumore P, et al: Lytic osseous destruction in vertebral sarcoidosis. N Y State J Med 92:213-214, 1992.
48. Sharma OP: Sarcoidosis: Clinical Management. London, Butterworths, 1984.
49. Sharma OP, Sharma AM: Sarcoidosis of the nervous system: A clinical approach. Arch Intern Med 151:1317, 1991.

50. Soskel NT, Fox R: Sarcoidosis or something like it. South Med J 83:1190, 1990.
51. State on Sarcoidosis: Joint Statement of the American Thoracic Society (ATS), the European Respiratory Society (ERS), and the World Association of Sarcoidosis and Other Granulomatous Disorders (WASOG) adopted by the ATS Board of Directors and the ERS Executive Committee, February 1999. Am J Respir Crit Care Med 160:736, 1999.
52. Sundaram M, Place H, Shaffer WO, et al: Progressive destructive vertebral sarcoid leading to surgical fusion. Skeletal Radiol 28:717-722, 1999.
53. Tannenbaum H, Rocklin RE, Schur PH, Sheffer AL: Immune function in sarcoidosis. Clin Exp Immunol 26:511, 1976.
54. Thomas PD, Hunninghake GW: Current concepts of the pathogenesis of sarcoidosis. Am Rev Resp Dis 135:747, 1987.
55. Wurm K, Rosner R: Prognosis of chronic sarcoidosis. Ann N Y Acad Sci 278:732, 1976.
56. Yeager J Jr, Williams MC, Beekman JF, et al: Sarcoidosis: Analysis of cells obtained by bronchoalveolar lavage. Am Rev Respir Dis 116:951, 1977.
57. Yee AMF, Pochapin MB: Treatment of complicated sarcoidosis with infliximab anti-necrosis factor-alpha therapy. Ann Intern Med 135:27-31, 2001.
58. Zener JC, Alpert M, Klainer LM: Vertebral sarcoidosis. Arch Intern Med 11:696, 1963.

RETROPERITONEAL FIBROSIS

CAPSULE SUMMARY

	LOW BACK	NECK
Frequency of spinal pain	Uncommon	Not applicable (NA)
Location of spinal pain	Lower back and lower abdomen	NA
Quality of spinal pain	Dull pain	NA
Symptoms and signs	Weight loss, fever, decreased urine output, abdominal masses, peripheral edema	NA
Laboratory tests	Impaired renal function, increased erythrocyte sedimentation rate	NA
Radiographic findings	Intravenous pyelogram—ureteral obstruction Magnetic resonance imaging—extent of fibrous plaque	NA
Treatment	Ureterolysis, corticosteroids	NA

PREVALENCE AND PATHOGENESIS

Retroperitoneal fibrosis is a disease of unknown cause that causes fibrosis of the retroperitoneum and renal dysfunction secondary to ureteral obstruction. A grayish plaque of fibrosis envelops the retroperitoneum from the level of the renal arteries to the pelvic brim and laterally to the psoas margins. The structures enveloped in the fibrosis include the aorta, inferior vena cava, ureters, and spinal nerves.

Albarran was the first to describe the disease, in 1905.[1] However, Ormond in 1948 described the disease in two patients so that it was recognized as a distinct clinical entity.[51] Retroperitoneal fibrosis has been associated with a variety of names including *Ormond's diseases*, *nonspecific retroperitoneal inflammation*, *sclerosing retroperitonitis*, *retroperitoneal vasculitis*, *periureteritis fibrosa*, and *periaortitis*.

Epidemiology

The prevalence of retroperitoneal fibrosis is about 1 per 200,000 population.[13] Although the literature contains reports that review large numbers of patients with retroperitoneal fibrosis, it is an uncommon disorder, with approximately 800 reported cases.[29,31,42] Patients develop the disease between the fifth and seventh decades, with an average age at diagnosis of 50 years. The male-to-female ratio for retroperitoneal fibrosis is 3:1.

Pathogenesis

The pathogenesis of retroperitoneal fibrosis is unknown. The association of vascular inflammation and panniculitis (Weber-Christian disease) has suggested an immunologic basis similar to that seen with other collagen vascular diseases. Patients with scleroderma, systemic lupus erythematosus, and retroperitoneal fibrosis have been reported.[23,34,35,52] Retroperitoneal fibrosis also has been described in patients with immune thrombocytopenia and those with polyserositis mimicking systemic lupus erythematosus.[43,68] Another possible cause is a disorder of uncontrolled fibrous proliferation.[18] Retroperitoneal fibrosis may occur in combination with other disorders, such as Dupuytren's contracture, Riedel's struma, or sclerosing cholangitis, which are associated with excessive fibrous proliferation in a number of organs.[25] Genetic factors may also play a role in light of a report of patients with HLA-B27 who developed retroperitoneal fibrosis.[72] However, retroperitoneal fibrosis has been reported in individuals with spondyloarthropathy who are HLA-B27 negative.[19,36]

Retroperitoneal fibrosis occurs near areas of atherosclerotic disease affecting large, elastic arteries. One postulated theory for fibrosis is based on the hypothesis that fibrosis develops in response to the leakage of insoluble lipid, ceroid.[10,53] Ceroid may be produced and deposited in atherosclerotic plaques by the oxidation of low-density lipoproteins. Immunoglobulins, particularly IgG, are deposited with ceroid in vessel plaques. Characterization of the inflammatory cells in patients with ceroid deposits and fibrosis identifies a variety of activated immune cells including B and helper T lymphocytes. Retroperitoneal fibrosis may be the result of an immune response to ceroid deposits. Fibrosis does occur in patients with abdominal aortic aneurysms.[33] However, this theory would not explain the presence of fibrosis in areas devoid of atherosclerotic disease.

Malignancy accounts for up to 10% of retroperitoneal cases.[29] In response to the presence of metastases, a desmoplastic response results in the production of fibrous tissue. A wide variety of tumors have been associated with fibrosis, including breast, lung, thyroid, genitourinary (including kidney), and cervix tumors and lymphomas.[16,58]

A number of drugs have been associated with retroperitoneal fibrosis. Methysergide, an ergot derivative, accounted for 12% of cases when it was frequently prescribed for migraine headache.[29] Methysergide is a strong, competitive antagonist of serotonin and causes an increase in the amount of endogenous serotonin. Fibrosis is thought to occur secondary to increased concentrations of serotonin. Other medications including other ergot derivatives that may affect blood vessel function have been implicated as initiators of fibrosis.[3] Beta-blocking agents have also been implicated.[14] Retroperitoneal fibrosis has also been reported subsequent to multiple celiac plexus anesthetic blocks.[54]

The largest group of patients with retroperitoneal fibrosis have idiopathic disease. Over two thirds of patients with this illness have no underlying explanation for the initiation of the fibrotic response in the retroperitoneum.

Approximately 44% of patients with retroperitoneal fibrosis have back pain as a presenting complaint. As the disease progresses, the back, flank, and abdominal lower quadrants become painful.[31]

CLINICAL HISTORY

The presenting symptom of patients with retroperitoneal fibrosis is pain located in the lower quadrants of the abdomen or the lumbosacral spine. The percentage of patients with flank pain and back pain is 42% and 32%, respectively.[5] Pain is insidious in onset, dull, and noncolicky. It may radiate, in the referred pain pattern of the ureter, from the flank to the periumbilical area and to the testes. Patients also may give a history of weight loss, anorexia, fever, and joint pain.[71] Symptoms of urologic compromise, hematuria or oliguria, occur in a later stage of the illness. Occasionally, patients may have spinal stiffness, muscle tenderness, and Raynaud's phenomenon as part of their symptom complex.

PHYSICAL EXAMINATION

The most common physical findings are masses found on abdominal and rectal examination. Compression of the inferior vena cava is associated with peripheral edema in the lower extremities. Patients may complain of pain with percussion over the lumbosacral spine. Hypertension may be noted in 68% of those with renal dysfunction. Testicular examination may reveal hydroceles, testicular atrophy, or scrotal edema. In rare circumstances, lower extremity weakness may be noted. If associated with sensory abnormalities, a lesion affecting the spinal cord or cauda equina should be suspected. A fibrotic epidural mass contiguous with the retroperitoneum may grow epidurally to compress neural elements.[59]

LABORATORY DATA

The most commonly abnormal laboratory finding associated with retroperitoneal fibrosis is an elevated erythrocyte sedimentation rate (ESR), which occurs in more than 90% of patients.[31] C-reactive protein may also be elevated. Less often, but still in a majority of patients (67%), a decrease in hematocrit and an elevation in blood urea nitrogen are noted. Antithyroid, anti-smooth muscle, and Coombs' antibodies have been reported.[34,61] Urinalysis may reveal a variety of abnormalities including proteinuria, microscopic hematuria, and pyuria. In two patients, elevated serum alkaline phosphatase level was associated with active retroperitoneal fibrosis. The serum abnormality returned to normal with corticosteroid therapy for the fibrosis.[6]

Pathology

On gross pathologic inspection, retroperitoneal fibrosis appears as a glistening, grayish-white, woody-hard, fibrous plaque that resembles a malignant retroperitoneal tumor.[13] The fibrosis envelops the retroperitoneal structures, including the aorta, vena cava, renal pedicle, ureters, and psoas muscle. The plaque usually is centered over the anterior surfaces of the fourth and fifth lumbar vertebrae. The tissue is adherent but does not invade the underlying structures. The process may involve the retroperitoneum and may spread as far as the mediastinum.[65]

Histologic specimens from biopsies of the retroperitoneum in patients with retroperitoneal fibrosis reveal dense fibrosis with distinct areas of chronic inflammation.[41,61,69] The chronic inflammation is centered on adipose tissue and blood vessels and is nonsuppurative. The inflammatory component includes lymphocytes, plasma cell, eosinophils, and polymorphonuclear leukocytes. Multinucleated giant cells and granulomas have been described. The inflammation has been associated with chronic inflammation of fibrofatty tissue, perivasculitis, vasculitis, necrotizing vasculitis, and fat necrosis.[31]

RADIOGRAPHIC EVALUATION

Roentgenograms

Radiographic techniques that demonstrate the location of retroperitoneal structures or obstruction of the genitourinary system help make the diagnosis. The classic triad of findings on intravenous pyelography (IVP) is bilateral ureteral narrowing at the level of the fifth lumbar vertebra; medial deviation of the ureters; and dilation of the calyces, pelvis, and ureter (Fig. 18-13). Ureteral stenosis may be

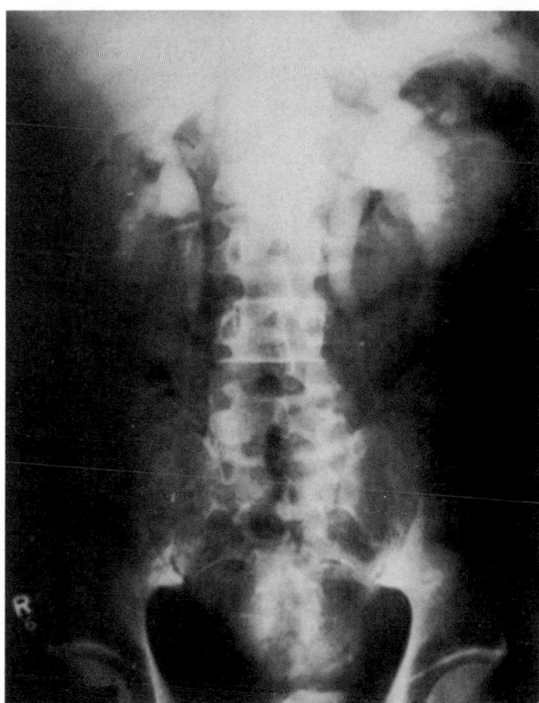

Figure 18-13 IVP of a 57-year-old man with acute onset of anuria with chronic, diffuse low back pain demonstrates dilation of the calices, pelvis, and ureter of both kidneys. Obstruction of the ureters is greatest at the level of L4 and L5 vertebral bodies. *(Courtesy of Arnold Kwart, MD.)*

limited to the L4 and L5 vertebral body level in a majority of ureters evaluated by IVP.[67] Retrograde pyelography may show ureteral obstruction. The sonographic appearance of the retroperitoneum in retroperitoneal fibrosis is one of a smooth-bordered echo-free mass over the sacrum.[60] Renal ultrasonography reveals a poorly marginated, periaortic mass associated with hydronephrosis. Lymphangiography is useful in distinguishing retroperitoneal fibrosis from lymphoma.[7] Gallium 67 imaging may be useful in measuring the state of inflammatory activity of fibrosis in the retroperitoneum. Gallium scan may identify an area of increased activity that would be an appropriate location for a diagnostic biopsy.[26]

Computed Tomography

In the past, CT was the most sensitive technique for evaluation of retroperitoneal fibrosis. CT scan is capable of detecting the presence and extent of the characteristic soft tissue mass as well as its relation to adjacent abdominal structures (Fig. 18-14).[15] However, CT scan is not able to identify the quality of soft tissue disease allowing the differentiation of the various causes of retroperitoneal fibrosis.[38] CT scan also may miss fibrosis that causes renal dysfunction in the form of obstructive uropathy but does not cause ureteral dilation.[63] In patients with renal failure, the use of contrast dye worsens kidney dysfunction. Unenhanced scanning makes it difficult to distinguish the aortic lumen from surrounding tissues in some patients. Neoplastic tissues may not be differentiated from benign fibrosis. CT-guided biopsy is a frequently used method for obtaining histologic specimens. CT is limited to the axial plane.[46]

Magnetic Resonance

MR is the radiographic technique of choice to evaluate retroperitoneal fibrosis.[3,73] T1-weighted images of fibrotic plaque have low to medium signal. T2-weighted images have high signal intensity. The presence of high signal intensity may be noted in patients with malignant fibrosis as well as those with an inflammatory stage of benign fibrosis because of high free-water content and hypercellularity.[30] The presence of low intensity signal on both T1 and T2 images suggests benign retroperitoneal fibrosis (Fig. 18-15).[4]

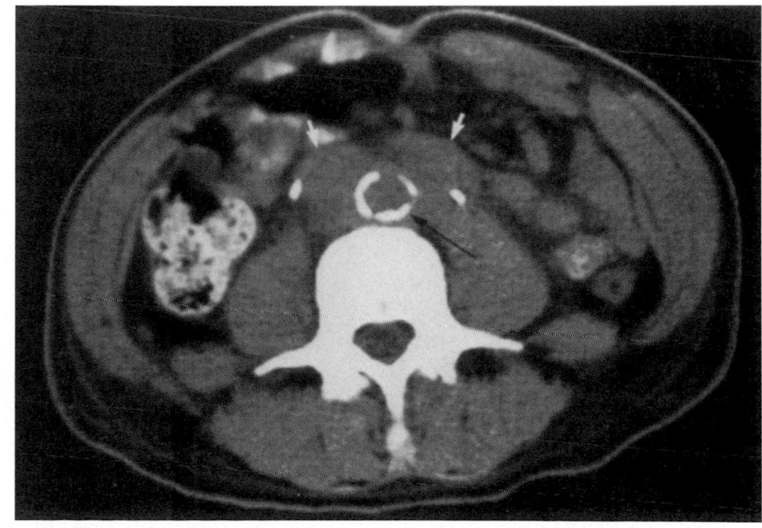

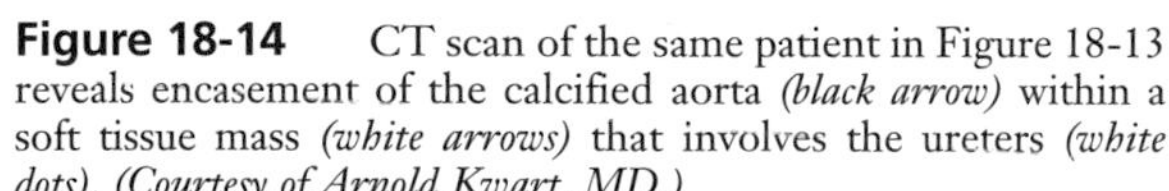

Figure 18-14 CT scan of the same patient in Figure 18-13 reveals encasement of the calcified aorta *(black arrow)* within a soft tissue mass *(white arrows)* that involves the ureters *(white dots)*. *(Courtesy of Arnold Kwart, MD.)*

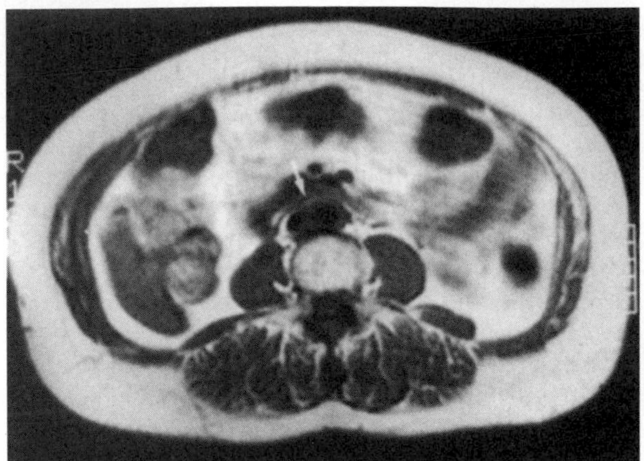

Figure 18-15 Retroperitoneal fibrosis. A 50-year-old woman with a history of lumbar laminectomy and fusion in 1983 who subsequently developed retroperitoneal fibrosis requiring right nephrectomy in 1988. In April 1992, an MR scan was obtained to determine the extent and activity of her fibrosis. The T2-weighted image demonstrated retroperitoneal fibrosis that had a slightly bright signal *(arrow)*, suggesting mild activity of her disease. Her erythrocyte sedimentation rate (ESR) was 85 mm/hr. She refused corticosteroid therapy. Over the following year, her ESR has fallen to 59 mm/hr and her renal function has been stable.

DIFFERENTIAL DIAGNOSIS

The diagnosis of retroperitoneal fibrosis can be suspected in a patient with back pain, constitutional symptoms, and evidence of genitourinary obstruction and is confirmed by biopsy of the retroperitoneum. There are many disease processes, including malignancy, trauma, infection, reactions to drugs, and connective tissue diseases, associated with retroperitoneal fibrosis (Table 18-6). Metastatic carcinoma from abdominal organs or breast may deposit in the retroperitoneum, causing ureteral obstruction and fibrosis.[64] Neoplastic diseases such as Hodgkin's disease, non-Hodgkin's lymphoma, and sarcomas may originate in the retroperitoneum and may produce extensive sclerotic reactions.[48] Rare tumors, such as teratomas, may present in adults and may mimic changes of retroperitoneal fibrosis.[9] Carcinoid tumors with increased production of serotonin have been associated with fibrosis.[44] Radiation therapy of the retroperitoneum given for the treatment of tumors may result in fibrosis.[45] The clinician must remember that retroperitoneal malignancy leaves subtle findings that are initially overlooked. Additional biopsies and close evaluation should elucidate those individuals with "idiopathic" retroperitoneal fibrosis who actually have fibrosis resulting from a malignant tumor.[32]

18-6 CAUSES OF RETROPERITONEAL FIBROSIS

Malignancy
- Periureteral metastatic disease
- Primary retroperitoneal tumors
- Carcinoid

Retroperitoneal injury
- Bleed (anticoagulants, clotting factor deficiency)
- Trauma (blunt, operative)
- Ruptured diverticulum
- Appendicitis
- Urinary extravasation
- Radiation

Infection agents
- Genitourinary tract
- Histoplasmosis

Drugs
- Methysergide
- Amphetamines

Collagen vascular disease
- Vasculitis
- Weber-Christian panniculitis
- Mesenteric panniculitis
- Systemic lupus erythematosus
- Scleroderma

Miscellaneous
- Sclerosing fibrosis

Modified from Lepor H, Walsh PC: Idiopathic retroperitoneal fibrosis. J Urol 122:1, 1979.

Trauma to the retroperitoneum may result in subsequent fibrosis. Examples of trauma include bleeding into the retroperitoneum secondary to a clotting factor deficiency or anticoagulant therapy.[57] Bleeding from Henoch-Schönlein purpura and abdominal aneurysm may also cause fibrosis. Trauma to the suprapubic area with hematoma formation may produce retroperitoneal fibrosis.[70] Inflammatory bowel disease that extends beyond the walls of the gut into the retroperitoneum may initiate fibrosis.[21]

Infections in the genitourinary tract may cause fibrosis. Infection may spread through the lymphatics from the bladder to the retroperitoneum and cause fibrosis in periureteral tissues.[47] Specific infections such as tuberculosis, syphilis, actinomycosis, and histoplasmosis have been implicated as causes of retroperitoneal fibrosis.[3]

Drugs are associated with the development of retroperitoneal fibrosis. Methysergide (Sansert), a drug used in the treatment of migraine headaches, has been implicated as a cause.[66] Amphetamines have been blamed in a much smaller number of patients. Other drugs implicated for causing fibrosis include beta-blockers, methyldopa, and hydralazine.[3]

Retroperitoneal fibrosis also may be caused by connective tissue diseases. Weber-Christian disease, a connective tissue disease associated with panniculitis (fat inflammation), causes fibrosis in the retroperitoneum and lymph gland inflammation in the abdomen.[40] Retroperitoneal fibrosis has been associated with vasculitis, including polyarteritis nodosa.[22]

TREATMENT

Treatment for retroperitoneal fibrosis may include surgery to remove ureteral obstruction and/or the administration of corticosteroids (Fig. 18-16).

Surgery

Ureterolysis, freeing the ureters from the retroperitoneum and placing them laterally or intraperitoneally, is essential to relieve obstruction and preserve renal function.[61] Surgical intervention allows for open biopsy to exclude malignancy and relieve mechanical obstruction.[50] Other surgical techniques, such as autorenal transplantation, or ureteral reimplantation are possible if ureterolysis is not successful.[39] To prevent the reinvolvement of the ureters, they may be

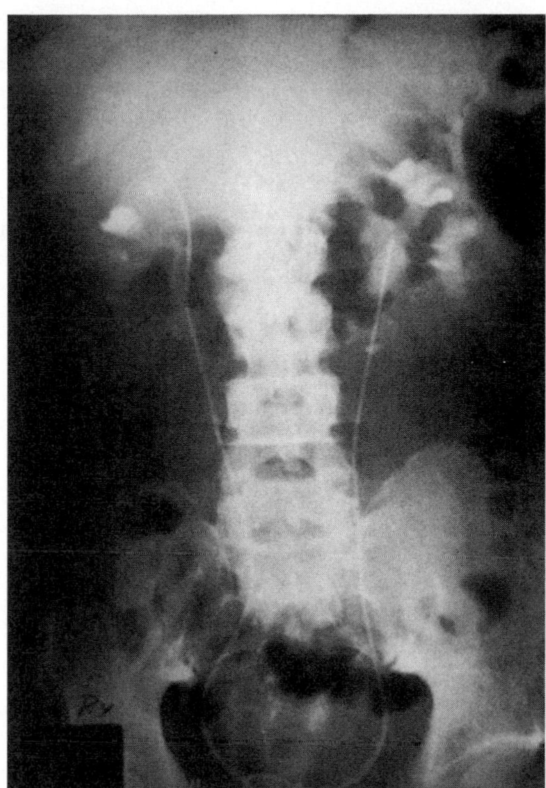

Figure 18-16 In the same patient as in Figure 18-13, ureteral catheters have been threaded up both ureters to relieve obstruction caused by retroperitoneal fibrosis. *(Courtesy of Arnold Kwart, MD.)*

placed in an intraperitoneal location or wrapped with omentum. These surgical procedures also may relieve back pain and normalize both the hematocrit and the ESR.

Corticosteroids

Corticosteroids are useful in the early stages of the illness before dense fibrosis is encountered and for relapses of obstruction after initial ureterolysis (Fig. 18-17).[49] The optimum dose of corticosteroid to be employed has not been established. Most patients are treated with moderate doses of prednisone, 60 to 80 mg/day. Pulse therapy also may be considered.[5] Most urologists are reluctant to use corticosteroids alone as the primary therapy for retroperitoneal fibrosis because of the risk of mismanaging a potentially malignant process. However, nonmalignant, early disease typically responds to corticosteroids in 7 to 10 days by relieving ureteral obstruction.[24] The use of MR should be helpful in identifying the benign nature of the fibrosis and the response to therapy. A course of corticosteroid therapy (initially methylprednisolone [Solu-Medrol] 60 mg on alternate days for 2 months, then tapering to 5 mg over 6 weeks, with 5 mg every day dose for maintenance) continued for a 2-year period is associated with remission of disease in 75% of patients.[28]

Immunosuppressives

A preliminary report has suggested that immunosuppressive therapy, in the form of azathioprine over a 6-week course, may resolve ureteral obstruction.[12] A subsequent report has confirmed the use of azathioprine therapy for retroperitoneal fibrosis.[37] Methotrexate 7.5 mg/week may also offer long-term control.[62] Mycophenolate mofetil (2 g/day) and prednisone (50 mg/day) may be effective therapy to reverse advanced fibrosis.[20]

Tamoxifen

The efficacy of tamoxifen, a selective estrogen receptor modulator, in pelvic desmoid tumors prompted the use in retroperitoneal fibrosis despite the absence of estrogen receptors in fibrous tissue. Tamoxifen inhibits protein kinase C, a mediator of cell proliferation. Tamoxifen increases the synthesis and secretion of transforming growth factor-beta, an inhibitory growth factor.[2] Tamoxifen has been used successfully to reverse retroperitoneal fibrosis.[11] The therapy may be effective in a majority of patients; however, the drug is associated with increased risk of thromboembolism and ovarian cancer.[42]

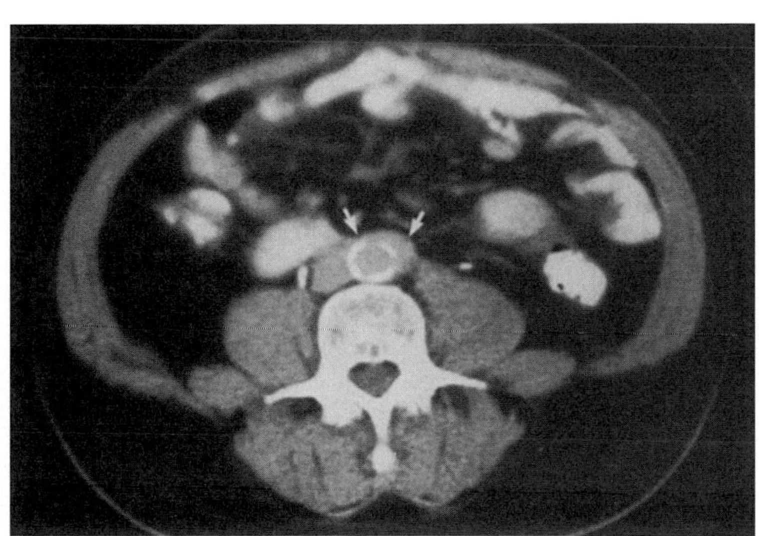

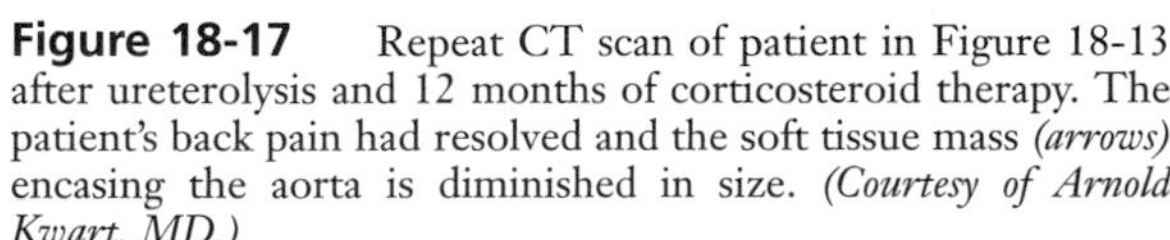

Figure 18-17 Repeat CT scan of patient in Figure 18-13 after ureterolysis and 12 months of corticosteroid therapy. The patient's back pain had resolved and the soft tissue mass *(arrows)* encasing the aorta is diminished in size. *(Courtesy of Arnold Kwart, MD.)*

PROGNOSIS

The prognosis and course of retroperitoneal fibrosis are variable. Cases of spontaneous remissions have been reported.[55] Other patients have had resolution of the disease after surgical biopsy of the lesion.[23] An essential part of therapy is to relieve the obstruction of the ureters. The relief of obstruction may be the key element to allow for spontaneous resolution of the fibrosis.[56] Patients who are anemic at initial presentation have a poorer prognosis.[61] Patients who are older or who have more renal failure have a higher mortality.[5] Patients with early disease treated with surgery and corticosteroid therapy have the potential to achieve a complete remission of their illness.[27] However, short courses of corticosteroids less than 6 months may allow a recurrence of the illness. These patients require a more prolonged course of corticosteroid therapy.[17] The course of the illness and the resolution of inflammation and fibrosis may be followed by serial MR scans.[8,73]

References

Retroperitoneal Fibrosis

1. Albarran J: Retention renale par petriureterite: Liberation externe de l'uretere. Ass Fr Urol 9:511, 1905.
2. Al-Salman J, Makhdomi AR: Treatment of retroperitoneal fibrosis with tamoxifen. South Med J 95:947, 2002.
3. Armis ES Jr: Retroperitoneal fibrosis. AJR Am J Roentgenol 157:321, 1991.
4. Arrive L, Hricak H, Tavares NJ, Miller TR: Malignant versus nonmalignant retroperitoneal fibrosis: Differentiation with MR imaging. Radiology 172:139, 1989.
5. Baker LR, Mallinson WJ, Gregory MC, et al: Idiopathic retroperitoneal fibrosis: A retrospective analysis of 60 cases. Br J Urol 60:497, 1987.
6. Barrison IG, Walker JG, Jones C, Snell ME: Idiopathic retroperitoneal fibrosis—is serum alkaline phosphatase a marker of disease activity? Postgraduate Med J 64:239, 1988.
7. Bookstein JJ, Schroeder KF, Batsakis JG: Lymphangiography in the diagnosis of retroperitoneal fibrosis: Case report. J Urol 95:99, 1966.
8. Brooks AP, Reznek RH, Webb JA: Magnetic resonance imaging in idiopathic retroperitoneal fibrosis: Management of T1 relaxation time. Br J Radiol 63:842, 1990.
9. Bruneton JN, Diard F, Drouillard JP, et al: Primary retroperitoneal teratoma in adults. Radiology 134:613, 1980.
10. Bullock N: Idiopathic retroperitoneal fibrosis [Editorial]. BMJ 297:240, 1988.
11. Clark CP, Vanderpool D, Preskitt JT: The response of retroperitoneal fibrosis to tamoxifen. Surgery 109:502, 1991.
12. Cogan E, Fastrez R: Azathioprine: An alternative treatment for recurrent idiopathic retroperitoneal fibrosis. Arch Intern Med 145:753, 1985.
13. Debruyne FM, Bogman MJ, Ypma AF: Retroperitoneal fibrosis in the scrotum. Eur Urol 8:45, 1982.
14. Demko TM, Diamond JR, Groff J: Obstructive nephropathy as a result of retroperitoneal fibrosis: A review of its pathogenesis and associations. J Am Soc Nephrol 8:684-688, 1997.
15. Feinstein RS, Gatewood OM, Goldman SM, et al: Computerized tomography in the diagnosis of retroperitoneal fibrosis. J Urol 126:255, 1981.
16. Fromowitz FB, Miller F: Retroperitoneal fibrosis as host response to papillary renal cell carcinoma. Urology 38:259, 1991.
17. Gilkeson GS, Allen NB: Retroperitoneal fibrosis: A true connective tissue disease. Rheum Dis Clin North Am 22:23-38, 1996.
18. Gleeson MH, Taylor S, Dowling RH: Multifocal fibrosclerosis. Proc R Soc Med 63:1309, 1970.
19. Golbach P, Mohsenifar Z, Salick AI: Familial mediastinal fibrosis associated with seronegative spondyloarthropathy. Arthritis Rheum 26:221, 1983.
20. Grotz W, Zedwitz IV, Andre M, et al: Treatment of retroperitoneal fibrosis by mycophenolate mofetil and corticosteroids. Lancet 352:1195, 1998.
21. Harlin HC, Hamm FC: Urologic disease resulting from nonspecific inflammatory conditions of the bowel. J Urol 68:383, 1952.
22. Hautekeete ML, Bakerabany G, Marcellin P, et al: Retroperitoneal fibrosis after surgery for aortic aneurysm in a patient with periarteritis nodosa: Successful treatment with corticosteroids. J Intern Med 228:533, 1990.
23. Hellstrom HR, Perez-Stable EC: Retroperitoneal fibrosis with disseminated vasculitis and intrahepatic sclerosing cholangitis. Am J Med 40:184, 1966.
24. Higgins PM, Bennett-Jones DN, Naish-Aber GM: Non-operative management of retroperitoneal fibrosis. Br J Surg 75:573, 1988.
25. Hoffman WW, Trippel OH: Retroperitoneal fibrosis: Etiologic considerations. J Urol 86:222, 1961.
26. Jacobson AF: Gallium-67 imaging in retroperitoneal fibrosis: Significance of a negative result. J Nucl Med 32:521, 1991.
27. Jones JH, Ross EJ, Matz LR, et al: Retroperitoneal fibrosis. Am J Med 48:203, 1970.
28. Kardar AH, Kattan S, Lindstedt E, et al: Steroid therapy for idiopathic retroperitoneal fibrosis: Dose and duration. J Urol 168:550-555, 2002.
29. Koep L, Zuidema GD: The clinical significance of retroperitoneal fibrosis. Surgery 81:250, 1977.
30. Lee JK, Glazer HS: Controversy in the MR imaging appearance of fibrosis. Radiology 177:21, 1990.
31. Lepor H, Walsh PC: Idiopathic retroperitoneal fibrosis. J Urol 122:1, 1979.
32. LeVine M, Schwartz S, Allen A, Narciso FV: Lymphosarcoma and periureteral fibrosis. Radiology 82:92, 1964.
33. Lindell OI, Sariola HV, Lehtonen TA: The occurrence of vasculitis in perianeurysmal fibrosis. J Urol 138:727, 1987.
34. Lipman RL, Johnson B, Berg G, Shapiro AP: Idiopathic retroperitoneal fibrosis and probable systemic lupus erythematosus. JAMA 196:1022, 1966.
35. Mansell MA, Watts RWE: Retroperitoneal fibrosis and scleroderma. Postgrad Med J 56:730, 1980.
36. Martinez FD, Gil JG, Veiga FG, et al: The association of idiopathic retroperitoneal fibrosis and ankylosing spondylitis. J Rheumatol 19:1147, 1992.
37. McDougal WS, MacDonell RC Jr: Treatment of idiopathic retroperitoneal fibrosis by immunosuppression. J Urol 145:112, 1991.
38. Megibow AJ, Mitnick JS, Bosniack MA: The contribution of computed tomography to the evaluation of the obstructed ureter. Urol Radiol 4:95, 1982.
39. Mikkelsen D, Lepor H: Innovative surgical management of idiopathic retroperitoneal fibrosis. J Urol 141:1192, 1989.
40. Milner RD, Mitchinson MJ: Systemic Weber-Christian disease. J Clin Pathol 18:150, 1965.
41. Mitchinson MJ: The pathology of idiopathic retroperitoneal fibrosis. J Clin Pathol 23:681, 1970.
42. Monev S: Idiopathic retroperitoneal fibrosis: Prompt diagnosis preserves organ function. Cleve Clin J 69:160-166, 2002.
43. Morad N, Strongwater SL, Eypper S, Woda BA: Idiopathic retroperitoneal and mediastinal fibrosis mimicking connective tissue disease. Am J Med 82:363, 1987.
44. Morin LJ, Zuerner RT: Retroperitoneal fibrosis and carcinoid tumor. JAMA 216:1647, 1971.
45. Moul JW: Retroperitoneal fibrosis following radiotherapy for stage I testicular seminoma. J Urol 147:124, 1992.
46. Mulligan SA, Holley HC, Koehler RE, et al: CT and MR imaging in the evaluation of retroperitoneal fibrosis. J Comput Assist Tomogr 13:277, 1989.
47. Mulvaney NP: Periureteritis obliterans: A retroperitoneal inflammatory disease. J Urol 79:410, 1958.
48. Niz GL, Hewitt CB, Straffon RA, et al: Retroperitoneal malignancy masquerading as benign retroperitoneal fibrosis. J Urol 103:46, 1970.
49. Ochsner MG, Brannan W, Pond HS, Goodlet JS Jr: Medical therapy in idiopathic retroperitoneal fibrosis. J Urol 114:700, 1975.
50. Onuigbo M, Lawrence K, Park S: Retroperitoneal fibrosis: Unusual cause of low back pain. South Med J 94:735-737, 2001.
51. Ormond JK: Bilateral ureteral obstruction due to envelopment and compression by an inflammatory retroperitoneal process. J Urol 59:1072, 1948.

52. Ormond JK: Idiopathic retroperitoneal fibrosis: A discussion of the etiology. J Urol 94:385, 1965.
53. Parums D, Choudhury RP, Shields SA, Davies AH: Characterization of inflammatory cells associated with "idiopathic retroperitoneal fibrosis." Br J Urol 67:564, 1991.
54. Pateman J, Williams MP, Filshie J: Retroperitoneal fibrosis after multiple coeliac plexus blocks. Anesthesia 45:309, 1990.
55. Perlow S: Obstruction of the iliac artery caused by retroperitoneal fibrosis. Am J Surg 105:285, 1963.
56. Pierre S, Cody PE, Razvi H: Retroperitoneal fibrosis: A case report of spontaneous resolution. Clin Nephrol 57:314-319, 2002.
57. Popham BK, Stevenson TD: Idiopathic retroperitoneal fibrosis associated with a coagulation defect (factor VII deficiency): Report of a case and review of the literature. Ann Intern Med 52:894, 1960.
58. Rivlin ME, McGehee RP, Bakerower JD: Retroperitoneal fibrosis associated with carcinoma of the cervix: Review of the literature. Gynecol Oncol 41:95, 1991.
59. Sa JD, Pimentel J, Carvalho M, et al: Spinal cord compression secondary to idiopathic retroperitoneal fibrosis. Neurosurgery 26:678, 1990.
60. Sanders RC, Duffy T, McLoughlin MG, Walsh PC: Sonography in the diagnosis of retroperitoneal fibrosis. J Urol 118:944, 1977.
61. Saxton HM, Kilpatrick FR, Kinder CH, et al: Retroperitoneal fibrosis: A radiological and follow-up study of fourteen cases. Q J Med 38:159, 1969.t
62. Scavelli AS, Spadaro A, Riccieri V, et al: Long-term follow-up of low-dose methotrexate therapy in one case of idiopathic retroperitoneal fibrosis. Clin Rheumatol 14:481-484, 1995.
63. Spital A, Valvo JR, Segal AJ: Nondilated obstructive uropathy. Urology 31:478, 1988.
64. Usher SM, Brendler H, Ciavarra VA: Retroperitoneal fibrosis secondary to metastatic neoplasm. Urology 9:191, 1977.
65. Utz DC, Henry JD: Retroperitoneal fibrosis. Med Clin North Am 50:1091, 1966.
66. Utz DC, Rooke ED, Spittell JA Jr, Bartholomew IG: Retroperitoneal fibrosis in patients taking methysergide. JAMA 191:983, 1965.
67. Wagenknecht LV, Auvert J: Symptoms and diagnosis of retroperitoneal fibrosis: Analysis of 31 cases. Urol Int 26:185, 1971.
68. Wallach PM, Flannery MT, Adelman HM, et al: Retroperitoneal fibrosis accompanying immune thrombocytopenia. Am J Hematol 37:204, 1991.
69. Webb AJ: Cytological studies in retroperitoneal fibrosis. Br J Surg 54:375, 1967.
70. Webb AJ, Dawson-Edwards P: Malignant retroperitoneal fibrosis. Br J Surg 54:505, 1967.
71. Wicks IP, Robertson MR, Murnaghan GF, Bertouch JV: Idiopathic retroperitoneal fibrosis presenting with back pain. J Rheumatol 15:1572, 1988.
72. Willscher MK, Novicki DE, Cwazka WF: Association of HLA-B27 antigen with retroperitoneal fibrosis. J Urol 120:631, 1978.
73. Yuh WTC, Barloon TJ, Sickels WJ, et al: Magnetic resonance imaging in the diagnosis and followup of idiopathic retroperitoneal fibrosis. J Urol 141:602, 1989.

Section IV

Therapy

Therapy for pain in the low back or neck has been based on such diverse foundations as double-blind, placebo-controlled randomized trials, clinical experience, anecdotes, fads, and "scientific" articles in weekly magazines bought at grocery store checkout counters. For example, the following headline appears from time to time in one of the weekly tabloid papers: "Sex Cures Arthritis, Prevents Back Pain and Many Killer Diseases." The amount of scientific data that supports the use of sex as a treatment for back pain, as well as that for a wide range of other therapeutic interventions used in this disorder, is meager. However, the number of scientific trials that have proven efficacy and inefficacy of a variety of treatments for spinal pain has increased. For example, The Cochrane Collaboration monitors the medical literature to determine the number of well-designed studies that support the efficacy of therapies for clinical disorders, including low back and neck pain.[20] Some physicians have used the absence of studies to propose that recommended therapies should be exclusively limited to those that have been proved effective in controlled clinical trials. Some older drug therapies (oral corticosteroids) are unlikely to be studied in clinical trials because of the absence of a monetary incentive. Oral corticosteroids are beneficial for the treatment of specific cohorts of patients with spinal pain with inflammatory disorders or radiculopathy. Other physicians take a more nonchalant attitude and use the patient's response "I feel better" as adequate evidence of efficacy. Physicians should realize that therapies that have been demonstrated to be ineffective for spinal pain in controlled trials have benefits that are probably related to placebo response exclusively. The placebo response has powerful effects on patient improvement over the short term. Effective therapies should be the first choice offered to patients with spinal disorders. The difference of opinion regarding the degree of proof of efficacy should not preclude the use of therapies that have not been investigated in controlled trials but are believed to be safe and effective for spinal pain in individual patients; on the other hand, one should not be satisfied with the recommendation of unproven spinal pain therapy for large populations of patients until the therapy has been shown to be effective scientifically.

There is no single form of therapy that is effective for all forms of spinal pain. The various therapies that are effective treatment for specific diseases have been listed in Section III. Section IV concentrates on a more detailed review of the component parts of therapy. The indications for the use of the specific therapies and the toxicities and complications associated with each are discussed. Whenever possible, recommendations are based on published clinical trials. Recommendations based on personal clinical experience are also given and are stated as such as "Our Recommendation." Medical treatment in general and specific therapeutic regimens that have been used successfully in the care of patients with uncomplicated spinal disorders are presented in Chapter 19. Chapter 20 describes the indications and expected results from spinal surgery. The success of surgery is based on careful selection of patients; the patient's physician can help the surgeon decide whether the individual is an appropriate candidate from a general medical, musculoskeletal, and psychological standpoint.

Decisions regarding therapy for patients with low back or neck pain are arduous and taxing. The level of misunderstanding has not necessarily improved with the multiple sources of information available to patients from the Internet. Physicians must remain focused on the goals of therapy despite the many distractions that may arise from patients, insurance companies, and workers' compensation carriers, for example. They need to keep the following axioms of therapy in mind to provide appropriate care to their patients with spinal pain.

AXIOMS OF THERAPY

1. Most spinal pain is mechanical in origin.
2. Most mechanical spinal pain resolves by the end of 2 months.
3. Common sense is the most important part of therapy. Both the patient and physician should use it as much as possible during the course of treatment.
4. The goals of therapy must be the same for the patient and physician.
5. The physician must clearly state the goals at the start of therapy. Inform the patient.
6. Do the patient no harm. Limit the patient's exposure to medications with excessive toxicities and operative procedures of questionable benefit.
7. Accept the placebo response (an endogenous opiate effect) as an effective part of therapy.
8. Modify the therapeutic regimen according to changes (improvement or deterioration) in the patient's condition.
9. Improving the patient's general physical condition is an important component of spinal therapy.
10. Consider improved physical function, increased self-reliance, and improved self-esteem as good outcomes of patient therapy.

In general, therapy for spinal pain is directed at controlling pain in the acute situation. Control of acute pain can prevent the development of chronic pain with the attended modifications of membrane nociceptive receptors, loss of inhibitory interneurons, and modifications of the cerebral cortex. In patients with mechanical causes of spinal pain, restoration of normal physiology (i.e., muscle length and strength) should commence as pain is relieved. Patients who are at risk for continuous "injuries" that result in spinal dysfunction (e.g., muscle strain in computer programmers) should be instructed in appropriate body mechanics (good posture, appropriate work stance, correct sitting positions) to help prevent recurrent episodes of spinal pain.[6] Patients who do not follow these recommendations may improve in any case or may develop chronic pain that can persist despite healing of the acute injury.

Another important component of medical therapy for spinal pain is the prevention of injury to the axial skeleton. For example, diving accidents are a common cause of cervical spine injury in young adults.[12] Approximately 50% of individuals were intoxicated with alcohol at the time of their accidents. Many of these individuals were injured at their homes in backyard pools. Additionally, osteoporosis is a preventable cause of lumbar spine fracture.[15]

A number of components of therapy have been evaluated by scientific study. Controversies exist for most therapies utilized for patients with spinal pain. Conservative therapy limited to those components shown to be statistically significantly better than placebo include activity as tolerated, cyclooxygenase-2 (COX-2) inhibitors, and back school.[9,11,14,18] Some physicians believe that most spinal pain is psychological in origin and that controlling life stress or anxiety is the best way of treating spinal pain. Others believe that spinal pain is an inability to cope with one's social environment. This predicament is not made better with oral therapies but with coming to grips with the environment and treating yourself.[7] This outlook on spinal disorders excludes the axial skeleton from the same vicissitudes that occur in other portions of the musculoskeletal system. Why the spine with its muscles, ligaments, tendons, bones, joints, cartilage, and nerves should be excluded from injury or disease in a way different from the appendages is implausible. The need to know the exact structure that is disordered is not necessary to treat. The requirement to visualize components of the spine with radiographs or rapid MR scans does not result in improved care.[10] However, the predicament is that visualization with radiographic techniques is unable to detect the physiologic alterations in the structures resulting in dysfunction, not that the dysfunction is fictitious. In the past, some disorders were thought to be psychological in origin and were thought not to exist (e.g., fibromyalgia). Recent studies of functional MR images of the brain have demonstrated the differences in the processing of nociceptive signals in patients with fibromyalgia from control subjects.[5] Further investigations of spinal pain may also document abnormalities of musculoskeletal and neural function that explain the clinical complaints of our patients. The goal of the treating physician is to return the patient with spinal pain to a less painful state, with improved function with only the necessary degree of diagnostic investigation and the most effective, least invasive, and safest therapy. Placebo response is a powerful component of therapy.[16] When the placebo response is blocked by naloxone or psychological interventions, the efficacy of a therapy is diminished. Conversely, the belief that a therapy will be effective has a positive result on the efficacy of an agent that has no inherent therapeutic benefit.[1]

In a study similar to a report concerning lumbar spine disease, the Quebec Task Force published a review concerning the diagnosis and treatment of whiplash-associated disorders.[19] Few scientific studies are available to demonstrate the efficacy of therapeutic interventions in the course of this cervical injury. Of a review of 1204 studies, only 62 were found to be scientifically valid. Recommendations of rest and the use of a cervical collar may be counterproductive and may slow improvement in some individuals with whiplash injuries. Some of the recommendations for increasing movement in cases of whiplash may be applicable to therapy for other neck disorders. However, an approval of all the recommendations for other forms of cervical spine disorders should not be assumed. Additional research is required to determine the efficacy of a wide range of therapeutic interventions for neck pain. The clinician should use therapies that improve functional capacity of the patient, in the absence of scientific data, when exposure to harm associated with a specific intervention is limited.

The appropriate selection of patients for surgical intervention is debated in the literature. Intervertebral disc herniation may be treated effectively by nonoperative interventions.[13] Studies suggest that abnormal physical findings (positive straight leg–raising test) correlate with anatomic abnormalities seen at surgery, but outcome is best related to the psychological health of the patient.[17] If taken to an extreme, surgical intervention might be limited to the most severely affected individuals with marked neurologic compromise. Controversy exists in regard to the efficacy of surgical lumbar fusion in the treatment of patients requiring laminectomies or decompression procedures.[8] Increased morbidity and mortality may occur in older patients who undergo decompression procedures.[3] Controversy also exists in regard to the appropriate use of surgery in the therapy for cervical spine disorders. The rates of cervical spine surgery have been increasing from 1979 to 1990, increasing more than 70% during this period.[2] There are wide variations in the rate of cervical spine surgery within different geographic areas.[4] Reasons for the rate of increase of neck procedures include an increase in the incidence of cervical spine disease, increasing numbers of physicians available to perform surgery, a lower threshold for surgical treatment, and altered patient expectations for treatment. Additional data are needed to determine the efficacy of these invasive procedures and whether the rate of spinal surgery is appropriate.

When is the risk associated with surgery outweighed by the benefit in quality of life associated with improved physical function? In this setting of conflicting studies and personal testimonials, thoughtful, unbiased clinical judgment must be the guide to the therapy for spinal pain. In a time of increasing pressures on health care providers to deliver cost-effective care, thoughtful evaluation of the efficacy of the therapies we use for spinal pain is essential. Our goal is to return the patient to full function. A variety of therapies may be needed to reach that goal. The choice for the physician is to pick those that are effective for that specific patient while exposing that individual to the least risk.

Our recommendations at the end of discussions in Section III are made for the usual patient with low back and neck pain. Patients with spinal pain should receive therapies that are effective with limited toxicities. Therapies with no proven efficacy or excessive risks should not be given to the usual patient with spinal pain.

References

1. Bratton RL, Montero DP, Adams KS, et al: Effect of "ionized" wrist bracelets on musculoskeletal pain: A randomized, double-blind, placebo-controlled trial. Mayo Clin Proc 77:1164-1168, 2002.
2. Davis H: Increasing rates of cervical and lumbar spine surgery in the United States, 1979-1990. Spine 19:1117-1123, 1994.
3. Deyo RA, Cherkin DC, Loeser JD, et al: Morbidity and mortality in association with operations on the lumbar spine: The influence of age, diagnosis, and procedure. J Bone Joint Surg Am 74A:536-543, 1992.

4. Einstadter D, Kent DL, Fihn SD, et al: Variation in the rate of cervical spine surgery in Washington State. Med Care 31:711-718, 1993.
5. Gracely RH, Petzke F, Wolf JM, et al: Functional magnetic resonance imaging evidence of augmented pain processing in fibromyalgia. Arthritis Rheum 46:1333-1343, 2002.
6. Grandjean E: Fitting the Task to the Man: A Textbook of Occupational Ergonomics, 4th ed. London: Taylor & Francis, 1988.
7. Hadler NM: MRI for regional back pain: Need for less imaging, better understanding. JAMA 289:2863-2864, 2003.
8. Hanley EN, David SM: Lumbar arthrodesis for the treatment of back pain. J Bone Joint Surg Am 81A:716-730, 1999.
9. Hurri H: The Swedish back school in chronic low back pain: I. Benefits. Scand J Rehabil Med 21:33-40, 1989.
10. Jarvik JG, Hollingworth W, Martin B, et al: Rapid magnetic resonance imaging vs radiographs for patients with low back pain: A randomized controlled trial. JAMA 289:2810-2818, 2003.
11. Katz N, Ju WD, Krupa DA, et al: Efficacy and safety of rofecoxib in patients with chronic low back pain: Results from two 4-week, randomized, placebo-controlled, parallel-group, double-blind trials. Spine 28:851-859, 2003.
12. Kluger Y, Jarosz D, Paul DB, et al: Diving injuries: A preventable catastrophe. J Trauma 36:349-35, 1994.
13. Komori H, Shinomiya A, Haro H, et al: Contrast-enhanced magnetic resonance imaging in conservative management of lumbar spine disc herniation. Spine 22:67-73, 1998.
14. Malmivaara A, Hakkinen U, Aro T, et al: The treatment of acute low back pain: Bed rest, exercises, or ordinary activity. N Engl J Med 332:351-355, 1995.
15. Margolis KL, Ensrud KE, Schreiner PJ, et al: Body size and risk for clinical fractures in older women. Ann Intern Med 133:123-127, 2000.
16. Rowbotham DJ: Endogenous opioids, placebo response, and pain. Lancet 357:1901-1902, 2001.
17. Spengler DM, Ouelette EA, Battie M, et al: Elective discectomy for herniation of a lumbar disc: Additional experience with an objective method. J Bone Joint Surg Am 72A:230-237, 1990.
18. Spitzer WO, LeBlanc FE, Dupuis M, et al: Scientific approach to the assessment and management of activity-related spinal disorders. Spine 12(Suppl):S1-S59, 1987.
19. Spitzer WO, Skovron ML, Salmi LR, et al: Scientific monograph of the Quebec Task Force on whiplash-associated disorders: Redefining "whiplash" and its management. Spine 20:S1-S73, 1995.
20. Van Tulder MW, Scholten RJPM, Koes BW, et al: Nonsteroidal anti-inflammatory drugs for low back pain: A systematic review within the framework of the Cochrane Collaboration Back Review Group. Spine 25:2501-2513, 2000.

CHAPTER 19

MEDICAL THERAPY

CONTROLLED PHYSICAL ACTIVITY (BED REST)

Patients with acute spinal pain have difficulty ambulating. Certain positions, particularly sitting and standing, exacerbate their pain. These patients spontaneously take to their bed to relieve their symptoms. The amount of scientific evidence to prove, in an objective manner, that bed rest is effective is small. Data exist documenting short duration bed rest (2 days) as appropriate therapy for low back pain. In the past, bed rest or "controlled physical activity" (a more honest term, because many patients find staying in bed for 10 to 14 days very boring and stand or sit during this period) was a mainstay of therapy.[23,24,30] Currently, limiting bed rest to a short period of time is preferred and more effective.[13] The limitation of controlled physical activity is particularly applicable to individuals with localized neck or low back pain. Patients experiencing leg or arm pain associated with intervertebral disc herniation do obtain some relief of appendicular pain with bed rest but do not have improved outcomes compared with individuals who continue activities of daily living, as tolerated.[27] Individuals who remain at bed rest decondition their muscles and become weaker. The degree of decline in cardiovascular and physical work capacity associated with 3 weeks of bed rest is greater than that with aging 30 years, as demonstrated in a study of five healthy men.[14] To return to normal function, they have to strengthen these muscles to return to their baseline status. The less the patients become deconditioned, the more rapidly they can recover.

Cervical Spine

Patients with acute neck pain have difficulty walking, particularly with arm radiculopathy. Decreased physical activity is recommended for therapy for a variety of patients with neck pain. Upright positions exacerbate their pain, with an increase in their neck, arm, and head discomfort. Patients with a herniated cervical intervertebral disc with radiculopathy may find that bed rest with a supporting, appropriately fitted, cervical pillow relieves their neck and arm pain (Fig. 19-1). Upright positions exacerbate their pain, with an increase in their neck, arm, and head discomfort. These patients spontaneously take to bed to relieve their symptoms.

A number of patients with neck pain describe difficulty sleeping or finding comfort in bed because of their pillow. Patients can start with rolling a towel lengthwise and placing it on their regular pillow. In studies of pillows, a soft pillow with support of the cervical lordosis is preferred.[22] Other studies have reported decreased sleeping duration with a roll pillow compared with a water-based pillow.[10] An alternative to a cervical pillow is the arrangement of two pillows in a V with the apex located cranially, with a third pillow placed across the apex of the V. This allows mild traction on the neck and internal rotation of the shoulder, resulting in decreased traction on the cervical nerve roots.[19] Patients should avoid lying prone. No one pillow fits all. Attempting a few different varieties may be necessary before finding the best match.

The amount of scientific evidence to prove these clinical observations is relatively small. No studies have been reported that evaluate the independent effect of rest on mechanical neck pain.[26] Data determining the appropriate duration of bed rest are also limited. In general, cumulative evidence suggests that *prolonged* periods of bed rest are detrimental to recovery of patients. Prolonged immobilization promotes decreased neck motion.[15-17] A systematic review of clinical trials involving limited versus active motion in whiplash injuries revealed improved outcomes for the active therapies.[21]

In fact, patients who are busy rarely stay at bed rest for even a day unless their neck pain is severe. Most patients, however, strictly limit their recreational activities and try to minimize their time at work. An explanation of the appropriate role of controlled physical activity is important at the outset of therapy. Informing patients of the benefits of rest and gradual mobilization results in their understanding the basic components of the treatment program. Bed rest may be poorly tolerated by older patients, including those with trauma to the cervical spine.[12] Prolonged bed rest may result in a number of detrimental alterations in physiologic function, including decreased pulmonary and cardiac function.[9]

Lumbar Spine

Patients with lumbar herniated discs may obtain comfort by assuming a supine position. The biomechanical rationale for bed rest was that the lowest intradiscal pressures were recorded in the supine position.[20] However, other measurements have documented increased intradiscal pressures in the supine position compared with sitting.[31] The semi-Fowler position with the knees and hips flexed is even more helpful in reducing symptoms.[2] The semi-Fowler position also may be comfortable for patients with apophyseal joint disease. These individuals experience less pain secondary to flattening of the lumbar lordosis by decreasing pressure on joint structures.

Patients with radicular pain are prescribed bed rest at home as long as family members or friends are available to aid them. The patient's position in bed is one of comfort. The patient lies on his or her back with hips and knees flexed to a moderate degree. Pillows behind the knees help to relieve pressure on the sciatic nerve (Fig. 19-2). Lying on either side with legs drawn up in the fetal position also affords comfort (Fig. 19-3). The only positions to be avoided are lying prone (face down), which hyperextends the spine, and sitting for prolonged periods, which increases intradiscal pressure and increases sciatica in patients with a herniated disc.[2] Patients should be out of bed to use the bathroom. A bedside commode may be an alternative if walking is severely limited by pain. Each patient is followed carefully and is not allowed complete mobility with exercising until objective signs of a list or paravertebral spasm disappear. As symptoms abate, patients are encouraged to take short walks but to do as little sitting as possible. Increased physical activity is prescribed to increase mobility without incurring a return of symptoms.[28] Periods of bed rest longer than 2 weeks have a deleterious effect on the body in general. Patients with herniated discs will rarely stay at complete bed rest for longer than 2 weeks.

Scientific evidence demonstrating the efficacy of bed rest for low back pain unrelated to disc herniations has reported conflicting results.[4,8,11,30] Garfin and Pye demonstrated some improvement for patients who used firm mattresses compared with softer mattresses, waterbeds, and foam on waterbeds.[8] Lidstrom and Zachrisson[11] compared heat therapy with rest and traction, finding that the rest and traction group had greater improvement. Wiesel and colleagues reported on an experience with military recruits who developed nonradiating back pain.[30] Those who were ordered to bed rest had less pain and a faster return to full duty compared with those who remained ambulatory. The response to bed rest may be rapid, with improvement seen after 2 days, according to Deyo and co-workers.[4] In a comparison of patients with nonradiating back pain who received 2 days and 7 days of bed rest, patients with 2 days of bed rest did as well as those assigned 7 days at 3-week and 3-month follow-up evaluations. The results of this study suggest that patients may be able to return to work more quickly, with a reduction in lost productivity. In a French study of 287 patients with low back pain, individuals with sedentary jobs who received bed rest as therapy had a greater number of sick days over the next 6 months compared with those treated with activity as tolerated.[25] Other studies have reported improvement of muscle strain and herniated intervertebral discs with sciatica with decreased physical activity.[5,29]

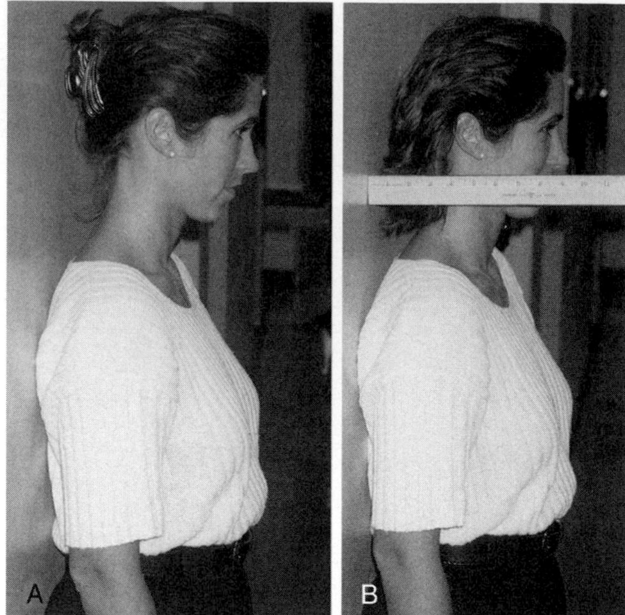

Figure 19-1 Correctly measuring height of cervical pillow. *A*, Patient stands against the wall with head in a comfortable position. *B*, The recommended height of a cervical pillow is the distance from the wall to the base of the skull. *(Courtesy of Tom Welsh, RPT.)*

Another frequently asked question involves the best resting surface (mattress) for controlled physical activity. The amount of clinical trial data involving mattresses is small. One study described improvement with air mattresses compared with regular mattresses for 30 patients with chronic back pain.[18] There are no adequate data to recommend one form of surface over another. General guidelines regarding firmness can be made regarding preference for a maintenance of lordosis (hard surface) versus flattened lordosis (softer surface).[1]

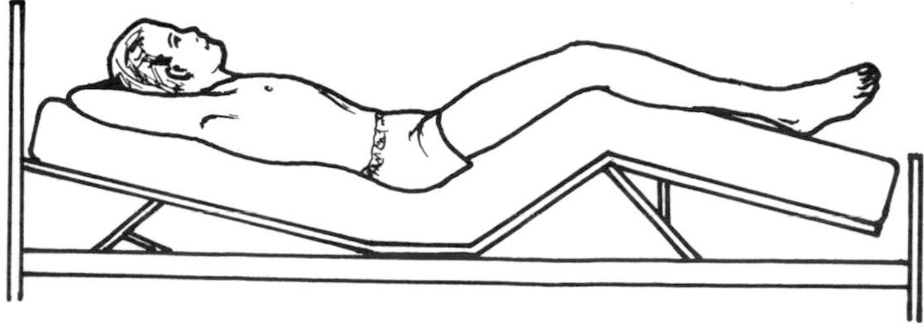

Figure 19-2 The preferred bed rest position for patients with low back pain. If a hospital bed is unavailable, pillows or wedges may be used to obtain the appropriate position for the patient. Pillows placed under the bed sheets remain more securely on the bed. The bed should be firm. A bed board (1 inch thick) may be inserted under the mattress to add support.

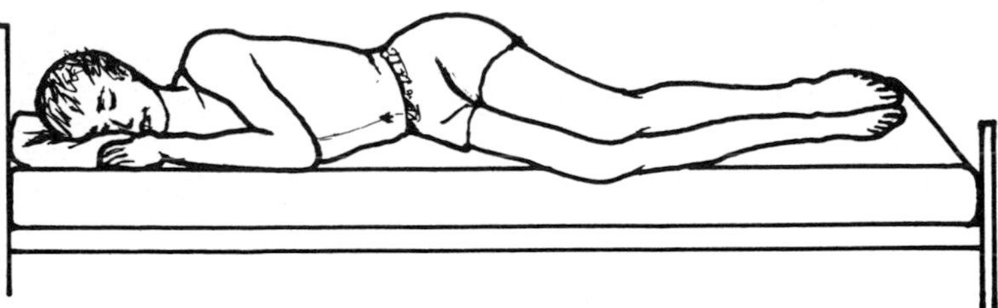

Figure 19-3 Lateral bed rest position with hips and knees flexed. This body orientation is the starting position for getting out of bed. Patients may use their arms to push themselves upright while maintaining a slightly flexed position of the lumbar spine. Patients should not flex the lumbar spine while coming to a straight sitting-up position with legs extended.

In realistic terms, busy patients rarely stay at bed rest for even a day unless their back pain is severe. Most patients will strictly limit their recreational activities and try to minimize time on their job. Explaining the importance of the appropriate amount of controlled physical activity as a component of conservative therapy cannot be overemphasized. It is essential for patients to understand the limited benefits of bed rest for pain relief. Those patients with acute low back pain who do limit their time in bed will have a faster return to normal function and are much less likely to experience recurrent, and eventually chronic, pain and limitation of function.

Recommendations regarding the balance between rest and activity must be based on good clinical judgment. During the acute phase of mechanical back pain, reduced physical activity is helpful. The recommendation should be to increase activity as tolerated. Too lengthy a time of bed rest can be detrimental. In one study, 60 of 171 (35%) patients had prescriptions for bed rest that were too prolonged.[7] Extended bed rest has physiologic implications that are detrimental, particularly for geriatric patients. In the elderly, a number of organs, including the cardiovascular, musculoskeletal, respiratory, gastrointestinal, and urinary systems, are affected. Some of the abnormalities associated with prolonged bed rest include decreased cardiac output, orthostatic instability, atelectasis, muscle atrophy, decreased aerobic capacity, joint contracture, constipation, renal calculi, pressure sores, and impaired ambulation.[9]

On the other hand, patients with chronic back pain should not be immobilized in bed even for short periods of time.[6] They should be encouraged to ambulate as much as possible. Activities can be selected that avoid specific tasks that increase the load on the spine without increasing pain. Increased activity may help bone and muscle strength, improve nutrition to intervertebral discs and cartilage, and increase endorphin levels and decrease sensitivity to pain. With these positive effects in mind, patients with chronic back pain should be encouraged to be active. Physicians remain unaware of the detriments of bed rest for chronic low back pain. In a survey of 1200 responding physicians regarding treatment of chronic low back pain, no consensus on rest was elicited.[3] However, many physicians continued to prescribe bed rest as a primary therapy for low back pain. This perception must be modified to understand the benefits of continued activity.

Our Recommendation

Encourage activity as tolerated that does not exacerbate pain. Patients with radiculopathy should limit time in bed to maintain function.

References

Controlled Physical Activity (Bed Rest)

1. Borenstein D: Back In Control: A Conventional and Complementary Prescription for Eliminating Back Pain. New York, M Evans, 2001, pp 188-189.
2. Cailliet R: Low Back Pain Syndrome. Philadelphia, FA Davis, 1981, pp 80-81.
3. Cherkin DC, Deyo RA, Wheeler K, et al: Physician views about treating low back pain: The results of a national survey. Spine 20: 1-20, 1995.
4. Deyo RA, Diehl AK, Rosenthal M: How many days of bed rest for acute low back pain? A randomized clinical trial. N Engl J Med 315:1064-1070, 1986.
5. Ellenberg M, Reina N, Ross M, et al: Regression of herniated nucleus pulposus: Two patients with lumbar radiculopathy. Arch Phys Med Rehabil 70:842 844, 1989.
6. Fast A: Low back disorders: Conservative management. Arch Phys Med Rehabil 69:880-891, 1988.
7. Frazier LM, Carey TS, Lyles MF, et al: Lengthy bed rest prescribed for acute low back pain: Experience at three general medicine walk-in clinics. South Med J 84:603-606, 1991.
8. Garfin SR, Pye SA: Bed design and its effect on chronic low back pain—a limited controlled trial. Pain 10:87-91, 1981.
9. Harper CM, Lyles YM: Physiology and complications of bed rest. J Am Geriatr Soc 36:1047-1054, 1988.
10. Lavin RA, Pappagallo M, Kuhlemeier KV: Cervical pain: A comparison of three pillows. Arch Phys Med Rehabil 78:193-198, 1997.
11. Lidstrom A, Zachrisson M: Physical therapy on low back pain and sciatica. An attempt at evaluation. Scand J Rehabil Med 2:37-42, 1970.
12. Lieberman IH, Webb JK: Cervical spine injuries in the elderly. J Bone Joint Surg Br 76B:877-881, 1994.
13. Malmivaara A, Hakkinen U, Aro T, et al: The treatment of acute low back pain: bed rest, exercises, or ordinary activity. N Engl J Med 332:351-355, 1995.
14. McGuire DK, Levine BD, Williamson JM, et al: A 30-year follow-up of the Dallas bedrest and training study: II. Effect of age on cardiovascular adaptation to exercise training. Circulation 104:1358-1366, 2001.
15. McKinney LA: Early mobilization and outcome in acute sprains of the neck. BMJ 299:1006-1008, 1989.
16. McKinney LA, Dornan JO, Ryan M: The role of physiotherapy in the management of acute neck sprains following road-traffic events. Arch Emerg Med 6:27-33, 1989.
17. Mealy K, Brennan H, Fenelon GC: Early mobilization of acute whiplash injuries. BMJ 292:656-657, 1986.
18. Monsein M, Corbin TP, Culliton PD, et al: Short-term outcomes of chronic back pain patients on an airbed vs innerspring mattresses. Med Gen Med 2(3):E36, 2000.
19. Murphy MJ, Lieponis JV: Nonoperative treatment of cervical spine pain. In The Cervical Spine Research Society Editorial Committee: The Cervical Spine, 2nd ed. Philadelphia, JB Lippincott, 1989, pp 670-677.
20. Nachemson A: The load on lumbar discs in different positions of the body. Clin Orthop 45:107, 1966.
21. Peeters GG, Verhagen AP, de Bie RA, et al: The efficacy of conservative treatment in patients with whiplash injury: A systematic review of clinical trials. Spine 26:E64-E73, 2001.
22. Persson L, Moritz U: Neck support pillows: A comparative study. J Manipulative Physiol Ther 21:237-240, 1998.
23. Quinet RJ, Hadler NM: Diagnosis and treatment of backaches. Semin Arthritis Rheum 8:261-287, 1979.

24. Rowe ML: Low back pain in industry: A position paper. J Occup Med 11:161-169, 1969.
25. Rozenberg S, Delval C, Rezvani Y, et al: Bed rest or normal activity for patients with acute low back pain: A randomized controlled trial. Spine 27:1487-1493, 2002.
26. Spitzer WO, Skovron ML, Salmi LR, et al: Scientific monograph of the Quebec Task Force on whiplash-associated disorders: Redefining "whiplash" and its management. Spine 20:S1-S73, 1995.
27. Vroomen PCAJ, DeKrom MCTFM, Wilmink JT, et al: Lack of effectiveness of bed rest for sciatica. N Engl J Med 340:418-423, 1999.
28. Wagner CJ: Williams's flexion regime in the treatment of low back pain. J Int Coll Surg 18:69, 1952.
29. Weinert AM Jr, Rizzo TD Jr: Nonoperative management of multilevel lumbar disk herniations in an adolescent athlete. Mayo Clin Proc 67:137-141, 1992.
30. Wiesel SW, Cuckler JM, DeLuca F, et al: Acute low-back pain: An objective analysis of conservative therapy. Spine 5:324-330, 1980.
31. Wilke H, Need P, Caimi M, et al: New in vivo measurements of pressures in the intervertebral disc in daily life. Spine 24:755-762, 1999.

TRACTION

Traction is a nonstandardized conservative treatment modality for spinal pain and radiculopathy that has been used over the centuries.[17] The basic premise of traction is that unloading the components of the spine by stretching muscles, ligaments, and functional spinal units will decrease intradiscal pressure, thereby relieving symptoms. When applied correctly, spinal traction can cause distraction or separation of vertebral bodies and facet joints, tensing of ligamentous spinous structures, widening of the intervertebral foramen, straightening of spinal curves, and stretching of spinal musculature. Traction plays a more significant role in the cervical spine compared with the lumbar spine.

Cervical Spine

Cervical traction is a nonstandardized conservative treatment modality for neck pain and radiculopathy. Traction has been suggested as a therapeutic intervention to relieve symptoms associated with nerve root compression, osteoarthritis of the zygapophyseal joints, and contracted cervical muscles. Patients with radiculopathy seem to benefit most from traction. Local muscle spasm is less responsive to traction.[19] The basic premise of traction is unloading the components of the spine by stretching muscles, ligaments, and functional spinal units. This stretching results in distraction of articular surfaces, prevention and lysis of adhesions within the dural sleeves, relief of nerve root compression within the neural foramen, decreased pressure within the intervertebral discs, relief of tonic muscle contraction, and improved vascular status within the epidural space and perineural structures.[29]

There are many forms of cervical spinal traction. Traction may be applied manually or mechanically. The tension may be intermittent or continuous. The patient may be upright or supine when tension is applied. Intermittent traction is best applied to the supine patient. The most effective intermittent traction consists of the greatest force and longest duration that causes the least discomfort to the patient's jaw and chin. The force may vary from 5 to 50 pounds for 15 seconds' duration, with 7 seconds' rest, for a 5- to 20-minute period. The weight and duration are increased corresponding to patient tolerance.[33] Intermittent traction may be most helpful for osteoarthritis or muscular strain associated with spondylosis.[36] This form of traction should not be continued if the patient experiences an exacerbation of neck pain.

Continuous traction is less well tolerated than other forms of traction secondary to the constant pressure on the chin and jaw. During an acute phase, maximum traction is limited to 5 pounds for a brief duration of 5 minutes. The maximum tolerated weight is 50 pounds for 15 minutes. If applied correctly, this form of therapy straightens the cervical spine and enlarges the intervertebral foramina. This therapy may be applied at home by the patient (Fig. 19-4).

The force and duration of traction vary with patient and condition. If posterior vertebral separation is desired, a weight of 25 to 45 pounds is required.[36] An increased degree of neck flexion (20 to 30 degrees) is associated with greater elongation of the cervical spine. Angles of 24 degrees are associated with the most effective widening of the intervertebral foramina.[5] Greater angles of traction increase muscle tension.[8]

Manual traction allows the therapist to control the amount of force applied to the neck at varying angles of cervical flexion, extension, and rotation. The application of the hands to the neck allows the therapist a continuous

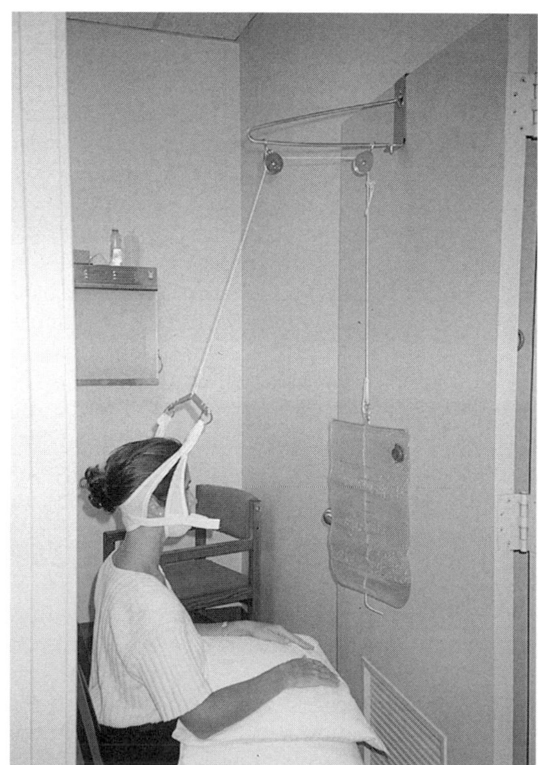

Figure 19-4 Overhead traction. The patient sits facing the door with arms resting on two pillows. Head harness is adjusted to apply pressure to the back of the head and only slightly under the chin. A resting mandibular splint in a form of gauze or moldable wax may increase comfort on the chin. A 30-degree angle of tension is desired with a weight of 8 to 12 pounds for 15 minutes. Traction is applied twice daily for pain relief and three times weekly for maintenance. *(Courtesy of Tom Welsh, RPT.)*

assessment of the extent of muscle spasm and joint movement associated with stretching. Traction is applied to the supine patient after moist heat is applied to the cervical musculature to promote relaxation.

Contraindications for cervical traction include a variety of disorders. A partial list of examples includes rheumatoid arthritis, spondyloarthropathies, osteomyelitis, malignancies, myelopathy, hypermobility, torticollis, and structural scoliosis.

Special concern is also given to patients with temporomandibular joint dysfunction. Patients with temporomandibular joint dysfunction may develop pain in the jaw that radiates to anterior and posterior locations in the cervical spine, including the sternocleidomastoid and trapezius muscles. Individuals involved in rear-end automobile accidents may develop injury to discs and ligaments of these joints as the head is thrown posteriorly and the jaw moves anteriorly. The masseter and temporalis muscles are tender and firm to palpation. Attempts to open the jaw result in ear and jaw pain.[13] Patients with temporomandibular joint dysfunction are not candidates for cervical traction. They also may not tolerate cervical orthoses.

A study by Zylbergold and Piper reported on a comparison of three types of cervical traction.[38] Groups given static traction, intermittent traction, and manual traction were compared with a control group given no traction. All groups received education, heat treatments, and exercises. Patients receiving traction (25 pounds at 25 degrees for 15 minutes) had greater range of motion and less need for medication. The authors advocate the use of intermittent traction.[38]

Patients receiving traction must continue with exercises to maintain the benefit of traction. Mechanical traction may be used if active modalities and manual traction have failed.[33] The patient should be supine when therapy is applied by a therapist.[7] This position improves patient comfort and relaxation. Therapy should be given three times a week for 10 to 15 sessions.[29] For home use, a simple pulley system attached over the door is useful. This home system is limited by patient compliance.

The authors believe that cervical traction is helpful for patients with cervical spine pain and radiculopathy. Critical reviews of clinical trials examining traction for neck pain have been marginal in demonstrating efficacy. The failure of the studies to demonstrate efficacy is related to the use of multiple therapies, inadequate study design, and modest treatment effects.[15,18]

Lumbar Spine

Lumbar spine traction was a popular therapy at a time when admission to the hospital was less carefully scrutinized. Patients would be placed in traction for low back or leg pain with the expectation that stretching of the lumbar area would result in distraction of the structural elements and resolution of the pain. This therapy was frequently prescribed, but the best form of traction and the extent of its benefits were not studied.

There are many forms of spinal traction:

1. Continuous traction uses light weights applied for several hours at a time. This form of traction is not effective because patients cannot tolerate the amount of weight necessary to distract the spine for that length of time.
2. Sustained (static) traction uses a steady amount of weight for periods of up to 30 minutes. Heavier weights are tolerated for this shorter period of time. Force may be generated by hanging weights or a mechanical device that generates the pounds of traction force for the specified time. This form of traction is more effective if a split table is utilized, reducing friction.
3. Intermittent mechanical traction is frequently used in the United States and employs a mechanical device that applies and releases traction every few seconds.[14]
4. Manual traction is applied by a therapist who manually grasps the patient to generate the force. The traction can be in the form of a steady pull for a few seconds or a quick thrust.
5. Positional traction is applied by placing the patient in a variety of positions to obtain a longitudinal pull on spinal structures; this is usually used to stretch one side of the spine.
6. In autotraction, a patient lies with flexed hips and knees and generates traction by pulling on a harness that is attached to an encircling belt. Sessions may last up to an hour.[21]
7. Gravity lumbar traction uses the force of gravity to stretch the spine in a patient who is suspended vertically by a harness or in an inverted position hanging by ankle boots.[27,32]

The application of traction to the lumbar spine is used most often for patients with a herniated nucleus pulposus. The rationale for this therapy is that the stretching of the lumbar spine results in distraction of the vertebrae so that protruded discs return to a more normal anatomic position.

Friction hinders the transmission of force to the back. A force equal to 50% of body weight is required to move the body horizontally. The lower half of the body needs to be moved before any force is transmitted to the lumbar spine. Since 50% of the body weight lies beneath L3, 25% of applied force to the lumbar spine is lost overcoming friction. Therefore, a patient in a horizontal position in a conventional bed will receive effective traction only at weights equal to 25% to 50% of body weight. Weights over 50% of body weight will cause the patient to slide, whereas less than 25% will not overcome friction.

Another factor that must be overcome is the elasticity of muscles. A muscle pulled by a minimal force will behave as an elastic body; and as the force increases, the elongation of the muscle will be limited by a stretch reflex. Traction forces in the range of hundreds of pounds may be necessary to overcome this effect in the muscles that protect the lumbar spine. The application of pulley traction with conventional weights on a regular bed over a prolonged period is no more beneficial than bed rest because there is little distraction of the spine.[37] The efficacy of applying force to the lumbar spine is increased by the use of a split table, which eliminates lower body resistance. Traction on the spine will increase stature. Increased stature will occur when traction with one third of body weight is placed on the lumbar spine. The increase in stature, measured in millimeters, was greatest within the first 15 minutes. This form of traction was more effective at increasing spine length than lying in a fetal position for a similar length of time. The clinical importance of this therapeutic intervention remains to be determined.[3]

Mathews used epidurography to study the effect of lumbar traction on returning protruded lumbar discs to their normal position.[23] Disc protrusion was reversed by the application of traction to the lumbar spine with vertebral distraction of 2 mm per disc. However, the amount of weight required to obtain this effect was 120 pounds and the duration of traction was between 30 and 38 minutes. The effect on the disc was of short duration with reappearance of disc prolapse within 14 minutes after the discontinuance of the traction forces. Gupta also demonstrated reduction of disc herniation with epidurography with associated clinical improvement in 9 of 12 patients given traction for 4 hours with 80 pounds for 10 to 15 days.[12]

Another rationale for the use of traction is reduction of intradiscal pressure. Nachemson and Elfstrom studied the reduction of intradural pressure in normal individuals placed in traction using a pelvic and thoracic harness, a split table, and 30 kg of tractive force for 3 seconds with 5-second intervals.[26] Intradiscal pressure was reduced by only 20% to 30%.

A number of therapeutic trials have been undertaken to study the efficacy of traction for the treatment of lumbar spine pain.[6,16,22,24] Many of the studies have design flaws that limit their scientific validity.[9] Weber undertook a controlled trial of effective weight traction (one third body weight) versus control weight traction (weight to tighten the harness) in patients with radiographically confirmed nerve root compression. Traction was given for 20-minute sessions. Clinical assessment of the two groups revealed no significant difference.[35] Mathews and Hickling completed a study of patients with sciatica with dural tension signs, limited back movement, and pain who underwent lumbar traction with a minimum of 45 kg sustained for 30 minutes compared with a control group of infrared heat treatments for 15 minutes.[24] Traction relieved pain but did not have a long-lasting effect. Traction was not thought to be more helpful than heat treatments except for women younger than 45 years of age with sciatica.

The role of traction for the treatment of nonspecific low back pain without sciatica was studied by Beurskens and colleagues in a clinical trial of high-dose (12 times for 20 minutes per session in 5 weeks) versus sham traction involving 151 patients.[2] The sham patients felt pressure without distraction of the structures of the lumbar spine. At 3 and 6 months, no difference was found with regard to severity of pain, functional status, range of motion, work absence, or medical treatment between the treatment groups.

Traction is not totally without benefit, however. In a later study, Weber found a positive psychological effect in regard to the patient's expectations for recovery while in traction. However, the beneficial effect may have been more closely related to the enforcement of bed rest than to the tractive force on the spine.[34] Larsson and associates found autotraction to be better than corsets for patients with low back pain.[21] The benefits of the autotraction system are that (1) the patient controls the amount of traction; (2) the device is portable and can be used at home; and (3) the device is relatively inexpensive. Autotraction is done for 15-minute periods, 2 to 5 times daily. This technique may be more beneficial for patients with muscle spasm as opposed to a herniated disc.[20] Andersson and co-workers measured disc pressures in patients who underwent active (autotraction) and passive traction.[1] Patients using autotraction contracted their thoracic muscles and had increased intradiscal pressure in comparison with those who received passive traction with disc pressures that decreased, remained unchanged, or, occasionally, rose. Unilateral traction may be of benefit in patients with lumbar scoliosis associated with muscle spasm and unassociated with nerve root irritation. A constant, gentle pull on the muscles may relax the muscle, breaking the spasm cycle.[30]

Gravity techniques, which use the body's weight, have been proposed as a means of generating tractive forces. The Sister Kenney Institute Gravity Lumbar Reduction Therapy Program utilizes a harness placed under the ribs and a tilt bed to generate gravitational forces on the lumbar spine.[4] The patient needs to be hospitalized for a 10- to 14-day period. The program requires very close scrutiny by the health care professional caring for the patient, making the program labor intensive.

Inversion therapy also uses gravity to provide traction. Inversion may be accomplished by using special boots clipped to an overhead bar or by kneeling over thigh platforms.[27,28] Gianakopoulos and Waylonis evaluated a number of gravity techniques.[11] Patients experienced improvement in symptoms and distraction of the lumbar spine of 0.3 to 4.0 mm. However, side effects included elevated systolic and diastolic blood pressure, decreased heart rate, periorbital and pharyngeal petechiae, headache, blurred vision, nasal stuffiness, and conjunctival infection. Other potential complications are retinal detachment, bleeding from berry aneurysms, and gastrointestinal reflux.[10] One other potential hazard is equipment failure. Unless therapy is done in the presence of another individual, the patient may fall on his or her head or cervical spine, sustaining spinal cord injury. The side effects of this therapy far outweigh its benefits.

In summary, the scientific proof for the efficacy of traction is sparse. The benefit of traction is most likely related to bed rest in patients with disc disease. Patients with muscle spasm may benefit from traction, but it must be given in the setting of a comprehensive program for back pain. New forms of traction using technologically advanced systems that offer vertebral axial decompression at a more expensive cost do not offer a unique intervention despite reported excellent results of relieving pain.[31] In a time of limited medical financial resources, the option of admitting a patient to the hospital for traction is gone. Traction, if used at all, is an outpatient therapeutic option. Patients with cervical radiculopathy are the best candidates for this therapy.

Our Recommendation

Cervical traction decreases arm pain in patients with cervical radiculopathy. Lumbar traction is not helpful for lumbar radiculopathy.

References

Traction

1. Andersson GBJ, Schultz HB, Nachemson AL: Intervertebral disc pressures during traction. Scand Rehab Med (Suppl)9:88-91, 1983.
2. Beurskens AJ, de Vet HC, Koke AJ, et al: Efficacy of traction for nonspecific low back pain: 12-week and 6-month results of a randomized clinical trial. Spine 22:2756-2762, 1997.
3. Bridger RS, Ossey S, Fourie G: Effect of lumbar traction on stature. Spine 15:522-524, 1990.
4. Burton CV: The Sister Kenney Institute Gravity Lumbar Reduction Therapy Program. In Finneson BE (ed): Low Back Pain, 2nd ed. Philadelphia, JB Lippincott, 1981, pp 277-280.
5. Colachis SC Jr, Strohm BR: A study of tractive forces and angle of pull on vertebral interspaces in the cervical spine. Arch Phys Med 46:820, 1965.
6. Coxhead CE, Inskip H, Meade TW, et al: Multicentre trial of physiotherapy in the management of sciatic symptoms. Lancet 1:1065-1068, 1981.
7. Deets D, Hands KL, Hopp SS: Cervical traction: A comparison of sitting and supine positions. Phys Ther 57:255-261, 1977.
8. DeLacerda FG: Effect of angle of traction pull on upper trapezius muscle activity. J Orthop Sports Phys Ther 1:205, 1980.
9. Deyo RA: Conservative therapy for low back pain: Distinguishing useful from useless therapy. JAMA 250:1057-1062, 1983.
10. Friberg TR, Weinreb RN: Ocular manifestations of gravity inversion. JAMA 253:1755-1757, 1985.
11. Gianakopoulos G, Waylonis GW, Grant PA, et al: Inversion devices: Their role in producing lumbar distraction. Arch Phys Med Rehab 66:100-102, 1985.
12. Gupta R, Ramarao S: Epidurography in reduction of lumbar disc prolapse by traction. Arch Phys Med Rehabil 59:322-327, 1978.
13. Hodges J: Managing temporomandibular joint syndrome. Laryngoscope 100:60-66, 1990.
14. Hood L, Chrisman D: Intermittent pelvic traction in the treatment of the ruptured intervertebral disc. Phys Ther 48:21-30, 1968.
15. Hoving JL, Gross AR, Gasner D, et al: A critical appraisal of review articles on the effectiveness of conservative treatment for neck pain. Spine 26:196-203, 2001.
16. Jayson MIV, Sims-Williams H, Young S, et al: Mobilization and manipulation for low back pain. Spine 6:409 416, 1981.
17. Judovich B: Lumbar traction therapy. JAMA 159:549, 1955.
18. Kjellman GV, Skargren EI, Oberg BE: A critical analysis of randomized clinical trials on neck pain and treatment efficacy: A review of the literature. Scand J Rehabil Med 31:139-152, 1999.
19. Klaber-Moffett JA, Hughes GI, Griffiths P: An investigation of the effects of cervical traction: II. The effects on the neck musculature. Clin Rehabil 4:287, 1990.
20. Lancort JE: Traction techniques for low back pain. J Musculoskel Med 3(4):44, 1986.
21. Larsson U, Choler U, Lidstrom A, et al: Auto-traction for treatment of lumbago-sciatica. Acta Orthop Scand 51:791-798, 1980.
22. Lidstrom A, Zachrisson M: Physical therapy on low back pain and sciatica: An attempt at evaluation. Scand J Rehabil Med 2:37-42, 1970.
23. Mathews JA: Dynamic discography: A study of lumbar traction. Ann Phys Med 9:275-279, 1968.
24. Mathews JA, Hickling J: Lumbar traction: A double-blind controlled study for sciatica. Rheumatol Rehabil 14:222-225, 1975.
25. Mathews JA, Mills SB, Jenkins VM, et al: Back pain and sciatica: Controlled trials of manipulation, traction, sclerosant and epidural injections. Br J Rheumatol 26:416-423, 1987.
26. Nachemson A, Elfstrom G: Intravital dynamic pressure measurements in lumbar discs: A study of common movements, maneuvers, and exercises. Scand J Rehabil Med (Suppl) 1:1-40, 1970.
27. Nosse L: Inverted spinal traction. Arch Phys Med Rehabil 59: 367-370, 1978.
28. Oudenhoven RC: Gravitational lumbar traction. Arch Phys Med Rehabil 59:510-512, 1978.
29. Rath W: Cervical traction: A clinical perspective. Orthop Rev 13:29, 1984.
30. Saunders H: Unilateral lumbar traction. Phys Ther 61:221, 1981.
31. Sherry E, Kitchener P, Smart R: A prospective randomized controlled study of VAX-D and TENS for the treatment of chronic low back pain. Neurol Res 23:780-784, 2001.
32. Swezey RL: The modern thrust of manipulation and traction therapy. Semin Arthritis Rheum 12:322-331, 1983.
33. Tan JC, Nordin M: Role of physical therapy in the treatment of cervical disk disease. Orthop Clin North Am 23:435-449, 1992.
34. Weber H: Lumbar disc herniation: A prospective study of prognostic factors including a controlled trial: I. J Oslo City Hosp 28:33-61, 1978.
35. Weber H: Traction therapy in sciatica due to disc prolapse: Does traction treatment have any positive effect on patients suffering from sciatica caused by disc prolapse? J Oslo City Hosp 23:169-176, 1973.
36. Welsh TM: Physical therapy, ergonomics, and rehabilitation. In Wiesel SW, Boden SD, Borenstein DG, Feffer HL (eds): Neck Pain. Charlottesville, VA, The Michie Co, 1992, pp 377-453.
37. Youel MA: Effectiveness of pelvic traction. J Bone Joint Surg Am 49A:2051, 1967.
38. Zylbergold RS, Piper MC: Cervical spine disorders: A comparison of three types of traction. Spine 10:867-871, 1985.

PHYSICAL MODALITIES

In addition to exercises, physical therapists may use various physical modalities to relieve patient symptoms. Treatment methods may include ice massage, hot packs, whirlpool, diathermy, ultrasound, transcutaneous electrical nerve stimulation (TENS), and high-voltage electrical stimulation. All of these counterirritant modalities offer transient relief of symptoms but do not alter the underlying physical abnormality. Modalities may be used in conjunction with other therapies (e.g., exercises) that allow for greater motion and decreased post-activity symptoms.

Cold (Cryotherapy)

Patients with acute low back or neck pain may experience analgesia with ice massage and cold packs. Therapeutic cold will reduce pain, swelling, and muscle spasm during the acute phase of an injury within the first 48 hours. Cold also reduces local metabolic activity, decreases muscle spindle activity, and slows nerve conduction.[7,14] Cold vasoconstricts peripheral vessels of the skin, resulting in increased blood flow to deeper vessels and tissues, increased muscle tone, reduced swelling, increased patient tolerance to deep massage, and enhanced voluntary motion.[18]

Cervical Spine

Initially, the patient experiences a burning sensation, which dissipates as the application is continued. The ice is applied in a stroking direction following the course of the muscle fibers. A cold pack is used first if a patient cannot tolerate ice massage. The cold pack may be placed in a wet towel to limit contact with the skin. Cold packs with silica gel can be refrozen and used again in patients who experience continued pain. Vapor-coolant spray, fluoromethane or ethyl chloride, is another form of cryotherapy. Fluoromethane is nonvolatile and does not irritate the skin as much as ethyl chloride. For neck muscles, a cold pack or chipped ice wrapped in a terry cloth towel, applied for 15 minutes, may be the best choice.[1] A comparison of ice massage and cold packs reveals that ice massage cools the skin to a greater degree than the underlying muscle and may facilitate alpha motor neuron discharge.[5] Clinically, this explains the occasional patient who experiences increased muscle spasm with ice massage.

The anesthetic effect of cold increases patients' tolerance of stretching of contracted neck muscles by the physical therapist. The "spray and stretch" technique may be particularly helpful for patients with contracted paracervical muscles. The skin is sprayed with repeated parallel sweeps over the length of the muscle in the radiation of the neck pain.[17] The neck should be positioned to allow maximal stretching of the injured muscle, with the onset of analgesia associated with application of the spray. A spray period of 3 seconds is sufficient to allow for deep massage and active assisted stretching. If the skin reddens after deep massage, the patient's circulatory status is normal. Persistence of blanching suggests decreased circulatory capacity and potential toxicity from cold application. The duration of relief from pain and spasm is longer with cold than with superficial heat. Cryotherapy should not be used in patients with Raynaud's phenomenon, impaired circulation, peripheral vascular disease, loss of thermal sensitivity, or extreme sensitivity of the skin to temperatures. Cryotherapy is also not indicated for patients with long-standing contracted muscles. For these patients, cryotherapy facilitates the return of shortened muscles to their contracted length after lengthening with stretching exercises.

Lumbar Spine

In evaluating forms of pain therapy in patients with chronic low back pain, Melzack and colleagues found that over two thirds of affected individuals experienced a 33% reduction in pain following ice massage.[11] Cold should not be used as the sole treatment for spinal pain. Cold is used as an adjunct to facilitate the benefit of other therapies, such as exercises.

In general, the number of studies documenting the benefit of ice massage for neck or low back pain are few. This includes studies of acute or serial applications of cryotherapy.[3] No consensus exists regarding the duration, frequency, and use of barriers between ice and skin from a variety of sources, including textbooks.[8] We recommend ice application in patients who have localized neck or back pain. The patient is proactive in his or her therapy and controls the duration of the application at an acceptable expense.

Heat (Thermotherapy)

Heat is useful in easing pain and reducing muscle spasm. Heat cannot be used in patients with impaired mental status, diminished circulation, or decreased sensation because thermal damage to the skin can occur if heat is applied for an excessive period of time. Heat also is not indicated in patients with low back or neck pain secondary to trauma where swelling may increase with heating. Heat causes vasodilatation with increased blood flow. It also increases the elastic properties of connective tissue. In addition, heat decreases gamma fiber activity, decreasing muscle spindle excitability and resting muscle tension. Heat to both skin and deeper structures will have the beneficial effects of decreasing pain through counterirritant mechanisms and by decreasing muscle ischemia associated with increased muscle spasm. Hot packs have been reported to reduce muscle spasms.[4]

Superficial Heat. Superficial heat provides mild heating of less than 40°C and penetrates to the level of the subcutaneous tissues. Hydrocollator packs, heating pads, infrared heat, and whirlpools generate superficial heat. Hydrocollator packs (heated to 65°C) are wrapped in two towels and placed on the prone patient's spine (not underneath to prevent skin burn) for 15 to 20 minutes. Whirlpool baths provide massaging effects as well as heat. A warm shower may also offer temporary heating to the neck and shoulder region, allowing for greater compliance with range of motion exercises. For all forms of superficial heat, the maximal safe exposure is 30 minutes at 45°C applied directly to the skin.

Infrared Heating. Infrared heating allows the therapist to observe the area as it is treated. The amount of heat applied to the skin is determined by the size of the bulb generating the infrared radiation and its distance from the skin. Thirty minutes is the duration of therapy.

Topical Agents. Another form of superficial heating is generated through the application of topical agents. Capsaicin excites nociceptive fibers to release substance P. Prolonged application of this agent depletes substance P from nociceptive fibers, resulting in inhibition of pain sensation. Application of capsaicin to the neck four times a day may result in pain relief in those individuals unable to tolerate other forms of medical therapy.[9]

Topical heat in the form of thin wraps (40°C) that are directly placed on the skin for prolonged application to the neck or low back are as effective as simple analgesics for pain relief. In a study of 371 patients with acute nonspecific low back pain treated with acetaminophen, ibuprofen, or topical heat wraps, the heat treatment was more effective than drug therapy for pain relief and improved function for the 4 days of the study.[12] Overnight use of heat wraps may also offer improved pain relief.[13]

Whirlpool. Whirlpool therapy is difficult to use in patients with back pain. They may have difficulty getting in and out of the tub, and these movements may exacerbate their symptoms.

Deep Heat. Deep heat penetrates to structures below the subcutaneous tissues. Diathermy and ultrasound generate deeper heat.

Shortwave Diathermy. Shortwave diathermy penetrates the soft tissues and delivers heat to deeper structures, such as muscle, bone, and ligaments. Although diathermy has been shown to be effective in decreasing pain in trigger points including the low back, other heat modalities have been used in its place for deep heat therapy.[10] Microwave diathermy uses electromagnetic waves to transfer heat.

Ultrasound. Ultrasound delivers heat more deeply than diathermy. It is not used in the acute situation, in which heat will cause additional swelling to the traumatized area. Ultrasound is used for 20-minute sessions three times a week for 2 to 3 weeks. Therapy is delivered to paraspinous structures but not over the spinal cord itself or gas-containing organs. It is contraindicated for patients with bleeding disorders.

The benefits of ultrasound are debated in the literature. Concerns exist about the evidence that proves the in vivo biophysical effects of ultrasound. A number of clinical trials have called into question the benefits of ultrasound for musculoskeletal disorders.[2,16]

A patient with spinal pain may participate in a home program that may include a hydrocollator, hot showers with a thick towel around the neck, an electric moist heating pad, or topical heat wraps applied to the neck or low back. Hydrocollators are less expensive than electric pads but are less convenient. Deep heat should not be applied to the spine for longer than 30 minutes because of the risk of increased blood flow with resultant swelling and stiffness.

Chronic Spinal Pain

Questions remain concerning the relative utility of heat and/or cold in the therapy for chronic spinal pain. Roberts and co-workers studied the effects of cold packs and ice massage versus hot packs in 36 patients with chronic back pain 1 hour after therapy.[15] Ice massage gave the greatest amount of immediate post-treatment pain relief. At 1 hour after therapy, a significant difference remained between the ice massage patients and the other groups, although pain had increased for all groups in comparison to the immediate post-treatment period. Ice massage should be considered for chronic low back pain. Landon also reported his experience with temperature counterirritant therapy in 117 patients with back pain. In acute conditions, patients treated with heat had shorter hospital stays than those treated with ice application. Cryotherapy was more effective than heat therapy in chronic conditions.[6]

Our Recommendation

Physical modalities that are convenient and inexpensive are useful adjuncts to spinal therapy. Expensive temperature modalities offer little additional benefit and are not cost effective.

References

Physical Modalities

1. Belitsky RB, Odam SJ, Hubley-Kozey C: Evaluation of the effectiveness of wet ice, dry ice, and cryogen packs in reducing skin temperature. Phys Ther 67:1080-1084, 1987.
2. Ebenbichler GR, Erdogmus CB, Resch KL, et al: Ultrasound therapy for calcific tendonitis of the shoulder. N Engl J Med 340:1533-1338, 1999.
3. Ernst E, Fialka V: Ice freezes pain? A review of the clinical effectiveness of analgesic cold therapy. J Pain Symptom Manage 9:56-59, 1994.
4. Fountain FP, Gersten JW, Sengu O: Decrease in muscle spasm produced by ultrasound, hot packs and infrared radiation. Arch Phys Med Rehabil 41:293, 1960.
5. Hartviksen K: Ice therapy in spasticity. Acta Neurol Scand 38(Suppl 3):79, 1962.
6. Landon BR: Heat or cold for the relief of low back pain? Phys Ther 47:1126, 1967.
7. Lehman JF, Delateur BJ: Diathermy and superficial heat, laser, and cold therapy. In Kottke FJ, Lehman JF (eds): Kausen's Handbook of Physical Medicine and Rehabilitation, 4th ed. Philadelphia, WB Saunders, 1990, pp 283-367.
8. MacAuley D: Do textbooks agree on their advice on ice? Clin J Sport Med 11:67-72, 2001.
9. Mathias BJ, Dillingham TR, Zeigler DN, et al: Topical capsaicin for chronic neck pain. Am J Phys Med Rehabil 74:39-44, 1995.
10. McCray RE, Patton NJ: Pain relief at trigger points: A comparison of moist heat and shortwave diathermy. J Orthop Sport Phys Ther 5:175, 1984.
11. Melzack R, Jeans ME, Straford JG, Monks RC: Ice massage and transcutaneous electrical stimulation: Comparison of treatment of low back pain. Pain 9:209-217, 1980.
12. Nadler SF, Steiner DJ, Erasala GN, et al: Continuous low-level heat wrap therapy provides more efficacy than ibuprofen and acetaminophen for acute low back pain. Spine 27:1012-1017, 2002.
13. Nadler SF, Steiner DJ, Petty SR, et al: Overnight use of continuous low-level heatwrap therapy for relief of low back pain. Arch Phys Med Rehabil 84:335-342, 2003.
14. Ottoson D: The effects of temperature on the isolated muscle spindle. J Physiol 180:636-648, 1965.
15. Roberts DJ, Walls CM, Carlile JA, et al: Relief of chronic low back pain: Heat versus cold. In Aronoff GM (ed): Evaluation and Treatment of Chronic Pain. Baltimore: Urban & Schwarzenberg, 1985, pp 263-266.
16. Robertson VJ, Baker KG: A review of therapeutic ultrasound: Effectiveness studies. Phys Ther 81:133-150, 2001.
17. Travell JG, Simons DG: Myofascial Pain and Dysfunction, The Trigger Point Manual: The Upper Extremities. Baltimore, Williams & Wilkins, 1983, p 66.
18. Welsh TM: Physical therapy, ergonomics, and rehabilitation. In Wiesel SW, Boden SD, Borenstein DG, Feffer HL (eds): Neck Pain, 2nd ed. Charlottesville, VA, The Michie Co, 1992, pp 377-453.

LUMBAR CORSETS AND BRACES

The rationale for the use of external supports arises from the work of Bartelink, who proposed the theory that increased intra-abdominal pressure imparts force against the diaphragm and thoracic spine, decreasing the load on the lumbar spine.[2] Part of the load may be transmitted to transverse and oblique abdominal muscles. Nachemson and Morris have demonstrated a decrease of 25% in intradiscal pressure to a value intermediate between the supine and standing position by the use of an inflatable corset that increased intra-abdominal pressure and/or decreased the compressive force of the iliopsoas on the lumbar spine.[13]

In regard to decreasing movement of the spine, lumbar braces may actually increase lumbar motion during ambulation.[9,20] The increase in motion is true for all standard braces, even those that stretch from the sacral area to the thoracolumbar junction.[14] The gross range of motion of the lumbar spine is decreased while individual segments have continued motion.[4]

According to a national survey, the use of corsets and braces by orthopedists is common, with only 1% never using the appliances in low back pain, despite a paucity of clinical controlled trials.[3,8,12,15] The rationales cited for use of braces included restriction of lumbosacral motion, abdominal support, and postural correction, although the previously cited studies challenge these concepts. In a review of the mechanisms of action of lumbar supports during lifting, reduced trunk motion for flexion-extension and lateral bending was the only mechanism substantiated.[17] In addition, the use of external supports may cause disuse atrophy of those muscles that specifically support the lumbar spine.[5]

The choice of a brace or corset is based on construction. The brace with its metal stays is built more sturdily, has less surface contact with the patient, and is therefore cooler. Otherwise there is no particular benefit of a brace over a corset. Corsets come in many forms. One that has been readily accepted by patients is an elastic cinch with a slot for a heat-molded rigid plastic lumbosacral insert that is custom fitted to the patient (Figs. 19-5 and 19-6).[16] Some patients prefer a narrow elastic band (sacroiliac trochanteric belt), which is prescribed more for a sense of security than for mechanical support.

External supports are indicated for only a short period in the average patient's recovery. Willner reported that patients who had pain relief when bent forward or in the supine position had pain relief with a rigid brace.[21] However, many patients with low back pain of unknown cause had no improvement with braces that decreased lumbar lordosis. A properly fitted corset will allow the patient to regain mobility faster. As recovery continues, the corset is abandoned in favor of an active exercise program.

Excessively obese patients with weak abdominal muscles who have poor posture may benefit from long-term bracing. Realistically, these patients are very hard to fit in braces and may not be able to wear them for extended periods. Another group who may obtain greater benefit from bracing are elderly patients with multilevel degenerative disease who do not tolerate exercises and those with vertebral compression fractures. These patients may feel more comfortable and secure in a brace, although there is no scientific evidence to support its utility.

It should be remembered that bracing is a major part of therapy in idiopathic or genetic scoliosis. These patients may benefit from Milwaukee braces or other similar appliances that slow the progression of scoliosis. Other individuals who may specifically benefit from a brace are those with spondylolisthesis. Also, a thermoplastic antilordotic low back brace along with muscle-strengthening exercises may be beneficial for individuals with spondylolisthesis.[11]

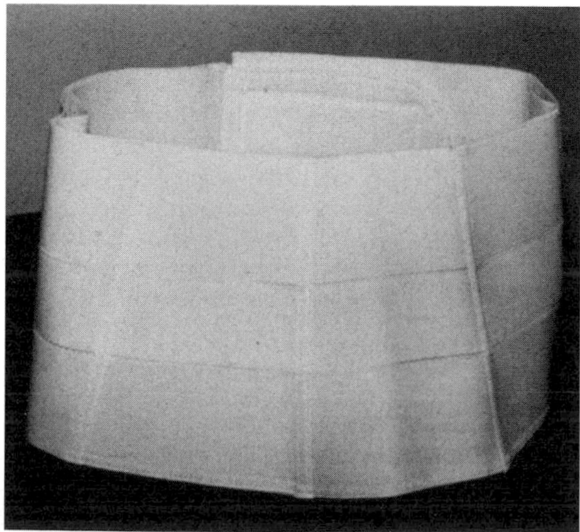

Figure 19-5 Flexible corset with pocket for removable plastic insert.

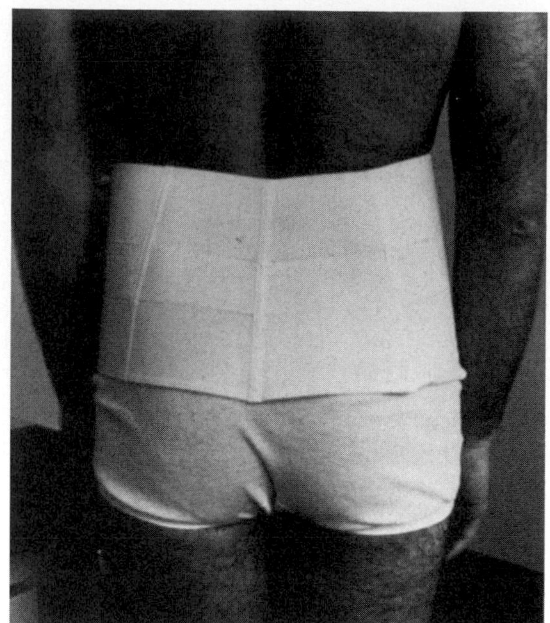

Figure 19-6 Placement of flexible corset for low back strain.

Alaranta and Hurri completed a study of 113 patients prescribed corsets for chronic low back pain.[1] In this compliance study, 37% of respondents described excellent or good results from wearing the brace. Only 60% had worn the brace during the preceding month. Men preferred the low, semirigid, elastic models, whereas women preferred the high semirigid corset. To improve compliance, a thorough explanation of the use and purpose of the corset is helpful.

Lumbar Supports in the Occupational Setting

For those who are returning to heavy labor, a corset will keep the worker aware of his or her back and prevent the application of maximum stress to the lumbosacral spine during work. After work is completed, the corset is removed. The patient who wears a corset at work is encouraged to perform strengthening exercises of the abdominal and paravertebral muscles. Once the patient feels confident, the corset can be removed while working. Patients may find leaving the corset off for the first half of the day and wearing it in the afternoon after fatigue sets in a way to wean themselves from the external support.

Van Poppel and colleagues completed a randomized, controlled trial of lifting education and lumbar support, versus education, versus lumbar support, versus control in 282 manual airport workers over a 6-month period.[18] Education consisted of three sessions of proper lifting mechanics. The lumbar corset had easy-release fasteners, flexible stays, and no shoulder straps. Compliance with wearing the support was 43% of the eligible time. Back pain incidence and number of sick days was 36% and 0.4 day with lumbar supports versus 34% and 0.4 day without. In a subgroup with back pain at baseline, lumbar supports reduced the number of days with low back pain per month (1.2 vs. 6.5). Although lumbar supports and education did not prevent low back pain, the use of a corset did decrease the degree of pain in those workers with lumbar pain at the onset of the study.

Another large study reported by Wassell and coworkers failed to demonstrate any benefit of the use of a back belt in a large cohort of material-handling workers in retail merchandise stores.[19] Of a total of 9377 workers, 6311 (67%) completed a questionnaire concerning back pain after a 6-month treatment interval. Neither frequent back belt use nor a belt-requirement store policy was associated with a decreased incidence of back pain (rate ratio: 1.22 belt-wearers vs. 0.95 controls). As opposed to the van Poppel and colleagues' study, individuals with previous back pain did not have fewer subsequent episodes of back pain with using a belt. In an accompanying editorial, Hadler and Carey suggest that low back pain as a regional musculoskeletal disorder afflicts individuals independent of their work exposure.[6] The disability of the disorder is more directly associated with the ability to cope than the amount lifted. On the other hand, biomechanical models exist demonstrating the effects of back pain on spine loading and the increased risk of muscle fatigue and injury.[10] Are back belts being worn appropriately to offer support of the spine? Wassell and colleagues observed a small subset of individuals for a brief period to determine correct positioning of the belts. Observations were not completed at the end of the study. In the setting of the workplace, a back belt may be considered for the individual with a prior history of back pain who participates in heavy manual labor. The questions regarding the correct model for the development of spinal pain in the workplace continue to be debated.

Jellema and colleagues reviewed the scientific literature regarding the efficacy of lumbar supports for the prevention and treatment of low back pain.[7] No evidence suggests the ability of supports to prevent back pain primarily or secondarily. Lumbar supports do offer some limited therapeutic benefit but are no more effective than other forms of therapy for low back pain.

Our Recommendation

External supports for the usual patient with low back pain have limited benefit. A lumbar corset reminds individuals to lift with their legs not their back.

References

Lumbar Corsets and Braces

1. Alaranta H, Hurri H: Compliance and subjective relief by corset treatment in chronic low back pain. Scand J Rehab Med 20:133-136, 1988.
2. Bartelink DL: Role of abdominal pressure in relieving pressure on lumbar intervertebral discs. J Bone Joint Surg 39:718, 1957.
3. Coxhead CE, Inskip H, Meade TW, et al: Multicentre trial of physiotherapy in the management of sciatic symptoms. Lancet 1:1065-1068, 1981.
4. Fidler MW, Plasmans CMT: The effect of four types of support on the segmental mobility of the lumbosacral spine. J Bone Joint Surg Am 65A:943-947, 1983.
5. Hadler NM: Diagnosis and treatment of backache. In Hadler NM (ed): Medical Management of the Regional Musculoskeletal Diseases. Orlando, FL, Grune & Stratton, 1984, pp 3-52
6. Hadler HM, Carey TS: Back belts in the workplace. JAMA 284:2780-2781, 2000.
7. Jellema P, van Tulder MW, van Poppel MNM, et al: Lumbar supports for prevention and treatment of low back pain: A systematic review within the framework of the Cochrane back review group. Spine 26:377-386, 2001.
8. Laisson U, Choler U, Lidstrom A, et al: Auto-traction for treatment of lumbago-sciatica: A multicentre controlled investigation. Acta Orthop Scand 51:791-798, 1980.
9. Lumsden RM, Morris JM: An in vivo study of axial rotation and immobilization at the lumbosacral joint. J Bone Joint Surg Am 52A:1591-1602, 1968.
10. Marras WS, Davis KG, Ferguson SA, et al: Spine loading characteristics of patients with low back pain compared with asymptomatic individuals. Spine 26:2566-2574, 2001.
11. Micheli LJ, Hall JE, Miller ME: Use of modified Boston brace for back injuries in athletes. Am J Sports Med 8:351-356, 1980.
12. Million R, Nilsen KH, Jayson MIV, Baker RD: Evaluation of low back pain and assessment of lumbar corsets with and without back supports. Ann Rheum Dis 4:449-454, 1981.
13. Nachemson A, Morris JM: In vivo measurement of intradiscal pressure: Discometry, a method for the determination of pressure in the lower lumbar discs. J Bone Joint Surg Am 46A:1077, 1964.
14. Norton PL, Brown T: The immobilizing efficiency of back braces. J Bone Joint Surg Am 39A:111, 1957.
15. Perry J: The use of external support in the treatment of low-back pain: Report of the subcommittee on prosthetic orthotic education, National Academy of Sciences, National Research Council. J Bone Joint Surg Am 52A:1440-1442, 1970.
16. Russek AS: Biomechanical and physiological basis for ambulatory treatment of low back pain. Orthop Rev 4:21, 1976.
17. van Poppel MNM, de Looze MP, Koes BW, et al: Mechanisms of action of lumbar supports: A systematic review. Spine 25:2103-2113, 2000.
18. van Poppel MNM, Koes BW, van der Ploeg T, et al: Lumbar supports and education for the prevention of low back pain in industry: A randomized controlled trial. JAMA 279:1789-1794, 1998.
19. Wassell JT, Gardner LI, Landsittel DP, et al: A prospective study of back belts for prevention of back pain and injury. JAMA 284:2727-2732, 2000.
20. Waters RL, Morris JM: Effect of spinal supports on the electrical activity of muscles of the trunk. J Bone Joint Surg Am 50A:51-60, 1970.
21. Willner S: Effect of a rigid brace on back pain. Acta Orthop Scand 50:40-42, 1985.

CERVICAL ORTHOSES

Prescriptions for cervical orthoses must consider the biomechanics and pathophysiology of the disease being treated.[6] Spinal bracing affects the movement and stability of the cervical spine. The major reasons for the need to decrease motion are to decrease or control pain, protect the unstable spine, and limit damage to the traumatized cervical spine.[19] Cervical orthoses also have additional biomechanical effects of transferring partial weight of the head to the trunk when an individual is upright. While decreasing pain, cervical bracing has detrimental effects on the cervical spine structures. Muscle atrophy and weakness occur secondary to reducing the muscular activity necessary to support the skull. Decreased motion associated with the use of cervical braces promotes contracture of soft tissue structures. Psychological dependence and increased energy expenditures are also potential complications.[6]

Studies in whiplash patients demonstrated less pain improvement and range of motion in those individuals who wore a collar as opposed to those who continued neck motion as tolerated.[3,8] Cervical orthoses (collars and braces) have been used to decrease the motion of the cervical spine and head since the 5th Egyptian dynasty (from about 2750 BC).[20]

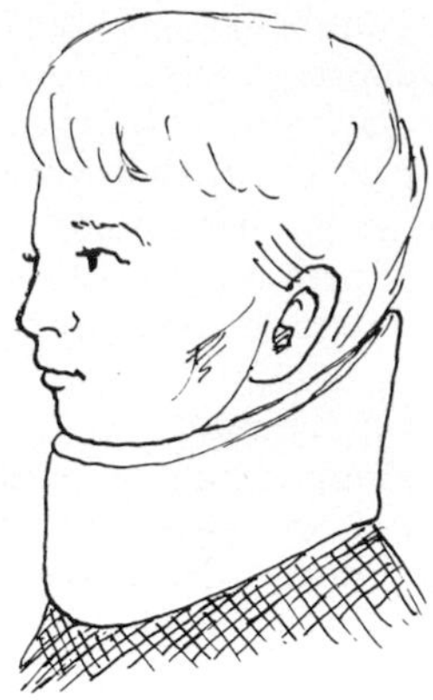

Figure 19-7 Soft cervical collar is the most comfortable orthosis. The soft collar is ineffective at limiting neck motion.

Cervical Motion

The planes of motion of the cervical spine are flexion-extension and rotation and lateral bending and are the greatest of all portions of the entire spinal column. Flexion and extension are coupled with rotation in the cervical spine. Most axial rotation occurs between C1 and C2, with the remainder occurring between segments C4 and C7. Considerable flexion and extension occur between the occiput and C1, with the remainder from the lower segments of the cervical spine. Most lateral bending occurs in the middle portion of the cervical spine at C2 to C6.[18]

Types

Cervical orthoses come in four categories: (1) cervical (CO) (soft, rigid); (2) head-cervical (HCO) (molded, poster); (3) head-cervical-thoracic (HCTO) (molded, poster); and (4) halo. These categories range from least restrictive to most restrictive. In general, cervical orthoses are most effective in limiting flexion and extension and limiting lateral bending by 50% and rotation by 20%.[6] As opposed to lumbar supports that have contact over the entire lumbar spine, cervical orthoses must control motion by contact between the mandible and the thorax. Cervical orthoses should fit snugly but not so tight as to cause discomfort. If fitted too tightly, pressure on soft tissue structures causes pain.[5] Ill-fitted cervical collars can also cause pressure sores over the occiput.[17] Cervical collars are available that decrease the risk of these complications.

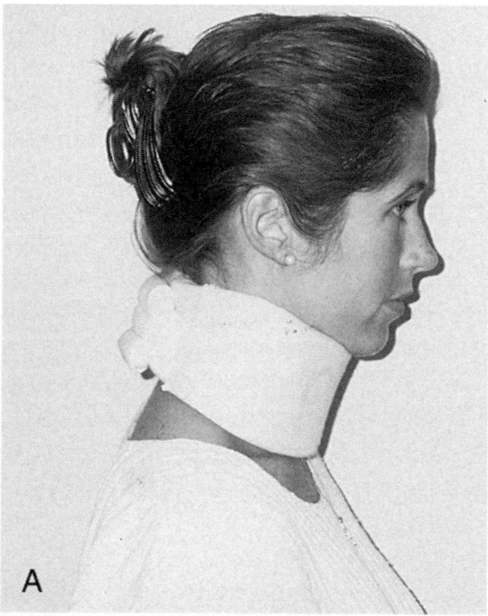

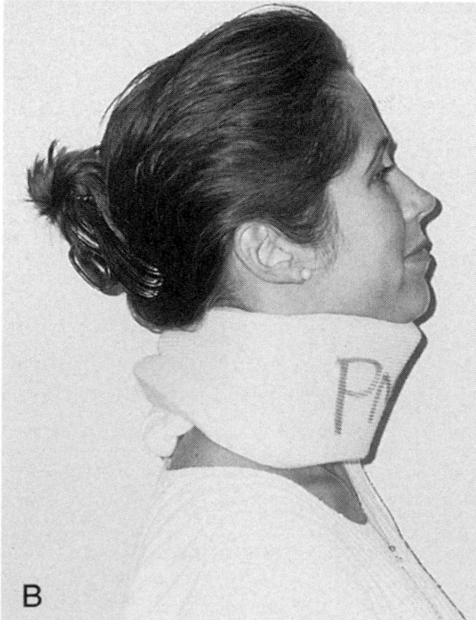

Figure 19-8 Fitting of soft cervical collar. *A*, The width of the collar should allow the neck to be in a slightly forward position. *B*, A collar that is too wide can cause pain secondary to excessive extension. In this circumstance, the collar should be reversed and fastened in front. A smaller collar should be obtained if extension of the spine cannot be corrected. *(Courtesy of Tom Welsh, RPT.)*

Soft Collar

For mild neck pain, the soft cervical collar is the most commonly prescribed orthosis (Fig. 19-7). The collar is made of firm foam covered with cotton that is held together with a Velcro closure. The foam may vary in thickness or firmness. The soft collar is the least effective orthosis for reducing motion, but it provides comfort and warmth surrounding the neck.[21] The soft collar reduces motion in the sagittal plane by 26% but does not limit rotation or lateral bending.[12] The restriction of motion is mediated through sensory feedback and a reminder to limit head and neck motion more than an actual restriction of motion (Fig. 19-8). Sleep may be the ideal time for the use of a soft collar. The collar may limit awkward positions of the head. The hard collars (polyethylene) may have occipital and mandibular projections for added support. The Thomas collar has adjustments in height with foam edges. It decreases 75% of sagittal motion but does not restrict other planes of motion.[10] A higher anterior part of the collar results in decreased flexion, and a higher posterior part results in decreased extension. Scientific evidence demonstrating the efficacy of soft cervical collars is generally lacking.[4,11] However, significant decrease in neck pain associated with the use of a cervical collar has been reported on occasion.[2,15] Variability of results may be related to patient compliance.

Head-Cervical Orthoses

HCO collars support the occipital and chin regions.[9] The most common HCO collar is the Philadelphia collar (Fig. 19-9). The collar consists of two pieces of Plastazote foam, with sides reinforced by rigid thermoplastic with Velcro closures. The orthosis may be less irritating to the skin by placing cloth padding under the chin support. The Philadelphia collar limits sagittal movement to 30% of normal.[7] The collar may also be extended along the thorax and thoracic spine, with a strap around the thorax at the xiphoid level for increased support (Fig. 19-10). Other forms of this collar include the Aspen, Stifneck, Miami J, and Neoloc. Different collars are reported to offer different levels of patient comfort while limiting cervical spine motion.[1,16]

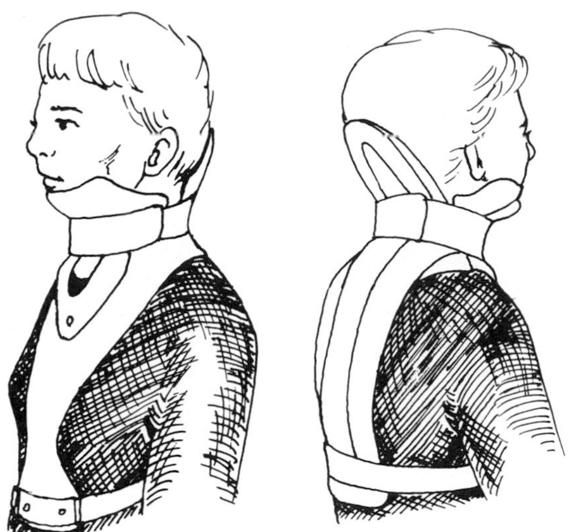

Figure 19-10 Molded cervicothoracic orthosis.

Head-Cervical-Thoracic Orthoses

HCTO collars are rigid poster-type supports with two or four upright supports. The four-post collar limits sagittal motion to 5% to 21% of normal, rotation to 27% of normal, and lateral bending to 46% of normal.[12] The Guilford brace has an anterior and posterior support but may be less effective at limiting lateral bending (Fig. 19-11). These orthoses offer less warmth to the neck than closed orthoses.

Another form of HCTO is the sternal-occipital-mandibular immobilizer (SOMI) brace (Figs. 19-12 and 19-13). This brace consists of a broad chest piece that extends down the xiphoid and is hung on shoulder straps that attach behind to an encircling chest strap. The support may attach under the chin or solely to the occiput. The main advantage of this brace is the fitting of supine patients and the ease of adjustment. This brace is effective in immobilizing the upper cervical spine (C1-C5) in flexion. The SOMI brace allows 28% of normal sagittal motion, 34% of rotation, and 66% of lateral bending.[19] It is used after surgical fusions, to immobilize stable fractures of the neck, and to wean patients from bony-contact orthoses like the halo vest.

Halo Vest

The halo vest consists of a steel band encircling the head and secured to the skull with metal pins with attachments to a plastic thoracic vest with upright supports (Fig. 19-14). It requires expert fitting but offers the greatest restriction of cervical motion while the patient remains ambulatory. The vest reduces motion to 4% of sagittal motion, 1% of rotation, and 4% of lateral bending.[12] However, individual cervical segments may move in the lower cervical spine (snaking phenomenon).[13] A Minerva

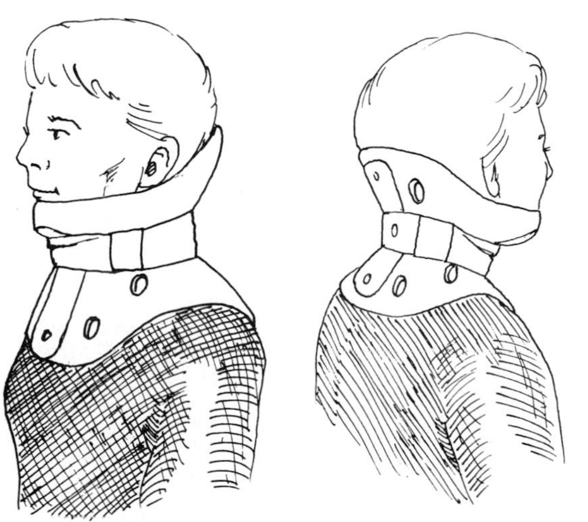

Figure 19-9 Philadelphia collar.

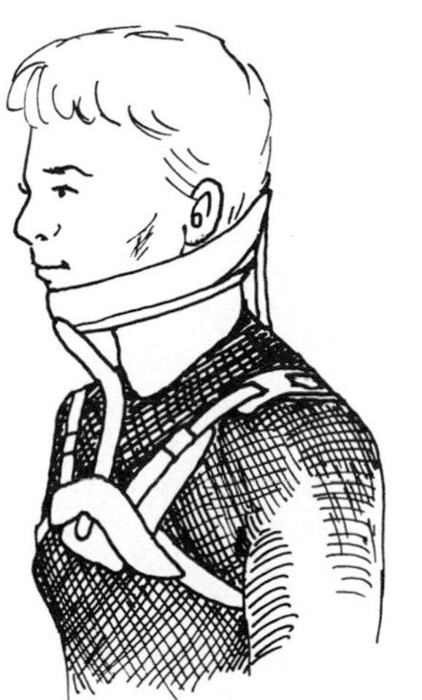

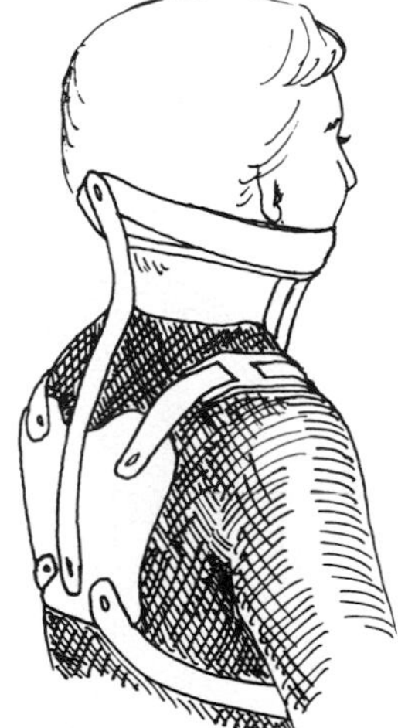

Figure 19-11 Guilford brace.

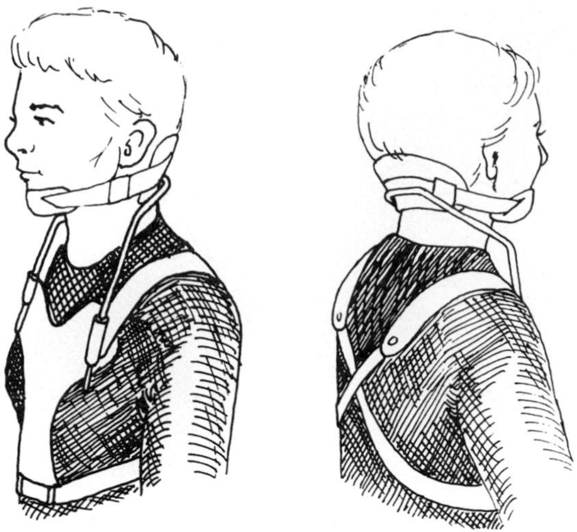

Figure 19-12 Sternal-occipital-mandibular immobilizer orthosis with mandibular support.

jacket consists of a body jacket with a chin, occipital, and forehead support. Movement of individual segments is decreased with the Minerva jacket compared with the halo vest. The Minerva jacket is also more comfortable than the halo vest.[14]

The most effective orthoses for control of sagittal motion are the halo vest and Minerva jacket. Rotation is also controlled with these orthoses. No orthosis offers total control of lateral bending. The halo vest limits lateral bending to 4% or less.

In conclusion, the selection of an orthosis must balance the comfort of the patient with the need for restriction of cervical motion. The CO collar is tolerated better than more restrictive braces. The soft collars should be used for a limited time. The patient should be encouraged to remove the collar at every opportunity. The only orthosis that effectively controls motion between the occiput and C1 is the halo vest; it is required for patients with instability of the upper cervical spine. For patients with lower cervical spine instability, the HCO or SOMI braces are adequate. The more serious conditions associated with neurologic symptoms require more restrictive orthoses. Orthoses should be selected to offer the appropriate restriction of motion at the proper intervertebral level. In complicated patients, an orthotist can be helpful in selecting the correct brace.

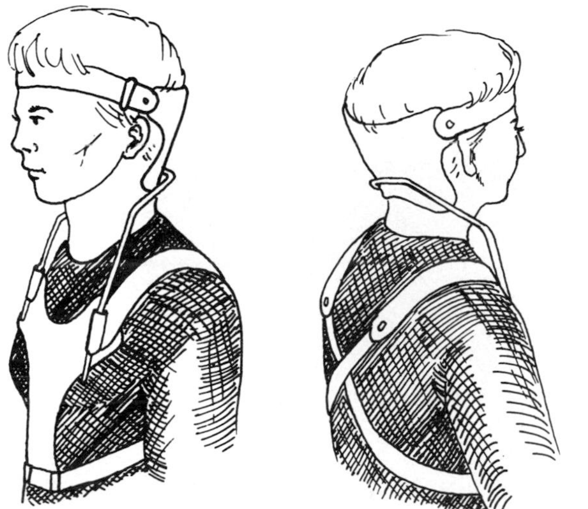

Figure 19-13 Sternal-occipital-mandibular immobilizer orthosis with occipital support.

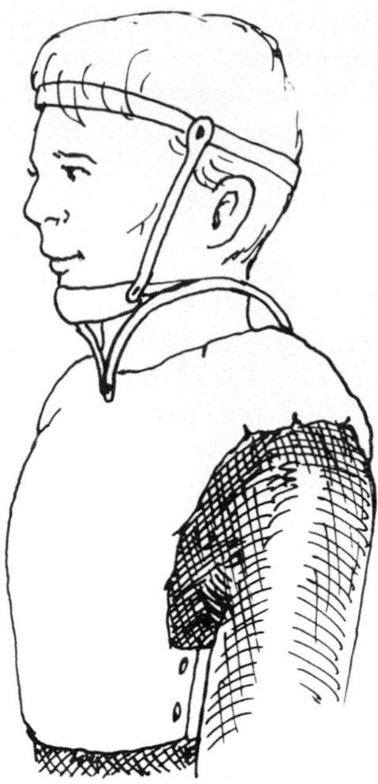

Figure 19-14 Halo vest.

Our Recommendation

Cervical soft collars are useful to stabilize the neck to improve sleep. Hard cervical collars are used most commonly in postsurgical patients. The halo vest offers the greatest degree of stability for the cervical spine but is reserved for those at risk for spinal cord damage.

References

Cervical Orthoses

1. Askins V, Eismont FJ: Efficacy of five cervical orthoses in restricting cervical motion: A comparison study. Spine 22:1193-1198, 1997.
2. Barnes MP, Saunders M: The effect of cervical mobility on the natural history of cervical spondylitic myelopathy. J Neurol Neurosurg Psychiatry 47:17-20, 1984.
3. Borchgrevink GE, Kassa A, McDonagh D, et al: Acute treatment of whiplash neck sprain injuries: A randomized trial of treatment during the first 14 days after a car accident. Spine 23:25-31, 1998.
4. British Association of Physical Medicine: Pain in the neck and arm: A multicentre trial of the effects of physiotherapy. BMJ 1:253, 1966.
5. Fisher SV: Proper fitting of the cervical orthoses. Arch Phys Med Rehabil 59:505-507, 1978.
6. Fisher SV: Spinal orthoses. In Kottke FJ, Lehmann JF (eds): Krusen's Handbook of Physical Medicine and Rehabilitation, 4th ed. Philadelphia, WB Saunders, 1990, pp 593-601.
7. Fisher SV, Bowar JF, Awad EA, et al: Cervical orthoses effect on cervical spine motion: Roentgenographic and goniometric method of study. Arch Phys Med Rehabil 58:109-115, 1977.

8. Gennis P, Miller L, Gallagher EJ, et al: The effect of soft cervical collars on persistent neck pain in patients with whiplash injury. Acad Emerg Med 3:568-573, 1996.
9. Harris JD: Cervical orthoses. In Redford JB (ed): Orthotics, etcetera, 3rd ed. Baltimore, Williams & Wilkins, 1986, pp 100-121.
10. Hartman JT, Palumbo F, Hill BJ: Cineradiography of the braced normal cervical spine: A comparative study of five commonly used orthoses. Clin Orthop 109:97-102, 1975.
11. Huston GJ: Collars and corsets. BMJ 296:276, 1988.
12. Johnson RM, Hart DL, Simmons EF, et al: Cervical orthoses. J Bone Joint Surg Am 59A:332-339, 1977.
13. Lind B, Sihlbolm H, Nordwall A: Forces and motions across the neck in patients treated with halo-vest. Spine 13:162-167, 1988.
14. Maiman D, Millington P, Novak S, et al: The effect of the thermoplastic Minerva body jacket on cervical spine motion. Neurosurgery 25:363-367, 1989.
15. Naylor JR, Mulley GP: Surgical collars: A survey of their prescription and use. Br J Rheumatol 30:282-284, 1991.
16. Plaisier B, Gabram SG, Schwartz RJ, et al: Prospective evaluation of craniofacial pressure in four different cervical orthoses. J Trauma 3:714-720, 1994.
17. Powers J: A multidisciplinary approach to occipital pressure ulcers related to cervical collars. J Nurs Care Qual 12:46-52, 1997.
18. Punjabi MM, Vasavada A, White AA: Cervical spine biomechanics. Semin Spine Surg 5:10, 1993.
19. Redford JB, Patel AT: Orthotic devices in the management of spinal disorders. Phys Med Rehabil 9:709, 1995.
20. Smith GE: The most ancient splints. BMJ 1:732, 1908.
21. Wolf JW Jr, Johnson RM: Cervical orthoses. In The Cervical Spine Research Society Editorial Committee: The Cervical Spine, 2nd ed. Philadelphia, JB Lippincott, 1989.

PHYSICAL THERAPY AND EXERCISES—LUMBAR SPINE

Physical therapy in conjunction with personal exercise regimens is recommended to many patients with low back pain. In the past, it was common practice to tear off an exercise instruction sheet (usually for flexion exercises) and give it to any patient with low back pain without further explanation. The therapeutic results of these exercises were varied: some patients had improvement; some had exacerbation of symptoms; some would follow the instructions incorrectly; and some would not do them at all. The results of this haphazard attempt at physical therapy exercises left some physicians skeptical of their benefit. The timing of physical therapy is key to its success. Increased physical exercises beyond activities of daily living in the early stages of an acute pain episode may exacerbate symptoms. The same exercises completed later in the course of an acute event may result in an improved outcome. Many of the exercises listed in this chapter are for those individuals who are resolving an acute event, have chronic pain, or are attempting to improve general physical conditioning.

Goals of Therapy

The goals of the exercise regimens vary greatly. Some strengthen lumbar spine extensors, whereas others strengthen abdominal muscles. Other exercises concentrate on lengthening contracted muscles. Physicians frequently choose a course of exercises for a patient based on a general concept of strengthening muscles, whether paraspinous or abdominal, as the goal of exercise. They do not individualize the patient's regimen to the underlying disease or the associated abnormality in the musculoskeletal structures of the lumbosacral spine, and, consequently, the maximum benefit of therapy may not be achieved. For example, an ideal exercise program requires individualized therapy, which may include flexion or extension exercises that concentrate on strengthening and/or lengthening back muscles.

Rationale for Physical Therapy

In a two-part article, Jackson and Brown point out many of the fallacies and misconceptions associated with exercises and low back pain.[24,25] The reasons for prescribing exercises for patients with low back pain are listed in Table 19-1.

Many theories have been proposed to explain how low back exercises result in pain relief. Williams postulated that back and leg pain resulted from compression of radicular nerves as they passed through the intervertebral foramen. Flexion exercises purportedly opened the foramen, relieving nerve root compression.[56,57] In opposition to the flexion theory, McKenzie proposed that radicular pain was related to disc protrusion and that repeated extension exercises shifted extruded disc material anteriorly, relieving compression.[37] Flexion and extension exercises are not helpful in all patients with back pain. For example, neither of these exercise methods has been proved to be effective in relieving sciatic pain. Nerve compression is associated with numbness, not pain. It is the inflammation associated with chronic compression that causes pain. Neither flexion nor extension exercises relieve nerve inflammation or sciatic pain. Therefore, the potential for these exercises to significantly reduce radicular pain, acutely, is minimal. In regard to shifting disc material, both anterior and posterior compressive forces on the disc are associated with movement of nuclear material.[28] If pain is related to disc compression of nerve roots and exercises cause nuclear material to return to normal anatomic position, pain relief may gradually occur as the forces on the nerves are reduced. Flexion exercises commenced early in an episode of low back pain may not improve outcome. In a study of flexion exercises, a total of 473 Dutch patients with low back pain were divided into three groups with exercise instruction (eight flexion exercises) with advice for daily life activities, placebo ultrasound

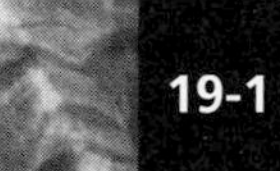

19-1 REASONS FOR THE PRESCRIPTION OF EXERCISES FOR PATIENTS WITH LOW BACK PAIN

Decrease pain
Strengthen weak muscles*
Stretch contracted muscles
Decrease mechanical stress to spinal structures
Improve fitness to prevent injury*
Stabilize hypermobile segments
Improve posture
Improve mobility
As a last resort

*Proven effective therapy.
Modified from Jackson CP, Brown MD: Analysis of current approaches and a practical guide to prescription of exercise. Clin Orthop 176:46, 1983.

therapy, or care by a general practitioner, including analgesics and patient education.[14] The outcomes were similar at 2 and 4 weeks and at 12 months in all groups except for shorter duration of pain recurrences in the exercise group. The early intervention with exercise may have biased the results of this investigation.

Pain relief has been proposed as a beneficial component of aerobic exercise. Strenuous aerobic exercise is associated with increased endorphin levels, a sense of euphoria, and the potential for pain relief. Unfortunately, increases in levels of endorphins peripherally are not necessarily correlated with increased central nervous system levels.[20] Generalized pain relief cannot be obtained through generalized strenuous aerobic exercise and probably does not play a role in pain relief associated with exercises in back patients. In general, aggressive exercise programs are more successful in improving functional status, such as return to work, than in significantly relieving pain.[39] However, improved function may decrease the anxiety associated with fear of exacerbation of back pain. This decrease in anxiety may have beneficial psychological effects. Early return to work after an aggressive exercise program is not associated with an increased rate of recurrence of low back pain.[36]

Strengthening of back muscles has been advocated as a beneficial aspect of exercise programs that are a part of a comprehensive program to control back pain.[2] Patients who have acute low back pain do not exhibit extensor muscle weakness.[5,48] In contrast, those patients with chronic back pain of a month or longer do exhibit muscle weakness.[44] In these patients with chronic pain, trunk extensors are weakened to a greater degree than flexors.[1,38] This is in stark contrast to normal individuals without back pain who have stronger extensor muscles.[10,52] In normal individuals, extensor strength is typically 30% greater than flexor strength.[6]

The paraspinous muscles are involved not only in job-related tasks but also in the maintenance of posture. The role of muscle weakness in the development of postural back pain was studied by De Vries.[12] Patients with back pain and bad posture had abnormalities on electromyographic (EMG) analysis of paraspinous muscles not elicited from normal controls without pain. He suggested that muscular deficiency was a cause of back pain and that this category of back pain was amenable to endurance exercises.

Posture also may play a role in causing pain in patients with occupations that require assuming one position for an extended period of time. The strength of the back muscles is important for completing certain tasks (lifting, carrying) but may not prevent the development of back pain in an individual who lacks the muscular endurance to maintain a certain posture.[33] Those workers who lack adequate strength or endurance relative to their work are at greater risk of developing back injury.[51] These findings suggest that abnormalities in strength or endurance of paraspinous muscles may act independently as sources of pain. Over time, back pain causes decreased muscle strength. In addition, the lack of muscle endurance may add to the perpetuation of back pain. A return of full muscle strength, joint movement, and endurance is necessary for a complete recovery of function. Back strength is more closely related to ability to work than to the degree of pain. Parnianpour and co-workers developed a device that can measure motor output (torque) and movement pattern (angular position and velocity profile) in three dimensions associated with work-related tasks that generated isoinertial forces. Isoinertial forces are generated by muscles contracting against a constant load. In a study, workers were asked to use maximum effort lifting a constant load.[45] With increasing fatigue, greater range of motion was noted in planes other than flexion and extension associated with the lifting task. The inability of the primary muscles to complete the task resulted in the recruitment of secondary muscle groups. The recruitment of these secondary muscles loaded the spine in a more injury-prone pattern. Fatigued muscles were less capable of compensating for any perturbation in the lifted load. The implication of this study is that endurance of back muscles related to a job task is a more useful predictor of the incidence of back pain than is the absolute strength of these muscles.

A number of studies have demonstrated the relationship between mechanical stress and low back pain.[23,53] The relative benefit of flexion versus extension versus isotonic exercises in the relief of back pain remains controversial.[21,42,57] Whether specific exercises can be used to reduce mechanical loads on the spine and whether increased intradiscal stress on normal discs is necessarily associated with back pain remain to be determined.

Good general fitness is associated with decreased incidence of back injuries and decreased duration of incapacity with a back injury according to a prospective study of 1652 firefighters.[8] This study is strong evidence for improved fitness to prevent injuries but does not have relevance to those patients in poor physical condition with concurrent back pain.

Exercises directed at stabilizing a hypermobile or hypomobile spinal segment by increasing muscle strength do not work. Paraspinous muscles lack the voluntary control to allow for specific segment strengthening. Patients must be evaluated for imbalances in muscle strength and length. Strengthening and lengthening the paraspinous, psoas, and hamstring muscles to achieve normal physiologic balance of the lumbosacral spine and its supporting structures give patients a greater chance of decreasing pain than does concentrating on strengthening an isolated area.[43]

Exercises to improve structural postural abnormalities are not effective. The degree of structural lordosis is unrelated to abdominal or back extensor muscle strength or to hip or trunk flexibility.[17] Flexion or isometric exercises that attempt to correct these postural abnormalities have been ineffective in altering nonpathologic structural back anatomy.[11,19]

Although adequate mobility is necessary for normal function of the spine, the total range that has the greatest mechanical efficiency, tissue nutrition for discs and cartilage, and adequate facet joint motion has not been determined. Too little motion (less than 30 degrees) may limit flexibility, whereas too much can excessively load the spine.[15] Exercises that attempt to increase spinal mobility beyond normal ranges of motion are not necessarily beneficial.

Exercise programs are occasionally prescribed for patients with chronic low back pain as a last resort after other therapies have failed. Exercise programs can have a beneficial effect even if the patient's physical condition is not dramatically altered. The active involvement of patients in their exercise program is an essential part of therapy. Exercise may decrease stress and foster better sleep habits and may also improve the patient's self-image and self-esteem.[7,9,40]

Lumbar Spine Exercise Programs

Therapeutic exercise can be defined as structural and controlled body movement to correct an impairment, improve musculoskeletal function, or maintain a state of well-being. Exercises can increase muscle strength, elasticity, range of motion, and endurance. A prescription for physical therapy must have a specified objective. The program of exercises may be modified as a patient's condition is altered and may include passive, active-assisted, active, or active-resistive exercises.

Exercise Regimens

Passive exercise is produced entirely by an external force without any voluntary contraction of muscles by the patient. The exercises maintain range of motion and elasticity of soft tissue. Active-assisted exercises, which require muscular contraction to move a portion of the body without an external force, maintain flexibility and decrease potential for muscle atrophy. Isometric, isotonic, and isokinetic exercises are classified as active-resistive. Isometric contraction is associated with increased muscle tension without change in muscle length. Strength is increased only at the length of muscle contraction; contraction at different muscle lengths is needed to increase generalized muscle strength. Isotonic exercise decreases fiber length without a change in muscle tension. Strengthening occurs through maximal effort of motion. Isokinetic exercises move body parts through ranges of motion at a constant speed. This kind of therapy is done with a Cybex machine.

Which is the best exercise program for patients with low back pain? Kendall and Jenkins studied three types of treatment: (1) mobility and strengthening exercises, (2) lumbar isometric flexion exercises, and (3) hyperextension exercises. At the end of the 3-month study, the isometric group had a statistically significant improvement in symptoms.[26] In contrast, Davies found that patients assessed at 4 weeks of treatment described greater improvement with extension exercises than with isometric exercises or heat. The period of time to return to work was shorter in the extension and control groups (2 weeks) than in the isometric group.[11] Data demonstrating the greater efficacy of one type of exercise over another are not available. The physician must decide whether flexion, extension, isometric, or general fitness exercises are best for specific problems their patients are experiencing.

Flexion Exercises

Flexion exercises are used to open intervertebral foramina and facet joints, to stretch hip flexors and back extensors, to strengthen abdominal and gluteal muscles, and to mobilize the posterior fixation of the lumbosacral articulation.[56,57] Williams' exercises have been modified over the years but basically consist of partial sit-ups in the hook-lying position (feet on floor, knees flexed, head slightly raised) to strengthen abdominal muscles, pelvic tilts to flatten lumbar lordosis, knees to chest, and stretching hip flexors (Fig. 19-15).

These exercises are designed to increase intra-abdominal pressure to stabilize the spine. The muscles that actually generate abdominal pressure are the internal and external oblique muscles, which are involuntary muscles in the generation of abdominal pressure.[3] Voluntary efforts to increase pressure, such as contracting the rectus abdominis during a Valsalva maneuver, increase the load on the intervertebral discs and may be counterproductive. Exercises to increase strength in the oblique muscles without participation of the rectus abdominis include rotating the thorax on the pelvis, posterior pelvic tilt while standing, and hip roll.[46] The desired effect may also be obtained by lifting a shoulder during a modified sit-up in the hook-lying position.[22]

Other components of flexion exercises such as posterior pelvic tilts while supine, bilateral straight leg–raising, and toe touches either have no benefit or increase intradiscal pressures.[24] In particular, flexion exercises are not indicated in patients with acute disc prolapse, immediately after periods of prolonged rest with hyperhydrated discs that are susceptible to injury, postural low back pain secondary to flexion, or lateral trunk list.[24]

Extension Exercises

Extension exercises may be attempted with paraspinous extensors in a flexed or neutral position with the goal of improving motor strength and endurance or attempted in the hyperextended position with the goal of improving mobility, strengthening the back extensors, or promoting a shift of nuclear material to a normal position (Fig. 19-16). People with strong paraspinous extensors have less postural fatigue and pain, greater capacity to lift weights and to withstand axial compression, and better overall physical fitness. Evidence exists demonstrating the effects of extension exercises on strengthening lumbar extensor muscles.[49] The primary functions of the paraspinous extensors are maintaining posture and controlling the descent of the trunk during flexion.[18,41] Maximum trunk extensor movement occurs in 40 to 45 degrees of flexion, and that is the range in which the muscles should be exercised. By positioning themselves at the edge of a table on their stomachs, patients can exercise the extensors by lifting and lowering their trunk without extending the lumbar spine. EMG studies of paraspinous muscles indicate that hyperextension exercises are the most effective for strengthening the extensor muscles.[47] Other components of a hyperextension exercise program include press-ups in the prone position and strengthening and stretching of hip extensors (hamstrings and gluteal muscles) (see Fig. 19-16).[16]

Patients with low back pain often have tight hamstring muscles. Exercises to stretch and strengthen the hip extensors are an important component of an extension program. Stretching from a flexed, sitting posture may have limitations by hyperflexing the spine, increasing intradiscal pressure, and straining paraspinous muscles.[31] Unilateral hamstring stretches may be a safer alternative for improving hamstring muscle function without straining other lumbar structures.

Although extension exercises have been associated with relief of low back symptoms, not all patients benefit from them.[50] Patients who have an acute disc prolapse, have undergone multiple back operations, have limited flexion because of paraspinous scarring, or have facet joint disease (spinal stenosis) may have exacerbation of symptoms with extension exercises.[24]

Isometric Flexion Exercises

Others propose isometric flexion exercises as the most appropriate for back patients.[21,27] These exercises eliminate hyperextension and encourage contraction of trunk muscles and strengthening of abdominal muscles. The exercises are done in a supine position, although the same maneuvers may be attempted while sitting or standing. A sequence of active contractions involve the abdominal muscles; the gluteal muscles; the abdominal and gluteal muscles, resulting in a pelvic tilt; and, finally, contraction of the hip adductors. The contractions are held for 5 to 15

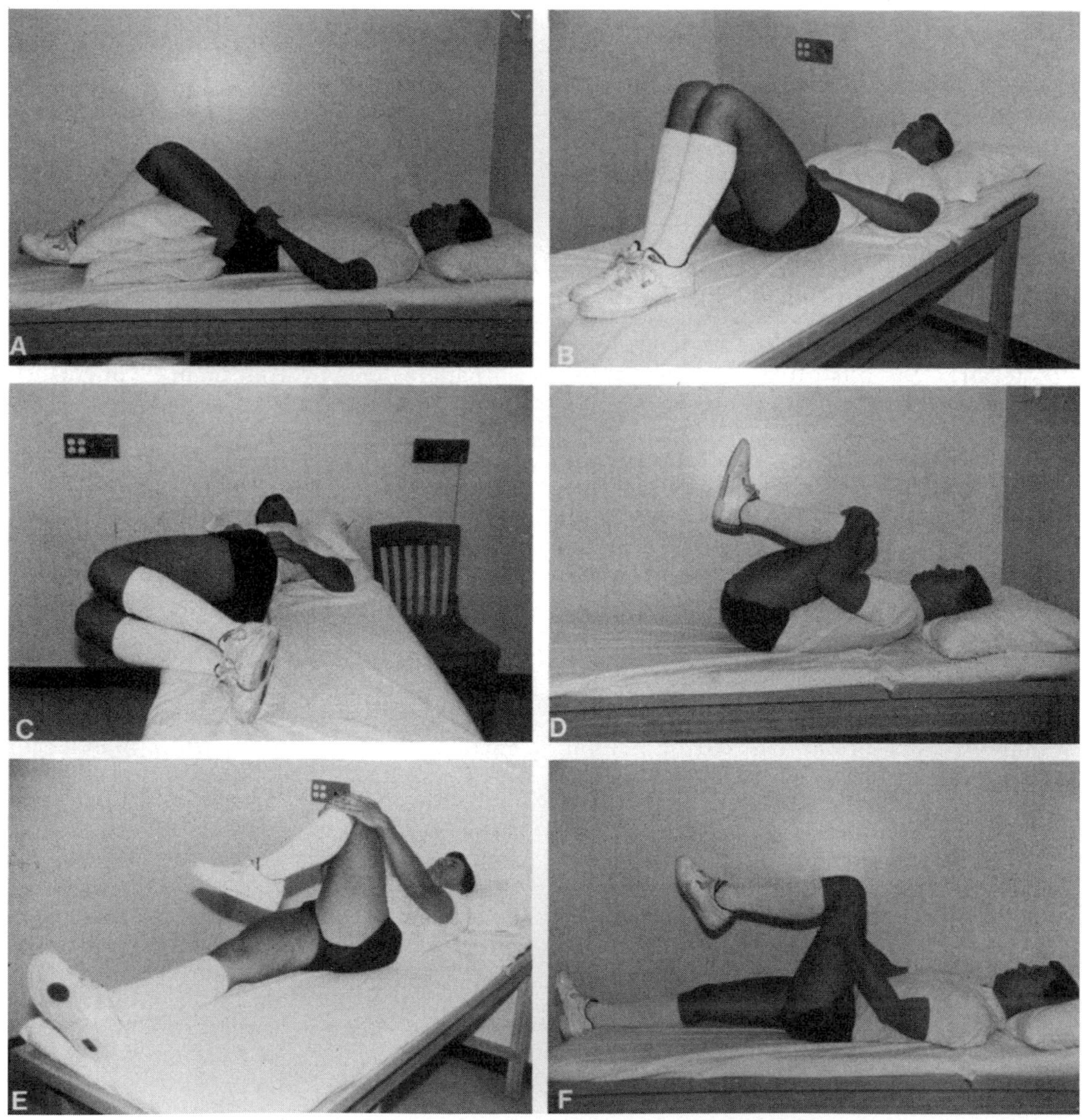

Figure 19-15 Flexion exercises. *A* to *C*, Acute (relaxation) phase. *A*, Resting position—hips flexed with pillows under knees. This flattens the lumbar spine. Duration: 15 minutes. *B*, Resting position without pillows. *C*, Back rotation—shoulders remain on the table while the pelvis is turned to one side to the patient's tolerance. This exercise stretches and strengthens the internal and external obliques. Duration: 1 minute. Patient alternates side to side. (These exercises promote relaxation of muscles.) *D* and *E*, Stretching phase. *D*, Knees to chest while raising the pelvis. This exercise stretches the paraspinous muscles. *E*, Crossover leg exercise—the heel is placed on the contralateral knee and the bent knee is pulled to tolerance toward the contralateral shoulder. Duration: The position is held to a count of 3, and the leg is rested in the neutral position for a count of 6. The legs are alternated with 10 repetitions. (These exercises stretch the paraspinous and hip abductor muscles.) *F* to *I*, Stretching and strengthening phase. *F*, Hamstring stretch with hip flexed, knee flexed.

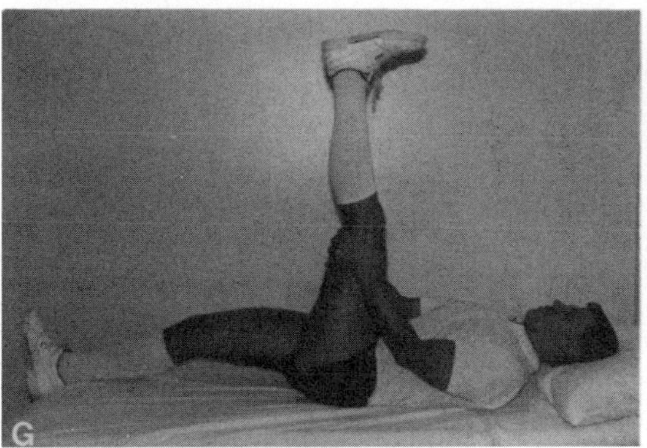

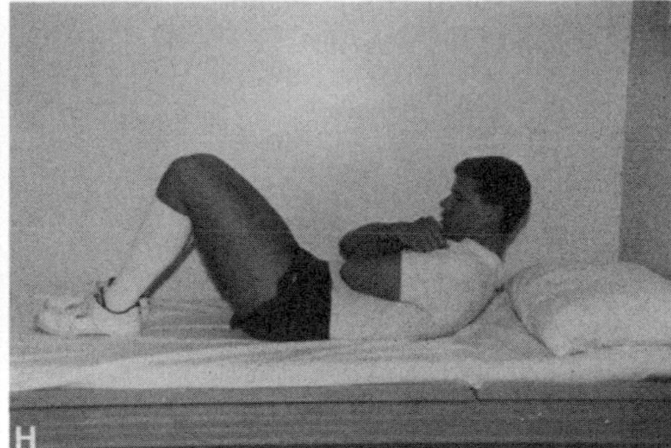

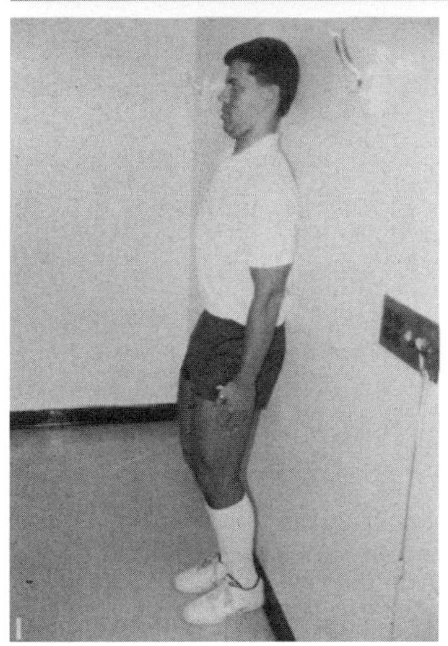

Figure 19-15, cont'd *G,* Hamstring stretch—fully extended knee. Duration: Hold for a count of 3, then count to 6 with the leg in the neutral position. *H,* Partial sit-up—strengthens the abdominal muscles. Duration: Hold for a count of 3, then rest for a count of 6 for 25 repetitions. *I,* Pelvic tilt in standing position—back flattened against the wall, knees flexed. Duration: Count of 3, done hourly. (These exercises stretch and strengthen the paraspinous and hamstring muscles and strengthen the abdominal muscles.) *(Courtesy of Thomas Welsh.)*

seconds. The exercises are done frequently, for short periods, during the day. Progress is measured by increased duration and number of exercise completions. In a study comparing conventional physical therapy with mobilizing and strengthening exercises versus isometric flexion versus controls in 62 outpatients with sciatica, Lidstrom and Zachrisson demonstrated significantly greater improvement in the isometric group than in the other two groups. Patients in the isometric group had decreased mobility.[30]

Elnaggar and coworkers studied the efficacy of flexion versus extension exercises in 56 patients with chronic mechanical low back pain for 3 months or longer.[13] Each patient received six therapist sessions and eight self-directed sessions over a 2-week period. Patients repeated the flexion or extension exercises two to three times over a 30-minute period. At the end of the 2-week exercise period, both groups experienced a significant decrease in low back pain. The flexion groups demonstrated increased sagittal motion compared with the extension group. This study points out the importance of exercise, in general, as a means to improve the function of patients with low back pain.

Aerobic Exercises

Jackson and Brown suggest a general aerobic program for patients with back pain who have been medically screened for cardiovascular disease.[24] Exercise sessions, which involve large muscle groups, include a warm-up and cool-down period, last 30 to 40 minutes, and are completed three times a week. Temperature extremes should be avoided. Walking and swimming are probably the best aerobic exercises for the majority of patients with back pain.

Mannion and co-workers reported the benefits of an aerobic exercise program compared with physical therapy and isoinertial exercise machines.[35] In 148 patients divided into three groups, aerobic exercise consisting of 1 hour of low impact aerobics supplemented with whole-body stretching was better and more cost effective than a 12-week 1-hour exercise machine program and a physical therapy program with active exercises and passive modalities. All three active therapies were equally efficacious in their effect on reducing pain intensity, pain frequency, and disability in tasks of daily living. Lumbar mobility was increased with aerobics and devices to a greater degree than physiotherapy. The cost of physiotherapy was three times greater, and the cost of exercise devices four times

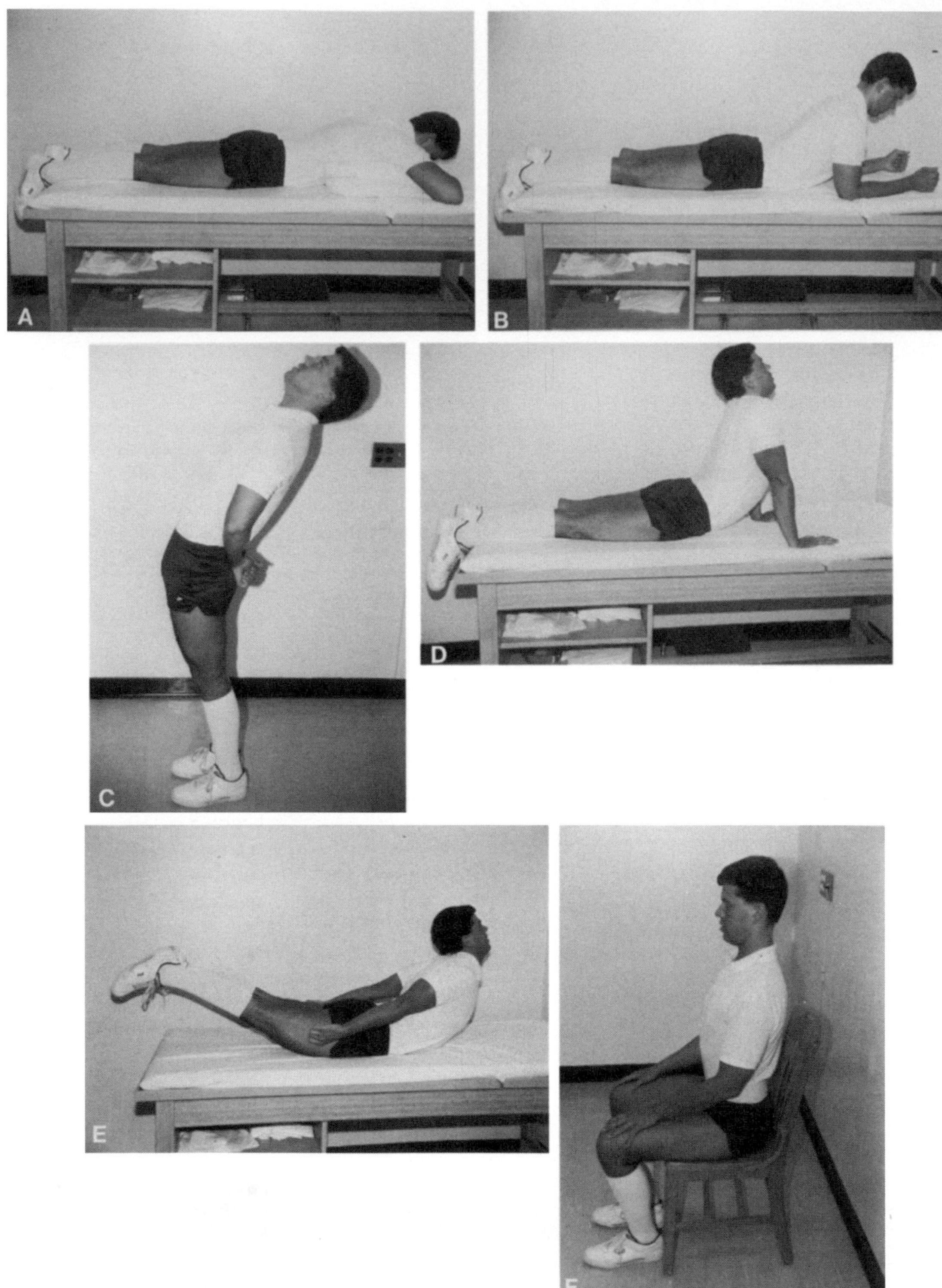

Figure 19-16 Extension exercises. *A,* Acute (relaxation) phase. Prone position resting on pillows. Additional pillows are used to patient's tolerance. Duration: 15 minutes. (This exercise promotes relaxation of paraspinous muscles.) *B* to *D,* Stretching phase. *B,* Patient is propped up on bent elbows. Duration: Hold to a count of 3, then rest for a count of 6. *C,* Extension of the lumbar spine in standing position. Duration: Hold for a count of 3, then rest for a count of 6. This exercise is done hourly. *D,* Full extension. Duration: Hold for a count of 10, with 10 repetitions. (These exercises stretch the paraspinous muscles.) *E* to *F,* Strengthening phase. *E,* Full extension with arms extended and legs lifted to tolerance. Duration: Hold for a count of 3, then rest for a count of 6. *F,* Extension—seated position. (Maintenance of lumbar lordosis.) *(Courtesy of Thomas Welsh.)*

greater than the aerobic exercise program. Administration of aerobics as an efficacious therapy for chronic low back pain has the potential to offer a useful cost-effective intervention to a wide range of individuals with limited access to health care.

Exercise Prescription

Just as there is no single therapy for all cases of back pain, there is no one physical therapy program for all patients with lumbosacral disease.[54] Some patients benefit from flexion, some from extension, and some from isometrics (Fig. 19-17); some do not improve at all. Listening carefully to the patient's symptoms and observing the movements that cause pain help the physician decide which physical therapy program has the greatest chance for success in an individual patient (Tables 19-2 and 19-3). It must be reiterated that the therapy program is not cast in stone. Communication among the patient, therapist, and physician is essential. As the patient improves, increasingly stressful tasks may be added to the exercise program in an attempt to increase endurance and strength in preparation for return to work. If symptoms increase, exercises may be discontinued or reduced, to be reinitiated once the patient's symptoms return to baseline. Individualizing exercise programs to patient symptoms leads to greater patient compliance and improved outcome.

Exercise Outcomes

The aggressiveness of the exercise program will have an effect on the degree of pain the patient experiences. Manniche and co-workers completed a study of 105 patients with low back pain divided into three exercise groups.[34] One group received 30 sessions of intensive dynamic back extensor exercises over a 3-month period.

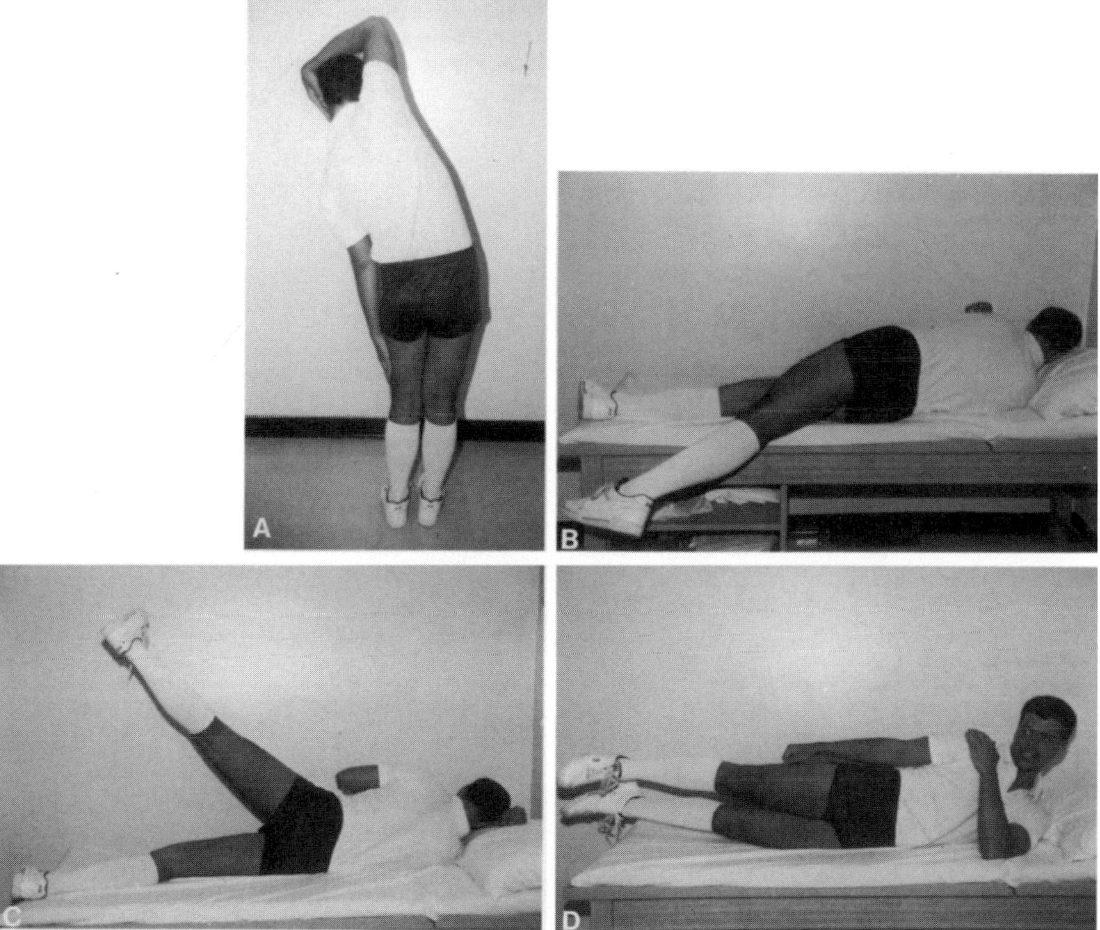

Figure 19-17 Two weeks after the start of flexion or extension exercises, the following set of exercises is initiated. *A*, Lateral bending in standing position. Duration: Hold for a count of 10 done hourly. (This exercise stretches the latissimus dorsi and the quadratus lumborum on the side with the list.) *B*, Hip abductor stretch. This exercise lengthens the side with the shortened iliotibial band. *C*, Hip abductor strengthening for the muscle opposite the shortened side. *D*, Oblique muscle strengthening and stretching. The oblique and latissimus dorsi muscles on the down side are lengthened while the muscles on the up side are strengthened. (These exercises restore muscle balance to the patient with back list.) *(Courtesy of Thomas Welsh.)*

19-2 INDICATIONS FOR FLEXION EXERCISES

Pain relief on:
 Sitting
  and with:
 Repeated forward bending
 Increased lumbar lordosis
 Fixed lumbar lordosis with bending
Pain exacerbation on:
 Walking
 Standing
  and with:
 Sustained forward bending
 Repeated backward bending
 Sustained backward bending
 Extreme range of backward bending
Pain unchanged on:
 Stooping

Another group received six sessions of similar exercises over a 3-month period. The final group received massage and mild exercises. The treatment group that received the intensive exercise program had increased discomfort during the first month but felt better during the second and third months than did the individuals in the other study groups. Benefits from exercise can be long lasting. The physician should encourage the patient to continue with the exercise program even if there is some increase in discomfort initially. Most patients recognize the meaning of the saying "no pain, no gain." The full benefit of improved physical conditioning occurs after the initial phases of exercise that are more painful.[4]

Ljunggren and colleagues reported on a 12-month study of an exercise program utilizing conventional flexion and extension exercises or an exercise apparatus for 153 Norwegian individuals with low back pain. Over the 12-month period, absenteeism from work was reduced by 80% with either regimen.[32]

Exercises have the potential to prevent back pain in asymptomatic individuals. As compared with educational strategies, mechanical supports, and risk factor modification, exercises that strengthen back and abdominal muscles are the intervention associated with decreased frequency and duration of low back pain.[29]

19-3 INDICATIONS FOR EXTENSION EXERCISES

Pain relief on:
 Lying
 Walking
  and with:
 Repeated backward bending
 Decreased lumbar lordosis
Pain exacerbation on:
 Sitting
 Driving
 Arising from chair
 Stooping
 Bending
  and with:
 Forward bending
 Repeated forward bending

In summary, the positive benefit of exercise in the treatment of low back pain may depend on the duration of the pain, the host, the job setting, and the form of exercise.[55]

Exercises for Inflammatory Arthropathies

Patients with nonmechanical back pain may also benefit from physical therapy and exercises. Patients with a spondyloarthropathy need to be involved in a regular home exercise program that includes chest expansion, range of motion, and strengthening exercises for the lumbosacral and cervical spine. Once again, the exercise program must be individualized, and this is best achieved under the direction of a physical therapist who communicates with both the patient and the physician.

Our Recommendation

Exercises are recommended as a component of therapy after the initial stages of recovery from an acute back pain episode. Physical therapy is recommended to improve function in those individuals who have become deconditioned or immobilized from chronic pain.

References

Physical Therapy and Exercises—Lumbar Spine

1. Addison R, Schultz A: Trunk strengths in patients seeking hospitalization for chronic low back disorders. Spine 5:539-544, 1980.
2. Alston W, Carlson KE, Feldman DJ, et al: A quantitative study of muscle fatigue in the chronic low back syndrome. Ann Surg 80:762, 1950.
3. Andersson GBJ, Ortengren R, Nachemson AL: Intradiscal pressure, intra-abdominal pressure and myoelectric back muscle activity related to posture and loading. Clin Orthop 129:156-164, 1977.
4. Balogun JA, Olokungbemi AA, Kuforji AR: Spinal mobility and muscular strength: Effects of supine- and prone-lying back extension exercise training. Arch Phys Med Rehabil 73:745-751, 1992.
5. Beckson M, Schultz A, Nachemson AL, Andersson GBJ: Voluntary strengths of adults with acute low back syndrome. Clin Orthop 129:84-95, 1977.
6. Beimborn DS, Morrissey MC: A review of the literature related to trunk muscle performance. Spine 13:655-660, 1988.
7. Browman CP: Sleep following sustained exercise. Psychophysiology 17:577-580, 1980.
8. Cady LD, Bischoff DP, O'Connell ER, et al: Strength and fitness and subsequent back injuries in firefighters. J Occup Med 21:269-272, 1979.
9. Collingwood TR: The effects of physical training upon behavior and self attitude. J Clin Psychol 28:583-585, 1972.
10. Davies G, Gould J: Trunk testing using a prototype Cybex II isokinetic dynamometer stabilization system. J Orthop Sports Phys Ther 3:164, 1982.
11. Davies JE, Gibson R, Tester L: The value of exercises in the treatment of low back pain. Rheumatol Rehabil 18:243-247, 1979.
12. De Vries H: EMG fatigue nerve in postural muscles: A possible etiology for idiopathic low back pain. Am J Phys Med 47:175, 1968.
13. Elnaggar IM, Nordin M, Sheikhszadeh A, et al: Effects of spinal flexion and extension exercises on low-back pain and spinal mobility in chronic mechanical low-back pain patients. Spine 16:967-972, 1991.
14. Faas A, Chavannes AW, van Eijk JTHM, et al: A randomized, placebo-controlled trial of exercise therapy in patients with acute low back pain. Spine 18:1388-1395, 1993.
15. Farfan HF: The biomechanical advantage of lordosis and hip extension for upright activity. Spine 3:336-342, 1978.

16. Farfan HF, Cassette JW, Robertson GH, et al: The effect of torsion in the production of disc degeneration. J Bone Joint Surg Am 52A:468-497, 1970.
17. Flint MM: Lumbar posture: A study of roentgenographic measurement and the influence of flexibility and strength. Res Q 34:15, 1963.
18. Floyd WF, Silver PHS: The function of the erector spinae muscles in certain movements and postures in man. J Physiol 129:184, 1955.
19. Fox MG: The relationship of abdominal strength to selected postural faults. Res Q 22:141, 1951.
20. Fraioli F, Moretti C, Paolucci D, et al: Physical exercise stimulates marked concomitant release of beta-endorphin and adrenocorticotropic hormone (ACTH) in peripheral blood in man. Experientia 36:987-989, 1980.
21. Hadler NM: Diagnosis and Treatment of Backache. In Hadler NM: Medical Management of the Regional Musculoskeletal Diseases. Orlando, FL, Grune & Stratton, 1984, pp 3-52.
22. Halpern A, Bleck EE: Sit-up exercises: An EMG study. Clin Orthop 145:172-178, 1979.
23. Hirsch C: Studies on the pathology of low back pain. J Bone Joint Surg Br 41B:237, 1959.
24. Jackson CP, Brown MD: Analysis of current approaches and a practical guide to prescription of exercise. Clin Orthop 179:46-54, 1983.
25. Jackson CP, Brown MD: Is there a role for exercise in the treatment of patients with low back pain? Clin Orthop 179:39-45, 1983.
26. Kendall PH, Jenkins JS: Exercise for backache: A double-blind controlled trial. Physiotherapy 54:154, 1968.
27. Kendall PH, Jenkins JM: Lumbar isometric flexion exercises. Physiotherapy 54:158, 1968.
28. Kramer J: Pressure dependent fluid shifts in the intervertebral disc. Orthop Clin North Am 8:211-216, 1977.
29. Lahad A, Malter AD, Berg AO, et al: The effectiveness of four interventions for the prevention of low back pain. JAMA 272:1286-1291, 1994.
30. Lidstrom A, Zachrisson M: Physical therapy on low back pain and sciatica: An attempt at evaluation. Scand J Rehabil Med 2:37, 1970.
31. Liemohn W: Exercises and the back. Rheum Dis Clin North Am 16:945-970, 1990.
32. Ljunggren AE, Weber H, Kogstad O, et al: Effect of exercise on sick leave due to low back pain: A randomized, comparative long-term study. Spine 22:1610-1617, 1997.
33. Magora A: Investigation of the relation between low back pain and occupation: VI. Medical history and symptoms. Scand J Rehabil Med 6:81-88, 1974.
34. Manniche C, Hesselsoe G, Bentzen L, et al: Clinical trial of intense muscle training for chronic low back pain. Lancet II:1473-1476, 1988.
35. Mannion AF, Muntener M, Taimela S, et al: 1999 Volvo award winner in clinical studies: A randomized clinical trial of three active therapies for chronic low back pain. Spine 24:2435-2448, 1999.
36. Mayer TG, Gatchel RJ, Mayer H, et al: A prospective two-year functional restoration in industrial low back pain injury. JAMA 258:1763-1767, 1987.
37. McKenzie RA: The Lumbar Spine: Mechanical Diagnosis and Therapy. Waikanae, New Zealand: Spinal Publications, 1981.
38. McNeill T, Warwick D, Andersson GBJ, Schultz A: Trunk strengths in attempted flexion, extension and lateral bending in healthy subjects and patients with low back disorders. Spine 6: 529-238, 1980.
39. Mitchell RI, Carmen GM: Results of a multicenter trial using an intensive active exercise program for the treatment of acute soft tissue and back injuries. Spine 15:514-521, 1990.
40. Morgan WP, Hortsman DH: Anxiety reduction following acute physical activity. Arch Phys Med 52:422-425, 1971.
41. Morris JM, Benner G, Lucas BD: An EMG study of the intrinsic muscles of the back in man. J Anat 96:509, 1962.
42. Nachemson AL: The load on lumbar disc in different positions of the body. Clin Orthop 45:107-122, 1966.
43. Nachemson AL: The possible importance of the psoas muscle for stabilization of the lumbar spine. Acta Orthop Scand 39:47-57, 1968.
44. Nachemson AL, Lindh M: Measurement of abdominal and back muscle strength with and without low back pain. Scand J Rehabil Med 1:60-63, 1969.
45. Parnianpour M, Nordin MA, Kahanovitz N, Frankel V: The triaxial coupling of torque generation of trunk muscles during isometric exertions and the effect of fatiguing isoinertial movement on the motor output and movement. Spine 13:982-992, 1988.
46. Partridge M: Participation of the abdominal muscles in various movements of the trunk in man: An EMG study. Phys Ther Rev 39:791, 1959.
47. Pauley J: EMG analysis of certain movements and exercise: Some deep muscles of the back. Anat Rec 155:223, 1966.
48. Pedersen OF, Peterson R, Staffeldt ES: Back pain and isometric back muscle strength of workers in a Danish factory. Scand J Rehabil Med 7:125, 1975.
49. Pollock ML, Leggett SH, Graves JE, et al: Effect of resistance training on lumbar extension strength. Am J Sports Med 17:624-629, 1989.
50. Ponte DJ, Jensen GJ, Kent BE: A preliminary report on the use of the McKenzie protocol versus Williams protocol in the treatment of low back pain. J Orthop Sports Phys Ther 6:130, 1984.
51. Poulsen E: Back muscle strength and weight limits in lifting. Spine 6:73-75, 1981.
52. Schmidt GL, Amundson LR, Dostal WF: Muscle strength at the trunk. J Orthop Sports Phys Ther 1:665, 1980.
53. Schultz A, Andersson GBJ: Analysis of loads on the lumbar spine. Spine 6:76-82, 1981.
54. Sikorski JM: A rationalized approach to physiotherapy for low-back pain. Spine 10:571-579, 1985.
55. Van Tulder M, Malmivarra A, Esmail R, et al: Exercise therapy for low back pain: A systematic review within the framework of the Cochrane Collaboration Back Review Group. Spine 25:2784-2796, 2000.
56. Williams PC: Lesions of the lumbosacral spine: I. J Bone Joint Surg 19:343, 1937.
57. Williams PC: Lesions of the lumbosacral spine: II. J Bone Joint Surg 19:690, 1937.

PHYSICAL THERAPY AND EXERCISES —CERVICAL SPINE

Physical therapy together with personal exercise regimens are recommended to many patients with neck pain. Similar to the scenario for low back pain, patients with neck pain received a sheet of neck exercises without much instruction. The course of events and therapeutic results of these exercises, given to patients without physicians' instructions, were the following: some had improvement; some had exacerbation of symptoms; some would follow the instructions incorrectly; and some would not do the exercises at all. The wide range of effects would usually have the physicians skeptical of the benefit of this component of treatment. One size does not fit all patients with neck pain. The onset and type of exercise prescribed can have a marked effect on the potential benefit of the intervention.

Cervical Spine Exercise Programs

Exercise Regimens

Therapeutic exercise may be defined as structural and controlled body movement to correct an impairment, improve musculoskeletal function, or maintain a state of well-being. Exercises can increase muscle strength, elasticity, range of motion, and endurance. A prescription for physical therapy must have a specified objective. The program of exercises may be modified as a patient's condition is altered. Therapeutic programs may include passive, active-assisted, active, or active-resistive exercises. Passive exercise is produced entirely by an external force without any voluntary contraction of muscles by the patient. These exercises maintain range of motion and elasticity of soft tissue. Active-assisted exercises require muscular contraction to move a part of the body without an external force. These exercises maintain flexibility and decrease potential for muscle atrophy. Isometric, isotonic, and isokinetic exercises are classified as active-resistive. Isometric contraction is associated with increased muscle tension without change in muscle length. Strength is increased only at the length of muscle contraction. Different lengths of contraction are needed to increase generalized muscle strength. Isotonic exercise decreases fiber length without a change in muscle tension. Strengthening occurs through maximal effort of motion. Isokinetic exercises move body parts through ranges of motion at a constant speed. This kind of therapy is given through the use of a Cybex machine.

Exercise Goals

The purpose of physical therapy and exercises is to relieve pain and to regain normal movement of the cervical spine.[8] The choice of therapy must correspond to the phase of the neck injury. During the initial stage, pain may be too severe to allow for increased movement. Patients may wear a soft collar to decrease pain. As the initial pain decreases, the collar is removed and range of motion exercises are completed while the patient is supine, with the neck supported by a pillow (Fig.19-18). Range of motion exercises performed by the patient are encouraged to decrease the possibility of cervical contractures. Stretching exercises are performed by a therapist on a patient. As the patient improves with more tolerable neck pain, the cervical spine is exercised to the limits of mobility and pain. The spine is then returned to the neutral position. With improvement, additional pressure may be applied to the occiput to increase neck movement. Isometric exercises are accomplished by applying external force that prevents movement of the neck, thereby limiting pain (Fig.19-19). These exercises maintain the strength of agonist-antagonist muscles; they are essential to counteract the atrophy associated with the use of cervical collars. These exercises may be used while patients remain in cervical orthoses.[7] Isokinetic and isotonic exercises are not as helpful for the cervical spine as for other portions of the axial skeleton. In the final stages of improvement, the seated patient starts postural exercises with maximum range of motion (Fig. 19-20).

Exercises are continued as pain decreases and motion improves. Exercises should be discontinued if severity or radiation of pain increases in a manner other than the expected discomfort or stiffness associated with normal exercise. One new exercise should be added per day to better assess the effect of the intervention on the damaged structures. In the early stages of an exercise program, the sessions should be limited to 5 minutes. Patients who are overly aggressive with exercise should be cautioned to limit duration of exercise sessions so that pain is not increased. Postural exercises should be performed five to six times per day for 1 month or until posture is improved. Subsequently, postural and prevention exercises should be done twice per day to maintain improvement (Fig. 19-21).

General aerobic exercises, such as cycling, walking, and swimming, should be encouraged to limit general deconditioning. However, limits should be placed on activities involving continuous extension or persistent rotation of the neck. A snorkel may decrease neck movement associated with swimming. Exercises should begin as soon as severe pain decreases.

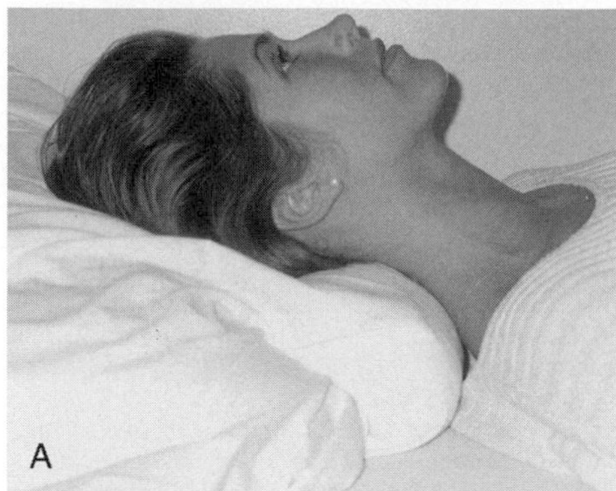

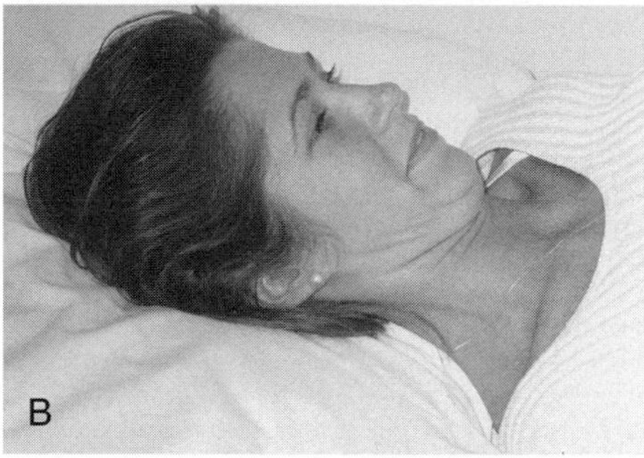

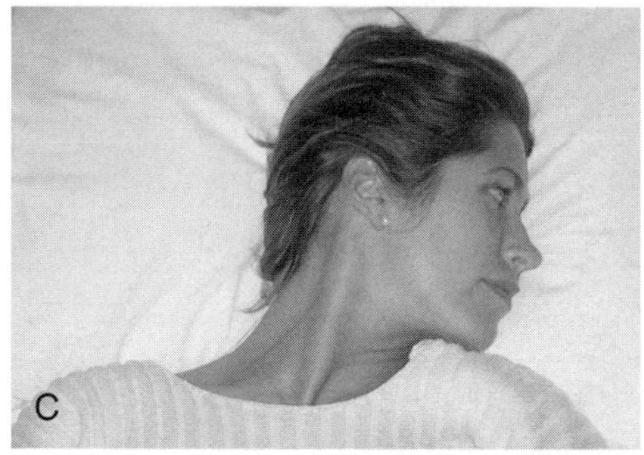

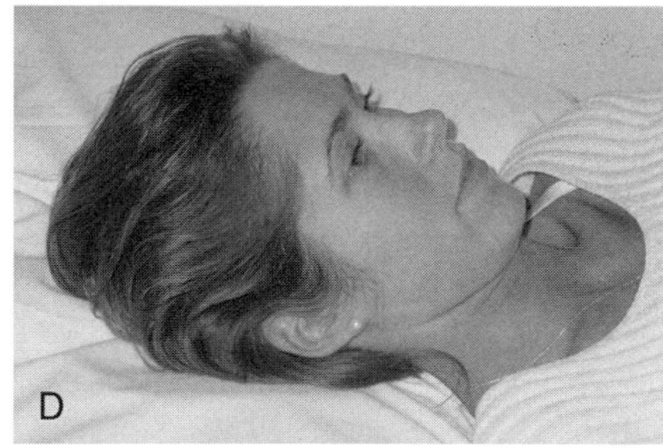

Figure 19-18 Therapeutic exercises, stage 1. *A*, Begin in a supine position with a pillow. *B*, Tuck the chin downward toward the collar bone and at the same time force the back of the head into contact with the pillow. Perform slowly and do not hold the contraction. Perform 10 times, 3 times per day. *C*, Lie on back with small flat pillow under the head. Tuck chin downward and gently rotate head and neck to the left and return to original position. Perform 5 times. Perform same procedure to opposite side 5 times. To prevent added pain, do not overturn. Perform 3 times per day. *D*, Lie on back with or without a pillow. Take a deep breath with upper chest and keep shoulders back. Slowly inhale through the nose and exhale through the mouth. Perform 10 times, 3 times per day. *(Courtesy of Tom Welsh, RPT.)*

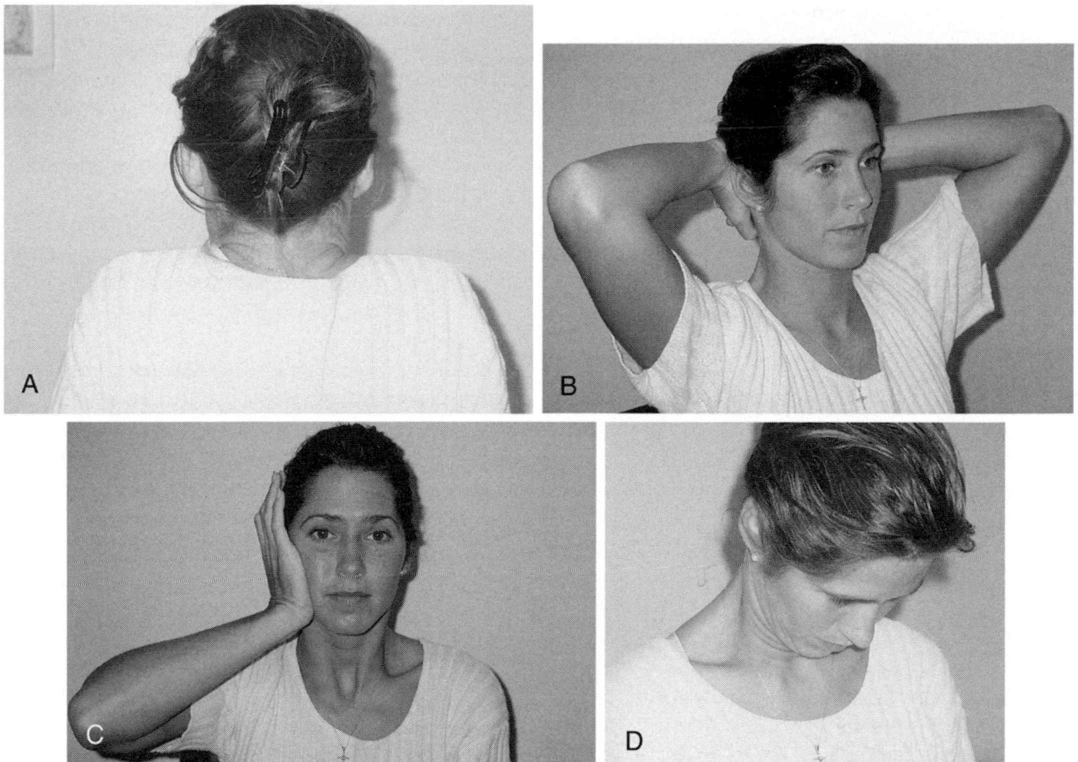

Figure 19-19 Therapeutic exercises, stage 2. *A*, In a seated position with the head in good posture, perform shoulder shrugs by raising shoulders up toward ears. Hold for a count of 3 and rest. Perform 10 times. Repeat hourly. Isometric exercises for sitting or standing position for anterior, posterior, and lateral neck muscles (do not be overaggressive). Perform 3 times per day. *B*, Place both hands behind the head on occiput and apply equal force to backward motion of the head and neck. Hold for a count of 5 and relax for a count of 3. Perform 5 times. *C*, Place the right hand against right side of face and apply equal forces of pressure from hands against lateral bending with rotation of the head and neck. Hold for a count of 5 and relax for a count of 3. Perform 5 times. Perform same procedure on the left side and on the forehead (not shown). *D*, In a seated position, bend the head and neck toward chest without forcing the movement if there is pain. If there is no pain or stiffness, apply overpressure with hands at end of movement. Perform 10 times hourly. *(Courtesy of Tom Welsh, RPT.)*

Exercise Prescription

Just as there is no single therapy for all causes of neck pain, there is no one physical therapy program for all patients with cervical spine disease. Some patients benefit from range of motion exercises, some from stretching, some from isometrics, and some do not improve at all from exercises. Listening carefully to the patient's symptoms and observing the movements that cause pain help the physician decide which physical therapy program has the greatest chance for success in an individual patient. To increase patient compliance, neck exercises should be simple and easily accomplished. Patients should be supervised to ensure achievement of maximum improvement. Exercise programs should be explained with visual aids, including the number of repetitions, duration, time of exercise, and sequence of progression.[2] No therapy program is

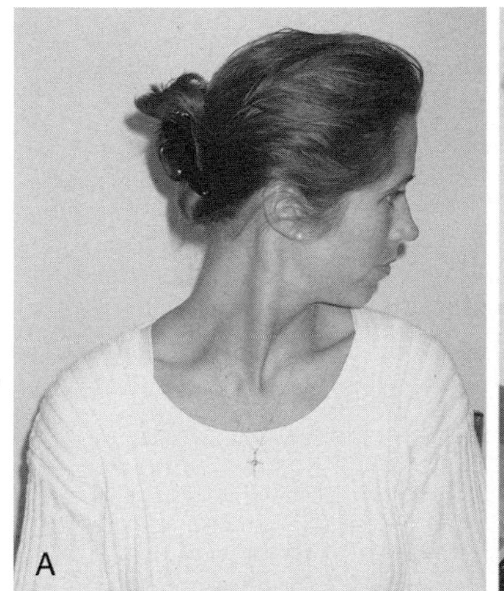

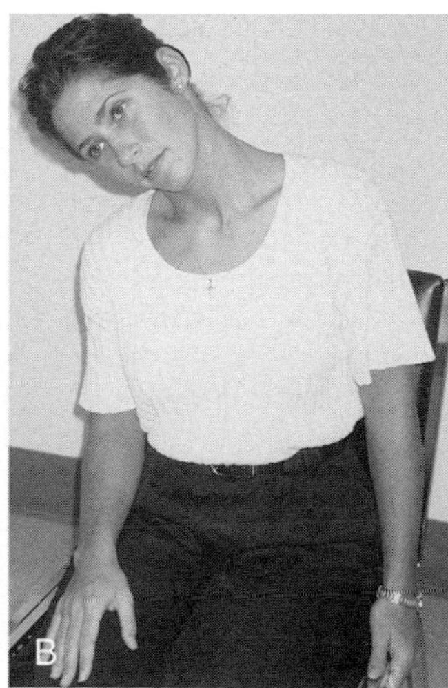

Figure 19-20 Therapeutic exercises, stage 3 (discontinue stage 1 exercises, continue stage 2, and add one exercise daily as tolerated). Lie on back with flat pillow under the neck, raise head off pillow, and bring chin to chest (not shown). Try 1 time and assess pain. Perform 5 times if tolerable. If there is no pain the next day, add one repetition until 10 raises can be performed comfortably. Perform 3 times per day. *A*, In a seated position, keep chin in and rotate head to look over the left shoulder within pain tolerance, hold for a count of 3, and return to center. Perform same procedure to right side. Perform 10 times hourly. *B*, In seated position, keep chin in and bend head and neck laterally so that right ear moves toward right shoulder. Do not raise shoulder. If there is stiffness and no pain, gentle overpressure may be applied with right hand. Perform same procedure to left side. Perform 10 times hourly. *(Courtesy of Tom Welsh, RPT.)*

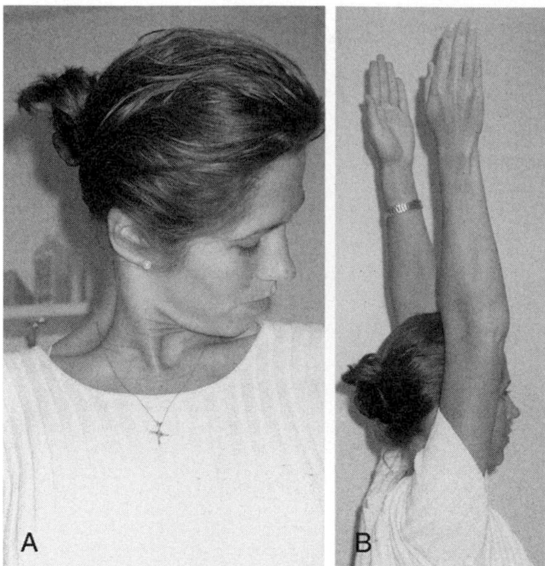

Figure 19-21 Therapeutic exercises, stage 4. A, In a seated position, tuck chin in and rotate head and neck toward the right shoulder. Bend neck laterally so that right ear moves toward chest. Apply overpressure with right hand if comfortable. Hold for a count of 3 and relax for a count of 3. Perform 5 times. Perform same procedure for left side. B, In a standing or seated position, raise arms straight toward ceiling. Do not look up. Hold arms up for a count of 3. Perform 10 times. In a standing or seated position, tuck chin in and hold head and neck in good alignment. Bend elbows and raise both arms out to the side so that they are parallel to the ground. Rapidly, move arms backward with elbows moving toward each other behind back. Perform these movements for 10 seconds (not shown). In a standing position with back to wall, tuck chin in and try to flatten the back of the neck against the wall. Hold for a count of 3 (not shown). *(Courtesy of Tom Welsh, RPT.)*

unchanging. Communication between the patient, therapist, and physician is essential in optimizing an exercise program. As patients improve, increasingly stressful tasks may be added to the program in an attempt to increase endurance and strength in preparation for return to work. If symptoms increase, exercises may be discontinued or reduced and reinitiated once the patient's symptoms return to baseline. Conforming exercise programs to patient symptoms results in greater patient compliance and possibilities of improved outcome.

Exercises for Inflammatory Arthropathies

Patients with nonmechanical neck pain may also benefit from physical therapy and exercises. Patients with a spondyloarthropathy need a regular exercise program they can do at home. Therapy may include chest expansion, range of motion, and strengthening exercises for the lumbosacral and cervical spine. The program must be individualized for each patient. This is best achieved under the direction of a physical therapist who communicates with the patient and the physician.

Ergonomics

Ergonomics is a discipline that integrates psychology, physiology, physics, medicine, and engineering to address problems regarding the preservation of health and efficiency at work, in daily living, and in recreation.[1] Ergonomics is concerned with the match between machine, task operations, and work environment and human capacities and limitations. Individuals who are interested in ergonomics include industrial engineers, occupational safety officers, and physical therapists.

Workers may experience fatigue, muscle tension, and postural discomfort even with effective workstation design. An ergonomics team may be able to design modifications of the task to match physical capabilities to limit fatigue and strain.

Occupations that require coordination of visual and hand tasks along with a great amount of concentration or stress often result in postural pain problems involving the neck, shoulders, and upper and lower back. Fatigue may continue, resulting in a stressful work environment. Improvement of the work environment may avoid worker injury.

The worker needs to be observed in both dynamic and static tasks. During the dynamic muscular activity, the muscles contract and relax rhythmically. Walking, climbing stairs, and loading boxes are examples of dynamic activity. Static muscle activity supports a weight without movement but with a steady consumption of energy. Examples of static activities include neck posture in front of a computer screen, lateral neck flexion to hold a telephone, or neck posture in painting a ceiling. Some tasks have components of both activities.

Of the two activities, static activity results in overfatigue and muscle strain. Decreased blood flow to muscle and soft tissue during tonic contractions may result in relative anoxia and pain. Dynamic tasks are fatiguing only after duration of many hours. Dynamic tasks allow for persistent blood flow to exercising tissues. A brief set of dynamic exercises at the workstation may help the individual with static tasks to increase muscular blood flow and decrease neck pain. These exercises may include deep breathing, shrugging shoulders, moving lower extremities, flattening the lumbar spine, flexion of the lumbar spine, and straightening the cervical spine.[5,7]

Improvement of posture, workstation (through engineering), and body mechanics may decrease the risk for worker injury (Fig. 19-22).

Good posture is achieved by balancing the head and spine over the center of gravity. Poor posture is fatiguing and may result in instability, falls, and related accidents. The proper position of the head and neck is an angle of 20 to 30 degrees of flexion. Tilting the head backward should be avoided. A range of eye movement within 15 degrees above and below the normal line of sight is most comfortable.[1] The visibility distance between the eye and object should be 1 ft. Continuous deviations from this range may result in neck muscle fatigue and pain. Sitting posture is also important in maintaining static positions that are painless. Knees should be slightly higher than the hips, arm rests and chair back should support arms and spine, and reclined postures are acceptable with adequate support of the head (Table 19-4). Work should be at the same height as the elbows.[3]

Engineering of workstations is important in limiting worker fatigue and pain. Placement of machines in awkward places may increase stress on the worker's musculoskeletal system. Evaluation of the components and order of a task may suggest more appropriate placement of machines. Neck stress and upper back pain may develop if the head is held too far forward or backward with sedentary activities. The appropriate placement of visual display terminals may limit the stress on the cervical spine by taking into account the capabilities and limitations of the worker. The head should also not be rotated or bent for any extended period. The work surface should be easily accessible.

A functional capacity evaluation measures the physical capacities of individuals. The evaluation measures strength, maximum effort, ranges of motion, walking pace, squatting ability, and posture.[4] The requirements of job tasks should be assessed. Abilities and preferences of the worker are compared with job demands and modifications made to diminish the risk of re-injury to the worker.

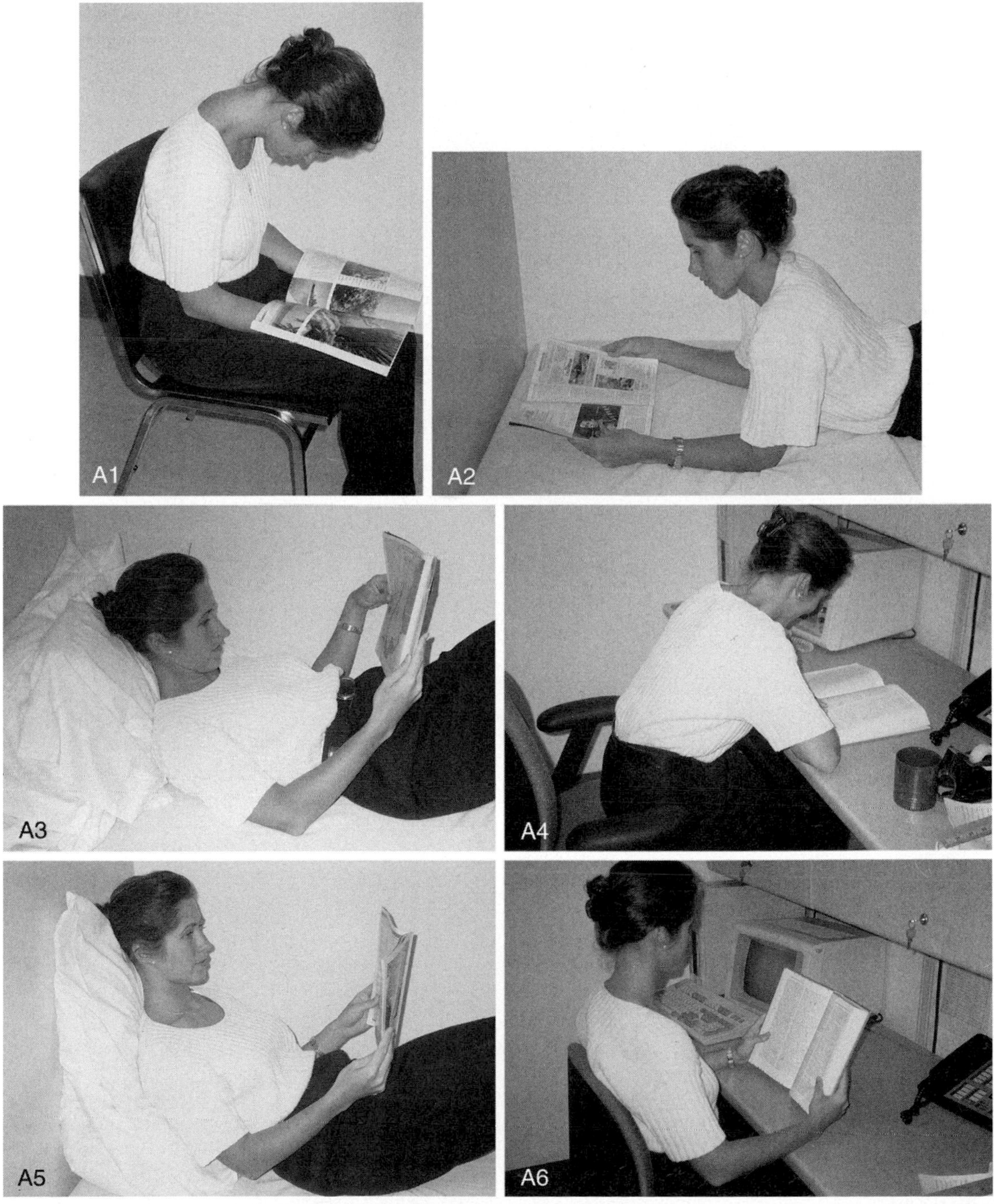

Figure 19-22 Postures for preventing neck pain. **Reading positions**. Incorrect: *A(1)*, Avoid reading position that encourages prolonged forward head posture. *A(2)*, Avoid prolonged extension of the neck. *A(3)*, Avoid pillows under head only. This position promotes stretch in the posterior neck structures. *A(4)*, Avoid excessive flexion of the neck. Correct: *A(5)*, Reading in bed, pillows should support the back, shoulders, and neck. *A(6)*, Reading material should be at appropriate level to maintain normal cervical lordosis.

Continued

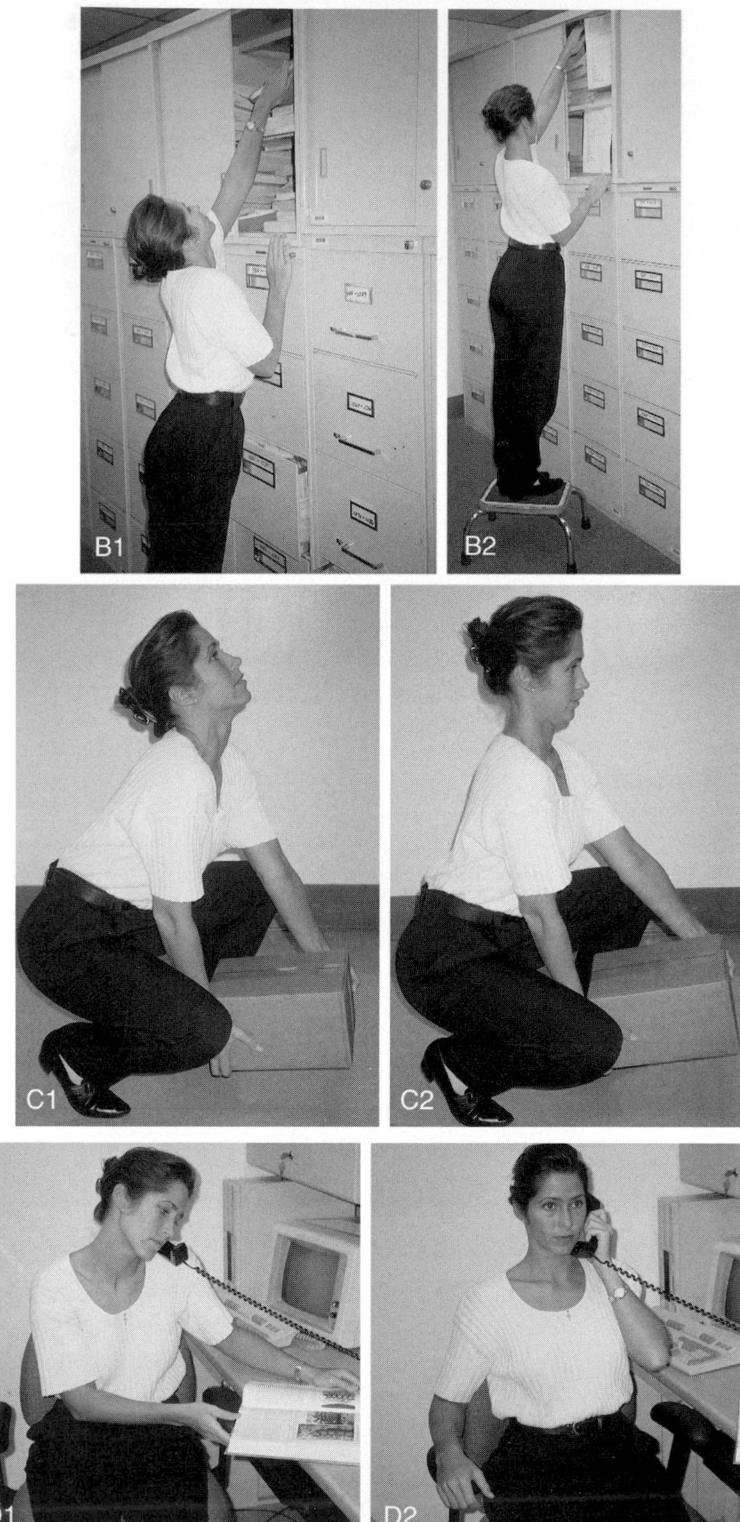

Figure 19-22, cont'd **Overhead work**. Incorrect: *B(1)*, Avoid continuously reaching overhead and extending neck to look up. Correct: *B(2)*, Use a stool to keep objects to be reached at chest level. **Stooping and lifting**. Incorrect: *C(1)*, Avoid extending and lifting quickly. Correct: *C(2)*, Keep chin down and neck muscles fixed. Lift with legs and shoulders. **Telephone use**. Incorrect: *D(1)*, Avoid cradling the phone between shoulder and ear. Use a receiver cradle to maintain appropriate neck position. Correct: *D(2)*, Head should be maintained in midline position. Use headset if both hands are required for desk tasks.

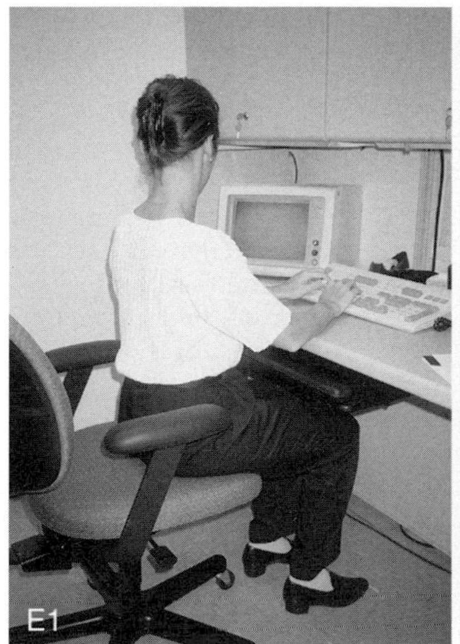

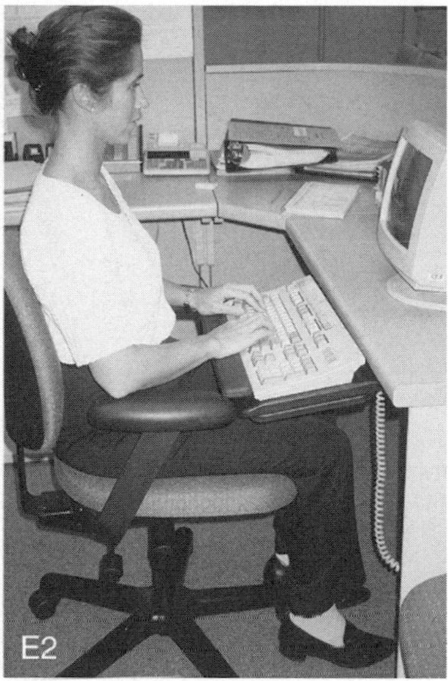

Figure 19-22, cont'd **Computer use**. Incorrect: *E(1)*, Avoid unsupported back and rotation of the neck. Correct: *E(2)*, Low back is supported with head erect with elbows resting comfortably at sides. *(Courtesy of Tom Welsh, RPT.)*

Neck School

Patient education in a variety of forms may be helpful in informing individuals of their physical capabilities and limitations. Neck school is patterned after the back school concept.[7] Patients receive information on the anatomy and biomechanics of the cervical spine. A group discussion allows presentation of practical techniques for relaxation, exercises, and activities of daily living. Neck school may inform patients but may be too general to help individuals prevent neck pain in the workplace.[7] Cervicothoracic stabilization training is another method of strengthening the cervical spine to improve stability and flexibility and to decrease neck pain.[6]

19-4 SELECTION OF ERGONOMICALLY APPROPRIATE CHAIR

1. Back and seat components should be contoured for maximum comfortable support.
2. The chair should have a flexible tilt for better support and variety of movement.
3. Seat and back components should be independently adjustable. The angle between the seat and back should be greater than 90 degrees. The height of support for the thighs should also be greater than 90 degrees.
4. Upholstery of the chair should consist of a porous, rough-textured material to dissipate heat, facilitate circulation, and reduce static pressure.
5. A high back rest is preferable for office work to support the trunk and should be concave to support the head.
6. The back rest should be angled at 10 to 15 degrees from vertical.
7. An adjustable seat height allows the appropriate placement of the feet on the floor and elbows on the arm rests to allow for correct tension in the cervical musculature. Adequate support of the feet and arms allows for the correct position of the cervical spine to decrease fatigue.
8. Adjustable seat depth allows for correct thigh support and avoidance of pressure on the lower leg.
9. Seat width should allow for movement.
10. A five-spur, swivel pedestal chair with casters allows for stability and mobility.

Modified from Abdel-Moty E, Khalil TM, Rosomoff RS, et al: Ergonomic considerations and interventions. In Tollison CD, Satterthwaite JR (eds): Painful Cervical Trauma: Diagnosis and Rehabilitative Treatment of Neuromusculoskeletal Injuries. Baltimore, Williams & Wilkins, 1992, pp 214-229.

Our Recommendation

Exercises are recommended as a component of therapy after the initial stages of recovery from an acute neck pain episode. Physical therapy is recommended to improve function in those individuals who have become deconditioned or immobilized from their pain.

References

Physical Therapy and Exercises—Cervical Spine

1. Abdel-Moty E, Khalil TM, Rosomoff RS, et al: Ergonomic considerations and interventions. In Tollison CD, Satterthwaite JR (eds): Painful Cervical Trauma: Diagnosis and Rehabilitative Treatment of Neuromusculoskeletal Injuries. Baltimore, Williams & Wilkins, 1992, pp 214-229.
2. Glossop ES, Goldenberg E, Smith DS, et al: Patient compliance in back and neck pain. Physiotherapy 68:225, 1982.
3. Grandjean E: Fitting the Task to the Man: A Textbook of Occupational Ergonomics, 4th ed. London: Taylor & Francis, 1988.
4. Khalil TM, Goldberg ML, Asfour SS, et al: Acceptable maximum effort (AME): A psychophysical measure of strength in back pain patients. Spine 12:372, 1987.
5. Sundelin G, Hagberg M: The effects of different pause types on neck and shoulder EMG activity during VDU work. Ergonomics 32:527, 1989.

6. Sweeney T: Neck school: Cervicothoracic stabilization training. Occup Med 7:43, 1992.
7. Tan JC, Nordin M: Role of physical therapy in the treatment of cervical disk disease. Orthop Clin North Am 23:435, 1992.
8. Welsh TM: Physical therapy, ergonomics, and rehabilitation. In Wiesel SW, Boden SD, Borenstein DG, Feffer HL (eds): Neck Pain, 2nd ed. Charlottesville, VA, The Michie Co, 1992, pp 377-453.

INJECTION THERAPY

Local and regional analgesia, either applied topically or injected locally or regionally, is part of the therapeutic regimen for patients with low back or neck pain. The basic premise on which this therapy is based is that nociceptive input can be interrupted at its source by blocking the function of nociceptive sensory fibers in the peripheral nerve supplying the "injured" area as well as by interrupting the afferent limb of abnormal reflexes that increase muscle tension, which also contributes to pain. Depending on the type of agent used (topical cooling spray vs. short-acting analgesic vs. corticosteroid), the concentration of the medicine, and the site of application, the peripheral and central nervous systems can be affected in a number of ways. For example, low concentrations of local anesthetics can block the unmyelinated C and B fibers and small myelinated A-delta fibers without affecting A-alpha or motor fibers. If motor function must be blocked to decrease muscle spasm, this effect can be obtained through the use of an appropriate anesthetic at an increased concentration.

Bonica has suggested that blocks not only are therapeutic but also have diagnostic and prognostic indications (Table 19-5).[7] One must be careful in ascribing too much diagnostic importance to a response to an injection. The clinician should not confuse a response to an anesthetic with a definite diagnosis of the cause of spinal pain. Certainly, a response to an injection with relief of pain suggests that the area treated has been the source of nociceptive input, but referred pain may improve from an injection as well. The physician must continue to observe the patient who receives a therapeutic injection. An initial beneficial response may wane if a more sinister problem than local muscle strain is the cause of the pain.

19-5 INDICATIONS FOR NERVE BLOCKS WITH LOCAL ANESTHETICS

DIAGNOSTIC BLOCKS
Aid in the identification of the site(s) and cause(s) of pain.
Identify nociceptive pathways (specific peripheral nerve).
Determine mechanism of chronic pain syndromes.
Determine patient's reaction to pain relief.

PROGNOSTIC BLOCKS
Determine potential response to permanent blocks or neurosurgery.
Allow patients to experience the sensation and side effects of permanent procedures on a temporary basis (decision concerning surgery).

THERAPEUTIC BLOCKS
Relieve acute postoperative pain and pain from self-limited diseases.
Prolong pain relief by breaking reflex mechanisms.
Provide temporary relief to allow the onset of action of other therapies with delayed effects.

Modified from Bonica JJ: Local anesthesia and regional block. In Wall PD, Melzack R. (eds): Textbook of Pain. Edinburgh, Churchill Livingstone, 1984, p 541.

Soft Tissue Injections

A variety of topical and injectable anesthetics are available for use in patients with acute and chronic pain. All have advantages and disadvantages in specific circumstances. A brief review of their characteristics will help the clinician decide which agent is most appropriate for a given patient.

Mechanism of Action

The local anesthetics produce their effects by blocking the depolarization of nerves inhibiting the flux of sodium ions across membranes. The local anesthetic blocks the mouth of the sodium channel and does this to a greater degree in nerves that are actively conducting impulses than in nerves that are inactive.[20] The sensitivity of nerves to local anesthetics relates to fiber size and myelination. Fibers that are thicker and myelinated transmit nerve impulses faster and are more resistant to local blockade than thin, unmyelinated fibers. The minimum amount of anesthetic that blocks impulse transmission (Cm) varies for each nerve and each agent. The Cm of A-alpha fibers (motor—greatest velocity) is approximately twice that of A-delta fibers (pain and temperature). B fibers (preganglionic autonomic nervous system) are the most sensitive of all fibers despite their thin myelination and have a Cm about one third that of unmyelinated C fibers (pain).[20] Agents also have different onsets of action correlated with diffusion capacity. Agents with greater lipophilic action (increased binding to tissue) have a slower onset of action. The characteristics of the most common local anesthetics are listed in Table 19-6.

Toxicities

Side effects of local anesthetic agents are uncommon but potentially serious. Systemic reactions occur when these agents are injected directly into the bloodstream. Locally injected anesthetics slowly diffuse into the bloodstream over time. Hypersensitive patients may develop systemic allergic reactions to locally injected medications. The neurologic toxicities range from slight dizziness to grand mal seizures, which occur when high concentrations of anesthetic reach the central nervous system. This complication can be prevented by using low doses of anesthetic, aspirating the area before injection, and injecting at a slow rate. Other toxicities include hypersensitivity reactions and cardiac toxicity in the form of conduction delays.[21,45] Repeated injections of anesthetic into the same location may cause local irritation and muscle spasm.

Neurolytic Agents

Some patients with chronic pain obtain only short-term relief with short-acting anesthetics. These patients may benefit from injection with neurolytic agents, which destroy nerve fibers and produce prolonged, or sometimes permanent, nerve blockade. This procedure is reserved for patients with intractable pain who are not candidates for

19-6 CLINICAL CHARACTERISTICS AND DOSAGE OF LOCAL ANESTHETICS

	Procaine (Novocain)	**2-Chlorprocaine (Nesacaine)**	**Lidocaine (Xylocaine)**	**Mepivacaine (Carbocaine)**	**Prilocaine (Citanest)**	**Tetracaine (Pontocaine)**	**Bupivacaine (Marcaine)**	**Etidocaine (Duranest)**
Onset of action	Moderate	Fast	Fast	Moderate	Moderate	Very slow	Fast	Very fast
Dispersion	Moderate	Marked	Marked	Moderate	Moderate	Poor	Moderate	Moderate
Duration of action	Short	Very short	Moderate	Moderate	Moderate	Long	Long	Long
Optimal concentration (%)								
Local	0.5	0.5	0.25	0.25	0.25	0.05	0.05	0.1
Spinal nerve	1.5-2.0	1.0-2.0	0.5-1.0	0.5-1.0	0.5-1.0	0.1-0.2	0.25-0.5	0.5-1.0
Maximum safe dose (mg/kg)	12	15	6	6	6	2	2	2

Modified from Bonica JJ: Local anesthesia and regional block. In Wall PD, Melzack R (eds): Textbook of Pain. Edinburgh, Churchill Livingstone, 1984, p 541.

peripheral nerve section. The agents injected include 12% phenol in Renografin, 50% alcohol, 10% ammonium sulfate, and hypertonic saline.[36,80] These agents may act on C pain fibers only or on the entire peripheral nerve. The choice of agent and its concentration will have variable effects on the degree of destruction of the peripheral nerve. These drugs are administered by an anesthesiologist.

Techniques of Injection

Identification of those patients who would benefit from injection is essential for a successful outcome. Patients who describe localized areas of muscle or ligamentous tenderness are candidates for local anesthetic therapy. These patients must be reliable; that is, they must be able to limit their activities to avoid increased tissue damage in areas with blocked reflex action. If there is any doubt in our minds, we will not inject the patient.

Trigger Points

The area of tenderness may be secondary to localized trauma or strain or may be a myofascial trigger point. Travell and Simons popularized the theory of localized areas of muscle damage. The increased metabolism and decreased circulation in these areas cause accumulation of products that result in painful contracted muscles.[96] Active myofascial trigger points are those that are painful at rest, prevent full lengthening of muscles, weaken the muscle, refer pain on direct palpation, and cause a local twitch response in the muscle band containing the trigger point. Latent trigger points are those that are tender only on compression.[89]

Whether undertaken to relieve pain associated with trigger points or, as some prefer to consider, local areas of muscle trauma, the use of local anesthetics is helpful in the treatment of paraspinous muscle pain. The procedure is started by identifying the area to be treated. Two cutaneous coolants are available: ethyl chloride, which is flammable and very cold when applied, and Fluori-Methane, which is nonflammable and the preferred coolant. The spray is applied in sweeps in one direction only to match the pattern of referred pain. This procedure is used to stretch muscles that are foreshortened due to trigger points. The muscle is gradually stretched after the spray is applied.[96]

In many patients, local cooling with stretching is inadequate and injection of medication is needed to control local areas of pain. The skin must be cleansed with a suitable antiseptic and sterile technique must be utilized. Patients are questioned about any prior sensitivity to injected anesthetics. Also, the possibility of vasovagal reaction is raised. If the patients have had vagal reactions in the past, they should be premedicated with atropine or placed in a supine position to limit potential hemodynamic effects. The choice of anesthetic depends on the desired effect (see Table 19-6).

Travell and Simons advocate the use of procaine for trigger point injections because this agent has less systemic and local toxicity, in addition to its vasodilator effect.[96] Swezey and Clements have proposed the use of 2 to 5 mL of 1% lidocaine in combination with a depository form of corticosteroid.[94] Raj has used a mixture of 0.5% etidocaine and 0.375% bupivacaine for prolonged analgesia (the former for motor blockade and the latter for sensory blockade).[79] Bonica has advocated using lower concentrations of anesthetics (0.25% lidocaine, 0.05% bupivacaine) because these concentrations are effective for local injections.[7] A Japanese double-blind study confirmed better efficacy and less injection pain of a mixture of 1% lidocaine in sterile distilled water at a ratio of 1:3 compared with 1% lidocaine alone.[46,47]

The use of corticosteroids, in addition to anesthetics, is advisable for patients with soft tissue inflammation or with postinjection soreness, according to Travell and Simons.[96] Swezey and Clements have advocated the use of triamcinolone in conjunction with anesthetics.[94] Raj prefers 4 mg (1 mL) of soluble dexamethasone in 9 mL of local anesthetic. He reports no untoward effects other than a burning sensation in the area of the injection, which lasts 24 to 48 hours. We have used betamethasone sodium phosphate suspension (6 mg/mL), 1 mL per 3 to 4 mL of anesthetic solution with good success.

After allowing the antiseptic to dry, the area to be injected is wiped clean with a sterile alcohol swab and anesthetized with coolant spray. The skin is entered and injection is started only after the area has been aspirated to ensure that the tip of the needle is not in a blood vessel. Fingers are placed on the skin surface to try to localize the point of maximum tenderness. A small amount of solution is injected. If the appropriate area has been entered, the patient will experience an increase in pain before the analgesic effects of the injected solution commence. The tip of the needle is moved in a fanlike pattern to cover the entire painful area. During the injection, we test for tenderness over the injected area to be sure that the medication has been placed in the appropriate location. After removal of the needle, the patient is reminded of the potential for burning and redness over the area. Patients are instructed to call if symptoms persist or increase over the next 24 to 48 hours. It should be noted that dry needling or the injection of saline without anesthetic into trigger points also has been associated with decreased pain.[89] Some physicians believe that the benefits of these injections are related to the process of needling the area, independent of the injection of any fluid.[54]

After injection, patients may commence stretching exercises to maximize the length of contracted muscles. Additional modalities, including heat, or massage, may be utilized to maximize normal activity in the muscle, allowing adequate blood flow and return of muscle strength.

If pain continues, repeat injections may be necessary. These may be done on a weekly basis for three to four additional sessions. If the pain still continues, other therapies are indicated because repeated injections cause local irritation and muscle spasm.

Lumbar Spine Trigger Points

In the lumbar spine, trigger points are located in the iliocostalis and longissimus muscles of the multifidus. Pain from these points may radiate down toward the buttock and then down the lateral thigh in the distribution of the tensor fasciae latae. The quadratus lumborum may also cause localized back pain. Trigger points are present in the muscle body that radiate pain to the sacroiliac joint area or the lateral thigh near the greater trochanter.[83,95] Trigger points have also been described in the gluteal muscles with radiation down the leg below the knee. The injection sites that correlate with trigger areas (which also correspond to acupuncture points) include the sciatic outlet, deep in the gluteus maximus; the mid-belly of the gluteus medius between the greater trochanter and the iliac crest; and midway up the quadratus lumborum between the iliac crest and lower ribs.[63]

CLINICAL TRIALS

In regard to the efficacy of local injections, Garvey and coworkers reported the results of a double-blind, randomized study of trigger point injection therapy for localized low back pain. A total of 63 patients with muscle strain with local, nonradiating pain, normal neurologic findings, and normal lumbar spine roentgenograms were treated with an injection of lidocaine, lidocaine with corticosteroids, acupuncture (dry needling), or vapocoolant spray with acupressure after 4 weeks of no response to conservative therapy. The percentage of improvement after therapy was 40% lidocaine alone, 45% lidocaine and corticosteroids, 61% acupuncture, and 67% acupressure and vapocoolant spray. The sole measure of outcome of this study was subjective patient response to improvement, a significant shortcoming of the study. Nevertheless, the benefit of injection may be related to pressure over the painful area similar to the mechanism implicated for counterirritant therapies including acupuncture.[34]

Cummings and White reviewed 23 papers concerning trigger point injections. None of the study designs was of sufficient quality to document efficacy in the treatment of trigger point or myofascial pain.

In general, local injections are more effective for acute low back pain. Individuals with subacute or chronic low back pain are less likely to obtain a benefit from injection therapy. Randomized clinical trials documenting improvement in these patients are lacking.[68]

Cervical Spine Trigger Points

In the cervical spine, trigger points are located in the trapezius and splenius muscles. Pain from these points may radiate to the neck, head, and shoulder. The locations for injection that correlate with trigger areas, which parenthetically correspond with acupuncture points, include the upper border of the trapezius and the medial portion of the neck near its base.[96]

Botulinum Toxin Injections

Clostridium botulinum is the source of the neurotoxin. Types A and B enzymatically cleave different proteins at the cholinergic junctions at the motor endplate, inhibiting release of acetylcholine. Botulinum toxin is not thought to modify sensory nerves.[64] Botulinum toxin type A and type B are approved in the United States for the treatment of blepharospasm, strabismus, and cervical dystonia (spasmodic torticollis).[35] This toxin has also been approved for the removal of glabellar lines (wrinkles). Cervical dystonia is a sustained or intermittent, painful, involuntary neck muscle contraction. Once injected into a muscle, botulinum toxin causes focal weakness within a few days. The benefit lasts 3 months. In cervical dystonia, botulinum toxin injections help 80% of patients.[64] Dysphagia from the injection is a frequent toxicity if the incorrect dose is injected. Systemic side effects are rare.[55]

Injections of the toxin are given into the muscle exhibiting tonic contraction. The injection contain 50 to 100 units. A maximum dose of 360 units can be given 12 weeks apart.[14]

Clinical trials have demonstrated benefits for myofascial pain syndromes in the lumbar spine. Foster and colleagues reported on a randomized trial of patients with chronic low back pain who received 40 units/site at five paraspinal lumbar levels. A total of 73% of the botulinum A toxin group had more than 50% pain relief versus 25% of the saline group. Improvement was maintained at 3 and 8 weeks.[32] The benefits of botulinum toxin for unilateral myofascial neck pain have not been documented. Wheeler and colleagues reported on the response of 33 patients injected with 50 or 100 units of botulinum toxin type A or normal saline.[100] All groups demonstrated improvement.

Botulinum toxin is available in 100-unit vials. Each vial costs hundreds of dollars. Complications of these injections include dysphagia, aspiration, and generalized weakness.

Botulinum injections are being used for over 50 different disorders, including palmer hyperhidrosis, focal limb dystonia, sialorrhea, and anal fissures.[49] This therapy is not approved for the diagnosis of myofascial pain. Any patient who receives this therapy must be informed of the potential benefits and detriments of the therapy and the absence of approval by the U.S. Food and Drug Administration (FDA) for low back or neck pain.

Epidural Corticosteroid Injection

The injection of epidural corticosteroids has been tried in patients in whom conservative therapy for lumbar nerve root compression has failed. The theory supporting the use of corticosteroids in the epidural space is the increased anti-inflammatory effect on the nerve root and its surrounding connective tissue in comparison with oral corticosteroids. The injections are given for radicular pain. Very little evidence exists supporting the benefit of epidural injections for low back pain.[72]

Technique, Frequency, and Interval between Injections

The caudal approach places a needle through the sacral hiatus into the caudal canal, which is continuous with the lumbar epidural space.[90] With the causal approach, the corticosteroid is spread over the caudal canal before reaching the lumbar region. This approach may be most useful for those who have had prior lumbar spine surgery. The lumbar approach utilizes the same technique as a lumbar puncture but uses an epidural needle and advances the needle only to the level of the epidural space. The volume of the injection is 10 mL of saline mixed with 80 mg of methylprednisolone.

The number of injections in a series has been limited to three. A study reported no greater benefit with more than three injections.[10] Repeated injections were thought to increase the risk of toxicity. If one injection provides complete relief, additional injections in the series are not indicated. After the initial round of injections is completed, patients with a herniated intervertebral disc and sciatica do not usually receive a second course.

Injection Interval

The course of therapy includes three injections at variable intervals (days to weeks). The minimum interval between injections is usually 14 days. On occasion, a patient in severe pain may have an additional injection in 7 days. The interval between injections may be months in patients with spinal stenosis. The usual course of a series of injections involves a total of 240 mg of methylprednisolone administered over a 6-month period. The rationale for the longer interval between injections for spinal stenosis follows the pathophysiology of the disorder. As opposed to herniated intervertebral discs, spinal stenosis has no tissue that can be resorbed. The tissues become repeatedly swollen with resumption of symptoms. The intermittent injections allow for decreased swelling of tissues, improving function.

Lumbar Spine

Clinical Trials

Dilke's double-blind, controlled study of 100 patients demonstrated a significant difference in pain relief and resumption of usual activity at 3 months in patients receiving an extradural injection of 80 mg of methylprednisolone in 10 mL of saline versus an injection of 10 mL of saline into the interspinous ligaments as a control.[23] In contrast, White and colleagues reported a study of patients who received epidural corticosteroids that did little to alter the course of the disease.[101] Cuckler and co-workers reported their experience with epidural corticosteroids, which showed no significant difference between the medicated and control groups.[19] In this double-blind study of 73 patients, epidural corticosteroids plus procaine were no better than epidural procaine alone in the reduction of symptoms secondary to acute herniated nucleus pulposus or spinal stenosis. A second injection was not associated with greater improvement. Power and co-workers described a study of 16 patients with sciatica who received epidural injection.[76] Patients were evaluated at 1 and 7 days after injection. Response was minimal and the 16 patients underwent surgical intervention for discectomy. Patients received only one injection. A retrospective study of 40 patients who received one to four epidural injections reported 50% of patients had temporary, acute relief of sciatic symptoms secondary to intervertebral disc herniation.[85] Long-term relief occurred in less than 25% of patients.

Other reports of epidural corticosteroid injections have appeared in the medical literature that have described beneficial effects from these injections. Ridley and co-workers completed a double-blind outpatients' injection study of 39 patients comparing epidural injection of 80 mg of methylprednisolone with an interspinous injection of 2 mL of saline.[84] Of the 35 patients who completed the study, 19 received active drug treatment. Seventeen of 19 (90%) patients had improvement in rest and walking pain during the blinded observation period of 1 month at the start of the study. Only 19% of the placebo group improved during this same time period. Fourteen patients in the placebo group were crossed over to the corticosteroid group. Approximately 38% of these patients were improved after corticosteroid injection. At 6 months, only 11 of 17 patients who responded favorably to active injection maintained their improvement. Fifty-seven percent of patients received pain relief from injection. Poor response was associated with previous sciatica and neurologic deficits. The benefits of injection are short term.

Bush and Hillier also completed a study of epidural injection in sciatica patients.[11] A total of 23 patients with radiculopathy were entered into a study without radiographic corroboration of nerve impingement. In this 1-year, double-blind, placebo-controlled trial, patients received two caudal injections of corticosteroids or saline at a 2-week interval. Patients were assessed at baseline, 4 weeks, and 1 year. At 4 weeks, the corticosteroid group demonstrated significant improvement in pain and motion. At 1 year, both groups demonstrated improvement. Straight leg–raising was the only objective measurement that improved to a greater degree in the corticosteroid group at 1 year. In the discussion of this report, the authors suggest that previous studies that described little benefit of epidural injection assessed improvement too soon after injection.[19] Pain relief may occur 2 weeks or longer after injection. Mathews and associates also reported greater improvement in patients who received epidural injections 3 months after injection compared with control subjects.[60] Hickey reviewed his experience of 250 patients with sciatica treated with epidural injections. He reported a better response in individuals who received epidural injection early in the course of sciatic pain.[38] Multiple injections improved the success rate of relieving pain.

Over a 40-month period, 78 patients with sciatica with herniated disc received three epidural injections with 80 mg of methylprednisolone acetate versus 80 patients who received three injections of 1 mL of saline.[12] Carette and colleagues reported at 3 weeks that the Oswestry disability score was improved in the corticosteroid group compared with control subjects. The patients who were given corticosteroids also had greater improvement in finger-to-floor distance and sensory deficits. At 6 weeks, leg pain was less in the group who were given corticosteroids. At 3 months, there was no significant differences between the groups. Approximately 55% of each group reported very marked or marked improvement at 3 months. Withdrawal from the study for inefficacy during the first 6 weeks occurred in 5% of the patients taking corticosteroids and 14% of control subjects. At 12 months, the cumulative probability of having back surgery was 25.8% in the corticosteroid group versus 24.8% with placebo. This surgical rate was significantly greater than the 10% to 15% stated in the literature, suggesting that these patients had more severe disease than the usual patients with herniated discs.

NEEDLE PLACEMENT

The correct placement of the injection needle is another reason that epidural injections may not always be effective in reducing sciatic pain. Renfrew and co-workers reported that the placement of the epidural needle during a caudal injection was correct in 48% to 62% of procedures, depending on the experience of the physician.[82] In 9% of injections, the needle was placed intravenously. El-Khoury also reported the benefit of utilizing fluoroscopic control with a limited epidurogram to corroborate the location of the needle in the epidural space.[29] The blind placement of caudal epidural needles may be correct in upward of 90% of patients if appropriate landmarks are used. Results are improved if anatomic landmarks are easily identified and no air is palpable subcutaneously over the sacrum during the injection.[93] If an injection is unsuccessful, radiographic corroboration of needle placement may be required before assessing the lack of efficacy of the procedure.

COMPLICATIONS

The procedure is safe if meticulous technique is used.[4] However, complications include tuberculous meningitis, arachnoiditis, aseptic meningitis, and sclerosing spinal pachymeningitis,[26] and these risks must be considered in light of the 40% response rate to injection. One proposed mechanism explaining toxicities associated with epidural injection may be related, in part, to the presence of polyethylene glycol that gains access to the central nervous system and causes a sterile meningitis.[69] In a study with epidural injection of depot corticosteroids in rabbits, there was no evidence of meningitis or inflammatory response in the meninges or nerve roots. This study concluded that corticosteroids were not associated with detrimental effects on neural tissues.[16] Infection, in the form of epidural abscesses, is a rare but serious complication of epidural injection.[59]

Another concern is the safety of epidural injections in individuals consuming nonsteroidal anti-inflammatory drugs (NSAIDs), including low-dose aspirin. Horlocker and colleagues reviewed their experience with hemorrhagic complications in 1035 individuals undergoing 1214 epidural injections.[41] Bruising or bleeding occurred in 155 of individuals. NSAIDs were consumed by 383 patients, with aspirin most common in 158 individuals. No spinal hematomas were reported. Minor hemorrhagic complications (blood in needle or catheter) occurred in 63 (5.2%). NSAIDs did not increase the frequency of bleeding. Increased age, needle gauge, number of needle attempts, needle insertion at multiple interspaces, volume of injection, and dural punctures were associated with minor complications.

The frequency of epidural corticosteroid injections in the therapy for radiculopathy was reported by Fancuillo and co-workers.[30] Descriptive data from 25,479 selected patients with spinal and radicular pain were reviewed. Epidural injections were recommended to 2022 (7.9%) patients. Patients with lumbar pain had injections 12.6% of the time. Injections were recommended for 3.7% and 1.8% of cervical and thoracic lesions, respectively. Patients who received injections were more likely to have pain radiation, dermatomal pain distribution, and neurologic signs. They also had more co-morbidities and were older.

Koes and co-workers reviewed all randomized clinical trials of epidural injections between 1966 and 1993.[56] Twelve studies met requirements for their evaluation. Of these, six indicated that epidural corticosteroid injections were more effective than reference therapy (i.e., noninjection, medical therapy), and six were no more effective than reference therapy. Until larger studies are conducted, epidurally administered corticosteroid injections are an unproven therapy for lumbar radiculopathy. Epidural injections may be effective in some subgroups of patients with radiculopathy, but their characteristics have not been described. In patients who have continued pain and are poor candidates for surgical intervention, epidural corticosteroid injections may be considered.[7a]

In the past, corticosteroids, chymopapain, or collagenase was injected directly into disc spaces, but this technique has lost favor and is no longer done.[31] The benefit of chymopapain injection for herniated disc is very limited. Chymopapain injection may have little effect on modifying the physical appearance of intervertebral disc herniations 3 months after injection when viewed by CT scan.[8] Although chymopapain injection may be associated with relief of sciatic pain in some patients, it is a form of injection therapy with potential toxicities that have limited its use. Most physicians recommend a small laminectomy, as opposed to a chymopapain injection, as the preferred procedure to remove herniated disc material.[1,67]

Cervical Spine

TECHNIQUE

The procedure is safe when the cervical spine anatomy is considered.[97] The cervical spinous processes form an angle of 45 degrees with the axis of the cervical spine. The C7-T1 interspace is the largest, making access relatively easy.[75] The cervical cord is narrowest at the C7 level. The negative pressure in the cervical epidural space is most pronounced at the C7-T1 level, corresponding to its proximity to the thorax. The C7-T1 and C6-C7 interspaces are the usual locations for epidural injections. A total of 10 to 12 mL of fluid (anesthetic and Depo-Medrol) injected into the C7-T1 interspace spreads cephalad to C2 and caudad to T4. The injection should avoid the subdural space.

CLINICAL TRIALS

In a study of 58 patients, good or excellent results were reported in 35 (60.7%) as long as 6 months after a single injection.[15] The maximum effects of the injection may require 7 to 10 days to appear. The ideal frequency of injections for sustained relief of pain is not established. Single injections may be adequate to diminish cervical pain.[15] The course of therapy includes up to three injections at varying intervals (days to weeks) between injections. After the course of injections is completed, patients usually do not receive a second course of injections.

COMPLICATIONS

Complications are associated with cervical epidural injections (Table 19-7). Subdural hematoma is a rare, but life-threatening complication of cervical epidural injections.[81] Patients should not have cervical epidural injections while

19-7 COMPLICATIONS OF CERVICAL EPIDURAL INJECTIONS

INITIAL

Intravascular injection (seizures, cardiac arrest)
Vasovagal syncope
Subdural injection
  Total spinal block
  Postinjection headache
Cervical spinal cord damage
High cervical block with hypotension, bradycardia
Transient neurologic deficits

LATE

Epidural hematoma
Anterior spinal artery thrombosis
Superficial infection
Epidural abscess
Neck stiffness
Abdominal distention

Modified from Parris WCV: Nerve blocks and invasive therapies. In Tollison CD, Satterthwaite JR (eds): Painful Cervical Trauma: Diagnosis and Rehabilitative Treatment of Neuromusculoskeletal Injuries. Baltimore, Williams & Wilkins, 1992, pp 134-143.

sedated. Hodges and co-workers reported two cases of individuals who were sedated at the time of their injections who sustained intrinsic cervical cord damage associated with persistent neurologic deficits.[40] These complications are not frequent but must be considered in reference to the specific patient to evaluate the relative benefit of the injection. Until larger studies are conducted, epidurally administered corticosteroid injections are an unproven therapy for cervical radiculopathy. In patients who have continued pain and who are poor candidates for surgical intervention, epidural corticosteroid injections may be considered.

Facet Joint Injection

Patients with facet joint arthritis may develop pain that simulates radicular pain. If these patients do not respond to conservative therapy, they may benefit from facet joint anesthesia. Each facet joint receives sensory innervation from two spinal segment levels. Therefore, facets both at and above the level of the involved joint must be blocked or denervated to obtain adequate analgesia.

Procedure

The procedure requires radiographic surveillance for placement of the spinal needle. Diagnostic block at the initial step employs 2 mL of 1% lidocaine at each level to confirm responsiveness. Patients then receive a solution of methylprednisolone (20 mg) in up to 4 mL of bupivacaine at each level to be blocked. In the cervical spine, the volume is limited to 2 mL to limit extravasation and blockade of the cervical spinal nerve root.[74] If neurolytic therapy is being used, phenol in a contrast solution is given.[6] Repeat injections may be given every 2 to 4 weeks for three sessions.

The mechanism by which injections cause improvement (anti-inflammatory, neurolytic, or sclerosant action) is not apparent. Patients are told that symptoms will be aggravated before they improve.

Low Back Studies

Jackson and co-workers studied the effects of facet joint blocks in 454 patients.[48] The placement of the injecting needle was confirmed by facet joint arthrography. In this study, 30 (7.7%) patients had total pain relief after injection. Mean pain relief for all patients was 29%. No unique historic or physical examination characteristics would identify responsive patients. The characteristics of the patients who did respond included older age; history of back pain; normal gait; and absence of leg pain, muscle spasm, and aggravation of pain with Valsalva maneuver. Many questions remained that were not answered by the Jackson study. The long-term benefit of the injections was not assessed. "Facet syndrome" patients were not exclusively studied. Some patients had discogenic disease that would not respond to joint injection.

Another large study using facet joint corticosteroid injections was completed by Carette and co-workers.[13] Patients who responded to local analgesic facet joint blocks were randomized to corticosteroid or placebo injections. At 1 month, there was no difference in 190 treatment and placebo patients. The corticosteroid group had 42% of patients improved. The placebo group had 33% improved. At 6 months, the corticosteroid group had greater pain relief, but the results of the study were clouded by the use of concurrent interventions.

Revel and co-workers measured the benefit of one facet joint injection with anesthetic versus placebo for painful facet joints. Forty-three individuals with back pain with five of seven criteria associated with facet joint pain were compared with 37 people who met fewer than five criteria.[82a] The criteria included pain not exacerbated by coughing, forward flexion, rising from flexion, hyperextension, or extension-rotation; age of greater than 65 years; and pain relieved with recumbency. Lidocaine injection provided greater pain relief than placebo.

The use of facet joint blocks remains controversial in the treatment of patients with low back pain. Selection of patients for injection is essential for increasing the probability of success. Facet joint injections should be limited to patients with localized back pain that is exacerbated by extension of the spine, who have pain with ipsilateral bending, and who have had no response to other components of conservative management.

Cervical Spine Studies

Uncontrolled studies of facet joint blocks with corticosteroid have reported improvement in neck pain.[25,28,42,86,98] Barnsley and colleagues reported on a double-blind injection study comparing bupivacaine with betamethasone for chronic pain associated with cervical zygapophyseal joints.[3] The corticosteroid therapy was no better than anesthetic at 1 week and 1 month with regard to relief of pain. Less than 50% of patients reported pain relief of more than 1 week's duration. Facet joint blocks in the cervical spine can be considered to offer only short-term improvement for neck pain.

Denervation Procedures

Facet joint denervation may be attempted with neurolytic techniques (chemical—phenol, heat—radiofrequency generator, cold—nitrous oxide cryoprobe). The major advantage of this procedure is that all afferent stimuli from the posterior elements of the vertebral segments are blocked. Success rates of up to 60% have been reported in patients receiving chemoneurolysis with phenol or corticosteroids.[39,65]

Cryolysis

Brechner reported on the effect of percutaneous cryolysis of facet joint nerves. She used the cryoprobe in patients who had pain for 6 months or longer, who were between 25 and 35 years old, and who had radiation of pain in a sciatic distribution but not below the knee. These patients had 75% relief of pain with local facet injection.[9] The probe is placed with fluoroscopic guidance. A local anesthetic is injected for diagnostic purposes to locate the appropriate facet joint. The cryoprobe is placed near the facet joint until the patient's low back pain is elicited. If the probe is on the spinal nerve, radicular pain is produced and the needle is repositioned. One-minute freeze-thaw cycles are performed two to three times at two or three levels. At 1-week follow-up, patients had 70% pain relief, but at 3 months, low back pain had recurred at its original level of intensity. Cryolysis must be considered a temporary measure for the control of facet pain.

Radiofrequency Neurolysis

Mehta reported his experience with a 1-year follow-up study of facet joint denervation associated with radiofrequency-induced heat lesions.[62] Approximately 50% of patients had an initial response to therapy. However, at 1-year follow-up, only 25% of the initial group of patients had continued relief of symptoms. North and colleagues reported a 50% reduction in pain in 45% of patients at a mean follow-up of 3.2 years.[70] Response to temporary injections did not predict who would obtain long-term pain relief.

Lord and colleagues reported on a study of percutaneous radiofrequency neurotomy of 24 patients with chronic cervical zygapophyseal joint pain of a 34 months' median duration.[58] Patients who responded to local temporary injections were eligible for the study. Patients who received active therapy reported 263 days before the return of 50% of their pain versus 8 days for the placebo group. Another study documented a response to a second procedure if the pain recurred.[61]

Denervation of the facet joint has been documented to offer pain relief measured in months but not years. At this time, denervation should be offered to patients only after conservative methods have failed and with the recognition that there may be no long-term benefit.

Peripheral Nerve Blocks

The technique of differential nerve block is useful in the diagnosis of chronic pain and is discussed in Chapter 8. In addition to blockade of the conus medullaris and cauda equina, individual spinal nerves may be blocked. Not infrequently, patients with tumors may develop intractable pain if peripheral nerves are invaded. These patients may benefit from blockade of specific nerves such as the sciatic, femoral, obturator, or lateral femoral cutaneous nerve.[66] By accurately placing the needle with the aid of CT guidance before injection, paravertebral injection can be helpful in decreasing chronic peripheral nerve pain.[78] Injected medications may spread in an area beyond the local site of the injection. Radiographic guidance is warranted when longer-lasting neurolytic injections are utilized for pain control.

Complex Regional Pain Syndrome

Patients with radicular pain secondary to nerve root irritation of any cause and those with neurogenic pain of peripheral nerve origin may develop, in addition, a component of sympathetic nerve pain. *Causalgia* is the term used to describe this pain, which is of a burning, agonizing quality. The pain is constant and is not relieved by changing positions. The affected area also shows alteration in sweating and temperature function along with loss of motor power. Patients with complex regional pain syndrome also develop dysesthesias in the affected area so that the slightest touch causes unpleasant sensations. Complex regional pain syndromes can occur in patients with postherpetic neuralgia; carcinomatous invasion of nerves; trauma, including nerve root damage, associated with subsequent scarring; and phantom limb pain. Sympathetic blockade is most often used for arterial disease of the lower extremities.

Cervical Spine Technique

If patients do not respond to physical therapy and a course of oral medication, including NSAIDs and/or corticosteroids, paravertebral or regional sympathetic blockade (e.g., stellate ganglion blockade) with local anesthetics or other medications is indicated.[5,43,88,91] The procedure can be carried out on an outpatient basis. A series of three injections is usually given to obtain continued blockade. The location for the injection in the cervical spine is the C6 transverse process (cricoid cartilage) to minimize the risk of pneumothorax.[75] The needle is inserted to contact with the transverse process and then withdrawn 2 mm. Aspiration for blood is essential to prevent the injection of anesthetic directly into the vertebral arteries. An injection of up to 10 mL of bupivacaine has sufficient volume to anesthetize the sympathetic ganglion. Three injections are usually given to obtain continued blockade. The efficacy of the blockade can be assessed by the development of Horner's syndrome (ptosis, miosis, and enophthalmos). Complications associated with stellate blocks include vertebral artery injection with convulsions, neuralgias, pneumothorax, intradural injections, phrenic nerve blockade, and hematoma. Bilateral injections are not done to prevent the possibility of airway compromise. Patients who have pain secondary to sympathetic nerve irritation notice a change in their pain within 12 to 24 hours of the injection. Increased physical activity is encouraged once pain relief starts. By increasing "normal activity" in the peripheral and central nervous system, the opportunity for "abnormal activity" to predominate in sensory pathways is diminished.

Lumbar Spine Technique

Two to three 22-gauge, 8-cm needles are used to make a tract 5 to 6 cm lateral to the spinous processes of L2, L3, and L4.[92] A 20-gauge 15-cm sympathectomy needle is introduced at an angle of 10 degrees from the parasagittal plane to contact the transverse process. Fluoroscopy is used to advance the needle to the anterolateral portion of the vertebral body and into the retroperitoneal space for the injection of anesthetic. A complication of the injection is the development of genitofemoral neuralgia in 15% of patients.

Compression Syndrome Injections

Nerve blocks may also be given to relieve symptoms associated with compression of peripheral nerves. Areas around the suprascapular, greater occipital, median, and lateral femoral cutaneous nerves are injected with a combination of anesthetic and corticosteroid. The reduction of swelling and inflammation results in relief of pain in the distribution of the compressed nerve.[75]

Iliac Donor Site Injections

One additional area that may be benefited by local analgesic injection is the harvest site for bone for spinal fusion. Banwart and co-workers reviewed the frequency of iliac crest bone donor site complications.[2] Of 180 patients, complications occurred in 88 individuals (49%) and in 90 of 195 (47%) donor sites. Major complications (10%) included suture rejection with chronic drainage, scar revision, and chronic bone pain. In the remaining patients, mild complications included dysesthesias and scar formation. These areas of bone where the periosteum has been removed may remain painful long after the operative site has healed. Neuromas also may form in these locations. If these sites remain painful, injection therapy can be helpful in decreasing pain. Longer-acting agents may be used if short-acting agents only provide temporary relief.

Periradicular Injections

Periradicular injections involve infiltration around the spinal nerve root in the neural foramen. A 25-gauge spinal needle is used to place 0.5 mL of contrast medium to identify the nerve root and subsequently 2 mL for L4 and L5 and 3 mL for S1 injections of corticosteroids and anesthetic. A randomized, double-blind trial of 160 patients with sciatica received an injection with a methylprednisolone/bupivacaine combination (n = 80) versus placebo (n = 80).[51] In this study, the corticosteroid group had improved pain relief at 2 weeks but had greater pain than the placebo group at 3 and 6 months. By 1 year, 18 patients in the corticosteroid group and 15 in the saline group had surgery. Periradicular infiltration may decrease pain in the early stage of radiculopathy and is most beneficial for contained herniations.[52] Patients with extruded discs have a rebound phenomenon and less pain relief.

Intervertebral Disc Injections (IDET Procedure)

A new therapy for chronic discogenic back pain involves the use of an electric catheter that heats and congeals the internal components of the disc. This procedure is proposed in place of interbody fusion with plates or cages for symptomatic disc disease. The technique involves the placement of a catheter with a temperature-controlled thermal resistive coil near the inner posterior annulus of the intervertebral disc.[87] Discography is the method used to determine the symptomatic levels. The catheter temperature is raised to 90°F over 13 minutes, maintained for 4 minutes creating an annular temperature of 60°F to 65°F, followed by an injection of 20 mg of cefazolin. In an initial study of 25 patients with follow-up over 7 months, 80% reported a reduction of at least 2 points in a visual analogue pain scale and improvement in sitting tolerance as well as reduction or discontinuation of analgesic medication in 72%. No major complications occurred in this initial group of 25. Additional patients have undergone the procedure with similar results with follow-up at 1 and 2 years and have been reported in the literature by the same authors.[99] Karasek and Bogduk reported on 35 patients followed for 12 months who underwent an IDET procedure.[50] A total of 60% of the patients had a significant benefit from the procedure. Other studies have not documented benefits of the IDET procedure.[33] Among a group of 79 patients treated with IDET procedure, 48% had significant pain relief. Obesity was the characteristic most closely associated with failed IDET procedures.[17]

Complications have been described in IDET patients, including vertebral osteonecrosis.[27] Another complication includes the risk of developing a disc herniation at the level of the injection.[18] The long-term effects of modifying the collagen in intervertebral discs have not been determined. A major question that remains regarding IDET is who is the ideal candidate for this procedure. The problem is the identification of the patient with discogenic pain. Does discogenic pain exist? Is the disc the source of pain or are the surrounding structures? The answers to these questions need to be answered to determine whether this procedure has any benefit for back pain. At this time, the procedure has not been approved by the FDA and is experimental.

Sclerosant (Prolotherapy) Injection

Ligamentous structures play a significant role in supporting the lumbar spine. Damage to these structures in the form of ligamentous strain is one mechanism of developing low back pain. Inflammation in these structures may result in pain and tenderness over the damaged area. The healing process may result in shortening of these ligamentous supporting structures, resulting in stiffness and decreased motion. Attempts at increasing motion may result in recurrent re-injury and chronic inflammation. If this description of soft tissue injury is correct, optimal treatment of lumbar spine pain requires mobilization of stiffened structures while strengthening supporting connective tissue. This is the rationale for the use of sclerosant or prolotherapy. This therapy uses a chemical irritant to induce fibroblastic hyperplasia, resulting in increased collagen formation. The increased strength of hyperplastic normal tissue results in improved stability of spinous structures. Therefore, the goal of prolotherapy is the deposition of increased amounts of normal (not scar) collagenous material in ligament, tendon, or fascia by provoking a controlled inflammation at the injection site.[24] According to the theory supporting the use of prolotherapy, sclerosant injections in the lumbar spine supporting ligaments reestablish the proper alignment of vertebrae, relieving pressure on the intervertebral discs.[37]

In the 1930s, prolifcrant injection therapy was reported to be successful in decreasing back pain in 82% of treated patients with low back pain.[73] The inadvertent injection of these agents (psyllium seed oil and zinc sulfate) into the subarachnoid space resulted in cases of paralysis and deaths, halting the enthusiasm for this form of therapy in the 1960s.[44,53] A dextrose-glycerine-phenol solution used for varicose veins was substituted as a sclerosant solution. Different components of the solution cause direct chemical tissue injury and attract neutrophils (phenol) and local tissue damage by bursting cells with osmotic shock (dextrose, glycerin).[24] As part of sclerosant therapy, mobilization of the stiff joint to maximize motion is given before therapy, with flexion exercises encouraged after injection.

Clinical Trials

Sclerosant therapy has been studied in clinical trials. In a double-blind study of 81 patients with chronic low back pain, injection therapy with dextrose-glycerine-phenol solution and flexion exercises resulted in a statistically significant decrease in disability compared with the 41 controls who received saline injections with exercises.[73] In another study by Mathews and colleagues, sclerosant therapy was associated with decreased low back pain.[60] However, the number of patients was small and no specific conclusions could be drawn from the investigation. A group of 74 patients with chronic back pain received prolotherapy with lignocaine in the form of three once-weekly injections versus an injection with lignocaine alone. There were no differences between the groups in regard to pain relief or improvement of function at the 6-month follow-up.[22] Prolotherapy has also been utilized for chronic neck pain, but randomized clinical trials documenting the benefit of this therapy do not exist.

Prolotherapy has been advocated for Ehlers-Danlos syndrome patients with the intent of decreasing the excess motion of joints. Because prolotherapy is purported to cause hypertrophy of "normal" connective tissue, the benefit of these injections to produce stability in excessively elastic ligaments is not clear. If one location becomes stiff, areas that are not treated may experience increased stresses with excess motion.

Prolotherapy may cause toxicities if the injection affects nonconnective tissues.

Case Study 19-1

C.M. is a 49-year-old man with left-sided low back and leg pain. He had a history of low back pain that had been resistant to initial nonsteroidal therapy. He received a sclerosant injection into the left buttock for presumed sacroiliac joint pain. The injection was inadvertently injected into the vicinity of the left sciatic nerve. He experienced persistent burning pain in the buttock, numbness in the left leg, and weakness in the calf. The burning pain increased over a period of months and became chronic. The pain was eventually controlled with a combination of NSAIDs, muscle relaxants, gabapentin, and non-narcotic analgesics.

Prolotherapy should be given only by physicians familiar with the appropriate sites for injection, the side effects of the injected sclerosants, and the necessary course of exercises needed to maximize return of physical function. Even in the hands of an experienced practitioner, this therapy cannot be recommended as therapy for spinal pain.

Implantable Devices

Patients who have undergone multiple surgical spinal procedures without pain relief suffer with a failed back syndrome. These individuals endure intractable pain that is resistant to many conventional therapies. These individuals may be candidates for implantable devices in the spinal column to offer pain relief. These devices include spinal cord stimulators and intrathecal drug delivery systems.[77] Spinal cord stimulation has been an available therapy since 1967. More precise epidural placement and multichannel programmable systems have improved the benefit of these devices. However, the benefits of stimulators versus reoperation continues to be debated.[71] These therapies can offer pain relief and are cost effective. Implantable pumps utilize epidural catheters to deliver a steady, or programmable, concentration of analgesic medications. These devices can be helpful to patients with malignant or nonmalignant disorders. In a study of 67 failed back syndrome patients, the 23 patients who received a programmable drug delivery pump had a 5-year cumulative cost in Canadian dollars of $29,410 versus $38,000 for the conventional therapy patients. The Oswestry disability index scores showed a 27% improvement in the intrathecal group versus 12% in the control group.[57]

In summary, the role of injection therapy in the treatment of spinal pain remains controversial.[68] From the standpoint of scientific proof, a few series of studies proving efficacy have appeared in the literature. Prime examples, in the setting of epidural injections, of studies that have shown no efficacy were poorly designed, measuring therapeutic effects of injections before the active agent had time to work or, at times, distant to the initial injection, when intervening events could alter responses. These studies cannot be used to prove or disprove the efficacy of this mode of therapy despite their presence in the medical literature. On the basis of pathophysiologic mechanisms, correctly placed injection therapy should have an effect on decreasing pain.

Our Recommendation

In the patient who fails initial conservative management with activity as tolerated, physical modalities, and oral medications, injection therapy should be considered. Local injections are useful for acute paraspinous pain. Epidural injections are useful for patients with radiculopathy resistant to oral medications. Facet joint blocks are reserved for patients who have pain responsive to local anesthetic injections. Prolotherapy is not recommended. IDET procedures should be considered experimental.

References

Injection Therapy

1. Alexander AH, Burkus JK, Mitchell JB, et al: Chymopapain versus surgical discectomy in a military population. Clin Orthop 244:158, 1989.
2. Banwart JC, Asher MA, Hassanein RS: Iliac crest bone graft harvest donor site morbidity: A statistical evaluation. Spine 20:1055-1060, 1995.
3. Barnsley L, Lord SM, Wallis BJ, et al: Lack of effect of intraarticular corticosteroids for chronic pain in the cervical zygapophyseal joints. N Engl J Med 330:1047, 1994.
4. Barry PJC, Kendall PH: Corticosteroid infiltration of the extradural space. Ann Phys Med 6:267, 1962.
5. Benzon HT, Chomka CM, Brunner EA: Treatment of reflex sympathetic dystrophy with regional intravenous reserpine. Anesth Analg 59:500, 1980.
6. Boas RA: Facet joint injections. In Stanton-Hicks M, Boas R (eds): Chronic Low Back Pain. New York, Raven, 1982, pp 199-211.
7. Bonica JJ: Local anaesthesia and regional blocks. In Wall PD, Melzack R (eds): Textbook of Pain. Edinburgh, Churchill Livingstone, 1984, p 541.

7a. Borenstein D: Are epidural corticosteroid injections effective for sciatica? Curr Prac Med 1:19-21, 1998.

8. Boumphrey FRS, Bell GR, Modic M, et al: Computed tomography scanning after chymopapain injection for herniated nucleus pulposus: A prospective study. Clin Orthop 219:120, 1987.
9. Brechner T: Percutaneous cryogenic neurolysis of the articular nerve of Luschka. Reg Anaesth 6:18, 1981.
10. Brown FW: Management of discogenic pain using epidural and intrathecal steroids. Clin Orthop 129:72-78, 1977.
11. Bush K, Hillier S: A controlled study of caudal epidural injections of triamcinolone plus procaine for the management of intractable sciatica. Spine 16:572, 1991.
12. Carette S, LeClaire R, Marcoux S, et al: Epidural corticosteroid injections for sciatica due to herniated nucleus pulposus. N Engl J Med 336:1634-1640, 1997.
13. Carette S, Marcoux S, Truchon R, et al: A controlled trial of corticosteroid injections into facet joints for chronic low back pain. N Engl J Med 325:1002, 1991.
14. Childers MK: Use of Botulinum Toxin Type A in Pain Management. Columbia, MO, Academic Information Systems, 1999, pp 1-127.
15. Cicala RS, Thoni K, Angel JJ: Long-term results of cervical epidural steroid injections. Clin J Pain 5:143, 1989.
16. Cicala RS, Turner R, Moran E, et al: Methylprednisolone acetate does not cause inflammatory changes in the epidural space. Anesthesiology 72:556, 1990.
17. Cohen SP, Larkin T, Abdi S, et al: Risk factors for failure and complications of intradiscal electrothermal therapy: A pilot study. Spine 28:1142-1147, 2003.
18. Cohen SP, Larkin T, Polly DW Jr: A giant herniated disc following intradiscal electrothermal therapy. J Spinal Disord Tech 15:537-541, 2002.
19. Cuckler JM, Bernini PA, Wiesel SW, et al: The use of epidural steroids in the treatment of lumbar radicular pain: A prospective, randomized double blind study. J Bone Joint Surg Am 67A:63, 1985.
20. de Jong RH: Local anesthetics. In Raj PP (ed): Practical Management of Pain. Chicago, Year Book Medical, 1986, pp 539-556.
21. de Jong RH, Ronfeld RA, DeRosa RA: Cardiovascular effects of amide local anesthetics. Anesth Analg 61:3, 1982.
22. Dechow E, Davies RK, Carr AJ, et al: A randomized, double-blind, placebo-controlled trial of sclerosing injections in patients with chronic low back pain. Rheumatology 38:1255-1259, 1999.
23. Dilke TFW, Burry HC, Grahame R: Extradural corticosteroid injection management of lumbar nerve root compression. BMJ 2:635, 1973.
24. Dorman TA: Refurbishing ligaments with prolotherapy. Spine St Arts Rev 9:509-516, 1995.
25. Dory MA: Arthrography of the cervical facet joints. Radiology 148:379, 1983.
26. Dougherty JH Jr, Fraser RAR: Complications following intraspinal injection of steroids: Report of two cases. J Neurosurg 48:1023, 1978.
27. Drurasovic M, Glassman SD, Dimar JR II, et al: Vertebral osteonecrosis associated with the use of intradiscal electrothermal therapy: A case report. Spine 27:E325-328, 2002.
28. Dussault RG, Nicolet VM: Cervical facet joint arthrography. J Can Assoc Radiol 36:79, 1985.
29. El-Khoury G, Ehara S, Weinstein JN, et al: Epidural steroid injection: A procedure ideally performed with fluoroscopic control. Radiology 168:554, 1988.
30. Fanciullo GJ, Hanscom B, Seville J, et al: An observational study of the frequency and pattern of use of epidural steroid injection in 25,479 patients with spinal and radicular pain. Reg Anesth Pain Med 26:5-11, 2001.
31. Feffer HL: Regional use of steroids in the management of lumbar intervertebral disc disease. Orthop Clin North Am 6:249, 1975.
32. Foster L, Clapp L, Erickson M, et al: Botulinum toxin A and chronic low back pain: A randomized, double-blind study. Neurology 56:1290-1293, 2001.
33. Freeman BJC, Fraser RD, Cain CMJ, et al: A randomized double-blind controlled efficacy study: Intradiscal electrothermal therapy (IDET) versus placebo. Presented at the ISSLS 30th Annual Meeting, abstract 11. Vancouver, British Columbia, May 13-17, 2003.
34. Garvey TA, Marks MR, Wiesel SW: A prospective, randomized, double-blind evaluation of trigger-point injection therapy for low back pain. Spine 14:962, 1989.
35. Greene P, Kang U, Fahn S, et al: Double-blind, placebo-controlled trial of botulinum toxin injections for the treatment of spasmodic torticollis. Neurology 40:1213-1218, 1990.
36. Gregg RV, Constantini CH, Ford DJ, et al: Electrophysiologic and histopathologic investigation of phenol in Renografin as a neurolytic agent. Anesthesiology 63:A239, 1985.
37. Hauser RA: Prolo Your Pain Away: Curing Chronic Pain with Prolotherapy. Oak Park, IL, Beulah Land Press, 1998, pp 71-85.
38. Hickey RF: Outpatient epidural steroid injections for low back pain and lumbosacral radiculopathy. N Z Med J 100:594, 1987.
39. Hickey RFJ, Fregonning GD: Denervation of spinal facet joints for treatment of chronic low back pain. N Z Med J 85:96, 1977.
40. Hodges SD, Castleberg RL, Miller T, et al: Cervical epidural steroid injection with intrinsic spinal cord damage: Two case reports. Spine 23:2137-2142, 1998.
41. Horlocker TT, Bajwa ZH, Ashraf Z, et al: Risk assessment of hemorrhagic complications associated with nonsteroidal anti-inflammatory medications in ambulatory pain clinic patients undergoing epidural steroid injection. Anesth Analg 95:1691-1697, 2002.
42. Hove B, Gyldensted C: Cervical analgesic facet joint arthrography. Neuroradiology 32:456, 1990.
43. Hughes-Davies DF, Redman LR: Chemical lumbar sympathectomy. Anaesthesiology 31:1068, 1976.
44. Hunt WE, Baird WC: Complications following injections of sclerosing agent to precipitate fibro-osseous proliferation. J Neurosurg 18:461, 1961.
45. Incaudo G, Schatz M, Patterson R, et al: Administration of local anesthetics to patients with a history of prior adverse reaction. J Allergy Clin Immunol 61:339, 1978.
46. Iwama H, Akama Y: The superiority of water-diluted 0.25% to neat 1% lidocaine for trigger-point injection in myofascial pain syndrome: A prospective, randomized, double-blinded trial. Anesth Analg 91:408-409, 2000.
47. Iwama H, Ohmori S, Kaneko T, et al: Water-diluted anesthetic for trigger-point injection in chronic myofascial pain syndrome: Evaluation of types of local anesthetic and concentrations in water. Reg Anesth Pain Med 26:333-336, 2001.

48. Jackson RP, Jacobs RR, Montesano PX: Facet joint injection in low-back pain: A prospective statistical study. Spine 13:966, 1988.
49. Jost WH, Kohl A: Botulinum toxin: Evidence-based criteria in rare indications. J Neurol 248 (Suppl):39-44, 2001.
50. Karasek M, Bogduk N: Twelve-month follow-up of a controlled trial of intradiscal thermal annuloplasty for back pain due to internal disc disruption. Spine 25:2601-2607, 2000.
51. Karppinen J, Malmivarra A, Kurunlahti M, et al: Periradicular infiltration for sciatica: A randomized controlled trial. Spine 26:1059-1067, 2001.
52. Karppinen J, Ohinmaa A, Malmivarra A, et al: Cost effectiveness of periradicular infiltration for sciatica: Subgroup analysis of a randomized controlled trial. Spine 26:2587-2595, 2001.
53. Keplinger JE, Bucy PC: Paraplegia from treatment with sclerosing agents—report of a case. JAMA 73:1333, 1960.
54. Kim PS: Role of injection therapy: Review of indications for trigger point injections, regional blocks, facet joint injections, and intra-articular injections. Curr Opin Rheumatol 14:52-57, 2002.
55. Klein AW: Complications and adverse reactions with the use of botulinum toxin. Dis Mon 48:336-356, 2002.
56. Koes BW, Scholten RJ, Mens JM, et al: Efficacy of epidural steroid injection for low back pain and sciatica: A systemic review of randomized clinical trials. Pain 63:279-288, 1995.
57. Kumar K, Hunter G, Demeria DD: Treatment of chronic pain by using intrathecal drug therapy compared with conventional pain therapies: A cost-effectiveness analysis. J Neurosurg 97:803-810, 2002.
58. Lord SM, Barnsley L, Wallis BJ, et al: Percutaneous radio-frequency neurotomy for chronic cervical zygapophyseal-joint pain. N Engl J Med 335:1721-1726, 1996.
59. Mamourian AC, Dickman CA, Drayer BP, et al: Spinal epidural abscess: Three cases following spinal epidural injection demonstrated with magnetic resonance imaging. Anesthesiology 78:204, 1993.
60. Mathews JA, Mills SB, Jenkins VM, et al: Back pain and sciatica: Controlled trials of manipulation, traction, sclerosant and epidural injections. Br J Rheumatol 26:416, 1987.
61. McDonald GJ, Lord SM, Bogduk N: Long-term follow-up of patients treated with cervical radiofrequency neurotomy for chronic neck pain. Neurosurgery 45:61-67, 1999.
62. Mehta M, Sluijter MF: The treatment of chronic back pain. Anaesthesia 34:768, 1979.
63. Melzack R, Stillwell DM, Fox EV: Trigger points and acupuncture points for pain: Correlations and implications. Pain 3:3, 1977.
64. Misra VP: The changed image of botulinum toxin: Its unlicensed use is increasing dramatically ahead of robust evidence. BMJ 325:1188, 2002.
65. Mooney V, Robertson J: The facet syndrome. Clin Orthop 115:149, 1976.
66. Murphy TM, Raj PP, Stanton-Hicks M: Techniques of nerve blocks—spinal nerves. In Raj PP (ed): Practical Management of Pain. Chicago, Year Book Medical Publishers, 1986, pp 597-636.
67. Nachemson Al, Rydevik B: Chemonucleolysis for sciatica: A critical review. Acta Orthop Scand 59:56, 1988.
68. Nelemans PJ, deBie RA, deVet HC, et al: Injection therapy for sub-acute and chronic benign low back pain. Spine 26:501-515, 2001.
69. Nelson DA: Dangers from methylprednisolone acetate therapy by intraspinal injection. Arch Neurol 45:804, 1988.
70. North RB, Han M, Zahurak M, et al: Radiofrequency lumbar facet denervation: Analysis of prognostic factors. Pain 57:77-83, 1994.
71. North RB, Wetzel FT: Spinal cord stimulation for chronic pain of spinal origin: A valuable long-term solution. Spine 27:2584-2591, 2002.
72. O'Neill C, Derby R, Kenderes L: Precision injection techniques for diagnosis and treatment of lumbar disc disease. Semin Spine Surg 11:104-118, 1999.
73. Ongley MJ, Klein RG, Dorman TA, et al: A new approach to the treatment of chronic low back pain. Lancet 2:143, 1987.
74. Pappas JL, Kahn CH, Warfield CA: Facet block and neurolysis. In Waldman SD, Winnie AP (eds): Interventional Pain Management. Philadelphia, WB Saunders, 1996, pp 284-303.
75. Parris WCV: Nerve blocks and invasive therapies. In Tollison CD, Satterthwaite JR (eds): Painful Cervical Trauma: Diagnosis and Rehabilitative Treatment of Neuromusculoskeletal Injuries. Baltimore, Williams & Wilkins, 1992, pp 134-143.
76. Power RA, Taylor GJ, Fyfe IS: Lumbar epidural injection of steroid in acute prolapsed intervertebral discs. Spine 17:453, 1992.
77. Prager JP: Neuraxial medication delivery: The development and maturity of a concept for treating chronic pain of spinal origin. Spine 27:2593-2605, 2002.
78. Purcell-Jones G, Pither CE, Justins DM: Paravertebral somatic nerve block: A clinical, radiographic, and computed tomographic study in chronic pain patients. Anesth Analg 68:32, 1989.
79. Raj PP: Myofascial trigger point injection. In Raj PP (ed): Practical Management of Pain. Chicago, Year Book Medical, 1986, pp 569-577.
80. Raj PP, Denson DD: Neurolytic agents. In Raj PP (ed): Practical Management of Pain. Chicago, Year Book Medical, 1986, pp 557-565.
81. Reitman CA, Watters W III: Subdural hematoma after cervical epidural steroid injection. Spine 27:E174-E176, 2002.
82. Renfrew DL, Moore TE, Kathol MH, et al: Correct placement of epidural steroid injections: Fluoroscopic guidance and contrast administration. AJNR Am J Neuroradiol 12:1003, 1991.
82a. Revel M. Poiraudeau S, Auleley GR, et al: Capacity of the clinical picture to characterize low back pain relieved by facet joint anesthesia. Proposed criteria to identify patients with painful facet joints. Spine 23:1972-1977, 1998.
83. Reynolds MO: Myofascial trigger point syndromes in the practice of rheumatology. Arch Phys Med Rehabil 62:111, 1981.
84. Ridley MG, Kingsley GH, Gibson T, et al: Outpatients lumbar epidural corticosteroid injection in the management of sciatica. Br J Rheumatol 27:295, 1988.
85. Rosen CD, Kahanovitz N, Bernstein R, et al: A retrospective analysis of the efficacy of epidural steroid injections. Clin Orthop 228:270, 1988.
86. Roy DF, Fleury J, Fontaine SB, et al: Clinical evaluation of cervical facet joint infiltration. Can Assoc Radiol J 39:118, 1988.
87. Saal JS, Saal JA: Management of chronic discogenic low back pain with a thermal intradiscal catheter: A preliminary report. Spine 25:382-388, 2000.
88. Schutzer SF, Gossling HR: The treatment of reflex sympathetic dystrophy syndrome. J Bone Joint Surg Am 66A:625, 1984.
89. Simons DG, Travell JG: Myofascial pain syndromes. In Wall PD, Melzack R (eds): Textbook of Pain. Edinburgh, Churchill Livingstone, 1986, pp 263-276.
90. Spaccarelli KC: Lumbar and caudal epidural corticosteroid injections. Mayo Clin Proc 71:169-178, 1996.
91. Stanton-Hicks M, Abram SE, Nolte H: Sympathetic blocks. In Raj PP (ed): Practical Management of Pain. Chicago, Year Book Medical, 1986, pp 661-681.
92. Stanton-Hicks M: Lumbar sympathetic nerve block and neurolysis. In Waldman SD, Winnie AP (eds): Interventional Pain Management. Philadelphia, WB Saunders, 1996, pp 353-359.
93. Stitz MY, Sommer HM: Accuracy of blind versus fluoroscopically guided caudal epidural injections. Spine 24:1371-1376, 1999.
94. Swezey RL, Clements PJ: Conservative treatment of back pain. In Jayson MIV (ed): The Lumbar Spine and Back Pain, 3rd ed. Edinburgh, Churchill Livingstone, 1987, pp 299-314.
95. Travell JG: The quadratus lumborum muscle: An overlooked cause of low back pain. Arch Phys Med Rehabil 57:566, 1976.
96. Travell JG, Simons DG: Myofascial Pain and Dysfunction, The Trigger Point Manual: The Upper Extremities. Baltimore, Williams & Wilkins, 1983.
97. Waldman SD: Cervical epidural nerve block. In Waldman SD, Winnie AP (eds): Interventional Pain Management. Philadelphia, WB Saunders, 1996, pp 275-283.
98. Wedel DJ, Wilson PR: Cervical facet arthrography. Reg Anesth 10:7, 1985.
99. Wetzel FT, McNally TA, Phillips FM: Intradiscal electrothermal therapy used to manage chronic discogenic low back pain: New directions and intervention. Spine 27:2621-2626, 2002.
100. Wheeler AH, Goolkasian P, Gretz SS: A randomized, double-blind, prospective pilot study of botulinum toxin injection for refractory, unilateral, cervicothoracic, paraspinal, myofascial pain syndrome. Spine 23:1662-1666, 1998.
101. White AH, Derby R, Wynne G: Epidural injections for the diagnosis and treatment of low-back pain. Spine 5:78, 1980.

NSAIDS, ANALGESICS, AND NARCOTICS

A number of drugs have been advocated for the treatment of low back pain on a short- or long-term basis. NSAIDs and analgesics, both non-narcotic and narcotic, have been used in the therapy for back and neck pain. In general, the scientific evidence demonstrating efficacy of NSAIDs in spinal pain is small compared with the frequency of their use. Nevertheless, NSAIDs play a useful role in the control of pain and inflammation in these patients.

A number of factors need to be considered when deciding whether to prescribe NSAIDs or analgesics for spinal pain. The natural history of acute low back and neck pain is one of resolution over a short period of time in 80% to 90% of patients. Patients may go through this period using physical measures (activity as tolerated and physical therapy) alone. On the other hand, the pain the patients experience may be diminished through the use of NSAIDs or analgesics. In making the decision to use these drugs, the physician must remember not to exacerbate the condition or cause serious toxicities while the patient's back or neck pain resolves. The clinical correlate of this prohibition is that NSAIDs and non-narcotic analgesics are appropriate agents in some patients with acute spinal pain, but short-acting narcotic analgesics are reserved for only a very small group of patients with documented anatomic abnormalities (postsurgical, compression fractures) for specified brief periods of time. Long-acting narcotic therapy in patients with chronic spinal pain is reserved for individuals who have failed other non-narcotic analgesics in whom sustained-release analgesia will result in improved function.

NSAIDs

NSAIDs have analgesic properties when given in single doses and are anti-inflammatory and analgesic when given chronically in larger doses. Pure analgesics have no anti-inflammatory effect, whereas corticosteroids have anti-inflammatory but no analgesic effects except for those mediated through reduction of inflammation.

Whereas narcotic analgesics act on the endorphin system in the central nervous system, NSAIDs act at the site of peripheral injury where peripheral nerves send nociceptive impulses to the cortex. Prostaglandins do not cause pain by themselves, but rather sensitize nociceptive nerve fibers to environmental chemical factors (bradykinin, histamine). In the presence of prostaglandins, small amounts of these chemical factors initiate nociceptive impulses. Cyclooxygenase inhibition by NSAIDs with decreased production of prostaglandins seems to play a role in the analgesic action of these agents.

Cyclooxygenase-1/Cyclooxygenase-2

Both the therapeutic effects and effects and potential toxicities of NSAIDs are related to the inhibition of the synthesis of prostaglandins by the cyclooxygenase (COX) enzyme. A single COX enzyme was once thought to regulate the production of prostaglandins for the maintenance of organ function (gastric mucosal integrity) and the promotion of an inflammatory response. However, understanding of the mechanism of action of the NSAIDs has been advanced by the identification of two forms of the COX enzyme.

COX-1 is a constitutive form that produces prostaglandins that maintain organ function. COX-1 is inhibited by most of the available NSAIDs (e.g., ketoprofen, aspirin, indomethacin). Inhibition of COX-1 activity induced by the NSAIDs is associated with increased risk of gastrointestinal toxicity, potential renal dysfunction in at-risk patients, and decreased aggregation of platelets associated with increased risk of bleeding.[54] COX-2 is an inducible enzyme that develops at inflammatory sites with the stimulation of inflammatory cytokines, growth factors, and endotoxin.[10] COX-2 is also inhibited by the same number of NSAIDs. COX-3 is a variant of COX-1 and is found in the brain and heart of humans. This enzyme is selectively inhibited by analgesic/antipyretic drugs such as acetaminophen. Inhibition of this enzyme may be the mechanism by which acetaminophen exerts its analgesic effects without causing the toxicities associated with COX-1/COX-2 inhibitors.[8]

The two isoforms of the COX enzymes differ in the shape of their active sites. The active site of COX-1 has a linear configuration, whereas the COX-2 active site is located in a side pocket off the main channel of the enzyme. The original NSAIDs had chemical forms that easily fit into both active sites. A new class of COX-2 inhibitors have side chains that fit into the COX-2 active site, inhibiting the production of inflammatory prostaglandins. The same side chain physically excludes COX-2 drugs from entering the COX-1 active site. The clinical result of COX-2 inhibition is the control of inflammation and pain to a degree similar to that measured with COX-1/COX-2 inhibitors, with a significant decrease in associated toxicity in the gastrointestinal tract and platelets. For example, COX-2 inhibitors do not affect bleeding time, a measurement of platelet function. Also, patients on COX-2 therapy are able to take their medication up to the time of their invasive procedures without the exacerbation of disease associated with the discontinuation of their NSAID.

Other mechanisms must also act in the production of analgesia associated with these drugs because the potency of the NSAIDs as prostaglandin inhibitors does not necessarily correlate with their efficacy as analgesics. NSAIDs also have significant effects on other components of the inflammatory response, including oxidative phosphorylation, superoxide production, and cellular activation.[1]

Pharmacokinetics

The pharmacokinetics and clinical pharmacology of these agents have little direct bearing on their time course of action; that is, the onset of analgesia does not parallel the peak plasma level. Agents that are rapidly absorbed do not necessarily have more rapid onset of analgesic effect. Determinations of peak plasma levels are not obtained clinically because they have little bearing in predicting qualitative or quantitative responses to a medication. Patient response to medications seems to be individualized and cannot be predicted by the pharmacokinetics of a drug.[11]

The duration of anti-inflammatory effect of a medication may be different from that of the analgesic effect. An example given by Huskisson is that of piroxicam with a plasma half-life of 38 hours.[24] The anti-inflammatory effect of this drug lasts for 24 hours with a once-a-day dose, whereas the analgesic effect is only 6 hours in duration, similar to that of aspirin. A drug should be used until it reaches a steady-state level (five half-lives) before determining efficacy.

Although the NSAIDs are all weak organic acids, except nabumetone, a prodrug that is administered as a base, they belong to different chemical groups (Table 19-8). The drugs may be divided by their chemical grouping in a variety of ways depending on the complexity of the classification.[37,44] For example, aspirin may be considered a salicylate or a heterocarboxylic acid. These groups include the salicylates (heterocarboxylic acids), propionic acid derivatives (phenylacetic acid, naphthaleneacetic acid, oxazolepropionic acid, benzeneacetic acid), acetic acid derivatives (indoleacetic acid, pyrrole acetic acid), fenamates (anthranilic acids or heterocarboxylic acids), oxicams, naphthylalkanone derivatives, pyrrolo-pyrrole derivative, pyrazolones (pyrazolidinediones), and COX-2 inhibitors (sulfonamide and sulfone derivatives). Within these groups are agents with a short half-life and rapid onset of action and others with a longer half-life and slower onset of action. In general, the half-life of the drug plays a greater role in selection of a specific NSAIDs than the chemical grouping. However, when an NSAID is ineffective, the choice of the subsequent NSAID is usually one from a different chemical group with a similar half-life.

Analgesic NSAIDs

NSAIDs that are used as analgesics include aspirin, diflunisal, fenoprofen, ibuprofen, mefenamic acid, naproxen, naproxen sodium, piroxicam, ketoprofen, ketorolac tromethamine, etodolac, diclofenac potassium, celecoxib, rofecoxib, and valdecoxib. In general, the dosage needed for the production of the analgesic effect of these agents is lower than that required for anti-inflammatory effects. The daily doses required for analgesic effects are aspirin, 2600 mg; diflunisal, 1000 mg; ibuprofen, 1600 mg; naproxen, 500 mg; ketorolac tromethamine, 30 mg; etodolac, 900 mg; diclofenac potassium, 100 mg; celecoxib, 400 mg; rofecoxib, 25 mg; or valdecoxib, 20 mg.

Most of the NSAIDs, when used as analgesics, must be given every 4 to 6 hours (ibuprofen). Other NSAIDs and COX-2 inhibitors may be used every 12 to 24 hours (diflunisal, piroxicam, naproxen sodium, or rofecoxib). The analgesic effect of diflunisal lasts up to 12 hours, so the drug should be given only twice a day. Although the analgesic effect of piroxicam lasts for 6 hours, the drug has a long half-life, which limits its use to once a day because of gastrointestinal intolerance. Therefore, piroxicam is not a first-line agent for analgesia. Naproxen sodium should be given every 8 hours at a maximum. Rofecoxib at a dose of 25 mg to 50 mg may be dosed once a day for 24-hour analgesia. If an agent helps for a portion of the day but then loses effect, an additional dose at the end of the day might be appropriate.

When the NSAIDs are used as anti-inflammatory agents, higher doses are necessary to obtain adequate anti-inflammatory effects. In addition, when the drugs are used for chronic diseases, the rapid onset of action is not as important as the drug's eventual efficacy for that individual patient. Examples of the daily dosages of drugs that may be required for therapy for the spondyloarthropathies or rheumatoid arthritis are aspirin, 5300 mg; sulindac, 400 mg; naproxen, 1500 mg; ibuprofen, 3600 mg; diclofenac sodium, 225 mg; nabumetone, 2000 mg; etodolac, 1600 mg; oxaprozin, 1800 mg; celecoxib, 400 mg; rofecoxib, 25 mg; or valdecoxib, 20 mg. For osteoarthritis, lower doses of NSAIDs may be used to limit toxicity while decreasing pain and local synovial inflammation. Examples of therapy for patients with osteoarthritis may include daily doses of aspirin, 2200 mg; sulindac, 300 mg; naproxen, 500 mg; ibuprofen, 1600 mg; diclofenac sodium, 100 mg; nabumetone, 1000 mg; etodolac, 800 mg; oxaprozin, 1200 mg; meloxicam, 7.5 mg; celecoxib, 200 mg; rofecoxib, 12.5 mg; or valdecoxib, 10 mg. Although acetaminophen has been suggested as adequate therapy for osteoarthritis, no study has demonstrated the consistent benefit of this drug for patients with osteoarthritis of the spine.[6] In fact, many patients try acetaminophen for back pain before seeking medical attention. In many circumstances, they see a physician because acetaminophen was inadequate for decreasing their pain. Acetaminophen may be used as an adjunctive therapy along with an NSAID or COX-2 inhibitor for additional pain relief.

NSAIDs Toxicities

The toxicities of the NSAIDs are predominantly gastrointestinal and renal. Aspirin ingestion has been associated with acute gastrointestinal bleeding.[30] Other NSAIDs have also been associated with bleeding.[21,23] The enteric-coated salicylates and sulindac are less likely to cause acute gastric damage according to endoscopic studies in normal volunteers.[29] Approximately 10% of patients develop gastrointestinal toxicity, usually dyspepsia.[45] Nabumetone has been cited as being milder but not devoid of gastrointestinal tract toxicity.[5] Corticosteroids have a low risk of causing gastrointestinal bleeding because of gastrointestinal ulceration.[7] It is more likely that the illness for which the corticosteroids are being given causes gastrointestinal injury (head trauma). Patients taking corticosteroids are admitted to the hospital more frequently for gastrointestinal bleeding than normal population controls.[34] The increased risk was related to concomitant medications and the underlying disorders for which the corticosteroids were administered. However, the combination of NSAIDs and corticosteroids does increase the risk of injury.[38] Patients who receive both classes of drugs must be warned of the potential complications so that they can inform their physician of any alteration in gastrointestinal function. The COX-2 inhibitors have a decreased risk of causing gastrointestinal toxicity including obstruction, perforation, and bleeding. A variety of studies have reported a 50% decreased in the risk of significant gastrointestinal bleeding.[2,14]

Another major toxicity associated with NSAIDs is related to renal dysfunction.[9] A small group of patients develop an idiosyncratic reaction with interstitial nephritis. A larger group develop reversible renal failure secondary to

19-8 NONSTEROIDAL ANTI-INFLAMMATORY DRUGS

(Chemical Class) Drug	Trade Name	Tablet/Capsule Size (mg)	Dose (mg/day)	Frequency (Times/Day)	Onset (hr)	Half-Life (hr)
(Salicylates)						
Aspirin	Bayer	325	Up to 5200	4-6	1-2	4
Enteric coated	Ecotrin	325	5200	4-6	1-2	4
	Easprin	975	3900	4	1-2	
Time release	Zorprin	800	3200	2	2	4
(Substituted Salicylates)						
Diflunisal	Dolobid	250,500	500-1500	2-3	1 (with loading dose)	11
Salsalate	Disalcid	500,750	3000	2	2	4
Choline magnesium trisalicylate	Trilisate	500,750,1000, liquid (500 mg/5 mL)	3000	2	2	4
Choline salicylate	Arthropan	650 mg/mL	1950	4-6	1	4
Magnesium salicylate	Magan	545	3270	3-4	2	4
Sodium salicylate	Uracel	325	3900	3-6	1	4
Aspirin/antacids	Ascriptin	325	5200	4-6	2	4
(Propionic Acid Derivatives)						
Ibuprofen	Motrin	200	1200-3600	4-6	1-2	1-3
	Rufen	400				
	Advil	600				
	Medipren	800				
	Nuprin	200				
Naproxen	Naprosyn	250,375,500	500-1500	2-3	3	13
Sodium naproxen	Anaprox	275,550	550-1100	2	1-2	13
Fenoprofen calcium	Nalfon	200,300,600	600-3000	3-4	3	2-3
Ketoprofen	Orudis	25,50,75	150-300	3-4	2	3-4
	Oruvail	200 SR				
Flurbiprofen	Ansaid	50,100	300	2-3	1-2	6
Oxaprozin	Daypro	600	1800	1-2	3-5	25
(Pyrrole Acetic Acid Derivatives)						
Sulindac	Clinoril	150,200	300-450	2-3	2	18
Indomethacin	Indocin	25,50,75 SR, 50 suppositories	75-225	1-3	2	1-4
Tolmetin sodium	Tolectin	200,400	600-1600	4	1	1-4
(Benzeneacetic Acid Derivative)						
Diclofenac sodium	Voltaren 100 XR	25,50,75	75-225	2-3	2-3	2
Diclofenac potassium	Cataflam	25,50	100-150	2-3	1	2
Diclofenac sodium + misoprostol	Arthrotec	50+200,75+200	150-200	2-3	2-3	2
(Oxicam)						
Piroxicam	Feldene	10,20	20	1	5	38-45
Meloxicam	Mobic	7.5,15	7.5-15	1	3	15-20
(Pyranocarboxylic acid)						
Etodolac	Lodine	200,300,400 400 XL	800-1600	2-4	2	6
(Fenamate)						
Meclofenamate sodium	Meclomen	50,100	200-400	4	1	4
Mefenamic acid	Ponstel	250	1000	4	3	4
(Pyrrolo-pyrrole)						
Ketorolac tromethamine	Toradol	10	10-40	4	1	4-6
(Naphthylalkanone)						
Nabumetone	Relafen	500,750	1000-2000	1-2	4	26
(Pyrazolones)						
Phenylbutazone	Butazolidin, Azolid	100	400	4	2 (with loading)	72
(COX-2) Coxibs						
Celecoxib	Celebrex	100,200 400	200-800	1-2	3	11
Rofecoxib	Vioxx	12.5,25,50 12.5/5mL, 25/5 mL (liquid)	12.5-50	1	1	18
Valdecoxib	Bextra	10,20	10-40	1	1	11
(Investigational Drugs)						
Etoricoxib	Arcoxia	30,60,90		1		
Lumiracoxib	Prexige	400		1		

bid, twice daily; BM, bone marrow; CNS, central nervous system; COX, cyclooxygenase; G, gastrointestinal; NSAIDS, nonsteroidal anti-inflammatory drugs; qd, four times daily; R, renal; SR, slow-release; XR/XL, extended release.
Modified from The Medical Letter 42:58, 2000.

Metabolism	Excretion	Major Toxicity	Cost ($/Month)	Comments
Liver	Kidney	G, R	8.80 (5200 mg) (generic)	Less expensive than other NSAIDs
Liver	Kidney	G, R	50.40 (4000 mg)	Less G upset than aspirin
Liver	Kidney	G, R	20.39 (3900 mg) (generic)	Less G upset than aspirin
Liver	Kidney	G, R	76.80 (3200 mg)	Less G upset than aspirin
Liver	Kidney	G, R	47.62 (1000 mg) (generic)	Loading dose for rapid onset of action; long half-life bid dosing
Liver	Kidney	G, R	25.20 (4000 mg) (generic)	Less G upset than aspirin
Liver	Kidney	G, R	51.60 (3000 mg) (generic)	Less G upset than aspirin
Liver	Kidney	G, R	40.45 (1950 mg)	Ease of swallowing
Liver	Kidney	G, R	43.13 (3270 mg)	Magnesium toxicity with impaired renal function
Liver	Kidney	G, R	8.80 (5400 mg)	Simple analgesic, less effective than aspirin; increased sodium intake
Liver	Kidney	G, R	18.85	Antacids do not buffer gastric acid adequately
Liver	Kidney	G, R	9.99 (3200 mg) (generic—Motrin)	Need larger doses for anti-inflammatory effect (rheumatoid arthritis)
Liver	Kidney, stool	G, R	21.00 (1000 mg) (generic)	Effective in a number of musculoskeletal disorders
Liver	Kidney, stool	G, R	10.94 (825 mg) (generic)	Onset of action more rapid than naproxen
Liver	Kidney	G, R	32.40 (2400 mg) (generic)	Associated with renal toxicity more often than other nonsteroidals
Liver	Kidney, stool	G, R	38.40 (300 mg) (generic)	Newer nonsteroidal (extended release)
Liver	Kidney	G, R	38.40 (200 mg) (generic)	More powerful form of ibuprofen
Liver	Kidney, stool	G, R	43.80 (1200 mg)	Convenient qd dosing
Liver	Kidney, stool	G	27.00 (400 mg) (generic)	Effective in a number of musculoskeletal disorders; less renal toxicity
Liver	Kidney, stool	G, R CNS, BM	17.10 (150 mg) (generic) 26.70 (150 mg SR)	Drug of choice for spondylitis; greatest CNS toxicity of all NSAIDs
Liver	Kidney	G, R	40.50 (1200 mg) (generic)	Cross reactivity with zomepirac sodium (Zomax)
Liver	Kidney, stool	G, R	46.20 (150 mg) (generic)	Effective in a number of musculoskeletal conditions
Liver	Kidney, stool	G, R	55.54 (100 mg) (generic)	Potassium salt associated with more rapid onset of analgesia
Liver	Kidney, stool	G, R	126.90 (200 mg)	Decreased G ulcers
Liver	Kidney	G, R	31.80 (20 mg) (generic)	Substantial G toxicity; long duration of action, which extends toxicity
Liver	Kidney	G, R	59.70	Inhibits COX-2 more than COX-1, no effect on platelet aggregation
Liver	Kidney	G, R	47.70 (1200 mg) (generic)	Multiple dosage form allows for specific amounts for different disorders
Liver	Kidney, stool	G, R	63.60 (400 mg) (generic)	Diarrhea in one third of patients
Liver	Kidney, stool	G, R	32.34 (1000 mg) (generic)	Dysmenorrhea
Liver	Kidney	G, R	77.96 (30 mg)	Effective, rapid onset analgesic
Liver	Kidney, stool	G, R	71.40 (1000 mg)	Only basic NSAID, less toxic to G tract
Liver	Kidney, stool	G, R, BM	Unavailable	Bone marrow toxicity limits utility in most back pain patients, limited availability
Liver	Kidney	R	84.00 (400 mg)	Decreased G toxicity
Liver	Kidney	R	72.00 (25 mg)	Decreased G toxicity
Liver	Kidney	R	88.19 (20 mg)	Decreased G toxicity
Liver	Kidney			
Liver	Kidney			

diminished renal prostaglandins, which are directly associated with diminished renal blood flow. Sulindac, a drug with fewer active metabolites in the renal circulation, has less effect on renal blood flow and is rarely the cause of this form of renal toxicity.[9] The COX-2 inhibitors decrease COX-2 prostaglandins produced in the kidney that sustain renal blood flow when function is compromised. COX-2 inhibitors have similar renal toxicities as traditional NSAIDs. Other forms of NSAID toxicity include neurologic, hematologic, and hepatic complications.[11] Dermatologic and hypersensitivity reactions also are associated with these drugs.[5]

The clinician should take into account the characteristics of both the patient and the drug in deciding on the best agent for a particular individual (Table 19-9). Of greatest importance is efficacy. When choosing an agent for acute back or neck pain, one with rapid onset of action is preferred once its efficacy has been established. Most of the NSAIDs have similar safety profiles. The COX-2 inhibitors are most effective in limiting gastrointestinal toxicity in those individuals at greatest risk of bleeding (past history of gastrointestinal hemorrhage, elderly, concomitant aspirin).[2] Most individuals tolerate the NSAIDs. Geriatric patients may require smaller doses because drug metabolism slows with age. If patients cannot take the COX-2 inhibitors and take a traditional NSAID that is an effective agent but develop gastric toxicity, alternative means of taking the medication may be tried (e.g., with meals). Alterations in other habits (alcohol, coffee consumption, smoking) or adding antacids or antiulcer medications (H_2-receptor antagonists, cytoprotective agents, e.g., misoprostol) may be useful in increasing tolerability of an effective drug.[52] Misoprostol should be given in small doses (100 μg twice daily) initially. The drug must be given with meals to minimize the major complication of diarrhea. Eating allows the drug to remain in the stomach and out of the small intestine where the prostaglandin will cause diarrhea. As the patient tolerates the agent, the frequency of administration should be increased to three to four times a day with meals. In general, agents that require ingestion of fewer tablets are associated with greater patient compliance. Flexibility in the amount of drug per tablet and of the total dose needed to attain and maintain efficacy is useful. Some patients will obtain adequate analgesia at low doses of a drug, whereas others require larger amounts to obtain pain relief. Some patients prefer aspirin because of its lower cost (see Table 19-9).

19-9 FACTORS IN CHOICE OF A NONSTEROIDAL ANTI-INFLAMMATORY DRUG

Drug Characteristics	Patient Characteristics
Efficacy	Individual variations
Safety	Nature of the disease
Tolerance	Other drugs
Compliance potential	Age
Dose	Severity of disease
Formulation	Time factors
Cost	Pregnancy

Patient Characteristics

In regard to patient characteristics, it is impossible to predict which chemical class will be effective in an individual patient. Patients with mechanical problems improve with the analgesic effects of NSAIDs, whereas those with spondyloarthropathies require the anti-inflammatory action of these drugs. Drug interactions may limit choices. Shorter half-life drugs may be safer in older patients who have a diminished capacity to metabolize drugs. COX-2 inhibitors are safer in older individuals who are at greater risk of gastrointestinal bleeding. Some patients have difficulty swallowing pills and prefer liquid forms of NSAIDs. The combination of all these factors should be considered before the physician chooses an NSAID for a particular patient.

Most patients obtain significant pain relief with an NSAID and are able to stop the drug when resolution of their spinal pain occurs. Occasionally after an initial recovery, a patient will experience intermittent recurrent attacks or complain of a chronic neck or backache. These patients benefit from a maintenance dose of an NSAID. Medication should be taken on a regular schedule. Delaying medication until pain is present is not an appropriate way to take an NSAID. The drugs work better before pain is maximum. Patients should take medicine for a set time until pain is resolved and then discontinue the drug a few days later.

Clinical Trials

Some of the NSAIDs have been studied in patients with acute and chronic low back pain. Indomethacin was found no better than a placebo in patients with sciatica.[15] Naproxen and diflunisal had greater efficacy than placebo in relieving chronic back pain according to patient opinion.[3] Diflunisal was also preferred to acetaminophen in another study of back pain.[22] Wiesel demonstrated a small preference for aspirin compared with acetaminophen and phenylbutazone that was not statistically significant in a study of acute back pain.[53] Mefenamic acid at high dose (500 mg) was better than low-dose mefenamic acid, low-dose salicylate, and placebo in controlling chronic low back pain.[32] A double-blind study of piroxicam and indomethacin demonstrated efficacy of both NSAIDs in patients with back pain.[51]

Van Tulder and colleagues systematically reviewed the NSAID studies for treatment of acute low back with or without radiation. Of 51 trials and 6057 patients, 16 (31%) trials were of high quality. The pooled relative risk for global improvement after 1 week was 1.24 and for additional analgesic use was 1.29, indicating a statistically significant but small effect in favor of NSAIDs as compared with placebo.[49] No specific NSAID offered greater benefit than another in the treatment of spinal pain. COX-2 inhibitors were not included in this review.

Studies demonstrating the efficacy of COX-2 inhibitors in the treatment of acute pain, osteoarthritis, and rheumatoid arthritis are in the medical literature, but the efficacy of COX-2 inhibitors in the spondyloarthropathies remains to be reported.[4,26,31,46] In general, doses effective for rheumatoid arthritis are also useful for the control of spinal inflammation associated with spondyloarthropathies.

A review of NSAID studies for chronic low back pain has not been completed because of a lack of clinical trials. A COX-2 inhibitor (rofecoxib) has been examined in chronic low back pain and was superior to placebo in initial studies of 690 patients.[27] A dose of rofecoxib, 25 mg, was as effective as 50 mg compared with placebo with fewer adverse events. Clinical trials of other COX-2 inhibitors for chronic low back pain are ongoing and have demonstrated efficacy in preliminary studies.

Oral Corticosteroids

In rare circumstances, patients who are resistant to epidural injection may be considered for a short course (7 days or less) of oral corticosteroid therapy.[16] Dexamethasone (Medrol Dosepak) is the form of corticosteroids most frequently used for this purpose. The highest dose administered is 40 to 60 mg for 1 or 2 days at most, and the drug is rapidly tapered over the next 5 to 6 days. Oral corticosteroids have been reported to be helpful in decreasing radicular pain.[18] Other studies have found no significant relief of pain with dexamethasone compared with placebo.[17] The potential toxicity of the drug (hyperglycemia, fluid retention, hypertension, and infection) must be balanced against the potential benefit. In addition, the possibility of developing avascular necrosis of bone with 60 mg doses of dexamethasone must be considered.[13] The relationship between short courses of corticosteroids and the development of toxicities, such as osteonecrosis, remains controversial. If there is any doubt, the high dose of corticosteroid should not be given.

Lower doses of corticosteroids (5 to 30 mg daily) may be considered for patients who are resistant to other therapies or who have experienced toxicities to other drugs. Oral corticosteroids may be used before epidural injections in patients resistant to spinal injections. The dose of 20 to 30 mg is continued until radicular pain has improved or for a duration of 6 weeks. Patients who have improvement have their doses gradually tapered over a period of weeks as spinal nerve function improves. Those who receive no benefit have their doses rapidly tapered over days. The benefits of oral corticosteroids for radicular pain associated with a herniated disc or spinal stenosis have not been proven in a double-blind, placebo-controlled trial. The monetary cost of this therapy is minimal, and the risks of therapy are small as long as the oral doses are limited. Therefore, we believe this therapy to be worthwhile for patients with radiculopathy. Low-dose corticosteroids (prednisone, 5 mg) may be helpful with minimal toxicity in older individuals with spinal stenosis. Patients must be fully informed of the benefits and risks of therapy and must be followed carefully for the development of any corticosteroid-associated toxicities.

Analgesics

Non-narcotic Analgesics

The analgesic medications are divided into non-narcotic (acetaminophen, tramadol) and narcotic (codeine, oxycodone, meperidine, morphine) groups. Patients who are unable to tolerate the NSAIDs may benefit from a non-narcotic analgesic such as acetaminophen or tramadol.

ACETAMINOPHEN

Acetaminophen, a paraphenol derivative, is a pure analgesic with antipyretic but without anti-inflammatory effects. Acetaminophen inhibits central nervous system prostaglandin production but not peripheral production; this corresponds to its activity as an analgesic and antipyretic and its lack of effect as an anti-inflammatory agent. The drug is given in doses of 500 to 650 mg every 4 hours. Acetaminophen is packaged in an extended-release form. In this form, it is slowly released for 8 hours, allowing for a more sustained analgesic effect. Acetaminophen is probably a little less effective as an analgesic than aspirin but there is no gastrointestinal bleeding as there may be with acetylsalicylic acid. In addition, no cross-tolerance exists between NSAIDs and acetaminophen. Added analgesic effects can be demonstrated in patients who take both agents simultaneously. Acetaminophen should be considered as initial therapy for patients with osteoarthritis of the spine. For elderly patients, this drug has less toxicity than NSAIDs. However, many patients have tried acetaminophen before consulting a physician. In this circumstance, acetaminophen may be used in conjunction with an NSAID. The concomitant use of acetaminophen allows for a lower dose of NSAID to be effective for analgesia because both drugs have a synergistic effect for pain relief. The maximum dose of acetaminophen per day is 4000 mg. Hepatic damage is mainly due to a single toxic metabolite, *N*-acetyl-*p*-benzoquininemine, formed by oxidation of the drug. Glutathione conjugates and inactivates the metabolite. Ethanol induces the enzymes that oxidizes acetaminophen. Chronic alcohol intake depletes glutathione stores and induces the enzyme that oxidizes acetaminophen. This places chronic alcohol drinkers at risk from acetaminophen at high doses. Short-term studies of alcohol drinkers who have ingested acetaminophen in controlled trials have demonstrated no toxicity.[28] However, patients have claimed liver damage requiring liver transplantation related to the concomitant use of acetaminophen and ethanol. The lowest dose with constant monitoring should be used if individuals imbibe alcohol.

TRAMADOL

Tramadol HCl is a non-NSAID drug with analgesic properties that is equipotent to acetaminophen and codeine preparations. The drug has no prostaglandin inhibition and does not cause gastrointestinal bleeding. Tramadol is a pure, weak opioid agonist that also inhibits reuptake of serotonin and norepinephrine at the level of the dorsal horn, increasing neurotransmitter concentrations while downregulating central pain pathways. Tramadol is available as 50-mg tablets. It may be given at a total dose of 100 mg every 6 hours. The common toxicities of tramadol include nausea, dizziness, somnolence, and headaches. Tramadol may also decrease seizure threshold in individuals with epilepsy.

Tramadol has been studied compared with placebo in 380 patients with chronic low back pain.[41] In the design of the study, discontinuation was the primary outcome measure. The therapeutic failure rate of tramadol at a dose of

200 to 400 mg was 20.7% versus 51.3% in the placebo group. The pain score was significantly less in the tramadol (3.5 cm on a 10-cm scale) group versus placebo group (5.1 cm). Tramadol may also result in improved analgesia, allowing for dose reduction of concomitant NSAID therapy.[42] A combination tablet containing tramadol (37.5 mg) and acetaminophen (325 mg) is available. The agent offers the benefit of two complementary analgesics. In a 4-week study of tramadol/acetaminophen versus codeine/acetaminophen (30 mg/300 mg) for the treatment of chronic low back pain or osteoarthritis in 462 patients, the tramadol/acetaminophen combination was comparable to the other analgesic but with less somnolence and constipation.[33]

Narcotic Analgesics

The role of narcotic analgesics in the therapy for spinal disorders has changed since the last edition of this book. Previously, narcotics were avoided at all costs, with the fear of habituation being the overriding concern. This view overlooked the benefits of pain relief on physical and mental function that can be sustained with the appropriate choice of medication in the compliant patient. Many individuals with chronic low back pain have sources of pain that are related to permanent alterations of the spine or neural tissues (arachnoiditis). Some of these individuals have a neuropathic component to their chronic pain. The use of long-acting narcotics as a component of therapy decreases pain, increases function, and improves quality of life without drug seeking or tolerance.

Patients who experience an acute herniated nucleus pulposus may develop severe low back and radicular pain that is not relieved by NSAIDs alone. These patients may obtain analgesia with the use of codeine, 60 mg, every 4 to 6 hours in combination with acetaminophen or aspirin. These medications are given in conjunction with a therapeutic program of activities as tolerated and temperature modalities. Patients may require oral narcotic therapy (hydrocodone, oxycodone) in the acute situation to maintain function. Patients are given strict parameters for the use of these short-acting medicines. Inefficacy of the analgesic therapy must be reported to the physician so that appropriate interventions (injection therapy) are instituted as opposed to the continued escalation of narcotic dose of a short-acting drug.

In rare circumstances, parenteral narcotics (meperidine, morphine) are required (sickle cell crisis, vertebral compression fractures). These drugs are given on a regular basis, in adequate doses to relieve acute pain, while the patient receives other therapies. The chance of developing addiction to narcotics during a short course of therapy is small. Therefore, physicians should prescribe sufficient doses of narcotics to provide adequate analgesia.[48] Ketorolac is an effective parenteral or oral analgesic with potency similar to some narcotics.[35] Intramuscular ketorolac (60 mg) has comparable pain relief to intramuscular meperidine (1 mg/kg) for the treatment of acute low back pain with less sedation and gastrointestinal toxicities in the emergency department.[50] Hydrocodone (7.5 mg) and ibuprofen (200 mg) are available in a combination tablet. This combination of drugs is as effective as a more potent narcotic with acetaminophen. In a study of 147 patients with acute low back pain treated for up to 8 days, the combination of hydrocodone (7.5 mg) and ibuprofen (200 mg) was as effective as that of oxycodone (5 mg) and acetaminophen (325 mg) with similar frequencies of toxicity.[36] As pain decreases, non-narcotic analgesics are substituted for the more potent narcotic analgesics.

Patients with chronic spinal pain need to be treated in an effective manner to improve their quality of life. Patients with metastatic cancer to the spine, osteoporotic vertebral compression fractures, failed back surgery, or severe end-stage inflammatory arthritis of the spine are examples of individuals who benefit from tonic control of spinal pain. In these patients, regular narcotic therapy, such as morphine sulfate in a controlled release form, may allow pain relief so that the patient is functional.[20] Patients may find other oral sustained-release forms of narcotics (oxycodone) most helpful. Patients with chronic pain may find transdermal administration of a narcotic a preferable mode of administration of a drug (Table 19-10). Methadone has a long plasma half-life of 24 hours but an intermediate length of action of 4 to 8 hours for analgesia. The once-a-day dosing would not be appropriate for pain therapy. Patients should be informed that they are not addicts if they require long-term narcotic therapy for pain relief. They become physically dependent. They rarely become tolerant and do not require increasing doses of medicine once they reach their maintenance dose. The number of individuals who become addicted to narcotics after exposure to the drug is minimal. For example, a large survey of inpatients, the Boston Collaborative Drug Surveillance Project, identified only four cases of addiction among 11,882 hospitalized patients with no history of substance abuse.[39]

Narcotic therapy has been shown to be effective for individuals with chronic spinal pain. In a study of 25,479 patients with spinal pain, 3.4% had opioids included in their therapeutic regimen. These individuals had symptoms longer than 3 months and a greater incidence of objective findings.[12]

In a study of 36 patients with low back pain treated with naproxen, set-dose oxycodone, or titrated-dose oxycodone and sustained-release morphine sulfate, patients with the titrated sustained-release narcotic had less pain and emotional distress than the other groups. Little difference was noted with activity or hours asleep. Only one participant showed signs of abuse behavior. However, once tapered off narcotics, no long-term benefit was noted.[25] As reported by Hale and colleagues, controlled-release oxycodone given every 12 hours is comparable to immediate-release oxycodone given four times daily in a study of 57 adult outpatients with chronic back pain.[19] The sustained-release oxycodone dose was below 40 mg in 68% of patients. Schofferman reported on 28 patients who received long-term opioid analgesic therapy and were followed for a mean of 32 months versus 5 patients who discontinued the narcotics because of intolerable side effects followed for the same period of time.[43] Twenty-one patients were able to tolerate the drug and improved in regard to pain relief and improved function. The doses remained stable (methadone, levorphanol, sustained-release morphine), and no illicit drug abuse occurred.

19-10 NARCOTIC DRUGS*

Drug	Brand Name	Route	Size	Frequency	Half-Life	Duration
Morphine	MSIR	Oral	15/30 mg 20 mg/mL	q4h	2-3 hr	3-6 hr
Morphine CR	MS Contin	Oral	15, 30, 60, 100, 200 mg	q12h	2-3 hr	8-12 hr
Morphine SR	Kadian	Oral	20, 30, 50, 60, 100 mg	q24h	2-3 hr	24 hr
	Avinza	Oral	30, 60, 90, 120 mg	q24h	2-3 hr	24 hr
Oxycodone	OxyIR	Oral	5 mg 20 mg/mL		2-3 hr	3-6 hr
	Oxycontin	Oral	10, 20 mg	q12h	2-3 hr	8-12 hr
Fentanyl	Duragesic	Transdermal	25, 50, 75, 100 μg	q48-72h	13-22 hr	48-72 hr
	Actiq	Transmucosal (cancer RX)	200, 400, 600, 800, 1200, 1600 mg	q6h	7 hr	6-12 hr

*This is only a partial listing.

Transdermal fentanyl is another form of long-acting opioid therapy that is effective for chronic pain of spinal origin. Simpson and colleagues reported on 50 patients with chronic pain with between one to five spinal surgeries with inadequate control of pain with oral narcotic medications.[47] The doses were titrated to 25 μg (n = 40), 50 μg (n = 6), 75 μg (n = 3), or 100 μg (n = 1) in this open-label study. Fentanyl was continued for 1 month and then the oral narcotic therapy was resumed. Pain and disability were significantly reduced in 86% of patients compared with oral narcotic therapy. A fentanyl patch should be considered for patients with chronic spinal pain resistant to other narcotic medications. Fentanyl patches were also effective in improving quality of life and pain at rest in 61% of patients with back pain associated with vertebral osteoporosis.[40]

Our Recommendation

NSAIDs are a mainstay of therapy for patients with acute or chronic low back or neck pain. The smallest effective dose should be used. Long-acting NSAIDs have the convenience of once-a-day dosing but must have adequate analgesic effects to be effective. The toxicities of the NSAIDs remain a concern in the sustained use of these drugs. The COX-2 inhibitors are a better choice in individuals with increased risk of gastrointestinal toxicities. The use of analgesics is appropriate to limit acute pain. The selection of a narcotic for a patient is appropriate when additional analgesia is required to improve function and quality of life.

References

NSAIDs, Analgesics, and Narcotics

1. Abramson SB, Weissmann G: The mechanisms of action of nonsteroidal anti-inflammatory drugs. Arthritis Rheum 32:1, 1989.
2. Baigent C, Patrono C: Selective cyclooxygenase 2 inhibitors, aspirin, and cardiovascular disease: A reappraisal. Arthritis Rheum 48:12-20, 2003.
3. Berry H, Bloom B, Hamilton EBD, Swinson DR: Naproxen sodium, diflunisal, and placebo in the treatment of chronic back pain. Ann Rheum Dis 41:129, 1982.
4. Bombardier C, Laine L, Reicin A, et al: Comparison of upper gastrointestinal toxicity of rofecoxib and naproxen in patients with rheumatoid arthritis. VIGOR study group. N Engl J Med 343:1520-1528, 2000.
5. Borda IT, Koff RS: NSAIDs: A Profile of Adverse Effects. Philadelphia, Hanley & Belfus, 1992, p 240.
6. Brandt KD: Should osteoarthritis be treated with nonsteroidal anti-inflammatory drugs? Rheum Dis Clin North Am 19:697, 1993.
7. Carson JL, Strom BL, Schinnar R, et al: The low risk of upper gastrointestinal bleeding in patients dispensed corticosteroids. Am J Med 91:223, 1991.
8. Chandrasekharan NV, Dai H, Lamar Tureu Roos K, et al: COX-3, a cyclooxygenase-1 variant inhibited by acetaminophen and other analgesic/antipyretic drugs: Cloning, structure, and expression. Proc Natl Acad Sci U S A 99:13926-13931, 2002.
9. Clive DM, Stoff JS: Renal syndrome associated with nonsteroidal anti-inflammatory drugs. N Engl J Med 310:563, 1984.
10. Crofford LJ, Lipsky PE, Brooks P, et al: Basic biology and clinical application of specific cyclooxygenase-2 inhibitors. Arthritis Rheum 43:4-13, 2000.
11. Dahl SL: Nonsteroidal anti-inflammatory agents: Clinical pharmacology/adverse effects/usage guidelines. In Willkens RF, Dahl SL (eds): Therapeutic Controversies in the Rheumatic Diseases. Orlando, FL, Grune & Stratton, 1987, pp 27-68.
12. Fanciullo GJ, Ball PA, Girault G, et al: An observational study on the prevalence and pattern of opioid use in 25,479 patients with spine and radicular pain. Spine 27:201-205, 2002.
13. Fast A, Alon M, Weiss S, et al: Avascular necrosis of bone following the short-term dexamethasone therapy for brain edema. J Neurosurg 61:983, 1984.
14. Feldman M, Mc Mahon AT: Do cyclooxygenase-2 inhibitors provide benefits similar to those of traditional nonsteroidal anti-inflammatory drugs, with less gastrointestinal toxicity? Ann Intern Med 132:134-143, 2000.
15. Goldie I: A clinical trial with indomethacin (Indomee) in low back pain and sciatica. Acta Orthop Scand 39:117, 1968.
16. Green LN: Dexamethasone in the management of symptoms due to herniated lumbar disc. J Neurol Neurosurg Psychiatry 38:1211, 1975.
17. Haimovic IC, Beresford HR: Dexamethasone is not superior to placebo for treating lumbosacral radicular pain Neurology 36:1593-1594, 1986.
18. Hakelius A: Prognosis in sciatica: A clinical follow-up of surgical and nonsurgical treatment. Acta Orthop Scand 129 (Suppl):1, 1970.
19. Hale ME, Fleischmann R, Salzman R, et al: Efficacy and safety of controlled-release versus immediate-release oxycodone: Randomized, double-blind evaluation in patients with chronic back pain. Clin J Pain 15:179-183, 1999.
20. Hanks GW, et al: Controlled-release morphine tablets: A double-blind trial in patients with advanced cancer. Anesthesia 42:840, 1987.
21. Hart FD: Naproxen and gastrointestinal hemorrhage. BMJ 2:51, 1974.

22. Hickey RFJ: Chronic low back pain: A comparison of diflunisal with paracetamol. N Z Med J 95:312, 1982.
23. Holdstock DJ: Gastrointestinal bleeding: A possible association with ibuprofen. Lancet 1:541, 1972.
24. Huskisson EC: Non-narcotic analgesics. In Wall PD, Melzack R (eds): Textbook of Pain. Edinburgh, Churchill Livingstone, 1984, pp 505-513.
25. Jamison RN, Raymond SA, Slawsby EA, et al: Opioid therapy for chronic noncancer back pain: A randomized prospective study. Spine 23:2591-2600, 1998.
26. Katz N: Coxibs: Evolving role in pain management. Semin Arthritis Rheum 32(Suppl 3):15-24, 2002.
27. Katz N, Ju WD, Krupa DA, et al: Efficacy and safety of rofecoxib in patients with chronic low back pain: Results from two 4-week, randomized, placebo-controlled, parallel-group, double-blind trials. Spine 28:851-859, 2003.
28. Kuffner EK, Dart RC, Bogdan GM, et al: Effect of maximal daily doses of acetaminophen on the liver of alcoholic patients: A randomized, double-blind, placebo-controlled trial. Arch Intern Med 161:2247-2252, 2001.
29. Lanza FL: Endoscopic studies of gastric and duodenal injury after the use of ibuprofen, aspirin, and other nonsteroidal anti-inflammatory agents. Am J Med 77:19, 1984.
30. Levy M: Aspirin use in patients with major upper gastrointestinal bleeding and peptic ulcer disease. N Engl J Med 290:1158, 1974.
31. Miceli-Richard C, Dougados M: NSAIDs in ankylosing spondylitis. Clin Exp Rheumatol 20(Suppl 28):S65-S66, 2002.
32. Moore RA, McQuay HJ, Carroll O, et al: Single and multiple dose analgesic and kinetic studies of mefenamic acid in chronic back pain. Clin J Pain 2:39, 1986.
33. Mullican WS, Lacy JR; TRAMAP-ANAG-600 study group: Tramadol/acetaminophen combination tablets and codeine/acetaminophen combination capsules for the management of chronic pain: A comparative trial. Clin Ther 23:1429-1445, 2001.
34. Nielsen GL, Sorensen HT, Mellemkjoer L, et al: Risk of hospitalization resulting from upper gastrointestinal bleeding among patients taking corticosteroids: A register-based cohort study. Am J Med 111:541-545, 2001.
35. O'Hara DA, Fragen RJ, Kinzer M, et al: Ketorolac tromethamine as compared with morphine sulfate for treatment of postoperative pain. Clin Pharmacol Ther 41:556, 1987.
36. Palangio M, Morris E, Doyle RT Jr, et al: Combination hydrocodone and ibuprofen versus combination oxycodone and acetaminophen in the treatment of moderate or severe low back pain. Clin Ther 24:87-99, 2002.
37. Paulus HE, Bulpitt KJ: Nonsteroidal anti-inflammatory agents and corticosteroids. In Schumacker HR Jr (ed): Primer of the Rheumatic Diseases, 10th ed. Atlanta, Arthritis Foundation, 1993, pp 298-303.
38. Piper JM, Ray WA, Daugherty JR, et al: Corticosteroid use and peptic ulcer disease: Role of nonsteroidal anti-inflammatory drugs. Ann Intern Med 114:735, 1991.
39. Porter J, Jick H: Addiction rare in patients treated with narcotics [Letter]. N Engl J Med 302:123, 1980.
40. Ringe JD, Faber H, Bock O, et al: Transdermal fentanyl for the treatment of back pain caused by vertebral osteoporosis. Rheumatol Int 22:199-203, 2002.
41. Schnitzer TJ, Gray WL, Paster RZ, et al: Efficacy of tramadol in treatment of chronic low back pain. J Rheumatol 27:772-778, 2000.
42. Schnitzer TJ, Kamin M, Olson WH: Tramadol allows reduction of naproxen dose among patients with naproxen-responsive osteoarthritis pain: A randomized, double-blind, placebo-controlled study. Arthritis Rheum 42:1370-1377, 1999.
43. Schofferman J: Long-term opioid analgesic therapy for severe refractory lumbar spine pain. Clin J Pain 15:136-140, 1999.
44. Shaw J, Brooks PM, McNeil JJ, et al: Therapeutic usage of the nonsteroidal anti-inflammatory drugs. Med J Aust 149:203, 1988.
45. Simon LS, Mills JS: Drug therapy: Nonsteroidal anti-inflammatory drugs. N Engl J Med 302:1179, 1237, 1980.
46. Simon LS, Weaver AL, Graham DY, et al: Anti-inflammatory and upper gastrointestinal effects of celecoxib in rheumatoid arthritis: A randomized, controlled trial. JAMA 282:1921-1928, 1999.
47. Simpson RK, Edmondson EA, Constant CF, et al: Transdermal fentanyl as treatment for chronic low back pain. J Pain Symp Manag 17:218-224, 1999.
48. Stimmel B: Pain, analgesia, and addiction: An approach to the pharmacologic management of pain. Clin J Pain 1:14, 1985.
49. van Tulder MW, Scholten RJPM, Koes BW, et al: Nonsteroidal anti-inflammatory drugs for low back pain: A systematic review within the framework of the Cochrane Collaboration Back Review Group. Spine 25:2501-2513, 2000.
50. Veenema KR, Leahey N, Schneider S: Ketorolac versus meperidine: ED treatment of severe musculoskeletal low back pain. Am J Emerg Med 18:404-407, 2000.
51. Videman T, Osterman K: Double-blind parallel study of piroxicam versus indomethacin in the treatment of low back pain. Ann Clin Res 16:156, 1984.
52. Walt RP: Misoprostol for the treatment of peptic ulcer and anti-inflammatory drug-induced gastroduodenal ulceration. N Engl J Med 327:1575, 1992.
53. Wiesel SW, Cuckler JM, DeLuca F, et al: Acute low back pain: An objective analysis of conservative therapy. Spine 5:324, 1980.
54. Wolfe MM, Lichtenstein DR, Singh G: Gastrointestinal toxicity of nonsteroidal anti-inflammatory drugs. N Engl J Med 340:1888-1899, 1999.

MUSCLE RELAXANTS

Although muscle relaxants have been employed in the treatment of spinal pain for a number of years, their use has remained controversial. Not all physicians believe that these agents have a therapeutic role in the care of patients with spinal pain. There are a number of reasons why this is the case (Table 19-11). Muscle spasm in the low back or neck may have a number of causes, including local pathologic processes and referred mechanisms. No one therapy is effective in all forms of muscle spasm. Muscle relaxants do not relieve spasm in all patients with tonic muscle contraction. Some physicians believe muscle spasm to be a natural, protective mechanism by which the body heals itself; consequently, the dissipation of spasm should occur naturally as the underlying lesion heals and should not be speeded up with medications. Others do not believe that patients with spinal pain actually experience muscle spasm, since muscles are not damaged in this disorder. The anatomic abnormality is in the annular fibers of the disc. Therefore, muscle relaxants are not useful in improving the condition, because the medications have no effect on healing the disc disorder.

Other reasons for resistance to using muscle relaxants involve their site of action. Many of these drugs do not work on the muscles themselves but instead act on the central nervous system to modify muscle tone. Differences of opinion exist in regard to the concentration of medication needed in the bloodstream to achieve muscle relaxation. Some physicians believe that the concentration obtained in the blood is adequate to affect muscle spindle function.

19-11 REASONS CITED FOR RESISTANCE TO THE USE OF MUSCLE RELAXANTS IN LOW BACK PAIN
Multiple causes of low back spasm (posture, arthritis, referred pain from viscera)
Muscle spasm as "natural protective mechanism"
Drug effect: central nervous system—sedation
Drug toxicity: addiction, depression (diazepam)
Few scientific studies demonstrating efficacy

Others think that blood concentration is sufficient to cause sedation only by effects on the central nervous system. In other words, these physicians view muscle relaxants as sedatives rather than relaxants and consider them to be ineffective in the therapy for this muscle disorder. In addition, some of these agents have serious potential toxicities including addiction (diazepam). The use of benzodiazepines causes depression, which compounds the difficulties of patients with chronic spinal pain who are already depressed from long-term pain and disability. Finally, the number of scientific studies that have investigated the role of these agents in the care of patients with low back or neck pain, acute or chronic, is relatively small,[1,4,8,17,18,20,21,27,37] and the number of studies that actually demonstrate efficacy is even smaller.[13] Therefore, anecdotal evidence and clinical experience are often offered as proof of efficacy, but to some physicians that evidence is inadequate to justify the use of muscle relaxants.[19]

Some of these criticisms of muscle relaxants are valid. These agents are not indicated for all patients with spinal pain. However, they do seem to relieve symptoms in carefully selected patients and should not be condemned outright.[20] In our experience, the combination of a muscle relaxant and an NSAID has been effective in decreasing symptoms and improving function, including return to work.[5] Patients with the combination of low back pain and involuntary, chronic muscle contraction benefit from a course of an NSAID and a muscle relaxant. In a study of patients with acute low back pain and tonic muscle contraction, the combination of naproxen and cyclobenzaprine was more effective than naproxen alone in decreasing pain.[7] A similar study using diflunisal and cyclobenzaprine also demonstrated a beneficial effect by day 4 of the combination therapy compared with placebo.[2]

Pathophysiology of Muscle Spasm

The interrelation of the sensory and motor systems is clearly recognized at the level of the spinal cord. This relationship involves the classic reflex arc in which stretching of a tendon (afferent-sensory input) results in a reflex contraction of the corresponding muscle (efferent-motor output). Adding to this simple arc are inputs from other levels of the spinal cord, the brain stem, and the cerebral cortex, which alter the threshold of the reflex arc. Increased muscle tension may occur as a consequence of intramuscular (trauma, fatigue), perimuscular (arthritis, bone fracture), or referred pain (kidney stone) processes.

Local trauma to muscles may cause reflex spasm. Tissue damage activates nociceptive (unmyelinated) nerve fibers that are distributed through tendons, fascial sheaths, and adventitial sheaths of intramuscular blood vessels. Increased muscle tension decreases muscle movement and allows for the damaged area to heal, usually in a contracted position.[22] In addition to the nociceptive input derived from tissue damage, pain sensations may be generated through muscle fatigue associated with tonic contraction. Muscles that are chronically fatigued become locally painful and tender. This process may occur secondary to chronic contraction associated with trauma or to hyperactivity of muscles associated with poor posture and occupational or sports activities.[32] Muscle spasm may continue while the patient sleeps, as measured by nocturnal EMG recordings.[15] The pain associated with chronic fatigue may be related to the inadequate blood flow that accompanics muscle hyperactivity.[26] That component of muscle pain related to overuse may be relieved with rest and increased blood flow promoted by heat or massage.

Muscle spasm may also occur in response to disease processes in structures to which muscles and tendons attach. Inflammatory processes affecting joints in the axial skeleton can result in reflex muscle spasm, which limits mobility. Patients with spondyloarthropathies are prime examples of this mechanism. Patients with sacroiliitis may develop piriformis syndrome with contraction of that muscle and compression of the sciatic nerve. Therapy directed at decreasing joint inflammation, and thereby muscle spasm, decreases the symptoms of this syndrome. Patients who experience vertebral compression fractures develop severe spasm in paraspinous muscles. The muscles contract to splint the fractured bone, limiting painful motion. Once the fracture is diagnosed and pain is relieved, muscle spasm diminishes. Continued spasm is not necessary for healing of the fracture. Patients with spondylitis of the neck may experience associated paracervical muscle spasm. Relief of spasm while the patient limits activities is appropriate and decreases pain.

Spasm that is secondary to sensory input from organs with common innervation results from the common connections of these nerve fibers in the spinal cord.[24] Abnormalities in the gastrointestinal, genitourinary, and vascular systems may cause reflex spasm in the lumbosacral or cervical spine. Therapy must be given to alleviate the primary disorder for muscle spasm to be relieved.

Action of Muscle Relaxants

The exact mechanism of action of the muscle relaxants is not known. Depression of polysynaptic, to a greater degree than monosynaptic, reflexes has been reported in animal studies.[30,33] These effects are mediated through the central nervous system. The area of the central nervous system affected is the lateral reticular area of the brain stem, which monitors the facilitative and inhibitory nerve pathways that affect the activity of the muscle stretch reflexes.[16] The effects of these agents may be mediated through enhanced stimulation of gamma-aminobutyric acid (GABA) neurons, which play a significant role in the inhibition of tonic facilitative input from supraspinal sources on motor neurons, both alpha and gamma. This effect on GABA receptors has been associated with the action of benzodiazepines (diazepam).[34] The oral doses of the muscle relaxants are below the levels needed in animal studies to achieve muscle relaxation. As mentioned, this fact has been used by some investigators to conclude that the beneficial effect of muscle relaxants is, in fact, sedation. Clinically, sedation is noted by some but not all patients who ingest any of the members of this group of agents. It should be noted, however, that some patients obtain muscle relaxation without associated sedation. Sedation was not associated with the beneficial effect of muscle relaxation in a study of 1405 patients with acute low back and neck muscle spasm treated with cyclobenzaprine at 10 mg, 5 mg, or 2.5 mg three times a day.[6]

The oral muscle relaxants have been shown to be better than placebo in acute muscle spasm. There are fewer studies demonstrating efficacy in chronic muscle spasm. Combinations of muscle relaxants and analgesics are more effective than their individual components in the control of muscle spasm.[14] The Drug Efficacy and Safety Implementation Program of the Food and Drug Administration has categorized all such combination products as possibly effective. The muscle relaxants alone do not provide analgesia, although cyclobenzaprine, 5 mg and 10 mg, three times a day alone was associated with pain relief in acute muscle spasm of the neck or low back.[6]

The drugs included in the oral muscle relaxant group are cyclobenzaprine (Flexeril), chlorphenesin (Maolate), orphenadrine citrate (Norflex), chlorzoxazone (Paraflex, Parafon Forte DSC), methocarbamol (Robaxin), metaxalone (Skelaxin), carisoprodol (Soma), and diazepam (Valium). Combinations of these agents with analgesics include the drugs Norgesic, Parafon Forte, Robaxisal, Soma Compound, and Soma Compound with Codeine (Table 19-12).

Clinical Trial Outcomes

Muscle relaxants have been studied and found to be better than placebo in both acute and chronic muscle spasm. Both carisoprodol and chlorphenesin were effective in acute but not chronic disorders.[11,23,36,38] In studies of acute pain, chlorzoxazone, metaxalone, and methocarbamol were also effective.[12,28,35] Cyclobenzaprine was compared with placebo in chronic disorders and was found to be superior.[3,4,8] Diazepam was not better than placebo in acute and chronic pain in hospitalized patients.[3] In unspecified musculoskeletal disorders, chlorphenesin, chlorzoxazone, and methocarbamol were found better than placebo but diazepam was not.[25,29,31,37] Cyclobenzaprine offers improvement with acute muscle spasm that appears early in the course of treatment.[9]

Studies comparing muscle relaxants have been completed but the results do not demonstrate the clear superiority of any one agent.[14] Combination tablets appear to be more effective than single agents alone. However, no difference among the combination products was noted.[14]

Borenstein and Korn reported on two placebo-controlled trials of the treatment of acute muscle spasm of the low back or neck with cyclobenzaprine at 10 mg, 5 mg, or 2.5 mg three times a day versus placebo.[6] The primary efficacy measures were patient-rated clinical global impression of change, medication helpfulness, and relief from starting muscle ache. Neither study allowed an NSAID or analgesic as an active control. A total of 1405 patients (study 1, n = 737; study 2, n = 668) were studied, with two thirds having back pain and one third having neck pain. Over the 7-day study, cyclobenzaprine, 5 mg three times a day, was equally effective as 10 mg three times a day (2.5 mg was ineffective) and had fewer adverse events (including sedation) compared with 10 mg.

Cherkin and co-workers conducted a longitudinal observational study of the efficacy of medications at 7 days for the treatment of acute low back pain.[10] A total of 219 patients with back pain who made a visit to the Puget Sound Health Maintenance Organization were contacted by telephone 1 week after the appointment to assess symptom severity and physical dysfunction. The drugs prescribed included none in 21%, NSAIDs in 69%, muscle relaxants in 35%, narcotics in 12%, and acetaminophen in 4%. Patients who received medications had more pain below the knee, less than 3 weeks of pain before the visit, more severe symptoms, greater dysfunction, or a desire for medication. Almost 50% of the patients took medication before the visit to the physician. Almost 90% of those reporting self-medication were taking NSAIDs. Those receiving medications had less severe symptoms after 1 week than did patients who received no medication. Patients receiving a muscle relaxant and an NSAID had the best outcome. Although this study lacked a double-blind, placebo-controlled design, the study reported the utility of NSAIDs and muscle relaxants in the therapy for acute low back pain.

Toxicities

The major side effect of these agents is drowsiness. Other central nervous system effects include headache, dizziness, and blurred vision. Cyclobenzaprine causes dry mouth. Nausea and vomiting occur rarely with all these agents. Orphenadrine may have a direct depressant and anticholinergic effect on the heart, which may cause arrhythmias and cardiac arrest at lethal doses of 2 to 3 g. Carisoprodol is metabolized to meprobamate, an anxiolytic, that is a controlled substance. Chronic use of carisoprodol may be associated with tolerance for the drug. Patients may ask for increasing doses of the medicine for the same muscle relaxing effect. The medicine may also cause severe drowsiness and dizziness.

Diazepam is a muscle relaxant that is not used with our patients with spinal pain. While the evidence for efficacy of this agent in back spasm is meager, its toxicities are real and troublesome. One cannot predict which patients with acute spinal pain will go on to develop chronic low back or neck pain and depression. Diazepam will only worsen the depression and drug dependence of these patients. The drug is not indicated in this disorder.

The sedation that occurs in some patients occurs in a minority. The sedation associated with the drug usually appears early at the initiation of the drug. This sedative effect diminishes over time with continued use of the drug. The drug is continued for up to 2 weeks in patients with acute spasm. Patients are easily tapered off the medicine without any withdrawal symptoms. If there is no response to cyclobenzaprine, then chlorzoxazone, orphenadrine, methocarbamol, or carisoprodol may be substituted (see Table 19-12). Higher dosages and more frequent administration are necessary to achieve adequate levels of these other medications. These agents belong to different chemical groups, and, as with the NSAIDs, a lack of response to one agent does not equate with inefficacy of the whole group of drugs. A series of agents may be tried before an efficacious and well-tolerated agent is found. The total dose of medication and frequency of administration must

19-12 ORAL MUSCLE RELAXANTS

Drug	Brand Name	Tablet/Capsule Size (mg)	Dose (mg/day)	Frequency (times/day)	Onset (hr)	Duration (hr)	Half-Life	Major Toxicity	Excretion	Comments
Cyclobenzaprine hydrochloride	Flexeril	10/5	15-60	1-3	1-2	12-24	1-3 days	Drowsiness, dry mouth, dizziness	Kidney, stool	5 or 10 mg 2 hours before sleep may be adequate dose with half-life; Caution: angle-closure glaucoma, prostatic hypertrophy, myocardial infarction
Chlorphenesin carbamate	Maolate	400	1600-2400	3-4	3	4-6	5 hr	Drowsiness, dizziness	Kidney	
Orphenadrine citrate	Norflex Norgesic	100 30 mg/dL	200	2	2	4-6	14 hr	Blurred vision, dry mouth, urinary retention	Kidney, stool	Intravenous form for therapy for acute spasm (Norgesic includes aspirin and caffeine)
Chlorzoxazone	Paraflex Parafon Forte DSC	250 500	1500-3000	3-4	1	3-4	1 hr	Drowsiness, dizziness	Kidney	Parafon Forte includes acetaminophen Contraindicated—history of liver disease
Methocarbamol	Robaxin Robaxisal	500, 750 100 mg/dL	6000	4-6	1	3	2 hr	Dizziness, blurred vision	Kidney, stool	Intravenous form for acute spasm, tetanus (Robaxisal includes aspirin)
Metaxalone	Skelaxin	400/800	2400-3200	3-4	1	4-6	2-3 hr	Drowsiness	Kidney	
Carisoprodol	Soma	350	1400	4	1	4-6	8 hr	Drowsiness	Kidney	Extreme weakness Temporary loss of vision (rare) Mild withdrawal symptoms with abrupt cessation Contraindicated—acute intermittent porphyria (Soma compound includes aspirin)
Diazepam	Valium	2, 5, 10 (5 mg/mL, 15 slow release)	4-40	4	1	8-12	24 hr	Drowsiness	Kidney	Withdrawal symptoms with abrupt cessation Depression with prolonged use

be individualized. Occasionally, combination tablets (Parafon Forte, Robaxisal) are used. These preparations are convenient because the muscle relaxant and analgesic are in the same tablet, but the amount of medicine is fixed, limiting the flexibility in dosage that some patients require.

Use with Spondyloarthropathies

The use of muscle relaxants is not limited to traumatic muscle strain alone. Patients with arthritic conditions, particularly the spondyloarthropathies, may benefit from long-term use of a muscle relaxant. The following case is presented as an example of a patient with a spondyloarthropathy who had greater mobility because of the use of a muscle relaxant.

Case Study 19-2

J.A. is a 46-year-old man admitted to the hospital because of neck, right buttock, left index finger, left great toe, and right heel pain that developed over a 3-week period after a fall from a 2-foot garden wall. The patient had marked limitation of cervical motion in all directions, associated with marked paravertebral muscle spasm. Swollen joints included the right knee, ankle, heel and left great toe, and index finger. The diagnosis of incomplete Reiter's syndrome was made and the patient was started on indomethacin, 50 mg three times a day, which was increased to 75 mg slow-release three times a day. The patient's lower and upper extremity arthritis improved, but severe muscle spasm of the cervical spine continued. Cyclobenzaprine, 10 mg twice daily, was added and the patient had gradual improvement in his neck motion. There was an exacerbation of symptoms after discharge from the hospital. Cyclobenzaprine was increased to 30 mg/day, and prednisone, 10 mg/day, was added. Over the next 2 months, the patient's symptoms gradually resolved. One year after discharge, the patient was able to discontinue prednisone therapy. Attempts at reducing cyclobenzaprine were associated with decreased neck motion. The patient remains on indomethacin, 75 mg twice daily, and cyclobenzaprine, 10 mg, at night. He is active and is able to complete a full day's work without difficulty. He volunteers the fact that he believes that the muscle relaxant played a substantial role in his recovery.

An anecdotal case report does not prove efficacy scientifically. However, clinical observation is a reasonable means to study the effects of therapeutic interventions. Other patients with spondyloarthropathies have been placed on muscle relaxants and have noted decreased pain and improved motion with the addition of a muscle relaxant to the NSAID. Muscle relaxants are not indicated for all patients with spinal pain. In the carefully chosen patient, however, their use can relieve symptoms while the natural course of healing unfolds.

Our Recommendation

Muscle relaxants are useful in patients who, on examination, have palpable evidence of muscle spasm or who have difficulty sleeping because of muscle pain. These patients may be experiencing spasm, although their primary symptom is pain.[15] While superior efficacy has not been demonstrated for any one muscle relaxant, the chemical properties of cyclobenzaprine are very useful in the clinical setting. The drug is not combined with any analgesic, so it can be used with any of the NSAIDs or analgesics. Its long half-life equates with once-a-day dosing in many patients. The medication is given 2 hours before sleep; this time interval allows the medicine to build up in the bloodstream so that the patient is sleepy at the appropriate time if he or she develops somnolence. The patient awakens the next day feeling rested and not drowsy. Recent studies have demonstrated the efficacy of the 5-mg tablet as an adequate dose for many patients.

References

Muscle Relaxants

1. Baratta RR: A double-blind comparative study of carisoprodol, propoxyphene, and placebo in the management of low back syndrome. Curr Ther Res 20:233, 1976.
2. Basmajian JV: Acute back pain and spasm: A controlled multicenter trial of combined analgesic and antispasm agents. Spine 14:438, 1989.
3. Basmajian JV: Cyclobenzaprine hydrochloride effect on skeletal muscle in the lumbar region and neck: Two double-blind controlled clinical and laboratory studies. Arch Phys Med Rehabil 59:58, 1978.
4. Bercel NA: Cyclobenzaprine in the treatment of skeletal muscle spasm in osteoarthritis of the cervical and lumbar spine. Curr Ther Res Clin Exp 22:462, 1977.
5. Borenstein D, Feffer H, Wiesel S: Low back pain (LBP): An orthopedic and medical approach. Clin Res 33:757A, 1985.
6. Borenstein DG, Korn S: Efficacy of a low-dose regimen of cyclobenzaprine hydrochloride in acute skeletal muscle spasm: Results of two placebo-controlled trials. Clin Ther 25:1056-1073, 2003.
7. Borenstein DG, Lacks S, Wiesel SW: Cyclobenzaprine and naproxen versus naproxen alone in the treatment of acute low back pain and muscle spasm. Clin Ther 12;125, 1990.
8. Brown BR, Womble J: Cyclobenzaprine in intractable pain syndromes with muscle spasm. JAMA 240:1151, 1978.
9. Browning R, Jackson JL, O'Malley PG: Cyclobenzaprine and back pain: A meta-analysis. Arch Intern Med 161:1613-1620, 2001.
10. Cherkin DC, Wheeler KJ, Barlow W, et al: Medication use for low back pain in primary care. Spine 23:607-614, 1998.
11. Cullen AP: Carisoprodol (Soma) in acute back conditions: A double-blind randomized, placebo-controlled study. Curr Ther Res Clin Exp 20:557, 1976.
12. Dent RW, Ervin DK: A study of metaxalone (Skelaxin) vs placebo in acute musculoskeletal disorders: A cooperative study. Curr Ther Res Clin Exp 18:433, 1975.
13. Deyo RA: Conservative therapy for low back pain: Distinguishing useful from useless therapy. JAMA 250:1057, 1983.
14. Elenbaas JK: Centrally acting oral skeletal muscle relaxants. Am J Hosp Pharm 37:1313, 1980.
15. Fischer AA, Chang CH: Electromyographic evidence of paraspinal muscle spasm during sleep in patients with low back pain. Clin J Pain 1:147, 1985.
16. Ginzel KH: The blockade of reticular and spinal facilitation of motor function by orphenadrine. J Pharmacol Exp Ther 154:128, 1966.
17. Gordon EF: Carisoprodol in the treatment of musculoskeletal disorders of the back. Am J Orthop 5:106, 1963.
18. Gready DM: Parafon Forte versus Robaxisal in skeletal muscle disorders: A double-blind study. Curr Ther Res 20:666, 1976.
19. Hadler NM: Diagnosis and treatment of backache. In Hadler NM (ed): Medical Management of the Regional Musculoskeletal Diseases. Orlando, FL, Grune & Stratton, 1984, pp 3-52.
20. Hindle TH: Comparison of carisoprodol, butabarbital, and placebo in treatment of the low back syndrome. Calif Med 117:7, 1972.
21. Hingorani K: Diazepam in backaches: A double-blind controlled trial. Ann Phys Med 8:303, 1966.

22. Jarvinen TAH, Kaarianen M, Jarvinen M, et al: Muscle strain injuries. Curr Opin Rheumatol 12:155-161, 2000.
23. Jones AC: Role of carisoprodol in physical medicine. Ann N Y Acad Sci 86:226, 1960.
24. Kerr FWL: Neuroanatomical substrates of nociception in the spinal cord. Pain 1:325, 1975.
25. Kolodny AL: Controlled clinical evaluation of a new muscle relaxant—chlorphenesin carbamate. Psychosomatics 4:161, 1963.
26. Kuroda E, Klissouras V, Mulsum JH: Electrical and metabolic activities and fatigue in human isometric contraction. J Appl Physiol 29:358, 1970.
27. McGuinnes BW: A double-blind comparison in general practice of a combination tablet containing orphenadrine citrate and paracetamol (Norgesic) with paracetamol alone. J Int Med Res 11:42, 1983.
28. Ogden HD, Shackett L: Controlled studies of chlorzoxazone and chlorzoxazone-acetaminophen in treatment of myalgia associated with headache. South Med J 53:1415, 1960.
29. Payne RW, Xorenson EJ, Smalley TK, Brandt EN Jr: Diazepam, meprobamate, and placebo in musculoskeletal disorders. JAMA 188:229, 1964.
30. Roszkowski AP: A pharmacological comparison of therapeutically useful centrally-acting skeletal muscle relaxants. J Pharmacol Exp Ther 129:75, 1970.
31. Schiener JJ: Evaluation of combined muscle relaxant-analgesic as an effective therapy for painful skeletal muscle spasm. Curr Ther Res Clin Exp 14:168, 1972.
32. Simons DG: Muscle pain syndrome: II. Am J Phys Med 55:15, 1976.
33. Smith CM: Relaxants of skeletal muscle. In Root WS, Hoffman FG (eds): Physiological Pharmacology, vol II. New York, Academic, 1965, pp 1-96.
34. Study RE, Barker JL: Cellular mechanisms of benzodiazepine action. JAMA 247:2147, 1982.
35. Tisdale SA, Ervin DK: A controlled study of methocarbamol (Robaxin) in acute painful musculoskeletal conditions. Curr Ther Res Clin Exp 17:525, 1975.
36. Turner R, Rockwood CA: Chlorphenesin carbamate (Maolate) in the relief of muscle pain. Mil Med 132:371, 1967.
37. Valtonen EJ: A double-blind trial of methocarbamol versus placebo in painful muscle spasm. Curr Med Res Opin 3:382, 1975.
38. Waltham-Weeks CD: The analgesic properties of chlorphenesin carbamate in the treatment of osteoarthrosis. Ann Phys Med 9:197, 1967-1968.

ANTIDEPRESSANTS

During the past 30 years, tricyclic antidepressants (TCAs) have been widely used for the treatment of chronic pain in patients with or without depression (Table 19-13).[1,6] The mechanism of action that results in pain relief remains unknown, although a number of theories have been proposed. In addition, the factors that might better predict a beneficial response to these drugs by patients with chronic pain remain to be determined.[19]

Mechanism of Action

The basis for a response of pain to TCAs seems to be related to alterations in the central nervous system associated with chronic pain. Sternbach postulated that chronic pain results in depression, which is associated with depletion of serotonin in the brain. TCAs, which increase serotonin levels, might therefore be associated with pain relief.[18] This hypothesis was tested in a study using fenfluramine, a drug that causes a relatively selective release of serotonin, at a dose of 40 mg/day. This drug transiently reduced both chronic pain and depression in some patients, supporting this hypothesis.[3]

Another popular theory involves the activation of the endogenous opiate system in the central nervous system by TCAs. TCAs can exert analgesic effects either directly or indirectly on the endogenous opiate system.[17] TCAs can increase the low levels of endogenous opiates in patients with organic pain.[20]

As a neurotransmitter, serotonin may also play an important role as an inhibitor of pain. The pain inhibitory pathway descends from the raphe nuclei in the brain stem via the lateral columns of the dorsal spinal cord to the superficial laminae (substantia gelatinosa) of the dorsal horn.[12] Antinociceptive effects are generated by the application of serotonin and norepinephrine to the substantia gelatinosa in animal models.[8] From anatomic and neurophysiologic data, serotonergic pathways significantly modify transmission of nociceptive impulses.

Reduction of anxiety and relief of muscle tension may also decrease low back and neck pain. Amitriptyline, a sedating antidepressant, has been associated with pain relief in individuals with chronic muscle tension.[11]

Pain relief by antidepressants also may be ascribed to therapy for masked depression. Pain may be a part of the symptom-complex of the depressed patient. Although this may play a part in the resolution of symptoms, studies have demonstrated improvement in pain but not depression in depressed patients with chronic pain treated with TCAs.[21]

TCAs work by inhibiting the uptake of serotonin and/or norepinephrine by the nerve terminal that released them, thereby increasing the concentration of the neurotransmitter in the synapse. Increased neurotransmitter concentrations amplify the tone in corresponding neural pathways where these substances are neurotransmitters. TCAs that have been associated with potentiation of serotonin and related pain relief include imipramine, amitriptyline, doxepin, and desipramine.

Clinical Trials

A few clinical studies have investigated the use of TCAs in patients with chronic low back pain. Two double-blind studies comparing imipramine and placebo generated conflicting results. In a study using low-dose imipramine for a 4-week period, no difference was noted between imipramine and placebo.[10] In contrast, a study using higher doses for an 8-week period found statistically significant improvement with imipramine compared with placebo.[1] Doxepin has been found to be effective in reducing pain compared with placebo in clinical studies. Hameroff and associates showed antidepressant doses of doxepin to be superior to placebo.[6]

In Ward's study, 60% of patients experienced pain reduction with doxepin and desipramine.[19] The findings supported the hypothesis of low serotonin concentrations being associated with chronic pain. Those patients who responded to fenfluramine were the same ones who were more likely to have pain relief with either antidepressant. Levels of endorphins, pain tolerance, and EMG findings were unaltered by the medications. Sedation was not a key factor in that the nonsedating drug (desipramine) was as effective as the sedating agent (doxepin). Patients, with or without depression, or with or without physical trauma, responded equally well. Doxepin has also been shown to be effective in patients with spinal pain who have failed other therapies.[5]

Amitriptyline, the agent with the greatest serotonergic activity, is also associated with pain relief in patients with chronic back pain. In a double-blind study, amitriptyline was associated with a significant decrease in the use of analgesics but no measurable change in activity level in patients with low back pain.[13] Nortriptyline may work as an analgesic for chronic pain for individuals who are not depressed. In a randomized, double-blind, placebo-controlled 8-week trial of nortriptyline between 50 to 150 mg, mean pain reduction was 1.68 with a 22% reduction with nortriptyline versus 9% on placebo.[2] Reduction in disability favored nortriptyline but other quality of life measures were not improved.

The use of TCAs in the treatment of chronic back pain is not totally benign. In one study, 100% of patients taking TCAs developed side effects, however minor.[14] The toxicities of these agents are nicely summarized by Hart[7]:

> [The TCAs] should be used with extreme caution in cardiovascular disease, liver disorders, epilepsy, patients with known suicidal tendencies, conditions where an anticholinergic agent would be undesirable, for example, glaucoma, urinary retention and pyloric stenosis, prostatic hypertrophy, pregnancy. Barbiturates alter the pharmacologic effects of tricyclic antidepressants, which can in turn alter the action of other drugs administered concurrently including other antidepressants (especially MAOIs); alcohol; some antihypertensives, for example methyldopa and guanethidine; anticholinergics and local anaesthetics with noradrenaline.

These toxicities are particularly troublesome in the elderly, who are more prone to the diseases and to drug-related complications.[16]

In contrast to the use of TCAs in depression, the dose for analgesia should be kept low and raised slowly in light of the patient's clinical response.[9] Reaching antidepressant levels of 150 mg of amitriptyline has not been necessary in patients with chronic pain. The drug is taken as a single dose, 2 hours before bedtime. Ten milligrams of amitriptyline is the initial dose, which may be increased to 25 mg within 2 to 3 weeks. Over the following 8 weeks, the dose may be increased to 75 to 100 mg. It is rare to use larger doses unless the patient is clinically depressed. The therapeutic ranges of the TCAs are listed in Table 19-13. Blood levels of antidepressant do not correlate with pain efficacy. Obtaining drug levels is not necessary unless the treatment of depression is also targeted and a therapeutic concentration is required.[4]

In a review of nine randomized controlled trials including 504 patients with chronic low back pain, antidepressant treatments (imipramine, amitriptyline, desipramine, doxepin, trazodone, nortriptyline, maprotiline, paroxetine) have improved pain relief but not improved activities of daily living compared with placebo. This improvement comes at an expense of increased toxicities.[15]

Non-tricyclic antidepressants—fluoxetine, sertraline, paroxetine, and bupropion—are effective for treating depression, but their efficacy for pain relief similar to the tricyclic antidepressants has not been established. The antinociceptive effect of the selective serotonin reuptake inhibitors (SSRIs) is less than that of the TCAs.[4] Studies in the future may demonstrate efficacy in patients with spinal pain, making SSRIs a worthwhile addition to the therapy for chronic spinal pain.

Venlafaxine is a potent inhibitor of neuronal serotonin and norepinephrine reuptake and a weak inhibitor of dopamine reuptake. It is an antidepressant used for depression and generalized anxiety. Venlafaxine is a drug that is useful in patients who are experiencing chronic pain and depression and is also helpful in patients with fibromyalgia. The beginning dose is 37.5 mg/day. Many patients find this dose adequate to relieve symptoms. The maximum daily dose is 75 mg/day.

Our Recommendation

The TCAs are relatively safe at the doses that are effective in patients with chronic pain. In patients with spinal pain who have failed other therapies, a trial of TCAs is indicated. The choice of agent is determined by the physician's familiarity with the individual TCAs and the need for sedation (amitriptyline). The trial should be continued for a number of weeks unless toxicity intervenes.

19-13 SELECTED ANTIDEPRESSANTS

Class	Pain Dose (mg)	Depression Dose (mg)	Sedation (Grades 1–4)
TRICYCLIC TERTIARY AMINES			
Imipramine (Tofranil)	10-75	300	3+
Amitriptyline (Elavil)	10-100	300	4+
Doxepin (Sinequan)	10-100	300	4+
Clomipramine (Anafranil)	25-100	250	3+
TRICYCLIC SECONDARY AMINES			
Desipramine (Norpramin)	10-100	300	1+
Nortriptyline (Pamelor)	10-100	250	3+

References

Antidepressants

1. Alcoff J, Jones E, Rust P, Newman R: Controlled trial of imipramine for chronic low back pain. J Fam Pract 14:841, 1982.
2. Atkinson JH, Slater MA, Williams RA, et al: A placebo-controlled randomized clinical trial of nortriptyline for chronic low back pain. Pain 76:287-296, 1998.
3. Clineschmidt BV, Zacchei AG, Totaro JA, et al: Fenfluramine and brain serotonin. Ann NY Acad Sci 305:222, 1978.
4. Fishbain D: Evidence-based data on pain relief with antidepressants. Ann Med 32:305-316, 2000.
5. Hameroff SR, Cork RC, Weiss JL, et al: Doxepin effects on chronic pain and depression: A controlled study. Clin J Pain 1:171, 1985.
6. Hameroff SR, Crago BR, Cork RC, et al: Doxepin effects on chronic pain, depression, and serum opioids. Anesth Analg 61:187, 1982.
7. Hart FD: The use of psychotropic drugs in rheumatology. J Int Med Res 4(Suppl 2):15, 1976.
8. Headley PM, Duggan AW, Griersmith BT: Selective reduction by noradrenaline and 5-hydroxytryptamine of nociceptive responses of cat dorsal horn neurons. Brain Res 145:185, 1978.
9. Hollister LE: Treatment of depression with drugs. Ann Intern Med 88:78, 1978.
10. Jenkins DG, Ebbutt AF, Evans CD: Tofranil in the treatment of low back pain. J Int Med Res 4(Suppl 2):28, 1976.
11. Lance JW, Curran DA: Treatment of chronic tension headache. Lancet 1:1236, 1964.
12. Oliveras JL, Bourgoin S, Hery F, et al: The topographical distribution of serotonergic terminals in the spinal cord of the cat: Biochemical mapping by the combined use of microdissection and microassay procedures. Brain Res 138:393, 1977.
13. Pheasant H, Bursk A, Goldfarb J, et al: Amitriptyline and chronic low-back pain: A randomized double-blind crossover study. Spine 8:552, 1983.
14. Pilowsky I, Hallett EC, Basset DL, et al: A controlled study of amitriptyline in the treatment of chronic pain. Pain 14:169, 1982.
15. Salerno SM, Browning R, Jackson JL: The effect of antidepressant treatment on chronic back pain: A meta-analysis. Arch Intern Med 162:19-24, 2002.
16. Shillcutt SD, Easterday JL, Anderson RJ: Geriatric pharmacology: I. Antidepressant medications. Hosp Formul 19:941, 1984.
17. Spiegel K, Kalb R, Pasternak GW: Analgesic activity of tricyclic antidepressants. Ann Neurol 13:462, 1983.
18. Sternbach RA: The need for an animal model of chronic pain. Pain 2:2, 1976.
19. Ward NG: Tricyclic antidepressants for chronic low back pain: Mechanisms of action and predictors of response. Spine 11:661, 1986.
20. Ward NG, Blood VL, Dworkin S, et al: Psychobiological markers in coexisting pain and depression: Toward a unified theory. J Clin Psychiatry 43:8(Sec 2)32, 1982.
21. Watson CP, Evans RJ, Reed K, et al: Amitriptyline versus placebo in postherpetic neuralgia. Neurology 32:671, 1982.

MISCELLANEOUS MEDICATIONS

Anticonvulsant Drugs

Anticonvulsant drugs (ACDs) are agents that have been used in the treatment of chronic pain syndromes for decades.[8] ACDs are adjunct therapies for chronic neuropathic pain. Neuropathic pain is pain due to dysfunction of the nervous system in the absence of ongoing tissue damage. Once nerves are damaged there is a potential disruption in the balance between excitatory (glutamate) and inhibitory (GABA) neurotransmitters. The result of this imbalance is hyperexcitability of the sodium and calcium channels, resulting in the ectopic firing of the nerve.[10] The ACDs have a variety of actions, many of which modify the functionality of sodium- and calcium-dependent channels and GABA metabolism.

Tricyclic antidepressants (imipramine, 10 to 100 mg) are effective for neuropathic pain but may have limited utility secondary to toxicities. Low doses of some of the ACDs offer additional benefits without significantly increasing toxicity. These levels are subtherapeutic for treatment of epilepsy. Monitoring drug levels is not useful. Older ACDs (phenytoin, 200 to 400 mg; carbamazepine, 200 to 400 mg; valproic acid, 250 mg) have hematologic and hepatic toxicities that temper enthusiasm for these agents.

Gabapentin

Gabapentin is an adjunctive therapy for partial seizures. In addition, gabapentin decreases pain in postherpetic neuralgia, diabetic neuropathy, and complex regional pain syndrome.[2,5,7] The mode of action of this drug is unknown. Gabapentin is postulated to increase GABA levels but does not interact with GABA receptors, is not converted to GABA, nor affects GABA metabolism. Patients receive analgesia at doses between 900 mg and 3200 mg in divided doses per day. The higher doses are indicated for postherpetic neuralgia. Of the newer ACDs, gabapentin appears to be most effective and best tolerated. Another advantage is the opportunity to use this agent with other drugs without adverse reactions.

Topiramate

Topiramate is an adjunctive therapy for partial seizures and generalized tonic-clonic seizures. The mechanism of action is related to blocking sodium channels, potentiating GABA inhibitory neurons, and blocking glutamate channels. Topiramate is used for pain related to intercostal neuralgia and other neuropathic pain states.[4] The usual dose of topiramate is 25 to 50 mg/day. A maximum dose is 200 mg twice a day. The most effective dose for neuropathic pain is unknown.

Alpha-2-Adrenergic Receptor Agonist (AARA)

AARA drugs are centrally acting muscle relaxants. These agents decrease excitatory input to alpha motor neurons. They are most frequently utilized to decrease spasticity associated with cerebral or spinal cord upper motor neuron disorders.[9] Tizanidine is an AARA drug. The dose ranges from 2 to 36 mg in divided doses. The maximal effects may not be seen for 4 weeks. Spasm frequency and clonus are reduced with this agent. Tizanidine has been studied in acute low back pain in conjunction with ibuprofen. In a study of 105 patients with acute low back pain given tizanidine (4 mg three times a day) plus ibuprofen (400 mg three times a day) or placebo plus ibuprofen (400 mg three times a day), earlier improvement was demonstrated with combination therapy.[3] Fewer gastrointestinal toxicities were recorded with the tizanidine plus ibuprofen combination than with ibuprofen alone. The effects of tizanidine on chronic pain are unknown. Patients with chronic pain (fibromyalgia) have described benefits with administration of tizanidine. Low doses of 2 to 12 mg are adequate to obtain improvement. The toxicities of the drug are sicca symptoms and somnolence. These are rarely causes to discontinue the drug. If other agents are ineffective, tizanidine may be added, particularly in the patient who may be hypertensive.

Topical Lidocaine Patch

Peripheral topical analgesics, lidocaine 5% patch, allows for targeted analgesia at the peripheral sites of pain. The affects are local, not central. Therefore, the risks for toxicities are less than compared with centrally acting analgesics. The potential for drug-drug interactions are less.

The lidocaine 5% patch is indicated for the treatment of postherpetic neuralgia. Pain and quality of life measures are improved with the patch in these patients.[6]

The lidocaine 5% patch has been tested in an open-label study in patients with acute, subacute, and chronic low back pain. Four Lidoderm patches were placed on areas of maximal pain every 24 hours in a 6-week study. A majority of the patients experienced some pain relief, but the full effects of the therapy were not reported.[1] The benefits of lidocaine patches for spinal pain patients are known. Randomized trials will need to be completed before efficacy can be determined. In the interim, the therapy has little toxicity other than local rash. In a patient who is resistant to oral therapies, topical therapies should be considered.

Our Recommendation

The anticonvulsants, alpha-2-adrenergic receptor agonists, and topical patches are additional therapies for the patient with chronic spinal pain. They should be added to a regimen of NSAIDs, analgesics, and muscle relaxants for additional pain relief.

References

Miscellaneous Medications

1. Argoff CE: Targeted topical peripheral analgesics in the management of pain. Curr Pain Head Rep 7:34-38, 2003.
2. Backonja M, Beydoun A, Edwards KR, et al: Gabapentin for the symptomatic treatment of painful neuropathy in patients with diabetes mellitus: A randomized controlled trial. JAMA 280:1831-1836, 1998.
3. Berry H, Hutchinson DR: Tizanidine and ibuprofen in acute low-back pain: Results of a double-blind multicentre study in general practice. J Int Med Res 16:83-91, 1988.
4. Chong MS, Libretto SE: The rationale and use of topiramate for treating neuropathic pain. Clin J Pain 19:59-68, 2003.
5. Dworkin RH, Schmader KE: Treatment and prevention of postherpetic neuralgia. Clin Infect Dis 36:877-882, 2003.
6. Galer BS, Rowbotham MC, Perander J, et al: Topical lidocaine patch relieves post-herpetic neuralgia more effectively than vehicle patch: Results of an enriched enrollment study. Pain 80:533-538, 1999.
7. Mellick GA, Mellick LB: Reflex sympathetic dystrophy treated with gabapentin. Arch Phys Med Rehabil 78:98-105, 1997.
8. Sindrup SH, Jensen TS: Efficacy of pharmacological treatments of neuropathic pain: An update and effect related to mechanism of drug action. Pain 83:389-400, 1999.
9. Wagstaff AJ, Bryson HM: Tizanidine: A review of its pharmacology, clinical effects, and tolerability in the management of spasticity associated with cerebral and spinal disorders.
10. Woolf CJ, Mannion RJ: Neuropathic pain: Aetiology, symptoms, mechanisms, and management. Lancet 353:1959-1964, 1999.

ELECTROTHERAPY

Transcutaneous Electrical Nerve Stimulation

Evidence has been reported suggesting that transcutaneous electrical nerve stimulation (TENS) therapy may alleviate chronic pain, including back pain. The exact mechanism by which electrical current decreases pain is unknown, although there are a number of hypotheses. Most reports have assumed that TENS activates larger-diameter afferent A-alpha nerve fibers. The input through these nerves presumably activates an intraneural network that presynaptically or postsynaptically inhibits ongoing transmission of nociceptive impulses supplied through the small C unmyelinated and alpha-D fibers or inhibits the C fibers directly.[7,32] TENS preferentially stimulates the low-threshold A-alpha fibers.[5] The effect of TENS on pain modulation does not seem to be directly related to endogenous opiates. Naloxone, an inhibitor of endogenous and exogenous opiates, failed to reverse the effect of high-frequency TENS in patients with acute and chronic pain.[1]

Electrical stimulation to the nerves may be accomplished by TENS using surface electrodes applied to the skin, subcutaneous implanted electrodes, or electrodes implanted directly on the nerve or dorsal column with stimulation applied directly to the spinal cord or through the dura. The transcutaneous stimulator is most frequently used.

The basic equipment for TENS therapy is an electrical pulse generator and transcutaneous electrodes. The pulses produced by the generator may be high frequency, low frequency, or variable frequency. The pulse generator feeds its output to an amplifier that increases the signal to a level that delivers current to the electrodes. The waveforms most commonly used are rectangular and spike. The rectangular waveform can be adjusted for amplitude and pulse width, while the spike form can be modified by amplitude alone. TENS therapy uses alternating current to limit the flow of material on the surface of the skin (electrode gel) into subdermal structures that results in irritation.

The electrodes receive the current and produce an electric field that excites the afferent fibers in the neighboring peripheral nerve. The current must be delivered without damaging the skin. The most widely used electrodes are silicone rubber impregnated with carbon particles. The electrodes are flexible and follow the contours of the body. An aquaphilic gel is needed to reduce skin resistance to facilitate current transmission, and the electrodes must be taped appropriately to maintain a tight fit with the underlying skin; poor contact may result in sparking and damage to the skin. Disposable and reusable electrodes that have preapplied gel and adhesive are available, but they are more expensive and detach from the skin more easily, particularly when the patient perspires.

The choice of electrode placement depends on the location of the pain. The electrodes may be placed directly over the area, within the dermatome or myotome, or over a superficial peripheral nerve. The optimal site of stimulation is proximal to the painful area. The closer the electrodes are to the nerve, the lower the current required to stimulate the appropriate nerve fibers. Patients with back and radicular pain may benefit from electrodes placed on the leg in the distribution of the radiated pain in addition to electrodes placed over the lumbosacral area (Fig. 19-23). It is not possible to predict the most effective site for electrode placement, and different locations may need to be tested before the optimal site is identified. Some patients will need bilateral stimulation even in the circumstance of unilateral pain.[23] For bilateral neck pain, crisscrossed electrode placement is preferred.[19]

Once the electrodes are placed, waveform parameters are altered to maximize pain relief. The parameters that can be modified are pulse rate, width, and amplitude. The rate regulates the number of electrical impulses delivered per second (pps). The range is from 2 to 200 pps, with 2 to 150 pps the most commonly used rates. The pulse width determines the duration of each impulse. A range of 50 to 250 μ/sec is commonly used. The amplitude of the signal is measured in milliamperes (mA).

Various combinations of rate, width, and amplitude will have a marked effect on the signal that reaches the stimulated area. The conventional mode of TENS therapy utilizes a high pulse rate (80 to 100 pps) and low pulse width (less than 100 μ/sec). The amplitude is increased until a tingling sensation is felt in the stimulated area. The aim is to activate large sensory myelinated fibers without producing muscle contraction or dysesthesias.

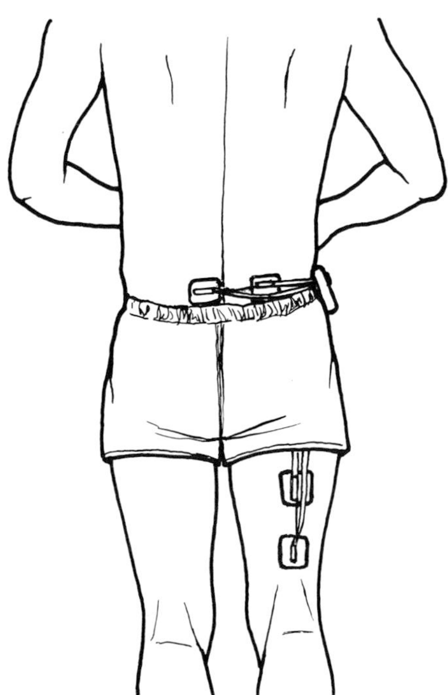

Figure 19-23 Electrode placement for low back pain radiating to the posterior aspect of the right thigh.

Other signal forms may be uncomfortable and are used only for short periods of time. High pulse width at low rates (2 to 4 pps) stimulates nerves at the superficial to deep levels and may cause muscle contraction. Like acupuncture, this form of TENS may stimulate endogenous opiate (endorphin) production.[25] Burst mode uses a low rate (4 pps) of a series of impulses (7 in number). The pulse width is wide and the amplitude high. In the burst mode, which is useful for chronic, deep pain,[13] rhythmic muscle contraction occurs. The subcutaneous and cutaneous nerves are stimulated with high rate, wide width, and high amplitude settings. Newer units allow the operator to alternate between modes that stimulate deep and superficial structures. This switching between modes may help prevent adaptation to TENS therapy. Once the effective mode is determined, that single mode is used, instead of multiple modes, to produce more lasting effects.[28]

The induction time for TENS to produce analgesia ranges from immediately to several hours, the average time being 20 minutes. The effect of TENS therapy may be cumulative in patients with chronic pain. Patients may not experience pain relief if duration of stimulation is limited to 30 minutes or less.[31] Therefore, TENS therapy should be used for a minimum of 30 minutes at a time. TENS should be given at 2-hour intervals, with a maximum of 8 hours per day. This regimen should be given for 3 weeks, with a reduction of the time of the time of application of TENS during the next 12 weeks.[28] The pain relief from TENS may be present only during the stimulation or may last for an extended period of time.[20]

TENS therapy may be indicated for patients with acute or chronic pain. It has been used to decrease postoperative pain in patients who have undergone lumbar spine operations.[26] Patients with chronic pain from back conditions or neurogenic injuries have had pain relief with TENS therapy as well.[3,8] Patients who have psychogenic pain not infrequently have increased discomfort with TENS therapy.[21] In treating patients with acute cervical pain, caution must be used so that electrodes are not placed over the carotid sinus or epiglottis.[27]

Is TENS therapy better than placebo for the treatment of spinal pain? Although TENS has been shown to be helpful in other pain conditions, few controlled trials have been reported.[6,10] TENS, like other forms of pain therapy, has a significant placebo component.[29] In the early stages of therapy, it produces 60% to 80% relief of chronic pain. The placebo effect portion of the response quickly falls off while the therapeutic efficacy of TENS decreases more slowly, so that between 20% and 30% continue to experience pain relief at 1 year.[3] Patients with radicular symptoms and sciatic pain may benefit from TENS therapy.[2] This modality may also be helpful in patients with back pain without sciatica. In a study of back pain using TENS therapy, a gradual reduction in efficacy occurred over a 2-month period.[16] TENS should be thought of as only a temporary therapy to be used while the patient tries to increase his or her physical status. TENS may cause a more rapid restoration of cervical mobility when used with other modalities in patients with acute cervical pain.[22]

Clinical Trials

In an attempt to answer the concerns about the efficacy of TENS for treatment of low back pain, Deyo and coworkers designed a randomly assigned, controlled trial of TENS therapy for 145 patients divided into four groups: TENS alone, 36 subjects; TENS plus exercise, 37; sham TENS alone, 36; and sham TENS plus exercise, 36.[11] TENS therapy was employed over the maximum point of tenderness for 45 minutes, three times a day. The exercise program consisted of 13 exercises, including relaxation, stretching, and bending. Measurement of outcome included functional status, physical measures, and the use of medical services. Improvement was demonstrated in all four groups during the 4-week study but was diminished at the 3-month follow-up period. Exercise was the factor that was most closely associated with improvement. TENS was not a significant factor in improvement. Criticisms of this study have raised a number of issues, including the improper placement of electrodes and improper machine settings. Jenkner suggests that for optimal results TENS must be set for monophasic pulses, using a frequency of 20 to 60 pps, with unequal size electrodes on specific locations without modifications by the patient.[16] Other criticisms included inadequacy of blinding patients when physical therapies are involved. Deyo has responded to these criticisms, suggesting that controls were appropriate for the TENS study.[12]

Brosseau and colleagues reviewed the randomized clinical trials testing TENS as a treatment for chronic low back pain.[6] Only five trials were of adequate quality to be included. The outcome measures were variable as were the techniques of applying TENS. The analysis demonstrated no benefit for TENS compared with placebo. The authors conclude that additional studies with standardized measures of outcome are necessary to determine the true efficacy of TENS.

Percutaneous Electrical Nerve Stimulation

Percutaneous electrical nerve stimulation (PENS) is a method using acupuncture-like needle probes to deliver electrical pulses to peripheral sensory nerves at dermatomal levels corresponding to local pathologic processes. In a study of 29 men and 31 women with back pain secondary to degenerative disc disease, four therapeutic modalities (PENS, sham-PENS, transcutaneous electrical nerve stimulation, and exercise) were each administered for a period of 30 minutes 3 times a week for 3 weeks in a random progression over a 15-week period.[14] At the conclusion of the study, PENS was found to be more effective than the other modalities at decreasing pain as measured by a visual analogue scale. The use of nonopioid analgesics was decreased to a greater degree in the PENS group. Percutaneous electrical nerve stimulation was the preferred therapy to decrease pain in 91% subjects. It was more effective in improving physical activity, quality of sleep, and sense of well-being. Criticisms of the study include the absence of a true comparable control with known efficacy. The exercise program was not a serious attempt at physical intervention. The degree of improvement was relatively small. The therapy does take time and must be applied by another person.

Weiner and colleagues reported on a study of PENS and physical therapy with sham-PENS and therapy in community-dwelling older adults.[30] At baseline, 6 weeks, and 3 months, PENS and physical therapy resulted in significant reductions in pain intensity measures compared with placebo. Physical function was also improved. The study included 34 individuals.

Our Recommendation

TENS therapy is applied by our physical therapists to patients with localized, chronic low back pain of traumatic origin. It is most useful in patients who experience limitations at work because of pain. The use of TENS therapy allows these patients to complete a usual day's work with much less discomfort. They can also use the units during recreational activities or activities of daily living. These patients use the units on an intermittent basis and have found this to be a way to sustain the beneficial effects of the therapy. Patients are always advised to rent, not buy, units initially. Only after a period of months of sustained pain relief should they buy their units. Whether through a placebo effect or direct effect on the nervous system, TENS therapy does help patients with back pain become more functional. However, in patients with chronic back pain who respond to TENS, the beneficial effect may not last.

TENS should be limited to individuals who have chronic spinal pain who have achieved inadequate pain relief with other effective therapies. It should be offered as a means of improving function with specific goals.

Iontophoresis

Iontophoresis, also called common ion transfer, uses direct current, as opposed to the alternating current of TENS, to induce the transfer of an ion across a body surface. A variety of medications including corticosteroids, epinephrine, and local anesthetics may enter soft tissue without an injection. A study by Russo and colleagues demonstrated that patients derived an equal amount of analgesia from an injection of lidocaine and lidocaine iontophoresis.[24] Harris reported on 50 patients with inflammatory musculoskeletal conditions; about 76% had marked relief of pain with iontophoresis of a solution composed of lidocaine and dexamethasone.[15] This technique may be of benefit to a patient with localized areas of pain that are irritated by injection. Pain may be diminished by iontophoresis with the instillation of a local anesthetic (lidocaine 4% solution) alone or in combination with a soluble corticosteroid. The effectiveness of iontophoresis continues to be studied. The beneficial effect of the therapy may not rely solely on the medication but also on the effects of direct electrical current on tissues.[9]

Advances are being made in the administration of drugs through the skin with or without electrical current. New technologies are able to store medications in reservoirs that are slowly leeched into the skin. Medications that are available with transcutaneous delivery include clonidine, scopolamine, estradiol, fentanyl, nitroglycerin, and nicotine.[4]

Our Recommendation

Iontophoresis is a useful technique for the placement of medication at a locally painful site when injection is not preferred or contraindicated.

High-Voltage Stimulation

High-voltage stimulation is a form of TENS that utilizes high-voltage, monophasic pulses of short duration to stimulate soft tissue structures in the lumbosacral spine. High-voltage stimulation may be particularly helpful in eliminating persistent muscle spasm. Repeated electrical stimulation relaxes protective muscle spasm, thereby decreasing muscle fatigue. Patients may be able to exercise or stretch the muscle in spasm once electrical stimulation has been applied to the superficial area over the muscle. Electrical stimulation of muscles may maintain strength and endurance. In a 4-week controlled study, electrical muscle stimulation increased trunk endurance and strength in healthy women.[17] The ability of electrical muscle stimulation to increase strength of injured muscle requires additional study. This form of therapy may be considered only an adjunct to a therapy program, including active strengthening exercises.

Another proposed electrical therapy for low back pain is laser therapy. Lasers emit coherent photons that interact with biologic molecules to produce chemical reactions in the body. The use of laser in chronic back pain was no better than exercises alone in the treatment of pain.[18]

Our Recommendation

High-voltage stimulation has marginal benefit.

References

Electrotherapy

1. Abrams SE, Reynolds AC, Cusick JF: Failure of naloxone to reverse analgesia from transcutaneous electrical stimulation in patients with chronic pain. Anaesth Analg 60:81, 1981.
2. Anderson SA: Pain control by sensory stimulation. In Bonica JJ, Liebeskind JC, Albe-Fessard DG (eds): Advances in Pain Research and Therapy, vol 3. New York, Raven Press, 1979, pp 569-585.
3. Bates JAV, Nathan PW: Transcutaneous electrical nerve stimulation for chronic pain. Anaesthesia 35:817, 1980.
4. Berti JJ, Lipsky JJ: Transcutaneous drug delivery: A practical review. Mayo Clin Proc 70:581-586, 1995.
5. Bloedel J, McCreery D: Organization of peripheral and central pain pathways. Surg Neurol 4:65, 1975.
6. Brosseau L, Milne S, Robinson V, et al: Efficacy of the transcutaneous nerve stimulation for the treatment of chronic low back pain: A meta-analysis. Spine 27:596-603, 2002.
7. Campbell JN, Taub A: Local analgesia from percutaneous electrical stimulation. Arch Neurol 28:347, 1973.
8. Cauthen JC, Renner EJ: Transcutaneous and peripheral nerve stimulation for chronic pain states. Surg Neurol 4:102, 1975.
9. Chantraine A, Ludy JP, Berger D: Is cortisone iontophoresis possible? Arch Phys Med Rehabil 67:38, 1986.
10. Deyo RA: Conservative therapy for low back pain: Distinguishing useful from useless therapy. JAMA 250:1057, 1983.
11. Deyo RA, Walsh NE, Martin DC, et al: A controlled trial of transcutaneous electrical nerve stimulation (TENS) and exercise for chronic low back pain. N Engl J Med 322:1627, 1990.
12. Deyo RA, Walsh NE, Schoenfeld LS, et al: Can trials of physical treatments be blinded? The example of transcutaneous electrical stimulation for chronic pain. Am J Phys Med Rehabil 69:6, 1990.
13. Eriksson MB, Sjolund BH, Nielzen S: Long term results of peripheral conditioning stimulation as an analgesia measure in chronic pain. Pain 6:335, 1979.
14. Ghoname E, Craig WF, White PF, et al: Percutaneous electrical stimulation for low back pain: A randomized crossover study. JAMA 281:818-823, 1999.
15. Harris PR: Iontophoresis: Clinical research in musculoskeletal inflammatory conditions. J Orthop Sports Phys Ther 4:109, 1982.
16. Jenkner FL: TENS—an international perspective. Phys Ther 73:64, 1993.
17. Kahanovitz N, Nordin M, Verderame R, et al: Normal trunk muscle strength and endurance in women and the effect of exercises and electrical stimulation: II. Comparative analysis of electrical stimulation and exercises to increase trunk muscle strength and endurance. Spine 12:112, 1987.
18. Klein RG, Eek BC: Low-energy laser treatment and exercise for chronic low back pain: Double-blind controlled trial. Arch Phys Med Rehabil 71:34, 1990.
19. Mannheimer JS: Transcutaneous electrical nerve stimulation: Its uses and effectiveness with patients in pain In Ecternach JL (ed): Pain. New York, Churchill Livingstone, 1987 pp 213-254.
20. Meyer GA, Fields HL: Causalgia treated by selective large fiber stimulation of peripheral nerves. Brain 95:163, 1972.
21. Nielzen S, Sjolund BH, Eriksson MB: Psychiatric factors influencing the treatment of pain with peripheral conditioning stimulation. Pain 13:365, 1982.
22. Nordemar R, Thorner C: Treatment of acute cervical pain: A comparative group study. Pain 10:93, 1981.
23. Picaza J, Cannon BW, Hunter SE, et al: Pain suppression by peripheral nerve stimulation: I. Observation with transcutaneous stimuli. Surg Neurol 4:105, 1975.
24. Russo J Jr, Lipman AG, Comstock TJ, et al: Lidocaine anesthesia: Comparison of iontophoresis, injection, and swabbing. Am J Hosp Pharm 37:843, 1980.
25. Sjolund B, Eriksson M: Endorphins and analgesia produced by peripheral conditioning stimulation. In Bonica JJ, Liebeskind JC, Albe-Fessard DG (eds): Advances in Pain Research and Therapy, vol 3. New York, Raven, 1979, pp 587-591.
26. Solomon RA, Viernstein MC, Long DM: Reduction of postoperative pain and narcotic use by transcutaneous electrical nerve stimulation. Surgery 87:142, 1980.
27. Soric R, Devlin M: Role of physical medicine In Tollison CD (ed): Handbook of Chronic Pain Management. Baltimore, Williams & Wilkins, 1988, pp 147-162.
28. Tan JC, Nordin M: Role of physical therapy in the treatment of cervical disk disease. Orthop Clin North Am 23:435, 1992.
29. Thorsteinsson G, Stonnington HH, Stillwell GK, Elveback LR: The placebo effect of transcutaneous electrical stimulation. Pain 5:31, 1978.
30. Weiner DK, Rudy TE, Glick RM, et al: Efficacy of percutaneous electrical nerve stimulation of the treatment of chronic low back pain in older adults. J Am Geriatr Soc 51:599-608, 2003.
31. Wolf SL, Gersh MR, Rao VK: Examination of electrode placement and stimulating parameters in treating chronic pain with conventional transcutaneous electrical nerve stimulation (TENS). Pain 11:37, 1981.
32. Woolf CJ: Transcutaneous and implanted nerve stimulation. In Wall PD, Melzack R (eds): Textbook of Pain. Edinburgh, Churchill Livingstone, 1986, pp 679-690.

PATIENT EDUCATION

Education is an essential part of the therapy for the spinal pain patient. Understanding the problem makes the patient an active partner in the treatment plan. Patients who know that spinal pain usually resolves over a short period of time have less stress regarding their condition. They are able to improve more rapidly.

In a study conducted by Cherkin and colleagues, 321 people with acute low back pain of 7 days or less to an exercise program supervised by physical therapists, to manipulation treatments given by chiropractors, or to an educational booklet about low back pain.[2] In the first month of the study, the people in the exercise and manipulation programs had less pain. However, at 1 year, no differences could be found concerning days lost from work or the frequency of additional attacks of low back pain among the groups. The cost of the educational booklet was one third of the expense of the exercise and manipulation therapies. The patients informed about their back pain with the educational booklet needed to go to the doctor less frequently than those who received no information.

In another study from the same group, 293 patients with low back pain were randomly allocated to usual care, an education booklet, or a 15-minute session with a clinic nurse, including the booklet and a follow-up telephone call.[3] At the end of 7 weeks, the knowledge and functional capacity of the groups was not significantly different. Education is helpful but must be reinforced to be effective.

Educational materials written for the general public or courses led by lay people have as much or greater success at improving low back pain as regular medical care. In one study, 255 patients with low back pain were assigned either to a self-management group intervention administered by a non-physician trained to implement a structured program or to usual care.[9] At 12 months, the self-management regimen had less apprehension, greater positive attitudes toward self-care, and greater function.

Many resources are available for patients who are interested in learning about their disorder. The Arthritis Foundation has pamphlets and books that discuss common musculoskeletal disorders, including low back pain. *Back in Control: A Conventional and Complementary Prescription for Eliminating Back Pain*[1] by David Borenstein, MD, is another example of a book specifically written in a format that the public can understand. The premise of this book is that individuals have the ability to play an active role in the resolution of their back problem. The book offers components of care that are key elements of cognitive-behavioral therapy.

Cognitive-Behavioral Therapy

Cognitive and behavioral therapies (CBT) are training programs that utilize operant conditioning, communication, stress management, and relaxation techniques. CBT have in common (1) the assumption that an individual's behaviors are influenced by his or her thoughts; (2) techniques to help patients identify, monitor, and change maladaptive thoughts, feelings, and behaviors; and (3) teaching skills that patients can apply to a variety of problems.[8]

CBT are most applicable to patients who suffer chronic low back or neck pain. When diagnostic techniques fail to identify a specific abnormality causing pain, clinicians should discuss the rehabilitation model of maximizing function versus pain relief with the patient. Psychosocial influences on the patient's pain behaviors need to be considered. These include significant anxiety or depression, disability in excess of objective findings, and excess use of pain medications. Physicians should inquire about patients' beliefs regarding the cause of their pain, beliefs about what helps and harms them, how activities have changed because of pain, responses of family members to pain behaviors, area of stress, symptoms of anxiety and depression, drug and alcohol use, and work and liability issues.[8] The second stage of therapy is to have the patient accept the condition as one that will run its course without the need for invasive medical therapy. Self-management offers the best chance for improvement. If a medication is to be used, the drug is given on a time-contingent, not pain-contingent, basis. The medicine is prescribed for a specific period of time whether pain is present or not to maximize function. This empowers the patient to use therapies for pain but also for improving their quality of life in general.

CBT has been studied in patients with acute and chronic spinal pain. Studies of the effects of CBT on acute neck and low back pain demonstrate modest effects. Individuals may have less pain or sickness at 6 to 12 months after the initiation of therapy compared with those receiving traditional treatments.[4,7] Patients with chronic spinal pain benefit from CBT. Nicholas and colleagues reported greater improvement in pain and disability in patients who received CBT plus physiotherapy versus those who received physiotherapy alone.[5,6] A major concern regarding CBT is whether individual or group sessions are equally effective in changing patient behavior. Physicians have a limited amount of time (8 to 15 minutes) to interact with a patient. Proficiency at self-management techniques is important for the success of the program. Applicability of CBT to the general population of spinal pain patients is limited by the time physicians have with patients and the availability (number of programs) and accessibility (insurance coverage) to CBT programs.

Our Recommendation

Patient education is an important component of spinal care. Educational materials should be in language understood by the public. The benefits of education can be as effective as other components of spinal care. CBT is an important part of a therapeutic regimen for individuals with chronic low back or neck pain.

References

Patient Education

1. Borenstein D: Back in Control: A Conventional and Complementary Prescription for Eliminating Back Pain. New York, M Evans, 2001, pp 1-208.
2. Cherkin DC, Deyo RA, Battie M, et al: A comparison of physical therapy, chiropractic manipulation, and provision of an educational booklet in the treatment of patients with low back pain. N Engl J Med 339:1021-1029, 1998.
3. Cherkin DC, Deyo RA, Street JH, et al: Pitfalls of patients education: Limited success of a program for back pain in primary care. Spine 21:345-355, 1996.
4. Fordyce WE, Brockway JA, Bergman JA, et al: Acute back pain: A control-group comparison of behavioral vs traditional management methods. J Behav Med 9:127-140, 1986

5. Nicholas MK, Wilson PH, Goyen J: Comparison of cognitive-behavioral group treatment and an alternative non-psychological treatment for chronic low back pain. Pain 48:339-347, 1992.
6. Nicholas MK, Wilson PH, Goyen J: Operant-behavioural and cognitive-behavioural treatment for chronic low back pain. Behav Res Ther 29:225-238, 1991.
7. Phillips HC, Grant L, Berkowitz J: The prevention of chronic pain and disability: A preliminary investigation. Behav Res Ther 29:443-450, 1991.
8. Turner JA: Educational and behavioral interventions for back pain in primary care. Spine 21:2851-2859, 1996.
9. Von Korff M, Moore JE, Lorig K, et al: A randomized trial of a lay person-led self-management group intervention for back pain patients in primary care. Spine 23:2608-2615, 1998.

BACK SCHOOL

As part of the nonsurgical management of patients with back pain, back schools have been developed to educate patients to be better able to manage their own back problems. The modern back school was developed in 1969 in Sweden by Zachrisson-Forssell.[16] The basic concept behind the school was that if patients understand the anatomic, epidemiologic, and biomechanical factors that give rise to low back pain, they will be better able to control their back problems in activities of daily living. Education will help patients take responsibility for management of their spine problems. In patients with back pain, particularly those with chronic pain whose daily activities are curtailed, the encouragement to take responsibility for treatment of their back problems is an essential part of therapy.

Back schools may be used to prevent initial episodes of back pain or as part of a treatment program to prevent recurrent attacks; most schools deal primarily with prevention of recurrences. The goals of the back school in the short run are to reduce pain, encourage appropriate rest, and emphasize the good prognosis of most back pain problems. Teaching patients proper body mechanics, to develop coping skills for episodes of pain, to accept shared responsibility for their recovery, and to improve their general physical condition to help prevent recurrent back pain are the long-range goals.[1]

The methods used by back schools to teach patients may be cognitive (classroom instruction of basic facts), physical (demonstrations of appropriate exercises and work habits), and motivational (encouragement to be an active participant in their own care). A number of back schools have been developed that utilize a combination of these methods.

Swedish Back School

The Swedish Back School is designed as a general information program for patients with acute and chronic pain who can use knowledge about their back to be more active in their treatment program. The program also emphasizes the prevention of recurrences.[15] The school consists of four 45-minute lessons, given over a 2-week period. There are eight patients in a class, which is taught by a physiotherapist. The initial lesson, utilizing audiovisual materials, includes information on epidemiology, anatomy, function of the back, treatment modalities, and positions for resting. Subsequent lessons cover back strain associated with poor posture and work activities, ways to decrease physical strain, and general methods to improve physical conditioning.

Canadian Back School

The Canadian Back School is oriented toward the treatment of chronic low back pain through psychological approaches to encourage patients to assume responsibility for their own health.[5] The faculty of the Canadian school includes an orthopedist, physiotherapist, psychiatrist, and psychologist who give 90-minute lectures on four successive weeks to 20 patients. The content of the initial 2 weeks of classes is similar to that of the Swedish school. During the third week, the psychiatrist explains emotional aspects of chronic pain and amplifies the interconnection among anxiety, muscle tension, and pain. The last class reviews physical therapy methods for relaxation and improved muscle strength.

California Back School

The California Back School is directed primarily at the patient with acute low back pain.[10] The teachers are a physiotherapist and a consulting orthopedic surgeon. An essential component of the California program is an obstacle course that is used the first day to measure physical performance in an objective manner. The goals of the obstacle course are to identify postures or motions that produce pain that may alter the stated diagnosis of the patient; provide objective measurement of performance of standardized activities to be matched against a control population and as a baseline; demonstrate proper body mechanics; and correct specific job-related body mechanics problems.[14] The obstacle course consists of a number of motions and tasks that exert the lumbar spine. The course proper consists of three weekly 90-minute visits, with a fourth visit 1 month later with four patients in each class. The developers of the California school believe that the small classes foster group participation while allowing for individual instruction for specific mechanical problems. The first class includes the obstacle course and basic education on the natural history, anatomy, and physiology of back pain along with a review of activities to be avoided. The second class concentrates on training in the tasks included in the obstacle course, review of body mechanics, and a home exercise program. A retest on the obstacle course and a test on the information given during the course are given at the third class. At follow-up 1 month later, individual mechanical problems are discussed.

The back school programs are only as good as the educational materials (slides, tapes, pamphlets) used and, most importantly, the expertise and enthusiasm of the instructors. The ability to motivate course participants and answer their questions seems most closely associated with a good outcome for the patients.

Outcomes

Do back schools help patients decrease pain and prevent recurrences? Berquist-Ullman and Larsson did a controlled prospective study of 217 Volvo employees with acute low back pain who were randomly assigned to physiotherapy, back school, and placebo.[2] The duration of symptoms was shorter for the physiotherapy and back school groups than for the placebo group. Back school patients were off work during the initial episode for a shorter period of time than the physiotherapy and placebo groups. The investigators concluded that back school was as effective as physiotherapy and was cost effective since one therapist treated a number of patients at the same time. The course of pain and the number of days lost from work during the first year due to recurrences were the same for each group.

Hall and Iceton reported on 6418 participants in the Canadian program. Back pain improvement occurred in 64%, and 97% rated the program helpful.[5] The outcome was not adversely affected by previous back surgery or severity of pain, but use of a large number of consulting physicians and multiple physical therapy modalities before enrollment in the course had a negative prognostic value.

Mooney reported on his behavioral modification program at Rancho Los Amigos Hospital in Downey, California.[11] Approximately 75% of patients reported decreased pain and increased activity and 62% returned to work.

The California Back School has also reported similar success rates. A review of the first 300 patients with acute low back pain revealed 89% needed no further medical treatment, 95% resumed normal activities, and 64% had no change in lifestyle.[10]

How do back schools benefit patients? The goals of the various programs are to inculcate independence and self-reliance into their patients. This is accomplished through instruction by individuals who are considered authorities on back pain. Fisk and colleagues propose the notion that it is the influence of these authority figures and the promotion of self-sufficiency that account for the efficacy of back schools, rather than the actual educational or training procedures themselves.[4] Patients who have a close working relationship with a health care professional may be able to substitute that interaction for a formal school setting. What is important is the stress placed on self-reliance and better understanding of the way the back works and how to prevent recurrences. These methods can be helpful for the patient with acute or chronic back pain who is motivated to improve his or her condition. Back school is most effective when used as a part of a broader treatment program consisting of the modalities discussed in this section.

Back school is as effective as other conservative therapies. In a study designed by Hseih and colleagues, 200 patients with low back pain were randomly assigned to back school, joint manipulation, myofascial therapy, or combined manipulation and myofascial therapy.[6] Patients were assessed at baseline, 3 weeks of therapy, and 6 months after the completion of therapy. All groups demonstrated improvement at 3 weeks but no further benefit at 6 months. Back school was as effective as all three manual therapies. Lonn and colleagues also demonstrated the benefit of back school with decreased recurrences and longer period of time to develop a new episode of pain.[8]

The benefits of back school are improved when patients interact. In a study of 108 patients who attended a back school course, 54 were included in a treatment group that included physical exercise and interaction with other members of the group and 54 were selected as a control group.[13] Both groups improved in perceived functional capacity and life quality. At 6 months, the groups that interacted had improved statistically significantly more in life quality than the controls. Social interaction increases the beneficial effects of education.

Back school programs are not as effective in the workplace. In two studies, one from Canada and the other from the United States, back school did not result in fewer episodes of pain or decreased days off work. Leclaire and colleagues described a Canadian experience with physical therapy (n = 86) versus physical therapy and back school (n = 82).[7] Both groups returned to work at 33 days and had similar compensated recurrence rates (10 vs. 14/yr). In the United States, Daltroy reported on 4000 postal workers trained about low back pain in a back school taught by experienced physical therapists.[3] In a comparison with control groups, the back school patients did not have a reduction in rate of back injury, the median cost per injury, time off work per injury, or rate of repeated injury. The only factor improved was the subject's knowledge of safe behavior.

In a systematic review of back school studies, Maier-Riehle and Harter evaluated 18 controlled back school studies involving 1682 participants.[9] Studies evaluated 14 outcome criteria and four time categories. Although the knowledge of course content was greater in the back school group, the intervention had only small effects on health economic variables and no effects on pain intensity. This meta-analysis concludes that the effectiveness of back school depends on the outcome criterion reviewed and the time of measurement.

Our Recommendation

Back school is an effective means of educating patients with acute and chronic low back pain. Back school has less impact when it is the sole therapy. It works best when it is one of a variety of therapies given for low back pain. Back school may be given after the patient's episode of pain has resolved or as a component of a multifaceted therapeutic program. The information given must be adapted to the needs of the participants. All the staff of the school must give consistent information to the patients. Patients with chronic low back pain will gain little from a program directed solely at acute problems.[12] The benefits are greatest when individuals with spinal pain are able to interact with one another.

References

Back School

1. Andersson GBJ: Back schools. In Jayson MIV (ed): The Lumbar Spine and Back Pain, 3rd ed. Edinburgh, Churchill Livingstone, 1987, pp 315-320.
2. Berquist-Ullman M, Larsson U: Acute low back pain in industry. Acta Orthop Scand (Suppl) 170:73, 1977.

3. Daltro LH, Iversen MD, Larson MG, et al: A controlled trial of an educational program to prevent low back injuries. N Engl J Med 337:322-328, 1997.
4. Fisk JR, DiMonte P, Courington SM: Back schools: Past, present, and future. Clin Orthop 179:18, 1983.
5. Hall H, Iceton JA: Back school. Clin Orthop 179:10, 1983.
6. Hseih CY, Adams AH, Tobis J, et al: Effectiveness of four conservative treatments for subacute low back pain: A randomized clinical trial. Spine 27:1142-1148, 2002.
7. Leclaire R, Esdaile JM, Suissa S, et al: Back school in a first episode of compensated acute low back pain: A clinical trial to assess efficacy and prevent relapse. Arch Phys Med Rehabil 77:673-679, 1996.
8. Lonn JH, Glomsrod B, Soukup MG, et al: Active back school: Prophylactic management for low back pain: A randomized, controlled, 1-year follow-up study. Spine 24:865-871, 1999.
9. Maier-Riehle B, Harter M: The effects of back schools: A meta-analysis. Int J Rehabil Res 24:199-206, 2001.
10. Mattmiller AW: The California back school. Physiotherapy 66:118, 1980.
11. Mooney V: Alternative approaches for the patient beyond the help of surgery. Orthop Clin North Am 6:331, 1975.
12. Nordin M, Cedraschi C, Balague F, et al: Back schools in prevention of chronicity. Clin Rheumatol 6:685, 1992.
13. Penttinen J, Nevala-Puranen N, Airaksinen O, et al: Randomized controlled trial of back school with and without peer support. J Occup Rehabil 12:21-29, 2002.
14. White AH: Back School and Other Conservative Approaches to Low Back Pain. St. Louis, CV Mosby, 1983.
15. Zachrisson-Forssell M: The back school. Spine 6:104, 1981.
16. Zachrisson-Forssell M: The Swedish back school. Physiotherapy 66:112, 1980.

WORK-RELATED EDUCATIONAL PROGRAMS

Another component of patient education and physical therapy is job assessment, functional capacity evaluation, and work hardening.[2] These components of therapy are directed at returning the patient to the workplace. The prevention of back pain can be obtained when the ergonomics of a specific task are evaluated in relationship to the prevention of spinal pain. Some factors associated with occupational risk for back pain include heavy physical labor, sustained trunk posture, prolonged sitting, frequent twisting with lifting, and whole-body vibration. Modifications of the workplace to decrease exposure to these physical risks decrease the potential for back injuries. Education of workers in regard to proper body mechanics also can be helpful in decreasing injuries. After injury, workers may be evaluated in regard to their physical capabilities in relationship to the requirements of the work tasks. Exercises (work hardening) may be given to strengthen those physical characteristics that are inadequate to complete the work tasks. The age of workers, days of sick leave, connection to the work force, and back pain intensity have been identified as characteristics of workers affecting improved functional outcome independent of the treatment they receive.[1] Vocational rehabilitation may be considered for those patients who have inadequate physical abilities to safely participate in their former employment. These individuals need to be retrained for jobs associated with less physically demanding work. Functional restoration programs work best within 4 to 8 months after the work-related injury. Individuals who receive interventions at 18 months may receive benefit but, more commonly, have had spinal surgery in the interim.[3] Work-hardening programs can have similar benefits for individuals with work-related cervical spine injuries.[4]

Our Recommendation

Individuals with spinal pain should be encouraged to return to an improved functional status. Programs that enable individuals to return to work are cost effective.

References

Work-Related Educational Programs

1. Bendix AF, Bendix T, Haestrup C: Can it be predicted which patients with chronic low back pain should be offered tertiary rehabilitation in a functional restoration program: A search for demographic, socioeconomic, and physical predictors. Spine 23:1775-1783, 1998.
2. Halpern M: Prevention of low back pain: Basic ergonomics in the workplace and the clinic. Clin Rheumatol 6:705, 1992.
3. Jordan JD, Mayer TG, Gatchel RJ: Should extended disability be an exclusion criterion for tertiary rehabilitation? Socioeconomic outcomes of early versus late functional restoration in compensation spinal disorders. Spine 23:2110-2117, 1998.
4. Wright A, Mayer TG, Gathcel RJ: Outcomes of disabling cervical spine disorders in compensation injuries: A prospective comparison to tertiary rehabilitation response for chronic lumbar spinal disorders. Spine 24:178-183, 1999.

COMPLEMENTARY (ALTERNATIVE) THERAPIES

The term *complementary* implies that such therapies are used in concert with conventional therapies. *Alternative* therapies are those that are utilized exclusively without any other form of therapy.

In 1997, an estimated 629 million visits were made to practitioners of alternative medicine. In contrast, 388 million visits were made to primary care physicians.[3] Four of 10 Americans use complementary therapies to some extent. Patients with spinal pain visit chiropractors, acupuncturists, massage therapists, and yoga or Pilates instructors. Complementary therapies are popular among those who have a condition with a variable response. They are considered free of risk and less expensive than conventional therapy. The total out-of-pocket expenditures for complementary therapy in 1997 was estimated to be $27 billion. This amount is comparable to the out-of-pocket expenditures for all physician services.[1]

In a survey of 2055 adults with low back or neck pain during 2002, Wolsko and colleagues found 37% utilized conventional providers whereas 54% had used complementary therapies.[4] Chiropractic, massage, and relaxation techniques were the most commonly used complementary treatments for low back or neck pain (20%, 14%, and 12%, respectively). These therapies were rated as very helpful by back or neck pain users (61%, 65%, and 43%, respectively). Conventional therapy was rated very helpful by 27% of users. A total of 203 million of the 629 million visits to complementary practitioners in 1997 were for back or neck pain.

Many patients are undergoing complementary therapies but will not inform their primary care physician unless asked. Physicians should ask about complementary therapies. Not all complementary and herbal therapies are benign.[2] Complementary therapies are too widely used to be ignored.

References

Complementary (Alternative) Therapies

1. Eisenberg DM, Davis RB, Ettner SL, et al: Trends in alternative medicine use in the United States, 1990-1997: Results of a follow-up national survey. JAMA 280:1569-1575, 1998.
2. Ernst E: Complementary and alternative medicine in rheumatology. Balliere's Clin Rheumatol 14:731-749, 2000.
3. Rao JK, Mihaliak K, Kroenke K, et al: Use of complementary therapies for arthritis among patients of rheumatologists. Ann Intern Med 131:409-416, 1999.
4. Wolsko PM, Eisenberg DM, Davis RB, et al: Patterns and perceptions of care for treatment of back and neck pain: Results of a national survey. Spine 28:292-297, 2003.

MANIPULATION

Spinal manipulation—movement of parts of the axial skeleton through the use of external force—is controversial, since in the United States this therapy is associated with the practice of chiropractic. Manipulation has been used for deformities of the spine since Greek medicine as described by Hippocrates.[1] Spinal manipulation is based on the assumption that subluxation of the vertebra precipitates low back or neck complaints and that these symptoms can be reduced with correction of the subluxation. Subluxation in chiropractic parlance connotes a functional and not necessarily an anatomic entity.[34] In conflict with the basic premise of pain associated with malposition are studies of large groups of patients that have shown no relationship between vertebral malalignment and spinal pain.[30,35] Manipulation may also include massage or stretching techniques to relax muscles that are shortened and in spasm. Other explanations for benefits of manipulation include reduction of posterior disc herniations by tightening the posterior longitudinal ligament and freeing of adhesions around a prolapsed disc, mechanically stimulating large A-alpha fibers, and blocking nociceptive input.[28,32] While Mathews and Yates demonstrated a reduction of small lumbar disc protrusions,[32] another study of 39 patients examined by myelography failed to demonstrate any persistent disc reduction after manipulation.[9,8]

The terminology used by chiropractors must be defined. Mobilization is a less aggressive maneuver than manipulation. Mobilization starts where the active range of motion ends at the physiologic extreme of normal motion of the anatomic structure. Between the physiologic barrier and an anatomic barrier is the movement associated with manipulation. Chiropractors use the term *adjustment* for both maneuvers. Mobilization goes past the active range of a joint and stretches the elastic tissues in the joint capsule, resulting in increased range of motion. With manipulation, a high-velocity, short-amplitude force is applied to stretch structures such as the capsule and ligaments. The cracking sound is caused by the negative pressure (vacuum) produced, resulting in the sudden production of joint nitrogen. Adjustments are directed at one specific joint with force applied in a specific direction.[39] A variety of concepts of pathophysiologic abnormalities have been proposed as explanations of the benefits of chiropractic intervention.[49] The Maitland concept suggests articular derangements of vertebral segments as the cause of pain. The Maigne concept suggests manipulation in the direction or opposite to the direction of limitation of motion depending on the abrupt limitation of movement with spinal palpation. The Sohier concept suggests abnormalities in articular structures and muscle tension.

Evaluation of patients considered for manipulation therapy involves measurement of active joint motion, passive joint motion, and accessory movements.[36] This evaluation is necessary to determine whether distraction, nonthrust, or thrust movements should be used. The manipulations may be given with varying force from different positions[36] but are always done in the direction that causes no pain for the patient. Manipulation does not require a forceful action to be effective. Patients are told to relax and are taken through a maximum range of passive motion. A gentle thrust at this point takes the joint or muscle to its maximum range of motion.

Contraindications

Absolute contraindications for mobilization include malignancy, osteomyelitis, osteoporosis, fracture, ruptured ligaments, acute arthritis, herniated nucleus pulposus, neurologic dysfunction, hypermobility, anticoagulant therapy, pregnancy in the first trimester, and acquired bleeding disorders.[36]

In the setting of intervertebral disc herniation, no evidence is available to demonstrate the reversibility of disc herniation with manipulation therapy.[5]

Complications

Spinal manipulation is not a benign procedure. Significant mechanical damage can result from physical force applied to the vertebral column.[38] These complications include cauda equina compression, disc herniation, and vertebral pedicle fracture.[11,16] The most frequent complications are minor (local discomfort) and transient but occur in half the patients.[48] The complications with chiropractic manipulation are rare compared with the number of treatments given, but the kinds of injuries are significant when they occur.[23,43,45] Complications of cervical manipulation have been reported at a range of frequency from 1 per 400,000 to two to three cases per million treatments.[12,13,48] There have been 138 cases of extracranial vascular injury associated with cervical manipulation.[40] Many complications are severe, associated with arterial injuries, stroke, and death.[14] Of the complications associated with spinal manipulation, 81.2% were associated with cervical manipulation.[38] Quadriplegia has been reported in misdiagnosed individuals with cervical vertebral osteomyelitis.[31]

Cerebral artery dissection has been reported after single or multiple manipulations. The onset of a new headache should be a cause of evaluation. Other patients with a partial dissection may seek manipulation therapy, at which point any form of movement results in ischemia, particularly in the vertebrobasilar system.[22]

The risk-benefit ratio for cervical manipulation for patients with neck pain remains significantly high. Most patients with neck pain improve spontaneously. Any severe complication is unacceptable for a benign condition. Other conservative modalities have the opportunity to improve neck pain with less serious toxicities. Mobilization, not manipulation, by a physiotherapist has been recommended for the treatment of whiplash patients by the Quebec Task Force.[47]

Low Back Manipulation

Manipulation has been recommended for uncomplicated acute and chronic low back pain, sciatica without neurologic deficit, sequestrated discs, facet syndrome, sacroiliac strain, piriformis syndrome, psoas syndrome, spondylolisthesis, and spinal stenosis.[21] The ideal patient for manipulative therapy is one with a degree of joint fixation or hypomobility. Absolute contraindications to manipulation include malignancy, osteomyelitis, osteoporosis, fracture, ruptured ligaments, acute arthritis, neurologic dysfunction, hypermobility, and pregnancy in the first trimester.

Neck Manipulation

Patients with decreased range of cervical motion are considered for spinal manipulation. Short-levered, high-velocity thrust therapy is used most often. A course of therapy is given for 4 to 12 weeks. Treatment is given daily for 2 weeks; then manipulation is administered three times per week for the remainder of the course. To prevent recurrence, one treatment per month is recommended.

Manipulation Studies

A number of studies have investigated the benefit of manipulation for low back pain.[19,24,28,44] A review published by the Rand Corporation tabulated the benefits of spinal manipulation from 58 published articles including 25 controlled trials.[41] The majority of studies reported only a brief effect in relieving pain. The difficulty in determining the benefits of manipulation from these studies is the lack of definition of the specific therapies given in each study. Manipulation may mean a variety of therapies were given to a patient, including modalities and exercises in addition to manipulation. It is difficult to determine the component of therapy that is effective when a number of therapies may be given as a part of a manipulative adjustment. Other methodologic problems included absence of placebo groups, inadequate blinding of patients, inadequate measurements of effects of therapy, small patient groups, and reasons for lack of response (patient dropouts). In general, spinal manipulation is associated with transient benefit, lasting hours. Evaluation at periods of 3 months or longer does not show any significant difference among patients who have received manipulation and a variety of other therapeutic modalities. Patients who seem to benefit most are those who have a shorter history of pain. These findings may correlate with the spontaneous resolution of low back pain.[28] Many of the studies of manipulation are flawed by inappropriate control groups, indefinite entry criteria, and variable outcome measures.[17] In a study of 54 patients with low back pain, subjects were divided into those with pain for less than 2 weeks and those with pain for 2 to 4 weeks. No benefit was noted by either group immediately after the treatment. However, by day 3, patients with pain for 2 to 4 weeks seemed to receive significant benefit from manipulation. The groups did not receive identical therapies. Those treated with manipulation seemed to have a more rapid response.[20]

In a study done in Utah, a comparison of physicians and chiropractors was undertaken to determine their effectiveness in the care of back pain patients.[29] Patients expressed confidence in both groups but were more satisfied with the therapy and explanations of the chiropractor. The chiropractors tended to spend more time talking to the patients and gave them emotional support. It seems that anyone "who is responsive to the emotional needs of the patient could achieve equal results in the vast majority of uncomplicated low back pain patients."[29] The essential beneficial factor in manipulation may not be the thrust but the conversation before and after the manipulation. Similar results were reported in a group of 467 patients with back pain of 2 weeks' duration who were treated by a family physician or a chiropractor. Overall satisfaction was three times greater with the chiropractors than with the physicians. Physicians were perceived as being less concerned about the patient's condition and pain. Physicians were also perceived as being less confident about the cause of the patient's pain. Patients who went to the chiropractor reported fewer days of limited activity associated with back pain.[7]

Another study reported the results of a 2-year study contrasting the results of private chiropractic therapy to hospital outpatient physical therapy.[33] Patients who received chiropractic therapy reported consistently greater benefit. However, the groups were not comparable, and the number of therapies were not equal. The recommendations of the authors included adding chiropractic treatment to the National Health Service in England.

Chiropractic therapy may also be cost effective when evaluating the total cost of a back injury. The Utah State Workmen's Compensation System calculated the total cost of medical therapy and days lost from work for patients with low back pain treated by chiropractors and physicians. The total cost for chiropractic treatment was less than for physician's treatment for the same diagnostic codes.[27] However, another report revealed the costs associated with 1020 episodes of back pain associated with 8825 health care provider (general practitioner, orthopedist, chiropractor) visits.[42] Chiropractors, who saw 40% of the patients with low back pain, had the greatest number of visits per episode and the highest mean outpatient cost. In another study comparing the costs of primary care physicians, chiropractors, and orthopedic surgeons, primary care physicians provide the least expensive care for acute low back pain.[6] All of these factors must be considered when considering the recommendation for treatment of a patient with low back pain by a chiropractor. As with any other professional, some practitioners are excellent and have great experience; others do not. A relationship between a physician and another well-trained professional for appropriate referrals may be of benefit to a specific group of patients with acute low back pain and hypomobility.

Only six studies of manipulation therapy for neck pain have been reported.[35] Some studies used passive mobilization only. Two trials demonstrated significant improvement 1 week after mobilization was initiated but did not analyze the benefit after this period. Another study found no significant difference in treated patients compared with control subjects after 3 and 12 weeks.[4,26,46]

Different groups of patients visit a chiropractor versus a medical physician. Cote and co-workers studied individuals from Saskatchewan, Canada, who had neck or back pain who visited a health care provider in the past month.[10] Twenty-five percent of individuals with neck or back pain visited a health care provider. Compared with medical patients, fewer chiropractic patients lived in rural areas or reported arthritis. Patients who seek care have worse health status than those who do not seek care. Patients consulting chiropractors alone report fewer comorbidities and are less limited in the activities than those consulting medical doctors.

Manual Therapy

Manual therapy has similarities with chiropractic manipulation but does not utilize high-velocity, short-amplitude thrusts.[18] Manual therapy uses "hands-on" techniques for muscular mobilization, articular mobilization, and stabilization. Osteopathic manual therapy may involve mobilization exclusively depending on the practitioner. A manual therapist will interact frequently with the spinal pain patient to maximize motion through the use of massage, stretching, and postural control.

Manual therapy clinical trials have reported improvement in pain and function compared with other modalities, including physical therapy and standard care by a general practice physician. Andersson and colleagues reported on the similar outcomes of osteopathic spinal treatments and standard care for patients with subacute low back pain (3 weeks' to 6 months' duration). Both groups had 90% satisfaction with their care, with the osteopathic group requiring less medication.[2]

Manual therapy has also been shown to be effective for neck pain of 3 months' duration or less. Manual therapy had a better outcome than physical therapy and care by a general practitioner in a Dutch study.[25] As mentioned in an accompanying editorial, the applicability of these techniques to other locations is questionable.[37] The frequency of interactions may play a significant role in the benefits of therapy. Manual therapy in this study may contain different interventions than manual therapy in a different country. However, this form of therapy has shown beneficial effects on neck pain and function that go beyond the bounds of physical measurements of motion. Patients are pleased with the therapy and demonstrate outcomes equal to accepted, effective interventions.

Massage

Massage of back muscles provides mechanical stimulation of tissues that offers relaxation of contracted muscles along with increased circulation to the massaged areas. Massage techniques are numerous, ranging from light superficial touch to deep stretching movements (rolfing).[3] The exact mechanism of benefit is not known, although the hypothesis of counterirritant therapy and release of endorphins seems plausible.[49] The psychological benefits of the therapy cannot be overlooked. Many patients mention the relaxation associated with massage as a significant component of this therapy. Massage may be beneficial for patients with subacute or chronic nonspecific low back pain, especially when combined with exercises and education.[15] Other studies describe benefits that are sustained for months related to massage treatments given over weeks that are independent of other therapeutic interventions.[8] Massage therapy is more effective than spinal manipulation and acupuncture for chronic back pain. Massage also may decrease the cost of treatment after the initial course of therapy.

Demonstrating the benefit of massage therapy is difficult because it is used as part of placebo treatment in a variety of studies.[49] Therefore, although some patients state "they cannot get through the week without their massage," this form of therapy must be used in the setting of a total, conservative therapeutic program involving other forms of treatment.

Our Recommendation

Chiropractic manipulation of the lumbar spine is a complementary intervention for those individuals who need a stimulus to increase range of motion of the spine. Osteopathic therapy may also offer improved motion with less drug therapy. Massage therapy of the low back and neck is a cost-effective therapy if practitioners of massage are available.

References

Manipulation

1. Adams F (trans): The Genuine Works of Hippocrates. Huntington, NY, Robert E. Krieger, 1972, pp 238-239.
2. Andersson GBJ, Lucente T, Davis AM, et al: A comparison of osteopathic spinal manipulation with standard care for patients with low back pain. N Engl J Med 341:1426-1431, 1999.
3. Borenstein D: Back in Control! A Conventional and Complementary Prescription for Eliminating Back Pain. New York, M Evans, 2001, pp128-129.
4. Brodin H: Cervical pain and mobilization. Med Phys 6:67, 1983.
5. Bronfort G, Haldeman S: Spinal manipulation in patients with lumbar disc disease. Semin Spine Surg 11:97-103, 1999.
6. Carey TS, Garrett J, Jackman A, et al: The outcome and costs of care for acute low back pain among patients seen by primary care practitioners, chiropractors, and orthopedic surgeons. N Engl J Med 333:913-917, 1995.
7. Cherkin DC, MacCornack FA: Patient evaluations of low back pain care from family physicians and chiropractors. West J Med 150:351, 1989.
8. Cherkin DC, Sherman KJ, Deyo RA, et al: A review of the evidence for the effectiveness, safety, and cost of acupuncture, massage therapy, and spinal manipulation for back pain. Ann Intern Med 138:898-906, 2003.
9. Chrisman OD, Mittnacht A, Snook GA: A study of the results following rotary manipulation in the lumbar intervertebral disc syndrome. J Bone Joint Surg Am 46A:517, 1964.
10. Cote P, Cassidy JD, Carroll L: The treatment of neck and low back pain: Who seeks care? Who goes where? Med Care 39:956-967, 2001.

11. Dan NG, Saccasan PA: Serious complications of lumbar spinal manipulation. Med J Aust 2:672, 1983.
12. Dvorak J, Orelli P: How dangerous is manipulation to the cervical spine? Manual Med 2:1, 1985.
13. Fitzgerald PB: Manipulation and mobilization. In Tollison CD, Satterthwaite JR (eds): Painful Cervical Trauma: Diagnosis and Rehabilitative Treatment of Neuromusculoskeletal Injuries. Baltimore, Williams & Wilkins, 1992, pp 120-133.
14. Ford RF, Clark D: Thrombosis of the basilar artery with softening of the cerebellum and brain stem due to manipulation in the neck. Johns Hopkins Hosp Bull 98:37, 1956.
15. Furlan AD, Brosseau L, Imamura M, et al: Massage for low-back pain: A systematic review within the framework of the Cochrane Collaboration Back Review Group. Spine 27:1896-1910, 2002.
16. Gallinaro P, Cartesegna M: Three cases of lumbar disc rupture and one of cauda equina associated with spinal manipulation (chiropro-sis) [Letter to the Editor]. Lancet 1:411, 1983.
17. Godfrey CM, Morgan PP, Schatzker J: A randomized trial of manipulation of low-back pain in a medical setting. Spine 9:301, 1984.
18. Gross AR, Aker PD, Quartly C: Manual therapy in the treatment of neck pain. Rheum Dis Clin North Am 22:579-598, 1996.
19. Hadler NM: Diagnosis and treatment of backache. In Hadler NM (ed): Medical Management of the Regional Musculoskeletal Diseases. Orlando, FL, Grune & Stratton, 1984, pp 3-52.
20. Hadler NM, Curtis P, Gillings DB, et al: A benefit of spinal manipulation as adjunctive therapy for acute low-back pain: A stratified controlled trial. Spine 12:703, 1987.
21. Haldeman S: Spinal manipulative therapy in the management of low back pain. In Finneson BE (ed): Low Back Pain, 2nd ed. Philadelphia, JB Lippincott, 1981, pp 245-275.
22. Haldeman S, Kohlbeck FJ, McGregor M: Unpredictability of cerebrovascular ischemia associated with cervical spine manipulation therapy: A review of sixty-four cases after cervical spine manipulation. Spine 27:49-55, 2002.
23. Haldeman S, Rubinstein SM: Cauda equina syndrome in patients undergoing manipulation of the lumbar spine. Spine 17:1469, 1992.
24. Hoehler FK, Tobis JS, Buerger AA: Spinal manipulation for low back pain. JAMA 245:1835, 1981.
25. Hoving JL, Koes BW, de Vet HCW, et al: Manual therapy, physical therapy, or continued care by a general practitioner for patients with neck pain: A randomized, controlled trial. Ann Intern Med 136:713-722, 2002.
26. Howe DH, Newcombe RG, Wade MT: Manipulation of the cervical spine: A pilot study. J R Coll Gen Pract 33:574, 1983.
27. Jarvis KB, Phillips RB, Morris EK: Cost per case comparison of back injury claims of chiropractic versus medical management for conditions with identical diagnostic codes. J Occup Med 33:847, 1991.
28. Jayson MI, Sims-Williams H, Young S, et al: Mobilization and manipulation for low back pain. Spine 6:409, 1981.
29. Kane RL, Leymaster C, Olsen D, et al: Manipulating the patient: A comparison of the effectiveness of physician and chiropractor care. Lancet 1:411, 1983.
30. LaRocca H, Macnab I: Value of pre-employment radiographic assessment of the lumbar spine. Can Med Assoc J 101:383, 1969.
31. Lewis M, Grundy D: Vertebral osteomyelitis following manipulation of spondylitic necks: A possible risk. Paraplegia 30:788, 1992.
32. Mathews JA, Yates DAH: Reduction of lumbar disc prolapse by manipulation. BMJ 3:692, 1969.
33. Meade TW, Dyer S, Browne W, et al: Low back pain of mechanical origin: Randomized comparison of chiropractic and hospital outpatient treatment. BMJ 300:1431, 1990.
34. Meeker WC, Haldeman S: Chiropractic: A profession at the crossroads of mainstream and alternative medicine. Ann Intern Med 136:216-227, 2002.
35. Nachemson A: A long term follow-up study of non-treated scoliosis. Acta Orthop Scand 39:466, 1968.
36. Paris SV: Spinal manipulative therapy. Clin Orthop 179:55, 1983.
37. Posner J, Glew C: Neck pain. Ann Intern Med 136:758-759, 2002.
38. Powell FC, Hanigan WC, Olivero WC: A risk/benefit analysis of spinal manipulation therapy for relief of lumbar or cervical pain. Neurosurgery 33:73, 1993.
39. Raftis K, Warfield CA: Spinal manipulation for back pain. Hosp Pract 24:89, 1989.
40. Robertson JT: Neck manipulation as a cause of stroke. Stroke 12:260, 1987.
41. Shekelle PG, Adams AH, Chassin MR, et al: Spinal manipulation for low-back pain. Ann Intern Med 117:590, 1992.
42. Shekelle PG, Markovich M, Louie R: Comparing the costs between provider types of episodes of back pain care. Spine 20:221-227, 1995.
43. Shvartzman P, Abelson A: Complications of chiropractic treatment for back pain. Postgrad Med 83:57, 1988.
44. Sims-Williams H, Jayson MI, Young SMS, et al: Controlled trial of mobilization and manipulation for low back pain: Hospital patients. BMJ 2:1318, 1979.
45. Slater RNS, Spencer JD: Central lumbar disc prolapse following chiropractic manipulation: A call for audit of "alternative practice." J R Soc Med 85:637, 1992.
46. Sloop PR, Smith DS, Goldenberg E, et al: Manipulation for chronic neck pain: A double-blind controlled study. Spine 7:532, 1982.
47. Spitzer WO, Skovron ML, Salmi LR, et al: Scientific monograph of the Quebec Task Force on whiplash-associated disorders: Redefining "whiplash" and its management. Spine 20:1, 1995.
48. Stevinson C, Ernst E: Risks associated with spinal manipulation. Am J Med 112:566-570, 2002.
49. Tan JC, Roux EB, Dunand J, et al: Role of physical therapy in the management of common low back pain. Clin Rheumatol 6:629, 1992.

MAGNETS/BRACELETS

Magnets have been proposed as offering benefits for musculoskeletal pain by normalizing electrical forces in the body. Collacort and colleagues conducted a randomized, double-blind, placebo-controlled, pilot study of 20 individuals with chronic low back pain of a mean duration of 19 years.[2] Real and sham bipolar permanent magnets were applied on alternate weeks, for 6 hours per day, 3 days per week, for 1 week, with a 1-week washout period between two treatment weeks. The outcome measures included a visual analogue scale, the McGill Pain Questionnaire, and range of motion measurements. No significant difference was noted in any of the outcome measures between the groups. The study was criticized because of the small number of patients, the types of magnets, the duration of active therapy, and the type of back conditions. Some patients remain convinced that magnets are helpful to their pain. It is not clear whether it is the holder for the magnets that offers counterirritant therapy as much as the magnets that results in decreased pain. This form of therapy has no toxicities.

Bratton and co-workers reported on the benefits of "ionized" bracelets for the treatment of low back, neck, and other musculoskeletal pain. The bracelets allow a natural flow of Chi by restoring the balance of ions in the body. In a study of 610 patients, 305 wore an "ionized" bracelet and 305 wore an identical placebo bracelet for 4 weeks.[1] In the placebo group 83.6% and in the active group 76.6% thought that the bracelets "worked." The benefits of the bracelets were almost immediate, with 23% improvement on day 1 in both groups and 29% by the fourth week. The bracelets have no toxicities. The bracelets offer a means of harnessing the placebo effect for improved analgesia with no side effects. However, they should not be recommended as proven, effective therapy.

Our Recommendation

Magnets and bracelets cannot be recommended other than for their decorative value.

References

Magnets

1. Bratton RL, Montero DP, Adams KS et al: Effect of "ionized" wrist bracelets on musculoskeletal pain: A randomized, double-blind, placebo-controlled trial. Mayo Clin Proc 77:1164-1168, 2002.
2. Collacott EA, Zimmerman JT, White DW, et al: Bipolar permanent magnets for the treatment of chronic low back pain: A pilot study. JAMA 283:1322-1325, 2000.

ACUPUNCTURE

Acupuncture is based on the theory that the production of brief, moderate pain in specific locations will abolish severe, chronic pain. The same principle has been used in many forms over the years, including cupping, scarification, and cauterization. These counterirritant therapies have been referred to by Melzack as "hyperstimulation analgesia."[24] Acupuncture points can be stimulated by heat, cold, pressure, electricity, ultrasound, or lasers. The most common method of stimulation is insertion of tiny needles into acupuncture points.[23]

Mechanism

The efficacy of acupuncture in diminishing pain is related to endorphin release and to stimulation of large myelinated fibers blocking nociceptive transmission from small unmyelinated C fibers. Stimulation of large fiber mechanoreceptors in a dermatome will inhibit the small fiber pain input in the ipsilateral or contralateral dermatome by "closing the gate" in the spinal cord that allows nociceptive impulses to reach the cerebral cortex.[8,27] This mechanism would explain the lack of effect of acupuncture in disorders involving large fiber destruction, such as postherpetic neuralgia.[19] The importance of afferent transmission to achieve analgesia is also demonstrated by observations that the analgesic effect is blocked by procaine infiltration of acupuncture points. Acupuncture may also produce analgesia by stimulating a location distant to the site of pain. Acupuncture causes the release of endorphins, the endogenous opiates.[33] The effect of acupuncture analgesia can be partially abolished by injection of naloxone, an opiate antagonist.[1,22] Opiate antagonists may prevent the beneficial effect on nociceptive reflexes when injected before acupuncture. The opiate antagonist fails to suppress the beneficial effect of acupuncture on nociceptive reflexes if given after the cessation of therapy. The hypothesis is that acupuncture causes the release of endorphins that set up a cascade effect that is not dependent on endorphins for sustained effect.[23] The long-term relief of pain associated with acupuncture may occur by two mechanisms: (1) normal physiologic activity may resume in a stimulated area with reestablishment of normal large fiber proprioceptive input, which blocks nociceptive input[25] and (2) pain, which may be a learned response or part of memory, is "forgotten" with brief intense stimulation.[24] Evidence also supports the role of acupuncture stimulating increased gene expression of neuropeptides.[9]

The response to acupuncture may result, in part, to the frequency of activation of the sensory system.[23] Low-frequency electrical stimulation results in the secretion of enkephalins from the midbrain that inhibit primary afferent fibers via the dorsolateral funiculus to the spinal cord and endorphins from the hypothalamus that bind to opiate receptors that cause generalized analgesia. High-frequency electrical activation enhances serotonin/norepinephrine descending inhibitory fibers that induce regional analgesia.

Technique

Acupuncture analgesia is obtained by stimulation of particular areas of the skin with fine needles (30-gauge steel, silver, or gold), which are slowly twisted after insertion. The specific areas to be stimulated follow specific meridians (14 in all) that have been plotted on charts.[5] The most effective acupuncture points are often located where nerves enter muscle.[11] The location of acupuncture points and the location for nerve blocks are similar.[15] Acupuncture points may have greater concentrations of pain fibers and vascular structures, which explains the enhanced sensitivity of these points. Most points are at or near the site of pain and a few are distant from it. The needles are left in place for 20 to 40 minutes. The needle insertion feels like a small prick, followed by an ache, numbness, and warmth in the area.[23] Electrical stimulation that directs current with a square or spike wave with variable frequency, pulse width, and voltage may be applied to the needles in situ. Low-frequency electrical stimulation increases the efficacy of the acupuncture procedure.[31]

Contraindications/Toxicities

Patients who are overanxious or who have visceral pain should not receive acupuncture.[21] Potential complications of acupuncture include hemorrhage, pneumothorax, hepatitis, and endocarditis.[7,10,21] In general, acupuncture has few toxicities when administered by an experienced practitioner.

Low Back Pain

Acupuncture has been studied in the treatment of low back pain. In a placebo-controlled, double-blind, crossover study of low back pain, acupuncture was no better than placebo in relieving low back pain.[28] Meta-analysis of studies of acupuncture for the treatment of acute and chronic back pain have revealed contradictory results depending on the entity being studied.[14] Systematic reviews of acute and chronic back pain have reported superiority of acupuncture to various control interventions.[6] However, the efficacy of acupuncture beyond placebo effect has not been demonstrated in a number of analyses.[2,16,38] Acupuncture may not be better than massage for chronic low back pain.[3] In a review of 13 chronic neck and back pain acupuncture studies, Smith reported 5 as positive and 8 as negative.[13] The confusion in the medical community regarding the benefits of acupuncture may be explained in part by the variable findings of efficacy in different studies.

Acupuncture should be considered adjunctive therapy for patients with chronic low back pain. Patients should be considered candidates for this therapy even if they have not responded to TENS therapy. Acupuncture of the body and/or ear may be tried. Obviously, the availability of this therapy depends on the accessibility of an experienced acupuncturist. Electroacupuncture has been tested against paracetamol and was more effective for control of low back pain. A specialized unit that locates acupuncture points on the skin by virtue of properties of altered electrical resistance was helpful in identifying appropriate points of stimulation for patients.[18] Although this study of 40 patients is useful, the applicability of electroacupuncture to a wide range of patients with chronic back pain has not been demonstrated.

Neck Pain

Acupuncture has been studied in the treatment of neck pain. In a placebo-controlled, double-blind, crossover study of neck pain, acupuncture demonstrated an 80% remission rate of neck pain compared with a placebo rate of 33%.[4] Teng and colleagues reported the efficacy of acupuncture in combination with physical therapy in the treatment of cervical spondylosis.[36] Tan and Nordin reported long-term beneficial effects of electroacupuncture on 64.9% of patients with chronic neck and shoulder pain.[35]

Acupuncture Regimen

How often should treatments be given? The first treatment may produce only a few hours of relief. Subsequent visits result in more lasting benefit. A chronic condition requires 5 to 7 treatments given weekly or biweekly. This regimen may result in 60% pain relief over a 6-month period.[21] The patient should be made aware that acupuncture also may increase pain.[34] Too strong a stimulus may result in tenderness that may last 48 hours or longer.

The placement of needles and the frequency of acupuncture may differ depending on the preferences of the acupuncturist. A study was designed to determine the consistency of treatment regimens for back pain. A single patient was evaluated by seven acupuncturists. Diagnostic agreement was found among most of the practitioners, but no consensus was developed regarding the selection of acupuncture points for the patient with chronic back pain.[13] Experience of the practitioner may be essential in obtaining benefit from acupuncture treatments.

Acupuncture and Pregnancy

Acupuncture has been demonstrated to be effective for back pain in pregnant women. In a study of 60 women treated with physiotherapy or acupuncture, pain relief and function were improved to a greater degree in the pregnant group with no serious adverse events. Acupuncture should be considered in those woman with back pain who have concerns with oral medications.[39]

Auricular Acupuncture

Auriculotherapy is acupuncture of the auricle. Nogier has proposed that an inverted homunculus is represented on the auricle.[29] In a double-blind study, Oleson and associates were able to find abnormalities in other parts of the body by detecting areas of increased skin conductivity and tenderness over the ear.[30] Areas of the body that have been injured have altered conductivity of electrical current. Electrical current will follow the path of least resistance and will bypass injured areas. Diseased areas of the body may be located by measuring the electrical conductivity of the skin over suspicious areas, including the auricle, with an ohmmeter.[23] A hypothesis also has been proposed that visceral disorders may be discovered by identification of abnormal electroconductivity in specific meridians corresponding to individual organs. The explanation for this phenomenon is the viscero-skin-sympathetic nerve reflex. Abnormalities in the viscera are transmitted to the spinal cord and are reflected onto the skin via the efferent sympathetic nerves as longitudinal areas of electrical resistance. Electrostimulation of areas of the auricle has been demonstrated to increase cerebrospinal fluid endorphin levels.[32] Others have not been able to reproduce these results.[24] The efficacy of this therapy may be related to anatomic organization of the nervous system. Inputs from the ear project to central nervous system structures that play a role in referred sensation. Low-frequency versus high-frequency electroacupuncture may have a differential effect on the type of neurotransmitters (low-frequency endogenous opioids, high-frequency nonopioid neurotransmitters) resulting in analgesia.[18] Whether specific auricular stimulation or placebo stimulation alone accounts for analgesia with auriculotherapy remains to be determined. In their study, Katz and Melzack were unable to demonstrate any increased benefit of stimulating "Nogier" points compared with placebo points in the auricle.[15] However, about a third of patients reported warmth and other sensations in distant parts of the body with ear stimulation. This suggests that referred sensations are generated by ear stimulation.[15] Kovacs and co-workers reported benefits of "neuroreflexotherapy" (epidermal tacks) in specific locations in the ear and lumbar spine in patients with chronic low back pain. The beneficial effects lasted at least 45 days.[17] Acupuncture of the ear is associated with toxicities including auricular chondritis that is resistant to therapy.[37]

The same mechanism that results in analgesia with acupuncture also may cause the pain relief associated with TENS, ice massage, and needle effect (dry needling of trigger points). The counterirritation of superficial structures may have analgesic effects of short, intermediate, or prolonged duration.[20,26]

The amount of unconventional medicine utilized in the United States is significant.[12] Approximately 33% of people surveyed described visiting an acupuncturist or chiropractor for their medical problems. Unconventional therapy was used for chronic, non–life-threatening conditions. Approximately 83% of individuals also sought advice from their medical doctor for the same condition, and, of these, 72% did not tell their physician that they had seen another health care provider. Medical physicians should ask their patients about the use of unconventional therapy when they obtain a medical history.

Our Recommendation

Acupuncture is a complementary therapy that is passive, time consuming, and invasive. It is a therapy to be considered for individuals with chronic spinal pain resistant to conventional therapies, such as may occur in pregnant women.

References

Acupuncture

1. Chapman CR, Colpitts YM, Beneditti C, et al: Evoked potential assessment of acupunctural analgesia: Attempted reversal with naloxone. Pain 9:183, 1980.
2. Cherkin DC, Eisenberg D, Sherman KJ, et al: Randomized trial comparing traditional Chinese medical acupuncture, therapeutic massage, and self-care education for chronic low back pain. Arch Intern Med 161:1081-1088, 2001.
3. Cherkin DC, Sherman KJ, Deyo RA, et al: A review of the evidence for the effectiveness, safety, and cost of acupuncture, massage therapy, and spinal manipulation for back pain. Ann Intern Med 138:898-906, 2003.
4. Coan RM, Wong G, Coan PL: The acupuncture treatment of neck pain: A randomized controlled study. Am J Chin Med 9:326, 1982.
5. Duke M: Acupuncture: The Meridians of Ch'i. New York, Pyramid House, 1972.
6. Ernst E: Complementary and alternative medicine in rheumatology. Balliere's Clin Rheumatol 14:731-749, 2000.
7. Evans D: Acupuncture. In Raj PP (ed): Practical Management of Pain, 2nd ed. St. Louis, Mosby–Year Book, 1992, pp 934-944.
8. Fitzgerald M: The contralateral input to the dorsal horn of the spinal cord in the decerebrate spinal rat. Brain Res 236:275, 1982.
9. Gao M, Wang M, Li K, et al: Brain substrates activated by electroacupuncture (EA) of different frequencies: II. Role of Fos/Jun proteins in EA-induced transcription of preproenkephalin and preprodynorphin genes. Brain Res Mol Brain Res 43:167-173, 1996.
10. Gilbert JG: Auricular complication of acupuncture. N Z Med J 100:142, 1987.
11. Gunn CC: Motor points and motor lines. J Acupunc 6:55, 1978.
12. Hyodo M: Modern scientific acupuncture as practiced in Japan. In Lipton S, Miles J (eds): Persistent Pain: Modern Methods of Treatment. Orlando, FL, Grune & Stratton, 1985, pp 129-156.
13. Kalauokalani D, Sherman KJ, Cherkin DC: Acupuncture for chronic low back pain: Diagnosis and treatment patterns among acupuncturists evaluating the same patient. South Med J 94:486-492, 2001.
14. Kaptchuk TJ: Acupuncture: Theory, efficacy, and practice. Ann Intern Med 136:374-383, 2002.
15. Katz J, Melzack R: Referred sensations in chronic pain patients. Pain 28:51, 1987.
16. Kent GP, Brondum J, Keenlyside RA, et al: A large outbreak of acupuncture-associated hepatitis B. Am J Epidemiol 127:591, 1988.
17. Kovacs FM, Abraira V, Pozo F, et al: Local and remote sustained trigger point therapy for exacerbations of chronic low back pain: A randomized, double-blind, controlled, multicenter trial. Spine 22:786-797, 1997.
18. Lee JH, Beitz AJ: Electroacupuncture modifies the expression of c-fos in the spinal cord induced by noxious stimulation. Brain Res 577:80, 1992.
19. Levine JD, Gormley J, Fields HL: Observations on the analgesic effects of needle puncture (acupuncture). Pain 2:149, 1976.
20. Lewit K: The needle effect in the relief of myofascial pain. Pain 6:83, 1979.
21. MacDonald AJR: Acupuncture analgesia and therapy. In Wall PD, Melzack R (eds): Textbook of Pain, 2nd ed. Edinburgh, Churchill Livingstone, 1989, pp 906-919.
22. Mayer DJ, Price DD, Raffi A: Antagonism of acupuncture analgesia in man by the narcotic antagonist naloxone. Brain Res 121:368, 1977.
23. McLean B, Fives HE: Stimulation-induced analgesia. In Warfield CA (ed): Principles and Practice of Pain Management. New York, McGraw-Hill, 1993, pp 413-425.
24. Melzack R: Folk medicine and the sensory modulation of pain. In Wall PD, Melzack R (eds): Textbook of Pain, 2nd ed. Edinburgh, Churchill Livingstone, 1989, pp 897-905.
25. Melzack R: Prolonged relief of pain by brief, intense transcutaneous somatic stimulation. Pain 1:357, 1975.
26. Melzack R, Jeans ME, Stratford JG, Monks RC: Ice massage and transcutaneous electrical stimulation: Comparison of treatment for low-back pain. Pain 9:20, 1980.
27. Melzack R, Wall PD: Pain mechanisms: A new theory. Science 150:971, 1965.
28. Mendelson G, Selwood TS, Kranz H, et al: Acupuncture treatment of chronic back pain: A double-blind, placebo-controlled trial. Am J Med 74:49, 1983.
29. Nogier PFM: Treatise of Auriculotherapy. Maisonneuve, France: Moulin-les-Metz, 1972.
30. Oleson TD, Kroening RJ, Bressler DE: An experimental evaluation of auricular diagnosis: The somatotopic mapping of musculoskeletal pain at ear puncture points. Pain 8:217, 1980.
31. Omura Y: Electro-acupuncture: Its electrophysiologic basis and criteria for effectiveness and safety: I. Acupunct Electrother Res 1:157, 1975.
32. Pert A, Dionne R, Ng L, et al: Alterations in rat central nervous system endorphins following transauricular electroacupuncture. Brain Res 224:83, 1981.
33. Pomerantz B, Chiu D: Naloxone blockade of acupuncture analgesia: Endorphin implicated. Life Sci 19:1757, 1976.
34. Scheel O, Sundsfjord A, Lunde P, Andersen BM: Endocarditis after acupuncture and injection—treatment by a natural healer. JAMA 267:56, 1992.
35. Tan JC, Nordin M: Role of physical therapy in the treatment of cervical disk disease. Orthop Clin North Am 23:435, 1992.
36. Teng C, Liu T, Chang W: Effect of acupuncture and physical therapy in the management of cervical spondylosis. Arch Phys Med Rehabil 54:601, 1973.
37. Ter Riet G, Kleijnen J, Knipschild P: Acupuncture and chronic pain: A criteria-based meta-analysis. J Clin Epidemiol 43:1191, 1990.
38. van Tulder MW, Cherkin DC, Berman B, et al: The effectiveness of acupuncture in the management of acute and chronic low back pain: A systematic review within the framework of the Cochrane Collaboration Back Review Group. Spine 24:1113-1123, 1999.
39. Wedenberg K, Moen B, Norling A: A prospective randomized study comparing acupuncture with physiotherapy for low-back and pelvic pain in pregnancy. Acta Obstet Gynecol Scand 79:331-335, 2000.

MIND-BODY THERAPIES

Behavioral treatment has a place in the treatment of chronic low back and neck pain. Systematic reviews of these therapies have demonstrated improvement in pain intensity and functional status.[7,22] The characteristics of the patients who benefit most from these therapies have not been elucidated.

Cognitive-Behavioral Therapy

Cognitive-behavioral therapy (CBT) is derived from learning theory. CBT aim to modify maladaptive behaviors directly through the application of learning techniques.[21] Maladaptive behaviors are theorized to be learned behaviors that can be modified. Cognitive processes (thoughts, attributions, beliefs, appraisals) are recognized as mediators of individuals' emotional and behavioral responses to environmental events. CBT teaches coping skills that identifies and corrects negative distortions of themselves and their environment. The advantages of CBT are that it is effective in 6 to 12 sessions with groups or individuals with a variety of chronic pain problems, including arthritis.[10] The disadvantage is that the patient must be an active participant and must practice the techniques.

Fundamental characteristics of CBT include the following[21]:

1. The assumption that an individual's feelings and behaviors are influenced by his or her thoughts (cognitions)
2. An emphasis on using active, structured techniques aimed at teaching patients how to identify, monitor, and change maladaptive thoughts, feelings, and behaviors ("This pain is awful, and will never get better.")
3. A focus on helping patients acquire skills in applying such techniques on their own in a variety of life problems (coping)
4. A collaborative approach to therapy, in which the patient and therapist work as a team to help the patient learn and apply skills that are most relevant to the patient's unique situation
5. A relatively brief course of therapy

Patients may believe that referral to CPT is an admission that the pain is psychological and not real. These patients can benefit from the effects of CBT on stress management. Stress increases muscle tension and increases pain. Methods to control stress can have a beneficial effect on muscle tension. CBT can improve the interactions with vocation, family, marital, and social relationships that are hindered by chronic pain. Coping skills can also decrease pain and stress. Some of these techniques include relaxation, imagery, and coping self-statements (i.e., "Relax. I can cope. Focus on what you have to do.").

CBT is an effective therapy in spinal disorders. In a study of nurses, Linton and co-workers demonstrated the benefits of CBT in secondary prevention for back pain.[9] Benefits included less pain intensity, anxiety, stress, fatigue, and helplessness than the controls on the waiting list. Turner and Jensen demonstrated the benefits of CBT in a group of 102 patients with chronic low back pain patients.[20] Cognitive therapy, relaxation therapy, or a combination of the two had potential benefits for decreased pain compared with controls.

Systematic reviews of randomized controlled trials for CBT have demonstrated efficacy for specific disorders. CBT may not be effective in all chronic pain problems. It is effective for chronic low back pain for up to a period of 12 months.[14] Another review reported the benefit of CBT on a self-report measure of disability improvement.[19]

The limitation of CPT is the availability of instructors to teach the techniques. Lay people can be taught the methods if an accomplished practitioner is in the community. CPT is effective therapy administered to an individual or to groups of people.[17] It is one of the therapies shown to be effective for patients with spinal pain. CBT should be considered in patients with chronic pain who is willing to learn techniques to improve their coping skills.

Biofeedback

Chronic pain is associated with the development of a depressed or vegetative state. Pain, when associated with change in personality and mentation, may persist despite resolution of the physical trauma associated with the initial pain. In these circumstances, therapies directed only at relieving pain without attempting to modify the psychological state of the patient may not be successful.

A number of techniques are available to alter the psychological state of patients with chronic pain. Biofeedback is a technique by which alterations in biologic processes are demonstrated by a proportional change in a sensory signal (visual or auditory). The biologic processes measured include muscle tension measured by electromyograms (EMGs), skin temperature, pulse volumes, and waveforms on electroencephalograms. Biofeedback techniques are valuable in reducing anxiety and stress, emphasizing self-control, and manifesting the mind-body relationship. Biofeedback treatment is based on the premise that patients with spinal pain have elevated levels of muscular tension, particularly in the paraspinal muscles.[5,23] EMG biofeedback has been tried in chronic low back pain with mixed results. Nouwen reported increased paraspinal muscle EMG activity in patients with chronic pain.[15] A 3-week treatment period was associated with a decrease in EMG activity compared with controls but was not associated with decreased pain. Melzack reported decreased pain in patients using biofeedback who felt in greater control of their symptoms.[13] Kravitz was unable to demonstrate a correlation between paraspinal EMG reduction and pain reduction in patients with chronic low back pain.[8]

Patients who may have the best outcomes from biofeedback were studied by Keefe. These individuals initially rated their pain as severe, were less likely to be receiving disability payments, had fewer years of continuous pain, and had fewer surgical procedures.[2]

The efficacy of biofeedback in low back pain remains to be determined. The reliance on control of a physiologic function ignores the complex psychological, affective, and behavioral components of the pain experience. CBT may offer greater benefit to prevent chronicity than biofeedback in individuals with sciatica.[6] Biofeedback may work by allowing the patient to improve focused thinking, resulting in increased relaxation.[1]

Biofeedback requires several weeks of training. It is indicated only in patients who have persistent chronic pain, and patient motivation must be high. In many circumstances, biofeedback is used in conjunction with relaxation training for control of pain.

Relaxation

The basic premise of this form of therapy is that elicitation of the relaxation response will result in an altered state of consciousness associated with a sense of well-being and peace of mind and concomitant decrease in oxygen consumption, respiratory rate, and heart rate.[23] Blue-collar workers show elevated psychological stress levels, which are higher than those with more flexible work arrangements.[11] These stress levels may cause increased muscle contraction and pain. The proposed mechanisms of benefit of relaxation include increased endorphin levels and presence of increased alpha waves on electroencephalography.[2] The scientific data to support these proposed mechanisms are inconclusive. The relaxation response leads to generalized decreased sympathetic nervous system activity. This response may be mediated by an area in the hypothalamus.[3] More than one relaxation technique is able to elicit the relaxation response.[4]

Relaxation may be induced by a simple technique as proposed by Beary and Benson.[1] The instructions are as follows:

1. Sit quietly with eyes closed.
2. Relax all your muscles starting with the feet and progressing to the head. Keep all muscles deeply relaxed.
3. Breathe through the nose. Say the word "one" silently after each breath. Continue for 20 minutes. Eyes are opened to check the time, but no alarm is used. After 20 minutes, rest with eyes closed, then opened.
4. Do not attempt within 2 hours of any meal.

This technique may be used alone or in conjunction with biofeedback or hypnosis to achieve the desired response.

Other relaxation techniques besides deep breathing also may be effective in achieving an appropriate relaxation response. Progressive muscle relaxation training will decrease muscular tension and pain. Mindfulness meditation uses imagery techniques to focus on distinguishing pain from other sensations.[18] Few studies have been completed comparing the efficacy of relaxation techniques with other therapies. Progressive muscle relaxation is effective and superior to placebo in the therapy for low back pain.[12] Relaxation techniques may not be proven better than placebo but are relatively cost effective and lack lasting harmful side effects. Although the specific physiologic mechanisms resulting in pain relief are unproven, relaxation reduces muscle tension, decreases sympathetic nervous system tone, and provides a cognitive distraction from distress.

Hypnosis

Hypnosis is an altered state of awareness in which the patient experiences increased suggestibility. The hypnotic state narrows attention to exclude extraneous stimulation. Chronic pain is not purely a physical phenomenon. It is associated with emotions and thoughts that alter the patient's perceptions. Through its effects on emotions and thoughts, hypnosis can alter the perception of pain.

Hypnotic suggestion may decrease pain in a number of ways. Patients may attain a level of deep relaxation. The pain may be directly diminished by suggestion or by transfer to another part of the body. The quality of the pain may be altered to tingling or numbness. Patients may be distracted from the pain or told to think of a time before the onset of pain.[16] Hypnotic therapy is most useful if the patient can be taught self-hypnosis, eliminating the need for a hypnotherapist on a continuing basis.

Our Recommendation

Mind-body therapies are complementary techniques that may improve the psychological status of patients with chronic spinal pain. They are helpful for only a small minority of patients who are motivated and have access to experienced therapists.

References

Mind-Body Therapies

1. Beary JF, Benson H: A simple psychophysiologic technique which elicits the hypometabolic changes of the relaxation response. Psychosom Med 36:115, 1974.
2. Benson H, Pomeranz B, Kutz I: The relaxation response and pain. In Wall PD, Melzack R (eds): Textbook of Pain. Edinburgh, Churchill Livingstone, 1984, pp 817-822.
3. Benson H, Arns P, Hoffman J: The relaxation response and hypnosis. Int J Clin Exp Hypn 29:259, 1981.
4. Domar AD, Friedman R, Benson H: Behavioral therapy. In Warfield CA (ed): Principles and Practice of Pain Management. New York, McGraw-Hill, 1993, pp 437-444.
5. Evaskus DS, Laskin DM: A biochemical measure of stress in patients with myofascial dysfunction syndrome. J Dent Res 51:1464, 1972.
6. Hasenbring M, Ulrich HW, Hartmann M, et al: The efficacy of a risk factor-based cognitive behavioral intervention and electromyographic biofeedback in patients with acute sciatic pain: An attempt to prevent chronicity. Spine 24:2525-2535, 1999.
7. Karjalainen K, Malmivaara A, van Tulder M, et al: Multidisciplinary biopsychosocial rehabilitation for neck and shoulder pain among working age adults: A systematic review within the framework of the Cochrane Collaboration Back Review Group. Spine 26:174-181, 2001.
8. Kravitz E, Moore ME, Glaros A: Paralumbar muscle activity in chronic low back pain. Arch Phys Med Rehab 62:172, 1981.
9. Linton SJ, Bradley LA, Jensen I, et al: The secondary prevention of low back pain: A controlled-study with follow-up. Pain 36:197-207, 1989.
10. Lorig K, Mazonson P, Holman H: Evidence suggesting that health education for self-management with chronic arthritis has sustained health benefits while reducing health care costs. Arthritis Rheum 36:439-446, 1993.
11. Lundberg U: Stress responses in low-status jobs and their relationship to health risk: Musculoskeletal disorders. Ann N Y Acad Sci 896:162-172, 1999.
12. McCauley JD, Thelen M, Frank R, et al: Hypnosis compared to relaxation in the outpatient management of chronic low back pain. Arch Phys Med Rehabil 64:548, 1983.
13. Melzack R, Perry C: Self-regulation of pain: The use of alpha feedback and hypnotic training for the control of chronic pain. Exp Neurol 46:452, 1975.
14. Nielson WR, Weir R: Biopsychosocial approaches to the treatment of chronic pain. Clin J Pain 17 (4 Suppl):S114-S127, 2001.
15. Nouwen A: EMG biofeedback used to reduce standing levels of paraspinal muscle tension in chronic low back pain. Pain 17:353, 1983.
16. Pawlicki RE, Wester WC II: Hypnosis. In Raj PP (ed): Practical Management of Pain. Chicago, Year Book Medical, 1986, pp 829-833.
17. Rose MJ, Reilly JP, Pennie B, et al: Chronic low back pain rehabilitation programs: A study of the optimum of treatment and a comparison of group and individuals therapy. Spine 22:2246-2253, 1997.
18. Syrjala KL: Relaxation techniques. In Bonica JJ (ed): The Management of Pain, 2nd ed. Philadelphia: Lea & Febiger, 1990, pp 1742-1750.
19. Turner JA: Educational and behavioral interventions for back pain in primary care. Spine 21:2851-2859, 1996.
20. Turner JA, Jensen MP: Efficacy of cognitive therapy for chronic low back pain. Pain 52:169-177, 1993.
21. Turner JA, Romano JM: Cognitive-behavioral therapy for chronic pain. In Loeser JD (ed): Bonica's Management of Pain, 3rd ed. Philadelphia, Lippincott Williams & Wilkins, 2001, pp 1751-1758.
22. van Tulder MW, Ostelo R, Vlaeyen JW, et al: Behavioral treatment for chronic low back pain: A systematic review within the framework of the Cochrane Collaboration Back Review Group. Spine 26:270-281, 2001.
23. Wallace RK: Physiological effects of transcendental meditation. Science 167:1751, 1970.

HOMEOPATHY

Homeopathic remedies are among the most frequently prescribed complementary therapies. The first principle of homeopathy is "like cures like," meaning that a particular pattern of complaints can be cured by a drug that produces the same pattern of complaints in a healthy person.[2] The second principle is that remedies retain biologic activity if diluted in series and agitate between each dilution. Dilutions have been taken below Avogadro's number with continued potency. The efficacy of homeopathic therapy may be based on placebo or artifact.[1] The third principle is that remedies are most effective when re-creating the total characteristics of the illness. Musculoskeletal disorders are one of the 10 most common ailments treated by homeopathic treatments.[4] In studies of arthritis, the evidence from controlled trials is inconclusive.[3]

References

Homeopathy

1. Jacobs J, Chapman EH, Crothers D: Patients characteristics and practice patterns of physicians using homeopathy. Arch Fam Med 7:537-540, 1998.
2. Jonas WB, Kaptchuk TJ, Linde K: A critical overview of homeopathy. Ann Intern Med 138:393-399, 2003.
3. Jonas WB, Linde K, Ramirez G: Homeopathy and rheumatic disease. Rheum Dis Clin North Am 26:117-123, 2000.
4. Maddox J, Randi J, Stewart WW: "High-dilution" experiments a delusion. Nature 334:267-291, 1988.

HERBAL THERAPIES/NUTRITIONAL SUPPLEMENTS

In the 1997 survey of adults and the use of alternative therapies, 12.1% had used an herbal medicine in the previous 12 months.[6] A number of herbal preparations are used to treat musculoskeletal symptoms. Some of these herbal and nutritional therapies include S-adenosylmethionine, methylsulfonylmethane, glucosamine, ginger, devil's claw, and willow bark, among others.[7] Few of these therapies have been subjected to clinical trials to determine their efficacy or toxicities. A manufacturer of a herbal preparation is permitted to claim that a product affects the structure or function of the body as long as there is no claim of effectiveness for the prevention or treatment of a specific disease.[5] The production of preparations may vary from lot to lot. Herbs contain complex mixtures of constituents that may require specific ratios of ingredients to be effective. These preparations are not approved by a government agency to guarantee consistency. The purity of the preparations must also be questioned.[11] Contaminants can include other botanicals, microorganisms, microbial toxins, pesticides, fumigation agents, toxic metals, or drugs.[5] Many over-the counter herbal supplements have interactions with prescription drugs that are potentially harmful (St. John's wort, ginkgo, ginseng, kava, ephedra).[1]

Willow Bark

Willow bark is the source for salicin, the prodrug of salicylate derivatives. Interest in willow bark has returned, with the expectation that toxicities may be less with herbal preparations. Chrubasik and colleagues completed a placebo-controlled study of 210 patients with back pain with 120 mg or 240 mg of salicin, with tramadol as the sole rescue medication in a 4-week study.[3] The outcome measure was the proportion of patients pain free for 5 days during the final week without tramadol therapy. The consumption of 240 mg of salicin is bioequivalent to 50 mg of aspirin. Patients who received high-dose salicin (39%) had a greater response than the low-dose salicin (21%) and placebo (4%) in the reduction of low back pain. The frequency of adverse reactions was rare and was more commonly related to tramadol. The ideal study would be aspirin versus high-dose salicin versus placebo. The equivalency of salicin was not established with this study.

Devil's Claw

Devil's claw *(Harpagophytum procumbens)* comes from an African plant with fruit with bumpy hooks. The tubers from this plant contain harpagoside, a chemical with analgesic properties. Harpagoside is available as a proprietary extract (Doloteffin) given in daily doses of up to 60 mg. Chrubasik and colleagues reported the results of a randomized double-dummy, double-blind pilot study of Doloteffin (60 mg) versus rofecoxib (12.5 mg) in patients with chronic low back pain.[4] Devil's claw was given to 43 patients and rofecoxib to 36 patients. At 6 weeks, 10 patients taking devil's claw and 5 taking rofecoxib reported no pain without rescue medicine for at least 5 days in the final week of the trial. However, tramadol, the rescue medicine, was used by 21 devil's claw patients versus 13 rofecoxib patients. Adverse events occurred in both groups. This study was unable to demonstrate the benefits of the herbal preparation over the COX-2 inhibitor.

Glucosamine

Glucosamine is glucose with an added amino group. After being acetylated, glucosamine is a major constituent of glycosaminoglycans within connective tissues. Glucosamine in in vitro and ex vivo models inhibits interleukin-1–induced increases in aggrecanase activity and nitric oxide production. Glucosamine increases proteoglycan synthesis, which may be mediated through increased gene expression.[13] Glucosamine is used for symptomatic osteoarthritis. Studies have reported benefits in regard to lower extremity joints.[10] When benefits occur, they are delayed in onset, requiring 2 to 3 months to appear. Systematic reviews of studies of glucosamine have concerns regarding the quality of research protocols.[8] The studies report preservation of cartilage with these supplements.[9] Controversy remains concerning the most accurate radiographic means of measuring cartilage preservation. The benefits of glucosamine sulfate and chondroitin sulfate may also be related to the sulfate they share, as opposed to other components of the molecule. Another concern is the relationship between pain relief and the preservation of cartilage.

Low back and neck pain have not been areas of active research with glucosamine. Clinical trials have not been completed using this supplement. Preliminary trials have been presented at meetings but have not been published. In my own practice, patients who have reported improvement from glucosamine for osteoarthritis of the knee or hip have described, contemporaneously, no benefit for their osteoarthritis of the spine.

S-Adenosylmethionine (SAM-e)

SAM-e is formed by the combination of the essential amino acid methionine and adenosine triphosphate. It is involved with methylation of a variety of compounds that control neurotransmitter and cartilage production.[2] SAM-e is a supplement that has been tested in osteoarthritis. In 11 controlled trials of 1442 patients treated for 10 to 84 days, SAM-e (400 to 1200 mg/day) is more effective in reducing functional limitations than reducing pain in osteoarthritis compared with placebo.[12] SAM-e was as effective as NSAIDs over this short trial. Only 24 patients were treated for longer than 1 month. The continued efficacy over a period of months was not established. The cost of SAM-e compared with generic NSAIDs or acetaminophen is substantial.

The initial dose is 400 mg twice a day. The maximal dose is 1600 mg per day in divided doses. SAM-e is reported to have fewer adverse reactions than NSAIDs. However, a byproduct of SAM-e metabolism is homocysteine, a metabolite that is detrimental to cardiac health when increased. Another limitation of SAM-e is its cost.

Methylsulfonylmethane (MSM)

MSM is a derivative of dimethyl sulfoxide (DMSO), the chemical used to treat interstitial cystitis. DMSO is a solvent passing molecules across the skin. DMSO is easily absorbed. It leaves a bad taste in the mouth and gives off a garlic aroma. MSM has none of these bad characteristics and no garlic aroma. MSM has not been tested in patients with spinal pain and its benefits in these individuals are unknown.

References

Herbal Therapies/Nutritional Supplements

1. Bauer S, Stormer E, Johne A, et al: Alterations in cyclosporin A pharmacokinetics and metabolism during treatment with St John's wort in transplant patients. Br J Clin Pharmacol 55:203-211, 2003.
2. Bottiglieri T: *S*-Adenosyl-L-methionine (SAMe): From the bench to bedside: Molecular basis of a pleiotrophic molecule. Am J Clin Nutr 76:1151S-1157S, 2002.
3. Chrubasik S, Eisenberg E, Balan E, et al: Treatment of low back pain exacerbations with willow bark extract: A randomized double-blind study. Am J Med 109:9-14, 2000.
4. Chrubasik S, Model A, Black A, et al: A randomized double-blind pilot study comparing Doloteffin and Vioxx in the treatment of low back pain. Rheumatology 42:141-148, 2003.
5. De Smet P: Herbal remedies. JAMA 347:2046-2056, 2002.
6. Eisenberg DM, Davis RB, Ettner SL, et al: Trends in alternative medicine use in the United States, 1990-1997: Results of a follow-up national survey. JAMA 280:1569-1575, 1998.
7. Ernst E: Complementary and alternative medicine in rheumatology. Bailliere's Clin Rheumatol 14:731-749, 2000.
8. McAlindon TE, LaValley MP, Gulin JP, et al: Glucosamine and chondroitin for treatment of osteoarthritis: A systematic quality assessment and meta-analysis. JAMA 283:1469-1475, 2000.
9. Pavelka K, Gatterova J, Olejarova M, et al: Glucosamine sulfate use and delay of progression of knee osteoarthritis: A 3-year, randomized, placebo-controlled, double-blind study. Arch Intern Med 162:2113-2123, 2002.
10. Reginster JY, Deroisy R, Rovati LC, et al: Long-term effects of glucosamine sulphate on osteoarthritis progression: A randomized, placebo-controlled clinical trial. Lancet 357:251-256, 2001.
11. Slifman NR, Obermeyer WR, Musser SM, et al: Contamination of botanical dietary supplements by digitalis lanata. N Engl J Med 339:806-811, 1998.
12. Soeken KL, Lee WL, Bausell RB, et al: Safety and efficacy of *S*-adenosylmethionine (SAMe) for osteoarthritis. J Fam Pract 51:425-430, 2002.
13. Towheed TE, Anastassiades TP: Glucosamine and chondroitin for treating symptoms of osteoarthritis: Evidence is widely touted but incomplete. JAMA 283:1483-1484, 2000.

TRYPTOPHAN

The rationale for using L-tryptophan in the treatment of chronic pain is related to the role of serotonin in the central nervous system (CNS). L-Tryptophan is a precursor to serotonin. Ingested tryptophan is absorbed in increased quantities by the CNS and is converted to serotonin. Increased serotonin heightens the tone in the serotonergic inhibitory nerve pathway. L-Tryptophan also potentiates opiate analgesia.[6]

Clinical studies of L-tryptophan have been completed in a small number of patients with chronic pain of maxillofacial origin.[8] Patients who received L-tryptophan in a double-blind study showed statistically greater reduction in pain than the patients taking placebos. Similar findings were reported by Brady and colleagues, who measured pain relief in 10 patients with chronic pain, including 2 with back pain, who were treated with L-tryptophan.[1]

Therapy with L-tryptophan requires a high-carbohydrate, low-fat, low-protein diet in addition to oral administration of 4 g of the drug. Dietary alterations are needed to favor CNS absorption of L-tryptophan over that of other neutral amino acids.[2] This therapy should be considered in patients with chronic pain who are willing to alter their diet as well as ingest 4 g of the medication.

Eosinophilia-Myalgia Syndrome

The use of tryptophan as a therapy for pain has been severely curtailed because of the association of the amino acid with eosinophilia-myalgia syndrome.[5] The source of tryptophan in the United States was a Japanese manufacturer. This tryptophan was thought to have a contaminant that caused the eosinophilia-myalgia syndrome.[3,10] The abnormal metabolism of tryptophan resulted in eosinophil activation and release of eosinophil-derived toxic proteins into the extracellular space.[9] The disorder is characterized by peripheral eosinophilia, myalgias, rash, edema, dyspnea, neuropathies, and myopathies.[11] Patients with neurologic involvement have a poor prognosis.[7] Pathologic findings include inflammatory infiltrates in muscle, connective tissue, small blood vessels, nerves, and septa of subcutaneous adipose tissue.[4] The most effective method for controlling this disorder was the removal of tryptophan from the market, which has resulted in no additional cases. This amino acid is not available as a separate therapy for analgesia for patients with low back pain.

References

Tryptophan

1. Brady JP, Cheatle MD, Ball WA: A trial of L-tryptophan in chronic pain syndrome. Clin J Pain 3:39, 1987.
2. Fernstrom JD, Wurtman RJ: Brain serotonin content: Physiological regulation by plasma neutral amino acids. Science 189:414, 1972.
3. Henning KJ, Jean-Baptiste E, Singh T, et al: Eosinophilia-myalgia syndrome in patients ingesting a single source of L-tryptophan. J Rheumatol 20:273, 1993.
4. Herrick MK, Chang Y, Horoupian DS, et al.: L-Tryptophan and the eosinophilia-myalgia syndrome: Pathologic findings in eight patients. Hum Pathol 22:12, 1991.
5. Hertzman PA, Blevins W, Mayer J, et al.: Association of the eosinophilia-myalgia syndrome with the ingestion of L-tryptophan. N Engl J Med 322:864, 1990.
6. Ho Sobuchi Y, Lamb S, Bascom D: Tryptophan loading may reverse tolerance to opiate analgesia in humans: A preliminary report. Pain 9:161, 1980.
7. Krupp LB, Masur DM, Kaufman LD: Neurocognitive dysfunction in the eosinophilia-myalgia syndrome. Neurology 43:931, 1993.
8. Seltzer S, Dewart D, Pollack RL, Jackson E: The effects of dietary tryptophan on chronic maxillofacial pain and experimental pain tolerance. J Psychiatr Res 17:181, 1982-1983.
9. Silver RM, Heyes MP, Maize JC, et al.: Scleroderma, fasciitis, and eosinophilia associated with the ingestion of tryptophan. N Engl J Med 322:874, 1990.
10. Silver RM, McKinley K, Smith EA, et al.: Tryptophan metabolism via the kynurenine pathway in patients with the eosinophilia-myalgia syndrome. Arthritis Rheum 35:1097, 1992.
11. Swygert LA, Maes EF, Sewell LE, et al.: Eosinophilia-myalgia syndrome: Results of national surveillance. JAMA 264:1698, 1990.

RECOMMENDED THERAPEUTIC REGIMEN—SPINAL PAIN

With so many different recommended forms of therapy, it is clear that there is no one therapeutic intervention that is effective for the universe of patients with spinal pain (Table 19-14). The physician faced with this myriad of therapeutic options should refer back to the axioms of treatment that introduced this section for the basic considerations in deciding on a specific treatment program. These guidelines will help the physician decide on the forms of appropriate therapy for each specific patient with spinal pain.

The choice of effective therapies for spinal pain can be made based on personal experience, case reports, and evidence-based medicine. In the setting of developing recommendations for large populations of patients with spinal pain, evidence-based studies have the greatest validity. In the case of the individual patient, all forms of information should be

19-14 RECOMMENDED THERAPEUTIC REGIMEN

ACUTE LOW BACK PAIN

1. Controlled physical activity: bed rest with access to bathroom (maximum of 2 days)
2. Physical modalities:
   a. Cryotherapy—ice pack *or*
   b. Thermotherapy—hot towel in plastic bag
3. Nonsteroidal anti-inflammatory drugs
   a. Analgesic nonsteroidals:
      Aspirin, 650 mg qid, *or* ketorolac, 10 mg qid, *or* diflunisal, 500 mg bid (after loading with 1000 mg), *or* diclofenac potassium, 50 mg bid, *or* flurbiprofen, 100 mg bid, *or* naproxen sodium, 550 mg bid, *or* etodolac, 300 mg tid, *or* ibuprofen, 800 mg qid. COX-2 inhibitors (rofecoxib, 25 to 50 mg/day; celecoxib, 400 mg bid; valdecoxib, 40 mg/day) for patients with past history of gastrointestinal events
   b. Muscle relaxants (palpable spasm or difficulty sleeping):
      Cyclobenzaprine, 10 or 5 mg 2 hours before bedtime increased to 10 mg tid as needed and tolerated
      If ineffective, not tolerated: orphenadrine citrate, 100 mg bid, *or* chlorzoxazone, 500 mg qd to qid, *or* metaxalone, 400 mg qd to qid as tolerated
4. Injection therapy: anesthetic with/without corticosteroids
5. Optional therapy—prevent recurrence: exercises or Back School

CHRONIC LOW BACK PAIN

1. Physical modalities:
   a. Cryotherapy or thermotherapy
2. Nonsteroidal anti-inflammatory drugs:
   a. Aspirin, 650 mg qid, *or* diclofenac sodium, 75 mg tid, *or* nabumetone, 1000 mg bid, *or* oxaprozin, 1200 mg qd, *or* sulindac, 200 mg bid, *or* naproxen, 500 mg bid, *or* etodolac, 400 mg qid, *or* piroxicam, 20 mg qd, *or* ketoprofen, 200 mg qd
   b. Other choices—ibuprofen, indomethacin, COX-2 inhibitors (rofecoxib, 25 to 50 mg qd; celecoxib, 400 mg bid; valdecoxib, 40 mg qd) for patients with past history of gastrointestinal events
3. Muscle relaxants (palpable spasm or difficulty sleeping):
   a. Cyclobenzaprine, 10 or 5 mg qd; increase to tid as tolerated
   b. If ineffective: amitriptyline, 10 mg, increasing to 100 mg qhs, *or* doxepin, 10 mg, increasing to 100 mg qhs (less sedating)
4. Physical therapy:
   a. Exercises: flexion or extension or isometric
   b. Modalities: temperature (with exercise), TENS
   c. Work hardening: determination of job capabilities
   d. Complementary therapy: massage
   e. Cognitive-behavioral therapy

PERSISTENT CHRONIC LOW BACK PAIN

Pain clinic

considered. A physician's experience needs to be used to convince the patient of the potential for success of the therapeutic regimen. Common sense plays a significant role in making choices for patients. Make use of it constantly.

Acute Spinal Pain

Acute spinal pain of any cause is usually a self-limited illness in most circumstances. Educating the patient on this point is an essential part of treatment. The time spent with the patient increases the confidence the patient places in the physician's recommendations and facilitates the therapeutic process. The patient is told that he or she will improve. Patients with acute pain of short duration can experience total relief of his or her pain and should expect to return to usual activities. The physician will be correct 80% to 90% of the time. During the initial period of pain, individuals should maintain their non-exercise daily activities as tolerated. Any period of time with controlled physical activity (bed rest) should be kept to a minimum. Non-narcotic analgesics in the form of aspirin or other rapid-onset NSAIDs (diflunisal, naproxen sodium, ibuprofen, ketorolac, diclofenac potassium) should be added to decrease pain. Cyclooxygenase-2 inhibitors are preferred in those individuals who have a history of gastrointestinal bleeding or who are on low-dose aspirin for cardioprotection. Ketorolac may be used in the patient with acute pain, particularly when evaluated in the emergency department. An intramuscular injection is very effective for controlling pain without the need for narcotics. If anti-inflammatory therapy is needed, however, another NSAID should be chosen because ketorolac has a relatively mild anti-inflammatory effect with an increased risk of gastrointestinal bleeding compared with other NSAIDs. If patients experience muscle spasm, which is noted on physical examination, or develop difficulty sleeping because of muscle tightness, muscle relaxants, which are nonaddictive, are indicated. These agents may cause sedation. Lower dose formulations of these agents decrease this toxicity. Instructing the patient to take the muscle relaxant 2 to 3 hours before bedtime decreases the likelihood of somnolence the following morning. The patient should be cautioned about driving and the use of heavy machinery when initially starting these agents. Therapeutic modalities in the form of cold, initially, or heat, subsequently, may be applied to the painful area while the patient is at home.

With resolution of spinal pain, the patient may resume usual activities with or without additional education. A session in a back school or with a physical therapist is useful for those patients interested in learning to improve physical function with exercises and possibly prevent recurrence of pain.

Patients who do not improve on this regimen are candidates for additional therapy, which may take the form of local injection of painful sites. A change in NSAIDs and/or muscle relaxant after a trial of 2 to 3 weeks may be warranted if pain continues. If the patient had a partial response to the NSAID without toxicity, the dose of the drug should be increased to the maximum.

Patients who have improved but who will resume strenuous physical activities are candidates for physical therapy. Exercises will improve their general physical condition and prepare them for increased strain on the spine. Patients should learn how to lift and carry objects. They may also need to learn how to sit appropriately in a stress-free manner in front of their computers. Support in the form of a lumbar corset or a neck brace makes the patient mindful of the back and neck, respectively, limiting exposure to potentially damaging stresses encountered during work. These external supports should be only given with a course of strengthening exercises and the admonition for use only during working hours. Patients should be weaned from these external supports as quickly as their clinical improvement allows.

Patients who are concerned about returning to physically demanding work may benefit from a functional capacity evaluation, quantifying their ability to complete tasks associated with their work in a controlled environment. If the patient is "weak" in comparison to the tasks required, a work-hardening program is worthwhile. In a work-hardening program, the patient "goes to work" at the work-hardening center. Over the 2- to 3-week period, the patient is given increasingly difficult physical tasks associated with work. By the end of the session, the patient has retrained for the work-associated tasks so that there is less risk of having a recurrence of injury when returning to work.

Chronic Spinal Pain

The therapy for chronic spinal pain patients is more difficult. The goal of therapy for these patients is maximal physical function despite continued pain. The general internist or family practitioner may offer therapies that diminish but not abolish discomfort. The patients must understand, from the outset, the goal for therapy and the likelihood of only partial pain relief. Chronic pain is an illness of its own. Alterations of the spinal cord and brain with upregulation of NMDA receptors and loss of inhibitory interneurons, for example, may not be reversed despite healing of the original source of pain. This understanding is an essential part of therapy. If these patients do not accept these goals and outcomes, they will be quickly disappointed, frustrated, and depressed and will not improve.

Patients are instructed at the initial meeting with the physician that maximal function and return to work is the goal of therapy. Pain may continue and may be exacerbated at times but this is not necessarily indicative of past or present disease-associated damage. Patients can be functional despite pain. Patients with organic pain readily accept these goals. Malingerers are frequently disappointed with this regimen and miss appointments.

Patients with chronic spinal pain are treated with NSAIDs, muscle relaxants, and/or injection therapy when indicated. Other medications of the same class will be substituted for the initial agents if they prove to be ineffective. Low-dose tricyclic antidepressants may be added for patients with a partial response to the initial regimen. Tricyclic antidepressants may work whether or not the individual has clinical symptoms of depression. Other pain-relieving medications that have benefits for inhibition of pain in the central nervous system include gabapentin, topiramate, or tizanidine. These agents are used on series in low doses to limit toxicity while maximizing effects.

Analgesics also play a role in the treatment of chronic pain. Non-narcotic therapies should be prescribed as an adjunct to other medications (NSAIDs). Acetaminophen, tramadol, and tramadol/acetaminophen combination are non-narcotic analgesics with efficacy synergistic with the NSAIDs. The role of narcotic analgesics has evolved since the first edition of this book. Originally, narcotic therapy was prohibited as a component of chronic pain therapy. Our understanding of narcotics and their role in chronic pain management has increased over the past decade (see Chapter 3). Long-acting narcotic therapy can decrease pain and improve function without the development of tolerance or addiction. Physical dependence should not be confused with addiction or drug-seeking behavior. Patients with chronic spinal pain can reach a steady dose level without the need for increasing levels of narcotic medication.

Referral to a physical therapist is made for exercises to improve general conditioning as well as to correct any imbalance in the spine with stretching and strengthening exercises of the flexion, extension, or isometric variety.

Patients who continue to experience pain should try counterirritant therapy. Some patients prefer topical heat packs that are applied to the low back or neck. TENS units can be used to improve involvement with daily activities. Patients are fitted with the machine by the therapist, and those who find the unit useful can rent it for varying periods of time. Patients should buy units only if they obtain benefit from the TENS machine over a period of months.

Referral to a pain clinic should be considered for patients who continue to experience pain after receiving these therapies. Pain clinics offer a multidisciplinary approach to pain, employing neurosurgeons, anesthetists, psychiatrists, physical therapists, vocational rehabilitation counselors, and other professionals interested in the therapy of chronic pain. A number of invasive procedures (nerve ablation, spinal cord stimulators) are available for individuals with unrelenting pain. The number of people who require this type of therapy in comparison with those who present with low back or neck pain is extremely small. However, the opportunity for this group of patients with chronic pain to improve without this combined therapeutic approach is limited.

CHAPTER 20

SURGICAL THERAPY

Surgical intervention, when indicated, provides predictable and gratifying results. Despite areas of minor controversies, the indications for surgical procedures have been well established. Judicious selection of patients who require lumbar or cervical spine surgery results in rewarding outcomes for both patient and physician. There is no place for exploratory operations, which are associated with poor outcomes and persistent pain and complications.

With the establishment of strict criteria for patient selection, results ranging from good to excellent can approach 90% to 95% in most cases. Lumbar spine surgery is more straightforward than cervical spine surgery and has less risk of damaging the spinal cord. Surgery on the cervical spine is not as easily mastered, and the complications, when present, can be quite serious. The purpose of this chapter is not to detail the surgical procedures but to provide a general discussion of the selection of surgical patients and the role of surgery in the treatment of axial skeletal disorders. The potential complications of surgical intervention are reviewed.

INDICATIONS FOR CERVICAL SPINE SURGERY

Surgery on the cervical spine is performed to relieve pain (usually radicular or arm pain), bony instability, and neural element compression (spinal cord and nerve roots). The procedures performed may be grouped into one of three categories: decompression (with or without disc excision), stabilization (fusion or bony ankylosis), or both. Furthermore, the cervical spine surgeon must decide whether the problem area in the spine should be approached anteriorly or posteriorly and in one or two stages.

CERVICAL HERNIATED NUCLEUS PULPOSUS

Indications for Surgery

When nonoperative therapeutic measures have proven unsuccessful in managing the patient with symptoms from an acute herniated disc, surgical intervention can and should be considered.[7,12] This occurs in 10% to 15% of all cases. Patients with a cervical herniated disc can present predominantly with neck pain, lower extremity dysfunction, arm pain, or a combination of all three.

Neck Pain

Failure of nonoperative treatment is not an indication for operative treatment for patients mainly with neck pain associated with a cervical disc. The results of surgery are much less predictable than those associated with relief of arm pain. Disc surgery for neck pain alone is unpredictable and should be undertaken with great caution.

Profound Spinal Cord Impingement

The most dramatic, but fortunately the most rare, presentation of a cervical herniated nucleus pulposus is sudden and profound neurologic loss produced by a large central disc displacement. This disc displacement produces a profound or progressive acute myelopathy with quadriparesis or quadriplegia below the level of the herniation. If not decompressed urgently, the potential for lasting weakness, spasticity, loss of bowel and bladder function, and sexual dysfunction is increased.[17] In some cases, even prompt treatment does not reverse the spinal cord damage thought to be the result of lack of blood supply. Once this clinical condition is identified, the patient should undergo emergent myelography or magnetic resonance (MR) scan, followed by decompression of the offending disc by anterior discectomy and interbody fusion. Despite the potential lack of total recovery, the surgery often prevents further damage to the spinal cord and loss of neurologic function.

Progressive Neurologic Deficit

If the physician can document a worsening in a patient's neurologic examination, prompt surgical intervention should be considered. Commonly, a patient presents with arm pain radiating into the index and long fingers. A diminished brachioradialis and possibly a diminished biceps reflex are noted on initial examination. Conservative treatment is instituted and the patient is later reevaluated. Subsequent evaluation might reveal a further loss in the arm reflexes associated with demonstrable motor weakness in the biceps muscle. This constellation of findings represents a progressive neurologic deficit. Because this is usually not reversible with medications and rest, and the surgeon wants to prevent further permanent nerve damage, surgical decompression should be done once confirmatory evidence of the location of the lesion is provided by computed tomography (CT) (with myelography) or MR evaluation.

The more common patient presentation is one of an acute stable neurologic deficit. If the deficit is profound with significant motor weakness, for example, complete paralysis of the hand intrinsic muscles (C8 and T1), surgical intervention is a viable option and most spine surgeons consider it mandatory.[13] Although often difficult to quantitate, clinical experience suggests that the more prolonged and severe the pressure on a spinal nerve, the less likely the nerve is to recover function. Unfortunately, there are no good prospectively controlled series to document the recovery of cervical nerve root function. Every spine surgeon remembers cases in which the return was noted within days and those in which it never improved or even worsened. Presently, recommendations for surgery have to be individualized for each patient, based on the clinical picture and the significance of the neurologic findings.

It is an even more difficult clinical judgment when the patient presents with a partial neurologic lesion (weakness) or the clinical situation is subacute. A stable neurologic finding, by itself, is not a good criterion for surgery because it is unpredictably reversed. One must keep in mind the temporal relationship because acute or subacute pain may not correlate with the patient's neurologic findings. Previous medical records and examination are often helpful in making this decision.

Unrelenting Radicular Arm Pain (Brachialgia)

Occasionally an acute episode of brachialgia without neurologic deficit fails to respond to conservative treatment. The exact timing of surgical treatment varies from patient to patient, depending on individual pain tolerance, socioeconomic factors, and emotional stability. In most instances, if a patient has an abnormal electromyogram, has an abnormal myelogram or MR scan, and has not improved with a minimum of 6 weeks of nonoperative treatment, the patient may be considered for surgery. However, if some improvement is realized, waiting up to an additional 6 weeks may result in continued resolution of symptoms. The results of surgery are not as predictable as with those of neurologic deficits, but they can be dramatic.

Recurrent Episodes of Arm Pain

A small group of patients with arm or radicular pain have recurrent episodes of incapacitating pain. Most often the arm or radicular pain is low grade or smoldering between the incapacitating episodes, suggesting chronic cervical spondylosis. The time between episodes is tolerable for the patient. If the recurrent acute pain episodes are within the patient's tolerance and minimally affect activities of daily living, nonoperative therapy should be provided. Less commonly, the frequency and intensity of the pain are severe enough to interfere with the patient's employment and avocational endeavors such that surgery should be considered. As a guideline, if the patient experiences three or more episodes in a year, surgery should be offered if the confirmatory tests of nerve compression are positive.

The relief of the painful condition requires that the surgeon find evidence of a physical or organic cause of the patient's pain. This means that, ideally, mechanical compression of the suspicious nerve root is demonstrable from either a bony spur (also known as a hard disc) or a soft tissue abnormality such as a herniated disc (soft disc). On the contrary, if one undertakes to decompress a nerve root that is not the focus of a mechanical or organic lesion, the results are no better than a placebo (about 50%). The so-called exploratory spinal operation should be avoided for pain relief.

When the patient with brachialgia is considered for surgery, the following three criteria should be met if an excellent result is to be anticipated: (1) clear radicular pain pattern, (2) neurologic deficit, and (3) positive confirmatory test (myelogram or MR).[24] The results of surgery cannot be expected to be excellent unless the patient has at least a neurologic examination and a correlative MR or myelogram showing abnormalities.

Patient Factors

The key to a successful outcome in any surgery, especially spine surgery, is patient selection. Even the most expertly performed surgical procedure if done in an inappropriate patient is doomed to an unfavorable outcome. A patient's emotional, psychological, and socioeconomic condition must be considered. A patient's concern or depression about his or her condition should not be misinterpreted; physical and psychological factors interrelate. In a patient with a complicated clinical situation, organic problems may coexist with psychological difficulties.

The emotional factor is difficult to quantitate; it is a subjective measure best ascertained by patient interview. The Minnesota Multiphasic Personality Inventory, a questionnaire that measures relative levels of hysteria, depression, and hypochondriasis, among others, may be of use preoperatively in predicting the surgical outcome. If the patient presents with minor complaints and a paucity of physical findings but has a significant emotional overlay or even overt depression, continued nonoperative treatment is warranted. If, on the other hand, definite physical findings are present (e.g., a neurologic deficit) and emotional problems preexist, a psychiatric consultation is recommended. The patient may need to have optimal medical and psychiatric management before surgery or, as is often the case, once the psychological overlay is treated, the symptoms improve enough that surgery is no longer required. As a rule, emotional and psychological factors should be addressed and treated before surgical intervention.

Socioeconomic factors include litigation and work-related injury. Patients with cervical spine problems who were involved in an automobile accident (usually minor) or injured at work are some of the most difficult patients to treat successfully.[25] These patients, unlike those with psychological overlays, do not exhibit emotional problems. It is often difficult to pinpoint a reason for their less than optimal response to treatment. Unless these patients have a profound or progressive neurologic condition with objective findings that warrants emergency surgery, the wisest course is to continue conservative treatment until the litigation or compensation is settled. Although these problems are not as prominent in cervical spine disease as in lumbar spine disease, their presence should not be overlooked or underemphasized. Finally, a small group of patients, usually women who have domestic problems, warrants special mention. These patients may have been injured at home or may have spouse-related problems but do not have compensation or litigation claims. They have so-called domestic neuroses. The secondary factors that preclude a good response to surgery are the patient's home environment and marital problems, resulting in varying levels of emotional overlay and depression.

Selection of Surgical Method

The goals of surgery for cervical disc herniation are to decompress the spinal nerve by removing the mechanical impingement on the nerve root and to relieve the patient's radicular arm pain. Two surgical options of nearly equal efficacy can be undertaken in patients with a posterolateral disc herniation.[24] The first involves a partial removal of the offending facet through a posterior approach and is called a "keyhole" foraminotomy.

The second surgical procedure is the anterior disc excision with bony fusion. This procedure involves an anterior or frontal approach to the cervical spine and directly addresses the problem.[2,9] This procedure is clearly superior in a true central disc herniation with acute spinal cord compression. In general, the anterior approach provides about a 90% to 95% chance of good-to-excellent results in relief of the radicular arm pain (Fig. 20-1). The long-term results of this operation have been documented to a greater degree in the literature than results of the posterior approach.

In general, the authors favor an anterior procedure for two reasons: (1) the procedure approaches the offending problem most directly and (2) the long-term results, excluding bone graft donor site pain, are slightly better. Donor site pain may affect up to a third of patients.[19,20,28] Either procedure is adequate for treating radicular arm pain and may be chosen based on the surgeon's preference and experience. Anterior surgery, however, is clearly the procedure of choice for central disc herniation.

Herkowitz and colleagues designed a prospective study to compare anterior fusion versus laminotomy-foraminotomy in patients with cervical disc herniation.[23] The success rate for anterior fusion was 85% versus 75% for laminotomy. Zeidman and Ducker described their experience with posterior cervical laminoforaminotomy for radiculopathy.[35] A success rate of 97% was reported for 172 patients with cervical radiculopathy, but follow-up was limited.

CERVICAL SPONDYLOSIS/STENOSIS

Indications for Surgery

Cervical spondylosis, or chronic cervical disc degeneration, produces pathologic changes in the diameter of the cervical spinal canal or neural foramina, or both. The reduction in area can compress the spinal cord and either directly or secondarily, owing to spinal cord ischemia, lead to spinal cord damage or myelopathy. Once myelopathy has been diagnosed, surgery should be considered.[8,26] The goals of surgery are to relieve the pressure on the spinal cord and thereby prevent the progression of the myelopathic symptoms. Improvement of myelopathy is harder to achieve and relates to the duration and severity of the spinal cord compression. Neck pain relief is not a goal of the surgery but fortunately not a significant part of the clinical symptoms either. Furthermore, the patient must understand that myelopathy, unlike radicular arm pain, is less predictable in its response to decompression.

Routine radiographs of the cervical spine are helpful in cervical spine stenosis because they reveal degenerative disc space narrowing, spur formation, and a diminished spinal canal diameter. Unfortunately, the mere presence of these findings does not explain the patient's clinical picture; further confirmation is required. A CT scan with small amounts of intrathecal water-soluble dye (CT/myelogram) aids in the diagnosis as an alternative to plain myelography or MR scanning.

Selection of Surgical Method

The goal of an operation for cervical spinal stenosis is to remove all pressure from the neural elements completely. The type of problem dictates the nature and extent of the decompression required. If a large, central, soft disc herniation is encroaching on the spinal canal, the herniation must be removed. More commonly, anterior spondylotic or bony spurs (hard discs) compress the neural elements, which are further exacerbated by the posterior changes in the ligamentum flavum and facet joints. Unlike in the lumbar spine, complete removal of all the offending elements is not possible or even necessary to provide an adequate decompression.

When cervical spinal stenosis involves four or more levels, a posterior laminectomy or laminoplasty is favored. If radicular symptoms coexist from foraminal narrowing, foraminal decompression at the appropriate level is also done. If more than two foraminotomies are required, they may best be done anteriorly despite the need for a large bone graft, which incorporates slowly. On the other hand, if the spinal canal stenosis involves three or fewer adjacent vertebral levels, anterior disc fusion without removal of posterior osteophytes is favored. Anterior cervical discectomy without fusion results in decompression but may result in a risk of 50% of patients developing autofusion in kyphosis. The results of the surgery in cervical spinal stenosis are satisfactory in about 80% of cases, with the anterior procedures providing slightly better results.[22]

RESULTS OF OPERATIVE TREATMENT

A general statement regarding the results of cervical spine surgery is not possible. Each category of cervical degenerative disc disease and inflammatory cervical processes has its own peculiar problems that influence the end results.

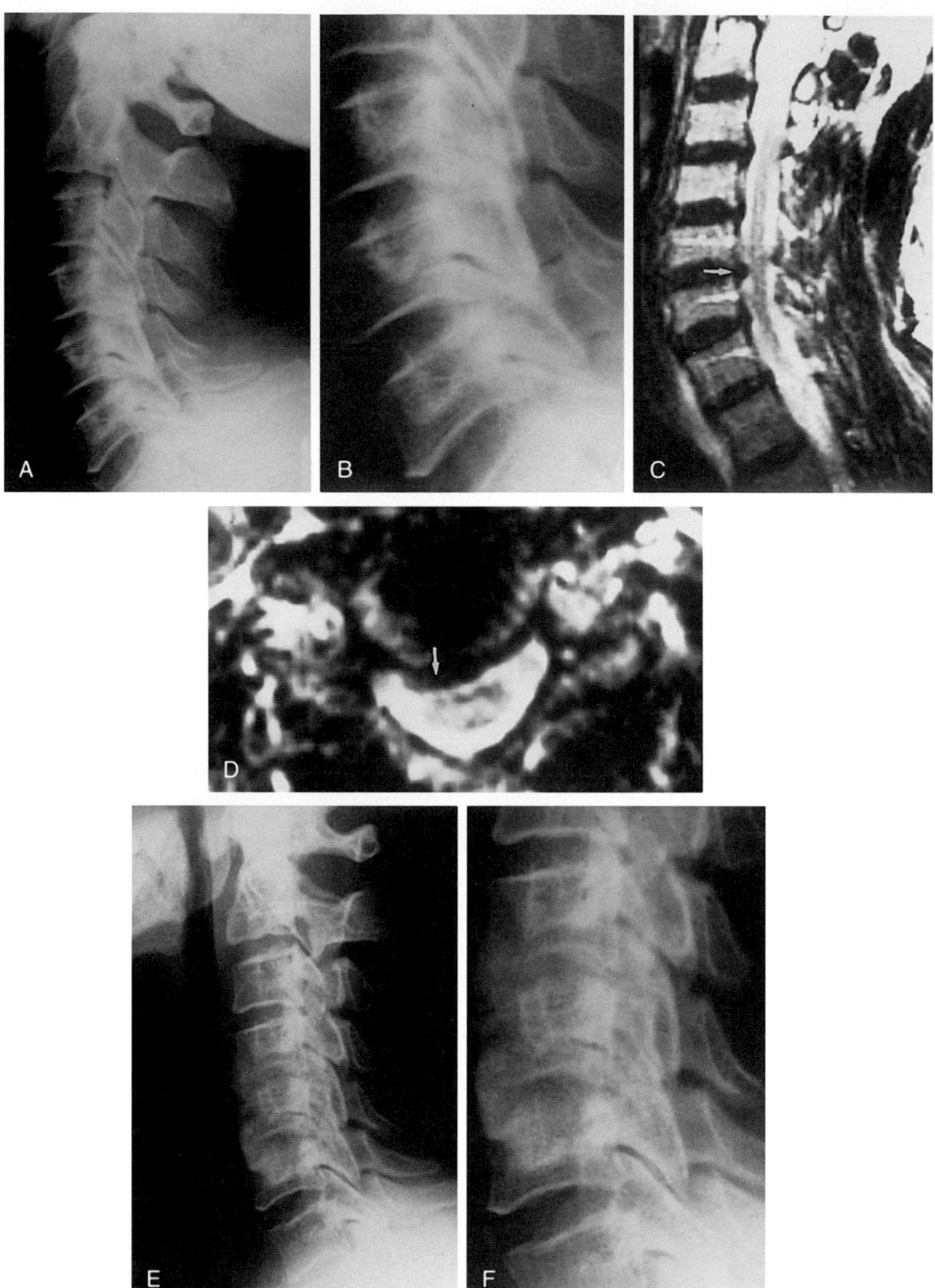

Figure 20-1 Herniated cervical disc. A patient presented with right arm pain in a C6 dermatomal pattern and neck pain suggestive of discogenic pain in a C4-C5 distribution. Lateral views *(A* and *B)* of the cervical spine: preoperative views on plain roentgenograms do not reveal significant discogenic disease. Preoperative magnetic resonance sagittal *(C)* and axial *(D)* views reveal a herniated nucleus pulposus at the C5-C6 level *(arrows)*. Postoperative roentgenograms *(E* and *F)* were taken after anterior cervical discectomy and fusion with autogenous iliac crest bone graft from C4-C5 to C5-C6. The patient had total postoperative relief of arm and neck pain.

The results of cervical spine surgery for acute herniated disc with radicular arm pain, cervical spondylosis with neck pain only, cervical spondylosis with myelopathy and myeloradiculopathy, and cervical instability in rheumatoid arthritis are reviewed.

Cervical Herniated Disc

Surgery for acute cervical herniated disc has been moving slowly from the posterolateral keyhole foraminotomy to the anterior disc excision with fusion. The results of these two procedures are similar in long-term reviews, but the anterior approach with discectomy and fusion is slightly better, despite requiring bone grafting. If proper indications are followed in the appropriate patient population, one can expect a 90% chance of good-to-excellent results. This is the most common type of surgery performed on the cervical spine.[23]

Cervical Spondylosis without Radiculopathy

Surgery for cervical spondylosis with neck pain only is much less satisfactory and unpredictable. Good or excellent results were achieved only in 63% of these patients. The quality of the result does not deteriorate with time, and older patients tend to have a higher percentage of satisfactory results.

Cervical Myelopathy

Results of decompressive laminectomy for cervical spondylosis are variable. The goal is mainly prophylactic—to prevent further neurologic deficit. On occasion, improvement of the clinical state present 6 months before surgery can be achieved, and sometimes more dramatic recovery occurs. The procedure has yielded a rate of 70% to 85% satisfactory (good to excellent) results.

Cervical Instability—Rheumatoid Arthritis

Rheumatoid arthritis (RA) commonly involves the neck but infrequently requires surgery. RA patients with atlantoaxial subluxation with posterior atlantodental intervals of 14 mm or less are candidates for posterior arthrodesis from the first to second cervical vertebrae. Patients with atlantoaxial subluxation and 5 mm of basilar invagination are candidates for posterior arthrodesis of the occiput to the second cervical vertebra after halo traction to reduce subluxation.[5] The results of surgery in RA are not as good as for cervical degenerative disc disease. In large part, this is explained by the nature of the systemic progressive rheumatoid process. These patients tend to be quite ill, and the perioperative mortality rate is about 10%. At 2 years, the mortality rate may reach 27% of RA postsurgical patients. The deaths are related to the RA and not the surgical intervention.[30] A second problem is the severe bone loss and erosion that are a consequence of RA and disuse osteoporosis. The bones of the neck are weak and do not hold instrumentation well. Fusion fails to occur in 20% to 50% of cases. Patients are also at risk of infection.[10] Other complications of surgery of the rheumatoid cervical spine include wound dehiscence, wire breakage, nonunion, and late subaxial subluxation below a fused segment.[4]

Long-Term Results

Surgery for acute herniated cervical disc provides satisfactory long-term results in 90% of cases, whereas surgery for myelopathy provides satisfactory long-term results in 70% to 80% of cases. Surgery for patients with cervical disc disease with neck pain only has the worst rate, with long-term satisfactory results of about only 60%. Finally, in RA patients, the results are not always satisfactory, with high rates of perioperative morbidity with persistent neurologic deficits, pseudarthrosis, and mortality.[27]

INTRAOPERATIVE AND POSTOPERATIVE COMPLICATIONS

Intraoperative Complications

Even with meticulous surgical exposure and the surgeon's intimate knowledge of anatomy, complications occur during cervical spine surgery.[21] Some complications are unique to the anterior or posterior approach; others are common to both. The overall complication rate is estimated at 3% to 4%, and the frequency of neurologic complications is 1% to 2%. Although the anterior approach has a lower rate of neurologic complications (less than 1%) than the posterior approach (1% to 2%), it is associated with a higher rate of complications related to the bone graft used for fusion (1% to 5%). In a study of 384 surgical patients with cervical myelopathy, 21 (5.5%) sustained neurologic deterioration related to spinal cord or nerve root dysfunction.[33] Surgical failure may occur if inadequate decompression is obtained in patients with multiple levels of neurologic compression. Complete decompression with adequate stabilization with fusions is necessary in these patients with multilevel disease.[16]

Anterior Approach

Intraoperative complications unique to the anterior approach include complications associated with soft tissue manipulation, including perforation of the pharynx, trachea, and esophagus, which can be devastating if unrecognized during surgery.[29] Vascular injury to the carotid artery, jugular vein, vertebral artery, and thoracic duct must be avoided.[11] The most frequent neurologic complication is injury to the recurrent laryngeal nerve, but injury to the spinal cord, nerve roots, and sympathetic chain may also occur. Injury to the recurrent laryngeal nerve may be related to endotracheal tube pressure and placement of retractors during the anterior approach procedure. Release of pressure and re-inflation during the operation results in a decrease of temporary paralysis from 6.4% to 1.69%.[1] Complications associated with the autogenous iliac crest bone graft include improper graft positioning with cervical canal compromise, anterior extrusion of the graft, and graft donor site problems such as injury to the lateral femoral cutaneous nerve and hematoma.

Posterior Approach

Intraoperative complications associated with the posterior approach include injury to the spinal cord or nerve roots, most frequently those of C5. Late instability or kyphosis due to aggressive decompression without fusion may occur. The most common complications of posterior cervical fusion include wire pull-out and pseudarthrosis.

Postoperative Complications

Postoperative complications that are common to both approaches include hematoma, cerebrospinal fluid leakage from dural tears, infection, and failure of fusion with subsequent kyphosis. The anterior approach may also rarely be complicated by discitis. Pulmonary atelectasis, deep venous thrombosis, and intestinal ileus may occur. Positioning of the patient with cervical instability in the appropriate manner and intubation with the patient awake limits the postoperative complications of increased extrinsic cord compression during induction of general anesthesia.[3] The sitting position is beneficial for decreasing bleeding, but it increases the risk for venous air embolism.[14] The preferred prone position is not associated with the complication of air embolism, but it may cause venous engorgement and retinal artery thrombosis secondary to increased intraocular pressure.[29] Most of these complications can be prevented or at least minimized if recognized and treated early. Longer complex operative procedures may increase the risk of ophthalmologic abnormalities.[25a,27a]

Some patients do not improve after surgery because their condition is the result of two diseases. Approximately 10% of patients with cervical spondylosis have concomitant lumbar spinal stenosis associated with lower extremity symptoms.[15] Central nervous system diseases (multiple sclerosis and spinal cord tumors) have symptoms and signs similar to those of compressive myelopathy. These primary neurologic disorders need to be considered in the differential diagnosis of the patient with cervical myelopathy.

Patients who undergo decompression and fusion may develop progressive symptoms during the next 12 to 24 months secondary to the breakdown of the fusion mass.[6] Pseudarthrosis rates vary from 0% to 26%.[31,32] A variety of salvage surgery techniques are available to stabilize the cervical spine in those patients who experience nonunion of their grafts.[18,34]

References

Indications for Cervical Spine Surgery

1. Apfelbaum RI, Kriskovich MD, Haller JR: On the incidence, cause, and prevention of recurrent laryngeal nerve palsies during anterior cervical spine surgery. Spine 25:2906-2912, 2000.
2. Aronson NI: The management of soft disc protrusions using the Smith-Robinson approach. Clin Neurosurg 20:253, 1973.
3. Blair J, Garfin S: Complications of cervical laminectomy in degenerative disorders of the cervical spine. Semin Spine Surg 7:52, 1995.
4. Boden SD: Rheumatoid arthritis of the cervical spine: Surgical decision making based on predictors of paralysis and recovery. Spine 19:2275, 1994.
5. Boden SD, Dodge LD, Bohlman HH, Rechtine GR: Rheumatoid arthritis of the cervical spine. J Bone Joint Surg 75A:1282, 1993.
6. Brodsky AE, Khalil MA, Sassard WR, et al: Repair of symptomatic pseudoarthrosis of anterior cervical fusion: Posterior versus anterior repair. Spine 17:1137, 1992.
7. Brodsky AE: Management of radiculopathy secondary to acute cervical disc degeneration and spondylosis by the posterior approach. In Sherk HH, Dunn EJ, Eismont FJ, et al (eds): The Cervical Spine. Philadelphia, JB Lippincott, 1989, pp 617-624.
8. Clark CR: Cervical spondylitic myelopathy: History and physical findings. Spine 13:847, 1988.
9. Clements DH, O'Leary PF: Anterior cervical discectomy and fusion. Spine 15:1023, 1990.
10. Conaty JP, Mongan ES: Cervical fusion in rheumatoid arthritis. J Bone Joint Surg Am 63A:1218, 1981.
11. Curylo LJ, Mason HC, Bohlman HH, et al: Tortuous course of the vertebral artery and anterior cervical decompression: A cadaveric and clinical case study. Spine 25:2860-2864, 2000.
12. DePalma AF, Rothman RH: The Intervertebral Disc. Philadelphia, WB Saunders, 1970, p 225.
13. DePalma AF, Rothman R, Lewinnek G, et al: Anterior interbody fusion for severe cervical disc degeneration. Surg Gynecol Obstet 134:755, 1972.
14. Ducker T, Zeidman S: The posterior operative approach for cervical radiculopathy. Neurosurg Clin N Am 4:61, 1993.
15. Edwards W, LaRocca SH: The developmental segmental sagittal diameter in combined cervical and lumbar spondylosis. Spine 10:42, 1985.
16. Emery SE, Bohlman HH, Bolesta MJ, et al: Anterior cervical decompression and arthrodesis for the treatment of cervical spondylotic myelopathy: Two to seventeen-year follow-up. J Bone Joint Surg Am 80A:941-951, 1998.
17. Fager CA: Results of adequate posterior decompression in the relief of spondylitic cervical myelopathy. J Neurosurg 38:684, 1973.
18. Fellrath RF Jr, Hanley EN Jr: The causes and management of pseudoarthrosis following anterior cervical arthrodesis. Semin Spine Surg 7:43, 1995.
19. Fernyhough JC, Schimandle JJ, Weigel MC, et al: Chronic donor site pain complicating bone graft harvesting from the posterior iliac crest for spinal fusion. Spine 17:1474-1480, 1992.
20. Goulet JA, Senunas LE, DeSilva GL, et al: Autogenous iliac crest bone graft: Complications and functional assessment. Clin Orthop 339:76-81, 1997.
21. Graham JJ: Complications of cervical spine surgery. In Sherk HH, et al: The Cervical Spine, 2nd ed. Philadelphia, JB Lippincott, 1989, pp 831-837.
22. Herkowitz HN: A comparison of anterior cervical fusion, cervical laminectomy, and cervical laminoplasty for the surgical management of multiple level spondylotic radiculopathy. Spine 13:774, 1988.
23. Herkowitz HN, Kurz LT, Overholt DP: Surgical management of cervical soft disc herniation: A comparison between the anterior and posterior approach. Spine 15:1026, 1990.
24. Herkowitz HN, Simeone FA, Blumberg KD, Dillin WH: Surgical management of cervical disc disease. In Rothman RH, Simeone FA: The Spine, 3rd ed. Philadelphia, WB Saunders Co, 1992, pp 597-639.
25. MacNab I: The "whiplash" syndrome. Orthop Clin North Am 2:389, 1971.
25a. Myers MA, Hamilton SR, Bogosian AJ, et al: Visual loss as a complication of spine surgery: A review of 37 cases. Spine 22:1325-1329, 1997.
26. Nurick S: The natural history and the results of surgical treatment of the spinal cord disaster associated with cervical spondylosis. Brain 95:101, 1972.
27. Peppelman WC, Kraus DR, Donaldson WF, Agarwal A: Cervical spine surgery in rheumatoid arthritis: Improvement of neurologic deficit after cervical spine fusion. Spine 18:2375, 1993.
27a. Stevens WR, Glazer PA, Kelley SD, et al: Ophthalmic complications after spinal surgery. Spine 22:1319-1324, 1997.
28. Summers BN, Eisenstein SM: Donor site pain from the ilium: A complication of lumbar spine fusion. J Bone Joint Surg Br 71B:677-680, 1989.
29. Ullman JS, Camins MB, Post KD: Complications of cervical disk surgery. Mt Sinai J Med 61:276, 1994.
30. Van Asselt KM, Lems WF, Bongartz EB, et al: Outcome of cervical spine surgery in patients with rheumatoid arthritis. Ann Rheum Dis 60:448-452, 2001.
31. White A, Southwick W, Deponte R, et al: Relief of pain by anterior cervical spine fusion for spondylosis. J Bone Joint Surg Am 55A:525, 1973.
32. Whitecloud TS, LaRocca SH: Fibular strut graft in reconstruction surgery of the cervical spine. Spine 1:33, 1976.
33. Yonenbu K, Hosono N, Iwasaki M, et al: Neurologic complications of surgery for cervical compression myelopathy. Spine 16:1277, 1991.
34. Zdeblick TA, Hughes SS, Riew KD, et al: Failed anterior cervical discectomy and arthrodesis: Analysis and treatment of thirty-five patients. J Bone Joint Surg Am 79A:523-532, 1997.
35. Zeidman SM, Ducker TB: Posterior cervical laminoforaminotomy for radiculopathy: Review of 172 cases. Neurosurgery 33:356, 1993.

INDICATIONS FOR LUMBAR SPINE SURGERY

Accepted guidelines exist for the selection of patients for lumbar spine surgery. These criteria are similar to those of the cervical spine. They also contain considerations specific to the lumbar spine. When these selection criteria are followed, good surgical outcomes can be expected.

LUMBAR HERNIATED NUCLEUS PULPOSUS

Indications for Surgery

A herniated disc can present clinically with varying degrees of severity, each with its corresponding indications for surgery.

Cauda Equina Compression

The most dramatic presentation of an acute disc herniation is the profound or progressive neurologic deficit referred to as a cauda equina compression (CEC) syndrome.[11] Affected patients may have loss of all neurologic function below the level of the lesion, including bowel and bladder control. It is a true surgical emergency. If bowel and bladder function are to be preserved, immediate surgical decompression of the cauda equina is imperative. The longer the delay, the less recovery can be expected; in view of the complex interplay of compression, edema, and vascular insult to these delicate nerve roots, prediction of surgical results is difficult. These patients may fail to recover fully even with the most expeditious treatment. Surgical intervention for cauda equina decompression is best accomplished within 48 hours of symptom onset.[1,34]

Progressive Neurologic Deficit

The other indication for early surgical intervention is a progressive neurologic deficit. For example, a patient who was first seen with an absent Achilles reflex is then noted to be gradually losing muscle strength in the legs. Such patients must be kept under close observation, because if the trend cannot be reversed an operation may be the only way to prevent further progression. This presentation is unusual but must be kept in mind because of the serious risk of further neurologic impairment.

Sciatica

Occasionally an acute attack of sciatica will fail to respond to all forms of conservative treatment. The exact time when surgery should be recommended will vary from patient to patient according to pain tolerance, emotional stability, and socioeconomic factors. In general, the authors do not recommend consideration of surgery in acute sciatica until 4 to 6 weeks have elapsed. On the other end of the spectrum if there has been little or no improvement by 12 weeks, surgery should be done because further procrastination might adversely affect the end result.[28]

After an initial successful course of conservative treatment, certain individuals will have recurrent sciatica that becomes incapacitating. Symptoms may be completely absent between episodes, or what begins as low-grade pain may become increasingly severe. If the recurrent episodes are not too disabling and if the intensity of the symptoms is within the patient's tolerance, then continued conservative management is indicated. However, if the frequency and intensity of attacks are severe enough to interfere with the individual's ability to pursue gainful employment and enjoy the normal activities of daily living, then surgery should be seriously considered. In general, the authors would consider surgery after the third episode, but in this regard there is some difference of opinion.

In most instances, surgery is performed to relieve sciatic pain, and the effectiveness of the procedure will depend on the identification and relief of pressure on the neural elements. Ideally, a mechanical nerve root compression will be found whenever an operation is done to relieve sciatica. Diagnosis of mechanical root compression requires (1) either a positive tension sign or a neurologic deficit and (2) radiologic confirmation by MR or CT with/without myelography. With the availability of MR, which is noninvasive, it would be most unusual to undertake surgery without preoperative confirmation of the lesion. A variety of procedures for herniated discs exist, and each is briefly discussed.

Stable Neurologic Deficit

It is more common, however, for patients to present with an acute, stable neurologic deficit. If it is profound, such as complete paralysis of the quadriceps muscles of the thigh or the dorsal flexors of the foot, surgery is a viable option and in some centers is considered mandatory.[35] Some believe that the more prolonged the pressure on the spinal nerves and the more intense the compression, the less likely is return of function. There have been no controlled studies that have prospectively compared the return of nerve function with and without surgery. Anecdotes abound of "miraculous" return to full function after surgery was delayed or refused, so the final decision about surgical intervention is often predicated on the quality of the surgery available.

Uncertainty concerning the need for surgical intervention is even greater when motor weakness is less severe or when the situation is subacute. A stable neurologic deficit is not in and of itself an indication for surgery because an operation does not necessarily lead to a return of function. One should also keep in mind that the deficit may not have any temporal relevance; that is, it could very well be a residuum of a prior attack. A well-documented history can be a great help in these situations.

Weber, in an excellent prospective study, took a group of patients with stable neurologic deficits and operated on half of them.[37] After 3 years of follow-up, the neurologic residua were similar in both the surgically and conservatively treated groups. In a stable situation, the aim of surgery is to relieve pain, not to regain neurologic function. The stable deficit should not be used as an excuse for inadequate conservative management and premature intervention. Sensory loss and reflex change are helpful in terms of diagnosis, but they are not in themselves indications for surgical intervention. They have no prognostic value in terms of the ultimate outcome.

Selection of Surgical Method

Open (conventional) discectomy has proved to be safe and efficient in treating patients with herniated discs who have failed to respond to appropriate conservative therapy. With proper patient selection, conventional discectomy can be expected to initially provide good to excellent results in 90% to 95% of cases, but the long-term success rate in these patients may decrease to 70% over the subsequent decade owing to recurrence or scarring.[13] It is estimated that conventional discectomy has a 0.03% mortality rate, with an incidence of neurologic complications of less than 0.5% and minor complications in 4.7% of cases.[15] Although acute lumbar disc herniation in the elderly is not a common problem, surgery yields a high rate of satisfactory results in selected patients older than age 60 years.[21] With a high percentage of successful results and a low morbidity, this procedure has stood the test of time; other procedures must show definitive advantages before open discectomy can be abandoned in their favor.

Microsurgical discectomy involves the use of a small incision (2.5 to 3 cm), the operating microscope for high magnification, and intense illumination of the operative field. Its theoretical technical advantages are improved visualization of microanatomy, preservation of epidural fat, meticulous hemostasis, minimal nerve root trauma, and minimal dissection of paravertebral muscles.[23] An apparent economic advantage over conventional discectomy is the decreased hospital stay, although postoperative recovery time is similar.[17] At the extreme, ambulatory microsurgery for lumbar discs also has been reported.[3] However, retrospective studies have unfairly compared the length of hospitalization for microsurgical discectomies with that for open discectomies performed in the 1970s—a time when the average stay for all surgical procedures was much longer than it is today.

Most reports claim at least a 90% success rate for microsurgical discectomy at relieving leg pain and somewhat less success at relieving back pain.[25,36] Concerns with this technique include the relatively high recurrence rate reported in some series[25] and an excessive number of dural tears.[29] A case of bowel perforation after microsurgical lumbar discectomy also has been reported.[33] In comparison with other techniques, the success rate of microsurgical discectomy appears to be superior to that of chemonucleolysis[22,40] and comparable to that of conventional discectomy.[26,29,32] However, no prospective, randomized investigations with standardized monitoring of postoperative pain have been conducted.

Many surgeons, including the authors, are not convinced that the theoretical technical advantages and apparent cost savings with microsurgical discectomy are worth compromising surgical exposure.[8] The microsurgical technique does not facilitate adequate assessment or treatment of stenosis of the nerve root canal (which may coexist with disc protrusion), nor does it ensure visualization of disc fragments that may be forced above or below the disc level—two common reasons for re-operation. The authors agree that a technique that decreases hospital stay and lost work days is attractive; however, these advantages must definitively be proved in a prospective, randomized study with long-term follow-up.

Percutaneous discectomy is another technical method of removing a disc. By mechanically decompressing the disc, percutaneous lumbar discectomy may have the beneficial effects of chymopapain without the associated complications. Various posterolateral and lateral approaches have been reported, usually with manual removal of disc material with forceps after confirmation of location with fluoroscopy. The reported complications include leg dysesthesia and paraspinal muscle spasm. Early trials indicate that this treatment was effective in 65% to 75% of patients, but these positive results were too optimistic.[5,12]

Onik and co-workers have described their experience with automated percutaneous discectomy.[27] The advantage of their technique is the introduction of a specially designed nucleotome through a narrow cannula (2.8 mm) to aspirate disc material without anterior perforation of the annulus. They reported an 86% success rate in 36 patients who met stringent clinical and radiographic criteria for surgery; those who had radiographic evidence of a free disc fragment or facet disease were excluded. When the procedure was performed under local anesthesia with fluoroscopic guidance, no neurologic complications occurred. As with chemonucleolysis, it is difficult to envision that removal of the nucleus pulposus will relieve pressure on neural elements caused by a large protrusion of disc material into the spinal canal. In a randomized, controlled trial of 71 individuals with a contained herniated disc, automated percutaneous lumbar discectomy in 31 individuals was matched against lumbar microdiscectomy in 40 individuals. In procedures completed by the same surgeons, the percutaneous procedure produced 29% with satisfactory results, whereas the microdiscectomy procedure resulted in an 80% satisfactory result rate. These results suggest that automated percutaneous lumbar discectomy is an ineffective procedure in the treatment of a contained lumbar disc herniation.[4a]

Other percutaneous techniques are under investigation that attempt to remove the offending herniated disc fragment, rather than just the center of the disc. These techniques use a larger working cannula often with endoscopic guidance and flexible instruments to retrieve contained posterolateral disc fragments. Preliminary reports on the results of endoscopic procedures suggest success similar to more established techniques.[39] Additional studies are required to determine if these less invasive techniques result in the same favorable results as those associated with more established techniques.

LUMBAR SPINAL STENOSIS

Indications for Surgery

Lumbar spinal stenosis is the narrowing of the spinal canal because of degeneration of the facet joints as well as the intervertebral disc spaces. If the narrowing is severe, constriction of the neural contents within the spinal canal will develop and cause symptoms, which may vary significantly from patient to patient and can be manifested by back pain, leg pain, or both. When pain constantly interferes with ambulation, surgery should be considered. Unlike the clinical syndrome associated with an acute disc herniation, there may be no objective clinical findings in canal stenosis; consequently, a carefully constructed history is particularly important and the patient's description of his or her discomfort should be carefully noted.

Routine roentgenograms are quite helpful in canal stenosis and show disc space narrowing as well as facet joint arthritis and decreased spinal canal diameter.[7] Similar findings also can be observed on a CT scan. Unfortunately, many asymptomatic patients will show these same radiologic findings, so a surgical decision cannot be based solely on these findings: the clinical and radiologic data must be compatible if a satisfactory operative result is to be expected. The patient must also be aware that the aim of surgery is to relieve leg pain; relief of back pain is less predictable.

SPONDYLOLISTHESIS

Indications for Surgery

Spondylolisthesis is the forward slipping of one vertebral body on another (horizontal translation). Routine roentgenograms are all that is necessary to make the diagnosis, but this is a relatively common condition that may be unrelated to the back pain in question and such an incidental radiologic finding can on occasion confuse the diagnostic process. Assuming that low back pain symptoms are due to the related instability, the spondylolisthesis can usually be treated successfully by limiting stressful activities and by bracing and exercises. Most people with spondylolisthesis do not require surgery.

In the majority of cases, once a patient becomes symptomatic, some form of job modification becomes necessary, because, regardless of treatment, heavy work will always be a problem. Surgery should be considered only after an adequate trial of conservative treatment has failed.[14] Most of these patients will complain of mechanical back pain with or without leg pain. It should be appreciated that surgery will relieve the pain but will not return these patients to unrestricted activity.

SPINAL FUSION

Indications for Surgery

The exact indications for spinal fusion are as yet unknown and will not be determined until the completion of long-term, prospective studies in which patients within specific diagnostic categories are treated in a controlled, randomized fashion. From what is known today, the authors believe that a spinal fusion should be considered only for the following indications:

1. The presence of surgical instability created during decompression with bilateral removal of the facet joints.
2. The presence of neural arch defects (spondylolysis or spondylolisthesis).
3. The presence of a symptomatic and radiographically demonstrable segmental instability that can be objectively identified by weight-bearing lateral flexion and extension roentgenograms. Instability can be assumed when there is more than a 3.5-mm horizontal translation, a reversal of the intervertebral angle at a specific interspace, or both.

Technique of Laminectomy and Fusion

The surgical excision of a herniated disc is straightforward. It is designed to minimize the postoperative recovery time yet effectively treat the source of nerve root compression.[38]

The operation may be performed with the patient under spinal or general anesthesia. The patient is placed in a kneeling position so that the abdomen is free and intra-abdominal pressure is reduced. A straight incision is made over the desired interspace and carried down to the lamina. The ligamentum is removed as well as bone from the adjacent lamina. The goal is to visualize the involved nerve root, which is retracted medially, and remove the disc. The procedure usually takes between 1 and 2 hours. There should be very little blood loss. Postoperatively, the patient may stand immediately and walk. Prolonged sitting is avoided for the first 6 weeks to decrease pressure on the involved disc space.

A lumbar fusion or arthrodesis of the spine is a more involved procedure. The anesthesia and position are the same. The object of the operation is to place bone between the transverse processes of the adjacent vertebrae to be fused. This is termed a *bilateral lateral fusion*. The fusion site has to first be decorticated and the bone harvested from one of the posterior iliac crests. There is significant blood loss, and 2 to 4 units need to be reserved for the patient. The use of fusion for a variety of lumbar operations remains an area of active investigation. Studies have described no improved benefit from fusion with or without segmental fixation, compared with decompression alone.[10] Nutritional status is an important issue for individuals who undergo spinal fusion. Those who are malnourished at the time of surgery (low albumin, lymphopenia) are at greater risk for postoperative infections.[19]

Postoperatively the patients experience a great deal of pain. This is due to the decorticated surfaces of the fusion site and graft site. It may take as long as 12 months for fusion to occur, and some form of brace is usually prescribed.

COMPLICATIONS OF LUMBAR SPINAL SURGERY

Low back surgery is not without risks and should be undertaken only for the proper indications.[31] During the operation the most frequent problem is injury to the neural elements; this can involve just an isolated nerve root or the cauda equina itself. Another intraoperative complication is injury to the major vascular or visceral structures. This usually occurs during removal of the disc when an instrument violates the anterior longitudinal ligament.

Postoperative complications include wound infection, cauda equina syndrome, and urinary retention. These patients need to be watched very carefully for the first 48 hours. Possible causes of immediate postsurgical failure include insufficient surgical decompression, surgery at the wrong level, and traumatization of the nerve root. Incorrect diagnoses, such as lateral spinal stenosis, recurrent or persistent disc herniation, arachnoiditis, central canal stenosis, or epidural fibrosis, are additional causes of immediate failure. Incorrect diagnoses can also be a cause of delayed failure. Epidural fibrosis as a cause of back and leg pain remains controversial. Studies have reported radicular pain in individuals with MR evidence of epidural fibrosis.[30] Because of the severity of the complications it should again be stressed that low back surgery should not be undertaken without due consideration and there is no place today for exploratory surgery.

RESULTS OF SURGERY

If the expected pathologic process is found at surgery, the results of low back surgery are quite rewarding.[16] The average age of patients subjected to lumbar disc surgery is 40 years. In individuals with surgery on the L5-S1 disc space, 15% have persistent back pain postoperatively, 7% have persistent sciatica, and 14% have both back and leg pain. The results are essentially the same when the operation is done at the L4-5 interspace.

Preoperative physical findings such as muscle spasm, tenderness, limitation of motion, and positive straight leg–raising test disappear in 90% of patients. Neurologic deficits clear less frequently. Reversal of preoperative motor and sensory deficits can be expected in 50% of patients, and lost reflexes will return to normal in only 25%. Individuals with chronic psychological distress before surgery may not have as good a response to surgical intervention.[4]

OTHER SURGICAL PROCEDURES

A number of disorders may benefit from surgical interventions. Many of these are traumatic in origin and are beyond the scope of this book. A number of resources are available for review of these topics.[9] Patients who have sustained severe trauma to the axial skeleton can be stabilized with surgical intervention (Fig. 20-2). Surgical procedures are also available for patients who have osteolysis of the spine related to malignancy (Fig. 20-3) or osteoporosis (Fig. 20-4).

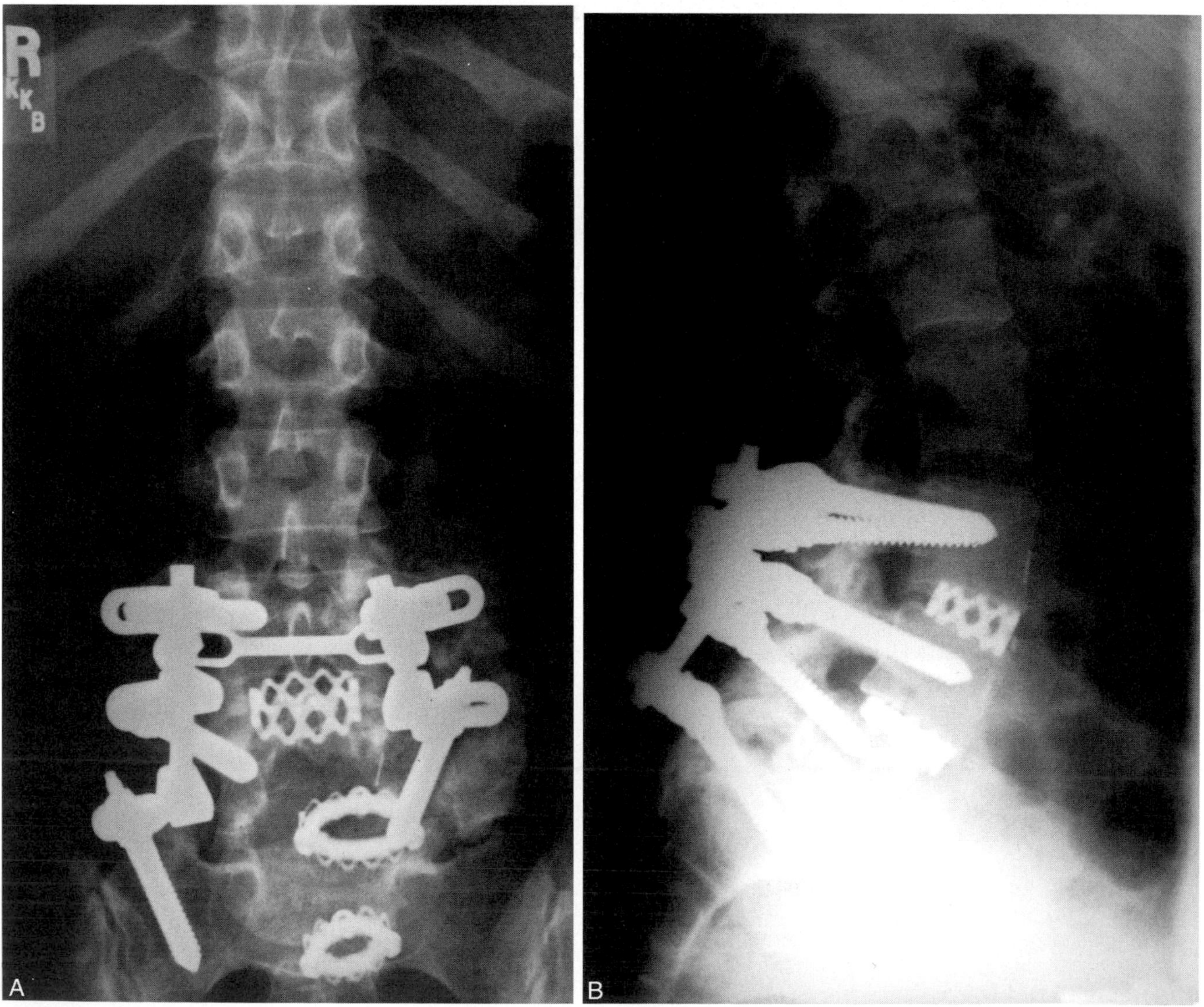

Figure 20-2 Post-traumatic lumbar spine. A 38-year-old woman was involved in two motor vehicle accidents. The second accident resulted in marked spinal instability. Anteroposterior *(A)* and lateral *(B)* views of the lumbar spine with three disc spacers and four-level spinal screw placement are shown.

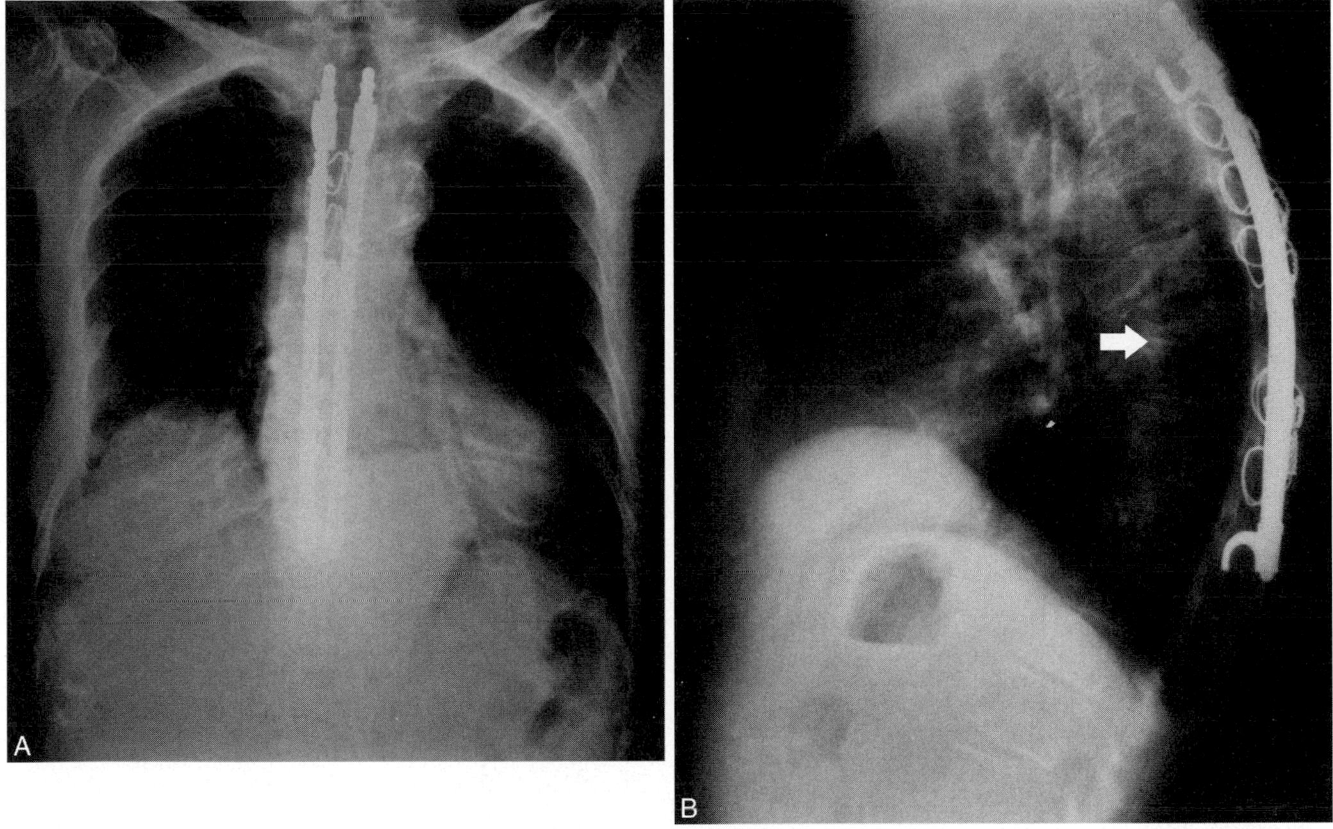

Figure 20-3 Metastatic breast cancer. A 55-year-old woman had breast cancer that metastasized to the thoracic spine and resulted in vertebral body collapse *(white arrow)*. Anteroposterior *(A)* and lateral *(B)* views of the thoracic spine show rod placement for spinal stability.

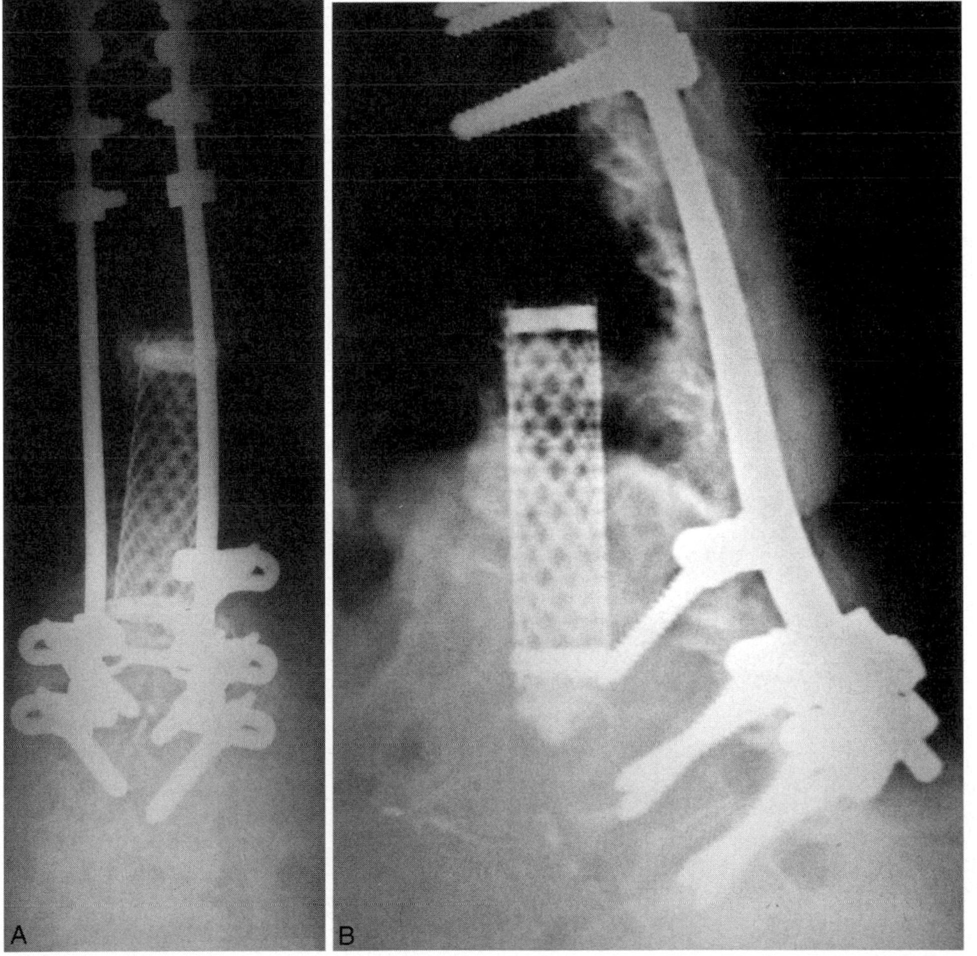

Figure 20-4 Corticosteroid-induced osteoporosis. A 39-year-old woman with connective tissue disease with vasculitis required large, sustained doses of corticosteroids. She developed increasing osteoporosis with compression fractures despite medical therapy. Her spine became unstable. Anteroposterior *(A)* and lateral *(B)* views of the thoracolumbar spine demonstrate a metal cylinder replacement for four vertebral bodies. Spinal rods were required for adequate spinal stability.

In summary, if the appropriate indications for low back surgery are followed, one can expect 90% overall satisfaction with the operation. Although relief from leg pain is reasonably predictable, only 80% of patients achieve a satisfactory result as far as their back pain is concerned.

NEW ADVANCES

A number of surgical innovations are being actively investigated. Improved means of obtaining bone fusion is being advanced through the use of bone morphogenetic proteins.[2] Minimally invasive spinal surgical procedures allow the opportunity to do little damage to nonpathologic tissues.[6] Questions remain whether limited exposure allows for adequate decompression.[24] Total disc replacements, nucleus replacement, and procedures for annulus repair are being studied for individuals with severe intervertebral disc disease.[18,20]

References

Indications for Lumbar Spine Surgery

1. Ahn UM, Ahn NU, Buchowski JM, et al: Cauda equina syndrome secondary to lumbar disc herniation: A meta-analysis of surgical outcomes. Spine 25:1515-1522, 2000.
2. Boden SD, Kang J, Sandhu H, et al: Use of recombinant human bone morphogenetic protein-2 to achieve posterolateral lumbar spine fusion in humans: A prospective, randomized clinical pilot trial: 2002 Volvo award in clinical studies. Spine 27:2662-2673, 2002.
3. Cares HL, Steinberg RS, Robertson ET, et al: Ambulatory microsurgery for ruptured lumbar discs: Report of ten cases. Neurosurgery 22:523, 1988.
4. Carragee EJ: Psychological screening in the surgical treatment of lumbar disc herniation. Clin J Pain 17:215-219, 2001.

4a. Chatterjee S, Foy PM, Findlay GF: Report of a controlled clinical trial comparing automated percutaneous lumbar discectomy and microdiscectomy in the treatment of contained lumbar disc herniation. Spine 15:734-738, 1995.

5. Davis GW, Onik G: Clinical experience with automated percutaneous lumbar discectomy. Clin Orthop 238:98, 1989.
6. Ditsworth DA: Endoscopic transforaminal lumbar discectomy into the spinal canal. Surg Neurol 49:588-597, 1998.
7. Epstein BS, Epstein JA, Jones MD: Lumbar spinal stenosis. Radiol Clin North Am 15:227, 1977.
8. Fager CA: Lumbar microdiscectomy: A contrary opinion. Clin Neurosurg 33:419, 1986.
9. Fardon DF, Garfin SR, Abitol J, et al (eds): Orthopaedic Knowledge Update: Spine 2. Rosemont, IL, American Academy of Orthopaedic Surgeons, 2002, p 530.
10. Fischgrund JS, Mackay M, Herkowitz HN, et al: Degenerative lumbar spondylolisthesis with spinal stenosis: A prospective, randomized study comparing decompressive laminectomy and arthrodesis with and without spinal instrumentation. Spine 22:2807-2812, 1997.
11. Floman Y, Wiesel SW, Rothman RH: Cauda equina syndrome presenting as a herniated lumbar disc. Clin Orthop 147:234, 1980.
12. Friedman WA: Percutaneous discectomy: An alternative to chemonucleolysis? Neurosurgery 13:542, 1983.
13. Frymoyer JW: Back pain and sciatica. N Engl J Med 318:291, 1988.
14. Henderson ED: Results of the surgical treatment of spondylolisthesis. J Bone Joint Surg Am 48A:619, 1966.
15. Hill GM, Ellis EA: Chemonucleolysis as an alternative to laminectomy for the herniated lumbar disc: Experience with patients in a private orthopedic practice. Clin Orthop 225:229, 1987.
16. Hirsch C: Efficiency of surgery in low back disorder. J Bone Joint Surg Am 47A:991, 1965.
17. Kahanovitz N, Viola K, Muculloch J: Limited surgical discectomy and microdiskectomy: A clinical comparison. Spine 14:79, 1989.
18. Klara PM, Ray CD: Artificial nucleus replacement: Clinical experience. Spine 27:1374-1377, 2002.
19. Klein JD, Hey LA, Yu CS, et al: Perioperative nutrition and postoperative complications in patients undergoing spinal surgery. Spine 21:2676-2682, 1996.
20. Lemaire JP, Skalli W, Lavaste F, et al: Intervertebral disc prosthesis: Results and prospects for the year 2000. Clin Orthop 337:64-76, 1997.
21. Maistrelli GL, Vaughn PA, Evans DC, et al: Lumbar disc herniation in the elderly. Spine 12:63, 1987.
22. Maroon JC, Abla A: Microdiscectomy versus chemonucleolysis. Neurosurgery 16:644, 1985.
23. Maroon JC, Abla A: Microlumbar discectomy. Clin Neurosurg 33:407, 1986.
24. McAfee PC, Regan JR, Zdeblick T, et al: The incidence of complications in endoscopic anterior thoracolumbar spinal reconstructive surgery: A prospective multicenter study comprising the first 100 consecutive cases. Spine 20:1624-1632, 1995.
25. Mixter WJ, Barr JS: Rupture of the intervertebral disc with involvement of the spinal canal. N Engl J Med 211:210, 1934.
26. Nystrom B: Experience of microsurgical compared with conventional technique in lumbar disc operations. Acta Neurol Scand 76:129, 1987.
27. Onik G, Maroon J, Helms C, et al: Automated percutaneous diskectomy: Initial patient experience. Radiology 162:129, 1987.
28. Postacchini F: Results of surgery compared with conservative management for lumbar disc herniations. Spine 21:1383-1387, 1996.
29. Rogers LA: Experience with limited versus extensive disc removal in patients undergoing microsurgical operations for ruptured lumbar discs. Neurosurgery 22:82, 1988.
30. Ross JS, Robertson JT, Frederickson RC, et al: Association between peridural scar and recurrent radicular pain after lumbar discectomy: Magnetic resonance evaluation: ADCON-L European study group. Neurosurgery 38:855-861, 1996.
31. Rothman RH, Simeone FA: The Spine, 2nd ed. Philadelphia, WB Saunders, 1982.
32. Sachdev VF: Microsurgical lumbar discectomy: A personal series of 300 patients with at least 1 year of follow-up. Microsurgery 7:55, 1986.
33. Schwartz AM, Brodkey JS: Bowel perforation following microsurgical lumbar discectomy. A case report. Spine 13:104, 1988.
34. Shapiro S: Medical realities of cauda equina syndrome secondary to lumbar disc herniation. Spine 25:348-352, 2000.
35. Spangfort EV: The lumbar disc herniation—a computerized analysis of 2,504 operations. Acta Orthop Scand (Suppl) 142:52, 1972.
36. Thomas AM, Afshar F: The microsurgical treatment of lumbar disc protrusion. J Bone Joint Surg Br 69B:696, 1987.
37. Weber H: Lumbar disc herniation: A prospective study of prognostic factors including a controlled trial. J Oslo City Hosp 28:33, 1978.
38. Wiesel SW, Bernini P, Rothman RH: The Aging Lumbar Spine. Philadelphia, WB Saunders, 1982.
39. Yeung AT, Tsou PM: Posterolateral endoscopic excision for lumbar disc herniation: Surgical technique, outcome, and complications in 307 consecutive cases. Spine 27:722-731, 2002.
40. Zieger HE: Comparison of chemonucleolysis and microsurgical discectomy for the treatment of herniated lumbar disc. Spine 12:796, 1987.

MULTIPLE OPERATIONS ON THE LUMBAR SPINE

Continued pain after low back surgery is a difficult problem. Fifteen percent of all patients who undergo an initial surgical procedure will have significant discomfort and disability.[7] The inherent complexity of these cases necessitates a method of problem solving that is precise and unambiguous.

The best possible solution for preventing recurrent symptoms is to avoid inappropriate initial surgery whenever possible.[8] Again, it must be stressed that proper surgical indications should be strictly adhered to for the first procedure. The idea of "exploring" the low back when the necessary objective criteria are not present is no longer acceptable. In fact, even when there are objective findings but the patient is psychologically unstable or there are compensation litigation factors, the outcome of low back surgery is uncertain. Thus, the initial decision to operate is the most important one. Once the situation of recurrent pain after surgery arises, the potential for a solution is limited at best.

The physician must differentiate the patient with symptoms secondary to a mechanical lesion from one with some other problem. Recurrent herniated disc, spinal instability, and spinal stenosis are the principal mechanical lesions and are amenable to surgical intervention. Scar tissue (arachnoiditis or perineural fibrosis), psychosocial instability, or a systemic medical disease is the nonmechanical problem commonly found in the patient who has undergone multiple low back operations; none of these entities can be relieved by additional surgery.

Successful treatment for these patients is dependent on obtaining an accurate diagnosis. This essential step is often omitted, and inappropriate care is rendered. The goals of this section are to review the major points in the evaluation of low back pain that continues after multiple back operations and to present an algorithm (Fig. 20-5) for obtaining a specific diagnosis.

EVALUATION

The evaluation of the patient who has continuing low back pain after surgery can be quite confusing. The history, physical examination, and roentgenographic studies need to be assessed in a standardized fashion.[5] With accurate information, a diagnosis usually can be obtained.

First, it should be determined if the patient's complaint is based on a medical cause such as pancreatitis or an abdominal aneurysm. Thus, a thorough general medical examination should be routinely performed. In addition, if there is any indication of psychosocial instability, evidenced by alcoholism, drug dependence, or depression, a thorough psychiatric evaluation is necessary. Persons with profound emotional disturbances do not derive any observable benefit from additional surgery. In many cases, once a patient's underlying psychosocial problem has been treated successfully, his or her somatic back complaints and disability will disappear.

If the lumbar spine is the probable source of the patient's complaints, three specific historical points need clarification. The first is the number of previous lumbar spine operations the patient has undergone. It has been shown that with every subsequent operation, regardless of the diagnosis, the likelihood of a good result decreases. Statistically, the second operation has a 50% chance of success, and beyond two operations patients are more likely to be made worse than better.

The next important historical point is determination of the pain-free interval after the patient's previous operation. If the patient awoke from surgery with pain still present, the nerve root may not have been properly decompressed or the wrong level may have been explored. If the pain-free interval was longer than 6 months, the patient's recent pain may be due to recurrent disc herniation at the same or a different level. If the pain-free interval was between 1 and 6 months, the diagnosis most often is arachnoiditis or infection.

Finally, the patient's pain pattern must be evaluated. If leg pain predominates, a herniated disc or spinal stenosis is most likely. If back pain is the main complaint, instability, tumor, infection, and arachnoiditis are the major considerations. If both back and leg pain are present, spinal stenosis and arachnoiditis are the possibilities.

Physical examination is the next major step in the evaluation of the patient in whom previous back surgery has failed to relieve pain. The neurologic findings and existence of a tension sign, such as a positive straight leg–raising test or sitting root test, are noted. It is most important to have the results of a dependable previous examination so a comparison can be made between the preoperative and postoperative states. If the preoperative neurologic picture is unchanged and the tension sign is negative, mechanical compression is unlikely. If, however, there is a new neurologic deficit or the tension sign is positive, pressure on the neural elements is possible.

Roentgenographic studies are an important part of the patient's work-up. Again, it is most helpful to have a previous set of plain roentgenograms, MR images, CT scans, and myelograms for comparison of the preoperative and postoperative situations. The plain roentgenograms are evaluated for the extent and level of previous laminectomy(ies) and for evidence of spinal stenosis. Weight-bearing lateral flexion-extension films of the lumbar spine are examined to see if instability is present. An unstable spine may be the result of the patient's intrinsic disease or secondary to a previous surgical procedure.

Water-soluble myelography and CT play a limited role in evaluating the multiply operated lumbar spine. While these tests can identify extradural compressions, they cannot distinguish between disc material and epidural scar. The major use of these two tests in combination is for confirmation of arachnoiditis when the diagnosis is otherwise uncertain.

MR is perhaps the most valuable diagnostic test in these complicated patients. With the administration of an intravenous paramagnetic contrast material (gadolinium-diethylenetriaminepentaacetic acid/dimeglutamine [Gd-DTPA]), a recurrent disc herniation may be distinguished from epidural scar. A herniated disc is avascular and will not enhance (light up) immediately after the injection of intravenous contrast material; scar tissue, on the other hand, is vascular and will enhance with contrast agent administration. MR is also extremely helpful in identifying inflammatory processes such as discitis, which demonstrates a decreased signal intensity on T1-weighted images.

ALGORITHM FOR BACK PAIN AFTER MULTIPLE OPERATIONS

A specific diagnosis is necessary if an additional operation on the spine is to succeed.[9] Basically, the physician is trying

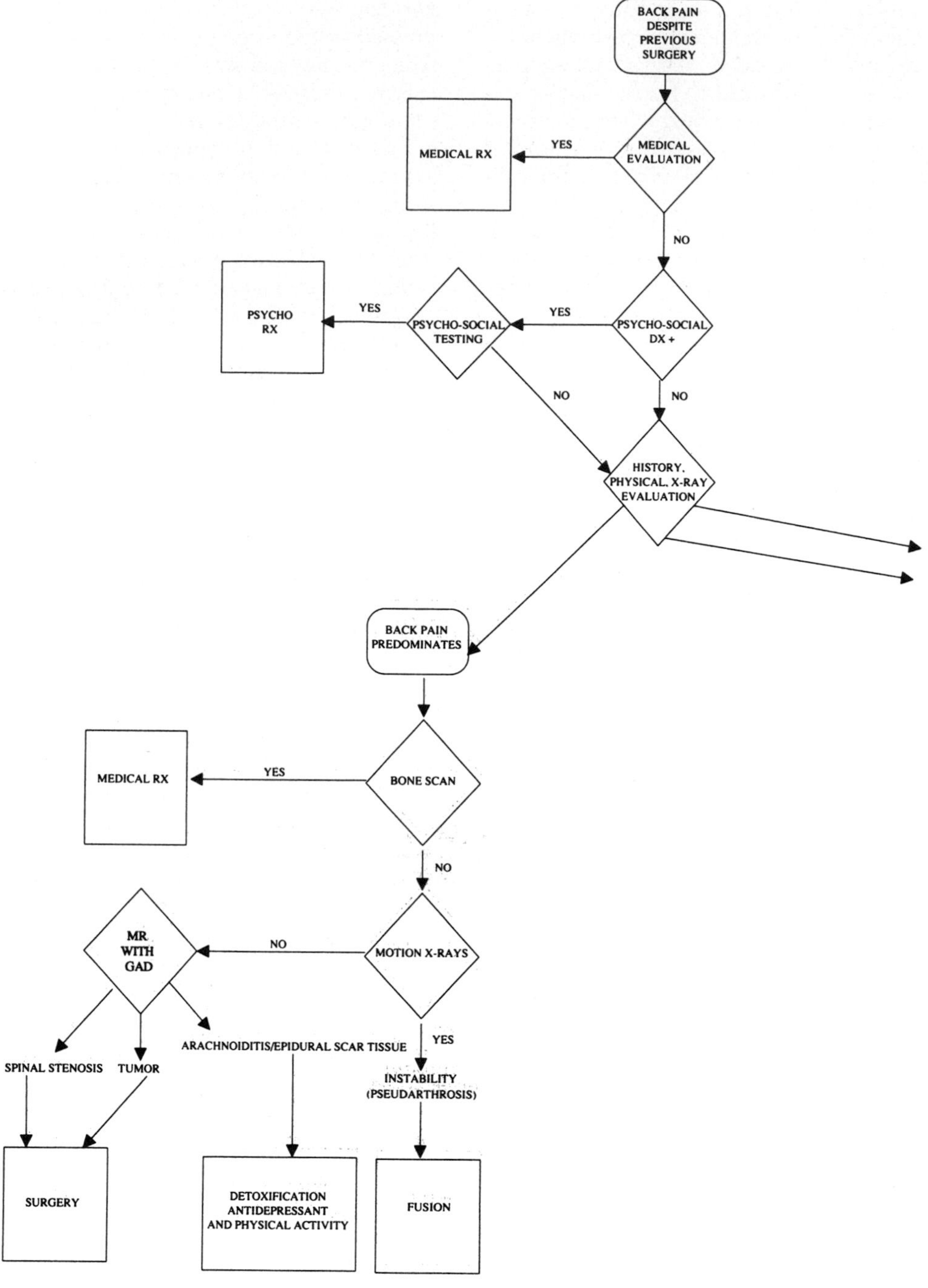

Figure 20-5 Algorithm for lumbar pain after multiple operations.

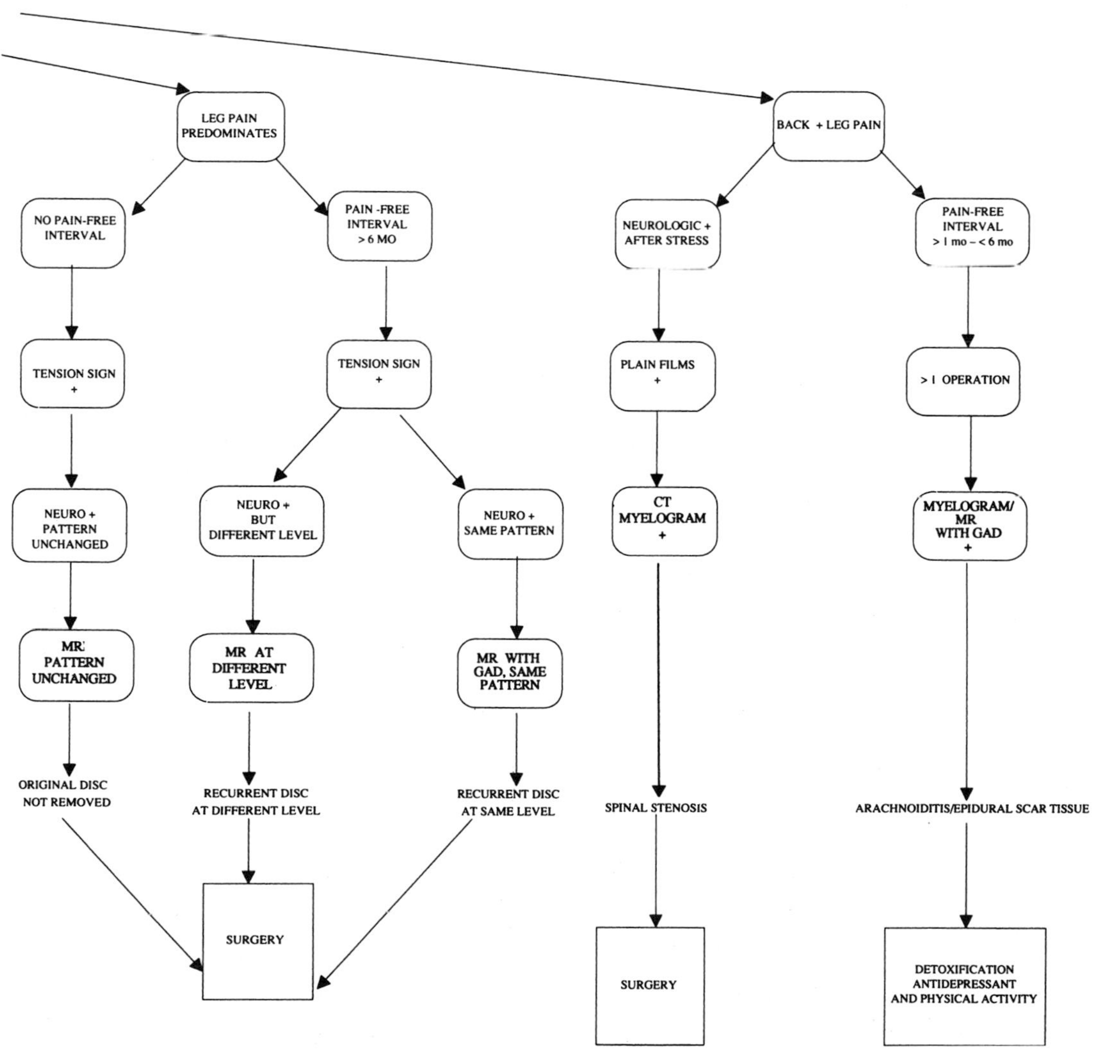

Figure 20-5, cont'd

20-1 DIFFERENTIAL DIAGNOSIS FOR BACK PAIN AFTER MULTIPLE OPERATIONS

History/ Physical Findings	Original Disc Not Removed	Recurrent Disc at Same Level	Recurrent Disc at Different Level	Spinal Instability	Spinal Stenosis	Arachnoiditis	Epidural Scar Tissue	Discitis
Previous operations						>1		
Pain-free interval	None	>6 mo	>6 mo			>1 mo but <6 mo	>1 mo gradual onset	
Predominant pain (leg vs. back)	Leg pain	Leg pain	Leg pain	Back pain	Back and leg pain	Back and leg pain	Back and/or leg pain	Back pain
Tension sign	+	+	+			May be positive	May be positive	±
Neurologic examination	+ same pattern	+ same pattern	+ different level		+ after stress			
Plain x-ray films	+ if wrong level			+				
Lateral motion x-ray films				+				
Metrizamide myelogram	+ but unchanged	+ same level	+ different level		+	+	+	
CT scan	+	+	+		+		+	
MR	+	+	+		+		+	+

to differentiate the patients whose symptoms have mechanical causes (e.g., recurrent herniated disc) from those who have pain secondary to scar tissue.

Each pathologic entity has associated specific symptoms, signs, and radiographic appearance (Table 20-1), and this information can be reformatted into an algorithmic form (see Fig. 20-5). Each of the pathologic problems that respond to surgery can be differentiated from scar tissue, which is not amenable to an invasive procedure.[16] It must be stressed that the number of operative patients will always be much lower than that of nonoperative patients.

Three possibilities exist if the patient's pain is caused by a herniated disc. First, the disc that caused the original symptoms may not have been satisfactorily removed. This can happen if the wrong level was decompressed, if the laminectomy performed was not adequate to free the neural elements, or if a fragment of disc material was left behind. Such patients will continue to have pain because of mechanical pressure on and irritation of the same nerve root that caused their initial symptoms. They will complain predominantly of leg pain, and their neurologic findings, tension signs, and radiographic patterns will remain unchanged from the preoperative state. The distinguishing feature is that they will report no pain-free interval; they will have awakened from the operation complaining of the same preoperative pain. Patients in this group will be aided by a technically correct laminectomy.

A second possibility is that there is a recurrent herniated intervertebral disc at the previously decompressed level. These patients complain of sciatica and have unchanged neurologic findings, tension signs, and radiographic studies. The distinguishing characteristic here is a pain-free interval of greater than 6 months. Another operative procedure is indicated in these patients provided that an MR image with gadolinium can demonstrate herniated disc material rather than just scar tissue.

Finally, a herniated disc can occur at a completely different level. Such patients generally will suffer sudden onset of recurrent pain after a pain-free interval of more than 6 months. Sciatica predominates, and tension signs are positive. However, a neurologic deficit, if present, and the radiographic signs will be seen at a different level from that on the original studies. A repeat operation for these patients will be beneficial.

Lumbar instability is another condition causing pain on a mechanical basis in the multiply operated back patient. Instability is the abnormal or excessive movement of one vertebra on another, causing pain. The cause may be the patient's intrinsic back disease or an excessively wide bilateral laminectomy.[7,8] Pseudarthrosis resulting from a failed spinal fusion is included in this category, because the pain is caused by the instability created by the failed fusion.

Patients with instability will complain predominantly of back pain, and their physical examinations may be negative. Sometimes the key to diagnosis of these patients is the weight-bearing lateral flexion-extension film; however, it is often difficult to precisely define the anatomic origin of back pain in the presence of radiographic instability. Relative flexion-sagittal plane translation of more than 8% of the anteroposterior diameter of the vertebral body or a relative flexion-sagittal plane rotation of more than 9 degrees between segments is the most commonly cited guideline for instability of the lumbar spine.[12,17] At the lumbosacral junction the criteria are slightly different: relative translation of more than 6% or rotation of more than 1 degree is significant. These criteria are based on maximum displacements on a single flexion or extension view; however, calculation of relative dynamic translation and rotation from flexion to extension may prove to be a more reliable indication of true instability.[1]

Unfortunately, there is little information to explain why some patients with segmental instability develop back pain while others do not. If there is radiographic evidence of instability in symptomatic patients, spinal fusion (or repair of the pseudarthrosis) may be considered.[10,15] Additional confirmatory evidence to determine the precise level of origin of the patient's symptoms may be gathered from facet injections and discography; however, these tests have a substantial rate of false-positive results.[6]

Spinal stenosis in the multiply operated back patient can mechanically produce both back and leg pain. The cause may be secondary to progression of the patient's inherent degenerative spine disease, a previous inadequate decompression, or overgrowth of a previous posterior fusion. The physical examination is often inconclusive, although a neurologic deficit may occur following exercise; with reproduction of the patient's symptoms this phenomenon is termed a *positive stress test*.

The plain films can be suggestive and may display facet degeneration, decreased interpedicular distance, decreased sagittal canal diameter, or disc degeneration. A CT scan will demonstrate bony encroachment on the neural elements; this is especially helpful in evaluating the lateral recesses and neural foramina. A myelogram or MR image will show compression of the dural sac at the involved levels. It should be appreciated that spinal stenosis and scar tissue can co-exist.[4] Good results can be expected from surgery in at least 70% of properly selected cases, but if there has been a previous laminectomy and spinal fusion, surgery will be less successful. If there is definite evidence of bony compression, a laminectomy is indicated; however, if substantial scar tissue is present, the degree of pain relief the patient can anticipate is uncertain.

Scar tissue (arachnoiditis or epidural fibrosis) and discitis are nonmechanical causes of recurrent pain in the multiply operated back patient. Whereas the etiologies and specific locations of these lesions are different, they are discussed in the same section because none of them will respond to another surgical procedure.

Postoperative scar tissue can be divided into two main types based on anatomic location. Scar tissue that occurs beneath the dura is commonly referred to as arachnoiditis. Scar tissue also can form extradurally, either directly on the cauda equina or around a nerve root.

Arachnoiditis is strictly defined as an inflammation of the pia arachnoid membrane surrounding the spinal cord or cauda equina.[2] The condition may be present in varying degrees of severity, from mild thickening of the membranes to solid adhesions. The scarring may be severe enough to obliterate the subarachnoid space and block the flow of contrast agents.

This condition has been attributed to many factors: lumbar spine surgery and previous injections of intrathecal contrast material seem to be the most frequent precipitating factors.[13] This problem is much less common since the advent of water-soluble contrast dyes. Postoperative infection also may play a role in the pathogenesis. The exact mechanism by which arachnoiditis develops from these events is not clear.

There is no uniform clinical presentation for arachnoiditis. Statistically, the history will reveal more than one previous operation and a pain-free interval of between 1 and 6 months. Often these patients will complain of back and leg pain. Physical examination is not conclusive; alterations in neurologic status may be due to a previous operation. As mentioned earlier, myelography, CT, and MR can be helpful in confirming the diagnosis.

At present there is no effective treatment for arachnoiditis. Surgical intervention has not proved effective in eliminating the scar tissue or significantly reducing the pain. Along with much needed encouragement, there are various nonoperative measures that can be employed. Epidural corticosteroids, transcutaneous nerve stimulation, spinal cord stimulation, operant conditioning, bracing, and patient education have all been tried. None of these will lead to a complete cure, but when used judiciously they can provide symptomatic relief for varying periods of time. Patients should be detoxified from all narcotics, placed on amitriptyline (Elavil), and encouraged to do as much physical activity as possible. Treating these patients is a challenge, and the physician must be willing to devote time and patience to achieve optimal results.

Formation of scar tissue outside the dura on the cauda equina or directly on nerve roots is a relatively common occurrence.[14] This *epidural scar tissue* acts as a constrictive force about the neural elements and frequently can cause postoperative pain. However, although most patients have some epidural scar tissue, only an unpredictable few become symptomatic.

Patients with epidural scarring may present with symptoms from several months to 1 or 2 years after surgery. They may complain of back pain or leg pain, or both. Commonly there are no new neurologic findings, but there may be a positive tension sign purely on the basis of scar formation around a nerve root. Epidural fibrosis is best differentiated from a recurrent herniated disc using gadolinium-enhanced MR.

As with arachnoiditis, there is no definitive treatment for epidural scar tissue. Prevention may be the best answer, and a free fat graft is sometimes used as an interposition membrane to minimize epidural scar tissue after laminectomy.[11] Use of too thick a fat graft may result in absorption of blood and swelling of the graft; there have been anecdotal reports of postoperative cauda equina syndrome associated with large fat grafts. Once scar has formed, surgery is not successful because scarring will often re-form in greater quantity. The treatment program should be similar to that already described for arachnoiditis.

Discitis is an uncommon but debilitating complication of lumbar disc surgery. Its pathogenesis is postulated to be direct inoculation of the avascular disc space but is not completely understood.[3] The onset of symptoms usually occurs about 1 month after surgery, and most patients will complain of severe back pain. Physical examination will sometimes reveal fever, a positive tension sign, and, occasionally, a superficial abscess.

If discitis is suspected from the history and physical examination, an erythrocyte sedimentation rate, blood cultures, and plain radiographs should be obtained. Plain films may not demonstrate the changes of disc space narrowing and end-plate erosion in the early stages. MR should confirm the diagnosis.

Effective treatment has been controversial.[3] The authors recommend placing the patient at bed rest acutely with immobilization of the lumbar spine using a brace or corset. If the patient experiences progressive pain after adequate immobilization or has constitutional symptoms, a needle aspiration biopsy should be performed. If a bacterial organism is identified, 6 weeks of intravenous antibiotics is indicated. There is no need for open disc space biopsy provided the patient responds to conservative therapy. With improvement of symptoms and laboratory findings the patient may ambulate as tolerated.

References

Multiple Operations on the Lumbar Spine

1. Boden SD, Wiesel SW: Lumbosacral segmental motion in normal individuals. Spine 15:571, 1990.
2. Burton CV: Lumbosacral arachnoiditis. Spine 3:24, 1978.
3. Dall BE, Rowe DE, Odette WG, et al: Postoperative discitis: Diagnosis and management. Clin Orthop 224:138, 1987.
4. Epstein BS: The Spine. Philadelphia, Lea & Febiger, 1962.
5. Grauer JN, Patel TC, Bell GR: Evaluation of the failed back. Semin Spine Surg 13:176-183, 2001.
6. Grubb SA, Lipscomb HJ, Gilford WB: The relative value of lumbar roentgenograms, metrizamide myelography, and discography in the assessment of patients with chronic low-back syndrome. Spine 12:282, 1987.
7. Hopp E, Tsou PM: Postdecompression lumbar instability. Clin Orthop 227:143, 1988.
8. Johnsson KE, Willner S, Johnsson K: Postoperative instability after decompression for lumbar spinal stenosis. Spine 11:107, 1986.
9. Karch MM, Tannoury TY, Lauerman WC, et al: The multiply operated low back: An algorithmic approach. Semin Spine Surg 13:201-215, 2001.
10. Laasonen EM, Soini J: Low-back pain after lumbar fusion: Surgical and computed tomographic analysis. Spine 14:210, 1989.
11. Langenskydd A, Kiviluoto O: Prevention of epidural scar formation after operations on the lumbar spine by means of free fat transplants. Clin Orthop 115:92, 1976.
12. Posner I, White AA, Edwards WT, et al: A biochemical analysis of the clinical stability of the lumbar and lumbosacral spine. Spine 7:374, 1982.
13. Quiles M, Marchisello PJ, Tsairis P: Lumbar adhesive arachnoiditis: Etiologic and pathologic aspects. Spine 3:45, 1978.
14. Rothman RH, Simeone FA: The Spine, 2nd ed. Philadelphia, WB Saunders, 1982.
15. Sidhu KS, Graziano GP, Abitol JJ: Fusion strategies in the previously operated spine. Semin Spine Surg 13:220-231, 2001.
16. Stambough JL: Failed back: Etiologies. Semin Spine Surg 13: 162-175, 2001.
17. White AA, Panjabi MM, Posner I, et al: Spinal stability: Evaluation and treatment. American Academy of Orthopaedic Surgeons Instructional Course Lectures, vol. XXX. St. Louis, CV Mosby, 1981, pp 457-483.

APPENDIX A

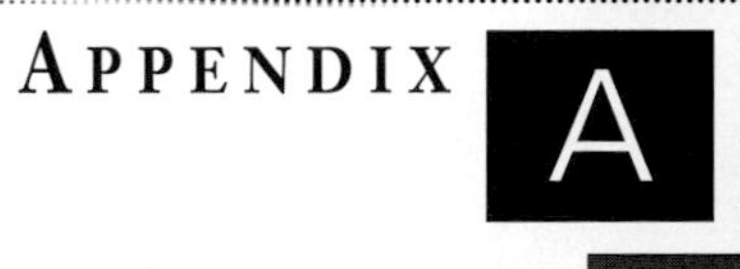

LOW BACK PAIN

Disease Entity	Back Pain: *Character*	Back Pain: *Location*	Back Pain: *Radiation*	Additional History	Physical Examination
MECHANICAL					
Cauda equina compression syndrome (deep somatic)	Sharp	Low back	Anteromedial thighs	Loss of bowel and/or bladder control	Saddle anesthesia Decreased reflexes in legs Decreased rectal tone
Muscle strain (deep somatic)					
Mild	Sharp (acute) Ache (chronic)	Low back	Buttocks Posterior thigh	None	Point tenderness
Moderate	Sharp (acute) Ache (chronic)	Low back	Buttocks Posterior thigh	None	Point tenderness Spasm Decreased range of motion
Severe	Sharp	Low back	Buttocks Posterior thigh	None	Point tenderness Spasm Inability to walk Decreased range of motion
Herniated nucleus pulposus (HNP) (radicular)					
L3-4 (L4 nerve root)	Sharp pain with numbness	Low back	Posterolateral aspect of thigh Across patella Along anteromedial aspect of leg	None	Weak knee extensor Quadriceps muscle atrophy Decreased patellar reflex
L4-5 (L5 nerve root)	Sharp pain with numbness	Low back	Anteromedial aspect of leg and foot to big toe	None	Weakness of great toe Dorsiflexion of foot Anterior tibial muscle atrophy Straight leg–raising test positive No reflex change
L5-S1 (S1 nerve root)	Sharp pain with numbness	Low back	Posterolateral aspect of leg to lateral toes	None	Weakness of plantarflexion of foot Calf atrophy Straight leg–raising test positive Decreased ankle reflex
Lumbar spondylosis (deep somatic)	Ache	Low back		Pain increases with activity, especially standing	Decreased range of motion
Spinal stenosis (deep somatic, radicular)	Ache	Low back	One or both legs with ambulation	Intermittent episodes of low back pain	May be normal Stress test positive or negative
Spondylolysis (deep somatic)	Ache	Low back	Legs	Trauma	Point tenderness
Spondylolisthesis (deep somatic)	Ache	Low back	Legs	Trauma	Increased lordosis Point tenderness
Adult scoliosis (deep somatic)	Ache	Low back	None	Deformity	Spinal deformity
RHEUMATOLOGIC					
Ankylosing spondylitis	Sharp (acute) Ache (chronic)	Bilateral sacroiliac joint Midline	Posterior thigh	Male predominance Morning stiffness Pseudoclaudication	Decreased distance on Schober's test Decreased motion of lumbosacral spine in all planes Percussion tenderness

Laboratory Abnormalities	Radiographs	Diagnosis	Therapy	Comments
Normal	Compression of cauda equina	Clinical history Physical examination CT-myelogram/MR	Emergency surgery	Rapid surgical decompression necessary to prevent incontinence within 48 hours
Normal	Normal	Clinical history Physical examination	Controlled physical activity NSAIDs Muscle relaxants	Pain relief in 3-4 days
Normal	Normal	Clinical history Physical examination	Controlled physical activity NSAIDs Muscle relaxants	Pain relief in 7-10 days
Normal	Normal	Clinical history Physical examination	Controlled physical activity NSAIDs Muscle relaxants	Pain relief in 2 weeks
Normal	L3-L4 disc herniation	Clinical history Physical examination Radiographs are confirmatory	Initial: rest, NSAIDs, oral low-dose steroids After 4-6 weeks with no response: epidural steroids Continued pain: surgery	70%-80% of patients with an HNP should respond to noninvasive therapy Tumor necrosis factor inhibitors may be beneficial
Normal	L4-L5 disc herniation	Clinical history Physical examination Radiographs are confirmatory	Initial: rest, NSAIDs, oral low-dose steroids After 4-6 weeks with no response: epidural steroids Continued pain: surgery	70%-80% of patients with an HNP should respond to noninvasive therapy Tumor necrosis factor inhibitors may be beneficial
Normal	L5-S1 disc herniation	Clinical history Physical examination Radiographs are confirmatory	Initial: rest, NSAIDs, oral low-dose steroids After 4-6 weeks with no response: epidural steroids Continued pain: surgery	70%-80% of patients with an HNP should respond to noninvasive therapy Tumor necrosis factor inhibitors may be beneficial
Normal	Disc space and joint space narrowing	Clinical history Physical examination Radiographs	Controlled physical activities NSAIDs	Facet syndrome in minority
Normal	Spinal canal narrowing	Clinical history Radiographs are confirmatory	Controlled physical activities, NSAIDs, back support No response: epidural steroids No response: possible surgery	Majority of patients do well without surgery Interval between epidural steroid injections 2 months or more
Normal	Lytic lesion in pars	Plain roentgenograms	Controlled physical activity Back support	Few need surgery
Normal	Displacement of vertebral bodies	Plain roentgenograms	Surgery for grades III and IV Controlled physical activity, back support for grades I and II A few will need surgery	Surgery will not return people to full activity, just decreases pain
Normal	Scoliotic curves	Plain roentgenograms	Bracing Progression or lack of response: surgery	Mild scoliosis in lumbar area usually asymptomatic—consider other diagnosis
Increased ESR HLA-B27 90%	Bilateral sacroiliitis Marginal syndesmophytes	Clinical history Plain roentgenograms (HLA)	Exercises NSAIDs Muscle relaxants Tumor necrosis factor inhibitors	Pain improved with motion Iritis HLA confirmatory, not diagnostic

Continued

Disease Entity	Back Pain: Character	Back Pain: Location	Back Pain: Radiation	Additional History	Physical Examination
Reactive arthritis (deep somatic)	Ache	Unilateral or bilateral sacroiliac joint Midline	Posterior thigh	Male predominance Morning stiffness Conjunctivitis Urethritis Skin lesions	Unilateral or bilateral sacroiliac joint tenderness Decreased motion of lumbasacral spine in all planes
Psoriatic spondylitis (deep somatic)	Ache	Unilateral or bilateral sacroiliac joint Midline	Posterior thigh	Morning stiffness Skin lesions	Psoriatic plaques Unilateral or bilateral sacroiliac joint tenderness Decreased motion of lumbosacral spine in all planes
Enteropathic arthritis (deep somatic, referred)	Ache	Bilateral sacroiliac joint Midline	Posterior thigh	Morning stiffness Abdominal pain Cramps	Abnormal abdominal examination Joint tenderness Decreased motion of lumbosacral spine in all planes
Behçet's syndrome (deep somatic)	Ache	Unilateral or bilateral sacroiliac joint	Posterior thigh	Morning stiffness Oral and genital ulcers Iritis Meningitis	Ulcerations Unilateral or bilateral sacroiliac joint tenderness
Whipple's disease (deep somatic)	Ache	Unilateral or bilateral sacroiliac joint	Posterior thigh	Gastrointestinal symptoms of malabsorption, fever, mental status changes	Hyperpigmentation Lymphadenopathy Percussion tenderness over sacroiliac joints Decreased motion of lumbosacral spine in all planes
Familial Mediterranean fever (deep somatic)	Ache	Unilateral or bilateral sacroiliac joint	Posterior thigh	Male predominance Episodic peritonitis	Normal between attacks
Hidradenitis suppurativa (deep somatic)	Ache	Unilateral or bilateral sacroiliac joint Midline	Posterior thigh	Skin disease precedes arthritis frequently	Axillary and inguinal disease Dissecting cellulitis Scalp lesions Acne conglobata
Rheumatoid arthritis (deep somatic)	Ache	Diffuse	Posterior thigh	Disease of long duration	Generalized involvement of hands and feet Lumbosacral spine tenderness
Diffuse idiopathic skeletal hyperostosis (DISH) (deep somatic)	Mild ache	Midline	None	Dysphagia	Mild limitation of lumbosacral spine motion
Vertebral osteochondritis (deep somatic)	Ache	Midline	Hip Paravertebral muscles	Spinal angulation	Thoracic kyphosis Pain on palpation
Osteitis condensans ilii (deep somatic)	Dull ache	Bilateral or unilateral sacroiliac joint	Buttock	Pregnancy Postpartum	Sacroiliac joint percussion tenderness
Polymyalgia rheumatica (deep somatic)	Muscle soreness	Shoulders Thighs	Arms Legs	Severe morning stiffness No muscle weakness	Muscle tenderness on palpation
Fibromyalgia (deep somatic)	Ache	Generalized	Tender points	Morning stiffness Fatigue Sleeplessness	Localized pain (tender points)

Laboratory Abnormalities	Radiographs	Diagnosis	Therapy	Comments
Increased ESR HLA-B27 80%	Unilateral or bilateral sacroiliitis Nonmarginal syndesmophytes Heel periostitis	History of clinical triad (HLA)	Exercises NSAIDs Antibiotics	Spondylitis may occur in absence of sacroiliitis
Increased ESR HLA-B27 60%	Unilateral or bilateral sacroilitis Nonmarginal syndesmophytes	Clinical history Rash Plain roentgenograms (HLA)	Exercises Topical skin care NSAIDs Methotrexate Tumor necrosis factor inhibitors	Spondylitis may precede skin manifestations by many years Spondylitis may occur in absence of sacroiliitis
Increased ESR Blood in stool HLA-B27 50%	Bilateral sacroiliitis Marginal syndesmophytes	Clinical history Gastrointestinal radiographs, biopsy	Exercises NSAIDs Tumor necrosis factor inhibitors	Activity of bowel and axial skeletal disease do not correlate
Increased ESR	Unilateral or bilateral sacroiliitis	Clinical history	Corticosteroids Thalidomide Colchicine	Ulcerations are painful
Decreased Hct Abnormal intestinal absorption studies	Unilateral or bilateral sacroiliitis	Small bowel biopsy PCR of *T. whipplei* in tissues	Procaine penicillin G Streptomycin Trimethoprim-sulfamethoxazole	Pathogenic organism—*T. whipplei*
Increased WBC Increased ESR with attacks	Unilateral or bilateral sacroiliitis	Clinical history	Colchicine	
Decreased Hct Increased ESR	Unilateral or bilateral sacroiliitis Asymmetrical syndesmophytes	Rash Plain roentgenograms	Antibiotics Incision and drainage Corticosteroids Isotretinoin	Arthritis parallels activity of skin disease Sacroiliitis 80%
Decreased Hct Increased ESR Rheumatoid factor 80%	Sacroiliitis without sclerosis Lumbar spine malalignment	Clinical history Plain roentgenograms RA factor positive Anemia	Exercises NSAIDs Antirheumatics Corticosteroids Tumor necrosis factor inhibitors Anti-IL-1 inhibitors	
None	Flowing calcification on anterolateral aspect of four contiguous vertebral bodies	Plain roentgenograms	NSAIDs Exercises	
None	Vertebral body wedging Irregular endplates Limbus vertebrae	Roentgenograms	Exercises Bracing Surgery	Surgery for severe kyphosis, respiratory insufficiency
None	Triangular sclerosis on iliac side of sacroiliac joint	Roentgenograms	Exercises Firm mattress	Sacroiliac joint changes confused with ankylosing spondylitis
Increased ESR Isolated increased alkaline phosphatase	None	Clinical history	Corticosteroids	Diagnosis by exclusion
None	None	Clinical history	Rest Graduated exercises NSAIDs Antidepressants	Diagnosis by exclusion

Continued

Disease Entity	Back Pain: Character	Back Pain: Location	Back Pain: Radiation	Additional History	Physical Examination
INFECTIONS					
Lumbosacral osteomyelitis (deep somatic) Bacterial	Sharp	Area infected	Paraspinous muscles	Extraosseous source of infection Fever	Percussion tenderness over involved bone Decreased motion
Tuberculous	Sharp	Area infected	Buttock	Low-grade fever Weight loss	Angular deformity Localized tenderness
Fungal	Sharp	Area infected	Buttock	Low-grade fever	Localized tenderness
Spirochetal	Ache or none	Area infected	Buttock	Rash or ulcers	Localized tenderness
Parasitic	Ache or none	Area infected	Buttock	Geographic exposure	Localized tenderness
Discitis (deep somatic)	Severe, sharp	Disc infected	Flank Abdomen Lower extremity	Male predominance	Localized tenderness Marked limitation of motion
Pyogenic sacroiliitis (deep somatic)	Severe, sharp	Sacroiliac joint	Buttock Thigh Calf	Male predominance Muscle spasm	Localized tenderness Patrick test positive Soft tissue abscess Fever
Herpes zoster (superficial somatic, radicular)	Burning	Dermatomal		Fever Malaise	Vesicular dermatomal rash
Lyme disease (deep somatic, radicular)	Ache	Lumbar spine	Legs	Tick bite Erythema migrans	Rash Radicular pain
TUMORS AND INFILTRATIVE DISEASE					
Benign					
Osteoid osteoma (deep somatic)	Boring	Affected bone	Paravertebral muscles	Male predominance Young Nocturnal pain	Localized tenderness Scoliosis
Osteoblastoma (deep somatic)	Dull ache	Affected bone	Paravertebral muscles Posterior thigh	Male predominance Young	Localized tenderness and swelling scoliosis
Osteochondroma (deep somatic)	Mild ache	Affected bone	Paravertebral muscles	Male predominance Slowly progressive	Restricted spinal motion
Giant cell (deep somatic)	Intermittent ache	Affected bone		Female predominance Neurologic dysfunction	Localized bone tenderness and swelling Rectal mass with sacral involvement

Laboratory Abnormalities	Radiographs	Diagnosis	Therapy	Comments
Elevated ESR Blood cultures (50%) Bone cultures (60%)	Subchondral bone loss Endplate loss Narrow disc space Contiguous endplate erosion	Positive culture Radiographs	Antibiotics Immobilization	Severe pain exacerbated by motion Hip pain Abdominal pain Meningeal signs
Bone biopsy: granulomas Cultures Positive PPD	Subchondral bone loss Endplate loss Narrow disc space Paravertebral soft tissue abscess	Positive culture Roentgenograms	Antibiotics Immobilization	Radiographic changes occur less rapidly than with bacterial infection
Bone biopsy: granulomas Cultures	Anterior and posterior elements of vertebral body Spares disc	Positive culture Roentgenograms	Antifungals Immobilization	Indolent course
Positive FTA	Localized lysis and sclerosis Marked dissolution	Serology Bone pathology	Antibiotics	Charcot spine Painless
	Expansive osteolytic lesion containing trabeculae	Radiographs	Antihelminthics	
Increased ESR Increased WBC Blood culture Disc culture	Decreased disc height Reactive sclerosis adjoining vertebral bodies	Positive culture	Antibiotics Immobilization	Pain exacerbated with motion Severe muscle spasm Bone scan positive before plain roentgenograms MR positive before bone scan
Increased ESR Increased WBC Blood cultures (50%) Fluid culture	Blurred joint margins Erosions Sclerosis MR positive early	Positive synovial fluid culture	Antibiotics Surgical drainage if necessary	Unilateral involvement
Increased CSF WBC (33%)	Normal	Clinical history Physical examination	Analgesics Corticosteroids Antivirals	Occult malignancy Often lymphoreticular
Elevated ESR *Borrelia* antibodies CSF pleocytosis	None	History Erythema migrans	Antibiotics: early disease—oral; late disease—IV	Lyme antibodies are confirmatory, not diagnostic
Bone biopsy: nidus of osteoid, fibrous tissue, thickened cortical bone	Lytic area surrounded by sclerotic border Bone scan: hot spot	Bone biopsy	Excision Aspirin	Increased noctural pain Concave side scoliosis
Bone biopsy: osteoblasts, osteoid, giant cells	Posterior vertebral body expansile, well delineated, with periosteal new bone	Bone biopsy	Excision	Confused with osteosarcoma, but no cartilage or anaplastic cells in osteoblastoma
Bone biopsy: cartilage cap, woven bone with nests of cartilage	Posterior vertebral body well-demarcated sessile or pedunculated bone with cartilage cap	Radiographs Normal laboratory findings	Excision	Nerve impingement requires decompression Malignant degeneration with multiple osteochondromas
Bone biopsy: osteoclastic giant cells, mono-nuclear stromal cells, thin-walled vessels	Anterior vertebral body expansile lesion Thin cortical margin No bony reaction	Radiographs Bone biopsy	En bloc excision	Recurrence common with partial excision Malignant transformation rare

Continued

Disease Entity	Back Pain: *Character*	Back Pain: *Location*	Back Pain: *Radiation*	Additional History	Physical Examination
Aneurysmal bone cyst (deep somatic)	Acute onset Increasing severity	Affected bone		Female predominance Young	Localized bone tenderness Skin erythema and warmth
Hemangioma (deep somatic)	Throbbing	Affected bone		Mid-life onset	Localized bone tenderness Limitation of motion with muscle spasm
Eosinophilic granuloma (deep somatic)	Persistent ache	Affected bone		Male predominance Young	Nontender swelling
Gaucher's disease (deep somatic)	Persistent ache	Affected bone		Abdominal distention Generalized fatigue Protracted course Intermittent exacerbations	Localized bone tenderness Abdominal organomegaly
Sacral lipoma (deep somatic)	Ache	Unilateral	Buttock Anterior thigh Lower extremity	Increased pain with compression (sleeping) Limited motion 40 years or older	Tender nodules over sacroiliac joints Flexion increases pain Obese
Malignant					
Multiple myeloma (deep somatic, radicular)	Mild ache (onset) Acute pain (fractures)	Affected bone	Radicular	Generalized bone pain Generalized fatigue Nausea, vomiting Mental status alterations Renal dysfunction (40 years or older)	Diffuse bone tenderness Fever Pallor
Chondrosarcoma (deep somatic, radicular)	Mild discomfort	Affected bone	Radicular	Male predominance (40-60 yr)	Painless swelling Rectal mass
Chordoma (deep somatic, radicular)	Dull or sharp Persistent	Sacral Lumbar	Hip Knee Groin	Male predominance (40-70 yr) Constipation Urinary dysfunction	Presacral mass on rectal examination Muscle flaccidity

Laboratory Abnormalities	Radiographs	Diagnosis	Therapy	Comments
Bone biopsy: cystic cavities lined with fibroblasts, osteoid, multinucleated giant cells	Posterior vertebral body osteolytic expansile lesion Thin demarcated periosteal shell of bone	Radiographs	En bloc excision	Local recurrence with partial excision Pathologic fracture
Bone biopsy: increased capillary and venous vessels with sparse trabecular tissue	Anterior vertebral body prominent vertical striations with unchanged body configuration	Radiographs	Radiation therapy for symptomatic lesions	Most lesions asymptomatic Surgical excision for neural compression
Peripheral eosinophilia (10%) Increased ESR Bone biopsy: eosinophils, benign pleomorphic histiocytes	Osteolytic areas without sclerosis Vertebra plana Epidural extension on MR	Bone biopsy	Curettage	Bone biopsy findings confused with Hodgkin's disease
Pancytopenia Increased nonprostatic acid phosphatase Decreased leukocyte glucocerebrosidase Bone marrow: Gaucher cells	Vertebral body radiolucency: accentuated vertical trabeculae Vertebra plana	Decreased leukocyte Glucocerebrosidase	Alglucerase	Accumulation of ceramide glucoside
Lipoma 1-5 cm, Fibrous capsule containing normal adipose tissue	None	Clinical history Physical examination	Local injection Surgical removal	Patients diagnosed with psychogenic rheumatism when lipoma unrecognized
Decreased Hct Increased WBC Decreased platelets Coombs' test positive Increased ESR Increased calcium Increased uric acid Increased creatinine M-protein positive Bence-Jones proteinuria	Diffuse vertebral body osteolysis without reactive sclerosis Spares posterior elements CT scan more sensitive	Abnormal plasma cells M-protein Electrophoresis	Chemotherapy Decompressing laminectomy and/or local radiotherapy for cord compression	Most common primary malignant tumor Bone scan does not identify bone lesion
Decreased Hct Increased ESR (late in course) Bone biopsy: verifying degree of malignant chondrocyte atypia with abnormal matrix production	Expansile, interior fluffy or lobular calcifications Thickened cortex CT scan: soft tissue extension	Bone biopsy	En bloc resection	Grade 1—slowly progressive Grade 3—more malignant, locally invasive
Decreased Hct Increased ESR (late in course) Bone biopsy: gelatinous tumor, physaliphorous cells interspersed in fibrous tissue	Osteolysis with calcific soft tissue mass Vertebral body without disc involvement initially	Bone biopsy	En bloc resection Radiotherapy for inaccessible tumors	Unpredictable clinical course, slow and indolent or rapid and destructive, 10 year survival 10-40%

Continued

Disease Entity	Back Pain: *Character*	Back Pain: *Location*	Back Pain: *Radiation*	Additional History	Physical Examination
Lymphoma (deep somatic, radicular)	Persistent ache	Affected bone	Radicular	Male predominance Pain increases with recumbency or alcohol ingestion	Localized tenderness and swelling
Skeletal metastases (deep somatic, radicular)	Gradual onset with increasing intensity	Affected bone	Radicular	Increased pain with recumbency, cough, motion Prior malignancy (over 50 years old)	Tenderness with palpation Limited motion Fever
Intraspinal neoplasms Extradural (deep somatic, radicular)	Increasing intensity Unrelenting	Affected bone	Radicular	Increased with recumbency or activity Unresponsive to mild analgesics	Tenderness with palpation Abnormal neurologic signs with compression
Intradural-extramedullary (deep somatic, radicular)	Slowly progressive	Back and leg	Radicular	Increased with recumbency, not by activity Neurofibromatosis	Gait disturbance Sensory changes Muscle atrophy Incontinence
Intramedullary	Painless			Sensory deficits Weakness Incontinence	Abnormal pain and temperature sensation Hyperreflexia Spasticity
ENDOCRINOLOGIC AND METABOLIC					
Osteoporosis (deep somatic)	Acute (fractures) Dull (chronic)	Midline	Flank Posterior thigh Abdomen	Pain increases with motion Generalized bone pain Corticosteroids	Bone pain with spine percussion Paraspinous spasm Ileus
Osteomalacia (deep somatic)	Diffuse ache	Midline	Paravertebral muscles	Pain increases with activity and standing Muscle weakness and spasm	Bone pain with spine percussion Kyphoscoliosis Proximal muscle weakness
Parathyroid Hyperparathyroidism (deep somatic)	Diffuse ache Acute (fractures) Colic (stones)	Midline		Female predominance Gastrointestinal symptoms Genitourinary symptoms Mental status changes	Bone pain with spine percussion Kyphosis

Laboratory Abnormalities	Radiographs	Diagnosis	Therapy	Comments
Decreased Hct Immunoglobulin abnormalities Disseminated disease	Osteolytic (75%) Sclerotic (15%) Mixed (5%) Periosteal (5%) Vertebral body compression fracture Spares disc space	Bone biopsy	Chemotherapy and/or radiotherapy	Potential for cure if diagnosed before extensive disease
Decreased Hct Increased ESR Urinalysis: RBC Increased alkaline phosphatase, prostatic acid phosphatase Bone biopsy: may or may not show characteristics of primary tumor	Osteolytic: lung, kidney, breast, thyroid Osteoblastic: prostate, breast, colon, bronchial carcinoid Spares disc Bone scan: 85% both symptomatic and asymptomatic areas Myelography: cord compression MR: most sensitive test	Bone biopsy if no primary neoplasm is identified	Palliative Radiotherapy Corticosteroids Decompressive laminectomy for spinal cord compression	Most common malignant lesion of the spine
Decreased Hct Increased ESR Bone biopsy: metastasis	Rapid bone destruction, body or posterior elements Myelogram: complete block, varying densities, displaces cord MR: contrast increases sensitivity	Lesional biopsy	Radiotherapy Corticosteroids Decompressive laminectomy	Metastatic lesions
Increased cerebrospinal fluid protein	Posterior scalloping of vertebral bodies Uniform dilatation of neural foramen Myelogram: sharp, smooth outline of lesion MR: contrast increases sensitivity	Radiographs	Surgical removal	Neurofibromas Meningiomas
	Myelogram: fusiform enlargement MR: infiltrative lesion	Lesional biopsy	Surgical removal	Ependymomas Gliomas
Primary: normal Secondary: decreased Hct, increased ESR Pyridinolines	Diffuse vertebral involvement Endplate "fish vertebrae" Compression fractures DEXA scan—decreased bone mineral	Clinical history Confirmed by bone biopsy	Calcium Vitamin D SERMS Calcitonin Bisphosphonates Parathyroid hormone Kyphoplasty	Women 65 years old 50% asymptomatic osteoporosis, 3% disabling Back pain with fracture may persist indefinitely
Decreased serum calcium, vitamin D, phosphate Increased alkaline phosphatase Decreased urinary calcium Increased parathyroid hormone Bone biopsy: increased osteoid, inadequate mineralization	"Cod-fish" vertebrae Scoliosis "Hot spots" on bone scan—Looser's zones	Clinical history confirmed by bone biopsy	Vitamin D Calcium Phosphate	
Increased serum calcium Decreased phosphate Increased chloride Increased alkaline phosphatase Increased serum parathyroid hormone	Resorption at symphysis pubis, sacroiliac joints Wedge vertebrae "Rugger-jersey" spine Schmorl's nodes	Surgical removal of abnormal parathyroid tissue	Surgery in symptomatic patients NSAIDs Braces	Clinical diagnosis: Hypercalcemia Secondary forms—renal osteodystrophy

Continued

Disease Entity	Back Pain: *Character*	Back Pain: *Location*	Back Pain: *Radiation*	Additional History	Physical Examination
Hypoparathyroidism (deep somatic)	Stiffness	Midline		Female predominance Muscle spasm Mental status changes	Tetany Decreased spine motion
Pituitary (deep somatic)	Ache	Midline	Lower leg	Headache Visual disturbances Muscle weakness Carpal tunnel syndrome 20-40 years old	Bone pain with spine percussion Normal range of motion Kyphosis Coarsened facial features
Microcrystalline Disease (Deep Somatic)					
Gout	Acute (sharp) Chronic (ache)	Sacroiliac joint Midline		Chronic peripheral gouty arthritis Male predominance	Straightening lumbosacral spine Tophi
Calcium pyrophosphate dihydrate disease	Acute (sharp) Chronic (ache)	Sacroiliac joint Midline		Male predominance	Straightening lumbosacral spine Loss of motion
Ochronosis (deep somatic)	Ache	Midline		Peripheral joint arthritis Dark urine	Lumbosacral spine Loss of motion Percussion tenderness Dark pigmentation of nose, ears, sclerae
Fluorosis (deep somatic)	Ache	Midline		Hand pain Weakness	Loss of motion in lumbosacral spine Generalized osteophytes Discolored teeth
GENETIC DISORDERS					
Marfan syndrome (deep somatic)	Chronic ache	Diffuse low back	None	Family history Myopia Hypermobility	Arachnodactyly Scoliosis Aortic murmur
Mucopolysaccharidoses Morquio's syndrome (deep somatic)	Chronic ache	Diffuse		Onset in childhood Decreased hearing Normal intelligence	Short stature Kyphoscoliosis Clouded corneas Ligamentous laxity Hepatomegaly
HEMATOLOGIC DISORDERS					
Hemoglobinopathies (deep somatic)	Pressure ache	Midline	Flank	Black predominance Repeated episodes of bone pain Cholelithiasis Pulmonary infarcts Pneumonia	Bone tenderness increased with palpation Fever with crises
Myelofibrosis (deep somatic)	Severe sharp	Midline		Weakness Weight loss Abdominal pain or fullness 50 years old	Bone tenderness Splenomegaly
Mastocytosis (deep somatic)	Ache	Midline		Hyperpigmentation Urticaria Diarrhea Flushing	Bone tenderness Hepatosplenomegaly Skin pigmentation

Laboratory Abnormalities	Radiographs	Diagnosis	Therapy	Comments
Decreased serum calcium Increased serum phosphate Normal alkaline phosphatase	Osteosclerosis Calcification of longitudinal ligaments	Serum parathyroid hormone decreased	Vitamin D Calcium	
Increased growth hormone, somatomedin-C, phosphate, glucose, alkaline phosphatase	Anterior and lateral osteophytes Posteriorly scalloped vertebral bodies Increased disc space Disc calcification	Nonsuppressible increased growth hormone concentrations	Ablation of pituitary tumor Bromocriptine Octreotide	Progressive degenerative back changes despite normalization of growth hormone concentrations
Monosodium urate monohydrate crystals Increased serum uric acid	Sacroiliac joint erosions Marginal sclerosis	Monosodium urate monohydrate crystals	Colchicine NSAIDs Corticosteroids (acute) Uricosurics Xanthine oxidase inhibitors (chronic)	
Calcium pyrophosphate dihydrate crystals	Disc calcification and narrowing Osteophytes	Calcium pyrophosphate dihydrate crystals	NSAIDs Colchicine (33%)	Secondary forms: Hyperparathyroidism Hemochromatosis Hypothyroidism Wilson's disease Ochronosis
Dark alkalinized urine	Disc narrowing and calcification Osteophytes Bone scan—spinal whiskering	Homogentisic acid in urine	Rest NSAIDs Analgesics	Homogentisic acid oxidase deficiency Bony overgrowth Confused with ankylosing spondylitis
Increased urinary fluoride, serum alkaline phosphatase	Osteosclerosis Osteophytes Calcification of soft tissues, including entheses, ligaments	Urinary fluoride Radiographs Bone biopsy	Limit fluoride exposure and intake	Fluoride exposure: drinking water, insecticides
None	Posterior scalloping Double curve scoliosis Spinal canal enlargement	Clinical criteria	Bracing Operative stabilization of scoliosis	Abnormal fibrillin gene chromosome 15
Increased urinary keratan sulfate	Platyspondyly Central beaking of vertebral bodies Increased kyphosis	Increased keratan sulfate	Bracing	Galactosamine-6-sulfate sulfatase deficiency Mild form of β-galactosidase deficiency
Decreased Hct Increased WBC Increased serum bilirubin	Coarsened trabeculae Osteoporosis "Fish-mouth" vertebrae Bone sclerosis	Hemoglobin Electrophoresis	Hydration Analgesics Hydroxyurea	Sickle cell anemia most common form
Decreased Hct Increased WBC Increased uric acid Bone marrow biopsy: fibrosis, hypocellularity	Osteosclerosis of inferior and superior endplates	Bone marrow biopsy	Transfusions Analgesics Radiation therapy Bone marrow transplant	Acute myelogenous leukemia (20%)
Decreased Hct Increased WBC Increased mast cells Bone marrow biopsy: fibrosis, bone matrix increased	Admixture of osteosclerosis and osteoporosis	Bone marrow biospy	Transfusions Analgesics H_2 blockers H_1 blockers Cromolyn	Mast cells mistaken for granulomas in bone marrow biopsy

Continued

Disease Entity	Back Pain: *Character*	Back Pain: *Location*	Back Pain: *Radiation*	Additional History	Physical Examination
NEUROLOGIC AND PSYCHIATRIC DISORDERS					
Neuropathy (femoral, radicular)	Burning	Paraspinous	Thigh Knee	Episodes of lancinating pain, increased at night Pain not increased with cough	Pelvic girdle and thigh weakness Absent knee reflex
Psychogenic rheumatism Depression (psychogenic)	Dull ache	Low back		Listlessness Sleepiness Anorexia Constipation	Normal
Malingering (psychogenic)	Severe constant	Entire back	Nondermatomal	No relief with any therapy Job-related	Inconsistent abnormalities Nondermatomal sensory loss Pain with head compression
REFERRED PAIN					
Vascular (Visceral-Referred)					
Abdominal aortic aneurysm	Dull constant (chronic)	Left paraspinous	Hips Thighs	White men 60-70 years old Claudication Epigastric pain Hypertension Diabetes Smoking	Pulsatile abdominal mass Bruits Hypotension with rupture
Genitourinary (Visceral-Referred)					
Kidney stone	Dull persistent and/ or sharp cramping	Costovertebral angle (CVA)	None *or* genitalia	20-60 years old History of gout Acute severe pain Writhing with nausea and vomiting	Tender costovertebral angle Paraspinous spasm Acute scoliosis
Pyelonephritis	Dull persistent	CVA	None	Female 20-60 years old Diabetic Urinary tract infection in childhood Foul-smelling urine Chills Neurogenic bladder	Tender CVA Fever
Ureteropelvic junction obstruction	Dull persistent Sharp	CVA	None	Flank pain with fluid intake or diuretics	Tender CVA
Renal infarction	Acute sharp	CVA	None	Heart disease Atrial fibrillation Vascular disease Hypertension	Tender CVA Ileus
Renal cancer	None Dull Sharp	CVA	None	Gross hematuria	Abdominal mass Abdominal flank tenderness
Ureter					
Stone in upper ureter	Colicky Sharp	Flank Paraspinous	Genitalia Lower quadrant	20-60 years old Stone Gout Acute-onset nausea and vomiting	CVA tenderness Abdominal tenderness Paraspinous spasm Acute scoliosis
Stone in lower ureter	Colickly Sharp	Lower quadrant	Genitalia	Writhing with episode Frequency Urgency	

Laboratory Abnormalities	Radiographs	Diagnosis	Therapy	Comments
Hyperglycemia Elevated CSF protein	Normal	Clinical examination Slowed nerve conduction	Analgesics Glucose control Mexiletene Gabapentin	Diabetes common cause
Normal	Normal	History	Antidepressants	
Normal	Normal	History Physical examination	Psychiatric	
Normal or decreased Hct	Cross-table lateral: curvilinear calcification CT scan or sonogram: vessel enlargement	Radiographic visualization	Surgical excision	Femoral nerve entrapment with retroperitoneal bleeding
Microscopic hematuria	KUB: stone IVP: confirms location, rules out obstruction	History Physical examination Urinalysis KUB IVP	Observation Extracorporeal shock wave lithotripsy Percutaneous removal	Open surgery has become less frequent
Pyuria WBC casts Culture positive	IVP: renal swelling Sonogram: enlarged kidney Gallium scan positive	History Urinalysis	Antibiotics	Obstruction Abscess must be ruled out
Normal urine	IVP: dilated renal pelvis, hydronephrosis Sonogram: same findings Renal scan: obstruction	History Radiologic studies	Surgical repair Observation Nephrectomy	Often asymptomatic and diagnosed incidentally Capsular distention
Normal urine	IVP: kidney not seen Sonogram: normal Renal scan: no flow Arteriogram: identifies location	History Radiologic studies	Surgical after <24 hours observation	Diagnosis often delayed, resulting in kidney loss
Hematuria	IVP: mass Sonogram: solid mass CT scan: solid mass, nodes, tumor, clot Arteriogram: mass, tumor, clot	History Radiologic studies	Radical nephrectomy	Incidentally found Commonly classic triad: flank pain, hematuria, abdominal mass
Microscopic hematuria	KUB: calcium stone IVP: stone site, obstruction	History Urinalysis Radiographs	Analgesics Antiemetics Extracorporeal shock wave lithotripsy Transurethral stone manipulation Percutaneous stone removal	Surgical removal infrequently indicated

Continued

Disease Entity	Back Pain: *Character*	Back Pain: *Location*	Back Pain: *Radiation*	Additional History	Physical Examination
Vesicoureteral reflux	Dull	Flank, unilateral or bilateral	None	Female pyelonephritis Flank pain with voiding Urinary tract infection in childhood	Negative
Bladder					
Urinary retention	Dull	Sacral	None	Male older than 60 Difficulty voiding Incontinence	Lower abdominal midline mass Prostatic enlargement
Urinary infection	Dull	Sacral	None	Sexually active women Frequency Urgency Afebrile	Tender lower abdomen Tender bladder on pelvic examination
Prostate					
Chronic prostatitis	Dull	Lumbosacral	None	Prior nongonococcal urethritis Discharge Urinary irritation Testicular perineal pain	Normal or lumpy, bumpy prostate
Carcinoma	Dull insidious Sharp focal	Vertebral bodies	Legs	Difficulty voiding Urinary frequency	Focal vertebral tenderness Rock-hard prostate
Testis					
Cancer	Dull	Lumbar	None	Testicular fullness Weight loss Gynecomastia	Testicular mass Abdominal mass Percussion tenderness along spine
Uterus					
Leiomyomas	Ache Pressure	Sacrum	Thigh	Abdominal heaviness +/– Abnormal menses	Palpable masses
Retroverted	Pressure	Sacrum	Thigh	Dysmenorrhea Dyspareunia	Retroverted uterus
Prolapsed	Pulling	Sacrum			Cervical descent to vulva
Endometriosis	Cyclic cramping	Sacrum	Thigh	Dysmenorrhea	Beading of uterosacral ligaments
Pregnancy	Ache Pulling	Sacroiliac joints Pubis	Thigh	Increases with duration of pregnancy	Hyperlordosis
Fallopian Tube					
Pelvic inflammatory disease	Acute, sharp	Sacrum	Thigh	Fever Discharge	Pelvic tenderness on motion of cervix and adnexa
Ectopic pregnancy	Pressure Pain	Sacrum	Thigh	Missed menses	Adnexal tenderness, mass
Ovary					
Benign neoplasm	Pressure Ache	Sacrum			Adnexal masses
Malignant neoplasm	Ache	Paraspinous	Thigh	Weight loss Increased abdominal girth	Adnexal mass Ascites

Laboratory Abnormalities	Radiographs	Diagnosis	Therapy	Comments
Renal impairment in minority	Cystogram: reveals reflux IVP: dilated ureters, renal atrophy	History Cystogram	Ureteral reimplantation Observation Antibiotics	Ureteral reimplantation eliminates pyelonephritis
Renal impairment in minority	IVP: post-void residual, hydronephrosis Sonogram: bladder distention, hydronephrosis	Physical examination Radiographs	Catheterization Prostatectomy	Clinical presentation: slow progression
Hematuria Pyuria Positive culture	None	History Physical examination	Antibiotics Bladder analgesics	Usually respond in 24 hours, otherwise complicating factors
Inflammation in prostatic secretion	None	History Prostatic secretion	Antibiotics Massage	Prostate is most frequently normal Secretion is obtained by massage Commonly overlooked cause of back pain
Elevated acid phosphatase Prostatic specific antigen	Bone scan: uptake in blastic lesions	Physical examination Radiographs	Hormonal therapy Observation	30-40% of prostatic cancer patients present with metastatic disease Acute paraplegia is rare complication
Elevated tumor markers: alpha-fetoprotein, beta-hCG	IVP: Deviated ureter CT scan: abdominal mass	Physical examination Radiographs	Orchiectomy Chemotherapy Surgery	Back pain is reflection of bulky retroperitoneal disease
Decreased Hct	Sonography: uterine masses	Sonography Physical examination	Surgery	
None	Sonography: posterior position	Physical examination	Surgery	
None	Sonography: prolapsed position	Physical examination	Surgery	
None	Normal	Physical examination Laparoscopy	Hormonal supplementation Surgery	Rare episodes of sciatica
None	Normal	Physical examination Laparoscopy	Support Exercises Delivery	Relaxation of uterosacral ligaments, pain with increased load and strain
Gram stain Cultures	Normal	Culture	Antibodies	
Pregnancy test positive	Sonography: adnexal enlargement	Laparoscopy	Surgery	
None	Sonography: mass	Physical examination Laparoscopy	Hormonal supplementation Surgery	
Decreased Hct CEA positive	Sonography: mass	Physical examination Biopsy	Surgery Chemotherapy	Ovarian carcinoma with extension causes back pain

Continued

Disease Entity	Back Pain: *Character*	Back Pain: *Location*	Back Pain: *Radiation*	Additional History	Physical Examination
GASTROINTESTINAL (VISCERAL-REFERRED)					
Pancreas					
Pancreatitis Acute	Severe, sharp	Midline (L1)	From epigastrium	Alcoholism Gallstone Hypertriglyceridemia	Fever Tachycardia Hypotension Abdominal tenderness
Chronic	Boring, constant	Midline (L1)	From epigastrium	Anorexia Weight loss New-onset diabetes Greasy stools Jaundice Male predominance	Abdominal mass (pseudocyst)
Tumor	Dull or sharp Episodic or continuous	Midline	From epigastrium	Anorexia Weight loss Jaundice	Abdominal mass
Biliary Tree/Gallbladder					
Acute cholecystitis	Severe Colicky	Right paraspinous	From right upper quadrant	Nausea Vomiting Female predominance 40 years old	Fever Abdominal guarding
Hollow Viscus Stomach/Duodenum					
Gastric ulcer Duodenal ulcer	Boring Burning	Midline (L1)	From epigastrium	Alcohol Caffeine Drugs Smoking	Epigastric tenderness
Colon					
Diverticulitis	Persistent cramp	Sacrum	From left lower quadrant	Change in bowel habits	Tender left lower quadrant Decreased bowel sounds Rectal or lower quadrant mass
Cancer	Ache	Sacrum	Legs	Weight loss	Hard, nontender rectal or abdominal mass
MISCELLANEOUS DISORDERS					
Paget's disease (deep somatic, radicular)	Deep, boring	Affected bone	Legs	40 years or older Pain with walking Increasing skull size Deafness	Decreased spine motion Percussion tenderness with bone fracture Scalp veins Angioid streaks
Endocarditis (deep somatic, radicular)	Diffuse ache	Low back	Legs	Fever Chills Anorexia Arthralgias Myalgias	Heart murmur Peripheral arthritis Rash

Laboratory Abnormalities	Radiographs	Diagnosis	Therapy	Comments
Increased trypsin, amylase, lipase	Pleural effusions Sentinel loop CT scan or sonogram: diffusely enlarged pancreas	Increased trypsin and amylase Compatible sonogram or CT scan	Hydration Nasogastric suction Treat complication: shock, renal or pulmonary insufficiency, abscesses	Pain lasts for days Increased in supine position, decreased in forward flexion Head—right of spine, tail—left of spine
Decreased Hct Decreased trypsinogen Increased alkaline phosphatase	CT scan or sonogram: pancreatic calcification, pseudocyst	Decreased trypsinogen Compatible CT scan or sonogram	Enzyme replacement Insulin Pseudocyst drainage	Common cause: alcoholism, biliary tract disease
Decreased Hct Increased alkaline phosphatase Increased bilirubin	CT scan or sonography: pancreatic mass, liver metastases, enlarged intra-abdominal lymph glands	Needle biopsy or laparotomy	Pancreatectomy Diversion-bypass procedure	
Increased WBC Increased bilirubin Increased amylase	Scintiscan: nonvisualization of gallbladder Sonography: stones	Scintiscan Sonography	Fluids Analgesics Antibiotics Nasogastric suction Surgery: perforation, abscess	Pain begins abruptly, subsides gradually Chronic cholecystitis and choledocholithiasis have similar clinical patterns Episodic pain
Decreased Hct Increased amylase	Posterior ulcer	Endoscopy	Histamine receptor antagonists Surface agents Antacids	Pancreatitis with duodenal penetration
Increased WBC Abnormal urinalysis	Localized diverticulosis Microperforations Obstructive gas pattern	Barium studies	Antibiotics Surgical drainage of abscesses	
Decreased Hct Hemoccult positive stools Increased ESR	Abnormal barium enema	Colonoscopy Flexible sigmoidoscopy Biopsy	Surgery	
Increased alkaline phosphatase, urinary hydroxyproline Bone biopsy: increased osteoclastic activity with mosaic and woven bone osteoblastic response	Lytic and sclerotic areas in vertebrae "Picture frame" appearance Enlarged "ivory" vertebrae Scintiscan: increased bone activity	Laboratory abnormalities Biopsy rarely	NSAIDs Calcitonin Bisphosphonates	Bone involvement Asymptomatic in many Cauda equina syndrome rare Slow virus infection
Decreased Hct Increased WBC Increased ESR Rheumatoid factor positive after 6 weeks	Abnormal chest roentgenogram	Blood cultures New murmur	Antibiotics	Delay in diagnosis Worse prognosis in those with musculoskeletal symptoms Vertebral osteomyelitis, radicular "disc-like" symptoms in minority

Continued

Disease Entity	Back Pain: Character	Back Pain: Location	Back Pain: Radiation	Additional History	Physical Examination
Vertebral sarcoidosis (deep somatic)	Intermittent stabbing Dull	Involved bone	Thighs	Black men Cough Dyspnea Anorexia Weight loss	Percussion tenderness Limitation of motion Rash Lymphadenopathy Abnormal breath sounds
Retroperitoneal fibrosis	Dull Insidious	Lumbar spine, flank	None	Over 40 years old Weight loss Decreased urine output Low-grade fever	Abdominal rectal examination Empty bladder Percussion tenderness over costovertebral angles and paravertebral areas

Laboratory Abnormalities	Radiographs	Diagnosis	Therapy	Comments
Increased calcium Increased alkaline phosphatase Increased gamma globulins Increased angiotensin converting enzyme Increased ESR Cutaneous anergy Biopsy: noncaseating granuloma	Bone lysis with marginal sclerosis Vertebral body collapse Paravertebral ossification Disc space narrowing	Bone biopsy	Corticosteroids Surgical decompression	Patients with extrathoracic disease have worse prognosis
Impaired renal function No urine production Increased ESR	IVP: medial deviation of ureters Retrograde study: same CT scan: mass, ureteral and vascular encasement MR—extent and activity of fibrosis	Radiographs (biopsy)	Ureteral stents Ureterolysis Corticosteroids	Rare entity: may have idiopathic or neoplastic etiology

A-1 DIFFERENTIAL DIAGNOSIS OF LOW BACK PAIN

Evaluation	Back Strain	Herniated Nucleus Pulposus	Spinal Stenosis	Spondylolisthesis/ Instability	Spondy- loarthropathy	Infection	Tumor	Metabolic	Hematologic	Visceral
Predominant pain (back vs. leg)	Back	Leg (below knee)	Back/leg	Back	Back	Back	Back	Back	Back	Back (buttock, thigh)
Constitutional symptoms					+	+	+	+	+	+
Tension sign		+		+/–						
Neurologic examination		+/–	+/– after stress							
Plain roentgenograms			+	+	+	+/–	+/–	+	+	
Lateral motion roentgenograms				+						
CT/MR		+	+			+	+			+
Myelogram		+	+							
Bone scan					+	+	+	+	+	
ESR					+	+	+		+	+
Serum chemistries							+	+	+	+

+/–, positive in only some patients with the condition; CT, computed tomography; MR, magnetic resonance; ESR, erythrocyte sedimentation rate.

APPENDIX B

NECK PAIN

Disease Entity	Neck Pain: *Character*	Neck Pain: *Location*	Neck Pain: *Radiation*	Additional History	Physical Examination
MECHANICAL					
Muscle strain (deep somatic)					
Mild	Sharp (acute) Ache (chronic)	Neck	Interscapular Top of shoulders	None	Point tenderness
Moderate	Sharp (acute) Ache (chronic)	Neck	Interscapular Top of shoulders	None	Point tenderness Spasm Decreased range of motion of neck
Severe	Sharp	Neck	Interscapular Top of shoulders	Tension headache	Point tenderness Spasm Decreased range of motion of neck
Herniated nucleus pulposus (radicular) C3-C4 (C4 nerve root)	Sharp pain with numbness	Neck	Levator scapulae Anterior chest	Associated headaches	Decreased range of motion Point tenderness Normal neurologic
C4-C5 (C5 nerve root)	Sharp pain with numbness	Neck	Tip of shoulder Anterior chest	Associated headaches	Decreased range of motion Point tenderness Sensory change: deltoid area Motor deficit: deltoid, biceps Reflex change: biceps
C5-C6 (C6 nerve root)	Sharp pain with numbness	Neck	Shoulder Medial border of scapula Lateral arm Dorsal forearm	None	Decreased range of motion Point tenderness Sensory change: thumb, index finger Motor deficit: biceps Reflex change: biceps
C6-C7 (C7 nerve root)	Sharp pain with numbness	Neck	Shoulder Medial border of scapula Lateral arm Dorsal forearm	None	Decreased range of motion Point tenderness Sensory change: middle and ring finger Motor deficit—triceps Reflex change—triceps
C7-T1 (C8 nerve root)	Sharp pain with numbness	Neck	Shoulder Lateral forearm	None	Decreased range of motion Point tenderness Sensory change: ring and little finger Motor deficit—hand muscles Reflex change—none
Cervical spondylosis (deep somatic)	Ache	Neck		Pain increases with activity, especially rotation of the neck	Decreased range of motion
Myelopathy (radicular)	Ache	Neck	Interscapular and into one or both arms	Difficulty walking, associated with clumsiness and weakness	Decreased range of motion Long tract signs in lower extremities
Hyperextension injuries: whiplash (deep somatic)	Ache	Neck	Interscapular Shoulders	Headaches Pain with motion	Decreased range of motion Muscle spasm

Laboratory Abnormalities	Radiographs	Diagnosis	Therapy	Comments
Normal	Normal	Clinical history Physical examination	Controlled physical activity NSAIDs Collar (intermittent), limited use Muscle relaxants	Pain relief in 3-4 days
Normal	Normal	Clinical history Physical examination	Controlled physical activity NSAIDs Collar (intermittent), limited use Muscle relaxants	Pain relief in 7-10 days
Normal	Normal	Clinical history Physical examination	Controlled physical activity NSAIDs Collar (limited use) Muscle relaxants	Pain relief in 2 weeks
Normal	C3-C4 disc herniation	Clinical history Physical examination Radiographs are confirmatory	Initial: Rest, NSAIDs, oral low dose steroids After 4-6 weeks with no response: epidural steroids Continued pain: surgery	Up to 70% of patients with an HNP should respond to noninvasive therapy Tumor necrosis factor inhibitors may be beneficial
Normal	C4-C5 disc herniation	Clinical history Physical examination Radiographs are confirmatory	Initial: Rest, NSAIDs, oral low dose steroids After 4-6 weeks with no response: epidural steroids Continued pain: surgery	Up to 70% of patients with an HNP should respond to noninvasive therapy Tumor necrosis factor inhibitors may be beneficial
Normal	C5-C6 disc herniation	Clinical history Physical examination Radiographs are confirmatory	Initial: Rest, NSAIDs, oral low dose steroids After 4-6 weeks with no response: epidural steroids Continued pain: surgery	Up to 70% of patients with an HNP should respond to noninvasive therapy Tumor necrosis factor inhibitors may be beneficial
Normal	C6-C7 disc herniation	Clinical history Physical examination Radiographs are confirmatory	Initial: Rest, NSAIDs, oral low dose steroids After 4-6 weeks with no response: epidural steroids Continued pain: surgery	Up to 70% of patients with an HNP should respond to noninvasive therapy Tumor necrosis factor inhibitors may be beneficial
Normal	C7-T1 disc herniation	Clinical history Physical examination Radiographs are confirmatory	Initial: Rest, oral low dose steroids After 4-6 weeks with no response: epidural steroids Continued pain: surgery	Up to 70% of patients with an HNP should respond to noninvasive therapy Tumor necrosis factor inhibitors may be beneficial
Normal	Disc space and facet joint narrowing	Clinical history Physical examination Radiographs	Controlled physical activity Collar (intermittent), limited use NSAIDs	Majority of patients have resolution of symptoms
Normal	Compression of spinal cord	Clinical history Physical examination Radiographs are confirmatory	Surgery: decompress neural elements	Goal of surgery to prevent further neurologic deficit; many patients do recover some neural function
Normal	None	Clinical history Physical examination	NSAIDs Muscle relaxants Collar (intermittent, limited use) Physical therapy	Majority of patients improve but may take an extended period of therapy to recover

Continued

Disease Entity	Neck Pain			Additional History	Physical Examination
	Character	*Location*	*Radiation*		
RHEUMATOLOGIC					
Rheumatoid arthritis (deep somatic)	Ache	Neck	Interscapular	Headaches	Generalized involvement of hands and feet Decreased range of motion Positive long tract signs with neural compression
Ankylosing spondylitis (deep somatic)	Sharp (acute) Ache (chronic)	Neck	Interscapular	Male predominance: morning stiffness, back pain	Decreased range of motion Entire spine
Psoriatic spondylitis (deep somatic)	Ache	Neck	Interscapular	Morning stiffness Skin lesions	Psoriatic plaques Decreased motion of cervical spine in all planes
Reactive arthritis (deep somatic)	Ache	Neck	Interscapular	Conjunctivitis Urethritis Male predominance	Decreased range of motion Cervical spine
Enteropathic arthritis (deep somatic, referred)	Ache	Neck	Interscapular	Morning stiffness Abdominal pain Cramps	Abnormal abdominal examination Joint tenderness Decreased motion of cervical spine in all planes
Diffuse idiopathic skeletal hyperostosis (deep somatic)	Mild ache	Midline	None	Dysphagia	Mild limitation of cervical spine motion
Polymyalgia rheumatica (deep somatic)	Muscle soreness	Shoulders Thighs	Arms Legs	Severe morning stiffness No muscle weakness	Muscle tenderness on palpation
Fibromyalgia (deep somatic)	Ache	Generalized	Tender points	Morning stiffness Fatigue Sleeplessness	Localized pain (tender points)
INFECTIONS					
Vertebral osteomyelitis (deep somatic) Bacterial	Sharp	Area infected	Paraspinous muscles	Extraosseous source of infection Fever	Percussion tenderness over involved bone Decreased motion
Meningitis (deep somatic)	Sharp ache	Neck Occiput	Head Lower spine	Fever	Neck rigidity Brudzinski's sign
Discitis (deep somatic)	Severe, sharp	Disc infected	Shoulder	Male predominance	Localized tenderness Marked limitation of motion
Herpes zoster (superficial somatic, radicular)	Burning	Dermatomal		Fever Malaise	Vesicular dermatomal rash
Lyme disease (deep somatic, radicular)	Ache	Cervical	Arms	Tick bite Erythema migrans	Rash Radicular pain

Laboratory Abnormalities	Radiographs	Diagnosis	Therapy	Comments
Decreased Hct level Increased ESR Rheumatoid factor 80%	C1-C2 subluxation MR + neural compression	Clinical history Physical examination RA factor + anemia Plain roentgenograms	NSAIDs Antirheumatics Corticosteroids Surgery: significant neural compression Tumor necrosis factor inhibitors IL-1-inhibitors	Most patients do not require surgery Subluxation: atlantoaxial basilar invagination Subaxial instability
Increased ESR HLA-B27 90%	Marginal syndesmophytes Bilateral sacroiliitis	Clinical history Plain roentgenograms (HLA)	Exercises NSAIDs Muscle relaxants Surgery: instability Tumor necrosis factor inhibitors	Pain improved with motion Iritis HLA confirmatory: not diagnostic
Increased ESR HLA-B27 60%	Nonmarginal syndesmophytes Unilateral or bilateral sacroiliitis +/–	Clinical history Skin rash Plain roentgenograms (HLA)	Exercises Topical skin care NSAIDs Methotrexate Tumor necrosis factor inhibitors	Spondylitis may precede skin manifestations by many years Spondylitis may occur in absence of sacroiliitis
Increased ESR HLA-B27 75%	Nonmarginal syndesmophytes Unilateral or bilateral sacroiliitis +/–	History Plain roentgenograms (HLA)	Exercises NSAIDs Muscle relaxants Methotrexate	Cervical spine involvement is uncommon
Increased ESR Blood in stool HLA-B27 50%	Marginal syndesmophytes Bilateral sacroiliitis	Clinical history Gastrointestinal radiographs, biopsy	Exercises NSAIDs Tumor necrosis factor inhibitors	Activity of bowel and axial skeletal disease do not correlate
None	Flowing calcification on anterolateral aspect of four contiguous vertebral bodies	Plain roentgenograms	NSAIDs Exercises	Surgical removal for severe dysphagia
Increased ESR Isolated increased alkaline phosphatase	None	Clinical history	Corticosteroids	Diagnosis by exclusion
None	None	Clinical history	Rest Graduated exercises NSAIDs Antidepressants	Diagnosis by exclusion
Elevated ESR Bone cultures (50%) Bone cultures (60%)	Subchondral bone loss Endplate loss Narrow disc space Contiguous endplate erosion	Positive culture Radiographs	Antibiotics Immobilization	Severe pain exacerbated by motion Meningeal signs
CSF leukocytosis + Gram's stain	Parameningeal focus	Positive culture	Antibiotics	Rapid diagnosis essential for good prognosis
Increased ESR Increased WBC Blood culture Disc culture	Decreased disc height Reactive sclerosis adjoining vertebral bodies	Positive culture	Antibiotics Immobilization	Pain exacerbated with motion Severe muscle spasm Bone scan positive before plain radiograph MR positive before bone scan
Increased CSF WBC (33%)	Normal	Clinical history Physical examination	Analgesics Corticosteroids Antivirals	Occult malignancy Often lymphoreticular
Elevated ESR Borrelia antibodies CSF pleocytosis	None	History Erythema migrans	Antibiotics: early disease—oral; late disease—IV	Lyme antibodies are confirmatory, not diagnostic

Continued

Disease Entity	Neck Pain			Additional History	Physical Examination
	Character	*Location*	*Radiation*		
TUMORS AND INFILTRATIVE DISEASE					
Benign					
Osteoblastoma (deep somatic)	Dull ache	Affected bone	Paravertebral muscles Shoulders	Male predominance Young	Localized tenderness and swelling, scoliosis
Osteochondroma (deep somatic)	Mild ache	Affected bone	Paravertebral muscles	Male predominance Slowly progressive	Restricted spinal motion
Giant cell (deep somatic)	Intermittent ache	Affected bone		Female predominance Neurologic dysfunction	Localized bone tenderness and swelling
Aneurysmal bone cyst (deep somatic)	Acute onset Increasing severity	Affected bone		Female predominance Young	Localized bone tenderness Skin erythema and warmth
Hemangioma (deep somatic)	Throbbing	Affected bone		Midlife onset	Localized bone tenderness Limitation of motion with muscle spasm
Eosinophilic granuloma (deep somatic)	Persistent ache	Affected bone		Male predominance Young	Nontender swelling
Malignant					
Multiple myeloma (deep somatic, radicular)	Mild ache (onset) Acute pain (fractures)	Affected bone	Radicular	Generalized bone pain Generalized fatigue Nausea, vomiting Mental status alterations Renal dysfunction (40 years of age and older)	Diffuse bone tenderness Fever Pallor
Chondrosarcoma (deep somatic, radicular)	Mild discomfort	Affected bone	Radicular	Male predominance (40-60 years of age)	Painless swelling

Laboratory Abnormalities	Radiographs	Diagnosis	Therapy	Comments
Bone biopsy: osteoblasts, osteoid, giant cells	Posterior vertebral body expansile, well delineated, with periosteal new bone	Bone biopsy	Excision	Confused with osteosarcoma, but no cartilage or anaplastic cells in osteoblastoma
Bone biopsy: cartilage cap, woven bone with nests of cartilage	Posterior vertebral body well-demarcated sessile or pedunculated bone with cartilage cap	Radiographs Normal laboratory findings	Excision	Nerve impingement requires decompression Malignant degeneration with multiple osteochondromas
Bone biopsy: osteoclastic giant cells, mononuclear stromal cells, thin-walled vessels	Anterior vetebral body expansile lesion Thin cortical margin No bony reaction	Radiographs Bone biopsy	En bloc excision	Recurrence common with partial excision Malignant transformation rate
Bone biopsy: cystic cavities lined with fibroblasts, osteoid, multinucleated giant cells	Posterior vertebral body expansile lesion Thin demarcated periosteal shell of bone	Radiographs	En bloc excision	Local recurrence with partial excision Pathologic fracture
Bone biopsy: increased capillary and venous vessels with sparse trabecular tissue	Anterior vertebral body prominent vertical striations with unchanged body configuration	Radiographs	Radiation therapy for symptomatic lesions	Most lesions asymptomatic Surgical excision for neural compression
Peripheral eosinophilia (10%) Increased ESR Bone biopsy: eosinophils, benign pleomorphic histiocytes	Osteolytic areas without sclerosis Vertebra plana Epidural extension on MR	Bone biopsy	Curettage	Bone biopsy findings confused with Hodgkin's disease
Decreased Hct level Increased WBC Decreased platelets Coombs's test positive Increased ESR Increased calcium Increased uric acid Increased creatinine M-protein positive Bence-Jones proteinuria	Diffuse vertebral body osteolysis without reactive sclerosis Spares posterior elements CT scan more sensitive	Abnormal plasma cells M-protein Electrophoresis	Chemotherapy Decompressing laminectomy and/or local radiotherapy for cord compression	Most common primary malignant tumor Bone scan does not identify bone lesion
Decreased Hct level Increased ESR (late in course) Bone biopsy: verifying degree of malignant chondrocyte atypia with abnormal matrix production	Expansile, interior fluffy or lobular calcifications Thickened cortex CT scan: soft tissue extension	Bone biopsy	En block resection	Grade 1—slowly progressive Grade 3—more malignant, locally invasive

Continued

Disease Entity	Neck Pain: *Character*	Neck Pain: *Location*	Neck Pain: *Radiation*	Additional History	Physical Examination
Chordoma (deep somatic, radicular)	Dull or sharp Persistent	Cervical	Shoulder	Male predominance (40-70 years of age)	Muscle flaccidity
Lymphoma (deep somatic, radicular)	Persistent ache	Affected bone	Radicular	Male predominance Pain increases with recumbency or alcohol ingestion	Localized tenderness and swelling
Skeletal metastases (deep somatic, radicular)	Gradual onset with increasing intensity	Affected bone	Radicular	Increased pain with recumbency, cough, motion Prior malignancy (older than 50 years of age)	Tenderness with palpation Limited motion Fever
Intraspinal neoplasms Extradural (deep somatic, radicular)	Increasing intensity Unrelenting	Affected bone	Radicular	Increased with recumbency or activity Unresponsive to mild analgesics	Tenderness with palpation Abnormal neurologic signs with compression
Intradural-extramedullary (deep somatic, radicular)	Slowly progressive	Neck and arm	Radicular	Increased with recumbency, not by activity Neurofibromatosis	Sensory changes Muscle atrophy
Intramedullary	Painless			Sensory deficits Weakness	Abnormal pain and temperature sensation Hyperreflexia Spasticity
ENDOCRINOLOGIC AND METABOLIC					
Microcrystalline Disease (deep somatic)					
Gout	Acute (sharp) Chronic (ache)	Neck Midline		Chronic peripheral gouty arthritis Male predominance	Straightening cervical spine Tophi
Calcium pyrophosphate dihydrate disease	Acute (sharp) Chronic (ache)	Neck Midline	Secondary forms: Hyperparathyroidism	Male predominance	Straightening cervical spine Loss of motion
GENETIC DISORDERS					
Mucopolysaccharidoses Morquio's syndrome (deep somatic)	Chronic ache	Diffuse		Onset in childhood Decreased hearing Normal intelligence	Short stature Kyphoscoliosis Clouded corneas Ligamentous laxity Hepatomegaly

Laboratory Abnormalities	Radiographs	Diagnosis	Therapy	Comments
Decreased Hct level Increased ESR (late in course) Bone biopsy: gelatinous tumor, physaliphorous cells interspersed in fibrous tissue	Osteolysis with calcific soft tissue mass Vertebral body without disc involvement initially	Bone biopsy	En bloc resection Radiation therapy for inaccessible tumors	Unpredictable clinical course, slow and indolent or rapid and destructive, 10-year survival 10%-40%
Decreased Hct level Immunoglobulin abnormalities Disseminated disease	Osteolytic (75%) Sclerotic (15%) Mixed (5%) Periosteal (5%) Vertebral body compression fracture Spares disc space	Bone biopsy	Chemotherapy and/or radiotherapy	Potential for cure if diagnosed before extensive disease
Decreased Hct level Increased ESR Urinalysis: RBC Increased alkaline phosphatase, prostatic acid phosphatase Bone biopsy: may or may not show characteristics of primary tumor	Osteolytic: lung, kidney, breast, thyroid Osteoblastic: prostate, breast, colon, bronchial carcinoid Spares disc Bone scan: 85% symptomatic and asymptomatic areas Myelography: cord compression MR: most sensitive test	Bone biopsy if no primary neoplasm is identified	Palliative Radiotherapy Corticosteroids Decompressive laminectomy for spinal cord compression	Most common malignant lesion of the spine
Decreased Hct level Increased ESR Bone biopsy: metastasis	Rapid bone destruction, body or posterior elements Myelogram: complete block, varying densities, displaces cord MR: contrast agent increases sensitivity	Lesional biopsy	Radiotherapy Corticosteroids Decompressive laminectomy	Metastatic lesions
Increased cerebrospinal fluid protein	Posterior scalloping of vertebral bodies Uniform dilatation of neural foramen Myelogram: sharp, smooth outline of lesion MR: contrast agent increases sensitivity	Radiographs	Surgical removal	Neurofibromas Meningiomas
	Myelogram: fusiform enlargement MR positive	Lesional biopsy	Surgical removal	Ependymomas Gliomas
Monosodium urate monohydrate crystals Increased serum uric acid	Vertebral erosions Marginal sclerosis	Monosodium urate monohydrate crystals	Colchicine NSAIDs Corticosteroids (acute) Uricosurics Xanthine oxidase inhibitors (chronic)	
Calcium pyrophosphate dihydrate crystals	Disc calcification and narrowing Osteophytes	Calcium pyrophosphate dihydrate crystals	NSAIDs Colchicine (33%)	Secondary forms: Hyperparathyroidism Hemochromatosis Hypothyroidism Wilson's disease Ochronosis
Increased urinary keratan sulfate	Platyspondyly Central beaking of vertebral bodies Increased kyphosis	Increased keratan sulfate	Bracing	Galactosamine-6-sulfate sulfatase deficiency Mild form of beta-galactosidase deficiency

Continued

Disease Entity	Neck Pain: *Character*	Neck Pain: *Location*	Neck Pain: *Radiation*	Additional History	Physical Examination
NEUROLOGIC AND PSYCHIATRIC DISORDERS					
Neuropathy (radicular)	Burning	Paraspinous	Arm Hand	Episodes of lancinating pain, increased at night Pain not increased with cough	Arm or hand weakness Absent biceps reflex
Psychogenic rheumatism (psychogenic)	Dull ache	Neck Shoulder		Listlessness Sleepiness Anorexia Constipation	Normal
Malingering (psychogenic)	Severe, constant	Entire neck and back	Nondermatomal	No relief with any therapy Job-related	Inconsistent abnormalities Nondermatomal sensory loss Pain with head compression
REFERRED PAIN					
Vascular (Visceral Referred)					
Myocardial infarction	Crushing	Anterior neck	Arm—C8 distribution	Angina, hypertension increased with exertion	Diaphoresis Abnormal cardiac sounds
Carotid artery dissection	Sharp constant	Unilateral neck	Head	Smoking Fibromuscular dysplasia	Focal neurologic deficits Carotid bruits
Thoracic aortic dissection	Tearing	Chest	Lateral posterior neck	Older male Arteriosclerotic cardiovascular disease	Hypotension with proximal dissections
Biliary Tree/Gallbladder					
Acute cholecystitis	Severe Colicky	Right paraspinous Right scapula	From right upper quadrant	Nausea Vomiting Female predominance 40 years of age	Fever Abdominal guarding
Hollow viscus Esophagus diverticulum	Ache	Throat	Lateral neck	Dysphagia, regurgitation	Local neck mass
Esophageal cancer	Ache	Chest	Upper neck	Dysphagia Weight loss	Local neck mass
MISCELLANEOUS DISORDERS					
Paget's disease (deep somatic, radicular)	Deep, boring	Affected bone	Shoulders	40 years of age and older Pain with walking Increasing skull size Deafness	Decreased spine motion Percussion tenderness with bone fracture Scalp veins Angioid streak
Vertebral sarcoidosis (deep somatic)	Intermittent stabbing Dull	Involved bone	Shoulders	Black males Cough Dyspnea Anorexia Weight loss	Percussion tenderness Limitation of motion Rash Lymphadenopathy Abnormal breath sounds

CK, creatine kinase; CSF, cerebrospinal fluid; CT, computed tomography; ESR, erythrocyte sedimentation rate; Hct, hematocrit; HLA, human leukocyte antigen; HNP, herniated nucleus pulposus; MR, magnetic resonance; NSAIDs, nonsteroidal anti-inflammatory drugs; RBC, red blood cell; WBC, white blood cell.

Laboratory Abnormalities	Radiographs	Diagnosis	Therapy	Comments
Abnormal nerve conduction electromyogram	Normal	Clinical examination Slowed nerve conduction	Analgesics Mexiletene Gabapentin	Carpal tunnel most common form
Normal	Normal	History	Antidepressants	
Normal	Normal	History Physical examination	Psychiatric	
Electrocardiogram: ischemia	Angiogram Stenosis	Angiogram Elevated creatine kinase	Reversal of stenosis	Cervical disc may mimic myocardial infarction
Normal	Arteriogram: dissection	Arteriogram	Heparin	Vertebral artery dissection has similar abnormalities affecting posterior circulation
Normal	Aortograph: dissection	Aortography	Control hypertension Surgical repair	
Increased WBC count Increased bilirubin Increased amylase level	Scintiscan: nonvisualization of gallbladder Sonography: stones	Scintiscan Sonography	Fluids Analgesics Antibiotics Nasogastric suction Surgery: perforation, abscess	Pain begins abruptly, subsides gradually Chronic cholecystitis and choledocholithiasis have similar clinical patterns Episodic pain
Normal	Barium esophagogram	Esophagogram	Surgical removal	Esophagoscopy contraindicated: perforation
Decreased Hct level	Barium esophagogram	Biopsy	Diversion: bypass procedure	Neck pain poor prognostic sign
Increased alkaline phosphatase, urinary hydroxyproline Bone biopsy: increased osteoclastic activity with mosaic and woven bone osteoblastic response	Lytic and sclerotic areas in vertebrae "Picture frame" appearance Enlarged "ivory" vertebrae Scintiscan: increased bone activity	Laboratory abnormalities Biopsy rarely	NSAIDs Calcitonin Bisphosphonates	Bone involvement Asymptomatic in many Slow virus infection
Increased calcium Increased alkaline phosphatase Increased gamma globulins Increased angiotensin converting enzyme Increased ESR Cutaneous anergy Biopsy: noncaseating granuloma	Bone lysis with marginal sclerosis Vertebral body collapse Paravertebral ossification Disc space narrowing	Bone biopsy	Corticosteroids Surgical decompression	Patients with extrathoracic disease have worse prognosis

B-1 DIFFERENTIAL DIAGNOSIS OF NECK PAIN

Evaluation	Neck Strain	Herniated Nucleus Pulposus	Instability	Degenerative Disc Disease	Myelopathy	Tumor	Spondylo-arthropathy	Infection	Visceral
Predominant pain (arm vs. neck)	Neck	Arm	Neck	Neck	Neck	Neck	Neck	Neck	Neck/Throat
Constitutional symptoms						+	+	+	+/–
Compression test		+							
Neurologic examination		+	+/–		+	+/–			+/–
Plain roentgenograms			+/–	+	+/–	+/–	+	+/–	
Lateral motion roentgenograms			+						
Bone scan				+/–		+	+	+	
CT scan		+		+/–	+	+		+	+
Myelogram		+			+				
MR scan		+		+	+	+		+	+
ESR						+	+	+	+/–
Serum chemistries						+			

+/–, positive in only some patients with the condition; CT, computed tomography; MR, magnetic resonance; ESR, erythrocyte sedimentation rate.

Index

Page numbers followed by f indicate figures; page numbers followed by t indicate tables.

A

D

E

F

G

J

K

L

M

O

P

W

Y

Z